# Rapid-Sequence Intubation*

1. Preoxygenate with 100% oxygen
2. Apply cricoid pressure
3. Induction: etomidate (0.3 mg/kg), propofol (0.5–2 mg/kg) or ketamine (2 mg/kg) IV push
4. Neuromuscular blockade: succinylcholine 1.5 mg/kg IV push
5. Wait 30–45 sec
6. Intubate when optimal conditions achieved

*Consider pretreatment with fentanyl (2–3 $\mu$g/kg) IV push and lidocaine (1.5 mg/kg) IV push if concern for increased intracranial pressure or severe hypertension
*Consider defasciculating dose of paralytic if concern for increased intracranial pressure (see table for dosage)
*Atropine: 0.02 mg/kg IV push (for children <5 yr old)

## Neuromuscular Blocking Agents

| Agent | Dosage (paralytic) | Dosage (fas pro*) | Onset | Duration |
|---|---|---|---|---|
| Succinylcholine | RSI: 1–2 mg/kg | | 30–60 sec | 4–6 min |
| Rocuronium | RSI: 0.6–1.2 mg/kg<br>M: 0.6 mg/kg | 0.06 mg/kg | 2 min | 30 min |
| Vecuronium | RSI: 0.015–0.25 mg/kg<br>M: 0.1 mg/kg | 0.01 mg/kg | 2.5–5 min | 25–40 min |
| Atracurium | M: 0.4 mg/kg | 0.04 mg/kg | 3–5 min | 20–35 min |
| Pancuronium | M: 0.1 mg/kg | 0.01 mg/kg | 3–5 min | 45–60 min |

*fas pro, fasciculation prophylaxis/defasciculating dose; RSI, rapid-sequence intubation; M, maintenance dose.

## Sedative and Induction Agents

| Sedative | Dosage IVP | Onset | Duration |
|---|---|---|---|
| Etomidate | 0.2–0.6 mg/kg | 60 sec | 3–5 min |
| Fentanyl | Induction: 2–10 $\mu$g/kg<br>Sedation (titrate): 2–4 $\mu$g/kg | 60 sec | 30–60 min |
| Ketamine | 2 mg/kg | 30–60 sec | 15 min |
| Midazolam | Induction: 0.07–0.3 mg/kg<br>Sedation (titrate): 0.02–0.04 mg/kg | 2 min | 1–2 hr |
| Propofol | 0.5–2 mg/kg IVP | 30 sec | 3–10 min |
| Thiopental | 3–5 mg/kg | 20–40 sec | 5–10 min |

# Pediatric Vital Signs and Resuscitation Equipment Sizes

| | Term | 6 mo | 1 yr | 2 yr | 5 yr | 10 yr |
|---|---|---|---|---|---|---|
| Approximate weight | 2–4 kg | 8 kg | 10 kg | 13 kg | 20 kg | 35 kg |
| Vital signs | | | | | | |
|   BP (systolic) mm Hg | 60 ± 10 | 89 ± 29 | 96 ± 30 | 99 ± 25 | 99 ± 20 | 112 ± 19 |
|   HR | 125 | 130 | 125 | 115 | 100 | 75 |
|   RR | 40 ± 10 | 38 ± 10 | 39 ± 11 | 28 ± 4 | 27 ± 6 | 21 ± 4 |
| Resuscitation | | | | | | |
|   Defibrillation | 8 J | 16 J | 20 J | 26 J | 40 J | 70 J |
|   Cardioversion | 2–4 J | 4–8 J | 5–10 J | 7–13 J | 20–40 J | 25–70 J |
|   Suction catheter | 8F | 8–10F | 8–10F | 10F | 10F | 12F |
| Airway | | | | | | |
|   Laryngoscope blade | 1 (st) | 1–2 (st) | 1–2 (st) | 2 (st/c) | 2 (st/c) | 2–3 (st/c) |
|   Endotracheal tube (mm) | 3.0–3.5 | 3.5–4.0 | 4.0–4.5 | 4.5 | 5.0–5.5 | 6.5 |
|   Lip–tip length (mm) | 10.5 | 12 | 12 | 13.5 | 16.5 | 19.5 |
| Tubes | | | | | | |
|   Nasogastric tube | 5/6 | 8 | 10 | 10 | 10–12 | 12 |
|   Urinary catheter | 5 feeding tube | 5–8 feeding tube | 8 feeding tube | 10 Foley | 10 Foley | 10 Foley |
|   Chest tube (Fr) | 10–12 | 14–20 | 16–20 | 14–24 | 20–28 | 28–32 |

# Temperature Conversion: Celsius ↔ Fahrenheit

| Celsius | Fahrenheit | Celsius | Fahrenheit |
|---|---|---|---|
| 34.2 | 93.6 | 38.6 | 101.4 |
| 34.6 | 94.3 | 39.0 | 102.2 |
| 35.0 | 95.0 | 39.4 | 102.9 |
| 35.4 | 95.7 | 39.8 | 103.6 |
| 35.8 | 96.4 | 40.2 | 104.3 |
| 36.2 | 97.1 | 40.6 | 105.1 |
| 36.6 | 97.8 | 41.0 | 105.8 |
| 37.0 | 98.6 | 41.4 | 106.5 |
| 37.4 | 99.3 | 41.8 | 107.2 |
| 37.8 | 100.0 | 42.2 | 108.0 |
| 38.2 | 100.7 | 42.6 | 108.7 |

$$°F = 9/5 × °C + 32$$

# Weight Conversion: Pounds ↔ Kilograms

| | | | |
|---|---|---|---|
| 10 lb | 4.53 kg | 110 lb | 49.89 kg |
| 20 lb | 9.07 kg | 120 lb | 54.43 kg |
| 30 lb | 13.60 kg | 130 lb | 58.96 kg |
| 40 lb | 18.14 kg | 140 lb | 63.50 kg |
| 50 lb | 22.68 kg | 150 lb | 68.04 kg |
| 60 lb | 27.21 kg | 160 lb | 72.57 kg |
| 70 lb | 31.75 kg | 170 lb | 77.11 kg |
| 80 lb | 36.28 kg | 180 lb | 81.64 kg |
| 90 lb | 40.82 kg | 190 lb | 86.18 kg |
| 100 lb | 45.36 kg | 200 lb | 90.72 kg |

$$kg = lb × 2.2$$

# Rosen & Barkin's
# 5-Minute Emergency Medicine Consult

## 4TH EDITION

**Jeffrey J. Schaider, MD**
Associate Professor of Emergency Medicine
Rush Medical College
Chairman
Department of Emergency Medicine
Cook County Health and Hospital System
Chicago, Illinois

**Roger M. Barkin, MD**
Clinical Professor of Pediatrics
University of Colorado School of Medicine
Emergency Physician
CarePoint/Rose Medical Center
Denver, Colorado

**Stephen R. Hayden, MD**
Professor of Clinical Medicine
Program Director, Residency Program
Department of Emergency Medicine
University of California San Diego
Editor-in-Chief, Journal of Emergency Medicine
Medical Center
San Diego, California

**Richard E. Wolfe, MD**
Associate Professor
Division of Emergency Medicine
Harvard Medical School
Chief of Emergency Medicine
Beth Israel Deaconess Medical Center
Boston, Massachusetts

**Adam Z. Barkin, MD, MPH**
Clinical Instructor
Department of Emergency Medicine
University of Colorado School of Medicine
Aurora, Colorado
Attending Physician
Emergency Medicine
Rose Medical Center
Denver, Colorado

**Philip Shayne, MD**
Associate Professor
Vice Chair for Education and Residency
  Program Director
Department of Emergency Medicine
Emory University School of Medicine
Atlanta, Georgia

**Peter Rosen, MD**
Senior Lecturer Medicine
Harvard University
Attending Physician
Beth Israel Deaconess Hospital
Boston, Massachusetts
Visiting Professor
University of Arizona
Tucson, Arizona

# Rosen & Barkin's
# 5-Minute Emergency Medicine Consult

## 4TH EDITION

Jeffrey J. Schaider, MD

Roger M. Barkin, MD

Stephen R. Hayden, MD

Richard E. Wolfe, MD

Adam Z. Barkin, MD, MPH

Philip Shayne, MD, FACEP

Peter Rosen, MD

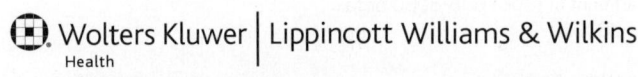 Wolters Kluwer | Lippincott Williams & Wilkins
Health

Philadelphia · Baltimore · New York · London
Buenos Aires · Hong Kong · Sydney · Tokyo

Acquisitions Editor: Frances DeStefano
Product Manager: Julia Seto
Production Manager: Bridgett Dougherty
Senior Manufacturing Manager: Benjamin Rivera
Marketing Manager: Angela Panetta
Design Coordinator: Teresa Mallon
Production Service: Aptara, Inc.

**Library of Congress Cataloging-in-Publication Data**

Rosen & Barkin's 5-minute emergency medicine consult / [edited by]
Jeffrey J. Schaider ... [et al.].—4th ed.
    p. ; cm.
    Other title: 5-minute emergency medicine consult
    Other title: Rosen and Barkin's 5-minute emergency medicine consult
    Includes bibliographical references and index.
    Summary: "This best-selling emergency department reference is now in its thoroughly updated Fourth Edition. The foremost authorities provide practical information on over 600 clinical problems in a fast-access two-page outline format that's perfect for on-the-spot consultation during care in the emergency department. Coverage of each disorder includes clinical presentation, pre-hospital, diagnosis, treatment, disposition, and ICD-10 coding. Icons enable practitioners to quickly spot the information they need. This edition provides up-to-date information on topics such as emerging infections, new protocols, and new treatments"—Provided by publisher.
    ISBN-13: 978-1-60831-630-4
    ISBN-10: 1-60831-630-0
    1. Emergency medicine—Handbooks, manuals, etc.  2. Medical emergencies—Handbooks, manuals, etc.
I. Rosen, Peter, 1935-  II. Schaider, Jeffrey.  III. Title: 5-minute emergency medicine consult.
IV. Title: Rosen and Barkin's 5-minute emergency medicine consult.
    [DNLM: 1. Emergency Medicine—Handbooks.  2. Emergency Medical Services—Handbooks.
3. Emergency Treatment—Handbooks.  WB 39]
    RC86.8.A14 2011
    616.02'5—dc22                                                    2010030437

To purchase additional copies of this book, call our customer service department at (800) 638-3030 or fax orders to (301) 223-2320. International customers should call (301) 223-2300.

Visit Lippincott Williams & Wilkins on the Internet: at LWW.com. Lippincott Williams & Wilkins customer service representatives are available from 8:30 am to 6 pm, EST.

10 9 8 7 6 5 4 3 2 1

# PREFACE

Rosen and Barkin's 5-Minute Emergency Medicine Consult continues to reflect the unique nature of our clinical emergency medicine practices. Emergency medicine provides unique challenges to the clinician, reflecting a remarkable breadth of clinical conditions that are encountered, as well as the time constraints of an acute illness, frequently modified by environmental considerations along with the logistical demands of concurrent priorities and multiple patients. Time is of the essence, and this book is truly designed to meet the needs of clinicians working in settings providing urgent and emergent care. When the database conflicts with the clinical assessment, the clinician must rely upon judgment and "gestalt" along with further evaluation and intervention; it is often too easy to endow laboratory numbers with infallibility, and to ignore pertinent clinical findings. To look for a diagnosis, one must think of it, and the very nature of the emergency department (ED) is discouraging to prolonged deliberation. Nevertheless, it must become instinctive to think about the statistically rare, but clinically serious entity, rather than to just reach for the statistically probable but non–life-threatening diagnosis.

The focus of the book is to provide concise formatted information that will allow the busy clinician to respond to challenges appropriately. The book is meant to be readily available in the ED, and frequently used in the trenches. It is written and edited by practicing clinicians for their colleagues to use readily and repeatedly. The book is written with the intent to synthesize a mountain of information into tightly formatted chapters that stimulate analysis and subsequent assessment, serving to awaken a key memory with which to proceed with the care of a patient.

We have attempted to integrate the data bank our authors have acquired through many years of practice onto the pages of this book. The book is not meant to be a diagnostic engine, but rather a place to turn to confirm a diagnosis that is supported by the clinical presentation and the subjective and objective evidence that supports our clinical judgment.

Our very experienced authors discuss each topic from the perspective of the information needed in a busy ED, trying to give a precise and clinically relevant summary useful in caring for the patient as well as providing a structure for a student or resident to approach the problem encountered. We are indebted to them for their commitment to this task.

The book is intended to be accurate, focused and readily integrated into practice, rather than being definitive and all encompassing. This new edition incorporates new information and approaches to management, while allowing us to modify topics that reflect some of the new challenges we face.

We are delighted to welcome two new editors to the book, Drs. Adam Barkin and Phil Shayne, representing a new generation of emergency physicians who will become the leaders of our profession in the decades ahead.

We hope that Rosen and Barkin's 5-Minute Emergency Medicine Consult will be useful to both novices in emergency medicine and experienced clinicians. The information and organization is designed to be easily used within the "chaos" that surrounds our clinical settings.

Clinical acumen, judgment, and experience remain as the foundations for our clinical practice. It is our hope that this book will serve students, nurses, emergency medical personnel, residents, and practicing emergency physicians as a useful and readily used resource in this critical process, and enhance the fulfillment of practicing emergency medicine for our readers.

JEFFREY J. SCHAIDER
ROGER M. BARKIN
STEPHEN R. HAYDEN
RICHARD E. WOLFE
ADAM Z. BARKIN
PHILIP SHAYNE
PETER ROSEN

# ACKNOWLEDGMENTS

The dedication of our authors and the input of our readers is appreciated and forms the foundation for this book. Julia Seto of Lippincott Williams & Wilkins held our hands throughout the production.

To my wife Anna and sons Jacob and Isaac—thank you for your continued support and inspiration. Thanks to the Cook County Emergency Medicine Attendings and Residents for their contributions to the book and to enhancing my knowledge and understanding of our unique field.

J.J.S.

I am most appreciative for my family's support. Suzanne Barkin, MD is an exemplary clinician and has been a remarkable model and teacher for the residents she has trained. It has been an honor and pleasure to watch Adam Barkin, MD become an outstanding practicing emergency physician and educator. Michael, Jill, and Jacob remind us all of the importance of our roles as clinicians and reaffirm our commitment to excellence.

The emergency medicine staff of Rose Medical Center, Denver continue to be supportive, providing an environment in which to practice our specialty. It is also important to acknowledge and thank our colleagues nationally and internationally who continue to teach each of us on an ongoing basis and will hopefully find this book useful in their daily practices.

R.M.B.

To my wife Marina, and my children Connor, Maia, and Kenny; without your support and understanding, my involvement in academic emergency medicine and this book would be not possible. To my current residents and past graduates; I hope the information in this book helps guide your clinical decisions and prompts you to always maintain your intellectual curiosity.

S.R.H.

To my wife Alice whose unflagging support, patience, and humor provide the support for these efforts.

R.W.

Thanks to Jill who has been ever patient and supportive. To Jacob, you were born halfway through production of this book, and we already cannot imagine life without you. To Roger, you have taught me so much about the practice of medicine and fatherhood.

A.Z.B

I want to express my appreciation to both my families for their support in allowing me the freedom to work on this book. To my family at home—Helen, Dylan, and David— and to my family at work—Sharon, Sheryl, Todd, Ted, and Melissa—thank you.

P.S.

# CONTRIBUTORS

James Adams, MD
Professor and Chair
Department of Emergency Medicine
Northwestern University Feinberg School
    of Medicine
Northwestern Memorial Hospital
Chicago, Illinois

Leon Adelman, MD
Resident
Department of Emergency Medicine
Beth Israel Deaconess Medical Center
Boston, Massachusetts

Mitchell Adelstein, MD
Assistant Professor
Department of Emergency Medicine
St. Luke's Hospital
New York, New York

Spencer A. Adoff, MD
Research Fellow
Department of Emergency Medicine
Pennsylvania State Hershey
    Medical Center
Hershey, Pennsylvania

Steven Aks, DO
Associate Professor
Department of Emergency Medicine
Rush Medical College
Director, The Toxicon Consortium, Section
    of Toxicology
Department of Emergency Medicine
John H. Stroger Hospital of Cook County
Chicago, Illinois

Nadeem Al-Duaij, MD, MPH
Instructor
Emergency Medicine
Harvard Medical School
Boston, Massachusetts
Staff Physician
Cambridge Health Alliance
Cambridge, Massachusetts

Paul J. Allegretti, DO, FACOEP
Associate Professor and Program Director
Emergency Medicine
Midwestern University/Chicago College
    of Osteopathic Medicine
Downers Grove, Illinois
Attending Physician
Emergency Medicine
Provident Hospital of Cook County
Chicago, Illinois

Marilyn Althoff, MD
Faculty
Department of Medicine
Morristown Memorial Hospital
Morristown, New Jersey

Christopher E. Anderson, MD
Resident Physician
Emergency Medicine
Mayo Clinic
Rochester, Minnesota

Phillip D. Anderson, MD
Assistant Professor
Department of Emergency Medicine
Harvard Medical School
Attending Physician
Department of Emergency Medicine
Beth Israel Deaconess Medical Center
Boston, Massachusetts

Jonathon S. Anderson, MD
Senior Resident
Emergency Medicine
Harvard University
Senior Resident
Emergency Department
Beth Israel Deaconess Medical Center
Boston, Massachusetts

L. Kristian Arnold, MD
Chief Medical Officer
ArLac Global Health Services
Lexington, Massachusetts
Medical Director
Boston Police Department
Boston, Massachusetts

Hany Y. Atallah, MD
Assistant Professor
Department of Emergency Medicine
Emory University
Assistant Medical Director
Emergency Department
Grady Memorial Hospital
Atlanta, Georgia

Veronique Au, MD
Physician
Emergency Department
Straub Hospital and Clinics
Honolulu, Hawaii
Emergency Department
Novato Community Hospital
Novato, California

Ann Azcuy, MD, MS
Resident
Emergency Medicine
Emory University
Atlanta, Georgia

Brandon H. Backlund, MD
Assistant Professor
Department of Emergency Medicine
University of Colorado School
    of Medicine
Attending Physician
Department of Emergency Medicine
Denver Health Medical Center
Denver, Colorado

John Bailitz, MD
Assistant Professor of Emergency
    Medicine
Rush Medical College
Assistant Program Director
Department of Emergency Medicine
Cook County Hospital
Chicago, Illinois

Kevin M. Ban, MD
Assistant Clinical Professor
Department of Medicine
Harvard Medical School
Attending Physician
Department of Emergency Medicine
Beth Israel Deaconess Medical Center
Boston, Massachusetts

Adam Z. Barkin, MD, MPH
Clinical Instructor
Department of Emergency Medicine
University of Colorado School of
    Medicine
Aurora, Colorado
Attending Physician
Emergency Medicine
Rose Medical Center
Denver, Colorado

Roger M. Barkin, MD
Clinical Professor of Pediatrics
University of Colorado School of
    Medicine
Emergency Physician
CarePoint/Rose Medical Center
Denver, Colorado

Suzanne Z. Barkin, MD
Associate Professor of Radiology
  (Pediatrics)
Department of Radiology
Denver Health Medical Center
Denver, Colorado

David Barlas, MD
Assistant Professor
Department of Emergency Medicine
Cornell University-Weill College
  of Medicine
New York, New York
Associate Residency Director
Department of Emergency Medicine
New York Hospital Queens
Flushing, New York

Erik D. Barton, MD, MBA
Associate Professor
Department of Surgery
Division Chief
Department of Emergency Medicine
University of Utah
Salt Lake City, Utah

Beverly Bauman, MD, FAAP, FACEP
Assistant Professor
Department of Emergency Medicine
Oregon Health and Sciences
  University
Portland, Oregon

Todd Baumbacher, MD, MS
Physician
Department of Emergency Medicine
University of California San Diego
San Diego, California

Jamil D. Bayram, MD
Assistant Professor
Department of Emergency Medicine
Rush University Medical Center
John H. Stroger Hospital of Cook
  County
Chicago, Illinois

B.J. Beck MSN, MD
Clinical Instructor
Department of Psychiatry
Harvard Medical School
Clinical Assistant
Department of Psychiatry
Massachusetts General Hospital
Boston, Massachusetts

Kyan J. Berger, MD, FAAEM
Emergency Physician
Department of Emergency Medicine
Beverly Hospital and Addison Gilbert
  Hospital
Beverly, Massachusetts

Matthew R. Berkman, MD
Assistant Professor
Clinical Emergency Medicine
University Medical Center
Tucson, Arizona

Ajay Bhatt, MD
Emergency Medicine Physician
Department of Emergency Medicine
Emory University School of Medicine
Atlanta, Georgia

Colleen M. Birmingham, MD
Chief Resident
Harvard Affiliated Emergency Medicine
  Residency
Beth Israel Deaconess Medical Center
Boston, Massachusetts

Matthew D. Bitner, MD
Assistant Professor
Division of Emergency Medicine
Department of Surgery
Duke University School of Medicine
Durham, North Carolina

Herbert G. Bivins, MD
Clinical Professor
Department of Emergency
  Medicine
University of California at Fresno
Assistant Program Director
Department of Emergency Medicine
University Medical Center
Fresno, California

Matthew J. Bivens, MD
Resident
Department of Emergency Medicine
Beth Israel Deaconess Medical Center
Boston, Massachusetts

Guy M. Bizek, MD
Chief Resident
Department of Emergency Medicine
University of California San Diego
San Diego, California

Adam Black, MD
Assistant Director
Department of Emergency Medicine
St. Elizabeth's Hospital
Chicago, Illinois

Paul Blackburn, DO, FACOEP,
FACEP
Attending Physician
Department of Emergency Medicine
Maricopa Medical Center
Phoenix, Arizona

Alexander Blau, MD
Resident Physician
Division of Emergency Medicine
Stanford/Kaiser Emergency Medicine
  Residency
Stanford, California

Keith S. Boniface, MD
Associate Professor
Associate Residency Director
Department of Emergency Medicine
Director, Emergency Ultrasound
Assistant Medical Director
Maritime Medical Access
The George Washington University
Washington, D.C.

Michael J. Bono, MD, PhD
Professor, Associate Director
Department of Emergency Medicine and
  Emergency Medicine Residency
  Program
Eastern Virginia Medical School
Norfolk, Virginia

Steven H. Bowman, MD
Assistant Professor
Department of Emergency Medicine
Rush Medical College
Program Director
Department of Emergency Medicine
Cook County Stroger Hospital
Chicago, Illinois

Jefferson D. Bracey, DO
Clinical Assistant Professor
Department of Surgery
University of Nevada School
  of Medicine
Assistant Medical Director
Department of Emergency Medicine
St. Rose Dominican Hospitals
Las Vegas, Nevada

Andrea Bracikowski, MD
Associate Professor
Departments of Emergency Medicine and
  Pediatrics
Vanderbilt University Medical Center
Attending Physician
Department of Pediatric Emergency
  Medicine
Vanderbilt Children's Hospital
Nashville, Tennessee

Harminder Brar, MD
Department of Emergency Medicine
Baptist Memorial Hospital
Memphis, Tennessee

**Nicholle D. Bromley, MD**
Emergency Medicine Resident
Emergency Medicine
University of California San Diego
Emergency Medicine Resident
Emergency Medicine
University of California San Diego
  Hospital
San Diego, California

**David F. M. Brown, MD, FACEP**
Associate Professor
Division of Emergency Medicine
Harvard Medical School
Vice Chair
Department of Emergency Medicine
Massachusetts General Hospital
Boston, Massachusetts

**Lance Brown, MD, MPH**
Associate Professor of Emergency
  Medicine and Pediatrics
Department of Emergency Medicine
Loma Linda University
Chief, Division of Pediatric Emergency
  Medicine
Department of Emergency Medicine
Loma Linda University Medical Center and
  Children's Hospital
Loma Linda, California

**Brian J. Browne, MD, FACEP**
Professor
Department of Emergency Medicine and
  Medicine
Chairman
Department of Emergency Medicine
University of Maryland Medical Center
Baltimore, Maryland

**G. Richard Bruno, MD**
Clinical Assistant Professor
Department of Surgery
University of Hawaii
Honolulu, Hawaii
Chairman
Department of Emergency Medicine
Castle Hospital
Kailua, Hawaii

**Sean M. Bryant, MD**
Assistant Professor
Emergency Medicine
Rush Medical College
Attending Physician/Medical
  Toxicologist
Emergency Medicine, Division of
  Toxicology
Cook County Stroger Hospital
Chicago, Illinois

**Gary Bubly, MD, FACEP**
Clinical Associate Professor
Emergency Medicine and Medicine
Alpert Medical School of Brown
  University
Associate Director
Emergency Department
The Miriam Hospital
Providence, Rhode Island

**Ann M. Buchanan, MD**
Trauma Medical Director
Department of Emergency Medicine
St. David's Medical Center
Austin, Texas

**Robert G. Buckley, MD, MPH, FACEP**
Captain, Medical Corps, US Navy
Chief of Staff
Fort Belvoir Community Hospital
Fort Belvoir, Virginia

**Kevin Buford, MD**
Resident
Emergency Medicine
University of California San Diego
San Diego, California

**Colleen J. Buono, MD**
Emergency Medical Services Fellow
Department of Emergency Medicine
University of California, San Diego
Clinical Faculty
Department of Emergency Medicine
University of California, San Diego Medical
  Center
San Diego, California

**David W. Callaway**
Clinical Instructor
Medicine
Harvard Medical School
Attending Physician
Emergency Medicine
Beth Israel Deaconess Medical Center
Boston, Massachusetts

**Colleen Campbell, MD**
Associate Professor of Emergency
  Medicine
Department of Emergency Medicine
University of California San Diego
San Diego, California

**Taylor Y. Cardall, MD**
Prehospital Medical Director
Department of Emergency Medicine
Scottsdale Healthcare
Scottsdale, Arizona

**Keri L. Carstairs, MD**
Attending Physician
Department of Emergency Medicine
Naval Medical Center, San Diego
San Diego, California

**Shaun D. Carstairs, MD**
Attending Physician
Department of Emergency Medicine
Naval Medical Center, San Diego
San Diego, California

**Ingrid D. Carter**
Coral Springs, Florida

**Wallace A. Carter, MD**
Associate Professor of Emergency
  Medicine
Weill Medical College of Cornell
  University
Associate Professor of Clinical Medicine
Columbia University College of Physicians
  and Surgeons
Program Director, Emergency Medicine
  Residency
New York Presbyterian Hospital
New York, New York

**Austen Chai, MD**
Assistant Professor, Department of
  Emergency Medicine
Rush Medical College
Department of Emergency Medicine
John H. Stroger Hospital of Cook County
Chicago, Illinois

**Theodore C. Chan, MD**
Associate Professor of Medicine
Department of Medicine
Medical Director
Department of Emergency Medicine
University of California, San Diego
San Diego, California

**Andrew K. Chang, MD**
Associate Professor
Department of Emergency Medicine
Albert Einstein College of Medicine
Attending Physician
Department of Emergency Medicine
Montefiore Medical Center
Bronx, New York

**Danielle Chase, MD**
Chief Resident
Emergency Medicine
Texas Tech University Health Sciences
  Center
El Paso, Texas

Navneet Cheema, MD
Emergency Medicine Resident
Emergency Medicine
Northwestern University
Emergency Medicine Resident
Emergency Medicine
Northwestern Memorial Hospital
Chicago, Illinois

Peter J. Chen, MD
Resident
Department of Emergency Medicine
New York Presbyterian Hospital
New York, New York

Stephen L. Chesser, PharmD
Clinical Pharmacist, Emergency
    Department
Department of Pharmacy Services
Summa Health Systems
Akron, Ohio

Michele Chetham, MD
Emergency Pediatrician
Emergency Medicine
Swedish Medical Center
Denver, Colorado

Gordon S. Chew, MD
Assistant Chief
Emergency Department
Kaiser Permanente Medical Center
Napa/Solano, California

Alan T. Chiem, MD, MPH
Resident
Department of Emergency Department
Emory University School of Medicine
Atlanta, Georgia

Hong K. Choi, MD
Assistant Professor
Department of Emergency Medicine
Albert Einstein College
Attending Physician
Montefoire Medical Center
Bronx, New York

Yi-Mei Chng, MD, MPH
Department of Emergency Medicine
Kaiser Permanente
Santa Clara Medical Center
Santa Clara, California

Jeremy T. Chou, MD
Resident
Emergency Medicine
Emory University School of Medicine
Resident
Emergency Care Center
Grady Memorial Hospital
Atlanta, Georgia

Gregory Ciottone, MD
Director, International Section
Department of Emergency Medicine
Harvard Medical School
Director, Division of Disaster Medicine
Department of Emergency Medicine
Beth Israel Deaconess
    Medical Center
Boston, Massachusetts

Brian Clyne, MD
Assistant Professor
Department of Emergency Medicine
Brown University
Residency Program Director
Department of Emergency Medicine
Rhode Island Hospital
Providence, Rhode Island

Michael Cocchi, MD
Instructor of Medicine
Harvard University Medical School
Attending Physician
Emergency/Critical Care Medicine
Beth Israel Deaconess Medical Center
Boston, Massachusetts

Stewart R. Coffman, MD, FACEP
Clinical Assistant Professor
    of Surgery
Division of Emergency Medicine
UT Southwestern Medical School
Chief Medical Officer
Questcare Partners
Dallas, Texas

Christopher B. Colwell, MD, FACEP
Associate Professor
Department of Surgery
University of Colorado Health Sciences
    Center
Associate Director
Department of Emergency Medicine
Denver Health Medical Center
Denver, Colorado

James Comes, MD
Associate Clinical Professor
Department of Emergency Medicine
University of California Fresno
Program Director
Department of Emergency Medicine
University Medical Center
Fresno, California

Matthew D. Cook, MD
Attending Physician
Emergency Medicine
Lehigh Valley Health Network
Allentown, Pennsylvania

Marco Coppola, DO, FACEP
Adjunct Clinical Professor of Emergency
    Medicine
University of North Texas Health Science
    Center
Fort Worth, Texas
Regional Director of Medical Education
Questcare Partners
Dallas, Texas

Kelly Corrigan, MD
Department of Emergency Medicine
Beth Israel Deaconess Medical Center
Boston, Massachusetts

Brian N. Corwell, MD
Assistant Professor
Department of Emergency Medicine
University of Maryland Medical Center
Baltimore, Maryland

Linda C. Cowell, MD
Newton Wellesley Hospital
Norfolk, Massachusetts

Richard A. Craven, MD, FACOEM
Associate Professor
Department of Family Medicine
Eastern Virginia Medical School
Norfolk, Virginia

Jennifer Cullen, MD
Resident
Department of Emergency Medicine
University of California San Diego
San Diego, California

Kirk L. Cumpston, DO
Assistant Professor
Emergency Medicine
Virginia Commonwealth University
Virginia Commonwealth University Health
    System
Emergency Medicine
Medical College of Virginia Hospital
Richmond, Virginia

Liesel A. Curtis, MD, FACEP
Assistant Professor
Department of Emergency Medicine
Georgetown University Hospital
Washington, DC

Rita K. Cydulka, MD, MS
Associate Professor
Department of Emergency Medicine
Case Western Reserve University School
    of Medicine
Associate Chair
Department of Emergency Medicine
Metrohealth Medical Center
Cleveland, Ohio

**Jamila Danishwar, MD, MS**
Physician Resident
Emergency Department
University of California San Diego Medical
  Center
San Diego, California

**Daniel Davis, MD**
Associate Clinical Professor of Medicine
Department of Emergency Medicine
Faculty Physician
Department of Emergency Medicine
University of California, San Diego

**Michelle Davitt, MD**
Assistant Professor
Department of Emergency Medicine
Albert Einstein College of Medicine
Attending Physician
Montefoire Medical Center
Bronx, New York

**Peter M.C. DeBlieux, MD**
Professor of Clinical Medicine
Department of Emergency Medicine
Director of Resident and Faculty
  Development
Section of Emergency Medicine
LSUHSC New Orleans
New Orleans, Louisiana

**David Della-Guistina, MD**
Clinical Assistant Professor
Department of Medicine
University of Washington
Seattle, Washington
Chairman
Department of Emergency Medicine
Madigan Army Medical Center
Tacoma, Washington

**Paul H. Desan, MD, PhD**
Assistant Professor
Department of Psychiatry
Yale University School of Medicine
Director
Psychiatric Consultation Service
Yale New Haven Hospital
New Haven, Connecticut

**Paul L. DeSandre, DO**
Assistant Professor
Department of Emergency Medicine
Albert Einstein College of Medicine
Bronx, New York
Department of Emergency Medicine
Beth Israel Medical Center
New York, New York

**Diane DeVita, MD, FACEP**
Department of Emergency Medicine
Madigan Army Medical Center
Tacoma, Washington

**Chirag A. Dholakia, MD**
Clinical Instructor
General Surgery
University of California Irvine Medical Center
Orange, California

**Michael K. Doney, MD, MS, MPH**
Medical Officer
Centers for Disease Control and Prevention
Atlanta, Georgia

**Michael Donnino, MD**
Assistant Professor of Medicine
Harvard University Medical School
Attending Physician
Emergency/Critical Care Medicine
Beth Israel Deaconess Medical Center
Boston, Massachusetts

**Erica Douglass, MD**
Resident
Emergency Medicine
Denver Health Medical Center
Denver, Colorado

**Jeffrey Druck, MD**
Assistant Professor
Emergency Medicine
University of Colorado
Denver, Colorado
Assistant Head, Education
Emergency Medicine
University of Colorado Hospital
Aurora, Colorado

**Susan Dufel, MD**
Associate Professor
Traumatology and Emergency Medicine
University of Connecticut
Farmington Connecticut
Residency Director
Hartford Hospital
Hartford, Connecticut

**Susan Echemandia-Writh, MD**
Attending Physician
Department of Emergency Medicine
St. Vincent's Hospital
New York, New York

**Kathryn C. EcKstein, MD**
Child and Adolescent Psychiatry Fellow
Department of Psychiatry
Massachusetts General Hospital
Boston, Massachusetts

**Kamryn T. Eddy, PhD**
Instructor of Psychology
Harvard Medical School
Assistant in Psychology
Psychiatry
Massachusetts General Hospital
Boston, Massachusetts

**Jonathan A. Edlow, MD**
Associate Professor
Department of Medicine
Harvard Medical School
Associate Chief
Department of Emergency Medicine
Beth Israel Deaconess Medical Center
Boston, Massachusetts

**Arunachalam Einstein, MD**
Clinical Instructor of Medicine
University of Washington
Seattle, Washington
Emergency Physician
Emergency Medicine
Providence Regional Medical Center
Everett, Washington

**Robert Eisenstein, MD**
Associate Professor and Vice Chairman
Department of Emergency Medicine
UMDNJ/Robert Wood Johnson Medical
  School
Chief
Ambulatory Service/Division of Emergency
  Care
Robert Wood Johnson University Hospital
New Brunswick, New Jersey

**Tala R. Elia, MD**
Assistant Professor
Department of Emergency Medicine
Tufts University
Assistant Professor
Department of Emergency Medicine
Baystate Medical Center
Springfield, Massachusetts

**Norbert Elsner, MD, MA**
Assistant Professor
Department of Emergency Medicine
Albert Einstein College of Medicine
Associate Director
Department of Emergency Medicine
Jacobi Medical Center
Bronx, New York

**Janet Eng, DO**
Emergency Medicine Attending
  Physician/Toxicologist
Ingham Regional Medical Center
Lansing, Michigan

**Stephen K. Epstein, MD, MPP**
Instructor
Department of Emergency Medicine
Harvard Medical School
Department of Emergency Medicine
Beth Israel Deaconess Medical Center
Boston, Massachusetts

Timothy B. Erickson, MD, FACEP
FAACT, FACMT
Professor
Emergency Medicine
University of Illinois at Chicago
Head
Emergency Department and Division of
    Medical Toxicology
University of Illinois Medical Center
Chicago, Illinois

Barnet Eskin, MD, PhD
Clinical Assistant Professor
Department of Surgery
UMDNJ-New Jersey Medical School
Newark, New Jersey
Attending Emergency Physician
Department of Emergency Medicine
Morristown Memorial Hospital
Morristown, New Jersey

Tamara Espinoza, MD
Chief Resident
Department of Emergency Medicine
Cook County Hospital
Chicago, Illinois

Brian D. Euerle, MD
Associate Professor
Emergency Medicine
University of Maryland School
    of Medicine
Attending Physician
Emergency Medicine
University of Maryland Medical
    Center
Baltimore, Maryland

Saleh Fares, MD, FRCPC, FACEP
Fellow
Disaster Medical Section
Harvard Medical School
Fellow
Department of Emergency Medicine
Beth Israel Deaconess Medical
    Center
Boston, Massachusetts

David Feldman, MD
Department of Emergency Medicine
Sutter Delta Medical Center
Antioch, California

James Feldman, MD, FACEP
Associate Professor of Emergency
    Medicine
Department of Emergency Medicine
Boston University School of Medicine
Research Director
Department of Emergency Medicine
Boston Medical Center
Boston, Massachusetts

Robert Feldman, MD
Assistant Professor
Department of Emergency Medicine
Rush Medical College
Attending Physician
Department of Emergency Medicine
John H. Stroger Hospital of Cook County
Chicago, Illinois

Ian Glen Ferguson, DO
Attending Physician/Clinical Faculty
Department of Surgery/Division of
    Emergency Medicine
Stanford University Medical Center
Palo Alto, California
Vice Chairman
Department of Emergency Medicine
Santa Clara Valley Medical Center
San Jose, California

Maggie Ferng, MD
Department of Emergency Medicine
John H. Stroger Hospital of Cook County
Chicago, Illinois

Christopher Fischer, MD
Instructor
Department of Emergency Medicine
Beth Israel Deaconess Medical Center
Boston, Massachusetts

Jonathan Fisher, MD, MPH
Emergency Medicine
Beth Israel Deaconess Medical Center
Boston, Massachusetts

Michael A. Fogel, MD, PhD
Clinical Fellow
Department of Medicine
Harvard University
Resident
Department of Emergency Medicine
Beth Israel Deaconess Medical Center
Boston, Massachusetts

Kelly Anne Foley, MD, FACEP
Associate Professor
Department of Emergency Medicine
Eastern Virginia Medical School
Norfolk, Virginia

Samantha Foy, MD
Resident
Emergency Medicine
Beth Israel Deaconess Medical Center
Boston, Massachusetts

Nicole M. Franks, MD, FACEP
Assistant Professor
Emergency Medicine
Emory School of Medicine
Associate Medical Director
Emergency Medicine
Emory University Hospital Midtown
Atlanta, Georgia

Jessica Freedman, MD
Department of Emergency Medicine
Mt. Sinai School of Medicine
New York, New York

Franklin D. Friedman, MS, MD
Assistant Professor
Emergency Medicine
Tufts University School of Medicine
Director of Prehospital Care and
    Emergency Preparation
Emergency Medicine
Tufts Medical Center
Boston, Massachusetts

Steven Furer, MS, FACEP
Attending Physician
Department of Emergency Medicine
The Medical Center of Aurora
South Aurora, Colorado

Richard Gabor, MD
Assistant Professor of Emergency
    Medicine
Bay State Medical Center
Western Campus of Tufts University
    School of Medicine
Director
Pediatric Emergency Department
Department of Emergency Medicine
Baystate Medical Center
Springfield, Massachusetts

Benjamin Z. Galper, MD, MPH
Resident
Department of Medicine
Columbia University
Columbia Presbyterian Hospital
New York, New York

Theresa Gandor, MD
Resident
Department of Emergency Medicine
Cook County Stroger Hospital
Chicago, Illinois

Charles Garcia, DO
Resident
Department of Emergency Medicine
University of Nevada School of
    Medicine
University Medical Center
Las Vegas, Nevada

Rajender Gatt MD, MRCP
Assistant Professor of Pediatrics
Division of Pediatric Emergency
    Medicine
University of Maryland School of
    Medicine
Baltimore, Maryland

Nicholas Genes, MD, PhD
Informatics Fellow
Department of Emergency Medicine
Mount Sinai School of Medicine
Clinical Instructor
Department of Emergency Medicine
The Mount Sinai Hospital
New York, New York

Delaram Ghadishah, MD
Staff Physician
Emergency Department
Kaiser Permanente
West Los Angeles, California

Hina Zafar Ghory, MD
Chief Resident
Emergency Medicine
New York Presbyterian Hospital
New York, New York

Brandon Giberson, BS, WEMT-I
Clinical Research Coordinator
Cardiac Arrest Center
Beth Israel Deaconess Medical Center
Boston, Massachusetts

Colleen Gibson, MD
Resident
Department of Emergency Medicine
University of Maryland School of Medicine
Baltimore, Maryland

Bret E. Ginther, MD
Assistant Medical Director
Emergency Medicine
Inland Valley Medical Center
Wildomar, California

Robyn Heister Girard, MD
Kaiser Permanente
Redwood City, California

Judd L. Glasser, MD
Clinical Instructor
Department of Emergency Medicine
University of California San Diego
Attending Staff
Department of Emergency Medicine
Tri-City Medical Center
Oceanside, California

Laura B. Glicksman, MS, DMD
Private Practice
Needham, Massachusetts

Donald C. Goff, MD
Professor of Psychiatry
Harvard Medical School
Director
Schizophrenia Program
Massachusetts General Hospital
Boston, Massachusetts

Katja Goldflam, MD
Harvard Affiliated Emergency Medicine
    Resident
Massachusetts General Hospital/
    Brigham & Women's Hospital
Boston, Massachusetts

Dolores Gonthier, MD
Consultant
MD2 Healthcare Consulting, Inc.
Wexford, Pennsylvania

J. Scott Goudie
Carolina Health Specialists
Myrtle Beach, South Carolina

Deepi G. Goyal, MD
Assistant Professor
Mayo Clinic
Associate Residency Director
Mayo Emergency Medicine Residency
Rochester, Minnesota

Matthew N. Graber, MD, PhD
Assistant Professor
Department of Emergency Medicine and
    Department of Biochemistry
Emory University School of Medicine
Atlanta, Georgia

Ruth Granlund, MD
Physician
Department of Emergency Medicine
Feather River Hospital
Paradise, California

Siobhan Gray, MD
Emergency Medicine Resident
Department of Emergency Medicine
University of California San Diego
Resident
Department of Emergency Medicine
University of California San Diego Medical
    Center
San Diego, California

Ian Greenwald, MD
Assistant Professor
Department of Emergency Medicine
Emory University
Atlanta, Georgia

Samuel C. Gross, MD
Resident
Department of Emergency Medicine
Beth Israel Deaconess Medical Center
Boston, Massachusetts

Shamai A. Grossman, MD, MS
Assistant Professor of Medicine
Emergency Medicine
Harvard Medical School
Director, Cardiac Emergency Center and
    CDU
Emergency Medicine
Beth Israel Deaconess Medical Center
Boston, Massachusetts

Ian R. Grover, MD
Associate Clinical Professor of Medicine
Emergency Medicine
University of California San Diego
Medical Director
Hyperbaric Medicine Center
University of California San Diego
San Diego, California

Kama Guluma, MD
Assistant Clinical Professor
Department of Emergency Medicine
University of California San Diego
San Diego, California

Atul Gupta, DO, FAAEM
Chairman
Department of Emergency Medicine
Long Beach Memorial Medical Center
Long Beach, California

David A. Guss, MD
Professor and Chair
Department of Emergency Medicine
University of California San Diego School
    of Medicine
San Diego, California

Marilyn M. Hallock, MD
Assistant Professor
Department of Emergency Medicine
Rush University Medical Center
Chicago, Illinois

Robert S. Hamilton, MD, FAAEM
Volunteer Clinical Faculty
University of California, Davis
Medical Director, Emergency Services
Mercy Medical Center, Redding
Redding, California

Jeremy B. Hammel, MD
Resident Physician
Emergency Medicine
Loma Linda University Medical Center
Loma Linda, California

Allan V. Hansen, MD
Emergency Ultrasound Fellow
Emergency Medicine
University of California San Diego
San Diego, California

Brenden L. Hansen, MD
Resident Physician
Emergency Medicine
Loma Linda University Medical Center
Loma Linda, California

Kohei Hasegawa, MD
Harvard Affiliated Emergency Medicine
    Resident
Massachusetts General Hospital/
    Brigham & Women's Hospital
Boston, Massachusetts

**Jeanette Haslett, MD**
Resident
Department of Emergency Medicine
Cook County Stroger Hospital
Chicago, Illinois

**Stephen R. Hayden, MD**
Professor of Clinical Medicine
Program Director, Residency Program
Department of Emergency Medicine
University of California San Diego
Editor-in-Chief, Journal of Emergency
    Medicine
Medical Center
San Diego, California

**Benjamin S. Heavrin, MD**
Assistant Professor
Emergency Medicine
Vanderbilt University
Nashville, Tennessee

**Tarlan Hedayati, MD**
Assistant Professor
Department of Emergency Medicine
Rush Medical College
Attending Physician
Department of Emergency Medicine
Stroger Hospital of Cook County
Chicago, Illinois

**Timothy D. Heilenbach, MD**
Assistant Professor
Department of Medicine
University of Chicago
Chicago, Illinois
Attending Physician
Division of Emergency Medicine
Northshore University Health System
Evanston, Illinois

**Robin R. Hemphill, MD, MPH**
Associate Professor
Department of Emergency Medicine
Emory University School of Medicine
Atlanta, Georgia

**Sean O. Henderson, MD**
Vice Chair
Emergency Medicine
Keck School of Medicine of the University
    of Southern California
Los Angeles, California

**Gregory W. Hendey, MD, FACEP**
Professor
Emergency Medicine
University of California San Francisco
    School of Medicine
San Francisco, California
Vice Chair and Research Director
Emergency Medicine
University of California San Francisco
    Fresno Medical Education Program
Fresno, California

**Daniel J. Henning, MD**
Resident
Department of Emergency Medicine
Beth Israel Deaconess Medical Center
Boston, Massachusetts

**Patricia C. Henwood, MD**
Clinical Fellow in Medicine
Harvard Affiliated Emergency Medicine
    Residency
Brigham and Women's Hospital
Massachusetts General Hospital
Boston, Massachusetts

**David B. Herzog, MD**
Professor of Psychiatry (Pediatrics)
Department of Psychiatry
Harvard Medical School
Director, Eating Disorders Unit, Child
    Psychiatry Services at Massachusetts
    General Hospital
Department of Psychiatry
Massachusetts General Hospital
Boston, Massachusetts

**Braden J. Hexom, MD**
Instructor
Department of Emergency Medicine
Mount Sinai School of Medicine
Attending Physician
Department of Emergency Medicine
Mount Sinai Medical Center
New York, New York

**Colleen N. Hickey, MD**
Assistant Professor
Department of Emergency Medicine
Rush University
Attending Physician
Department of Emergency Medicine
John H. Stroger Jr. Hospital of Cook County
Chicago, Illinois

**Ra'ed A. Hijazi**
Assistant Professor
Department of Emergency Medicine
King Saud University of Health Sciences
Deputy Chairman, Emergency Department
Division Head, Trauma and Critical Care
Director of Disaster Medicine
Medical Director, Emergency Medical
    Services
King Abdulaziz Medical City, National
    Guard
Riyadh, Saudi Arabia

**Lisa G. Lowe Hiller, MD, MPH**
Department of Emergency Medicine
University of California San Diego Medical
    Center
San Diego, California

**Doodnauth Hiraman**
Assistant Professor of Medicine
Weill Medical College of Cornell University
Department of Emergency Medicine
New York Presbyterian Hospital
New York, New York

**Christanne M. Hoffman, MD**
Resident
Emergency Medicine
University of California, San Diego
San Diego, California

**Michael Homeyer, MD**
Assistant Clinical Professor
School of Allied Health
Loma Linda University
Resident Physician
Emergency Medicine
Loma Linda University Medical
    Center
Loma Linda, California

**Jason Hoppe, DO**
Assistant Professor
Department of Emergency Medicine
University of Colorado
Aurora, Colorado

**Erin R. Horn, MD**
Resident
Department of Emergency Medicine
Harvard Affiliated Emergency Medicine
    Residency
Resident
Department of Emergency Medicine
Beth Israel Deaconess Medical Center
Boston, Massachusetts

**Gudrun T. Hoskuldsdttir, MD**
Resident
Department of Emergency Medicine
Landspitali University Hospital
Reykjavik, Iceland

**Mark A. Hostetler, MD**
Department of Emergency Medicine
Phoenix Children's Hospital
Phoenix, Arizona

**John E. Houghland, MD**
Resident Physician
Emergency Medicine
Denver Health Medical Center
Denver, Colorado

**J.C. Huffman, MD**
Assistant Professor of Psychiatry
Harvard Medical School
Department of Psychiatry
Massachusetts General Hospital
Boston, Massachusetts

Peter L. Hulsey, DO
Resident
Department of Emergency Medicine
Baystate Medical Center
Springfield, Massachusetts

James Hwang, MD
Department of Emergency Medicine
Brigham and Women's Hospital
Boston, Massachusetts

Wender Hwang, MD
Department of Emergency Medicine
Loma Linda University Medical
  Center
Loma Linda, California

Jason Imperato, MD, MBA
Assistant Professor, Medicine
Medicine
Harvard Medical School
Boston, Massachusetts
Attending Physician
Department of Emergency Medicine
Mount Auburn Hospital
Cambridge, Massachusetts

Kelly E. Irwin, MD
Clinical Fellow
Psychiatry
Harvard Medical School
Resident, Psychiatry
Massachusetts General Hospital
Boston, Massachusetts

Paul Ishimine, MD
Associate Clinical Professor
Departments of Medicine and
  Pediatrics
University of California San Diego
La Jolla, California
Fellowship Director, Emergency Pediatric
  Medicine
Department of Emergency Medicine
University of California San Diego
San Diego, California

Kenneth Jackimczyk, MD
Attending Physician
Department of Emergency medicine
Maricopa Medical Center
Phoenix, Arizona

Lisa Jacobson, MD
Emergency Department
Georgetown University
Attending Physician
Emergency Department
Washington Hospital Center
Washington, DC

Irving Jacoby, MD, FACEP, FACP
Professor of Medicine
Department of Medicine
University of California, San Diego School
  of Medicine
Attending Physician
Department of Emergency Medicine
University of California, San Diego
San Diego, California

Gabrielle A. Jacquet, MD
Resident Physician
Emergency Medicine
University of Colorado Hospital
Aurora, Colorado
Emergency Medicine
Denver Health
Denver, Colorado

Liudvikas Jagminas, MD, FACEP
Vice Chair and Associate Professor
Emergency Medicine
Yale School of Medicine
Director of Clinical Operations
Emergency Medicine
Yale New Haven Hospital
New Haven, Connecticut

Thea James, MD
Department of Emergency Medicine
Boston University School of Medicine
Boston, Massachusetts

Gregory D. Jay, MD, PhD
Professor of Medicine and Emergency
  Medicine
The Warren Alpert School of Medicine at
  Brown University
Associate Chair for Research
Department of Emergency Medicine
Rhode Island Hospital
Providence, Rhode Island

David Jerrard, MD
Associate Professor
Emergency Department
University of Maryland
Baltimore, Maryland

Albert Jin, MD
Department of Emergency Medicine
Mission Hospital, Laguna Beach
Laguna Beach, California

Gary A. Johnson, MD, FACEP
Interim Chairman
Emergency Medicine
Upstate Medical University
Chief of Service
University Hospital
Syracuse, New York

Mary Beth Johnson, MD
Assistant Clinical Professor
Department of Emergency Medicine
University of California San Diego
Attending Physician
Department of Emergency Medicine
University of California San Diego Medical
  Center
San Diego, California

Madeline M. Joseph, MD
Associate Professor
Emergency Medicine and Pediatrics
Assistant Chair for Pediatrics and Division
  Chief
University of Florida Health Science Center
Jacksonville, Florida

Alfred Joshua, MD
Resident Physician
Department of Emergency Medicine
University of California San Diego
San Diego, California

Maureen L. Joyner, MD, FACEP
Assistant Professor
Emergency Medicine
Emory University
Atlanta, Georgia

Tarina Lee Kang, MD
Instructor
Department of Emergency Medicine
Harvard Medical School
Department of Emergency Medicine
Beth Israel Deaconess Medical Center
Boston, Massachusetts

Harry C. Karydes, DO
Toxicology Fellow
Department of Emergency Medicine
Cook County Hospital
Chicago, Illinois

A. Antoine Kazzi, MD, FAAEM
Chief of Service
Emergency Medicine Medical Director
The Emergency Unit
The American University of Beirut
Beirut, Lebanon

Ziad N. Kazzi, MD, FAAEM
Assistant Professor
Department of Emergency Medicine
Emory University School of Medicine
Atlanta, Georgia

Matthew T. Keadey, MD, FACEP
Assistant Professor
Department of Emergency Medicine
Emory University School of Medicine
Chief of Service
Emergency Department
Emory University Hospital
Atlanta, Georgia

**Samuel M. Keim, MD, MS**
Professor
Emergency Medicine
University of Arizona
Vice Head and Residency Director
Emergency Medicine
University Medical Center
Tucson, Arizona

**Elicia Sinor Kennedy, MD**
Assistant Professor Clinical Faculty
Department of Emergency Medicine
University of Arkansas for Medical
    Sciences
Little Rock, Arkansas

**Joseph H. Khan, MD**
Associate Professor
Emergency Medicine
Boston University School of Medicine
Director of Medical Student
    Education
Emergency Medicine
Boston Medical Center
Boston, Massachusetts

**James P. Killeen, MD**
Associate Professor
Department of Emergency Medicine
University of California, San Diego
Clinical Faculty
Department of Emergency Medicine
University of California, San Diego Medical
    Center
San Diego, California

**Grace Kim, MD**
Assistant Professor
Department of Emergency Medicine
Loma Linda University
Attending Physician
Department of Emergency Medicine
Division of Pediatric Emergency
    University
Loma Linda University Medical
    Center
Loma Linda, California

**Ronald E. Kim, MD**
Attending Physician
Department of Emergency Medicine
Cook County Stroger Hospital
Chicago, Illinois

**Renee A. King, MD, MPH**
Senior Instructor
Emergency Medicine
University of Colorado, Denver
Denver, Colorado

**Matthew A. Kippenhan, MD**
Assistant Professor
Department of Emergency Medicine
Northwestern University Feinberg School
    of Medicine
Attending Physician
Department of Emergency Medicine
Northwestern Memorial Hospital
Chicago, Illinois

**Kellie Kirkpatrick, MD**
Chicago, Illinois

**Jessica H. Klausmeier, MD, MPH**
Resident
Emergency Medicine
Beth Israel Deaconess Medical Center
Boston, Massachusetts

**Barry J. Knapp, II, MD, FACEP**
Associate Professor
Department of Emergency Medicine
Eastern Virginia School of Medicine
Norfolk, Virginia

**H. Samuel Ko, MD, MBA**
Emergency Medicine Resident Physician
Department of Emergency Medicine
Loma Linda University Medical Center
Loma Linda, California

**Leo Kobayashi, MD**
Assistant Professor
Department of Emergency Medicine
Brown Medical School
Attending Physician
Department of Emergency Medicine
Rhode Island Hospital
Providence, Rhode Island

**Paul Kolecki, MD, FACEP**
Associate Professor
Emergency Medicine
Thomas Jefferson University
    Hospital
Philadelphia, Pennsylvania

**Jennifer L. Kolodchak, MD**
Clinical Instructor
Department of Emergency Medicine
Rush Medical College
Attending Physician
Department of Emergency Medicine
Rush University Medical Center
Chicago, Illinois

**Amy V. Kontrick, MD**
Assistant Professor
Department of Emergency Medicine
Northwestern University, Feinberg School
    of Medicine
Chicago, Illinois

**Richard S. Krause, MD**
Residency Program Director
Department of Emergency Medicine
University of Buffalo School of Medicine
    and Biomedical Sciences
Buffalo, New York

**Joel Kravitz, MD, FACEP, FRCPSC**
Department of Emergency Medicine
Albert Einstein Medical Center
Philadelphia, Pennsylvania

**Lara K. Kulchycki, MD**
Attending Physician
Department of Emergency Medicine
Beth Israel Deaconess Medical Center
Boston, Massachusetts

**Alan M. Kumar, MD**
Clinical Instructor
Department of Medicine
University of Chicago
Attending Physician
Department of Emergency Medicine
Lutheran General Hospital
Park Ridge, Illinois

**Amanda J. Lamond, MD**
Resident Physician, Third Year
Emergency Medicine
University of California San Diego Medical
    Center
San Diego, California

**Owen Lander, MD**
Director of Clinical Research
Department of Emergency Medicine
Robert C. Byrd Health Sciences Center
West Virginia University
Morgantown, West Virginia

**Brooks T. Laselle, MD**
Clinical Instructor
Emergency Medicine
University of Washington
Seattle, Washington
Director, Ultrasound Fellowship
Department of Emergency Medicine
Madigan Army Medical Center
Tacoma, Washington

**Emi Latham, MD**
Assistant Clinical Professor of
    Medicine
Emergency Medicine
University of California, San Diego
San Diego, California

**Denise S. Lawe, MD**
Assistant Professor
Department of Emergency Medicine
Emory School of Medicine
Atlanta, Georgia

Minh V. Le, MD
Clinical Instructor
Family Medicine
University of California San Diego
Emergency Medicine
Kaiser Permanente Zion Hospital
San Diego, California

James M. Leaming, MD
Assistant Professor
Department of Emergency Medicine
Tufts School of Medicine
Attending Physician
Department of Emergency Medicine
Tufts–New England Medical Center
Boston, Massachusetts

JiWon E. Lee, MD
Department of Emergency Medicine
Medical Center of Lewisville
Lewisville, Texas

Moses S. Lee, MD, FACEP, FAAEM
Assistant Clinical Professor
Department of Emergency Medicine
Rush Medical College
Senior Attending Physician
Department of Emergency Medicine
John H. Stroger Hospital of Cook County
Chicago, Illinois

Donald J. Lefkowits, MD, FACEP
Assistant Clinical Professor
Family Medicine
Univers of Colorado Denver School of
   Medicine
Medical Director
Emergency Department
Rose Medical Center
Denver, Colorado

Eric Legome, MD
Chairman
Department of Emergency Medicine
St. Vincent's Hospital, Manhattan
New York, New York

Steven Lelyveld, MD
Associate Professor
Departments of Medicine and Pediatrics
University of Chicago Pritzker School of
   Medicine
Medical Director
University of Chicago Occupational
   Medicine
University of Chicago Medical Center
Chicago, Illinois

Amy LePage, MD
Department of Emergency Medicine
Benefits Healthcare
Great Falls, Montana

Roneet Lev, MD
Clinical Faculty
Emergency Medicine
University of California, San Diego
Director of Operations
Emergency Department
Scrips Mercy Hospital
San Diego, California

William J. Lewander MD
Professor of Emergency Medicine and
   Pediatrics
The Warren Alpert School of Medicine
   of Brown University
Director, Pediatric Emergency
   Medicine
Hasbro Children's Hospital
Providence, Rhode Island

Trevor Lewis, MD, FACEP
Assistant Professor
Department of Emergency Medicine
Rush Medical College
Medical Director
Department of Emergency Medicine
Cook County Hospital
Chicago, Illinois

Lazaro Lezcano, MD, FAAP
Assistant Professor
Pediatrics
Albert Einstein College of Medicine
Director, Division of Neonatology
Pediatrics
St. Barnabas Hospital
Bronx, New York

Richard Lichenstein, MD
Associate Professor
Pediatric Emergency Medicine
University of Maryland School
   of Medicine
Director, Pediatric Emergency Medicine
   Research
Pediatric Emergency Medicine
University of Maryland Hospital for
   Children
Baltimore, Maryland

Alexander T. Limkakeng, Jr., MD
Department of Emergency Medicine
Duke University Health System
Durham, North Carolina

Ming Valerie Lin, MD
Medicine Resident
Department of Internal Medicine
University of Pennsylvania
Resident
Department of Internal Medicine
Pennsylvania Hospital
Philadelphia, Pennsylvania

David A. Listman, MD
Assistant Professor
Pediatrics
Albert Einstein College of Medicine
Director, Pediatric Emergency Medicine
Department of Pediatrics
St. Barnabas Hospital
Bronx, New York

Jean C.Y. Lo, MD, MS
Toxicology Fellow
Department of Emergency Medicine
University of California San Diego
San Diego, California
Emergency Department
California Hospital
Los Angeles, California

Frank Lovecchio, MD
Assistant Clinical Professor of Medicine
Emergency Medicine
University of California San Diego
San Diego, California

Jenny J. Lu, MD
Assistant Professor
Department of Emergency Medicine
Rush Medical College
Attending Physician
Department of Emergency Medicine
Division of Toxicology
Cook County Hospital
Chicago, Illinois

Binh T Ly, MD
Associate Clinical Professor of medicine
Department of Surgery
University of California, San Diego
Director, Emergency Medicine Residency
   Program
Director, Toxicology Fellowship Program
University of California San Diego Medical
   Center
San Diego, California

Gene Ma, MD, FACEP
Voluntary Assistant Clinical Professor
School of Medicine
University of California San Diego
San Diego, California
Chairman
Emergency Medicine
Tri-City Medical Center
Oceanside, California

John MacKay, Jr., MD
Assistant Professor and Clership
Director
Department of Emergency Medicine
Texas Tech University
Attending Physician
Department of Emergency Medicine
Thomson Hospital
El Paso, Texas

Laura Macnow, MD
Instructor
Department of Emergency Medicine
Harvard Medical School
Attending Physician
Department of Emergency Medicine
Beth Israel Deaconess Medical Center
Boston, Massachusetts

Bo E. Madsen, MD
Instructor in Medicine
Emergency Medicine
Harvard Medical School
Attending Physician
Emergency Medicine
Beth Israel Deaconess Medical
    Center
Boston, Massachusetts

John Mahoney, MD
Associate Professor
Department of Emergency Medicine
University of Pittsburgh School of
    Medicine
Attending Physician
Department of Emergency Medicine
UPMC Presbyterian
Pittsburgh, Pennsylvania

Mamta Malik, MD
Department of Emergency Medicine
Rush Medical Center
Chicago, Illinois

Gerald Maloney, Jr., DO
Assistant Professor
Department of Emergency Medicine
Case Western Reserve School of
    Medicine
Cleveland, Ohio

Mark Mandell, MD
Chairman
Department of Emergency Medicine
Morristown Memorial hospital
Morristown, New Jersey

Brian V. Maneevese, MD
Resident Physician
Emergency Medicine
Texas Tech University Health Sciences
    Center
Resident Physician
Emergency Medicine
University Medical Center El Paso
El Paso, Texas

Francesco Mannelli, MD, PhD
Chief
Emergency Department
Pediatric Meyer Hospital
Florence, Italy

Jeffrey A. Manko, MD
Assistant Professor
Department of Emergency Medicine
New York University
Program Director, Emergency Medicine
    Residency
Department of Emergency Medicine
New York University/Bellevue Medical
    Center
New York, New York

Jon D. Mason, MD
Associate Professor
Departments of Emergency Medicine and
    Pediatrics
Eastern Virginia Medical School
Attending Physician
Department of Emergency Medicine
Sentara Norfolk General Hospital
Norfolk, Virginia

Brandon Maughan, MD
Resident
Department of Emergency Medicine
Rhode Island Hospital
Providence, Rhode Island

Suzan Mazor, MD
Departments of Toxicology and
    Emergency Medicine
Seattle Children's Hospital
Seattle, Washington

Christopher M. McCarthy, II, MD
Morristown Memorial Hospital
Morristown, New Jersey

Robert F. McCormack, MD
Clinical Chief of Emergency Medicine,
Attending Physician, Buffalo General
    Hospital
Buffalo, New York

Daniel C. McGillicuddy, MD
Instructor of Medicine
Internal Medicine
Harvard Medical School
Assistant Residency Director
Beth Israel Deaconess Medical Center
Boston, Massachusetts

Anthony J. Medak, MD
Department of Emergency Medicine
University of California, San Diego
San Diego, California

Timothy J. Meehan, MD, MPH
Senior Fellow
Toxikon Consortium
Clinical Instructor of Emergency Medicine
Department of Emergency Medicine
University of Illinois at Chicago Medical
    Center
Chicago, Illinois

Moss Mendelson, MD
Associate Professor
Emergency Medicine
Eastern Virginia Medical School
Norfolk, Virginia

Eduardo J. Menjivar, MD
Attending Physician
Emergency Medicine
Sentara Careplex
Hampton, Virginia

Mary K. Meyer, MD
Resident
Department of Emergency Medicine
Mayo Clinic
Rochester, Minnesota

Nathan Mick, MD
Attending Physician
Department of Pediatric Emergency
    Medicine
Maine Medical Center
Portland, Maine

Alexander D. Miller, MD
Clinical Instructor
Department of Emergency Medicine
University of California San Diego
Attuning Physician
Department of Emergency Medicine
University of California San Diego Medical
    Center
San Diego, California

Scott A. Miller, MD
Clinical Instructor
Department of Emergency Medicine
Rush University Medical Center
Chicago, Illinois

Shayle Miller, MD, FACEP
Voluntary Attending Physician
Department of Emergency Medicine
Cook County Stroger Hospital
Chicago, Illinois

Trevor J. Mills, MD, MPH
Associate Professor of Emergency
    Medicine
Louisiana State University Health Sciences
    Center
New Orleans, Louisiana
Chief of Emergency Medicine
VA Northern California Health Care System
Sacramento, California

Andrew Milstein, MD, MS, FACEP
Division of Emergency Medicine
University of Maryland
Baltimore, Maryland
Department of Emergency Medicine
Baltimore Washington Medical Center
Glen Burnie, Maryland

Elizabeth L. Mitchell, MD
Clinical Associate Professor
Department of Emergency Medicine
Boston University
Boston, Massachusetts

Christy Rosa Mohler, MD, FACEP, FAAEM
Emergency Physician
Department of Emergency Medicine
Scripps Mercy Hospital Chula Vista
Chula Vista, California

Robert C. Montana
Everette, Washington

Maria E. Moreira, MD
Assistant Professor, Surgery
University of Colorado Denver School of Medicine
Aurora, Colorado
Attending Physician
Emergency Medicine
Denver Health Medical Center
Denver, Colorado

Daniel Morris, MD
Resident Physician
Emergency Medicine
University of California San Diego Medical Center
San Diego, California

Nicholas C. Mosely, MD
Chief Resident
Department of Emergency Medicine Academic
Emory University School of Medicine
Chief Resident
Department of Emergency Medicine
Grady Memorial Hospital
Atlanta, Georgia

Jarrod Mosier, MD
Chief Resident
Emergency Medicine
University of Arizona
University Medical Center
Tucson, Arizona

Jordan Moskoff, MD
Clinical Instructor
Department of Emergency Medicine
Rush University Medical College
Department of Emergency Medicine
John H. Stroger Hospital of Cook County
Chicago, Illinois

Matthew B. Mostofi, DO
Assistant Professor
Department of Emergency Medicine
Tufts University School of Medicine
Attending Physician
Department of Emergency Medicine
Tufts-New England Medical Center
Boston, Massachusetts

Linda Mueller, MD
Department of Emergency Medicine
Edward Hospital
Naperville, Illinois

David W. Munter, MD, MBA
Associate Clinical Professor of Emergency Medicine
Eastern Virginia Medical School
Norfolk, Virginia
Associate Professor of Emergency Medicine
Edward Via Virginia College of Osteopathic Medicine
Blacksburg, Virginia
Medical Director, Emergency Medical Department
Sentara Obici Hospital
Suffolk, Virginia

Michael S. Murphy, MD
Medical Director for Pre-Hospital Care
Department of Emergency Medicine
South Shore Hospital
South Weymouth, Massachusetts

Mark B. Mycyk, MD
Associate Professor
Department of Emergency Medicine
Boston University School of Medicine
Department of Emergency Medicine
Boston Medical Center
Boston, Massachusetts

Antonio Napolitano, MD
Assistant Professor
Department of Emergency Medicine
Albert Einstein College of Medicine
Attending Physician
Montefiore Medical Center
Bronx, New York

Kathleen Nasci, MD
Medical Director
Department of Emergency Medicine
Pennsylvania Hospital
Philadelphia, Pennsylvania

Isam F. Nasr, MD, FACEP
Assistant Professor
Department of Emergency Medicine
Rush Medical College
Attending Physician
Department of Emergency Medicine
Cook County Stroger Hospital
Chicago, Illinois

Sean-Xavier Neath, MD, PhD
Assistant Professor
Department of Emergency Medicine
University of California, San Diego
San Diego, California

James A. Nelson, MD
Assistant Professor, non-salaried
Emergency Medicine
University of California San Diego
San Diego, California
Attending Physician
Emergency Medicine
Pioneers Memorial Hospital
Brawley, California

Edward Newton, MD
Professor and Chair
Department of Emergency Medicine
Keck School of Medicine, University of Southern California
Chairman
Department of Emergency Medicine
Los Angeles California and University of Southern California Medical Center
Los Angeles, California

Vinh D. Ngo, MD
Senior Resident
Emergency Medicine
Emory University
House Staff
Emergency Medicine
Grady Memorial Hospital
Atlanta, Georgia

Ann P. Nguyen, MD
Attending Physician
Department of Emergency Medicine
Bellevue Hospital Center and New York Medical Center
New York, New York

Michael W. Nielson
Department of Emergency Medicine
University of California San Diego Medical Center
San Diego, California

Sean Patrick Nordt, MD, PharmD
Assistant Professor
Department of Emergency Medicine
University of Southern California
LAC and USC Medical Center
Los Angeles, California

Charles W. O'Connell, MD
Resident
Department of Emergency Medicine
University of California San Diego
San Diego, California

Francis J. O'Connell, MD
Resident
Emergency Medicine
Beth Israel Deaconess Medical Center
Boston, Massachusetts

Neil O'Connor, MD, FACEP
Medical Director
CarePoint PC
Denver, Colorado

**Carol R. Okada, MD**
Instructor
Department of Pediatrics
University of Colorado at Denver
Pediatric Hospitalist
Department of Pediatrics
Denver Health Medical Center
Denver, Colorado

**Yasuharu Okuda, MD**
Associate Clinical Professor
Emergency Medicine and Medical
    Education
Mount Sinai School of Medicine
Director, Assistant Vice President
Institute for Medical Simulation and
    Advanced Learning
NYC Health and Hospitals Corporation
New York, New York

**Jonathan S. Olshaker, MD**
Professor and Chairman
Department of Emergency Medicine
Boston University School of Medicine
Chief, Department of Emergency Medicine
Boston Medical Center
Boston, Massachusetts

**Ben Osborne, MD**
Assistant Professor
Department of Emergency Medicine
Tufts University School of Medicine
Boston, Massachusetts
Associate Residency Director
Department of Emergency Medicine
Baystate Medical Center
Springfield, Massachusetts

**Seth M. Oskie, MD**
Emergency Medicine Resident
Department of Emergency Medicine
Loma Linda University Medical Center
Loma Linda, California

**Leslie C. Oyama, MD**
Assistant Clinical Professor
Emergency Medicine
University of California San Diego
San Diego, California

**David Palafox, MD**
Department of Emergency Medicine
Thomason General Hospital
El Paso, Texas

**Lynne M. Palmisciano, MD**
Assistant Professor, Emergency Medicine
The Warren Alpert School of Medicine of
    Brown University
Attending Physician, Pediatric Emergency
    Medicine
Hasbro Children's Hospital
Providence, Rhode Island

**Peter S. Pang, MD**
Assistant Professor
Emergency Medicine and Medicine
Northwestern University
Associate Chief
Department of Emergency Medicine
Northwestern Memorial Hospital
Chicago, Illinois

**Rajan Parikh, MD**
Resident
Department of Emergency Medicine
Cook County Stroger Hospital
Chicago, Illinois

**Jennifer M. Park, MD**
Instructor
Department of Psychiatry
Harvard Medical School
Boston, Massachusetts
Staff Psychiatrist
Walter Reed Army Medical Center
Washington, DC

**Lawrence T. Park, MD**
Assistant Professor
Department of Psychiatry
Harvard Medical School
Boston, Massachusetts

**Peter J. Park, MD**
Attending Physician
Department of Emergency Medicine
Naval Medical Center San Diego
San Diego, California

**Robert A. Partridge, MD, PPH, DTM, FACEP**
Associate Professor
Department of Emergency Medicine
Brown Medical School
Attending Physician
Department of Emergency Medicine
Rhode Island Hospital
Providence, Rhode Island

**Hetal Bharat Patel, MD**
Resident
Emergency Medicine
University of California San Diego
San Diego, California

**David A. Peak, MD**
Instructor
Department of Emergency Medicine
Harvard Medical School
Staff Physician
Department of Emergency Medicine
Massachusetts General Hospital
Boston, Massachusetts

**Phillips Perera, MD, RDMS, FACEP**
Assistant Clinical Professor
Emergency Medicine
Columbia University Medical Center/
    New York Presbyterian Hospital
New York, New York

**David A. Perstein, MD**
Assistant Professor, Pediatrics
Albert Einstein College of Medicine
Medical Director, Pediatrics
St. Barnabas Hospital
Bronx, New York

**Angela Pham, MD**
Resident
Department of Emergency Medicine
University of California San Diego
Resident
Department of Emergency Medicine
University of California San Diego Medical
    Center
San Diego, California

**Yalonda L. Phillips, DO**
Resident
Emergency Medicine
Baystate Medical Center
Springfield, Massachusetts

**Matthew J. Pirotte, MD**
Resident
Department of Emergency Medicine
Northwestern Memorial Hospital
Chicago, Illinois

**Stephen Roy Pitts, MD, MPH**
Associate Professor
Emergency Medicine
Emory University
Attending Physician
Emergency Department
Grady Memorial Hospital
Atlanta, Georgia

**Charles V. Pollack, Jr., MA, MD, FACEP, FAAEM, FAHA**
Professor and Chairman
Department of Emergency Medicine
Pennsylvania Hospital, University of
    Pennsylvania
Philadelphia, Pennsylvania

**Jennifer V. Pope, MD**
Instructor
Department of Emergency Medicine
Harvard Medical School
Assistant Program Director
Department of Emergency Medicine
Beth Israel Deaconess Medical Center
Boston, Massachusetts

**Janet M. Poponick, MD**
Assistant Professor
Department of Emergency Medicine
Case Western Reserve University
MetroHealth Medical Center
Cleveland, Ohio

**William Porcaro, MD**
Department of Emergency Medicine
University of Massachusetts Memorial
    Healthcare
Worcester, Massachusetts

Jason J. Prystowski, MD, MPH
Department of Emergency Medicine
Ronald Reagan UCLA Medical Center
Los Angeles, California

Yanina A. Purim-Shem-Tov, MD, MS, FACEP
Assistant Professor
Medical Director of Chest Pain Center
Director of Research, Department of
    Emergency Medicine
Rush University Medical Center
Chicago, Illinois

Arun V. Raghavan, MD, FACEP
Clinical Adjunct Assistant Professor
Division of Emergency Services
University of North Texas Health Science
    Center
Medical Director and Chairman
Division of Emergency Services
Plaza Medical Center of Fort Worth
Fort Worth, Texas

Vittorio Raho, MD
Department of Emergency Medicine
Beverly Hospital
Beverly, Massachusetts

Kelley Ralph, MD, MS
Resident
Emergency Medicine
Emory University
Atlanta, Georgia

Harish Raj Seetha Rammohan, MD, MRCP
Postgraduate Resident, YR-1
Internal Medicine
Pennsylvania Hospital of the University
    of Pennsylvania Health System
Philadelphia, Pennsylvania

Niels K. Rathlev, MD
Professor and Chair
Emergency Medicine
Tufts University School of Medicine
Boston, Massachusetts; Chair
Emergency Medicine
Baystate Medical Center
Springfield, Massachusetts

Neha P. Raukar, MD, MS
Assistant Professor
Department of Emergency Medicine
The Warren Alpert Medical School
Brown University
Attending Physician
Department of Emergency Medicine/
    Primary Care Sports Medicine
The Rhode Island Hospital and the Miriam
    Hospital
Providence, Rhode Island

Ian Reilly, MD
Department of Emergency Medicine
Scripps Memorial Hospital, La Jolla
La Jolla, California

James W. Rhee, MD
Departments of Emergency Medicine and
    Medical Toxicology
Loma Linda University Medical Center
Loma Linda, California

Shada A. Rhouhani, MD
Harvard Affiliated Emergency Medicine
Resident
Massachusetts General Hospital/
    Brigham & Women's Hospital
Boston, Massachusetts

Mark Richmond, MD
Department of Emergency Medicine
Santa Barbara Cottage Hospital
Santa Barbara, California

Steven T. Riley, MD
Clinical Assistant Professor
Pediatrics and Emergency Medicine
Vanderbilt University School of Medicine
Nashville, Tennessee

Jaime B. Rivas, MD
Physician
Department of Emergency Medicine
Palomar and Pomerado Hospitals
Escondido, California

Jonathon Roberts, MD
Harvard Medical School
Resident Physician
Department of Emergency Medicine
Beth Israel Deaconess Medical
    Center
Boston, Massachusetts

Matthew Robinson, MD
Department of Emergency Medicine
University of Missouri Medical center
Columbia, Missouri

Colleen N. Roche, MD
Assistant Professor
Department of Emergency Medicine
The George Washington University
Washington, DC

E. Jedd Roe, MD, MBA, MSF
Residence Director
Associate Professor
Department of Emergency Medicine
University of Alabama at Birmingham
Birmingham, Alabama

Joshua L. Roffman, MD
Assistant Professor of Psychiatry
Harvard Medical School
Department of Psychiatry
Massachusetts General Hospital
Boston, Massachusetts

Carlo L. Rosen, MD
Associate Professor
Department of Medicine
Harvard Medical School
Program Director and Vice Chair for
    Education
Emergency Medicine
Beth Israel Deaconess Medical Center
Boston, Massachusetts

Noah K. Rosenberg, MD
Resident
Department of Emergency Medicine
Brown University
Resident
Department of Emergency Medicine
Rhode Island Hospital
Providence, Rhode Island

Alix L. Rosenstein, MD
Department of Emergency Medicine
Case Western Reserve School of
    Medicine
Cleveland, Ohio

Lucas C. Rociere, MD
Resident Physician
Department of Emergency Medicine
Northwestern University Feinberg School
    of Medicine
Chicago, Illinois

Christopher Ross, MD, FAAEM, FRCPC
Assistant Professor
Department of Emergency Medicine
Rush Medical College
Assistant Program Director
Department of Emergency Medicine
John H. Stroger Hospital of Cook County
Chicago, Illinois

Ethan M. Ross, MD
Resident
Emergency Medicine
Beth Israel Deaconess Medical Center
Boston, Massachusetts

David H. Rubin MD
Clinical Professor of Pediatrics
Albert Einstein College of Medicine
Chairman and Program Director
Department of Pediatrics
St. Barnabas Hospital
Bronx, New York

**Gary S. Sachs, MD**
Associate Professor of Psychiatry
Department of Psychiatry
Massachusetts General Hospital
Director of Bipolar Clinic and Research
  Program
Harvard Medical School
Boston, Massachusetts

**Anthony C. Salazar, MD**
Chief Resident
Department of Emergency Medicine
University of California San Diego
Chief Resident
Department of Emergency Medicine
University of California San Diego Medical
  Center
San Diego, California

**Erich Salvacion, MD**
Hospitalist
Department of Internal Medicine
Kaiser Permanente
Downey, California

**Leon D. Sanchez, MD, MPH**
Assistant Professor
Emergency Medicine
Harvard Medical School
Attending Physician
Emergency Medicine
Beth Israel Deaconess Medical Center
Boston, Massachusetts

**Arthur B. Sanders, MD**
Professor
Emergency Medicine
University of Arizona College of Medicine
Attending Physician
Emergency Medicine
University Medical Center
Tucson, Arizona

**Kathy M. Sanders, MD**
Assistant Professor
Psychiatry
Harvard Medical School
Psychiatrist
Massachusetts General Hospital
Boston, Massachusetts

**Scott R. Sanderson, MD**
Madigan Army Medical Center
Department of Emergency Medicine
Tacoma, Washington

**Marcelo Sandoval, MD**
Assistant Professor
Department of Emergency Medicine
Albert Einstein College of Medicine
Bronx, New York
Department of Emergency Medicine
Beth Israel Medical Center
New York, New York

**John P. Santamaria, MD**
Affiliate Professor of Pediatrics
University of South Florida School of
  Medicine
Tampa, Florida

**Sally Santen, MD**
Associate Professor
Department of Emergency Medicine
Emory University School of Medicine
Atlanta, Georgia

**John Santoro, MD**
Assistant Professor, Department of
  Emergency Medicine
Tufts University School of Medicine
Boston, Massachusetts
Vice Chair, Department of Emergency
  Medicine
Baystate Medical Center
Springfield, Massachusetts

**Elaine Sapiro, MD, MPH**
Assistant Clinical Professor
Emergency Medicine
University of California, San Diego
San Diego, California

**Davut J. Savaser, MD, MPH**
Emergency Medicine Resident
Department of Emergency Medicine
University of California San Diego
Resident
Emergency Medicine
University of California San Diego Medical
  Center
San Diego, California

**Daniel L. Savitt, MD**
Associate Professor of Medicine and
  Emergency Medicine
Warren Alpert School of Medicine of Brown
  University
Medical Director
Emergency Medicine
The Miriam Hospital
Providence, Rhode Island

**Assad J. Sayah, MD**
Harvard Medical School
Chief
Emergency Department
Cambridge Health Alliance
Boston, Massachusetts

**Shari Schabowski, MD**
Assistant Professor
Department of Emergency Medicine
Rush Medical College
Senior Attending Physician
Department of Emergency Medicine
Cook County Hospital
Chicago, Illinois

**Jeffrey J. Schaider, MD**
Associate Professor of Emergency
  Medicine
Rush Medical College
Chairman
Department of Emergency Medicine
Cook County Health and Hospital System
Chicago, Illinois

**Michael Schmidt, MD**
Assistant Professor
Department of Emergency Medicine
Northwestern University Feinberg School
  of Medicine
Department of Emergency Medicine
Northwestern Memorial Hospital
Chicago, Illinois

**Jeffrey I. Schneider, MD**
Assistant Professor
Department of Emergency Medicine
Boston University School of Medicine
Attending Physician
Boston Medical Center
Boston, Massachusetts

**Hugh A. Schuckman, MD**
Clinical Professor
Emergency Medicine
North East Ohio Universities College
  of Medicine
Rootstown, Ohio
Attending Physician
Emergency Medicine
Summa Health Systems
Akron, Ohio

**Suzanne Schuh, MD, FRCP(C)**
Professor
Paediatrics
University of Toronto
Staff and Research Director
Paediatric Emergency Medicine
The Hospital for Sick Children
Toronto, Canada

**Theresa Schwab, MD**
Department of Emergency Medicine
Christ Medical Center
Oak Lawn, Illinois

**Rebecca Wilks Schwartz, MD**
Affiliate Assistant Professor
Emergency Department
Oregon Health & Sciences University
Portland, Oregon
Attending Physician
Emergency Department
Kaiser Sunnyside Medical Center
Clackamas, Oregon

Gary Schwartz, MD
Assistant Professor
Department of Emergency Medicine
Vanderbilt University Medical
    Center
Nashville, Tennessee

James L. Scott, MD
Dean
School of Medicine and Health
    Sciences
The George Washington University
Professor
Department of Emergency Medicine
The George Washington University
Washington, DC

Michelle Sergel, MD
Assistant Professor
Assistant Residency Director
Department of Emergency medicine
Rush University Medical Center
Attending Physician
Department of Emergency Medicine
John H. Stroger Hospital of Cook
    County
Chicago, Illinois

Fred Severyn, MD, FACEP
Assistant Professor of Emergency
    Medicine
University of Colorado, Denver
Assistant Professor of Emergency
    Medicine
University of Colorado Hospital
Denver, Colorado

Purvi D. Shah, MD
Assistant Professor
Emergency Medicine
Albert Einstein College of Medicine
Assistant Director
Emergency Medicine
Montefiore Medical Center
Bronx, New York

Nathan Shapiro, MD, MPH
Assistant Professor
Harvard Medical School
Research Director
Beth Israel Deaconess Medical Center
Boston, Massachusetts

Philip Shayne, MD
Associate Professor
Vice Chair for Education and Residency
    Program Director
Department of Emergency Medicine
Emory University School of Medicine
Atlanta, Georgia

Ghazala Q. Sharieff, MD, FAAEM,
FACEP
Clinical Professor
University of California San Diego
Division Director
Emergency Department
Rady Children's Hospital Emergency Care
    Center
San Diego, California

Scott C. Sherman, MD
Associate Professor
Department of Emergency Medicine
Rush University Medical School
Assistant Program Director
Department of Emergency Medicine
Cook County Stroger Hospital
Chicago, Illinois

Chet Shermer, MD
Clinical Assistant Professor
Department of Emergency Medicine
University of Mississippi Medical Center
Staff Physician
Department of Emergency Medicine
Mississippi Baptist Medical Center
Jackson, Mississippi

Patricia Shipley, MD
Rush University Medical Center
Chicago, Illinois

Robert Sidman, MD
Chief, Emergency Services
William Backus Hospital
Providence, Rhode Island

Christine Tsien Silvers, MD, PhD
Research Affiliate
Children's Hospital Informatics Program
Children's Hospital
Boston, Massachusetts
Attending Physician
Emergency Medicine
Caritas Good Samaritan Medical Center
Brockton, Massachusetts

Alison K. Sisitsky
Attending Physician
Department of Emergency Medicine
Newton Wellesley Hospital
Newton, Massachusetts

Carl G. Skinner, MD
Emergency Physician & Medical
    Toxicologist
Madigan Army Medical Center
Department of Emergency Medicine
Tacoma, Washington

Christian M. Sloan, MD
Assistant Clinical Professor
Department of Emergency Medicine
University of California San Diego medical
    Center
San Diego, California

Michael D. Smith, MD
Assistant Professor
Department of Emergency Medicine
Case Western Reserve University
Attending Physician
Department of Emergency Medicine
MetroHealth Medical Center
Cleveland, Ohio

Felicia A. Smith, MD
Instructor
Department of Psychiatry
Harvard Medical School
Department of Psychiatry
Massachusetts General Hospital
Boston, Massachusetts

James L. Smith, Jr, MD
Department of Emergency Medicine
Gwinnett Medical Center
Lawrenceville, Georgia

Lauren M. Smith, MD
Assistant Professor
Emergency Medicine
Rush Medical College
Attending Physician
Emergency Medicine
John H. Stroger Hospital of Cook County
Chicago, Illinois

Rebecca Smith-Coggins, MD
Associate Professor
Department of Surgery/Emergency
    Medicine
Stanford University
Stanford, California

Brian K. Snyder
Associate Clinical Professor of Medicine
Department of Emergency Medicine
University of California, San Diego
San Diego, California

Devin R. Sokolowski, MD
Department of Emergency Medicine
Warren Alpert Medical School of Brown
    University
Rhode Island Hospital
Providence, Rhode Island

Julia H. Sone, MD
Attending Physician
General, Colon and Rectal Surgery
INOVA Fairfax Hospital
Falls Church, Virginia
Virginia Hospital Center
Arlington, Virginia

Arash Soroudi, MD
Resident
Emergency Department
University of California San Diego Medical
    Center
San Diego, California

Zachary P. Soucy, DO
Resident
Emergency Medicine
Mayo Clinic
St. Mary's Hospital
Rochester, Minnesota

Matthew T. Spencer, MD
Associate Professor
Department of Emergency Medicine
University of Rochester School of Medicine
    and Dentistry
Rochester, New York

Linda L. Spillane, MD
Associate Professor
Department of Emergency Medicine
University of Rochester School of Medicine
    and Dentistry
Department of Emergency Medicine
Strong Memorial Hospital
Rochester, New York

Dale W. Steele, MD
Associate Professor
Departments of Emergency Medicine and
    Pediatrics
Brown Medical School
Attending Physician and Fellowship
    Director
Department of Pediatric Emergency
    Medicine
Hasbro Children's Hospital
Providence, Rhode Island

James M. Stephen, MD
Assistant Professor
Department of Emergency Medicine
Tufts University School of Medicine
Department of Emergency medicine
Tufts-New England Medical Center
Boston, Massachusetts

T.A. Stern, MD
Psychiatric Consultation Service
Massachusetts General Hospital
Harvard Medical School
Boston, Massachusetts

Lori Stolz, MD
Resident
Department of Emergency Medicine
University of Arizona
Resident
Department of Emergency Medicine
University Medical Center
Tucson, Arizona

Julie L. Story, MD
Resident
Department of Emergency Medicine
Vanderbilt Medical Center
Nashville, Tennessee

Shannon Straszewski, MD
Resident Physician
Emergency Medicine
Harvard Affiliated EM Residency
Resident Physician
Emergency Medicine
Beth Israel Deaconess Medical Center
Boston, Massachusetts

Helen Straus, MD, MS
Assistant Professor
Department of Emergency Medicine
Rush Medical School
Attending Physician
Department of Emergency Medicine
Cook County Hospital
Chicago, Illinois

John Sullivan, MD
Attending Physician and Core Faculty
Department of Emergency Medicine
Jackson Memorial Hospital
Miami, Florida

Patrick H. Sweet, III, MD
Lieutenant
Medical Corps
United States Navy
General Medical Officer
USS Makin Island
United States Third Fleet

Paul A. Szucs, MD
Associate Residency Program Director
Assistant Clinical Professor
Morristown Memorial Hospital
Morristown, New Jersey

Brad Talley, MD
Resident
Emergency Medicine
Denver Health Medical Center
Denver, Colorado

David A. Tanen, MD
Residency Director
Department of Emergency Medicine
Naval Medical Center
San Diego, California

Christopher Tedeschi, MD, MA
Assistant Clinical Professor of Medicine
Department of Medicine
Columbia University
Attending Physician
New York-Presbyterian Hospital
Columbia University Medical Center
New York, New York

Elizabeth Temin, MD
Instructor
Department of Emergency Medicine
Harvard Medical School
Attending Physician
Department of Emergency Medicine
Massachusetts General Hospital
Boston, Massachusetts

Brigham R. Temple, MD
Clinical Instructor of Emergency Medicine
Emergency Medicine
University of Chicago
Chicago, Illinois
Emergency Medicine
North Shore University Health System
Evanston, Illinois

Lisa E. Thomas, MD
Harvard Affiliated Emergency Medicine
    Resident
Massachusetts General Hospital/
    Brigham & Women's Hospital
Boston, Massachusetts

Kristine Thompson, MD
Department of Emergency Medicine
St. Luke's Hospital
Jacksonville, Florida

Trevonne M. Thompson, MD
Assistant Professor
Department of Emergency Medicine
Associate Director, Medical Toxicology
University of Illinois at Chicago College of
    Medicine
Chicago, Illinois

Stephen L. Thornton, MD
Assistant Professor
Department of Emergency Medicine
University of Kansas
Attending
Department of Emergency Medicine
University of Kansas Hospital
Kansas City, Kansas

Carrie Tibbles, MD
Associate Residency Director
Department of Emergency Medicine
Harvard Affiliated Emergency Medicine
    Residency
Physician
Beth Israel Deaconess Medical Center
Boston, Massachusetts

Aleksandr M. Tichter, MD
Assistant Professor
Emergency Medicine
Columbia University
Attending Physician
Emergency Medicine
New York-Presbyterian Hospital
New York, New York

Vaishal M. Tolia, MD, MPH
Assistant Professor
Emergency Medicine
University of California San Diego
San Diego, California

Mercedes Torres, MD
Department of Emergency Medicine
University of Maryland Medical Center
Baltimore, Maryland

Susan P. Torrey, MD, FACEP
Assistant Professor
Department of Emergency Medicine
Tufts University School of Medicine
Boston, Massachusetts
Associate Residency Director
Department of Emergency Medicine
Baystate Medical Center
Springfield, Massachusetts

Heather D. Torrez, MD
Department of Emergency Medicine
Loma Linda University Medical Center
Loma Linda, California

Jason Tracy, MD
Instructor in Medicine
Harvard Medical School
Boston, Massachusetts
Chief of Emergency Services
Nashoba Valley Medical Center
Ayer, Massachusetts

Brandon C. Tudor, MD
Chief Resident
Emergency Medicine
Cook County Hospital
Chicago, Illinois

Edward Ullman, MD
Attending Physician
Department of Emergency Medicine
Beth Israel Deaconess Medical Center
Boston, Massachusetts

Thomas A. Utecht, MD, FACEP
Associate Professor
Department of Emergency Medicine
University of California San Francisco
   School of Medicine
San Francisco, California
Chief Quality Officer
Community Medical Centers
Fresno, California

Sami H. Uwaydat, MD
Department of Ophthalmology
Harvey and Bernice Jones Eye Institute
University of Arkansas for Medical
   Sciences
Little Rock, Arkansas

Carla C. Valentine, MD
Attending Physician
Department of Emergency Medicine
Santa Barbara Cottage Hospital
Santa Barbara, California

Matthew Valento, MD
Toxikon Consortium
Stroger-Cook County Hospital
Chicago, Illinois

Karen D. Van Hoesen, MD
Clinical Professor of Medicine
Department of Emergency Medicine
University of California, San Diego
San Diego, California

Arjun K. Venkatesh, MD
Harvard Affiliated Emergency Medicine
   Resident
Massachusetts General Hospital/
   Brigham & Women's Hospital
Boston, Massachusetts

Gary M. Vilke, MD
Professor of Clinical Medicine
Emergency Medicine
University of California San Diego
Director of Clinical Medicine
Emergency Medicine
University of California San Diego Medical
   Center
San Diego, California

Deborah Vinton, MD
Resident
Emergency Medicine
Denver Health Medical Center
Denver, Colorado

Robert Vissers, MD, FACEP
Adjunct Associate Professor
Oregon Health and Sciences University
Director
Department of Emergency Medicine
Legacy Emanual Hospital
Portland, Oregon

Kathryn A. Volz, MD
Resident
Department of Emergency Medicine
Beth Israel Deaconess Medical Center
Boston, Massachusetts

Michael Wahl, MD, FACEP
Clinical Instructor
Division of Emergency Medicine
University of Chicago
Medical Director
Illinois Poison Center
Metropolitan Chicago Healthcare Council
Chicago, Illinois

James S. Walker, DO, FACEP,
FACOEP, FAAEM
Clinical Professor of Surgery
Department of Surgery
University of Oklahoma Health Sciences
Center
Oklahoma City, Oklahoma
Medical Director
Department of Emergency Medicine
Logan Medical Center
Guthrie, Oklahoma

Jonathan B. Walker, DO
Physician
Emergency Department
Indian Health Service: Phoenix Indian
   Medical Center
Phoenix, Arizona

Kevin R. Weaver, DO
Residency Program Director
Emergency Medicine
Lehigh Valley Health Network
Allentown, Pennsylvania

Joseph M. Weber, MD
Assistant Professor
Emergency Medicine
Rush Medical College
EMS Director
Emergency Medicine
Cook County Stroger Hospital
Chicago, Illinois

Bruce Webster, MD, PhD
Emergency Medicine
Swedish Medical Center
Seattle, Washington

Scott G. Weiner, MD, MPH
Assistant Professor
Department of Emergency Medicine
Tufts University School of Medicine
Director of Clinical Research
Department of Emergency Medicine
Tufts Medical Center
Boston, Massachusetts

Matthew A. Wheatley, MD, FACEP
Assistant Professor
Department of Emergency Medicine
Emory University
Medical Director
Clinical Decision Unit
Grady Memorial Hospital
Atlanta, Georgia

Melissa H. White, MD, MPH
Assistant Professor
Emergency Medicine
Emory University
Atlanta, Georgia

Patrick M. Whiteley, MD
Medical Toxicology Fellow
Emergency Medicine, Division of
    Toxicology
Cook County Hospital (Stroger)
Chicago, Illinois

Herbert Neil Wigder, MD, FACEP
Clinical Associate Professor
Section of Emergency Medicine
Department of Internal Medicine
University of Chicago
Chicago, Illinois
Vice Chair
Department of Emergency Medicine
Advocate Lutheran General Hospital
Park Ridge, Illinois

Jessa Williams, MD
Department of Emergency Medicine
Madigan Army Medical Center
Tacoma, Washington

George C. Willis, MD
Chief Resident/Faculty Development
    Fellow
Department of Emergency Medicine
University of Maryland Medical Center
Attending Physician
Department of Emergency Medicine
Mercy Medical Center
Baltimore, Maryland

Kelvey R. Wilson, MD, MS
Department of Emergency Medicine
Tufts University
Boston, Massachusetts
Department of Emergency Medicine
Baystate Medical Center
Springfield, Massachusetts

Michael P. Wilson, MD, PhD
Department of Emergency Medicine
University of California, San Diego
San Diego, California

Joanne C. Witsil, PharmD, RN, BCPS
Adjunct Clinical Assistant Professor
Department of Pharmacy Practice
University of Illinois at Chicago
Clinical Pharmacist
Department of Emergency Medicine
Cook County Hospital
Chicago, Illinois

Jeanette M. Wolfe, MD, FACEP
Clinical Assistant Professor
Department of Emergency Medicine
Tufts University School of Medicine
Department of Emergency Medicine
Baystate Hospital
Springfield, Massachusetts

Richard E. Wolfe, MD
Associate Professor
Division of Emergency Medicine
Harvard Medical School
Chief of Emergency Medicine
Beth Israel Deaconess Medical
    Center
Boston, Massachusetts

Daniel T. Wu, MD
Assistant Professor
Department of Emergency Medicine
Emory University School of Medicine
Atlanta, Georgia

Lynne M. Yancey, MD
Assistant Professor
Department of Emergency Medicine
University of Colorado School of
    Medicine
Denver, Colorado

Bradley N. Younggren, MD
Assistant Professor
Department of Medicine
University of Washington
Seattle, Washington
Assistant Chief
Emergency Medicine
Madigan Army Medical Center
Fort Lewis, Washington

Richard D. Zane, MD, FAAEM
Associate Professor, Harvard Medical
    School
Vice Chair, Department of Emergency
    Medicine
Brigham and Women's Hospital
Boston, Massachusetts

Michelle Zell-Kanter, PharmD
Coordinator, Toxikon Consortium
Emergency Medicine
Cook County Hospital
Chicago, Illinois

Julie Zeller, MD
Department of Emergency Medicine
Grand Strand Regional Medical
    Center
Myrtle Beach, South Carolina

Beth A. Zelonis, MD
Resident
Emergency Medicine
University of California San Diego
San Diego, California

Aviva Jacoby Zigman, MD
Attending Physician
Department of Emergency
    Medicine
Portland Adventist Medical Center
Portland, Oregon

Andrew B. Ziller, MD
Staff Physician
Emergency Department
Rose Medical Center
Denver, Colorado

Gary D. Zimmer, MD
Assistant Professor
Drexel University
Philadelphia, PA
Chairman
Emergency Medicine
St. Mary Medical Center
Langhorne, PA

Karen P. Zimmer, MD
Assistant Professor
Pediatrics
Johns Hopkins University
Baltimore, Maryland
Pediatrics
Thomas Jefferson University Hospital
Philadelphia, Pennsylvania

David N. Zull, MD, FACEP, FACP
Associate Professor
Departments of Medicine and Emergency
    Medicine
Northwestern University
Co-Director, Emergency Department
    Observation Unit
Department of Emergency Medicine
Northwestern Memorial Hospital
Chicago, Illinois

# CONTENTS

# TOPICAL TABLE OF CONTENTS

## Metabolic Emergencies

# Rosen & Barkin's
# 5-Minute Emergency Medicine Consult

**4TH EDITION**

# ABDOMINAL AORTIC ANEURYSM

Daniel J. Henning
Jason Imperato
Carlo L. Rosen

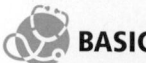 **BASICS**

## DESCRIPTION

- Focal dilation of the aortic wall with an increase in diameter by at least 50% (>3 cm)
- 95% are infrarenal.
- Rapid expansion or rupture causes symptoms.
- Rupture can occur into the intraperitoneal or retroperitoneal spaces.
- Intraperitoneal rupture is usually immediately fatal.
- Average growth rate of 0.2–0.5 cm/yr
- Of ruptures:
  - 90% overall mortality
  - 80% mortality for patients that reach the hospital
  - 50% mortality for patients that undergo emergency repair

### Geriatric Considerations

- Risk increases with advanced age.
- Present in:
  - 4–8% of all patients older than 65 yr
  - 5–10% of men 65–79 yr old
  - 12.5% of men 75–84 yr old
  - 5.2% of women 75–84 yr old

## ETIOLOGY

- Risk factors:
  - Male gender
  - Age >65 yr old
  - Family history
  - Cigarette smoking
  - Atherosclerosis
  - HTN
  - Diabetes mellitus
  - Connective tissue disorders:
    - Ehlers-Danlos syndrome
    - Marfan syndrome
- Uncommon causes:
  - Blunt abdominal trauma
  - Congenital aneurysm
  - Infections of the aorta
  - Mycotic aneurysm secondary to endocarditis

- Rupture risk factors:
  - Size (annual rupture rates):
    - Aneurysms 5.0–5.9 cm = 4%
    - Aneurysms 6.0–6.9 cm = 7%
    - Aneurysms 6.9–7.0 cm = 20%
  - Expansion:
    - A small aneurysm that grows >0.5 cm in 6 mo is at high risk for rupture.
  - Gender:
    - For aneurysms 4.0–5.5 cm, women have 4x higher risk of rupture compared to men with similar sized aneurysms.

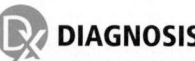 **DIAGNOSIS**

## SIGNS AND SYMPTOMS

### History

- Abdominal, back, or flank pain:
  - Vague, dull quality
  - Constant, throbbing, or colicky
  - Acute, severe, constant
  - Radiates to chest, thigh, inguinal area, or scrotum
  - Flank pain radiating to the groin in 10% of cases
- Lower extremity pain
- Syncope, near-syncope
- Unruptured are most often asymptomatic

### Physical Exam

- Unruptured:
  - Abdominal mass or fullness
  - Palpable, nontender, pulsatile mass
  - Intact femoral pulses
- Ruptured:
  - Classic triad (only 1/3 of cases):
    - Pain
    - Hypotension
    - Pulsatile abdominal mass
  - Systemic:
    - Hypotension
    - Tachycardia
    - Evidence of systemic embolization

- Abdomen:
  - Abdominal, back, or flank pain
  - Pulsatile, tender abdominal mass
  - Flank ecchymosis (Grey-Turner's sign) indicates retroperitoneal bleed.
  - Only 75% of aneurysms >5 cm are palpable.
  - Abdominal tenderness
  - Abdominal bruit
  - Gastrointestinal (GI) bleeding
- Extremities:
  - Diminished or asymmetric pulses in the lower extremities
- Complications:
  - Large emboli: Acute painful lower extremity
  - Microemboli: Cool, painful, cyanotic toes ("blue toe syndrome")
  - Aneurysmal thrombosis: Acutely ischemic lower extremity
  - Aortoenteric fistula: GI bleeding

## ESSENTIAL WORKUP

- Unstable patients:
  - Bedside abdominal US
  - Explorative surgery without further ancillary studies
- Stable, symptomatic patients:
  - Abdominal CT

## DIAGNOSTIC TESTS & INTERPRETATION

### Lab

- Type and cross-match blood
- CBC
- Creatinine
- Urinalysis
- Coagulation studies

### Imaging

- Plain radiographs:
  - Abdominal or lateral lumbar radiographs
  - Only if other tests are unavailable
  - Curvilinear calcification of the aortic wall or a paravertebral soft-tissue mass indicates abdominal aortic aneurysm (AAA) in 75% of patients.
  - Cannot identify rupture
  - Negative study does not rule out AAA.

- Abdominal ultrasound:
  - 100% sensitive and 92–99% specific for detecting AAA prior to rupture
  - In emergent setting, useful to determine presence of AAA.
  - Ultrasound findings consistent with AAA are enlarged aorta >3 cm or focal dilatation of the aorta.
  - Sensitivity has been reported as low as 10% following rupture.
  - Indicated in the unstable patient
- Abdominal CT scan:
  - Contrast is not necessary.
  - Will demonstrate both aneurysm and site of rupture (intraperitoneal versus retroperitoneal)
  - Allows more accurate measurement of aortic diameter
  - Indicated in stable patients only
- Aortography:
  - No use in emergent evaluation
  - The presence of mural thrombi can lead to underestimation of the size of the aorta.

## DIFFERENTIAL DIAGNOSIS
- Other abdominal arterial aneurysms (ie, iliac or renal)
- Aortic dissection
- Renal colic
- Biliary colic
- Musculoskeletal back pain
- Pancreatitis
- Cholecystitis
- Appendicitis
- Bowel obstruction
- Perforated viscus
- Mesenteric ischemia
- Diverticulitis
- GI hemorrhage
- Aortic thromboembolism
- Myocardial infarction
- Addisonian crisis
- Sepsis
- Spinal cord compression

 TREATMENT

### PRE-HOSPITAL
- Establish 2 large-bore IV lines
- Rapid transport to the nearest facility with surgical backup
- Alert ED staff as soon as possible to prepare the following:
  - Operating room
  - Universal donor blood
  - Surgical consultation

### INITIAL STABILIZATION/THERAPY
- 2 large-bore IV lines
- Crystalloid infusion
- Cardiac monitor
- Early blood transfusion

### ED TREATMENT/PROCEDURES
For patients suspected of symptomatic AAA:
- Avoid overaggressive fluid resuscitation; this leads to increased bleeding.
- Emergent surgical consult and operative intervention
- Laparotomy versus Endovascular Aortic Repair (EVAR) by vascular surgeon
- Diagnostic tests should not delay definitive treatment.

 FOLLOW-UP

### DISPOSITION
*Admission Criteria*
All patients with symptomatic AAA require emergent surgical intervention and admission.

*Discharge Criteria*
Asymptomatic patients only

### FOLLOW-UP RECOMMENDATIONS
- Close vascular surgery follow up must be arranged prior to discharge
- Instructions to return immediately for:
  - Any pain in the back, abdomen, flank, or lower extremities
  - Any dizziness or syncope

## PEARLS AND PITFALLS
- AAA should be on the differential for any patient presenting with pain in the abdomen, back, or flank
- Symptomatic AAA requires immediate treatment. Do not delay definitive care for extra studies.
- A hemodynamically unstable (ie, hypotensive) patient should not be taken for CT scan

## ADDITIONAL READING
- Bessen HA. Abdominal aortic aneurysms. In Marx JA, et al, eds. *Rosen's emergency medicine: concepts and clinical practice*. 5th ed. St. Louis, MO.: Mosby, 2002:1176–1186.
- Ernst CB. Abdominal aortic aneurysm. *N Engl J Med*. 1993;328.1167–1172.
- Rogers RL, McCormack R. Aortic disasters. *Emerg Med Clin N Am*. 2004;22:887–908.
- Bentz S, Jones J. Accuracy of emergency department ultrasound in detecting abdominal aortic aneurysm. *Emerg Med J*. 2006 Oct;23(10):803–804.
- The United Kingdom Small Aneurysm Trial Participants. Long-term outcomes of immediate repair compared with surveillance of small abdominal aortic aneurysms. *N Engl J Med*. 2002 May 9;346(19):1445 1452.
- Tibbles C, Barkin A. The Aorta. In Cosby K, Kendall J. *Practical Guide to Emergency Ultrasound*. Philadelphia, PA; Lippincott, WilLiams, & Williams, 2006:219–236.

### See Also (Topic, Algorithm, Electronic Media Element)
- Aortic Dissection
- Peripheral Artery Disease

## CODES

ICD9
- 441.3 Abdominal aneurysm, ruptured
- 441.4 Abdominal aneurysm without mention of rupture

# ABDOMINAL PAIN

*Richard E. Wolfe*
*Saleh Fares*

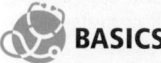 **BASICS**

## DESCRIPTION

- Parietal pain:
  - Irritating material causing peritoneal inflammation
  - Pain transmitted by somatic nerves
  - Exacerbated by changes in tension of the peritoneum
  - Pain characteristics:
    - Sharp
    - Well localized
    - Abdominal tenderness
    - Involuntary guarding
    - Rebound tenderness
    - Exacerbated by movement and coughing
- Visceral pain:
  - Distention of a viscous or organ capsule or spasm of intestinal muscularis fibers
    - Pain is generally poorly localized.
    - Colicky with intestinal distention
    - Constant with a distended gallbladder or kidney
  - Inflammation:
    - Initially the pain is poorly localized.
    - Focal tenderness develops as the inflammation extends to the peritoneum or localizers.
  - Ischemia from vascular disturbances:
    - Pain is severe and diffuse with catastrophic vascular emergencies.
    - The pain is disproportional to the abdominal examination.
- Referred pain:
  - Felt at distant location from diseased organ
  - Due to an overlapping supply by the affected neurosegment to the perceived location of pain
- Abdominal wall pain:
  - Constant
  - Aching
  - Muscle spasm
  - Involvement of other muscle groups

## ETIOLOGY

- Peritoneal irritants:
  - Gastric juice
  - Fecal material
  - Pus
  - Blood
  - Bile
  - Pancreatic enzymes
- Visceral obstruction:
  - Small intestines
  - Large intestines
  - Gallbladder
  - Ureters and kidneys
  - Visceral ischemia
  - Intestinal
  - Renal
  - Splenic

- Visceral inflammation:
  - Appendicitis
  - Inflammatory bowel disorders
  - Cholecystitis
  - Hepatitis
  - Peptic ulcer disease
  - Pancreatitis
  - Pelvic inflammatory disease
  - Pyelonephritis
- Abdominal wall pain
- Referred pain:
  - The possibility of intrathoracic disease must be considered in every patient with abdominal pain.

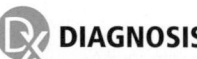 **DIAGNOSIS**

## SIGNS AND SYMPTOMS

- General:
  - Anorexia
  - Malaise
  - Tachycardia
  - Hypotension
  - Fever
  - Nausea
  - Vomiting
- Abdominal:
  - Diarrhea
  - Constipation
  - Distended abdomen
  - Abnormal bowel sounds:
    - High-pitched rushes with bowel obstruction
    - Absence of sound with ileus or peritonitis
    - Often unreliable
  - Pulsatile abdominal mass
  - Rovsing's sign:
    - Palpation of left lower quadrant causes pain in right lower quadrant (RLQ).
    - Suggestive of appendicitis
  - McBurney's point tenderness associated with appendicitis:
    - Palpation in RLQ 2/3 distance between umbilicus and right anterior superior iliac crest causes pain.
  - Murphy's sign:
    - Pause in inspiration while examiner is palpating under liver
    - Suggestive of cholecystitis
  - Psoas sign:
    - Pain on extension of the thigh
    - Suggests inflammation around psoas muscle
  - Obturator sign:
    - Pain on rotation of the flexed thigh, especially internal rotation
    - Inflammation around internal obturator muscle
  - Tender or discolored hernia site
  - Rectal and pelvic examination:
    - Tenderness with pelvic peritoneal irritation
    - Cervical motion tenderness
    - Adnexal masses
    - Rectal mass or tenderness
    - Guaiac positive stool

- Genitourinary:
  - Flank pain
  - Dysuria
  - Hematuria
  - Vaginal bleeding
  - Tender adnexal mass on pelvis
  - Testicular pain:
    - May be referred from renal or appendiceal pathology
  - Testicular swelling
  - High-riding testes
  - Transverse lie of testis
- Extremities:
  - Shoulder pain above the collar bone (Kehr's sign)
  - Pulse deficit or unequal femoral pulses
- Skin:
  - Jaundice
  - Herpes zoster
  - Cellulitis

## ESSENTIAL WORKUP

Historical characteristics:

- Nature of onset of pain
- Time of onset and duration of pain
- Location of pain initially and at presentation
- Extraabdominal radiations
- Quality of pain (sharp, dull, crampy)
- Palliative or provocative factors
- Relation of associated finding to onset of pain
- Changes in bowel habits
- History of trauma or visceral obstruction
- Gynecologic history

## DIAGNOSTIC TESTS & INTERPRETATION

### Lab

- CBC:
  - WBC is a poor predictor of surgical disease.
- Urinalysis
- Serum lipase:
  - More sensitive and specific than serum amylase
- hCG (age reproductive women)
- Serum electrolytes and glucose
- LFTs

### Imaging

- EKG:
  - Consider if risk factors for coronary artery disease are present
- KUB and Upright:
  - Air fluid levels and intestinal distention
  - Foreign bodies
- Upright CXR:
  - Pneumoperitoneum
  - Intrathoracic disease causing referred abdominal pain
- US:
  - Biliary abnormalities
  - Hydronephrosis
  - Intraperitoneal fluid
  - Aortic aneurysm

- Abdominal CT:
  - Spiral CT without contrast:
    - Renal Colic
    - AAA
    - Retroperitoneal hemorrhage
    - Appendicitis
  - CT with intravenous contrast only:
    - Vascular rupture suspected in a stable patient
    - Ischemic bowel
  - CT with IV and oral contrast:
    - Indicated when there is a suspicion of a surgical etiology involving bowel
    - History of inflammatory bowel disease
    - Thin patients (low BMI)
  - CT with rectal contrast only:
    - Used occasionally in appendicitis and diverticulitis
- IVP:
  - Indicated in patients with suspected ureteral calculi
  - More time-consuming than spiral CT
- Barium enema:
  - Intussusception
  - Volvulus
- MRI:
  - If concerns for radiation exposure or nephrotoxicity
  - Contraindicated in patients with metallic implants

## DIFFERENTIAL DIAGNOSIS
- Abdominal aortic aneurysm
- Appendicitis
- Boerhaave's syndrome
- Diverticulitis with perforation or abscess
- Ruptured ectopic pregnancy
- Ruptured ovarian cyst
- Pancreatitis
- Perforated peptic ulcer
- Perforated viscus
- Splenic rupture
- Visceral pain:
  - Abdominal epilepsy
  - Abdominal migraine
  - Adrenal crisis
  - Early appendicitis
  - Bowel obstruction
  - Cholecystitis
  - Constipation
  - Depression
  - Diabetic ketoacidosis
  - Diverticulitis
  - Dysmenorrhea
  - Ectopic pregnancy
  - Esophagitis
  - Endometriosis
  - Fecal impaction
  - Fitz-Hugh–Curtis syndrome
  - Gastroenteritis
  - Hepatitis

  - Hirschsprung's disease
  - Incarcerated hernia
  - Inflammatory bowel disease
  - Intussusception
  - Irritable bowel syndrome
  - Ischemic bowel
  - Lactose intolerance
  - Lead poisoning
  - Meckel's diverticulitis
  - Neoplasm
  - Ovarian torsion
  - Ovarian cysts (hemorrhagic)
  - Pancreatitis
  - Pelvic inflammatory disease
  - Peptic ulcer disease
  - Renal/ureteral calculi
  - Renal Infarction
  - Sickle cell crisis
  - Spider bite (Black widow)
  - Splenic infarction
  - Spontaneous abortion
  - Testicular torsion
  - Tubo-ovarian abscess
  - Urinary tract infection
  - Volvulus
- Referred pain:
  - Myocardial infarction
  - Pneumonia
- Abdominal wall pain:
  - Abdominal wall hematoma or infection
  - Black widow spider bite
  - Herpes zoster

### Pediatric Considerations
- Under 2 yr:
  - Hirschsprung's disease
    Incarcerated hernia
  - Intussusception
  - Neoplasm
    Sickle cell crisis
  - Volvulus
  - Foreign body ingestion
- 2–5 yr:
  - Appendicitis
  - Incarcerated hernia
  - Meckel's diverticulitis
  - Neoplasm
  - Sickle cell crisis
  - Henoch-Schönlein purpura (HSP)

## TREATMENT

### INITIAL STABILIZATION/THERAPY
Emergent laparotomy:
- Patients who are hemodynamically unstable with suspected vascular rupture

### ED TREATMENT/PROCEDURES
- Antiemetics are important for comfort.
- Narcotics or analgesics should not be withheld.
- Antibiotics are needed in potential perforation and in peritonitis.
- Surgical consultation based on suspected etiology

## MEDICATION
- Compazine: 10 mg IV q3–4h PRN
- Fentanyl: 1–2 μg/kg IV qh
- Morphine sulfate: 0.1 mg/kg IV q4h PRN
- Ondansetron: 4 mg IV
- Prochlorperazine: 0.13 mg/kg IV/PO/IM q6h PRN nausea; 25 mg PR q6h in adults
- Promethazine: 1 mg/kg IM/PO/PR

 **FOLLOW-UP**

### DISPOSITION
#### Admission Criteria
- Surgical intervention
- Peritoneal signs
- Patient unable to keep down fluids
- Lack of pain control
- Medical cause necessitating in-house treatment (MI, DKA)
- IV antibiotics needed

#### Discharge Criteria
No surgical or severe medical etiology found in patient who is able to keep fluid down, has good pain control, and is able to follow detailed discharge instructions

### FOLLOW-UP RECOMMENDATIONS
The patient should return with any warning signs:
- Vomiting
- Blood or dark/black material in vomit or stools
- Yellow skin or in the whites of the eyes
- No improvement or worsening of pain within 8–12 hr
- Shaking chills, or a fever >100.4°F (38°C)

## PEARLS AND PITFALLS
- Elderly patients are more likely to present with atypical presentations and life threatening etiologies requiring admission.
- Only consider constipation if there is stool in the rectal vault.
- Etiology requiring surgical intervention is less likely when vomiting precedes the onset of pain.

## ADDITIONAL READING
- Kamin RA, et al. Pearls and pitfalls in the emergency department evaluation of abdominal pain. *Emerg Med Clin North Am*. 2003;21(1):61–72, vi
- McCollough M, Sherieff GQ. Abdominal pain in children. *Pediatr Clin North Am*. 2006;53(1):107–137, vi
- Yeh EL, McNamara RM. Abdominal pain. *Clin Geriatr Med*. 2007;23(2):255–270.

# ABDOMINAL TRAUMA, BLUNT

*Stewart Coffman*

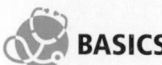

## BASICS

### DESCRIPTION
- Injury results from a sudden increase of pressure to abdomen.
- Solid organ injury usually manifests as hemorrhage.
- Hollow viscus injuries result in bleeding and peritonitis from contamination with bowel contents.

### ETIOLOGY
- 60% result from motor vehicle collisions.
- Solid organs are injured more frequently than hollow viscus organs.
- The spleen is the most frequently injured organ (25%), followed by the liver (15%), intestines (15%), retroperitoneal structures (13%), and kidney (12%).
- Less frequently injured are the mesentery, pancreas, diaphragm, urinary bladder, urethra, and vascular structures.

#### Pediatric Considerations
- Children tend to tolerate trauma better because of the more elastic nature of their tissues.
- Owing to the smaller size of the intrathoracic abdomen, the spleen and liver are more exposed to injury because they lie partially outside the bony rib cage.

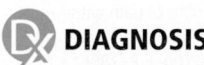

## DIAGNOSIS

### SIGNS AND SYMPTOMS
- Spectrum from abdominal pain, signs of peritoneal irritation, to hypovolemic shock
- Nausea or vomiting
- Labored respiration from diaphragm irritation or upper abdominal injury
- Left shoulder pain with inspiration (Kehr sign) from diaphragmatic irritation owing to bleeding
- Delayed presentation possible with small-bowel injury

### ESSENTIAL WORKUP
- Evaluate and stabilize airway, breathing, and circulation (ABCs).
- Primary objective is to determine need for operative intervention.
- Examine abdomen to detect signs of intra-abdominal bleeding or peritoneal irritation.
- Injury in the retroperitoneal space or intrathoracic abdomen is difficult to assess by palpation.
- Remember that the limits of the abdomen include the diaphragm superiorly (nipples anteriorly, inferior scapular tip posteriorly) and the intragluteal fold inferiorly and encompass entire circumference.
- Abrasions or ecchymoses may be indicators of intra-abdominal injury:
  - Roll the patient to assess the back.
  - Lap belt abrasions can be indicative of significant intra-abdominal injuries.
- Bowel sounds may be absent from peritoneal irritation (late finding).
- Foley catheter (if no blood at the meatus, no perineal hematoma, and normal prostate exam) to obtain urine and record urinary output
- Plain film of the pelvis:
  - Fracture of the pelvis and gross hematuria may indicate genitourinary injury.
  - Further evaluation of these structures with retrograde urethrogram, cystogram, or IVIV pyelogram
- CT most useful in assessing need for operative intervention and for evaluating the retroperitoneal space and solid organs:
  - Patient must be stable enough to make trip to scanner.
  - Also useful for suspected renal injury
- FAST (focused abdominal sonography for trauma) to detect intraperitoneal fluid:
  - US is rapid, requires no contrast agents, and is noninvasive.
  - Operator dependent
- Diagnostic peritoneal lavage (useful for revealing injuries in the intrathoracic abdomen, pelvic abdomen, and true abdomen) primarily indicated for unstable patients:
  - Positive with gross blood, RBC count of >100,000/mm³, WBC count of 500/mm³, or presence of bile, feces, or food particles

### DIAGNOSTIC TESTS & INTERPRETATION
#### Lab
- Hemoglobin/hematocrit, which initially may be normal owing to isovolemic blood loss
- Type and screen is essential. Cross-match PRBC units for unstable patients.
- Urinalysis for blood:
  - Microscopic hematuria in the presence of shock is an indication for genitourinary evaluation.
- ABG:
  - Base deficit may suggest hypovolemic shock and help guide the resuscitation.

#### Imaging
See Essential Workup.

#### Diagnostic Procedures/Surgery
See Essential Workup.

### DIFFERENTIAL DIAGNOSIS
Lower thoracic injury may cause abdominal pain.

**TREATMENT**

**PRE-HOSPITAL**
- Titrate fluid resuscitation to clinical response. Target SBP of 90–100 mm Hg
- Normal vital signs do not preclude significant intra-abdominal pathology.

**INITIAL STABILIZATION/THERAPY**
- Ensure adequate airway:
  – Intubate if needed.
  – $O_2$ 100% by non-rebreather face mask
- 2 large-bore IV lines with crystalloid infusion
- Begin infusion of PRBCs if no response to 2 L of crystalloid.
- If patient is in profound shock, consider immediate transfusion of O-negative blood.

**ED TREATMENT/PROCEDURES**
- Continue stabilization begun in field.
- Nasogastric tube to evacuate stomach, decrease distention, and decrease risk of aspiration:
  – May relieve respiratory distress if caused by a herniated stomach through the diaphragm

**MEDICATION**
- Tetanus toxoid booster: 0.5 mL IM for patients with open wounds
- Tetanus immunoglobulin: 250 units IM for patients who have not had complete series
- IV antibiotics: Broad-spectrum aerobic with anaerobic coverage such as a 2nd-generation cephalosporin

**Pediatric Considerations**
- Crystalloid infusion is 20 mL/kg if patient in shock.
- PRBC dose is 1 mL/kg.

 **FOLLOW-UP**

**DISPOSITION**
**Admission Criteria**
- Postoperative cases
- Equivocal findings on diagnostic peritoneal lavage, FAST exam, or CT
- Many blunt abdominal trauma patients benefit from admission, monitoring, and serial abdominal exams.

**Discharge Criteria**
No patient in whom you suspect intra-abdominal injury should be discharged home without an appropriate period of observation, despite negative exam or imaging studies.

## PEARLS AND PITFALLS

- Do not delay blood products when patient is in obvious shock despite normal Hct.
- Avoid overaggressive resuscitation with crystalloids.
- Obtain a pregnancy test in all females of childbearing age.
- Do not transport unstable patients to CT for diagnostic imaging.

## ADDITIONAL READING

- American College of Surgeons Committee on Trauma. Abdominal Trauma. In: *ATLS student course manual*, 8th ed. American College of Surgeons, 2008.
- Amoroso TA. Evaluation of the patient with blunt abdominal trauma: An evidence based approach. *Emerg Med Clin North Am*. 1999;17:63–75.
- Holmes JF, et al. Performance of helical CT without oral contrast for the detection of gastrointestinal injuries. *Ann Emerg Med*. 2004;43(1):120–128.
- Kendall JL, Faragher J, Hewitt GJ, et al. Emergency department ultrasound is not a sensitive detector of solid organ injury. *West J Emerg Med*. 2009;10(1):1–5.
- Stengel D, Bauwens K, Sehouli J, et al. Systematic review and meta-analysis of emergency ultrasonography for blunt abdominal trauma. *Br J Surg*. 2001;88:901–912.

 **CODES**

**ICD9**
868.00 Injury to unspecified intra-abdominal organ without mention of open wound into cavity

# ABDOMINAL TRAUMA, IMAGING

Hina Ghory
Phillips Perera

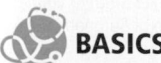 **BASICS**

## DESCRIPTION
These are diagnostic procedures; the basis for their use will vary with the results of exam.

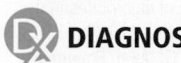 **DIAGNOSIS**

## SIGNS AND SYMPTOMS
- Abdominal trauma may be seen in a spectrum of patients ranging from those with isolated abdominal injury to multisystem trauma.
- Abdominal trauma can be divided into blunt and penetrating injuries. Penetrating abdominal injuries are further divided into stab wounds and gunshot wounds.
- Assessment of abdominal trauma begins with an evaluation of the patient's hemodynamic status. Most unstable patients will require early surgical management, while many stable patients with abdominal trauma may be managed nonoperatively.

### History
- History should include mechanism of injury, restraint use and type, airbag or helmet use, prehospital vital signs, initial mental status and change in mental status, any prehospital treatments performed and their effect on patient status.
- AMPLE history (allergies-to-medications and radiographic contrast agents, medications taken, past medical and surgical history, last meal, events leading up to the injury)

### Physical Exam
- A comprehensive physical exam should include full exposure of the patient and careful palpation of all abdominal quadrants.
- Caution should be taken because the physical exam is accurate in determining serious abdominal injury in only 45–50% of cases.
- The abdominal physical exam is frequently misleading in intoxicated and multisystem trauma patients.

## ESSENTIAL WORKUP
- See "Abdominal Trauma (Blunt)" and "Abdominal Trauma (Penetrating)."
- All trauma patients should be initially managed with the ABCDE survey, IV access, oxygen and cardiac monitoring.

## DIAGNOSTIC TESTS & INTERPRETATION
General approach to imaging in abdominal trauma:
- Unstable trauma patients:
  - Unstable patients should have a bedside ultrasound performed immediately as part of the primary survey (circulation). A positive FAST suggests that intra-abdominal bleeding is the source of hypotension. A negative FAST suggests either a retroperitoneal bleed, blood loss in the field, bleeding from an unstable pelvic fracture, or hemorrhage into another body cavity.
- A surgeon should be consulted immediately to prepare for definitive operative care of the patient:
  - Stable trauma patients: The 3 main modes of diagnosing the extent of injury in hemodynamically stable abdominal trauma patients include:

- US: Initial screening test of choice for hemodynamically stable patients. A positive US in the stable trauma patient warns the clinician about the possibility of impending hemodynamic deterioration. CT scan and surgical consult should be rapidly facilitated in this group of patients.
- CT scan: The definitive test for stable abdominal trauma patients. CT scanning will diagnose both solid organ and retroperitoneal injuries better than ultrasound. CT imaging allows a determination of whether an embolization procedure is warranted for hemorrhage control. It is indicated in all stable patients with stab wounds. It is also indicated in patients with gross hematuria, to look for renal injury.
  - Diagnostic peritoneal lavage: Currently used infrequently as there has been a shift to increased reliance on CT scanning in the diagnosis of abdominal trauma.
- Local wound exploration: While frequently used in the past in penetrating abdominal trauma to look for violation of the fascia, it has now also been replaced with CT scanning in the majority of patients (see Diagnostic Tests & Interpretation).

### Lab
- Blood type and screen
- CBC
- Electrolytes and creatinine
- Lipase
- UA
- EKG

### Imaging
- US:
  - Advantages:
    - Rapid
    - Noninvasive
    - Can be performed at the patient's bedside concurrent with evaluation and initial resuscitation
    - Does not require contrast agents or ionizing radiation
    - Can be repeated in the case of changes in the patient's hemodynamic status or physical exam
  - Disadvantages:
    - Operator dependent
    - Does not reliably identify solid organ or retroperitoneal injuries. May be negative with pelvic fractures despite significant hemorrhage. Not sensitive for bowel injury.
  - Contraindications:
    - Absolute: None
    - Relative: Obesity; subcutaneous emphysema
  - Positive test:
    - Demonstration of free fluid or obvious solid organ injury. ~600 mL free fluid required in adults for a positive right upper quadrant Morison's pouch view. ~150 mL is required for a positive pelvic/suprapubic view (optimally performed prior to Foley placement).
    - Adequate exam includes visualization of the right upper quadrant, left upper quadrant, suprapubic/pelvis, and cardiac areas.

- CT scan:
  - Advantages:
    - Sensitivity of 85–98%, PPV (for detecting need for laparotomy) of 85%
    - Provides specific and detailed organ injury information
    - Fosters a nonoperative approach to solid organ injuries, which may frequently be managed with observation or interventional radiology mediated embolectomy.
    - Allows imaging of adjacent spinal structures to diagnose fracture.
  - Disadvantages:
    - Costly
    - Possible risk: Up to 1 in 2,000 increase in risk of fatal cancer from radiation
    - Requires IV/IV contrast (with risk of acute contrast reactions and renal toxicity).
    - Isolated diaphragmatic, pancreatic, bowel injuries may be missed, especially if performed immediately after injury.
  - Indications:
    - Hemodynamically stable patients
  - Contraindications:
    - Absolute: Preexisting indication for exploratory laparotomy; hemodynamic instability; previous contrast reaction
  - Considerations:
    - Many institutions now manage multisystem trauma patients with the "pan-scan," which includes CT imaging of the head, C-spine, chest, and abdomen/pelvis in 1 session.
    - IV contrast is sufficient in the abdominal trauma patient. Oral and rectal contrast is not needed.

### Diagnostic Procedures/Surgery
- Diagnostic peritoneal lavage:
  - Advantages:
    - Rapid
  - Helpful in detecting mesenteric and hollow organ injuries
  - May be considered in patients with pelvic fractures and hemorrhage
  - Relatively simple to perform
  - Sensitivity 87–92%, specificity 82%, PPV 52%, NPV 87%:
    - Low complication rate
- Disadvantages:
  - Invasive
  - Largely replaced by bedside US
  - Does not identify specific organ injury
  - 1–2% complication rate
  - May miss retroperitoneal injuries and intraperitoneal bladder rupture
  - High false-positive rates
- Possible Indications:
  - Hemodynamically unstable patients
  - Patients requiring emergent surgery for other conditions (eg, craniotomy for epidural hematoma)
  - Pelvic fractures
- Contraindications:
  - Absolute: Pre-existing indication for exploratory laparotomy
  - Relative: Previous abdominal surgery, severe abdominal distention, pregnancy, pediatric patients

- Considerations:
  – Foley catheter and nasogastric tube placement is recommended before beginning the procedure.
- Contraindications:
  – Blood at urethra
  – High riding prostate
- Positive test:
  – Aspiration of >10 mL of blood, bile, bowel contents, or urine
  – Diagnostic peritoneal lavage fluid in the urine or chest tube
  – Blunt trauma with >100,000 erythrocytes/mm$^3$
  – Penetrating trauma >1,000 erythrocytes/mm$^3$

## DIFFERENTIAL DIAGNOSIS
See "Abdominal Trauma (Blunt)" and "Abdominal Trauma (Penetrating)."

 **TREATMENT**

## PRE-HOSPITAL
All patients with a significant mechanism of injury or suspicion of major trauma should be triaged to a designated trauma center (preferably a Level 1 Center as certified by the American College of Surgeons).

### Pediatric Considerations
- Pediatric patients should be triaged to a pediatric trauma center or to an adult trauma center equipped to manage children.
- CT scan should be considered the diagnostic test of choice in children, as a greater percentage of injuries in children will be managed nonoperatively.

## INITIAL STABILIZATION/THERAPY
- In unstable patients, management of the airway, breathing, and circulation with resuscitation of hypovolemic shock and rapid control of major hemorrhage must take precedence.
- See "Abdominal Trauma (Blunt)" and "Abdominal Trauma (Penetrating)."

## ED TREATMENT/PROCEDURES
- See "Abdominal Trauma (Blunt)" and "Abdominal Trauma (Penetrating)."
- Crystalloid IV therapy is generally warranted with significant abdominal injury.
- 2 large bore IV catheters should be placed.
- Blood transfusion is indicated for all hemodynamically unstable abdominal trauma patients. Consider unmatched blood if needed expediently. O negative blood should be used in women of child-bearing age. O negative or O positive blood can be used in males and women beyond child-bearing age.
- Hemodynamically unstable trauma patients with altered mental status and inability to protect airway will usually need endotracheal intubation prior to transfer to operating suite.

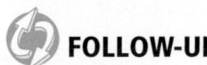 **FOLLOW-UP**

## DISPOSITION
### Admission Criteria
- All unstable trauma patients require admission to the hospital and most will require surgical management.
- Most multisystem trauma patients who also have abdominal trauma will need admission.

- Pregnant women >24 wk gestation should be admitted for fetal–maternal monitoring.
- Stable trauma patients can be divided into 3 classes:
  – Gun shot wounds to abdomen: Almost all will require admission. Rate of surgical exploration is high in this category due to elevated risk of organ injury.
  – Stab wounds to abdomen: Patients with penetration of fascia and entry into abdominal compartment will require admission. US, CT, and/or physical exam will define the subset of patients who need operative management.
  – Blunt abdominal trauma: US, CT, and/or physical exam will define subset of patients who need admission.

### Discharge Criteria
- Patients with stable hemodynamics during their ED course with a negative evaluation and reliable follow-up may be considered for discharge.
- Patients with inability to travel back to the hospital or to contact EMS for aid in case of deterioration must be considered for admission.

## FOLLOW-UP RECOMMENDATIONS
A small subset of discharged patients may have an undiagnosed injury (most commonly intestinal or pancreatic). Patients must be instructed to return to the ED with worsening abdominal pain, distention, vomiting or rectal bleeding.

## PEARLS AND PITFALLS
- US has a role in both unstable and stable trauma patients and can be immediately performed at the bedside concurrent with initial evaluation and stabilization.
- Consider serial US exams. This is especially important if at any point during the ED evaluation, there is a change in the patient's hemodynamic status or physical exam.
- CT has become indispensable in all classes of stable abdominal trauma. Many stable adult and pediatric trauma patients with significant injuries are now being managed nonoperatively with embolization and/or close observation after grading of injury on CT scan.
- "Pan CT scan" decreases missed injury rate but at a cost of increasing lifetime risks of radiation exposure.
- With increased use of US and CT, DPL and local wound exploration have become less useful in the evaluation of abdominal trauma.
- Repeat physical exams are important in managing trauma patients, as delayed presentations of intestinal injuries may be seen.
- Pitfalls include:
  – Not immediately sending type and screen or checking a pregnancy test
  – Sending pregnant women >24 wk gestation home without fetal–maternal monitoring

## ADDITIONAL READING
- Amoroso TA. Evaluation of the patient with blunt abdominal trauma: An evidence based approach. *Emerg Med Clin North Am.* 1999;17:63–75.
- Bifflm WL, et al. Management of patients with anterior abdominal stab wounds: A western trauma association multicenter trial. *J Trauma.* 2009;66:1294–1301.

- Branney SW, et al. Quantitative sensitivity of ultrasound in detecting free intraperitoneal fluid. *J Trauma Crit Care.* 1995;39(2):375–380.
- Chiquito PE. Blunt abdominal injuries. Diagnostic peritoneal lavage, ultrasonography and computed tomography scanning. *Injury.* 1996;27:117–124.
- Cothren CC, Moore EE, Warren PA, et al. Local wound exploration remains a valuable triage tool for the evaluation of anterior abdominal stab wounds. *Am J Surg.* 2009;198:223–226.
- Goodman CS, Hur JY, Adajar MA, et al. How well does CT predict the need for laparotomy in hemodynamically stable patients with penetrating abdominal injury? A review and meta-analysis. *AJR.* 2009;193.
- Griffin XL, et al. Are diagnostic peritoneal lavage or focused abdominal sonography for trauma safe screening investigations for hemodynamically stable patients after blunt abdominal trauma? A review of the literature. *J Trauma.* 2007;62:779–784.
- Ma OJ, Kefer MP, Mateer JR, et al. Evaluation of hemoperitoneum using a single- vs. multiple-view ultrasonographic examination. *Acad Emerg Med.* 2008;2(7):581–586. Epub ahead of print.
- Melniker LA, et al. Randomized controlled clinical trial of point-of-care, limited ultrasonography for trauma in the emergency department: The first Sonography Outcomes Assessment Program Trial. *Ann Emerg Med.* 2006;48(3):227–235.
- Pryor JP, Reilly PM, Dabrowski GP, et al. Nonoperative management of abdominal gunshot wounds. *Ann Emerg Med.* 2004;43(3):344–353.
- Ramirez RM, Cureton EL, Ereso AQ, et al. Single contrast computed tomography for the triage of patients with penetrating torso trauma. *J Trauma.* 2009;67:583–588.
- Rose JS. Ultrasound in abdominal trauma. *Emerg Med Clin North Am.* 2004;22(3):581–599.
- Stengel D, Bauwens K, Sehouli J, et al. Emergency ultrasound-based algorithms for diagnosing blunt abdominal trauma. *Cochrane Database Syst Rev.* 2005;18(2):cd004446.
- von Kuenssberg D, et al. Sensitivity in detecting free intraperitoneal fluid with the pelvic views of the FAST exam. *Am J Emerg Med.* 2004;24(6):476–478.

### See Also (Topic, Algorithm, Electronic Media Element)
- Abdominal Trauma, Blunt
- Abdominal Trauma, Penetrating

 **CODES**

ICD9
- 868.00 Injury to unspecified intra-abdominal organ without mention of open wound into cavity
- 868.10 Injury to unspecified intra-abdominal organ, with open wound into cavity

# ABDOMINAL TRAUMA, PENETRATING

*Stewart R. Coffman*

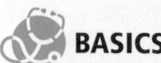

## BASICS

### DESCRIPTION
- Solid organ injury usually results in hemorrhage.
- Hollow viscus injury can lead to spillage of bowel contents and peritonitis.
- Associated conditions:
  – Injury to both thoracic and abdominal structures occurs in 25% of cases.

### ETIOLOGY
80% of gunshot wounds and 20–30% of stab wounds result in significant intra-abdominal injury. Commonly injured structures include:
- Liver (37%)
- Small bowel (26%)
- Stomach (19%)
- Colon (17%)
- Major vessel (13%)
- Retroperitoneum (10%)
- Mesentery/omentum (10%)
- Other:
  – Spleen (7%)
  – Diaphragm (5%)
  – Kidney (5%)
  – Pancreas (4%)
  – Duodenum (2%)
  – Biliary (1%)

## DIAGNOSIS

### SIGNS AND SYMPTOMS
- Penetrating wound from knife, gun, or other foreign object
- Spectrum of presentation ranging from localized pain to peritoneal signs:
  – High-velocity projectile can cause extensive direct tissue damage.
  – Secondary missiles and temporary cavitation of effected structures
  – Exit wound may be larger than entrance wound, but small entrance and exit wounds can conceal massive internal damage.
- Remember the borders of the abdomen: Superior from the nipples (anteriorly) or inferior tip of scapula (posteriorly) to inferior gluteal folds.

### ESSENTIAL WORKUP
- Diagnosis of intra-abdominal injury from gunshot wounds to the abdomen are made by laparotomy in the operating room.
- Locally explore stab wounds to anterior abdomen:
  – If the wound penetrates anterior fascial layer, the patient should undergo diagnostic peritoneal lavage or bedside US.
- Diagnostic laparoscopy is useful in diagnosing diaphragmatic injury and spleen and liver lacerations:
  – May help avoid unnecessary surgery.
- CT is useful in the evaluation of patients with a suspected retroperitoneal injury:
  – Not reliable for detection of hollow viscus or diaphragmatic injuries
- If 10,000 RBC/mm$^3$ or more are found in the diagnostic peritoneal lavage fluid, the patient should undergo laparotomy.
- If <10,000 RBC/mm$^3$ are present, the patient should be observed for 8–24 hr for the development of peritoneal signs.

### DIAGNOSTIC TESTS & INTERPRETATION
*Lab*
- Hemoglobin or hematocrit:
  – Repeated measurements to assess for ongoing hemorrhage
- Urinalysis for blood to assess for possible genitourinary tract damage
- ABG:
  – Base deficit may be helpful in assessing hypovolemia and guide volume resuscitation.
- Type and cross-match for all patients with significant intra-abdominal injuries.

*Imaging*
- Plain films:
  – Obtain after placement of markers for localization of foreign bodies, missiles, associated fractures, and free air.
- IV pyelogram:
  – For possible renal injury
- Bedside abdominal US (FAST: Focused abdominal sonography for trauma):
  – May reveal intraperitoneal blood or fluid
- CT with IV contrast in experienced facilities and with stable patients:
  – For possible retroperitoneal and solid organ injuries

### DIFFERENTIAL DIAGNOSIS
- In cases of upper abdominal wounds, consider the possibility of intrathoracic injury.
- In cases of wounds to the lower thoracic area, consider the possibility of intra-abdominal injury.

## TREATMENT

### PRE-HOSPITAL
- Controversies:
  – Military antishock trousers (MAST) should not be used.
  – Titrate fluid resuscitation to clinical response.
- Caution:
  – Apply sterile dressings to open wounds and moistened sterile dressings to eviscerated bowel.
  – Secure impaled foreign objects in place; do not remove them.

### INITIAL STABILIZATION/THERAPY
- 2 large-bore IV lines with crystalloid infusion
- If no response to 2 L of crystalloid, infuse 2–4 units packed red blood cells:
  – May use O-negative blood initially if patient unstable
  – Type-specific and cross-matched blood when it becomes available
- 100% oxygen by nonrebreather face mask

*Pediatric Considerations*
- Children in hypovolemic shock should receive 20-mL/kg boluses of crystalloid.
- Children in severe hypovolemic shock should receive 1 mL/kg of packed red blood cells.
- Age <8 yr is a relative contraindication for diagnostic peritoneal lavage.

## ED TREATMENT/PROCEDURES

- Nasogastric tube placement:
  - Will decrease aspiration risk
  - Place nasogastric tube before performing diagnostic peritoneal lavage to decompress stomach and reduce risk of iatrogenic injury.
  - May relieve respiratory distress in cases of diaphragmatic injury with herniated abdominal contents in the thorax
- Foley catheter placement:
  - Insert after ruling out urethral injuries
  - Facilitates rapid assessment of genitourinary injury
  - Assists in monitoring of urinary output
- Tetanus toxoid if appropriate; tetanus immunoglobulin if primary tetanus series not administered

## MEDICATION

- Tetanus toxoid: 0.5 mL IM
- Tetanus immunoglobulin: 250 units IM for patients who have not had a complete series
- IV antibiotics: Broad-spectrum aerobic with anaerobic coverage such as 2nd generation cephalosporin

 **FOLLOW-UP**

## DISPOSITION

### Admission Criteria

- Patients requiring abdominal surgery
- Observe the following patients for at least 8 hr:
  - Patients with negative findings on diagnostic peritoneal lavage, CT, or US. During hospitalization, the following are necessary:
    ○ Frequent abdominal exam
    ○ Repeated hematocrit levels at regular intervals

### Discharge Criteria

Patients with stab wounds without fascial penetration may be discharged after observation in the ED.

## PEARLS AND PITFALLS

Permissive hypotension is gaining support as a resuscitative principle:

- Avoid normal or near normal BP.
- Avoid overaggressive resuscitation with crystalloids.
- Completely exposing the patient will minimize overlooking an injury.
- Spinal immobilization is unnecessary unless there is an obvious spinal cord injury.

## ADDITIONAL READING

- Goodman CS, Hur JY, Adajar MA, et al. How well does CT predict the need for laparotomy in hemodynamically stable patients with penetrating abdominal injury? A review and meta-analysis. *AJR Am J Roentgenol.* 2009;193(2):432–437.
- Kirkpatrick AW, et al. The hand-held ultrasound examination for penetrating abdominal trauma. *Am J Surg.* 2004;187:660–665.

- Nicholas JM, Rix EP, Easley KA, et al. Changing patterns in the management of penetrating abdominal trauma: The more things change, the more they stay the same. *J Trauma.* 2003;55(6):1095–1108; discussion 1108–1110.
- Richards CF, Mayberry JC. Initial management of the trauma patient. *Crit Care Clin.* 2004;20(1):1 11.
- Sebesta J. Special lessons learned from Iraq. *Surg Clin North Am.* 2006;86(3):711–726.
- Thal ER. Evaluation of peritoneal lavage and local exploration in lower chest and abdominal stab wounds. *J Trauma.* 1979;17:642.

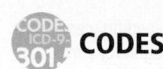 **CODES**

### ICD9

868.10 Injury to unspecified intra-abdominal organ, with open wound into cavity

# ABORTION, SPONTANEOUS
*Aviva Jacoby Zigman*

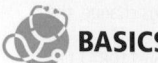 **BASICS**

## DESCRIPTION
- Spontaneous termination of a <20-wk intrauterine pregnancy
- Occurs in up to 20–25% of recognized pregnancies
- Vaginal bleeding in the 1st trimester seen in about 20% of pregnant patients:
  – 50% of these women will eventually miscarry.
- Definitions:
  – *Threatened abortion:* Vaginal bleeding, cervical os is closed, viable intrauterine pregnancy confirmed:
    ○ 50% of women seen in the ED for threatened abortion will eventually miscarry
  – *Inevitable abortion:* Vaginal bleeding, cervical os is open; products of conception (POC) have not been expelled
  – *Incomplete abortion:* Vaginal bleeding, cervical os is open with partial passage of some POC and some retained POC
  – *Complete abortion:* Vaginal bleeding, cervical os closed, complete passage of POC; no surgical or medical intervention
  – *Missed abortion:* Fetal demise with no uterine activity to expel
  – *Septic abortion:* Spontaneous abortion complicated by intrauterine infection
  – *Recurrent spontaneous abortion:* 3 or more consecutive pregnancy losses

## ETIOLOGY
- Chromosomal abnormalities of the fetus
- Uterine abnormalities
- Risk factors include:
  – Increased age of both the mother and father
  – Increased parity
  – Alcohol use
  – Cigarette smoking
  – Cocaine use
  – Conception within 3–6 mo after delivery
  – Chronic maternal disease:
    ○ Poorly controlled diabetes
    ○ Autoimmune disease
    ○ Celiac disease

– Intrauterine device
– Maternal infections:
  ○ Bacterial vaginosis
  ○ Mycoplasmosis
  ○ Herpes simplex
  ○ Toxoplasmosis
  ○ Listeriosis
  ○ Chlamydia/gonorrhea
  ○ HIV
  ○ Syphilis
  ○ Parvovirus B19
  ○ Malaria
  ○ CMV
  ○ Rubella
– Medications:
  ○ Misoprostol
  ○ Methotrexate
  ○ NSAIDs
– Multiple previous elective abortions
– Previous spontaneous abortion
– Toxins
– Uterine abnormalities

 **DIAGNOSIS**

## SIGNS AND SYMPTOMS
### History
- Last menstrual period (LMP)
- Obstetric history:
  – Parity
  – Risk factors of abortion
  – Prenatal care
- Abdominal pain, cramping
- Vaginal bleeding:
  – Duration
  – Amount of bleeding (quantify by number of pads used, compare with normal menstrual period for patient)
  – Passage of clots
- Dizzy, syncope

### Physical Exam
- Determine hemodynamic status of patient:
  – Pregnant patients in late first trimester have an increased blood volume.
  – Can lose substantial amount of blood before having abnormal vital signs
- Pelvic exam:
  – Determine whether the internal cervical os is opened or closed
  – Amount of bleeding
  – Presence of POC
  – Presence of adnexal tenderness or peritoneal irritation can be consistent with an ectopic pregnancy.

- Bimanual exam to determine the size of the uterus:
  – Size of an orange: 6–8 wk
  – Fundus at the symphysis pubis: 12 wk
  – Fundus at the umbilicus: 16–20 wk
  – Confirm pregnancy with urine or serum testing.
  – Rapid hemoglobin determination: Type and Rh

## ESSENTIAL WORKUP
- Pregnancy test as below
- Imaging as below

## DIAGNOSTIC TESTS & INTERPRETATION
### Lab
- Confirm pregnancy with a urine or serum test:
  – Urine pregnancy test: Most are positive at $\beta$-hCG levels of 25–50 mIU/mL ~1 wk gestational age and remain positive 2–3 wk after induced or spontaneous abortions.
- CBC, type and Rh
- Type and cross-match for woman with low Hct or signs of active blood loss
- Quantitative $\beta$-hCG if indicated (see below)
- Any POC passed should be sent to pathology for confirmation.

### Imaging
- Transvaginal ultrasound (TVS):
  – Gestational sac seen at 5 wk
  – Cardiac activity seen at 6.5 wk
- Transabdominal ultrasound (TAS):
  – Gestational sac at 6 wk
  – Cardiac activity seen at 8 wk
- Discriminatory zone: Level of $\beta$-hCG where a normal IUP should be detected:
  – 1,500–2,000 for TVS
  – 6,500 for TAS

## DIFFERENTIAL DIAGNOSIS
- Positive pregnancy test with vaginal bleeding:
  – Cervicitis
  – Ectopic pregnancy
  – Trauma
  – Septic abortions
  – Molar pregnancy
  – Subchorionic hemorrhage
- 2nd- and 3rd-trimester vaginal bleeding:
  – Placenta previa
  – Placental abruption

**TREATMENT**

### PRE-HOSPITAL
Cautions:

- Patients with SAB/vaginal bleeding can have severe hemorrhage and present in shock, especially at >12 wk.
- BP drops during the 2nd trimester of pregnancy with an average of 110/70.
- IV fluids, oxygen, and cardiac monitor

### INITIAL STABILIZATION/THERAPY
- Stable patients:
  - IV
  - Pelvic exam
- Unstable patients:
  - Oxygen, IV fluids via 2 large-bore IVs, cardiac monitor
  - Transfuse PRBC if patient does not stabilize after 2–3 L of crystalloid.
  - Gynecologic consultation immediately
  - Oxytocin or methylergonovine may be necessary to control hemorrhage.
  - These patients are at high risk for having ruptured ectopic pregnancies and may need emergent operative intervention.

### ED TREATMENT/PROCEDURES
- Threatened abortion:
  - Pelvic rest, close follow-up with obstetrics
  - Patients <6.5 wk pregnant with no documented cardiac activity by vaginal US need to be followed with serial $\beta$-hCG to assess the viability of the fetus and to rule out ectopic pregnancy.
- Inevitable and incomplete abortions:
  - Dilation and curettage or evacuation, removal of POC at the cervical os to help decrease bleeding and cramping
  - The confirmation of POC by pathology rules out ectopic pregnancy.
- Complete abortion:
  - May treat with methylergonovine or oxytocin if bleeding is heavy
  - If quantitative $\beta$-hCG is <1,000 and the US is negative, may follow-up with obstetrics for serial $\beta$-hCG to confirm the levels are decreasing

- Missed abortion:
  - These patients are at risk for disseminated intravascular coagulation (DIC), especially if fetus is retained >4–6 wk.
  - Obtain CBC, PT/PTT, fibrin-split products (FSP), and fibrinogen levels.
  - These patients may be followed closely as outpatients if stable with an early, confirmed IUP and no evidence of DIC.
  - Patients may choose to have a dilation and curettage at a later date or miscarry at home with no intervention; this decision should be made in consultation with OB/Gyn.

### MEDICATION
#### First Line
- RHO immunoglobulin in Rh-negative women:
  - 50 $\mu$g for women with threatened or complete abortion at <12 wk
  - 300 $\mu$g for women with threatened or complete abortion at $\geq$12 wk
- Patients need RhoGAM administration within 72 hr to prevent future isoimmunization.

#### Second Line
Usually given in consultation with OB/Gyn:

- Oxytocin: 20 IU in 1,000 mL of NS at a rate of 20 mIU/min titrated to decrease bleeding; may repeat for a max dose of 40 mIU/min
- Methylergonovine: 0.2 mg IM/PO q.i.d. bleeding

 **FOLLOW-UP**

### DISPOSITION
#### Admission Criteria
- Suspected unstable ectopic pregnancy (see "Ectopic Pregnancy")
- Hemodynamically unstable patients with hypovolemia or anemia
- DIC
- Septic abortions
- Suspected gestational trophoblastic disease

#### Discharge Criteria
- Dilation and curettages can be done in the ED for incomplete and inevitable abortions, and patients may be discharged home if stable after 2–3 hr.
- Some early inevitable miscarriages can be discharged to complete their miscarriages at home without a D&C. Discharge with pain medications and close OB/Gyn follow-up.
- Patients with threatened abortions should be told to avoid strenuous activity.
- Pelvic rest (ie, "nothing in the vagina" during active bleeding; may increase risk of infection)
- Patients should be instructed to return to the ED for any increase in bleeding, dizziness, or temperature >100.4°F.
- Patients and their partners should be told that early miscarriages are common and that they are not anyone's fault.

### FOLLOW-UP RECOMMENDATIONS
Patients with positive pregnancy tests and vaginal bleeding with or without abdominal pain should be followed by OB/Gyn.

## PEARLS AND PITFALLS
- Recognize the possibility of ectopic pregnancy.
- Patients with spontaneous abortion may have clinically significant blood loss.

## ADDITIONAL READING
- Griebel CP, Halvorsen J, Gloemon TB, et al. Management of spontaneous abortion. *Am Fam Physician.* 2005;72:1243–1250.
- Juliano M, Dabulis S, Heffner A. Characteristics of women with fetal loss in symptomatic first trimester pregnancies with documented fetal cardiac activity. *Ann Emerg Med.* 2008;52:143–147.
- Marx JA, Hockberger RS, Walls RM, et al. *Rosen's Emergency Medicine: Concepts and Clinical Practice.* 7th ed. St. Louis, MO: Mosby; 2009.

### See Also (Topic, Algorithm, Electronic Media Element)
- Ectopic Pregnancy
- Vaginal Bleeding

# ABRUPTIO PLACENTAE

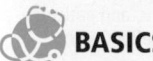

*Rebecah W. Schwartz*

## 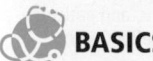 BASICS

### DESCRIPTION
- Hemorrhage at the decidual-placental interface leading to complete or partial separation of the normally implanted placenta before delivery of the fetus
- Incidence/prevalence:
  - ~1% of all pregnancies
  - 30% of bleeding episodes in the second half of pregnancy
  - 15% of all fetal deaths
  - Neonatal death in 10–30% of cases
  - 6% of all maternal mortality
- Synonym(s): Placental abruption, Accidental hemorrhage (in UK)

### ETIOLOGY
- Primary cause unknown
- Vascular injury with dissection of blood into the decidua basalis or mechanical shearing between the placenta and uterus leading to bleeding and clot formation
- More severe cases lead to:
  - Development of disseminated intravascular coagulation (DIC)
  - Maternal-fetal compromise
- Recent research suggests the majority of abruptions are due to chronic processes:
  - Inflammatory changes in the placenta
  - Manifestation of ischemic placental disease
- Acute abruption can occur due to:
  - Trauma
  - Rapid uterine decompression
  - Placenta implantation over a uterine anomaly or fibroid
- Multiple known risk factors:
  - Previous abruption (10–20% recurrence risk)
  - Maternal hypertension (>140/90) and preeclampsia
  - Increased parity and maternal age
  - Multiple gestation
  - Fibroids or other uterine/placental abnormalities
  - Tobacco use
  - Cocaine abuse
  - Trauma
  - Premature rupture of membranes, particularly if associated with chorioamnionitis or oligohydramnios
  - Rapid uterine decompression:
    - Polyhydramnios with membrane rupture
    - Rapid delivery of 1st twin
  - Elevated 2nd trimester maternal serum alpha-fetoprotein

- Thrombophilias:
  - Factor V Leiden
  - Prothrombin gene mutations
  - Antithrombin III
  - Protein C or S deficiency
  - Antithrombin deficiency
  - Lupus anticoagulant
  - Anticardiolipin antibodies
  - Methyltetrahydrofolate reductase deficiency
- Maternal race:
  - More common among African American and Caucasian women
  - Incidence increasing more rapidly among African American women

##  DIAGNOSIS

### SIGNS AND SYMPTOMS
#### History
- Typically in 2nd half of pregnancy
- Vaginal bleeding (>80%, usually painful)
- Abdominal or back pain (>50%)
- Uterine cramps, tenderness, frequent contractions, or tetany
- Nausea, vomiting
- Otherwise unexplained preterm labor
- History of recent trauma should be elicited
- Recent drug use, particularly cocaine or other sympathomimetics
- Prior abruption or other risk factors
- Estimated gestational age
- Prenatal care

#### Physical Exam
- Signs of *hypotensive shock* may be present.
- Uterine tenderness frequently but not always
- Vaginal bleeding (absent in 20–25%)
- Petechiae, bleeding, and other signs of DIC or coagulopathy
- Decreased fetal heart tones and movement
- Fetal bradycardia or nonreassuring fetal heart rate tracings

### ALERT
Sterile vaginal examination must be performed with great caution to avoid tissue injury, especially if placenta previa suspected:
- Consider sterile vaginal examination:
  - Assess for presence of amniotic fluid (Nitrazine paper turns blue; ferning of fluid on glass slide)
  - Evaluate for vaginal or cervical lacerations

### ESSENTIAL WORKUP
- Large bore IV access
- Blood type, Rh, and cross-match
- Rapid hemoglobin determination
- Determine fetal heart tones by Doppler
- Fetal monitoring to detect signs of early fetal distress
- Uterine tocographic monitoring

### DIAGNOSTIC TESTS & INTERPRETATION
#### Lab
- Blood type and Rh
- CBC, platelets
- PT/PTT
- Fibrinogen levels (normally 450 in latter half of pregnancy)
- Fibrinogen <200 mg/dL and platelets <100,000/$\mu$L highly suggestive of abruption
- Fibrin-split products:
  - Kleihauer-Betke if mother Rh-negative (significant fetal-to-maternal hemorrhage more likely in traumatic abruption)

#### Imaging
- US demonstrates evidence of abruption in only 50% of cases.
- False-negative US is common.
- MRI sensitive but impractical

### DIFFERENTIAL DIAGNOSIS
- Placenta previa
- Vasa previa
- Bleeding during labor
- Vaginal or cervical lacerations
- Uterine rupture
- Preterm labor
- Ovarian torsion
- Pyelonephritis
- Cholelithiasis/cholecystitis
- Appendicitis
- Preeclampsia complications
- Other blunt intra-abdominal or pelvic injuries

**TREATMENT**

**PRE-HOSPITAL**
- Patients with abruption may be in shock and need full resuscitative measures.
- Transport in the left lateral recumbent position

**INITIAL STABILIZATION/THERAPY**
- Airway, breathing, circulation (ABCs), oxygen
- Cardiac monitor
- Placement of large-bore IVs
- IV crystalloid resuscitation

**ED TREATMENT/PROCEDURES**
- Maternal cardiac and tocographic monitoring
- Continuous fetal monitoring
- Transfuse PRBCs, fresh frozen plasma (FFP), cryoprecipitate, and platelets as indicated
- Immediate OB/Gyn consultation
- Foley catheter for close monitoring of urine output
- Tocolysis is generally contraindicated, particularly in severe abruption with coagulopathy or fetal compromise.
- If abruption is suspected in the setting of trauma, maternal stabilization is of primary importance:
  - All indicated radiographs should be performed as needed.

**MEDICATION**
*First Line*
- Rh-immunoglobulin in Rh-negative women.
  - 300 μg IM in women at ≥12 wk gestation
  - Higher doses if indicated by results of Kleihauer-Betke test
- Blood products as indicated

*Second Line*
Consider with obstetrician recommendation:
- Magnesium sulfate if tocolysis indicated
- Steroids for fetal lung maturation if gestational age between 24 and 34 wk

 **FOLLOW-UP**

**DISPOSITION**
*Admission Criteria*
- Patients with abruptio placenta must be admitted for maternal and fetal monitoring.
- Admit to ICU if DIC, amniotic fluid embolism, or significant hemorrhage (known or suspected)
- Victims of multiple trauma with abruption should be admitted and managed in accordance with trauma protocols.
- Transportation to higher trauma or obstetric level of care is appropriate if the patient is stable for transfer or appropriate care unavailable at existing facility.

*Discharge Criteria*
- Trauma patients with no evidence of abruption or other significant injury may be discharged after 4–6 hr of normal maternal and fetal monitoring.
- Discharge instructions include pelvic rest, no intercourse, no heavy lifting, no prolonged standing
- Discharge decision should be made in consultation with OB/Gyn and include close follow-up.

*Issues for Referral*
All cases of confirmed or suspected abruption require immediate obstetric consultation.

## PEARLS AND PITFALLS

- Primarily a clinical diagnosis: No single test reliably confirms or rules out abruptio placenta.
- Hypotension typically occurs late in the course of hypovolemic shock in pregnancy.
- Anticipate a consumptive coagulopathy and consider the need for blood products early in presentation.
- Abruption may be associated with severe preeclampsia, causing a hypovolemic patient to be normotensive:
  - Maintain a high index of suspicion for preeclampsia in patients with severe abruption and no obvious cause.

## ADDITIONAL READING

- Ananth CV, Oyelese Y, Yeo L, et al. Placental abruption in the United States, 1979 through 2001: Temporal trends and potential determinants. *Am J Obstet Gynecol*. 2005;192:191–198.
- Ananth CV, Kinzler WL. Clinical features and diagnosis of placental abruption. *UpToDate*. 2009;17:2.
- Elasser DA, Ananth CV, Prasad V, et al. Diagnosis of placental abruption: Relationship between clinical and histopathological findings. *Eur J Obstet Gynecol Repro Biol*. 2009.
- Oyelese Y, Ananth CV. Management and outcome of pregnancies complicated by placental abruption. *UpToDate*. 2009;17:2.
- Oyelese Y, Ananth CV. Placental abruption. *Obstet Gynecol*. 2006;108:1005–1016.
- Sakornbut E, Leeman L, Fontaine P. Late pregnancy bleeding. *Am Fam Physician*. 2007;75:1199–1206.

**See Also (Topic, Algorithm, Electronic Media Element)**
- Placenta Previa
- Pregnancy, Trauma in
- Vaginal Bleeding in Pregnancy

# ABSCESS, SKIN/SOFT TISSUE
*Neal O'Connor*

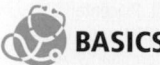 **BASICS**

## DESCRIPTION
- A localized collection of pus surrounded and walled off by inflamed tissue. Abscesses can occur on any part of the body.
- Furuncle:
  - Arises from infected hair follicle
  - Most common on back, axilla, and lower extremities
- Carbuncle:
  - Larger and more extensive than furuncle
- Dog/cat bite:
  - Usually polymicrobial
- Breast:
  - Puerperal:
    - Usually during lactation
    - Located in peripheral wedge
    - Usually staphylococci
  - Duct ectasia:
    - Caused by ecstatic ducts
    - Periareoloar location
    - Usually polymicrobial
- Hiradenitis suppurativa:
  - Chronic abscess of apocrine sweat glands
  - Groin and scalp
  - *Staph aureus* and *staph viridans* are common
  - *E. coli* and *proteus* may be present in chronic disease
- Pilonidal abscess:
  - Epithelial disruption of gluteal fold over coccyx
  - Staphylococcal species are most common
  - May be polymicrobial
- Bartholin's abscess:
  - Obstruction of Bartholin duct
- Perirectal abscess:
  - Originates in anal crypts and extends though ischiorectal space
  - Inflammatory bowel disease and diabetes are predisposing factors
  - *Bacteroides fragilis* and *E. coli* are most common
  - Requires operative drainage
- Muscle (pyomyositis):
  - Typically in the tropics
  - *Staph aureus* is most common
- IV drug abuse:
  - Staph species are most common
  - MRSA is common
  - May be sterile
- Paronychia:
  - Infection around nail fold
  - Usually *Staph aureus*
- Felon:
  - Closed space abscess in distal pulp of finger
  - Usually *Staph aureus*

## ETIOLOGY
- Abscess formation typically occurs due to a break in the skin, obstruction of sebaceous or sweat glands, or inflammation of hair follicles. The collection may be classified as bacterial or sterile:
- Bacterial: Most abscesses are bacterial with the microbiology reflective of the microflora of the involved body part:
  - *Staph aureus* is the most common causative organism
  - Community-acquired MRSA increasingly common
- Sterile: More associated with intravenous drug abuse and injection of chemical irritants.
- Risk factors for abscess formation:
  - Immunosuppression
  - Soft-tissue trauma
  - Mammalian/human bites
  - Tissue ischemia
  - IV drug use
  - Crohn disease (perirectal)

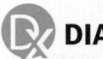 **DIAGNOSIS**

## SIGNS AND SYMPTOMS
- Local:
  - Erythema
  - Tenderness
  - Heat
  - Swelling
  - Fluctuance
  - May be associated with surrounding cellulitis
  - Regional lymphadenopathy and lymphangitis may occur.
- Systemic:
  - Often absent
  - Patients with extensive soft tissue involvement, necrotizing fasciitis, or underlying bacteremia may present with signs of sepsis including:
    - Fever
    - Rigors
    - Hypotension
    - Altered mentation

## History
- Previous episodes: Raise concern for CA-MRSA
- Immunosuppression
- Medications:
  - Chronic steroids, chemotherapy
- IVDU
- History of mammalian bite

## Physical Exam
- Location and extent of infection
- Presence of:
  - Associated cellulitis
  - Subcutaneous air
  - Deep structure involvement
- Involvement of specialty area:
  - Perirectal
  - Hand
  - Face/Neck

## ESSENTIAL WORKUP
- History and physical examination.
- Gram stain unnecessary for simple abscesses in healthy patients
- Wound cultures:
  - Not indicated in simple abscesses
  - May help guide therapy if systemic treatment is planned
  - May be useful in confirming community-acquired MRSA in patients with recurrent abscesses
  - May guide specific therapy in a compromised host, abscesses of the central face or hand, and treatment failures

## DIAGNOSTIC TESTS & INTERPRETATION
### Lab
- Routine laboratory tests are not typically indicated.
- Glucose determination may be useful if:
  - Underlying undiagnosed diabetes is a concern
  - There is a concern for associated DKA
- For febrile patients who appear septic, systemically ill, or have recent IVDU the following labs are indicated:
  - Blood cultures
  - Lactate
  - Renal function
  - CK if myositis suspected

### Imaging
- Bedside US can be helpful distinguishing cellulitis from abscess.
- CT/MRI can be helpful determining deeptissue involvement.
- Plain films may reveal gas in tissue planes

## DIFFERENTIAL DIAGNOSIS
- Cellulitis
- Necrotizing fasciitis
- Aneurysm (especially with IV drug abusers)
- Cysts
- Hematoma

**TREATMENT**

## PRE-HOSPITAL
Caution: Septic patients may require rapid transport with intravenous access and volume resuscitation.

## INITIAL STABILIZATION/THERAPY
Septic patient:
- Immediate IV access
- Oxygen
- Crystalloid volume resuscitation
- Blood cultures/lactate
- Early antibiotic therapy—broad spectrum to include MRSA coverage.
- Rapid source control (abscess drainage)
- If patient remains hypotensive after volume resuscitation consider:
  - Central venous pressure monitoring
  - Mixed venous sampling

## ED TREATMENT/PROCEDURES
- Incision and drainage are the mainstays of treatment.
  - Incision should be deep enough to allow adequate drainage
  - Elliptical incision prevent early closure
  - Break loculations with gentle exploration
  - Irrigate cavity after expressing all pus
  - A loose packing should be placed in the cavity to promote drainage and prevent premature closure.
- Routine antibiotics are not indicated.
- Antibiotics are indicated for the following conditions:
  - Sepsis/systemic illness
  - Facial abscesses drained into the cavernous sinus
  - Concurrent cellulitis (see "Medication")
  - Mammalian bites
  - Immunocompromised hosts
- Perirectal abscess requires treatment in the operating room.
- Hand infections that may require surgical intervention:
  - Deep abscesses
  - Fight bite abscesses
  - Associated tenosynovitis/deep fascial plane infection

### Pediatric Considerations
Incision and drainage are painful procedures that often require procedural sedation and analgesia.

## MEDICATION

### ALERT
Know your local Suseptability patterns
- Oral Antibiotics (moderate associated cellulitis):
  - Amoxicillin/clavulanate:
    - Use: Mammalian bites/MSSA/Strep Species
    - Adult dose: 500–875 mg (peds 40 80 mg/kg/day div q12h) PO q12h
  - TMP-SMX:
    - Use: MRSA
    - Adult Dose: 160/800 mg (peds 4–5 mg/kg) PO b.i.d.
  - Clindamycin:
    - Use: MRSA
    - Adult dose: 300–450 mg (peds 4–8 mg/kg) PO q8h
  - Doxycycline:
    - Use: MRSA
    - Adult dose: 100 mg(peds over 8 yr: 1.1 mg/kg) PO q12h
  - Cephalexin:
    - Use: MSSA/Strep species
    - Adult dose: 250–500 mg (peds 25–50 mg/ day div q6h) PO q8h
  - Erythromycin:
    - Use: MSSA/Strep species
    - Adult dose: 250–500 mg (peds 10 mg/kg) PO q6–8h
- IV antibiotics (Systemic illness or extensive associated cellulitis):
  - Ampicillin/sulbactam
    - Uses: Human/mammalian bites and facial cellulitis
    - Adult Dose: 1.5–3.0 g (peds <40 kg, 75 mg/kg; ≥40 kg, adult dose) IV q6h (max = 12 g/day)
  - Vancomycin:
    - Use: MRSA
    - Adult Dose: 15 mg/kg IV q12h (peds 10–15 mg/kg/day div q6–8 h) (max = 2,000 mg/day)
  - Daptomycin:
    - Use MRSA
    - Adult dose: 4 mg/kg IV q24h
  - Linezolid:
    - Use: MRSA
    - Adult Dose: 600 mg IV/PO q12h (peds 30 mg/kg/day div q8h)
  - Clindamycin:
    - Use: MRSA
    - Adult dose: 600 mg (peds 10–15 mg/kg) IV q8h

 **FOLLOW-UP**

## DISPOSITION
In accordance with abscess type and severity of infection

### Admission Criteria
- Sepsis/systemic illness
- Immunocompromised host with moderate/large cellulitis
- Perirectal involvement
- Any abscess requiring incision and debridement in the operating room

### Discharge Criteria
Most patients with uncomplicated abscesses can be treated with incision and drainage and close follow-up.

## FOLLOW-UP RECOMMENDATIONS
- Recheck in 24–48 hr for packing removal and wound check.
- Warm soaks for 2–3 days after packing removal

## PEARLS AND PITFALLS

- Consider CA-MRSA in recurrent abscesses
- Pain control is essential during incision and drainage of abscesses
- Beware of tenosynovitis and deep fascial space infections

## ADDITIONAL READING

- Hankin A, Everett W. Are antibiotics necessary after incision and drainage of a cutaneous abscess? *Ann Emerg Med.* 2007;50:49–51.
- Jayal V, Hasan N, et al. The effect of soft-tissue ultrasound on the management of cellulitis in the emergency department. *J Acad Emer Med.* 2006;13: 384–388.
- Buescher ES. Community-acquired methicillin-resistant *Staphylococcus aureus* in pediatrics. *Curr Opin Pediatr.* 2005;17:67–70.
- Alison DC, Miller T, Holtom P, et al. Microbiology of upper extremity soft tissue abscesses in injecting drug abusers. *Clin Orth Related Res.* 2007;461: 9–13.

### See Also (Topic, Algorithm, Electronic Media Element)
- Bartholin's abscess
- Bite, Animal
- Cellulitis
- CA-MRSA
- Hand infection
- Mastitis
- Paronychia

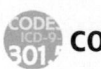 **CODES**

### ICD9
682.9 Cellulitis and abscess of unspecified sites

# ABUSE, ELDER
*Helen Straus*

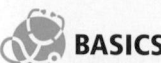 **BASICS**

## DESCRIPTION
Elder abuse may include the following:

- Emotional abuse:
  - Insults
  - Humiliation
  - Threats to institutionalize or abandon
- Physical and/or sexual abuse:
  - Hitting
  - Slapping
  - Pushing
  - Burning
  - Inappropriate restraining
  - Forced sexual activity
- Material exploitation:
  - Stealing or coercion involving patient monies or property
- Neglect:
  - Behaviors by a patient or caregiver that compromise the patient's health or safety
  - Failure to provide adequate food, shelter, hygiene, and/or medical attention

## EPIDEMIOLOGY
### Incidence and Prevalence Estimates
- In the U.S., 1 million known cases annually (estimated 5 million cases); 2% reported by physicians
- 9% verbal mistreatment:
  - Verbal mistreatment is more likely in women and those with physical vulnerabilities and less likely for Latinos than for Caucasians.
- 3.5% financial mistreatment:
  - More likely for African Americans than for Caucasians; less likely for Latinos than for Caucasians
  - Less likely for those with partners than for those without partners
- 0.2% physical mistreatment

## ETIOLOGY
- Caregiver stress, dependency, or psychopathology
- Victim dependency or diminishment of ability to perform activities of daily living

 **DIAGNOSIS**

## SIGNS AND SYMPTOMS
Variable, possibly inconsistent, history or physical findings

### History
- Not willing or able to obtain adequate food/clothing/shelter
- Not providing for personal hygiene/safety
- Delay in obtaining medical care/previously untreated medical condition
- Vague (or implausible/inappropriate) explanations
- Disparities between histories given by patient and caregiver
- Caregiver who insists on giving the patient's history
- Medication difficulties:
  - Incorrect doses
  - Lost medications
  - Unfilled prescriptions
- Altered interpersonal interactions:
  - Withdrawn
  - Indifferent
  - Demoralized
  - Fearful
  - Substance abuse
- Caregiver with:
  - Financial dependence on patient
  - Substance abuse or psychiatric or violence history
  - Controlling behavior (may refuse to leave elder alone with physician) or poor knowledge
  - Significant life stressors
  - Relationship issues
  - Financial difficulties
  - Legal problems

### Physical Exam
- Inconsistent findings:
  - Patterns or variable-age bruises, burns, lacerations/abrasions
  - Unusual sites of bruising (inner arm, torso, buttocks, scalp)
  - Poor hygiene (inadequate care of skin, nails, teeth)
- Unexplained injuries:
  - Bruised or bleeding genital or rectal area
  - Wrist or ankle lesions suggestive of restraint use
- Findings that may be consistent with neglect or delay in seeking/obtaining medical attention:
  - Dehydration
  - Weight loss
  - Decubitus ulcer
  - Malnutrition

## DIAGNOSTIC TESTS & INTERPRETATION
Perform any examination and laboratory or radiographic studies as indicated by the patient's condition.

## ESSENTIAL WORKUP
- Obtain history without family members/caregivers present:
  - Abused elders may fear institutionalization if they report caregivers.
  - Many may feel embarrassment and responsibility for abuse.
  - Frequently will not volunteer information
  - Ask patient specifically about abuse or neglect (in private)
- Patient's medical condition may influence quality of history obtained
- Obtain history from caregivers/other relatives/friends/neighbors
- Document a clear and detailed description of findings including the following:
  - Statements of the patient as they pertain to the abuse
  - Psychosocial history:
    ○ Family and other social relationships
    ○ Caregiver burdens/coping mechanisms
    ○ Drug/ethanol (EtOH) use
    ○ Prior adult protective services reports
  - Skin and other physical findings:
    ○ Photographic documentation
    ○ Safety assessment

## DIAGNOSTIC TESTS & INTERPRETATION
### Lab
As appropriate for medical condition(s)

### Imaging
As appropriate for medical condition(s)

*Diagnostic Procedures/Surgery*
As appropriate for medical condition(s)

## DIFFERENTIAL DIAGNOSIS

- Patient may present with any chief complaint:
  – Potential differential diagnosis is nonspecific.
  – Abuse best identified by asking patient directly in a setting apart from caregivers/family and correlating with risk factors and provider findings
- Differentiate findings consistent with other disease entities from abuse/neglect:
  – Dehydration
  – Ill-fitting dentures
  – Burns
  – Ecchymoses
  – Insomnia
  – Medication noncompliance
  – Dementia
  – Depression

 TREATMENT

## PRE-HOSPITAL

Observe details of the patient's environment that may not be immediately available to the hospital care team, including the following:

- Interpersonal interactions at the scene:
  – Embarrassment
  – Shame
  – Fear of reprisal, abandonment, and/or institutionalization
- Conditions in the physical environment that present a potential danger

## INITIAL STABILIZATION/THERAPY

- ABCs
- Treat life-threatening medical/traumatic conditions as appropriate.

## ED TREATMENT/PROCEDURES

- May require separation of the patient and the caregiver or family member
- Social work referral:
  Safety planning
  – Respite planning for caregiver
  – Adult protective services referral

- Competent elder patients are free to accept or decline treatment or disposition despite risks they may incur.
- General measures appropriate to the medical/traumatic conditions identified, including:
  – Fluids
  – Medications
  – Surgery
  – Diet
  – Activity
  – Nursing care
  – Physical therapy

 FOLLOW-UP

## DISPOSITION

Disposition determined by medical condition and home environment

### Admission Criteria

- Medical condition requiring admission
- Abuse or neglect renders home conditions unsafe.
- Need for more information or time to enhance objective decision-making and patient management

### Discharge Criteria

- Medical condition(s) addressed
- Safe environment available
- Abuse or neglect successfully countered by social services and/or law enforcement

### Issues for Referral

- Many states have mandatory reporting requirements:
  – Comply with area legal requirements.
- Alcohol/drug treatment as appropriate
- Notify adult protective services.

### FOLLOW-UP RECOMMENDATIONS

As appropriate for medical condition(s)

## PEARLS AND PITFALLS

- Entertaining the possibility of abuse or neglect in an elder patient offers the best possibility of diagnosis and successful intervention.
- Only ~1/3 of healthcare providers identified a case of elder abuse in the past year.
- Current data are inconclusive about the effectiveness of interventions for diminishing recurrence of elder abuse.
- Obtain the aid of social work, physicians trusted by the patient, even an ethics consultant, should a vulnerable competent elder seek to decline an elder abuse/neglect investigation.

## ADDITIONAL READING

- Clarke ME, Pierson W. Management of elder abuse in the emergency department. *Emerg Med Clin North Am.* 1999;17:631–644.
- Cooper C, Selwood A, Livingston G. Knowledge, detection, and reporting of abuse by health and social care professionals: A systematic review. *Am J Geriatr Psychiatry.* 2009;17(10):826–838.
- Lachs MS, Pillemer K. Elder abuse. *Lancet.* 2004;364:1263–1272.
- Laumann EO, Leitsch SA, Waite LJ. Elder mistreatment in the United States; prevalence estimates from a nationally representative study. *J Gerontol B Psychol Sci Soc Sci.* 2008 July;63(4): S248–S254.
- Levine JM. Elder neglect and abuse—a primer for primary care physicians. *Geriatrics.* 2003;58(10): 37–40, 42–44.
- Marshall CE, Benton D, Brazier JM. Elder abuse: Using clinical tools to identify clues of mistreatment. *Geriatrics.* 2000;55:42–50.
- Ploeg J, Fear J, Hutchison B, et al. A systematic review of interventions for elder abuse. *J Elder Abuse Negl.* 2009;21(3):187–210.

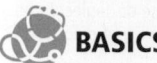

## BASICS

### DESCRIPTION
- Child abuse impacts up to 14 million or 2–3% of U.S. children each year.
- 1,200–1,400 children die of maltreatment each year in the U.S. Of these, 80% <5 yr and 40% <1 yr.
- Mandated reporters of suspected abuse or neglect include all health care workers.
- Risk factors:
  - Child: Usually <4 yr, often handicapped, retarded or special needs ("vulnerable child"), premature birth, or multiple birth
  - Abusive parent: Low self-esteem, abused as child, violent temper, mental illness history, rigid and unrealistic expectations of child, or young maternal age
  - Family: Monetary problems, isolated and mobile, or marital instability
  - Poor parent–child relationship, unwanted pregnancy
  - Abuse crosses all religious and socioeconomic groups

## DIAGNOSIS

### SIGNS AND SYMPTOMS
*History*
- History and mechanism inconsistent with the injury or illness:
  - Unexplained death, apnea, and injury
  - Unexplained ingestion or toxin exposure
  - Recurrent injury
  - Parent/caregiver reluctant to give information or denies knowledge of how injury occurred
  - Discrepancy among different caregivers
  - Developmentally, child unable to experience mechanism
  - Inappropriate response to injury or illness; delay in seeking care
  - If alleged anogenital/sexual abuse, history credible
- Munchausen by proxy:
  - Recurrent illness without medical explanation
  - Unexplained metabolic disorder suspicious for poisoning
- Failure to thrive:
  - Inadequate caloric intake secondary to poor maternal bonding/neglect
  - Review of past ED encounters and contact with the patient's primary care physician may be helpful.

*Physical Exam*
- Cutaneous bruising/contusions:
  - Regular pattern, straight line of demarcation, regular angles, slap marks from fingers, dunking burns (stocking or glove burns or doughnut shaped on buttock), bites, strap, buckle, cigarette burns
  - Location: Buttocks, hips, face (not forehead), arms, back, thighs, genitalia, or pinna
  - Aging:
    ○ Often different ages of bruises
    ○ Yellow bruises are older than 18 hr
    ○ Red, blue and purple, or black color may occur from 1 hr after injury to resolution
    ○ Red may be present irrespective of age
    ○ Bruises of identical age and cause on the same person may appear to be different.
- Skeletal trauma:
  - Usually multiple, unexplained, various stages of healing
  - Metaphyseal or corner (classic metaphyseal lesions) fractures (pathognomonic)
  - Skull fractures that cross suture lines
  - Posterior rib fractures (rib fractures almost never occur in infants from CPR)
  - Spiral fractures of long bones
  - Subperiosteal new bone formation
  - Uncommon fractures (vertebrae, sternum, scapula, spinous process) without significant mechanism
- CNS:
  - Altered mental status or seizure
  - Head trauma is leading cause of death in child abuse.
  - Skull fracture: Must consider child abuse in children <1 yr
  - Subdural hematoma, subarachnoid hemorrhage
  - Shaken baby syndrome with shearing and rotational injury
- Ocular findings:
  - Retinal hemorrhage or detachment:
    ○ 53–80% of abusive head injury has retinal hemorrhage (commonly bilateral) while present in only 0–10% severe accidental trauma
  - Hyphema
  - Corneal abrasion/conjunctival hemorrhage
- Oral trauma
- Abdominal injuries:
  - Lacerated liver, spleen, kidney, or pancreas
  - Intramural hematoma (duodenal most common)
  - Retroperitoneal hematoma
- Anogenital/sexual abuse:
  - Contusion, erythema, open wounds, scarring, or foreign material (hair, debris, or semen)
  - Presence of STD or pregnancy in child <12 yr
- Death:
  - Unexplained death

### ESSENTIAL WORKUP
- Formal oral and written report to appropriate child welfare agency
- Family and environmental evaluation, usually in cooperation with responsible child welfare agency
- Diagram or photograph of bruises is helpful.

> **ALERT**
> When suspected, health professionals have a legal obligation to report their suspicion to the appropriate authorities.

### DIAGNOSTIC TESTS & INTERPRETATION
*Lab*
- Bleeding screen if there is a history of recurrent bruising or bruising is the prominent manifestation; may usually be done electively: CBC, platelets, PT/PTT, or bleeding time (or PFA collagen epinephrine)
- If significant blunt trauma, CBC, LFT, amylase, and urinalysis
- Toxicology, chemistry, and metabolic screens in children with altered mental status
- Consider other differential considerations.

*Imaging*
- Global assessment:
  - Indicated for children <2 yr to exclude unsuspected injuries
  - In children 2–5 yr, in selected cases where physical abuse is strongly suspected
  - In older children, radiographs of individual sites of injury suspected on clinical grounds
  - Radiographic skeletal survey:
    ○ Anteroposterior (AP) and lateral skull
    ○ Lateral cervical spine
    ○ AP and lateral thoracic and lumbar spine
    ○ AP and obliques of chest
    ○ AP pelvis
    ○ AP humerus, forearm, and hands (bilateral)
    ○ AP femur, tibia, and feet (bilateral)
  - If fracture identified, get at least 2 views, 90° to original view.
  - May need coned-down view of joints for visualization of classic metaphyseal lesions
  - Skeletal scintigraphy provides adjunctive screening if suspicion exists beyond skeletal survey.
- Visceral imaging:
  - Suspected thoracoabdominal injury:
    ○ Abdominal CT scan with IV and possibly oral contrast

- Neuroimaging:
  - Nonenhanced head CT with brain, subdural, and bone windowing
  - MRI:
    - Adjunctive in evaluation of acute, subacute, and chronic intracranial injury; useful for shear injuries, evolving hemorrhage, contusion, or secondary hypoxic/ischemic injury

## DIFFERENTIAL DIAGNOSIS

- General:
  - Trauma—accidental or birth/obstetrical
- Cutaneous:
  - Burn—accidental
  - Infection
  - Impetigo/cellulitis
  - Staphylococcal scalded skin syndrome
  - Henoch-Schönlein purpura
  - Purpura fulminans/meningococcemia
  - Sepsis
  - Dermatitis: Contact or photo
  - Hematologic/oncologic disorder (idiopathic thrombocytopenic purpura [ITP], leukemia)
  - Bleeding diathesis (hemophilia, von Willebrand)
  - Nutritional deficiency: Scurvy
  - Cultural healing practices (coining, cupping)
- Skeletal:
  - Osteogenesis imperfecta
  - Nutritional (rickets, copper deficiency, or scurvy)
  - Menkes syndrome
  - Peripheral sensory impairment (indifference to pain)
- Ocular:
  - Conjunctivitis
- Abdomen and GU tract:
  - GI disease (obstruction, peritonitis, or inflammatory bowel disease)
  - GU tract infection/anomaly
- CNS:
  - Intoxication, ingestion (CO, lead, or mercury)
- Infection:
  - Metabolic: Hypoglycemia
  - Epilepsy
- Death:
  - SIDS, apparent life-threatening event (ALTE)

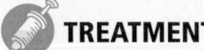

## TREATMENT

### PRE-HOSPITAL

- Diagnosis relies on physical evidence in child and inconsistency with the history and mechanism.
- Examination of the scene may be useful:
  - Evaluate validity of mechanisms.
  - General appearance of home
  - Consistency of history by multiple caregivers
  - Evaluation of parent–child interaction

### INITIAL STABILIZATION/THERAPY

As indicated by specific injury

### ED TREATMENT/PROCEDURES

- Medical and trauma management as required
- Mandatory reporting to local child welfare agency of any suspected child abuse to determine appropriate social disposition:
  - This does *not* imply or require 100% certainty of abuse.
  - Expedited family, environmental, and social evaluation
- Communication with family about report and primary concern is responsibility of child welfare.
  - Security may be required to protect child and staff.
- Siblings and other household children must be examined in appropriate time frame.

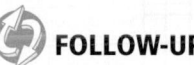

## FOLLOW-UP

### DISPOSITION

#### Admission Criteria

- Observation and intervention for traumatic injury
- Concerns about disposition or lack of availability of child welfare receiving site, if required
- Goal must always be to ensure safety of child and siblings.

#### Discharge Criteria

- Adequate ED evaluation and medical follow-up
- Safe setting for child must determine disposition
- Child (and siblings) may require placement in foster care.

#### Issues for Referral

All patients require referral to the appropriate child welfare agency.

## PEARLS AND PITFALLS

- A history inconsistent with the physical findings should lead to a suspicion of nonaccidental trauma.
- When child abuse is suspected, it must be reported.

## ADDITIONAL READING

- American Academy of Pediatrics, section of radiology. Diagnostic imaging of child abuse. *Pediatrics.* 2000;105:1345.
- American Academy of Pediatrics, Committee on Child Abuse and Neglect. Evaluation of suspected child physical abuse. *Pediatrics.* 2007;119:1232.
- Guenther E, Knight S, Olson LM, et al. Prediction of child abuse risk from emergency department use. *J Pediatr.* 2009;154:272–277.
- Hudson M and Kaplan R. Clinical response to child abuse. *Pediatr Clin North Am.* 2006;53:27–39.
- Kleinman PK, ed. *Diagnostic Imaging of Child Abuse.* 2nd ed. St. Louis, MO: Mosby; 1998.
- Togioka BM, Arnold MA, Bathurst MA, et al. Retinal hemorrhages and shaken baby syndrome: An evidence-based review. *J Emerg Med.* 2009;37: 98–106.

### See Also (Topic, Algorithm, Electronic Media Element)

Trauma, Multiple

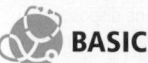

## BASICS

### DESCRIPTION
- Acetaminophen (APAP) is available alone, in combination with oral narcotics, and in >200 cold remedies:
  - One of the most common drugs implicated in intentional and unintentional poisonings
  - The number 1 reason for hepatic transplantation in the US
- *N*-acetyl-p-benzoquinoneimine (NAPQI) produced when APAP metabolized by cytochrome P-450:
  - NAPQI normally detoxified by glutathione
  - In overdose, glutathione is quickly depleted and NAPQI causes hepatic damage.
  - *N*-acetylcysteine (NAC) replenishes the liver's glutathione stores.

- Increased risk of toxicity:
  - Increased activity of cytochrome P-450 system (phenobarbital, rifampin)
  - Patients with poor nutrition have decreased glutathione stores.
- Pharmacokinetics:
  - APAP half-life:
    - 2.5–4 hr in a nonoverdose setting
    - >4 hr in overdose
  - Toxic dose >150 mg/kg acutely
  - Probable toxic level is 140 $\mu$g/mL at 4 hr postingestion (see Fig. 1 nomogram for acute intoxication).
  - Therapeutic plasma concentration is 5–20 $\mu$g/mL.

## DIAGNOSIS

### SIGNS AND SYMPTOMS
Acute overdose:
- Phase 1: 0.5–24 hr postingestion:
  - Nausea, vomiting, malaise
  - Occurs with large overdoses
  - May not be present with smaller toxic doses
- Phase 2: 24–72 hr postingestion:
  - Decreased GI symptoms
  - Hepatic damage is occurring.
  - Right upper quadrant pain and tenderness
  - Elevation of liver enzymes, PT/INR, bilirubin
  - Oliguria
  - Prolonged (>4 hr) APAP half-life implies hepatic toxicity.
- Phase 3: 72–96 hr postingestion:
  - Critical time period in the prognosis
  - Peak liver function abnormalities
  - Hepatic encephalopathy develops.
  - If the PT/INR continues to rise and/or renal insufficiency develops beyond the 3rd day postingestion, there is high likelihood that the patient will require hepatic transplantation.
- Phase 4: 96 hr to 10 days postingestion:
  - Resolution of hepatic injury or progression to complete hepatic failure

### ESSENTIAL WORKUP
- Ingestion history of all APAP-containing products
- Time of ingestion
- APAP level:
  - Obtain 4-hr postingestion level or immediately on presentation if >4 hr postingestion.
  - Use Rumack-Matthew nomogram as therapeutic guide for single acute overdose (see Fig. 1).
  - Obtain level, but do not use nomogram for therapeutic guidance in chronic ingestions or very late ingestions (>24 hr).
- Call poison center ([800] 222-1222) or toxicologist.

### DIAGNOSTIC TESTS & INTERPRETATION
*Lab*
- APAP level
- Electrolytes, BUN, creatinine, and glucose
- Liver enzymes:
  - Elevated AST is the first abnormality detected.
  - AST/ALT levels may rise >10,000 in stage III of toxicity.
  - Bilirubin
- PT/INR
- Pregnancy test

### DIFFERENTIAL DIAGNOSIS
- Suspect APAP as coingestant with other drugs in overdose.
- Causes of acute onset hepatotoxicity:
  - Infectious hepatitis
  - Reye syndrome
  - *Amanita* sp. mushrooms toxicity
  - Herbal and dietary supplements
  - Other drug ingestions

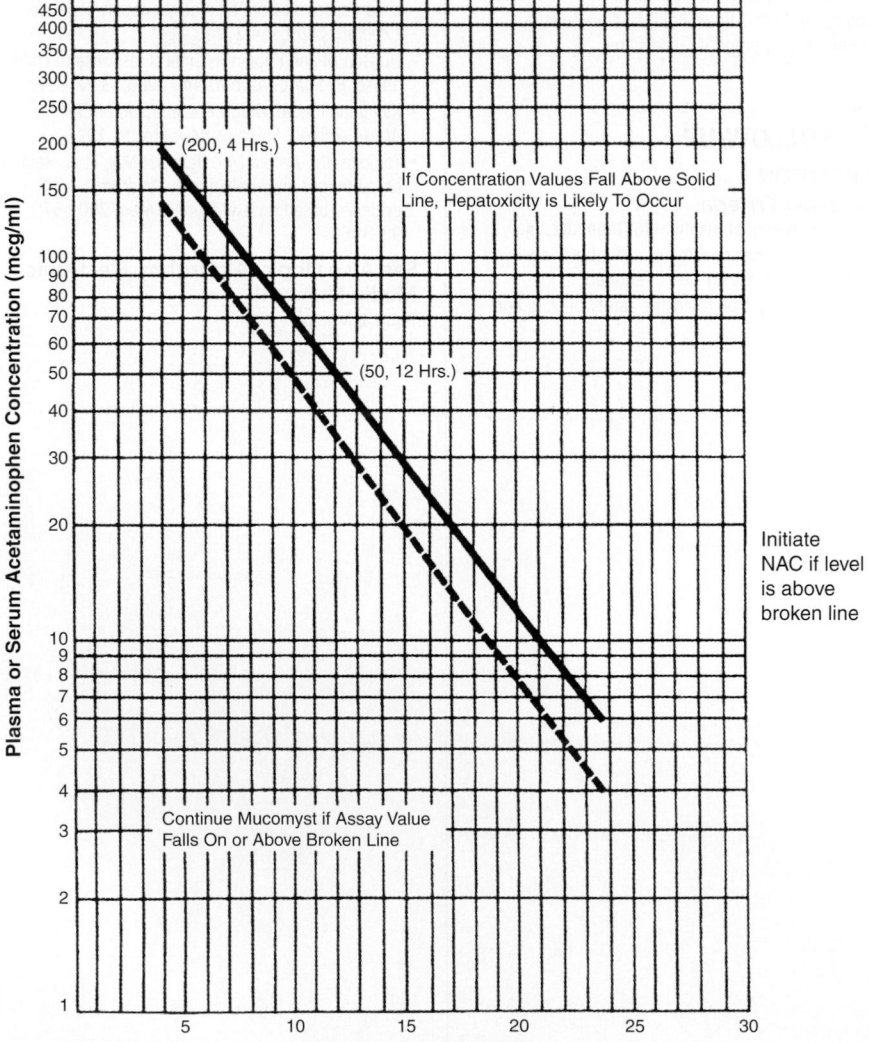

Rumack-Matthew nomogram. (Adapted from Rumack BH, Matthew H. Acetaminophen poisoning and toxicity. *Pediatrics.* 1975;55:871–876.)

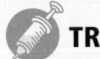

# TREATMENT

## PRE-HOSPITAL
- Transport all pill bottles/pills involved in overdose for identification in ED.
- OTC cold remedies often contain acetaminophen.

## INITIAL STABILIZATION/THERAPY
- Airway, breathing, circulation (ABCs)
- Administer supplemental oxygen.
- Administer naloxone, thiamine, D50 (or Accu-Chek) for altered mental status.

## ED TREATMENT/PROCEDURES
- Supportive care:
  - IV fluids
  - Antiemetics
- Gastric decontamination:
  - Administer a single dose of activated charcoal if recent ingestion.

### NAC Administration
- Administer if toxic level detected as defined by Rumack-Matthew nomogram.
- NAC virtually 100% hepatoprotective if initiated within 8 hr of an acute overdose
- NAC available in oral form or IV form
- <8 hr postingestion:
  - Check APAP level.
  - Initiate NAC if APAP level will not be available within 8 hr of ingestion and toxic ingestion suspected.
  - Discontinue NAC if APAP level nontoxic.
- ≥8 hr postingestion:
  - Initiate NAC immediately if suspected toxic ingestion.
  - Check APAP level.
  - Discontinue NAC if APAP level is nontoxic.
- >24 hr postingestion or chronic repeated APAP ingestion
  - Initiate NAC if:
    - Ingestion >150 mg/kg APAP
    - Symptomatic
    - Abnormal hepatic screening panel
    - Discontinue NAC if APAP falls to nondetectable level and no AST elevation occurs by 36 hr postingestion.
    - Call poison center (|800] 222-1222) or toxicologist for help.

### NAC Preparations
- Oral NAC:
  - Poor taste and odor:
    - Dilute to 5% with fruit juice or soft drink to increase palatability.
  - Use antiemetics (metoclopramide or ondansetron) liberally to facilitate PO administration.
  - If the patient vomits NAC within 1 hr of administration, repeat the dose.
  - Administer NAC as a drip through nasogastric (NG) tube if vomiting continues.
  - Given q4h

- IV NAC (2 options):
  - Acetadote infusion given per manufacturer's instructions
  - Oral NAC given by IV route if:
    - Oral form not tolerated because of vomiting
    - Acetadote not available
    - Contact local poison center or toxicologist for help.

### Pregnancy Considerations
- No teratogenicity with NAC
- NAC may be effective in protecting fetal liver:
  - Fetal liver metabolizes APAP to toxic NAPQI after 14 wk gestation.

## ALERT
A shortened oral NAC protocol may be considered with poison center or toxicology consultation.

## MEDICATION
- Activated charcoal: 1–2 g/kg PO
- Dextrose: $D_{50}W$ 1 amp (50 mL or 25 g; peds: $D_{25}W$ 2–4 mL/kg) IV
- Metoclopramide: Start with 10 mg (peds: 1 mg/kg) IV (1 mg/kg max)
- N-acetylcysteine (NAC): 140 mg/kg PO loading (adult and pediatric) followed by 70 mg/kg q4h for 17 additional doses
- Acetadote: 21-hr IV infusion (see package insert for dosing)
- Naloxone (Narcan): 0.4–2 mg (peds: 0.1 mg/kg) IV or IM initial dose
- Ondansetron: >80 kg, 12 mg; 45–80 kg, 8 mg (peds 0.15 mg/kg) IV
- Thiamine (vitamin $B_1$): 100 mg (peds: 50 mg) IV or IM

### Pregnancy Considerations
Treating the mother maximizes treatment for the fetus. NAC crosses the placenta and is considered safe PO or IV.

# FOLLOW-UP

## DISPOSITION

### Admission Criteria
- Hepatotoxic level of APAP requiring full course of NAC therapy (see "Treatment")
- LFT abnormalities in the setting of chronic ingestion or late presentation
- Nontoxic suicide attempt requiring psychiatric treatment

### Discharge Criteria
Asymptomatic patients with nontoxic ingestions not requiring full course of NAC therapy

### Issues for Referral
Evidence of significant hepatotoxicity at time of ED arrival warrants early evaluation by hepatology and/or transplant service.

### FOLLOW-UP RECOMMENDATIONS
- Substance abuse referral for patients with oral narcotic abuse
- Patients with unintentional (accidental) poisoning require poison prevention counseling.
- Patients with intentional (eg, suicide) poisoning require psychiatric evaluation.

## PEARLS AND PITFALLS
- Consider occult acetaminophen poisoning in patients evaluated for oral narcotic abuse.
- Do not use the nomogram for patients with chronic ingestion or late presentation.
- Do not stop NAC therapy until improvement or resolution of laboratory and clinical evidence of hepatotoxicity.

## ADDITIONAL READING
- Anker AL. Acetaminophen. In: Ford MD, Delaney KA, Ling LJ, et al., eds. Clinical Toxicology. Philadelphia: WB Saunders; 2001:265–274.
- Buckley NA, Whyte IM, O'Connell DL, et al. Oral or intravenous N-acetylcysteine: Which is the treatment of choice for acetaminophen (paracetamol) poisoning? J Toxicol Clin Toxicol. 1999;37(6): 759–767.
- Heard K. Acetylcysteine for acetaminophen poisoning. N Engl J Med. 2008;359(3):285–92.
- Rumack BH. Acetaminophen misconceptions. Hepatology. 2004;40(1):10–15.
- Smilkstein MJ, Knapp GL, Kulig KW, et al. Efficacy of oral n-acetylcysteine in treatment of acetaminophen overdose. Analysis of the national multicenter study. N Engl J Med. 1988;319:1557–1562.
- Yarema M, Johnson DW, Berlin RJ, et al. Comparison of the 20-hour intravenous and 72-hour oral acetylcysteine protocols for the treatment of acute acetaminophen poisoning. Ann Emerg Med. 2009;54(4):606–14.
- Yip L, Dart RC, Hurlbut KM. Intravenous administration of oral N-acetylcysteine. Crit Care Med. 1998;26:40–42.

# ACIDOSIS
*Matthew Robinson*

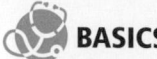 **BASICS**

## DESCRIPTION

Respiratory Acidosis

- Reduced pH owing to alveolar hypoventilation with elevated $PaCO_2$
- Defined as $PaCO_2$ >45 mm Hg or higher than expected for calculated respiratory compensation for metabolic acidosis
- Divided into 3 broad categories:
  - Primary failure in CNS drive to ventilate:
    ○ Sleep apnea
    ○ Anesthesia
    ○ Sedative overdose
  - Primary failure in transport of $CO_2$ from alveolar space:
    ○ COPD
    ○ Myasthenic crisis
    ○ Severe hypokalemia
    ○ Guillain-Barré syndrome
  - Primary failure in transport of $CO_2$ from tissue to alveoli:
    ○ Severe heart failure/pulmonary edema

Metabolic Acidosis

- Process that reduces serum pH by decreasing plasma bicarbonate levels
- Primarily caused by:
  - Accumulation of a strong acid through ingestion or metabolism
  - Loss of bicarbonate from the body
- Metabolic acidosis is clinically evaluated by dividing into 2 main groups:
  - Elevated anion gap metabolic acidosis:
    ○ Bicarbonate reduced through buffering of added strong acid
    ○ Anion gap is increased owing to retention of the unmeasured anion from the titrated strong acid.
  - Normal anion gap metabolic acidosis owing to:
    ○ Kidneys fail to reabsorb or regenerate bicarbonate.
    ○ Losses of bicarbonate from GI tract (diarrhea)
    ○ Ingestion or infusion of substances that release hydrochloric acid
  - No anion gap is observed owing to the absence of any unmeasured anion of a titrated acid and secondary chloride retention with $HCO_3^-$ loss.

## ETIOLOGY

- Respiratory acidosis:
  - Inhibition of respiratory center:
    ○ Cardiac arrest
    ○ Drugs (opiates, benzodiazepines, etc)
    ○ Meningitis/encephalitis
    ○ CNS lesions (mass, CVA)
  - Impaired gas exchange:
    ○ Pulmonary edema
    ○ Asthma/COPD
    ○ Pneumonia
    ○ Interstitial lung disease
    ○ Obesity
    ○ Pulmonary contusion
  - Neuromuscular disease:
    ○ Diaphragmatic paralysis
    ○ Guillain-Barré syndrome
    ○ Myasthenia gravis
    ○ Muscular dystrophy
    ○ Spinal cord injury
    ○ Hypokalemia/hypophosphatemia
    ○ MS
  - Obstructive:
    ○ Congenital lesions (laryngomalacia)
    ○ Foreign body aspiration
    ○ Vascular ring
    ○ Infectious (epiglottitis, croup, abscess)
- Anion gap acidosis: Mnemonic *A CAT PILES MUD*:
  - Alcohol ketoacidosis
  - Carbon monoxide or cyanide
  - Aspirin
  - Toluene
  - Paraldehyde
  - Iron/isoniazid
  - Lactic acidosis
  - Ethylene glycol
  - Starvation
  - Methanol
  - Uremia
  - Diabetic ketoacidosis
- Increased osmolar gap: Mnemonic *ME DIE*:
  - Methanol
  - Ethylene glycol
  - Diuretics (mannitol; no acidosis)
  - Isopropyl alcohol (no acidosis)
  - Ethanol
- Nonanion gap metabolic acidosis:
  - GI losses of bicarbonate:
    ○ Diarrhea
    ○ Villous adenoma
    ○ Removal of small bowel, pancreatic or biliary secretions
    ○ Tube drainage
    ○ Small bowel/pancreatic fistula
  - Anion exchange resins (ie, cholestyramine)
  - Ingestion of calcium chloride or magnesium chloride

- Type I renal tubular acidosis (distal): Hypokalemic hyperchloremic metabolic acidosis:
  ○ Decreased ability to secrete hydrogen
  ○ Serum $HCO_3$ <15 mEq/L when untreated
  ○ Potassium low
  ○ Renal stones common
- Type II renal tubular acidosis (proximal): Hypokalemic hyperchloremic metabolic acidosis:
  ○ Decreased proximal reabsorption of $HCO_3^-$
  ○ Acidosis limited by reabsorptive capacity of proximal tubule for $HCO_3^-$
  ○ Serum $HCO_3$ typically 14–18 mEq/L
  ○ Low/normal potassium
- Type IV renal tubular acidosis (hypoaldosteronism): Hyperkalemic hyperchloremic acidosis:
  ○ Aldosterone deficiency or resistance causing decreased $H^+$ secretion
  ○ Serum bicarb >15 mEq/L
  ○ Normal/elevated potassium
- Carbonic anhydrase inhibitors
- Tubulointerstitial renal disease
- Hypoaldosteronism
- Addition of hydrochloric acid such as:
  ○ Ammonium chloride
  ○ Arginine hydrogen chloride
  ○ Lysine hydrogen chloride

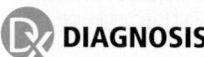 **DIAGNOSIS**

## SIGNS AND SYMPTOMS

- Nonspecific findings
- Vital signs:
  - Tachypnea or Kussmaul respirations with metabolic acidosis
  - Hypoventilation with respiratory acidosis
  - Tachycardia
- Somnolence
- Confusion
- Altered mental status ($CO_2$ narcosis)
- Myocardial conduction and contraction disturbances

## ESSENTIAL WORKUP

- Electrolytes, BUN, creatinine, and glucose:
  - Decreased bicarbonate with metabolic acidosis
  - Hyperkalemia and hypercalcemia with severe metabolic acidosis
- Arterial blood gases:
  - pH
  - $CO_2$ retention in respiratory acidosis
  - CO level

Check the degree of compensation by calculating the expected values and comparing them to the observed laboratory values as follows:

- Respiratory acidosis:
  - Acute: Expected $HCO_3^-$ increased by 1 mEq/L for every 10 mm Hg increase in $PaCO_2$
  - Chronic: Expected $HCO_3^-$ increased by 4 mEq/L for every 10 mm Hg increase in $PaCO_2$

- Calculate anion gap: $Na^+ - (HCO_3^- + Cl^-)$:
  - Correct anion gap for hypoalbuminemia:
    - For every 1 g/dL decrease in albumin (from 4.0 g/dL), add 2.5 points to calculated anion gap.
  - Do not correct sodium concentration when calculating the anion gap in the setting of marked hyperglycemia because hyperglycemia affects the concentration of chloride and bicarbonate, as well as sodium.
  - Normal range = $5$–$12 \pm 3$ mEq/L
  - Anion gap >25 mEq/L is seen only with:
    - Lactic acidosis
    - Ketoacidosis
    - Toxin-associated acidosis
- Calculate the degree of compensation:
  - Expected $PaCO_2 = 1.5[HCO_3^-] + 8$
  - If $PaCO_2$ inappropriately high, patient has a concomitant respiratory acidosis and/or inadequate compensation.
- Evaluate the delta gap:
  - For every 1-point increase in anion gap, $HCO_3^-$ should decrease by 1 mEq/L in simple acid–base disorder.
- Evaluate by comparing the change in the anion gap ($\Delta AG$) with the change in the $HCO_3^-$ ($\Delta HCO_3^-$) from normal:
  - If $\Delta AG > \Delta HCO_3^-$, then patient has a concomitant metabolic alkalosis.
  - If $\Delta HCO_3^- > \Delta AG$, then patient has concomitant nonanion gap acidosis.

### DIAGNOSTIC TESTS & INTERPRETATION
#### Lab
- ABG: See interpretation above.
- VBG:
  - Obvious benefit is less patient discomfort and ease in acquiring sample
  - pH varies by <0.04 units when compared to arterial sampling.
  - Correlation between venous $pCO_2$ lacking
  - Useful in simple acid–base disorders
- Urinalysis for glucose and ketones
- Measure serum osmolality:
  - Calculated serum osmolality = 2 Na + glucose/18 + BUN/2.8
- Osmolal gap = difference between calculated and measured osmolality:
  - Normal = <10
  - Elevated osmolar gap may indicate toxic alcohol as etiology of acidosis.
  - Absence of an osmolar gap should never be used to rule out toxic ingestions:
    - Osmolar gap imprecisely defined
    - Delayed presentations may have normal gap
    - Large variance in gap among normal patients
- Toxicology screen:
  - Methanol, ethylene glycol, ethanol, and isopropyl alcohol if increased osmolality gap
  - Aspirin or iron levels for suspected ingestion
- Co-oximetry for CO exposure
- Serum ketones or $\beta$-hydroxybutyrate level
- Serum lactate

#### Imaging
CXR:
- May identify cardiomyopathy or CHF
- Underlying pneumonia

#### Diagnostic Procedures/Surgery
ECG:
- May identify regional wall motion abnormalities or valvular dysfunction
- Evaluate for conduction disturbances

### DIFFERENTIAL DIAGNOSIS
- Anion gap acidosis:
  - Mnemonic *A CATPILES MUD*
- Increased osmolar gap:
  - Mnemonic *ME DIE*

 **TREATMENT**

### INITIAL STABILIZATION/THERAPY
Airway, breathing, and circulation (ABCs):
- Early intubation for severe metabolic acidosis with progressive/potential weakening of respiratory compensation
- Naloxone, $D_{50}W$ (or Accu-Chek), and thiamine if mental status altered

### ED TREATMENT/PROCEDURES
- Respiratory acidosis:
  - Treat underlying disorder.
  - Provide ventilatory support for worsening hypercapnia.
  - Identify and correct aggravating factors (pneumonia) in chronic hypercapnia.
- Metabolic acidosis:
  - Identify if concurrent osmolal gap.
  - Treat underlying disorder:
    - Diabetic ketoacidosis
    - Lactic acidosis
    - Alcohol ketoacidosis
    - Ingestion
  - Correct electrolyte abnormalities.
- IV Fluids:
  - Rehydrate with 0.9% normal saline if patient hypovolemic.
  - Consider hemodialysis

### MEDICATION
- Dextrose: $D_{50}W$ 1 amp (50 mL or 25 g); (peds: $D_{25}W$ 4 mL/kg) IV
- Naloxone (Narcan): 2 mg (peds: 0.1 mg/kg) IV or IM initial dose
- Thiamine (vitamin $B_1$): 100 mg (peds: 50 mg) IV or IM

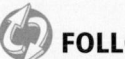 **FOLLOW-UP**

### DISPOSITION
#### Admission Criteria
Consider ICU admission if:
- pH <7.1 or if altered mental status
- Respiratory acidosis
- Hemodynamic instability
- Dysrhythmias
- Electrolyte abnormalities

#### Discharge Criteria
Resolving or resolved anion gap metabolic acidosis

## PEARLS AND PITFALLS
- Failure to appreciate acidosis in mixed acid–base disorders
- Failure to appreciate inadequate respiratory compensation for metabolic acidosis and need for ventilatory support
- Clues to the presence of a mixed acid–base disorder are normal pH with abnormal $PCO_2$ or $HCO_3^-$, when the $HCO_3^-$ and $PCO_2$ move in opposite directions, or when the pH changes in the direction opposite that expected from a known primary disorder.

## ADDITIONAL READING
- Kellum JA. Clinical Review: Reunification of acid-base physiology. *Crit Care.* 2005;9(5): 500–507.
- Kellum JA. Determinants of plasma acid-base balance. *Crit Care Clin.* 2005;21(2):329–346.
- Laski ME, Kurtzman NA. Acid base disorders in medicine. *Dis Mon.* 1996;42(2):51–125.
- Swenson ER. Metabolic acidosis. *Respir Care.* 2001;46:342.
- Whittier WL, Rutecki GW. Primer on clinical acid-base problem solving. *Dis Mon.* 2004;50:122.

**See Also (Topic, Algorithm, Electronic Media Element)**
Alkalosis

# ACROMIOCLAVICULAR JOINT INJURY

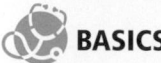

Aleksandr M. Tichter
Wallace A. Carter

 **BASICS**

## DESCRIPTION
- The acromioclavicular (AC) joint is formed by the articulation of the distal clavicle and the scapular acromion.
- It is stabilized by the acromioclavicular (AC) ligament, coracoclavicular (CC) ligament, and attachments from deltoid and trapezius muscles.

## ETIOLOGY
- Injury most commonly seen in young, active males
- Injury often occurs in contact sports
- Most common mechanism is direct trauma to superior or lateral shoulder while arm is adducted
- May also occur indirectly via a fall on an outstretched hand or elbow, with transmission of force to the AC joint

## DIAGNOSIS

### SIGNS AND SYMPTOMS
- Diagnosis of AC joint injury is made clinically.
- Pain to anterior or superior aspect of the shoulder
- Pain exacerbated by moving arm across the chest, behind the back, or overhead
- Rockwood Classification (sequential injury pattern):
  - Type 1:
    - Sprained AC ligament (AC joint tender)
    - No CC ligament injury
    - No deltoid or trapezius injury
    - No radiographic abnormality
  - Type 2:
    - Ruptured AC ligament (AC joint tender)
    - Sprained CC ligament (CC ligament tender)
    - Minimal deltoid and trapezius injury
    - Radiographs show slight widening of AC joint (normal <5 mm).
    - Normal coracoclavicular space (11–13 mm)
  - Type 3:
    - Ruptured AC ligament (AC joint tender)
    - Ruptured CC ligament (CC ligament tender)
    - Detached deltoid and trapezius
    - Radiographs show widening of AC joint.
    - Increased CC space, with distal clavicle above superior aspect of acromion (100% displaced)

- Types 4, 5, and 6:
  - Cause more significant pain then types 1, 2, and 3
  - Best visualized on lateral/axillary radiographs
  - All require operative treatment.
  - Greater risk for prolonged disability
- Type 4:
  - Identical ligamentous/muscular injury pattern to type 3
  - Clavicle is displaced *posteriorly* into trapezius muscle.
  - Posteriorly displaced clavicle may be palpable on exam.
  - May cause tenting of skin posteriorly
- Type 5:
  - Rare
  - Identical ligamentous/muscular injury pattern to type 3
  - Clavicle is displaced *superiorly* above the trapezius (100–300% increase in CC space).
  - Shoulder droops severely.
  - Clavicle may be palpated subcutaneously.
  - May cause tenting, ischemia, or disruption of skin
- Type 6:
  - Usually associated with severe trauma
  - Identical ligamentous/muscular injury pattern to type 3
  - Clavicle is displaced *inferiorly* into subacromial or subcoracoid location.
  - Shoulder appears flattened.
  - Associated neurovascular injury is common.

### Pediatric Considerations
- AC joint injury rarely occurs in isolation in the pediatric population.
- Pediatric clavicle encased in periosteal tube:
  - Coracoclavicular ligament within tube
  - Acromioclavicular ligament external to tube (more vulnerable)
- When injury does occur, usually is type 1, 2, or 3.
- Distal clavicular fractures are more common than AC joint dislocations in children.

### History
- Mechanism/force (will dictate injury pattern)
- Cervical spine symptoms
- Associated neurovascular symptoms

### Physical Exam
- Exam in standing or sitting position as supine position can mask joint instability.
- Sequential palpation of sternoclavicular joint, length of clavicle, AC joint, CC ligament, coracoid process, scapular spine, and proximal humerus
- Careful cervical spine exam for radiculopathy or referred pain
- Cross-body adduction test:
  - Pain caused when arm adducted 90 degrees and elbow flexed 90 degrees is brought across patient's body
  - Can confirm AC injury by specifically compressing the joint
- Complete distal neurovascular exam

### ESSENTIAL WORKUP
- History to seek mechanisms that commonly cause AC joint injury and associated force
- Physical exam to exclude other causes of pain
- Radiographic evaluation as outlined below

### DIAGNOSTIC TESTS & INTERPRETATION
#### Imaging
- Specific AC joint radiograph:
  - Recommended if AC injury suspected
  - Should include bilateral AC joints (for comparison)
  - Standard shoulder views will over penetrate AC joint and may obscure subtle injuries.
  - Stress views no longer recommended
  - Zanca view (10–15 degree cephalic tilt) for limited initial views
  - Axillary view for type III–VI injuries to determine position of distal clavicle
- US may be used to exclude AC joint inflammation.
- CT can be useful (especially in trauma cases) to evaluate bony abnormalities and fractures.
- MRI is very effective for evaluating soft tissue injuries:
  - MR angiography (MRA) may be used to evaluate associated vascular injuries.

### DIFFERENTIAL DIAGNOSIS
- Shoulder dislocation
- Osteoarthritis
- Osteomyelitis
- Fractures of acromion or clavicle
- Rotator cuff injury
- Tendinitis
- Capsulitis
- Cervical radiculopathy

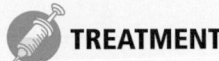 **TREATMENT**

### PRE-HOSPITAL
- Ice packs
- Sling immobilization
- Cervical spine immobilization if indicated

### INITIAL STABILIZATION/THERAPY
- Ice packs
- Sling immobilization
- Cervical spine immobilization if indicated
- Analgesia (NSAIDs, other analgesics)

### ED TREATMENT/PROCEDURES
- Types 1 and 2:
  - Rest, ice, analgesics
  - Brief sling immobilization (typically 3–7 days)
  - Range of motion (ROM) and strengthening exercises as soon as can be tolerated
  - Resume normal activities once ROM and strength have returned (2–4 wk).
- Type 3:
  - Rest, ice, analgesics
  - Sling immobilization and early (within 72 hr) orthopedic referral
  - Treatment plan is controversial.
  - Best available data demonstrate similar functional outcome for conservative vs. surgical management.
  - Which approach is chosen may depend on general health of patient, level of activity, occupation, hand dominance, and risk for re-injury.
- Types 4, 5, and 6:
  - Rest, ice, analgesics
  - Sling immobilization and immediate orthopedic referral
  - Require early surgical intervention
- Special circumstance: Potential future complication of AC joint injury is arthritis of the joint.
- Presents as impingement syndrome, which causes pain at extremes of abduction

### Pediatric Considerations
- Types 1 and 2:
  - Conservative management (rest, ice, analgesics, sling)
  - Should heal without major sequelae
- Type 3:
  - Age <15 yr, conservative management
  - Age ≥15 yr may require more aggressive treatment.
- Types 4, 5, and 6:
  - Operative repair

### MEDICATION
- Ibuprofen: 600 mg (peds: 4–10 mg/kg) PO q.i.d.
- Ketorolac: 30 mg (peds: 0.5 mg/kg up to 30 mg if >6 mo) IM/IV q6h (15 mg IM/IV q6h if >65 yr or <50 kg)

 **FOLLOW-UP**

### DISPOSITION
#### Admission Criteria
- Open injury
- Types 4, 5, and 6 require admission for operative repair.

#### Discharge Criteria
- Types 1 and 2 can be discharged with orthopedic referral.
- Type 3 should have urgent orthopedic referral.

### FOLLOW-UP RECOMMENDATIONS
- Type I & II: Orthopedic follow-up within 2–4 wk
- Type III: Early (within 72 hr) orthopedic follow-up
- Type IV–VI: Immediate orthopedic referral
- All pediatric injuries should have prompt orthopedic follow-up, with type IV–VI injuries requiring immediate referral

## PEARLS AND PITFALLS
- Type I & II AC injuries:
  - No increase in CC space
  - Conservative management with rest, ice, sling, and ROM/strength exercises
- Type III injuries:
  - 100% superior displacement of distal clavicle
  - Management somewhat controversial
  - Data advocate for initial conservative management with early orthopedic follow-up.
- Type IV–VI injuries:
  - Identical ligamentous and muscular injuries to Type III
  - Difference according to position of distal clavicle
  - Operative management is standard of care.

## ADDITIONAL READING
- Bossart PJ, Joyce SM, et al. Lack of efficacy of weighted radiographs in diagnosing acute acromioclavicular separation. *Ann Emerg Med.* 1988;17:47–51.
- Dumonski M, Mazzocca AD, Rios C, et al. Evaluation and management of acromioclavicular joint injuries. *Am J Orthop.* 2004;33(10):526–532.
- Mazzocca AD, Arciero RA, Bicos J. Evaluation and treatment of acromioclavicular joint injuries. *Am J Sports Med.* 2007;35(2):316–329.
- Simovitch R, Sanders B, Ozbaydar M, et al. Acromioclavicular joint injuries: Diagnosis and Management. *J Am Acad Ortho Surg.* 2009;17:207–219.
- Skinner HB. Acromioclavicular injury. In: *Current diagnosis and treatment in orthopedics,* 4th ed. [online]. 2006.
- Spencer EE. Treatment of grade III acromioclavicular joint injuries: A systematic review. *Clin Orthop Relat Res.* 2006;445:38–44.

### See Also (Topic, Algorithm, Electronic Media Element)
- Clavicle Fracture
- Shoulder Dislocation
- Sternoclavicular Joint Injury

 **CODES**

### ICD9
- 810.03 Closed fracture of acromial end of clavicle
- 840.0 Acromioclavicular (joint) (ligament) sprain

# ACUTE CORONARY SYNDROME: CORONARY VASOSPASM

Shamai A. Grossman
Benjamin Z. Galper

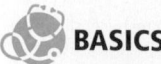 BASICS

## DESCRIPTION

- Spontaneous episodes of chest pain due to coronary artery vasospasm in absence of increase in myocardial oxygen demand in either normal or diseased coronary vessels
- Also known as Prinzmetal angina or variant angina
- Most common in younger patients and men
- Occurs in patients without other cardiac risk factors
- Risk factors:
  - Smoking
  - Hyperinsulinemia
  - Insulin resistance
  - Cocaine use
- Associated with minimal coronary artery disease

## ETIOLOGY

- Abnormal vasodilator function in coronary arteries
- Focal coronary artery vasospasm often adjacent to or at the site of fixed stenoses
- Unopposed alpha sympathetic stimulation
- Sympathetic stimulation by endogenous hormones may cause vasoconstriction.
- Hypersensitivity of coronary arteries due to mediators of vasoconstriction
- Endothelial dysfunction possibly from genetic mutations in nitric oxide synthase
- May or may not be associated with a fixed coronary lesion

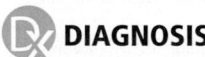 DIAGNOSIS

## SIGNS AND SYMPTOMS

- Chest pain:
  - Retrosternal
  - Radiates to neck, jaw, left shoulder, or arm
  - Occurs at rest
- Palpitations
- Presyncope or syncope
- Associated with migraine headaches and Raynaud disease in a minority of patients
- May occur during cold weather or stress
- May be prolonged in duration compared to typical angina
- May be elicited by hyperventilation
- May be relieved by exercise
- Circadian pattern, most commonly in early morning

## History

May mimic angina, but ask about association with cold weather or stress and relief with exercise.

## Physical Exam

Physical examination is nondiagnostic.

## ESSENTIAL WORKUP

- Must include an ECG
- Use of other tests depends on history.

## DIAGNOSTIC TESTS & INTERPRETATION

- ECG:
  - Transient ST-segment elevation is characteristic
  - May be followed by ST depression or T-wave inversion
  - May have associated dysrhythmia during coronary spasm
  - Heart block with right coronary artery spasm
  - Ventricular tachycardia with LAD spasm
  - In rare cases can present with sudden death during prolonged vasospasm period

## Lab

- CK-MB and troponin I or T
- Toxicology screen:
  - Helpful if cocaine is suspected as etiology of chest pain

## Imaging

- CXR:
  - May be helpful to rule out other etiologies such as pneumonia, pneumothorax, or aortic dissection
- Thallium scintigraphy may be useful to localize area of spasm.

## Diagnostic Procedures/Surgery

- Exercise stress testing:
  - Helpful only if there are underlying fixed stenoses
- Coronary angiography:
  - Mild atherosclerosis is often the norm.
  - Provocative test with ergonovine, acetylcholine, or hyperventilation will induce coronary spasm.

## DIFFERENTIAL DIAGNOSIS

- Angina pectoris
- Anxiety and panic disorders
- Aortic dissection
- Esophageal rupture
- Esophageal spasm
- Esophagitis
- GERD
- Mitral valve prolapse
- Musculoskeletal chest pain
- MI
- Peptic ulcer disease
- Pericarditis
- Pneumothorax
- Pulmonary embolism

 TREATMENT

## PRE-HOSPITAL

Treat as any other acute coronary syndrome.

## INITIAL STABILIZATION/THERAPY

- IV access
- Oxygen
- Cardiac monitoring
- Vital signs and oxygen saturation

## ED TREATMENT/PROCEDURES

- All patients with chest pain in which cardiac ischemia is a consideration should receive an aspirin upon arrival to the ED:
  - Possibility of actually increasing severity of episodes in Prinzmetal angina due to inhibiting biosynthesis of naturally-occurring coronary vasodilator prostacyclin
- Nitroglycerin should then be administered and is appropriate to help relieve both ischemic and vasospastic chest pain.
- A trial of calcium channel blockers is indicated if clinical history is consistent with coronary vasospasm.
- Heparin and β-blockers are not helpful:
  - β-blockers may actually be detrimental due to unopposed α-mediated vasoconstriction.

## MEDICATION
- Aspirin: 325 mg PO
- Diltiazem: 30–60 mg PO
- Nitroglycerin, either:
  - 0.4 mg sublingual
  - 10–20 mcg/min IV, titrating to effect
  - 1–2 in of nitro paste
- Verapamil: 40–80 mg PO

### First Line
Diltiazem/verapamil:
- >40% of patients will have recurrence of vasospastic angina despite calcium-channel blocker therapy

### Second Line
- α-blocking agents
- Fluvastatin in studies in conjunction with calcium channel blockers reduced recurrence
- Percutaneous intervention with stenting of fixed lesions in area of vasospasm controversial; can lead to spasm in other areas of coronary tree
- Pacemaker placement for patients with recurrent syncope or AV nodal block from vasospastic angina

 FOLLOW-UP

## DISPOSITION
### Admission Criteria
- New-onset chest pain
- Rest chest pain (by definition most patients with coronary vasospasm)
- Accelerated chest symptoms

### Discharge Criteria
Stable (chronic chest pain)

## FOLLOW-UP RECOMMENDATIONS
Usually will need periodic cardiology follow up

## PEARLS AND PITFALLS
- 95% survival at 5 yr
- Patients typically without traditional coronary risk factors other than smoking.
- Calcium channel blockers are 1st-line therapy.
- 40% of patients will have recurrent vasospastic angina.
- β-blockers can lead to worsening of vasospasm due to unopposed alpha vasoconstriction.
- Patients with prolonged vasospasm can present with ST elevation MI, ventricular arrhythmias, and sudden death.

## ADDITIONAL READING
- Crea F, Kaski JC, Maseri A. Key references on coronary artery spasm. *Circulation*. 1994;89: 2442–2446.
- Harding MB, Leithe ME, Mark DB. Ergonovine maleate testing during cardiac catheterization: A 10-year perspective in 3,447 patients without significant coronary artery disease or Prinzmetal's variant angina. *J Am Coll Cardiol*. 1992;20: 107–111.
- Lanza GA, Sestito A, Sgueglia GA. Current clinical features, diagnostic assessment and prognostic determinants of patients with variant angina. *Int J Cardiol*. 2006;118:41–47.

- Ogawa T, Komukai K, Ogawa K. High incidence of repeat anginal attacks despite treatment with calcium-channel blockers in patients with coronary spastic angina. *Circ J*. 2009;73(3):512–515. Epub 2009 Feb 3.
- Prinzmetal M, Kennamer R, Merliss R. A variant form of angina pectoris. *Am J Med*. 1959;27:375–388.
- Stern S, Bayes de Luna A. Coronary artery spasm: A 2009 update. *Circulation*. 2009;119(18): 2531–2534.
- Tani S, Nagao K, Anazawa T. Treatment of coronary spastic angina with a statin in addition to a calcium channel blocker: A pilot study. *J Cardiovasc Pharmacol*. 2008;52(1):28–34.

### See Also (Topic, Algorithm, Electronic Media Element)
ACS Unstable Angina, ACS Myocardial Infarction

# ACUTE CORONARY SYNDROME: DRUG-INDUCED

Shamai A. Grossman
Michael A. Fogel

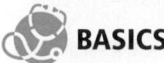 **BASICS**

## DESCRIPTION
Imbalance in myocardial blood supply and oxygen requirement

## ETIOLOGY
- Sympathomimetics are associated with myocardial oxygen mismatch due to induced vasoconstriction:
  - Cocaine
  - Cocaethylene is a toxic compound formed by hepatic transesterification of alcohol and cocaine further exacerbates the sympathomimetic effects of cocaine.
  - Amphetamines (crank)
  - Ephedrine (dietary supplement), pseudoephedrine (decongestant)
  - Ma huang (herbal diet supplement)
  - Dipivefrin (glaucoma eye drop)
  - Phenylpropanolamine (nasal decongestant)
  - Epinephrine
  - Methylene 3,4 dioxymethamphetamine (ecstasy)
- Cocaine-induced chest pain also caused by:
  - Increased myocardial workload
  - Accelerated atherosclerosis
  - Activation of platelets and promotion of thrombosis
- Antimigraine therapy—sumatriptan, methysergide, ergotamine, and isometheptene:
  - Vasoconstrictors
  - Particularly with cardiac risk factors or known coronary disease
- Calcium channel blockers—nifedipine:
  - Reflex tachycardia and vasoconstriction
- β-blockers (metoprolol and propranolol):
  - α-adrenergic mediated coronary vasospasm
- Carbon monoxide found with gas heaters, smoke inhalation, furniture stripping with methylene chloride:
  - Decreasing oxygen-carrying capacity
  - Shifting the oxyhemoglobin dissociation curve to the left
  - Binding to myoglobin
- Bromocriptine:
  - Vasoconstrictor
  - Used for acromegaly, Parkinson disease, hyperprolactinemia, amenorrhea/galactorrhea, lactation cessation
  - Risk increased by predisposing conditions:
    ○ Pregnancy-induced HTN
    ○ Other vasospastic conditions (Raynaud disease or migraine headaches)
- Other dopaminergic agents (dopamine):
  - Vasoconstriction and vasospasm

- Sildenafil:
  - Vasodilatory properties
  - Transient decreases in supine BP
  - Increase the risk of cardiac event during sexual activity
- Oral contraceptives:
  - Prothrombotic
  - Higher incidence of MI in young women with concomitant smoking
- Allergic reactions (Kounis syndrome):
  - Presumed secondary to inflammatory mediators and histamine leading to vasospasm, plaque rupture, or thrombus
  - Obtain ECG in all allergic reactions
  - Treat allergic reaction and ACS, caution with epinephrine
- Other agents in case-reports: Sorafenib (chemotherapeutic), Prostaglandin E, Paclitaxel, cannabis, Venlafaxine, Sibutramine (amphetamine-like), capecitabine (carrier for 5-FU)

 **DIAGNOSIS**

## SIGNS AND SYMPTOMS
- Chest pain
- Substernal pressure
- Heaviness
- Squeezing
- Burning sensation
- Tightness
- Sympathomimetic toxidrome symptoms:
  - Agitation
  - Tremulousness
  - Tachypnea
  - Tachycardia
  - HTN
  - Hyperthermia
  - Moist skin
  - No urine retention

### History
- Recent ingestion of medication/drug that induces coronary vasospasm
- Cardiac risk factors or known cardiac disease

### Physical Exam
- Physical exam is usually unrevealing
- BP is usually elevated during symptoms

## ESSENTIAL WORKUP
History is critical in diagnosing and differentiating drug-induced and unusual causes of acute coronary syndromes.

## DIAGNOSTIC TESTS & INTERPRETATION
- ECG:
  - Normal ~50% of the time
  - Compare to prior tracings
  - New ST-segment changes or T-wave inversions
  - 1-mm depression of the ST-segment below the baseline
  - 80 ms from the J point
  - Helpful in diagnosing other etiologies
- ECG in carbon monoxide poisoning:
  - Premature ventricular contractions
  - Dysrhythmias
  - Tachycardia
  - Nonspecific ST-T wave abnormalities
  - Acute MI: ST elevation or depression

### Lab
- Serial cardiac enzymes
- Troponin may be more helpful.
- Creatine kinase may be elevated in cocaine-induced rhabdomyolysis.
- Carboxyhemoglobin level for suspected carbon monoxide (CO) toxicity
- Serum toxicology screening

### Imaging
- CXR:
  - Usually normal
  - May show cardiomegaly
  - CHF
  - May identify other etiologies of chest pain such as pneumonia
- Exercise stress testing: Can identify underlying atherosclerosis
- Technetium Tc-99m perfusion scan can identify myocardial damage/MI
- ECG: May identify wall motion abnormalities

### Diagnostic Procedures/Surgery
- Gold standard: Cardiac catheterization
- Most patients will have angiographically normal coronary arteries.

## DIFFERENTIAL DIAGNOSIS
- Anxiety
- Aortic dissection
- Biliary colic
- Costochondritis
- Esophageal reflux
- Esophageal spasm
- Herpes zoster
- Hiatal hernia

- Mitral valve prolapse
- MI
- Panic disorder
- Peptic ulcer disease
- Pneumonia
- Psychogenic
- Pulmonary embolus
- Unstable angina

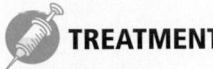 TREATMENT

### PRE-HOSPITAL
- Remove patient from contaminated environment if carbon monoxide toxicity is a consideration.
- IV access
- Oxygen
- Cardiac monitoring
- Sublingual nitroglycerin for symptom relief

### ALERT
- All chest pain should be treated and transported as a possible life-threatening emergency.
- Avoid $\beta$-adrenergic antagonists in cases of suspected cocaine use.

### INITIAL STABILIZATION/THERAPY
- Place patient on a monitor.
- IV access should be obtained.
- $O_2$: 100% oxygen
- Nitrates

### ED TREATMENT/PROCEDURES
- Aspirin
- $\beta$-adrenergic blockers should be avoided in patients who are suspected to have used cocaine.
- Benzodiazepines: 1st line for cocaine use
- Nitrates or phentolamine. 2nd line after cocaine use
- Goal to reduce BP and heart rate
- Decreasing myocardial oxygen demand
- Heparin or enoxaparin
- Thrombolytics: Use with caution in suspected vasospasm induced acute coronary syndrome
- Cardiac catheterization: Diagnostic or therapeutic
- Carbon monoxide toxicity:
  - 100% $O_2$
  - Hyperbarics if:
    - Carboxyhemoglobin level is >25–40%.
    - Any period of coma
    - Neurologic deficits
    - Persistent metabolic acidosis
    - Pregnant and carboxyhemoglobin level is >15%.
    - Cardiac instability
    - Acute MI, unless hemodynamically unstable
  - Half-life of carboxyhemoglobin:
    - Room air: 300 min
    - 100% $O_2$: 90 min
    - Hyperbaric chamber at 3 ATM: 20 min

### MEDICATION
- Aspirin: 160–325 mg PO
- Enoxaparin (Lovenox): 1 mg/kg SC q12h
- Heparin: 80 U/kg IV bolus, then 18 U/kg/hr
- Labetalol: 20 mg IV or 100 mg PO
- Lorazepam: 1–2 mg IV
- Phentolamine: 1 mg IV, q5min
- Metoprolol: 5 mg IV q5min–q15min followed by 25–50 mg PO starting dose as tolerated (note: $\beta$-blockers contraindicated in cocaine chest pain)
- Morphine: 2 mg IV, may titrate upward in 2-mg increments for relief of pain assuming no respiratory deterioration and SBP >90 mm Hg
- Nitroglycerin: 0.4 mg sublingual
- Nitroglycerin: IV drip at 5–10 $\mu$g/min
- Nitropaste: 1–2 in transdermal
- Tenecteplase: For 60-kg person, 30 mg; >60–69 kg, 35 mg; 70–79 kg, 40 mg; 80–89 kg, 45 mg, ≥90 kg, 50 mg given IV; or Reteplase, 10 U IV over 2 min, repeat in 30 min

 FOLLOW-UP

### DISPOSITION
#### Admission Criteria
- Similar to patients with acute coronary syndromes of atherosclerotic origin
- New-onset chest pain
- Rest chest pain
- Accelerated chest pain symptoms

#### Discharge Criteria
Chronic stable chest pain

### FOLLOW-UP RECOMMENDATIONS
- Risks of further drug use should be explained to the patient and family
- Referral if possible to a drug treatment program

## PEARLS AND PITFALLS

Thrombolytics and $\beta$-adrenergic blockers should be used with caution if drug induced cardiac ischemic is suspected.

## ADDITIONAL READING

- Honderick et al. A prospective, randomized, controlled trial of benzodiazepines and nitroglycerine or nitroglycerine alone in the treatment of cocaine-associated acute coronary syndromes. *Am J Emerg Med*. 2003;21(1):39–42.
- Lai TI, Hwang JJ, Fang CC, et al. Methylene 3,4 dioxymethamphetamine-induced acute myocardial infarction. *Ann Emerg Med*. 2003;42(6):759–762.
- Lange RA, Hillis LD. Cardiovascular complications of cocaine use. *N Engl J Med*. 2001;345:351–358.
- Manini AF, Kabrhel C, Thomsen Acute myocardial infarction after over-the-counter use of pseudoephedrine. *Ann Emerg Med*. 2005;45(2): 213–218.
- Marius-Nunez AL. Myocardial infarction with normal coronary arteries after acute exposure to carbon monoxide. *Chest*. 1990;97:491–494.
- McCord et al. Management of cocaine-associated chest pain and myocardial infarction: A scientific statement from the American Heart Association Acute Cardiac Care Committee of the Council on Clinical Cardiology. *Circulation*. 2008;117(14): 1897–907.
- Ottervanger JP, Wilson JH, Stricker BH. Drug-induced chest pain and MI. Reports to a national center and review of the literature. *Eur J Clin Pharmacol*. 1997;53:105–110.
- Qasim A, Townend J, Davies MK. Esctasy induced myocardial infarction. *Heart*. 2001;85(6):E10.
- Ridella et al. Kounis syndrome following beta-lactam antibiotic use: Review of literature. *Inflamm Allergy Drug Targets*. 2009;8(1):11–6.
- Tanis BC, van den Bosch MA, Kemmeren JM, et al. Oral contraceptives and the risk of myocardial infarction. *N Engl J Med*. 2001;345:187–1793.
- Wasson S, Jayam VK. Coronary vasospasm and myocardial infarction induced by oral sumatriptan. *Clin Neuropharmacol*. 2004;27(4):198–200.

# ACUTE CORONARY SYNDROME: MYOCARDIAL INFARCTION

Shamai A. Grossman
Ethan M. Ross

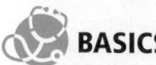 **BASICS**

## DESCRIPTION
- Imbalance in myocardial blood supply and oxygen requirement
- Acute cardiac ischemia encompasses a spectrum of disease processes:
  - Unstable angina pectoris
  - Acute myocardial infarction (AMI)
  - ST elevation myocardial infarction (STEMI)
  - Non-STEMI

## ETIOLOGY
- Atherosclerotic narrowing of coronary vessels
- Vasospasm (Prinzmetal or variant angina)—although this is usually at rest and considered unstable if new onset
- Microvascular angina or abnormal relaxation of vessels with diffuse vascular disease
- Plaque disruption
- Thrombosis
- Arteritis:
  - Lupus
  - Takayasu disease
  - Kawasaki disease
  - Rheumatoid arthritis
- Prolonged hypotension
- Anemia/stress ischemia:
  - Hemoglobin <8 g/dL
- Elevations in carboxyhemoglobin
- Coronary artery gas embolus
- Thyroid storm
- Structural abnormalities of coronary arteries:
  - Radiation fibrosis
  - Aneurysms
  - Ectasia
- Cocaine- or amphetamine-induced vasospasm
- Cardiac risk factors include:
  - Hypercholesterolemia
  - DM
  - HTN
  - Smoking
  - Family history in a 1st-degree relative less than 55 yr old
  - Men, age >55 yr
  - Postmenopausal women

## DIAGNOSIS

### SIGNS AND SYMPTOMS
- Chest pain:
  - Most common presentation of MI
  - Substernal pressure
  - Heaviness
  - Squeezing
  - Burning sensation
  - Tightness
- Anginal equivalents (MI without chest pain):
  - Abdominal pain
  - Syncope
  - Diaphoresis
  - Nausea or vomiting
  - Weakness
- May localize or radiate to arms, shoulders, back, neck, or jaw
- Associated symptoms:
  - Dyspnea
  - Syncope
  - Fatigue
  - Diaphoresis
  - Nausea
  - Vomiting
- Symptoms are usually reproduced by exertion, eating, exposure to cold, or emotional stress.
- Symptoms commonly last 30 min or more.
- Symptoms may occur with rest or during exertion.
- Often preceded by crescendo angina
- May be improved or relieved with rest or nitroglycerin
- Symptoms generally unchanged with position or inspiration
- Positive Levine sign or clenched fist over chest is suggestive of angina.
- BP is usually elevated during symptoms.

### Physical Exam
- Physical exam is usually unrevealing.
- Occasional physical findings include:
  - S3 or S4 due to left ventricular systolic or diastolic symptoms
  - Papillary muscle dysfunction resulting in mitral regurgitation
  - Diminished peripheral pulses
  - Physical findings of decompensated CHF

## ESSENTIAL WORKUP
History is critical in differentiating MI from noncardiac etiologies.

### DIAGNOSTIC TESTS & INTERPRETATION
#### Lab
- Electrolytes
- Calcium, magnesium
- Cardiac enzymes:
  - Especially for type II 2nd- and 3rd-degree blocks
- Digoxin level

#### Imaging
- CXR:
  - May identify cardiomyopathy or CHF

#### Diagnostic Procedures/Surgery
- ECG:
  - STEMI
  - Differentiate from non ischemic causes of ST elevation
    - Pericarditis
    - Benign early repolarization
    - Left ventricular hypertrophy with strain
    - Prior MI with left ventricular aneurysm
    - Hyperkalemia
  - Findings in non-STEMI
- Echo:
  - May identify regional wall motion abnormalities or valvular dysfunction

### DIFFERENTIAL DIAGNOSIS
- Aortic dissection
- Anxiety
- Biliary colic
- Costochondritis
- Esophageal spasm
- Esophageal reflux
- Herpes zoster
- Hiatal hernia
- Mitral valve prolapse
- Peptic ulcer disease
- Psychogenic symptoms
- Panic disorder
- Pericarditis
- Pneumonia
- Pulmonary embolus

# TREATMENT

## PRE-HOSPITAL
- IV access
- Aspirin
- Oxygen
- Cardiac monitoring
- Sublingual nitroglycerin for symptom relief
- 12-lead ECG, if possible, with transmission or results relayed to receiving hospital

## INITIAL STABILIZATION/THERAPY
- IV access
- Oxygen
- Cardiac monitoring
- Oxygen saturation
- Continuous BP monitoring and pulse oximetry

## ED TREATMENT/PROCEDURES
- STEMI requires reperfusion therapy as soon as possible:
  - Percutaneous coronary intervention (PCI) is preferred diagnostic and therapeutic modality if available.
- Goal is primary PCI within 90 min of 1st medical contact.
  - Thrombolytics should be given if percutaneous coronary intervention is not readily available within 90 min of 1st medical contact (see "Reperfusion Therapy, Cardiac").
- Goal is thrombolytic therapy within 30 min of presentation if PCI not available within 90 min.
- Patients with non-STEMI, benefit from administration of a glycoprotein IIb/IIIa inhibitor if planned PCI with stent within 48-hr timeframe.
- Aspirin should be administered first to all patients with suspected MI unless the patient has a known allergy.
- If BP is >90–100 mm Hg systolic, administer sublingual nitroglycerin, nitropaste, or IV nitroglycerin assuming no ECG criteria or clinical evidence of right ventricular infarct:
  - Symptoms that persist after 3 sublingual nitroglycerin tablets are strongly suggestive of AMI or noncardiac etiology.
- β-blockers should be initiated within 1st 24-hr if no contraindications (eg, heart block, heart rate <60, signs of heart failure, evidence of low output state, increased risk for cardiogenic shock, hypotension, or obstructive pulmonary disease) are present.
- Morphine may be given to relieve pain, anxiety, and increase oxygen carrying capacity.
- Enoxaparin or heparin is generally appropriate as the next line of therapy.
- ACE inhibitors should be started and continued indefinitely in all patients recovering from STEMI unless contraindicated.
- If non-STEMI is clearly the clinical diagnoses, a glycoprotein IIb/IIIa inhibitor should be started.
- Clopidogrel should be added to standard therapy regardless of whether PCI or reperfusion therapy is planned.

- Statin therapy reduces clinical events in patients with stable coronary artery disease, this may also extend to patients experiencing an acute ischemic coronary event.
- If patient is in cardiogenic shock, patient should be transported to a cardiac catheterization laboratory for angioplasty and intra-aortic balloon pump as soon as possible (see "Congestive Heart Failure").
- Ventricular dysrhythmias:
  - See "Ventricular Tachycardia"
- Bradydysrhythmia associated with hypotension should be treated with atropine or external pacing.
- Conduction disturbances:
  - 1st-degree aortic valve (AV) block and Mobitz I (Wenckebach) are often self-limited and do not require treatment.
  - Mobitz II, complete heart block, new right bundle branch block (RBBB) in anterior MI, RBBB plus left anterior branch block or left posterior fascicular block, left bundle branch block plus 1st-degree AV block may require a temporary transvenous pacemaker.

## MEDICATION
- Amiodarone: 150 mg IV over 5 min then 0.5 mg/min
- Aspirin: 160–325 mg PO
- Clopidogrel (Plavix): 300–600 mg PO load, 75 mg PO per day
- Enoxaparin (Lovenox): 1 mg/kg SC q12h
- Glycoprotein IIb/IIIa inhibitors:
  - Eptifibatide (Integrilin): 180 μg/kg IV over 1–2 min, followed by continuous infusion of 2 μg/kg/min up to 72 hr
  - Tirofiban (Aggrastat): 0.4 μg/kg/min for 30 min, then 0.1 μg/kg/min for 48–108 hr
  - Abciximab (ReoPro) for use prior to PCI only: 0.25 mg/kg IV bolus
- Heparin 60 units/kg IV bolus (max 4,000 U), then 12 U/kg/h (max 1,000 U/hr)
- Lidocaine: 1.5 mg/kg IV bolus, infusion of 2–4 mg/kg/min
- Magnesium: 2 g bolus IV
- Metoprolol: 5 mg IV q5min–q15min followed by 25–50 mg PO starting dose as tolerated (note: β-blockers contraindicated in cocaine chest pain)
- Morphine: 2 mg IV, may titrate upward in 2-mg increments for relief of pain assuming no respiratory deterioration and SBP >90 mm Hg
- Nitroglycerin: 0.4 mg sublingual q5min for maximum 3 doses
- Nitroglycerin: IV drip at 5–10 μg/min
- Nitropaste: 1–2 in transdermal
- Thrombolytics: See "Reperfusion Therapy, Cardiac," for dosing

# FOLLOW-UP

## DISPOSITION
### Admission Criteria
- Patients with an AMI require hospital admission.
- If the diagnosis is unclear, admission to the hospital or an ED observation unit may be useful for serial cardiac enzymes, ECGs, and exercise stress testing and/or cardiac catheterization.

### Discharge Criteria
No patient with an AMI should be discharged from the ED.

### Issues for Referral
If PCI is unavailable in the treating institution, and particularly if the patient is in cardiogenic shock, patients should be transported to another hospital if PCI can be initiated within 90 min of 1st medical contact.

## PEARLS AND PITFALLS
- Goal of reperfusion therapy is primary PCI within 90 min of 1st medical contact. Transfer to a PCI capable facility when this window can be accomplished.
- Goal of thrombolytic therapy is a 30 min door to needle time if PCI not possible.

## ADDITIONAL READING

- Chen ZM, Pan HC, Chen YP, et al. Early intravenous then oral metoprolol in 45,852 patients with acute myocardial infarction: Randomised placebo-controlled trial. *Lancet.* 2005;366:1622–1632.
- Kushner FG, Hand M, Smith SC, et al. ACC/AHA guidelines for the management of patients with ST-elevation myocardial infarction (updating the 2004 guideline and 2007 focused update) and ACC/AHA/SCAI guidelines on percutaneous coronary intervention (updating the 2005 guideline and 2007 focused update). *Circulation.* 2009;120:2271–2306.
- Sabatine MS, Cannon CP, Gibson CM, et al. CLARITY-TIMI 28 Investigators. Addition of clopidogrel to aspirin and fibrinolytic therapy for myocardial infarction with ST-segment elevation. *N Engl J Med.* 2005;352(12):1179–1189.
- Smith SC Jr., Allen J, Blair SN, et al. AHA/ACC guidelines for secondary prevention for patients with coronary and other atherosclerotic vascular disease: 2006 update. *J Am Coll Cardiol.* 2006;47:2130–2139.
- White HD, Braunwald E, Murphy SA, et al. Enoxaparin vs. unfractionated heparin with fibrinolysis for ST-elevation myocardial infarction in elderly and younger patients: Results from ExTRACT-TIMI 25. *Eur Heart J.* 2007;28:1066–1071.

## See Also (Topic, Algorithm, Electronic Media Element)
- Cardiac Testing
- Reperfusion Therapy
- Unstable Angina

# ACUTE CORONARY SYNDROME: NON–Q-WAVE (NON-ST ELEVATION) MI

David F. M. Brown
Shada A. Rouhani

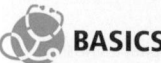

## BASICS

### DESCRIPTION
- Non-ST-elevation myocardial infarction (NSTEMI) is a part of a clinical syndrome that includes unstable angina.
- Probable cause is the generation of a subtotal coronary occlusion or functional collateral circulation:
  - Often indicates an incomplete ischemic event
- Coronary plaque disruption:
  - Endothelial disruption exposes subendothelial collagen and other platelet-adhering ligands, von Willebrand factor (vWF), and fibronectin.
  - Release of tissue factors activates factor VII and extrinsic pathway.
- Thrombus generation:
  - Platelet adhesion via glycoprotein (GP) Ia/IIa to collagen; GP Ib to vWF:
    - Platelet activation: Release of ADP, thromboxane $A_2$, and serotonin alters the platelet GP IIb/IIIa receptor; also causes local vasoconstriction
    - Platelet aggregation: GP IIb/IIIa receptor binds fibrinogen molecules, cross-links platelets forming local platelet plug
  - Platelet stabilization: Thrombin converts fibrinogen to fibrin, provides fibrin mesh, stabilizes platelet aggregate

### ETIOLOGY
- Coronary thrombosis
- Coronary artery spasm, idiopathic or cocaine induced
- In situ thrombosis/hypercoagulable states
- Embolic event
- Arteritis

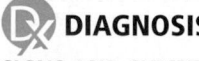

## DIAGNOSIS

### SIGNS AND SYMPTOMS
#### History
- Pain:
  - Pressure or tightness or heaviness
  - Substernal, epigastric
  - +/– radiation to arm, jaw, back
- Nausea, vomiting
- Diaphoresis
- Cough
- Dyspnea
- Anxiety
- Light-headedness
- Syncope
- Recent cocaine or amphetamine use
- Family history of coronary disease

### Geriatric Considerations
Geriatric patients may present with atypical symptoms or silent ischemia.

#### Physical Exam
- HTN
- Hypotension
- Arrhythmias
- S4 heart sound

### ESSENTIAL WORKUP
ECG, cardiac markers, CXR

### DIAGNOSTIC TESTS & INTERPRETATION
#### Lab
- Cardiac markers:
  - Troponins: Specific indicators of myocardial infarction, rises within 3–6 hr after MI, peaks at 9–10 days
  - Creatine kinase (CK): Rises within 4–8 hr, peaks at 18–24 hr, subsiding at 3–4 days; isoenzyme CK-MB more specific for cardiac origin
  - Myoglobin: Rises within 2–6 hr, returns to baseline within 24 hr, highly sensitive but very nonspecific
  - LDH: Rises within 24 hr, peaks at 3–6 days, returns to baseline at 8–12 days
- CBC
- Serum electrolytes including magnesium
- PT/PTT/INR for patients on warfarin
- NT-ProBNP: Higher levels correlate with increased mortality in NSTEMI patients.

#### Imaging
- ECG:
  - ST-segment depression or transient elevation indicates increased risk.
  - T-wave inversion in regional patterns does not increase risk but helps differentiate cardiac pain from non cardiac pain.
  - Deep (>2 mm) precordial T-wave inversion suggests cardiac ischemia.
- CXR:
  - To assess heart size, pulmonary edema/congestion or identify other causes of chest pain
- ECG:
  - To identify wall motion abnormalities and assess ventricular function
- Radionuclide studies:
  - Thallium or sestamibi scanning: Identifies viable myocardium
  - Technetium 99: Identifies recently infarcted myocardium

### Diagnostic Procedures/Surgery
Coronary angiography, typically as an inpatient, depending on patient's risk of ischemia

### DIFFERENTIAL DIAGNOSIS
- ST-elevation myocardial infarction
- Pulmonary embolus
- Aortic dissection
- Acute pericarditis
- Pneumothorax
- Pancreatitis
- Pneumonia
- Esophageal spasm/gastroesophageal reflux
- Esophageal rupture
- Musculoskeletal pain (diagnosis of exclusion)

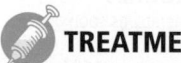

## TREATMENT

### PRE-HOSPITAL
- IV access
- Oxygen administration
- 12-lead EKG, cardiac monitoring, and treatment of arrhythmias
- Aspirin, analgesia, anxiolytics

### INITIAL STABILIZATION/THERAPY
- Oxygen administration
- IV access
- 12-lead EKG, cardiac monitoring, and treatment of arrhythmias

### ED TREATMENT/PROCEDURES
- Anti-ischemic therapy to reduce myocardial demand and increase myocardial supply of oxygen:
  - β-Blockers: IV if hypertensive with ongoing pain, else use orally within 24 hr; contraindicated in heart failure
  - Nitrates: Contraindicated with critical AS, suspicion of RV infarct or recent use of phosphodiesterase inhibitors (eg, sildenafil)
  - Oxygen
  - Morphine sulfate
  - Calcium channel blockers (nondihydropyridines—eg, diltiazem, verapamil) may be used in patients with ongoing ischemia and contraindications to β-blockade: Contraindicated in heart failure
- Antiplatelet therapy to decrease platelet aggregation:
  - Aspirin
  - Clopidogrel

- GP IIb/IIIa inhibitors (eptifibatide, tirofiban):
  - Only if ongoing ischemia, positive cardiac markers and PCI planned; may be deferred to inpatient setting
- Anticoagulation therapy to prevent thrombus propagation:
  - Unfractionated heparin or enoxaparin are 1st-line therapies.
  - Fondaparinux (factor 10A inhibitor) is a reasonable alternative, especially for medically managed patients; may have reduced bleeding risk.
  - Reserve bivalirudin (direct thrombin inhibitor) for patients with known heparin-induced thrombocytopenia
- Anxiolytics to suppress sympathomimetic release

### MEDICATION
#### First Line
- Aspirin 162–325 mg PO per day
- β-Blockers:
  - Atenolol: Start 5 mg IV over 5 min, then 5 mg IV 10 min later, then 50–100 mg PO per day (1–2 hr after IV doses).
  - Esmolol: 100 mcg/kg/min IV infusion (titrate by increasing 50 mcg/kg/min q15min until effect—to max dose 300 mcg/kg/min)
  - Metoprolol: Start 5 mg IV q5min × 3, after 15 min begin 25–50 mg PO q6h.
  - Propranolol: 0.5–1 mg IV then 40–80 mg PO q6–8h
- Clopidogrel: 300–600 mg PO × 1, then 75 mg/d
- Heparins:
  - Enoxaparin: 1 mg/kg SC q12h, can give 30 mg IV bolus before SC dose (beware of enoxaparin in patients with renal dysfunction)
  or
  - Unfractionated heparin: 60 U/kg IV bolus then 12 U/kg/hr infusion (max bolus 4,000 U, max infusion rate 1,000 U/hr (goal is aPTT 50–75 sec)
- Morphine sulfate: 1–5 mg IV q5–30min PRN pain
- Nitroglycerin: 0.3–0.6 mg SL or 0.4 mg by spray q5min followed by IV infusion beginning at 10–20 mcg/min if pain persists (max. dose 200 mcg/min)
- GP IIb/IIIa inhibitors:
  - Abciximab (only just prior to PCI): 0.25 mg/kg IV bolus then 0.125 mcg/kg/min infusion (max 10 mcg/min) for 12–24 hr
  - Eptifibatide: 180 mcg/kg IV bolus then 2 mcg/kg/min infusion for 72–96 hr
  - Tirofiban: 0.4 mcg/kg/min IV × 30 min, then 0.1 mcg/kg/min infusion for 48–96 hr

#### Second Line
- Calcium channel blockers:
  - Diltiazem: Start 0.25 mg/kg IV bolus, then 0.35 mg/kg IV after 15 min if needed then 30 mg PO q6h
  - Verapamil: Start 5–10 mg IV, repeat after 30 min if needed, then 80–160 mg PO q8h
- Lorazepam: 1–2 mg IV PRN anxiety
- Anticoagulation (instead of unfractionated heparin or enoxaparin):
  - Fondaparinux: 2.5 mg SC once a day
  or
  - Bivalirudin (only prior to PCI): 0.75 mg/kg IV bolus, then 1.75 mg/kg/hr IV for up to 4 hr, then 0.2 mg/kg/hr IV for up to 20 hr

## 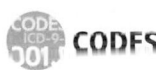 FOLLOW-UP

### DISPOSITION
#### Admission Criteria
- All patients with positive cardiac markers or significant clinical probability of acute coronary syndrome
- Intensive care unit for monitoring unstable patients

#### Discharge Criteria
Only those who are ruled out for acute coronary syndrome/non–Q-wave infarction can be safely sent home.

### FOLLOW-UP RECOMMENDATIONS
Only patients ruled out for acute coronary syndrome can be safely discharged:
- Discharged patients should follow up in 1–2 days with their primary care physician or cardiologist.
- Outpatient stress tests should be done within 72 hr.

## PEARLS AND PITFALLS

- EKG should be done in all patients with chest pain on arrival to the ED.
- Early medical therapy can reduce mortality in NSTEMI
- Pitfalls:
  - Do not rule out infarction based on initial or single set of cardiac markers, particularly if the time from symptom onset is <4–6 hr.
  - Do not fail to screen for amphetamine or cocaine use.
  - Do not fail to ask about use of sildenafil, vardenafil, or tadalafil before giving nitroglycerin.

## ADDITIONAL READING

- Anderson J, et al. ACC/AHA 2007 guidelines for the management of patients with unstable angina/non-ST-elevation myocardial infarction. *J Am Coll Cardiol* 2007;50:e1–157.
- Bonaca M, et al. Antithrombotics in acute coronary syndromes. *J Am Coll Cardiol* 2009;54(11): 969–984.
- Doshi A, et al. Evaluation and management of non-ST-segment elevation acute coronary syndromes in the emergency department. *Emerg Med Pract.* 2010;12(1):1–26.
- DeFilippi CR. Evaluating the chest pain patient. Scope of the problem. *Cardiol Clin.* 1999;17(2): 307–326.
- Fesmire F, et al. Clinical policy: Critical issues in the evaluation and management of adult patient with non-ST-segment elevation acute coronary syndromes. *Ann Emerg Med.* 2006;48(3):270–301.
- Pollack C, et al. 2007 Update to the ACC/AHA Guidelines for the Management of Patients with Unstable Angina and Non-ST-Segment Elevation Myocardial Infarction: Implications for Emergency department practice. *Ann Emerg Med.* 2008;51(5):591–606.
- Wackers FJ Th. Chest pain in the emergency department: Role of cardiac imaging. *Heart.* 2009;95(12):1023–1030.

### See Also (Topic, Algorithm, Electronic Media Element)
- Acute Coronary Syndromes
- Cardiac Testing
- Chest Pain

## CODES

**ICD9**
411.1 Intermediate coronary syndrome

# ACUTE CORONARY SYNDROME: STABLE ANGINA

*Shamai A. Grossman*
*Daniel J. Henning*

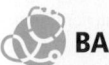 **BASICS**

## DESCRIPTION
- Chest discomfort that is <u>predictable in nature</u>, occurs with exertion, and <u>improves with rest</u>
- Imbalance in myocardial blood supply and oxygen requirements
- Canadian Cardiovascular Classification—class I: Ordinary physical activity does not cause symptoms.
- Canadian Cardiovascular Classification—class II: Symptoms that slightly limit normal activity such as:
  - Walking
  - Climbing stairs
  - Emotional stress
  - Cold

## ETIOLOGY
- Cardiac risk factors include:
  - Hypercholesterolemia
  - DM
  - HTN
  - Smoking
  - Family history
  - <u>Men: Age >35 yr</u>
  - Postmenopausal women
- <u>Atherosclerotic narrowing of coronary vessels</u>
- Vasospasm, although this is usually at rest and considered unstable if new onset
- Microvascular angina or abnormal relaxation of vessels with diffuse vascular disease
- <u>Arteritis:</u>
  - Lupus
  - Takayasu disease
  - Kawasaki disease
  - Rheumatoid arthritis
- <u>Anemia:</u> Hemoglobin <8 g/dL
- Hyperbarism or elevations in carboxyhemoglobin
- Structural abnormalities of coronary arteries:
  - Radiation fibrosis
  - Aneurysms
  - Ectasia
- Cocaine- or amphetamine-induced vasospasm

## DIAGNOSIS

### SIGNS AND SYMPTOMS
*History*
- Chest pain:
  - Substernal pressure
  - Heaviness
  - Squeezing
  - Burning sensation
  - Tightness
- May localize or radiate to arms, shoulders, back, neck, or jaw
- May be associated with dyspnea, syncope, fatigue, diaphoresis, nausea, or vomiting
- Usually reproduced by exertion, eating, exposure to cold, or emotional stress
- <u>Symptoms last <20 min,</u> but more than a few sec.
- Recurrent symptoms of ≥2 mo duration
- Usually relieved with <u>rest or nitroglycerin</u>
- Symptoms generally unchanged with position or inspiration
- No changes in pattern or frequency of symptoms
- Occasional anginal equivalents include:
  - Abdominal pain
  - Syncope
  - Diaphoresis
  - Nausea or vomiting
  - Weakness

*Physical Exam*
- Positive <u>Levine sign</u> or clenched fist over chest is suggestive of angina.
- BP is usually elevated during symptoms.
- Physical exam is usually unrevealing.
- Occasional symptoms include:
  - S3 or S4 due to left ventricular systolic or diastolic symptoms
  - Mitral regurgitation or pansystolic murmur
  - Diminished peripheral pulses

### ESSENTIAL WORKUP
- History is critical in differentiating stable and unstable angina.
- ECG:
  - Will be normal minimally 50% of the time
  - ST-segment changes or T-wave inversions most often will be unchanged from previous tracings.
  - Must be compared to prior tracings if available
  - New ST-segment changes or T-wave inversions are suspicious for unstable angina.
  - Serial ECG tracings that remain unchanged may assist in differentiating stable from unstable angina.
  - 1-mm depression of the ST-segment below the baseline, 80 ms from the J point, is characteristic of angina.
- ECG may be helpful in diagnosing other causes of chest pain:
  - Pericarditis is suggested by diffuse ST elevations followed by T-wave inversions and pulse rate depression.
  - Pulmonary embolism is suggested by an S1, Q3, T3 pattern; unexplained tachycardia; and signs of right heart strain.

### DIAGNOSTIC TESTS & INTERPRETATION
*Lab*
<u>Cardiac enzymes</u> should not be elevated and are not indicated unless the history is suspicious for acute myocardial infarction (AMI).

*Imaging*
- Chest radiograph:
  - Usually normal
  - May show cardiomegaly
  - CHF is suggestive of unstable angina.
  - May identify other etiologies of chest pain, such as pneumonia
- Coronary CTA:
  - Can be obtained as dedicated Coronary CTA or as part of "Triple Rule-out" CTA (TRO-CTA)
  - Useful if history is inconclusive in defining symptoms as stable angina
  - High negative predictive value to rule out ACS in low- to intermediate-risk patients
  - As TRO-CTA, may also identify other chest pain etiologies, eg, pneumothorax or pulmonary embolus
  - Absence of coronary atherosclerosis or stenosis suggests noncardiac etiology for chest pain.

### Diagnostic Procedures/Surgery

Exercise stress testing may help establish the diagnosis of stable angina and provide prognostic information:

- 1-mm depression of the ST segment below the baseline, 80 ms from the J point, in 3 consecutive beats and 2 consecutive leads is characteristic of cardiac ischemia.
- Early positive (within 3 min) stress tests are worrisome for unstable angina.
- 6 min of exercise utilizing a standard Bruce protocol suggests an excellent prognosis.
- Exercise stress testing with ECG alone has a sensitivity of 68% and specificity of 77%.
- Exercise stress testing with ECG has a sensitivity of 85% and specificity of 77%.
- Exercise stress testing with thallium-201 or technetium Tc-99m sestamibi has a sensitivity of 87% and specificity of 64%.

### DIFFERENTIAL DIAGNOSIS

- Anxiety
- Aortic dissection
- Biliary colic
- Costochondritis
- Esophageal reflux
- Esophageal spasm
- Herpes zoster
- Hiatal hernia
- Mitral valve prolapse
- MI
- Panic disorder
- Peptic ulcer disease
- Pneumonia
- Psychogenic
- Pulmonary embolus
- Unstable angina

 TREATMENT

### PRE-HOSPITAL

- IV access
- Oxygen
- Cardiac monitoring
- Sublingual nitroglycerin for symptom relief
- Aspirin

### INITIAL STABILIZATION/THERAPY

- IV access
- Oxygen
- Cardiac monitoring
- Oxygen saturation

### ED TREATMENT/PROCEDURES

- Aspirin
- Sublingual nitroglycerin:
  - Symptoms that persist after 3 sublingual nitroglycerines are strongly suggestive of unstable angina, AMI, or noncardiac etiology.
- May require adjustment of patient's outpatient medical regimen including adding or changing the dosage of a $\beta$-blocker

### MEDICATION

- Aspirin: 160–325 mg
- Nitroglycerin: 0.4 mg sublingual
- Isosorbide mononitrate: 20 mg PO b.i.d. or isosorbide dinitrate 5–40 mg PO t.i.d. or Nitropatch 1–2 in 10–14 hr daily
- Metoprolol: 25–50 mg PO starting dose
- Clopidogrel, in conjunction with standard therapy for ST-segment elevation myocardial infarction, was shown to reduce the odds of AMI patients having another occluded artery or a 2nd heart attack or death by 36% after 1 wk of hospitalization.
- Statin therapy reduces clinical events in patients with stable coronary artery disease; this may also extend to patients experiencing an acute ischemic coronary event.

 FOLLOW-UP

### DISPOSITION

#### Admission Criteria

- Patients with stable angina generally do not require hospital admission.
- If the diagnosis is unclear, admission to the hospital or an ED observation unit may be useful for serial cardiac enzymes, ECGs, and exercise stress testing.
- Patients who require additional adjustment of medication or angioplasty to reduce symptoms and improve quality of life may also benefit from admission.

#### Discharge Criteria

By definition, patients who meet diagnostic criteria of stable angina are safe to discharge.

### FOLLOW-UP RECOMMENDATIONS

Patients with stable angina should follow up with a cardiologist as well as their PCP.

### PEARLS AND PITFALLS

- History is the most useful factor in differentiating stable from unstable angina.
- All ED patients with chest pain or symptoms suggestive of an acute coronary syndrome require an immediate ECG.
- Patients with chest pain, even with stable angina, should receive a daily aspirin unless otherwise contraindicated (ie, allergy or active bleed).
- A single set of negative cardiac enzymes in a patient with chest pain may not rule out ACS.
- Female and diabetic patients frequently present with atypical symptoms of ACS, and require a low threshold for ACS workup.

### ADDITIONAL READING

- Ben-Dor I, Battler A. Treatment of stable angina. *Heart*. 2007;93:868–874.
- Hollander JE, Chang AM, et al. One-year outcomes following coronary computerized tomographic angiography for evaluation of emergency department patients with potential acute coronary syndrome. *Acad Emerg Med*. 2009;16(8):693–698.
- Pope JH, Selker HP. Acute coronary syndromes in the emergency department: Diagnostic characteristics, tests, and challenges. *Cardiol Clin*. 2005;23(4): 423–451.

#### See Also (Topic, Algorithm, Electronic Media Element)

- Acute Coronary Syndrome: Cardiac Testing
- Acute Coronary Syndrome: Myocardial Infarction
- Acute Coronary Syndrome: Unstable Angina

*Shamai A. Grossman*
*Jessica H. Klausmeier*

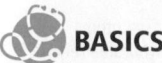

## BASICS

### DESCRIPTION

- Angina = myocardial ischemia = imbalance in myocardial blood supply and oxygen requirement:
  - Reversible (unlike infarction which is permanent myocardial damage due to prolonged ischemia)
  - Classification of severity
    - Class I: New onset, severe, or accelerated
    - Class II: Angina at rest and subacute (no anginal episodes within the preceding 48 hr)
    - Class III: Angina at rest and acute (angina within the preceding 48 hr)
- Unstable angina:
  - New onset angina ≥ class III in severity
  - Increase in frequency, duration, or lower threshold for developing symptoms
  - Angina occurs at rest, is prolonged >20 min
- Unstable angina is associated with an increased risk of transmural myocardial infarction and cardiac death.
- Very rarely is initial presentation of CAD—usually occurs in setting of chronic angina

### ETIOLOGY

- Chronic atherosclerotic narrowing of coronary vessels leads to insufficient myocardial perfusion during exertion, which causes stable angina.
- Disruption of a chronic, stable plaque leads to symptoms with less exertion or at rest.
- Atherosclerosis (and ACS) risk factors include:
  - Age
  - Male sex
  - Postmenopausal status (for women)
  - Hypercholesterolemia
  - DM
  - HTN
  - Smoking
  - Family history in a 1st-degree relative less than age 55
  - Postmenopausal women

### ALERT

In the ED, cardiac risk factors are poor predictors of cardiac risk for ACS (most useful in risk-stratification of asymptomatic individuals).

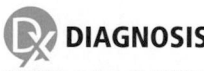

## DIAGNOSIS

### SIGNS AND SYMPTOMS

- Positive "Levine sign" or clenched fist over chest is classic for angina.
- Pain is visceral in origin and poorly localized.
- Chest pain is the most common presentation of myocardial ischemia for those ≤65 years old:
  - Substernal pressure, heaviness, squeezing, burning sensation, tightness
  - May localize or radiate to arms, shoulders, back, neck, or jaw

- Frequent anginal equivalents:
  - Dyspnea
  - Epigastric discomfort
  - Dyspepsia
  - Weakness/fatigue
  - Diaphoresis
  - Nausea or vomiting
- Occasional anginal equivalents:
  - Abdominal pain
  - Syncope
- Anginal symptoms are:
  - Usually reproduced by exertion, eating, exposure to cold, or emotional stress
  - Commonly last 15 min or more
  - Usually improved or relieved with rest or nitroglycerin
  - Generally unchanged with position or inspiration
- BP may be elevated during an anginal attack.

### Geriatric Considerations

- Women and elderly more likely to have atypical symptoms. Prognosis for people with atypical symptoms is worse than for those with typical symptoms.
- ACS often develops in elderly patients with acute comorbid illness (pneumonia, sepsis, fall, COPD), may lead to confusing picture and delayed diagnosis

### History

- Pain: Severity, location, radiation, duration, quality
- Associated symptoms: Nausea, diaphoresis, SOB
- Onset and duration, precipitant activities
- Frequency of symptoms
- Change in symptoms over time?
- PMHx:
  - CAD risk factors
  - Prior MI or interventions
  - History of prior stress test

### Physical Exam

- Physical exam is usually unrevealing.
- Patients may appear deceptively well.
- Patients may have pallor, cyanosis, diaphoresis, or tachypnea.
- Occasional physical findings include:
  - S3 or S4
  - Papillary muscle dysfunction resulting in mitral regurgitation/new murmur (ominous sign)

### ESSENTIAL WORKUP

ECG:

- Standard of care is the initial 12-lead ECG be obtained and read within 10 min of presentation for patients with acute chest pain or other symptoms concerning for myocardial ischemia
- Main utility is to detect acute MI, is less helpful in detecting unstable angina
- Must be compared to prior ECGs if available
- New ST segment changes or T-wave inversions are suspicious for unstable angina:
  - T-wave flattening or biphasic T waves
  - ≤1-mm depression of the ST segment below the baseline, 80 msec from the J point, is characteristic in angina
  - May see evidence of old ischemia, strain, or infarction: old TWI, Q waves, ST depression

- ST-segment changes or T-wave inversions most often will be unchanged from previous tracings.
- ECG may be helpful in diagnosing other etiologies of chest pain:
  - Pericarditis (diffuse ST elevations followed by T-wave inversions and PR depression)
  - Pulmonary embolism (S1, Q3, T3 pattern and sinus tachycardia)

### ALERT

Patients with a normal or nonspecific ECG have a 1–5% incidence of AMI and 4–23% incidence of unstable angina.

### DIAGNOSTIC TESTS & INTERPRETATION

#### Lab

- CK-MB and troponin I or T
  - <50% of patients with unstable angina will have low levels of troponin elevation.
  - CK-MB peaks in 12–24 hr, back to baseline in 2–3 days
  - Troponin peaks in 12 hr, back to baseline in 7–10 days
- Hematocrit—anemia increases risk of ischemia
- Coagulation profile
- Electrolytes: Pay particular attention to Cr and K+

#### Imaging

- CXR:
  - Usually normal
  - May show cardiomegaly or signs of CHF:
    - CHF is common in patients with unstable angina.
  - May identify other etiologies of chest pain such as pneumonia or pneumothorax
- Coronary CTA: Good only for patients with no known CAD and low risk for atherosclerosis—rules out ischemia as etiology of pain in patients with no coronary artery stenosis on CTA
- Bedside echo may detect severe wall motion abnormalities, can help rule out other causes of shock, and look for pericardial effusion or pneumothorax.
- Technetium Tc-99 sestamibi (rest):
  - Radionucleotide taken up by myocardium in varying amounts dependent on perfusion
  - Can compare perfusion during symptomatic episodes to determine whether the symptoms are due to myocardial ischemia
- Exercise stress testing may help establish the diagnosis of angina and provide prognostic information when the clinical presentation is equivocal:
  - Not appropriate if ongoing chest pain with moderate to high likelihood of ischemia
  - Imaging stress test (sestamibi, thallium, or echo) needed for patients with baseline EKG abnormalities
  - Early positive (within 3 min) stress tests are worrisome for unstable angina

## DIFFERENTIAL DIAGNOSIS

- Other nonatherosclerotic causes of cardiac ischemia:
  - Coronary artery spasm (spontaneous or drug induced—often happens with cocaine)
  - Coronary artery embolus
  - Congenital coronary disease
  - Coronary dissection
  - Coronary artery vasculitis
  - Valvular disease: AS, AI, pulmonary stenosis, mitral stenosis with pulmonary HTN
  - Congenital heart disease: Congenital valvular disease, coarctation, cyanotic heart disease
- Other cardiovascular:
  - Acute MI
  - Aortic dissection
  - Pericarditis, myocarditis
  - Mitral valve prolapse
- Pulmonary:
  - Pulmonary embolus
  - Pneumonia
  - Spontaneous pneumothorax
- GI:
  - Biliary colic
  - Esophageal reflux, spasm, or rupture
  - Peptic ulcer disease
- Other:
  - Costochondritis
  - Herpes zoster
  - Anxiety, panic, or conversion disorder

 **TREATMENT**

### PRE-HOSPITAL

- IV access
- Aspirin
- Oxygen
- Cardiac monitoring
- 12-lead EKG, if capability exists
- Sublingual nitroglycerin for symptom relief

### ALERT

All chest pain should be treated and transported as a possible life-threatening emergency.

### INITIAL STABILIZATION/THERAPY

- IV access
- Oxygen
- Cardiac monitoring, continuous $O_2$ sat

### ED TREATMENT/PROCEDURES

- Serial ECGs are essential to recognizing an evolving MI which may initially present as unstable angina.
- Oxygen therapy
- Pain control
- Anticoagulation

### MEDICATION

#### First Line

- Aspirin should be administered 1st to all patients with suspected unstable angina (unless true allergy):
  - 81 mg × 4 (chewed) or 325 mg chewed for fastest action
  - OK to give 1 dose in patients with history of GIB/gastritis from aspirin/NSAIDs
  - Clopidogrel 300 mg if aspirin allergic

- Nitroglycerin:
  - 0.4 mg sublingual, 1–2 in paste, or IV drip at 5–10 $\mu$g/min
  - Symptoms that persist after 3 doses of sublingual nitro is strongly suggestive of unstable angina, acute MI, or noncardiac etiology.
  - Beware giving nitro in patients without IV access (can severely drop BP)
  - Beware in patients with history of erectile dysfunction and use of phosphodiesterase inhibitors like sildenafil or tadalafil (Viagra or Cialis) in last 48 hr
  - Hold for hypotension, concern for RV infarction (preload dependent):
    - Q in II, III, and aVF, STE in R-sided V3, V4
- Morphine:
  - May be given to relieve pain not controlled by nitrates
  - 4 mg IV. Titrate upward in 4-mg increments for relief of pain assuming no respiratory deterioration and SBP >90 mm Hg
- Consider starting beta blocker therapy:
  - Metoprolol: 25–50 mg PO starting dose. Can use 5 mg IV q5–15min as tolerated for refractory HTN and tachycardia
  - Contraindications: Active RAD, signs of CHF, bradycardia, hypotension, heart block, cocaine use
  - Current data suggests that this occur within 1st 24 hr of AMI (not necessarily in ED for morbidity/mortality benefit)

#### Second Line

Anticoagulation:

- Enoxaparin (Lovenox): 1 mg/kg SC q12h or q24h for patients with Cr clearance <30 mL/min
- Heparin: 60 U/kg IV bolus, then 12 U/kg/hr (with goal ptt 50–70)
- Glycoprotein IIb/IIIa inhibitors
  - Eptifibatide (Integrilin): 180 $\mu$g/kg IV over 1–2 min, followed by continuous infusion of 2 $\mu$g/kg/min up to 72 hr
  - Tirofiban (Aggrastat): 0.4 $\mu$g/kg/min for 30 min, then 0.1 $\mu$g/kg/min for 48–108 hr
  - Abciximab (ReoPro): 0.25 mg/kg IV bolus, then 0.125 $\mu$g/kg/min
- Other options: Bivalirudin, fondaparinux (may be better for patients at high risk for bleeding: elderly, female, anemic, CKD)

#### Geriatric Considerations

Elderly patients have more frequent episodes of significant bleeding as with anticoagulation.

 **FOLLOW-UP**

### DISPOSITION

#### Admission Criteria

- Patients with unstable angina require hospital admission.
- If CK-MB and/or troponin are significantly elevated, the patient has persistent angina, or hemodynamic instability, mortality will likely be decreased by early intervention (cardiac cath).
- If the diagnosis is unclear, admission to the hospital or an ED observation unit may be useful for serial cardiac enzymes, ECGs, and exercise stress testing and/or cardiac catheterization.

#### Discharge Criteria

No patient with unstable angina should be discharged from the ED.

## PEARLS AND PITFALLS

- Many patients with true ACS will present with normal ECGs and atypical symptoms.
- It is important not to miss subtle anginal equivalents (weakness, nausea) especially in the elderly.
- Serial ECGs are essential for any patient being worked up for ACS.
- Should work closely with in-house cardiologist and interventionalist to determine anticoagulation regimen choice (may vary institution to institution)

## ADDITIONAL READING

- Alexander KP, Newby LK, Cannon CP, et al. Acute coronary care in the elderly, part 1: Non-ST-segment-elevation acute coronary syndromes: A scientific statement for healthcare professionals from the American Heart Association Council on Clinical Cardiology: In Collaboration with the Society of Geriatric Cardiology. *Circulation.* 2007;115: 2549–2569.
- Hollander JE. Acute coronary syndromes: Acute myocardial infarction and instable angina. *Tintinalli's Emergency Medicine: A Comprehensive Study Guide,* 6e. New York: McGraw-Hill; 2004.
- O'Donoghue M, Boden WE, Braunwald E, et al. Early invasive v conservative treatment strategies in women and men with unstable angina and non ST-segment elevation myocardial infarction. A meta-analysis. *JAMA.* 2008;300(1).71–80.
- Pollack CV, Braunwald E. Update to the ACC/AHA Guidelines for the management of patients with unstable angina and non-ST-segment elevation myocardial infarction: Implications for emergency department practice. *Ann Emerg Med.* 2007;51(5): 591–606.

### See Also (Topic, Algorithm, Electronic Media Element)

Cardiac Testing; Myocardial Infarction; Reperfusion Therapy; Stable Angina

# ADRENAL INSUFFICIENCY

*Rita Cydulka*
*Michael D. Smith*

 **BASICS**

## DESCRIPTION
- Inadequate hydrocortisone secretion to meet body's stress requirement
- Adrenal deficiency:
  - Inadequate cortisol
  - Unresponsive to stimulation with adrenocorticotropic hormone (ACTH)
- Functional hypoadrenalism:
  - Inadequate cortisol
  - Partial responsive to stimulation with ACTH
- Addisonian crisis (acute adrenal insufficiency):
  - Life-threatening emergency
  - Precipitated by intensification of:
    - Chronic adrenal insufficiency
    - Acute adrenal hemorrhage
    - Rapid steroid withdrawal
    - Treatment of hypothyroidism with unrecognized adrenal disease
    - Steroid-dependent patient under stress owing to pregnancy, surgery, trauma, infection, or dehydration

## ETIOLOGY
### Primary Adrenal Failure
- Adrenal dysgenesis/impaired steroidogenesis:
  - Congenital hypoplasia
  - Allgrove syndrome:
    - ACTH resistance
    - Achalasia
    - Alacrima
  - Glycerol kinase deficiency:
    - Psychomotor retardation
    - Hypogonadism
    - Muscular dystrophy
- Congenital hyperplasia
- Aldosterone synthetase deficiency
- Mitochondrial disease

- Adrenal destruction:
  - Autoimmune:
    - Autoimmune polyglandular syndrome types 1 and 2 (alopecia universalis, chronic mucocutaneous candidiasis, hypoparathyroid, thyroid autoimmunity, diabetes, celiac disease, pernicious anemia)
    - Adrenoleukodystrophy
  - Infectious:
    - Granulomatous: TB
    - Protozoal and fungal: Histoplasmosis, coccidioidomycosis, and candidiasis
    - Viral: Cytomegalovirus, herpes simplex virus, and HIV
    - Bacterial
  - Infiltration:
    - Sarcoid
    - Neoplasm
    - Hemochromatosis
    - Amyloidosis
    - Iron depletion
- Postadrenalectomy
- Hemorrhage:
  - Sepsis: Particularly meningococcemia, *Pseudomonas* infection
  - Birth trauma/anoxia
  - Pregnancy
  - Seizures
  - Anticoagulants
  - Rhabdomyolysis
- Pharmacologic inhibition:
  - Etomidate
  - Herbal medications
  - Ketoconazole
  - Metyrapone
  - Suramin

### Secondary Adrenal Failure
- Pituitary insufficiency
- Sepsis
- Head trauma
- Hemorrhage
- Infarction (Sheehan syndrome)
- Infiltration: Neoplasm, amyloid, sarcoid, and hemochromatosis
- Adrenocorticotropic hormone deficiency
- Pharmacologic: Glucocorticoid administration, herbal medications

### Tertiary Adrenal Failure
- Hypothalamus insufficiency
- Sepsis
- Infiltrative: Neoplasm, amyloid, sarcoid, and hemochromatosis
- Head trauma

 **DIAGNOSIS**

## SIGNS AND SYMPTOMS
- Symptoms:
  - Depression
  - Lethargy
  - Malaise
  - Myalgias
  - Anorexia
  - Abdominal pain
  - Nausea
  - Vomiting
  - Dehydration (found in primary adrenal insufficiency only)
  - Salt craving
- Signs:
  - Fever or hypothermia
  - Mental status changes
  - Tachycardia
  - Orthostatic BP changes or frank shock
  - Weight loss
  - Goiter
  - Hypogonadism
  - Hyperkalemia
  - Sodium depletion
  - Eosinophilia
  - Hyperpigmentation (found in primary adrenal insufficiency only)
  - Vitiligo
- Addisonian crisis:
  - Hypotension and shock
  - Hyponatremia
  - Hyperkalemia
  - Hypoglycemia

## ESSENTIAL WORKUP

- Laboratory confirmation of diagnosis not possible in emergency department
- Adrenal crisis: Life-threatening condition:
  - High degree of suspicion should prompt initiation of therapy before definitive diagnosis.
- Plasma cortisol level $<20$ $\mu$g/dL accompanied by shock suggests adrenal insufficiency.
- Electrolytes:
  - Potassium
  - Sodium
- BUN, creatinine:
  - Elevated owing to dehydration
- Serum glucose levels may be low.

## DIAGNOSTIC TESTS & INTERPRETATION

### Lab

- CBC with differential:
  - Anemia
  - Eosinophilia
  - Lymphocytosis
- Arterial blood gases:
  - Hypoxemia
  - Acidosis
- Cosyntropin stimulation test:
  - Adrenal deficiency:
    - Random serum cortisol $<20$ $\mu$g/dL (while stressed)
    - ACTH stimulation unresponsive
  - Functional hypoadrenalism:
    - Random serum cortisol $= 20$ $\mu$g/dL (while stressed)
    - 60 min post ACTH stimulation $<30$ $\mu$g/dL or delta cortisol (60 min – baseline) $= 9$ $\mu$g/dL
- Search for underlying infection.

### Imaging

CRX:

- Look for infection or edema

### Diagnostic Procedures/Surgery

ECG:

- Evaluate for electrolyte disturbances

## DIFFERENTIAL DIAGNOSIS

- Sepsis
- Shock (any cause)
- Acute abdominal emergency

# TREATMENT

## INITIAL STABILIZATION/THERAPY

- Airway, breathing, and circulation management (ABCs)
- Cardiac monitor
- BP support for hypotension:
  - Normal saline (0.9%) IV fluids 500 mL–1 L (peds: 20 mL/kg) bolus
  - Avoid pressors (if possible):
    - May precipitate dysrhythmias
- Supplemental oxygen to meet metabolic needs
- Correct hyperthermia:
  - Initiate cooling measures.

## ED TREATMENT/PROCEDURES

- Glucocorticoid replacement:
  - IV hydrocortisone or dexamethasone
  - Dexamethasone will not interfere with results of cosyntropin stimulation tests.
- Volume expansion:
  - $D_5W$ 0.9% NS at rate of 500–1,000 mL/hr for 1st 3–4 hr
  - Care should be taken to note patient's age, volume, and cardiac and renal function.
- For hypoglycemia:
  - $D_{50}W$
- Treat life-threatening dysrhythmias secondary to hyperkalemia with calcium, bicarbonate, and insulin/glucose.
- Identification and correction of underlying precipitant

## MEDICATION

- Dexamethasone: 4 mg (peds: 0.15 mg/kg per dose) q12h
- Dextrose: 50–100 mL $D_{50}$ (peds: 2 mL/kg of $D_{10}$ over 1 min) IV
- Hydrocortisone: 100 mg (peds: 1–2 mg/kg per dose) IV q6h
- Insulin (regular): 10 U by IV push
- Sodium bicarbonate: 1–2 mEq/kg IV

# FOLLOW-UP

## DISPOSITION

### Admission Criteria

- All patients with acute adrenal insufficiency
- ICU admission for patients with unstable or potentially unstable cases

### Discharge Criteria

Normal laboratory evaluation with treated adrenal insufficiency

## FOLLOW-UP RECOMMENDATIONS

- Should have primary care physician follow-up within a few weeks depending on symptoms.
- May benefit from endocrinology referral

## PEARLS AND PITFALLS

- The benefit of steroids for relative adrenal insufficiency in septic shock is limited to the role of shock refractory to vasopressive treatment. Even then, the mortality benefit and clinical effect is questionable.
- The clinical consequence of single dose etomidate for rapid sequence intubation is controversial. Studies show biochemical adrenal suppression. The potential for adrenal suppression must be weighed against using agents with other undesirable properties while securing an emergent airway.

## ADDITIONAL READING

- Chang SS, Liaw SJ, Bullard MJ, et al. Adrenal insufficiency in critically ill emergency department patients: A Taiwan preliminary study. *Acad Emerg Med*. 2001;8:761–764.
- Oelkers W. Adrenal insufficiency. *N Engl J Med*. 1996;355:1206–1212.
- Rivers E, Blake HC, Dereczyk B, et al. Adrenal dysfunction in hemodynamically unstable patients in the emergency department. *Acad Emerg Med*. 1999;6:626–630.
- Rivers E, Gaspari M, Saad GA, et al. Adrenal insufficiency in high-risk surgical ICU patients. *Chest*. 2001;119:889–896.
- Sprung CL, Annane D, Keh D, et al. Hydrocortisone therapy for patients with septic shock. *N Engl J Med*. 2008;358(2):111–124.
- Ten S, New M, Noel M. Clinical review 130: Addison's disease 2001. *J Clin Endocrinol Metab*. 2001;86:2909–2922.

## See Also (Topic, Algorithm, Electronic Media Element)

Cushing Syndrome

# AIRWAY MANAGEMENT

*Scott G. Weiner*
*Carlo L. Rosen*

 **BASICS**

## DESCRIPTION

- Techniques that ensure adequate oxygenation of a patient
- Oral and nasopharyngeal airways:
  - Lift tongue off hypopharynx
  - Facilitate bag-valve-mask ventilation
  - Insert when gag reflex is absent
- Rapid sequence intubation (RSI):
  - Preferred method for ED oral intubation (minimizes aspiration risk)
  - Rapid induction of anesthesia and paralysis
  - Contraindicated in patients who should not be paralyzed
  - A preformulated backup strategy with alternative airway techniques is essential.
- Oral awake intubation:
  - Oral intubation with sedation only
  - Ketamine is the most common agent used for this purpose:
    - Although traditionally contraindicated in head injured patients, growing evidence shows that Ketamine may be neuroprotective in head trauma.
    - Use with benzodiazepines
    - Indicated when paralysis is contraindicated
- Gum elastic bougie:
  - Airway adjunct used when vocal cords are not well visualized
  - Placement confirmed by feeling bougie bump against tracheal rings
  - Slide endotracheal tube (ET) over bougie, then remove bougie
- Alternative airway devices:
  - Extraglottic devices:
    - Inserted blindly into oropharynx and inflated
    - Laryngeal mask airway (LMA) forms a seal around glottic structures in hypopharynx.
    - LMA offers less protection against aspiration than ET tube.
    - Intubating LMA can be used to place an ET tube.
    - Combitube occludes the esophagus and ventilates the hypopharynx.
  - Video laryngoscopes:
    - Fiberoptic camera on the tip of laryngoscope blade or LMA to visualize tube placement
  - Fiberoptic intubating stylets:
    - Fiberoptic camera on the tip of a stylet which holds ET tube

- Classic fiberoptic intubation:
  - ET tube placed over bronchoscope
  - Nasotracheal or orotracheal approach
  - Indications:
    - Anatomic limitations to glottis visualization
    - Limited mobility of mandible or cervical spine
    - Unstable cervical spine injury
  - Contraindications:
    - Need for immediate airway management
    - Significant oropharyngeal blood
- Nasotracheal intubation:
  - Indications:
    - Oral access impaired
    - Unsuccessful oral intubation
    - Paralysis is contraindicated
    - Limited cervical mobility
  - Contraindications:
    - Apnea (only absolute)
    - Anticoagulation
    - Massive facial, nasal, or head trauma
    - Upper airway abscess
    - Epiglottitis
    - Penetrating neck trauma
- Cricothyrotomy:
  - Definitive treatment for a failed airway
  - Incision in cricothyroid membrane
  - Tracheostomy tube inserted percutaneously into the airway
  - Indications:
    - Other airway attempts have failed
    - Massive facial trauma
    - Total upper airway obstruction
  - Contraindications:
    - Laryngeal crush injury
    - Tracheal transection
    - Expanding zone II or III hematoma
- Percutaneous translaryngeal ventilation (PTV):
  - Percutaneous placement of 12- or 14-gauge catheter through cricothyroid membrane
  - Intermittent ventilation via high-pressure oxygen source
  - Indications:
    - Failed oral or nasal intubation until cricothyrotomy is complete
  - Contraindications:
    - Upper airway obstruction preventing expiration
- Retrograde intubation:
  - Retrograde advancement of guidewire through translaryngeal catheter
  - ET tube advanced over wire once it comes out of the mouth

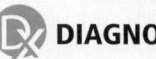 **DIAGNOSIS**

## SIGNS AND SYMPTOMS

Clinical conditions requiring airway management:

- Failure to maintain or protect the airway:
  - Oropharyngeal swelling
  - Absent gag reflex
  - Inability to clear secretions, blood
  - Stridor
- Hypoxia or ventilatory failure:
  - Shortness of breath
  - Altered mental status
  - Status epilepticus
- Anticipated clinical course:
  - Ventilatory control for head injury or tricyclic overdose
  - Sedation for diagnostic or therapeutic procedures
  - Early management if the airway might become compromised

## ESSENTIAL WORKUP

- Recognition of a difficult airway:
  - Anatomic considerations:
    - Short mandible, thick neck, narrow mouth, large tongue, and protruding teeth
    - Congenital syndromes, acromegaly
    - Obesity
  - Disease states:
    - Angioedema
    - Rheumatoid arthritis and other arthropathies that decrease cervical spine mobility
    - Goiter
    - Laryngeal–tracheal tumors
    - History of radiation therapy to the neck
    - Infections (epiglottitis, supraglottitis, croup, intraoral abscess, retropharyngeal abscess, Ludwig angina)
    - Profuse upper gastrointestinal hemorrhage
    - Trauma (facial, neck, cervical spine, laryngeal–tracheal, burns)
  - Mallampati criteria (increasing difficulty):
    - Class I: Soft palate, uvula, fauces, pillars visible
    - Class II: Soft palate, uvula, fauces visible
    - Class III: Soft palate visible
    - Class IV: Hard palate only
  - Rule of 3-3-2 (difficult airway if met):
    - Mouth opens <3 fingerbreadths
    - Horizontal length of mandible <3 fingerbreadths
    - Thyromental distance <2 fingerbreadths

- Verification of correct tube placement:
  - Visualization of tube passing through the vocal cords
  - Auscultate over stomach, axillae, and anterior lung fields
  - Observe chest wall movement
  - Condensation in the tube during ventilation End-tidal $CO_2$ colorimetric device:
    - Changes color if $CO_2$ is sensed, indicating tracheal placement
    - Color change may not be seen in cardiac arrest

## DIAGNOSTIC TESTS & INTERPRETATION
### Lab
- Pulse oximetry should rise after tracheal intubation
- Arterial blood gas to manage ventilator settings after intubation

### Imaging
CXR:
- To exclude mainstem bronchus intubation or pneumothorax
- Does not rule out esophageal intubation

### Diagnostic Procedures/Surgery
Direct visualization of the ET tube through the cords is gold standard.

## DIFFERENTIAL DIAGNOSIS
- Esophageal intubation
- Right or left mainstem bronchus intubation
- Extratracheal placement through tear in pyriform sinus or trachea
- Pneumothorax

 **TREATMENT**

### PRE-HOSPITAL
Options for patients in respiratory arrest for advanced life support (ALS) providers:
- Bag–valve management (BVM) ventilation followed by definitive airway management in the ED
- Orotracheal intubation
- Esophageal–tracheal tubes (eg, Combitube)
- LMA

### INITIAL STABILIZATION/THERAPY
- Maintain in-line cervical spine immobilization in trauma
- Oxygen, monitor, IV

### ED TREATMENT/PROCEDURES
- Rapid sequence intubation
- Prepare equipment:
  - Suction, BVM, various sizes of ET tubes and laryngoscope blades, stylets, and medications
- Preoxygenation:
  - 100% $FIO_2$ for 3 min
- Pretreatment:
  - Prevents physiologic sequelae of intubation
  - Performed 2–3 min prior to paralytic
  - Defasciculating dose of nondepolarizing agent
  - Fentanyl and lidocaine may minimize ICP rise and hemodynamic response to intubation in head-injured patients.
  - Lidocaine decreases airway irritability in reactive airway disease.

- Paralysis with induction:
  - Administration of induction agent (eg, etomidate or thiopental)
  - Rapidly followed by administration of paralytic agent (eg, succinylcholine)
    - Succinylcholine is relatively contraindicated with anticipated difficult oral intubation, open globe injury, organophosphate poisoning, burns >3 days old, denervation syndromes, myopathies, and suspected hyperkalemia.
    - Nondepolarizing agents (eg, rocuronium) can be used as an alternative to succinylcholine.
- Positioning:
  - Head extension, with midline cervical stabilization if trauma patient
  - Apply cricoid pressure (Sellick maneuver) to occlude esophagus and prevent aspiration
- Placement of tube:
  - After muscle tone is lost (45–60 sec after succinylcholine)
  - Use a stylet with the ET tube
  - Place tube through vocal cords
  - Inflate cuff
  - Begin ventilation
  - Confirm correct ET tube placement
- Postintubation:
  - Benzodiazepines, opiates, or propofol used for continued sedation
  - Vecuronium may be used for continued paralysis.

### Pediatric Considerations
- Estimation of ET tube size: 4 + age/4
- Uncuffed ET tubes may be used in patients <8 yr old.
- Straight Miller blade is preferred in patients <3 yr old.
- Cricothyrotomy contraindicated in patients <12 yr old; PTV is preferred
- Use atropine as pretreatment to reduce secretions and attenuate vagal effect.
- A defasciculating neuromuscular blocking agent is unnecessary for children <5 yr old

## MEDICATION
- Atracurium: 0.4–0.5 mg/kg IV
- Atropine: 0.02 mg/kg IV
- Diazepam: 2–10 mg (peds: 0.2–0.3 mg/kg) IV
- Etomidate: 0.3 mg/kg IV
- Fentanyl: 3 µg/kg IV
- Ketamine: 1–2 mg/kg IV or 4–7 mg/kg IM
- Lidocaine: 1.5 mg/kg IV
- Midazolam: 1–5 mg IV (0.07–0.30 mg/kg for induction)
- Propofol: 2–2.5 mg/kg IV
- Pancuronium: 0.01 mg/kg IV (defasciculating dose); 0.1 mg/kg IV (paralyzing dose)
- Rocuronium: 1 mg/kg IV
- Succinylcholine: 1.5 mg/kg (peds: 2 mg/kg) IV; 2.5 mg/kg IM/SC
- Thiopental: 3 mg/kg IV
- Vecuronium: 0.01 mg/kg IV (defasciculating dose); 0.1 mg/kg IV (paralyzing dose)

 **FOLLOW-UP**

## DISPOSITION
### Admission Criteria
Almost all intubated patients should be admitted to an ICU.

### Discharge Criteria
Rarely, certain ED patients who have been intubated for airway protection or to facilitate diagnostic workup may be extubated in the ED after a period of observation and then discharged.

## PEARLS AND PITFALLS
Respect the airway. Failure to intubate and ventilate is a life-threatening condition:
- Assess each patient for the possibility of difficult intubation.
- Prepare and familiarize yourself with all needed equipment and medications (including contraindications and side effects).
- ALWAYS formulate your backup plan in the case of a crash airway or failed standard orotracheal intubation before beginning the procedure.

## ADDITIONAL READING
- Murphy MF. Airway management. In: Wolfson AB, et al., eds. *Harwood-Nuss' Clinical Practice of Emergency Medicine*. 5th ed. Philadelphia: Lippincott Williams & Wilkins, 2009.
- Reardon RF, Mason PE, Clinton JE. Basic airway management and decision-making. In: Roberts JR, Hedges JR, eds. *Clinical Procedures in Emergency Medicine*. 5th ed. Philadelphia: WB Saunders, 2009.
- Walls RM. Airway. In: Marx JA, et al., eds. *Rosen's Emergency Medicine: Concepts and Clinical Practice*. 7th ed. St. Louis, MO: Mosby, 2009.

### See Also (Topic, Algorithm, Electronic Media Element)
Rapid Sequence Intubation

# ALCOHOL POISONING

*Timothy J. Meehan*
*Mark B. Mycyk*

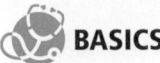 **BASICS**

## DESCRIPTION
- Alcohol is the most commonly abused recreational agent among emergency department patients.
- Alcohol is commonly associated with ED injury evaluations.

## ETIOLOGY
- Alcohol intoxication:
  - Directly depresses CNS function
  - Blood alcohol levels drop by 15–40 mg/dL/hr depending on individual variables and chronicity of alcohol use.
- Alcohol withdrawal:
  - Occurs in chronic alcohol abusers after partial or complete alcohol abstinence
  - May occur despite a serum alcohol level >100 mg/dL (eg, "intoxicated")
  - Profound CNS excitation
  - Increased catecholamine release and adrenergic tone
  - Decreased inhibitory activity

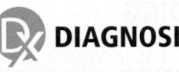 **DIAGNOSIS**

## SIGNS AND SYMPTOMS
### Acute Alcohol Intoxication
- Relaxation
- Euphoria
- Sedation
- Memory loss
- Impaired judgment
- Ataxia
- Slurred speech
- Nausea/vomiting
- Obtundation/coma

### Alcohol Withdrawal Syndrome
- Early or minor withdrawal:
  - <8 hr after last drink:
    - Symptoms of a hangover
    - Headache
    - Nausea/vomiting
  - 12 hr after last drink:
    - Mild tremors/anxiety
    - Anorexia, nausea, vomiting
    - Weakness
    - Myalgias
    - Vivid dreams/nightmares
  - 12–36 hr after last drink:
    - Irritability/agitation
    - Tachycardia/HTN
    - Tremors in hands and tongue

- 24–48 hr after last drink: Alcoholic hallucinosis:
  - Visual hallucinations most common (bug crawling)
  - Auditory hallucinations (buzz, clicks)
  - Present in minor and major withdrawal
- Alcoholic withdrawal seizures:
  - 8–12 hr after last drink
  - Brief, spontaneously abating tonic-clonic activity
  - Precedes delirium tremens (DTs)
- Late alcohol withdrawal or major withdrawal:
  - 48 hr after last drink
  - Delirium Tremens (DTs):
    - Clouded consciousness and delirium
    - Confusion/disorientation
    - Agitation/combativeness
    - Tachycardia/HTN
    - Hyperpyrexia
    - Diaphoresis

### History
- Often provided by EMS, family, or friends
- Beware the "frequent flyer" in the ED:
  - Can sometimes have other causes of AMS:
    - Hepatic disease/encephalopathy
    - Seizures (post-ictal)
    - Hypoglycemia
    - Head injury or intracranial bleeding

### Physical Exam
- Vital signs:
  - Acute Intoxication: Normal or depressed
  - Withdrawal: Usually elevated
- Mental status:
  - Acute Intoxication: Somnolent, obtunded, or comatose
  - Withdrawal: Hyperalert, agitated
- Signs of hepatic injury:
  - Jaundice
  - Icterus
  - Spider angiomata
  - Asterixis
  - Hepatomegaly
- Signs of malnutrition:
  - Alopecia
  - Poor dentition
  - Poor muscle mass
  - Abdominal wasting
  - Temporal wasting

### ESSENTIAL WORKUP
- Obtain accurate alcohol drinking and abstinence history.
- Investigate for life-threatening causes of seizures:
  - Hypoglycemia (get rapid bedside glucose)
  - Intracranial hemorrhage
  - CNS infection
  - Electrolyte abnormalities
- Evaluate for occult trauma
- Monitor all vital signs frequently:
  - Elevated temperature predicts poorer outcomes

## DIAGNOSTIC TESTS & INTERPRETATION
### Lab
- Alcohol level if abnormal mental status
- Urine toxicology screen to exclude coingestants
- Electrolytes, BUN, creatinine, and glucose
- CBC
- Magnesium, calcium, and phosphate
- PTT, PT/INR if coagulopathy suspected
- LFTs if liver disease suspected
- Ammonia level if hepatic encephalopathy suspected
- Urinary ketones or serum acetone if alcoholic ketoacidosis suspected

### Imaging
- CT of head if:
  - Alteration in mental status is out of proportion to expected AMS based on serum alcohol level
  - Suspected head trauma
  - Signs of increased intracranial pressure or focal findings on neurologic exams
  - New-onset seizure
  - Unimproved or deteriorating level of consciousness
- EEG differentiates alcohol withdrawal seizures from idiopathic epilepsy.
- Chest radiograph if suspected aspiration or pneumonia

## DIFFERENTIAL DIAGNOSIS
- Acute alcohol intoxication:
  - Hypoglycemia
  - Carbon dioxide narcosis
  - Mixed-drug overdose
  - Ethylene glycol, methanol, or isopropanol poisoning
  - Hepatic encephalopathy
  - Psychosis
  - Severe vertigo
  - Psychomotor seizure
- Alcohol withdrawal and seizures:
  - Sedative–hypnotic withdrawal
  - Acute intoxication or poisoning:
    - Carbon monoxide
    - Isoniazid (especially if prolonged seizures not responding to standard therapy)
    - Amphetamine
    - Anticholinergic
    - Cocaine
  - Secondary seizure disorders:
    - Infection
    - Meningitis
    - Encephalitis
    - Brain abscess
  - Trauma
  - Intracranial hemorrhage
  - CVA
  - Tumor
  - Anticonvulsant noncompliance
  - Thyroid disorder

# TREATMENT

## PRE-HOSPITAL
- Administer benzodiazepines for seizures.
- Give naloxone, oxygen, and dextrose for comatose individuals.
- Intubate as necessary for airway protection to prevent aspiration.
- C-spine immobilization if suspected trauma

## INITIAL STABILIZATION/THERAPY
- Airway, breathing, circulation (ABCs)
- Evaluate C-spine if suspected trauma.
- Initial IV rehydration with 0.9 NS, then D5 0.45 NS
- Administer naloxone, thiamine, and glucose (or Accu-Chek) if altered mental status.
- Benzodiazepines if seizing (may require large doses)

### Pediatric Considerations
- Young children have decreased hepatic glycogen reserves.
- Cannot mount an appropriate response to increased glucose needs
- Rapid bedside glucose (Accu-Chek) is ESSENTIAL:
  - Replace dextrose with D5 (10 mL/kg), D10 (5 mL/kg), or D25 (2 mL/kg) depending on age and size.

## ED TREATMENT/PROCEDURES
- Alcohol intoxication:
  - Rehydrate with IV fluids.
    Correct electrolyte abnormalities:
    - Magnesium
    - Potassium
    - Folate
    - Thiamine
    - Multivitamins
- Alcoholic ketoacidosis
  - Aggressive rehydration with D5 0.9 NS
  - Exclude other causes of wide anion-gap metabolic acidosis
- Alcohol withdrawal syndrome:
  - Benzodiazepines are agent of choice (diazepam, lorazepam, or chlordiazepoxide):
    - Cross-tolerant with alcohol
    - Increases GABA$_A$-mediated transmission
    - Anticonvulsant effect
    - Large, frequent doses required with significant withdrawal
    - May halt progression to DTs
  - Barbiturates (phenobarbital):
    - Cross-tolerant with alcohol
    - Anticonvulsant effect
    - Useful if severe withdrawal or DTs refractory to large doses of benzodiazepines
  - Propofol:
    - Agent of choice for intubated patients
    - Completely suppresses seizure activity
    - Requires intubation/ventilation
    - Caution if hypotensive

- β-blocker (labetalol, esmolol, or metoprolol):
  - Normalizes vital sign abnormalities
  - Does *not* treat CNS complications of alcohol use or withdrawal
- α-Agonist (clonidine):
  - Centrally acting $\alpha_2$-adrenergic agonist
  - Normalizes vital sign abnormalities
  - Does *not* treat CNS complications of alcohol use or withdrawal
- Phenytoin:
  - Not indicated in alcohol withdrawal seizures
  - Indicated if seizures secondary to idiopathic epilepsy, posttraumatic, or status epilepticus

## MEDICATION
- Chlordiazepoxide (Librium): 25–100 mg, PO or IV q6h
- Dextrose: D$_{50}$W 1 amp (50 mL or 25 g; peds: D$_{25}$W 2–4 mL/kg) IV
- Diazepam (Valium): 5–10 mg IV q5min–q10min until patient calm
- Lorazepam (Ativan): 0.5–4 mg IV/IM q5min–q10min until patient calm
- Naloxone (Narcan): 0.4–2 mg (peds: 0.1 mg/kg) IV or IM initial dose
- Phenobarbital: 10–20 mg/kg IV (loading dose)
- Phenytoin: 15–18 mg/kg at 50 mg/min IV:
  - May give Fosphenytoin at 15–20 mgPF/kg at a maximum rate of 150 mgPE/min
- Propofol: 0.5–1.0 mg/kg IV (loading dose), then 5–50 $\mu$g/kg/min (maintenance dose)
- Thiamine (vitamin B$_1$): 100 mg (peds: 50 mg) IV or IM

# FOLLOW-UP

## DISPOSITION

### Admission Criteria
- Inability to control seizures or withdrawal symptoms with oral medications
- Hepatic failure, infection, dehydration, malnutrition, cardiovascular collapse, cardiac dysrhythmia, or trauma
- Hallucinations, abnormal vital signs, severe tremors, or extreme agitation
- Wernicke encephalopathy
- Confusion or delirium

### Discharge Criteria
- Clinically sober
- Seizure free for 6 hr (with negative workup if 1st seizure)

### Issues for Referral
Discuss with social work and/or police and/or department of family services for pediatric patients.

### FOLLOW-UP RECOMMENDATIONS
Substance abuse referral for patients with recurrent alcohol intoxication/use

## PEARLS AND PITFALLS
- Failure to appreciate AMS due to nonalcoholic causes in chronic alcoholics:
  - Serum levels should drop by 15–40 mg/dL/h
  - If MS not improving (or worsening), need to investigate further
- Failure to adequately treat with benzodiazepines:
  - May require massive doses (eg, 200–300 mg of diazepam) to control
  - If unable to control, consider other GABAergic agents (phenobarbital, propofol).
- Failure to appreciate hypoglycemia as a common entity in these patients:
  - Can masquerade as "intoxication"
  - Can result in poor outcomes
  - Frequently occurs in chronic alcoholics and children

## ADDITIONAL READING
- Chiang C, Wax P. Withdrawal syndromes. In: Ford MD, Delaney KA, Ling LJ, et al., eds. *Clinical Toxicology*. Philadelphia: WB Saunders. 2001; 582–586.
- D'Onofrio G, Degutis LC. Preventive care in the emergency department: Screening and brief intervention for alcohol problems in the emergency department: A systematic review. *Acad Emerg Med*. 2002;9:627–638.
- D'Onofrio G, Rathlev NK, Ulrich AS, et al. Lorazepam for the prevention of recurrent seizures related to alcohol. *N Engl J Med*. 1999;340:915–919.
- Kosten TR, O'Connor PG. Management of drug and alcohol withdrawal. *N Engl J Med*. 2003;348: 1786–1795.
- Mayo-Smith MF. Pharmacological management of alcohol withdrawal. *JAMA*. 1997;278:144–151.
- McMicken DB, Freedland ES. Alcohol-related seizures. *Emerg Med Clin North Am*. 1994;12: 1057–1079.

## See Also (Topic, Algorithm, Electronic Media Element)
- Ethylene Glycol, Poisoning
- Methanol, Poisoning

# ALCOHOLIC KETOACIDOSIS

Jefferson D. Bracey
Charles Garcia

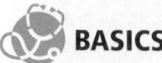 **BASICS**

## DESCRIPTION
- Increased production of ketone bodies due to:
  - Malnourished and hypovolemic patient
  - Depleted glycogen stores in the liver
  - Elevated ratio of NADH/NAD due to ethanol metabolism
  - Increased free fatty acid production
- Elevated NADH/NAD ratio leads to the predominate production of β–hydroxybutyrate (BHB) over acetoacetate (AcAc)

## ETIOLOGY
- Malnourished, chronic alcohol abusers following a recent episode of heavy alcohol consumption:
  - Develop nausea, vomiting, or abdominal pain
  - Leading to the cessation of alcohol ingestion
- Presentation usually occurs within 12–72 hr

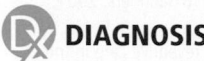 **DIAGNOSIS**

## SIGNS AND SYMPTOMS
- Dehydration
- Fever absent unless there is an underlying infection
- Tachycardia (common) due to:
  - Dehydration with associated orthostatic changes
  - Concurrent alcohol withdrawal
- Tachypnea:
  - Common
  - Deep, rapid, Kussmaul respirations frequently present
- Nausea and vomiting
- Abdominal pain (nausea, vomiting, and abdominal pain are most common symptoms):
  - Usually diffuse with nonspecific tenderness
  - Epigastric pain common
  - Rebound tenderness, abdominal distension, hypoactive bowel sounds uncommon
  - Mandates a search for an alternative, coexistent illness
- Decreased urinary output from hypovolemia
- Mental status:
  - Minimally altered as a result of hypovolemia and possibly intoxication
  - Altered mental status mandates a search for other associated conditions such as:
    - Head injury, cerebrovascular accident (CVA), or intracranial hemorrhage
    - Hypoglycemia
    - Alcohol withdrawal
    - Encephalopathy
    - Toxins
  - Visual disturbances:
    - Reports of isolated visual disturbances with AKA common

## History
Chronic alcohol use:
- Recent binge
- Abrupt cessation

## Physical Exam
- Findings of dehydration most common
- May have ketotic odor
- Kussmaul respirations
- Palmar erythema (alcoholism)

## ESSENTIAL WORKUP
- Presence of an increased anion gap metabolic acidosis secondary to the presence of ketones
- Differentiate from toxic alcohol ingestion and other causes of anion gap metabolic acidosis.

## DIAGNOSTIC TESTS & INTERPRETATION
### Lab
- Acid–base disturbance:
  - Increased anion gap metabolic acidosis hallmark
  - Mixed acid–base disturbance common:
    - Respiratory alkalosis
    - Metabolic alkalosis secondary to vomiting and dehydration
    - Hyperchloremic acidosis
  - Mild lactic acidosis common
    - Due to dehydration and the direct metabolic effects of ethanol
    - Profound lactic acidosis should prompt a search for other disorders such as seizures, hypoxia, and shock.
  - Positive urine and serum nitroprusside reaction tests for ketoacids
    - May not reflect the severity of the underlying ketoacidosis, since BHB predominates and is not measured by this test.
    - May become misleadingly more positive during treatment as more AcAc is produced.
- Electrolytes:
  - Decreased serum bicarbonate
  - Hypokalemia due to vomiting
  - Hypocalcemia
  - Hypophosphatemia
  - Hypomagnesemia
- Glucose:
  - Usually mildly elevated
  - Should be monitored frequently as per DKA
  - Hypoglycemia may be present
- Alcohol level may be elevated or normal
- BUN and creatinine mildly elevated due to dehydration

- CBC:
  - Mild leukocytosis
  - Thrombocytopenia and anemia commonly due to chronic alcoholism
- Urinalysis:
  - Ketonuria without glucosuria
- Amylase/lipase:
  - Elevated with associated pancreatitis
- LFTs:
  - Mildly elevated LFTs
- Osmolal gap:
  - May be elevated
  - Elevation >20 mOsm/kg should prompt evaluation for other ingestions (methanol and ethylene glycol)
  - Correct for ethanol level in osmolal gap by dividing ethanol level by 4.6

### Imaging
- CXR if suspect associated pneumonia
- Abdominal films for free air if an acute abdomen is present
- CT scan of the head if associated trauma or unexplained altered mental status

## DIFFERENTIAL DIAGNOSIS
- Elevated anion gap metabolic acidosis: *ACAAT MUDPILES:*
  - **A**lcoholic ketoacidosis
  - **C**yanide, CO, H₂S, others
  - **A**cetaminophen:
    - Rare in acute ingestion
    - Rare in chronic ingestion
    - Fulminant hepatic failure
  - **A**ntiretrovirals (NRTI)
  - **T**oluene
  - **M**ethanol, metformin
  - **U**remia
  - **D**iabetic ketoacidosis
  - **P**araldehyde, phenformin, propylene glycol
  - **I**ron, INH
  - **L**actic acidosis
  - **E**thylene glycol
  - **S**alicylate, acetylsalicylic acid (ASA; aspirin), starvation ketosis
- Hypovolemia:
  - GI bleeding
  - Sepsis
- Abdominal pain:
  - Pancreatitis
  - GI bleeding
  - Gastritis
  - Hepatitis
  - Perforated ulcer
  - Alcohol withdrawal

**TREATMENT**

### PRE-HOSPITAL

- Supportive measures including IV access with 0.9 NS, oxygen, and cardiac monitoring
- Search for historical clues that may suggest other etiologies such as toxic ingestions or diabetic history, consider scene search
- Attend to other possible coexistent illnesses such as GI bleeding.

### INITIAL STABILIZATION/THERAPY

- Cardiac monitor and supplement oxygen
- Naloxone, thiamine, and dextrose if altered mental status
- Initiate 0.9 NS IV fluids
  - 500 cc–1 L bolus
  - Resuscitation as necessary
  - Promotes renal excretion of ketone bodies

### ED TREATMENT/PROCEDURES

- Antiemetic for vomiting—ondansetron, promethazine, or prochlorperazine
- Benzodiazepines for symptoms of alcohol withdrawal
- Start dextrose containing solutions ($D_5NS$):
  - More rapid resolution of the metabolic abnormalities than saline alone
  - Rate higher than maintenance as tolerated until acidosis resolves
  - Avoid with significant hyperglycemia Repletes glycogen stores
  - Decreases production of ketone bodies by stimulating the production of endogenous insulin
- Thiamine repletion (IV) prior to glucose administration to avoid precipitating Wernicke encephalopathy
- Sodium bicarbonate rarely indicated:
  - Consider in severe acidosis with associated cardiovascular dysfunction or irritability

- Electrolyte replacement:
  - Hypokalemia occurs with treatment and should be anticipated.
  - Hypophosphatemia may occur with treatment.
  - Magnesium replacement as indicated for both hypomagnesemia and hypokalemia
- Insulin is not indicated and may precipitate hypoglycemia.

### MEDICATION

- $D_{50}W$: 1 ampule of 50% dextrose (25 g) IVP
- Lorazepam (benzodiazepine): 2 mg IV and titrate to effect
- Narcan: 2 mg IVP
- Ondansetron: 4–8 mg IVP
- Prochlorperazine: 5–10 mg IVP
- Promethazine: 12.5–25 mg IVP
- Thiamine: 100 mg IVP

## FOLLOW-UP

### DISPOSITION

#### Admission Criteria

- Persistent metabolic acidosis
- Persistent orthostatic hypotension
- Persistent nausea and vomiting
- Abdominal pain of uncertain etiology
- Co-morbid illness requiring admission for treatment
- Monitored bed due to electrolyte abnormalities requiring continued treatment

#### Discharge Criteria

- Many patients can be managed in observation unit over 12–24 hr.
- Tolerating oral fluids well
- Resolution of metabolic abnormalities
- No other associated illnesses requiring additional therapy

### FOLLOW-UP RECOMMENDATIONS

Counseling regarding alcohol cessation

## PEARLS AND PITFALLS

- Aggressive volume repletion with dextrose containing fluid is key.
- Thiamine repletion
- Monitor electrolytes before and after treatment.
- Unrecognized increased osmolal gap
- Inadequate monitoring of glucose levels
- Must be placed on monitor:
  - Cases of sudden death in AKA:
    ○ Possible alcoholic cardiomyopathy
    ○ Dysrhythmias
    ○ Electrolyte derangements

## ADDITIONAL READING

- Diltoer M, Troubleyn J, Lauwers R, et al. Ketosis and cardiac failure: Common signs of a single condition. *Eur J Emerg Med.* 2004;11(3):172–175.
- McGuire L, Cruickshank A, Munro P. Alcoholic ketoacidosis. *Emerg Med J.* 2006;23:417–420.
- Wrenn KD, Slovis CM, et al. The syndrome of alcoholic ketoacidosis. *Am J Med.* 1991;91(2): 119–128.
- Yanagawa Y, Kiyozumi T, et al. Reversible blindness associated with alcoholic ketoacidosis. *Am J Opthalmology.* 2003;137(4):775–777.
- Yanagawa Y, Sakamoto T, et al. Six cases of sudden cardiac arrest in alcoholic ketoacidosis. *Internal Medicine.* 2008;47(2):113–117

### See Also (Topic, Algorithm, Electronic Media Element)

- Acidosis
- Diabetic Ketoacidosis

# ALKALOSIS
*Matthew Robinson*

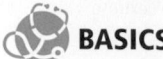 **BASICS**

## DESCRIPTION
- Respiratory alkalosis:
  - Elevated serum pH secondary to alveolar hyperventilation and decreased $PaCO_2$
  - Hyperventilation occurs through stimulation of 2 receptor types:
    - Central receptors—located in the brainstem and respond to decreased CSF pH
    - Chest receptors—located in aortic arch and respond to hypoxemia
  - Increased alveolar ventilation secondary to:
    - Disorders causing acidosis
    - Hypoxemia *or*
    - Nonphysiologic stimulation of those receptors by CNS or chest disorders
  - Rarely life threatening with pH typically <7.50
- Metabolic alkalosis:
  - Primary increase in serum $HCO_3^-$ secondary to loss of $H^+$ or gain of $HCO_3^-$
  - Pathogenesis requires an initial process that generates the metabolic alkalosis with a secondary or overlapping process maintaining the alkalosis.
- Generation occurs through one of the following mechanisms:
  - Gain of alkali through ingestion or infusion
  - Loss of $H^+$ through the GI tract or kidneys
  - Shift of hydrogen ions into the intracellular space
  - Contraction of extracellular fluid (ECF) volume with loss of $HCO_3^-$-poor fluids
- Renal maintenance is required to sustain a metabolic alkalosis secondary to the kidney's enormous ability to excrete $HCO_3^-$. This occurs through the following:
  - Decreased GFR (renal failure, ECF depletion)
  - Elevated tubular reabsorption of $HCO_3^-$ secondary to hypochloremia, hyperaldosteronism, hypokalemia, ECF depletion
- Mortality 45% if pH >7.55 and 80% if pH >7.65

## ETIOLOGY
- Respiratory alkalosis:
  - CNS:
    - Hyperventilation syndrome
    - Pain
    - Anxiety/psychosis
    - Fever
    - Cerebrovascular accident (CVA)
    - CNS infection (meningitis, encephalitis)
    - CNS mass lesion (tumor, trauma)
  - Hypoxemia:
    - Altitude
    - Anemia
    - Shunt
  - Medications/drugs:
    - Progesterone
    - Methylxanthines
    - Salicylates
    - Catecholamines
    - Nicotine
  - Endocrine:
    - Hyperthyroidism
    - Pregnancy

- Chest stimulation:
  - Pulmonary embolism
  - Pneumonia
  - Pneumothorax
- Other:
  - Sepsis
  - Hepatic failure
  - Heat exhaustion
- Metabolic alkalosis:
  - GI loss of $H^+$:
    - Vomiting
    - Nasogastric suctioning
    - Bulimia
    - Antacid therapy
    - Chloride losing diarrhea (villous adenoma)
  - Renal loss:
    - Diuretics (loop and thiazide)
    - Postchronic hypercapnia
    - Mineralocorticoid excess
    - Hyperaldosteronism
    - Drug/medication (carbenicillin)
    - Glucocorticoid excess (Cushing disease)
    - Gitelman syndrome
    - Hypercalcemia
    - Milk-alkali syndrome
    - Low chloride intake
    - Bartter syndrome
  - Intracellular $H^+$ shift:
    - Hypokalemia
    - Refeeding
  - Contraction alkalosis:
    - Diuretics
    - Sweat loss in CF
    - Gastric losses
  - $HCO_3^-$ retention:
    - $NaHCO_3$ infusion
    - Blood transfusions

 **DIAGNOSIS**

## SIGNS AND SYMPTOMS
- Signs and symptoms secondary to:
  - Arteriolar vasoconstriction
  - Hypocalcemia secondary to decreased ionized calcium from increased calcium binding to albumin
  - Associated hypokalemia
  - Underlying cause
- Weakness
- Seizures
- Altered mental status
- Tetany
- Chvostek sign
- Trousseau sign
- Arrhythmias
- Myalgias
- Carpal-pedal spasm
- Perioral tingling/numbness
- Hypoxemia
- Dehydration

## ESSENTIAL WORKUP
- Electrolytes:
  - Elevated $HCO_3^-$ with metabolic alkalosis
  - Evaluate for hypokalemia and hypocalcemia.
- BUN/creatinine:
  - Evaluate for renal failure or dehydration.
- Arterial blood gases:
  - pH
  - $PCO_2$ decreased in respiratory alkalosis
  - $PO_2$ for hypoxemia
- Calculate compensation to identify mixed acid–base disorders:
  - Acute respiratory alkalosis:
    - $HCO_3^-$ decreases secondary to intracellular shift and buffering within 10–20 min.
    - Expected $HCO_3^-$ decreased by 2 mEq/dL for each 10 mm Hg decrease in $PCO_2$.
  - Chronic respiratory alkalosis:
    - $HCO_3^-$ decreased secondary to renal secretion of $HCO_3^-$
    - Requires 48–72 hr for maximal compensation
    - Expected $HCO_3^-$ decreased by 5 mEq/dL for each 10 mm Hg decrease in $PCO_2$.
    - If $HCO_3^-$ greater than predicted, concomitant metabolic alkalosis
    - If $HCO_3^-$ less than predicted, concomitant metabolic acidosis
  - Metabolic alkalosis:
    - Expected $PCO_2 = 0.9 [HCO_3^-] + 9$
    - If $PCO_2$ greater than predicted, concomitant respiratory acidosis
    - If $PCO_2$ less than predicted, concomitant respiratory alkalosis
- Urine chloride:
  - More accurate marker than urine $Na^+$ for patient's volume status:
    - $UCl^-$ <20 mEq/L in volume depletion
    - $UCl^-$ >40 mEq/L in euvolemia or edematous states
  - Useful in therapy for determining saline-responsive vs. saline-resistant causes of metabolic alkalosis

## DIAGNOSTIC TESTS & INTERPRETATION
### Lab
- Glucose
- Ionized calcium
- Magnesium level
- Urine pregnancy
- Additional labs to evaluate underlying cause:
  - CBC, blood cultures for sepsis
  - LFT for hepatic failure
  - Aspirin level
  - Urine toxicology screen
  - Urine diuretics screen (bulimia)
  - Urine diuretic screen (surreptitious diuretic abuse)
  - Renin level
  - Cortisol level
  - Aldosterone level
  - TSH, T4
  - D-dimer

## Imaging
CXR:

- May identify cardiomyopathy or CHF
- Underlying pneumonia

### Diagnostic Procedures/Surgery
ECG:

- May identify regional wall motion abnormalities or valvular dysfunction
- Evaluate for conduction disturbances.

## DIFFERENTIAL DIAGNOSIS
- Respiratory alkalosis:
  - It is essential to rule out organic disease prior to diagnosing hyperventilation syndrome or anxiety states.
- Metabolic alkalosis:
  - Saline responsive (urine Cl$^-$ <20 mEq/dL):
    - Loss of gastric secretions
    - Chloride-losing diarrhea
    - Diuretics
    - Postchronic hypercapnia
    - CF
  - Saline resistant:
    - Hyperaldosteronism
    - Cushing syndrome
    - Bartter syndrome
    - Exogenous mineralocorticoids or glucocorticoids
    - Gitelman syndrome
    - Hypokalemia
    - Hypomagnesemia
    - Milk-alkali syndrome
    - Exogenous alkali infusion/ingestion
    - Blood transfusions

 TREATMENT

### INITIAL STABILIZATION/THERAPY
Airway, breathing, circulation (ABCs):

- Early intubation and airway control for obtundation or altered mental status
- IV, oxygen, and cardiac monitor
- Naloxone, D$_{50}$W (or Accu-Chek), and thiamine for altered mental status

## ED TREATMENT/PROCEDURES
- Respiratory alkalosis:
  - Treat underlying disorder.
  - Rarely life threatening
  - Sedation/anxiolytics for anxiety, psychosis, or drug overdose
  - Rebreathing mask bag for hyperventilation syndrome (used cautiously)
- Metabolic alkalosis: Examination of the urine chloride allows etiologies to be divided into saline responsive or saline resistant causes:
  - Urine chloride <20 mEq/L indicates volume depletion:
    - Rehydration with 0.9% saline lowers serum HCO$_3^-$ by increasing renal HCO$_3^-$ excretion
    - Saline responsive causes are associated with volume depletion.
  - Urine chloride >20 mEq/L indicates saline resistant etiology. Treat underlying disorder:
    - Potassium supplementation in hypokalemic states
    - Antagonism of aldosterone with spironolactone
    - Acetazolamide to increase renal HCO$_3^-$ excretion in edematous states
  - Other:
    - Infusion of dilute HCl in severe cases of metabolic alkalosis
    - Antiemetics for vomiting
    - Proton pump inhibitors for patients with nasogastric (NG) suction
    - Follow ventilatory status closely.
    - Correct electrolyte abnormalities.
    - Consider hemodialysis for severe electrolyte abnormalities.

## MEDICATION
- Dextrose: D$_{50}$W 1 amp (50 mL or 25 g; peds: 2% dextrose and water 2–4 mL/kg) IV
- KCl (K-Dur, Gen-K, Klor-Con): 20–120 mEq PO daily
- Naloxone: 2 mg (peds: 0.1 mg/kg) IV or IM initial dose
- Thiamine (vitamin B$_1$): 100 mg (peds: 50 mg) IV or IM
- 0.1–0.2N HCl (100–200 mEq/L): Infuse over 24–48 hr at rate not faster than 0.2 mmol/kg/hr

 FOLLOW-UP

### DISPOSITION
#### Admission Criteria
- ICU admission if:
  - pH >7.55 or altered mental status
  - Dysrhythmias
  - Severe electrolyte abnormalities
  - Hemodynamic instability
- Coexisting medical illness requiring admission

#### Discharge Criteria
Resolving or resolved alkalosis

## PEARLS AND PITFALLS
- Increased minute ventilation is the primary cause of respiratory alkalosis, characterized by decreased PaCO$_2$ and increased pH.
  - Metabolic alkalosis is usually caused by an increase in HCO$_3^-$, reabsorption secondary to volume, potassium, or Cl$^-$ loss.
  - Contraction alkalosis can result from extracellular volume reduction, with a consequent increase in the plasma HCO$_3^-$ concentration.
  - Clues to the presence of a mixed acid–base disorder are normal pH with abnormal PCO$_2$ or HCO$_3^-$, when the HCO$_3^-$ and PCO$_2$ move in opposite directions, or when the pH changes in the direction opposite that expected from a known primary disorder.

## ADDITIONAL READING
- Adrogue H. Management of life-threatening acid-base disorders. New Engl J Med. 1998; 338:107.
- Khanna A. Metabolic alkalosis. Respir Care. 2001; 46:354.
- Khanna A, Kurtzman NA. Metabolic alkalosis. J Nephrol. 2006;Suppl 9:S86–96.
- Laski ME, Sabatini S. Metabolic alkalosis, bedside and bench. Semin Nephrol. 2006;26(6):404–421.
- Whittier W. Primer on clinical acid-base problem solving. Dis Mon. 2004;50:117.

### See Also (Topic, Algorithm, Electronic Media Element)
Acidosis

# ALTERED MENTAL STATUS

*David F. M. Brown*
*Lisa E. Thomas*

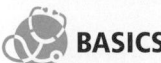 **BASICS**

## DESCRIPTION
- Dysfunction in either the reticular activating system in the upper brainstem or a large area of one or both cerebral hemispheres
- Definitions:
  - Confusion: A behavioral state of reduced mental clarity, coherence, comprehension, and reasoning
  - Drowsiness: The patient cannot be easily aroused by touch or noise and cannot maintain alertness for some time.
  - Lethargy: Depressed mental status in which the patient may appear wakeful but has depressed awareness of self and environment globally; cannot be aroused to full function
  - Stupor: The patient can be awakened only by vigorous stimuli, and an effort to avoid uncomfortable or aggravating stimulation is displayed.
  - Coma: The patient cannot be aroused by stimulation and no purposeful attempt is made to avoid painful stimuli.
  - Delirium: Acute onset of fluctuating cognition with impaired attention and consciousness, ranging from confusion to stupor.

## ETIOLOGY
- Hypoxic:
  - Severe pulmonary disease
  - Anemia
  - Shock
  - Intracardiac shunting (especially in pediatrics)
- Metabolic:
  - Hypoglycemia; hyperglycemia
  - Diabetic ketoacidosis
  - Nonketotic hyperosmolar coma
  - Hyponatremia; hypernatremia
  - Hypocalcemia; hypercalcemia
  - Hypomagnesemia; hypermagnesemia
  - Hypophosphatemia
  - Acidosis; alkalosis
  - Dehydration
  - Deficiency: Thiamine, folic acid, B12, niacin
  - Hyperammonemia (hepatic encephalopathy)
  - Uremia (renal failure)
  - $CO_2$ narcosis
- Toxicologic:
  - Toxic alcohols
  - Salicylates
  - Sedatives and narcotics
  - GHB (gamma-hydroxy-butyrate)
  - Anticonvulsants
  - Psychotropics
  - Isoniazid
  - Heavy metals
  - Carbon monoxide
  - Cyanide
  - Toxic plants (jimsonweed, mushrooms, etc.)
  - Sympathomimetics
  - Anticholinergic, cholinergic
  - Antiemetics
  - Antiparkinsonian medications
  - Withdrawal (especially alcohol, sedatives)
- Infectious:
  - UTI (especially in elderly)
  - Pneumonia
  - Sepsis; bacteremia
  - Meningitis, encephalitis, brain abscess

- Endocrine:
  - Myxedema coma
  - Thyrotoxicosis
  - Hypothyroidism
  - Addison disease
  - Cushing disease
  - Pheochromocytoma
  - Hyperparathyroidism
- Environmental:
  - Hypothermia
  - Hyperthermia; heat stroke
  - High-altitude cerebral edema
  - Neuroleptic malignant syndrome
  - Malignant hyperthermia
- Vascular:
  - Hypertensive encephalopathy
  - Cerebral vasculitis
  - TTP, DIC, hyperviscosity
  - MI
- Primary Neurologic:
  - Seizures, nonconvulsive status epilepticus, and postictal state
  - Head trauma, concussion
  - Diffuse axonal injury
  - Structural brain lesions:
    ○ Hemorrhage (subdural, epidural, subarachnoid, intraparenchymal)
    ○ Infarction
    ○ Tumors
    ○ Demyelination disorders
  - Intracranial hypertension (pseudotumor)
  - HIV-related encephalopathy
  - Autoimmune/inflammatory encephalitis
  - Carcinoid meningitis
  - Primary neuronal or glial disorders:
    ○ Creutzfeldt-Jakob disease
    ○ Marchiafava-Bignami disease
    ○ Adrenoleukodystrophy
    ○ Gliomatosis cerebri
    ○ Progressive multifocal leukoencephalopathy
- Trauma; burns
- Porphyria
- Psychiatric
- Multifactorial (especially in elderly)

 **DIAGNOSIS**

## SIGNS AND SYMPTOMS
### Confusion
- Difficulty in maintaining a coherent stream of thinking and mental performance:
  - Remember to consider level of education, language, and possible learning disabilities.
- Inattention
- Memory deficit:
  - Inability to recall any of the following:
    ○ The date, inclusive of month, day, year, and day of week
    ○ The precise place
    ○ Items of universally known information
    ○ Why the patient is in the hospital
    ○ Address, telephone number, or Social Security number

- Impaired mental performance:
  - Difficulty retaining seven digits forward and four backward
  - Difficulty naming ordinary objects
  - Serial calculations: 3-from-30 subtraction test
- Disorganized and rambling language:
  - May be mistaken for aphasia
  - **Findings That Suggest an Underlying Cause**
- Fever:
  - Infectious etiologies, drug toxicities, endocrine disorders, heat stroke
- Severe hypertension & bradycardia
  - Cushing reflex-suggests intracranial lesion
- Hypotension:
  - Infectious, toxicologic etiologies, decreased cardiac output
- Eye movements:
  - Ocular bobbing:
    ○ Cyclical brisk conjugate caudal jerks of the globes followed by a slow return to midposition
    ○ Seen in bilateral pontine damage, metabolic derangement, and brainstem compression
  - Ocular dipping:
    ○ Slow, cyclical, conjugate, downward movement of the eyes followed by a rapid return to midposition
    ○ Seen in diffuse cortical anoxic damage
- Pupil examination:
  - Nearly all toxic and metabolic causes of coma leave the pupillary reflexes sluggish but bilaterally intact.
- Focal findings (indicative of CNS process):
  - Hemiparesis
  - Hemianopsia
  - Aphasia
  - Myoclonus
  - Convulsions
  - Nuchal rigidity
- Asterixis:
  - Arrhythmic flapping tremor (almost always bilateral)
  - Seen in hepatic failure or severe renal failure

### History
- Ask witnesses, family, prehospital personnel
- Baseline mental status
- Medical history (immunosuppressed, liver failure, depression, or chronic conditions)
- Recent events: Trauma, fever, illness
- Detailed medication list
- Substance abuse history

### Physical Exam
- Vital signs
- Head: Signs of trauma, pupils
- Fundoscopic exam: Hemorrhage, papilledema
- Neck: rigidity, bruits, thyroid enlargement
- Heart and lungs
- Abdomen: Organomegaly, ascites
- Extremities: Cyanosis
- Skin: Diaphoretic/dry, rash, petechiae, ecchymoses, splinter hemorrhages, needle tracks
- Neurologic exam
- Mental status exam

## DIAGNOSTIC TESTS & INTERPRETATION
### Lab
- Dextrostix and glucose
- CBC
- Electrolytes (including Ca, Mg, Phos)
- Blood urea nitrogen, creatinine
- Toxicologic screen (including toxic alcohols)
- ECG
- Urinalysis
- Blood and urine cultures (suspected infection)
- PT, PTT (anticoagulated, liver failure patients)
- Consider LFTs, thyroid function tests, ammonia, serum osmolarity, arterial blood gas
- Consider B12, folic acid, RPR, urine porphobilinogen, heavy metal screening

### Imaging
- Head CT scan:
  - Noncontrast only to rule out hemorrhage and mass effect
- Chest Radiograph: To diagnose pneumonia
- MRI (if available):
  - Indicated when suspicious of ischemic stroke or other CNS abnormality
  - May be deferred when admitting the patient as part of the inpatient work-up

### Diagnostic Procedures/Surgery
- Lumbar puncture (LP):
  - Indicated when the etiology remains unclear after laboratory and CT scan
  - Empiric antibiotics should be given before LP to avoid any delay in therapy in patients with suspected meningitis.
- EEG (inpatient): For suspected seizure, nonconvulsive status epilepticus
- Caloric stimulation of the vestibular apparatus to assess unresponsive patients:
  - Contraindications: tympanic membrane perforation and cerumen impaction.
  - Irrigate auditory canal with 10 cc of ice-cold water after head is elevated 30 degrees.
  - Bilateral tonic deviation of the eyes toward the stimulus indicates an intact brainstem.
  - Nystagmus-like quick corrective phases indicates intact cerebral hemispheres.
  - A normal response in an unresponsive patient raises the suspicion of psychogenic coma.

## DIFFERENTIAL DIAGNOSIS
- Locked-in syndrome:
  - Rare disorder caused by damage to the corticospinal, corticopontine, and corticobulbar tracts resulting in quadriplegia and mutism with preservation of consciousness.
  - Communication may be established through eye movements (maintain vertical eye movements).
- Psychogenic unresponsiveness:
  - Conversion reactions
  - Catatonia
  - Malingering
  - Akinetic mutism (abulic state)
- Dementia:
  - Multiple progressive cognitive deficits
  - Attention is preserved in the early stages.

 **TREATMENT**

### PRE-HOSPITAL
- Airway management if loss of airway patency
- IV access, supplemental oxygen, cardiac monitor
- Spine immobilization if possibility of trauma
- "Coma cocktail":
  - Dextrose
  - Naloxone
  - Thiamine
- Look for signs of an underlying cause.
  - Medications, medic alert bracelets
  - Document a basic neurologic examination, GCS, pupils, extremity movements
  - Gross signs of trauma
- CONTROVERSIES
  - Empirical dextrose should not be withheld or delayed if Dextrostix is not available
    - Glucose can be safely administered before thiamine.

### INITIAL STABILIZATION/THERAPY
- IV D50
- Naloxone
- Thiamine

### ED TREATMENT/PROCEDURES
- Consider empiric use of antibiotics for altered mental status of undetermined etiology:
  - Broad spectrum with good CSF fluid penetration such as ceftriaxone and vancomycin
- Urgent CT if suspected intracranial bleed
- Empiric treatment if a toxic ingestion is suspected:
  - Activated charcoal
  - Alcohol drip or fomepizole if methanol or ethylene glycol is suspected
- Correct body temperature.
  - Warmed humidified O2 and IV fluids if hypothermic
  - Ice packs and forced air movement over exposed moistened skin if severe hyperthermia
- Specific therapy directed at underlying cause
  - (ie, IV fluids for dehydration, oxygen for hypoxia)

### MEDICATION
- Ceftriaxone: 2 g (peds: 50–75 mg/kg) IV
- Dextrose: 1–2 mL/kg of D50W (peds: 2–4 mL/kg D25W) IV
- Diazepam: 0.1–0.3 mg/kg slow IV (max 10 mg/dose) q10min–q15min × three doses
- Lorazepam: 0.05–0.1 mg/kg IV (max 4 mg/dose q10min–q15min)
- Mannitol: 0.5–1 g/kg IV
- Naloxone: 0.01–0.1 mg/kg IV/IM/SC/ET
- Thiamine: 100 mg IM or 100 mg thiamine in 1,000 mL of IV fluid wide open
- Vancomycin 1 g (peds: 10 mg/kg) IV

 **FOLLOW-UP**

### DISPOSITION
### Admission Criteria
All patients with acute and persistent changes in mental status require admission.

### Discharge Criteria
- Treated hypoglycemia related to insulin therapy with resolved symptoms
- Chronic altered mental status (eg, dementia) without change from baseline
- Acute drug intoxication with return of patient's mental status to baseline with observation and drug has no potential for delayed toxicity

### FOLLOW-UP RECOMMENDATIONS
Primary care follow-up to manage etiology which led to altered mental status (ie, adjust medication dosing, drug abuse treatment referral)

## PEARLS AND PITFALLS
- Consider reversible causes
  - Hypoglycemia (check glucose, give dextrose)
  - Opiate overdose (trial of naloxone)
  - Thiamine deficiency (trial of thiamine)
  - Address abnormal vital signs (IV fluids for hypotension, O2 for hypoxia, warming for hypothermia)
- Consider head CT for any patient with unclear etiology or neurologic abnormality
- Consider empiric antibiotics in patients with fever or unclear etiology

## ADDITIONAL READING
- Kanich W, Brady WJ, Huff JS, Perron AD, Holstege C, Lindbeck G, Carter CT. Altered mental status: evaluation and etiology in the ED. *Am J Emerg Med*. 2002;20:613–617.
- Leong LB, Jian KHW, Vasu A, Seow E. Prospective study of patients with altered mental status: clinical features and outcome. *Int J Emerg Med*. 2008;1: 179–182.
- Wilber S. Altered mental status in older emergency department patients. *Emerg Med Clin N Am*. 2006; 24:299–316.
- Young GB. Disorders of consciousness: Coma. *Ann NY Acad Sci*. 2009;1157:32–47.

### See Also (Topic, Algorithm, Electronic Media Element)
Coma

## CODES

### ICD9
- 298.9 Unspecified psychosis
- 780.09 Alteration of consciousness, other
- 780.97 Altered mental status

# AMEBIASIS

*Ann P. Nguyen*

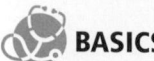

## BASICS

### DESCRIPTION
- Invasive parasitic infection with both intestinal and extraintestinal manifestations
- Endemic in developing countries
- Populations at risk:
  - Travelers to, citizens of, and immigrants from endemic areas
  - Institutionalized persons
  - Practitioners of anal sexual activity
- Risk factors for increased severity of disease and complications:
  - Corticosteroid use
  - Malignancy
  - Malnutrition
  - Pregnancy/postpartum state
  - Extremes of age

### ETIOLOGY
- *Entamoeba histolytica*, a nonflagellated protozoa
- Fecal–oral transmission:
  - Humans are sole reservoir.
- Ingested organisms cause invasive colitis.
- Extraintestinal spread is hematogenous.

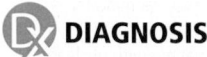

## DIAGNOSIS

### SIGNS AND SYMPTOMS
- Intestinal disease:
  - Onset 1 wk to 1 mo postexposure
  - Acute diarrhea (nondysenteric colitis):
    ○ 80% of cases
    ○ Afebrile
    ○ Occult blood in stool
    ○ Benign abdominal exam
  - Classic dysentery:
    ○ Bloody mucoid diarrhea
    ○ Abdominal pain
    ○ Tenesmus
    ○ Weight loss
    ○ Fever (rare)
    ○ Benign abdominal exam
  - Fulminant colitis:
    ○ Toxic-appearing patient
    ○ Rigid abdomen (25%)
    ○ Fever
    ○ Severe bloody diarrhea
    ○ Rapid progression to perforated bowel and frank peritonitis
    ○ >40% mortality
  - Toxic megacolon:
    ○ Toxic-appearing patient
    ○ Profuse diarrhea (>10 stools per day)
    ○ Fever
    ○ Distended, tympanitic abdomen with signs of peritonitis
    ○ Associated with corticosteroid use
    ○ High mortality

- Ameboma:
  ○ Intraluminal granulated mass
  ○ Tender palpable mass on exam
- Amebic strictures:
  ○ Owing to chronic inflammation and scarring
  ○ Crampy abdominal pain
  ○ Nausea and vomiting (may be feculent)
  ○ Presents as partial or complete bowel obstruction
- Chronic amebic colitis:
  ○ Mild recurrent episodes of bloody diarrhea, abdominal cramping, and tenesmus
  ○ Weight loss
  ○ May persist for years
- Extraintestinal disease:
  - Amebic liver abscess:
    ○ Most frequent extraintestinal manifestation (3–9% of cases)
    ○ Single abscess in right lobe (50–80%)
    ○ May develop months to years postexposure (median of 3 mo)
    ○ Fever
    ○ Right upper quadrant pain
    ○ Hepatomegaly with point tenderness
    ○ Rales at right lung base
    ○ Concurrent diarrhea unusual (20–33%)
    ○ Complication: Rupture into pleural cavity (10–20%), peritoneum or pericardium (rare)
    ○ Increased risk of rupture if >5 cm in diameter or left lobe location
  - Extrahepatic amebic abscess:
    ○ Brain
    ○ Lung
    ○ Perinephric
    ○ Splenic
    ○ Vaginal/cervical/uterine
  - Cutaneous amebiasis:
    ○ Perineum and genitalia
    ○ Painful, irregularly shaped ulcers
    ○ Purulent exudate

### Pediatric Considerations
Fulminant colitis is more likely

### Pregnancy Considerations
Fulminant colitis is more likely

### History
- Possible sources of exposure
- Membership in high-risk group

### Physical Exam
- Identify evidence of peritonitis, sepsis, or shock.
- Tender abdominal mass mandates workup for liver abscess or ameboma.
- Digital rectal exam shows gross or occult blood in >70% of patients.

## DIAGNOSTIC TESTS & INTERPRETATION
### Lab
- CBC:
  - Leukocytosis in amebic liver abscess and peritonitis
- Alkaline phosphatase and ALT:
  - Elevated in amebic liver abscess
- Serum electrolytes, BUN/creatinine if prolonged diarrhea or evidence of dehydration
- Stool PCR is diagnostic gold standard:
  - 100% sensitive and specific
- Stool ELISA for *E. histolytica*–specific antigen:
  - 74–95% sensitive, 93–100% specific
- Serum for anti-*E. histolytica* antibodies:
  - Essential if suspecting liver abscess as these patients rarely shed parasites in their stool
  - 90–100% sensitive in amebic liver abscess
  - 70–90% sensitive in amebic colitis
- Stool microscopy is <60% sensitive and no longer the test of choice.
- Fecal leukocytes and culture:
  - To rule out infection owing to enteroinvasive bacteria
  - Negative in amebiasis

### Imaging
- Abdominal US:
  - 58–90% sensitive for liver abscess
  - Evaluate abscess for increased risk of rupture (>5 cm or located in left lobe)
- Abdominal CT or MRI:
  - Equivalent to US for delineating liver abscesses
  - Superior to US for detecting abscesses in other organs
- Head CT or MRI:
  - Suspect amebic brain abscess if patient with known amebiasis has altered mental status or focal neurologic findings.
  - Irregular nonenhancing lesions
- CXR:
  - Elevated right hemidiaphragm and/or right pleural effusion in liver abscess

### Diagnostic Procedures/Surgery
- Colonoscopy with biopsy:
  - Provides definitive diagnosis of amebic dysentery, colitis, ameboma, and amebic stricture.
- Percutaneous fine-needle aspiration of liver abscess:
  - To exclude bacterial abscess if nondiagnostic serology or antiamebic therapy fails
  - Not for primary treatment of liver abscesses

## DIFFERENTIAL DIAGNOSIS

- Intestinal amebiasis:
  - Enteroinvasive bacterial infection (*Staphylococcus, E. coli, Shigella, Salmonella, Yersinia, Campylobacter*)
  - Inflammatory bowel disease
  - Ischemic colitis
  - Arteriovenous malformation
  - Abdominal aortic aneurysm
  - Perforated duodenal ulcer
  - Intussusception
  - Diverticulitis
  - Pancreatitis
  - Colorectal carcinoma
- Amebic abscess:
  - Bacterial abscess
  - Tuberculous cavity
  - Echinococcal cyst
  - Malignancy
  - Cholecystitis
- Cutaneous amebiasis:
  - Carcinoma
  - STDs (condyloma acuminata, chancroid, syphilis)

 TREATMENT

### INITIAL STABILIZATION/THERAPY
- Airway, breathing, circulation (ABCs)
- IV 0.9 NS if signs of significant dehydration or shock

### ED TREATMENT/PROCEDURES
- Oral fluids for mild dehydration
- Avoid antidiarrheal agents.
- Correct serum electrolyte imbalances.
- Stool sample for *E. histolytica* PCR or ELISA, plus serology for anti–*E. histolytica* antibodies
  If stool or serum is positive for *E. histolytica*:
  - Metronidazole or tinidazole is 1st-line drug for systemic amebiasis (90% cure rate)
  - Chloroquine is an alternative systemic agent
  - Always follow systemic therapy with a luminal agent to eradicate intestinal colonization (erythromycin, iodoquinol, nitazoxanide, paromomycin, or tetracycline).
  - Do not use the luminal agents alone
- If stool or serum is negative for *E. histolytica*:
  - Refer to gastroenterologist for colonoscopy with biopsy.
  - Repeat serology in 7 days.
  - Consider empiric course of metronidazole if high suspicion for amebiasis and patient is critically ill.
- If evidence of peritonitis or sepsis:
  - Add IV antibiotic directed against anaerobic and gram-negative bacteria.
  - Surgery if toxic megacolon or colonic perforation
- If liver abscess is suspected:
  - US or CT of hepatobiliary system with concurrent amebic serology
  - If imaging demonstrates an abscess but serology is negative, treat with amebicidals and repeat serology in 7 days.
  - Consider abscess drainage by surgeon or interventional radiologist in conjunction with amebicidal therapy.
  - If symptoms do not improve after 5–7 days of empiric amebicidal therapy, consider fine-needle aspiration to rule out bacterial abscess or hepatoma.

### Pregnancy Considerations
- Use metronidazole with caution in 1st-trimester pregnancy, but do not withhold if patient has fulminant colitis or amebic abscess.
- Use erythromycin or nitazoxanide as intestinal amebicides along with metronidazole.
- Erythromycin or nitazoxanide may be used alone for mild dysentery in 1st-trimester pregnancy.
- Chloroquine, iodoquinol, paromomycin, tetracycline, and tinidazole are contraindicated.

### MEDICATION
#### First Line
- Metronidazole: 500–750 mg (peds: 30–50 mg/kg/24 hr) PO/IV q8h for 5–10 days
- Tinidazole: 2 g/day (peds: 50–60 mg/kg/day) PO for 3–6 days

#### Pregnancy Considerations
Tinidazole is contraindicated

#### Second Line
- Chloroquine: 1,000 mg/day PO for 2 days then 500 mg/day PO for 14 days; or 200 mg IM for 10–12 days
- Erythromycin: 250–500 mg (peds: 30–50 mg/kg/24 hr) PO q6h for 10–14 days
- Iodoquinol: 650 mg PO q8h for 20 days
- Nitazoxanide: 500 mg (peds: 100 mg for ages 2–3 yr, 200 mg for ages 4–11 yr) PO b.i.d. for 3 days (10 days if liver abscess)
- Paromomycin: 500 mg (peds: 25–30 mg/kg/24 hr) PO q8h for 5–10 days
- Tetracycline: 250–500 mg (peds: 25–50 mg/kg/24 hr) PO q6h for 10 days

#### Pediatric Considerations
- Chloroquine and iodoquinol are contraindicated.
- Tetracycline contraindicated in children 8 yr of age and under

#### Pregnancy Considerations
Use erythromycin or nitazoxanide only.

 FOLLOW-UP

### DISPOSITION
#### Admission Criteria
- Shock, sepsis, or peritonitis
- Hypotension or tachycardia unresponsive to IV fluids
- Children with >10% dehydration
- Severe electrolyte imbalance
- Patients unable to maintain adequate oral hydration:
  - Extremes of age, cognitive impairment, significant co-morbid illness
- Fulminant colitis or toxic megacolon
- Bowel obstruction
- Extraintestinal abscesses
- Failure of outpatient regimen

#### Discharge Criteria
- Nontoxic presentation of acute or chronic dysentery
- Able to maintain adequate oral hydration and medication compliance
- Dehydration responsive to IV fluids

### Issues for Referral
Consult surgery if evidence of peritonitis, toxic megacolon, colonic perforation, or liver abscess.

### FOLLOW-UP RECOMMENDATIONS
- Gastroenterology and infectious disease follow-up in 7 days for repeat serology and possible endoscopic evaluation.
- Physical examination in 14 days to assess for treatment effectiveness and for development of complications or extraintestinal disease.

## PEARLS AND PITFALLS
- Avoid antidiarrheal medications
- Always give double therapy with both a systemic amebicidal (metronidazole, tinidazole, or chloroquine) plus an intestinal amebicidal (erythromycin, iodoquinol, nitazoxanide, paromomycin, or tetracycline) unless contraindicated.
- Always be vigilant for high-mortality complications such as fulminant colitis or extraintestinal disease.

## ADDITIONAL READING
- Chavez-Tapia NC, Hernandez-Calleros J, Tellez-Avila FI, et al. Image-guided percutaneous procedure plus metronidazole versus metronidazole alone for uncomplicated amoebic liver abscess. *Cochrane Database of Systematic Reviews.* 2009;Issue1.Art. No.:–CD004886.DOI:10.1002/14651858. CD004886.pub2.
- Escobedo AA, Almirall P, Alfonso M, et al. Treatment of intestinal protozoan infections in children. *Arch Dis Child.* 2009;94:478–482.
- Fotedar R, Stark D, Beebe N, et al. Laboratory diagnostic techniques for *Entamoeba* species. *Clin Microbiol Rev.* 2007;20:511–532.
- Gonzalez MLM, Dans LF, Martinez EG. Antiamoebic drugs for treating amoebic colitis. *Cochrane Database of Systematic Reviews.* 2009;Issue2.Art.No:–CD006085.DOI:10.1002/14651858.CD006085.pub2.

### See Also (Topic, Algorithm, Electronic Media Element)
- Diarrhea
- Gastroenteritis

# AMENORRHEA

*Christy Rosa Mohler*

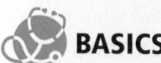 **BASICS**

## DESCRIPTION
- Absence of menstruation
- Primary amenorrhea:
  - No spontaneous uterine bleeding by age 14 yr in the absence of the development of secondary sexual characteristics or by age 16 yr with otherwise normal development
- Secondary amenorrhea:
  - Absence of menstrual bleeding for 6 mo in a woman with prior regular menses or for 12 mo in a woman with prior oligomenorrhea
  - More common than primary amenorrhea
  - Pregnancy is most common cause.

## ETIOLOGY
- Primary:
  - Gonadal dysgenesis
  - Chromosomal abnormalities
  - Imperforate hymen
  - Turner's syndrome
- Secondary:
  - Pregnancy, breast-feeding, or postpartum
  - Asherman syndrome (intrauterine adhesions)
  - Dysfunction of the hypothalamic-pituitary-ovarian axis
  - Endocrinopathies
  - Obesity, starvation, anorexia nervosa, or intense exercise
  - Drugs:
    - Oral contraceptives, antipsychotics, antidepressants, calcium channel blockers, chemotherapeutic agents, digitalis, or marijuana
  - Autoimmune disorders
  - Ovarian failure
  - Menopause

 **DIAGNOSIS**

## SIGNS AND SYMPTOMS
### History
- Menarche and menstrual history
- Sexual activity
- Exercise, weight loss
- Chronic illness
- Previous CNS radiation or chemotherapy
- Family history
- Infertility

### Physical Exam
- Low estrogen:
  - Atrophic vaginal mucosa
  - Mood swings, irritability
- High androgen:
  - Truncal obesity
  - Hirsutism
  - Acne
  - Male-pattern baldness
- Thyroid exam
- Pelvic/genital exam
- Tanner staging

## ESSENTIAL WORKUP
Pregnancy test

## DIAGNOSTIC TESTS & INTERPRETATION
### Lab
- If pregnancy test is negative, no further testing is needed emergently.
- May send TSH, prolactin, LH, FSH for follow-up by gynecology or primary care physician

*Imaging*
None needed emergently unless concern for ectopic pregnancy or other emergency as directed by patient's presentation

*Diagnostic Procedures/Surgery*
None needed emergently

## DIFFERENTIAL DIAGNOSIS
Pregnancy

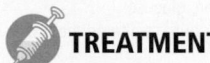 ## TREATMENT

### PRE-HOSPITAL
If amenorrhea is the result of pregnancy, stabilize patient as appropriate for pregnancy.

### ED TREATMENT/PROCEDURES
Reassurance and referral for follow-up

### MEDICATION
Defer for gynecology evaluation.

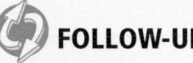 **FOLLOW-UP**

### DISPOSITION
*Admission Criteria*
No need for admission unless concern for ectopic pregnancy

*Discharge Criteria*
Discharge with appropriate referral.

*Issues for Referral*
Referral to gynecology

### FOLLOW UP RECOMMENDATIONS
Gynecology follow-up is recommended.

## PEARLS AND PITFALLS
- Pregnancy is the most relevant etiology of amenorrhea in the emergency department.
- Anorexia nervosa is an important consideration in patients with amenorrhea, particularly in adolescents.

## ADDITIONAL READING
- Berek JS, ed. *Berek & Novak's Gynecology*, 14th ed. Philadelphia: Lippincott Williams & Wilkins, 2007.
- Katz VL, Lentz G, Lobo RA, et al. *Comprehensive Gynecology*, 5th ed. St. Louis: Mosby; 2007.
- Master-Hunter T, Heiman DL. Amenorrhea: Evaluation and treatment. *Am Fam Physician*. 2006;73:1374–1382.
- Warren MP, Hagey AR. The genetics, diagnosis and treatment of amenorrhea. *Minerva Ginecol*. 2004; 56:437  455.

# AMPHETAMINE POISONING

*Seth M. Oskie*
*James W. Rhee*

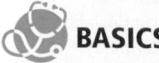 **BASICS**

## DESCRIPTION
- Increased release of norepinephrine, dopamine and serotonin
- Decreased catecholamine reuptake
- Direct effect on $\alpha$- and $\beta$-adrenergic receptors

## ETIOLOGY
- Prescription drugs:
  - Amphetamine (Benzedrine)
  - Dextroamphetamine (Dexedrine)
  - Diethylpropion (Tenuate)
  - Fenfluramine (Pondimin)
  - Methamphetamine
  - Methylphenidate (Ritalin)
  - Phenmetrazine (Preludin)
  - Phentermine
- "Designer drugs":
  - Variants of illegal parent drugs
  - Often synthesized in underground laboratories
  - "Crystal," "Ice":
    - Crystalline methamphetamine hydrochloride
    - Smoked, insufflated, or injected
    - Rapid onset; duration several hours
  - "Crank"
  - "Ecstasy" (3,4,- methylenedioxymetham-phetamine, MDMA, XTC, E):
    - Often used at dances and "rave" parties
    - Dehydration can lead to hyperthermia, hyponatremia, fatality.
  - MDA (3,4,-methylenedioxyamphetamine)
  - Methcathinone ("cat," "Jeff," "mulka"):
    - Derivative of cathinone, found in the evergreen tree *Catha edulis*
    - Frequently synthesized in home laboratories
    - Does not show up on urine toxicology screens

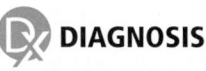 **DIAGNOSIS**

## SIGNS AND SYMPTOMS
- CNS:
  - Agitation
  - Delirium
  - Hyperactivity
  - Tremors
  - Dizziness
  - Mydriasis
  - Headache
  - Choreoathetoid movements
  - Hyperreflexia
  - Cerebrovascular accident
  - Seizures and status epilepticus
  - Coma
- Psychiatric:
  - Euphoria
  - Increased aggressiveness
  - Anxiety
  - Hallucinations (visual, tactile)
  - Compulsive repetitive actions

- Cardiovascular:
  - Palpitations
  - Hypertensive crisis
  - Tachycardia or (reflex) bradycardia
  - Dysrhythmias (usually tachydysrhythmias)
  - Cardiovascular collapse
- Other:
  - Rhabdomyolysis
  - Myoglobinuria
  - Acute renal failure
  - Anorexia
  - Diaphoresis
  - Disseminated intravascular coagulation (DIC)

## History
- Determine the type, amount, timing, and route of amphetamine exposure
- Assess for possible coingestions
- Evaluate for symptoms of end organ injury:
  - Chest pain
  - Shortness of breath
  - Headache, confusion and vomiting

## Physical Exam
- Common findings include:
  - Agitation
  - Tachycardia
  - Diaphoresis
  - Mydriasis
- Severe intoxication characterized by:
  - Tachycardia
  - HTN
  - Hyperthermia
  - Agitated delirium
  - Seizures
  - Diaphoresis
- Hypotension and respiratory distress may precede cardiovascular collapse.
- Evaluate for associated conditions;
  - Cellulitis and soft tissue infections
  - Diastolic cardiac murmurs or unequal pulses
  - Examine carefully for trauma
  - Pneumothorax from inhalation injury
  - Focal neurological deficits

## ESSENTIAL WORKUP
- Vital signs:
  - Temperature >40°C:
    - Core temperature recording essential
    - Peripheral temperature may be cool.
    - Indication for urgent cooling
    - Ominous prognostic sign
  - BP:
    - Severe hypertension can lead to cardiac and neurologic abnormalities.
    - Late in course, hypotension may supervene.
- ECG:
  - Signs of cardiac ischemia
  - Ventricular tachydysrhythmias
  - Reflex bradycardia

## DIAGNOSTIC TESTS & INTERPRETATION
### Lab
- Urinalysis:
  - Blood
  - Myoglobin
- Electrolytes, BUN/creatinine, glucose:
  - Hypoglycemia may contribute to altered mental status.
  - Acidosis may accompany severe toxicity.
  - Rhabdomyolysis may cause renal failure.
  - Hyperkalemia—life-threatening consequence of acute renal failure
- Coagulation profile to monitor for potential DIC:
  - INR, PT, PTT, platelets
- Creatine phosphokinase (CPK):
  - Markedly elevated in rhabdomyolysis
- Urine toxicology screen:
  - For other toxins with similar effects (eg, cocaine)
  - Some amphetaminelike substances (eg, methcathinone) may not be detected.
- Aspirin and acetaminophen levels if suicide attempt a possibility
- Arterial blood gas (ABG)

### Imaging
- Chest radiograph:
  - Adult respiratory distress syndrome
  - Noncardiogenic pulmonary edema
- Head CT for:
  - Significant headache
  - Altered mental status
  - Focal neurologic signs
  - For subarachnoid hemorrhage, intracerebral bleed

### Diagnostic Procedures/Surgery
Lumbar puncture for:
- Suspected meningitis (headache, altered mental status, hyperpyrexia)
- Suspected subarachnoid hemorrhage and CT normal

## DIFFERENTIAL DIAGNOSIS
- Sepsis
- Thyroid storm
- Serotonin syndrome
- Neuroleptic malignant syndrome
- Pheochromocytoma
- Subarachnoid hemorrhage
- Drugs that cause delirium:
  - Anticholinergics:
    - Belladonna alkaloids
    - Antihistamines
  - Tricyclic antidepressants
  - Cocaine
  - Ethanol withdrawal
  - Sedative/hypnotic withdrawal
  - Hallucinogens
  - Phencyclidine

- Drugs that cause HTN and tachycardia:
  - Sympathomimetics
  - Anticholinergics
  - Ethanol withdrawal
  - Phencyclidine
  - Caffeine
  - Phenylpropanolamine
  - Ephedrine
  - Monoamine oxidase inhibitors
  - Theophylline
  - Nicotine
- Drugs that cause seizures:
  - Carbon monoxide
  - Carbamazepine
  - Cyanide
  - Cocaine
  - Cholinergics (organophosphate insecticides) Camphor
  - Chlorinated hydrocarbons
  - Ethanol withdrawal
  - Sedative/hypnotic withdrawal
  - Isoniazid
  - Theophylline
  - Hypoglycemics
  - Lead
  - Lithium
  - Local anesthetics
  - Anticholinergics
  - Phencyclidine
  - Phenothiazines
  - Phenytoin
  - Propoxyphene
  - Salicylates
  - Strychnine

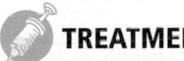 **TREATMENT**

### PRE-HOSPITAL
- Patient may be uncooperative or violent.
- Secure IV access.
- Protect from self-induced trauma.

### INITIAL STABILIZATION/THERAPY
- ABCs
- Establish IV 0.9% NS access.
- Cardiac monitor
- Naloxone, dextrose (or Accu-Chek), and thiamine if altered mental status

### ED TREATMENT/PROCEDURES
- Decontamination:
  - Gastric lavage:
    ○ Consider if recent (within 1 hr) or life-threatening ingestion.
    ○ Instill activated charcoal through large-bore orogastric tube both before and after lavage.
  - Administer activated charcoal with sorbitol:
    ○ Consider if recent ingestion
  - Whole-bowel irrigation with polyethylene glycol solution for body packers

- Hypertensive crisis:
  - Initially administer benzodiazepines if agitated.
  - Alpha-blocker (phentolamine) as second-line agent
  - Nitroprusside for severe, unresponsive hypertension
  - Avoid $\beta$-blockers, which may exacerbate hypertension.
- Agitation, acute psychosis:
  - Administer benzodiazepines.
- Hyperthermia:
  - Benzodiazepines if agitated
  - Active cooling if temperature >40°C:
    ○ Tepid water mist
    ○ Evaporate with fan.
  - Paralysis:
    ○ Indicated if muscle rigidity and hyperactivity contributing to persistent hyperthermia
    ○ Nondepolarizing agent (eg, vecuronium)
    ○ Avoid succinylcholine.
    ○ Intubation; mechanical ventilation Apply cooling blankets.
- Rhabdomyolysis:
  - Administer benzodiazepines.
  - Hydrate with 0.9% NS.
  - Maintain urine output at 1–2 mL/min.
  - Hemodialysis (if acute renal failure and hyperkalemia occur)
- Seizures:
  - Maintain airway.
  - Administer benzodiazepines.
  - Phenobarbital if unresponsive to benzodiazepines
  - Phenytoin contraindicated

### MEDICATION
- Activated charcoal: 1–2 g/kg up to 100 g PO
- Dextrose: D$_{50}$W 1 amp: 50 mL or 25 g (peds: D$_{25}$W 2–4 mL/kg) IV
- Diazepam (benzodiazepine): 5–10 mg (peds: 0.2–0.5 mg/kg) IV
- Lorazepam (benzodiazepine): 2–6 mg (peds: 0.03–0.05 mg/kg) IV
- Nitroprusside: 1–8 μg/kg/min IV (titrated to BP)
- Phenobarbital: 15–20 mg/kg at 25–50 mg/min until cessation of seizure activity
- Phentolamine: 1–5 mg IV over 5 min (titrated to BP)
- Sorbitol: 1–2 g/kg to a max. of 100 g PO mixed in the activated charcoal slurry (peds: >1 yr old: 1–1.5 g/kg as a 35% solution to a max. of 50 g); avoid repeat doses of sorbitol.
- Vecuronium: 0.1 mg/kg IVP

 **FOLLOW-UP**

### DISPOSITION
#### Admission Criteria
- Hyperthermia
- Persistent altered mental status
- Hypertensive crisis
- Seizures
- Rhabdomyolysis
- Persistent tachycardia

#### Discharge Criteria
- Asymptomatic after 6 hr observation
- Absence of above admission criteria

### FOLLOW-UP RECOMMENDATIONS
Patients may need referral for chemical dependency rehab and detoxification.

## PEARLS AND PITFALLS
- Admit patients with severe or persistent symptoms.
- Monitor core temperature:
  - Hyperthermia >40°C may be life threatening.
  - Treat with aggressive sedation and active cooling.
  - Recognize rhabdomyolysis and hyperkalemia.
  - Avoid physical restraints in agitated patients if possible.
- Consider associated emergency conditions:
  - Patients with chest pain should be evaluated for acute coronary syndromes and treated accordingly.
  - Consider infection in altered patients with fevers and history of IV drug use.
  - Methamphetamine abuse frequently associated with traumatic injury
- Benzodiazepines are 1st-line therapy in symptomatic methamphetamine intoxication.

## ADDITIONAL READING
- Callaway CW, Clark RF. Hyperthermia in psychostimulant overdose. *Ann Emerg Med*. 1994;24:68–75.
- Chan P, Chen JH, Lee MH, et al. Fatal and nonfatal methamphetamine intoxication in the intensive care unit. *Clin Toxicol*. 1994;32:147–155.
- Christophersen AS. Amphetamine designer drugs – An overview and epidemiology. *Toxicol Lett*. 2000;112–113:127.
- Doyon S. The many faces of ecstasy. *Curr Opinion Pediatr*. 2001;13:170–176.
- Gray SD, Fatovich DM, McCoubrie DL, et al. Amphetamine-related presentations to and inner-city tertiary emergency department: A prospective evaluation. *Med J Aust*. 2007;186:336.
- Turnipseed SD, Richards JR, Kirk JD, et al. Frequency of acute coronary syndrome in patients presenting to the emergency department with chest pain after methamphetamine use. *J Emerg Med*. 2003;24(4): 369–373.

### See Also (Topic, Algorithm, Electronic Media Element)
- Sympathomimetic Poisoning
- Tricyclic Antidepressant Poisoning

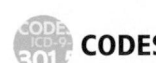 **CODES**

ICD9
969.72 Poisoning by amphetamines

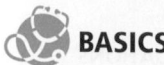 **BASICS**

## DESCRIPTION

- Partial amputations have tissue connecting the distal and proximal parts and are treated by revascularization.
- Complete amputations have no connecting tissue and may be treated by replantation.
- Both of the above are treated the same from an emergency standpoint.

## ETIOLOGY

Traumatic amputations result from machinery, powered hand tools, household appliances, lawnmowers, getting caught between objects, motor vehicle collisions, crush injuries, blast injuries, gunshot wounds, knives, degloving injuries to digits (ring avulsions), and animal bites.

 **DIAGNOSIS**

## SIGNS AND SYMPTOMS

### History

- Exact time of injury critical, as ischemia time predicts success for replantation:
  - Irreversible muscle necrosis begins at 6 hr of ischemia.
  - The amount of muscle present in the tissue predicts the tolerable ischemia time.
  - The temperature also affects the tolerable ischemia time.
  - Amputated digits have little muscle:
    ○ Can tolerate warm ischemia time of 6–8 hr
    ○ Can tolerate cool ischemia time of as much as 30 hr
  - Amputated limbs have more muscle mass:
    ○ Can tolerate warm ischemia time of 4–6 hr
    ○ Can tolerate cold ischemia time of 10–12 hr
- Mechanism of injury:
  - Clean-cut or "guillotine" amputations have better prognosis for replantation than crush or avulsion injuries.
- Comorbid illnesses that hinder successful replantation:
  - Diabetes, peripheral vascular disease, rheumatologic disease

### Physical Exam

- Assessment and documentation of injured extremity is crucial.
- Signs of neurologic compromise:
  - Loss of sensation and 2-point discrimination
  - Loss of active range of motion
- Signs of vascular compromise in partial amputations:
  - Distal part dusky or cyanotic
  - Delayed capillary refill (>2 sec)
  - Diminished or absent pulses (Doppler or palpation)
  - Use Allen test in hand injuries.
  - Pulse oximetry may be helpful.
- Soft tissue: Assess skin, muscle, tendon, and nail bed integrity.
- Identify exposed bone and fractures (gross deformity, tenderness, crepitus).

## ESSENTIAL WORKUP

ED workup includes obtaining an accurate history and physical, stabilizing the patient and injured part, and consultation or transfer if replantation is an option.

## DIAGNOSTIC TESTS & INTERPRETATION

### Lab

Preoperative lab studies if needed

### Imaging

Radiographs of both amputated part and stump are important, but should not delay transport.

### Diagnostic Procedures/Surgery

Determined by surgical consultant for replantation

## DIFFERENTIAL DIAGNOSIS

- Involves neurologic, vascular, and soft tissue integrity and potential for replantation/revascularization
- Do not miss other major injuries with concurrent trauma.

 **TREATMENT**

## PRE-HOSPITAL

- Collect all amputated body parts, including pieces of bone, tissue, and skin.
- See "Initial Stabilization" for care of amputated parts during transport.
- Transport patient and body parts to the nearest microvascular replantation center unless other major injuries require transport to the nearest trauma center:
  - Air transport from remote locations should be considered if ischemia time is of concern.

## INITIAL STABILIZATION/THERAPY

- Consult surgical specialist as early as possible.
- Establish IV access.
- Limit blood loss:
  - Elevate injured limb.
  - Direct pressure using bulky pressure dressing or pressure points if ineffective.
  - Use tourniquet if above methods fail to give desired hemostasis (BP cuff 30 mm Hg > systolic BP [SBP]).
  - Partial amputations bleed more because of lack of both retraction and spasm of blood vessels.
- Avoid further damage to injured part:
  - Avoid vascular clamps, cautery, vessel ligation, or débridement.
  - Avoid repeated exams of the stump or amputated part.
- Care of amputated part (complete and partial):
  - Remove gross contamination/foreign material.
  - Gently irrigate with saline (avoid antiseptics).
  - Wrap in gauze moistened with saline.
  - Place in clean, dry plastic bag or specimen cup.
  - Place sealed bag/cup in ice water (half water, half ice) or refrigerate at 4°C.
  - Never place directly onto ice or into ice water.
  - Avoid dry ice to prevent freezing.
- Care of the stump:
  - Irrigate with saline and cover with saline dampened gauze.
  - Splint if necessary; keep partial amputations as near anatomic position as possible.
- Maintain normal blood volume with IV fluids or blood products if necessary.

## ED TREATMENT/PROCEDURES

- Tetanus prophylaxis
- Adequate IV analgesia
- Patient NPO
- Prophylactic antibiotics if devitalized tissue, exposed bone, or contamination:
  - First-generation cephalosporin
- All patients are candidates for surgical repair until a specialist deems otherwise.
- Limit ischemia time of the amputated part (ie, early transfer if necessary).
- Patient considerations in decision to replant:
  - Age
  - Occupation/handedness
  - Degree of motivation
  - General physical condition and underlying diseases

- Indications for replantation (no absolute indications):
  - Thumb, any level (supplies 40% of hand function)
  - Multiple digits
  - Hand amputations through the palm and distal wrist
  - Individual digit distal to flexor digitorum superficialis tendon insertion and proximal to distal interphalangeal joint (DIP)
  - Some single-digit ring avulsion injuries
  - Arm proximal to midforearm (if sharp or moderately avulsed)
  - Virtually all pediatric amputations (younger patients have lower success rates but better functional outcomes)
- Contraindications to replantation:
  - Severely crushed or mangled parts
  - Injuries at multiple levels
  - Psychotic patients who willfully self-amputated the part
  - Single-digit amputations proximal to the flexor digitorum superficialis muscle insertion
  - Amputated parts with tendons avulsed from musculotendinous junctions
  - Lower extremities rarely attempted and usually in children
  - Unstable patients secondary to other serious injuries or diseases
  - Older patients or those with contraindications to general anesthesia
    Inappropriately prolonged ischemia time
- Fingertip amputations: Most common type of upper extremity amputation:
  - Distal to DIP joint
  - Primary goals of treatment:
    - Maintenance of length
    - Good soft-tissue coverage
    - Painless fingertip with durable and sensate skin
    - Nail preservation
  - Dorsal better prognosis than ventral
  - No exposed phalanx:
    - Irrigate with saline, apply petrolatum-soaked gauze and allow to heal by secondary intention (best result in wounds <1 cm²).
  - Small amount of exposed phalanx:
    - Shorten bone with rongeur below level of the tissue and close by primary intention or allow to heal by secondary intention.
    - Any bone left exposed requires additional operative procedures and consultation.
    - Replantation is an option for cosmetic reasons or for occupational consideration (eg, musicians).

- Considered open fractures if phalanx exposed, thus antibiotics are indicated.
  - Preserve nail bed and nail to optimize function and cosmesis.
  - Treat subungual hematomas.
  - Splint to prevent trauma to healing fingertip.
  - Consultation required if significant loss of bone or soft tissue for possible graft or flap
- Nonlimb amputations (penis, ear, nose): Amputated parts should be cared for similarly as above and emergently referred to a specialist for replantation:
  - Penile amputations: Most often secondary to self mutilation and psychiatric illness
  - Successful replantation unlikely beyond 24 hr of cold ischemia or 6 hr of warm ischemia
  - Ear amputations: Should be considered for replantation by appropriate specialist
  - Nose amputations: Replantation has been successfully performed with variable results.

### Pediatric Considerations
- All pediatric amputations considered for replantation
- Fingertip amputations often left to heal by secondary intention:
  - Spontaneous regeneration of fingertip occurs in children even with volar fingertip amputations.
  - Pediatric fingertip amputations distal to the lunula of the fingernail can be successfully replanted (unlike adults).

### Geriatric Considerations
Advanced age not an absolute contraindication to replantation; however, underlying medical problems often make older patients poor surgical candidates.

### MEDICATION
Cefazolin: 0.5–1.5 g IV or IM q6h–q8h (peds: 25–100 mg/kg/d divided q8h, max. 6 g/d)

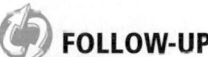 **FOLLOW-UP**

#### DISPOSITION
##### Admission Criteria
Hospitalization is required for all patients undergoing replantation or revascularization.

#### Discharge Criteria
- Mild fingertip amputations or mild degloving injuries with adequate repair and stable vasculature
- Close surgical or orthopedic follow-up is required.

#### FOLLOW-UP RECOMMENDATIONS
Patients discharged but with significant skin loss should be considered for skin grafting and have close surgical follow-up.

### PEARLS AND PITFALLS
- Replantation success is largely dependent on the skill of the surgeon and the replantation team.
- Expeditious consultation or transfer to appropriate surgeon and team is paramount.
- All multitrauma victims must have all life-threatening injuries stabilized prior to replantation.

### ADDITIONAL READING
- Bandi G, et al. Controversies in the management of male external genitourinary trauma. *J Trauma.* 2004;56(6):1362–1370.
- Boris AE, et al. Digit and hand replantation. *Arch Orthop Trauma Surg.* 09 December 2009 [Epub ahead of print].
- Hattori Y, et al. Fingertip replantation. *J Hand Surg.* 2007;32(4):548–555.
- Lyn ET, Mailhot T. Hand. In: Marx J, et al. *Rosen's emergency medicine: Concepts and clinical practice,* 7th ed. Philadelphia: Mosby/Elsevier; 2010:576–619.
- Soucacos PN. Indications and selection for digital amputation and replantation. *J Hand Surg.* 2001;26(6):572–581.

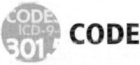 **CODES**

#### ICD9
- 885.0 Traumatic amputation of thumb (complete) (partial), without mention of complication
- 886.0 Traumatic amputation of other finger(s) (complete) (partial), without mention of complication
- 887.0 Traumatic amputation of arm and hand (complete) (partial), unilateral, below elbow, without mention of complication

# AMYOTROPHIC LATERAL SCLEROSIS

*Richard S. Krause*

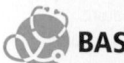 **BASICS**

## DESCRIPTION

- Progressive, presently incurable disease of adults
- Neurodegenerative disease of the motor system at all levels
- Some patients have associated dementia
- Manifestations:
  – Muscle weakness
  – Wasting
  – Fasciculations
  – Babinski's sign
  – Hyperreflexia
- Variants with predominately upper or lower motor neuron manifestations also occur.
- Also known as "Lou Gherig's Disease" after the famous baseball player who was affected.
- Eventually leads to respiratory compromise secondary to weakness of diaphragm and other muscles of respiration.
- 80% of cases begin between ages 40 and 70 yr.
- Death (usually from respiratory paralysis) typically occurs within 3–5 yr of the diagnosis.
- 50% die within 3 yr.
- ~10% ALS patients live 10 yr or more.
- Males > Females

## ETIOLOGY

- Etiology of amyotrophic lateral sclerosis (ALS) is unknown.
- ~10% of affected patients have another affected family member.
- Pathologically, there is loss of both upper and lower motor neuron cells.
- Predilection for the motor system and sparing of other neurons.

 **DIAGNOSIS**

## SIGNS AND SYMPTOMS

- Asymmetric limb weakness is the most common presentation of ALS (80%).
- May begin in either the arms (cervical onset) or the legs (lumbar onset):
  – Later all limbs are affected.
- Bulbar ALS:
  – Usually presents with dysarthria or dysphagia
  – 2nd most common presentation
- Both lower motor neuron (weakness and wasting with fasciculation) and upper motor neuron signs (Babinski sign with hyperreflexia) occur.
- Respiratory muscles and the vocal cords are affected late.
- Muscle fasciculation is common, but may not be apparent to the patient.
- Extraocular muscles, sphincters, cognition, and sensation are spared.
- 80% of cases begin between ages 40 and 70 yr.
- Death (usually from respiratory paralysis) typically occurs within 3–5 yr of the diagnosis.
- ~10% ALS patients live 10 yr or more.

### History

- Most ED patients with ALS will present with an established diagnosis.
- History should focus on clues regarding acute medical issues and functional decline.
- When the diagnosis of ALS is suspected due to a complaint of "weakness" consider that this occurs with many illnesses.
- These include pulmonary or cardiac disease, joint disease, anemia, depression, other neurological disease, etc.
- Differentiate true weakness from: shortness of breath, chest pain, joint pain, fatigue, poor exercise tolerance, etc.

- True weakness often leads to complaints of inability to perform specific tasks:
  – Bulbar palsy:
    ○ Facial weakness
    ○ Weakness and fasciculation of tongue
    ○ Dysarthria
  – Cervical onset ALS:
    ○ Difficult with washing hair, using comb
    ○ Impaired pincer grip
  – Lumbar onset ALS:
    ○ Frequent trips secondary to foot drop
    ○ Difficulty walking up stairs

### Physical Exam

- A detailed and thorough neurological exam is the key to diagnosis but is not typically performed in the ED.
- Upper motor neuron disease causes slow uncoordinated movements and stiffness.
- Lower motor neuron disease causes weakness accompanied by atrophy and muscle cramps are common.
- Common findings:
  – Brisk reflexes
  – Fasiculations
  – Muscle wasting
- Exam should focus on excluding or confirming other conditions.

## ESSENTIAL WORKUP

- Previously undiagnosed ALS:
  – Diagnosis of ALS is clinical and rarely made in the ED:
    ○ Recognition of the possibility of this disease is sufficient and mandates referral for workup.
  – If ALS is suspected, forced vital capacity (FVC) should be performed.
- Known ALS patient:
  – Patients with known disease and progressive symptoms:
    ○ Evaluate potentially treatable complications with lab and imaging studies.

- FVC is a sensitive indicator of respiratory muscle weakness:
  ○ FVC <50% of predicted is considered a sign of advanced disease.
  ○ FVC <50% usually requires ventilatory support.
  ○ Compare with the patient's previous baseline.
- CXR may reveal aspiration or pneumonia or co-morbid conditions such as CHF.
- Pulse oximetry and blood gas analysis aid in the diagnosis of respiratory failure.
- Electrolytes and other blood chemistry tests may reveal a treatable cause of increasing weakness.

### DIAGNOSTIC TESTS & INTERPRETATION
*Lab*
- In cases of undifferentiated weakness, consider CPK measurement along with blood chemistry:
  - Elevated CPK is associated with myopathy.
- Electrolyte abnormalities such as hypokalemia, hypercalcemia, etc. may cause generalized weakness but this is typically in association with other signs and symptoms.
- CBC, UA may be indicated to look for source of infection.

*Imaging*
Cervical spine, other skeletal radiography, or head CT may be needed in case of falls (common in ALS) or to rule out other conditions.

*Diagnostic Procedures/Surgery*
- Check forced vital capacity (FVC)
- Electromyography (EMG) may help confirm the diagnosis.

### DIFFERENTIAL DIAGNOSIS
- Cervical cord compression:
  - Similar symptoms but usually acute onset with pain and sensory changes
  - Spinal MRI or myelography for diagnosis
- Thyrotoxicosis may mimic ALS.
  - Usually marked systemic symptoms
- Heavy metal poisoning (lead, mercury, arsenic)
- Syphilis and Lyme disease
- Lymphoma may have an associated lower motor neuron syndrome, which mimics ALS.
- Bulbar ALS:
  - Esophageal cancer
  - Myasthenia gravis

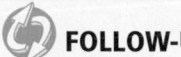

## TREATMENT

- There is no specific therapy for ALS.
- Recently, the drug riluzole, a glutamate release inhibitor, has been shown to extend survival in ALS patients for an average of a few months.
- Treatment issues in the ED revolve around symptomatic therapy and identification and treatment of complications.

### PRE-HOSPITAL
Controversies:
- Many patients will have advanced directives:
  - Unless immediate intervention is essential, intubation should be avoided until directives have been ascertained.
  - Noninvasive means of ventilatory support may be tried 1st.

### INITIAL STABILIZATION/THERAPY
- Respiratory insufficiency or failure:
  - Ascertain any advanced directives.
  - Noninvasive ventilatory support
  - Intubation as indicated
- Weaning off the ventilator is very difficult.
  - Average survival after institution of ventilation is 19 mo.

### ED TREATMENT/PROCEDURES
- Sedation and pain control as indicated:
  - Joint pain may respond to NSAIDs.
- Insomnia from pressure pain (owing to immobility) may respond to diphenhydramine or amitriptyline. Insomnia may also be treated with benzodiazepines.
- Aspiration or drooling may be treated with amitriptyline, atropine, or hyoscyamine (dries secretions).
- Muscle cramps may respond to baclofen or tizanidine.
- Constipation is related to immobility and diet:
  - Treated with laxatives, stool softeners, and dietary changes

### MEDICATION
- Amitriptyline: 25–100 mg PO QHS
- Atropine: 0.4 mg PO q4–6h
- Baclofen: 10–25 mg PO t.i.d.
- Diphenhydramine: 25–50 mg PO nightly at bedtime
- Tizanidine 2–4 mg PO b.i.d.

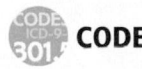

## FOLLOW-UP
### DISPOSITION
*Admission Criteria*
- Need for respiratory support
- Dehydration
- Unable to be cared for at home owing to progression of illness
- Complications (eg, infection) or other diagnosis that requires admission

*Discharge Criteria*
- *Suspected ALS:* Refer for outpatient evaluation if general condition permits and other serious conditions requiring admission are ruled out.
- *Complication of known ALS:* Discharge if outpatient treatment available and stable respiratory status.

### FOLLOW-UP RECOMMENDATIONS
If considering diagnosis of ALS, prompt follow-up with a neurologist should be arranged.

## PEARLS AND PITFALLS
- ALS is a progressive neurodegenerative disease affecting all components of the motor system.
- Many patients with ALS have advanced directives—inquire prior to any aggressive intervention.
- FVC <50% usually requires ventilatory support.

## ADDITIONAL READING

- Gregory SA. Evaluation and management of respiratory muscle dysfunction in ALS. *NeuroRehabilitation.* 2007;22:435–443.
- McGeer E, McGeer P. Pharmacologic approaches to the treatment of amyotrophic lateral sclerosis. *Biodrugs.* 2005;19:31–37.
- Mitchell JD, Borasio GD. Amyotrophic lateral sclerosis. *Lancet.* 2007;369:2031–2041.
- Servera E, Sancho J. Appropriate management of respiratory problems is of utmost importance in the treatment of patients with amyotrophic lateral sclerosis. *Chest.* 2005;127:1879–1882.

## CODES

ICD9
335.20 Amyotrophic lateral sclerosis

# ANAL FISSURE
*Julia Sone*

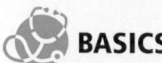 **BASICS**

## DESCRIPTION
- Hard stool passes and "cuts" anoderm
- Linear tear extends from dentate line to anoderm:
  – Posterior midline 95%
  – Anterior midline 5%
  – Externally: Forms skin tag or sentinel pile
  – Internally: Forms hypertrophied anal papilla
  – Chronic fissure may reveal fibers of internal sphincter with sentinel pile.

## ETIOLOGY
- Stress or an overly tight anal sphincter leads to local ischemia of posterior anoderm.
- Diarrhea or hard bowel movement tears anoderm.
- Local trauma from anal intercourse or sexual abuse may be cause.
- Lateral fissures indicate underlying causative systemic disease:
  – Crohn disease
  – Anal cancer
  – Leukemia
  – Syphilis
  – Previous anal surgery

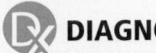 **DIAGNOSIS**

## SIGNS AND SYMPTOMS
- Bright red blood per rectum usually on toilet paper
- Sharp, cutting, throbbing or burning pain with bowel movement:
  – May last for hours
- Constipation; unable to pass stool owing to pain:
  – Hard, nondeformable stools

### History
- Passage of hard stool or constipation
- Episode(s) of diarrhea
- Bright red blood on toilet paper

### Physical Exam
Anal exam:
- Gently retract buttocks and have patient bear down to visualize the fissure.
- Severe pain usually prevents a manual or digital exam:
  – Use lidocaine jelly or ELA-Max5, a topical lidocaine ointment, before attempting digital rectal exam.
  – Need to exclude abscess or tumor

### Pediatric Considerations
A clear test tube may be used as an anoscope to visualize the anal canal/fissure.

## ESSENTIAL WORKUP
Careful rectal exam

## DIAGNOSTIC TESTS & INTERPRETATION
### Lab
Hematocrit if severe bleeding by history

### Imaging
CT pelvis:
- To exclude anal rectal abscess/tumor if palpable mass on rectal exam

## DIFFERENTIAL DIAGNOSIS
- Crohn disease
- Chronic ulcerative colitis
- Anorectal carcinoma
- Perirectal abscess
- Thrombosed hemorrhoid
- Sexual abuse
- TB
- Syphilis
- Lymphoma
- Leukemia
- Previous anal surgery

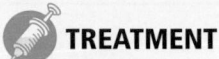

## TREATMENT

### PRE-HOSPITAL
Establish IV access for patients with significant rectal bleeding.

### INITIAL STABILIZATION/THERAPY
Administer pain medications for patients with significant pain.

### ED TREATMENT/PROCEDURES
- IV/IM/PO pain medications:
  - NSAIDs
    Acetaminophen
  - Muscle relaxants to relieve sphincter spasm:
    ○ Cyclobenzaprine
    ○ Diazepam
    ○ Diltiazem 2% ointment
    ○ Nifedipine ointment 0.3%
- Topical anesthetics:
  - ELA-Max5
  - Lidocaine jelly 2%
- Sitz baths (with warm water) to relieve sphincter spasm

### Diet
- High-fiber diet instruction:
  - Fiber/bran: 20 g/d
  - Psyllium seeds (Metamucil or Konsyl): 1–2 tsp (peds: 0.25–1 tsp/d) PO q24h
- Encourage consumption of 10–12 8-oz glasses of water per day.

### MEDICATION
- Cyclobenzaprine (Flexeril): 10 mg (peds: Not indicated) PO t.i.d.
- Diazepam (Valium): 5 mg (peds: 0.12–0.8 mg/kg/d) PO t.i.d. PRN for spasm
- Diltiazem 2% ointment: Apply to fissure b.i.d.
- Docusate sodium (Colace): 50–200 mg (peds: younger than 3 yr, 10–40 mg/d; 3–6 yr, 20–60 mg/d; 6–12 yr, 40–150 mg/d) PO q12h
- ELA-Max5 (5% lidocaine anorectal cream): Apply to perianal area q4h PRN pain (pediatric dose: Not for those younger than 12 yr)
- Ibuprofen: 400–600 mg (peds: 40 mg/kg/d)
- PO q6h
- Nifedipine ointment 0.3%: Apply to fissure t.i.d. with Q-tip (peds: Not indicated)
- Nitroglycerin ointment 0.2%: Apply to fissure b.i.d.–t.i.d. with cotton swab. (peds: Not indicated)

## FOLLOW-UP

### DISPOSITION

#### Admission Criteria
Severe abdominal pain/distention due to fecal impaction

#### Discharge Criteria
- Initial treatment is conservative therapy for acute anal fissures as an outpatient.
- Operative referral for chronic fissures

### FOLLOW-UP RECOMMENDATIONS
Colorectal or GI follow-up for patients with symptomatic fissures

## PEARLS AND PITFALLS
- Perform a careful physical examination of rectal area to delineate fissures and exclude other pathology.
- Provide combination of pain relief and muscle relaxants for patients with significant pain.
- Provide discharge medications/instructions to prevent constipation.

## ADDITIONAL READING
- Hyman H, Boyum J. Fissure-in-ano. *Semin Colon Rectal Surg.* 2003;14(2):107–110.
- Orsay C, Rakinic J. Practice parameters for the management of anal fissures (revised). *Dis Colon Rectum.* 2004;47:2003–2007.
- Rakinic J. Anal fissure. *Clin Colon Rectal Surg.* 2007;20(2):133–138.

### See Also (Topic, Algorithm, Electronic Media Element)
- Hemorrhoid
- Perirectal Abscess

# ANAPHYLAXIS

*Sean-Xavier Neath*

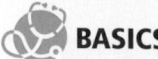 **BASICS**

## DESCRIPTION
- An acute, widely distributed form of shock that occurs within minutes of exposure to antigen in a sensitized individual
- ~500–1,000 deaths are attributed annually in the United States to anaphylaxis. There are approximately 10,000 ER visits per month for anaphylaxis in the U.S.
- Involves release of bioactive molecules such as histamine, leukotrienes, and prostaglandins from inflammatory cells:
  - Mediator release results in increased vascular permeability, vasodilation, smooth-muscle contractions, and increased epithelial secretion.
  - Physiologically, this is manifested in a decrease in total peripheral resistance, venous return, and cardiac output, as well as intravascular volume depletion.

## ETIOLOGY
- IgE-mediated:
  - Antibiotics, particularly penicillin family
  - Venoms, especially bee and wasp
  - Latex
  - Vaccines
  - Foodstuffs (shellfish, soybeans, peanuts, tree nuts, wheat, milk, eggs, nitrates/nitrites)
- Non-IgE mediated:
  - Iodine contrast media
  - Opiates
  - Vancomycin

### Pediatric Considerations
In children, foods are an important trigger for IgE-mediated anaphylaxis:
- Milk, egg, wheat, and soy (MEWS) are the most common food allergens.
- Peanut allergies are increasingly common and can be more potent; children can develop anaphylaxis from residual peanut in a candy bar.

 **DIAGNOSIS**

## SIGNS AND SYMPTOMS
- Symptoms begin within seconds to minutes after contact with an offending antigen.
- Anaphylactic reactions almost always involve the skin or mucous membranes. >90% of patients have some combination of urticaria, erythema, pruritus, or angioedema.
- Some patients may have an initial sensation of impending doom followed by more clearly definable symptomatology:
  - Respiratory: From sneezing and nasal congestion to frank bronchospasm and laryngeal edema
  - Cardiovascular: Hypotension, dysrhythmias, myocardial ischemia
  - Gastrointestinal: Nausea, vomiting, diarrhea
  - Ocular: Eye itching and tearing, conjunctival injection
  - Hematologic: Activation of intrinsic coagulation pathway sometimes leading to disseminated intravascular coagulation, thrombocytopenia
  - Neurologic: Seizures

### History
- The diagnosis of anaphylaxis is a clinical diagnosis.
- A brief history should include questions regarding a previous history of allergy or anaphylaxis, as well as exposure to potential new triggers.

### Physical Exam
- Usually will include alterations in a combination of any 2 or more of the following systems: cutaneous, respiratory, gastrointestinal or cardiovascular system
- Hypotension or airway compromise are not always present at onset.

## ESSENTIAL WORKUP
- Diagnosis is made based on clinical symptoms.
- It is important not to underestimate the potential severity of an allergic reaction in its early stages.
- ECG should be done in patients with previous cardiac history or ischemic symptoms; consider routinely in the elderly.

## DIAGNOSTIC TESTS & INTERPRETATION
### Lab
The diagnosis of anaphylaxis is made on clinical grounds; laboratory tests are usually not useful in aiding diagnosis in the acute setting. Tryptase levels remain elevated after an attack and can be useful for later confirmation of a suspected anaphylactic episode.

### Imaging
Hyperinflation can be seen on CXR.

## DIFFERENTIAL DIAGNOSIS
- Pulmonary embolism
- Acute MI
- Airway obstruction
- Asthma
- Tension pneumothorax
- NSAID reaction
- Vasovagal collapse
- Hereditary angioedema
- Serum sickness
- Systemic mastocytosis
- Pheochromocytoma
- Carcinoid syndrome

 **TREATMENT**

## PRE-HOSPITAL
- IV access, $O_2$, cardiac and pulse oximetry monitoring
- Early intubation based on the initial progression of disease and response to treatment:
  - Laryngeal edema and spasm can progress rapidly.
  - Laryngeal edema can be managed with racemic epinephrine prior to intubation.
- SC epinephrine can be administered en route even prior to establishment of an IV.

## INITIAL STABILIZATION/THERAPY

- ABCs
- Assure adequate ventilation
- Airway management:
  - Orotracheal intubation is the airway technique of choice.
  - If laryngeal edema, spasm, or soft tissue swelling present; consider using advanced airway adjuncts when available.
  - Consider blind nasotracheal intubation if soft tissue swelling prohibits an oral approach and there is absence of stridor.
  - Transtracheal jet insufflation or cricothyrotomy may be necessary to control the airway.
- Epinephrine IV/SC or endotracheal administration:
  - Direct injection into the venous plexus at the base of the tongue is an option.
- Volume resuscitation with crystalloids or colloids

## ED TREATMENT/PROCEDURES

- Continuous cardiac and vital sign monitoring until stable
- Persistent bronchospasm can be treated with $\beta_2$-agonist bronchodilators.
- Hypotension should be treated with volume repletion. Vasopressors can provide additional support.
- Antihistamines (both $H_1$ and $H_2$ blockers) have been shown to be helpful in preventing histamine interactions with target tissues.
- Corticosteroids help prevent the progression or recurrence of anaphylaxis.
- Glucagon is particularly useful in epinephrine-resistant anaphylaxis from $\beta$-adrenergic blocking agents.

## MEDICATION

### ALERT

A patient's concomitant use of a $\beta$-blocker may antagonize the effects of epinephrine. For these patients consider glucagon as it increases intracellular cyclic adenosine monophosphate levels by a mechanism that does not depend upon $\beta$-receptors.

### First Line

- Diphenhydramine: Adults—50 mg IV; (peds: 1–2 mg/kg) slow IVP
- Epinephrine: 0.3–0.5 mg; use 1:1,000 dilution for SC route and 1:10,000 for IV route (peds: epinephrine 0.01 mg/kg SC/IV)
- Hydrocortisone: Adults—500 mg IV (peds: 4–8 mg/kg/dose IV) OR
- Methylprednisolone: Adult—125 mg IV (peds: 1–2 mg/kg IV) OR
- Prednisone: Adult—60 mg PO (peds: 1 mg/kg PO)
- Albuterol: 0.5 mL of 0.5% solution in 2.5 mL of isotonic saline by nebulizer

### Second Line

- Racemic epinephrine: 2.25% solution (0.5 mL placed in a nebulizer in 2.5 mL of normal saline)
- Glucagon: Adults—1–2 mg IV/IM/SQ
- Ranitidine: Adult—50 mg IV or cimetidine 300 mg IV

 **FOLLOW-UP**

## DISPOSITION

### Admission Criteria

- Intubated patients or patients in respiratory distress should be admitted to an intensive care unit setting.
- A monitored inpatient bed may be necessary for the patient who has not had substantial response to initial therapy.
- Patients with significant generalized reactions and persistent symptoms should be admitted for observation for 24 hr. Biphasic or late phase reactions are known to occur.

### Discharge Criteria

Patients with complete resolution of symptoms may be discharged after several hours of ED observation.

### Issues for Referral

- Consultation with an allergist/immunologist is appropriate when desensitization to an antibiotic is being considered for the treatment of an infectious process.
- When a patient at high risk for contrast reaction needs a contrast study, consultation with the radiologist regarding pretreatment and choice of contrast agent is appropriate.

## FOLLOW-UP RECOMMENDATIONS

- Patients with allergic reactions should have a follow-up within 48 hr of discharge to evaluate effectiveness of outpatient therapy.
- Refer patients who are treated and released from the ED after an episode of anaphylaxis, angioedema, or urticaria to an allergist for follow-up skin testing and consideration for desensitization.
- Patients should be advised to carry some type of treatment that can be self-administered in the event of future reactions such as the prefilled syringe EpiPen.
- Patients with a known trigger should be counseled on strict avoidance of that trigger.

## PEARLS AND PITFALLS

- Failure to consider anaphylaxis early in presentation can lead to devastating hemodynamic compromise and airway collapse.
- Epinephrine given early is the most important intervention.
- Patients with a history of anaphylaxis should be educated about trigger avoidance and instructed in the correct use of epinephrine autoinjector pens.

## ADDITIONAL READING

- Barach EM, et al. Epinephrine for the treatment of anaphylactic shock. *JAMA.* 1984;251:2118.
- Simmons FER. Anaphylaxis: Recent advances in assessment and treatment. *J Allergy Clin Immunol.* 2009;124:625–636.
- Tang MLK, Osborne N, Allen K. Epidemiology of Anaphylaxis. *Curr Opin Allergy Clin Immunol.* 2009;9:351–356.
- Thomas M, Crawford I. Glucagon infusion in refractory anaphylactic shock in patients on beta-blockers. *Emerg Med J.* 2005;22:272–273.

### See Also (Topic, Algorithm, Electronic Media Element)

- Angioedema
- Urticaria

 **CODES**

### ICD9

- 989.5 Toxic effect of venom
- 995.0 Other anaphylactic shock, not elsewhere classified
- 995.60 Anaphylactic shock due to unspecified food

# ANEMIA
*Paul J. Allegretti*

 **BASICS**

## DESCRIPTION
- Reduction below normal in the mass of RBCs
- Measured by one or more of the major RBC components:
  - Hgb (hemoglobin): Concentration of the major oxygen-carrying component in whole blood
  - Hct (hematocrit): Percent volume of whole blood occupied by intact RBCs
  - RBC count: RBCs contained in a volume of whole blood
- Adult female: Hgb <12 g/dL or Hct <37%
- Adult male: Hgb <14 g/dL or Hct <42%
- Normal blood count values depend on age:
  - Birth: Hgb 16.5, Hct 51
  - 1 yr: Hgb 12, Hct 36
  - 6 yr: Hgb 12.5, Hct 37
  - Adult male: Hgb 14, Hct 42
  - Adult female: Hgb 12, Hct 37
- Hgb/Hct depends on oxygen pressure:
  - Increased in neonates and people living above 4,000 ft
- Hgb, Hct, and RBC count are concentrations:
  - Dependent on RBC mass and plasma volume
  - Values decrease if RBC mass decreases or plasma volume increases.
- Anemia is an indication of an underlying disorder or deficiency.

## ETIOLOGY
- Never a normal variant:
  - May be the first manifestation of a systemic disorder
  - Always seek a cause.
- Excessive blood loss (most common cause):
  - Trauma
  - GI bleed
  - Menstruation
- Hemolysis (increased RBC destruction, RBC lifespan <100 days):
  - Hypersplenism
  - Autoimmune hemolytic anemia
  - Mechanical trauma (prosthetic heart valves, vasculitis, thrombotic thrombocytopenic purpura [TTP], hemolytic uremic syndrome [HUS], or disseminated intravascular coagulation [DIC])
  - Toxins
  - Infections (malaria, babesiosis)
  - Membrane abnormalities
  - Intracellular RBC abnormalities (G6PD, sickle cell anemia, or thalassemia)
- Decreased RBC synthesis:
  - Classified by measurement of RBC size
  - Hypochromic/microcytic:
    - Iron deficiency
    - Thalassemia
    - Sideroblastic
    - Chronic disease
  - Normochromic/macrocytic:
    - Hypothyroidism
    - Folate deficiency
    - Vitamin B$_{12}$ deficiency
    - Liver disease
    - Myelodysplasia
    - Certain leukemias
  - Normochromic/normocytic:
    - Aplastic anemia
    - Chronic renal failure
    - Malignancy
    - Adrenal insufficiency
    - Hyperparathyroidism
    - Alcohol abuse
    - Acute blood loss

 **DIAGNOSIS**

## SIGNS AND SYMPTOMS
Depends on:
- Rapidity of onset:
  - Hypovolemia if acute
  - Asymptomatic if mild and chronic

### History
- Underlying disease
- Severity and type of anemia
- Fatigue
- Decreased exercise intolerance
- Shortness of breath
- Dyspnea on exertion
- Chest pain/angina
- Syncope
- Blood in stool/tarry black stools
- Irregular or heavy menses
- Easy bruising or history of excessive bleeding

### Physical Exam
- Cardiovascular:
  - Tachycardia, cardiomegaly, or murmurs
  - Postural hypotension
- Dermatologic:
  - Skin:
    - Cool
    - Pallor
    - Jaundice
    - Purpura
    - Telangiectasia
    - Petechiae
    - Ecchymosis
  - Spoon-shaped nails (koilonychia)
- Neurologic:
  - Neuropathy
  - Altered mental status
- Bone (especially sternal) or joint pain (sickle cell disease)
- Hepatomegaly, splenomegaly
- Lymphadenopathy
- Findings reflect underlying disease

## ESSENTIAL WORKUP
- CBC
- Vital signs/orthostatics
- Determine if:
  - Bleeding
  - Increased RBC destruction
  - Bone marrow suppression
  - Iron deficient

## DIAGNOSTIC TESTS & INTERPRETATION
### Lab
- CBC:
  - RBC indices:
    - Mean corpuscular volume (MCV; normal: 80–100 $\mu$m$^3$)
    - Mean corpuscular hemoglobin (MCH; normal: 27–34 pg/cell)
    - Mean corpuscular hemoglobin concentration (MCHC; normal: 33–36%)
  - Platelet count
- Thrombocytosis suggests:
  - Iron deficiency
  - Myeloproliferative disorders
  - Inflammation
  - Infection
  - Neoplasm
- Thrombocytopenia suggests:
  - Bone marrow malignancy
  - Hypersplenism
  - Sepsis
  - Vitamin B$_{12}$ or folate deficiency
  - Autoimmune disorders
- Reticulocyte count:
  - Normal 0.5–1.5% (reticulocytes/1,000 RBCs)
  - Increased retic count: Increased erythropoietic response to continued blood loss or hemolysis
  - Stable anemia with low retic count: Impaired RBC production
  - Active hemolysis or blood loss with low retic count: Concurrent disorder
  - Low retic count with pancytopenia: Aplastic anemia
  - Low retic count with normal WBC and platelets: Pure RBC aplasia
- Reticulocyte index (RI): Reticulocyte count (%) × (patient Hct/normal Hct):
  - RI <2% implies inadequate RBC production.
  - RI >2% implies increased RBC production with excessive RBC destruction or loss.
- WBC with differential and peripheral smear:
  - Leukopenia with anemia suggests bone marrow suppression, hypersplenism, or deficient vitamin B$_{12}$/folate
- Stool for occult blood
- Electrolytes, BUN, creatinine, glucose:
  - Chronic renal failure
- Urinalysis:
  - Hematuria
  - Hemoglobinuria in hemolytic anemia
- Workup strategy:
  - Hypochromic/microcytic anemias:
    - Iron
    - Total iron-binding capacity
    - Transferrin saturation
    - Ferritin
  - Macrocytic anemias:
    - Folate
    - Vitamin B$_{12}$
    - LFT
    - Thyroid function tests
  - Hemolytic anemia:
    - Rapid fall in Hgb
    - Reticulocytosis
    - Fragmented RBCs
    - Increased LDH
    - Increased indirect bilirubin
    - Decreased serum haptoglobin
    - Coombs positive

- Special tests:
  - Peripheral smear:
    - Helmet cells/schistocytes—microangiopathic hemolysis
    - Teardrop cells—myelofibrosis
    - Spherocytes—autoimmune hemolysis
    - Leukoerythroblastic pattern—bone marrow replacement
    - Bite cells—oxidative hemolysis
    - RBC parasites—malaria or babesiosis
    - Target cells—liver disease
    - Burr cells—uremia
    - Sideroblasts—alcoholism or myelodysplasia
    - Howell Jolly bodies—asplenia
  - Hgb electrophoresis for sickle cell/thalassemia
  - Iron, iron-binding capacity, transferrin saturation, ferritin:
    - Iron deficiency
    - Iron—decreased
    - Iron-binding capacity—increased
    - Transferrin saturation—decreased
    - Ferritin—decreased
  - Chronic disease:
    - Iron—decreased
    - Iron-binding capacity—decreased
    - Transferrin saturation—decreased/normal
    - Ferritin—normal/increased
  - Thalassemia:
    - Iron—normal
    - Iron-binding capacity—normal
    - Ferritin—normal
  - Sideroblastic anemia.
    - Iron—increased
    - Iron-binding capacity—normal
    - Ferritin—increased

### Diagnostic Procedures/Surgery
Bone marrow biopsy evaluates:
- Aplastic anemia
- Myelodysplasia
- Bone marrow malignancy
- Myeloproliferative disorders

### DIFFERENTIAL DIAGNOSIS
- Acquired versus inherited anemia
- Anemia of chronic disease
- Blood loss
- CHF
- Dilutional anemia
- Hemolysis
- Malignancy
- Nutritional deficiency/malabsorption
- Toxic bone marrow suppression

### Pediatric Considerations
Hemolytic anemia of the newborn:
- Rh antibody crosses placenta when Rh-negative mother has Rh-positive child.

### Pregnancy Considerations
Physiologic or dilutional anemia in 3rd-trimester pregnancy:
- 25% increase of RBC mass and 50% increase in plasma volume

### Geriatric Considerations
- Values for Hgb/Hct in healthy elderly are generally lower than in younger adults.
- This lower "normal" must be a diagnosis of exclusion.

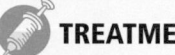

## TREATMENT

### PRE-HOSPITAL
Ongoing blood loss requires close assessment and rapid transport:
- Control bleeding
- Multiple large-bore IVs

### INITIAL STABILIZATION/THERAPY
- Airway, breathing, circulation (ABCs)
- Oxygen
- IV fluid resuscitation with 0.9% NS if ongoing loss/hypotension

### ED TREATMENT/PROCEDURES
- Depends on severity of anemia and acuteness of onset
- Transfusion for hemorrhage with unstable vital signs
- Most anemias seen in ED are chronic and do not require immediate intervention.
- Therapy for specific anemia:
  - Iron deficiency:
    - $FeSO_4$: 300 mg PO t.i.d.
    - Investigate underlying cause.
    - Increased Hgb expected in 2–3 wk
  - Renal failure:
    - Endogenous erythropoietin is diminished.
    - Replace with recombinant erythropoietin
  - Autoimmune hemolytic anemia:
    - Corticosteroids (prednisone 60 mg/d until response)
    - Immunosuppressive agents
    - Plasmapheresis
    - Splenectomy if splenic sequestration
  - Drug-induced hemolytic anemia: Stop offending agent.
  - Anemia of chronic disease: Treat underlying disease.
    Vitamin $B_{12}$ deficiency:
    - Vitamin $B_{12}$: 1,000 $\mu$g IM daily for 1 wk, then weekly for 1 mo, then monthly
    - Hematologic parameters normalize within 2 mo.
    - Neurologic symptoms present >6 mo may be permanent.
  - Folate deficiency:
    - Folic acid: 1 mg PO daily
  - Aplastic anemia
  - Antithymocyte globulin
  - Bone marrow transplantation:
    - Sickle cell anemia
    - Supportive care with oxygen, rehydration, analgesia
    - Treat precipitating cause.
  - Leukemia:
    - Bone marrow replacement

### MEDICATION
- Iron supplements
- Erythropoietin for renal failure
- Corticosteroids for autoimmune
- Vitamin $B_{12}$
- Folic acid (B9)

## FOLLOW-UP

### DISPOSITION
**Admission Criteria**
- Unstable vital signs
- Ongoing blood loss
- Symptomatic anemia—angina/dyspnea/syncope
- Pancytopenia
- Need for transfusion
- Need for aggressive evaluation
- Severe anemia
  - Initial, unexplained Hgb less than 8 g/dL
  - Major difficulty in obtaining outpatient care for patients whose Hgb are significantly low or when comorbidity is present

**Discharge Criteria**
Discharge vast majority of stable patients for outpatient workup.

### FOLLOW-UP RECOMMENDATIONS
Newly diagnosed anemic patients need to be worked up:
- If stable for discharge from the ED, provide follow-up options for workup

## PEARLS AND PITFALLS
- Anemia is an indication of an underlying disorder or deficiency.
- Severe or life-threatening cases require immediate correction via blood transfusion.
- Most cases seen in the ED are chronic and do not require immediate intervention.

## ADDITIONAL READING
- Beutler E. The definition of anemia: What is the lower limit of normal of the blood hemoglobin concentration? *Blood.* 2006.
- Fauci A, Braunwald E, et al. *Harrison's principles of internal medicine*, 17th Ed. New York: McGraw-Hill, 2008.
- Hoffman R, Furie B, et al. *Hematology: Basic principles and practice*, 5th Ed. New York: Churchill-Livingstone, 2009.
- McCullough J. *Blood and bone marrow pathology*. St. Louis, MO: Churchill, 2003.
- Schrier S. *Approach to the patient with anemia*. In: Basow DS (ed), *UpToDate*. Waltham, MA, 2009.

### See Also (Topic, Algorithm, Electronic Media Element)
- GI Bleeding
- Renal Failure
- Sickle Cell Disease

# ANGIOEDEMA
*Sean-Xavier Neath*

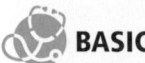

## BASICS

### DESCRIPTION
- Nonpruritic, well-demarcated, nonpitting edema of the dermis
- Due to the release of inflammatory mediators that cause dilation and increased permeability of capillaries and venules:
  - Mast cell-mediated
  - Kinin-related from the generation of bradykinin and complement-derived mediators
- Similar in pathologic basis to urticaria except that affected tissue lies deeper:
  - Urticaria affects superficial tissue and causes irritation to mast cells and nerves in the epidermis leading to intense itching.
  - Angioedema occurs in deeper layers, which have fewer mast cells and nerves, therefore causing less itching.
- Hereditary and acquired etiologies are due to deficiencies in the function of C1-INH rather than hypersensitivity reactions
- Hereditary angioedema (HAE):
  - An autosomal dominant disorder caused by a deficiency of C1-INH
  - The prevalence of hereditary angioedema is estimated to range from 1:10,000–1:150,000.
  - C1 INH has a regulatory role in the contact, fibrinolytic, and coagulation pathways.
  - Deficiency results in unregulated activity of the vasoactive mediators bradykinin, kallikrein, and plasmin.
  - More than 100 mutations of the C1-INH gene have been reported.
  - Type 1: Decreased expression of C1 INH
  - Type 2: Normal plasma levels of C1 INH but the protein is dysfunctional
  - Type 3: Mutation in coagulation factor XII resulting in increased kinin production:
    - Symptoms increased by estrogen-containing medications
  - Episodes occur in all 3 types when inflammation, trauma, or other factors lead to depletion of C1 INH.
- Acquired angioedema:
  - Normal quantities and function of C1-INH
  - Type 1 is associated with lymphoproliferative diseases and caused by consumption of the C1 INH protein by malignant cells.
  - Type 2 is autoimmune caused by circulating antibodies that inactivate C1 INH.
- ACE inhibitor–induced angioedema:
  - 0.1–2.2% of patients taking ACE inhibitors
  - Occurs in 25% during the 1st mo of taking the medication.
  - The 1st event may occur spontaneously after many years of use.

## ETIOLOGY
- Kinin-related etiologies:
  - Hereditary angioedema
  - Acquired angioedema:
    - Lymphoproliferative
    - Autoimmune
  - ACE inhibitor induced
- Mast cell-mediated etiologies:
  - Food allergies:
    - Additives
    - Nuts
    - Eggs
    - Shellfish
    - Soy
    - Wheat
    - Milk
  - Drug allergies:
    - Aspirin
    - NSAID
    - Antihypertensives
    - Narcotics
    - Oral contraceptives
  - Insect stings
  - Physically induced:
    - Cold
    - Heat
    - Vibration
    - Exercise
    - Trauma
    - Stress
    - UV light
- Cytokine-associated AE syndrome (Gleich syndrome)
- Hypereosinophilic syndrome
- Thyroid autoimmune disease
- Idiopathic recurrent AE

## DIAGNOSIS

### SIGNS AND SYMPTOMS
#### History
- A family history or history of recurrent episodes with the use of particular agents can be useful in the diagnosis.
- Abdominal pain associated with nausea, vomiting, and diarrhea
- Attacks of hereditary angioedema are not associated with hives.
- Emotional stress or physical trauma can trigger attacks.

#### Physical Exam
- The lesions of angioedema are large, swollen and nonpitting wheals.
- The eyelids and lips are frequently involved.
- Involvement of the pharynx and larynx may cause airway obstruction.

### ESSENTIAL WORKUP
- The diagnosis is made of clinical grounds based on the presentation of large nonpitting, nonpruritic wheals.
- A family history need not be present to diagnose the disease.

### DIAGNOSTIC TESTS & INTERPRETATION
#### Lab
- CBC with differential, ESR, ANA, rheumatoid factor
- Skin biopsy if an urticarial lesion is accessible

#### Diagnostic Procedures/Surgery
Measurement of C1-INH levels (not routinely available in EDs):
- Patients affected with hereditary angioedema type 1 have very low levels; carriers will have half-normal levels.
- C4 and C2 levels are low during attacks in both hereditary and acquired forms.

### DIFFERENTIAL DIAGNOSIS
- Edema:
  - SVC syndrome
  - Right heart failure
  - Constrictive pericarditis
  - Renal failure
  - Nephrotic syndrome
- Allergic contact dermatitis
- Blepharochalasis
- Facial cellulitis
- Facial lymphedema
- Edema secondary to autoimmune disorders:
  - Dermatomyositis
  - Lupus
  - Polymyositis
  - Sjögren syndrome
- Hypothyroidism

#### Pediatric Considerations
Recurrent angioedema presenting around puberty should raise suspicion of hereditary angioedema.

## TREATMENT

### PRE-HOSPITAL
- Establish IV access
- Early intubation may be necessary due to the rapid progression of laryngeal swelling.
- Administration of H1 blocker when available

## INITIAL STABILIZATION/THERAPY

- Active airway management and supportive measures are the primary goals of emergency treatment.
- Intubation may be necessary in severe cases:
  - Orotracheal intubation is the technique of choice but may be difficult because of laryngeal edema, spasm, or soft-tissue swelling.
  - Consider advanced airway adjuncts such as the gum elastic bougie to assist in securing endotracheal tube placement.
  - Blind nasotracheal intubation if soft tissue swelling prohibits an oral approach
  - Transtracheal jet insufflation or cricothyrotomy may be necessary to control the airway.
- Epinephrine, antihistamines, and steroids in obstructive airway swelling, although patient response can be variable.

## ED TREATMENT/PROCEDURES

- Airway management as above
- Acute angioedema with features of a type I hypersensitivity reaction:
  - Treat similarly to an allergic reaction with H1 and H2 blocker along with corticosteroids.
  - SC epinephrine should be used in refractory cases where the benefits outweigh the risks.
  - For abdominal attacks consider the addition of parenteral pain relief, antiemetics, and IV fluid replacement.
- Hereditary and acquired angioedema:
  - C1 inhibitors
  - Fresh frozen plasma (FFP) may be used as an alternative to C1 inhibitors.
  - The kallikrein inhibitor ecallantide (Kalbitor) was approved in 2009 for the treatment of acute attacks of HAE.
  - Tranexamic acid (Cyklokapron), an antifibrinolytic agent, are not as effective for acute attacks and are used

### ALERT

- C1 inhibition has been standard therapy in Europe for many years however the U.S. FDA has only recently been approving these medications for use in the United States therefore clinician and pharmacist recognition of the utility of these drugs may be limited.
- Therapy with FFP (as a source of nonpurified C1-INH) is advised with caution as it may paradoxically worsen some attacks due to its high concentration of complement components.
- Attenuated androgens, such as the anabolic steroids and gonadotropin inhibitor danazol, are used in the long-term prophylactic treatment. They may not have any effect for 24–48 hr in the acute setting.
- Angioedema associated with ACE inhibitors occurs in 0.1–0.2% of cases and requires immediate withdrawal of the ACE inhibitor and replacement with another antihypertensive medication. ACE inhibitor–related angioedema usually occurs within a week after starting ACE inhibitor therapy, but may occur at any time during the use of the medication.

## MEDICATION

- C1 inhibitors:
  - Cinryze: 1,000 U IV with additional 1,000 U if no improvement in 60 min
  - Berinert: 20 U/kg IV infused slowly not to exceed 4 mL/min
- Cimetidine: 300 mg IV
- Danazol: 400–600 mg PO up to 1 g/day
  *Contraindicated in children and pregnancy.*
- Diphenhydramine: Adult: 50 mg IV; peds: 1–2 mg/kg slow IVP
- Ecallantide: 30 mg SC
- Epinephrine: 0.3–0.5 mg (use 1:1,000 dilution for SC route, and 1:10,000 for IV route); peds: 0.01 mg/kg SC/IV
- Racemic epinephrine: 2.25% solution (0.5 mL placed in a nebulizer in 2.5 mL of NS)
- FFP (if C1-INH is unavailable): Adult: 2 U
- Hydrocortisone: Adult: 500 mg IV; peds: 4–8 mg/kg/dose IV.
- Methylprednisolone: Adult: 125 mg IV; peds: 1–2 mg/kg IV
- Prednisone: Adult: 60 mg PO; peds: 1 mg/kg PO
- Ranitidine: Adult: 50 mg IV
- Stanozolol: 2 mg PO up to 16 mg/day:
  - Discontinued in the U.S.
  - Contraindicated in children and in pregnancy
- Tranexamic acid: 1 g PO q3–4h for up to 48 hr if necessary
- Suspected HAE:
  - C1 inhibitors
  - Ecallantide
- Non-HAE:
  H1 blockers
  H2 blockers
  Corticosteroids

### Pediatric Considerations

Safety and efficacy of newer HAE treatment agents (such as C1 Inhibitors Cinryze and Berinert) have not been established in children as of this writing.

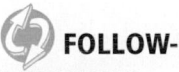 **FOLLOW-UP**

## DISPOSITION

### Admission Criteria

- Patients with systemic symptoms that do not resolve completely will need to be hospitalized for observation.
- A monitored bed is recommended for those with airway involvement.

### Discharge Criteria

- Patients presenting with minor symptoms of angioedema without progression after 4–6 hr of observation may be safely discharged home on a short course of steroids and antihistamines.
- Patients should be provided with an EpiPen and instructions in its use.

### Issues for Referral

Patients should be evaluated by an allergist/immunologist after the initial presentation, especially if there is a family history of angioedema, or if the angioedema is accompanied by abdominal pain, or triggered by trauma.

### FOLLOW-UP RECOMMENDATIONS

Patients without systemic symptoms who are stable for discharge should been seen in outpatient follow-up in a few days.

## PEARLS AND PITFALLS

- Early measures should be employed to maintain the patient's airway.
- Consider use of newer agents in HAE patients (eg, C1 Inhibitor and Kallikrein inhibition).

## ADDITIONAL READING

- Austen K. Allergies, anaphylaxis, and systemic mastocytosis. In: Fauci AS, Braunwald E, Kasper DL, et al., eds. *Harrison's Principles of Internal Medicine*, 17e. McGraw Hill; 2008.
- Gompels M, Lock R, Abinun M, et al. C1 inhibitor deficiency: Consensus document. *Clin Exp Imm.* 2005;139:379–408.
- Grattan C, Powell S, Humphreys F. Management and diagnostic guidelines for urticaria and angio-oedema. *Br J Dermatol.* 2001;144:708–714.
- Temiño VM, Stokes Peebles R. The spectrum and treatment of angioedema. *Am J Med.* 2008;121:282–286.
- Zuraw B. Hereditary Angioedema. *N Engl J Med.* 2008;359:1027–1036.

### See Also (Topic, Algorithm, Electronic Media Element)

- Anaphylaxis
- Urticaria

 **CODES**

### ICD9

- 277.6 Other deficiencies of circulating enzymes
- 995.1 Angioneurotic edema, not elsewhere classified

# ANKLE FRACTURE/DISLOCATION

Binh T. Ly
Leslie C. Oyama

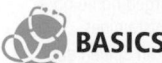 **BASICS**

## DESCRIPTION
Common mechanisms and injury patterns of the ankle:

- Mechanism of Injury:
  - Inversion injury:
    ○ Avulsion fracture of the lateral malleolus
    ○ Oblique fracture of the medial malleolus
  - Eversion injury:
    ○ Avulsion fracture of the medial malleolus
    ○ Oblique fracture of the fibula
  - External rotation injury:
    ○ Disruption of the tibiofibular syndesmosis, or a fibular fracture above the plafond
    ○ Anterior or posterior tibial fracture with separation of the distal tibia and fibula (unstable fracture)
  - Inversion and external rotation (Maisonneuve fracture):
    ○ Medial malleolus avulsion fracture or deltoid ligament tear
    ○ Disruption of the tibiofibular syndesmosis
    ○ Oblique fracture of the proximal fibula
  - Inversion and dorsiflexion (Snowboarders' fracture):
    ○ Fracture of the lateral process of the talus

### Pediatric Considerations
- Ankle fractures in children often involve the physis (growth plate):
  - May cause chronic deformity from growth plate injury
  - In children <10 yr of age, growth plate is weaker than epiphysis.

- *Tillaux fracture:* Salter–Harris type III injury of the lateral tibial epiphysis caused by eversion and lateral rotation.
- *Triplane fracture:* Unusual fracture of distal tibia with fracture lines in three distinct planes (coronal, transverse, sagittal):
  - Ottawa Ankle Rules. (Adapted from Bachmann LM. *Br Med J.* 2003;326:417) Available at http://bmj.bmjjournals.com/content/vol326/issue7386/images/large/bacl4176.f2.jpeg.

 **DIAGNOSIS**

## SIGNS AND SYMPTOMS
- History of trauma
- Local ankle pain, swelling, deformity
- Inability to bear weight
- Soft tissue injury, swelling, ecchymosis, skin tenting, skin blanching
- Neurovascular compromise:
  - Diminished capillary refill
  - Diminished posterior tibialis (PT) or dorsalis pedis (DP) pulses
- Limited range of motion

### History
- Discover the position of the ankle at the time of injury.
- Determine if patient was able to bear weight immediately or if he or she needed assistance to walk afterwards.
- Ask if the patient heard audible "pop" or "snap," as this may indicate partial or full tendon rupture.

### Physical Exam
- *Ottawa ankle rules* (Figure): Decision rules for ordering radiographs in patients with suspected injury to the ankle and midfoot:
  - Malleolar zone (if either finding is present, then *ankle* radiographs are indicated):
    ○ Bony tenderness at the posterior edge or distal 6 cm of either malleoli (points A and B)
    ○ Inability to bear weight for 4 consecutive steps both immediately after the injury and in ED
  - Midfoot zone (if either finding is present, then *foot* radiographs are indicated):
    ○ Bony tenderness at the base of the fifth metatarsal (point C)
    ○ Bony tenderness of the navicular medially (point D)
    ○ Inability to bear weight for 4 consecutive steps both immediately after the injury and in ED
- Assess the skin for disruption or ischemia.
- Careful evaluation of distal neurovascular status:
  - Capillary refill
  - Palpation or Doppler of dorsalis pedis and posterior tibialis pulses
- Palpate proximal fibula for tenderness, especially when medial malleolus or deltoid ligament tenderness is present:
  - Peroneal nerve is at risk for injury with a Maisonneuve fracture:
    ○ Wraps around the fibular head
    ○ Test anterior tibialis and extensor hallucis longus.
    ○ Assess sensation in first web space.
- Radiography:
  - Anteroposterior (AP), lateral, and mortise (leg internally rotated 20 degrees) views of the ankle if tenderness is elucidated in the malleolar zone
  - Evaluate the mortise view for widening of the medial clear space >4 mm and tibiofibular clear space >6 mm.
  - Consider radiographs for the following special circumstances:
    ○ Altered sensorium or diminished distal limb sensation
    ○ Multiple painful and distracting injuries
    ○ Injuries that occurred 10 days prior to evaluation

## DIAGNOSTIC TESTS & INTERPRETATION
### Imaging
- Unstable ankle fractures or dislocations require postreduction radiographs in all 3 planes after splinting.
- AP and lateral radiographs of the tibia and fibula are indicated if a Maisonneuve fracture is suspected clinically.
- Stress testing of the ligaments in a painful ankle is unnecessary in the ED if the patient will be re-examined in 3–7 days.
- Stress radiographs of the ankle are usually unnecessary acutely.
- CT scan or MRI:
  - Assess the degree of injury to the tibial plafond.

### Diagnostic Procedures/Surgery
N/A

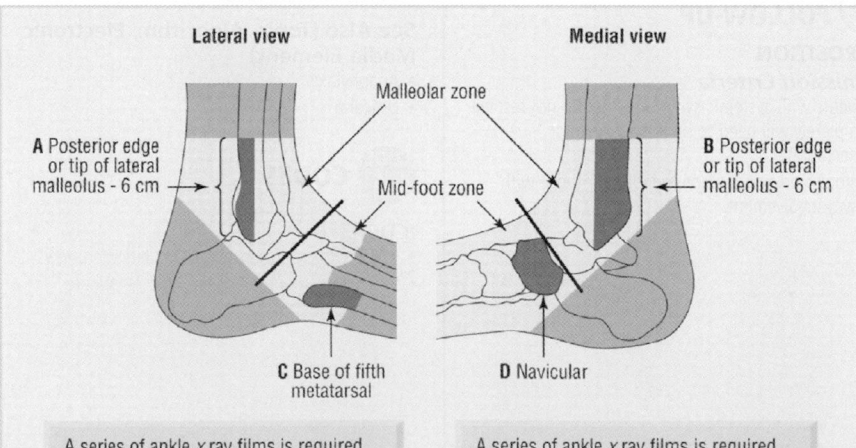

## DIFFERENTIAL DIAGNOSIS

- Ankle sprain
- Achilles tendon injury
- Os trigonum fracture
- Fifth metatarsal fracture (Jones fracture)
- Peroneal tendon dislocation or injury
- Talar fractures
- Talar dome fracture/lesion
- Subtalar dislocations
- Calcaneal fractures
- Foot fractures
- Ankle diastasis
- Rattlesnake envenomation

### Pediatric Considerations

- Injury to the growth plates may not be apparent on plain radiographs.
- Consider immobilization, non-weight-bearing status, and orthopedic referral if clinical suspicion warrants, even in the setting of negative radiographs.
- CT scan or MRI may be warranted to delineate the extent of the injury.
- Inform parents of the possibility of growth abnormalities in patients with injury to the physis.

 **TREATMENT**

### PRE-HOSPITAL

- Immobilize with soft splint to reduce pain, bleeding, and further injury.
- Cautions:
  - Traction devices are usually unnecessary:
    - Contraindicated with open injuries
  - Protruding bone should not be reduced; the wound should be covered with a clean dressing.

### INITIAL STABILIZATION/THERAPY

- Avoid weight bearing
- Ice
- Compression
- Elevation

### ED TREATMENT/PROCEDURES

- Ankle fracture:
  - All ankle fractures or dislocations require orthopedic consultation or referral.
  - Open ankle fractures:
    - Remove contaminants.
    - Apply moist sterile dressing.
    - Assess tetanus immunity.
    - Antibiotics
    - Emergent orthopedic consultation

- Closed ankle fractures:
  - Closed reduction if necessary
  - Immobilize with a posterior splint.
  - *Posterior splint* immobilizes the foot at a 90° angle with the application of bulky dressings and covered by volar (posterior) *and* coaptation (U-shaped stirrup) splinting material.
- *Stable injury* (injury to only one side of the ankle):
  - Isolated injury to the lateral malleolus without medial involvement is virtually always stable.
  - Apply posterior splint.
- *Unstable injury* (both sides of the ankle are injured):
  - Urgent orthopaedic consultation
  - Posterior splint as in stable injuries
  - May require open reduction and internal fixation (ORIF) emergently before significant swelling develops
- *Neurovascular injury* requires emergent orthopedic consultation.
- Ankle dislocations:
  - Closed reduction should be performed as rapidly as possible to minimize ischemia to the skin and reduce the risk of avascular necrosis of the talus.
  - Skin tenting and evidence of neurovascular compromise are indications for immediate reduction, even prior to radiographs.
  - Most ankle dislocations require ORIF.
  - After reduction, place a posterior splint.

### MEDICATION

- Closed fractures.
  - Primarily analgesics (opioids)
- Dislocations or displaced fractures requiring closed reduction:
  - Short-acting benzodiazepine (midazolam 0.05–0.1 mg/kg IV) or barbiturate (methohexital 1–1.5 mg/kg IV) with opioid analgesic
- Open fractures:
  - Cefazolin: 2 g loading dose (peds: 50 mg/kg) IV
  - Gentamicin: 5–7 mg/kg (peds: 2.5 mg/kg) IV
  - Vancomycin: 1-g loading dose (10 mg/kg in children) if penicillin allergic IV
  - Tetanus toxoid if indicated

 **FOLLOW-UP**

### DISPOSITION

#### Admission Criteria

- Unstable ankle fractures require urgent orthopedic consultation and may require admission.
- Open ankle fractures and dislocations should be admitted for debridement, irrigation, and IV antibiotics.
- Ankle dislocations that are treated with either open or closed reduction
- Concern for compartment syndrome or neurovascular injury

#### Discharge Criteria

Simple nondisplaced stable ankle fractures without neurovascular compromise may be splinted and the patient discharged.

#### FOLLOW-UP RECOMMENDATIONS

- Splinting
- Elevation of affected lower extremity
- Fitted for crutches and shown how to use them
- Placed on non-weight-bearing status of affected joint, until seen by orthopedist

## PEARLS AND PITFALLS

- To reduce dislocated ankle, partial flexion of knee of affected limb will decrease tension on Achilles' tendon and ankle.
- Differentiate between ankle fracture and subtalar fracture on physical exam: While the latter is rare, it is also rarely reducible.

## ADDITIONAL READING

- Bachmann LM, Kolb E, Koller MT, et al. Accuracy of Ottawa ankle rules to exclude fractures of the ankle and mid-foot: Systematic review. *Br Med J.* 2003;326:417.
- Duchesneau S, Fallat LM. The Maisonneuve fracture. *J Foot Ankle Surg.* 1995;34(5):422–428.
- Slimmon D, Brukner P. Sports ankle injuries: Assessment and management. *Aust Fam Physician.* 2010;39(1–2):18–22.
- Marsh JL, Saltzman CL. Ankle fractures. In: Bucholz RW, Heckman JD, eds. *Rockwood and Green's Fractures in Adults,* 5th ed. Philadelphia: Lippincott Williams & Wilkins, 2001;201–283.
- Moehring HD, Tan RT, Marder RA, et al. Ankle dislocation. *J Orthop Trauma.* 1994;8:167–172.
- Plint AC, Bulloch B, Osmond MH, et al. Validation of the Ottawa Ankle Rules in children with ankle injuries. *Acad Emerg Med.* 1999;6:1005–1009.
- Syed AA, Agarwal M, Dosani A, et al. Medial subtalar dislocation: Importance of clinical diagnosis in distinguishing from other dislocations. *Eur J Emerg Med.* 2003;10(3):232–235.

### See Also (Topic, Algorithm, Electronic Media Element)

Ottawa Ankle Rules Figure

 **CODES**

### ICD9

- 824.8 Unspecified fracture of ankle, closed
- 837.0 Closed dislocation of ankle

# ANKLE SPRAIN

*Taylor Y. Cardall*

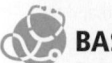 **BASICS**

## DESCRIPTION
- Injuries to ligamentous supports of the ankle
- Ankle joint is a hinge joint composed of the tibia, fibula, and talus.
- Injuries may range from stretching with microscopic damage (grade I) to partial disruption (grade II) to complete disruption (grade III).

## ETIOLOGY
- Forced inversion or eversion of the ankle
- Forceful collisions
- 85–90% of ankle sprains involve lateral ligaments:
  - Anterior talofibular (ATFL)
  - Posterior talofibular (PTFL)
  - Calcaneofibular (CFL)
  - Usually the result of an inversion injury
  - The ATFL is the most commonly injured.
  - If the ankle is injured in a neutral position, the CFL is often injured.
  - The PTFL is rarely injured alone.
- Injury to the deltoid ligament (connecting the medial malleolus to the talus and navicular bones) is usually the result of an eversion injury:
  - Often associated with avulsion at the medial malleolus or talar insertion
  - Rarely found as an isolated injury
  - Suspect associated lateral malleolus fracture or fracture of the proximal fibula (Maisonneuve fracture).
- Syndesmosis sprains (injury to the tibiofibular ligaments or the interosseous ligament of the leg):
  - Occur most commonly in collision sports
  - Syndesmosis injuries ("high ankle sprains") have a higher morbidity and potential for long-term complications.

### Pediatric Considerations
- Children <10 yr with traumatic ankle pain and no radiologic evidence of fracture most likely have a Salter-Harris I fracture.
- The ligaments are actually stronger than the open epiphysis.

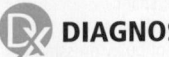 **DIAGNOSIS**

## SIGNS AND SYMPTOMS
### History
History may predict the type of injury found and should include:
- Time of injury
- Mechanism
- The presence of a "pop" or "crack"
- History of previous trauma
- Relevant medical conditions (eg, bone or joint disease)
- Treatments attempted prior to arrival
- Ability to bear weight subsequent to the injury at scene and ED

### Physical Exam
- Aimed at detecting joint instability and any associated injuries:
  - Note the presence or absence of bony tenderness at posterior edge of medial and lateral malleoli as well as at the base of the 5th metatarsal.
- Document neurovascular status distal to the injury.
- Assess range of motion and compare it with the uninjured side.
- Stress testing in the ED is often limited by pain and may impair detection of ligament injury.
- The squeeze test helps identify syndesmosis injuries:
  - Squeeze tibia and fibula together at the midcalf; pain felt in the ankle indicates a positive test.

## ESSENTIAL WORKUP
- The Ottawa Ankle Rules, a selective strategy for obtaining ankle radiographs in adults, suggest that foot or ankle radiographs are unnecessary except when any of the following are present:
  - Bony tenderness at the posterior edge of the distal 6 cm or tip of either malleolus
  - Bony tenderness along the base of the 5th metatarsal or navicular bone
  - Inability to take 4 unassisted steps both immediately after the injury and in the ED
- The rules have been prospectively validated by the original authors as well as independently by groups in the U.S., the U.K., France, and other countries.

## DIAGNOSTIC TESTS & INTERPRETATION
### Imaging
- Ankle injuries should be radiographed if there is concern for fracture.
- Stress radiographs are rarely useful in the ED and should not be routinely ordered unless requested by a consultant.

## DIFFERENTIAL DIAGNOSIS
- Ankle fracture (lateral, medial, or posterior malleolus) or dislocation
- Achilles tendon injury
- Maisonneuve fracture
- Os trigonum fracture
- 5th metatarsal fracture (Jones fracture)
- Transchondral talar dome fracture
- Peroneal tendon dislocation or injury

 **TREATMENT**

## PRE-HOSPITAL
Immobilize ankle as necessary.

## INITIAL STABILIZATION/THERAPY
- Prevent further injury; avoid weight-bearing if painful.
- RICE (rest, ice, compression, elevation)

## ED TREATMENT/PROCEDURES

- The goal of treatment is reduction of pain and return to normal activity without long-term pain or joint laxity.
- Existing evidence supports early mobilization and functional treatment:
  - Unstable ankles (ie, grade III) or those with severe pain may benefit from brief immobilization followed by early return to functional treatment.
- Grade I or II sprains can be treated with functional support (elastic bandage, air splint, gel splint, etc.):
  - Recent evidence suggests an elastic bandage dressing couple with an air stirrup splint is superior to other forms of immobilization.
- Grade III sprains can be treated by immobilization (sugar tong with posterior splint or elastic bandage dressing coupled with air stirrup splint) and early orthopedic consultation or referral.
- Crutches may be needed initially for comfort, but encourage weight-bearing as tolerated for grades I and II.
- Once acute pain and swelling have resolved, strengthening exercises and proprioceptive training (eg, balance board, small circle walking) improve ankle strength and function and prevent reinjury.
- Full sports activities may be resumed only when running and turning are pain free.
- Ankle taping, air splints, or gel splints reduce the risk of recurrent injury in high-risk sports such as basketball, volleyball, soccer, and running.

## MEDICATION

- NSAIDs are useful in treating acute pain:
  - Ibuprofen: 800 mg (peds: 5–10 mg/kg) PO t.i.d.
- Narcotic analgesics may be required for severe pain.

## 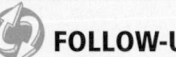 FOLLOW-UP

### DISPOSITION

#### *Admission Criteria*
An isolated ankle sprain should not require admission.

#### *Discharge Criteria*
An isolated ankle sprain may be safely discharged from the ED with appropriate treatment, prescriptions, aftercare instructions, and referrals.

#### *Issues for Referral*
Patient copies of any radiographs obtained may facilitate early follow-up.

### FOLLOW-UP RECOMMENDATIONS

- Patients with grades I and II sprains should be instructed to follow up with the primary care physician in 1–2 wk.
- Patients with grade III sprains and syndesmosis injuries should be referred to an orthopedic surgeon or sports medicine specialist within 7–10 days.

## PEARLS AND PITFALLS

- The Ottawa Ankle Rules may decrease the need for radiographs.
- Immobilization with an elastic bandage dressing coupled with an air stirrup splint followed by early functional therapy may shorten healing time.

## ADDITIONAL READING

- Beynnon BD, Renström PA, Haugh L, et al. A prospective, randomized clinical investigation of the treatment of 1st-time ankle sprains. *Am J Sports Med.* 2006;35:1401–1402.
- Ho K, Abu-Laban RB. Ankle and foot. In: Marx JA, ed. *Rosen's emergency medicine: Concepts and clinical practice*, 7th ed. Philadelphia: Mosby/Elsevier, 2010:670–697.
- Jones MH, Amendola AS. Acute treatment of inversion ankle sprains: Immobilization versus functional treatment. *Clin Orthop Relat Res.* 2007;455:169–172.
- Stiell IG, McKnight RD, Greenberg GH, et al. Decision rules for use of radiography in acute ankle injuries: Refinement and prospective validation. *JAMA.* 1993;269:1127–1132.

##  CODES

### ICD9
845.00 Unspecified site of ankle sprain

# ANKYLOSING SPONDYLITIS

Paul L. DeSandre

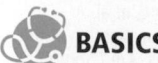 **BASICS**

## DESCRIPTION
- Inflammatory disorder, primarily spinal, with sacroiliac involvement universally:
  - SI joints 100%
  - Cervical spine 75%
  - Thoracic spine 70%
  - LS spine 50%
  - Hip joints 30%
  - Shoulder joints 30%
- *Spondylitis* (inflammation of vertebrae) of ankylosing spondylitis (AS) begins at the insertions of the outer fibers of the annulus fibrosus (enthesitis) of the vertebrae:
  - Ossification (syndesmophyte formation) may lead to complete fusion, *ankylosis*, of the vertebrae.
  - Extensive spinal involvement causes the radiographic appearance of the brittle cbamboo spine.d
- Onset 15–35 yr of age
- Male to female ratio is 3:1.

### ALERT
The brittle spine of AS patients significantly increases their risks for fracture and paralysis.

## RISK FACTORS
### Genetics
Strong genetic component. HLA-B27 gene contributes approximately 37% overall.

## ETIOLOGY
Disease is likely triggered by environmental factors in genetically predisposed individuals, such as trauma or infection.

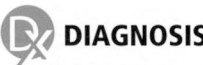 **DIAGNOSIS**

## SIGNS AND SYMPTOMS
- Spinal: Low back pain with sacroiliitis is the most common presentation:
  - Paralysis from minor spinal trauma or manipulation
  - Cauda equina syndrome
- Extraspinal inflammatory conditions (which may precede spinal symptoms):
  - Ocular (the most common):
    - Uveitis (40%)
  - Cardiac:
    - Proliferative endarteritis
    - Increased risk of CAD
    - Aortic (19%) and mitral (32%) regurgitation
  - Pulmonary:
    - Progressive restrictive lung disease due limited expansion and fibrosis
  - GI:
    - Possible inflammatory enteritis
  - GU:
    - Possible prostatitis
  - Enthesitis (inflammation at tendon or ligament insertion):
    - Often Achilles tendonitis or plantar fasciitis

## History
- Inflammatory low back pain >3 mo, radiating into gluteal areas from sacroiliac region, and progressing to involve entire spinal region:
  - Worse with rest and improved with mild activity.
  - Women may have more cervical and extraspinal manifestations than men.
- Possible prior history of uveitis, aortic or mitral valve disease, restrictive pulmonary disease, inflammatory enteritis, prostatitis, enthesitis, or hip or shoulder arthritis.

## Physical Exam
- Flattening of the normal lumbar lordosis
- Exaggeration of thoracic kyphosis
- Limitation of spinal movement
- Possible aortic or mitral valve regurgitation murmur
- Reduction in chest expansion

## Pediatric Considerations
- Juvenile ankylosing spondylitis (JAS) may mimic a septic process with fever and systemic signs.
- Onset of JAS is late childhood or adolescence (usually before age 16 yr); primarily boys.
- JAS may initially present as aortic regurgitation with fulminant aortitis and may have an association with Takayasu arteritis.
- JAS has a much greater predilection for extraspinal joints and entheses of the lower extremities; in addition to sacroiliac tenderness, examine for:
  - Asymmetrical arthritis of the joints of the lower extremities, especially hip
  - Enthesitis of the Achilles tendon attachment at the heel, the plantar fascia attachments to the sole of the foot, the patellar ligament attachment to the tibial tuberosity, and the quadriceps tendon attachments to the patella

## ESSENTIAL WORKUP
- Exclude fracture or neurologic injury in any patient with suspected AS for any new spinal pain (even without trauma).
- Exclude sepsis or septic joint if clinically indicated.
- Evaluate for sacroiliitis with pelvic rock test (compression) or Patrick test (sacroiliac distraction).

## DIAGNOSTIC TESTS & INTERPRETATION
### Lab
- CBC may show mild leukocytosis with slight to moderate anemia and thrombocytosis.
- BUN, creatinine, and electrolytes may be useful to assess renal involvement.
- Erythrocyte sedimentation rate (ESR) or C-reactive protein (CRP) may be elevated, but are of limited use in the ED.

## Imaging
- Pelvic radiograph: Should be done in any adult patient suspected of undiagnosed ankylosing spondylitis:
  - Sacroiliitis is essential to the diagnosis of AS; this is seen initially as subchondral bony erosions on the iliac side of the sacroiliac (SI) joint, which later manifest as bony proliferation and sclerosis.
- Lumbar, thoracic, and cervical spine radiographs to exclude fracture for complaint of new pain to these areas with or without trauma
- CT should be performed to further evaluate possible fractures on plain radiographs.
- MRI should be performed emergently on any patient with neurologic deficit.
- Chest radiograph may show patchy inflammatory infiltrates.

## Diagnostic Procedures/Surgery
- Electrocardiogram indications:
  - Symptoms of acute coronary syndrome (increased risk)
  - Symptomatic arrhythmia:
    - AV block (20%)
- Echocardiogram indications:
  - Severe acute valvulitis
    - Sudden heart failure with severe AR or MR murmur.

## DIFFERENTIAL DIAGNOSIS
- Juvenile ankylosing spondylitis:
  - Onset before age 16
  - More enthesites and extraspinal joint involvement.
- Reactive arthritis (formerly Reiter's syndrome):
  - Arthritis, urethritis, and conjunctivitis beginning about 1 mo after an episode of urethritis or enteritis.
- Enteropathic arthritis:
  - Crohn's disease or ulcerative colitis:
  - Primarily involves knee, elbow, ankle, or wrist, and usually exacerbated by flares of the bowel disease
- Psoriatic arthritis:
  - Psoriasis rash
  - Much greater predilection for the hands and feet.
- Septic arthritis:
  - Exclude with arthrocentesis if clinically suspected in single joint involvement.
- Mechanical low back pain:
  - Improved with rest and exacerbated by exercise without signs of systemic inflammatory process.
- Infectious low back pain:
  - More constant, unremitting, and typically associated with fever.
- Neoplastic low back pain:
  - Typically in patients older than 40, more constant and unremitting, and more characteristically at night.

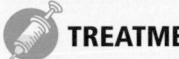 **TREATMENT**

### PRE-HOSPITAL

#### ALERT
- High risk of spinal injury from minor trauma.
- Spinal immobilization must avoid creating further injury:
  - Cushion stabilization and scoop board in position of comfort may be a better approach than cervical collar and/or backboard.
- Intubation difficulty
  - Cervical and TMJ restriction may limit success in all but fiberoptic techniques.
  - Consider alternative airway approaches such as LMA or bag valve mask with oral airway until definitive airway can be achieved safely (usually fiberoptic).
- Ventilation difficulty
  - Chest wall restriction from deformity and pulmonary fibrosis
- CPR, although unavoidable, may carry a higher likelihood of rib fractures

### INITIAL STABILIZATION/THERAPY
- Trauma: ABCs while maintaining safe immobilization
- Acute traumatic paralysis: Immediate high dose methylprednisolone IV and neurosurgical evaluation

### ED TREATMENT/PROCEDURES
- Exclude cord compression if clinically suspected (MRI is the study of choice).
- Exclude spinal fracture for any new spinal pain (CT may be necessary).
- Exclude infection if clinically suspected with laboratory analysis and arthrocentesis.
- Control pain and inflammation with NSAIDs

### MEDICATION
- Nonselective NSAIDs:
  - Ibuprofen: 35 mg/kg/d divided q.i.d., max. 50 mg/kg/d (adult: 300–800 mg PO t.i.d. or q.i.d.)
  - Indomethacin: 1–2 mg/kg/d divided b.i.d. or q.i.d., max. 4 mg/kg/d (adult: 25 mg PO b.i.d. or t.i.d.)
  - Naproxen: 10 mg/kg/d divided b.i.d., max. 1,000 mg/d (adult: 250–500 mg PO b i d)
- COX 2 inhibitors:
  - Cefelocoxib (adult: 100 mg–200 mg PO b.i.d)

### Pregnancy Considerations
- NSAIDs should be avoided in pregnancy.
  - Acetaminophen is first line
  - Opioids are second line

### Geriatric Considerations
NSAID use may increase risk in the elderly for cardiovascular disease, GI bleeding, renal function, and hypertension. Although effective in select patients, close follow-up is prudent.

#### ALERT
- High dose steroids for acute paralysis:
  - Methylprednisolone: 30 mg/kg bolus, then 5.4 mg/kg/h for 24 hr total
- NSAIDs:
  - GI bleeding risks
    - elderly, history of PUD, concurrent use of glucocorticoids, anticoagulants, low dose aspirin (<325 mg/day), smoking, alcohol use, and higher doses.
    - Consider celecoxib or adding an H2 blocker or PPI if patient is at higher risk for GI bleeding.

### Second Line
Consider if NSAIDs or acetaminophen are ineffective at appropriate doses:
- Opioid analgesics, muscle relaxants, or low-dose steroids.

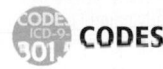 **FOLLOW-UP**

### DISPOSITION

#### Admission Criteria
- Acute neurologic impairment
- Pain is intractable.
- Sepsis or septic joint cannot be excluded.

#### Discharge Criteria
- No serious injuries or neurologic deficit
- Pain is manageable to the patient

#### Issues for Referral
- The patient should be encouraged to obtain a medical alert bracelet.
- Rheumatology:
  - Delay in diagnosis remains a challenge. Patients with sufficient evidence of a new diagnosis of AS should be considered for early referral to a specialist in Rheumatology.
  - TNFb1 blockers are an effective additional treatment in certain patients, and may be a consideration when referring for further outpatient management.
- Physical Medicine and Rehabilitation:
  - Resting splints for inflamed joints
  - Orthoses for enthesitis (such as heel cushion inserts to rest Achilles tendon attachment)

### FOLLOW-UP RECOMMENDATIONS
- Routine primary care reevaluation within 1–2 wk to assess response to treatment.
- Earlier follow-up in any patient with higher risk for adverse response to NSAIDs:
  - Elderly, hypertensive patients, and patients with higher GI bleeding risks.

## PEARLS AND PITFALLS
- Intubation is likely to be difficult and should avoid neck repositioning
  - Consider airway adjuncts (such as LMA) until a definitive airway (usually fiberoptic) can be safely assured.
- Immobilization must avoid creating additional injury
  - Consider cushion/tape stabilization in position of comfort rather than standard cervical collar and backboard
- Minor injuries in AS can result in spinal fracture and possible cord injury. Maintain a high clinical suspicion.

## ADDITIONAL READING

- Sidiropoulos PI, Hatemi G, Song IH, et al. Evidence-based recommendations for the management of ankylosing spondylitis: systematic literature search of the 3E Initiative in Rheumatology involving a broad panel of experts and practicing rheumatologists. Rheumatology 2008;47:355–361.
- McVeigh CM, Cairns AP. Diagnosis and management of ankylosing spondylitis. Br Med J 2006;333: 581–585.
- Song IH, Poddubnyy DA, Rudwaleit M, et al. Benefits and risks of ankylosing spondylitis treatment with nonsteroidal anti-inflammatory drugs. Arthritis & Rheumatism 2008;58:929–938.

### See Also (Topic, Algorithm, Electronic Media Element)
- http://www.spondylitis.org

**CODES**

### ICD9
720.0 Ankylosing spondylitis

# ANTERIOR CRUCIATE LIGAMENT INJURY

*Moss Mendelson*

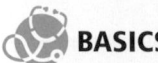

## BASICS

### DESCRIPTION
- The anterior cruciate ligament (ACL) inserts anterolaterally to the anterior tibial spine and to the posterior aspect of the lateral femoral condyle:
  - Portions are under tension (ie, at risk) in both flexion and extension.
- The ACL prevents excessive anterior movement, excessive internal rotation of the tibia on the femur, or hyperextension of the knee.
- Mechanism of injury is often deceleration with flexion and rotation:
  - Hyperextension can also occur.

### ETIOLOGY
The ACL is the most commonly injured ligament of the knee:
- Most injuries to the ACL are sports-related, especially to skiing and football.
- Noncontact injury is common: Plant-and-pivot or stop-and-jump mechanism.
- Female athletes are more susceptible to ACL injury.
- Sports in which cleats are used may result in higher incidence of ACL injury.

### *Pediatric Considerations*
- The ACL is the most frequently injured knee ligament in children.
- Tears of the ACL in children often occur at the insertion site of the ligament.

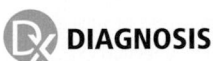

## DIAGNOSIS

### SIGNS AND SYMPTOMS
#### *History*
- Feeling knee "give way."
- Hearing a pop or feeling a tearing sensation at time of injury
- Pain most common complaint with ACL rupture
- Partial injury may not be particularly painful owing to paucity of pain fibers in ACL itself.
- Most patients report immediate knee dysfunction:
  - Some may ambulate despite complete ACL rupture because of stability from supporting structures.

#### *Physical Exam*
- *Immediate effusion* (hemarthrosis within 2–3 hr) usually indicates a significant intra-articular injury.
- About 70% of acute knee hemarthroses are caused by ACL injury.
- Lack of hemarthrosis does not rule out ACL injury:
  - Capsular disruption may allow extravasation of intra-articular blood.
- "Locking" may occur because of interposition of torn cruciate, associated torn menisci, or loose body:
  - Pseudolocking may be present from pain, effusion, or spasm.
- Stress testing—*always compare the injured to the uninjured side:*
  - Asymmetry is more reliable than absolute degree of laxity.
  - Pain and spasm can limit the utility of all stress testing in the acute phase.
  - *Lachman test* is most reliable:
    - Knee flexed 20 degrees, patient supine with thigh supported; tibia is brought forward on the femur, one hand holding proximal tibia, the other stabilizing the femur just above the patella.
    - Pain with no motion is probable grade 1 injury.
    - Pain with motion indicates partial tear or disruption.
    - Firm endpoint of motion suggests partial tear.
  - *Pivot shift test:* More specific for ACL injury but unreliable without anesthesia; use cautiously in acutely injured knee:
    - Patient supine, knee in full extension
    - Internal rotation of tibia via a hand on foot is applied simultaneously with valgus stress from the other hand.
    - With knee flexion to 20–30 degrees, the examiner notices a jerk at the anterolateral corner of the proximal tibia.
  - *Anterior drawer sign:* Not as sensitive or specific as Lachman test:
    - Knee flexed 90 degrees, patient supine, hip flexed 45 degrees, foot neutral and stabilized
    - Anterior motion is positive.

#### *Pediatric Considerations*
Children and adolescents show more laxity on exam than adults.

### ESSENTIAL WORKUP
- Neurovascular evaluation
- Exclusion of fractures/dislocations
- Valgus/varus stress at 20 degrees of flexion
- Extensor mechanism function
- Lachman test (as described above) is most important and sensitive test for ACL injury.
- Look for signs of associated ligament or meniscus injury:
  - Present in about half of patients with ACL injury

### DIAGNOSTIC TESTS & INTERPRETATION
#### *Lab*
- If cause of knee effusion is uncertain, synovial aspirate can be sent for cell count, Gram's stain, and culture and crystals:
  - Fat globules in aspirate suggest intra-articular fracture.
- Arthrocentesis is usually not indicated except to relieve symptoms from tense effusion.

#### *Imaging*
- Plain films have low rate of positive findings: Clinical decision rules can limit number of negative plain films obtained.
- Ottawa knee rules (apply to adults): Plain films required for patients with any of 5 findings:
  - Age $\geq 55$
  - Isolated tenderness of patella
  - Tenderness at head of fibula
  - Inability to flex 90°
  - Inability to bear weight both immediately and in ED (4 steps)
- *Lateral capsular sign* is lateral tibial plateau avulsion fracture, just below joint line:
  - Diagnostic for ACL rupture, but present in <10% of ACL injuries
- MRI is around 95% sensitive for ACL tears and even more specific, but it is rarely indicated emergently.

*Pediatric Considerations*
Ottawa knee rules do not apply to children.

## DIFFERENTIAL DIAGNOSIS
- Meniscal injury (present in up to 50% of ACL injuries)
- Collateral ligament injury
- Tibial plateau bony injury
- Transient knee dislocation

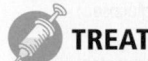 **TREATMENT**

## INITIAL STABILIZATION/THERAPY
- Document neurovascular function.
- Immobilize knee, apply ice, elevate.

## ED TREATMENT/PROCEDURES
- Injury is graded by severity:
  - Grade 3 is complete disruption of ligament.
  - Grade 2 represents severe stretching with partial tear of ligament.
  - Grade 1 is microscopic ligamentous damage with no clinical instability.
- General care:
  - First-degree injury may be treated with compressive wrap and weight bearing as tolerated.
  - More severe grades: Treat with immobilization and non-weight-bearing with crutches.
  - Ice for first 48 hr, elevation
  - Analgesics
  - Aspiration of a tense effusion (hemarthrosis) may relieve pain.

*Pediatric Considerations*
- Conservative treatment in children is generally associated with poor outcome.
- Controversy exists as to best surgical approach in children.

## MEDICATION
- NSAIDs or narcotic pain medications are mainstay.
- Ibuprofen: 400–600 mg (peds: 5–10 mg/kg) PO q.i.d.

 **FOLLOW-UP**

## DISPOSITION
### Admission Criteria
- Isolated ACL injury rarely requires emergent hospitalization.
- For suspected complete ruptures, definitive therapy is often surgical and orthopedic consultation is appropriate.

### Discharge Criteria
Most patients can be managed as outpatients with appropriate referral.

### Issues for Referral
- Re-examination is recommended at 48 hr if ED exam is inconclusive or if history suggests more significant injury than initial exam demonstrates (ie, severe symptoms, hearing "pop").
- Orthopedic referral within 1–2 wk is necessary if significant ligamentous injury is present.
- Surgical repair may be considered for patients wishing to return to sports or active lifestyles.

- Intra-articular reconstruction has gained popularity, though practice variation remains among orthopedists caring for ACL-injured patients.
- Physical therapy is a key part of treatment for most with ACL injury, coordinated by the referral MD.

## ADDITIONAL READING

- Atanda A Jr, Reddy D, Rice JA, et al. Injuries and chronic conditions of the knee in young athletes. *Pediatr Rev.* 2009;30(11):419–428.
- Beasley LS, Chudik SC. Anterior cruciate ligament injury in children: Update of current treatment options. *Curr Opin Pediatr.* 2003;15:45–52.
- Harmon K, Ireland M. Gender differences in noncontact anterior cruciate ligament injuries. *Clin Sports Med.* 2000;19(2):287–302.
- Roberts DM, Stallard TC. Emergency department evaluation and treatment of knee and leg injuries. *Emerg Med Clin North Am.* 2000;18(1):67–84, v–vi.
- Solomon DH, Simel DL, et al. Does this patient have a torn meniscus or ligament of the knee?. Value of the physical examination. *JAMA.* 2001;286:1610.
- Stiell IG, Greenberg GH, et al. Prospective validation of a decision rule for the use of radiography in acute knee injuries. *JAMA.* 1996;275:611.
- Zarins B, Adams M. Knee injuries in sports. *N Engl J Med.* 1988;318:950.

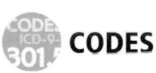 **CODES**

ICD9
- 717.83 Old disruption of anterior cruciate ligament
- 844.2 Sprain of cruciate ligament of knee

# ANTICHOLINERGIC POISONING

*Patrick M. Whiteley*

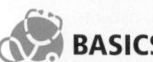 **BASICS**

## DESCRIPTION
- Central and peripheral cholinergic blockade
- Depending on the drug involved, antagonism occurs at muscarinic (most common), nicotinic, or both receptors.
- Onset of activity: 15–30 min after ingestion
- Duration of effect: 2–24 hr

## ETIOLOGY
- Many drugs contain anticholinergic properties:
  - Mild at therapeutic doses
  - Life threatening in overdose
- Anticholinergic substances:
  - Antihistamines
  - Belladonna alkaloids and synthetic congeners
  - Antiparkinsonian drugs
  - Cyclic antidepressants
  - Antipsychotics (neuroleptics)
  - Mydriatics
  - Skeletal muscle relaxants (orphenadrine, cyclobenzaprine)
  - Antispasmodics
  - Mushrooms—*Amanita muscaria, A. pantherina*
  - Plants—deadly nightshade, mandrake, henbane
  - Jimson weed—smoked or ingested

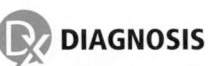 **DIAGNOSIS**

## SIGNS AND SYMPTOMS
### History
- Onset and duration of symptoms
- Type and extent of ingestion/exposure

### Physical Exam
- Classic toxidrome:
  - **"Mad as a hatter"**—altered mental status
  - **"Hot as a hare"**—hyperthermia
  - **"Red as a beet"**—flushed skin
  - **"Dry as a bone"**—dry skin and mucous membranes
  - **"Blind as a bat"**—blurred vision secondary to mydriasis
- General:
  - Hyperthermia
  - Altered mental status
- Ocular:
  - Unreactive mydriasis
  - Inability to accommodate
- Cardiovascular:
  - Sinus tachycardia
  - Dysrhythmias (rare except in massive ingestions)
  - Hypotension/HTN
  - Cardiogenic pulmonary edema
- Pulmonary:
  - Tachypnea
  - Respiratory failure
- GI:
  - Decreased/absent bowel sounds
  - Dysphagia
  - Decreased GI motility
  - Decreased salivation
- Genitourinary (GU):
  - Urinary retention
- Integument:
  - Decreased sweating
  - Flushed skin
  - Dry skin and mucous membranes
- CNS:
  - Altered mental status
  - Auditory or visual hallucinations
  - Coma
  - Seizures

## ESSENTIAL WORKUP
Diagnosis based on clinical presentation and an accurate history

## DIAGNOSTIC TESTS & INTERPRETATION
### Lab
- Urine toxicologic screen to exclude other ingestions
- Electrolytes, BUN, creatinine, and glucose
- CBC
- Creatine phosphokinase (CPK) if suspected rhabdomyolysis
- Urinalysis
- Acetaminophen level:
  - Detects occult ingestion (eg, Tylenol PM)

### Imaging
ECG:
- Sinus tachycardia most common
- QRS prolongation
- AV blockade
- Bundle branch block pattern
- Dysrhythmias

## DIFFERENTIAL DIAGNOSIS
- Sympathomimetic intoxication
- Withdrawal syndrome
- Acute psychiatric disorders
- Sepsis
- Thyroid disorder

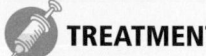 **TREATMENT**

### PRE-HOSPITAL
Transport all pills/pill bottles involved in overdose for identification in ED.

### INITIAL STABILIZATION/THERAPY
- Airway, breathing, and circulation (ABCs):
  - Airway control essential
  - Administer supplemental oxygen.
  - IV access
  - Cardiac monitor and pulse oximetry
- Naloxone, thiamine, $D_{50}$ (or Accu-Chek) if altered mental status

### ED TREATMENT/PROCEDURES
- Supportive care:
  - IV rehydration with 0.9% NS
  - Standard aggressive cooling measures for hyperthermia
  - Use benzodiazepines for treatment of agitation:
    - Avoid phenothiazines owing to anticholinergic effects.
  - Treat seizures with benzodiazepines and barbiturates.
  - Dysrhythmias:
    - Use standard antidysrhythmics.
    - Avoid class Ia antidysrhythmic owing to the quinidinelike effect of many anticholinergic drugs.
    - Sodium bicarbonate may reverse the quinidine-like effects.
- Decontamination:
  - Administer activated charcoal for oral ingestions.
  - Ocular lavage for eyedrop exposure
- Physostigmine (Antilirium):
  - Reversible acetylcholinesterase inhibitor that crosses the blood–brain barrier
  - Reverses both central and peripheral anticholinergic effects
  - Indicated in the presence of peripheral anticholinergic signs and the following:
    - Seizures unresponsive to conventional therapy
    - Uncontrollable agitation
  - Use with caution owing to risk of dysrhythmias (especially asystole), seizures, and cholinergic crises:
    - Place on cardiac monitor.
    - Observe for cholinergic symptoms.
  - Contraindications:
    - Cyclic antidepressant overdose (potentiates toxicity)
    - Cardiovascular disease
    - Asthma/bronchospasm
    - Intestinal obstruction
    - Heart block
    - Peripheral vascular disease
    - Bladder obstruction

### MEDICATION
- Activated charcoal: 1 mg/kg PO
- Dextrose: 50–100 mL $D_{50}$ (peds: 2 mL/kg of $D_{25}$ over 1 min) IV; repeat if necessary
- Diazepam: 5–10 mg (peds: 0.2–0.5 mg/kg) IV every 10–15 min
- Dopamine: 2–20 $\mu$g/kg/min with titration to effect
- Lorazepam: 2–4 mg (peds: 0.03–0.05 mg/kg) IV every 10–15 min
- Physostigmine: 0.5–2.0 mg (peds: 0.02 mg/kg) IV over 5 min; repeat if necessary in 30–60 min
- Phenobarbital: 10–20 mg/kg IV (loading dose)
- Thiamine (vitamin $B_1$): 100 mg (peds: 50 mg) IV or IM

### First Line
Lorazepam or Diazepam

### Second Line
Physostigmine (use with caution and consider consult with medical toxicologist)

 **FOLLOW-UP**

### DISPOSITION

### Admission Criteria
- ICU admission for moderate to severe anticholinergic symptoms (agitation control, temperature control, and observation for seizures or dysrhythmias)
- Any patient receiving physostigmine

### Discharge Criteria
Mild and improving symptoms of anticholinergic toxicity after 6–8 hr of ED observation

### Issues for Referral
- Substance abuse referral for patients with recreational anticholinergic abuse
- Patients with unintentional (accidental) poisoning require poison prevention counseling.
- Patients with intentional (eg, suicide) poisoning require psychiatric evaluation.

### FOLLOW-UP RECOMMENDATIONS
Appropriate psychiatric referral for intentional ingestions

## PEARLS AND PITFALLS
- Aggressively treat hyperthermia.
- Antipyretic medications are not effective in toxic hyperthermia.
- Use physostigmine cautiously and consult with medical toxicologist when available.

## ADDITIONAL READING
- Burns MJ, Linden CH, Graudins A, et al. A comparison of physostigmine and benzodiazepines for the treatment of anticholinergic poisoning. *Ann Emerg Med*. 2000;35:374–381.
- Ceha LJ, Presperin C, Young E, et al. Anticholinergic toxicity from nightshade berry poisoning responsive to physostigmine. *J Emerg Med*. 1997;15:65–69.
- Delaney KA. Anticholinergics and antihistamines (H1 antagonists). In: Ford MD, Delaney KA, Ling LJ, et al., eds. *Clinical Toxicology*. Philadelphia: WB Saunders. 2001;472–477.
- Hidalgo HA, Mowers RM. Anticholinergic drug abuse. *Ann Pharmacother*. 1990;24:40.
- Patel RJ, Saylor T, Williams SR, et al. Prevalence of autonomic signs and symptoms in antimuscarinic drug poisonings. *J Emerg Med*. 2004;26(1):89–94.
- Reilly KM, Chan L, Mehta NJ, et al. Systemic toxicity from ocular homatropine. *Acad Emerg Med*. 1996; 3:868–871.

# ANTIDEPRESSANT POISONING

*Gerald Maloney, Jr.*

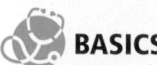 **BASICS**

## DESCRIPTION
- Newer antidepressants, including the atypical antidepressants and selective serotonin reuptake inhibitors (SSRIs), and atypical antipsychotics
- Most widely prescribed medications in U.S.
- Tricyclic antidepressants (TCAs) covered in separate chapter

## ETIOLOGY
Mechanism:
- SSRIs:
  - Inhibit the reuptake of serotonin at the 5HT1A receptor.
  - Older agents include fluoxetine (Prozac).
  - Newer agents include citalopram (Celexa) and escitalopram (Lexapro).
- Atypical antidepressants:
  - Activity on multiple receptor sites, including serotonin dopamine and norepinephrine reuptake
- Atypical antipsychotics:
  - Multiple receptor sites involved; serotonin, norepinephrine, anticholinergic and antihistaminic effects
  - Multiple drug–drug interactions
- Cardiotoxicity in these agents is owing to sodium and potassium channel blockade, similar to TCAs but less frequent.

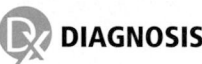 **DIAGNOSIS**

## SIGNS AND SYMPTOMS
- SSRIs:
  - Traditional SSRIs (fluoxetine, paroxetine):
    - Seizures
    - Serotonin syndrome
    - Rarely, QTc prolongation
    - Sedation
  - Citalopram:
    - Seizures
    - Sedation
    - QTc prolongation
    - Active metabolite is cardiotoxic: Exhibits *delayed* cardiotoxicity (up to 12 hr postingestion)
  - Escitalopram:
    - QTc and QRS prolongation
    - Sedation

- Atypical antidepressants:
  - Venlafaxine:
    - Seizures
    - QTc prolongation
    - Bupropion:
    - Sedation
    - Seizures
    - QRS/QTc prolongation
  - Trazodone:
    - Sedation
    - QTc prolongation
    - Hypotension
    - Priapism
  - Mirtazapine:
    - Sedation
    - QTc prolongation
    - Agranulocytosis (usually with chronic dosing)
- Atypical antipsychotics:
  - All have activity at dopamine receptors.
  - Fewer extrapyramidal symptoms (EPS) and tardive dyskinesias
  - Most have some $\alpha$-adrenergic antagonism as well
  - QTc prolongation common and increased risk for arrhythmias
  - Clozapine:
    - Sedation
    - Agranulocytosis (in up to 1% taking chronically)
    - Anticholinergic toxidrome
  - Olanzapine:
    - Fluctuating level of consciousness (LOC) with miosis
    - Pancreatitis
    - Diabetic ketoacidosis (DKA)
    - Only atypical clearly associated with neurologic malignant syndrome (NMS)
  - Quetiapine:
    - QTc prolongation
    - Sedation up to coma
    - Hypotension
  - Risperidone:
    - Sedation
    - QTc prolongation (rare)
    - Mild anticholinergic toxidrome
  - Ziprasidone:
    - Sedation
    - QRS/QTc prolongation
  - Aripiprazole:
    - Sedation most common effect
    - Some reports of NMS, prolonged neuro symptoms (altered mentation, clonus, tremors) lasting up to 36 hr

## ESSENTIAL WORKUP
- Determine agents ingested, dose, and time of ingestion:
  - Investigate for co-ingested drugs.
- Rapid bedside glucose (Accu-Chek) if altered mental status

## DIAGNOSTIC TESTS & INTERPRETATION
### Lab
- Specific drug levels rarely available and usually do not guide clinical management
- EKG:
  - For evaluation of QTc and QRS width
- Urine pregnancy:
  - In females of childbearing age
- Electrolytes, BUN, creatinine, glucose
- Serum osmolality:
  - Cannot rely on serum osmolality to rule out ingestion of other agents, such as toxic alcohols
- Routine toxicology screening:
  - Rarely alters clinical management
- Salicylate and acetaminophen levels
- Serum EtOH:
  - To exclude ethanol intoxication as a cause of altered mental status
  - Required if osmoles are measured
- Arterial/venous blood gases (ABG/VBG)
  - Check pH.

### Imaging
- CT of brain to evaluate for other causes of altered mentation
- CXR if intubated or hypoxic

## DIFFERENTIAL DIAGNOSIS
- Tricyclic antidepressant overdose
- Ethanol overdose
- Isoniazid overdose
- Hypoglycemia
- Hypoxemia
- Hyponatremia
- Hypocalcemia
- Withdrawal syndromes
- Serotonin syndrome
- Head trauma
- Opioid intoxication
- Sedative-hypnotic intoxication
- DKA

**TREATMENT**

### PRE-HOSPITAL
- In cases of suspected overdose, bring all medication bottles to hospital with patient.
- ABCs
- 0.9% NS IV fluids for BP stabilization
- Benzodiazepines for seizures
- In cases of wide-complex tachycardia, administer sodium bicarbonate IV fluid bolus to standard advanced cardiac life support (ACLS) measures.

### INITIAL STABILIZATION/THERAPY
- ABCs:
  - Administer oxygen.
  - Place on cardiac monitor and measure pulse oximetry.
  - Establish IV access with 0.9% NS.
  - Intubate as dictated for airway protection or respiratory status.
- Rapid bedside glucose determination
- Naloxone, thiamine, and $D_{50}W$ as indicated for altered mental status:
  - Flumazenil is not recommended for mixed-overdose patients, patients with underlying seizure disorder, or patients chronically on benzodiazepines.
- May give diphenhydramine 25–50 mg IM/IV or Cogentin 1 mg PO for EPS

### ED TREATMENT/PROCEDURES
- GI decontamination:
  - Do not attempt decontamination in a patient who does not have a stable airway.
  - Intubation solely for decontamination purposes, however, is not generally indicated.
  - Activated charcoal in a dose of 50–75 g PO or via nasogastric tube (NGT) if the patient is intubated may be beneficial in early presenting overdoses.
  - Gastric lavage is not generally indicated for patients with an isolated overdose of the agents listed in this chapter.
- For QRS widening, administer sodium bicarbonate IV bolus.
- Treat hypotension unresponsive to IV fluids with norepinephrine rather than dopamine owing to $\alpha_1$ receptor antagonism.
- Treat seizures with:
  - Initial therapy: Benzodiazepines
  - For refractory seizures: Phenobarbital and pyridoxine
- Treat symptoms of serotonin syndrome (fever, AMS, tachycardia, rigidity, hyperreflexia) with benzodiazepines, cooling, cyproheptadine.

### MEDICATION
- Activated charcoal: 50–75 g PO initial dose
- $D_{50}W$: 25 g (peds: 0.5 g/kg $D_{50}W$ if <50 kg; 0.5 g/kg $D_{25}W$ if >50 kg) IV for hypoglycemia
- Diazepam: 5–10 mg IV bolus (peds: 0.1 mg/kg IV bolus or 0.5 mg/kg rectal)
- Lorazepam: 2–4 mg (peds: 0.1 mg/kg) IV bolus
- Naloxone: 0.4–2 mg (peds: 0.1 mg/kg) initial bolus; may repeat up to a total of 10 mg
- Norepinephrine: 0.5–2 $\mu$g/kg IV infusion
- Phenobarbital: 15–20 mg/kg IV max. dose is 2 gm; caution: See respiratory depression with IV loading doses
- Pyridoxine: 5 g (peds: 50–100 mg) initial IV bolus unless known amount of isoniazid is given, in which case pyridoxine is gram:gram of INH
- Sodium bicarbonate: 1 mEq/kg IV bolus (adult 8.4%; peds: <50 kg, 4.2%)
- Thiamine: 100 mg (peds: 1 mg/kg) IV or IM
- Diphenhydramine 25–50 mg IM/IV (peds 1 mg/kg)
- Cogentin 1 mg PO

 **FOLLOW-UP**

### DISPOSITION
#### Admission Criteria
- Coma
- Altered mentation
- Symptoms of NMS
- Hemodynamic compromise
- EKG changes
- Suicidal patients should be on a 1:1 observation

#### Discharge Criteria
- Asymptomatic patients >12 hr postingestion may be medically cleared for psychiatric admission.
- Discharge only asymptomatic patients >12 hr postingestion who are not suicidal.

### FOLLOW-UP RECOMMENDATIONS
Psychiatry referral for patients with intentional overdose

## PEARLS AND PITFALLS
- For QRS widening, administer sodium bicarbonate IV bolus.
- Treat hypotension unresponsive to IV fluids with norepinephrine rather than dopamine owing to $\alpha_1$ receptor antagonism.

## ADDITIONAL READING
- Balit CR, Isbister GK, Hackett LP, et al. Quetiapine poisoning: A case series. *Ann Emerg Med*. 2003; 42(6):751–758.
- Cuenca PJ, Holt KR, Hoefle JD. Seizure secondary to citalopram overdose. *J Emerg Med*. 2004;26(2): 177–181.
- Flanagan RJ. Fatal toxicity of drugs used in psychiatry. *Hum Psychopharmacol*. 2008;23(1): 43–51.
- Isbister GK, Bowe SJ, Dawson A, et al. Relative toxicity of selective serotonin reuptake inhibitors (SSRIs) in overdose. *J Toxicol Clin Toxicol*. 2004; 42(3):277–285.
- Reilly TH, Kirk MA. Atypical antipsychotics and newer antidepressants. *Emerg Med Clin North Am*. 2007;25(2):477–497.
- Sarko J. Antidepressants, old and new. A review of their adverse effects and toxicity in overdose. *Emerg Med Clin North Am*. 2000;18(4):637–654. Review.
- Tann HH, Hoppe J, Heard K. A systematic review of cardiovascular effects after atypical antipsychotic medication overdose. *Am J Emerg Med*. 2009;27(5). 606–616.

### See Also (Topic, Algorithm, Electronic Media Element)
Tricyclic Antidepressant Poisoning

 **CODES**

### ICD9
- 298.9 Unspecified psychosis
- 311 Depressive disorder, not elsewhere classified

# AORTIC DISSECTION, THORACIC

*Jeffrey I. Schneider*
*Jonathan S. Olshaker*

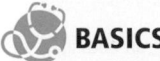 **BASICS**

## DESCRIPTION
- Aortic dissection begins when a jet of blood induces an intimal tear.
- Blood then dissects through the media under aortic systolic pressure.
- It is thought that hypertension is a major factor in the dissection process.
- Dissections can start proximally at the root and dissect distally to involve any or all branches of the aorta, such as the carotid and subclavian arteries.
- The dissection process can also proceed proximally to involve the aortic root, the coronary ostia, and the pericardium.
- Dissection that progresses proximally may lead to occlusion of the coronary ostia, aortic valve incompetence, or cardiac tamponade.
- Classification related to portion of aorta involved:
  - Stanford classification:
    ○ Type A: Ascending aorta
    ○ Type B: Distal to ascending aorta
  - DeBakey classification:
    ○ DeBakey I: Intimal tear in aortic arch or root
    ○ DeBakey II: Ascending aorta
    ○ DeBakey III: Distal to takeoff of left subclavian artery

## ETIOLOGY
Any process that affects the mechanical properties of the aortic wall can lead to dissection:
- Hypertension
- Congenital heart disease (bicuspid aortic valve, coarctation)
- Aortic wall connective tissue abnormalities (cystic medial necrosis)
- Connective tissue disease (Marfan disease, Ehlers-Danlos syndrome)
- Pregnancy
- Infectious/inflammatory conditions of the aorta (lupus, syphilis, endocarditis, giant cell arteritis)
- Tobacco use

## DIAGNOSIS

### SIGNS AND SYMPTOMS
#### History
- Chest pain:
  - May be absent in as many as 15% of patients
  - Substernal if type A dissection
  - Intrascapular is descending thoracic dissection
  - Lumbar if abdominal aorta involved
  - Starts abruptly
  - Usually described as sharp
  - Most severe at onset

- Back pain:
  - Commonly interscapular or lumbar
- Combination of chest, back, and abdominal pain
- Neurologic complaints:
  - Visual changes
  - Stroke symptoms
- Nausea, vomiting
- Peak age for occurrence:
  - Proximal dissection: 50–55 yr
  - Distal dissection: 60–70 yr

#### Pregnancy Considerations
Risk of dissection increases in presence of pregnancy:
- In woman <40 yr of age, 50% of dissections occur during pregnancy.

#### Physical Exam
- HTN:
  - 35–40% may be normotensive.
- Pulse deficits:
  - Discrepancies in BP between limbs
  - Usually in upper extremities
- Neurologic/spinal cord deficits
- Murmur of aortic regurgitation:
  - Occurs in up to 31% of patients
  - Musical, vibrating quality with variable intensity

### ESSENTIAL WORKUP
ECG:
- Useful in ruling in or out ST-elevation myocardial infarction (MI) or ischemia
- Dissection may involve coronary ostia and cause MI:
  - Inferior MI (right coronary artery lesion) is more common than left coronary artery territory.
- Useful for evaluating the presence of left ventricular hypertrophy
- A normal ECG in the presence of severe, acute-onset chest/back pain should heighten one's suspicion of an aortic dissection.

### DIAGNOSTIC TESTS & INTERPRETATION
#### Lab
- Leukocytosis
- Hematuria
- Elevated BUN and creatinine
- Elevated amylase secondary to bowel ischemia
- Elevated cardiac enzymes due to myocardial ischemia

#### Imaging
- CXR:
  - Useful in excluding other etiologies such as pneumothorax and pneumonia
  - In dissection, there may be a widened mediastinum or abnormal aortic contour.
  - An enlarged heart secondary to pericardial fluid (blood) may be present.
  - May be completely normal in as many as 12–18% of cases
- Echo—transthoracic or transesophageal:
  - Transthoracic:
    ○ Not very helpful in the diagnosis of aortic dissection
    ○ May be used to evaluate for complications of a known dissection such as tamponade, valvular incompetence, or MI (from ostial occlusion)
  - Transesophageal:
    ○ May be performed in the ED
    ○ Patients may require intubation.
    ○ Provides information regarding extent of dissection and complications
- CT:
  - Very useful in defining extent of dissection
  - May also be used in diagnosing clinical entities such as pulmonary embolism
  - Has a high sensitivity for the diagnosis of aortic dissection and is the diagnostic modality of choice in many centers
- MRI:
  - Highly sensitive and specific
  - Requires patient transport out of ED for extended period of time
  - Lack of immediate availability may be a problem
  - Study of choice in those with renal insufficiency or dye allergy
- Aortography:
  - High sensitivity and specificity
  - Useful for preoperative planning
  - Difficult to obtain in many centers
- Cardiac catheterization:
  - Due of overlap of symptomatology with cardiac ischemia, some patients may have diagnosis made by cardiac catheterization when an intimal flap is visualized.

### DIFFERENTIAL DIAGNOSIS
- Myocardial infarction/ischemia
- Unstable angina
- Pneumothorax
- Esophageal rupture
- Pulmonary embolism
- Pericarditis
- Pneumonia
- Musculoskeletal pain

 **TREATMENT**

### PRE-HOSPITAL
- Monitor
- IV access
- Oxygen

### INITIAL STABILIZATION/THERAPY
- 2 large-bore IV lines
- Continuous cardiac monitoring
- Pulse oximetry
- Oxygen
- Type and cross

### ED TREATMENT/PROCEDURES
- BP reduction to reduce shearing forces on aortic wall and slow down the dissection process
- Medications: IV $\beta$-blockade and nitroprusside
  - Medications are used to control HTN and cardiac contractility and decrease shearing forces.
  - Esmolol (IV) or labetalol (IV):
    - Contraindications: Bradycardia, COPD, hypotension
  - Nitroprusside (commonly used in conjunction with IV $\beta$-blocker)
  - Caution when using the above together: To prevent an initial increase in shear forces, $\beta$-blocker therapy should be started prior to the addition of nitroprusside therapy
- Emergent surgery:
  - Treatment of choice for type A dissection
  - Treatment for type B dissections in those who have failed medical therapy
- Medical management:
  - Treatment of choice for stable type B dissections

### ALERT
Symptoms of aortic dissection may be similar to those of cardiac ischemia/infarction and pulmonary embolus. Treatment with thrombolytics and anticoagulants may be harmful and potentially fatal if aortic dissection is present.

### MEDICATION
- Esmolol: 500 $\mu$g/kg bolus IV, then 25–50 mg/kg/min drip
- Labetalol: 10–20 $\mu$g IV q10–15min, then 2–4 mg/hr drip
- Nitroprusside: 0.5 $\mu$k/kg/min IV and titrate upwards to desired effect

 **FOLLOW-UP**

### DISPOSITION
#### Admission Criteria
- All patients with aortic dissection should be admitted to the intensive care unit.
- Emergency cardiothoracic surgery consultation should be obtained, especially in cases of type A dissection.

#### Discharge Criteria
None

### FOLLOW-UP RECOMMENDATIONS
Close follow-up with cardiology and/or cardiothoracic surgery is of paramount importance.

## PEARLS AND PITFALLS

- Untreated, nearly 75% of patients with ascending aortic dissection can be expected to die within 2 wk, with a mortality of 1–3%/hr in the 1st 48 hr.
- Majority of patients present with pain (90%) of severe intensity (90%) that occurred suddenly (84%).
- Although some recent literature has suggested a role for D-dimer testing, there is insufficient evidence to support its use as the sole screening test for aortic dissection.
- Should consider the diagnosis in patients with chest pain in whom conventional therapy (nitrates, $\beta$-blockers) are ineffective, and in those who have chest pain in addition to another complaint (extremity weakness, back pain, paresthesias, abdominal pain).

- Identification of risk factors is critical. These include:
  - HTN
  - Male gender
  - Cocaine use
  - Advanced age
  - Pregnancy
  - Connective tissue disorders, such as Marfan syndrome or cystic medial necrosis
  - Bicuspid aortic valve
  - Turner syndrome
  - Family history

## ADDITIONAL READING

- Erbel R, Alfonso F, Boileau C, et al. Diagnosis and management of aortic dissection. *Eur Heart J.* 2001;22(18):1642–1681.
- Hagan PG, Nienaber CA, Isselbacher EM, et al. The international registry of acute aortic dissection: New insights into an old disease. *JAMA.* 2000;283(7): 897–903.
- Khan IA, Nair CK. Clinical, diagnostic, and management perspectives of aortic dissection. *Chest.* 2002;122(1):311–328.
- Klompas M. Does this patient have an acute thoracic aortic dissection? *JAMA.* 2002;287:2262–2272.
- Mészáros I, Morocz J, Szlávi J, et al. Epidemiology and clinicopathology of aortic dissection. *Chest.* 2000;117(5):1271–1278.
- Moore AG, Eagel KA, Bruckman D, et al. Choice of computed tomography, transesophageal echocardiography, magnetic resonance imaging, and aortography In acute aortic dissection: International registry of acute aortic dissection, *Am J Cardiol.* 2002;89:1235–1238.
- Sutherland A, et al. D-dimer as the sole screening test for acute aortic dissection: A review of the literature. *Ann Emerg Med.* 2008;52(4):393–343.

 **CODES**

### ICD9
441.01 Dissection of aorta, thoracic

# AORTIC RUPTURE, TRAUMATIC (TAI)

*Arash Soroudi*

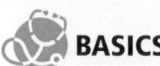 **BASICS**

## DESCRIPTION

- Traumatic aortic rupture (also referred to as traumatic aortic injury or TAI) is the cause of death in an estimated 20% of lethal motor vehicle collisions.
- An estimated 85% of patients with TAI die before reaching the hospital.
- Patients surviving to the ED usually have a contained rupture as aortic blood is tamponaded by the adventitia.
- Without proper treatment, of the 15% that survive the initial event, 49% will die within the 1st 24 hr, and 90% within 4 mo.
- Mean age of patients sustaining aortic rupture is 33 yr, and 70% are male.
- Most tears are transverse, not longitudinal.
- Tears may be partially or completely circumferential.

## ETIOLOGY

- Most commonly results from motor vehicle collisions >30 mph
- Unrestrained passengers, driver seat occupants (injuries from steering column and instruments), and ejected occupants are most at risk.
- Other mechanisms: Auto vs. pedestrian, airplane crashes, falls from height >10 ft, crush and blast injuries, direct blow to chest
- Proposed mechanisms of aortic injury:
  - Shear forces arising from unequal rates of deceleration of the relatively fixed descending aorta and the more mobile arch
  - "Bending" stress at the aortic isthmus may cause flexion of the aortic arch on the left mainstem bronchus and pulmonary artery.
  - Twisting of the arch forces it superiorly and causes it to stretch.
  - Osseous structures (eg, medial clavicles, manubrium, 1st rib) cause pinching of the trapped aorta as they strike the vertebral column.
  - "Waterhammer" fluid wave causes explosive rupture of aorta just distal to the aortic valve.

 **DIAGNOSIS**

## SIGNS AND SYMPTOMS

### ALERT
Despite the severe nature of the injury, clinical manifestations are often deceptively subtle or nonexistent as patients frequently present with multiple coexisting injuries. 1/3–1/2 of these patients do not have external signs of chest trauma.

### History
- Substernal chest pain is the most common symptom, but only present in ~25% of cases.
- Dyspnea, hoarseness, and stridor (tracheal compression from expanding hematoma) are less common.

### Physical Exam
- Neither sensitive nor specific for aortic injury
- Generalized HTN may occur from stimulation of sympathetic afferent nerves located near aortic isthmus.
- Harsh precordial or midscapular systolic murmur (1/3 of patients)
- Ischemic pain in lower extremities, oliguria/anuria, paraplegia from decreased aortic blood flow distal to aortic arch
- Swelling of base of neck (extravasation of blood)
- Acute coarctation syndrome (1/3 of patients): Upper extremity HTN with decreased pressures in low extremities, caused by periaortic hematoma compressing aortic lumen

## ESSENTIAL WORKUP
Plain CXR is the primary screening tool with ~90% sensitivity, but low specificity.

## DIAGNOSTIC TESTS & INTERPRETATION
### Lab
- CBC
- Chemistry
- Prothrombin time/partial thromboplastin time
- Type and cross-match (6–8 units PRBC)

### Imaging
- Plain CXR:
  - Findings suggestive of mediastinal hemorrhage, hematoma, or associated injuries:
    - Widening of the superior mediastinum at level of aortic arch (defined as >8 cm on a supine film, >6 cm in an upright PA film, or >0.25 mediastinum-width to chest-width ratio) is the most sensitive sign.
    - Obscuration of the aortic knob is also a sensitive sign.
    - More specific, but less sensitive signs include opacification of the aortopulmonary window, rightward displacement of nasogastric tube, widened paratracheal stripe, and widened right paraspinal interface.
  - 7–10% false-negative rate with normal mediastinum on x-ray; several authors recommend liberal use of helical chest CT with high-speed deceleration mechanisms.
  - In pediatric patients: The most common findings are a left apical cap, pulmonary contusion, aortic obscuration, and mediastinal widening.
- Helical chest CT-angiography:
  - Preferred confirmatory study in stable patients
  - Nearly 100% sensitivity and specificity for detecting aortic rupture with improved CT technology
  - Has largely eliminated need for aortography
  - Advantages over aortography include noninvasive, provides information on other thoracic structures, more rapid
- Aortography:
  - Still considered by some to be the gold standard for diagnosis of TAI
  - Provides precise anatomic localization of aortic tears, useful for aorta injured at >1 site (15–20% of cases)
  - Risk of further damage to aorta from catheter
  - Need for this modality is declining given advances in CT imaging quality.
- Transesophageal ECG (TEE):
  - Can be done rapidly in the ED
  - Can detect associated cardiac injuries (contusion, effusion, etc)
  - Reported 87–100% sensitivity and 98–100% specificity, so further studies needed if TEE is equivocal
  - Contraindicated in patients with cervical, maxillofacial, or esophageal injuries

- MRI:
  - High accuracy
  - Lengthy study time and difficulty monitoring patients limits use
- Intravascular US:
  - Newer modality, availability is limited
  - Preliminary data suggest high sensitivity and specificity.

### *Pediatric Considerations*
Presence of large thymus may make diagnosis of widened mediastinum difficult.

## DIFFERENTIAL DIAGNOSIS
- Supine CXR can lead to false positive for widened mediastinum; obtain upright PA if possible.
- Mediastinal hematoma owing to other causes
- Mediastinal lymphadenopathy or tumor
- Redundant aorta resulting from HTN

 ## TREATMENT

### PRE-HOSPITAL
Important information to retrieve at scene of injury:
- Vehicular speed
- Patient in driver or passenger seat
- Damage to steering column if driver is patient
- Ejection or use of seat belt

### INITIAL STABILIZATION/THERAPY
- Follow advanced trauma life support protocols.
- Life-threatening intracranial, peritoneal, and retroperitoneal injuries take precedence.

### ED TREATMENT/PROCEDURES
- Immediate trauma surgery consultation
- Immediate cardiothoracic or vascular surgery consultation (institution dependent)
- Avoid maneuvers that may result in a Valsalva-like response (eg, gagging, straining)
- Aggressive pharmacologic treatment of BP and heart rate, as emerging data suggest delaying surgical repair may lead to improved outcomes.

- Goal of medical therapy is to target heart rate 60 ± 5 bpm, systolic BP 100–120 mm Hg, and mean arterial BP 70–80 mm Hg to decrease risk of sudden free rupture and exsanguination:
  - β-Blockers such as esmolol and labetalol are 1st-line agents
  - Calcium channel blockers in patients with contraindications to β-blockade (CHF, COPD, 2nd- or 3rd-degree atrioventricular block)
  - Add vasodilator (nitroprusside) if needed to reach target BP and heart rate goals.
  - Antihypertensives are relatively contraindicated in acute coarctation syndrome.
- For significant hypotension, initiate rapid volume expansion, including blood.
- Vasopressors for refractory hypotension; norepinephrine and phenylephrine are preferred
- Central venous and arterial catheters

### ALERT
Only administer vasodilator after initiating negative inotrope (β-blocker or calcium channel blocker), as vasodilator alone can cause an increase in shearing forces on the intact aortic adventitia.

### MEDICATION
- Esmolol: 500 μg/kg bolus IV (peds. 100–500 μg/kg bolus), then 50–150 μg/kg/min IV infusion (peds: 25–100 μg/kg/min IV infusion)
- Labetalol: 20 mg IV, followed by additional doses of 40 mg and 80 mg (peds: 0.2–10 mg/kg per dose, max. 20 mg per dose) IV q10–15min, to 300 mg IV total; start infusion at 2 mg/min and titrate up to 10 mg/min (peds: 0.4–3 mg/kg/h infusion)
- Diltiazem. 20 mg (0.25 mg/kg) IV over 2 min; 2nd bolus 25 mg (0.35 mg/kg) in 15 min if needed; infusion 5–15 mg/hr
- Norepinephrine: Start with 0.5–1 μg/min and titrate to desired response; 8–30 μg/min is usual dose (peds: Start 0.05–0.1 μg/kg/min, max. 2 μg/kg/min)
- Phenylephrine. 0.1–0.5 mg IV boluses q10–15min, initial dose not to exceed 0.5 mg (peds: 5–20 μg/kg/dose q10–15min); 100–180 μg/min or 0.5 μg/kg/min titrated to desired effect (peds: 0.1–0.5 μg/kg/min, titrated to desired effect)

 ## FOLLOW-UP

### DISPOSITION
*Admission Criteria*
All patients with aortic injuries must be admitted to the ICU if not taken directly to the OR.

### FOLLOW-UP RECOMMENDATIONS
All patients with TAI are admitted to the hospital.

## PEARLS AND PITFALLS
- Maintain a high degree of suspicion for TAI in patients with injuries from significant deceleration mechanisms.
- Clinical signs and symptoms may be subtle or nonexistent, necessitating some reliance on radiologic imaging for diagnosis.
- Special attention should be given to assessment of the mediastinum on CXR in trauma patients.
- Early pharmacologic control of BP and heart rate is of utmost importance when diagnosis is confirmed.

## ADDITIONAL READING

- Burkhart HM, Gomez GA, Jacobson LE, et al. Fatal blunt aortic injuries: A review of 242 autopsy cases. *J Trauma.* 2001;50:113–115.
- Demetriades D, Velmahos GC, Scalea TM, et al. Blunt traumatic thoracic aortic injuries: Early or delayed repair—Results of an American Association for the Surgery of Trauma prospective study. *J Trauma.* 2009;66(4):967–973.
- Moore MA, Wallace EC, Westra SJ. The imaging of paediatric thoracic trauma. *Pediatr Radiol.* 2009;39(5):485–496. Epub 2009 Jan 17. Review.
- Ng CJ, Chen JC, Wang LJ, et al. Diagnostic value of the helical CT scan for traumatic aortic injury: Correlation with mortality and early rupture. *J Emerg Med.* 2006;30(3):277–282.
- O'Connor CE. Diagnosing traumatic rupture of the thoracic aorta in the emergency department. *Emerg Med J.* 2004;21:414–419.
- Parmley LF, Mattingly TW, Manion WJ, et al. Nonpenetrating traumatic injury of the aorta. *Circulation.* 1958;17:1086–1101.
- Pretre R, Chilcott M. Blunt trauma to the heart and great vessels. *New Engl J Med.* 1997;336:626–632.

 ## CODES

### ICD9
- 901.0 Injury to thoracic aorta
- 902.0 Injury to abdominal aorta

# APHTHOUS ULCERS
*Matthew R. Berkman*

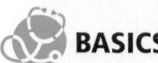 **BASICS**

## DESCRIPTION
Painful ovoid or round ulcerations on the mucous membranes of the mouth or genitals:
- Commonly referred to as "canker sores"

## ETIOLOGY
- Single etiology: Unknown
- Etiology likely multifactorial with some correlation with:
  - Immunologic dysfunction; activation of cell mediated immune system
  - Infection
  - Food hypersensitivities (ie, gluten)
  - Vitamin deficiency
  - Pregnancy
  - Menstruation
  - Trauma
  - Stress
  - Immunodeficiency
  - Medications: Beta-blockers, anti-inflammatory
- Epidemiology: Usually occurs in children and young adults (10–30 yr old), 20–30% of general population:
  - More common in women
  - Less common in smokers
  - May be familial

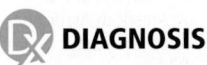 **DIAGNOSIS**

## SIGNS AND SYMPTOMS
- Minor aphthous ulcers:
  - 70–90% of all aphthae
  - <8 mm in diameter; up to five appear at a time
  - Painful, shallow ulcers with necrotic centers
  - Raised margins and erythematous halos
  - Gray-white pseudomembrane
  - Affect nonkeratinized mucosa of anterior oral cavity
    - Labial and buccal mucosa
    - Floor of mouth
    - Ventral surface of tongue
  - Rarely found on dorsum of tongue, hard palate, or gingiva
  - Last for 10–14 days; do not scar
  - Fever/constitutional symptoms rarely associated

- Major aphthous ulcers or Sutton disease:
  - 10–15% of all aphthae
  - Similar in appearance but more painful than minor form
  - >8 mm in diameter; 1–10 ulcers at a time
  - Deeper than minor form
  - Involve all areas of oropharynx including pharynx, soft/hard palate
  - Last for weeks to months, may heal with scarring
  - Often associated with underlying disease
  - Fever is rarely associated
- Herpetiform aphthous ulcers:
  - 7–10% of all aphthae
  - Multiple small clusters
  - 1–3 mm in diameter, 10–100 at any time, may coalesce into plaques
  - Herpetiform in nature, but herpes simplex virus cannot be cultured from lesions.
  - Last for 7–30 days; scarring could occur

### History
- Prodrome of burning or pricking sensation of oral mucosa 1–2 days prior to appearance of ulcers
- Inquire about family history of SLE, inflammatory bowel disease (IBD), Behçet disease, Reiter's disease
- Inquire about patient sexual history of syphilis or herpesvirus
- Inquire about patient medical history of SLE, HIV, IBD, Behçet disease, Reiter disease cancer
- Inquire about current medications:
  - NSAIDs
  - β-blockers

### Physical Exam
- See "Signs and Symptoms."
- Look for signs of dehydration:
  - Vital signs should be within normal limits.
  - Evaluate mucus membranes.
- Evaluate for signs of secondary infection.
- Evaluate for signs of systemic causes of ulcers (see "History").

## ESSENTIAL WORKUP
- Diagnosis is made by history and clinical presentation.
- Rule out oral manifestation of systemic disease:
  - More likely if persists >3 wk or associated with constitutional symptoms
- Focus on symptoms of eye, mouth, genitalia, skin, GI tract, allergy, and diet history and physical

## DIAGNOSTIC TESTS & INTERPRETATION
### Lab
Routine laboratory testing not indicated:
- Needed only when systemic etiologies causing ulcers are suspected
- Should be guided by history and physical:
  - CBC series
  - Rapid plasma reagin test
  - Fluorescent treponemal antibody-absorption test
  - Antinuclear antibody test
  - Tzanck stain: Inclusion giant cells (herpes virus)
  - Biopsy: Multinucleated giant cells (cytomegalovirus)
  - Fungal cultures

### Diagnostic Procedures/Surgery
An outpatient biopsy should be considered for any ulcer >3 weeks

## DIFFERENTIAL DIAGNOSIS
- Trauma:
  - Biting
  - Dentures
  - Braces
- Drug exposure:
  - NSAIDs
  - Nicorandil
  - β-blockers
- Infection:
  - Herpesvirus:
    - Vesicular lesions
    - Ulcers on attached mucosa
  - Cytomegalovirus:
    - Immunocompromised patient
  - Varicella virus:
    - Characteristic skin lesions
  - Coxsackievirus:
    - Ulcers preceded by vesicles
    - Hand, foot, and buttock lesions
  - Syphilis:
    - Other skin or genital lesions
  - Erythema multiforme:
    - Lip crusting
    - Lesions on attached and unattached mucosa skin lesions
  - *Cryptosporidium* infection, mucormycosis, histoplasmosis
  - Necrotizing gingivitis

- Underlying disease:
  - Behcet syndrome:
    - ○ Genital ulceration
    - ○ Uveitis
    - ○ Retinitis
  - Reactive arthritis (Reiter syndrome):
    - ○ Uveitis
    - ○ Urethritis
    - ○ HLA-B27-associated arthritis
  - Sweet syndrome:
    - ○ Fever
    - ○ Erythematous skin plaques/nodules
    - ○ In conjunction with malignancy
  - IBD:
    - ○ Bloody or mucous diarrhea
    - ○ GI ulcerations
    - ○ Weight loss
  - Lupus erythematosus:
    - ○ Malar rash
    - ○ ANA positive
  - Bullous pemphigoid/pemphigoid vulgaris:
    - ○ Vesiculobullous lesions on attached and unattached mucosa
    - ○ Diffuse skin involvement
  - Cyclic neutropenia:
    - ○ Periodic fever
  - Squamous cell carcinoma:
    - ○ Chronicity
    - ○ Head/neck adenopathy
- Immunocompromised patient:
  - HIV
  - Agranulocytosis
  - Malignancy

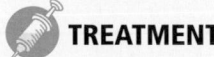

## TREATMENT

### ED TREATMENT/PROCEDURES
- Treatment guided by severity and duration of symptoms
- Goal is for symptomatic pain relief and reduction of inflammation.

### MEDICATION
- Mild to moderate disease:
  - Amlexanox 5% paste: 0.5 cm applied to ulcer q.i.d. after meals
  - Chlorhexidine gluconate aqueous mouthwash 0.12% (Peridex): q.i.d. until resolutions
  - Fluocinonide 0.05% gel: 0.5 cm applied to ulcer up to five times a day
  - Magnesium hydroxide/diphenhydramine hydrochloride 5 mg/5 mL in 1/1 mix swish
  - Triamcinolone dental paste 1% (Kenalog in Orabase): Apply to ulcer q.i.d. until healed and swallow q.i.d.
  - Topical OTC preparations (Orabase, Anbesol)
  - Viscous lidocaine 2%: Apply to ulcer as needed q.i.d.
- Severe disease:
  - Prednisone tablets: 40 mg PO per day × 7 days
  - Thalidomide: 50–200 mg PO per day × 4 wk

## FOLLOW-UP

### DISPOSITION
#### Admission Criteria
- Unable to eat or drink after appropriate analgesia
- Abnormal vital signs or evidence of dehydration

#### Discharge Criteria
- Tolerating fluids
- Adequate analgesia
- Normal vital signs

### Issues for Referral
Follow up with primary care physician if lesions have not resolved within 2 wk.

### FOLLOW-UP RECOMMENDATIONS
- Avoid oral trauma (hard foods) or acidic foods.
- Referral to a specialist if underlying disease suspected

## PEARLS AND PITFALLS

- The vast majority of aphthous ulcers are benign, self-limited, and treated symptomatically
- ED physicians must consider underlying systemic cause of ulcers.

## ADDITIONAL READING

- Akintoye SO, Greenberg MS. Recurrent aphthous stomatitis. *Dent Clin North Am*. 2005;49:31–47.
- Scully C. Aphthous ulceration. Clinical practice. *NEJM*. 2006;355:165–172.
- Scully C, Gorsky M, Lozada-Nur F. The diagnosis and management of recurrent aphthous stomatitis: A consensus approach. *J Am Dent Assoc*. 2003;134: 200–207.
- Wanda C, et al. Common Oral Lesion: Part I. Superficial Mucosal Lesions. *Am Fam Physician*. 2007;75:501–507.

# APNEA, PEDIATRIC
Carol R. Okada
James M. Stephen

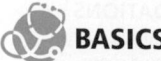 **BASICS**

## DESCRIPTION
- Absence of respiratory airflow for a period of 20 sec, with or without decreased heart rate:
  - Central apnea:
    - Disruption in the generation of propagation of respiratory signals in the brainstem and descending neuromuscular pathways
  - Obstructive apnea:
    - Respiratory effort is present, but there is no airflow.
    - Structural airway obstruction, often with paradoxical chest wall movement
    - Functional obstruction from airway collapse
  - Mixed
- Apparent life-threatening event (ALTE):
  - Episode that is associated with a combination of apnea, color change, change in tone, choking, or gagging
  - A clinical presentation, not a diagnosis

## ETIOLOGY
- Infection:
  - Sepsis
  - Meningitis or encephalitis
  - Pneumonia
  - Pertussis/chlamydia
  - RSV and other viral respiratory infections
- Respiratory:
  - Obstructive airway lesions
    - Enlarged tonsils and adenoids
    - Foreign body
    - Craniofacial abnormality
    - Choanal atresia or stenosis
  - Functional obstruction from airway collapse
  - Infection
  - Abnormal ventilatory response to hypoxia/hypercarbia
- Neurologic:
  - Seizure
  - Intracranial hemorrhage
  - Increased intracranial pressure
  - Tumor
  - Arnold Chiari or other CNS malformation
  - Ingestion
  - Toxin
  - Hypoxic injury
  - Neuromuscular disorder
  - Central hypoventilation syndrome

- Cardiac:
  - Dysrhythmia
  - Congenital heart disease
  - CHF
  - Myocarditis
  - Cardiomyopathy
- GI:
  - GERD
  - Volvulus
  - Intussusception
- Child abuse
- Endocrine/metabolic:
  - Hypoglycemia
  - Electrolyte disorders
  - Inborn errors of metabolism
- Other:
  - Transient choking episode
  - Laryngospasm
  - Periodic breathing
  - Breath-holding spell

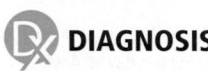 **DIAGNOSIS**

### ALERT
If the patient is apneic, treatment must commence at once.

## SIGNS AND SYMPTOMS
Apnea may be current, historical, or impending.

### History
- Duration of apnea
- State:
  - Asleep, awake, crying, relationship to feeds, supine, prone
- Respiratory effort:
  - None, shallow breathing, increased work of breathing, struggling to breathe, choking
- Presence and location of any color change
- Position of eyes
- Description of movements and muscle tone
- Interventions done by the caregiver
- Antecedent symptoms such as fever or cough
- Antecedent trauma
- Past medical history, including prematurity, cardiopulmonary, GI, or neurologic conditions
- Any past history of ALTEs in this patient or family members

## Physical Exam
- Vital signs with temperature
- Growth parameters:
  - Weight pattern
  - OFC pattern
- Pulse oximetry
- Examination of airway and lungs:
  - Assess impending apnea
  - Stridor or other evidence of upper airway obstruction
  - Fast or slow respirations
  - Use of accessory muscles
  - Adventitial lung sounds
- Examination of heart:
  - Irregular rhythm, tachycardia, or bradycardia
  - Murmur
  - Evidence of CHF
- Neurologic examination:
  - Assess mental status
  - Assess for trauma, seizure, or toxidrome
  - Muscle tone and reflexes
  - Funduscopic examination

## ESSENTIAL WORKUP
- Complete history and physical examination
- The historical factors and exam will direct the diagnostic evaluation and treatment.
- Check/clear out upper airway as appropriate.
- Remove or suction any obstruction as appropriate.
- Ensure proper head positioning with special consideration for occult trauma.

## DIAGNOSTIC TESTS & INTERPRETATION
### Lab
Perform as appropriate for presentation:
- Dextrostix
- CBC
- Urinalysis
- CSF studies
- Blood, urine, and CSF cultures
- Electrolytes (including calcium)
- BUN, creatinine
- Blood gas
- RSV and respiratory viral studies
- Pertussis and chlamydia tests
- Consider toxicologic screen (including toxic alcohols and acetaminophen)
- Consider LFTs and ammonia

*Imaging*
Perform as appropriate for presentation:
- CXR
- Head CT or MRI
- ECG
- UGI
- Polysomnography in follow-up in patient with suspected central or obstructive sleep apnea
- EEG in follow-up

## DIFFERENTIAL DIAGNOSIS
- Multiple etiologies as previously noted
- Special considerations:
  - Breath-holding spells:
    ○ Reflexive cessation of respiratory effort during expiration
    ○ Cyanotic and pallid types
    ○ Paroxysmal event occurring in 0.1–5% of healthy children 6 mo–6 yr of age
  - Periodic breathing may be seen in neonates:
    ○ 3 or more respiratory pauses lasting >3 sec with <20 sec of respiration between pauses
    ○ May be normal event

### ALERT
In a neonate, strongly consider occult sepsis.

# TREATMENT

## PRE-HOSPITAL
- High-flow oxygen if breathing resumes
- Check/clear out upper airway.
- Bag-mask ventilation with cricoid pressure
- Endotracheal intubation if continued apnea
- IV access, supplemental oxygen, cardiac monitor
- Look for signs of an underlying cause:
  - Medications
  - Document a basic neurologic examination:
    ○ GCS
    ○ Pupils
    ○ Extremity movements
  - Gross signs of trauma
  - Talk with family/prehospital personnel for information

## INITIAL STABILIZATION/THERAPY
- Establish unresponsiveness
- Check/clear out upper airway.
- Remove or suction any obstruction.
- Ensure proper head positioning.

## ED TREATMENT/PROCEDURES
- If currently apneic, ventilate with the bag-valve mask device and high-flow oxygen.
- Endotracheal intubation is required if apnea persists.
- Resuscitation medications and antibiotics as indicated

## MEDICATION
- Ceftriaxone: 50 mg/kg IV
- Vancomycin: 15 mg/kg IV
- Dextrose: 2–4 ml/kg $D_{25}W$ IV
  - Neonates: 1 mo 2–4 mL/kg $D_{10}W$ IV
- Naloxone: 0.01–0.1 mg/kg IV/IM/SC/ET. Caution: May precipitate withdrawal symptoms in patients with chronic opiate use.
- Flumazenil: 0.01 mg/kg IV titrate to effect. Caution: May precipitate seizures.

 FOLLOW-UP

## DISPOSITION
Patients who were or may become apneic should be admitted to an inpatient unit for appropriate monitoring. Those with continuing abnormal vital signs need intensive care monitoring.

Recommend referral for pediatric evaluation and follow-up as indicated. Interventions may include further studies, antireflux medications or caffeine, and home monitoring.

## PEARLS AND PITFALLS
- Consider occult sepsis, especially in a neonate
- Consider occult trauma

## ADDITIONAL READING
- De Piero A, Teach S, Chamberlain J. ED evaluation of infants after an apparent life-threatening event. *Am J Emerg Med*. 2004;22(2):83–86.
- Kahn A. Recommended clinical evaluation of infants with an apparent life-threatening event. Consensus document of the European Society for the Study and Prevention of Infant Death, 2003. *Eur J Pediatr*. 2004;163(2):108–115.
- McGovern MC, Smith MB. Causes of apparent life threatening events in infants: A systematic review. *Arch Dis Child*. 2004;89(11):1043–1048.

**See Also (Topic, Algorithm, Electronic Media Element)**
Sudden Infant Death Syndrome

# APPENDICITIS

Colleen N. Hickey
Jennifer L. Kolodchak

 **BASICS**

## DESCRIPTION
- Acute obstruction of appendiceal lumen results in distension followed by organ ischemia, bacterial overgrowth, and eventual perforation of the viscus.
- Pain migration:
  - Periumbilical pain: Appendiceal distension stimulates stretch receptors, which relay pain via *visceral* afferent pain fibers to tenth thoracic ganglion.
  - RLQ pain: As inflammation extends to surrounding tissues, pain occurs owing to stimulation of *parietal* nerve fibers and localizes to position of appendix.

### Pediatric Considerations
- 28–57% misdiagnosis in patients <12 yr (nearly 100% in patients <2 yr)
- 70–90% perforation rate in young children (<4 yr)
- Perforation correlates strongly with delayed diagnosis.

### Geriatric Considerations
- Decreased inflammatory response
- 3 times more likely to have perforation owing to anatomic changes
- Diagnosis often delayed owing to atypical presentations

### Pregnancy Considerations
- Slightly higher rate in 2nd trimester compared to 1st/3rd/postpartum periods
- Increased perforation rate (25–40%), highest in 3rd trimester
- RLQ pain remains most common symptom
- 7–10% fetal loss, up to 24% in perforated appendicitis

## ETIOLOGY
- Luminal obstruction of appendix
- Appendiceal lumen becomes distended, inhibiting lymphatic and venous drainage.
- Bacterial invasion of wall, with edema and blockage of arterial blood flow
- Perforation and spillage of contents into peritoneal cavity, causing peritonitis (usually 24–36 hr from onset)
- May wall off and form abscess
- Gram-negative rods and anaerobic organisms predominate

## DIAGNOSIS

### SIGNS AND SYMPTOMS
#### History
- Abdominal pain: Primary symptom:
  - Normal location:
    - RLQ pain
    - 35% of patients have appendix located within 5 cm of "normal" location.
  - Retrocecal appendix (28–68%):
    - Back pain
    - Flank pain
    - Testicular pain
  - Pelvic appendix (27–53%):
    - Suprapubic pain
    - Urinary or rectal symptoms
  - Long appendix (<0.2%):
    - Inflamed tip may cause pain in RUQ or LLQ.
    - Anorexia
    - Vomiting
- Change in bowel habits: Diarrhea (33%), constipation (9–33%)
- Classic presentation (<75% adults):
  - Initially periumbilical pain
  - Followed by anorexia (1st symptom in 95%) and nausea
  - Localizes to RLQ (1–12 hr after onset)
  - Finally, vomiting with fever

#### Pediatric Considerations
- Presentations often nonspecific and difficult to localize (<50% have classic presentation)
- Anorexia, vomiting, and diarrhea more common (half-eaten meal hours before complaints of pain may more accurately indicate duration of symptoms)
- Observe child before examination for subtle indicators of local inflammation:
  - Limping gait
  - Hesitation to move or climb
  - Flexed right hip

#### Physical Exam
- Vital signs:
  - Often normal
  - Fever: Normal to mild elevation (<1°F) initially, increases with perforation
- Abdominal exam:
  - Tenderness at McBurney point (1/3 of distance from right anterior iliac spine to umbilicus)
  - Guarding:
    - Voluntary guarding early owing to muscular resistance to palpation
    - Involuntary guarding (rigidity) later as inflammation progresses and perforation occurs
  - Rebound:
    - Pain with any rapid movement of peritoneum (eg, bumping stretcher)
  - Specific signs (less useful in pediatrics):
    - *Rovsing sign:* Pain in RLQ when palpating LLQ
    - *Psoas sign:* Increased pain on extension of right hip with patient lying on her or his left side, owing to inflamed appendix touching iliopsoas muscle.
    - *Obturator sign:* Pain with passive internal rotation and flexion of right hip

- Rectal exam:
  - Limited value: May localize tenderness/mass
- Pelvic exam:
  - Important to differentiate gynecologic disease
  - Vaginal discharge and/or adnexal tenderness or mass suggests gynecologic disease.
  - Cervical motion tenderness when present suggests PID, but can be seen in up to 25% of women with appendicitis
- Patient position:
  - Supine or decubitus with legs (particularly the right) drawn up
  - Prefer not to move
- Shuffling gait—known as "appy walk"

#### Pediatric Considerations
Almost all children have generalized abdominal tenderness with some rigidity.

#### Pregnancy Considerations
- Enlarging uterus displaces appendix upward and laterally.
- Hyperemesis gravidarum and other nonsurgical causes of vomiting should not cause abdominal tenderness.

#### Geriatric Considerations
Typical signs of peritonitis may be absent in elderly.

### ESSENTIAL WORKUP
- Suggestive history and physical exam sufficient to establish preoperative diagnosis and warrant surgical consultation.
- Tests listed below may be used to assist in diagnosis
- Atypical cases: Repeat serial exams in conjunction plus some of tests listed below is effective, with decreased rates of negative appendectomies and no increase in rates of perforation

### DIAGNOSTIC TESTS & INTERPRETATION
#### Lab
- CBC:
  - WBC >10,000, with left shift (80%)
  - Normal WBC does *not* exclude diagnosis.
- C-reactive protein:
  - Overall sensitivity 62%, specificity 66%
  - May not be elevated early (<12 hr)
  - Increased sensitivity with serial measurements
- Urinalysis:
  - Generally normal
  - Mild pyuria, bacteriuria, or hematuria (25–30%)
  - Pyuria present if inflamed appendix lies near ureter or bladder
- Pregnancy test for females of childbearing age

#### Imaging
- Unnecessary when diagnosis is clear
- Most helpful in female patients of childbearing age where diagnosis is often unclear
- Abdominal radiographs—not recommended
- US: Sensitivity 86–90%; specificity 92–95%:
  - Noncompressible appendix 6 mm anteroposterior (AP) diameter
  - Presence of appendicolith
  - Periappendiceal fluid/mass
  - Limited by obesity, bowel gas, retrocecal appendix, and operator
  - Negative study of limited use

- CT: Sensitivity 91–100%; specificity 94–97%:
  – Highest yield using oral and rectal contrast with focused appendiceal technique (5-mm cuts from 3 cm above cecum extending distally 12–15 cm)
  – Fat stranding (100%)
  – Appendix 6 mm in diameter (93%)
  – Focal cecal apical thickening
  – Defines appendiceal masses (phlegmon versus abscess)
  – Best study for finding alternative diagnoses
  – Nonvisualized appendix does not rule out appendicitis
- MRI: Sensitivity 97–100%, specificity 92–94%:
  – Appendix 7 mm in diameter
  – Periappendiceal fat stranding
  – Advantages: Lack of ionizing radiation, excellent safety profile of gadolinium contrast agents
  – Disadvantages: High cost, limited availability, lengthy examination, lack of radiologist familiarity in appendicitis
  – No gadolinium in early pregnancy (class C drug)

### Pediatric Considerations
American College of Radiology recommends US followed by CT as needed for suspected appendicitis.

### Diagnostic Procedures/Surgery
- Laparoscopy:
  – Diagnostic and therapeutic use
  – Gross pathology may be absent with positive microscopic findings.
- Open appendectomy
- Percutaneous drainage

## DIFFERENTIAL DIAGNOSIS
- Gastroenteritis
- Meckel diverticulum
- Epiploic appendagitis
- Crohn disease
- Diverticulitis
- Volvulus
- Abdominal aortic aneurysm
- Intestinal obstruction
- Urinary tract infection
- PID
- Ectopic pregnancy
- Ovarian cyst/torsion
- Tubo-ovarian abscess
- Endometriosis
- Renal stone
- Testicular torsion
- Sickle cell disease
- Mesenteric adenitis
- Henoch-Schönlein purpura
- Diabetic ketoacidosis
- Streptococcal pharyngitis (children)
- Biliary disease

 **TREATMENT**

### INITIAL STABILIZATION/THERAPY
- Airway, breathing, and circulation management (ABCs)
- Fluid resuscitation with LR or 0.9% NS

### ED TREATMENT/PROCEDURES
- IV fluids, correct electrolyte abnormalities
- Immediate surgical consult for convincing history and physical exam:
  Laparoscopic versus open technique
  – Negative appendectomy rate of 10% in males and 20% in females
  – Percutaneous drainage, IV antibiotics, bowel rest and possible interval appendectomy in 6–8 wk in appendiceal abscesses
- Peri-operative antibiotics
- NPO
- Order CT if palpable mass is present in RLQ to define phlegmon versus abscess
- If diagnosis is uncertain, send serial labs, observe, and repeat exams (6–10% negative appendectomy rate with observation protocols)
- Analgesics:
  – Administration of analgesics, including narcotics, does not adversely affect abdominal exam or mask pathology.

### MEDICATION
- Ampicillin/sulbactam: 3 g (peds: 100–200 mg ampicillin/kg/24 hr) IV q6h
- Cefoxitin: 2 g (peds: 80–100 mg/kg/24 hr) IV q6h
- Ceftriaxone: 1 g (peds: 50–100 mg/kg) IV q24h
- Ciprofloxacin: 400 mg (peds: 20–40mg/kg) IV q12h
- Ertapenem: 1 g IM/IV q24h
- Metronidazole: 500 mg (peds: 30–50 mg/kg/24 hr) IV q8–12h
- Morphine sulfate: 3–5 mg (peds: 0.1–0.2 mg/kg per dose q2h–q4h) IV, every 15 min titrated to effect
- Piperacillin/tazobactam: 3.375 g (peds: 150–300 mg/kg/d if <6 mo; 240–400 mg/kg/d if >6 mo) IV q6h

 **FOLLOW-UP**

### DISPOSITION
#### Admission Criteria
- Surgical intervention of acute appendicitis
- Observation or further diagnostic workup if diagnosis is uncertain

#### Discharge Criteria
Patients with abdominal pain thought not to be appendicitis may be discharged if they meet the following criteria:
- Resolved or resolving symptoms
- Minimal or no abdominal tenderness
- No laboratory/radiologic abnormalities
- Able to tolerate PO intake
- Adequate social support and able to return if symptoms worsen

#### Issues for Referral
Surgical consult for confirmed or suspected appendicitis

### FOLLOW-UP RECOMMENDATIONS
24–48 hr recheck for patients discharged from the ED with abdominal pain of unclear etiology for a recheck

## PEARLS AND PITFALLS
- Pediatric and geriatric patients present atypically and have increased perforation rates.
- Imaging is not required in a classic presentation of acute appendicitis.
- Appendicitis cannot be ruled out on any imaging modality if the appendix is not visualized.

## ADDITIONAL READING
- Basaran A, Basaran M. Diagnosis of acute appendicitis during pregnancy: A systematic review. Obstet Gynecol Surv. 2009;64(7):481–488.
- Cobben LP, Groot I, Haans L, et al. MRI for clinically suspected appendicitis during pregnancy. Am J Radiol. 2004;183:671–675.
- Kwok MY, Kim MK, Gorelick MH. Evidence-based approach to the diagnosis of appendicitis in children. Pediatr Emerg Care. 2004;20(10):690–701.
- Singh A, Danrad R, Hahn PF, et al. MR Imaging of the acute abdomen and pelvis: Acute appendicitis and beyond. Radiographics. 2007;27:1419–1431.
- Terasawa T, Blackmore CC, Bent S, et al. Systematic review: Computed tomography and ultrasonography to detect acute appendicitis in adults and adolescents. Ann Int Med. 2004;141(7):537–546.

### See Also (Topic, Algorithm, Electronic Media Element)
- Abdominal Pain
- Vomiting, Adult; Vomiting, Pediatric

# ARSENIC POISONING
*Gerald Maloney Jr.*

 **BASICS**

## DESCRIPTION
- Acute toxicity:
  - May be intentional ingestion, malicious poisoning, or medication error
- Chronic toxicity:
  - May be owing to occupational exposures, contamination of drinking water or food, or use of folk remedies containing arsenic
- Primarily owing to ingestion
- May also be inhalational toxicity from arsine gas

## ETIOLOGY
- Most arsenic poisonings seen in the ED setting are a result of intentional ingestion or malicious poisoning.
- Sodium arsenate, found in ant killer, is the most common acute exposure in the U.S.
- Overall, contaminated food/water supplies most common cause worldwide.
- Arsenic trioxide has been recently approved as chemotherapy for acute myelogenous leukemia (AML).
- Melarsoprol is used as antitrypanosomal agent in developing countries.
- Found in pesticides, certain folk remedies (herbal balls), preservatives in wood
- Also may be released as arsine gas from combustion of zinc- and arsenic-containing compounds

### Mechanism
- Arsenic exists in several forms: Gas (arsine, or lewisite), organic, elemental, and inorganic
- Inorganic forms most frequently encountered toxic exposure.
- Inorganic in trivalent (arsenite) or pentavalent (arsenate) forms:
  - Most pentavalent arsenic converted to trivalent arsenic in body, which is more toxic
  - Trivalent arsenic binds sulfhydryl groups and interferes in hemoglobin production.
  - Pentavalent arsenic uncouples oxidative phosphorylation.
  - Both function as cellular poisons.

## DIAGNOSIS

### SIGNS AND SYMPTOMS
- Cardiovascular:
  - Prolonged QTc interval
  - Hypotension
  - Dysrhythmias, primarily ventricular
  - Nonspecific ST segment changes
  - Noncardiogenic pulmonary edema
- CNS:
  - Altered mental status/encephalopathy
  - Peripheral neuropathy:
    - Acute: Sensory neuropathy
    - Subacute: Sensorimotor neuropathy
  - Peripheral dysesthesias:
    - Muscle weakness up to paralysis
  - Headache
  - Seizures
- GI:
  - Nausea, vomiting:
    - Protracted and may be refractory to antiemetics at usual doses
    - Can have hemorrhagic gastroenteritis; corrosive to GI tract
  - Rice water diarrhea
  - Abdominal pain
  - Garlic odor to breath, vomit, stools
  - Causes acute hepatitis; chronically, can cause portal HTN
- Miscellaneous:
  - Dermatitis (toxic erythroderma/hyperpigmented lesions)
  - Mee lines (white bands across the nails owing to growth arrest caused by arsenic)
  - Hemolytic anemia (more pronounced with arsine gas exposure)
  - Leukopenia (after several days)
  - Increased risk of carcinoma (liver/basal cell/squamous cell of skin/bronchogenic)
  - Acute rhabdomyolysis
  - Hypothyroidism (antagonizes thyroid hormone)
  - Patchy alopecia

### ESSENTIAL WORKUP
- Spot urine arsenic level
- CBC

## DIAGNOSTIC TESTS & INTERPRETATION
### Lab
- Spot urine arsenic level >1,000 $\mu$g/L may confirm diagnostic suspicion:
  - Peaks 10–50 hr postingestion
- Definitive test is 24-hr urine collection with speciation into organic and inorganic types of arsenic.
- Blood levels not routinely helpful owing to short half-life in serum (~2 hr)
- CBC to check for:
  - Anemia
  - Leukopenia
  - Basophilic stippling
- Electrolytes, BUN/creatinine and glucose
- Urinalysis to look for evidence of hemolysis/rhabdomyolysis
- Liver function tests
- Total creatine phosphokinase (CPK) for rhabdomyolysis
- Hair and nail arsenic levels:
  - Difficult to interpret and not helpful acutely
  - May help determine chronicity of exposure in select populations

### Imaging
- Plain abdominal radiographs to look for radiopaque foreign body
- Cranial CT/other studies as indicated by patient's condition

## DIFFERENTIAL DIAGNOSIS
- Other heavy metal intoxications
- Cyclic antidepressants
- Encephalopathy/Korsakoff syndrome
- Hyperemesis gravidarum
- Shock
- Guillain-Barré syndrome
- Addison disease
- Cholera
- Other neuropathies

**TREATMENT**

### PRE-HOSPITAL

#### ALERT
- If possible to do so safely, bring containers in suspected overdose/poisoning.
- Decontaminate skin.
- Support airway/breathing/circulation.
- Cardiac monitoring

### INITIAL STABILIZATION/THERAPY
- ABCs:
  - Cardiac monitor
  - Isotonic crystalloids as needed for hypotension
  - Vasopressors if refractory hypotension is present
- Naloxone, thiamine, and dextrose (D50W) as indicated for altered mental status
- Cardiovascular:
  - Avoid type 1A antidysrhythmics:
    - Exacerbate QTc prolongation
  - Continuous monitoring, as QTc prolongation is common
- Neurologic:
  - Treat seizures with benzodiazepines.
  - Assist ventilation as needed for respiratory insufficiency owing to neuromuscular weakness.
- Renal:
  - Urinary alkalinization for rhabdomyolysis
  - Hemodialysis for renal failure

### ED TREATMENT/PROCEDURES
- Decontamination:
  - If the patient presents within the 1st hr of ingestion, try orogastric lavage/aspiration.
  - Activated charcoal: Does not bind arsenic
  - If opacities seen on upright abdominal film, institute whole bowel irrigation at 1–2 L/hr of polyethylene glycol until abdominal films are clear.
  - If dermal exposure, decontaminate skin as 1st step in management.

- Ensure that no one else is contaminated and environment is evaluated.
- Evaluate need for chelation therapy, based on levels, acuity of exposure, symptoms:
  - Consultation with a medical toxicologist advised
  - Agents:
    - Dimercaprol (British anti-lewisite)
    - DMSA (succimer)
- Elimination:
  - Hemodialysis not routinely effective:
    - Consider for patient with renal failure
    - Must continue chelation through hemodialysis (HD)

### MEDICATION
- Dimercaprol (British anti-lewisite): 3 mg/kg IM q4h for 24 hr, then q6h for the next 24 hr, then q12h until able to tolerate PO:
  - Caution: Cannot use if patient has peanut allergy
- Dextrose 50%: 25 g (50 mL) (peds: 0.5 g/kg $D_{25}W$) IV for hypoglycemia
- DMSA (succimer): 10 mg/kg PO q8h for 5 days, then q12h for 14 days
- Sodium bicarbonate: 1 mEq/kg IV bolus, followed by infusion of 150 mEq in 1 L of $D_5W$ at 150 ml /hr:
  - Used to treat rhabdomyolysis
- Naloxone: 0.4–2.0 mg (peds: 0.1 mg/kg) IV, may repeat up to 10 mg for suspected opioid intoxication
- Thiamine: 100 mg IM or IV (peds: 1 mg/kg)

 **FOLLOW-UP**

### DISPOSITION
#### Admission Criteria
Symptomatic arsenic exposures should be admitted to an intensive care setting.

#### Discharge Criteria
- Asymptomatic patients with a spot urinary arsenic level <50 µg/L may be discharged.
- Suspected chronic exposures who do not require admission should be referred for outpatient evaluation and 24-hr urine collection.
- Ensure that home environment is safe for patient prior to discharge.

### FOLLOW-UP RECOMMENDATIONS
Psychiatric follow-up for intentional overdoses

## PEARLS AND PITFALLS
- Arsenic poisoning results in a myriad of signs and symptoms:
  - Suspect arsenic poisoning when patients present with these findings.
- Consult medical toxicologist regarding the need for chelation therapy.

## ADDITIONAL READING
- Ford M. Arsenic. In: *Goldfrank's toxicologic emergencies*, 8th ed. New York: McGraw-Hill, 2006.
- Graeme KA, Pollack CV. Heavy metal toxicity. Part I: Arsenic and mercury. *J Emerg Med*. 1998;16(1): 45–56.
- Tchounwou PB, Patlolla AK, Centeno JA. Carcinogenic and systemic health effects associated with arsenic exposure: A critical review. *Toxicol Pathol*. 2003;31(6):575–588.
- Vahidinia A, et al. Arsenic neurotoxicity: A review. *Hum Exp Toxicol* 2007;26(10):823–832.

 **CODES**

### ICD9
985.1 Toxic effect of arsenic and its compounds

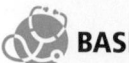

## BASICS

### DESCRIPTION

- Results when air bubbles enter the pulmonary venous return from ruptured alveoli, then propagate through the systemic vasculature:
  - Clinical manifestations depend on location of air bubbles in systemic vasculature system.
- Also known as dysbaric air embolism or cerebral air embolism
- Caused by overpressurization of lung tissue, causing pleural tear with air entering the vascular circulation:
  - Air bubbles tend to rise and enter the cerebral vessels, where they occlude vascular flow.
  - Boyle's law: At a constant temperature, pressure (P) is inversely related to volume (V):
    - $PV = K$ (constant) or $P_1V_1 = P_2V_2$
  - As pressure increases/decreases, volume decreases/increases.
  - Trapped air (in lungs with closed glottis) expands on diver ascent.

### ETIOLOGY

- Pulmonary atrioventricular (AV) shunts, or as paradoxical embolism via a patent foramen ovale (up to 30% of the adult population)
- Breath-holding during ascent:
  - Symptoms attributable to a shower of bubbles and multiple blood vessel involvement
- Iatrogenically during placement of central venous pressure (CVP) lines, cardiothoracic surgery, or hemodialysis
- Penetrating injuries to heart, with emergent repair of cardiac wound

## DIAGNOSIS

### SIGNS AND SYMPTOMS

- Cerebral:
  - Dive-related stroke
  - 2nd leading cause of dive-related death (after drowning)
  - 2 main presentations:
    - Apnea and full cardiopulmonary arrest
    - Any combination of neurologic deficits
  - Presentation depends on arterial distribution of gas embolism:
    - Change in level of consciousness (40%)
    - Sensory loss (20%)
    - Motor deficit (20%)
    - Paraplegia (10%)
    - Seizure (4%)
    - Visual changes
    - Aphasia
    - Paresthesias
  - Rapid onset:
    - 8.6% during ascent
    - 83.6% <5 min after surfacing
    - 7.8% between 5 and 10 min after surfacing
  - Spontaneous improvement minutes after initial deficits may occur:
    - High incidence of relapse
    - Improvement may be transiently related to postural changes that affect distribution of bubbles flowing to brain.
- Pulmonary:
  - Shortness of breath
  - Bloody, frothy sputum
  - SC air
- Cardiac:
  - MI owing to air in coronary vessels
  - Reduced cardiac output owing to air trapped in ventricle
  - Hamman sign: Crepitus on auscultation of heart
- Renal:
  - Renal infarction owing to air embolism

### History

Elicit time of symptom onset in relation to dive surfacing.

### Physical Exam

Careful neurologic exam owing to the wide variety of neurologic manifestations

### ESSENTIAL WORKUP

- Clinical diagnosis: Recognize risk factors and various clinical presentations.
- Inquire as to unusual circumstances during ascent:
  - Breath-holding
  - Panic/out-of-air situation
- Thorough neurologic exam must carefully document the extent of the deficits to the motor, sensory, cerebellar, and cranial nerves.

### DIAGNOSTIC TESTS & INTERPRETATION

#### Lab

- Serum creatinine kinase activity:
  - Marker of the severity of cerebral AGE
- CBC
- Electrolytes, BUN, creatinine, glucose
- ABG when respiratory symptoms are present

#### Imaging

- CXR:
  - For evidence of pneumothorax or mediastinal emphysema (both rare)
- EKG
- Echo:
  - Looking for evidence of patent foramen ovale
- CT head:
  - For altered mental status
  - Do not delay recompression for CT when AGE almost certain clinically.

### DIFFERENTIAL DIAGNOSIS

- Cerebrovascular accident (CVA) from causes unrelated to gas embolism
- Neurologic deficits owing to decompression sickness

**TREATMENT**

## PRE-HOSPITAL
- Cautions:
  - Patients who experience sudden neurologic recovery can relapse quickly as bubble positions change.
  - Recognize AGE as a potential diagnosis.
- Altered mental status within 10 min of surfacing from compressed air dive
- Sudden neurologic decompensation following placement of central line
- Controversies:
  - Trendelenburg positioning patients with suspected AGE is not effective:
    - Hypothesized that elevation of legs could cause air bubbles to migrate away from cerebral circulation and that increased hydrostatic pressure in brain will shrink bubbles
    - Trendelenburg positioning may in fact increase injury by increasing intracerebral pressure.

## INITIAL STABILIZATION/THERAPY
ABCs:
- 100% oxygen by tight-fitting mask
- Intubation for ventilation/protection of airway required
- IV access with volume augmentation

## ED TREATMENT/PROCEDURES
- Hyperbaric oxygen recompression therapy (see "Hyperbaric Oxygen Therapy"):
  - For all AGE
  - Arrange transportation to nearest hyperbaric facility.
  - Aircraft capable of cabin pressurization below 1,000 feet barometric pressure best suited for transfers
  - Prophylactic chest tube for simple pneumothorax to prevent conversion to tension pneumothorax during recompression
  - Fill endotracheal and Foley catheter balloons with water or saline to avoid shrinkage/damage during recompression.

- Divers Alert Network (DAN):
  - Based at Duke University Medical Center
  - Provides 24-hr emergency hotline for medical consultation on treatment of dive-related injuries and for referrals to hyperbaric chambers (telephone: [919] 684-8111)

 **FOLLOW-UP**

## DISPOSITION
### Admission Criteria
Admit all following initial hyperbaric therapy for observation and re-exam.

### Discharge Criteria
No AGE patients should be discharged from the ED.

## FOLLOW-UP RECOMMENDATIONS
Hyperbaric oxygen referral for patients with arterial case embolisms

# PEARLS AND PITFALLS

- Symptoms occur during ascent or within 10 min of reaching the surface.
- Patients who experience sudden neurologic recovery can relapse quickly as bubble positions change.
- Fill endotracheal and Foley catheter balloons with water or saline to avoid shrinkage/damage during recompression.

# ADDITIONAL READING

- Beckman TJ. A review of decompression sickness and arterial gas embolism. *Arch Fam Med*. 1997;6(5):491–494.
- Jerrard DA. Diving medicine. *Emerg Med Clin North Am*. 1992;10(2):329–338.
- Kizer KW. Diving medicine and arterial gas embolism. In: Auerbach PA, ed. *Wilderness medicine*. 4th ed. St. Louis: Mosby, 2001.
- Moon RE, Gorman DF. Treatment of decompression disorders. In: *The physiology and medicine of diving*, 5th ed. Philadelphia: WB Saunders, 2003.
- Smith RM, Neuman TS. Elevation of serum creatine kinase In divers with arterial gas embolism. *N Engl J Med*. 1994;330:19–24.
- van Hulst RA. Effects of hyperbaric treatment in cerebral air embolism on intracranial pressure, brain oxygenation, and brain glucose metabolism in the pig. *Crit Care Med*. 2005;33:841–846.

## See Also (Topic, Algorithm, Electronic Media Element)
- Barotrauma
- Decompression Sickness
- Hyperbaric Oxygen Therapy

 **CODES**

**ICD9**
958.0 Air embolism as an early complication of trauma

# ARTERIAL OCCLUSION

James M. Leaming
Spencer Adoff

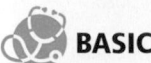

## BASICS

### DESCRIPTION
A sudden interruption in blood flow to a limb, with a resulting risk in tissue viability

### ETIOLOGY
- Thrombotic:
  - Low flow
  - Hypercoagulable states
  - Vascular grafts
  - Atherosclerosis
- Embolic:
  - Atrial fibrillation
  - MI
  - Valvular disease
  - Endocarditis
  - Proximal arterial aneurysm
  - Atherosclerotic plaques
  - Fat embolism
  - Cholesterol embolism
- Arterial injury:
  - Intimal flap
  - Dissection
  - Iatrogenic from arterial catheterization
  - Penetrating Trauma
  - Blunt Trauma

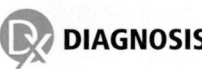

## DIAGNOSIS

### SIGNS AND SYMPTOMS
- The 6 Ps:
  - Pain
  - Pallor
  - Paresthesias
  - Paralysis
  - Pulseless (late finding)
  - Poikilothermia
- Blue toe syndrome:
  - Development of blue or violaceous discoloration in one or more toes
  - The affected digits are often painful.
  - The cyanosis initially blanches with pressure or leg elevation.

### History
- Claudication:
  - Reproducible discomfort of a defined group of muscles that is induced by exercise and relieved with rest
- Cramps
- Past medical history:
  - Risk factors for thrombosis:
    - Vascular grafts
    - Atherosclerosis
    - Hypercoagulable state
    - Low flow state
  - Risk factors for embolism:
    - Atrial fibrillation
    - MI
    - Endocarditis
    - Valvular disease
    - Atrial myxoma
    - Prosthetic valve
    - Patent foremen ovale and paradoxical embolus

### Physical Exam
- Sensory loss
- Muscle weakness
- Skin color changes
- Loss of pulse
- Signs of chronic arterial insufficiency:
  - Hair loss
  - Atrophic skin
- Ankle-brachial pressure index measurement:
  - Ratio of systolic BP in the lower legs to the brachial pressure in the arm:
    - Place cuff above malleoli to measure pressure in lower legs.
    - Use Doppler at posterior tibial or dorsalis pedis artery.
  - Chronic PVD <1.0
  - Acute arterial occlusion <0.5

### ESSENTIAL WORKUP
Acute arterial occlusion is a clinical diagnosis.

### ALERT
Elevation, cool compress or ice, or warm compress to the affected extremity is contraindicated.

## DIAGNOSTIC TESTS & INTERPRETATION

### Lab
- Electrolytes/anion gap
- BUN
- Creatinine
- CBC
- Creatine phosphokinase
- Specimen for type and screen:
  - Peripheral ischemic syndromes may result in changes in acid–base status (acidemia) and electrolyte derangement (hyperkalemia), which are acutely exacerbated on reperfusion.

### Imaging
- EKG
- Duplex US
- Angiography
- Plain films are of little use in the setting of peripheral vascular disease (PVD).
- MRI may be of some clinical benefit due to its high visual detail and can replace traditional arteriography.

### Diagnostic Procedures/Surgery
Arterial Doppler

### Classification
- Viable:
  - Needs attention, not in immediate danger:
    - No sensory loss, no muscle weakness, audible arterial Doppler
- Marginally threatened:
  - Needs immediate attention, tissue salvageable:
    - +/− sensory loss, no muscle weakness, +/− audible arterial Doppler
- Immediately threatened:
  - Needs immediate revascularization, tissue salvageable:
    - Sensory loss, muscle weakness, +/− no audible arterial Doppler
- Irreversible/nonviable:
  - Nonsalvageable tissue:
    - Sensory loss, muscle weakness (+/− paralysis), no audible arterial Doppler
    - Will require amputation

## DIFFERENTIAL DIAGNOSIS

- Lumbar spine disorders
- Back pain, mechanical
- Decreased cardiac output owing to advanced atherosclerotic disease
- Frostbite
- Peripheral neuropathy
- Aneurysm, abdominal
- Ankle injury, soft tissue
- Deep venous thrombosis
- Septic thrombophlebitis
- Superficial thrombophlebitis
- Trauma, peripheral vascular injuries

 **TREATMENT**

### PRE-HOSPITAL

Recognition of a potentially limb-threatening emergency

### ED TREATMENT/PROCEDURES

- Prompt consultation with vascular surgeon
- Heparin
- Intra-arterial thrombolytic agents vs. surgical revascularization depending on viability of limb
- Pain control

### MEDICATION

Heparin: Weight-based protocol anticoagulation with typical 80 IU/kg loading bolus; 18 IU/kg/hr IV

 **FOLLOW-UP**

### DISPOSITION

#### Admission Criteria

All patients with clinical diagnosis of acute arterial occlusion or (ABI <0.5) should be admitted after an emergency consultation with a vascular surgeon.

#### Discharge Criteria

- Patients with chronic occlusive disease, resolved pain, and stable ABI measurements
- No other acute medical issues (eg, new atrial fibrillation)
- Vascular surgical follow-up can be ensured.
- Patients should be instructed to return for any recurrent or progressive symptoms.

#### Issues for Referral

- PVD patents in which illness is not severe or acute as to require inpatient treatment may be discharged with appropriate follow-up with a vascular surgeon.
- Potential effects of various activities and medications on the course of their illness should be discussed.
- Education on smoking cessation, temperature extremes, and vasoconstricting medications should be considered.

## ADDITIONAL READING

- Feldman AJ. Acute extremity ischemia and thrombophlebitis. In: *Emergency Medicine: A Comprehensive Study Guide*. 4th ed.
- Howell JM, Haska ZJ, Hertzer NR, et al. Acquired diseases of the arteries and veins. *Emerg Med*. 1998:203–206.

- Hirsch AT, et al. ACC/AHA 2005 Practice Guidelines for the Management of Patients With Peripheral Arterial Disease (Lower Extremity, Renal, Mesenteric, and Abdominal Aortic). A collaborative report from the American Association for Vascular Surgery/Society for Vascular Surgery, Society for Cardiovascular Angiography and Interventions, Society for Vascular Medicine and Biology, Society of Interventional Radiology, and the ACC/AHA Task Force on Practice Guidelines (Writing Committee to Develop Guidelines for the Management of Patients With Peripheral Arterial Disease): endorsed by the American Association of Cardiovascular and Pulmonary Rehabilitation; National Heart, Lung, and Blood Institute; Society for Vascular Nursing; TransAtlantic Inter-Society Consensus; and Vascular Disease Foundation.*Circulation*. 2006;113(11):e463–e654.
- Hirschmann JV, Raugi GJ. Blue (or purple) toe syndrome. *J Am Acad Dermatol*. 2009;61(4): 727–728.
- Katzen BT. Clinical diagnosis and prognosis of acute limb ischemia. *Rev Cardiovasc Med*. 2002;3 (Suppl 2):S2–6.
- Tintinalli JE, Kelen GD, Stapczynski J, eds. *Emergency Medicine: A Comprehensive Study Guide*, 6th ed. New York: McGraw-Hill; 2004.

### See Also (Topic, Algorithm, Electronic Media Element)

Peripheral Vascular Disease

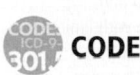 **CODES**

### ICD9

444.9 Embolism and thrombosis of unspecified artery

# ARTHRITIS, DEGENERATIVE

*Patrick H. Sweet, III*

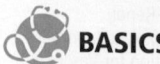 **BASICS**

## DESCRIPTION
- Degenerative arthritis or osteoarthritis (OA) is the most common progressive joint disease, with 20–30 million cases in the U.S.
- Found almost exclusively in the elderly

## ETIOLOGY
- Mechanism
- Repetitive stress to synovial joints associated with age
- May be seen in younger patients secondary to joint trauma
- Articular cartilage destruction:
  - Reactive changes in joint margin bone and subchondral sclerosis
- Risk factors include age, obesity, trauma, genetics, sex, and environment.

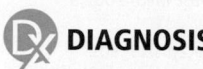 **DIAGNOSIS**

## SIGNS AND SYMPTOMS
- Chronic progressive joint pain:
  - Worse with weight bearing, improved with rest
- Asymmetric joint involvement:
  - Involves hand, foot, knee, hip, and spine joints
- Morning joint stiffness usually <30 min
- Joint deformity late in presentation with limited range of motion
- Heberden nodes at the distal interphalangeal joints
- Bouchard nodes at the proximal interphalangeal joints
- Absence of systemic symptoms
- Crepitus common

## ESSENTIAL WORKUP
- Thorough joint examination with assessment of range of motion and functional ability
- Radiographic examination helpful in diagnosis but is particularly indicated in the setting of trauma to exclude fracture. Typical findings in OA are decreased joint space, irregular bone at the joint margin, and osteophytes.
- Synovial fluid analysis in the setting of effusion may be therapeutic and diagnostic (see below), but is absolutely necessary if presents with warmth and erythema so as to rule out a septic joint or gout.
- Note: Arthrocentesis is contraindicated if a more superficial infection cannot be ruled out (eg, septic bursitis, cellulitis, etc.).

## DIAGNOSTIC TESTS & INTERPRETATION
### Lab
Synovial fluid examination typically reveals the following:
- Clear
- Elevated leukocyte cell count, but <4,000/mm$^3$
- <25% polymorphonuclear leukocytes
- Glucose level similar to blood levels (95–100%)

### Imaging
- Radiographs
- Joint space narrowing
- Osteophyte formation
- Marginal bone erosion
- Subchondral sclerosis

## DIFFERENTIAL DIAGNOSIS
- Gout or pseudogout
- Septic arthritis
- Rheumatoid arthritis
- Charcot joint
- Hemarthrosis

 **TREATMENT**

The general goal of treatment is to provide relief from symptoms. A patient may have significant radiographic evidence of disease but have very few symptoms. Therefore the treatment regimen is tailored to the patient's symptomatology.

## PRE-HOSPITAL
Immobilization of affected joint may be indicated until fracture is excluded.

## INITIAL STABILIZATION/THERAPY
- Pain management acutely
- Begin a daily medication that can by managed on follow-up with primary care physician.
- Instructions for gentle strengthening exercises
- Avoidance of unnecessary joint immobilization

## ED TREATMENT/PROCEDURES
Intra-articular (IA) arthrocentesis and injection:
- Shown to be an effective low-risk intervention for OA with or without effusion
- Though relatively rare in larger joints, dry tap is a possible complication due to anatomic abnormalities of the synovium and periarticular tissues found in OA.
- Careful attention must be given to aseptic technique.
- Comfortable positions that reduce muscle tension will allow for the most joint volume.
- Vapor coolant or lidocaine 1% or 2% can be used for local anesthesia.
- 22- or 18-gauge hypodermic needle should be used with one syringe for arthrocentesis and another for IA corticosteroid injection.
- If septic joint cannot be ruled out, corticosteroids should not be administered after arthrocentesis.

Corticosteroid dosing equivalents*:
- Small joints—wrist and foot:
  - Methylprednisolone 10–20 mg, triamcinolone 10 mg, betamethasone 0.75–1.5 mg
- Medium sized joints—elbow and ankle:
  - Methylprednisolone 40–80 mg, triamcinolone 20 mg, betamethasone 3–6 mg
- Large joints—knee and shoulder:
  - Methylprednisolone 80–120 mg, triamcinolone 40 mg; betamethasone 6–9 mg
- Some studies show triamcinolone to be more efficacious than other corticosteroids; the author recommends this, if available, over other preparations.

## MEDICATION

General guidelines:
- Acetaminophen is drug of choice initially as it has a safer medication profile compared with NSAIDs and has been shown to be as efficacious in some patients.
- If one class fails, consider another class (eg, salicylates versus COX-2 inhibitors).
- The two alternative medications below have been shown to have a small but positive effect by meta-analysis of recent studies and can be considered adjuncts.
- Patients at increased risk for gastrointestinal bleeding should be placed on COX-2 inhibitors or alternatively a proton pump inhibitor can be given with a nonselective COX inhibitor.

- NSAIDs:
  - Celecoxib (reversible COX-2–selective) 500 mg PO q24 or q12:
    - Note: Contraindicated in sulfonamide allergy
  - Ibuprofen (reversible nonselective COX): 400–600 mg PO q6h
  - Enteric-coated aspirin (irreversible nonselective COX): 325–650 mg PO q6h:
    - Note: Contraindicated if unable to rule out gout or patient has comorbid bleeding disorder
- Analgesics:
  - Acetaminophen: 650 mg PO q6h
  - Tramadol: 50 mg PO q4–6h:
    - Note: Use cautiously in elderly, patients with seizure disorders, concurrently using antidepressants, or in hepatic or renal dysfunction.
  - Other opioid narcotics rarely used
- Alternative therapies:
  - Glucosamine: 500 mg PO q8h
  - Chondroitin: 1200 mg PO q24h
  - *Some studies show more efficacy when chondroitin and glucosamine are used in combination.

 **FOLLOW-UP**

## DISPOSITION

### Admission Criteria
Rarely indicated in the absence of fracture

### Discharge Criteria
- Ambulatory and capable of activities of daily living
- Improvement in symptoms (ie, pain)

## ADDITIONAL READING

- Vangsness CT Jr, Spiker W, Erickson J. A review of evidence-based medicine for glucosamine and chondroitin sulfate use in knee osteoarthritis. *Arthroscopy.* 2009;25(1):86–94.
- National Center for Complimentary and Alternative Medicine. The NIH Glucosamine/Chondroitin Arthritis Intervention Trial (GAIT). *J Pain Palliat Care Pharmacother.* 2008;22(1):39–43.
- Hepper CT, Halvorson JJ, Duncan ST, et al. The efficacy and duration of intra-articular corticosteroid injection for knee osteoarthritis: A systematic review of level I studies. *J Am Acad Orthop Surg.* 2009;17(10):638–646.
- Frampton JE, Keating GM. Celecoxib: A review of its use in the management of arthritis and acute pain. *Drugs.* 2007;67(16):2433–2472.
- Marx JC, et al, eds. *Rosens's Emergency Medicine: Concepts and Clinical Practice.* 6th ed. Philadelphia: Mosby Elsevier, 2006:1776–1793.
- Stephens MB, Beutler AI, O'Connor FG. Musculoskeletal injections: A review of the evidence. *Am Fam Physician.* 2008;78(8):971–976.

 **CODES**

### ICD9
715.90 Osteoarthrosis, unspecified whether generalized or localized, involving unspecified site

# ARTHRITIS, JUVENILE IDIOPATHIC

*Jeannette M. Wolfe*

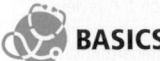 **BASICS**

## DESCRIPTION
- Previously called JRA
- JIA comprises persistent, unexplained arthritis lasting >6 wk, occurring <17 yr of age, and affecting a heterogeneous group of children.
- Prevalence up to 1 in 1,000 children
- Girls > boys for most forms
- New nomenclature by the International League of Associations for Rheumatology divides JIA into 7 subgroups: Systemic onset, polyarticular RF+, polyarticular RF, pauciarticular, psoriatic, enthesitis, other.
- Subtypes are based on number, type, and symmetry of joints involved; presence of systemic symptoms; skin involvement; family history; and lab values.
- Even with new nomenclature, ~20% of JIA patients remain unclassified or are classified in multiple categories.
- The natural course of the disease depends on the subtype (pauciarticular with overall best prognosis), but full resolution occurs in <50% of JIA patients.
- Many will have a fluctuating course and ongoing disease through adulthood.

## ETIOLOGY
Believed to be an autoimmune disease triggered by an unknown environmental trigger in a genetically susceptible host

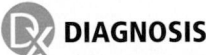 **DIAGNOSIS**

## SIGNS AND SYMPTOMS
- Systemic onset:
  - 10% of cases, girls = boys
  - Associated fever and arthritis:
    - Fever: diurnal (>39°C) of >2 wk duration, child looks ill during temperature spike
    - Arthritis: May involve any number of joints and may appear only wk to mo after onset of fever
  - In addition there must be one of the following:
    - Maculopapular, salmon-colored rash on trunk and axillae, fades with resolution of fever
    - Lymphadenopathy
    - Hepatosplenomegaly

### ALERT
- Systemic onset JIA patients are at risk for macrophage activation syndrome (MAS).
- MAS is a proliferation of macrophages causing a DIC-like picture with resultant fever, mucosal bleeding, neurologic changes and multisystem failure.
- MAS mortality is 8–22%.

- Pauciarticular:
  - 50% of cases
  - 80% girls, peak incidence 2–3-yr-olds
  - Insidious onset and child appears healthy
  - ≤4 joints involved at 6 mo:
    - Involves larger joints, *but hip rarely affected*
    - Joints swollen, mildly tender, with decreased range of motion (ROM), possible leg-length discrepancy
  - Uveitis in about 20%; no other systemic signs
  - Subset termed *extended* pauciarticular progresses to greater joint involvement after 6 mo and has worse prognosis
- Polyarticular:
  - 40% of cases, girls > boys, bimodal peaks: 2–5 and 10–14 yr
  - >4 joints involved at 6 mo:
    - Arthritis often symmetrical, small or large joints—commonly knees, wrists, and ankles
    - Decreased ROM of cervical and lumbar spine and temporomandibular joint (TMJ)
  - Systemic involvement rare except for fatigue and anemia
  - Older girls with RF+ often go on to develop typical adult rheumatoid arthritis (RA) and are placed in a separate subtype.
- Psoriatic:
  - Arthritis; asymmetric large joints of lower extremities and back
  - Psoriatic rash in patient or 2 of following; dactylitis, nail pitting, psoriatic rash in first-degree relative
  - Enthesitis-related (*enthesis* means pain at the insertion of a muscle or tendon)
  - Arthritis; asymmetric large joints of lower extremities
  - Boys > girls, age usually >6 yr
  - Sacroiliac (SI) joint pain
  - Limited flexion of lumbar spine
  - Uveitis
  - Often FH
- Otherwise unclassified:
  - Arthritis not fitting into any distinct category

## History
- Findings based on specific subtype
- New-onset systemic subtype most likely to use ED because they appear acutely ill, whereas other subtypes have a more insidious onset.

### ALERT
- Child with severe pain and red-hot joint probably does not have new-onset JIA.
- Rapid onset of polyarticular joint involvement is atypical for JIA; infectious or reactive cause of arthritis should be ruled out.
- Beware of occult infection in patients on immunosuppressants.

## Physical Exam
- Determine if child is systemically ill: Search for fever, rash or other nonarthritic involvement.
- Do careful joint evaluation, documenting the number of joints involved and noting whether they are red, warm and swollen or have limited ROM.

## ESSENTIAL WORKUP
- Rule out septic joint and malignant bone tumor.
- Rule out other identifiable causes of joint inflammation.
- Rule out complications from long-term drug therapy.

## DIAGNOSTIC TESTS & INTERPRETATION
### Lab
- CBC, ESR; if ill appearance, add blood cultures
- Other labs if suspicious of specific subtype: rheumatoid factor (RF), antinuclear antibodies (ANA), HLA-B27, LFTs:
  - Systemic—ESR often elevated, leukocytosis, thrombocytosis, anemia, minor AST/ALT elevations, positive RF or ANA rarely seen, MAS may be associated with elevated LFTs and abnormal clotting factors but will often have normal ESR
  - Pauciarticular—common to have positive ANA in young girls; other labs usually normal; if anemic or elevated ESR, are probably misclassified or pauciarticular extended subtype
  - Polyarticular—may be anemic; if positive RF more likely to go on to adult RA, ESR may be elevated
  - Enthesitis—more likely positive HLA; presence of positive RF or positive ANA specifically excludes enthesitis subtype
  - Psoriatic arthritis—usually seronegative RF
- Unfortunately, RF and ESR may also be elevated in acute infection unrelated to JIA.

### ALERT
- Consider additional labs focused on specific drug therapy toxicity.
- Consider adding Lyme titer if new joint swelling in endemic area.

### Imaging
- Joint radiograph:
  - Early presentation: Soft tissue swelling, joint effusion
  - Late presentation: Osteoporosis, joint destruction, early growth plate closure
- Ultrasound:
  - Evaluate for small effusion, especially if tap considered.

### Diagnostic Procedures/Surgery
Arthrocentesis if concern for septic arthritis:
- 5,000–8,000 WBC/mm$^3$ with negative Gram's stain and culture typical for JIA

### DIFFERENTIAL DIAGNOSIS
- Trauma
- Infection:
  - Septic arthritis, viral infection (especially parvovirus), Lyme disease, rheumatic fever, tuberculosis, subacute endocarditis, malaria, *Neisseria gonorrhoeae* infection

- Other rheumatic/connective tissue diseases:
  - Systemic lupus erythematosus, polyarteritis nodosa, Henoch-Schönlein purpura, sarcoid
  - Legg–Calvé–Perthes disease/slipped capital femoral epiphysis
- Neoplasm:
  - Be suspicious of neoplasm in a severely uncomfortable child with midshaft bone pain.
- Hematologic disease:
  - Sickle cell disease, hemophilia
- Drug reactions

 TREATMENT

### INITIAL STABILIZATION/THERAPY
Toxic-appearing children: IV access, $O_2$

### ED TREATMENT/PROCEDURES
- ED treatment is directed toward ruling out a septic joint and other causes of acute arthritis
- If the diagnosis of JIA is already established and the child presents with an acute flare, a treatment plan/medication adjustment should be coordinated with the child's rheumatologist.

### MEDICATION
- Medication in children with JIA is geared toward eliminating clinical signs of active disease, maximizing joint function, and preserving growth. (Chronic inflammation can make affected limb slightly longer.)
- Efficacy depends on JIA subtype and disease severity.
- Most pauciarticular JIA responds to NSAIDs and joint injections; polyarticular and systemic JIA usually require disease-modifying antirheumatic drug (DMARD) therapy and or biological agents.
- Antibiotics are indicated only if the joint is infected

### ALERT
As early aggressive therapy may prevent some of the long-term complications of JIA, it is now common for children to be placed on DMARDS and biological agents early in the disease course. These medications have serious potential side effects, including:
- Immunosuppression
- Decreased vaccine response (live vaccinations are contraindicated)
- Increased potential for malignancy

- NSAIDs:
  - Responsiveness differs within NSAID subtype
  - Used alone in mild JIA subtype or with other medications
  - Ibuprofen: 30–45 mg/kg divided t.i.d.–q.i.d.
  - Naproxen: 10–20 mg/kg divided b.i.d.
  - Side effects: gastritis, hepatitis, renal, headache, dermatitis
  - Intra-articular steroids: Triamcinolone hexacetonide: 1 mg/kg for large joints
  - Often provide long-term (6–18 mo) relief

- DMARDs:
  - Include corticosteroids, methotrexate, sulfasalazine
  - Corticosteroids:
  - Use judiciously because of long-term complications, but high-dose pulse therapy may be needed in acute attack.
  - Prednisone: 0.5–2 mg/kg PO
  - Methylprednisolone: 30 mg/kg daily IV up to 1 g for 1–5 days for high-dose pulse steroids
  - Side effects: gastritis, adrenal suppression, osteopenia, Cushing syndrome, infection
  - Methotrexate: 5–15 mg/m$^2$ PO/SC or IM per wk
  - Considered first-line DMARD, as most will respond
  - Side effects: GI, nausea, liver toxicity, teratogenic
  - Sulfasalazine: 30 mg/kg/d divided qid
  - Poorly tolerated in up to 30%
  - Side effects: GI, rash, anorexia
  - Biological agents—engineered to target specific key cytokines, very expensive
  - Tissue necrosis factor binders
- Etanercept: 0.8 mg/kg SC once a week
  - Adalimumab: < 30 kg: 20 mg, > 30 kg: 40 mg given q2wk
  - Side effects: Infection, injection-site reactions, inhibit T-cell activation Abatacept: 10 mg/kg infusion q4 wk
  - Side effects: Infusion reaction, HA, cough, nausea, infection
- Non-FDA-approved therapies:
- Remicade, rituximab, anakira, leflunamide IL-1 and IL-6 blockers
- Stem cell transplants are used rarely for severe cases unresponsive to medical treatment:
  - Treatment for MAS is nonstandardized but may include high-dose steroids, cyclosporine, cyclophosphamide, or intravenous immunoglobulin

 FOLLOW-UP

### DISPOSITION
#### Admission Criteria
Unclear diagnosis in ill-appearing child or if concern of secondary joint infection

#### Discharge Criteria
- No evidence of septic joint, systemic infection, or organ failure from drug therapy
- Patient appears comfortable.
- Appropriate follow-up has been arranged.

#### Issues for Referral
- Orthopedics if septic joint suspected
- Rheumatologist if meds need adjustment

### FOLLOW-UP RECOMMENDATIONS
- Children need long-term consults with a rheumatologist.
- Children with JIA need frequent eye exams to rule out uveitis (which is often asymptomatic until permanent damage has occurred).

## PEARLS AND PITFALLS
- Rule out acute joint infection (always consider Lyme disease in the appropriate geographic context).
- Consider systemic onset JIA in child with prolonged diurnal febrile illness that is unresponsive to antibiotics.
- Consider macrophage activation syndrome in systemic onset JIA patients who appear septic.
- Review patient's medications to identify potential side effects or immunosuppression.

## ADDITIONAL READING
- Beresford MW, Baildam EM. New advances in the management of juvenile idiopathic arthritis-1 Non-biological therapy. *Arch Dis Child Educ Pract Ed.* 2009;94:144–150.
- Beresford MW, Baildam EM. New advances in the management of juvenile idiopathic arthritis-2 The era of biologicals. *Arch Dis Child Educ Pract Ed.* 2009;94:151–156.
- Kahn P Juvenile idiopathic arthritis. Current and future therapies. *Bull NYU Hosp Joint Dis.* 2009;67:291–302.
- Lehman T. Clinical manifestations and diagnosis of systemic onset juvenile rheumatoid arthritis. *UpToDate.* Waltham, MA: UpToDate, May 1, 2009.
- Lehman T. Clinical manifestations and diagnosis of polyarticular onset juvenile rheumatoid arthritis. Uptodate 17.2 May 1, 2009
- Petty RE, Southwood TR, Manners P, et al. International League of Associations for Rheumatology classification of juvenile idiopathic arthritis: 2nd rev. *J Rheum.* 2004;31(2):390–392.

### See Also (Topic, Algorithm, Electronic Media Element)
- Septic Joint
- Lyme Disease

 CODES

ICD9
714.30 Chronic or unspecified polyarticular juvenile rheumatoid arthritis

# ARTHRITIS, MONOARTICULAR
*Paul Blackburn*

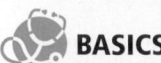 **BASICS**

## DESCRIPTION
- Localized to 1 joint
- Presence of 1 etiology does not exclude another.
- Infectious (septic) arthritis: Up to 46% have prior joint inflammation conditions:
  - Hematogenous spread
  - Contiguous extension (cellulitis, osteomyelitis)
  - Direct inoculation (puncture wound, joint surgery)
  - Predisposing factors:
    ○ Immunosuppression
    ○ IV drug use
    ○ Chronic illness
    ○ Local pathology (inflammatory arthritis, trauma, prosthetic joint)
- Crystalline: Crystal deposition in, around joint:
  - Gout: Uric acid crystals secondary to overproduction, underexcretion
  - Alcoholism, loop diuretics, renal failure, males 40–50, women >60
  - Pseudogout: Calcium pyrophosphate dihydrate (CPPD) crystals:
    ○ Most common monoarthritis in elderly; peak incidence females 60–70
    ○ Increased incidence in elderly, trauma, surgery, hyperparathyroidism, hemochromatosis, hypothyroidism patients
- Noninflammatory:
  - Osteoarthritis (nonspecific destructive process, cartilage or bone):
    ○ Loss of articular cartilage with reactive changes at joint margins
  - Greater incidence elderly men than women until 60 yr old, then ratio reverses
  - Morbidly obese
  - Congenital hip dysplasia: Hip pain in young
  - Trauma: Fracture, Charcot joint

## ETIOLOGY
- Most common pathogens in septic arthritis are gram-positive *Staphylococcus* and *Streptococcus*
- Gram-negative bacteria causative in up to 30% of cases
- Infectious, bacterial:
  - Knowledge of local microbiology
  - *Neisseria gonorrhea*
  - *Staphylococcus aureus:* Trauma, IV drug use
  - *Salmonella*: Sickle cell disease
  - Gram-negative organisms, anaerobes: Immunocompromised
- Infectious, spirochetal:
  - Tuberculosis
  - Lyme disease
- Infectious, viral:
  - More commonly polyarticular
- Infectious, fungal:
  - More commonly chronic
  - Immunosuppressed?
- Crystalline:
  - Gout (urate)
  - Pseudogout (CPPD)

- Inflammatory:
  - Diligent search for underlying conditions
  - Inflammatory bowel disease
  - Rheumatoid arthritis
  - Psoriatic
  - Reiter syndrome (seronegative spondyloarthropathy)
- Noninflammatory:
  - Osteoarthritis: Structural disease
  - Trauma: Fracture, internal derangement, neuropathic arthropathy
  - Tumor: Chronic effusion

### Pediatric Considerations
- Infectious (rare): Hip = knee:
  - Escherichia coli: Infants
  - Hemophiles influenzae: 6–24 mo
- Noninflammatory:
  - Congenital hip dysplasia
  - Legg-Calve-Perthes:
    ○ Spontaneous osteonecrosis femoral head
    ○ Age 4–9 yr
    ○ Bilateral 10% cases
  - Slipped capital femoral epiphysis in overweight adolescents

 **DIAGNOSIS**

## SIGNS AND SYMPTOMS
- Symptoms located to 1 joint:
  - Pain
  - Swelling
  - Warmth
  - Erythema
  - Decreased range of motion
  - Hyperacute presentation most typical
- Infectious (septic) arthritis:
  - Fever, chills, systemically ill
  - Large joints affected more often
  - Adults: Knee > hip > shoulder > ankle > wrist
  - Gonorrhea: Abdominal pain, genital discharge
  - Lyme disease:
    ○ Knees or shoulders most common
    ○ Nonspecific constitutional symptoms
    ○ Centrally clearing expanding skin eruption (erythema chronicum migrans)
- Crystalline:
  - Recurrent, self-limited inflammatory attacks, often of same joint
  - Tissue extension appears identical to cellulitis, septic arthritis
  - Gout: First metatarsophalangeal joint foot ("podagra") > ankle > tarsal joints > knee
  - Pseudogout: Knee > wrist > ankle = elbow
  - Tophi: Crystalline granulomas overlying affected joints
- Inflammatory:
  - Inflammatory bowel disease: Abdominal pain, bloody diarrhea with mucous, weight loss
  - Reiter syndrome: Conjunctivitis, urethritis, balanitis
  - Psoriatic arthritis: Characteristic skin plaques, "sausage digits"
  - Chronic: Infections (tuberculosis, fungi), tumors

- Noninflammatory:
  - Osteoarthritis:
    ○ Morning stiffness
    ○ Following activity (gelling)
    ○ Pain relieved by rest
  - Congenital hip dysplasia: Hip pain in young
  - Neuropathic: Charcot joint; swelling, effusion, little pain
  - Trauma: Pain, swelling

### History
See "Description," "Etiology," "Pediatric Considerations," and "Signs and Symptoms."

### Physical Exam
See "Description" and "Signs and Symptoms."

## ESSENTIAL WORKUP
- Complete history; any joint disorder is capable of presenting as monoarthritis:
  - Trauma
  - Surgery
  - STD exposure
  - IV drug abuse
  - Intra-articular injections
  - Immunosuppression
- Meticulous physical exam
- Establish truly monoarticular (vs. migratory); exacerbation vs. superimposed process
- Onset rapidity:
  - Seconds to minutes: Trauma, internal derangement
  - Hours to 2 days: Inflammatory; bacterial infection, crystalline
- Adjunctive diagnostic tests are supportive only.

## DIAGNOSTIC TESTS & INTERPRETATION
### Lab
- Arthrocentesis with joint fluid analysis:
  - The definitive procedure
  - Culture is definitive study of the fluid
  - WBC count with differential varies greatly, nonspecifically; interpret cautiously
  - Crystal analysis, Gram stain, glucose, viscosity
  - Serology never confirms a diagnosis:
    ○ WBC with differential
    ○ Blood cultures; panculture if suspected gonorrhea, sepsis
    ○ Acute phase reactant (ESR, CRP)
    ○ Uric acid can be normal under all conditions; not helpful
    ○ Consider glucose, chemistries, rheumatologic studies
- Microscopy with light helpful with gout; polarized light preferred

### Imaging
- Studies such as bone or gallium scans often not helpful initially in distinguishing between
- Infectious condition vs. inflammatory flare-up, particularly in the face of underlying chronic inflammation.
- Radiologically guided aspiration may be required for technically difficult joints, such as the hip or sacroiliac joints.

- Plain films a reasonable cost effective choice:
  - Infectious: Soft tissue swelling, osteoporosis, chondral erosion, joint margin destruction
  - Crystalline: Asymmetric bone erosions, reactive bone formation, soft-tissue calcification
- MRI detects bone necrosis or involvement:
  - Study of choice for occult fractures, obscured symptomatic conditions
- US: Presence of joint fluid, tissue perfusion, periarticular structures, aspiration guidance
- Nuclear medicine sensitive tool for deep joints difficult to examine, fibrocartilaginous joints, spine
- Bone and cartilage disorders: Asymmetric joint narrowing, osteophytes, subchondral cysts, loose bodies, fracture
- Synovium, bone biopsy:
  - Chronic, unexplained, monoarticular arthritis
  - Gonococcal, mycobacterial disease is suspected and no fluid available.

### Diagnostic Procedures/Surgery
- Urgent arthrocentesis for synovial fluid analysis
- Selective Imaging modalities tailored to joint involved, pretest probability
- Serological studies (see below)

## DIFFERENTIAL DIAGNOSIS
- See "Etiology" and "Pediatric Considerations."
- Rheumatoid arthritis most common inflammatory arthritis

 TREATMENT

### PRE-HOSPITAL
- Physical immobilization of the joint, medication for pain control
- Position of comfort
- IV placement, more rapid, titratable medication administration

### INITIAL STABILIZATION/THERAPY
- Urgent aspiration of the affected joints is required, concomitant antibiotic therapy.
- As dictated by severity of joint involvement, involved constitutional illnesses, traumatic etiologic component
- Management is growing in complexity with the advent of novel and antibiotic-resistant causative microorganisms and within the current climate of increased immunosuppression.
- Pain control

### ED TREATMENT/PROCEDURES
- See "Diagnostic Procedures."
- Septic arthritis:
  - Empiric, aggressive IV bactericidal antibiotics for anticipated organism may prevent joint destruction.
  - Antibiotic selection directed by history and physical
- Adults: Ceftriaxone, vancomycin to cover for staph, strep, and gonococcal arthritis:
  - Treatment: 2 wk IV followed by 2–6 wk of oral antibiotics
  - Shorter course acceptable only in gonococcal arthritis

- Knowledge of local microbiologic organisms is essential for effective empiric antibiosis.
- Methicillin resistance:
  - Gonorrhea
  - IV drug use
  - Prosthetic joints
  - Neonates, children <2 yr
- Surgery: Open vs. closed drainage, frequency of evaluation, treatment duration
- Crystalline:
  - NSAIDs (indomethacin)
  - Colchicine secondary choice to NSAIDs; do not use IV
  - Prednisone when NSAIDs, colchicine contraindicated
  - Adrenocorticotropic hormone (ACTH) for resistant cases, contraindications to NSAIDS
  - Allopurinol decreases uric acid production; avoid in acute therapy
  - Probenecid long-term; uricosuric
- Osteoarthritis:
  - NSAIDs, analgesics
  - Physical support, rehabilitation

## MEDICATION
- ACTH: 40–80 IU IM then 40 IU IM q6h–q12h until improvement
- Allopurinol: 200–600 mg q.d.
- Ceftriaxone: 1 g IV q.d.
- Colchicine: 1 tp 2 mg IV in 20 cc NS over 10 min; 0.5 mg PO q1h until asymptomatic, nausea diarrhea develop, or 10 doses
- Indomethacin: 75–200 mg per day, divided dosages
- Prednisone: 20–40 mg PO per day × 3–4 days
- Probenecid: 250 mg b.i.d. starting; maximum
- Vancomycin: 1 g IV q12h
- Antibiotics and dosage dependent on patient, infectious etiology, severity, duration

### First Line
- Pain control
- Antibiotics, medications required for systemic illness

 FOLLOW-UP

### DISPOSITION
#### Admission Criteria
- All septic arthritis:
  - General medical/surgical bed
  - Intensive care unit if generalized sepsis
- Crystalline:
  - Intractable pain
  - Intractable nausea, vomiting, diarrhea
  - Septic joint superimposed on other arthritides
- Any joint requiring surgical intervention (including serial washouts)
- Evidence systemic illness (sepsis)
- Unable to perform activities daily living

#### Discharge Criteria
- Crystalline tolerating oral NSAIDs
- Inflammatory unless admission required by overall disease, constitutional manifestations
- Osteoarthritis if pain controlled, fluid accumulation permits ambulation, activities of daily living

- Medication compliance: Capability to obtain meds (economically, logistically), compliant with indicated dosages, time intervals
- Timely follow-up arranged

### Issues for Referral
Immediate consultation and admission for suspected or proven infectious etiologies, intractable pain, poorly controlled comorbid illnesses, interference activities daily living

## FOLLOW-UP RECOMMENDATIONS
- As soon as practicable, with health care provider(s) specialty best suited for the etiologic agent, severity of involvement
- If unable to acquire the appropriate specialist in a timely manner, return to ED (safety net).

## PEARLS AND PITFALLS
- Consider septic arthritis in any patient with inflammatory arthritis who presents with a joint flare, particularly if 1 joint has flared more often than others.
- Fluid should be aspirated if the flare is more severe than usual, if there is a substantial loss of joint function, if the joint is red, or if the patient has systemic symptoms.
- Aspiration is the most important part of both diagnosis and management.
- Initiate empiric antibiotic therapy after aspiration, and narrow antimicrobial coverage once microbiology results are known.
- If septic arthritis is untreated, cartilage and bone destruction occurs in as little as 10 days. The end result is joint destruction and systemic sepsis.

## ADDITIONAL READING
- Kherani RB, Shojania K. Review: Septic arthritis in patients with prior inflammatory arthritis. CMAJ. 2007;176(11):1605.
- Li SF, Henderson J, Dickman E, et al. Laboratory tests in adults with monoarticular arthritis: Can they rule out a septic joint? Acad Emerg Med. 2004;11(3):276–280.
- Lin, Hm, Learch TJ, White EA, et al. Emergency joint aspiration: A guide for radiologists on call. Radiographics. 2009;29:1139–1158.
- Margaretten ME, Kohlwes J, Bent S. Does this adult patient have septic arthritis? JAMA. 2007;297: 1478–1488.
- Mathews CJ, Weston VC, Jones A, et al. Bacterial septic arthritis in adults. Lancet. 2010;375(9717): 846–855.

 CODES

### ICD9
716.60 Unspecified monoarthritis, site unspecified

# ARTHRITIS, RHEUMATOID

*Stephen R. Hayden*

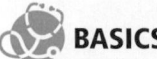 **BASICS**

## DESCRIPTION
- Chronic systemic inflammatory disorder that attacks the joints:
  - Nonsuppurative, proliferative synovitis
  - Destruction of the articular cartilage
  - Ankylosis of the joint
- Involvement of knee is common.
- Baker cysts may be seen in chronic disease.
- Involvement of spine is limited to cervical region:
  - May cause atlantoaxial subluxation
  - Rarely results in cord compression

### Pediatric Considerations
*Juvenile rheumatoid arthritis* (JRA) is a distinct entity (see "Arthritis, Juvenile Idiopathic").
- Genetics:
  - Genetic predisposition related to HLA-DR4
  - Female-to-male ratio is 3:1.
  - Typical age of onset is between 30 and 50.

## ETIOLOGY
- Etiology is unknown.
- Possible triggers include infection and autoimmune response.
- Prevalence is about 1% of both U.S. and world population.

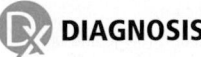 **DIAGNOSIS**

## SIGNS AND SYMPTOMS
- Malaise, fatigue
- Generalized musculoskeletal pain
- After weeks to months, patients develop swollen, warm, painful joints.
- Often worse in morning
- Joint involvement usually symmetric and polyarticular
- Starting in small joints of hands and feet:
  - Later wrists, elbow, and knees
- Distal interphalangeal (DIP) joints of hand generally not involved:
  - Presence of swelling in these joints should suggest another type of arthritis.
- Synovitis is typically gradual.
- Classic joint findings in long-standing disease:
  - Metacarpophalangeal (MCP) swelling with ulnar deviation
  - Swan neck and boutonniere deformities

- Extra-articular complications:
  - SC nodules
  - Vasculitis
  - Pericarditis or myocarditis
  - Pulmonary fibrosis
  - Pneumonitis
  - Sjögren syndrome
  - Mononeuritis multiplex
- Evidence of mild pericarditis on echocardiogram is found in up to 1/3 of patients.
- Patients usually present to ED owing to exacerbations of the disease or complication in other organ systems:
  - Airway obstruction from cricoarytenoid arthritis or laryngeal nodules
  - Heart block, constrictive pericarditis, pericardial effusion with possible tamponade or myocarditis
  - Pulmonary fibrosis, pleuritis, intrapulmonary nodules, or pneumonitis
  - Hepatitis
- Neurologic findings may result from cervical spine subluxation or ocular manifestations such as scleritis and episcleritis.
- Complications of chronic steroid use:
  - Infections
  - Steroid-induced osteopenia and fractures
- Patients may present with side effects related to chronic salicylate or NSAID use such as GI bleeding.
- Drugs such as methotrexate, gold, or d-penicillamine also have toxic side effects, most commonly GI.

## ESSENTIAL WORKUP
- Primary diagnosis of rheumatoid arthritis (RA) is rarely made in the ED.
- Synovitis should be present for at least 6 wk; a minimum of *four of the following seven criteria* as established by the American Rheumatism Association must be met to make the diagnosis:
  - Stiffness of the involved joints in the morning for at least 1 hr
  - Arthritis in 3 or more joints with effusion or soft tissue swelling
  - Arthritis of joint in hand (wrist, MCP, or proximal interphalangeal [PIP] joint)
  - Symmetric arthritis
  - Rheumatoid nodules on extensor surfaces or juxta-articular surfaces
  - Significantly elevated rheumatoid factor
  - Characteristic radiographic changes include erosions and decalcification (not attributable to osteoarthritis).

- Other pertinent history: Malaise, weakness, weight loss, myalgias, bursitis, tendonitis, fever of unknown cause
- Initial workup should focus on demonstrating that other causes of arthritis are not present, especially septic arthritis, reactive arthritis, or gout.
- Arthrocentesis of a joint effusion may be required.

## DIAGNOSTIC TESTS & INTERPRETATION
ECG, chest radiograph, C-spine or extremity radiograph, and hemoglobin testing are helpful if patient presents with complications of RA.

### Lab
- CBC: Mild anemia with leukocytosis and thrombocytosis
- Erythrocyte sedimentation rate (ESR): Often >30
- C-reactive protein correlates with erosive disease
- Antinuclear antibodies (ANA) 30–40% positive screening tool
- Rheumatoid factor: Elevated in ~70% of cases
- Joint fluid analysis:
  - Typically between 4,000 and 50,000 white cells
  - Neutrophil predominance
  - Microscopic Gram stain of fluid should show *no* organisms and *no* crystals.
- ECG: Conduction defects are rare, but heart block may be seen.

### Imaging
- Joint radiograph:
  - Joint effusion
  - Juxta-articular erosions and decalcification
  - Narrowing of joint space
  - Loss of cartilage
- MRI of joints can detect early inflammation before plain radiograph
- CXR reveal pulmonary fibrosis, pleural changes, nodular lung disease, or pneumonitis:
  - Cardiac silhouette may show changes related to myocarditis.
- Cervical spine radiograph:
  - Atlantoaxial joint subluxation may occur.

## DIFFERENTIAL DIAGNOSIS
- Osteoarthritis
- Septic arthritis
- Reactive arthritis
- Gonococcal arthritis
- Lyme disease
- Gout
- Connective tissue disorders
- Systemic lupus erythematosus (SLE), dermatomyositis, polymyositis, vasculitis, Reiter syndrome, and sarcoid
- Rheumatic fever
- Malignancy

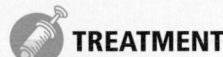

# TREATMENT

## PRE-HOSPITAL
Cervical spine immobilization and airway support as indicated

## INITIAL STABILIZATION/THERAPY
- ABCs:
  - Manage airway with attention to C-spine immobilization during intubation.
- Treat complications of RA as appropriate.

## ED TREATMENT/PROCEDURES
- Salicylates or NSAIDs are first-line treatment for RA:
  - If 1 NSAID fails, another NSAID from a different chemical class may work better.
- Early treatment of RA is important as joint changes may be most progressive during the 1st 18 mo.

## MEDICATION
- Glucocorticoids, methotrexate, and other second-line therapies should be initiated by a rheumatologist.
- Aspirin (ECASA): Adult: 900 mg PO q.i.d. (2.6–5.4 g/d); peds: 60–90 mg/kg/d q.i.d. up to 3.6 g
- Auranofin: 3–9 mg/d (peds: 0.15 mg/kg/d up to 9 mg) divided b.i.d.
- Celecoxib (Celebrex): 100–200 mg PO b.i.d.; peds: N/A
- Hydroxychloroquine: Adult: 200–600 mg/d divided b.i.d.; peds: 6 mg/kg/d up to 600 mg/d
- Ibuprofen (Ibuprin, Advil, Motrin): 200–800 mg (peds: 10 mg/kg) PO q6h
- Leflunomide (Arava): 100 mg PO daily for 3 days, then maintenance dose of 10–20 mg PO daily; peds: N/A
- Methotrexate (Rheumatrex): 0.2–0.4 mg/kg PO per week single dose

- Prednisone: Maintenance: 5–10 mg PO daily; acute exacerbations: 20–50 mg PO daily; peds: Maintenance: 0.1 mg/kg/d PO, acute exacerbations: 2–5 mg/kg/d PO
- Rofecoxib (Vioxx; *voluntary manufacturer withdraw*): 25 mg PO daily; peds: N/A
- Sulfasalazine: Adult: 500–1,000 mg PO b.i.d.; peds: 30–60 mg/kg/d q.i.d. up to 2 g
- Valdecoxib (Bextra): 10 mg PO daily; peds: N/A

## ALERT
Note: Recent studies have shown possibly increased risk of cardiovascular event with NSAID medications, particularly with COX-2 inhibitors.

# FOLLOW-UP

## DISPOSITION
### Admission Criteria
- Patients with severe or life-threatening presentations of RA and its complications should be admitted to hospital.
- Admission is warranted when diagnosis is unclear and serious illnesses such as septic joint or systemic vasculitis may be present or cannot be ruled out.
- Admission may be required for pain control.
- Admission may be required if patient has inadequate social supports and is unable to maintain activities of daily living.
- Pediatric patients with fever and arthritis should be strongly considered for admission.

### Discharge Criteria
Patients without serious complications may be managed as outpatients with appropriate medications and follow up.

### Issues for Referral
All patients should have primary physician for further therapy and care as well as appropriate specialty care referral such as rheumatologists, cardiologists, and orthopedics.

# PEARLS AND PITFALLS
- Recognize that symmetric arthritis is more consistent with RA.
- Even patients with RA can get septic arthritis.
- Consult rheumatologist rather than initiate steroids or TNF antagonists from ED.

# ADDITIONAL READING

- Smedslund G, Byfuglien MG, Olsen SU, et al. Effectiveness and safety of dietary interventions for rheumatoid arthritis: A systematic review of randomized controlled trials. *J Am Diet Assoc.* 2010;110(5):727–735.
- Imboden JB. The immunopathogenesis of rheumatoid arthritis. *Ann Rev Pathol.* 2009;4: 417–434.
- Bingham CO. Development and clinical application of COX-2 selective inhibitors for the treatment of osteoarthritis and rheumatoid arthritis. *Cleve Clin J Med.* 2002;69(suppl 1):SI5–12.
- The American College of Rheumatology Subcommittee on Rheumatoid Arthritis Guidelines. Guidelines for the management of rheumatoid arthritis 2002 update. *Arthritis Rheum.* 2002;46:328–346.
- Jain R, Lipsky P. Treatment of rheumatoid arthritis. *Adv Rheum.* 1997;81(1).57–84.
- King R. Arthritis, rheumatoid. Available at www.emedicine.com
- Sanders S, Harisdangkul V. Leflunomide for the treatment of rheumatoid arthritis and autoimmunity. *Am J Med Sci.* 2002;323(4):190–193.
- Smith JB, Haynes MK. Rheumatoid arthritis: A molecular understanding. *Ann Intern Med.* 2002;136(12):908–922.

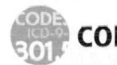

# CODES

**ICD9**
714.0 Rheumatoid arthritis

# ARTHRITIS, SEPTIC

*Ziad N. Kazzi*
*A. Antoine Kazzi*

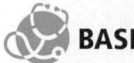 BASICS

## DESCRIPTION

- Bacteria can be introduced into a joint by:
  - Hematogenous spread (most common)
  - Invasive procedures
  - Contiguous infection (eg, osteomyelitis, cellulitis)
  - Direct inoculation such as plant thorns or nails
- Acute inflammatory process results in migration of WBCs into joint.
- Synovial hyperplasia, cartilage damage, and formation of a purulent effusion
- Irreversible loss of function in up to 50%

### Pediatric Considerations

- Hip infections are most common:
  - Often in patients with otitis media or upper respiratory tract infections
  - Complications of septic arthritis (SA) of hip in children: Avascular necrosis, epiphyseal separation, pathologic dislocation, and arthritis
- 50% occur in children <3 yr old.
- Infants present with irritability, fever, and loss of appetite.
- Older children present with a limp or refusal to bear weight or use joint.

## ETIOLOGY

- Risk factors:
  - Old age, infancy
  - Rheumatoid arthritis and degenerative joint disease
  - Intravenous drug user (IVDU), endocarditis
  - Females (gonococcal [GC] infection)
  - Immunosuppression (AIDS, diabetes, chemotherapy, steroid therapy)
  - Repeated joint injections, pre-existing joint diseases, trauma, or prosthesis
- No bacterial pathogen is identified in 10–20%.
- Most common organisms:
  - *Staphylococcus aureus* in adults, hip infections (80%), and patients with rheumatoid arthritis or diabetes
  - *Multi-drug-resistant S. aureus (MRSA)* has been noted in some studies to be the most common organism in community-onset adult septic arthritis.
  - *Neisseria gonorrhoeae* most common in young, healthy, sexually active patients (Incidence has decreased over the past decades due to a decrease in the incidence of mucosal GC infections)
- Other pathogens: Group A beta-hemolytic and group B, C, and G streptococci:
  - Gram-negative rods (eg, *Pseudomonas aeruginosa, Escherichia. coli*) in 10% of cases
- Common in old age, infancy, immunosuppression, and IVDU (*Pseudomonas*)
- Anaerobes: Diabetes, prosthetic joints
- Mycobacterial and fungal causes: Atypical (eg, in HIV); more indolent course

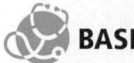 DIAGNOSIS

## SIGNS AND SYMPTOMS

- Presents abruptly as a single painful, swollen, warm, tender joint
- Common findings include:
  - Fever
  - A separate source of infection (eg, skin)
  - Extremely painful joint motion in all planes
  - A joint effusion (less evident in sacroiliac, hip, and shoulder)
- Any joint can be involved:
  - Typically a single joint is involved.
  - Most commonly knee, then hip, shoulder, and ankle
- Commonly seen in intravenous drug users (IVDUs): Sacroiliac costochondral and sternoclavicular joints:
  - Vertebral involvement such as lumbar facets possible
- Human and animal bites, local steroid therapy, and trauma may lead to infection in atypical locations.
- Polyarticular involvement in 10–20%:
  - Mostly with rheumatoid arthritis; delay in diagnosis from low suspicion and more subtle presentations (fever in only 50%)
  - Patients with sepsis
- GC SA features:
  - Develops in 1–3% of untreated gonorrhea and in 42–85% of disseminated GC infection:
- Typically monoarticular but commonly polyarticular
- Migratory polyarthralgia, tenosynovitis (present in 20% of patients with arthritis), and dermatitis:
  - Involves small joints (eg, fingers, wrist, elbow, ankle)
- Signs of urethral or vaginal GC infection may be present.
- Painless maculopapular lesions on trunk, arms, legs, and around affected joint

## ESSENTIAL WORKUP
### Arthrocentesis

- Perform joint aspiration in any suspected case.
- Send fluid for protein and glucose, cell count, Gram's stain, and culture.
- Typical SA findings:
  - A turbid, purulent, or serosanguineous fluid
  - A leukocytosis (50,000–150,000/mm$^3$) with a polymorphonuclear predominance (>75%)
  - Often a decreased glucose and elevated protein level

- The appearance of crystals does not rule out SA.
- Use special stain or culture media when indicated (eg, GC, anaerobes, fungus, mycobacterium)
- Intra-articular lidocaine reduces the sensitivity of subsequent cultures; immediate emptying of aspirated sample into a blood culture flask increases the yield.
- In non-GC SA, Gram's stain and culture are positive in 50% and 90% of cases, respectively:
  - Drops to nearly 10% and 50% in GC SA, respectively
- Fluoroscopic, sonographic, or CT guidance can be used in technically difficult aspirations.
- CT scan and MRI may aid in the diagnosis for joints such as the sacroiliac joint.
- Arthrocentesis is contraindicated whenever there is an underlying joint prosthesis or an overlying skin infection:
  - If cellulitis present, use an alternate approach through normal skin.

## DIAGNOSTIC TESTS & INTERPRETATION
### Lab

- Nonspecific serum leukocytosis (more common in children), left shift, and C-reactive protein (CRP) and ESR elevation are usually present.
- UA and culture can reveal a urologic source for the pathogen.
- Blood cultures may be useful: Positive in 50–70% of non-GC SA.
- Culture any potential focus of infection (pharynx, urine, cervix, or anus), particularly when suspecting GC.

### Imaging

- Plain radiographs to identify:
  - Effusion
  - Baseline status of the joint
  - Contiguous osteomyelitis
  - Concurrent rheumatologic diseases
  - Fractures or foreign body
  - Joint loosening (a late and nonspecific sign)
- US, CT, and MRI are more sensitive:
  - US may be used to guide aspiration of some joints (eg, hip) and to detect joint effusions.
- Scintigraphic techniques are sensitive and specific in diagnosis of SA:
  - Often not available through ED
- Other tests:
  - Bacterial DNA amplification techniques in early detection of organisms

## DIFFERENTIAL DIAGNOSIS
- Viral arthritis
- Rheumatoid arthritis
- Gout or pseudogout
- HIV-associated arthritis
- Reactive arthritis
- Lyme disease
- Osteomyelitis
- Endocarditis
- Trauma
- In children:
  - Juvenile rheumatoid arthritis
  - Slipped capital femoral epiphysis
  - Legg–Calvé–Perthes disease
  - Metaphyseal osteomyelitis
  - Transient synovitis

### Pediatric Considerations
- Because of vaccine, *Haemophilus influenzae* is no longer the most common agent.
- *S. aureus* is most common.
- Group B streptococcus, enterobacteria, and gram-negative rods in the newborn

 ## TREATMENT

### PRE-HOSPITAL
No specific considerations

### INITIAL STABILIZATION/THERAPY
- Patient may be septic and require resuscitation.
- If patient is toxic, do not delay antibiotics for aspiration results.

### ED TREATMENT/PROCEDURES
- Promptly aspirate joint fluid
- Obtain cultures.
- Start empiric antibiotics based on Gram's stain (if available) and age group or risk factors: Consider staphylococcal, streptococcal, and gram-negative coverage; consider MRSA in the appropriate setting—recommended duration of treatment is 2–4 wk:
  - Combine a beta-lactamase resistant penicillin (eg, nafcillin) with an aminoglycoside (eg, gentamicin) or a third-generation cephalosporin (eg, ceftriaxone).
  - Use vancomycin instead of penicillin when methicillin-resistant *S. aureus* or penicillin-resistant pneumococci are suspected.

- When suspecting GC, use a third-generation cephalosporin or a quinolone (eg, ceftriaxone, ciprofloxacin).
  - Treat patients with sickle cell disease using third-generation cephalosporin (ceftriaxone) and an antistaphylococcal drug (nafcillin, cloxacillin, clindamycin).
  - Intra-articular antibiotics are contraindicated.
- Early orthopedic consultation to evaluate eligibility for surgical drainage
- Pain control: Narcotics and moderately flexed splinting
- Immunologic therapies are experimental.
- Prosthesis: Some may try to preserve the limb unless it is loose on plain films.
- Patients should be at rest with joint maintained in optimal position to prevent damage.

### MEDICATION
- Cefazolin: 1–2 g IV q6h
- Cefotaxime: 1 g IV q8h; peds: 50 mg/kg q12h
- Ceftriaxone: 1 g IV qd; peds: 50 mg/kg
- Ciprofloxacin: 400 mg IV q12h
- Gentamicin: 2–5 mg/kg IV load
- Nafcillin: 2 g IV q4h; peds: 25 mg/kg q6h
- Piperacillin: 4 g IV q6h
- Tobramycin: 1 mg/kg IV q8h; peds: 2.5 mg/kg q8h
- Vancomycin: 1 g IV q12h; peds: 10 mg/kg q6h

### Pediatric Considerations
- Open surgical drainage is the method of choice in pediatric hip SA.
- Cover *H. influenzae* type B if prior immunization cannot be established.

 ## FOLLOW-UP

### DISPOSITION
#### Admission Criteria
- All patients with suspected SA should be admitted until SA is ruled out.
- May undergo drainage of joint, as indicated, by serial aspirations, arthroscopy, or arthrotomy

#### Discharge Criteria
Cases where suspected SA has been adequately ruled out

## PEARLS AND PITFALLS
It can be difficult to distinguish SA from toxic synovitis or crystal arthropathy; have a low threshold for arthrocentesis.

## ADDITIONAL READING
- Baker D, Schumacher HR. Acute monoarthritis. *N Engl J Med*. 1993;329:1013–1019.
- Frazee BW, Fee C, Lambert L. How common is MRSA in adult septic arthritis? *Ann Emerg Med*. 2009;54:695–700.
- Bardin T. Gonococcal arthritis. *Best Pract Res Clin Rheumatol*. 2003;17(2):201–208.
- Donatto KC. Orthopedic management of septic arthritis. *Rheum Dis Clin North Am*. 1998;24(2):275–286.
- Goldenberg D. Septic arthritis. *Lancet*. 1998;35:197–202.
- Greenspan A, Tehranzadeh J. Imaging of infectious arthritis. *Radiol Clin North Am*. 2001;39(2):267–276.
- Malleson P. Management of childhood arthritis. Part 1: Acute arthritis. *Arch Dis Child*. 1997;76:460–462.
- Shetty AK, Gedalia A. Management of septic arthritis. *Indian J Pediatr*. 2004;71:819–824.
- Shirtliff ME, Mader JT. Acute septic arthritis. *Clin Microbiol Rev*. 2002;15(4):527–544.

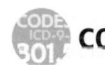 ## CODES

### ICD9
711.00 Pyogenic arthritis, site unspecified

# ASCITES
*Paul J. Allegretti*

 **BASICS**

## DESCRIPTION
- Pathologic accumulation of serous fluid in the peritoneal cavity
- Portal hypertension (>12 mm Hg) starts fluid retention.
- Avid sodium retention state
- Retained sodium and water increases plasma volume.
- Water excretion becomes impaired.
- Increased release of antidiuretic hormone (ADH)
- Urinary sodium retention, increased total body sodium, and dilutional hyponatremia
- Degree of hyponatremia correlates with disease severity; prognostic factor.
- Decreased plasma oncotic pressure from hypoalbuminemia
- Peritoneal irritation owing to infection, inflammation, or malignancy

## ETIOLOGY
- Parenchymal liver disease:
  - Cirrhosis and alcoholic hepatitis:
    ○ 80% of adult patients
  - Fulminant hepatic failure
- Hepatic congestion:
  - CHF
  - Constrictive pericarditis
  - Veno-occlusive disease and Budd-Chiari syndrome
- Malignancies:
  - Peritoneal carcinomatosis
  - Hepatocellular carcinoma or metastatic disease
- Infections:
  - TB, fungal, or bacterial peritonitis
- Hypoalbuminemic states:
  - Nephrotic syndrome
  - Malnutrition; albumin <2.0 g/dL
- Other conditions:
  - Pancreatic ascites
  - Biliary ascites
  - Nephrogenous ascites
  - Ovarian tumors
  - Chylous ascites from lymphatic leak
  - Connective tissue disease
  - Myxedema
  - Granulomatous peritonitis

### Pediatric Considerations
Most pediatric cases owing to:
- Malignancy (Burkitt lymphoma, rhabdomyosarcoma)
- Nephrotic syndrome
- Malnutrition

 **DIAGNOSIS**

## SIGNS AND SYMPTOMS
- Abdominal distention, discomfort
- Weight gain; sometimes weight loss
- Dyspnea
- Orthopnea
- Edema
- Abdominal hernias
- Muscle wasting
- Shifting dullness, flank fullness, fluid wave, puddle sign
- Signs and symptoms of underlying disease
- Stigmata of chronic liver disease

### History
- Risk factors for liver disease
- Description of onset of symptoms:
  - Distinguishes ascites from obesity
  - Patients less tolerant of rapid accumulation of ascitic fluid
- New-onset ascites in known cirrhotic signifies one of the following:
  - Progressive liver disease
  - Superimposed acute liver injury (alcohol, viral hepatitis)
  - Hepatocelluar carcinoma

### Physical Exam
- Detection difficult in obese patients
- Flank dullness is a prominent physical finding:
  - 500 mL for flank dullness
  - Fluid wave
  - Shifting dullness

## ESSENTIAL WORKUP
- Search for liver disease, CHF, TB, malignancy, and other systemic disorders.
- Abdominal paracentesis:
  - Necessary for:
    ○ New ascites
    ○ Worsening encephalopathy
    ○ Fever
    ○ Abdominal pain/tenderness
- Determine if fluid infected or presence of portal hypertension
- Test ascitic fluid for:
  - Cell count and differential:
    ○ Most helpful to determine infection quickly
    ○ Order on every specimen
  - Albumin
  - Protein
  - Gram stain
  - Culture twice in blood culture bottles with 10 mL of fluid
  - Lactate dehydrogenase (LDH)
  - Glucose
  - TB culture
  - Amylase
  - Triglyceride
  - Cytology
  - Bilirubin
  - Carcinoembryonic antigen

- Spontaneous bacterial peritonitis (SBP):
  - Ascitic fluid infection without an intra-abdominal surgically treatable source
  - Fever, abdominal pain/tenderness, altered mentation
  - Polymorphonuclear neutrophils (PMNs) >250 cells/mm$^3$
  - Ascitic fluid protein <1 g/dL
  - Low concentration of opsonins
- Secondary bacterial peritonitis:
  - Bacterial peritonitis from a surgically treatable intra-abdominal source
  - Gut perforation or intra-abdominal abscess (ie, perinephric abscess)
  - PMNs >250 cells/mm$^3$ with multiple micro-organisms on Gram stain plus 2 of the following found with secondary bacterial peritonitis:
    ○ Total protein >1 g/dL
    ○ Glucose <50 mg/dL
    ○ LDH greater than the upper limit of normal for serum

## DIAGNOSTIC TESTS & INTERPRETATION
### Lab
- CBC
- Basic chemistry
- LFTs
- PT, PTT, INR
- Arterial blood gas (ABG) or pulse oximeter
- Urinalysis
- Urine sodium
- Hepatitis panel
- Amylase/lipase
- Alpha fetoprotein
- TSH

### Imaging
- US:
  - Confirm ascites, especially if <500 mL
  - Evaluate liver, pancreas, spleen, and ovaries
  - Guides paracentesis
- Doppler study: Evaluate hepatic blood flow
- CT scan
- CXR: CHF, effusions, cavitary, or mass lesion
- ECG

### Diagnostic Procedures/Surgery
- Peritoneoscopy: Ascites of unknown cause; especially TB
- Paracentesis:
  - Clinical diagnosis of SBP without paracentesis is inadequate.
  - Safety of paracentesis:
    ○ 70% of ascitic patients have coagulopathy.
    ○ Benefits of a diagnostic paracentesis outweigh the risks.
    ○ Paracentesis is still indicated unless disseminated intravascular coagulation (DIC) is present.
    ○ Transfusion of plasma or platelets prior to paracentesis is not supported.

## DIFFERENTIAL DIAGNOSIS

- 1 of 5 "F" causes of abdominal swelling:
  - Fluid (including cysts)
  - Fat
  - Flatus
  - Fetus
  - Feces
  - Other: Organomegaly
- Serum-ascites albumin gradient (SAAG) = serum albumin − ascitic albumin:
  - Replaced ascitic fluid total protein in the differential diagnosis of ascites
    SAAG ≥ 1.1 g/dL.
    - 97% accurate in predicting portal hypertension
    - Cirrhosis
    - Alcoholic hepatitis
    - Cardiac
    - Liver metastases
    - Fulminant hepatic failure
    - Portal vein thrombosis
    - Veno-occlusive disease
    - Myxedema
    - Budd-Chiari
    - Fatty liver of pregnancy
    - Spontaneous bacterial peritonitis
  - SAAG <1.1 g/dL:
    - Peritoneal carcinomatosis
    - TB
    - Pancreatic ascites
    - Nephrotic syndrome
    - Bowel obstruction or infarction
    - Vasculitis
    - Postoperative lymphatic leak

## TREATMENT

### PRE HOSPITAL
Symptomatic hypotension:
- Airway, breathing, circulation (ABCs), IV 0.9 NS

### INITIAL STABILIZATION/THERAPY
Sudden increase in abdominal girth, pain, or fever requires urgent evaluation for possible complicating factor such as:
- Infection
- Hepatoma
- Obstruction of hepatic outflow
- Decompensated liver function

### ED TREATMENT/PROCEDURES
- Successful treatment depends on accurate diagnosis of underlying cause.
- Treat underlying cause.
- Minimize ascitic fluid and peripheral edema without causing intravascular volume depletion.
- Early detection of complications is necessary:
  - Spontaneous bacterial peritonitis:
    - High degree of suspicion
    - Low threshold for paracentesis
    - Prompt therapy
  - Tense ascites and hydrothorax:
    - Supplemental oxygen
    - Therapeutic paracentesis or thoracentesis for respiratory distress
  - Abdominal hernias:
    - Watch for incarceration, ulceration, or rupture.
    - Therapeutic paracentesis
    - Surgical consultation

- Persistent leak at paracentesis site:
  - Remove more fluid.
  - Stomal barrier device
- Meralgia paresthetica:
  - Owing to pressure on the lateral femoral cutaneous nerve
  - Relieve the pressure by paracentesis or diuresis.
- Large-volume paracentesis:
  - 5–10 L (100 mL/kg)
  - Performed safely in the ED with stable hemodynamics
  - Replace with IV albumin (5–10 g/L fluid removed) if >5 L removed.
  - Monitor the patient for 8 hr prior to discharge.
- Nonparacentesis reduction of ascites:
  - Strict sodium restriction:
    - <1 g/d
    - Restrict water if serum sodium <125 mEq/L
  - Spironolactone:
    - Works best for cirrhotic ascites
    - Alternatives: Amiloride or triamterene
  - Furosemide:
    - Works best for other causes of ascites
    - Add to spironolactone in cirrhotics at spironolactone/furosemide ratio of 100 mg/ 40 mg.
    - Add metolazone for less responsive cases.
  - Diuretic principles:
    - Administer diuretics as single morning dose.
    - Obtain spot-urine sodium to evaluate response.
    - Patients with urinary Na >10 mEq/L are more responsive to diuretics.
    - Diuretic-induced weight loss should not exceed 2 lb/d in patients without edema and 5 lb/d in patients with edema.
    - Monitor electrolytes and renal function.
    - Avoid hypokalemia.
    - Hypokalemia enhances renal ammonia production, precipitating hepatic encephalopathy.
  - Refractory ascites:
    - Accounts for 10% of patients
    - Ensure compliance with diet and medications.
    - Implement peritoneovenous shunt.
    - Transjugular intrahepatic portosystemic shunt
    - Liver transplantation
  - Avoid NSAIDs:
    - Diminish response to diuretics
    - Decrease renal plasma flow and GFR.
    - Cause sodium retention/reduces urinary Na excretion
  - Treat underlying cause of ascites owing to conditions other than cirrhosis:
    - TB, CHF

## MEDICATION

### First Line
- Albumin: 5–10 g/L of fluid removed if >5 L removed
- Cefotaxime: 2 g IV q8h
- Spironolactone: 100–400 mg/d (peds: 1–6 mg/kg) PO
- Furosemide: 40–160 mg/d (peds: 1–3 mg/kg) PO

### Second Line
- Amiloride: 10–40 mg/d PO
- Metolazone: 5 mg/d
- Triamterene: 100–300 mg/d PO

## FOLLOW-UP

### DISPOSITION
**Admission Criteria**
- Fulminant liver failure
- Hepatic encephalopathy
- Spontaneous bacterial peritonitis
- Hepatorenal syndrome
- GI bleeding
- Tense ascites not responding to ED treatment

**Discharge Criteria**
Patients responding to ED management

### FOLLOW-UP RECOMMENDATIONS
- GI for all new cases
- Primary doctor or GI for previously established cases

## PEARLS AND PITFALLS

- New cases need full workup and GI consultation for management.
- SBP symptoms are frequently vague.
- Must have a high suspicion and low threshold for paracentesis when considering SBP
- Benefits of confirming SBP outweigh risks of bleeding in a coagulopathic patient undergoing paracentesis.
- US guidance is helpful when performing paracentesis in lower volume ascites.

## ADDITIONAL READING

- Fauci A, Braunwald E, et al. *Harrison's Principles of Internal Medicine*, 17th ed. New York: McGraw-Hill, 2008.
- Feldman M. *Sleisenger and Fordtran's gastrointestinal and Liver Disease*, 8th ed. Philadelphia: WB Saunders, 2006.
- Runyon B. Management of adult patients with ascites caused by cirrhosis. *Hepatology.* 2004; 39:841.
- Runyon B, Such J. *Initial Therapy of Ascites in Patients with Cirrhosis.* UpToDate, 2009.

**See Also (Topic, Algorithm, Electronic Media Element)**
Cirrhosis

# ASTHMA, ADULT
*Melissa H. White*

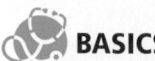 **BASICS**

## DESCRIPTION
- Increased expiratory resistance:
  - Bronchospasm
  - Airway inflammation
  - Mucosal edema
  - Mucous plugging
- Consequences:
  - Air trapping
  - Increased dead space
  - Hyperinflation
- Risk factors for life-threatening disease:
  - Prior intubations
  - Intensive care unit admissions
  - Chronic steroid use
  - Hospital admission for asthma during the past year
  - Inadequate medical management
  - Increasing age
  - Ethnicity (African Americans)
  - Lack of access to medical care

## ETIOLOGY
- Inflammatory process of the airways evidenced by episodic and reversible airflow obstruction and hyperresponsiveness with many cells and cellular elements contributing to the disease:
  - Neutrophils
  - Mast cells
  - Eosinophils
  - Macrophages
  - T lymphocytes
  - Epithelial cells
- Triggers:
  - Pollen
  - Dust mites
  - Molds
  - Animal dander
  - Other environmental allergens
  - Viral upper respiratory infections
  - Occupational chemicals
  - Tobacco smoke
  - Environmental change
  - Cold air
  - Exercise
  - Emotional factors
  - Drugs:
    - Aspirin
    - NSAIDs
    - $\beta$-blockers

# DIAGNOSIS

## SIGNS AND SYMPTOMS
- Wheezing
- Dyspnea
- Chest tightness
- Cough
- Tachypnea
- Tachycardia
- Respiratory distress:
  - Posture sitting upright or leaning forward
  - Use of accessory muscles
  - Inability to speak in full sentences
  - Diaphoresis
  - Poor air movement
- Altered mental status
- Pulsus paradoxus >18 mm Hg

## ESSENTIAL WORKUP
- Primarily a clinical diagnosis
- Measure and follow severity with peak expiratory flow rate (PEFR)
- Assess for underlying disease:
  - Pneumonia

## DIAGNOSTIC TESTS & INTERPRETATION
### Lab
- Arterial blood gas:
  - Not helpful during the initial evaluation
  - The decision to intubate should be based on clinical criteria.
  - Mild-moderate asthma: Respiratory alkalosis
  - Severe airflow obstruction and fatigue: Respiratory acidosis
- Pulse oximetry:
  - <90% is indicative of severe respiratory distress.
  - Patients with impending respiratory compromise may still maintain saturation above 90% until sudden collapse.
- WBC:
  - Leukocytosis is nonspecific
  - Pneumonia
  - Chronic steroid use
  - Stress of an asthma exacerbation
  - Demargination occurs after administration of epinephrine and steroids.

### Diagnostic Procedures/Surgery
- Peak expiratory flow rate:
  - Estimates the degree of airflow obstruction:
    - Normal peak flow in an adult is 400–600.
    - 100–300 indicates moderate airway obstruction.
    - <100 is indicative of severe airway obstruction.
    - Use serially as an objective measure of the response to therapy

- Forced expiratory volume (FEV):
  - More reliable measure of lung function than PEFR
  - More operator dependent
  - Difficult to use as a screening tool
  - Often unavailable in the ED
  - Severe airway obstruction: $FEV_1$ <30–50%
- CXR:
  - Indications:
    - Fever
    - Suspicion of pneumonia
    - Suspicion of pneumothorax or pneumomediastinum
    - Foreign body aspiration
    - 1st episode of asthma
    - Comorbid illness
    - Diabetes
    - Renal failure
    - AIDS
    - Cancer
  - Findings:
    - Hyperinflation
    - Scattered atelectasis
- ECG:
  - Indicated in patients at risk for cardiac disease:
    - Dysrhythmias
    - Myocardial ischemia
  - Transient changes in severe asthma:
    - Right axis deviation
    - Right bundle branch block
    - Abnormal P waves
    - Nonspecific ST-T wave changes

## DIFFERENTIAL DIAGNOSIS
- Allergic reaction
- Angioedema
- Bronchiolitis
- Bronchitis
- Carcinoid tumors
- Chemical pneumonitis
- Chronic cor pulmonale
- Chronic obstructive pulmonary disease
- CHF
- Croup
- Foreign body aspiration
- Immersion injury
- Myocardial ischemia
- Pneumonia
- Pulmonary embolus
- Smoke inhalation
- Upper airway obstruction
- Venous air embolus

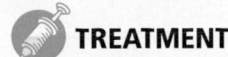

# TREATMENT

## PRE-HOSPITAL
- Recognize the "quiet chest" as respiratory distress.
- Supplemental oxygen
- Continuous nebulized $\beta$-agonist
- Administration of SC epinephrine

## INITIAL STABILIZATION/THERAPY
- Immediate initiation of inhaled $\beta$-agonist treatment
- Intubate for fatigue and respiratory distress.
- Steroids

## ED TREATMENT/PROCEDURES
$\beta$-adrenergic agonist:
- Mild-moderate asthmatic:
  - Administer every 20 min
- Severe asthmatic:
  - Continuous nebulized treatment
- Selective $\beta_2$-agonists (albuterol)
- SC $\beta$-agonist:
  - Severe exacerbations
  - Limited inhalation of aerosolized medicine
  - More side effects because of systemic absorption:
  - Terbutaline-longer acting $\beta$-2 agonist with bronchodilating effects equivalent to epinephrine in acute asthma.
  - Relative contraindications: age >40 yr and coronary disease
- Corticosteroids:
  - Reduce airway wall inflammation
  - Administered early
  - Onset of action may take 4–6 hr
  - Administer IV or PO
  - IV Solu-Medrol in the treatment of severe asthma exacerbation
  - Mild-moderate exacerbations may be treated with oral prednisone.
  - Inhaled corticosteroids are currently not recommended as initial therapy.
- Oxygen:
  - Maintain an oxygen saturation >90%
- Aminophylline:
  - Rare utility in acute management
  - Toxicity
  - Nausea
  - Tremor
  - Anxiety
  - Palpitations
  - Tachycardia
- Anticholinergic agents:
  - If minimal response to initial $\beta$-agonist treatment
  - Severe airflow obstruction
  - Inhaled anticholinergic agents should be used in conjunction with $\beta$-agonists.
- Magnesium sulfate:
  - No benefit in mild-moderate asthma
  - Benefit of magnesium remains unclear in severe asthma
- Heliox:
  - Mixture of helium and oxygen (80:20, 70:30, 60:40)
  - Less dense than air
  - Decrease airway resistance.
  - Decrease in respiratory exhaustion
  - Not currently recommended for routine use
- Consider in severe asthma

- Ketamine:
  - Bronchodilator and an anesthetic agent
  - Useful as an induction agent during intubation
  - Contraindications:
  - HTN
  - Coronary disease
  - Preeclampsia
  - Increased intracranial pressure
- Halothane:
  - Inhalation anesthetics are potent bronchodilators.
  - Refractory asthma in intubated patients
- Intubation of the asthmatic patient:
  - Rapid sequence intubation:
  - Lidocaine to attenuate airway reflexes
  - Etomidate or ketamine as an induction agent
  - Succinylcholine should be administered to achieve paralysis
  - A large endotracheal tube >7 mm should be used to facilitate ventilation.
  - May need to mechanically exhale for the patient
  - Permissive hypercapnia

## MEDICATION
- $\beta$-agonists
  - Albuterol: 2.5 mg in 2.5 mL NS q20min inhaled (peds: 0.1–0.15 mg/kg/dose q20min [minimum dose 1.25 mg])
  - Epinephrine: Adult: 0.3 mg (1:1,000) SC q0.5h–q1.0h × 3 doses (peds: 0.01 mg/kg up to 0.3 mg SC)
  - Terbutaline: 0.25 mg SC q0.5h × 2 doses (peds: 0.01 mg/kg up to 0.3 mg SC)
- Corticosteroids:
  - Methylprednisolone: 60–125 mg IV (peds: 1–2 mg/kg/dose IV or PO q6h × 24 hr)
  - Prednisone: 40–60 mg PO (peds: 1–2 mg/kg/d in single or divided doses)
- Anticholinergics
  - Ipratropium bromide: 0.5 mg in 3 mL NS q1h × 3 doses
- Magnesium: 2 g IV over 20 min
- Aminophylline: 0.6 mg/kg/h IV infusion
- Rapid sequence intubation:
  - Etomidate: 0.3 mg/kg, or ketamine: 1–1.5 mg/kg
  - Lidocaine: 1–1.5 mg/kg
  - Succinylcholine: 1.5 mg/kg

# FOLLOW-UP

## DISPOSITION
### Admission Criteria
**Medical Wards**
- PEFR <40% and minimal air movement
- Persistent respiratory distress:
  - Factors that should favor admission:
    ◦ Prior intubation
    ◦ Recent ED visit
    ◦ Multiple ED visits or hospitalizations
    ◦ Symptoms for more than 1 wk
    ◦ Failure of outpatient therapy
    ◦ Use of steroids
    ◦ Inadequate follow-up mechanisms
    ◦ Psychiatric illness

**Observation Unit**
- PEFR >40% but <70% of predicted
- Patients without subjective improvement
- Patients with continued wheeze and diminished air movement
- Patients with moderate response to therapy and no respiratory distress

### Discharge Criteria
- PEFR >70%
- Patient reports subjective improvement
- Clear lungs with good air movement
- Peak flow should be >300.
- Adequate follow-up within 48–72 hr

## FOLLOW-UP RECOMMENDATIONS
Encourage patients to contact their PMD or pulmonologist for asthma related problems over the next 3–5 days.

## PEARLS AND PITFALLS
- Altered mental status in asthma equals ventilatory failure.
- Patients should be able to demonstrate the correct use of their inhaler or nebulizer:
  - Discharge with a peak flow meter
- If no signs or symptoms of dehydration, no evidence that IVF will aid in clearing airway secretions.
- Antibiotics should generally be reserved for patients with purulent sputum, fever, pneumonia, or evidence of bacterial sinusitis.

## ADDITIONAL READING
- Fanta CH. Asthma. N Engl J Med. 2009;360:10.
- Holgate ST, Polosa R. The mechanisms, diagnosis, and management of severe asthma in adults. Lancet. 2006;368:780.
- Marx. Rosen's Emergency Medicine, 7th ed. Asthma. 2009
- National Asthma Education and Prevention Program Expert Panel Report 3. Guidelines for diagnosis and management of asthma. U.S. Dept of Health and Human Services, October 2007.
- National Center for Health Statistics. Asthma. Accessed at http://www.cdc.gov/nchc/fastats/asthma.htm. May 2009.
- Waltraud E, et al. The asthma epidemic. N Engl J Med. 2006;355:2226.
- The author gratefully acknowledges the contribution of Eric S. Nadel for the previous edition of this chapter.

# ASTHMA, PEDIATRIC

*Nathan Shapiro*
*Tarina Lee Kang*

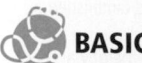 **BASICS**

## DESCRIPTION
- 2.7 million children (<18 yr) affected in the U.S.
- 850,000 ED visits per year in the U.S.
- Inflammatory events, usually viral, lead to bronchoconstriction:
  - Compounded by hyperreactivity of airways
  - Mediators of the inflammatory cascade exacerbate symptoms
- Airway obstruction produces increased airway resistance and gas trapping:
  - Mucosal edema
  - Bronchospasm
  - Mucous plugging
- Infants more vulnerable to respiratory failure:
  - Increased peripheral resistance
  - Decreased elastic recoil with early airway closure
  - Unstable rib cage
  - Mechanically disadvantaged diaphragm
- Family history of allergy
- Medical history of early injury to airway (bronchopulmonary dysplasia, pneumonia, intubation, croup, reflux, passive exposure to smoking), reactions to foods and drugs, other allergic manifestations
- Environmental exposures such as pets, smoke, carpets, or dust may trigger or exacerbate

## ETIOLOGY
### Precipitating/Aggravating Factors
- Infection:
  - Viral
  - Bacterial
- Allergic/irritant:
  - Environment: Pollens, grasses, mold, house dust mites, and animal dander
  - Occupational chemicals: Chlorine, ammonia—food and additives
  - Irritants: Smoke, pollutants, gases, and aerosols
  - Exercise
  - Cold weather
  - Emotional: Stress, phobia
  - Intoxication: $\beta$-blockers, aspirin, NSAIDs

# DIAGNOSIS

## SIGNS AND SYMPTOMS
### General
- Fatigue, somnolence
- Diaphoresis, agitation
- Hypoxia, cyanosis
- Tachycardia
- Dehydration
- Pulsus paradoxus

### Respiratory
- Wheezing, rales, rhonchi
- Cough, acute or chronic
- Tachypnea
- "Tight chest"
- Dyspnea, shortness of breath with prolonged expiratory phase
- Retractions, accessory muscle use, nasal flaring
- Hyperinflation
- Often a history of recurrent episodes and chronic restrictions
- Complications:
  - Recurrent pneumonia, bronchitis
  - Atelectasis
  - Pneumothorax, pneumomediastinum
  - Respiratory distress/failure/death

### History
- Precipitating events or known triggers
- Chronicity of symptoms
- Comorbid illnesses
- History of disease:
  - Previous hospitalizations for asthma
  - Previous intubations and intensive care

### Physical Exam
- Wheezing: Absence of wheezing may be associated with markedly impaired air movement and decreased breath sounds
- Signs of hypoxia
- Skin and nailbed color bluish
- Signs of respiratory fatigue:
  - Use of accessory muscles of respirations or retractions
  - Lethargy or confusion

## ESSENTIAL WORKUP
- Clinical diagnosis based primarily on physical exam and history; assess ventilation by observation for retractions and use of accessory muscles as well as auscultating for air exchange.
- Follow response to bronchodilator therapy with present illness and past episodes.
- Exclude other differential considerations.
- Pulse oximetry:
  - Initial SaO$_2$ <91% (sea level) associated with significant illness: Admission, relapse, prolonged course
- Peak flow meters in cooperative patients (usually >5 yr old)
  - <50–70% predicts moderate to severe obstruction.
  - >70–90% associated with mild to moderate obstruction
  - >90% considered normal

## DIAGNOSTIC TESTS & INTERPRETATION
### Lab
- Arterial blood gas (ABG) may be an adjunct to pulse oximetry to measure oxygenation and clinical exam to assess ventilation; not mandatory or routinely done.
- CBC as a nonspecific marker of infection
- Theophylline level: Only for patients on theophylline (not recommended)

### Imaging
Chest radiograph considered in the following patients:
- <1 yr of age to exclude foreign body or atelectasis
- First episode of significant wheezing (suggested to assess chronicity of illness and assist in excluding other conditions)
- Increasing respiratory distress or minimal response to therapy
- Respiratory distress/failure
- Shortness of breath in the absence of wheezing

### Diagnostic Procedures/Surgery
Peak flow measurement (see above)

## DIFFERENTIAL DIAGNOSIS
- Infection/inflammation:
  - Bronchiolitis: Clinically difficult to differentiate except by age and clinical history.
  - Pneumonia: Viral, bacterial, chemical, or hypersensitivity
  - Aspiration
  - Lymphadenopathy
  - Anaphylactic reaction
- Anatomic:
  - Pneumothorax
  - Foreign body

- Vascular disorder:
  - Compression of trachea by vascular anomaly
  - Pulmonary embolism
  - CHF
- Congenital disease:
  - Cystic fibrosis
  - Tracheoesophageal fistula
  - Bronchogenic cyst
  - Congenital heart disease
- Intoxication: Metabolic acidosis
- Neoplasm
- Vocal cord dysfunction (VCD)
- Pulmonary edema-cardiogenic or noncardiogenic

 TREATMENT

### PRE-HOSPITAL
- Oxygen and oxygen saturation monitoring
- Nebulized β-adrenergic agonist: Albuterol
- Intubate for respiratory failure or severe fatigue.
- IV fluids if evidence of dehydration
- Rapid transport and good communication with ED

### INITIAL STABILIZATION/THERAPY
- Maintain SaO₂ >90–95%.
- β-adrenergic nebulizer(s): Albuterol
- Intubate for respiratory failure.
- 20 mL/kg 0.9% NS bolus if evidence of dehydration.

### ED TREATMENT/PROCEDURES
- Assess patient for signs of potential respiratory failure:
  - Cyanosis
  - Severe anxiety or irritability
  - Lethargy, somnolence, fatigue
  - Persistent tachypnea
  - Poor air entry, ventilation
  - Severe retractions
- Monitor oxygenation, titrate oxygen saturation to SaO₂ >95% (sea level).
- β-adrenergic nebulizer: Albuterol:
  - Frequent or continuous for severe asthma
  - Levalbuterol may require less frequent dosing and be associated with less side effects.
- Ipratropium bromide may be added as adjunct to β-adrenergic agonists. Most effective when combined with 1st 3 doses of β-adrenergic agent in moderate to severely ill children
- Steroid therapy:
  - Oral for moderate exacerbations in those able to take oral meds
  - IV for severe exacerbations or in those unable to take oral meds
- SC epinephrine or terbutaline for severe or refractory asthma (rarely used)
- Magnesium sulfate may be useful in severe disease following standard therapy.
- Intubate for respiratory failure:
  - Ketamine is a useful induction agent.
- 20 mL/kg of 0.9% NS bolus if evidence of dehydration
- Heliox (oxygen and helium) may be useful but studies are inconclusive

### MEDICATION
- Albuterol (0.5% solution or 5 mg/mL):
  - Nebulizer: 0.15 mg/kg per dose, up to 5 mg per dose, q15–30min PRN
  - Metered-dose inhaler (MDI) (with spacer) (90 μg/puff): 2 puffs q5–10min, max. 10 puffs
  - Also available for nebulizer as 0.083% solution or 2.5 mg/3 mL
- Epinephrine (1:1,000) (1 mg/mL): 0.01 mg/kg SC, up to 0.35 mL per dose, q20min for 3 doses
- Ipratropium bromide: Nebulizer (0.02% inhaled sol 500 μg/2.5 mL), 250–500 μg per dose q6h
- Ketamine (for intubation): 1–2 mg/kg IV as induction agent
- Levalbuterol (0.63 and 1.25 mg vials): q6–8h by nebulizer
- Magnesium sulfate: 25 mg/kg per dose IV over 20 min; max. 1.2–2 g per dose
- Methylprednisolone: 1–2 mg/kg per dose IV q6h; max. 125 mg per dose
- Prednisolone: 1–2 mg/kg per dose PO q12h (available as 15 mg/5 mL)
- Prednisone: 1–2 mg/kg per dose PO q6–12h; max. 80 mg per dose
- Terbutaline/ (available as 1 mg/1 mL) (0.01%): 0.01 mL/kg SC q15–20min up to 0.25 mL per dose, q20min for 2 doses

### First Line
- Albuterol
- Steroids
- Ipratropium

### Second Line
- Epinephrine or terbutaline
- Magnesium sulfate

 FOLLOW-UP

### DISPOSITION
#### Admission Criteria
- Persistent respiratory difficulty:
  - Persistent wheezing
  - Increased respiratory rate/tachypnea
  - Retraction and use of accessory muscles
- SaO₂ <93% (sea level) on room air
- Peak expiratory flow rate (PEFR) <50–70% predicted levels
- Inability to tolerate oral medicines or liquids
- Prior ED visit in last 24 hr
- Comorbidity:
  - Congenital heart disease
  - Bronchopulmonary dysplasia
  - CF
  - Neuromuscular disease
- Concomitant illness:
  - Pneumonia
  - Severe viral infection

#### Intensive Care Unit Criteria
- Severe respiratory distress
- SaO₂ <90% or PaO₂ <60 mm Hg on 40% oxygen
- PaCO₂ >40 mm Hg
- Significant complications:
  - Pneumothorax
  - Dysrhythmia

#### Discharge Criteria
- Good response to therapy. Observe in ED 60 min after last treatment before discharging:
  - PEFR >70% predicted
  - SaO₂ >93% on room air (sea level)
  - Respiratory rate normal
  - No retractions
  - Clear or minimal wheezing
  - No or minimal dyspnea
- Good follow-up and compliance
- Discharge treatment:
  - Intensive β-adrenergic regimen for 3–5 days
  - Short course (3–5 days) of steroids (2 mg/kg/d) for those presenting with moderate symptoms with consideration of ongoing therapy using nebulized or MDI routes
  - Follow-up appointment 24–72 hr
  - Instructions to return for shortness of breath refractory to home regimen
  - Long-term therapy should be considered for children with recurrent episodes, persistent symptoms, or activity limitations.

### FOLLOW-UP RECOMMENDATIONS
Primary care physician for maintenance therapy, often including nebulized or MDI steroid therapy and education about acute rescue management.

### PEARLS AND PITFALLS
- Rapid treatment with continuous re-evaluation to detect any progression of disease is essential.
- When admitting patients, assure that β-adrenergic agent therapy is not interrupted.

### ADDITIONAL READING
- Robinson PD, Van Asperen P. Asthma in childhood. *Pediatr Clin North Am*. 2009;56(1):191–226.
- Rowe BH, Brezlaff JA, Bourdon C, et al. Intravenous magnesium sulfate treatment for acute asthma in the emergency department: A review of the literature. *Ann Emerg Med*. 2000;36:181–190.
- Sampayo EM, Chew A, Zorc JJ. Make an M'PACT on asthma: Rapid identification of persistent asthma symptoms in a pediatric emergency department. *Pediatr Emerg Care*. 2009;[Epub prior to print].
- Scarfone RJ, Friedlaender E. Corticosteroids in acute asthma: Past, present, and future. *Pediatr Emerg Care*. 2003;19(5):355–361.

### See Also (Topic, Algorithm, Electronic Media Element)
- Bronchiolitis, Pediatric
- Pneumonia, Pediatric

# ASYSTOLE

David F. M. Brown, MD
Kohei Hasegawa, MD

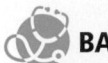 ## BASICS

### DESCRIPTION
- Absence of cardiac electrical activity
- End-stage cardiac rhythm

### ETIOLOGY
- May occur after progressive dysrhythmia:
  - Bradycardia
  - Prolonged ventricular fibrillation
  - Prolonged pulseless electrical activity
- Patient is extremely unlikely to survive when asystole occurs outside the hospital:
  - ~40% will have return of spontaneous circulation and survive to hospital admission, but <15% survive to hospital discharge.
- Prognosis is similarly poor for those patients who develop asystole after countershock for ventricular tachycardia/ventricular fibrillation (VF); <10% survive to hospital discharge.
- Potentially reversible causes include:
  - Hypoxia
  - Acidosis
  - Hyperkalemia
  - Hypokalemia
  - Drug overdose
  - Hypothermia
  - Pulmonary embolism
  - Myocardial infarction

 ## DIAGNOSIS

### SIGNS AND SYMPTOMS
- Unresponsive patient
- Pulseless
- No spontaneous respirations

### History
Lightheadedness or Syncope may precede

### ESSENTIAL WORKUP
- Confirm asystole in two limb leads to exclude ventricular fibrillation.
- Confirm lead and cable connections.
- Confirm monitor power is on.
- Confirm monitor gain is up.
- Identify reversible causes.

### DIAGNOSTIC TESTS & INTERPRETATION
### Lab
Arterial blood gas (potassium)

### Imaging
Cardiac US
- Confirm cardiac standstill

### DIFFERENTIAL DIAGNOSIS
Ventricular fibrillation

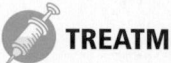 ## TREATMENT

### PRE-HOSPITAL
- No intervention should be made for patient with valid Do Not Resuscitate document.
- No intervention if patient can be verified as dead:
  - Rigor mortis
  - Dependent livedo
  - Injury incompatible with life (eg, decapitation)

### INITIAL STABILIZATION/THERAPY
- Initiate basic CPR.
- Confirm asystole with defibrillator.
- Place airway device and confirm placement.
- Establish IV access.
- Confirm asystole in two limb leads with monitor.
- Consider early transcutaneous pacing (within 3–5 min of onset of asystole).
- Epinephrine and atropine every 3–5 min.
- Vasopressin as a one-time dose (optional)
- Treat potentially reversible causes.
- Sodium bicarbonate if hyperkalemia or drug overdose suspected
- No proven benefit to an empiric single countershock.

## ED TREATMENT/PROCEDURES

- Consider induced hypothermia in comatose patients with return of spontaneous circulation
  - Target temperature 32–34°C for 12–24 hr
- Consider termination of resuscitation efforts if the following conditions are met:
  - Adequate CPR
  - Tracheal intubation
  - Effective ventilation
  - IV access
  - VF excluded
  - Epinephrine and atropine given:
    - Discuss indications of vasopressin versus epinephrine
  - Reversible causes corrected
  - Documented asystole despite 10 min of above interventions

## MEDICATION

- Atropine: 1 mg IV q3–5min:
  - Up to 3 mg total
- Epinephrine: 1 mg (peds: 0.01 mg/kg) IV q3–5 min
- Vasopressin: 40 U IV (single dose)
- Sodium bicarbonate: 1 mEq/kg IV only if:
  - Pre-existing acidosis
  - Hyperkalemia
  - Tricyclic antidepressant overdose is suspected.

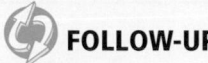 **FOLLOW-UP**

### DISPOSITION

#### Admission Criteria
All patients with return of spontaneous circulation

#### Discharge Criteria
None—all patients with return of spontaneous circulation need at least a period of monitored observation in the hospital.

### FOLLOW-UP RECOMMENDATIONS
Appropriate use of a permanent pacemaker may prevent primary asystole:
- High-grade heart block
- Sinus arrest

#### Patient Monitoring
ICU for cardiac monitoring and induced hypothermia as appropriate

## PEARLS AND PITFALLS

- Confirm asystole in 2 limb leads to exclude ventricular fibrillation
- Resuscitation is likely to be successful only if reversible causes corrected immediately

## ADDITIONAL READING

- Olasveengen TM, Sunde K, Brunborg C, et al. Intravenous drug adminisration during out-of-hospital cardiac arrest: a randomized trial. *JAMA*. 2009;302(20):2222–2229.
- 2005 American Heart Association Guidelines for Cardiopulmonary Resuscitation and Emergency Cadiovascular Care. Part 7.2: Management of Cardiac Arrest: 7.4: Monitoring and Medications: 7.5: Postresusciation Support. ECC Committee, Subcommittees and Task Forces of the American Heart Association. *Circulation*. 2005;112: (Suppl. 24):IV58–88.
- Cummins RO, Graves JR, Larsen MP, et al. Out-of-hospital transcutaneous pacing by emergency medical technicians in patients with asystolic cardiac arrest. *N Engl J Med*. 1993;328: 1377–1382.
- Wenzel V, Krismer AC, Arntz HR, et al. A comparison of vasopressin and epinephrine for out-of-hospital cardiopulmonary resuscitation. *N Engl J Med*. 2004;350(2):105–113.
- Bernard SA, Gray TW, Buist MD, Jones BM, et al. Treatment of comatose survivors of out-of-hospital cardiac arrest with induced hypothermia. *N Engl J Med*. 2002;346(8):557–563.

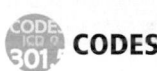 **CODES**

### ICD9
427.5 Cardiac arrest

# ATAXIA
*Lara K. Kulchycki*

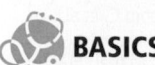 **BASICS**

## DESCRIPTION
- Inability to perform coordinated movements
- Often presents with unsteady gait

## ETIOLOGY
Usually cerebellar in origin, but may occur with sensory, motor, or vestibular dysfunction:
- Trauma
- Mass lesions
- Vascular disorders
- Infection or postinfectious process
- Toxins/drugs
- Metabolic/endocrine derangements
- Demyelinating disease
- Congenital malformations
- Hereditary disorders:
  - Inborn errors of metabolism
  - Progressive degenerative ataxias
- Nutritional deficiencies

 **DIAGNOSIS**

## SIGNS AND SYMPTOMS
### History
- A careful history is essential since gait changes may be caused by pain, weakness, lightheadedness, vertigo, or incoordination
- Onset
- Hours–days: Acute
- Weeks–months: Subacute
- Months–years: Chronic
- Symmetric or focal symptoms
- Presence of fever, mental status changes, weakness, sensory loss, or urinary incontinence
- Recent viral illness or immunizations
- History of trauma or toxic ingestion
- Family history of movement disorder

### Physical Exam
- Perform a complete physical exam, including neurological and gait testing.
- Assess for signs or symptoms of acute, life-threatening disorders such as hemorrhage, stroke, or CNS infection:
  - Altered mental status
  - Headache
  - Nausea/vomiting
  - Focal neurological deficits
  - Elevated intracranial pressure:
    - Bradycardia, HTN, abnormal respiratory pattern
    - Papilledema
    - Bulging fontanelles
  - Fever
  - Meningismus

- Cerebellar ataxia:
  - Wide-based, staggering gait
  - Test tandem gait to identify subtle ataxia
  - Ipsilateral limb ataxia often noted in hemispheric cerebellar lesions
  - Dysmetria: Under- or overshooting on finger-to-nose and heel-to-shin testing
  - Dysdiadochokinesis: Difficulty with rapid alternating movements
  - Staccato, scanning speech
  - Intention tremor
  - Titubation: Swaying of the head/trunk while at rest, occurs most commonly with midline cerebellar lesions
  - Nystagmus
  - Vertigo
- Sensory ataxia:
  - Cautious, steppage gait
  - Marked worsening of coordination with eyes closed:
    - A positive Romberg sign is the classic finding in sensory ataxia.
  - Loss of position/vibration sense
  - Difficulty with fine motor skills
- Motor ataxia:
  - Muscle weakness
  - May find diminished deep tendon reflexes or muscle tone
- Vestibular ataxia:
  - Vertigo:
    - Distinguish central from peripheral vertigo.
    - Peripheral vertigo is often severe and may be accompanied by ear pain, hearing loss, or tinnitus.
  - Nystagmus
  - Nausea/vomiting
  - Examine ears and perform provocative testing for nystagmus (Dix-Hallpike)
- Note the presence of intoxication or toxidromes in patients with suspected ingestion.

## ESSENTIAL WORKUP
A detailed history and physical exam will help determine which tests are necessary.

## DIAGNOSTIC TESTS & INTERPRETATION
### Lab
- Blood glucose level
- Serum electrolytes
- Toxicology screen
- Standard panels may not include the drugs of interest in the ataxic patient.
- Target any additional testing to likely exposures, such as anticonvulsants.
- Thyroid function testing in suspected hypothyroidism

### Imaging
- CT:
  - Head CT identifies mass, hemorrhage, subacute infarct, or hydrocephalus.
  - Consider CT with and without IV contrast if mass suspected.
  - CT angiography can be performed to evaluate neck vessels.
- MRI:
  - Excellent study to evaluate for acute ischemia, mass, demyelinating lesions, and vascular abnormalities
  - Superior for imaging the posterior fossa
  - MR angiography of head/neck may be indicated if vascular abnormality is suspected.
- EKG:
  - Not indicated as part of ED workup
  - May be used to evaluate for denervation of peripheral nerves

### Diagnostic Procedures/Surgery
Lumbar puncture:
- Rarely indicated unless CNS infection suspected
- May be of value in suspected cases of Guillain-Barré syndrome

## DIFFERENTIAL DIAGNOSIS
- Acute symmetric ataxia:
  - Head trauma
  - Drug use/toxic ingestion:
    - Alcohol
    - Lithium
    - Phenytoin
    - Barbiturates
    - Carbamazepine
    - Phenobarbital
    - Valproic acid
    - Benzodiazepines
    - Diphenhydramine
    - Dextromethorphan
  - Acute viral cerebellitis
  - Meningitis/encephalitis
  - Hydrocephalus
  - Postinfectious syndrome
  - Hypoglycemia
  - Hyponatremia
  - Severe heat stroke
- Acute focal ataxia:
  - Posterior circulation infarction
  - Anterior cerebral artery syndrome
  - Vertebrobasilar insufficiency (VBI)
  - Cerebellar hemorrhage
  - Subdural hematoma
  - Cerebellar abscess
  - Acute disseminated encephalomyelitis
  - Complicated migraine
  - Atypical seizure

- Subacute symmetric ataxia:
  - Drug use/toxic ingestion:
    - Mercury
    - Lead
    - Hydrocarbons
    - Glue sniffing
    - Cytotoxic chemotherapy
    - Organophosphates
  - Vitamin $B_1$ or $B_{12}$ deficiency
  - Paraneoplastic syndromes:
    - Breast/ovarian cancer
    - Hodgkin disease
    - Neuroblastoma
  - Lyme disease
  - Toxoplasmosis
  - Mycoplasma
  - Creutzfeldt-Jakob disease
- Subacute focal ataxia:
  - Cerebellar glioma
  - Metastatic tumors
    Lymphoma
  - MS
  - Guillain-Barré syndrome
  - AIDS-related progressive multifocal leukoencephalopathy
  - Syringomyelia
  - Cervical spondylosis
- Chronic ataxia:
  - Alcohol-related cerebellar degeneration
  - Stable gliosis
  - Inherited disorders:
    - Spinocerebellar ataxias
    - Friedreich's ataxia
    - Ataxia telangiectasia
    - Niemann-Pick disease
  - Hypothyroidism
  - Vitamin E deficiency
  - Tabes dorsalis
  - Congenital malformation:
    - Arnold Chiari
    - Dandy-Walker
- Disease states that cause peripheral vertigo can mimic the gait findings in ataxia:
  - Benign paroxysmal positional vertigo
  - Acute labyrinthitis
  - Ménière's disease

### Pediatric Considerations
- May present with a refusal to walk
- Acute ataxia in children is usually a benign, self-limited process:
  - 60% of cases caused by acute cerebellar ataxia or drug ingestion.
- Acute cerebellar ataxia:
  - Postinfectious cerebellar demyelination
  - Usually occurs in children 2–5 yr old
  - Onset 1–3 wk after triggering illness
  - Often linked to varicella but caused by many viral infections or immunizations
  - Normal mental status
  - No fever, focal deficits, or seizures
  - Mild cases may be managed at home, but require injury prevention counseling.
  - Most children recover completely within 3 mo without intervention.

- Drug/toxic ingestions:
  - Expect mental status changes.
  - Assess access to medications and order appropriate toxicological testing.
- Guillain-Barré syndrome:
  - 15% present with sensory ataxia.
  - Miller-Fisher variant: Clinical triad of ataxia, areflexia, and ophthalmoplegia
- Neoplasm:
  - More than 50% of childhood brain tumors occur in the brainstem or cerebellum.
  - Opsoclonus-myoclonus-ataxia syndrome:
    - Paraneoplastic autoimmune syndrome affecting cerebellum
    - Over 50% due to neuroblastoma
- Stroke:
  - Rare in children, but can occur in patients with sickle cell disease or hypercoagulable states

### Geriatric Considerations
- Gait disorders in the elderly are often multifactorial.
- Underlying cognitive deficits may make it difficult to distinguish presyncope, weakness, vertigo, and incoordination.
- Posterior circulation cerebrovascular syndromes, like VBI and stroke, are more common in the elderly and may present with vague symptoms, like dizziness.
- Evaluate for signs of orthostasis or extrapyramidal disorders, like Parkinsonism.

 TREATMENT

### PRE-HOSPITAL

**ALERT**
Acute onset of ataxia may be due to stroke or hemorrhage:
- Deterioration in mental status may warrant field endotracheal intubation.
- Cervical spine immobilization if traumatic etiology suspected

### INITIAL STABILIZATION/THERAPY
- ABCs
- IV access
- Supplemental oxygen
- Cardiac monitor
- Check fingerstick blood glucose:
  - Administer dextrose if hypoglycemic
  - Empiric thiamine in chronic alcoholics and malnourished patients

### ED TREATMENT/PROCEDURES
- Institute fall precautions
- Treatment must be tailored to the patient's presentation and underlying pathology.
- Cerebellar infarction can lead to significant edema with mass effect and herniation.
- Neurosurgery consultation may be needed for decompressive craniectomy.

### MEDICATION
- Dextrose: $D_{50}W$ 1 amp (50 mL or 25 g) (peds: $D_{25}W$ 2–4 mL/kg) IV
- Naloxone: 0.4–2 mg (peds: dose based on age) IV or IM initial dose
- Thiamine (vitamin $B_1$): 100 mg IV

 FOLLOW-UP

### DISPOSITION
#### Admission Criteria
- Acute and subacute ataxia, particularly if a benign etiology cannot be established
- Patients who cannot ambulate safely
- Admit patients with cerebellar hemorrhage or mass effect to the ICU.

#### Discharge Criteria
- Reversible or mild symptoms
- Normal mental status
- Able to ambulate safely

### FOLLOW-UP RECOMMENDATIONS
Follow up with primary care or neurology depending on likely etiology of symptoms.

## PEARLS AND PITFALLS
- Failure to distinguish true ataxia from other causes of gait instability
- Failure to note trauma in intoxicated patients
- Failure to realize the limitations of CT scan in evaluating the posterior fossa
- Failure to recognize the risk of herniation in cerebellar lesions, including stroke

## ADDITIONAL READING
- Friday, JH. Ataxia. In: Fleisher GR, Ludwig S, Henretig FM, et al., eds. *Textbook of Pediatric Emergency Medicine*, 5th ed. Philadelphia: Lippincott Williams & Wilkins; 2006:189–192.
- Savitz SI, Caplan LR. Vertebrobasilar disease. *N Engl J Med*. 2005;352:2618–2626.
- Sudarsky L. Gait and balance disorders. In: Fauci AS, Braunwald E, Kasper DL, et al., eds. *Harrison's Principles of Internal Medicine*, 17th ed. Philadelphia: McGraw-Hill; 2008:151–154.

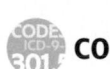 CODES

### ICD9
- 334.2 Primary cerebellar degeneration
- 781.3 Lack of coordination

# ATRIAL FIBRILLATION
*Edward Ullman*

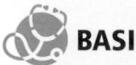 **BASICS**

## DESCRIPTION
- Dysrhythmia characterized by seemingly disorganized atrial depolarizations without effective atrial contraction
- Caused by multiple re-entrant waveforms within the atria
- Atrial rate ranges from 350–600 beats per minute (bpm).
- Results in loss of organized atrial contractions and rapid ventricular rate:
  - Decrease in cardiac output
  - Embolus formation
- Affects 2.2 million Americans
- Most common clinical arrhythmia:
  - Prevalence increasing with age
  - Men are at higher risk.

## ETIOLOGY
- Systemic disease:
  - HTN
  - Hyperthyroidism
  - Chronic pulmonary disease
  - Infection
  - Pulmonary embolus
  - Hypoxia
  - Drugs:
  - Sympathomimetics
  - Acute alcohol ingestion (holiday heart syndrome)
  - Obesity
- Underlying cardiac disease:
  - Cardiomyopathy
  - Coronary artery disease
  - Valvular disease:
    - Especially mitral
  - Pericarditis
  - Sick sinus syndrome
  - Myocardial contusion
  - CHF
  - Congenital heart disease
- Idiopathic:
  - Absence of any known etiologic factor
  - No clinical or echocardiographic evidence of heart disease

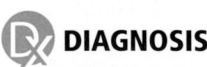 **DIAGNOSIS**

## SIGNS AND SYMPTOMS
- Decreased cardiac output:
  - Weakness
  - Light-headedness
  - Syncope
  - Hypotension
  - Angina
  - Pulmonary edema
  - Altered mental status
  - Lower-extremity edema
  - Hepatojugular reflex
- Embolus formation:
  - Acute neurologic injury
  - Mesenteric ischemia

### History
- Onset of symptoms
- Duration
- Inciting factors
- Prior episodes of fibrillation
- Prior heart disease

### Physical Exam
- Palpitations
- Irregularly irregular pulse
- Absence of *a* waves in the jugular venous pulse
- Pulse deficit with more rapid ventricular rates:
  - The auscultated or palpated apical rate is faster than the rate palpated at the wrist.

## ESSENTIAL WORKUP
- History and physical exam:
  - Assess for instability and need for immediate cardioversion.
  - Duration of symptoms >48 hr or <48 hr
  - Evidence of systemic disease or underlying cardiac disease
- ECG:
  - Absent P waves replaced by fibrillatory (f) waves:
    - 350 and 600 bpm
    - f waves vary in amplitude, morphology, and intervals
  - R-R intervals are irregularly irregular.
  - Ventricular rate ranges from 80–150 bpm:
    - If rate >200 associated with wide-irregular QRS, consider bypass tract.
  - Wide QRS complex suggests rate related bundle branch block or bypass tract.
  - Slower rate suggests abnormal AV node or presence of AV nodal blocking medication.
  - Usually marrow QRS complexes unless:
    - Functional aberration
    - Pre-existing bundle branch
    - Pre-excitation with ventricular activation via an accessory pathway

## DIAGNOSTIC TESTS & INTERPRETATION
### Lab
- CBC
- Electrolytes
- Cardiac enzymes—if ischemia is a concern
- Thyroid function
- Digoxin level—if patient is taking
- Urine drug screen

### Imaging
- CXR
- ECG

## DIFFERENTIAL DIAGNOSIS
- Atrial flutter with variable AV block
- Multifocal atrial tachycardia
- Sinus rhythm with frequent premature atrial contractions
- Atrial tachycardia with variable AV block

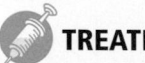 **TREATMENT**

## PRE-HOSPITAL
- IV access
- Monitor
- Oxygen
- Cardioversion:
  - In settings where patient is unstable

## INITIAL STABILIZATION/THERAPY
- IV
- Oxygen
- Monitor
- Immediate synchronized electrical cardioversion starting at 200 J if the patient is unstable

## ED TREATMENT/PROCEDURES
- Control rate:
  - Not necessary if rate <100 bpm or if rhythm spontaneously converts to sinus
  - AV nodal blockers (calcium channel blockers, $\beta$-blockers, and digoxin) contraindicated if bypass tract suspected
- Treat underlying cause if one is identified.
- Use procainamide to treat stable patients with a suspected bypass tract.
- Use electrical cardioversion for unstable patients.
- Calcium channel blockers:
  - Consider in patient with pulmonary disease
  - Use cautiously in patient with uncompensated CHF and 2nd- or 3rd-degree heart block
- $\beta$-Blockers:
  - Consider in patient with coronary artery disease (CAD)
  - Use cautiously in patient with uncompensated CHF, 2nd- or 3rd-degree heart block, and pulmonary disease
- Digoxin:
  - Consider in patient with pre-existing CHF
  - Do not give if concern for accessory pathway
- Rhythm control does not offer mortality benefit over rate control.
- However, may consider rhythm control for patients with symptomatic atrial fibrillation (AF) or those with their 1st episode.

- Synchronized electrical cardioversion:
  - Protocol depends on duration of AF.
  - <48 hr: Cardioversion. Consider IV heparin bolus prior.
  - >48 hr, delayed cardioversion: Anticoagulation (INR 2–3) for at least 3 wk, then cardioversion with 200–300 J, then anticoagulation for an additional 4 wk
  - >48 hr and requiring immediate cardioversion: IV heparin immediately, then transesophageal ECG to exclude atrial clot then cardioversion then anticoagulation for and additional 4 wk; if atrial clot noted on ECG, will have to defer to delayed cardioversion protocol
  - Consider pretreatment with antiarrhythmic drugs to increase likelihood of success of electrical cardioversion.
- Chemical cardioversion:
  - Choice of drug depends on history of CHF, high BP, LV hypertrophy, and CAD.
  - Medications may be proarrhythmic and should be used with caution.
  - As with electrical cardioversion, appropriate anticoagulation will be necessary depending on the duration and presence/absence of clot.
  - Ibutilide:
    - Requires a normal QTc, no history of torsades, and correction of hypokalemia
    - Posttreatment monitoring for at least 4 hr for possible Torsades de Pointes
  - Quinidine gluconate
  - Procainamide
  - Flecainide
  - Propafenone
  - Sotalol
- Anticoagulation determined by CHADS2 scoring:
  - Assign 1 point for each of the following:
    - History of cardiac failure
    - History of HTN
    - Age ≥75 yr
    - Diabetes
  - Assign 2 points for a history of stroke or TIA.
  - The adjusted annual stroke rate increases from 1.9% for a CHADS2 score of 0 to 18.2% for a CHADS2 score of 6.
  - CHADS2 score of 0:
    - 81–325 mg/day of aspirin
  - CHADS2 score of 1:
    - Either 81–325 mg/day of aspirin or adjusted dose warfarin with a target INR of 2.5
  - CHADS2 score >1:
    - Adjusted-dose warfarin with a target INR of 2.5 (range, 2.0–3.0)
- Aspirin:
  - Patients with contraindications to anticoagulation and unreliable individuals
  - Patients with low stroke risk

## MEDICATION

- Metoprolol: 5–10 mg slow IV push at 5-min intervals to total of 15 mg
- 25 mg–100 mg oral b.i.d.

- Diltiazem:
  - 0.25 mg/kg IV over 2 min; if unsuccessful, repeat in 15 min as 0.35 mg/kg IV over 2 min; an infusion of 5 mg/h is usually started after the initial dose to maintain rate control.
  - 120–300 mg oral daily
- Digoxin: 0.5 mg IV initially, then 0.25 mg IV q4h until desired effect
- Esmolol: 0.5 mg/kg over 1 min; maintenance infusion at 0.05 mg/kg/min over 4 min, then 0.1–0.2 mg/kg/min continuously
- Propranolol: 0.1 mg/kg IV divided into equal doses at 2–3-min intervals
- Verapamil:
  - 2.5–5 mg IV bolus over 2 min; may repeat with 5–10 mg q15–30min to max of 20 mg
  - 120–300 mg PO daily
- Amiodarone:
  - 5–7 mg/kg over 30–60 min, then 1.2–1.8 g/day continuous infusion or in divided PO doses until 10 g total
  - 600–800 mg/day divided dose until 10 g total, then 200–400 mg/day maintenance
- Procainamide: 15–18 loading dose administered as a slow infusion over 30 min. Max: 1.5 g. Then 2–6 mg/min infusion.
- Quinidine gluconate: 324–648 mg PO q8–12h
- Ibutilide: 1 mg IV for patients >60 kg; 0.01 mg/kg IV for patients <60 kg infused over 10 min; dose can be repeated once if sinus rhythm not restored within 10 min after infusion; patients must be monitored for 4 hr afterward for QT prolongation, Torsades de Pointes, and ventricular tachycardia.
- Flecainide: 2 mg/kg IV at 10 mg/min. Do not give in patients with structural heart disease.
- Propafenone: 1–2 mg/kg IV at 10 mg/min
- Sotalol: 1–1.5 mg/kg IV then infused at 10 mg/min
- Heparin: Load 80 IU/kg IV; infusion at 18 IU/kg/hr
- Low-molecular-weight heparin: 1 mg/kg SQ b.i.d.
- Warfarin sodium: 2.5–5 mg/day PO, dosage adjustments based on INR
- Aspirin: 50–325 mg/day

### ALERT
IV form for flecainide, propafenone, and sotalol not approved for use in U.S.; *must be infused slowly.*

 **FOLLOW-UP**

### DISPOSITION
#### Admission Criteria
- Unstable AF:
  - Inability to control rate
- High risk for stroke:
  - Prior cardiovascular accident
  - CHF
- Associated medical problems contributing to the AF that require inpatient management

#### Discharge Criteria
- Conversion to sinus rhythm if symptoms <48 hr
- Chronic AF with appropriate ventricular rate control and anticoagulation
- New-onset AF with rate control and anticoagulation

#### Issues for Referral
- Cardiology or an electrophysiologist
- Evaluation for outpatient cardioversion

### FOLLOW-UP RECOMMENDATIONS
- INR check if placed on warfarin
- The patient should return to the ED if feeling faint, dizzy, numbness or weakness of the face or limbs, or trouble seeing or speaking.

## PEARLS AND PITFALLS

- Mistaking f waves or u waves as P waves and misdiagnosing AF as a sinus rhythm
- Using calcium channel blockers, β-blockers, or digoxin in AF with a wide complex AF in a patient with an underlying bypass tract

## ADDITIONAL READING

- Falk RH. Atrial fibrillation. *N Engl J Med.* 2001;344(14):1067–1078.
- Fuster V, Ryden LE, Asinger RW, et al. ACC/AHA/ESC Guidelines for the Management of Patients with Atrial Fibrillation: Executive Summary a Report of the American College of Cardiology/American Heart Association Task Force on Practice Guidelines and the European Society of Cardiology. *Circulation.* 2006;148(4):e149–e246.
- Saxonhouse SJ, Curtis AB. Risk and benefits of rate control versus maintenance of sinus rhythm. *Am J Cardiol.* 2003;91(6A):27D–32D.
- Gage BF, Waterman AD, Shannon W. Validation of clinical classification schemes for predicting stroke. *JAMA.* 2001;285:2864.
- Crandall MA, Bradley DJ, Packer DL, et al. Contemporary management of atrial fibrillation: Update on anticoagulation and invasive management strategies. *Mayo Clin Proc.* 2009;84:643–662.

 **CODES**

### ICD9
427.31 Atrial fibrillation

# ATRIAL FLUTTER

*Liesl A. Curtis*

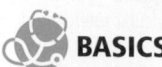

## BASICS

### DESCRIPTION
- Atrial dysrhythmia
- 200,000 new cases each year
- Male to female ratio 2:1
- A re-entrant circuit in the right atrium is thought to be the underlying mechanism.
- Most sensitive rhythm to cardioversion
- Seldom occurs in absence of organic heart disease
- Less common than supraventricular tachycardia (SVT) or atrial fibrillation
- Typically paroxysmal, lasting seconds to hours
- Occurs in ~25–35% of patients with atrial fibrillation
- Often reverts to sinus rhythm or atrial fibrillation
- Untreated, may promote cardiomyopathy

### ETIOLOGY
- Ischemic heart disease
- Valvular heart diseases
- CHF
- Myocarditis
- Cardiomyopathies
- Pulmonary embolus
- Other pulmonary disease
- Electrolyte abnormalities
- Alcoholism
- Postoperative following cardiac surgery (often in 1st postoperative week)
- Thyrotoxicosis

### *Pediatric Considerations*
- Occurs in children but is often asymptomatic
- Associated mortality is highest in the neonatal period.
- Associated with:
  – Congenitally acquired maternal antibodies
  – Congenital heart disease
  – Infectious etiologies, such as rheumatic fever or myocarditis
- Be sure to consider potential toxic ingestions in pediatric patients with new AV block

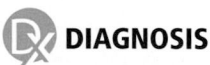

## DIAGNOSIS

### SIGNS AND SYMPTOMS
- Palpitations
- Syncope/presyncope
- Chest pain
- Fatigue
- Dyspnea
- Poor exercise capacity
- Tachycardia—heart rate >150 bpm:
  – Most often with a regular pulse
- Hypotension
- Heart failure

### *Pediatric Considerations*
- Infants do not tolerate atrial flutter well.
- The aortic valve (AV) node is capable of very rapid conduction.
- Extremely rapid ventricular rates can lead to shock or CHF.
- Atrial flutter can occur in the fetus and young infants without associated cardiac defects:
  – Often does not recur beyond neonatal period
- Most older children have an underlying cardiac abnormality:
  – More likely to recur, more difficult to control

### ESSENTIAL WORKUP
- EKG
- Labs
- CXR

### DIAGNOSTIC TESTS & INTERPRETATION
### *Lab*
- Electrolytes
- Calcium, magnesium
- Cardiac enzymes
- Digoxin level
- PT/PTT:
  – Useful to have baseline
  – Needed for patients who are anti-coagulated

### *Imaging*
- CXR:
  – May identify cardiomyopathy or CHF
- Echo:
  – May identify regional wall motion abnormalities or valvular dysfunction

### DIFFERENTIAL DIAGNOSIS
- SVT
- Sinus tachycardia
- Atrial fibrillation
- Multifocal atrial tachycardia
- Ventricular tachycardia

## TREATMENT

### PRE-HOSPITAL
- IV access
- Supplemental oxygen
- Cardiac monitoring
- Unstable patients should be cardioverted in the field:
  – Immediate synchronized cardioversion
  – Start with 50 J, then 100 J, 200 J, 300 J, and 360 J

### INITIAL STABILIZATION/THERAPY
- Oxygen
- Monitor
- IV access
- Immediate synchronized cardioversion starting at 50 J-min (monophasic) if the patient is unstable

## ED TREATMENT/PROCEDURES
- Rate control:
  – Rate control should be instituted prior to giving an antidysrhythmic to avoid risk of a 1:1 AV conduction ratio and hemodynamic collapse.
  – May be difficult to achieve
- Anticoagulation:
  – Same guidelines as for atrial fibrillation:
    ○ INR 2–3 for 3 wk prior to cardioversion if >48 hr or unknown duration
    ○ Recommended even if negative transesophageal ECG
    ○ Risk of thromboembolism ranges from 1.7–7%.
  – Patients at higher risk for thromboembolism include those patients with:
    ○ Valvular heart disease
    ○ Rhythms that alternate between atrial fibrillation and flutter
    ○ Left ventricular (LV) dysfunction
    ○ Prior stroke or thromboembolism
    ○ Longer symptom duration (>48 hr)
- Antiarrhythmic drugs:
  – Adenosine:
    ○ Unlikely to break atrial flutter
    ○ May aid in the diagnosis of atrial flutter by unmasking the flutter waves
  – Amiodarone:
    ○ Rate control in patients with pre-excited atrial arrhythmias (ie, WPW)
    ○ Preferable antiarrhythmic agent for patients with severely impaired heart function
    ○ Major adverse effects are hypotension and bradycardia, slower infusions can prevent this.
  – Calcium channel blockers:
    ○ Rate control
    ○ Verapamil has higher incidence of symptomatic hypotension than diltiazem.
    ○ Verapamil should only be used in narrow-complex arrhythmias (arrhythmias known to be supraventricular in origin).
  – β-Blockers:
    ○ Rate control
    ○ Added benefit of cardioprotective effects for patients with ACS
  – Magnesium sulfate:
    ○ Rate control
    ○ Low-level evidence
  – Digoxin:
    ○ Rate control
    ○ 3rd-line drug
    ○ Has inotropic properties so may be useful in patients with ventricular dysfunction
    ○ Longer onset to therapeutic effect
  – Procainamide:
    ○ Rhythm control
    ○ Drug of choice for patients with known pre-excitation syndromes (ie, WPW) and preserved ventricular function
    ○ Caution if patient has QT prolongation

- Sotalol:
  - Rhythm control
  - Not a 1st-line drug
  - For use in WPW and preserved ventricular function if duration of arrhythmia is ≤48 hr
- Ibutilide:
  - Rhythm control
  - For acute pharmacologic rhythm conversion in patients with preserved ventricular function (EF >30%) if duration of arrhythmia is ≤48 hr
  - Correct potassium and magnesium before use
  - Contraindicated if QTc >440 msec or in patients with severe structural heart disease
  - Efficacy rate of 38–76%
  - Mean time to conversion is 30 min.
  - Incidence of sustained polymorphic ventricular tachycardia (VT) 1.2–1.7%
  - Observe for 4–6 hr after administration for QT prolongation or VT.
- Cardioversion:
  - 50–360 J (25 J–100 J for most patients)
  - Sedation when possible
  - Safest and most effective means of restoring sinus rhythm
- Maintenance of sinus rhythm after cardioversion:
  - High recurrence rate: ~50% at 1 year; however, difficult to determine rate because data combines atrial fibrillation with atrial flutter
  - Amiodarone most effective
- Percutaneous catheter ablation:
  - Acute and long-term success rates exceed 90%.
  - Low complication rate
  - Candidates include:
    - Recurrent episodes of drug-resistant atrial flutter
    - Patients who are drug intolerant
    - Patients who do not desire long-term drug therapy

### Pediatric Considerations
- Verapamil is not recommended in infants and young children as it is associated with a low cardiac output and serious cardiovascular compromise.
- Digoxin is the 1st-line drug therapy for pediatric atrial flutter.
- Consider cardioversion as 1st-line therapy in neonates.

## MEDICATION
- Amiodarone: 150 mg IV over 10 min, then continuous infusion at 1 mg/min for 6 hr, then 0.5 mg/min infusion over 18 hr; supplemental 150-mg infusions can be dosed PRN to a maximum daily dose of 2.2 g (peds: 5 mg/kg IV loading dose over 20–60 min, may repeat to max of 15 mg/kg/day IV)
- Adenosine: 6 mg IV × 1. May give 12 mg IV q1–2 min × 2 if no conversion. Give all doses IV push

- Atenolol: 5 mg IV over 5 min, may repeat in 10 min if tolerated, then 50 mg PO q12h
- Digoxin: Loading dose 10–15 ug/kg lean body weight (peds: 8–12 $\mu$g/kg)
- Diltiazem: 0.25 mg/kg IV over 2 min followed in 15 min by 0.35 mg/kg IV over 2 min, maintenance infusion of 10–15 mg/hr titrated to heart rate
- Dofetilide: 8 ug/kg IV over 30 min
- Esmolol: 0.5 mg/kg over 1 min; maintenance infusion at 0.05 mg/kg/min; can repeat loading dose and increase in increments of 0.05 mg/kg/min q4min up to 0.3 mg/kg/min
- Flecainide: 2 mg/kg IV at 10 mg/min
- Ibutilide: 1 mg IV over 10 min for patients >60 kg; 0.01 mg/kg IV for patients <60 kg infused over 10 min; dose can be repeated once if normal sinus rhythm not restored within 10 min after infusion
- Magnesium sulfate: 1–2 g diluted in D5W over 5–60 min; slower rate preferable if patient is stable.
- Metoprolol: 5 mg IV push over 5 min at 5-min intervals to total of 15 mg, then 50 mg PO b.i.d.
- Procainamide: 20 mg/min until arrhythmia suppressed, hypotension, QRS prolongation of 50%, or total of 17 mg/kg; may be given at rate up to 50 mg/min (peds: 10–15 mg/kg IV over 15 min, then 20–80 $\mu$g/kg/min continuous infusion)
- Propranolol: 0.1 mg/kg in 3 equal doses by slow IV push at 2–3-min intervals, not faster than 1 mg/min (peds: 0.01–0.15 mg/kg/dose slow IV push over 5 min, max 1 mg/dose)
- Sotalol: 1–1.5 mg/kg then infused at 10 mg/min
- Verapamil: 2.5–5.0 mg IV bolus over 2 min; may repeat with 5–10 mg q15–30min to a max of 20 mg

 **FOLLOW UP**

### DISPOSITION
**Admission Criteria**
- New-onset atrial flutter requiring antidysrhythmics, rate control
- Symptomatic (ie, chest pain that warrants a rule out or cardioversion)
- CHF

**Discharge Criteria**
Chronic atrial flutter with good rate control and appropriate anticoagulation

### FOLLOW-UP RECOMMENDATIONS
Cardiologist:
- Radiofrequency ablation of atrial flutter emerging as treatment of choice for patients with symptomatic atrial flutter without identifiable reversible cause

## PEARLS AND PITFALLS
- Be aware of WPW:
  - Do not use adenosine, β-blockers, calcium channel blockers, and digoxin (Class III = can be harmful).
    - Can cause increased ventricular response, which can deteriorate to ventricular fibrillation
- Do not delay cardioversion in an unstable patient for IV placement.
- Use β-blockers with caution in patients with pulmonary disease or CHF.
- 4 major treatment issues in management of patients with atrial flutter:
  - Rate control
  - Prevention of systemic embolization
  - Reversion to sinus rhythm
  - Maintenance of sinus rhythm

## ADDITIONAL READING
- 2005 American Heart Association Guidelines for Cardiopulmonary Resuscitation and Emergency Cardiovascular Care. Part 7.3: Management of Symptomatic Bradycardia and Tachycardia. *Circulation*. 2005;112:IV-67–IV-77.
- Blomstrom-Lundqvist C, Scheinman MM, et al. ACC/AHA/ESC Guidelines for the Management of Patients with Supraventricular Arrhythmias–executive summary. *J Am Coll Cardiol*. 2003;42(8).1493–1531.
- Ghali WA, Wasil BI, Brant R, et al. Atrial flutter and the risk of thromboembolism: A systematic review and meta-analysis. *Am J Med*. 2005;118:101–107.
- Hood RE, Shorofsky SR. Management of arrhythmias in the emergency department. *Cardiol Clin*. 2006;24:125–133.
- Sunil D, Lidhoo P, Pooja MD, et al. Current concepts and management strategies in atrial flutter. *SMJ*. 2009;102(9):917–922.
- UpToDate.com: Overview of the evaluation and management of atrial flutter. Available at: www.utdol.com/online/content/topic.do?topicKey=carrhyth/56810&view=print. Accessed 01/24/10.

 **CODES**

ICD9
427.32 Atrial flutter

# ATRIOVENTRICULAR BLOCKS
*Colleen N. Roche*

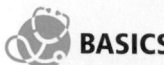 **BASICS**

## DESCRIPTION
- Impaired conduction between the atrium and the ventricle through the AV node or His-Purkinje system
- 1st-degree AV block:
  - Prolonged conduction through the AV node
  - Ventricular impulses are not lost.
  - Generally benign, and occurs in 1.6% healthy adults.
- 2nd-degree AV block:
  - Marked by a failure of some atrial impulses to reach ventricles
  - Mobitz Type I (Wenckebach):
    - Usually secondary to conduction deficit in AV node.
    - Progressive prolongation of the pulse-rate (PR) interval until a nonconducted P wave and a dropped QRS complex occur
    - Generally benign, but may be a complication of an inferior wall MI
  - Mobitz Type II:
    - Conduction deficit is usually below the level of the AV node.
    - PR intervals are constant until single or multiple beats are abruptly dropped.
    - High likelihood of progression to complete heart block
    - Worse prognosis if associated with an acute MI
    - Less common than type I
- 3rd-degree AV block:
  - Also known as complete heart block
  - All atrial impulses are unable to reach the ventricular conducting system; a ventricular escape pacemaker then takes over, resulting in AV dissociation.
  - Constant PP and RR intervals with variable PR intervals because PP and RR intervals are independent of each other.
  - More severe symptoms occur when the block is lower in the conducting system.
  - If secondary to toxicologic agents, often resolves upon omission of offending toxin
  - Never a benign condition

## ETIOLOGY
- Essentially due to:
  - A structural lesion
  - Increase in inherent refractory period
  - Marked shortening of the supraventricular cycle
- MI:
  - 1st-degree block and type I 2nd-degree AV block may be associated with an inferior wall MI:
    - These blocks are transient.
    - AV conduction usually returns to normal with no increased morbidity or mortality.
  - Type II 2nd-degree AV block may be associated with an anterior wall MI:
    - 5% anterior wall MIs are associated with AV blocks.
    - Increased mortality secondary to ventricular arrhythmias and left-heart failure

- Coronary artery disease:
  - Chronic ischemic injury can lead to fibrosis around the AV node
- Toxicologic:
  - Digoxin
  - $\beta$-Blockers
  - Calcium-channel blockers
  - Amiodarone
  - Procainamide
  - Class 1C agents: Propafenone, encainide, flecainide
  - Clonidine
- Congenital
- Valvular heart disease
- Surgical trauma:
  - S/P coronary artery bypass graft or valvular replacement
- Increased vagal tone
- Infectious:
  - Syphilis
  - Diphtheria
  - Chagas disease
  - TB
  - Toxoplasmosis
  - Lyme disease
  - Myocarditis
  - Endocarditis
  - Rheumatic fever
  - Abscess formation in interventricular septum
- Collagen vascular diseases
- Infiltrative diseases:
  - Sarcoidosis
  - Amyloidosis
  - Hemochromatosis
- Cardiomyopathy
- Electrolyte disturbances:
  - Hyperkalemia
- Myxedema
- Hypothermia

### Pediatric Considerations
- Occurs in children, but is often asymptomatic
- Associated mortality is highest in the neonatal period.
- Associated with:
  - Congenitally acquired maternal antibodies
  - Congenital heart disease
  - Infectious etiologies, such as rheumatic fever or myocarditis
- Be sure to consider potential toxic ingestions in pediatric patients with new AV block

 **DIAGNOSIS**

## SIGNS AND SYMPTOMS
### History
- 1st-degree AV block:
  - Asymptomatic
- Type I 2nd-degree AV block:
  - Pulse irregularities
- Type II 2nd-degree AV block and 3rd-degree block:
  - Exercise intolerance
  - Palpitations
  - Chest pain
  - Presyncope/syncope
  - Altered mental status
  - Dyspnea, orthopnea

### Physical Exam
- 1st-degree AV block:
  - No discrete physical exam findings
- Type I 2nd-degree AV block:
  - Regularly irregular pulse
- Type II 2nd-degree AV block and 3rd-degree block:
  - Irregular pulse
  - Hypotension
  - Mental status changes
  - Signs of heart failure:
    - Rales
    - Cyanosis
    - Jugular venous distention

## ESSENTIAL WORKUP
- A 12-lead EKG to determine the type of block and identify evidence of infarction
- 1st-degree AV block:
  - PR interval >0.20 sec
- 2nd-degree AV block:
  - Type I: Progressive prolongation of PR interval until there is a nonconducted P wave and a dropped QRS complex; occurs in repeated cycles; QRS is usually narrow.
  - Type II: PR interval remains constant; atrial impulses are not conducted intermittently, giving the appearance of an occasionally dropped ventricular beat; QRS may be prolonged depending on the level of the lesion.
- 3rd-degree AV block:
  - P waves occur at consistent intervals.
  - QRS complexes occur independently from P waves but also at consistent intervals.
  - QRS complexes are usually narrow unless there is an infranodal conduction disturbance or a ventricular escape rhythm.

## DIAGNOSTIC TESTS & INTERPRETATION
Additional studies aid in confirming the etiology of the identified AV block.

### Lab
- Electrolytes
- Calcium, magnesium
- Cardiac enzymes:
  - Especially for type II 2nd-degree and 3rd degree blocks
- Digoxin level, if patient has been exposed to this medication

### Imaging
- CXR:
  - May identify cardiomyopathy or CHF
- ECG:
  - May identify regional wall motion abnormalities or valvular dysfunction

## DIFFERENTIAL DIAGNOSIS
- Accelerated junctional rhythm
- Idioventricular rhythm
- Sinus bradycardia
- SA block

 TREATMENT

### PRE-HOSPITAL
- Transcutaneous pacing for unstable type II 2nd- or 3rd-degree block
- Atropine:
  - Avoid with type II 2nd-degree block because it may precipitate complete heart block
  - Contraindicated in 3rd-degree heart block with a widened QRS complex
- Attempts should be made to prevent increases in vagal tone

### INITIAL STABILIZATION/THERAPY
- Transcutaneous pacemaker:
  - Necessary for the unstable patient with signs of hypoperfusion:
    ○ Hypotension
    ○ Chest pain
    ○ Dyspnea
    ○ Mental status changes
- Atropine:
  - Can be administered in:
    ○ Complete heart block with a narrow QRS
    ○ Symptomatic sinus bradycardia

## ED TREATMENT/PROCEDURES
- 1st-degree AV block:
  - No treatment required
  - Avoid AV nodal blocking agents
  - Evaluate for associated MI, electrolyte abnormalities, medication excess in the appropriate clinical scenarios
- Type I 2nd-degree AV block:
  - Usually no treatment needed
  - If symptomatic, atropine will enhance AV conduction
- Type II 2nd-degree AV block:
  - Temporary transcutaneous or transvenous pacemaker
  - Atropine is not effective and should be avoided
- 3rd-degree AV block:
  - 1st line of treatment: Emergent pacemaker
  - May transiently respond to atropine with narrow QRS complexes
  - If block is identified to be toxin-mediated, specific treatments include:
    ○ Digoxin-specific antibodies (digoxin overdose)
    ○ Glucagon and calcium (β-blocker or calcium-channel blocker overdose)

## MEDICATION
- Atropine: 0.5–1.0 mg (peds: 0.01–0.03 mg/kg) IV q5min as necessary
- Digoxin-specific antibodies: 10 vials (380 mg) is an appropriate loading dose if digoxin toxicity is strongly suspected:
  - Serum level × weight (kg) = number of vials to be administered
- Glucagon: 5–10 mg (peds: 50 $\mu$g/kg) IV over 5 min
- Calcium chloride: 250–500 mg (peds: 20 mg/kg) IV

 FOLLOW-UP

### DISPOSITION
### Admission Criteria
Monitored bed:
- Type II 2nd-degree block
- 3rd-degree block

### Discharge Criteria
Asymptomatic 1st-degree and type I 2nd-degree blocks: Ensure follow-up for further outpatient workup.

## FOLLOW-UP RECOMMENDATIONS
Asymptomatic 1st-degree and type I 2nd-degree blocks can follow-up with a cardiologist on a routine outpatient basis.

## PEARLS AND PITFALLS
- Obtaining an EKG rapidly in symptomatic patients is paramount.
- Once a high-degree AV block has been diagnosed, initiate transcutaneous pacing immediately
- Obtain a complete history from all available resources; it may help you identify an offending toxin rapidly.
- Common pitfalls:
  - Failure to interpret EKG properly
  - Failure to diagnose AV block appropriately
  - Failure to initiate transcutaneous pacing in a timely fashion
  - Failure to consult cardiology for permanent pacemaker in a timely fashion

## ADDITIONAL READING
- Harrigan RA, Chan TC, Moonblatt S, et al. Temporary transvenous pacemaker placement in the emergency department. *J Emerg Med.* 2007;32(1):105–111.
- Olgin JE, Zipes DP. Specific arrhythmias: Diagnosis and treatment. Libby P, ed., *Braunwald's Heart Disease: A Textbook of Cardiovascular Medicine*, 8th ed. Philadelphia: Saunders Elsevier, 2008:913–923.
- Ufberg JW, Clark JS. Bradydysrhythmias and atrioventricular conduction blocks. *Emerg Med Clin North Am.* 2006;24(1):1–9.
- Yealy DM, Delbridge TR. Dysrhythmias. In Marx J, et al., eds. *Rosen's Emergency Medicine: Concepts and Clinical Practice*, 7th ed. St. Louis. CV Mosby, 2010:93–100.

### See Also (Topic, Algorithm, Electronic Media Element)
- Brady arrhythmias
- Cardiac Pacemakers

 CODES

### ICD9
- 426.11 First degree atrioventricular block
- 426.12 Mobitz (type) ii atrioventricular block
- 426.13 Other second degree atrioventricular block

# BABESIOSIS
*Philip D. Anderson*

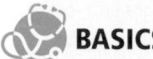 **BASICS**

## DESCRIPTION
- Tick-borne, malaria-like disease caused by Babesia a genus of protozoal piroplasms
- Babesia:
  - 2nd most common blood parasite of mammals
  - Exist in animal reservoirs:
    - Europe (cattle, rats)
    - U.S. (white-footed mouse, meadow voles, white-tailed deer)
  - Lacks an exoerythrocytic phase, so the liver is usually not affected
- Ixodid tick:
  - Most common vector for transmission of babesiosis to humans
  - Protozoa pass from tick salivary glands to mammalian bloodstream where they penetrate erythrocytes, mature and divide.
  - RBC membrane damage leads to lysis, hemolytic anemia and hemoglobinuria.
  - Damaged RBCs become less deformable, enhancing removal by spleen, but asplenic patients less able to clear infected RBCs, leading to more severe disease.
  - Damaged RBCs may result in microvascular stasis with secondary ischemic organ injury to liver, spleen, heart, kidney, or brain.
- Transmission via transfusion of red blood cells, platelets:
  - Rare
  - Low level parasitemia not visible on donor blood smears can transmit disease.
  - Parasites remain viable in banked blood even after freezing/thawing.
  - Symptoms usually develop 1–9 wk after transfusion.
- Asymptomatic infection:
  - 25% of adults and 50% of children
- Mild–moderate disease:
  - Gradual onset of flulike symptoms associated with fevers
  - Parasitemia levels are typically <4%.
  - Infections are usually self-limited or resolve with antibiotic therapy; asymptomatic parasitemia may persist in some patients.
  - Mortality in immune competent patients is usually <5%.
- Severe disease:
  - Defined as hospitalization >2 wk, >2 days in ICU, or leading to death.
  - Parasitemia levels typically >4%; may be up to 80%
  - Population at risk for severe disease:
    - Elderly
    - Asplenic
    - HIV coinfection
    - Immunosuppressive drug use
    - Malignancy
    - Mortality can be as high as 40%

## ETIOLOGY
- *B. microti*:
  - Most common species in the U.S.
  - Northeastern U.S. coastal regions and islands (estimates of seropositivity in population range from 4–21%)
  - Typically causes mild disease in immune competent patients
- *B. divergens*:
  - Most common species seen in Europe
  - Typically infects immune compromised patients and causes more severe disease
- *B. divergens*:
  - Midwest, West Coast U.S.
- *B. duncani*:
  - West Coast U.S.
- *B. venatorum*:
  - Europe

### Pediatric Considerations
Transmission can occur in utero and during delivery; youngest reported case was a 4-wk-old infant.

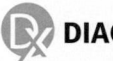 **DIAGNOSIS**

## SIGNS AND SYMPTOMS
Usually presents as a nonspecific febrile flulike illness; there can be a wide range of associated signs and symptoms; ranging from mild to severe; lasting from days to months including:
- Fever:
  - Intermittent or continuous
- Chills, sweats
- Fatigue, malaise, weakness
- Headache, stiff neck
- Myalgias, arthralgias, back pain
- Anorexia, nausea, vomiting, diarrhea, abdominal pain
- Cough, sore throat, shortness of breath
- Emotional lability, depression
- Weight loss
- Dark urine, jaundice

### History
- Flulike illness in patients who live in, or recently traveled to, an endemic area (especially during spring to summer months)
- Recent blood product transfusions
- Shock or sepsis presentation in patients with above history is suggestive of babesiosis (especially in presence of risk factors for severe disease):
  - Splenectomy, HIV, malignancy, immune suppressive drugs, age >50 yr, current or recent Lyme disease (borreliosis) or ehrlichiosis

### Physical Exam
- Fever
- Hepatosplenomegaly
- Jaundice
- Pharyngeal erythema
- Retinopathy with splinter hemorrhages
- Retinal infarcts
- Rash rarely found:
  - Ecchymosis
  - Petechiae
  - Erythema chronicum:
    - Suggestive of concurrent Lyme disease
- Severe disease:
  - Tachypnea
  - Hypoxia
  - Hypotension
  - Altered sensorium

## ESSENTIAL WORKUP
- Microscopy of thin blood smear should be performed in cases of suspected babesiosis.
- PCR is useful early in course of illness when parasitemia levels may be low.

## DIAGNOSTIC TESTS & INTERPRETATION
### Lab
- Microscopy (thin blood smear with Giemsa or Wright stain):
  - Intraerythrocytic parasites can be round, oval, or pear shaped.
  - Parasites in budding tetrad formation (Maltese cross) are pathognomonic for babesiosis, but not commonly seen.
  - Most common finding is intraerythrocytic round or oval (pyriform) rings with pale blue cytoplasm and red-staining nucleus.
  - Extracellular parasites may be seen with high levels of parasitemia.
  - Parasitemia levels may be <1% in early stages of disease, so multiple blood smears may be needed.
  - Ring forms may appear similar to *P. falciparum* (malaria); in babesiosis there are no pigment deposits (hemozoin) that are usually seen with malaria.
- PCR:
  - Amplification of babesial 18s rRNA gene
  - More sensitive than microscopy
  - Useful in cases with low levels of parasitemia
- Serology:
  - Indirect immunofluorescent antibody testing may be useful when microscopy and PCR testing are negative.
  - Serology alone not sufficient to make diagnosis as serum antibody titers usually do not rise until a few weeks after onset of symptoms
  - IgG titers ≥1:256 suggest active or recent infections; IgM titers ≥1:64 suggest acute infection.

- Nonspecific lab abnormalities that may be seen in babesiosis:
  - CBC (anemia, thrombocytopenia, mild leukopenia, atypical lymphocytosis)
  - LFTs (elevated alkaline phosphatase, transaminases, lactate dehydrogenase, bilirubin)
  - Urinalysis (hemoglobinuria, proteinuria)
  - Hemolysis profile (elevated reticulocyte count, decreased serum haptoglobin, hyperbilirubinemia, elevated lactate dehydrogenase, hemoglobinuria)
  - Elevated BUN, creatinine suggests renal insufficiency
  - Hyperkalemia may result from massive hemolysis

## DIFFERENTIAL DIAGNOSIS
- Malaria
- Other tickborne diseases:
  - Lyme disease (borreliosis)
  - Ehrlichiosis
  - Rocky Mountain spotted fever
  - Colorado tick fever
  - Q fever
  - Tularemia
  - Relapsing fever
- Typhoid fever
- Acute hemolytic anemia

 **TREATMENT**

### PRE-HOSPITAL
- Ensure a patent airway in patients with respiratory distress
- Provide supplemental oxygen and ventilatory assistance as needed.
- If patient presents in shock, establish IV access and administer a fluid bolus of 0.9% NS 500 ml (peds: 20 ml/kg) IV

### INITIAL STABILIZATION/THERAPY
- Airway management, ventilatory support for patients with acute respiratory distress
- IV access should be established in patients with evidence or risk factors for severe disease.
- IV fluids, pressor support for patients in shock
- Cardiac monitor: Patients with severe disease may develop cardiac ischemia, arrhythmias.

### ED TREATMENT/PROCEDURES
- Antipyretics for fever
- Start antibiotic therapy in symptomatic patients after confirming diagnosis on microscopy or PCR.
- Mild–moderate disease:
  - Oral atovaquone PLUS azithromycin for 7–10 days is regimen of choice.
  - Clindamycin PLUS quinine is effective alternative, but associated with significant side effects (tinnitus, gastroenteritis) that may require reduced dosing or stopping medication in up to a third of patients.

- Severe disease:
  - IV clindamycin PLUS oral quinine for 7–10 days is regimen of choice.
  - RBC exchange transfusion is indicated in patients with parasitemia >10%, hemoglobin <10 g/dL, as well as those with pulmonary, renal, or hepatic complications.
  - Persistent or relapsing disease may be seen in immunocompromised patients; these patients should receive antibiotic therapy for at least 6 wk, continuing for 2 wk after last positive blood smear; can use standard combinations (above).
- Asymptomatic infection:
  - Antibiotics are not indicated unless parasitemia on blood smears persists >3 mo.

## MEDICATION
- Acetaminophen: 325–1,000 mg (peds: 40–60 mg/kg/day) PO/PR q4–6h PRN
- Atovaquone: 750 mg (peds: 20 mg/kg; max 750 mg/dose) PO b.i.d. for 7 days
- Azithromycin: 500 mg (peds: 10 mg/kg; max 500 mg) PO on day 1, followed by 250 mg (peds: 5 mg/kg; max 250 mg) PO per day: 6 days
- Clindamycin: 300–600 mg (peds: 7–10 mg/kg q6–8h) IV q 6h; 600 mg (peds: 7–10 mg/kg q6–8h) PO q8h for 7–10 days
- Ibuprofen: 400 mg (peds: 20–40 mg/kg/day) PO q6–8h PRN
- Quinine: 650 mg (peds: 25 mg/kg/day) PO q8h for 7–10 days

 **FOLLOW-UP**

### DISPOSITION
#### Admission Criteria
- Patients with parasitemia >4%, severe anemia (hemoglobin <10 g/dL), significant symptoms or complications, or need for exchange transfusion require admission:
  - Respiratory distress
  - Hypotension or shock
  - New renal insufficiency or hepatic failure
  - Altered mental status
  - Severe hemolysis (jaundice, hematuria)
- Admission should also be considered in patients without any of the above, but who have risk factors for developing severe disease:
  - Immunodeficiency, asplenia, malignancy/chemotherapy
  - Elevated alkaline phosphatase, elevated WBC counts, and male gender have been associated with severe outcomes.

#### Discharge Criteria
- Patients with asymptomatic, mild or moderate disease
- Parasitemia <4%
- Intact spleen
- Able to tolerate oral medications

#### Issues for Referral
Immunodeficient patients are more likely to have persistent or relapsing disease following initial treatment and should be referred for infectious disease consultation.

### FOLLOW-UP RECOMMENDATIONS
Patients diagnosed with babesiosis should follow up with their primary care physician or infectious disease specialist for monitoring of parasitemia levels following completion of antibiotic course in symptomatic patients and at 3 mo in asymptomatic patients.

## PEARLS AND PITFALLS
- Consider babesiosis a life-threatening disease in asplenic patients.
- Consider babesiosis as a potential cause of respiratory distress/shock in patients with a travel history to an endemic area.
- Microscopy findings may not be present in early stages of disease when parasitemia levels are low.

## ADDITIONAL READING
- Gelfand JA, Vannier E. Clinical manifestations, diagnosis, treatment, and prevention of babesiosis. *UpToDate.* 2009.
- Leder K, Weller PF. Epidemiology and pathogenesis of babesiosis. *UpToDate.* 2009.
- Vannier E, Gewurz BE, Krause PJ. Human babesiosis. *Infect Dis Clin North Am.* 2008;22(3):469–488, viii–ix
- White DJ, Talarico J, Chang HG, et al., Human babesiosis in New York State: Review of 139 hospitalized cases and analysis of prognostic factors. *Arch Intern Med.* 1998;158(19):2149–2154.

### See Also (Topic, Algorithm, Electronic Media Element)
Lyme Disease

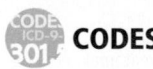 **CODES**

### ICD9
088.82 Babesiosis

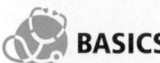 **BASICS**

## DESCRIPTION
- Low back pain (LBP):
  - Refers to pain in the area between the lower rib cage and the gluteal folds, often with radiation into the thighs
- Sciatica
  - Pain in the distribution of the lower lumbar spinal roots
  - May be accompanied by neurosensory and motor deficits
- Pain classification:
  - Acute: <6 wk
  - Subacute: 6–12 wk
  - Chronic: >12 wk

## ETIOLOGY
- Nonspecific musculoligamentous source including muscle, ligament, fascia (great majority)
- Herniation of the nucleus pulposus
- Degenerative joints or discs
- Spinal stenosis
- Anatomic abnormalities—especially spondylolisthesis
- Fractures from trauma and osteoporosis
- Underlying systemic diseases (minority):
  - Neoplasm
  - Infections
  - Vascular (dissection, aneurysm, and thrombosis)
  - Renal
  - GI
  - Pelvic organ pathology

 **DIAGNOSIS**

## SIGNS AND SYMPTOMS
- Musculoligamentous:
  - Poorly localized and dull back/gluteal pain without radiation past the knee
  - Usually there are no objective neurologic signs.
  - Back spasm is a variable and poorly reproducible finding.
- Sciatica:
  - Sharp, shooting, well-localized pain
  - Leg complaints often greater than back
  - May present with:
    - Asymmetric deep tendon reflexes
    - Decreased sensation in a dermatomal distribution
    - Objective weakness
- Massive central disc herniation (cauda equina syndrome):
  - Decreased perineal sensation
  - Urinary retention with overflow incontinence
  - Fecal incontinence

- Infectious processes:
  - Fever
  - Localized percussion tenderness of the vertebral bodies
- Bony lesion:
  - Continuous pain that does not change with rest
  - Constitutional symptoms
- Vascular etiology:
  - Severe, often "ripping or tearing" pain
  - May be associated with cold or insensate extremities

### History
- Can assist with focusing and narrowing differential diagnosis. Helps rule out concerning pathology for pain:
  - Intensity
  - Quality
  - Location and radiation
  - Onset
  - Exacerbating or remitting factors
  - Social or psychological factors
  - Response to previous therapy
- Risk factors for serious disease:
  - Fever
  - Constitutional symptoms
  - Trauma
  - Age >60 years
  - History of cancer:
    - Especially those that metastasize to bone
  - Chronic steroid use
  - IV drug use
  - Recent instrumentation or bacteremia
  - Night pain

### Physical Exam
- Fever
- Spasm or soft tissue tenderness is a poorly reproducible finding:
  - Vertebral tenderness sensitive but nonspecific for infection
- Straight leg raise—elevating the leg while supine reproduces sciatic symptoms:
  - Ipsilateral raise highly sensitive but not specific
  - Crossed leg raise highly specific but insensitive
- Ankle and great toe dorsiflexion and ankle plantar flexion (L5, S1 nerve roots)
- Ankle deep tendon reflexes (S1)
- Dermatomal sensory examination:
  - Assess for saddle anesthesia
- Rectal sphincter tone

## ESSENTIAL WORKUP
- Thorough history and physical, including detailed neurologic and vascular examination
- No specific tests are needed for musculoligamentous or sciatic pain without complicating factors.
- Rapid diagnostic testing and vascular consultation for pain concerning aortic etiology

## DIAGNOSTIC TESTS & INTERPRETATION
### Lab
- Urinalysis for suspected:
  - UTI
  - Pyelonephritis
  - Prostatitis
- ESR:
  - Very sensitive, though nonspecific for infectious or inflammatory etiologies
  - Used for screening if suspicion exists

### Imaging
- Lumbosacral radiograph:
  - Significant trauma
  - Age >50 yr
  - History or signs/symptoms of cancer
  - Fever
  - IV drug user
  - Pain at rest
  - Suspicion of ankylosing spondylitis or inflammatory etiology
  - Pain that does not improve after 4 wk
- Bedside US:
  - Full bladder suggests urinary retention
  - Abdominal aortic aneurysm
  - Abdominal CT if patient stable and abdominal aortic aneurysm is suspected
- MRI:
  - Suspicion of abscess:
    - Fever, immunocompromised, IVDA, history of bacteremia
  - Suspicion of metastatic tumor:
    - Systemic cancer, weight loss
  - Suspicion of hematoma:
    - Anticoagulation, recent spinal anesthesia
  - Rapidly progressing neurologic symptoms
  - Urinary retention or fecal incontinence associated with back pain
- CT:
  - Secondary modality for diagnosis of abscess, cancer or massive disc when MRI unavailable
  - Test of choice of imaging potential unstable fractures

## DIFFERENTIAL DIAGNOSIS
- Spinal origins—in the majority of patients no precise anatomic site is discovered:
  - Musculoligamentous (majority)
  - Discogenic
  - Fracture
  - Spondylolisthesis
  - Ankylosing spondylitis
  - Osteomyelitis
  - Epidural abscess/hematoma
  - Neoplasm
- Nonspinal causes:
  - AAA
  - Prostatitis
  - Upper UTI
  - Abdominal neoplasm
  - Renal colic
  - Aortic dissection

**TREATMENT**

### PRE-HOSPITAL
- Immobilization is not generally recommended for nontraumatic pain.
- Major trauma patients with acute back pain should be immobilized on a backboard until an unstable fracture can be ruled out.
- Rapid transport with IV access for any patient with concerns of vascular etiology

### ED TREATMENT/PROCEDURES
- APAP: Considered 1st-line therapy for mild to moderate pain
- NSAIDs:
  - Musculoligamentous pain
    Renal colic:
    ○ Similar benefits as APAP but less optimal side effect profile
- Muscle relaxants:
  - Cyclobenzaprine, methocarbamol, or carisoprodol
  - Possible benefits must be balanced by side effects, mostly sedation and dry mouth
- Benzodiazepines:
  - No clear evidence to prove or disprove utility
- Narcotics:
  - A reasonable course may be given for severe pain not relieved by anti-inflammatory or APAP.
- Corticosteroids:
  - No benefit in radicular or nonradicular back pain
- Spinal manipulation:
  - A short course (<2 wk) may be helpful in acute LBP without sciatica.
- Physical therapy/exercise:
  - No clear consensus for indications
  - May be helpful in symptomatic relief, preventing further episodes and teaching patients
- Acupuncture:
  - Controversial, probable benefit for chronic musculoskeletal pain
  - No clear benefit over other modalities
- Massage:
  - May be beneficial when combined with exercises and education
- Heat/cold therapy:
  - Limited evidence to support that heat wrap therapy may help reduce pain and disability for patients with back pain <3 mo
- Bed rest:
  - Unhelpful to speed recovery and may impede improvement. If patient requires bed rest acutely or is symptomatically improved, 1 or 2 days may be recommended.
- Back exercises:
  - Unlikely to be useful in acute phase; may assist with prevention of future episodes
- Expected recovery to pain-free state:
  - ~33% within 1 wk
  - ~90% within 6–8 wk
- Recurrence is common: ~40%.

### MEDICATION
#### First Line
- Acetaminophen: 650–1,000 mg PO q4–6h (peds: 15 mg/kg q6h)
- Hydrocodone/acetaminophen: 5/500 mg PO q4–6h
- Ibuprofen: 600–800 mg PO q6–8h (peds: 10 mg/kg q6h)
- Naproxen: 250–500 mg PO q12h
- Oxycodone/acetaminophen: 5/500 mg PO q4–6h

#### Second Line
- Cyclobenzaprine: 5–10 mg PO t.i.d.
- Methocarbamol: 500–1,500 PO q6h
- Valium: 5–10 mg PO q8h
- You may combine 1st- and 2nd-line therapies but the side effect profile will increase. 2nd-line therapy should not be prescribed as monotherapy.

 **FOLLOW-UP**

### DISPOSITION
#### Admission Criteria
- Severe pain with inability to ambulate
- Pain unresponsive to ED management
- Progressive neurologic deficits
- Signs of cauda equina syndrome
- Evidence of infectious, vascular, or neoplastic etiologies

#### Discharge Criteria
Uncomplicated presentation with ability to control pain and ambulate

#### Geriatric Considerations
- Maintain a high suspicion for serious disease including vascular etiology, neoplasm, or infection. Have a low threshold for imaging or diagnostic testing.

#### Pediatric Considerations
- Back pain is unusual in the pediatric patient; a high suspicion for an infectious etiology must be maintained.
- For musculoligamentous pain, a single trial found that Ibuprofen provides good pain control with a low side effect profile.

#### Pregnancy Considerations
Limited evidence suggests that tailored strengthening and pelvic tilt exercises combined with routine prenatal care may have some benefit if treating back pain; unclear if they prevent onset of pain.

#### Issues for Referral
Urgent neurosurgical or orthopedic consultation for definite diagnosis or high suspicion for abscess or lesion (disc, neoplasm or other) with rapidly progressive objective neurologic findings

### FOLLOW-UP RECOMMENDATIONS
- Uncomplicated back pain: PCP in 1–2 wk
- New sciatica without neurological findings: PCP or specialist in 7–10 days
- Complicated with sensory findings only or minimal motor symptoms: 24–48 hr
- Marked motor symptoms, rapidly progressive, or bowel/bladder findings warrant specialist consultation in the ED or transfer to a center with specialists available.

## PEARLS AND PITFALLS
- Consider MRI if there is a history of IV drug use to rule out epidural abscess.
- Elderly patients with minimal trauma may sustain fractures.
- Consider vascular etiology in elderly patients with first time presentation of back pain.
- Advise patients that this is often a prolonged course and they should not expect rapid resolution.

## ADDITIONAL READING
- Clark E, Plint AC, Correll R, et al. A randomized, controlled trial of acetaminophen, ibuprofen, and codeine for acute pain relief in children with musculoskeletal trauma. *Pediatrics*. 2007;119(6): 1271.
- Davies RA, Maher CG, Hancock MJ. A systematic review of paracetamol for non-specific low back pain. *Eur Spine J*. 2008;17:1423–1430.
- French SD, Cameron MC, Walker BF, et al. Superficial heat or cold for low back pain. *Spine* 2006;31(9):998–1006.
- Roelofs PDDM, Deyo RA, Koes BW, et al. Non-steroidal anti-inflammatory drugs for low back pain. *Spine*. 2008;33(16):1766–1774.
- Roger C, Huffman LH. Medications for acute and chronic low back pain: A review of the evidence for an American Pain Society/American College of Physicians Clinical Practice Guideline. *Ann Intern Med*. 2007;147:505–514.

**CODES**

### ICD9
- 724.2 Lumbago
- 724.5 Backache, unspecified

# BACTERIAL TRACHEITIS

*Gary Bubly*
*Noah H. Rosenberg*

 BASICS

## DESCRIPTION
- A tracheal infection potentially causing acute airway obstruction. Also known as bacterial croup and laryngotracheobronchitis.
- Usually secondary bacterial infection of trachea, complicating antecedent viral infection, or less commonly instrumentation
- Fatal in 0–20%
- Tracheal membrane formation, purulent discharge, subglottic edema, erosions, with normal epiglottis
- Classically presents with prodrome similar to croup followed by rapid deterioration and loss of airway patency
- Mean age 5 yr; rarely occurs in adults
- More common in children than epiglottitis, presumably due to success of *Haemophilus influenzae* immunization
- More frequent August–December

### ALERT
Patients may present with a fairly benign course, followed by rapid deterioration, with respiratory distress, toxic appearance, and acute airway obstruction.

## ETIOLOGY
- *Staphylococcus aureus* (with occ. MRSA)
- *Moraxella catarrhalis*
- *Streptococcus pneumoniae*
- *Group A streptococcal species*
- *Pseudomonas aeruginosa*
- *Haemophilus influenzae type B*
- *Escherichia Coli*
- Anaerobes
- *Klebsiella pneumoniae*
- Nocardia
- Associated with influenza A and B, parainfluenza, adenovirus, and RSV viral infections
- Aspergillus, HSV in immunocompromised hosts (HIV)

 DIAGNOSIS

## SIGNS AND SYMPTOMS
### History
Usually preceding viral infection with acute deterioration in course of illness

### Physical Exam
- Fever
- Cough
- Retractions
- Inspiratory/expiratory stridor
- Toxic appearance
- Hoarseness
- Cyanosis
- Nasal flaring
- Sore throat/neck pain
- Dysphonia (drooling uncommon)
- Complications:
  - Respiratory:
    - Airway obstruction
    - Subglottic stenosis
    - Pulmonary edema
    - Pneumothorax
    - ARDS
    - Endotracheal tube (ETT) plugging
  - Infection:
    - Septic shock
    - TSS
    - Pneumonia
    - Retropharyngeal cellulitis
  - Cardiopulmonary arrest
  - Renal failure

## ESSENTIAL WORKUP
- Clinical assessment and management of airway takes priority over diagnostic workup; secure airway, optimally in operating room under controlled conditions.
- Ensure adequate oxygenation before proceeding:
  - Pulse oximetry

## DIAGNOSTIC TESTS & INTERPRETATION
### Lab
- WBC variably elevated
- Blood cultures usually negative
- Request tracheal cultures from endoscopist/surgeon.

### Imaging
Radiographs of neck soft tissue:
- If done, perform in ED; accompany and monitor at all times.
- Intratracheal membranes
- Tracheal margin irregularities
- Subglottic narrowing
- Clouding of tracheal air column
- Irregular intratracheal densities
- Normal epiglottis

### Diagnostic Procedures/Surgery
- Flexible fiberoptic laryngoscopy:
  - Permits direct visualization of epiglottis
  - Mucosal edema
  - Subglottic edema, secretions, membrane
- Bronchoscopy:
  - Direct visualization of trachea
  - Laryngotracheal inflammation and erosions
  - Mucopurulent secretions
  - Membranes
  - Therapeutic stripping of membranes
  - Enables direct culture of material

## DIFFERENTIAL DIAGNOSIS
- Infection:
  - Croup
  - Epiglottitis
  - Peritonsillar abscess
  - Retropharyngeal abscess
  - Uvulitis
  - Laryngeal diphtheria
- Angioedema
- Intraluminal obstruction:
  - Foreign body aspiration
- Caustic ingestion
- Trauma

## TREATMENT

### PRE-HOSPITAL
- Assess airway/breathing:
  – Supplemental oxygen
  – Racemic epinephrine aerosol if easily tolerated
  – Reassurance; avoid agitating child
- Bag-valve-mask (BVM) ventilation if in respiratory failure
- Intubate if unable to maintain airway with BVM and other measures
- Immediate transport
- Notify receiving ED of airway status.

### INITIAL STABILIZATION/THERAPY
Airway management:
- Anticipate difficult airway.
- Intubation required in ~75% (40–100%) of patients. More frequently required in younger patients. Active airway management ensures stable airway and facilitates suctioning
- Intubation should ideally be performed in the operating room with surgical airway backup.
- Select an ETT 1–2 sizes smaller than usual for age/size.
- Meticulous ETT care and suctioning
- If BVM ventilation needed, use appropriately sized mask with 2-hand seal.
- Supplemental humidified oxygen

### ED TREATMENT/PROCEDURES
- Continue monitoring of ventilation and oxygenation.
- IV fluids, bolus, as necessary
- Bronchoscopy if not rapidly deteriorating:
  – Assess need for intubation
    Therapeutic stripping of membranes
- IV antibiotics to cover typical pathogens:
  – Ceftriaxone and nafcillin or vancomycin
  – Vancomycin or clindamycin for penicillin-allergic patients
  – Consider corticosteroid therapy

### MEDICATION
- Ceftriaxone: 50 mg/kg IV, max 2 g
- Nafcillin: 50 mg/kg IV; max 2 g
- Ampicillin/sulbactam: 50mg/kg; max 3 g
- Vancomycin: 15 mg/kg IV; max 1 g
- Clindamycin: 10 mg/kg IV; max 1 g
- Racemic epinephrine: 2.25% solution diluted 1:8 with water in doses of 2–4 mL via aerosol
- Dexamethasone: 0.6 mg/kg IV

### First Line
Ceftriaxone plus nafcillin

### Second Line
Vancomycin or clindamycin:
- Consider if penicillin allergic, and in areas of high prevalence of methicillin-resistant *staphylococcus aureus*

## FOLLOW-UP

### DISPOSITION
### Admission Criteria
All patients with suspected or documented bacterial tracheitis:
- Admit to PICU.
- PICU length of stay varies from 3–9 days.

### Discharge Criteria
None

### Issues for Referral
Critical care, otolaryngologist, or pulmonologist should be consulted.

### FOLLOW-UP RECOMMENDATIONS
Few long-term complications

## PEARLS AND PITFALLS
May be more severe in younger patients due to narrower tracheal diameters

## ADDITIONAL READING
- Hopkins A, Lahiri T, Salerno R, et al. Changing epidemiology of life-threatening upper airway infections: The re-emergence of bacterial tracheitis. *Pediatrics*. 2006;118:1418–1421.
- Huang YL, Peng CC, Chiu NC, et al. Bacterial tracheitis in pediatrics: 12 year experience at a medical center in Taiwan. *Pediatr Int*. 2009;51: 110–113.
- Salamone FN, Bobbitt DB, Myer CM, et al. Bacterial tracheitis reexamined: Is there a less severe manifestation? *Otolaryngol Head Neck Surg*. 2004;131:871–876.
- Tebruegge M, Pantadazidou A, Thorburn K, et al. Bacterial tracheitis: A multi-centre perspective. *Scan J Inf Dis*. 2009;41:548–557.

### See Also (Topic, Algorithm, Electronic Media Element)
Epiglottitis, Pediatric and Adult

# BARBITURATES POISONING

Shaun D. Carstairs
David A. Tanen

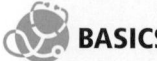 **BASICS**

## DESCRIPTION
- Class of sedative–hypnotic agents
- Derivatives of barbituric acid
- Mechanism:
  - Enhances activity of g-aminobutyric acid (GABA)
  - At high levels, directly opens GABA-A associated chloride channel
  - Leads to inhibition of vascular smooth muscle tone
  - May lead to direct myocardial depression

## ETIOLOGY
Overdose of barbiturates:
- Intentional or nonintentional

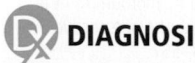 **DIAGNOSIS**

## SIGNS AND SYMPTOMS
- CNS:
  - Lethargy
  - Slurred speech
  - Incoordination
  - Ataxia
  - Coma (can mimic brain death)
  - Loss of reflexes
- Cardiovascular:
  - Hypotension
  - Bradycardia
- Ophthalmologic:
  - Miosis (generally associated with deep coma)
  - Nystagmus
  - Dysconjugate gaze
- Other:
  - Respiratory depression
  - Hypothermia
  - Bullae or "barb blisters"

### History
- Determine if this was an intentional overdose:
  - Pill bottles at the scene
  - History of depression or suicidal ideation
- Determine if there was a medication error:
  - What other medications was the patient taking?
  - Were there any recent changes in dose?
- Estimate how long the patient may have been unresponsive.

### Physical Exam
- CNS abnormalities:
  - Ataxia to coma
- Respiratory depression
- Cardiovascular:
  - Bradycardia and hypotension
- Ophthalmologic:
  - Miosis
  - Nystagmus
  - Dysconjugate gaze
- Hypothermia
- Bullae or "barb blisters"

## ESSENTIAL WORKUP
- Finger stick glucose
- Oxygen saturation monitor
- Monitor BP

### ALERT
Barbiturate poisoning can mimic brain death:
- Cannot pronounce a patient brain dead until barbiturate poisoning has been ruled out

## DIAGNOSTIC TESTS & INTERPRETATION
### Lab
- Electrolytes, BUN/creatinine, glucose:
  - Calculate anion gap
  - Assess for renal failure
- Urinalysis:
  - For myoglobin
  - For crystalluria (Primidone)
- Creatine phosphokinase for evidence of rhabdomyolysis
- Urine toxicology screen
- Obtain serum phenobarbital level (if suspected).
- Acetaminophen and salicylate levels if suspected suicide attempt
- TFTs

### Imaging
- CT scan of head for altered mental status
- CXR for evidence of aspiration

### Diagnostic Procedures/Surgery
- Non Con Head CT
- Lumbar puncture

## DIFFERENTIAL DIAGNOSIS
- Sedative–hypnotic poisoning (including $\gamma$-hydroxybutyrate [GHB] and its precursors)
- Carbon monoxide poisoning
- CNS infections
- Space-occupying lesions of the head
- Hypoglycemia
- Uremia
- Electrolyte imbalance (ie, hypermagnesemia)
- Postictal state following seizure
- Hypothyroidism
- Liver failure
- Psychiatric illness

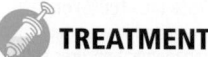 **TREATMENT**

## PRE-HOSPITAL
- Moderate to severe poisonings require paramedic transport.
- Intubation is often necessary because of respiratory depression or loss of gag reflex.
- IV access and supplemental oxygen:
  - IV fluid bolus for hypotension

## INITIAL STABILIZATION/THERAPY
- ABCs:
  - Administer supplemental oxygen.
  - Severe poisonings usually require endotracheal intubation.
- 0.9% NS:
  - Hypotensive patients require at least 1–2 L IV fluid resuscitation.
  - Pressor support may be necessary for refractory hypotension.
- Activated charcoal effectively binds barbiturates and may decrease systemic absorption.

## ED TREATMENT/PROCEDURES

- Administer 1 dose of activated charcoal:
  - Utility greatest if given within 1 hr of ingestion
  - Ensure patient is awake and alert (or airway protected) prior to administration.
  - Consider "gut dialysis" with repeated dose activated charcoal (without sorbitol) given q2–4h (as long as bowel sounds are present).
- Rewarm patient if hypothermic (see "Hypothermia" chapter).
- Treat hypotension resistant to IV fluid bolus with vasopressors (dopamine, norepinephrine, epinephrine).
- Alkalinize the urine for phenobarbital intoxication to increase excretion (not effective for shorter-acting barbiturates).
- Treat hyperkalemia (from muscle breakdown) with calcium, sodium bicarbonate, insulin and glucose, and/or potassium-binding agents.
- Repeat phenobarbital level in 2–4 hr to determine whether level is increasing.
- Consider hemodialysis if patient has:
  - Decreased or no renal function
  - Prolonged coma
  - Serum phenobarbital level >100 mg/dL
  - Refractory hypotension

## MEDICATION

### First Line

- Activated charcoal: 1 g/kg PO
- Dopamine: 5–10 mcg/kg/min titrating to desired effect (to max of 20 mcg/kg/min)
- Norepinephrine: 2–4 mcg/min titrating to desired effect (to max of 10 mcg/min)
- Sodium bicarbonate (in phenobarbital poisoning):
  - Bolus: 1–3 ampules (44 mEq/ampule) IV over 20–30 min (peds: 1–2 mEq/kg/dose)
  - Maintenance: 2–3 ampules (100–150 mEq) in 1 L D5W at 150–200 mL/h (peds: 2x maintenance fluid requirements) to achieve a blood pH of 7.45–7.50 and maintain urine output of 2 mL/kg/h

### Second Line

Epinephrine: 0.1 mcg/kg/min titrating to desired effect (to max of 1 mcg/kg/min)

##  FOLLOW-UP

### DISPOSITION

#### Admission Criteria

ICU admission for:

- Coma
- Respiratory depression
- Hypotension
- Hypothermia
- Rhabdomyolysis

#### Discharge Criteria

Asymptomatic after minimum of 6 hr of observation with 2 consecutive subtoxic phenobarbital levels before discharge

#### Issues for Referral

- If intentional overdose, will require psychiatric evaluation
- For nonintentional overdose, referral for adjustment in medications

### FOLLOW-UP RECOMMENDATIONS

For nonintentional overdose, may need referral for adjustment in medications or change of medications to agents with a greater therapeutic window.

## PEARLS AND PITFALLS

- Hypothermia may be pronounced:
  - Ensure core temperature is measured.
- Check for rhabdomyolysis, since the patient may have been down for a while.
- Barbiturate poisoning can cause prolonged coma:
  - Ensure medication effects have resolved prior to making diagnosis of brain death

## ADDITIONAL READING

- Buckley NA, McManus PR. Changes in fatalities due to overdose of anxiolytic and sedative drugs in the UK (1983–1999). *Drug Saf.* 2004;27:135–141.
- Lee DC. Sedative-hypnotic agents. In: Flomenbaum NE, et al., eds. *Goldfrank's toxicologic emergencies,* 8th ed. New York: McGraw-Hill, 2006;1098–1111.
- Pond SM, Olson KR, Osterloh J, et al. Randomized study of the treatment of phenobarbital overdose with repeated doses of activated charcoal. *JAMA.* 1984;251:3104–3108.

### See Also (Topic, Algorithm, Electronic Media Element)

- Benzodiazepine, Poisoning
- Coma
- Hypothermia
- Rhabdomyolysis

# BAROTRAUMA
*Peter J. Park*

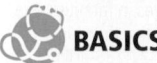

## BASICS

### DESCRIPTION
Injury resulting from the expansion or contraction of gases in an enclosed space

### ETIOLOGY
- Tissue damage results when a gas-filled space does not equalize its pressure with external pressure.
- Boyle's law: At a constant temperature, pressure (P) is inversely related to volume (V):
  – $PV = K$ (constant) or $P_1V_1 = P_2V_2$
  – As pressure increases/decreases, volume decreases/increases.
- Solid and liquid-filled spaces distribute pressure equally.
- Volume changes experienced during diver ascent are greatest in the few feet nearest the surface.
- Gas-filled cavities in the body are subject to expansion/contraction:
  – Middle ear:
    ○ Barotrauma of descent
    ○ Most common type of barotraumas
    ○ Seen in 30% of inexperienced divers and 10% of experienced divers
    ○ Inadequate equalization of pressure between middle ear and external ear canal
    ○ Eustachian tube provides sole route of pressure equalization for middle ear.
    ○ Inadequate clearance via eustachian tube leads to increasingly negative pressure gradient across tympanic membrane (TM).
  – External ear:
    ○ Barotrauma of descent
    ○ Pressure cannot equalize throughout canal because of blockage, and relative intracanal vacuum is created as pressure differential across obstruction increases.
  – Inner ear:
    ○ Barotrauma of descent
    ○ Results from forceful attempts at equalizing middle ear pressure (Valsalva, Frenzel maneuvers)
    ○ Increased middle ear pressure can raise intracranial pressure and cause rupture of round or labyrinth windows, allowing perilymph to enter middle ear.

– Paranasal sinus:
  ○ Barotrauma of descent
  ○ Nasal ostia act as valves to regulate sinus pressure.
  ○ If ostia fail to allow pressure equalization, congestion, edema, and hemorrhage can occur.
– External objects:
  ○ Air pockets in dive suit/mask expand and contract.
– Teeth:
  ○ Air trapped inside a filling
– GI:
  ○ Barotrauma of ascent
  ○ Swallowed air in GI tract expands as external pressure decreases.
– Pulmonary:
  ○ Barotrauma of ascent
  ○ Lungs expand against closed glottis (breath-holding).
  ○ Can lead to pulmonary rupture
  ○ Potential arterial gas embolism (see "Arterial Gas Embolism")
  ○ Divers with decreased lung compliance/increased lung volumes at increased risk (COPD, asthma)

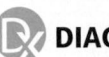

## DIAGNOSIS

### SIGNS AND SYMPTOMS
- Middle ear (barotitis media):
  – Begins as clogged sensation
  – Increasingly painful as pressure differential increases across TM
  – Progresses to rupture of TM
  – TM appearance:
    ○ Progresses from TM congestion to edema to hemorrhage to TM rupture
- External ear:
  – May result from tight-fitting hood, earplug, or earwax occluding canal
  – Auditory canal mucosa becomes edematous, then hemorrhagic, and ultimately tears
- Inner ear:
  – Sudden, severe vertigo
  – Tinnitus
  – Sensoneural hearing loss in affected ear

- Paranasal sinuses (barosinusitis):
  – Sinus congestion
  – Pain
  – Epistaxis
- Facial:
  – Occlusive dive mask: Conjunctival hemorrhage, facial edema, and swelling
- Extremities:
  – Tight-fitting dive suit: Edema and erythema of the skin at locations of air pockets
- Teeth (barodontalgia):
  – Severe tooth pain: Possible air trapped in fillings
- GI (aerogastralgia):
  – Excessive belching
  – Flatulence
  – Abdominal distention
- Pulmonary (pulmonary barotrauma [PBT], or pulmonary overpressurization syndrome):
  – Dyspnea: "The chokes"
  – Cough productive with frothy red sputum
  – Subcutaneous emphysema
  – Delayed symptoms include bull neck appearance, dysphagia, changes in voice character

### History
Onset of symptoms related to dive.

### Physical Exam
- HEENT for tympanic membrane rupture
- Lung for subcutaneous emphysema and pneumothorax
- Neurologic exam for imbalance/ataxia representing inner-ear pathology

### ESSENTIAL WORKUP
- HEENT exam with particular attention paid to TM and auditory canal to determine if rupture has occurred
- Pulmonary exam looking for signs of subcutaneous emphysema and pneumothorax
- Neurologic exam looking for signs of inner ear pathology

## DIAGNOSTIC TESTS & INTERPRETATION
### Lab
ABG for pulmonary symptoms
### Imaging
- Sinus imaging:
  - CT
  - Plain films
- CXR for pneumothorax
- Abdominal series (upright, decubitus) for free air from a ruptured viscus

## DIFFERENTIAL DIAGNOSIS
- Decompression sickness
- Otitis media
- Otitis externa
- Sinusitis

 TREATMENT

### PRE-HOSPITAL
- For barotrauma of descent, unless air-filled cavity has ruptured, no progression of disease on return to normal atmospheric pressure is to be expected.
- If patient requires air evacuation, maintain air cabin pressure at 1 atm or fly below 1,000 feet to avoid aggravating barotraumas.

### INITIAL STABILIZATION/THERAPY
Airway, breathing, and circulation management (ABCs):
- 100% oxygen for ill-appearing patients
- Intubation for patients with subcutaneous emphysema of neck
- Immediate needle thoracostomy for evidence of tension pneumothorax

## ED TREATMENT/PROCEDURES
- Establish IV access for unstable patients.
- Control bleeding from ear or nose.
- Decongestants for middle-ear or sinus congestion
- Antibiotics with TM or sinus rupture
- Analgesics

### MEDICATION
- Amoxicillin: 250–500 mg (peds: 40 mg/kg/24 h) PO t.i.d.
- Oxymetazoline 0.05% (Afrin): 2 or 3 drops/sprays per nostril b.i.d. for 3 days
- Pseudoephedrine (Sudafed): 60 mg (peds: 6–12 yr, 30 mg; 2–5 yr, 15 mg per dose) PO q4–6h
- Trimethoprim-sulfamethoxazole (Bactrim DS): 1 tablet double-strength (160 mg/800 mg) (peds: 40 mg/200 mg per 5 mL, 5 mL/10 kg per dose) PO b.i.d.

 FOLLOW-UP

### DISPOSITION
#### Admission Criteria
- Pulmonary barotraumas (PBTs)
- Inner-ear barotrauma with round window rupture or severe vertigo

#### Discharge Criteria
- Most non-PBT
- ENT follow-up for severe TM or sinus pathology

### FOLLOW-UP RECOMMENDATIONS
ENT referral for ruptured TM or inner-ear–related signs/symptoms

## PEARLS AND PITFALLS
- Watch closely for development of decompression sickness in patients who present with barotraumas.
- Perform careful lung exam for signs of pneumothorax.

## ADDITIONAL READING
- Becker GD, Parell GJ. Barotrauma of the ears and sinuses after scuba diving. *Eur Arch Otorhino* 2001;258(4):159–163.
- Kizer KW, van Hoesen KB. Diving medicine and barotrauma. In: Auerbach PA, ed. *Wilderness Medicine*, 5th ed. St. Louis: CV Mosby, 2007.
- Moon RE, Gorman DF. Treatment of decompression disorders. In: *The Physiology and Medicine of Diving*, 5th ed. Philadelphia: WB Saunders; 2003.
- O'Malley MR. Sudden hearing loss. *Otolaryngol Clin North Am*. 2008;41(3):633–649.
- Raymond LW. Pulmonary barotrauma and related events in divers. *Chest*. 1995;107:1648–1652.
- Tetzlaff K, et al. Risk factors for pulmonary barotrauma in divers. *Chest*. 1997;112(3):654–659.

### See Also (Topic, Algorithm, Electronic Media Element)
- Arterial Gas Embolus
- Decompression Sickness
- Hyperbaric Oxygen Therapy

 CODES

### ICD9
- 993.0 Barotrauma, otitic
- 993.1 Barotrauma, sinus
- 993.2 Other and unspecified effects of high altitude

# BARTHOLIN ABSCESS

*Marilyn Althoff*
*Mark Mandell*

 BASICS

## DESCRIPTION
- The Bartholin glands are located inferiorly on either side of vaginal opening:
  - Ducts open on sides of labial vestibule.
- Obstruction of duct produces a usually painless cyst:
  - Infection of cyst results in abscess formation.

## EPIDEMIOLOGY
### Prevalence
Most common in women aged 20–40 yr

## ETIOLOGY
- Anaerobic and aerobic microflora normally found in vagina:
  - Bacteroides species
  - *Peptostreptococcus* species
  - *Escherichia coli*
  - Other gram-negative organisms
- Occasionally *Neisseria gonorrhoeae* and *Chlamydia trachomatis*

 DIAGNOSIS

## SIGNS AND SYMPTOMS
- Swollen, painful labia
- Tender, fluctuant mass on posterolateral margin of vestibule of vagina
- Warmth, erythema

## History
Acute onset:
- Painful, unilateral labial swelling
- Pain with sitting, walking
- Dyspareunia

## Physical Exam
- Bartholin abscess:
  - Tender, fluctuant, unilateral labial mass
  - Surrounding erythema, warmth
  - Fever uncommon
- Bartholin cyst:
  - Painless, unilateral labial mass

## ESSENTIAL WORKUP
Diagnosis based on findings of tender, localized, fluctuant mass in region of Bartholin gland

## DIAGNOSTIC TESTS & INTERPRETATION
### Lab
- Culture material from abscess for gonorrhea and chlamydia.
- Culture cervix for gonorrhea and chlamydia.

### Imaging
Generally not indicated

## DIFFERENTIAL DIAGNOSIS
- Bartholin cyst
- Carcinoma of Bartholin gland (rare)
- Perineal hernia

 TREATMENT

## ED TREATMENT/PROCEDURES
- Prompt incision and drainage using local anesthesia with patient in lithotomy position
- Narcotic analgesia for patient comfort
- Alternative approaches include:
  - Simple incision and drainage
  - Word catheter method
  - Marsupialization
- Simple incision and drainage:
  - After local anesthesia, palpate abscess between thumb and index fingers.
  - Spread vulva apart and make stab incision on *mucosal* surface of abscess, parallel to hymenal ring.
  - When incising abscess, 2 tissue layers must be penetrated:
    ○ First the labial mucosa
    ○ Then abscess wall
    ○ Free flow of pus indicates penetration of abscess wall.
  - Pack wound with gauze.
  - Follow up in 24–48 hr for removal of packing.
  - Start sitz baths after 24 hr.
  - Consider referral for marsupialization to avoid recurrence.

- Word catheter method:
  - Use small, inflatable, bulb-tipped Word catheter to treat abscess.
  - May avoid recurrence and make marsupialization unnecessary
  - Stab wound is made as with simple incision and drainage:
    - It should be just large enough to easily admit catheter so that balloon does not fall out after inflation.
  - After inserting bulb tip of catheter, inflate balloon by injecting 2–4 mL water using 25-gauge needle (to minimize size of puncture):
    - Overinflation may cause patient discomfort
    - Remedied by withdrawing some water from balloon
  - Sitz baths may be started after 24 hr.
  - Follow-up in 2–4 days.
  - Leave catheter in place for 6–8 wk until epithelialization is complete; after device is removed, gland resumes normal function.
  - Common for catheter to fall out prematurely:
    - If this occurs, catheter may be reinserted or abscess can heal as with simple incision and drainage.
- Marsupialization:
  - Procedure allows for a permanent fistula by suturing wound edges of abscess cavity to edges of labial mucosa:
    - Technically more challenging in ED and better reserved for specialist.
  - Excise an ellipse of labial mucosa that overlays cyst cavity:
  - Incision and drainage of abscess
  - Evert edges of abscess and suture them to labial epithelium using absorbable suture:
    - Opening will shrink but remain patent.
    - Packing is not needed
  - Start sitz baths in 24–48 hr.
  - Follow up within 1 wk.

- Antibiotics not necessary after incision and drainage:
  - If mild cellulitis present or patient immunocompromised, broad-spectrum coverage may be started.
  - If sexually transmitted disease suspected, treat with antibiotics.

### MEDICATION

#### First Line
Broad-spectrum coverage:

- Amoxicillin/clavulanic acid: 500–875 mg PO b.i.d. for 5 days with metronidazole 500 mg PO b.i.d. for 5 days
- Ciprofloxacin: 500 mg PO b.i.d. for 5 days with metronidazole 500 mg PO b.i.d. for 5 days

#### Second Line
Treat for STD if indicated

 **FOLLOW-UP**

### DISPOSITION

#### Admission Criteria
- Sepsis
- Significant cellulitis
- Evidence of necrotizing infection

#### Discharge Criteria
Well-appearing patients may be discharged with designated follow-up plan.

#### Issues for Referral
Patients should have gynecologic follow-up:
- Follow up in 24–48 hr for removal of packing.
- Follow-up in 2–4 days after insertion of Word catheter.

### FOLLOW-UP RECOMMENDATIONS
Continue sitz baths for at least 72 hr.

## PEARLS AND PITFALLS

- Do not mistake a nontender Bartholin cyst, which does not require immediate treatment, for an inflamed abscess.
- Consider malignancy as an alternative cause of a mass, particularly in women >40 yr.
- Incision should be on mucosal surface of abscess.

## ADDITIONAL READING

- Patil S, Sultan AH. Bartholin's cysts and abscesses. *J Obstet Gynaecol.* 2007;27:241–245.
- Pundir J, Auld BJ. Review of management of diseases of Bartholin's gland. *J Obstet Gynaecol.* 2008;28:161–165.
- Word B. Office treatment of cyst and abscess of Bartholin's gland duct. *South Med J.* 1968;61:514–518.
- Zeger W, Holt K. Gynecologic infections. *Emerg Med Clin North Am.* 2003;21:631–648.

### See Also (Topic, Algorithm, Electronic Media Element)
- Treatment of Chlamydia
- Treatment of Gonococcal Disease

# BELL PALSY
Robert F. McCormack
Richard S. Krause

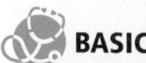 BASICS

## DESCRIPTION
- Acute, *idiopathic* peripheral CN VII (facial nerve) palsy
- Complete recovery in 85% of cases without treatment
- Degree of deficit correlates with prognosis:
  - Complete lesions have poorest prognosis.
  - Partial lesions often have excellent results.
- Recovery usually begins within 2 wk (often taste returns 1st) and is complete by 2–3 mo:
  - Advanced age and slow recovery are poor prognosticators.
- Affects men and women equally
- Age predominance between the 3rd and 5th decade (may occur at any age)
- Incidence 15–40 per 100,000 per year
- The most common cause of facial nerve palsy in children

## ETIOLOGY
- Idiopathic by definition, but viral cause (particularly herpes simplex) suspected
- Lyme disease, infectious mononucleosis (Epstein-Barr virus [EBV] infection), varicella-zoster infections, and others may cause peripheral 7th nerve palsy.
- Mechanism: Edema and nerve degeneration within stylomastoid foramen
- Innervation to each side of forehead is from both motor cortices:
  - Unilateral cortical processes do *not* completely disrupt motor activity of forehead.
- Only peripheral or brainstem lesion can interrupt motor function of just 1 side of forehead.

 DIAGNOSIS

## SIGNS AND SYMPTOMS
### History
Sudden onset of unilateral facial droop, incomplete eyelid closure, and loss of forehead muscle tone:
- Maximal deficit by 5 days in almost all cases (2 days in 50%)
- Tearing (68%) or dryness of eye (16%) and less frequent blinking on affected side
- Subjective "numbness" of the affected side
- Abnormal taste, drooling
- Hyperacusis (sensitivity to loud sounds)
- Fullness or pain behind mastoid
- Viral prodrome frequently reported

### Physical Exam
- Unilateral facial palsy including the forehead
- If forehead muscle tone is *not* lost, a central lesion is strongly implied (ie, this is *not* Bell palsy)
- Motor weakness isolated to 7th nerve distribution:
  - Involves both upper and lower face
- An otherwise normal neurologic exam including all cranial nerves and extremity motor function
- The Bell phenomenon (upward rolling of the eye on attempted lid closure) may be seen.

## ESSENTIAL WORKUP
Diagnosis is clinical and based on history and physical exam.

## DIAGNOSTIC TESTS & INTERPRETATION
### Lab
- Not helpful in diagnosis of Bell palsy
- Lyme titers are useful when Lyme disease is suspected or in endemic area
- Tests for mononucleosis (CBC, monospot) if EBV infection suspected

## DIFFERENTIAL DIAGNOSIS
- Brainstem events (mass, bleed, infarct) affecting CN VII almost always involve CN VI (abnormal EOM) and may affect long motor tracts:
  - There have been (rare) case reports of *isolated* CN VII palsy from brainstem disease.
- Lyme disease: History of tick bite, erythema migrans rash, or endemic area
- Zoster (Ramsay-Hunt syndrome): Look for herpetic vesicles, inquire about tinnitus or vertigo.
- Infectious mononucleosis: Look for pharyngitis, posterior cervical adenopathy
- Tumors: Parotid, bone, or metastatic masses, acoustic neuroma (deafness)
- Trauma: Skull fracture or penetrating facial injury may damage CN VII.
- Middle ear or mastoid surgery or infection, cholesteatoma
- Meningeal infection
- Guillain-Barré syndrome: Other neurologic deficits (eg, ascending motor weakness or diminished deep tendon reflexes [DTRs] present)
- Basilar artery aneurysm; other CN deficits should be present.
- Bilateral peripheral CN VII palsy: Consider multiple sclerosis, sarcoid, leukemia, and Guillain-Barré idiopathic (Bell) palsy may be bilateral in rare cases.
- Bell's palsy may reoccur; treatment is unchanged.

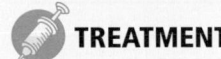

## TREATMENT

### PRE-HOSPITAL
None

### INITIAL STABILIZATION/THERAPY
Patients with an isolated peripheral CN VII palsy are stable.

### ED TREATMENT/PROCEDURES
- Corneal damage may result from incomplete eyelid closure:
  - Lubricating and hydrating ophthalmic preparations are essential
  - Eye patching at night
- Oral steroids may hasten recovery if started within 1 wk of onset:
  - Complications of therapy are rare and treatment is recommended.
- Antiviral therapy (acyclovir or valacyclovir) with steroids may be effective in improving functional nerve recovery:
  - Initiate within 72 hr of symptom onset.
  - No clear proven benefit.
  - May be indicated for severe palsy.
- Suspected Lyme disease should be treated with doxycycline or amoxicillin.
- Surgical decompression may be indicated for complete lesions that do not improve; this is controversial.

### MEDICATION
#### First Line
- Lacri-Lube: At bedtime and PRN; dryness/irritation in affected eye (or equivalent)
- Prednisone: 30–40 mg PO b.i.d. for 7 days, (peds: 2 mg/kg/day PO [max 60 mg])

#### Second Line
Valacyclovir 1 g PO t.i.d. for 7 days (peds: No data to support its use) may be useful in severe cases.

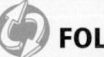

## FOLLOW-UP

### DISPOSITION
#### Admission Criteria
Isolated peripheral CN VII palsy does not require admission.

#### Discharge Criteria
Isolated peripheral CN VII palsy may be treated on outpatient basis.

### FOLLOW-UP RECOMMENDATIONS
Follow-up should be within 1 wk.

## PEARLS AND PITFALLS

- Motor weakness isolated to 7th nerve distribution:
  - Involves both upper and lower face
  - If tone is NOT lost on the forehead, it is *not* Bell's Palsy.
- An otherwise normal neurologic exam including all cranial nerves and extremity motor function
- Protect the eye with lacrilube.
- Steroids beneficial, antivirals controversial

## ADDITIONAL READING

- de Almeida JR, Al Khabori M, Guyatt GH, et al. Combined corticosteroid and antiviral treatment for Bell Palsy. *JAMA*. 2009;302:985–993.
- Gilden D. Bell's palsy. *N Engl J Med*. 2004;351: 1323–1331.

- Gilden DH, Tyler KL. Bell's palsy—Is glucocorticoid treatment enough? *N Engl J Med*. 2007;357: 1653–1655.
- Hato N, Yamada H, Kohno H, et al. Valacyclovir and prednisolone treatment for Bell's palsy: A multicenter, randomized, placebo-controlled study. *Otol Neurotol*. 2007;28:408–413.
- Sullivan FM, Swan IR, Donnan PT, et al. Early treatment with prednisolone or acyclovir in Bell's palsy. *N Engl J Med*. 2007;357:1598–1607.
- Engstrom M, Berg T, Stjernquist-Desatnik A, et al. Prednisolone and valaciclovir in Bell's palsy: A randomised, double-blind, placebo-controlled, multicentre trial. *Lancet Neurol*. 2008;7:993–1000.
- Wang C, Chang Y, Shih H, et al. Facial palsy in children: Emergency department management and outcome. *Pediatr Emerg Care*. 2010;26:121–125.

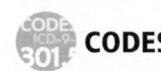

## CODES

### ICD9
351.0 Bell's palsy

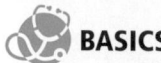 **BASICS**

## DESCRIPTION

- Acts to potentiate activity of $\gamma$-aminobutyric acid (GABA; major inhibitory neurotransmitter) by binding to its own specific site
- Facilitates GABA binding to its site
- Results in chloride influx, membrane hyperpolarization, and inhibition of cellular excitation:
  - Benzodiazepines (BZs) increase frequency of chloride channel opening.
  - Depression of spinal reflexes and reticular activating system
- Rapidly absorbed from GI tract:
  - Highly protein bound
  - Large $V_d$
  - Hepatic metabolism
  - Duration of action is inversely proportional to lipophilicity.
  - Duration of lorazepam > diazepam > midazolam.
  - Synergistic with other sedative-hypnotic medications (eg, ethanol, barbiturates, propofol)

 **DIAGNOSIS**

## SIGNS AND SYMPTOMS

- CNS:
  - Sedation/drowsiness
  - Slurred speech
  - Coma
  - Delirium
  - Midposition to small pupils
- Neuromuscular:
  - Incoordination
  - Slowed voluntary movements
  - Ataxia
  - Hypotension
  - Hyporeflexia/areflexia
- Cardiovascular:
  - Mild depression
  - Rarely lethal if ingested alone
- Respiratory:
  - Mild depression
  - Less depression versus barbiturates
  - Short acting and IV may produce depression

- GI:
  - Nausea, vomiting, diarrhea
- Other:
  - Hypothermia
  - Complications may include cerebral hypoxia, rhabdomyolysis, pressure-induced neuropathies.
  - No long-term organ toxicity

### *Pediatric Considerations*
Rarely may cause paradoxic restlessness, agitation

## ESSENTIAL WORKUP
Diagnosis based on:
- History of ingestion or recent injection
- Clinical findings associated with CNS depression
- No response to naloxone

## DIAGNOSTIC TESTS & INTERPRETATION
### *Lab*
- Pulse oximetry
- Electrolytes, BUN, creatinine, serum glucose
- Urinalysis (UA) for myoglobin when coma present
- ABG
- Qualitative urine screen:
  - Confirms exposure many times, but does not indicate or measure intoxication.
  - False-negative test results reported
  - Qualitative immunoassays detect only BZs that are metabolized to oxazepam.
  - Those that do not produce this metabolite (clonazepam, lorazepam, midazolam, alprazolam) are not detected on qualitative screen.
  - Does not correlate with clinical state
  - Serum levels not acutely practical
  - Clinical signs and symptoms more important than theoretic $LD_{50}$ or serum levels
- Alcohol(s) level
- Barbiturate level
- Acetaminophen and salicylate levels
- Pregnancy test

### *Imaging*
- EKG
- CXR for aspiration pneumonia

### *Diagnostic Procedures/Surgery*
Core body temperature

## DIFFERENTIAL DIAGNOSIS
- Drugs and toxins causing decreased level of consciousness:
  - Hypoglycemics
  - Other sedative-hypnotics (barbiturates)
  - Antidepressant-antipsychotic
  - Narcotics
  - Anticonvulsants
  - Carbon monoxide/cyanide
  - Alcohols
- Nontoxic medical condition:
  - Hypoxemia
  - Hypothermia
  - Head trauma (intracranial bleeding)
  - Infection (meningitis or encephalitis)
  - Electrolyte and metabolic disturbances

 **TREATMENT**

## PRE-HOSPITAL
- Attention to airway and breathing
- Cardiac monitor
- IV access
- Rapid glucose determination
- Bring in pill bottles/pills in suspected overdose.

## INITIAL STABILIZATION/THERAPY
- ABCs:
  - Secure airway and assist ventilation with supplemental oxygen to prevent hypoxemia and shock.
  - IV access with 0.9% NS
  - Cardiac monitor
- Administer naloxone, thiamine, and dextrose if altered mental status.

## ED TREATMENT/PROCEDURES
- Gastric lavage considered only when presents within 1 hr of life-threatening ingestion with protected airway
- Activated charcoal (AC) PO or via nasogastric tube (NGT)
- No role for diuresis, dialysis, or charcoal hemoperfusion

- Flumazenil (FZ):
  - Competitive BZ-receptor inhibitor
  - Rapidly reverses BZ-induced coma and respiratory depression
  - Onset within 1–2 min; peak at 6–10 min; duration 1–2 hr (repeated dosing may be indicated)
  - Efficacy dependent on dose of BZ being antagonized and dose of FZ used
  - Do not administer empirically as part of any standard protocol therapy or in unknown poisoned patient.
  - May help avert need of airway intubation
  - May be beneficial in shortening hospital stay or as diagnostic maneuver
  - Indications include isolated BZ overdose in nonhabituated user.
  - Useful to reverse iatrogenic poisoning (conscious sedation)
  - Contraindications include:
    - Coingestions that might lower seizure threshold (tricyclic antidepressants [TCAs])
    - Seizure activity
    - Allergy
    - Neuromuscular blockade
    - Do not use if hypotension, hypoxia, dysrhythmias, or increased intracranial pressure is present.
    - May precipitate withdrawal state including seizures

## MEDICATION

- Activated charcoal: 1–2 g/kg PO/NG (ideal 10:1 ratio)
- Dextrose: $D_{50}W$ 1 ampule: 50 mL or 25 g (peds: $D_{25}W$ 2–4 mL/kg) IV

- Flumazenil (Romazicon):
  - Initial: 0.2 mg IV over 30 sec (adult)
  - If no response: 0.3 mg IV after 30 sec
  - If still no response: 0.5 mg IV and repeat q1min if needed, to max. dose of 3 mg
  - Continuous infusion at 0.2–1.0 mg/hr if multiple repeated doses required to maintain response
  - Pediatric dosing not established; recommended starting dose is 0.01 mg/kg IV, titrate to max. dose of 1 mg, continuous infusion at 0.005–0.01 mg/kg/h
- Naloxone (Narcan): 2 mg (peds: 0.1 mg/kg) IV or IV Initial dose
- Thiamine (vitamin $B_1$): 100 mg IV/IM

 **FOLLOW-UP**

### DISPOSITION
#### Admission Criteria
- Persistent or profound CNS depression
- Cardiovascular or respiratory compromise
- Coingestants with potential delayed toxicity

#### Discharge Criteria
- Discharge after 4-hr observation period if no signs or symptoms of BZ poisoning develop.
- If flumazenil administered, observe for additional 2–4 hr for recurrent sedation.

#### Issues for Referral
Psychiatry consultation for intentional overdoses.

### FOLLOW-UP RECOMMENDATIONS
Habituated patients may experience BZ withdrawal after cessation:
- Autonomic instability, tremor, paresthesias, seizures

## PEARLS AND PITFALLS

IV formulations of certain BZs (eg, lorazepam) may contain propylene glycol diluent that can produce elevated anion gap metabolic acidosis.

## ADDITIONAL READING

- Farrell SE. Benzodiazepines. In: Ford MD, Delaney KA, Ling LJ, et al, eds. *Clinical toxicology*. Philadelphia: WB Saunders, 2001.
- Lee DC. Sedative-hypnotic agents. In: Goldfrank LR, ed. *Goldfrank's toxicologic emergencies*. New York: McGraw-Hill, 2006;1098–11.
- Leikin J, Paloucek F. Benzodiazepines, qualitative, urine. In: *Poisoning and toxicology handbook*. Hudson, OH: Lexi-Comp, 2002.
- Rasanen I, Ojanpera I, Vuori E. Quantitative screening for benzodiazepines in blood by dual-column gas chromatography and comparison of the results with urine immunoassay. *J Anal Toxicol*. 2000;24:46–53.
- Spivey WH, Roberts JR, Derlet RW. A clinical trial of escalating doses of flumazenil for reversal of suspected benzodiazepine overdose in the emergency department. *Ann Emerg Med*. 1993;22:1813–1821.

### See Also (Topic, Algorithm, Electronic Media Element)
Barbiturate Poisoning

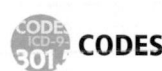 **CODES**

ICD9
969.4 Poisoning by benzodiazepine-based tranquilizers

# BETA-BLOCKER POISONING

*Janet Eng*

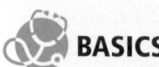 **BASICS**

## DESCRIPTION

### Normal Physiology
- Cardiovascular: $\beta_1$-receptors:
  - ATP converted to cAMP by adenyl cyclase with stimulation of $\beta$-receptors
  - cAMP activates protein kinase, which phosphorylates proteins of the sarcoplasmic reticulum.
  - Sarcoplasmic reticulum releases calcium.
  - Excitation-contraction coupling occurs.
- Effects of $\beta$-blockers:
  - Cardiovascular:
    ○ Decreased excitation/contraction
    ○ Membrane stabilizing activity
    ○ Sodium channel blockade causes a prolongation of the QRS complex (with some agents).
    ○ Prolongation of QTc interval leading to ventricular dysrhythmias (with some agents)
    ○ Intrinsic sympathomimetic activity
    ○ Partial agonist properties (with some agents)
  - Neurologic:
    ○ CNS effects with the lipophilic agents (propranolol, metoprolol, labetalol)

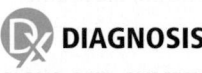 **DIAGNOSIS**

## SIGNS AND SYMPTOMS
- Cardiovascular:
  - Hypotension
  - Bradycardia
  - Cardiac conduction delays
  - Heart block
  - Heart failure
  - Electrical mechanical dissociation
  - Loss of $\beta$-selectivity in overdose settings
- Neurologic:
  - Coma
  - Seizures
- Pulmonary:
  - Bronchospasm
  - Pulmonary edema
- Metabolic:
  - Hypoglycemia

### History
- Inquire about risk of medication error.
- Inquire about risk of suicidal ideation with intent.
- Inquire about possible exposure to medications with a pediatric patient.

### Physical Exam
- Hypotension
- Bradycardia
- Dysrhythmias

## ESSENTIAL WORKUP
- With unknown ingestion: Suspect $\beta$-blocker poisoning with bradycardia/hypotension.
- ECG:
  - Conduction delays
  - 1st-, 2nd-, or 3rd-degree heart block
  - Bradycardia

## DIAGNOSTIC TESTS & INTERPRETATION
### Lab
- CBC
- Electrolytes, BUN, creatinine, glucose

## DIFFERENTIAL DIAGNOSIS
- Calcium-channel blocker toxicity
- Clonidine toxicity
- Digoxin toxicity
- Acute myocardial infarction with heart block

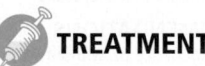 **TREATMENT**

## PRE-HOSPITAL
Transport pills and pill bottles when overdose suspected.

## INITIAL STABILIZATION/THERAPY
- ABCs:
  - Airway protection as indicated by mental status
  - Supplemental oxygen as needed
  - 0.9% NS IV access
  - Close hemodynamic monitoring
- Naloxone and thiamine if altered mental status
- Accu-Chek and treat hypoglycemia with $D_{50}W$.
- Treat prolonged seizures with benzodiazepines.

## ED TREATMENT/PROCEDURES
### Goals
- Heart rate >60 beats per minute
- Systolic BP >90 mm Hg
- Adequate urine output
- Improving level of consciousness

### GI Decontamination
- Syrup of ipecac: Contraindicated in the prehospital and ED setting.
- Consider lavage with Ewald tube if ingestion within 1 hr:
  - Propranolol may cause esophageal spasm producing difficulty with passage and removal of gastric lavage tube.
- Activated charcoal helpful especially in the presence of coingestants.

### Bradycardia/Hypotension
- Atropine:
  - Initial agent
  - Low success rate
- Glucagon:
  - Administer if atropine does not increase heart rate.
  - Promotes cAMP production through a receptor site other than the $\beta$-receptor
  - May cause nausea and vomiting
  - Mix with NS or $D_5W$
- IV fluids:
  - Administer cautiously in the hypotensive patient.
  - Swan-Ganz catheter or central venous pressure (CVP) monitoring to help follow volume status
- Amrinone:
  - Use in conjunction with glucagon to treat symptomatic sustained bradycardia.
- Pressor agents:
  - Initiate when symptomatic hypotension/bradycardia persists after atropine/glucagon.
  - Use invasive monitoring to help guide therapy.
  - Utility may be limited owing to $\beta$-blockade:
    ○ Higher doses may be required.
  - Isoproterenol (nonselective $\beta$-agonist):
    ○ Titrate for BP and heart rate.

- Epinephrine (potent $\alpha$- and $\beta$-receptor agonist):
  - BP increases as a result of direct myocardial stimulation, increase in heart rate, and vasoconstriction.
  - Use if no BP response with isoproterenol
  - High-dose dopamine
- Sodium bicarbonate:
  - In theory, this is used if there is evidence of prolongation of QRS >100 ms owing to some of the $\beta$-blockers also causing sodium channel blockade leading to a prolonged QRS.
  - Not routinely administered for all $\beta$-blocker toxicities
- Electrical pacing: When other treatment options have failed
- Insulin:
  - Promotes more efficient myocardial metabolism
  - May be considered as a treatment option

### Enhanced Elimination
- Hemodialysis helpful with water-soluble $\beta$-blocking agents:
  - Nadolol
  - Atenolol
  - Sotalol
- IV fat emulsion (20% Intralipid):
  - Potential treatment in the future

### MEDICATION
- Activated charcoal: 1 g/kg PO
- Amrinone: Loading dose 0.75 mg/kg; maintenance drip 2–20 $\mu$g/kg/min; titrate for effect
- Atropine: 0.5 mg (peds: 0.02 mg/kg) IV; repeat 0.5–1.0 mg IV (peds: 0.04 mg/kg)
- Dopamine: 2–20 $\mu$g/kg/min IV
- Dextrose: $D_{50}W$ 1 ampule (50 mL or 25 g; peds: $D_{25}W$ 2–4 mL/kg) IV

- Epinephrine: 2 $\mu$g/min (peds: 0.1 $\mu$g/kg/min); titrate to effect
- Glucagon: 3.5–5 mg IV over 1–2 min (peds: 0.03–0.1 mg/kg) bolus followed by 70-$\mu$g/kg/h infusion
- Isoproterenol: 5 $\mu$g/min IV and titrate for heart rate effect
- Naloxone (Narcan): 2 mg (peds: 0.1 mg/kg) IV or IM initial dose
- Sodium bicarbonate: 1 mEq/kg IVP
- Thiamine (vitamin $B_1$): 100 mg (peds: 50 mg) IV or IM

### First Line
- IV fluids
- Glucagon
- Pressor agents

### Second Line
- Sodium bicarbonate
- Hemodialysis

 **FOLLOW-UP**

### DISPOSITION
#### Admission Criteria
- ICU admission for decreased level of consciousness or hemodynamic instability (bradycardia, conduction delays, hypotension)
- Observation and monitoring for 24 hr for long-acting or sustained-release preparations owing to the potential delay in symptoms

#### Discharge Criteria
Asymptomatic 8–10 hr after ingestion of short- or immediate-release preparation

### FOLLOW-UP RECOMMENDATIONS
- Psychiatric evaluation for all suicidal patients
- Poison prevention guidance for parents of pediatric accidental ingestion

## PEARLS AND PITFALLS
- Consider $\beta$-blocker toxicity in patients who present with hypotension and bradycardia.
- Wide complex QRS dysrhythmias should be treated with sodium bicarbonate.

## ADDITIONAL READING
- Harvey M, Cave G. Intralipid infusion ameliorates propranolol-induced hypotension in rabbits. *J Med Tox.* 2008;4:71–76.
- Pfaender M, Casetti PG, Azzolini M, et al. Successful treatment of a massive atenolol and nifedipine overdose with CVVHDF. *Minerva Anestesiol.* 2008;74:97–100.
- Shepherd G. Treatment of poisoning caused by $\beta$-adrenergic and calcium-channel blockers. *Am J Health-Sys Pharm.* 2006;63:1828–1835.

### See Also (Topic, Algorithm, Electronic Media Element)
Calcium Channel Blocker, Poisoning

# BIOLOGIC WEAPONS
*Brigham R. Temple*

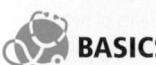 **BASICS**

## DESCRIPTION

- Defined as naturally occurring organisms or toxins that are purified and prepared for mass dissemination with intent of causing mass morbidity, mortality, and social disruption
- Organisms include bacteria, viruses, and fungi.
- Over 400 potential or actualized etiologic agents capable of being used as biological weapon:
  - Characterized by their relatively low cost compared with other weapons of mass destruction (WMD), high potency, and their ability to be delivered in a stealthy manner
  - Stealth quality of biologic weapons comes from organism's natural incubation period.
- Easy to conceal and difficult to detect:
  - Agents often invisible to naked eye, odorless, and tasteless
- Patients typically present to various health care facilities with host of common complaints, adding to delay in recognition of covert release of biologic weapon.
- Victims of biologic warfare agents are exposed either via direct cutaneous contact with agent, respiratory inhalation of aerosolized agent, or via GI tract after poisoning of food or water source.

## ETIOLOGY

- Bacteria:
  - Anthrax: *Bacillus anthracis*
  - Plague: *Yersinia pestis*
  - Cholera: infection from *Vibrio cholerae*:
    - Presents with severe GI symptoms and rapidly leads to profound dehydration
  - Tularemia: *Francisella tularensis*
  - Brucellosis: Organism in the *Brucella* genus
  - Q fever: *Coxiella burnetii*
- Viruses:
  - Smallpox: Variola virus
  - Viral encephalitides: Members of Alphavirus genus (Venezuelan equine encephalitis, Eastern equine encephalitis, and Western equine encephalitis)
  - Viral hemorrhagic fevers: From four families of viruses, includes illnesses such as Ebola, Marburg, Lassa, and dengue fever
- Toxins:
  - Ricin
  - Staphylococcal enterotoxin B
  - Botulinum toxin
  - Mycotoxins

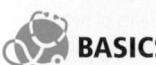 **DIAGNOSIS**

## SIGNS AND SYMPTOMS

- Health care providers need to be alert to detect illness patterns and diagnostic clues that indicate biologic weapon release.
- Indications of intentional release of agent include:
  - Geographic clustering of illnesses with individuals who live, work, or attended event in close proximity (if multiple people who work in same office develop pneumonia, it could potentially represent respiratory pathogen release)

- Unusual age distribution for common illness (chickenpox-like illness among adult patients could represent smallpox release)
- ≥2 patients presenting with similar unexplained illnesses (2 patients presenting with flaccid paralysis could represent botulinum toxin release)
- Single case of illness caused by uncommon agent (smallpox, inhalational anthrax)
- High volume of patients with similar presentation of symptoms associated with escalating morbidity and mortality

### Anthrax

- Inhalational anthrax:
  - Fever
  - Chills
  - Fatigue, malaise, lethargy
  - Cough, usually dry or minimally productive
  - Nausea or vomiting
  - Dyspnea
  - Diaphoresis
  - Chest pain
  - Myalgias
  - Tachycardia
  - Fever
  - Meningeal signs
- Cutaneous anthrax:
  - Skin lesion:
    - Painless pruritic papule
    - Turning into vesicle that ruptures forming necrotic ulcer
  - Black eschar
  - Surrounding gelatinous nonpitting edema

### Plague

- Abrupt onset
- Fever, chills
- Cough, hemoptysis, dyspnea
- Headache
- Vomiting
- Swollen tender lymph nodes (buboes)
- Skin lesions at site of inoculation (ie, flea bite)
- Confusion
- Abdominal pain
- Oliguria
- Obtundation
- Extensive ecchymosis
- Acral gangrene (digits, nose, penis)

### Tularemia

- See "Tularemia" chapter.
- Typhoidal:
  - Most likely form of disease when weaponized and delivered by aerosol
  - Fever, headache, malaise
  - Nonproductive cough
  - 35% mortality if untreated

### Q fever

- Incubation period 10–40 days
- Flulike symptoms and pleuritic chest pain for 2–10 days
- CXR shows patchy infiltrates.
- Definitively diagnosed serologically
- Mortality:
  - <1% even if untreated

### Smallpox

- Incubation period 7–17 days (average is 12 days)
- Flulike symptoms (fever, fatigue, myalgias, headache) for ~2–3 days followed by characteristic rash:
  - Progresses from macules to papules to pustular lesions and crusted lesions
  - Starts on face and extremities (including palms/soles) and spreads to trunk in 1 wk
  - Scabs over in 1–2 wk
- Mortality:
  - 30% if untreated

### Hemorrhagic Fevers

- See "Hemorrhagic Fever" chapter.
- Incubation period 1–3 wk
- Starts as flulike syndrome with fever, malaise, myalgias, headache, and sore throat
- Afterward, infectious gastroenteritis syndrome, rash, and renal/hepatic dysfunction
- Finally, hemorrhagic symptoms develop around the 5th day followed by shock and death:
  - Mortality in 50–90% for Ebola if untreated

## ESSENTIAL WORKUP

Suspect bioterrorism if:

- Multiple cases of relatively young, healthy patients who present with flulike syndrome and within days deteriorate rapidly
- Typical cutaneous lesions appear

## DIAGNOSTIC TESTS & INTERPRETATION

### Lab

- CBC
- Electrolytes, BUN, creatinine
- ABG
- Cerebrospinal fluid (CSF):
  - Anthrax: 50% with inhalation anthrax develop hemorrhagic meningitis.
- Coagulation studies:
  - Plague: Disseminated intravascular coagulation (DIC)
- Blood cultures
- Wound cultures
- Alert laboratory personnel to potential concerns of clinicians.

### Imaging

CXR:

- Anthrax: Mediastinal widening, pulmonary infiltrate/consolidation, pleural effusion
- Plague: Bronchopneumonia

## DIFFERENTIAL DIAGNOSIS

- Anthrax:
  - Influenza
  - Bacterial pneumonia
  - Bacterial meningitis
  - Brown recluse spider bite
  - Tularemia
  - Streptococcal/staphylococcal skin infection
- Plague:
  - Tularemia
  - Catscratch disease
  - Lymphogranuloma venereum
  - Chancroid
  - Tuberculosis
  - Streptococcal adenitis
  - Meningitis
  - Encephalitis
  - Sepsis

- Smallpox:
  - Varicella
  - Rash starts centrally on trunk and spreads outward:
    - Lesions in different stages of development
    - Rarely involves palms or soles
    - Disseminated molluscum contagiosum
  - Monkeypox
  - Drug eruptions
- Toxins:
  - Staphylococcal enterotoxin B:
    - Most common cause of food poisoning
    - Can be aerosolized in addition to being placed in food or water reservoir
    - When inhaled, produces febrile type of illness that can progress to septic shock picture
  - Ricin:
    - Plant protein derived from castor beans
    - Causes rapid progression from upper respiratory congestion to cardiopulmonary collapse
    - Ingestion is less toxic because GI tract does not absorb it well, but it can lead to local cytotoxic death, shock, and death.
  - Botulinum toxin:
    - Initially symptoms include cranial nerve dysfunction with descending paralysis that leads to respiratory failure.
  - Mycotoxins:
    - Highly toxic compounds produced by certain species of fungus
    - Dermal, respiratory, or GI contact can rapidly lead to multiorgan system failure and death.

 **TREATMENT**

### PRE-HOSPITAL
Universal precautions with N-95 mask

### INITIAL STABILIZATION/THERAPY
- ABCs
- 0.9% NS fluid bolus for hypotension
- Supplemental oxygen for hypoxemia
- Vasopressors for persistent hypotension.
- Respiratory and contact isolation for suspected cases

### ED TREATMENT/PROCEDURES
- All treatments include:
  - Control fever with acetaminophen.
  - Initiate therapy for specific disease.
- Anthrax:
  - Initiate antibiotics:
    - IV for inhalational or severe cutaneous
    - Antibiotic choice depends on susceptibility.
  - Antibiotic options:
    - Ciprofloxacin: 1st line
    - Doxycycline
    - Rifampin
    - Clindamycin
    - Vancomycin

- Plague:
  - Antibiotics initiated within 24 hr minimizes mortality.
  - 1st-line agents: Streptomycin or gentamicin
  - Add chloramphenicol if signs of meningitis or unstable patient
  - Prophylaxis: Doxycycline or ciprofloxacin
- Q fever:
  - Recovery occurs within 2 wk without treatment.
  - Doxycycline shortens duration of illness.
- Smallpox:
  - Supportive therapy
  - Vaccine given within 4 days of initial exposure decreases chances of contracting smallpox or developing severe symptoms.
  - Vaccinate medical staff caring for patient.
  - Treat secondary bacterial infection.
- Tularemia:
  - See "Tularemia."
- Hemorrhagic fevers:
  - See "Hemorrhagic Fever."

### MEDICATION
- Chloramphenicol: 25 mg/kg IV q6h
- Ciprofloxacin: 400 mg IV q12h or 500 mg PO b.i.d. (peds: 15 mg/kg b.i.d.)
- Clindamycin: 900 mg IV q12h
- Doxycycline: 100 mg (peds: ≥45 kg, 100 mg; if weight ≤45 kg, 2.2 mg/kg IV) PO/IV q12h
- Gentamicin: 5 mg/kg IM or IV q24h (peds: 2.5 mg/kg IV/IM q8h)
- Rifampin: 10 mg/kg IV not to exceed 600 mg/d
- Streptomycin: 1 g (peds: 15 mg/kg) IM q12h
- Vancomycin: 1 g IV q12h

 **FOLLOW-UP**

### DISPOSITION
#### Admission Criteria
- Decision to treat patient as inpatient vs. outpatient will have to be made in context of overall disaster.
- Toxic or hypoxic patients require admission.
- Respiratory isolation

#### Discharge Criteria
Mild, noncontagious illness

#### Issues for Referral
- Contact local and state health departments for suspected or confirmed illness related to biological weapons.
- Infectious disease and toxicology consult for suspected illness

### FOLLOW-UP RECOMMENDATIONS
- Post exposure prophylaxis and vaccinations should be continued based on the causative agent.
- Exposed staff should have follow-up with employee health and infection control prior to returning to work.

## PEARLS AND PITFALLS
- Early diagnosis is difficult, and a high index of suspicion is required.
- Failing to use personal protective equipment to protect self and staff is a pitfall.
- Suspect biological weapons etiology when there is geographic clustering of patients who live, work, or attended an event in close proximity.
- Initiate therapy or prophylaxis early in suspected illness.

## ADDITIONAL READING
- Centers for Disease Control and Prevention. Recognition of illness associated with the intentional release of a biologic agent. *MMWR Morb Mortal Wkly Rep.* 2001;50(11):893–897.
- Christopher GW, Eitzen EM, Kortepeter MG, et al. Biological weapons agents. In: Hogan DE, Burstein JL, eds. *Disaster medicine*, 2nd ed. Philadelphia: Lippincott Williams & Wilkins, 1997.
- Franz DR, Jahrling PB, Friedlander AM, et al. Clinical recognition and management of patients exposed to biological warfare agents. *JAMA.* 1997;278(5):399–411.
- Khan AS, Morse S, Lillibridge S. Public-health preparedness for biological terrorism in the USA. *Lancet.* 2000;356:1179–1182.
- US Army Medical Research Institute of Infectious Diseases. *Medical management of biological casualties handbook*, 6th ed. Fort Detrick, Frederick, MD: April 2005.

### Useful Web Sites
- emergency.cdc.gov/bioterrorism/
- sis.nlm.nih.gov/enviro/biologicalwarfare.html
- http://www.bordeninstitute.army.mil/published_volumes/chemBio/chembio.html

### See Also (Topic, Algorithm, Electronic Media Element)
- Botulism
- Hemorrhagic Fever
- Tularemia

# BIPOLAR DISORDER

Paul H. Desan
Gary S. Sachs

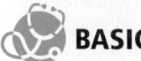 **BASICS**

## DESCRIPTION
- Mania:
  - Presentation is diverse and may be difficult to recognize as mania:
    - Simple irritability
    - Cheerfulness
    - Psychosis
    - Delirium
    - Agitation
  - Full extent of pathology often revealed only by outside informants
  - Onset gradual or acute, duration several weeks or months; rarely may be chronic
- Hypomania:
  - Milder symptoms without marked impairment
- Mixed mood:
  - Simultaneous symptoms of mania and depression
  - Treat in ED as for mania
- Bipolar disorder:
  - Formerly manic depressive disorder
  - Defined as one or more episodes of hypomanic, manic, or mixed mood
  - Possibly with episodes of depressed mood
  - Bipolar II is used to denote cases where hypomania has occurred in the course of the disorder but never mania.
  - Typically begins in the teens or 20s
  - Episodes of abnormal mood may be mild or severe, brief or prolonged, infrequent or chronic, chiefly elevated or chiefly depressed in character.
  - Bipolar disorder may be readily responsive to treatment or nearly intractable.
- Schizoaffective disorder:
  - Characterized by episodes of altered mood, but psychotic features present even when mood is normal

## ETIOLOGY
- Typically, a primary psychiatric disorder, with genetic association
- May be secondary to medical disorder (eg, drug toxicity, endocrine, neurological process)
- Particularly likely to be secondary if:
  - 1st episode
  - Patient older than 40 yr
  - Atypical or mixed presentation
  - Abnormal sensorium

## DIAGNOSIS

### SIGNS AND SYMPTOMS
*History*
- Psychiatric history:
  - Recent symptoms of mania (often collateral sources critical): Elevated, expansive, or irritable mood; increased energy and activity; decreased need for sleep; irresponsibility, disregard for negative consequences of actions; talkativeness; distractibility; fast thoughts; grandiosity, overconfidence
  - Past mania or depression
  - Noncompliance with mood stabilizer
  - Recent initiation or discontinuation of antidepressant
  - Recent substance abuse
  - Bipolar family history
- Medical history:
  - Endocrine, metabolic, or neurologic disorders
  - Current or recent medications

*Physical Exam*
- Appearance:
  - Hyperactive, if not agitated
  - Talkative, often with loud, rapid, or "pressured" speech
- Affect:
  - Irritable, argumentative, often multiple recent arguments or fights
  - Less commonly euphoric or expansive
  - Often labile with depressed or tearful intervals (may confound diagnosis)
  - Patient likely to describe mood as tense, irritable, or depressed rather than euphoric
- Neurovegetative:
  - Increased energy, engaged in multiple goal-directed activities many hours per day
  - Racing thoughts
  - Decreased sleep
- Thought process:
  - Rapid, distractible, may be incoherent, delirious
- Thought content:
  - Psychosis possible, either mood congruent (eg, delusions of grandeur or power) or mood incongruent (may be indistinguishable from other psychotic disorders)
- Judgment:
  - Inflated self-esteem, perhaps to grandiose or psychotic extent
  - Uncharacteristic, irresponsible behavior, such as financial or sexual indiscretions, with inability to recognize negative consequences of actions.
  - Substance abuse is frequent during mania.
- Sensorium:
  - Typically normal
  - Confusion or delirium possible

## ESSENTIAL WORKUP
- Physical and neurologic exam; vital signs
- Mania may present as delirium and need workup of full differential diagnosis of delirium.

## DIAGNOSTIC TESTS & INTERPRETATION
*Lab*
- Toxicology screen (urine or serum)
- Blood alcohol level
- Electrolytes
- Blood glucose
- CBC
- TSH
- Lithium, carbamazepine, valproate serum levels, if relevant
- Other tests as suggested by history or exam

*Imaging*
CT head only with suspicion of neurologic etiology

## DIFFERENTIAL DIAGNOSIS
- Primary mania of bipolar or schizoaffective disorder
- Psychosis
- Agitated depression
- Personality disorders:
  - Borderline
  - Narcissistic
  - Antisocial
- Attention deficit disorder
- Conduct or intermittent explosive disorders
- Organic brain syndrome
- Intoxication or withdrawal from alcohol or sedative hypnotics
- Intoxication with cocaine, amphetamines, phencyclidine, or other sympathomimetics
- Accidental or deliberate toxic overdose
- Treatment with antidepressants or electroshock therapy in susceptible individuals
- Recent discontinuation of antidepressant medication
- Corticosteroid or thyroid hormones
- Anticholinergics
- Treatment of Parkinson disease
- Cyclobenzaprine (Flexeril)
- Endocrine or metabolic disorders (particularly thyroid disease)
- Encephalitis
- Meningitis
- Postictal states
- MS
- Postcerebrovascular accident
- CNS tumors
- CNS vasculitis
- General paresis

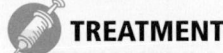

# TREATMENT

## INITIAL STABILIZATION/THERAPY

- High violence potential:
  - Quiet environment
  - Prompt evaluation
  - Nonconfrontational manner
  - Adequate security backup
    Physical restraint and sedation, as needed
- For cooperative, but agitated patient:
  - PO neuroleptics (eg, haloperidol, consider olanzapine or chlorpromazine as alternate) or PO benzodiazepines (eg, lorazepam)
- For uncooperative agitated patient:
  - Synergistic combination of IM, IV, or PO haloperidol and lorazepam widely used (some authorities favor monotherapy with benzodiazepine or neuroleptic):
    ○ Benztropine for prevention of acute dystonic reaction to haloperidol is not usually required when concurrent benzodiazepine is given.
  - Consider lorazepam, olanzapine, ziprasidone, or chlorpromazine IM as alternative.

## ED TREATMENT/PROCEDURES

- Outpatient management:
  - Neuroleptics for symptomatic treatment, on temporary or continuing basis
  - Agents for sleep
  - Discontinuation of antidepressant if related to present hypomania or mania
  - Initiation or restart of mood-stabilizer therapy:
    ○ Action of mood-stabilizing agents requires days or weeks, even after full serum level attained.
- Inpatient management:
  - Sedation or initiation of mood stabilizer in consultation with admitting psychiatrist

## MEDICATION

- Acute agitation:
  - Lorazepam: 2 mg PO/IM (lower dose in mild agitation or in frail or elderly); may repeat q30min, generally not to exceed 12 mg/24 hr
  - Haloperidol: 5 mg PO (lower dose in mild agitation or in frail or elderly); may repeat q30min, generally not to exceed 20 mg/24 hr (consider benztropine 1–2 mg PO q12h prophylaxis of dystonic reaction, particularly in continued neuroleptic treatment without benzodiazepine or in patients with history of dystonia); consider olanzapine 5–10 mg PO or chlorpromazine 50–100 mg PO as alternative to haloperidol
  - Synergistic combination of haloperidol, 5 mg IM/IV/PO plus lorazepam 1–2 mg IM/IV/PO, repeat q30min, as required (doses may be smaller in elderly or frail patients)

- Olanzapine 10 mg IM, ziprasidone 10 mg IM, or chlorpromazine 50 mg IM may be useful parenteral alternatives, perhaps at a lower dose in frail or elderly (avoid chlorpromazine in hypotension; ziprasidone may have more QT elongating effect than other neuroleptics but the clinical relevance of such effect at this dose is unclear).
- Typical outpatient medications:
  - Benztropine: 1 mg PO b.i.d.
  - Carbamazepine: 400–2,000 mg/d (often in div. doses or in sustained-release dose forms)
  - Clonazepam: 0.5–2 mg PO q.h.s. or 0.5–2 mg PO b.i.d.
  - Haloperidol: 0.5–5 mg PO b.i.d.
  - Lamotrigine: 25–200 mg/d in 1 or 2 div. doses (typically up to 100 mg/d in patients taking valproate, up to 500 mg/d in patients taking carbamazepine or certain other cytochrome inducers, but not valproate)

## ALERT

- Lamotrigine must be started by a gradual dose escalation schedule specified by manufacturer to avoid increased risk of severe dermatological reactions; if resumed after discontinuation for more than 5 half-lives (5–7 days), the gradual dose escalation schedule must be used again.
- Lithium: 600–3,000 mg/d (often in div. doses or in sustained-release dose forms; in acute mania, initiate at 300 mg PO t.i.d.)
- Olanzapine: 1.25–30 mg/d, q.h.s. or in div. doses
- Perphenazine: 4–16 mg PO b.i.d.
- Risperidone: 0.5–3 mg PO b.i.d.
- Valproate (eg, Depakote): 750–3,000 mg/d (often in div. doses, in acute mania, initiate at 250 mg PO t.i.d.)

## Pregnancy Considerations

The safety of psychotropic medications in pregnancy is a complex issue, but valproate and carbamazepine are Pregnancy Category D and may pose particular risks, highest in early pregnancy.

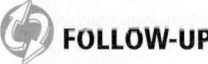

# FOLLOW-UP

## DISPOSITION

### Admission Criteria

- Involuntary hospitalization is required by danger to self:
  - Suicidal risk, especially if mixed or labile mood or psychotic
  - Unsafe behaviors due to impaired judgment
  - Medically unstable
  - Hospitalization diagnostically required
- Involuntary hospitalization also required by:
  - Risk of behaviors dangerous to others
  - Inability to care for self (unable to obtain basic needs, such as food, clothing, or shelter).

### Discharge Criteria

- Patients with mild symptoms may be discharged on medications noted above if:
  - Necessary supports to ensure safety are in place.
  - Patient is compliant with treatment plan.
  - Consultation with outpatient psychiatrist is available within 1–3 days.
- Some patients who are not legally committable may refuse treatment; explain availability of future treatment to patient and any involved friends or family.

## PEARLS AND PITFALLS

- Patients presenting with depression should be asked features suggesting mania and hypomania; 70% of bipolar patients have previously been misdiagnosed.
- Individuals with bipolar disorder are at risk for an addiction. This creates the problem of a dual diagnosis and, therefore, complicates treatment.
- Prompt recognition of the earliest signs of mania in a given individual allows a better likelihood of preventing a full episode.
- Bipolar disorder in children frequently manifests as behavioral disinhibition.
- Patients treated with atypical antipsychotic agents should be carefully monitored for development of metabolic syndromes.
- Remember that underlying medical conditions may mimic or aggravate psychotic features.

## ADDITIONAL READING

- Goodwin, GM, Consensus Group of the British Association for Psychopharmacology Evidence-based guidelines for treating bipolar disorder: Revised second edition—recommendations from the British association for psychopharmacology. *J Psychopharm.* 2009;23(4):346–388.
- Lukens TW, Wolf SJ, Edlow JA, et al. Clinical policy: Critical issues in the diagnosis and management of the adult psychiatric patient in an emergency department. *Ann Emerg Med.* 2006;47(1):79–99.
- Malhi GS, Adams D, Lampe I, et al. Clinical practice recommendations for bipolar disorder. *Acta Psychiatr Scand.* 2009;119(Suppl. 439):27–46.

### See Also (Topic, Algorithm, Electronic Media Element)

- Delirium
- Depression
- Dystonic Reaction
- Psychiatric Commitment
- Psychosis, Acute
- Psychosis, Medical vs. Psychiatric

# BITE, ANIMAL

*Daniel T. Wu*

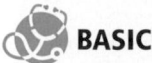 **BASICS**

## DESCRIPTION
- Most bites are from provoked animals.
- Dog bite wounds:
  - Large dogs inflict the most serious wounds (pit bulls cause the most human fatalities).
  - Most fatalities in children (70%) due to bites to face/neck
  - Dogs of family or friends account for most bites.
- Cat bite wounds:
  - Majority from pets known to victim
  - 50% infection rate in those seeking care
  - Puncture wounds most frequent due to sharp thin teeth causing deep inoculation of bacteria
- Cat-scratch disease (CSD):
  - 3 of the following 4 criteria:
    - Cat contact, with presence of scratch or inoculation lesion of the skin, eye, or mucous membrane
    - Positive CSD skin test result
    - Characteristic lymph node histopathology
    - Negative results of laboratory studies for other causes of lymphadenopathy
- Rat bite wounds:
  - Occur in laboratory personnel or children of low socioeconomic class
  - Infection rate
  - Rat bites rarely transmit rabies, and prophylaxis not routine

## ETIOLOGY
- Dog and cat bites:
  - *Pasteurella multocida* is the major organism in both:
    - Twice as likely to be found in cat bites than dog bites
    - Gram-negative aerobe found in up to 80% of cat infections
    - Infection appears in <24 hr
  - Staphylococcus or Streptococcus:
    - Infection appears in >24 hr
  - Other organisms include anaerobes and *Capnocytophaga canimorsus* (dogs).
- CSD:
  - Caused by *Bartonella henselae*
- Rat bites:
  - Caused by *Spirillum minus* and *Streptobacillus moniliformis*

 **DIAGNOSIS**

## SIGNS AND SYMPTOMS
- Distribution of mammalian bites:
  - Dog bites represent 80–90% of all bites.
  - Cat bites represent 5–15% of all bites.
  - Human bites represent 2–5% of all bites (see "Human Bite" chapter).
  - Rat bites represent 2–3% of all bites.
- Dog bites:
  - Appearance:
    - Crush injuries (most common), tears, avulsions, punctures, and scratches
  - Low rates of infection compared with cat and human bites
  - Infections usually present with:
    - Cellulitis
    - Malodorous gray discharge
    - Fever
    - Lymphadenopathy
- Cat bites:
  - Appearance:
    - Puncture wounds (most common)
    - Abrasions
    - Lacerations
  - High infection rates (30–50%) due to deeper puncture wounds
- CSD:
  - From the bite/scratch of a cat, dog, or monkey
  - Small macule or vesicle that progresses to a papule:
    - Begins several days (3–10) after inoculation
    - Resolves within several days or weeks
    - Regional lymphadenopathy occurs 3 wk postinoculation
    - Tender
    - Nonsuppurative
    - Resolves after 2–4 mo
  - Low-grade fever, malaise, headache

## History
- Animal's behavior, provocation, location, ownership
- Time since attack
- Past medical history: Conditions compromising immune function, allergies, and tetanus status

## Physical Exam
- Record the location and extent of all injuries.
- Document any swelling, crush injuries, or devitalized tissue.
- Note the range of motion of affected areas.
- Note the status of tendon and nerve function.
- Document any signs of infection, including regional adenopathy.
- Document any joint or bone involvement.

## DIAGNOSTIC TESTS & INTERPRETATION
### Lab
- Aerobic and anaerobic cultures from any infected bite wound
- Cultures not routinely indicated if wounds not clinically infected
- CSD:
  - Presence of elevated titers of *Bartonella (Rochalimaea) henselae*, or
  - Positive reaction to cat-scratch antigen (CSA):
    - Inject 0.1 mL CSA IM
    - Induration at the site 48–72 hr later equal to or exceeding 5 mm is positive

### Imaging
Plain radiograph indications:
- Fracture
- Suspect foreign body (eg, tooth)
- Baseline film if a bone or joint space has been violated in evaluating for osteomyelitis
- For infection in proximity to a bone or joint space

## DIFFERENTIAL DIAGNOSIS
- Human bite injuries: Human teeth cause crush injuries and animal teeth cause more punctures and lacerations.
- Bite injuries from other animals
- CSD-caused lymphadenopathy:
  - Reactive hyperplasia (leading cause of lymphadenopathy in children younger than 16 yr)
  - Infection, chronic lymphadenitis, drug reaction, malignancy, and congenital conditions

**TREATMENT**

## PRE-HOSPITAL
Apply pressure to any bleeding wound

## INITIAL STABILIZATION/THERAPY
- Achieve hemostasis on any bleeding wound.
- Airway stabilization if bite located on face or neck

## ED TREATMENT/PROCEDURES
- Wound irrigation:
  - Copious volumes of normal saline irrigation with an 18-gauge plastic catheter tip aimed in the direction of the puncture.
  - Avoid injection of saline through tissue planes due to force of irrigation.
- Débridement:
  - Remove foreign material, necrotic skin tags, or devitalized tissues.
  - Do not débride puncture wounds.
  - Remove any eschar present so underlying pus may be expressed and irrigated.

- Wound closure:
  - Closing wounds increases risk of infection and must be balanced with scar formation and effect of leaving wound open to heal secondarily.
  - Do not suture infected wounds or wounds >24 hr after injury.
  - Repair of wounds >8 hr: Controversial
  - Close facial wounds (warn patient of high risk of infection).
  - Infected wounds, those presenting >24 hr after the event, and deep hand wounds should be left open.
  - May approximate the wound edges with Steri-Strips and perform a delayed primary closure.
- Antibiotic indications:
  - Infected wounds
  - Cat bites
  - Hand injuries
  - Severe wounds with crush injury
  - Puncture wounds
  - Full-thickness puncture of hand, face, or lower extremity
  - Wounds requiring surgical débridement
  - Wounds involving joints, tendons, ligaments, or fractures
  - Immunocompromised patients
  - Wounds presenting >8 hr after the event
- Elevate injured extremity.
- Tetanus prophylaxis
- Rabies immunoprophylaxis:
  - Not required if rabies not known or suspected
  - Rodents (squirrels, hamsters, rats, mice) and rabbits rarely transmit the disease.
  - Skunks, raccoons, bats, and foxes represent the major reservoir for rabies.
  - See "Rabies" chapter for treatment guidelines.
- CSD:
  - Analgesics
    Apply local heat to affected nodes.
  - Avoid lymph node trauma.
  - Disease usually self-limiting
  - Antibiotics controversial, consider if severe disease is present or immunocompromised victim

## MEDICATION
### First Line
- Amoxicillin/clavulanic acid (Augmentin): 500/125 mg (peds: 40 mg/kg/24 hr) q8h PO
- Ampicillin-sulbactam (UniSyn): 3 g q6h IV
- Piperacillin-Tazobactam (Zosyn): 4.5 g q8h IV
- Ticarcillin-clavulanate (Timentin): 3.1 g q4h IV
- Ceftriaxone (Rocephin): 1 g/d PLUS:
  - Metronidazole (Flagyl): 500 mg q8h

### Second Line
- 2 drug therapy: 1 of the following below plus anaerobic coverage:
  - Trimethoprim-sulfamethoxazole (Septra DS): 1 tablet q12h (peds: 8 mg/kg trimethoprim and 40 mg/kg sulfamethoxazole per day divided into 2 daily doses) PO
  - Penicillin (Penicillin VK): 500 mg (peds: 50 mg/kg/24h) PO q6h
  - Ciprofloxacin (Cipro): 500–750 mg q12h PO or 400 mg q12h IV
  - Doxycycline: 100 mg PO b.i.d.
- PLUS (anaerobic coverage):
  - Clindamycin (Cleocin): 150–450 mg (peds: 8–20 mg/kg/24 hr) PO q6h or 600–900 mg (peds: 20–40 mg/kg/24 hr) IV q8h
  - Metronidazole (Flagyl): 500 mg PO t.i.d. (peds: 10 mg/kg per dose t.i.d.)

 **FOLLOW-UP**

## DISPOSITION
### Admission Criteria
- All bites:
  - Infected wounds at presentation
  - Severe/advancing cellulitis/lymphangitis
  - Signs of systemic infection
    Infected wounds that have failed to respond to outpatient (PO) antibiotics
- CSD:
  - Prolonged fever, systemic symptoms, and/or marked lymphadenopathy

### Discharge Criteria
- Healthy patient with localized wound infection:
  - Discharge on antibiotics with 24-hr follow-up.
- Noninfected wounds:
  - 48-hr follow-up

## FOLLOW-UP RECOMMENDATIONS
- Hand specialist referral/follow-up for infected hand wounds.
- Healthy patient with localized wound infection: Discharge on antibiotics with 24-hr follow-up.
- 48-hr follow up for noninfected wounds

## PEARLS AND PITFALLS

Animal bites must be reported to authorities in many localities.

## ADDITIONAL READING

- Baddour L. Soft tissue infections due to dog and cat bites. *UpToDate*. 2009.
- Brook I. Microbiology and management of human and animal bite wound infections. *Prim Care*. 2003;30(1):25–39.
- Galloway RE. Mammalian bites. *J Emerg Med*. 1998;6:325–331.
- Griego RD, et al. Dog, cat, and human bites: A review. *J Am Acad Dermatol*. 1995;33:1019–1029.
- Klein JD. Cat scratch disease. *Pediatr Rev*. 1994;15(9):348–353.
- Pickering L. *Red book: 2003 report of the committee on infectious diseases*, 26th ed. Amer Academy of Pediatrics, 2003.
- Smith PF, et al. Treating mammalian bite wounds. *J Clin Pharm Ther*. 2000;25.85–99.

### See Also (Topic, Algorithm, Electronic Media Element)
Rabies

# BITE, HUMAN

*Daniel T. Wu*

## BASICS

### DESCRIPTION
- 3rd most common bite (after dogs and cats)
- Most bites (up to 75%) occur during aggressive acts.
- 15–20% are related to sexual activity (love nips).
- 2 types of bites:
  - Occlusional bites: Laceration or crush injury to affected body part:
    ○ Occurs when human teeth bite into the skin
    ○ More prone to infection than animal bites
  - Clenched-fist injuries (CFIs): (CFIs; most serious type): Present as small wounds over metacarpophalangeal joints in dominant hand (fight bites):
    ○ Sustained from a clenched fist striking the mouth and teeth of another person
- With joint relaxation from the clenched position:
  - Puncture site sealed
  - Oral bacteria inoculated in the anaerobic setting within the joint
  - Bacterial inoculation carried by the tendons deeper into the potential spaces of the hand
  - Increases chances for a more extensive infection

### ETIOLOGY
- Aerobic and anaerobic organisms:
  - Most common:
    ○ *Streptococcus*
    ○ *Staphylococcus*
  - Others:
    ○ *Eikenella corrodens*
    ○ *Haemophilus influenzae*
    ○ *Peptostreptococcus*
    ○ *Corynebacterium*
    ○ *E. corrodens* exhibits synergism with *Streptococcus, Staphylococcus aureus, Bacteroides*, and gram-negative organisms
- Although rare, case reports of viral transmission via bites (hepatitis, HIV, and herpes)

## DIAGNOSIS

### SIGNS AND SYMPTOMS
- Location:
  - Upper extremities (60–75%)
  - Head and neck (15–20%)
  - Trunk (10–20%)
  - Lower extremities (~5%)
- Frequent complications:
  - Cellulitis
  - Serious deep-space infections (septic arthritis and osteomyelitis)
  - Fractures and tendon injuries
  - Hand bites have highest rates of infection.

### History
- Time of injury
- Patient allergies
- Relevant medical history (immune status)
- Last tetanus shot
- HIV, hepatitis B status of person inflicting bite

### Physical Exam
- Record the location and extent of all injuries.
- Document any swelling, crush injuries, or devitalized tissue.
- Note the range of motion of affected areas.
- Note the status of tendon and nerve function.
- Document any signs of infection, including regional adenopathy.
- Document any joint or bone involvement.

### ESSENTIAL WORKUP
Careful physical exam for involvement of deep structures and foreign bodies:
- Examine the deepest part of clenched-fist bites while putting the fingers through full range of motion to check for extensor tendon lacerations and joint violation.

### DIAGNOSTIC TESTS & INTERPRETATION
#### Lab
- Aerobic and anaerobic cultures from any infected bite wound
- Cultures not indicated if wounds not clinically infected
- CBC if signs of significant infection.
- Electrolytes, glucose, BUN, and creatinine:
  - For diabetic patients or those with significant infections

#### Imaging
- Generally not helpful
- Plain radiograph indications:
  - Fracture
  - Suspect foreign body (eg, tooth)
  - Baseline film if a bone or joint space has been violated in evaluating for osteomyelitis
  - For infection in proximity to a bone or joint space

### DIFFERENTIAL DIAGNOSIS
Bite injuries from animals:
- Sharper teeth cause more punctures and lacerations than human teeth, which usually cause more crush-type injuries.

### Pediatric Considerations
- In suspected sexual abuse:
  - Check for a central area of bruising or "hickey" from suction
- Linear abrasions or bruises on both the dorsal and palmar/plantar surfaces of the hand or foot:
  - Highly suggestive of bite marks
  - Lesions on one extremity should prompt a search for lesions on the other extremities.
- An intercanine distance of >3 cm indicates permanent dentition (present only if the attacker is older than 8 yr)
- If abuse suspected:
  - Rub a saline-moistened swab in the wound to collect any saliva and then place in a paper envelope for analysis.
  - Obtain photographs.
  - Notify authorities.

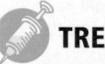

## TREATMENT

### PRE-HOSPITAL
Control bleeding with direct pressure.

### INITIAL STABILIZATION/THERAPY
ABCs: Ensure patent airway and adequate peripheral tissue perfusion

### ED TREATMENT/PROCEDURES
- Wound irrigation:
  - Copious volumes of normal saline irrigation with an 18-gauge needle or plastic catheter tip aimed in the direction of the puncture
  - Care should be taken not to inject fluid into the tissues.
- Débridement:
  - Remove any foreign material, necrotic skin tags, or devitalized tissues.
  - Do not débride puncture wounds.
  - Remove any eschar present so that underlying pus may be expressed and irrigated.
- CFIs:
  - Immobilize
  - Splint in a position of function that maintains the maximal length of ligaments and intrinsic muscles.
  - Use a bulky hand dressing.
  - Consultation with hand surgeon regarding operative irrigation/exploration of wound
  - Elevation for several days until any edema resolved
  - Sling for outpatients
  - Place the hand in a tubular stockinette attached to an IV pole for inpatients.
  - Administer antibiotics.
- Do not perform primary repair of avulsion wounds.

- Wound closure:
  - Closing wounds increases risk of infection and must be balanced with scar formation and effect of leaving wound open to heal secondarily.
  - Do not suture infected wounds or wounds >24 hr after injury.
  - Repair of wounds >8 hr after bite: Controversial
  - Close facial wounds up to 24 hr after bite (warn patient of high risk of infection).
  - Infected wounds and those presenting >24 hr should be left open.
  - May approximate the wound edges with Steri-Strips and perform a delayed primary closure
  - Do not suture CFIs.
- Prophylactic antibiotics controversial for low-risk bites
- Antibiotics for outpatients with:
  - Moderate to severe injuries with crush injury or edema
  - Involvement of the bone or a joint
  - Hand bites
  - Wounds near a prosthetic joint
  - Underlying disease (diabetes, prior splenectomy, or immunosuppression) that increases the risk of developing a more serious infection
- Tetanus prophylaxis
- Refer for possible testing/surveillance for HIV infection.

## MEDICATION
### First Line
- Amoxicillin/clavulanic acid (Augmentin): 500/125 mg (peds: 40 mg/kg/24h) q8h PO
- Ampicillin-sulbactam (UniSyn): 3 g q6h IV
- Piperacillin-Tazobactam (Zosyn): 4.5 g q8h IV
- Ticarcillin-clavulanate (Timentin): 3.1 g q4h IV
- Ceftriaxone (Rocephin): 1 g/day PLUS Metronidazole (Flagyl): 500 mg q8h

### Second Line
- 2 drug therapy: 1 of the following below plus anaerobic coverage:
  - Trimethoprim sulfamethoxazole (Septra DS): 1 tablet q12h (peds: 8 mg/kg trimethoprim and 40 mg/kg sulfamethoxazole per day divided into 2 daily doses) PO

- Penicillin (Penicillin VK): 500 mg (peds: 50 mg/kg/24 hr) PO q6h
  - Ciprofloxacin (Cipro): 500–750 mg q12h PO or 400 mg q12h IV
  - Doxycycline: 100 mg PO b.i.d.
- PLUS (anaerobic coverage):
  - Clindamycin (Cleocin): 150–450 mg (peds: 8–20 mg/kg/24 hr) PO q6h or 600–900 mg (peds: 20–40 mg/kg/24 hr) IV q8h
  - Metronidazole (Flagyl): 500 mg PO t.i.d. (peds: 10 mg/kg per dose t.i.d.)

 FOLLOW-UP

## DISPOSITION
### Admission Criteria
- Infected wounds at presentation
- Severe/advancing cellulitis/lymphangitis
- Signs of systemic infection
- Infected wounds that have failed to respond to outpatient (PO) antibiotics

### Discharge Criteria
- Healthy patient with localized wound infection:
  - Discharge on antibiotics with 24-hr follow-up.
- Noninfected wounds
  - 48-hr follow up

### Geriatric Considerations
- Human bite marks rarely occur accidentally; good indicators of inflicted injury.
- Consider elder abuse.

### Pediatric Considerations
- Human bite marks rarely occur accidentally; good indicators of inflicted injury.
- Consider child abuse.

### Issues for Referral
Suspected child abuse

## FOLLOW-UP RECOMMENDATIONS
- Hand specialist referral/follow-up for infected hand wounds
- Healthy patient with localized wound infection: Discharge on antibiotics with 24-hr follow-up.
- 48-hr follow-up for noninfected wounds

## PEARLS AND PITFALLS
- Examine the deepest part of clenched-fist bites while putting the fingers through full range of motion to check for extensor tendon lacerations and joint violation.
- Obtained hand consultation for operative irrigation for all patients with clenched-fist lacerations due to the high rate of infection.
- An intercanine distance of >3 cm indicates permanent dentition (present only if the attacker is older than 8 yr).

## ADDITIONAL READING
- Baddour L. Soft Tissue Infections due to Human bites. *UpToDate*, June 9, 2009.
- Broder J, et al. Low risk infection in selected human bites treated without antibiotics. *Amer J Emerg Med*. 2004;22(1):10–13.
- Brook I. Microbiology and management of human and animal bite wound infections. *Prim Care*. 2003;30(1):25–39.
- Medeiros I, et al. Antibiotic prophylaxis for Mammalian bites. *Cochrane Database Syst Rev*. 2001.
- Pickering L. *Red book: 2003 Report of the Committee on Infectious Diseases*, 26th ed. Amer Academy of Pediatrics, 2003.
- Smith PF, et al. Treating mammalian bite wounds. *J Clin Pharm Ther*. 2000;25:85–99.

### See Also (Topic, Algorithm, Electronic Media Element)
Bite, Mammal

# BLADDER INJURY

*Mary Beth Johnson*

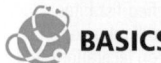 **BASICS**

## DESCRIPTION
- Blunt trauma is the most common mechanism.
- 10% of pelvic fractures have serious bladder injury.
- 80–90% of bladder ruptures have pelvic fracture.
- Mortality: 17–22% overall; 60% if combined intraperitoneal/extraperitoneal rupture

## ETIOLOGY
- Mechanism:
  - Trauma, 82%
  - Blunt trauma: Motor vehicle accident (MVA; 87%), falls (7%), assault (6%)
  - Penetrating: GSW (85%), stabbings (15%)
  - Iatrogenic 14%: TURP and urologic procedures, gynecologic procedures, obstetric procedures, abdominal procedures, hernia repair, intrauterine device (IUD), orthopedic hip procedures, biopsies, indwelling Foley
  - Intoxication 2.9%
  - Spontaneous <1%
- Classification:
  - Extraperitoneal bladder rupture (62%):
    - Associated with pelvic fractures
    - Caused by blunt force or fracture fragments
  - Intraperitoneal bladder rupture (25%):
    - Direct compression of distended bladder
    - Caused by rupture of the dome of the bladder
  - Combined extraperitoneal and intraperitoneal rupture (12%):
    - Highest mortality owing to associated injuries
  - Bladder contusion:
    - Damage to endothelial lining or muscularis layer with intact bladder wall
    - Gross hematuria after extreme physical activity (long-distance running)
    - Gross hematuria with normal imaging
    - Usually resolves without intervention

## Pediatric Considerations
- In children, the bladder is an intra-abdominal organ and descends into the pelvis by age 20 yr.
- Intraperitoneal rupture is more common in children than adults because the bladder is an abdominal organ.
- Bladder injury is more common in children than in adults because the pediatric bony pelvis is less rigid and transmits more force to adjacent structures.

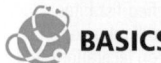 **DIAGNOSIS**

## SIGNS AND SYMPTOMS
Triad:
- Gross hematuria
- Suprapubic pain
- Difficulty voiding

### History
Establish potential mechanism.

### Physical Exam
Evaluate urethral meatus—if blood is present, do not insert Foley catheter until retrograde urethrogram (RUG) is performed (concomitant urethral and bladder injuries occur in 10–29% of patients).

## ESSENTIAL WORKUP
- History of trauma or procedures
- Evaluate urethral meatus for blood.
- Urinalysis (UA)
- Retrograde cystography

## DIAGNOSTIC TESTS & INTERPRETATION
### Lab
- Urinalysis:
  - Gross hematuria in 95–100% of patients with significant bladder or urethral trauma
  - Microscopic hematuria in 5%
- BUN and creatinine:
  - The BUN can be elevated from resorption of urine within the peritoneum.
- Electrolytes:
  - Hyperkalemia and hypernatremia may result from resorption of urine within the peritoneum.

### Imaging
- Retrograde cystography and retrograde CT cystography are the methods of choice to diagnose a ruptured bladder. Both studies have reported sensitivity and specificity of 95% and 100% respectively.
- If urethral injury is suspected, the cystogram is performed after a RUG.
- Cystography technique:
  - Kidneys/ureter/bladder (KUB) scout film
  - Infuse 100 mL of diluted contrast via Foley into bladder. Contrast material needs to be diluted: 30% or 6:1 saline; otherwise it is too dense.
  - Plane film is repeated to evaluate early extravasation.
  - If initial film is normal, fill rest of bladder with diluted contrast:
    - Minimum 300–350 mL total for adult
    - 3–5 mL/kg or 60 mL + (age in yr × 30) for children or until discomfort
  - It is essential to have a bladder full of contrast for diagnosis; it is not sufficient to place contrast and clamp Foley in antegrade fashion.
  - Cystogram films taken in AP, lateral, and oblique views (oblique may be difficult in trauma and CT is often used)
  - Empty bladder and obtain a postdrainage film unless CT cystography obtained.
  - Postdrainage film is essential without CT cystography—10% of bladder ruptures are seen only on postdrainage film; a distended bladder may hide extravasation.
- Cytography interpretation:
  - Extraperitoneal rupture: Tear drop- or star-shaped form
  - Intraperitoneal rupture: Outlining of bowel or contrast within the paracolic gutters

*Diagnostic Procedures/Surgery*
* FAST scan:
  – Free pelvic fluid should raise concern for bladder injury.

## DIFFERENTIAL DIAGNOSIS
* Peritoneal trauma
* Urethral trauma
* Renal or ureteric trauma

 # TREATMENT

### PRE-HOSPITAL
Do not attempt bladder catheterization in the field.

### INITIAL STABILIZATION/THERAPY
* ABCs
* Early urologic consultation

### ED TREATMENT/PROCEDURES
* Urologic consultation is needed when bladder rupture is diagnosed.
* Extraperitoneal nonpenetrating ruptures may be managed by catheter drainage:
  – 20 F Foley or larger for 14 days
  – 80% of lacerations will seal in 3 wk,
  – If patient is undergoing abdominal or pelvic surgery for other injury, surgical repair is recommended.
* Intraperitoneal ruptures require surgical exploration.
* Bladder contusions do not need any specific interventions.

### MEDICATION
Broad-spectrum antibiotics for intraperitoneal rupture

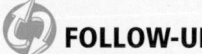 # FOLLOW-UP

## DISPOSITION
### Admission Criteria
* Concurrent major trauma requiring admission or observation
* Surgical intervention required

### Discharge Criteria
* Bladder contusion with no rupture or other major trauma requiring admission
* Most cases of bladder rupture will require admission; discharge only after clearance by urology and no other associated injuries.

### Issues for Referral
Any bladder injury managed as an outpatient should have urologic referral.

## FOLLOW-UP RECOMMENDATIONS
Follow-up to be arranged with urology:
* Extraperitoneal bladder rupture with Foley catheter management will have Foley removal in 14 days.

## PEARLS AND PITFALLS
* Any free fluid on CT or US exam should raise suspicion for bladder injury.
* Unresponsive, altered, and intoxicated patients warrant careful exam.
* Penetrating injuries to lower abdomen with any degree of hematuria warrant cystography.

## ADDITIONAL READING
* Marx JA, Hockberger RS, Walls RM, et al., eds. *Rosen's emergency medicine concepts and clinical practice*, 7th ed. St. Louis, MO: Mosby; 2009.
* Ramchadani P, Buckler PM. Imaging of genitourinary trauma. *Am J Roentgenol*. 200;192(6):1514–1523.
* Uptodate.com
* Wein AJ, Kavoussi LR, Novick AC, et al. eds. *Cambell-Walsh urology*, 9th ed. Philadelphia: WB Saunders, 2007.

### See Also (Topic, Algorithm, Electronic Media Element)
* Pelvic Fracture
* Urethral Trauma
* Trauma, Multiple

 # CODES

### ICD9
* 867.0 Injury to bladder and urethra without mention of open wound into cavity
* 867.1 Injury to bladder and urethra with open wound into cavity

# BLOW-OUT FRACTURE
*Shari Schabowski*

 **BASICS**

## DESCRIPTION
- Defined as an orbital floor fracture without orbital rim involvement
- Results from sudden blunt trauma to the globe:
  - Typically caused by the force of a projectile >half the size of the fist
- Force transmitted through the noncompressible structures of the globe to the weakest structural point: The orbital floor
- Transmitted force "blows out" or fractures the orbital floor.
- Orbital floor serves as roof to air-filled maxillary and ethmoid sinuses:
  - Communication between the spaces results in orbital emphysema.
- Orbit contains fat, which holds the globe in place:
  - Orbital floor fracture may result in herniation of the fat on the inferior orbital surface into the maxillary or ethmoid sinuses.
  - Leads to enophthalmos owing to orbital volume loss and sinus congestion and fluid collection may occur secondary to edema and bleeding.
- Infraorbital nerve runs through the bony canal 3 mm below the orbital floor:
  - Injury results in hypoesthesia of the ipsilateral cheek and upper lip.
  - To distinguish facial hypoesthesia related to local swelling from nerve injury: Test for sensation on the ipsilateral gingiva, which is within the infraorbital nerve distribution.
- Inferior rectus and the inferior oblique muscle run along the orbital floor:
  - Restriction of these extraocular muscles may occur because of entrapment within the fracture, contusion, or cranial nerve dysfunction.
  - Typically manifests as diplopia on upward gaze
  - Inability to elevate the affected eye normally on exam
- Medial rectus located above the ethmoid sinus:
  - Less commonly entrapped
  - Diplopia on ipsilateral lateral gaze

## ETIOLOGY
Caused by a projectile, which strikes the globe. The force is transmitted through the noncompressible structures of the globe to the weakest structural point: The orbital floor resulting in a blow out fracture.

### Pediatric Considerations
- Orbital roof fractures with associated CNS injuries more common
- Orbital floor fractures: Unlikely before 7 yr of age:
  - Orbital floor is not as weak a point in the orbit due to lack of pneumatization of the paranasal sinuses.
- Unfortunately fractures can occur in children and may result in unrecognized entrapment of the rectus muscle labeled the "white-eyed" fracture:
  - These children may present with marked nausea, vomiting, headache, and irritability suggestive of a head injury that commonly distracts from the true diagnosis.

 **DIAGNOSIS**

## SIGNS AND SYMPTOMS
- Periorbital tenderness, swelling, and ecchymosis
- Impaired ocular mobility or diplopia:
  - Restricted upward gaze owing to inferior rectus entrapment
  - Restricted ipsilateral lateral gaze with medial rectus entrapment
- Infraorbital hypoesthesia:
  - Caused by compression/contusion of infraorbital nerve
  - May extend to upper lip
- Enophthalmos:
  - Globe set back owing to orbital fat displaced through fracture
- Periorbital emphysema:
  - From the ethmoid or maxillary sinus
- Epistaxis
- Normal visual acuity:
  - If not, consider more extensive injuries
- No orbital rim step off

### Associated Severe Injuries
- Ocular injuries:
  - Ruptured globe:
    - Incidence up to 30% of blow-out fractures
    - Ophthalmologic emergency
  - Retrobulbar hemorrhage
  - Emphysematous optic nerve compression
- Cervical spine or intracranial injuries
- Commonly associated injuries:
  - Subconjunctival hemorrhage
  - Corneal abrasion/laceration
  - Hyphema
  - Traumatic mydriasis
  - Traumatic iridocyclitis (uveitis)
  - Less common:
  - Iridodialysis
  - Retinal detachment
  - Vitreous hemorrhage
  - Optic nerve injury
- Associated fractures:
  - Nasal bones
  - Zygomatic arch fracture
  - LeFort fracture
- Late complications:
  - Sinusitis
  - Orbital infection
  - Permanent restriction of extraocular movement
  - Enophthalmos

## History
Struck in the eye with a projectile. Paintball, handball, racquetball, baseball, rock, or possibly fist. Larger-sized projectiles will likely be blocked by the orbital rim. Seen frequently after MVC.

### Physical Exam
- Thorough ophthalmologic examination:
  - Palpate bony structures of the orbit for evidence of step off.
  - Careful attention not to place pressure on the globe until ruptured globe excluded:
    - Desmarres lid retractors may be necessary to evaluate the eye with swollen lid.
- Document pupillary response
- Visual acuity (should not be affected):
  - Handheld visual acuity Rosenbaum card is most useful with injuries.
- Test extraocular movements for disconjugate gaze or diplopia.
- Test sensation in inferior orbital nerve distribution.
- Examine lid and adnexa:
  - Orbital emphysema may be present.
- Slit-lamp and funduscopic examination to identify associated injuries
- Full physical exam to identify associated injuries and neurologic impairment

## DIAGNOSTIC TESTS & INTERPRETATION
### Lab
- Preoperative laboratory studies if indicated
- Pregnancy testing prior to radiography

### Imaging
- If CT unavailable or contraindicated, plain radiographs will provide important information:
  - Facial films
  - Orbits
  - Waters view and exaggerated Waters view:
    - Classic "teardrop sign" illustrates herniated mass of orbital contents in the ipsilateral maxillary sinus.
    - Opacification of or air fluid level in the ipsilateral maxillary sinus (less specific)
    - Orbital floor bony fracture
    - Lucency in orbits consistent with orbital emphysema
- CT-preferred modality:
  - Defines involved anatomy
  - Obtain axial and coronal 1.5-mm cuts:
    - Reconstruction of coronals not preferred but acceptable if positioning impossible

### Diagnostic Procedures/Surgery

Forced duction test:

- Distinguishes nerve dysfunction from entrapment
- Topical anesthesia applied to the conjunctiva on the opposite side, and the globe is pulled away from the expected point of entrapment; if the globe is not mobile, the test is positive—defining physical entrapment.

### Pediatric Considerations

- Orbital CT: Study of choice:
  - Plain films less helpful
- Essential to identify entrapment early as long-term outcome will likely be affected if left undiagnosed:
  - Early surgical intervention for entrapment may significantly improve outcome.

## DIFFERENTIAL DIAGNOSIS

- Cranial nerve palsy
- Orbital cellulitis
- Periorbital cellulitis
- Periorbital contusion/ecchymosis
- Retrobulbar hemorrhage
- Ruptured globe

 **TREATMENT**

## PRE-HOSPITAL

- Metal protective eye shield if possible globe injury
- Place in supine position.

## INITIAL STABILIZATION/THERAPY

Initial approach and immediate concerns:

- Assess for associated intracranial or cervical spine injuries.
- Rule out ruptured globe.
- Test visual acuity:
  - Decreased visual acuity suggestive of associated with more extensive injuries

## ED TREATMENT/PROCEDURES

- After globe rupture is excluded, apply cool compresses for the 1st 24–48 hr to decrease swelling to minimize or reverse herniation and avoid surgical intervention.
- Avoid Valsalva maneuvers and nose blowing to prevent compressive orbital emphysema.
- Prophylactic antibiotics to prevent infection
- Nasal decongestants if no contraindication
- Analgesics as needed
- Tetanus prophylaxis

## MEDICATION

- Antibiotics are recommended prophylactically to prevent sinusitis and orbital cellulitis:
  - Cephalexin 250 mg q6h for 10 days
- Systemic corticosteroids have been advocated to speed up the resorption of edema in order to more accurately assess any muscle entrapment and orbital damage:
  - Prednisone (60–80 mg/d) within 48 hr of the injury and continued for 5 days
- Nasal decongestants may be beneficial if not contraindicated:
  - Phenylephrine nasal spray b.i.d. for 2–4 days

 **FOLLOW-UP**

## DISPOSITION

### Admission Criteria

- Rarely indicated
- 85% resolve without surgical intervention.
- Consultation with facial trauma service in ED and consideration for admission if:
  - 50% of floor fractured
  - Diplopia or entrapment is identified
  - Particularly in children
  - Enophthalmos >2 mm or more

### Discharge Criteria

In most cases, observe for 10–14 days until swelling resolves, then follow up with facial trauma surgeon to determine need for surgical intervention.

## FOLLOW-UP RECOMMENDATIONS

Symptoms should improve over time:

- If at any point patient develops increased swelling, tenderness, redness or pain around the eye, they should return to ED for reevaluation.
- If any visual disturbance, visual loss, or increased eye pain return to ED for re-evaluation.

## PEARLS AND PITFALLS

- Be hypervigilant in checking pupillary response and visual acuity:
  - Abnormal results may be the 1st sign of serious complications:
    - Globe rupture
    - Optic nerve injury possibly stemming from emphysematous or retrobulbar compression
- Careful evaluation for entrapment:
  - Essential for all, but particularly children, to exclude white-eyed fracture and its long-term complications
- The oculocardiac (Aschner) reflex may be associated with this injury. It manifests as a decrease in pulse rate associated with traction applied to extraocular muscles and/or compression of the eyeball:
  - May be seen more commonly in children
  - Treated by release of pressure and in some cases may require atropine

## ADDITIONAL READING

- Burnstine M. Clinical recommendations for repair of isolated orbital floor fractures An evidence-based analysis. *Ophthalmology.* 2002;109(7):1207–1210.
- Cruz A, Antonio A, Eichenberger G. Epidemiology and management of orbital fractures. *Curr Opin Ophthalmol.* 2004;15(5):416–421.
- Hatton MP, Watkins LM, Rubin PA. Orbital fractures in children. *Ophthalmol Plast Reconstr Surg.* 2001;17(3):174–179.
- Linden JA, Renner GS. Trauma to the globe. *Emerg Med Clin North Am.* 1995;13(3):581–605.

### See Also (Topic, Algorithm, Electronic Media Element)

- Facial Fractures
- Globe Rupture
- Iritis
- Oculomotor Nerve Palsy
- Periorbital and Orbital Cellulitis

# BOERHAAVE SYNDROME
*Lauren M. Smith*

## 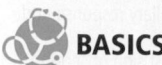 BASICS

### DESCRIPTION
- Spontaneous esophageal rupture:
  - From sudden combined increase in both:
- Intra-abdominal pressure
- Negative intrathoracic pressure
  - Causes complete, full-thickness (transmural), longitudinal tear in esophagus
- Esophagus has no serosal layer (which normally contains collagen and elastic fibers):
  - Results in weak structure vulnerable to perforation and mediastinal contamination
  - Esophageal wall is further weakened by conditions that damage mucosa (i.e. esophagitis is of various causes).
- Majority of perforations occur at left posterolateral wall of the lower third esophagus.
- Significant morbidity/mortality (most lethal GI tract perforation):
  - Owing to explosive nature of tear
  - Owing to almost immediate contamination of mediastinum with contents of esophagus

### ETIOLOGY
- Associated with:
  - Forceful vomiting and retching (most common)
  - Heavy lifting
  - Seizures
  - Childbirth
  - Blunt trauma
  - Induced emesis
  - Laughing
- Common in middle-aged men
- Medical procedures cause over 50% of all perforations.

### Pediatric Considerations
Described in female neonates but rarely seen

## 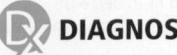 DIAGNOSIS

### SIGNS AND SYMPTOMS
#### History
- Often no classic symptoms
- Most common symptoms:
  - Chest or epigastric pain after vomiting/retching
- Mackler triad:
  - Vomiting/retching
  - Chest pain
  - Subcutaneous emphysema
- Retrosternal chest pain present in most patients:
  - Often pleuritic
  - Radiates to back or left shoulder
  - Worsens with swallowing
- Odynophagia
- Swallowing may precipitate coughing.

#### Physical Exam
- Dyspnea
- Diaphoresis
- SC emphysema in neck and chest wall
- Mediastinal crackling on auscultation (Hamman's crunch)
- Pleural effusions
- Tachypnea
- Fever
- Shock, in more severe cases
- If untreated, mediastinitis will develop and abscesses will form.
- Not usually associated with bleeding

### ESSENTIAL WORKUP
- Upright chest radiographs (preferably posteroanterior and lateral views if tolerated) evaluating for:
  - Pneumomediastinum
  - SC emphysema
  - Pleural effusion (left side)
  - Pneumothorax
  - Widened mediastinum
  - Hydropneumothorax
  - Empyema
  - Free peritoneal air
  - Naclerio "V" sign:
    - V-shaped radiolucency seen through the heart (air in left lower mediastinum)

- Contrast esophagram identifies leak in esophagus:
  - Controversy exists regarding contrast use, water-soluble vs. barium
  - Water-soluble contrast material was thought to be less toxic if extravasated into the mediastinum, however if aspirated may cause necrotizing pneumonitis.
  - Barium, more sensitive for diagnosing perforation, but more irritating to the mediastinum
  - If esophagus is intact, use barium contrast for better detail.
  - Aids in decision of which type of surgical approach

### DIAGNOSTIC TESTS & INTERPRETATION
#### Lab
- CBC
- PT/PTT
- Blood cultures
- Pleural effusion:
  - Amylase content
  - pH (<6)
  - Undigested food particles
- ECG

#### Imaging
- CXR
- Endoscopy:
  - Controversial
  - Can extend perforation and/or introduce air into mediastinum
- CT chest:
  - Sensitive for identifying free air, periesophageal fluid, mediastinal widening, but does not isolate lesion
  - Indicated if esophagram cannot be obtained
  - Evaluates other intrathoracic structures

### DIFFERENTIAL DIAGNOSIS
- Cholecystitis
- Dissecting aortic aneurysm
- Intestinal obstruction
- Lung abscess
- Mesenteric thrombosis
- Myocardial infarction
- Pneumothorax
- Pericarditis
- Pneumonia
- Pancreatitis
- Pulmonary thromboembolism
- Ruptured abdominal viscus
- Spontaneous pneumomediastinum (clinically benign)

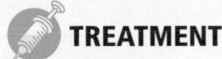

# TREATMENT

## PRE-HOSPITAL
- Airway control must be established if patient unresponsive or airway patency in jeopardy.
- Establish 2 large-bore intravenous catheters and treat hypotension with 0.9% NS.
- Avoid opiates until patient is in ED to avoid complication of hypotension.

## INITIAL STABILIZATION/THERAPY
- ABCs
- Airway control: 100% oxygen or intubate patient if unresponsive or airway patency is in jeopardy.
- Establish intravenous access and treat hypotension:
  - Administer 1 L (20 mL/kg) bolus with 0.9% NS (or lactated Ringer solution).
  - Initiate dopamine if blood pressure does not respond to fluids.
  - Central catheter placement if condition of patient remains unstable for more efficient delivery of fluids and monitoring of central venous pressure

## ED TREATMENT/PROCEDURES
- NPO
- Careful placement of a nasogastric tube to decompress the stomach
- Bladder catheter to monitor urine output
- Expedient diagnosis to decrease incidence of morbidity/mortality
- Prompt surgical consultation
- Definitive treatment:
  - Surgical repair of perforation
  - Adequate drainage
- Initiate broad-spectrum antibiotics directed against oral microflora and gastrointestinal pathogens:
  - Ampicillin/sulbactam plus gentamicin
  - Imipenem/Cilastatin

## MEDICATION
- Ampicillin/sulbactam: 3.0 g IV q6h
- Dopamine: 2–20 $\mu$g/kg/min IV per bolus
- Gentamicin: 2 mg/kg load, then 1.7 mg/kg IV q8h or 5.1 mg/kg IV qd (assuming normal renal function)
- Imipenem/cilastatin: 250–500 IV q6h

# FOLLOW-UP

## DISPOSITION
### Admission Criteria
All cases of Boerhaave syndrome must be admitted to surgical ICU:
- Cervical esophageal perforations may be treated by drainage alone.
- All thoracic and abdominal perforations require surgical intervention.

### Discharge Criteria
None

### Issues for Referral
Thoracic or general surgeon consult for admission and possible operative intervention.

## FOLLOW-UP RECOMMENDATIONS
As per surgeon recommendations

# PEARLS AND PITFALLS
- Chest radiographs done immediately after injury may be normal.
- Left pleural space involvement is usually associated with a distal esophageal perforation.
- Right pleural space involvement is usually associated with proximal esophageal perforations.

- Immediate surgical consultation is the keystone of management.
- If esophagram is negative and there is high suspicion, repeat with patient in left and right decubitus positions.

## ADDITIONAL READING
- Jagminas L, Silverman RA. Boerhaave syndrome presenting with abdominal pain and right hydropneumothorax. *Am J Emerg Med.* 1996;14:53–55.
- Ma G, Jacoby I. Spontaneous esophageal rupture. *J Emerg Med.* 2000;18:257–258.
- Singh H, Warshawrsky ME, Herman Shanies HM. Spontaneous esophageal rupture: Boerhaave's syndrome. *Clin Pulm Med.* 2003;10:177–182.
- Troum S, Lane CE, Dalton ML Jr. Surviving Boerhaave's syndrome without thoracotomy. *Chest.* 1994;106:297–298.
- Wu JT, Mattox KL, Wall MJ. Esophageal perforations: New perspectives and treatment paradigms. *J Trauma Inj Infect Crit Care.* 2007;63:1173–1184.
- Younes Z, Johnson DA. The spectrum of spontaneous and iatrogenic esophageal injury: Perforations, Mallory-Weiss tears, and hematomas. *J Clin Gastroenterol.* 1999;29:306–317.

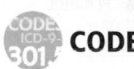 CODES

ICD9
530.4 Perforation of esophagus

# BOTULISM

Philip Shayne
Alan T. Chiem

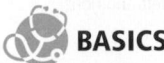 **BASICS**

## DESCRIPTION
- Rare in U.S., causing <200 cases/year; however, has significant bioterrorism potential.
- Caused by a polypeptide, heat-labile exotoxin produced by *Clostridium botulinum*:
  - Most potent poison known
- Toxin blocks neuromuscular transmission in cholinergic nerve fibers.
- Symptoms occur by inhibition of acetylcholine release from presynaptic nerve membranes:
  - Damage is permanent.
  - Recovery is by formation of new synapses through sprouting from the axon.
- Onset: 12–72 hr after exposure; may be up to 1 wk after exposure:
  - Death can occur 24 hr after onset of symptoms.
- Slow recovery; symptoms often persist for months
- Mortality:
  - Untreated: 60–70%
  - With supportive care: 3–10%
- 3 major types: Food-borne botulism, wound botulism, and infantile botulism (see "Pediatric Considerations")
- Food-borne botulism:
  - Occurs by ingestion of preformed toxin; improperly canned food facilitates the necessary anaerobic conditions.
  - Conditions required for exposure:
    - Food product contaminated with *C. botulinum* bacilli or spores
    - Proper conditions for germination of spores exist.
    - Time and conditions permit production of toxin before eating.
    - Food not heated sufficiently to destroy botulism toxin
    - Toxin-containing food ingested by susceptible host
- Wound botulism:
  - Clinical evidence of botulism after trauma with a resultant infected wound and no history suggestive of food-borne illness
  - Botulinum isolated in about 50%
  - Wounds usually contaminated with soil
  - Seen sporadically in chronic drug abusers, especially black-tar heroin users or "skin poppers"
- Other types:
  - Adult intestinal toxemia botulism:
    - Seen in adults with functional or structural GI abnormalities, or with prolonged antibiotic use
    - Predisposes to *Clostridial* colonization
    - May have sporadic or recurrent botulism with no known source and even after immunoglobulin treatment
  - Iatrogenic botulism:
    - Symptoms similar to those of classic botulism
    - Doses found in cosmetic applications are insufficient to cause systemic symptoms.
    - Doses for treatment of muscle movement disorders may cause systemic symptoms.
  - Inhalation botulism:
    - Aerosolization of toxin may have bioterrorism applications.

### Pediatric Considerations
- Infantile botulism occurs from the ingestion of *C. botulinum* spores, which germinate in the gut and produce the toxin.
- Accounts for 50–75% of botulism cases
- 90% occur in children younger than 6 mo:
  - Associated with patient or family exposure to soil, dust, or agricultural industry
  - May also be associated with weaning from breast milk, which may alter intestinal flora and increase susceptibility to *Clostridia* infection.
- Usually presents with change in stool pattern or constipation, progressing over several days to symptoms of bulbar weakness, then descending flaccid paralysis.
- Slower onset is attributed to the toxin being produced locally as opposed to being ingested in one dose.
- *C. botulinum* spores found in honey:
  - Honey not recommended for children younger than 1 yr.

## ETIOLOGY
- *C. botulinum* is a large spore-forming, usually gram-positive, strictly anaerobic bacilli ubiquitous in nature.
- Each strain produces antigenically distinct toxins, designated types A through G:
  - Types A, B, and E are responsible for most human cases.

 **DIAGNOSIS**

## SIGNS AND SYMPTOMS
### History
- Ingestions/food history for previous 4–5 days:
  - Exposures traditionally from home-processed fruit or vegetable products
- Immune status (AIDS, cancer, chronic illness)
- IV drug use
- Exposure to therapeutic/cosmetic use

### Physical Exam
- Food-borne botulism (classic botulism):
  - Bulbar weakness is invariably the initial presentation: Diplopia, dysphagia, dysarthria, and dysphonia
  - Subsequent symmetric, descending weakness or paralysis of the extremities (hallmark of the disease)
  - No sensory deficit
  - May have progressively diminishing deep tendon reflexes
  - Patient remains awake/alert; mentation unaffected
  - Ventilatory insufficiency from weakness of respiratory muscles

- Autonomic dysfunction (sympathetic and parasympathetic):
  - Dry mouth
  - Blurred vision
  - Orthostatic hypotension
  - Constipation
  - Urinary retention
- Nausea and vomiting with food-borne botulism only
- Afebrile
- Wound botulism:
  - Finding similar to food-borne botulism
  - May be febrile as a result of soft-tissue infection
- Infantile botulism:
  - Constipation
  - Weakness
  - Poor suck
  - Weak cry
  - Lethargy
  - Hypotonia
  - Flaccid facial expression
  - Respiratory difficulty
- Inhalation botulism:
  - Similar to food-borne with absence of GI symptoms

## ESSENTIAL WORKUP
- Diagnosis is entirely clinical.
- Workup focuses on differentiation from other conditions causing general paralysis.
- If diagnosis is suspected, immediately notify state health department or CDC.

## DIAGNOSTIC TESTS & INTERPRETATION
### Lab
- CBC
- Electrolytes, BUN/creatinine, and glucose:
  - Check for hypokalemia.
- Arterial blood gas (ABG):
  - For signs of respiratory insufficiency
- Confirmatory testing via mouse assay performed by select state and federal laboratories, using samples from:
  - Blood
  - Feces
  - Gastric contents
  - Suspected food and containers
- Anaerobic blood cultures:
  - May detect bacterium
- Nasal swab for ELISA test:
  - For inhalation botulism, as less reliably detected in sera and stool than other forms
  - Sample needs to be collected within 24 hr of exposure

### Imaging
CT/MRI of brain:
- Normal

### Diagnostic Procedures/Surgery
- CSF testing:
  - Normal
  - Helps differentiate from Guillain-Barré syndrome (which as markedly elevated CSF protein)
- Electrophysiologic studies:
  - Normal nerve conduction with diminished evoked muscle action potential
- Edrophonium testing may be positive, but not to the degree seen in myasthenia gravis.

### DIFFERENTIAL DIAGNOSIS
- Myasthenia gravis (less acute)
- Lambert-Eaton myasthenic syndrome (less acute)
- Polio (fever and asymmetric)
- Guillain-Barré (simultaneous sensory findings and elevated spinal fluid protein)
- Tick paralysis
- Magnesium intoxication
- Hypokalemic periodic paralysis
- Diphtheritic neuropathy
- Rare basilar stroke syndromes with bulbar palsy

### Pediatric Considerations
- Often misdiagnosed as dehydration, sepsis, or Reye syndrome
- Other diagnoses include: Inborn errors of metabolism, Guillain-Barré syndrome, and spinal muscle atrophy.

 TREATMENT

### ALERT
Death is invariably from progressive ventilatory failure:
- Intubate as soon as respiratory insufficiency noted, clinically or based on ABG.
- May require several weeks of ventilatory support

### PRE-HOSPITAL
- Transcutaneous pacing for unstable type II 2nd- or 3rd-degree block
- Atropine:
  - Avoid with type II 2nd-degree block because it may precipitate complete heart block
  - Contraindicated in 3rd-degree heart block with a widened QRS complex
- Attempts should be made at preventing increases in vagal tone.

### INITIAL STABILIZATION/THERAPY
- Early intubation and ventilatory support is the key to survival.
- Respiratory difficulties occur rapidly.

### ED TREATMENT/PROCEDURES
- Bivalent AB antitoxin:
  - IV administration as soon as the diagnosis is made, without waiting for laboratory confirmation
  - Before use assess hypersensitivity with skin test using horse serum or antitoxin
  - Using recommended dose <1% will have hypersensitivity reaction
- Nasogastric (NG) suctioning if ileus is profound
- If there is no evidence of ileus, use enema or cathartics to clear unbound toxin from GI tract.
- With wound botulism, perform wound débridement even if it appears to be healing.
- Antibiotics for specific infectious complications
- Standard precautions only; no evidence of person-to-person transmission

### MEDICATION
- ABE antitoxin formulations no longer used because of declines in titer to type E toxin
- FDA-approved:
  - Bivalent botulism equine-derived antitoxin: 1 vial (~10,000 IU each of types A, B) IV for adults
  - Baby BIG human-derived antitoxin to Type A and B: 50 mg/kg IV for pediatric patients

### Pediatric Considerations
- Baby BIG halves average hospital stay from 6–3 wk:
  - Adult equine antitoxin should not be used on pediatric patients
- Antibiotics:
  - Ineffective in eradicating organism from the intestine
  - Release of toxin in the gut through bacterial cell lysis may worsen neurologic symptoms.

### Second Line
Not FDA approved/investigational:
- Antitoxin to type E (available from CDC and CA Dept of Health Services)
- Heptavalent despeciated equine antitoxin (HE-BAT and Hfab-BAT, investigated by US Army Research Institute and CDC)

 FOLLOW-UP

### DISPOSITION
#### Admission Criteria
Admit patients with suspected botulism poisoning to monitored bed:
- ICU admission for any respiratory deficiency

#### Discharge Criteria
Clinical course of botulism poisoning is unpredictable; it can become rapidly progressive and fatal:
- Discharge only patients with a prolonged period of progressive recovery from symptoms.

### FOLLOW-UP RECOMMENDATIONS
- Physical medicine and rehabilitation:
  - Residual weakness can last for up to 1 yr
- Mental health:
  - Patients and their families often experience stress and depression with the prolonged recovery.

## PEARLS AND PITFALLS
- Botulism is a public health emergency; early consultation with state and federal health departments is required.
- Suspect botulism if there are more than 2 cases; other conditions on the differential do not produce outbreaks.
- Antitoxin does not reverse paralysis but only halts its progression. Therefore, administer antitoxin once diagnosis is suspected. Do not wait until signs of respiratory compromise are present.
- Initial signs of respiratory distress may not be clinically apparent secondary to paralysis.
- Bulbar palsy at presentation may be mistaken for altered mental status.

## ADDITIONAL READING
- CDC. Botulism. *Emergency Preparedness and Response*. Accessed on 11/02/09 from: http://emergency.cdc.gov/agent/botulism
- Dembek ZF, Smith LA, Rusnak JM. Botulism: Cause, effects, diagnosis, clinical and laboratory identification, and treatment modalities. *Disaster Med Public Health Preparedness*. 2007;1:122–134.
- Domingo RM, Haller JS, Gruenthal M. Infant botulism: Two recent cases and literature review. *J Child Neurol*. 2008;23:1336–1346.
- Robinson RF, Nahata MC. Management of botulism. *Ann Pharmacother*. 2003;37:127–131.
- Sobel J. Botulism. *Clin Inf Dis*. 2005;41:1167–1173.
- Wenham TN. Botulism: A rare complication of injecting drug use. *Emerg Med J*. 2008;25:55–56.

# BOWEL OBSTRUCTION
*Jenny J. Lu*

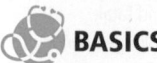 **BASICS**

## DESCRIPTION
- Obstruction of normal intestinal flow from mechanical or nonmechanical causes
- Obstruction leads to rapid increase in both anaerobic and aerobic bacteria, with resultant increase in methane and hydrogen production.
- Distended bowel becomes progressively edematous, and increased intestinal secretions cause further distention.
- Retrograde peristalsis causes vomiting.

## ETIOLOGY
- Small bowel obstruction (SBO):
  - Adhesions: Most common cause
  - Hernias
  - Neoplasms
  - Strictures: Inflammatory bowel
  - Trauma: Bowel wall hematoma
  - Miscellaneous: eg, ascaris infection
- Large bowel obstruction (LBO):
  - Carcinoma
  - Volvulus
  - Diverticular disease
  - Inflammatory bowel disease
  - Ischemic colitis

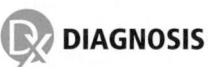 **DIAGNOSIS**

## SIGNS AND SYMPTOMS
### History
- Previous surgery, malignancy, constipation, or cathartic use
- Abdominal pain:
  - Intermittent when early
  - Constant with strangulated obstruction
- Vomiting:
  - Bile-stained emesis with proximal obstruction
  - Feculent emesis with distal obstruction
- Obstipation
- Stool caliber changes

## Physical Exam
- Vital signs:
  - Tachycardia, hypotension with significant volume depletion
  - Fever with strangulation or perforation
  - Hypothermia with sepsis
- Abdominal examination:
  - Distention
  - Variable tenderness, often diffuse
  - Hyperactive and high-pitched bowel sounds when early; hyperactive when late
  - Consider ischemic or gangrenous bowel if pain out of proportion to exam.
  - Peritoneal signs indicate strangulation or perforation.
- Hernia (ventral, inguinal, femoral)
- Rectal exam:
  - Rectal mass
  - Blood in stool, gross or occult

## Geriatric Considerations
- Abdominal pain variable in elderly, may be vague
- Nausea/vomiting and abdominal pain are common symptoms in elderly patients with acute myocardial infarctions:
  - Abdominal distention, obstipation, and colicky pain suggest GI cause.

## Pediatric Considerations
- Intussusception:
  - Leading cause of intestinal obstruction in infants
  - Most common between 3 and 12 mo of age
- Incarcerated inguinal/umbilical hernia
- Malrotation with volvulus:
  - Can occur as early as 3–7 days of age
  - Double bubble sign seen on plain radiograph owing to partial obstruction of duodenum, resulting in air in stomach and in first part of duodenum
- Pyloric stenosis:
  - Progressive, projectile, nonbilious, postprandial vomiting
  - Male/female ratio: 5:1 incidence
  - Onset usually 2–5 wk of age
- Other causes include duodenal atresia, Hirschsprung, and imperforate anus.

## ESSENTIAL WORKUP
Careful history and physical exam

## DIAGNOSTIC TESTS & INTERPRETATION
### Lab
- CBC:
  - Leukocytosis common
- Electrolytes, BUN/creatinine, glucose:
  - Hypokalemia
  - Hypochloremic metabolic alkalosis
  - Prerenal azotemia
- Urinalysis
- Amylase/lipase
- Lactate
- Stool heme test
- Type and cross-match
- PT/PTT
- Liver enzymes/function to exclude hepatic/biliary pathology
- ECG in patients at risk of coronary artery disease

### Imaging
- Upright CXR:
  - Evaluate for pulmonary pathology.
  - Check for free air beneath diaphragm.
- Plain abdominal radiographs, supine and upright (75% sensitivity):
  - Distended loops of bowel (normal small bowel <3 cm in diameter)
  - Distended cecum >13 cm indicates potential for perforation.
  - Air fluid levels
  - "String of pearls" sign if small bowel loops nearly completely fluid filled
- Abdominal CT:
  - Sensitivity:
    - 90% for SBO
    - 91% for LBO
  - Detects neoplastic causes and staging malignancy
  - Identify early strangulation (with IV contrast)
  - Exclude other incidental findings/causes
  - Has decreased use of contrast enemas due to ease of use
- US:
  - More sensitive and specific than plain films for small bowel obstruction but not as accurate as CT

### *Diagnostic Procedures/Surgery*
Upper GI/barium enema:
- If carcinoma or mass lesion suspected as cause
- Have decreased in use with availability of CT scan
- May be painful or difficult in sick patients

## DIFFERENTIAL DIAGNOSIS
- Paralytic ileus
- Pseudo-obstruction (Ogilvie)
- Perforated ulcer
- Pancreatitis
- Cholecystitis
- Colitis
- Mesenteric ischemia

 # TREATMENT

## PRE-HOSPITAL
Establish IV access for patients with dehydration, vomiting, or significant abdominal pain.

## INITIAL STABILIZATION/THERAPY
- ABCs
- 0.9% normal saline (NS) or lactated ringers (LR) IV fluid resuscitation for significant volume depletion and strangulated or perforated bowel:
  - Adults: 1 L bolus
  - Peds: 20 mL/kg bolus
- Correct electrolyte abnormalities, especially hypokalemia.

## ED TREATMENT/PROCEDURES
- IV fluids (IVFs)
- Nasogastric tube (NGT)
- Foley catheter to monitor urine output
- Surgical consultation
- Antibiotics for suspected strangulated/perforated bowel:
  - Antibiotic choices should cover gram-negative aerobic and anaerobic organisms:
  - Single agent:
    o Piperacillin/tazobactam
    o Ampicillin/sulbactam
    o Meropenem or imipenem
  - Combination regimen:
    o Metronidazole PLUS ciprofloxacin or ceftriaxone
- Analgesics:
  - Morphine sulfate
- Antiemetics:
  - Odansetron
  - Promethazine

## MEDICATION
- Antibiotic choices (broad spectrum, for suspected ischemia):
  - Piperacillin-tazobactam (Zosyn): 3.375 g (peds: 150–400 mg/kg/24 hr IV div. q6–8h) IV q4–6h
  - Ampicillin-sulbactam (Unasyn): 1.5–3 g (peds: 100–400 mg/kg/24 hr IV div. q6h) IV q6h
  - Meropenem (Merrem): Adult: 1 g (peds: 60–120 mg/kg/24 hr IV q8h) IV q8h
  - Imipenem-cilastatin (Primaxin/): 250–1,000 mg (peds: 50–100 mg/kg/24 hr IV q6–12h) IV q6–8h
  - Metronidazole (Flagyl): 1 g IV, then 500 mg IV q6h (peds: 7.5–30 mg/kg/24 hr IV div. q6–8h)
  - Ciprofloxacin (Cipro): 400 mg IV q12h
  - Ceftriaxone (Rocephin): 1–2 g (peds: 25–75 mg/kg/d IV up to 2 g div. q12–24h) IV q24h
- Analgesics:
  - Morphine: 2–10 mg/dose (peds: 0.1–0.2 mg/kg IV/IM/SC q2–4h) IV/IM/SC q2–6h PRN
- Antiemetics:
  - Odansetron (Zofran): 4 mg (peds: 0.1 mg/kg IV div. q8h) IV q4–8h PRN
  - Promethazine (Phenergan): 12.5–25 mg (peds: >2 yr: 0.25–1 mg/kg/d IV/IM/PR div. q4–6h PRN) IV/IM/SC q4h

 # FOLLOW-UP

## DISPOSITION
### *Admission Criteria*
All patients with suspected/confirmed intestinal obstruction should be admitted with early surgical consultation.

### *Discharge Criteria*
Normal laboratory/radiology results with resolution of symptoms and no further suspicion for intestinal obstruction.

### *Issues for Referral*
Surgery consult for patients with bowel obstruction

## FOLLOW-UP RECOMMENDATIONS
Discharged patients:
- Normal laboratory and radiological studies
- Timely appointment for re-evaluation
- Explicit instructions detailing signs/symptoms to return to emergency department

## PEARLS AND PITFALLS
- Carefully examine patient with history of vomiting for incarcerated hernias.
- Failure to diagnose bowel obstruction, bowel ischemia, and necrosis:
  - Symptoms potentially vague, nonspecific in very old and very young
- Failure to adequately replete fluid losses and electrolyte imbalances

## ADDITIONAL READING
- Blot S, DeWaele JJ. Critical issues in the clinical management of complicated intra-abdominal infections. *Drugs.* 2005;65(12):1611–1620.
- Jacob SE, Lee SH, Hill J. The demise of the instant/unprepared contrast enema in large bowel obstruction. *Colorectal Dis.* 2008;10(7):729–731.
- Moran BJ. Adhesion-related small bowel obstruction. *Colorectal Dis.* 2007;9(2):39–44.
- Sanson TG, O'Keefe KP. Evaluation of abdominal pain in the elderly. *Emerg Med Clin North Am.* 1996;14:615–627.
- Sivit C. Gastrointestinal emergencies in older infants and children. *Radiol Clin North Am.* 1997;35:865.

### See Also (Topic, Algorithm, Electronic Media Element)
- Abdominal Pain
- Gastric Outlet Obstruction
- Pyloric Stenosis
- Vomiting

# BRADYARRHYTHMIAS

*Julie L. Story*
*Benjamin S. Heavrin*

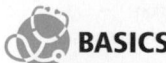 **BASICS**

## DESCRIPTION
- Ventricular heart rate <60 beats per minute:
  – Sinus bradycardia can be normal variant.
  – All other rhythms are pathogenic.
- May be asymptomatic or have hypotension, altered mental status, fatigue, nausea, syncope.
- Treatment varies based on ECG findings and clinical status.

## ETIOLOGY
- Idiopathic:
  – Healthy athletes
- Intrinsic cardiac disorders:
  – Sinus node dysfunction such as sick sinus syndrome (may alternate with tachycardia)
  – Atrioventricular block:
  – Junctional or ventricular escape rhythm
  – Infiltrative disease:
    ○ Amyloidosis, sarcoidosis, hemochromatosis
  – Collagen vascular disease:
    ○ SLE, scleroderma, rheumatoid arthritis
  – Anatomic abnormalities:
    ○ Congenital, postsurgical/posttransplant, postradiation
  – Muscular disorders:
    ○ Myotonic muscular dystrophy
  – Trauma with myocardial stunning
- Extrinsic disorders:
  – Cardiac injury and infarction:
    ○ RCA infarction can cause sinus bradycardia.
    ○ LAD infarction can cause high grade block.
  – Acidemia
  – Medication and toxin effects:
    ○ β-Blockers, calcium-channel blockers, digoxin, clonidine, antiarrhythmics, lithium, organophosphate
  – Electrolyte abnormalities:
    ○ Hypo-/hyperkalemia, hypoglycemia, hypo-/hypercalcemia, hypermagnesemia
  – Vital sign abnormalities:
    ○ Hypoxia, hypothermia, hypotension, HTN
  – Endocrine abnormalities:
    ○ Hypothyroidism
  – Infectious disease:
    ○ Lyme disease, Chagas disease, diphtheria, endocarditis, myocarditis
  – Neurologic disorders:
    ○ Increased intracranial pressure, increased vagal tone, carotid sinus hypersensitivity, spinal cord injury
    ○ Can be triggered by micturition, defecation, coughing, vomiting, ocular pressure, or other Valsalva maneuvers

### Pediatric Considerations
Hypoxia is the most common etiology in children.

### Pregnancy Considerations
Maternal systemic lupus erythematosus can result in congenital complete heart block.

## DIAGNOSIS

### SIGNS AND SYMPTOMS
- Often asymptomatic
- Lightheadedness, confusion, fatigue, decreased level of consciousness
- Dyspnea, cyanosis, pallor
- Chest pain/pressure, diaphoresis
- Hypotension, HR <60, syncope, cardiac arrest
- Hypothermia

### History
- Medication changes, especially cardiac
- Urine output:
  – Hypokalemia with diuretics
  – Hyperkalemia with renal failure
- Trauma:
  – Intracranial injury
  – Myocardial contusion
- Activity at time of symptom onset:
  – Increased vagal tone

### Physical Exam
- Respiratory status
- Perfusion status, pulses
- Regular vs. irregular cardiac rhythm
- Mental status, thorough neuro exam
- Body habitus, skin/hair/nails
- Temperature

### ESSENTIAL WORKUP
- ECG and continuous cardiac monitoring
- Pulse oximetry
- BP monitoring
- Glucose and electrolytes

### DIAGNOSTIC TESTS & INTERPRETATION
#### Lab
- Serum glucose
- Serum electrolytes
- BUN and creatinine
- Cardiac enzymes
- Digoxin level
- Thyroid function tests
- ANA, RF, other rheumatologic testing
- Lyme titers
- Iron levels

#### Imaging
CXR

### Diagnostic Procedures/Surgery
EKG:
- Sinus bradycardia:
  – P wave before every QRS, QRS after every P wave, usually narrow QRS
- Sinoatrial block: Abnormal conduction between sinus node and atrium
- Sinus arrest:
  – No sinus activity, no P waves
- Atrioventricular block: Abnormal conduction between atria and ventricles:
  – 1st degree: PR >0.2 sec, every P wave conducts a QRS complex
  – 2nd-degree type I, Mobitz I, Wenckebach: Progressive prolongation of PR interval and shortening of R-R interval with eventual dropped QRS, grouped beats
  – 2nd-degree type II, Mobitz II: Stable PR interval and intermittent dropped QRS, high risk of degeneration into 3rd-degree block
  – 3rd-degree, complete heart block: Complete dissociation of atrial and ventricular activity, constant P-P interval and constant R-R interval, but no relation between the 2, unstable rhythm
- Junctional rhythm:
  – Loss of atrial conduction, AV pacemaker "escapes" at 40–60 bpm
  – Retrograde P waves may occur before, during, or after QRS, and QRS can be any duration
- Idioventricular rhythm:
  – Loss of both SA and AV nodal activity, bundle of His or Purkinje network takes over at 30–40 bpm
  – QRS always >0.12 sec
  – Preterminal rhythm

### DIFFERENTIAL DIAGNOSIS
- Normal variant
- Cardiac ischemia
- Medication toxicity
- Pacemaker malfunction
- Hypoxia
- Hypothermia
- Electrolyte abnormality
- Renal failure
- Hypothyroidism
- Infection
- Rheumatologic disease
- Neuromuscular disease
- Increased intracranial pressure
- Myocardial contusion

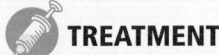
## TREATMENT

### PRE-HOSPITAL
- Treat the patient, not the heart rate
- Oxygen:
  - For all patients, especially pediatrics
- If hypothermic, warm the patient and give magnesium:
  - Do NOT pace; move patient gently as rough handling can induce v-fib.
- Atropine or epinephrine:
  - Only if hypotension or altered mental status
  - Often ineffective or harmful in 3rd-degree block
- Transcutaneous pacing:
  - If other measures ineffective

### INITIAL STABILIZATION/THERAPY
- ABCs
- Oxygen therapy
- Apply pacing pads and continuous cardiac monitoring
- IV access

### ED TREATMENT/PROCEDURES
- Asymptomatic bradycardia:
  - Monitor while continuing workup
- Symptomatic or unstable bradycardia:
  - Oxygen
  - Atropine:
    - Symptomatic sinus bradycardia and symptomatic 1st- and 2nd-degree type I AV blocks
    - Usually ineffective for high-grade AV blocks
  - Epinephrine
  - Transcutaneous pacing
  - Transvenous pacing if transcutaneous pacing unsuccessful
- Find and treat underlying cause:
  - Hypoglycemia:
    - D50
  - Hypocalcemia:
    - Calcium gluconate
  - Hypercalcemia:
    - NS +/− Lasix
  - β-Blocker or calcium channel blocker overdose:
    - Glucagon, calcium gluconate, insulin, D50
  - Hyperkalemia:
    - Calcium chloride or calcium gluconate, insulin, D50, albuterol, consider bicarb, Lasix, Kayexalate, dialysis
  - Hypokalemia:
    - Potassium
  - Digoxin toxicity:
    - Digibind (Digoxin Immune Fab)
  - MI:
    - ASA, Plavix, heparin, statin, cath lab
  - Hypothyroidism:
    - Levothyroxine
  - Hypothermia:
    - Warm $O_2$, warm IVF, Bair Hugger, blankets, warming lights, consider warm bladder and gastric irrigation, cardiopulmonary bypass
  - Infection:
    - Targeted antibiotics, antivirals, or antifungals
  - Myocardial contusion:
    - Supportive care
  - Increased intracranial pressure:
    - Mannitol, neurosurgical consult
  - Pacemaker malfunction:
    - Interrogate pacemaker, cardiology consult
  - Idiopathic:
    - Cardiology consult for ICU admission and pacemaker placement

### MEDICATION
- Atropine: 0.5–1 mg (peds: 0.02 mg/kg; min 0.1 mg) IV q3–5 min; max 3 mg or 0.04 mg/kg
- Calcium gluconate: 1,000 mg (peds: 60 mg/kg) IV q3–5 min, max 3 g
- $D_{50}$: 1–2 amps (peds: D10 or D25 2–4 mL/kg) IV
- Digoxin immune Fab: Dose varies with amount of digoxin ingested, average 6 vials (peds: Average dose, 1 vial) IV bolus; see package insert
- Epinephrine: 0.5–1 mg (peds: 0.01–0.03 mg/kg) IV q3–5min; infusion 2–10 mcg/min (peds: 0.1–1 mcg/kg/min) IV
- Glucagon: 3–5 mg (peds: 0.05 mg/kg) IV, can repeat once; infusion 1–5 mg/hr (peds: 0.07 mg/kg/hr) IV for BB or CCB overdose
- Insulin regular: 10 U (peds: 0.1 U/kg) IV × 1 with glucagon for BB or CCB overdose

### First Line
Atropine, epinephrine, pacing

### Second Line
Treatment for specific disorders

## FOLLOW-UP

### DISPOSITION
#### Admission Criteria
- ICU:
  - Hemodynamically unstable bradycardia
  - Transcutaneous or transvenous pacer
  - Pressors
  - Acute myocardial infarction or ischemia
- Telemetry:
  - Hemodynamically stable bradycardia

#### Discharge Criteria
Asymptomatic sinus bradycardia

#### Issues for Referral
- All patients without existing primary care physicians should be referred to a generalist for follow-up as needed.
- 1st- and 2nd-degree type I AV block need cardiology referral.
- Severe endocrine, rheumatologic, infectious, renal, or neurological disorders require appropriate specialty referral.

### FOLLOW-UP RECOMMENDATIONS
- Minor lab abnormalities that do not require admission require PCP follow-up.
- All patients except asymptomatic sinus bradycardia require cardiology follow-up.
- Specific disorders require appropriate specialty follow-up.

## PEARLS AND PITFALLS
- Asymptomatic sinus bradycardia is the ONLY potentially "normal" bradycardia. All others require treatment or follow-up.
- O2, O2 sat, IV, ECG, cardiac monitor for all patients
- Pediatric bradycardia is likely secondary to hypoxia.
- Have pacing pads available for all symptomatic patients.
- The most important treatment is of the underlying cause.

## ADDITIONAL READING
- Brady WJ, Harrigan RA. Evaluation and management of bradyarrhythmias in the emergency department. *Emerg Med Clin North Am*. 1998;16:361–388.
- Dovgalyuk J, Holstege C, Mattu A, et al. The electrocardiogram in the patient with syncope. *Am J Emerg Med*. 2007;25:688–701.
- Haro LH, Hess EP, Decker WW. Arrhythmias in the office. *Med Clin North Am*. 2006;90:417–438.
- Ufberg JW, Clark JS. Bradydysrhythmias and atrioventricular conduction blocks. *Emerg Med Clin North Am*. 2006;24:1–9.

### See Also (Topic, Algorithm, Electronic Media Element)
- Acute Coronary Syndrome
- β-Blocker Overdose
- Calcium Channel Blocker Overdose
- Digoxin Overdose
- Hyperkalemia
- Hypothermia
- Pacemaker

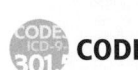
## CODES

### ICD9
427.89 Other specified cardiac dysrhythmias

# BRONCHIOLITIS

*Suzanne Schuh*

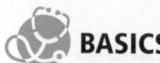 **BASICS**

## DESCRIPTION
Lower respiratory tract infection by airway inflammation and bronchoconstriction with wheezes/tachypnea and respiratory distress and upper respiratory prodrome

## ETIOLOGY
- Respiratory syncytial virus (RSV) in 85–90% of cases
- Influenza
- Parainfluenza
- Adenovirus
- Normally occurs during the winter months

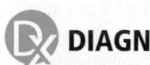 **DIAGNOSIS**

## SIGNS AND SYMPTOMS
- Age younger than 2 yr (usually 1 yr or younger)
- Nasal congestion, often with marked rhinorrhea
- Cough, sometimes associated with vomiting
- Wheezing
- Crackles, rhonchi
- Respiratory distress manifested by tachypnea, nasal flaring, retractions, grunting. Often progressive over a period of 1–3 days
- Fever usually <39.5°C
- Hypoxemia may be present (usually mild). Cyanosis rare
- Decreased fluid intake common, frank dehydration uncommon
- Apnea may occur, particularly in young infants with history of prematurity
- Synagis, an RSV specific immunoglobulin, may be administered IM monthly during winter months in high-risk children. This reduces risk of RSV infection.

## ESSENTIAL WORKUP
- Clinical diagnosis
- Defining viral cause may be useful for cohorting in hospital if admitted.
- Assess ventilation clinically.
- Pulse oximetry:
  – Confirms proper oxygenation on continuing basis
  – Follows trends over the course of illness

## DIAGNOSTIC TESTS & INTERPRETATION
### Lab
- Most patients need no specific tests beyond oximetry.
- Nasopharyngeal aspirate/wash:
  – Viral cultures
  – Fluorescent antibodies
  – Commercial kits are available.
  – Consider when:
    ○ Clinical symptoms suggestive of other cause (pertussis, chlamydia)
    ○ Critically ill child
    ○ Febrile child <3 mo old with bronchiolitis (consider UTI as coexistent cause of fever)
    ○ Coexisting signs suggesting bacterial sepsis (positive aspirate does not rule out coexisting bacterial sepsis)
    ○ Bronchopulmonary dysplasia or chronic lung disease
    ○ Coexistent cardiac disease
    ○ Prematurity
    ○ Other conditions warranting antiviral therapy (rare)

### Imaging
CXR:
- Usually hyperinflation, airway disease, atelectasis, variable infiltrate:
  – Atelectasis in young infants indicates more severe disease.
- Minority have airway plus airspace disease; pneumonia usually viral
- Rarely changes management acutely
- Consider when:
  – Need to exclude other diagnoses such as CHF, aspiration, congenital airway anomaly (rare)
  – Chronic course with lack of resolution over 2–3 wk
  – Critically ill infants with impending respiratory failure
  – Atypical presentation in toxic or deteriorating child
  – Not routinely indicated in typical clinical presentation

### Diagnostic Procedures/Surgery
- Septic workup in febrile bronchiolitis <28 days of age if respiratory status permits
- In febrile infants 1–3 mo of age, consider catheterized urine culture
- Oximetry during significant distress

## DIFFERENTIAL DIAGNOSIS
- Asthma/recurrent virus-induced wheezing: Severe bronchiolitis requiring hospitalization, and family history of atopy are risk factors for future asthma.
- Pertussis: No respiratory distress between coughing spasms, no wheezing
- Bacterial pneumonia: Often toxic appearance, no wheezing, isolated airspace disease (consolidation) with no airway abnormality on chest radiograph
- Foreign body: Sudden onset of symptoms, usually afebrile
- CHF: Pre-existing clinical red flags (failure to thrive [FTT], feeding problems)

 **TREATMENT**

### PRE-HOSPITAL

> **ALERT**
> - Young infants have limited respiratory reserve and decompensate rapidly with little warning.
> - Monitor cardiorespiratory status and oxygenation.
> - Supplemental oxygen if saturation <90–92% (sea level) and/or severe distress
> - Watch for apneic pauses:
>   – Greatest risk of developing high-risk outcomes in children younger than 7 wk, weight <4 kg, respiratory rate >80/min, heart rate >180/min, comorbidities, premature
>   – Bag-mask ventilation if recurrent apneas

### INITIAL STABILIZATION/THERAPY
- Pediatric advanced life support: Airway, ventilation, and fluid hydration
- Emergent intubation if recurrent apneas, impending respiratory failure

### ED TREATMENT/PROCEDURES
- Supplemental oxygen if oxygen saturation <90–92% (sea level)
- Parenteral hydration if dehydration or severe respiratory distress. Many children may improve their intake once respiratory status has improved.
- Many children with bronchiolitis do not benefit from pharmacotherapy.

- Bronchodilators (albuterol, racemic epinephrine, l-epinephrine, levalbuterol):
  - Should not routinely be used alone without determination of efficacy
  - Some clinicians administer on trial basis with 2–3 consecutive treatments in those with moderate to severe distress and continue as part of management if there is a clear decrease in the work of breathing.
  - Often utilized in significantly ill children
- Steroids:
  - On their own do not change clinical course or hospitalizations in the majority of patients without prior atopic or family history.
  - 2 doses of 1:1,000 l-epinephrine 30 min apart in the ED plus 6 daily doses of oral dexamethasone may be useful in moderate to severe distress—reduces admissions by 35% by day 7, shortens time to discharge and duration of symptoms
  - Conflicting evidence with another recent dexamethasone trial showing no benefit when used alone—synergy between steroids and epinephrine likely critical for efficacy
  - Often used empirically in children with past or family history of atopy. Prednisolone common for this usage.
  - Albuterol-dexamethasone combination efficacy not confirmed in a big trial.
  - Bronchodilators alone after discharge not effective unless there was demonstrated effectiveness prior to discharge.
- Antibiotics:
  - Not generally indicated since viral etiology
  - Consider if associated signs of focal bacterial disease (otitis, focal pneumonia), radiographic evidence of isolated lobar consolidation without airway disease (usually bacterial pneumonia rather than bronchiolitis), significant toxicity, sepsis
- Ribavirin.
  - No role in ED management and rarely used in the inpatient setting

## MEDICATION

- Albuterol: 2.5 mg/3 mL, 2–3 doses via nebulizer or 400 mcg via MDI/spacer 20–30 min apart in the ED. *A therapeutic trial can be considered but continue only if there is a clear improvement in the work of breathing. Does not change overall disease outcomes.*

- Levalbuterol: 1.25 mg/dose, 2–3 doses via nebulizer, 20–30 min apart in the ED. See above.
- l-Epinephrine: 3.0 mL (1:1,000 solution), 2 doses via nebulizer 30 min apart in the ED or with
- Dexamethasone: 1.0 mg/kg per dose PO in the ED, then 0.15 mg/kg daily for 5 days
- Prednisolone (15 mg/5 mL): 1–2 mg/kg/d PO b.i.d./3–5 days
- Comment: Most children require no medications. Bronchodilators *alone* rarely change outcomes. Initial trial of albuterol should be extended only if clear clinical improvement. Epinephrine-dexamethasone combination shown to decrease hospitalizations by day 7 and may warrant consideration.

##  FOLLOW-UP

### DISPOSITION

#### Admission Criteria

- Need for supplemental oxygen (oxygen saturation is <90–92% at sea level)
- Inability to self-hydrate
- Marked increase work of breathing (tachypnea with retractions or accessory muscle use)
- Apnea
- Severe underlying chronic lung disease or cardiac disease
- Persistent marked respiratory distress 4 hr after a trial of epinephrine and dexamethasone
- Significant comorbidity/suspicion of alternative diagnosis/underlying systemic disease/immunodeficiency or immunosuppressive therapy
- Strongly consider in infants younger than 7 wk, weight <4 kg, respiratory rate >80/min, heart rate >180/min, comorbidities, or prematurity
- Caretaker noncompliant or unable to monitor child closely

#### Discharge Criteria

- Feeding reasonably well
- Acceptable room air saturation
- Absence of significant respiratory distress
- Follow-up available within 24 hr
- Discharge Instructions:
  - Symptoms may persist for 2–3 wk.
  - Frequent small feeds
  - Bronchodilators after discharge not uniformly beneficial

### FOLLOW-UP RECOMMENDATIONS

Because of the progressive nature of bronchiolitis close follow-up is required, particularly early in the illness alerting parents to the likelihood of worsening respiratory distress, dehydration, and apnea.

## PEARLS AND PITFALLS

Infants with bronchiolitis often present with respiratory distress associated with hypoxia, dehydration, and/or apnea. Aggressive monitoring may be warranted.

## ADDITIONAL READING

- American Academy of Pediatrics Subcommittee on Diagnosis and Management of Bronchiolitis. Diagnosis and management of bronchiolitis. *Pediatrics.* 2006;118:1774–1793.
- Corneli HM, Zorc JJ, Mahajan P, et al. A multicenter, randomized, controlled trial of dexamethasone for bronchiolitis. *N Engl J Med.* 2007;257:331–339. [Erratum, *N Engl J Med* 2008;359:1972.]
- Kellner JD, Ohlsson A, Gadomski AM, et al. Bronchodilators for bronchiolitis. *Cochrane Databse Syst Rev.* 2000;(2):CD001266.
- Levine DA, Platt SL, Dayan PS, et al. Risk of serious bacterial infection in young febrile infants with respiratory syncytial visu infections. *Pediatrics.* 2004;113:1728–1734.
- Plint AC, Johnson DW, Patel H, et al. Epinephrine and dexamethasone in children with bronchiolitis. *N Engl J Med.* 2009;360:2079–2089.
- Schuh S, Coates AL, Binnie R, et al. Efficacy of oral dexamethasone in outpatients with acute bronchiolitis. *J Pediatr.* 2002;140:27–32.
- Schuh S, Lalani A, Allen U, et al. Evaluation of the utility of radiography in acute bronchiolitis. *J Pediatr.* 2007;150:429–433.

### See Also (Topic, Algorithm, Electronic Media Element)

Asthma, Pediatric

# BRONCHITIS
*Robin R. Hemphill*

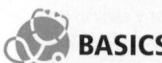 **BASICS**

## DESCRIPTION
- Hyperemia and edema of the mucous membranes
- Production of mucopurulent exudates
- Impairment of the productive function of the cilia, lymphatics, and phagocytes
- Airway obstruction from:
  - Edema
  - Secretions
  - Bronchial muscle spasm

## ETIOLOGY
- Viral infections are the primary cause of bronchitis:
  - Parainfluenza
  - Influenza A and B
  - Respiratory syncytial virus
  - Human meta pneumovirus
  - Echovirus
  - Coronavirus
  - Adenovirus
  - Coxsackievirus
  - Rhinovirus
  - Measles and herpes viruses (can cause severe viral bronchitis)
- Particularly severe or long-lasting bronchitis:
  - Mycoplasma pneumoniae
  - Chlamydia pneumoniae
  - Bordetella pertussis:
    ○ Rates of pertussis are increasing, even in the fully immunized population (little protection remains after 10 yr).
- Other bacteria have not been conclusively proven to cause bronchitis except in those with chronic lung disease.

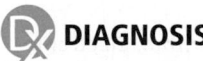 **DIAGNOSIS**

## SIGNS AND SYMPTOMS
### History
- Complaints that may precede upper respiratory tract infection (URTI) symptoms:
  - Malaise
  - Chills
  - Myalgias
  - Coryza
  - Sore throat
- Onset of URTI symptoms:
  - Mile dyspnea
  - Cough, initially dry and nonproductive
  - Cough, later becomes mucoid or mucopurulent
  - Chest pain or burning related to cough
  - Initial symptoms improve after 3–5 days, with 1–3 wk of residual cough and malaise

### Physical Exam
- Fever, not usually above 102°F (38.5°C)
- Tachypnea
- Mild hemoptysis
- Wheezing
- Rales
- Scattered rhonchi

## ESSENTIAL WORKUP
- Influenza A and B testing if identification of these organisms is required for treatment or reporting
- Evaluate for pertussis:
  - Acute cough illness lasting 14 days or more in a person with paroxysmal cough, posttussive vomiting, or inspiratory whoop
  - 14 days or more of cough within an outbreak setting

## DIAGNOSTIC TESTS & INTERPRETATION
### Lab
- Influenza A and B testing may help immediately confirm clinical suspicion.
- In most cases, no specific test will help make the diagnosis immediately.
- Viral or bacterial cultures are rarely helpful.
- CBC may show leukocytosis, but this is a nonspecific finding.
- Pertussis may be confirmed using PCR testing, but diagnosis will be delayed.

### Imaging
CXR:
- No evidence of consolidation
- Indications:
  - Shortness of breath
  - Hypoxia
  - Chest pain
  - Heart rate >100 beats/min
  - Respiratory rate ≥24 breaths/min
  - Temperature ≥38°C
  - Focal findings on chest examination
  - Elderly patient with multiple comorbid conditions
  - Hypoxia
  - 14 days or more of cough

### Diagnostic Procedures/Surgery
Pulmonary function tests are frequently abnormal.

## DIFFERENTIAL DIAGNOSIS
- Acute and subacute <8 wk:
  - Pneumonia
  - Reactive airway disease
  - Aspiration
  - Acute sinusitis
  - Bacterial tracheitis
  - Occupational exposure

- Chronic >8 wk:
  - Asthma
  - GERD
  - Chronic bronchitis
  - Bronchiectasis
  - ACE inhibitor use
  - Bronchogenic carcinoma
  - Carcinomatosis
  - Sarcoidosis
  - Left ventricular failure
  - Aspiration syndrome
  - Psychogenic/habit

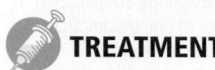 **TREATMENT**

## PRE-HOSPITAL
- Maintain adequate oxygenation
- Bronchodilators if wheezing is present

## INITIAL STABILIZATION/THERAPY
- Aggressive initial management of these patients is seldom required.
- Administer oxygen if the patient is hypoxic.
- Fluids may be administered if the patient is dehydrated.

## ED TREATMENT/PROCEDURES
- Bronchitis is usually a viral process, but may be bacterial and there is no practical test to distinguish between the 2:
  - Because this is usually a viral process, treatment is symptomatic:
    ○ Cough suppressants may be considered.
    ○ $\beta$-Adrenergic inhaler for patients with evidence of airflow obstruction
- Amantadine may be used in known outbreaks of influenza A, although local patterns of resistance should be reviewed.
- Oseltamivir (Tamiflu) and zanamivir ( Relenza ) may be considered in patients with recent onset of influenza.
- Antibiotics:
  - Generally, antibiotics are not indicated (even when secretions are purulent).
  - In healthy patients with no underlying lung disease, antibiotics may help some patients get better slightly faster, but weighed against the many people it does not help, cost, side effects, and resistance, antibiotics are not recommended.
  - Consider use in those patients who have recurrence of fever after initial improvement.
- Symptomatic control with antipyretics and analgesics

- Although patients should be encouraged to stop smoking, the use of tobacco is not an indication for antibiotics unless the patient has a known history of emphysema.

### ALERT
Be aware that respiratory viruses can cause significant morbidity in immunocompromised patients and their care should be discussed with their primary care physician.

### *Pediatric Considerations*
- Aggressive initial management of these patients is seldom required.
- Administer oxygen if the patient is hypoxic.
- Fluids may be administered if the patient is dehydrated.

### MEDICATION
- Albuterol Inhaler may be used for those with evidence of airflow obstruction.
- Amantadine: 100 mg/day PO, must be given within 48 hr of symptom onset
- Oseltamivir (Tamiflu) and zanamivir (Relenza) within 48 hr of symptom onset for influenza-related bronchitis:
  - Zanamivir: 10 mg inhalation q12h × 5 days (no pediatric dosing)
  - Oseltamivir: 75 mg PO b.i.d. (peds: 2 mg/kg) × 5 days
- Erythromycin should be given to proven cases of pertussis and to household contacts of those with proven pertussis.
- Yearly influenza vaccinations should be encouraged in health care providers and in the high-risk populations (elderly, immunocompromised, chronic lung disease).

### *Pediatric Considerations*
- Use of acetaminophen rather than aspirin for analgesia
- Antibiotic considerations are the same as in adults.
- Repeated bouts in children should lead to referral for complete evaluation of the respiratory tract.

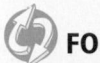 **FOLLOW-UP**

### DISPOSITION
### *Admission Criteria*
- Underlying significant cardiopulmonary compromise
- Significant hypoxia
- Ill patient with unclear diagnosis

### *Discharge Criteria*
- No pulmonary compromise should be present.
- Instruct patients, particularly high-risk patients, to return if no improvement or worsening of symptoms occurs.
- Bed rest
- Fluids
- Aspirin or acetaminophen

### FOLLOW-UP RECOMMENDATIONS
- No follow-up is needed in those patients that improved.
- Patients should be instructed to return to the ED for onset of shortness of breath and should see their doctor if not improved after 2–3 wk.

## PEARLS AND PITFALLS

Patients with high fever or significant pulmonary symptoms should be evaluated for pneumonia.

## ADDITIONAL READING

- Aagaard E, Gonzales R. Management of acute bronchitis. *Infect Dis Clinic N Am.* 2004;18: 919–937.
- Hirschmann JV. Antibiotics for common respiratory tract infections in adults. *Arch Intern Med.* 2002;162:256–264.
- Stephens MM, Nashelsky J. Do inhaled beta-agonists control cough in URIs or acute bronchitis? *J Fam Prac.* 2004;53:662–663.
- Smith SM, Fahey T, Smucny J, et al. Antibiotics for acute bronchitis. *Cochrane Database Syst Rev.* 2004;4(CD000245).
- Smucny J, Becker LA, Glazier R. Beta2-agonists for acute bronchitis. *Cochrane Database Syst Rev.* 2006;4(CD001726).
- Ward MA. Emergency department management of acute respiratory tract infections in adults. *Sem Resp Infec.* 2002;17:65–71.

### See Also (Topic, Algorithm, Electronic Media Element)
- Cough
- Dyspnea
- Pneumonia, Adult
- Pneumonia, Pediatric

 **CODES**

### ICD9
- 466.0 Acute bronchitis
- 490 Bronchitis, not specified as acute or chronic

# BUNDLE BRANCH BLOCKS

Keith S. Boniface
James Scott

 **BASICS**

## DESCRIPTION

- Blockage of intraventricular electrical impulses through the right and left bundles
- Complete bundle branch block:
  - Absence or delay of conduction down one bundle, with normal conduction down the other bundle
  - Affected ventricle depolarizes from muscle to muscle in a slower and more disorganized fashion.
  - Quasi-random signal (QRS) complex at 120 msec or longer
- Incomplete bundle branch block:
  - Delayed depolarization, but less than complete bundle branch block
  - QRS complex duration 100–120 msec
- Right bundle branch block (RBBB):
  - Delayed depolarization of the right ventricle
- Left bundle branch block (LBBB):
  - Delayed depolarization of the left ventricle
  - LBBB can be caused by delay of conduction in main left bundle or delay in both fascicles of the left bundle.
  - Causes early activation of the right side of the septum and the right ventricular myocardium (so explaining loss of "septal Q" on ECG)
  - Left bundle branches into 2 fascicles:
    - Left anterior fascicle: Initial septal activation proceeds inferiorly, anteriorly, and to the right.
    - Left posterior fascicle: Isolated blockage rare; activation begins in the midseptum and finishes in inferior and posterior walls.
- Bifascicular block:
  - Right bundle branch block with concomitant block of the left anterior or left posterior fascicle

## ETIOLOGY

- Myocardial infarction
- Cardiomyopathy
- Hypertension
- Age-related fibrosis of Purkinje fibers
- Valvular disease
- Exercise induced
- Congenital/atrial septal defect
- Brugada syndrome (right bundle branch block): Cause of sudden cardiac death in otherwise healthy patients.
- Chagas disease (especially Central/South America)
- Postoperative, following cardiac surgery
- Drugs:
  - Beta-blockers
  - Calcium blockers
  - Tricyclic antidepressants
  - Type Ia and Ic antiarrhythmics
  - Digitalis

 **DIAGNOSIS**

## SIGNS AND SYMPTOMS

- Asymptomatic
- RBBB: Split $S_2$ that persists with expiration
- LBBB: Reversed/paradoxical split $S_2$
- Syncope
- Chest pain

## ESSENTIAL WORKUP

ECG:

- RBBB:
  - Complete: QRS complex ≥0.12 sec
  - Incomplete: QRS complex duration 0.10–0.12 sec
  - rsr', rsR', rSR' in $V_1$ or $V_2$ (*M* shape)
  - Wide and deep S wave in $V_5$ through $V_6$
  - Brugada syndrome: RBBB and ST-segment elevation in $V_1$ through $V_3$

- LBBB:
  - Broad slurred R waves in leads $V_5$ through $V_6$, aVL, and I
  - Small/absent R wave in $V_1$ through $V_2$ and deep S waves
  - Absence of normal q waves in leads V5 through V6 and I
- Left anterior fascicular block:
  - QRS complex <120 msec, axis 45°–90°
  - Deep S wave in leads II, III, aVF, qR in leads aVL and I
- Left posterior fascicular block:
  - QRS <120 msec, axis ≥120°
  - RS waves in leads I and aVL, qR in leads II, III, and aVF
  - Exclusion of other things causing right axis deviation (right ventricle overload, right ventricular hypertrophy, lateral infarction)

## DIAGNOSTIC TESTS & INTERPRETATION
### Lab
- Potassium if hyperkalemia is suspected
- Cardiac enzymes if ischemia is suspected

### *Imaging*
- CXR:
  - May reveal cardiac enlargement or CHF
- Electrophysiologic testing:
  - Especially for unexplained syncope in patient with structural heart disease, as part of inpatient workup

## DIFFERENTIAL DIAGNOSIS
- Ventricular tachycardia
- MI:
  - Criteria for diagnosing MI with LBBB (Sgarbossa criteria) include any of following:
    - ST-segment elevation ≥1 mm concordant with QRS
    - ST-segment elevation ≥5 mm discordant with QRS
    - ST-segment depression ≥1 mm in leads $V_1$ through $V_3$
- Hyperkalemia
- Ventricular hypertrophy
- Drug effects (see "Etiology" section)

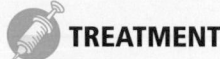

# TREATMENT

## PRE-HOSPITAL

Cautions:

- Monitor: Difficult to diagnose from single lead
- Avoid confusing with ventricular tachycardia or ischemia.
- Treat patient; bundle branch block requires no specific therapy.

## INITIAL STABILIZATION/THERAPY

- Standard treatment for symptoms of ischemia, dyspnea, and syncope
- Symptomatic bifascicular block and high-degree atrioventricular block:
  - Apply transcutaneous pacing pads to back and chest.
  - IV sedation and analgesia
  - Gradually increase current until capture is achieved.

## ED TREATMENT/PROCEDURES

- Asymptomatic: None
- Thrombolysis or cardiac catheterization for symptoms suggestive of myocardial infarction and new bundle branch block
- Transvenous pacemaker indications:
  - Bifascicular block and type II 2nd- or 3rd-degree atrioventricular block
  - Alternating LBBB and RBBB

# FOLLOW-UP

## DISPOSITION

### Admission Criteria

- Suspected myocardial ischemia
- Syncope
- Bundle branch block with high-degree atrioventricular block

### Discharge Criteria

Asymptomatic or incidental finding of bundle branch block

### Issues for Referral

At discharge, patient should be referred to cardiologist for evaluation of underlying disease.

## FOLLOW-UP RECOMMENDATIONS

- Reassure patients that usually no treatment is needed.
- Instruct patient to return or call for help if:
  - Dizziness
  - Fainting
  - Palpitations

# PEARLS AND PITFALLS

- Myocardial ischemia should be considered in all patients who develop new conduction abnormalities.
- Specific criteria can be used to diagnose cardiac ischemia in patients with a bundle branch block.

# ADDITIONAL READING

- Brignole M, Menozzi C, Moya A, et al. Mechanism of syncope in patients with bundle branch block and negative electrophysiological test. *Circulation*. 2001;104:2045–2050.
- Brugada J, Brugada R, Brugada P. Right bundle-branch block and ST-segment elevation in leads V1 through V3: A marker for sudden death in patients without demonstrable structural heart disease. *Circulation*. 1998;97:457–460.
- Epstein AE, DiMarco JP, Ellenbogen KA, et al. ACC/AHA/HRS 2008 guidelines for device-based therapy of cardiac rhythm abnormalities: A report of the American College of Cardiology/American Heart Association Task Force on Practice Guidelines. *JACC*. 2008;51:1–62.
- Tabas JA, Rodriguez RM, Seligman HK, et al. Electrographic criteria for detecting acute myocardial infarction in patients with left bundle branch block: A meta-analysis. *Ann Emerg Med*. 2008;52:329–336.

# CODES

## ICD9

- 426.2 Left bundle branch hemiblock
- 426.3 Other left bundle branch block
- 426.4 Right bundle branch block

B

# BURNS

Kevin Buford
Anthony J. Medak

 **BASICS**

## DESCRIPTION
Burn injuries represent an acute injury to the skin.

## ETIOLOGY
Burns can be classified into 7 categories:
- Scald: Hot liquids, grease, or steam
- Contact: Hot or cold surfaces
- Thermal: Fire or flames
- Radiation burns
- Chemical burns
- Electrical burns
- Friction burns: Road rash, rope burns

 **DIAGNOSIS**

## SIGNS AND SYMPTOMS
- Most burns will have external signs of integumentary damage.
- Inhalation injury:
  - Facial burns
  - Singed nasal hair/eyelashes
  - Carbonaceous sputum
  - Pharyngeal injection
  - Wheezing
  - Coughing
  - Tachypnea
- Electrical burns may have minimal external findings.

### History
- Information from EMS, family/friends, or witnesses may be helpful.
- Medical/surgical/social history, medications, allergies, tetanus immunization status
- Carbon monoxide (CO) poisoning (most common cause of death in fires) from exposure to wood based fires/combustion:
  - Pulse oximetry unreliable in CO poisoning
- Cyanide poisoning from burning wool, silk, nylon, and polyurethane found in furniture/paper

### Physical Exam
- Focus on airway/breathing 1st, then head-to-toe secondary survey for concurrent injuries.
- Evaluate face, oropharynx, and nares for signs of inhalation injury.
- Assess need for immobilization of cervical spine (ie, explosion/fall) while escaping fire.
- Eye exam for corneal burns
- Determine severity of partial- and full-thickness burns by assessing size/depth of burn:
  - Estimate surface area involved.

### Pediatric Considerations
Specific patterns of injury may indicate nonaccidental injury (stocking or glove appearance of wounds, cigarette burns, etc.).

## ESSENTIAL WORKUP
- The severity of the burn should be assessed by determining the size and depth of the burn.
- Size is reported as percent involvement of total body surface area (TBSA) in 1 of 3 ways:
- 1: Rule of nines:
  - TBSA of body parts is estimated by multiples of 9%; applies to adults only.
  - Adult estimates of percentage of TBSA:
    - Head and neck: 9
    - Arms: Right, 9; left, 9
    - Legs: Right, 18; left, 18
    - Trunk: Front, 18; back, 18
    - Perineum, palms: 1
  - In infants and children, the head contributes more to the percentage of TBSA and legs contribute less.
  - Infants/children:
    - Head and neck: 18
    - Arms: Right, 9; left, 9
    - Legs: Right, 14; left, 14
    - Trunk: Front, 18; back, 18
- 2: Lund and Browder chart; divides body into areas and assigns percentage of BSA based on age; produces more reliable results than rule of 9s
- 3: Palm surface area; patient's palm is ~1% of TBSA:
  - Estimate size in terms of number of patient's palms that cover burn.
  - Helpful in assessing irregular/scattered burns
- Depth of burn is superficial or 1st-degree (epidermis only) when: Local erythema, minimal swelling/pain, no blisters; healing occurs in several days
- Partial-thickness or 2nd-degree burns (epidermis and dermis): Divided into superficial partial-thickness and deep partial-thickness burns:
  - Superficial partial-thickness (epidermis and superficial dermis):
    - Often seen in scald injuries
    - Blister formation, underlying skin is pink, moist, painful, good capillary refill, sensation intact
    - Heals in 14–21 days
  - Deep partial-thickness burns (epidermis and deep dermis):
    - Skin may be blistered, with dermis white to yellow; absent capillary refill/pain sensation
    - Heals via epithelialization within 3–12 wk
- Full-thickness or 3rd-degree burns (epidermis and dermis, extends into subcutaneous tissue):
  - Skin is charred, leathery and pale, no blisters
  - Sensation absent
  - Will not heal spontaneously; needs surgical repair and skin grafting
- Full-thickness burns with damage to underlying muscle or 4th-degree burns:
  - Full-thickness plus involvement of underlying fascia, muscle, bone, and other tissues
  - Common when patient's clothes catch fire
  - Requires extensive debridement/grafting
  - Resultant disability

## DIAGNOSTIC TESTS & INTERPRETATION
### Lab
- For severe burns, obtain: CBC, serum electrolytes, glucose, BUN, creatinine, PT/PTT, type and cross-match, and pregnancy test (if indicated)
- Blood gas with carbon monoxide level for closed space or inhalation exposures
- Cyanide level (treat empirically if suspected)

### Imaging
CXR

### Diagnostic Procedures/Surgery
Bronchoscopy to assess for inhalation injury

## DIFFERENTIAL DIAGNOSIS
- Electrical injury
- Chemical injury
- Associated trauma or intoxication

 **TREATMENT**

## PRE-HOSPITAL
- Stop the burning process; remove smoldering/contaminated clothes/jewelry.
- Keep patient warm.
- Establish patent airway; frequent reassessment:
  - Early intubation for respiratory distress.
- Initiate early IV fluid therapy.
- Institute pain relief.
- Protect the wound with clean sheets.
- Transport to burn center (for major burns) if transport time <30 min.
- Immobilize spine if decreased sensorium, trauma, or blast injury.

## INITIAL STABILIZATION/THERAPY
- Airway control is paramount:
  - Early intubation for patients with signs of upper airway injury, significant nasolabial burns, or circumferential neck burns
- IV access, supplemental 100% oxygen, monitor, pulse oximetry
- Evaluation for concurrent injuries
- Provide adequate analgesia.
- Early fluid resuscitation is essential.

## ED TREATMENT/PROCEDURES
- Fluid resuscitation: Partial and full-thickness burns (>20% TBSA):
  - Parkland formula: 4 mL of lactated Ringer solution or normal saline (NS) per kilogram per percentage of BSA burned IV; 1/2 of this total is given in the 1st 8 hr and the remaining 1/2 over the next 16 hr:
    - Example: 70-kg patient with a 40% TBSA burn requires 4 mL × 70 kg × 40% = 11,200 mL over 24 hr, with 5,600 mL over 1st 8 hr or 700 mL/hr.
  - For large burns, >20% TBSA, IV fluid therapy should be guided by invasive hemodynamic monitoring or urine output; maintain urine output of 0.5 to 1.0 mL/kg/hr for adults and 1.0–1.5 mL/kg/hr for children.

- Escharotomy:
  - Circumferential burn eschar may lead to neurovascular compromise:
    - Monitor pulses; may need Doppler probe.
    - Elevate burned extremity.
    - If circulation is compromised, escharotomy incisions on extremities should be made medially and laterally along the long axis of the limb just superficial to the subcutaneous fat layer through the entire length of the burn eschar.
  - Circumferential chest wall burns may physically prevent adequate ventilation unless an escharotomy is performed:
    - Make longitudinal incisions at anterior axillary line from the 2nd rib to the level of the 12th rib; connect with 2 transverse incisions across the chest.
- Wound care:
  - Debride blisters, as they cause pressure necrosis.
  - Cover the wounds with Polysporin/bacitracin ointment and nonadherent dressings.
  - Use silver sulfadiazine in contaminated/dirty wounds (avoid if transferring to burn center as interferes with later assessment of burn).
  - Do not delay transfer to burn unit for wound care.
  - Prophylactic antibiotics are not indicated.
- Outpatient management of minor burns:
  - Sterile technique for cleansing and debridement
  - Remove loose, necrotic skin; debride broken, tense, or infected blisters.
  - Topical antibacterial agents: (eg, silver sulfadiazine, bacitracin, mafenide acetate) recommended in deep partial-thickness or full-thickness burns only
  - 3 layer burn dressings should keep the wound moist and absorb exudate.
    - Inner layer should be nonadherent porous mesh gauze saturated with a non-petroleum based lubricant, or use a mild ointment (eg, bacitracin or Polysporin) under a nonadherent porous gauze.
    - The next layer should be fluffed coarse mesh gauze.
    - The outer wrap should keep the dressing in place without constricting.
    - Dressings should be changed at least daily.
  - Silver wound dressings (Silverlon and Acticoat):
    - Thin coating of metallic silver applied to knitted fabric backing
    - Requires dressing to remain moist
    - May leave in place for up to 3 days

### Pediatric Considerations

- Parkland formula underestimates fluid requirements in children; the Galveston formula may be used instead: 5,000 mL/m$^2$ BSA burned plus 2,000 mL/m$^2$.
- TBSA of 5% dextrose in lactated Ringer solution IV over the 1st 24 hr, 1/2 in the 1st 8 hr and the other 1/2 over the next 16 hr:
  - Titrate to goal urine output of 1 cc/kg/hr
- Consider nonaccidental trauma, particularly with burns on the back of hands or feet, buttocks, perineum, and the legs.

- Avoid hypothermia:
  - Children have greater body surface area/mass ratio and lose heat more rapidly.
- Avoid hypoglycemia:
  - Children are more prone to hypoglycemia due to limited glycogen stores.

### Pregnancy Considerations

- Significant morbidity to mother and child
- Fluid requirements may exceed estimations.
- Fetal monitoring and early obstetric consultation recommended

## MEDICATION

- Bacitracin ointment: Apply to wound 1–4 times per day.
- Mafenide (Sulfamylon) acetate cream: Apply to wound 1 or 2 times per day.
- Morphine: 0.1–0.2 mg/kg titrated to effect for pain control after shock
- Silverlon and Acticoat: Cut sheet to size of burn; moisten with sterile water.
- Silver sulfadiazine cream: Apply to wound 1–2 times per day.
- Tetanus toxoid or immunoglobulin: 0.5 mL IM; 250 U IM once along with toxoid

 **FOLLOW-UP**

### DISPOSITION

#### Admission Criteria

- Injuries requiring admission:
  - Partial-thickness burns of noncritical areas (not including eyes, ears, face, hands, feet, or perineum) involving 10–20% of BSA in adults (>10 yr and <50 yr)
    Partial-thickness burns of noncritical areas involving 5–10% of BSA in children <10 yr
  - Suspicion of nonaccidental trauma
  - Patients unable to care for wounds in outpatient setting (eg, homeless patients)
- Injuries requiring transfer/admission to a burn center:
  - Partial-thickness or full-thickness burns involving ≥10% of BSA
  - Full-thickness burns involving >5% of BSA
  - Partial-thickness and full-thickness of face, hands, feet, genitalia, perineum, or major joints
  - Electrical burns, including lightning injury
  - Significant chemical injury
  - Inhalation injury
  - Burn injury in patients with preexisting illness that could complicate management
  - Burn injury in patients with concomitant trauma or social barriers

### Discharge Criteria

Partial-thickness burns of <15% of BSA in adults (<10% in children) involving noncritical areas only. Patients must be reliable, able to manage wounds as outpatients and obtain follow-up.

### Issues for Referral

Maintain low threshold for referral to burn specialist whenever there is raised concern regarding cosmesis, involvement of hands/face/eyes/perineum, or if burn is overlying a joint.

### FOLLOW-UP RECOMMENDATIONS

1–2 days after the injury to assess for early infection, saturation of dressings, pain control

## PEARLS AND PITFALLS

- Early IV fluid rehydration is essential.
- Intubate early for signs of respiratory distress; corollary is not recognizing potential for airway involvement and thus not controlling airway early.
- Debride blisters to avoid pressure necrosis.
- Monitor for hypoglycemia in children.
- Avoid silver sulfadiazine if transferring to burn center as it interferes with later assessment of the burn.

## ADDITIONAL READING

- Committee on Trauma, American College of Surgeons. Guidelines for the operation of burn units. Resources for Optimal Care of the Injured Patient; 2006:79–86.
- Holm C, et al. A clinical randomized study on the effects of invasive monitoring on burn resuscitation. *Burns.* 2004;30(8):798–807.
- Kavanagh S, et al. Care of burn patients in the hospital. *Burns.* 2004;30(8):A2–6.
- New Zealand Guidelines Group (NZGG). Management of burns and scalds in primary care. Wellington (NZ): Accident Compensation Corporation (ACC); 2007:116.
- Pham TN. American Burn Association practice guidelines burn shock resuscitation. *J Burn Care Res.* 2008;29(1):257–266.
- Schwartz LR. Thermal burns. In: Tintinalli JE, Kelen GD, Stapczynski JS. *Emergency medicine: A comprehensive study guide*, 6th ed. New York: McGraw-Hill, 2004:1220–1226.
- Tompkins D, et al. Care of out patient burns. *Burns.* 2004;30(8):A7–9.

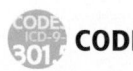 **CODES**

### ICD9

949.0 Burn of unspecified site, unspecified degree

# BURSITIS
*Patrick H. Sweet III*

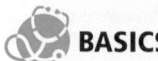 **BASICS**

## DESCRIPTION
- Bursae are synovial fluid-filled sacs:
  - ~150 are located between bones, ligaments, tendons, muscles, and skin.
- They provide lubrication to reduce friction during movement.
- Bursitis is inflammation of a bursa caused by trauma (acute or chronic), repetitive use, prolonged pressure, infection, crystal deposition, or systemic disease.
- Affected bursae display hypertrophy and villous hyperplasia.
- Affected joints:
  - Potentially any bursa may be affected.
  - Commonly affected joints:
    - Shoulder (subacromial)
    - Elbow (olecranon): Usually secondary to trauma
    - Wrist and hand
    - Hip (greater trochanter, ischial, iliopsoas): More common in elderly
    - Knee (prepatellar and pes anserine): Secondary to trauma or arthritis
    - Foot (calcaneal): Almost always secondary to improperly fitting shoes/heels

## ETIOLOGY
- Trauma (most common cause):
  - Specific traumatic event or repetitive use of associated joints
- Infection: Secondary to direct penetration; may be obvious or microscopic:
  - Higher risk with diabetes, chronic alcohol abuse, uremia, gout, immunosuppression
  - 90% caused by *Staphylococcus spp.*
- Crystal deposition: Calcium phosphate, urate
- Systemic disease: Rheumatoid arthritis, gout, ankylosing spondylitis, psoriatic arthritis, lupus, rheumatic fever

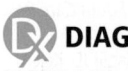 **DIAGNOSIS**

## SIGNS AND SYMPTOMS
### History
- Acute or chronic
- History of trauma, overuse, or prolonged pressure
- Pain with increased activity at respective joint or with pressure
- Functional complaints (eg, limping)
- History of localized swelling
- Screen for symptoms of systemic disease
- History of gout or pseudogout or rheumatologic disease
- In septic bursitis, a history of recent aspiration or corticosteroid injection

### Physical Exam
- Tenderness to palpation is absent to mild in nonseptic bursitis.
- Localized pain that worsens with movement of structures adjacent to affected bursae
- Often reduced active range of motion (ROM) with preserved passive ROM
- Localized swelling may be present with superficial bursal involvement (up to 40 mL).
- Skin trauma overlying bursa
- The constellation of erythema, warmth, swelling, and significant tenderness are common in septic bursitis.
- May be febrile in septic bursitis

## ESSENTIAL WORKUP
- Full assessment of adjacent musculoskeletal structures
- Any suspicion of infection warrants aspiration of bursae (especially olecranon and prepatellar bursae).
- Lateral approach to prevent a needle tract directly over lines of tension of the joint
- Aspiration of hip and other deep bursae may be guided in ED by US or deferred to interventional radiology, orthopedics, or rheumatology.

## DIAGNOSTIC TESTS & INTERPRETATION
### Lab
- Serum labs:
  - Suspected infection: CBC with differential
  - Evaluation of related systemic disease (eg, uric acid level for gout)
  - Send serum glucose if bursal fluid aspiration is done
- Bursal fluid analysis:
  - Send fluid for cell count with differential, glucose, total protein, crystal determination, Gram stain, and culture.
  - Because infection and inflammation may be difficult to differentiate, cultures must always be sent.
  - Normal fluid: Fluid is clear yellow with 0–200 WBCs, 0 RBCs, low protein, and glucose is same as serum.
  - Traumatic bursitis: Fluid is bloody/xanthochromic with <1,200 WBCs, many RBCs, low protein, and normal glucose.
  - Infective bursitis: Fluid is cloudy yellow with >50,000 WBCs, few RBCs, slightly increased protein, and decreased glucose; bacteria on Gram stain.
  - Rheumatoid and microcrystalline inflammation: Fluid is yellow, can be cloudy, and has 1,000–40,000 WBCs, few RBCs, slightly increased protein, and variable glucose; use polarizing microscope to identify crystals.

### Imaging
- Radiographs may demonstrate soft tissue swelling or adjacent chronic arthritic changes or calcium deposits:
  - Especially recommended when trauma is involved to rule out fracture or foreign body
- MRI and US may aid in diagnosis of deep bursitis and in defining the extent of septic bursitis.
- CT scans can also help differentiate septic from nonseptic bursitis.

## DIFFERENTIAL DIAGNOSIS
- Arthritides: Septic, inflammatory, rheumatoid and osteoarthritis
- Gout and pseudogout
- Tendonitis, fasciitis, epicondylitis
- Fracture, tendon/ligament tear, contusion, sprain
- Osteomyelitis
- Nerve entrapment
- Also in hips: Neuritis, lumbar spine disease, sacroiliitis

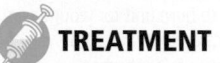 **TREATMENT**

## PRE-HOSPITAL
May be difficult to distinguish from fractures; suspicious joints should be immobilized, particularly in the setting of trauma.

## INITIAL STABILIZATION/THERAPY
- Immobilize joint if pain is severe.
- Shoulders should not be immobilized for >2–3 days because of the risk of adhesive capsulitis.

## ED TREATMENT/PROCEDURES
- Nonseptic bursitis:
  - Rest and removal of aggravating factors (eg, avoid direct pressure and repetitive use; protective padding where necessary)
  - Ice affected areas for 10 min, 4 times a day until improved; may alternate with heat.
  - NSAIDs for at least 7 days; best if continued for 5 days after improvement to help prevent recurrence
  - If fluctuant, then aspirate and place compression dressing
  - If no improvement within 5–7 days and infection has been ruled out (by culture), injection of lidocaine and corticosteroids may be considered:
    - Mix 2 mL of 2% lidocaine with appropriate depo-corticosteroid (see below) and inject 1–3 mL of this mixture into the bursa using sterile technique.
    - Steroid injections should not be repeated until 4 wk have passed, and no >2 injections per bursa should be performed without consultation.

- Septic bursitis:
  - Superficial bursae: Aspiration and antibiotics may be sufficient with close follow-up.
  - Other major bursae: Antibiotics and drainage of bursae (leaving in perforated drainage catheter can reduce period of treatment and avoid eventual bursectomy)
  - Febrile patients may need IV antibiotics.
  - Base antibiotic choice on the Gram stain:
    - Penicillinase-resistant antistaphylococcal drug may be used if Gram stain result is negative or shows gram-positive cocci.
    - If gram-negative organisms are found, blood cultures should be done and another primary source for the infection should be sought.
  - Antibiotics should be continued for 5–7 days beyond the sterilization of bursal fluid.
- Treat associated diseases as needed (eg, gout).

## MEDICATION
- NSAIDs (many choices; a few are listed here):
  - Diclofenac: 50 mg PO b.i.d./t.i.d.
  - Naprosyn: 500 mg PO q12h
  - Ibuprofen: 600 mg PO q6h (peds: 5–10 mg/kg PO q6h)
  - Ketorolac: 30 mg IV/IM q6h or 10 mg PO q4h–q6h
  - Piroxicam: 20 mg PO daily
- Corticosteroids for intrabursal injection:
  - Methylprednisolone acetate: 20–40 mg
  - Triamcinolone acetonide: 20–40 mg
  - Dexamethasone acetate/sodium: 8 mg

 **FOLLOW-UP**

### DISPOSITION
- Most patients may be treated as outpatients.
- Most patients respond to therapy in 3–4 days and may follow-up within 1 wk.
- Septic bursitis requires repeated bursal aspiration every 3–5 days until sterile.

### *Admission Criteria*
- Patients with high fevers, chills/rigors, large surrounding cellulitis, unable to take PO antibiotics, failed outpatient therapy, or immunosuppressed
- Unusual organisms, extrabursal primary site, or deep bursal involvement

### *Discharge Criteria*
- Able to tolerate pain
- Afebrile patients with septic bursitis are safe to discharge if appropriately treated.

### *Issues for Referral*
Rheumatology or orthopedic referral is recommended for patients who do not respond to intrabursal steroids or recurrent bursitis.

### FOLLOW-UP RECOMMENDATIONS
- Close follow-up for septic bursitis
- PRN to the emergency department for worsening symptoms but otherwise follow-up with primary care physician.

## PEARLS AND PITFALLS
- Examination alone may be unreliable in distinguishing between traumatic and septic bursitis:
  - Aspiration and fluid analysis may be the only method of distinguishing.
- Beware of risk for GI hemorrhage associated with PO NSAIDs.

- If presents with the 4 signs of infection— *humor, dolor, rubor,* and *calor*—then it is likely septic
- Beware of the potential of seeding organisms to adjacent joints when aspirating septic bursae.

## ADDITIONAL READING

- DeLee JC, Drez D, Miller MD, ed. *DeLee & Drez's orthopaedic sports medicine: Principles and practice,* 3rd ed. Philadelphia: Saunders Elsevier; 2010: 889–891, 1209–1212, 1246–1249, 1455–1458, 2030–2041.
- Fayad LM, Carrino JA, Fishman EK. Musculoskeletal infection: Role of CT in the emergency department. *Radiographics.* 2007;27(6):1723–1736.
- Larsson L, Baum J. The syndromes of bursitis. *Bull Rheum Dis.* 1986;36(1):1–8.
- Stephens MB, Beutler AI, O'Connor FG. Musculoskeletal injections: A review of the evidence. *Am Fam Physician.* 2008;78(8):971–976.

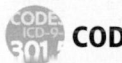 **CODES**

ICD9
727.3 Other bursitis disorders

# CALCIUM CHANNEL BLOCKER POISONING

*Janet Eng*

## BASICS

### DESCRIPTION
- 3 classes of calcium channel blockers (CCBs):
  - Phenylalkylamines (verapamil):
    - Vasodilation resulting in a decrease in BP
    - Negative chronotropic and inotropic effects: Reflex tachycardia not seen with a drop in BP.
  - Dihydropyridine (nifedipine):
    - Decreased vascular resistance resulting in a drop in BP
    - Little negative inotropic effect: Reflex tachycardia occurs.
  - Benzodiazepine (diltiazem):
    - Decreased peripheral vascular resistance leading to a decrease in BP
    - Heart rate (HR) and cardiac output initially increased
    - Direct negative chronotropic effect, which leads to a fall in HR
- Effects of calcium channel blockade
  - Calcium plays key role in cardiac and smooth muscle contractility.
  - CCBs prevent:
    - The entry of calcium, resulting in a lack of muscle contraction
    - The normal release of insulin from pancreatic islet cells, resulting in hyperglycemia

## DIAGNOSIS

### SIGNS AND SYMPTOMS
- Cardiovascular:
  - Hypotension
  - Bradycardia
  - Reflex tachycardia (dihydropyridine)
  - Conduction abnormalities/heart blocks
- Neurologic:
  - CNS depression
  - Coma
  - Seizures
  - Agitation
  - Confusion
- Metabolic:
  - Hyperglycemia

### History
- Inquire about risk of medication error.
- Inquire about risk of suicidal ideation with intent.
- Inquire about possible exposure to medications with a pediatric patient.

### Physical Exam
- Hypotension
- Bradycardia
- Skin may be warm instead of cool and clammy.

### ESSENTIAL WORKUP
ECG:
- Bradycardia (tachycardia with nifedipine)
- Conduction delays: QRS-complex prolongation
- Heart blocks

### DIAGNOSTIC TESTS & INTERPRETATION
### Lab
- Ionized calcium level when administering calcium
- Digoxin level if patient taking digoxin (dictate safety of calcium administration)
- CBC
- Electrolytes, BUN, creatinine, glucose:
  - Hyperglycemia/metabolic acidosis may occur.
- Toxicology screen if coingestants suspected

### DIFFERENTIAL DIAGNOSIS
- β-Blocker toxicity
- Clonidine toxicity
- Digitalis toxicity
- Acute myocardial infarction with heart block

## TREATMENT

### PRE-HOSPITAL
- Transport pill/pill bottles to ED.
- Calcium for bradycardic/unstable patient with confirmed CCB overdose

### INITIAL STABILIZATION/THERAPY
- ABCs:
  - Airway protection, as indicated
  - Supplemental oxygen, as needed
  - 0.9% NS IV access
- Hemodynamic monitoring

## ED TREATMENT/PROCEDURES
### Goals
- Heart rate >60 beats/min
- Systolic BP >90 mm Hg
- Adequate urine output
- Improving level of consciousness

### GI-Decontamination
- Syrup of ipecac: Contraindicated in the prehospital and ED setting
- Activated charcoal:
  - May be helpful, especially in the presence of coingestants
- Whole bowel irrigation:
  - Beneficial with ingestion of sustained-release preparations
  - Contraindicated in hemodynamically unstable patients

### Calcium
- 1st-line agent for CCB toxicity
- Calcium chloride (10%):
  - Contains 1.36 mEq $Ca^{2+}$/mL (3 times more calcium than calcium gluconate)
  - Can cause tissue necrosis and sloughing with extravasation
  - Very irritating to veins
- Calcium gluconate (10%):
  - Contains 0.45 mEq $Ca^{2+}$/mL
  - Does not cause tissue necrosis as calcium chloride does
  - Calcium gluconate: Preferred agent in an acidemic patient
- Follow serum calcium levels if repeated doses of calcium administered.
- Contraindicated in digoxin toxicity because calcium can produce serious adverse effects in digoxin toxicity

### Bradycardia Hypotension

- IV fluids:
  - Administer cautiously in the hypotensive patient.
  - Swan-Ganz catheter or central venous pressure (CVP) monitoring to help follow volume status
- Atropine usually ineffective
- Pressor agents:
  - No clear evidence that one agent is more effective than another
  - Institute invasive monitoring to help guide treatment.
  - Dopamine:
    - $\beta_1$-Receptor agonist at low doses, which causes a positive inotropic effect on the myocardium
    - $\alpha$-Receptor agonist at higher doses, which leads to vasoconstriction
  - Epinephrine:
    - Potent $\alpha$- and $\beta$-receptor agonist
- Glucagon:
  - Promotes cAMP production through a receptor site other than the $\beta$-receptor
  - May cause nausea and vomiting
  - Mix with NS or 5% dextrose in water.
- Amrinone:
  - Selective phosphodiesterase III inhibitor
  - Indirectly increases cAMP
- Electrical pacing: When other treatment options have failed
- Insulin:
  - Promotes more efficient myocardial carbohydrate metabolism
- Potential future therapies:
  - Hypertonic sodium bicarbonate
  - IV fat emulsion (20% Intralipid)

### MEDICATION

- Amrinone: Loading dose 0.75 mg/kg; maintenance drip 2–20 μg/kg/min; titrate for effect
- Atropine: 0.5 mg (peds: 0.02 mg/kg) IV; repeat 0.5–1.0 mg IV (peds: 0.04 mg/kg)
- Calcium chloride: 5–10 mL of 10% solution slow IVP (peds: 0.2–0.25 mL/kg; repeat in 10 min if necessary) followed by infusion 20–50 mg/kg/h
- Calcium gluconate: 10–20 mL of 10% solution slow IVP (peds: 1 mL/kg; may repeat in 10 min if necessary)

- Dextrose: 50 mL of 50% solution (peds: 0.25 g/kg of 25% solution)
- Dopamine: 2–20 μg/kg/min; titrate to effect
- Epinephrine: 1–2 μg/min (peds: 0.1 μg/kg/min); titrate to effect
- Glucagon: 3.5–5 mg (peds: 0.03–0.1 mg/kg) IV bolus followed by 70 μg/kg/h infusion
- GoLYTELY WBI: 2 L/h PO or by nasogastric tube (NGT) for 4–6 hr or until rectal effluent is clear (peds: 40 mL/kg/h)
- Insulin: 1 IU/kg bolus IV followed by 0.5–1.0 IU/kg/h titrated to clinical response
- Potassium: 40 mEq PO or IV

### First Line

- IV fluids
- Calcium
- Glucagon
- Dopamine
- Epinephrine
- Amrinone

### Second Line

High-dose insulin with dextrose and potassium:

- Should be considered if response to fluid resuscitation is inadequate
- Administer dextrose if blood glucose <200 mg/dL
- Administer potassium if serum potassium <2.5 mEq/L
- Approximate 24-hr insulin requirement: 1,500 U of regular insulin for adult patient

 **FOLLOW-UP**

### DISPOSITION

#### Admission Criteria

- Admit symptomatic patients to a monitored bed for hemodynamic monitoring.
- Admit all patients who ingested sustained-release CCBs for 24 hr of observation and monitoring owing to the potential delay in symptoms.

#### Discharge Criteria

Discharge asymptomatic patients 8 hr after ingestion of immediate-release preparation.

#### FOLLOW-UP RECOMMENDATIONS

- Psychiatric evaluation for all suicidal patients
- Poison prevention guidance for parents of pediatric accidental ingestion

## PEARLS AND PITFALLS

- Consider CCB toxicity in patients presenting hypotensive and bradycardic.
- Consider suicidal gesture in patients presenting with CCB toxicity.
- Consider high-dose insulin with dextrose and potassium if fluid resuscitation not effective.

## ADDITIONAL READING

- Greene S, Gawarammana I, Wood D, et al. Relative safety of hyperinsulinaemia/euglycaemia therapy in the management of calcium channel blocker overdose: A prospective observational study. *Intensive Care Med.* 2007;33:2019–2024.
- Shepherd G. Treatment of poisoning caused by β-adrenergic and calcium-channel blockers. *Am J Health-Syst Pharm.* 2006;63:1828–1835.
- Shepherd G, Klein-Schwartz W. High-dose insulin therapy for calcium-channel blocker overdose. *Ann Pharmacother.* 2005;39:923–930.

### See Also (Topic, Algorithm, Electronic Media Element)

β-Blocker, Poisoning

 **CODES**

ICD9
972.4 Poisoning by coronary vasodilators

# CANDIDIASIS, ORAL

Mary K. Meyer
Deepi G. Goyal

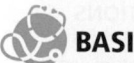

## BASICS

### DESCRIPTION
- Infection of oral mucosa with any species of *Candida*
- Up to 80% of isolates are *C. albicans,* (most common) *C. glabrata, and C. tropicalis.*
- *Candida* normally present as oral flora in 60% of the healthy population.
- Variations include pseudomembranous (thrush); chronic and acute atrophic candidiasis, angular cheilitis, and hyperplastic candidiasis.
- More common in neonates, elderly, and immunosuppressed individuals
- Usually benign course in healthy patients
- In immunocompromised patients, more likely to be recurrent and a non–*albicans* species
- May represent an early manifestation of AIDS in HIV-infected patients

### ETIOLOGY
- Usually overgrowth of *C. albicans* from alterations in intraoral environment
- May be medication induced—commonly antimicrobials, inhaled or systemic steroids, chemotherapy, immunosuppressive agents
- Immunocompromised patients: Congenital, HIV/AIDs, neutropenic, transplant, or on immunosuppressive medications
- Alterations or impairment of salivary flow:
  - Anticholinergic or psychotropic medications
  - Sjögren's disease
  - Head or neck radiation
- Presence of dentures or other orthodontics:
  - Occurs in up to 50–65% of denture wearers
  - Common etiology for chronic atrophic candidiasis
- Interruption of epithelial barrier (cheek biting)
- Endocrinopathies (diabetes, hypothyroidism)

### Pediatric Considerations
- Acute pseudomembranous candidiasis (thrush) is common in infancy likely because of immaturity of their immune system and lack of mature oral flora.
- Initial presentation may be feeding difficulty secondary to dysphagia.
- May have concurrent *Candida* diaper rash
- Consider maternal treatment if breastfeeding:
  - Maternal breast colonization may be cause for persistent thrush. Query maternal nipple pain, burning, itching, or cracked skin.

### Geriatric Considerations
- *Candida* organisms are normally present as oral flora from 65–88% of elderly or those in long-term care facilities.
- The presence of dentures or other orthodontic appliances can lead to *Candida* overgrowth.
- Angular cheilitis more common in the elderly secondary to facial wrinkling

## DIAGNOSIS

### SIGNS AND SYMPTOMS
- Pseudomembranous candidiasis (thrush):
  - Painless white mucosal plaques
  - Adherent but removable plaques
  - Erythematous base
  - May become confluent and curdlike
  - Anorexia, dysphagia
- Acute atrophic candidiasis:
  - Also referred to as erythematous candidiasis
  - Burning sensation in mouth or on tongue
  - Erythematous with few, if any white patches usually on the palate or dorsum of tongue
  - Tongue may be bright red in color—similar to nutritional deficiency.

- Chronic atrophic candidiasis:
  - Also referred as denture stomatitis
  - Irritation around denture-bearing mucosa
- Angular cheilitis:
  - Cracking or erythema at the corners of mouth
  - Lesion can be asymptomatic, pruritic, or painful
  - Superinfection with *Staphylococcus or Streptococcus* is common.
- Hyperplastic candidiasis:
  - Chronic, invasive ulcers
  - Typically on lateral borders of tongue or buccal mucosa
  - High incidence of malignant degeneration in tobacco users

### ESSENTIAL WORKUP
- Minimal workup needed in otherwise healthy infant. Diagnosis can be made clinically.
- Determine whether there is a cause for a breakdown of host factors.
- If no reason is found, evaluate for possible HIV infection or diabetes.
- Exclude a systemic infection.

### DIAGNOSTIC TESTS & INTERPRETATION
*Lab*
- Clinical diagnosis often sufficient
- CBC if suspect severe infection
- Glucose testing
- Potassium hydroxide (KOH)/fungal culture:
  - Obtain culture and sensitivity if failed first line treatment or high-risk individuals (HIV/AIDs, neutropenic, AIDs, transplant, etc.)

### DIFFERENTIAL DIAGNOSIS
- Hairy leukoplakia
- Lichen planus
- Squamous cell carcinoma
- Adherent food/milk

# TREATMENT

## ED TREATMENT/PROCEDURES
- IV fluids if dehydration and/or unable to tolerate PO fluids
- Topical analgesia: "Magic mouthwash:"
  - Mixture of equal parts 2% viscous lidocaine, Maalox, and diphenhydramine elixir
  - Swish for 1–2 min, then expectorate.
- Topical antifungal medications:
  - Suspension, troches, lozenges
  - Ointments (angular cheilitis)
- Systemic agents reserved for those with severe disease or resistant to topical therapy
- Provide oral hygiene education:
  - Instruct those using steroid inhalers to rinse mouth immediately after use.
  - Denture and orthodontic care

## MEDICATION
### Pediatric Considerations
- Dissolve troche in nipple of bottle.
- Mix suspensions with fruit juice and freeze into popsicle.
- Apply suspensions to affected areas with cotton-tipped swab.
- Instruct parents to disinfect or replace toothbrushes, pacifiers, bottle nipples.

### Geriatric Considerations
- Angular cheilitis: Treat with topical nystatin ointment
- Dentures: Remove, brush, and soak nightly. Consider overnight rinse with 2% chlorhexidine.

### First Line
- Nystatin: Oral suspension. Neonates 100,000 U, Older infants:200,000 U, children/adults:400,000–600,000 U. Swish and swallow q.i.d. for 7–14 days.
- Nystatin pastilles: 200,000 U PO q.i.d. for 7–14 days
- Clotrimazole troches: 10 mg PO 5 times per day for 7–14 days (children >3 yr)

### Second Line
- Oral fluconazole: Loading dose of 200 mg (peds: 6 mg/kg) on day 1, followed by 100 mg (peds: 3 mg/kg) PO daily for 7–14 days
- Ketoconazole: 200–400 mg (peds: >2 yr: 3.3–6.6 mg/kg/day) PO daily for 7–14 days
- Itraconazole solution: 200 mg daily (peds: 5 mg/kg) PO daily for 7–14 days

# FOLLOW-UP

## DISPOSITION
### Admission Criteria
- Inability to tolerate oral intake
- Newly diagnosed immunocompromised state
- Systemic infection

### Discharge Criteria
If the candidiasis does not threaten patient's hydration status, discharge to home.

## FOLLOW-UP RECOMMENDATIONS
Additional workup for immunodeficiency is warranted in older children and adults with unexplained candidiasis.

## PEARLS AND PITFALLS
- Failure to recognize immunodeficiency
- Failure to recognize other intra oral pathology such as squamous cell carcinoma

## ADDITIONAL READING
- Akpan A, Morgan R. Oral candidiasis. *Postgrad Med J.* 2002;78:455–459.
- Gonsalves W, Chi A, Neville B. Common oral lesions part I: Superficial mucosal lesions. *Am Fam Physician.* 2007;75:501–507.
- Krol D, Keels M. Oral conditions. *Pediatr Rev.* 2007;28:15–22.
- Pappas P, et al. Clinical practice guidelines for the management of candidiasis: 2009 update by the Infectious Diseases Society of America. *Clin Infect Dis.* 2009;48:503–535.

# CODES

**ICD9**
112.0 Candidiasis of mouth

C

# CARBAMAZEPINE, POISONING

Brenden L. Hansen
James W. Rhee

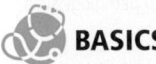 **BASICS**

## DESCRIPTION
- Therapeutic uses of carbamazepine:
  - Anticonvulsant
  - Treatment of chronic pain
  - Migraine prophylaxis
  - Mood stabilizer
- Mechanism:
  - Anticholinergic
  - Similarities to phenytoin and tricyclic antidepressants (TCAs)
  - Sodium channel blocker
  - Decreases synaptic transmission

## ETIOLOGY
Toxicity may occur from:
- Suicide attempt
- Accidental ingestion
- Supratherapeutic dosing
- Drug–drug interaction

 **DIAGNOSIS**

## SIGNS AND SYMPTOMS
- Neurologic manifestations common
- Cardiotoxicity rare, except in massive overdose
- CNS:
  - Ataxia
  - Dizziness
  - Drowsiness
  - Nystagmus
  - Hallucinations
  - Combativeness
  - Coma
  - Seizures
- Respiratory system:
  - Respiratory depression
  - Aspiration pneumonia
- Cardiovascular system:
  - Hypotension
  - Conduction disturbances (mostly in elderly)
  - Supraventricular tachycardia
  - Sinus tachycardia or bradycardia
  - ECG changes:
    - Prolongation of PR, QRS, and QTc intervals
    - T-wave changes

### Pediatric Considerations
Higher incidence of neurologic manifestations

## History
- Overdose of carbamazepine or extended release versions
- Time of ingestion
- Is the bottle available
- Accidental or intentional ingestion
- Coingestions

## Physical Exam
- May present with seizures or altered mental status
- May be combative or drowsy
- Sinus tachycardia (massive carbamazepine overdose)
- Bradydysrhythmia (often seen in elderly with mild increase in carbamazepine level)
- Anticholinergic manifestations:
  - Decreased bowel sounds
  - Mydriasis
  - Flushing
  - Urinary retention
- Neuromuscular changes:
  - Tremor
  - Slurred speech
  - Myoclonus
  - Choreiform and choreoathetoid movements

## ESSENTIAL WORKUP
- Continuous cardiac monitor
- Serum carbamazepine level:
  - Therapeutic, 6–12 μg/L
  - Levels >25–40 μg/mL associated with serious toxicity:
    - Coma
    - Seizures
    - Respiratory failure
    - Conduction defects
  - Serum levels do not clearly predict clinical toxicity:
    - Active metabolite carbamazepine 10, 11 epoxide not measured
    - Neurologic manifestations depend on CNS (not serum) level.
  - Serial levels may be needed owing to erratic absorption of carbamazepine.
- ECG:
  - Conduction delays:
    - Increased QRS interval
    - Increased PR interval
    - QTc prolongation
  - Dysrhythmias
- Serum acetaminophen level (to evaluate for coingestion in a suicide attempt)

## DIAGNOSTIC TESTS & INTERPRETATION
### Lab
- CBC:
  - Leukopenia or leukocytosis
- Electrolytes, BUN/creatinine, glucose:
  - Hyperglycemia
  - Hypokalemia
  - Hyponatremia
- Arterial blood gases (ABGs)
- Urinalysis:
  - Glucosuria
  - Ketonuria
- Pregnancy test
- ALT, AST, bilirubin, alkaline phosphatase:
  - May be mildly elevated
  - Usually not clinically significant

### Imaging
CXR:
- Aspiration pneumonia
- Pulmonary edema

## DIFFERENTIAL DIAGNOSIS
- Drugs that cause decreased mental status:
  - Alcohol
  - Anticholinergics
  - Barbiturates
  - Benzodiazepines
  - Lithium
  - Opiates
  - Phenothiazines
- Drugs that cause seizures:
  - Alcohol withdrawal
  - Anticholinergics
  - Camphor
  - Isoniazid
  - Lithium
  - Phenothiazines
  - Sympathomimetics:
    - Amphetamine
    - Cocaine
  - TCAs
- Drugs that cause abnormal movement:
  - Antihistamines
  - Butyrophenones
  - Caffeine
  - Cocaine
  - Levodopa
  - Meperidine
  - Phencyclidine
  - Phenothiazines
  - Phenytoin
  - TCAs

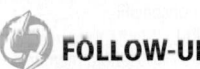 **TREATMENT**

### PRE-HOSPITAL
- Do *not* administer ipecac.
- Intubate if significant respiratory depression or airway compromise.
- Secure IV access.
- Get complete information about all products potentially ingested.

### INITIAL STABILIZATION/THERAPY
- ABCs
- IV access and fluid resuscitation if hypotensive
- Oxygen
- Cardiac monitor
- Naloxone, thiamine, $D_{50}W$ (or Accu-Chek) if altered mental status

### ED TREATMENT/PROCEDURES
- General management:
  - Gastric lavage:
    ○ Consider if recent ingestion (within 1 hr)
    ○ Few patients will need gastric lavage.
    ○ Instill activated charcoal through orogastric tube before and after lavage.
  - Activated charcoal:
    ○ Administer sorbitol with 1st dose (only) of activated charcoal.
    ○ Administer with caution if GI activity is decreased.
    ○ Contraindicated if bowel sounds are absent
  - Multidose activated charcoal:
    ○ Decreases mean half-life of carbamazepine
    ○ Binds unabsorbed drug in GI tract
    ○ Interrupts enterohepatic circulation
    ○ Do not give additional sorbitol.
  - Charcoal hemoperfusion/hemodialysis:
    ○ Removes small to moderate amount of ingested dose
    ○ Patients usually do well with supportive care without hemoperfusion or dialysis.
    ○ Indicated in cases of clinical deterioration or lack of improvement with good supportive care
- Respiratory depression:
  - Intubation
  - Ventilatory support
- Hypotension:
  - Bolus with IV isotonic crystalloid solution
  - Norepinephrine if unresponsive to IV fluids

- Seizures:
  - Diazepam (drug of choice)
  - Phenobarbital (if diazepam ineffective)
  - Phenytoin not effective in most toxic seizures
- Cardiac conduction delay:
  - QRS widening (>100 msec):
    ○ Sodium bicarbonate (to overcome sodium channel blockade)
- Psychiatric consultation if suicide attempt

### MEDICATION

> **ALERT**
> Only give sorbitol with the *1st* dose of activated charcoal.

#### First Line
- Activated charcoal (initial bolus): Slurry 1–2 g/kg up to 100 g PO mixed with sorbitol (below)
- Multidose activated charcoal: 25 g (peds: 0.25 g/kg) q2h PO after bolus dose (above), can also use 50 g q6h PO/NG
- Sorbitol: 1–2 g/kg to max. 100 g (peds: >1 yr old, 1–1.5 g/kg as 35% solution to max. 50 g) PO mixed with activated charcoal slurry (1st dose only)

#### Second Line
- Dextrose: $D_{50}W$ 1 ampule: 50 mL or 25 g (peds: $D_{25}W$ 2–4 mL/kg) IV
- Diazepam: 5–10 mg (peds: 0.2–0.5 mg/kg) IV
- Naloxone (Narcan): 2 mg (peds: 0.1 mg/kg) IV/IM initial dose
- Norepinephrine: 4–12 $\mu$g/min (peds: 0.05–0.1 $\mu$g/kg/min) IV titrated to effect
- Sodium bicarbonate: 1 or 2 amps IV push (peds: 1–2 mEq/kg)

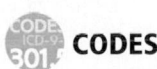 **FOLLOW-UP**

### DISPOSITION
#### Admission Criteria
- Decreased mental status at any time, even if resolving (tends to recur with fluctuating drug levels):
  - Observe at least 24 hr for late relapse.
- Seizures
- Cardiac dysrhythmias
- Lack of psychiatric clearance after suicidal ingestion

#### Discharge Criteria
- Asymptomatic after 6 hr of observation
- Normal mental status
- Normal or baseline ECG
- GI motility present
- Psychiatric clearance (after suicidal ingestion)

#### Issues for Referral
Suicidal patients need psychiatric evaluation referral.

### FOLLOW-UP RECOMMENDATIONS
Supratherapeutic dosing will need ongoing monitoring by physician treating underlying disorder.

## PEARLS AND PITFALLS

- Carbamazepine levels commonly rebound to higher levels during treatment. Obtain serial measurements for severe ingestions.
- Monitor closely for arrhythmias.
- Multidose charcoal may be needed for more serious ingestions.
- Paradoxical seizures may occur, use benzodiazepines to treat initially (diazepam is the drug of choice).

## ADDITIONAL READING

- Brahmi N, Kouraichi N, Thabet H, et al. Influence of activated charcoal on the pharmacokinetics and the clinical features of carbamazepine poisoning. *Am J Emerg Med*. 2006;24:440–443.
- Perez A, Wiley JF. Pediatric carbamazepine suspension overdose—Clinical manifestations and toxicokinetics. *Pediatr Emerg Care*. 2005;21(4): 252–254.
- Pilapil M, Petersen J. Efficacy of hemodialysis and charcoal hemoperfusion in carbamazepine overdose. *Clin Toxicol (Phila)*. 2008;46(4):342–343.
- Schmidt S, Schmitz-Buhl M. Signs and symptoms of carbamazepine overdose. *J Neurol*. 1995;242: 169–173.

**CODES**

ICD9
966.3 Poisoning by other and unspecified anticonvulsants

C

# CARBON MONOXIDE POISONING

*Trevonne M. Thompson*

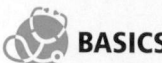

## BASICS

### DESCRIPTION
- Carbon monoxide (CO) is a colorless, odorless, nonirritating gas.
- Binds to hemoglobin to form carboxyhemoglobin:
  – Decreases $O_2$-carrying capacity
- Direct cellular toxin
- Impairs cellular $O_2$ utilization

### ETIOLOGY
- Endogenous:
  – Result of normal metabolism
- Incomplete combustion of carbonaceous fossil fuel:
  – Internal combustion engines
  – Natural gas
  – Heaters
  – Indoor grills
  – Fireplaces
  – Furnaces
  – Accidental fires
  – Tobacco smoke
- Methylene chloride:
  – Found in some solvents for paint removal and furniture stripping
  – Converted in vivo to carbon monoxide after exposure
  – Peak carboxyhemoglobin levels delayed after exposure
  – Half-life is approximately two times that of inhaled carbon monoxide.

## DIAGNOSIS

### SIGNS AND SYMPTOMS
*History*
- CNS:
  – Headache
  – Dizziness
  – Ataxia
  – Confusion
  – Syncope
  – Seizures
- GI:
  – Nausea
  – Vomiting
- Cardiovascular:
  – Chest pain
  – Palpitations
- Respiratory:
  – Dyspnea
- Ophthalmologic:
  – Decreased visual acuity

*Physical Exam*
- CNS:
  – Acute encephalopathy
  – Seizures
  – Coma
- Cardiovascular:
  – Tachycardia
  – Premature ventricular contractions
  – Dysrhythmias
  – Myocardial ischemia/infarction
- Respiratory:
  – Tachypnea
  – Noncardiogenic pulmonary edema
- Ophthalmologic:
  – Retinal hemorrhage
- Other:
  – Respiratory alkalosis
  – Rhabdomyolysis
  – Lactic acidosis

### ESSENTIAL WORKUP
- History:
  – Maintain a high index of suspicion.
  – Symptoms may be mild, nonspecific.
  – Inquire about the following:
    ○ Similar symptoms in other household members
    ○ Malfunctioning furnaces
    ○ Use of space heaters, open ovens for supplemental heat
    ○ Ill pets
- Arterial blood gas:
  – Normal $PaO_2$
  – Normal calculated $O_2$ saturation
  – Low measured $O_2$ saturation
  – Metabolic acidosis in severe cases

- Carboxyhemoglobin level:
  – Measure as soon as possible.
  – Level may not reflect clinical severity:
    ○ Patient may be critically ill despite unimpressive carboxyhemoglobin level.
    ○ May be misleadingly low if significant time has passed since exposure
    ○ Normal range is 0–3% (up to 10% in smokers).

### DIAGNOSTIC TESTS & INTERPRETATION
*Lab*
- Pulse oximetry:
  – Falsely elevated $SaO_2$ reading
  – Pulse oximeter cannot distinguish oxyhemoglobin from carboxyhemoglobin.
- Electrolytes:
  – Metabolic acidosis and elevated anion gap associated with increased clinical severity
- Cardiac enzymes:
  – When myocardial ischemia/infarction suspected
- Pregnancy test
- ECG:
  – CO may precipitate myocardial ischemia/infarction.
  – Dysrhythmias
  – Nonspecific ST-segment and T-wave abnormalities

*Imaging*
- Chest radiography:
  – Pulmonary edema
- CT scan of the head:
  – To evaluate for intracranial causes of altered mental status when indicated
  – Bilateral globus pallidus low-density lesions may be clue to CO poisoning in unclear cases.

### DIFFERENTIAL DIAGNOSIS
- Viral illness/viral syndrome
- Meningitis/encephalitis
- Intracranial hemorrhage
- Gastroenteritis
- Migraine headache
- Tension headache
- Ethanol intoxication
- Sedative–hypnotic overdose
- Cyanide poisoning
- Salicylate overdose
- Toxic alcohol exposure

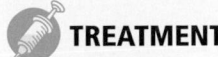 **TREATMENT**

### PRE-HOSPITAL
Administer 100% $O_2$

### INITIAL STABILIZATION/THERAPY
- ABCs
- Establish IV access
- 100% oxygen
- Cardiac monitor

### ED TREATMENT/PROCEDURES
- Oxygen:
  - Administer 100% normobaric $O_2$:
    - Via face mask or endotracheal tube
  - Continue $O_2$ therapy until carboxyhemoglobin level <10%.
  - Half-life of carboxyhemoglobin:
    - ~300 min in ambient air
    - ~90 min in 100% normobaric $O_2$
    - Approximately 20 min at 3 atm (hyperbaric $O_2$)
- Hyperbaric $O_2$:
  - Dose:
    - 100% $O_2$ at 3 atm
    - May be repeated
  - Benefits:
    - May reduce delayed neurologic sequelae
    - Decreases half-life of carboxyhemoglobin
  - Potential adverse effects:
    - Tympanic membrane rupture
    - Pneumothorax
    - Seizure
    - Decompression sickness
    - Pulmonary edema

- Indications for consulting hyperbaracist:
  - Altered mental status/coma
  - Focal neurologic deficits
  - Seizures
  - Cardiovascular compromise (infarction, persistent dysrhythmia)
  - Persistent metabolic acidosis
  - Carboxyhemoglobin level >25%
  - Pregnancy with carboxyhemoglobin level >10%

### Pregnancy Considerations
- Fetal hemoglobin has higher affinity for CO than adult hemoglobin.
- Fetal carboxyhemoglobin levels 10–15% higher than maternal levels
- Delayed clearance of fetal carboxyhemoglobin compared with maternal

 **FOLLOW-UP**

### DISPOSITION
### Admission Criteria
- Persistent symptoms after 4 hr of treatment with 100% oxygen
- Evidence of myocardial ischemia or cardiac instability
- Seizures
- Persistent metabolic acidosis
- Syncope

### Discharge Criteria
- Asymptomatic after 4 hr of observation
- Absence of aforementioned admission criteria
- Psychiatric clearance if suicidal exposure

### Issues for Referral
Need for hyperbaric oxygen therapy

### FOLLOW-UP RECOMMENDATIONS
Contact local fire department in cases of carbon monoxide home exposures.

## PEARLS AND PITFALLS
- Suspect CO poisoning in patients who present with headaches when home heaters are initiated.
- Suspect CO poisoning when family members living in the same enclosed space have similar symptoms.
- Administer 100% $O_2$ and transfer to hyperbaric facility if meets criteria described above.

## ADDITIONAL READING
- Kao LW, Nanagas KA. Carbon monoxide poisoning. *Emerg Med Clin North Am.* 2004;22(4):985–1018.
- Weaver LK, Hopkins RO, et al. Hyperbaric oxygen for acute carbon monoxide poisoning. *N Engl J Med.* 2002;347:1057–1067.
- Weaver LK. Carbon monoxide poisoning. *N Engl J Med.* 2009;360:1217–1225.

### See Also (Topic, Algorithm, Electronic Media Element)
Hyperbaric Oxygen

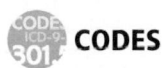 **CODES**

### ICD9
986 Toxic effect of carbon monoxide

# CARDIAC ARREST

Michael Donnino
Brandon Giberson
Michael Cocchi

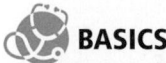 **BASICS**

## ALERT
- NOTE: The following information is based on 2005 ACLS Guidelines. Revisions made by the American Heart Association since then are not available at time of publication.
- Major ACLS Changes for the 2005 revision include:
  - Universal compression-to-ventilation ratio of 30:2 for 1 rescuer CPR of victims of all ages (except newborn infants).
  - Only 1 shock followed immediately by CPR instead of 3 stacked shocks for treatment of VT/VF.

## DESCRIPTION
- Sudden cardiac arrest is characterized by:
  - Unresponsiveness
  - Pulselessness
  - Little to no respiratory effort
- Factors affecting survival:
  - Initial rhythm
  - Total down time
  - Time to successful defibrillation

## ETIOLOGY
Contributing factors to cardiac arrest are outlined by the American Heart Association as:
- Hypovolemia
- Hypoxia
- Hydrogen ion (acidosis)
- Hypo-/hyperkalemia
- Hypoglycemia
- Hypothermia
- Toxins
- Tamponade, cardiac
- Tension pneumothorax
- Thrombosis
- Trauma

## Pediatric Considerations
- Sudden cardiac arrest in children is often of a respiratory rather than cardiac etiology.
- Follow current ACLS guidelines for pediatric cardiac arrest. Major differences between adult and pediatric cardiac arrest management include:
  - Depth of compressions for pediatric populations should be ~1/3 to 1/2 the depth of the chest.
  - AED use is not recommended for children <1 yr of age.
  - For two rescuer CPR, a 15:2 compression to ventilation rate is recommended.
  - Drug dosage differences: See "Medications" section.

## Pregnancy Considerations
Follow current ACLS guidelines for management of the pregnant cardiac arrest patient:
- Continuous cricoid pressure should be applied during PPV of the unconscious pregnant patient.
- Compressions should be performed at a higher location than conventional CPR, slightly above the center of the sternum.
- Follow Adult ACLS guidelines for defibrillation.
- Pre- or post-cardiac arrest pregnant patients should be placed in the left lateral recumbent position.
- To ensure a best possible outcome for the fetus, all efforts must be geared toward maternal survival.
- In the event of a failed maternal resuscitation, an emergent cesarean delivery must be considered.

 **DIAGNOSIS**

## SIGNS AND SYMPTOMS
- Unresponsiveness
- Pulselessness
- Shallow, gasping respirations may persist for a few minutes.
- Occasionally preceded by:
  - Chest pain
  - Dyspnea
  - Palpitations
  - Seizure activity
- Immediately prior to arrest:
  - Shock or hypotension
  - Impaired mentation

## ESSENTIAL WORKUP
- Assess airway, breathing, circulation
- Determine shockable vs. nonshockable rhythm and treat accordingly, per ACLS guidelines.

## DIAGNOSTIC TESTS & INTERPRETATION
### Lab
Indicated only when successful ROSC is achieved:
- Electrolytes
- BUN/creatinine
- Creatinine kinase with isoenzymes, cardiac troponin
- ABG
- CBC
- Therapeutic drug levels
- Toxicological testing
- Lactic acid levels

### Imaging
- EKG:
  - Evaluate for STEMI or ACS
- CXR:
  - Endotracheal tube position
  - Cardiac silhouette
  - Pneumothorax
- ECG:
  - Pericardial effusion
  - Wall motion abnormality
  - Valvular dysfunction
- Head CT scan (postresuscitation):
  - Rule out bleed/neurologic source

### Diagnostic Procedures/Surgery
- Suspected cardiac etiology:
  - Cardiac catheterization laboratory
  - Possible balloon pump
- EEG (postresuscitation)
  - Rule out status epilepticus.

## DIFFERENTIAL DIAGNOSIS
Sudden loss of consciousness with a palpable pulse:
- Syncope
- Seizure
- Acute stroke
- Hypoglycemia
- Acute airway obstruction
- Head trauma
- Toxins

**TREATMENT**

## PRE-HOSPITAL
- Prompt initiation of standard CPR
- Confirm underlying rhythm.
- Early defibrillation of ventricular tachycardia (VT) or ventricular fibrillation (VF):
  - Consider CPR before defibrillation in cases of unwitnessed/prolonged arrest.
- Secure airway and provide adequate respirations.
- Postresuscitation care:
  - Identify cause of arrest
  - 12-lead EKG
  - Monitor vital signs.

- Transport to the closest facility that is capable of handling postarrest patients:
  - Consider transport to center equipped for interventional cardiac care and those specializing in postarrest.
  - Pediatric critical care center for children

### INITIAL STABILIZATION/THERAPY

- Initiate advanced cardiac life support (ACLS)
- Perform standard CPR as long as no pulse is palpable:
  - Stop CPR only briefly to check pulse, cardiac rhythm, or defibrillate.
- Secure the airway.
- Obtain IV/IO access.
- Cardiac monitor
- Therapy is based on the underlying rhythm, according to ACLS protocols.

### ED TREATMENT/PROCEDURES

- Pulseless VT or VF:
  - Immediate defibrillation with 1 countershock:
    - Energy selection based on type of defibrillator for biphasic (if unknown use 200 J) or 360 J monophasic
  - If defibrillation is unsuccessful, continue CPR for 2 min and re-evaluate. When IV/IO access is established, consider:
    - Epinephrine
    - Vasopressin
  - If refractory to defibrillation and epinephrine, consider:
    - Amiodarone
    - Lidocaine
    - Magnesium for *torsades de pointes*
- Asystole:
  - Confirm in $\geq 2$ leads
  - Epinephrine
  - Atropine
  - May substitute vasopressin to replace 1st or 2nd dose of epinephrine
- Pulseless electrical activity:
  - Epinephrine
  - Atropine (for bradycardiac rhythm)
  - Treat for reversible cause of pulseless electrical activity/asystole.

- Postresuscitation:
  - Treat the underlying cause of the arrest.
  - EKG to establish presence of acute coronary syndrome:
    - Immediate catheterization for STEMI
    - Consider catheterization for non-STEMI with suspected ACS
  - Ventilatory support
  - Correct electrolyte abnormalities.
  - Initiate volume resuscitation and provide vasopressors/inotropic support as needed.
  - Induce hypothermia 32–34°C
  - Continuous EEG to rule out seizures

### MEDICATION

Medication administration should never interrupt CPR:

- Amiodarone: 300 mg (peds: 5 mg/kg to max 15 mg/kg) IVP
- Atropine: 1 mg (peds: 0.02 mg/kg up to 0.5 mg max. single dose) IV q3–5min
- Epinephrine: 1 mg (peds: 0.01 mg/kg) IVP q3–5min
- Lidocaine: 1–1.5 mg/kg 1st dose (peds 1 mg/kg) IVP, then 0.5–0.75 mg/kg (peds: 20–50 $\mu$g/min) IV, up to 3.0 mg/kg
- Magnesium: 1–2 g (peds: 25–50 mg/kg max of 2 g) slow IV
- Vasopressin: 40 U IVP (adults with VT/VF only)
- Sodium bicarbonate: 1 mEq/kg (peds: 1 mEq/kg) slow

 **FOLLOW-UP**

### DISPOSITION

#### Admission Criteria
Return of spontaneous circulation:

- Coronary care unit or ICU
- Postresuscitation care
- Treatment of underlying cause of arrest

#### Discharge Criteria
None

#### Issues for Referral
May consider referral to regional cardiac arrest center

Admission to ICU

### PEARLS AND PITFALLS

- Do not warm postarrest patients, but cool to 32–34°C.
- Expect recurrent cardiac arrest and provide close monitoring and appropriate postresuscitative treatment, which may consist of fluids and vasopressors.
- Get a cardiology consultation to determine if patient is candidate for cardiac catheterization.

### ADDITIONAL READING

- American Heart Association. Guidelines 2005 for cardiopulmonary resuscitation and emergency cardiovascular care. *Circulation*. 2005;v112, i24(Suppl):IV-1–IV-211.
- Hallstrom AP, Ornato JP, Weisfeldt M, et al. Public-access defibrillation and survival after out-of-hospital cardiac arrest. *N Engl J Med*. 2004;351:637–646.
- Nolan JP, Morley PT, Vanden Hoek TL, et al. Therapeutic hypothermia after cardiac arrest: An advisory statement by the advanced life support task force of the International Liaison Committee on Resuscitation. *Circulation*. 2003;108:118–121.
- Stiel IG, Hebert PC, Wells GA, et al. Vasopressin versus epinephrine for inhospital cardiac arrest: A randomised controlled trial. *Lancet*. 2001;358: 105–109.
- Wik L, Hansen TB, Fylling F, et al. Delaying defibrillation to give basic cardiopulmonary resuscitation to patients with out-of-hospital ventricular fibrillation: A randomized trial. *JAMA*. 2003;289:1389–1395.
- Zoll PM, Linenthal AJ, Gibson W, et al. Termination of ventricular fibrillation in man by externally applied electric countershock. *N Engl J Med*. 1956;254: 727–732.

 **CODES**

**ICD9**
427.5 Cardiac arrest

# CARDIAC PACEMAKERS
*Susan P. Torrey*

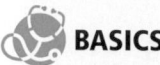 **BASICS**

## DESCRIPTION
- A device that uses electrical impulses to contract the heart muscles to regulate the beating of the heart
- Methods of cardiac pacing:
  - Percussive pacing:
    - Use of a closed fist, striking the sternum from a distance of 20–30 cm to induce a ventricular beat
    - Used only as a life-saving measure until an electrical pacemaker can be provided
  - Transcutaneous pacing:
    - 2 pads are placed on the chest in the anterior-lateral or anterior-posterior position.
    - The pacing current is gradually increased until electrical capturing occurs with a pulse.
    - Emergency therapy used only until transvenous pacing or another therapy can be applied
  - Temporary transvenous pacing:
    - A pacemaker wire is placed through central venous access into the right atrium (RA) or right ventricle (RV) and connected to an external pacemaker outside of the body.
    - Used as a bridge until a permanent pacemaker can be placed or there is no longer a need for a pacemaker
- Permanent, implanted pacemaker has 3 components:
  - A battery-powered energy source:
    - Lithium batteries last 7–10 yr
  - Generator:
    - A sophisticated computer with many programmable parameters
  - Leads connected to the RV/RA:
    - Typically sense electrical activity and pace the myocardium
- Pacemaker magnet:
  - Placed over pulse generator
  - Converts pacer to asynchronous mode
  - Useful if no pacer spikes on presenting ECG
  - A depleted battery will result in decrease in magnet rate by 10%.

### Pacemaker Terminology
- Fixed mode:
  - The pacemaker is set to fire at a set rate regardless of patient's underlying rhythm.
  - Occasionally seen in old pacers
- Demand mode:
  - The pacemaker fires only when necessary.
  - It senses the underlying rhythm.
  - It will only pace if the intrinsic rhythm is absent or less than a set rate.

- Sensing:
  - Refers to the pacemaker's ability to determine whether the heart is being intrinsically paced
- All pacemakers have a 5-letter code to describe their function.
- For ED purposes, only the 1st 3 letters of the code are necessary:
  - 1st letter in code indicates chamber being sensed by pacemaker:
    - **A: A**tria
    - **V: V**entricle
    - **D: D**ual (both chambers)
  - 2nd letter in code indicates chamber that can be paced:
    - **A: A**tria
    - **V: V**entricle
    - **D =** dual (both chambers)
  - 3rd letter in code describes pacemaker's response to sensed intrinsic complex:
    - **T: T**rigger (a sensed beat results in a pacing response as when a sensed atrial beat provokes a subsequent ventricular beat)
    - **I: I**nhibit (a sensed beat precludes pacemaker function)
    - **D: D**ual (a pacemaker is capable of both functions)
    - **O: N**o response
  - The most common pacemakers are VVI (single lead) and DDD (two leads).

## ETIOLOGY
- Pacemaker-associated infection:
  - Infection of pacemaker components often associated with endocarditis
  - *Staphylococcus epidermidis* and *S. aureus* account for >90% of infections.
  - Transesophageal ECG is the preferred diagnostic method.
- Venous thrombosis:
  - Very common (overall incidence 30–50%)
  - Symptomatic, acute obstruction is rare (<3%).
  - Pulmonary embolism is rare.
- Pacemaker failure to pace or discharge impulse:
  - Component failure is rare.
  - Battery depletion is rare with routine checks; it is not abrupt.
  - Lead fracture or disconnection
  - Oversensing of muscular activity or external electrical interference
- Pacemaker failure to capture myocardium:
  - Lead dislodgment is common.
  - Twiddler syndrome:
    - Unintentional manipulation of pacemaker generator, causing lead to dislodge from myocardium
  - Elevated myocardial threshold:
    - Hyperkalemia
    - Ischemia
  - Change in cardiac (QRS) morphology

- Pacemaker-mediated tachycardia:
  - Occurs with dual-chamber pacemakers
  - A re-entry rhythm using generator and intrinsic conduction system
  - Maximum rate typically 140 bpm due to built-in safeguards
- Runaway pacemaker:
  - Rare; triggered by battery depletion or component failure
  - Often rapid rates (>200 bpm) with hemodynamic compromise

 **DIAGNOSIS**

## SIGNS AND SYMPTOMS
- Pacemaker failure:
  - Bradycardia
  - Syncope
  - Hypotension, progressive to shock and hemodynamic collapse
  - Fatigue and weakness
  - Dyspnea on exertion or shortness of breath secondary to CHF
  - Ischemic chest pain
  - Altered level of consciousness
- Pacemaker-induced tachycardia:
  - Dyspnea
  - Ischemic chest pain
  - Lightheadedness
  - Syncope
- Pacemaker syndrome:
  - Symptoms related to asynchronous chamber contractions
  - Lightheadedness
  - Dyspnea
  - Palpitation
  - Syncope

### History
- Date of placement pacemaker
- Compliance with follow-up (battery checks)
- Type of pacemaker

### Physical Exam
General cardiac exam:
- Heart exam for murmurs
- Lung exam for CHF
- Chest wall exam at generator site

## ESSENTIAL WORKUP

- 12-lead EKG to assess whether there is any obvious evidence of pacemaker failure
- Metabolic workup to determine whether an acquired medical condition led to an elevated myocardial threshold
- EKG with pacer magnet:
  - Assess magnet rate.
  - Particularly useful when the baseline EKG does not reveal pacer spikes
  - The magnet activates asynchronous pacing mode.
  - Produces pacer spikes at a preprogrammed rate—regardless of the intrinsic rhythm
  - If the magnet rate equals the preprogrammed rate set at implantation, the pacer is okay.
  - If the magnet rate is >10% slower than at implantation, the battery is depleted.
  - If there are no pacer spikes, there is significant pacemaker malfunction.

## DIAGNOSTIC TESTS & INTERPRETATION

### Lab

- Serum potassium
- ABG
- Serum levels of antidysrhythmic drugs

### Imaging

CXR:

- Evaluate integrity of pacer lead(s) and position.
- Fractured lead
- Lead dislodgment:
  - Perforation

 **TREATMENT**

### PRE-HOSPITAL

Record rhythm strips for analysis

### INITIAL STABILIZATION/THERAPY

- Oxygen administered via 100% nonrebreather
- Intubation as needed
- IV access
- Advanced cardiac life support drugs as per usual protocol
- Defibrillation: Avoid placing paddles over generator.
- Transcutaneous pacemaker in hemodynamically unstable patients with pacemaker failure

## ED TREATMENT/PROCEDURES

- Pacemaker failure:
  - Transcutaneous pacemaker
  - Temporary transvenous pacemaker:
    - Obtain central IV access with a Cortis introducer.
    - Perform the procedure under fluoroscopy if possible.
    - Set the pulse generator to asynchronous mode.
    - Turn the output dial all the way up.
    - Advance the catheter through the central venous access Cortis until you see a QRS complex on the monitor.
    - Check the femoral pulse.
    - If you have a pulse and see a QRS complex, the pacer is "capturing."
    - Slowly turn the output dial down until you lose the QRS complex (capture threshold).
    - Turn the output dial up to 2 or 3 times the capture threshold.
    - Continuous EKG monitoring facilitates correct placement.
- Treat hyperkalemia (see "Hyperkalemia").
- Runaway pacemaker:
  - AV node blocking or reprogramming
  - In extreme situation, may need to disconnect lead from generator surgically

## MEDICATION

Adenosine: 6 mg IV bolus

 **FOLLOW-UP**

### DISPOSITION

### Admission Criteria

- Permanent pacemaker failure or malfunction
- Suspicion of infection involving pacemaker components

### Discharge Criteria

- Asymptomatic pacemaker malfunction
- A cardiologist has interrogated the pacemaker

### FOLLOW-UP RECOMMENDATIONS

Refer to cardiologist and/or pacemaker clinic

## PEARLS AND PITFALLS

- Always consider pacemaker failure in evaluation of cardiac decompensation, bradycardia, or syncope.
- Utilize pacemaker magnet to evaluate function.

## ADDITIONAL READING

- Cardall TY, Brady WJ, Chan TC, et al. Permanent cardiac pacemakers: Issues relevant to the emergency physician, parts I and II. *J Emerg Med*. 1999;17:479–489, 697–709.
- Griffin J, Smithline H, Cook J. Runaway pacemaker: A case report and review. *J Emerg Med*. 2000;19:177–181.
- McMullan J, Valento M, Attari M, et al. Care of the pacemaker/implantable cardioverter defibrillator patient in the ED. *Am J Emerg Med*. 2007;25(7):812–822.
- Scher D. Troubleshooting pacemakers and implantable cardioverter-defibrillators. *Curr Opin Cardiol*. 2004;19:36–46.
- Stone KR, McPherson CA. Assessment and management of patients with pacemakers and implantable defibrillators. *Crit Care Med*. 2004;32:155–165.

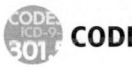 **CODES**

### ICD9

- V45.01 Cardiac pacemaker in situ
- 996.01 Mechanical complication due to cardiac pacemaker (electrode)
- 996.61 Infection and inflammatory reaction due to cardiac device, implant, and graft

# CARDIAC TESTING

Shamai A. Grossman
Matthew J. Bivens

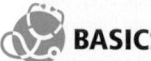

## BASICS

### DESCRIPTION
- Cardiac testing is indicated for emergency patients at risk for heart failure (HF) or acute coronary syndromes (ACS).
- These pathologies may be thought of as a spectrum: Unstable angina can evolve into MI, which in turn can cause heart failure:
  - ~20% of ED malpractice claims are due to missed diagnosis of ACS.
  - ~2% of patients with ACS are inappropriately discharged from an ED.
  - History, physical exam, and EKG are the critical elements in working up chest pain and ACS/HF.
  - History, physical, and EKG nevertheless miss 1–4% of all heart attacks.
  - Additional tools include imaging modalities and blood tests (eg, cardiac biomarkers)

### ETIOLOGY
ACS is caused by atherosclerotic narrowing of coronary vessels or by coronary vasospasm.

### Pregnancy Considerations
In the pregnant patient with chest pain and ischemic changes on EKG, also consider spontaneous coronary artery dissection.

## DIAGNOSIS

### SIGNS AND SYMPTOMS
#### History
- Symptoms usually are reproduced by exertion, eating, exposure to cold, or emotional stress; relieved by rest.
- ACS is less likely when chest pain is sharp, stabbing, pleuritic, or reproducible with palpation.
- Ischemia is still diagnosed in 13% of pleuritic chest pain and in 7% of chest pain reproducible with palpation.
- Nitroglycerin may relieve cardiac ischemia, but can also relieve pain in GI and aortic pathology.
- A "GI cocktail" of lidocaine and Maalox, or a proton-pump inhibitor such as omeprazole, may relieve GI pathology, but both can also relieve cardiac ischemia.
- Anginal symptoms last <20 min but longer than a few seconds.
- MI should be considered if symptoms last >20 min.

#### Physical Exam
Often unremarkable

### ESSENTIAL WORKUP
EKG:
- Per ACC/AHA guidelines, a 12-lead EKG should be performed on a patient with chest pain within 10 min of arrival to the ED:
  - A single EKG will miss 1/2 of acute MIs.
  - Hyperacute T waves (tall, broad-based, especially in anterior leads) may be earliest and only sign of AMI.

- During an MI, the EKG may evolve. Continuous EKG monitoring can identify an additional 16% of acute MIs not seen on initial ECGs. Absent continuous monitoring, consider a repeat EKG 15–60 min after the 1st.
- New ST-segment changes or T-wave inversions are suspicious for unstable angina.
- ST depressions of 1 mm are characteristic of angina; or, could be reciprocal changes, so check other leads.
- STEMI: ST elevation of >2 mm in ≥2 contiguous leads.
- New bundle branch block (left more commonly than right) is suggestive of AMI:
  - Old LBBB makes diagnosing AMI difficult: Apply Sgarbossa criteria: AMI is likely if LBBB and >1 mm ST elevation concordant with QRS, or ST depression >1 mm in leads V1, 2, or 3.
  - ST-segment elevations or depressions, or T-wave inversions, are often unchanged from previous tracings; EKG should be compared with prior tracings if available.
- Additional-lead EKGs: Standard 12 leads often miss infarcts in the posterior, right, and high lateral walls.
  - Right-sided EKG:
    - Move lead V4 to the right side of chest, midclavicular line, 5th intercostal space, and repeat EKG, to capture infarct in right ventricle.
    - A right-sided EKG is often performed in the setting of a STEMI in inferior leads (II, III, aVF) to diagnose a right ventricular (RV) infarct.
  - Posterior EKG:
    - Leads V7, V8, V9 are placed posterior thorax along 5th intercostal space: V7 at posterior axillary line, V8 at inferior angle of scapula, V9 paraspinal.
    - Performed in setting of inferior or lateral wall MI; or if ST depression in V1–V3. May identify a lateral or left circumflex infarct
  - 80-lead body surface mapping:
    - Provides a 27.5% increase in STEMI detection over a typical 12-lead
- EKG may be helpful in diagnosing other etiologies of chest pain:
  - Pericarditis is suggested by diffuse ST- elevations followed by T-wave inversions and P-R depression.
  - Pulmonary embolism is suggested by unexplained tachycardia, new-onset atrial fibrillation, or rarely with S1, Q3, T3 pattern.

### DIAGNOSTIC TESTS & INTERPRETATION
#### Lab
- Cardiac biomarkers:
  - Indicated if the history is suspicious for AMI
  - May be consistently normal in unstable angina
  - Should not be elevated and are not indicated in stable angina
- Troponin T and I: Starts to rise 2–3 hr after onset of chest pain of ACS and peaks in 8–12 hr. Remains elevated 7–14 days:
  - A single troponin has low sensitivity for ACS. (1 study of low-risk chest pain in patients with negative initial troponin: 2.3% rate of AMI and 1% rate of death at 30 days.)

- Timing of biomarker testing is critical: ACEP, supported by a single study, endorses with "moderate clinical certainty" that a single negative troponin can rule out AMI if drawn 8–12 hr after onset of symptoms.
- Newer, more sensitive assays may fully eliminate the need for a 2nd troponin.
- Minor troponin elevations may occur with renal failure, structural heart disease, CHF (acute or chronic), cardiac pacing, pulmonary embolism, sepsis, CVAs.
- False-negatives have been documented due to antitroponin antibodies; labs can run additional tests to clarify the result if a false-negative seems clinically unlikely.
- Lack of standardization among assays (particularly with troponin I) means values from 1 lab cannot always be compared to results from another.
- CK/CK-Mb: Less sensitive than troponin, rises more slowly. Little gained by using both CK-Mb and troponin assays.
- Myoglobin: Rises faster than standard troponin assays and thus able to detect AMI sooner, but maximum sensitivity is 70%.
- B-Type natriuretic peptide (BNP):
  - Release and synthesis activated by diastolic ventricular stretch
  - Useful for detecting heart failure
  - A cutoff of >100 pg/mL diagnosed HF with a sensitivity of 90% and specificity of 76%.
  - Unclear significance of elevated BNP in setting of ACS

#### Imaging
- CXR:
  - Usually normal
  - May show cardiomegaly
  - May show CHF
  - May identify other etiologies of chest pain, such as pneumonia or widened mediastinum of aortic dissection
- ECG (rest):
  - May identify ACS or AMI based on wall motion abnormalities; also can detect pump failure and valvular abnormalities
  - Rest ECG has a sensitivity of 70% and specificity of 87% for ACS.
  - Rest ECG has a sensitivity of 93% and specificity of 66% for AMI.
- Technetium$^{99m}$ sestamibi (rest):
  - Radioactive IV dye taken up by myocardium, and detected by single photon emission CT (SPECT) imaging. (Also known as myocardial perfusion imaging.)
  - Can be imaged at rest to detect low- or no-flow areas of myocardium; can also be imaged after exercise or pharmacologic stress.
  - Per 2009 AHA/ACC guidelines, reserve for intermediate- to high-risk patients.
  - Has a sensitivity of 81% and specificity of 73% for ACS
  - Has a sensitivity of 92% and specificity of 67% for AMI

- CT coronary angiography (CTCA):
  - Imaging to evaluate degree of coronary artery stenosis and calcium deposits
  - Negative predictive value between 97–100%, accuracy comparable to stress testing
  - Per 2007 AHA/ACC guidelines, CTCA can be "reasonable alternative" to stress testing.
- Exercise stress testing:
  - May help establish diagnosis of angina, provide prognostic information
  - 1-mm depression of the ST segment in 3 consecutive beats and two consecutive leads is characteristic of cardiac ischemia.
  - Early positive (within 3 min) stress tests are worrisome for unstable angina.
  - 6 min of exercise using a standard Bruce protocol suggests an excellent prognosis.
  - Exercise stress testing with EKG alone has a sensitivity of 68% and specificity of 77%.
  - Exercise stress testing with ECG has a sensitivity of 85% and specificity of 77%.
  - Exercise stress testing with technetium$^{99m}$ sestamibi has a sensitivity of 87% and specificity of 64%.
- Cardiac catheterization:
  - Considered the gold standard for evaluating coronary arteries.
  - A history of a negative catheterization does not exclude AMI.

### Diagnostic Procedures/Surgery
EKG, cardiac enzymes, echo, stress testing

### DIFFERENTIAL DIAGNOSIS
See ACS chapters.

## TREATMENT

### PRE-HOSPITAL
- Cardiac monitoring
- Out-of-hospital EKG:
  - Alone has a sensitivity of 76% and specificity of 88% for ACS
  - Alone has a sensitivity of 68% and specificity of 97% for AMI

### INITIAL STABILIZATION/THERAPY
- Cardiac monitoring
- Oxygen saturation

### ED TREATMENT/PROCEDURES
- See "Acute Coronary Syndrome: Stable Angina"; "Acute Coronary Syndrome: Unstable Angina"; and "Acute Coronary Syndrome: MI" for more detail.
- Guidelines for cardiac testing
- History suggestive of ACS:
  - Obtain ECG and 1st troponin (or other cardiac biomarkers).
- ECG or 1st troponin abnormal:
  - Admit; consider cardiology consult.
- Ongoing chest pain or pressure:
  - Obtain sestamibi or ECG.
  - Consider serial EKGs.

- Sestamibi, serial EKG or echo abnormal:
  - Admit; consider cardiology consult.
- Second troponin (or other cardiac biomarkers) abnormal:
  - Admit; consider cardiology consult.
  - History suggestive of ACS but EKG nondiagnostic, biomarkers normal?
- Ancillary testing:
  - Standard exercise testing (ETT): For low- to intermediate-risk patients:
    ○ If low-risk patient with good follow-up, ACC/AHA guidelines allow for outpatient stress testing within 72 hr.
    ○ Per 2007 AHA/ACC guidelines CTCA "reasonable alternative" to stress testing.
  - For abnormal or uninterpretable EKG: Stress EKG or sestamibi
  - For patient unable to exert self: Pharmacologic ETT (ie, dobutamine EKG or dipyridamole sestamibi)
  - Ancillary testing abnormal:
    ○ Admit or cardiology consult

### MEDICATION
Patient should not be started on new antianginal medication before stress testing in the ED.

 **FOLLOW-UP**

### DISPOSITION

### Admission Criteria
- History suggestive of cardiac etiology for chest pain
- Abnormal or changed EKG
- Positive cardiac biomarkers
- Positive rest imaging
- If the diagnosis is unclear, admission to the hospital or an ED observation unit may be useful for serial cardiac biomarkers, EKGs, and exercise stress testing.
- Early positive stress test:
  - If the patient has an otherwise positive stress test, the decision for admission should be made in consultation with the primary care physician or cardiologist.

### Discharge Criteria
Patients who meet the following criteria are safe to discharge:
- History not suggestive of cardiac etiology for chest pain
- Normal ECG
- Normal cardiac testing

### FOLLOW-UP RECOMMENDATIONS
- Abnormal stress test will require close follow-up with cardiology or PCP.
- Undifferentiated CP should have ED stress testing unless clear follow up is available.

## PEARLS AND PITFALLS

- Normal EKG or enzymes do not rule out CAD; repeat EKG or additional leads improve sensitivity.
- Most ED patients with undifferentiated chest pain will need some form of additional testing.
- Consider CT to rapidly rule out ACS in the ED.

## ADDITIONAL READING

- Cardiac Radionuclide Imaging Writing Group. Criteria for Cardiac Radionuclide Imaging. ACCF/ASNC/ACR/AHA/ASE/SCCT/SCMR/SNM 2009 Appropriate Use Criteria for Cardiac Radionuclide Imaging. Joint guideline of ACC/AHA.
- Hoekstra J, O'Neill BJ, Pride YB, et al. Acute detection of ST-elevation myocardial infarction missed on standard 12-lead EKG with a novel 80-lead real-time digital body surface map: Primary results from the multicenter OCCULT myocardial infarction trial. Ann Emerg Med. 2009;54(6): 779–788.
- Saenger A, et al. The use of biomarkers for the evaluation and treatment of patients with acute coronary syndromes. Med Clin N Am. 2007;91: 657–681.
- Tabas J, Rodriguez RM, Seligman HK, et al. Electrocardiographic criteria for detecting acute myocardial infarction in patients with left bundle branch block: A meta-analysis. Ann Emerg Med. 2008;52(4):329–336.
- Woo KC, Schneider J. High-risk chief complaints I: Chest pain—The big three. Emerg Med Clin N Am. 2009;27:685–712.

C

# CARDIAC TRANSPLANTATION COMPLICATIONS

*Jarrod Mosier*
*Samuel M. Keim*

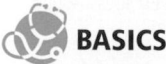 **BASICS**

## DESCRIPTION
- Cardiac transplant recipients are a unique population with increased risk for cardiac ischemia, heart failure, as well as general risks as an immunocompromised host.
- 2,200 cardiac transplants per year in the United States
- 1-yr survival 85–90%; 5-yr survival ~75%
- Typical immunosuppressive therapy to control rejection is a "triple-drug" regime often including steroids.
- Frequent biopsies are used initially to evaluate rejection; ECG often used in children.
- Complications occur most commonly in the 1st 6 wk after cardiac transplantation.

## ETIOLOGY
- Rejection:
  - Hyperacute rejection:
    ○ Occurs within minutes of transplantation
    ○ Rare, due to ABO or other graft/host major incompatibility
    ○ Aggressive and immediately fatal to graft
  - Acute rejection:
    ○ Lymphocyte infiltration and myocyte destruction
    ○ Most common in 1st 6 wk
    ○ May occur at any time
    ○ 75% prevalence
  - Chronic rejection:
    ○ Fibrosis and graft vascular disease
    ○ Long-term complication
    ○ Incompletely understood etiology
    ○ No effective therapy
- Cardiac allograft vasculopathy:
  - Analogous to accelerated coronary artery disease in native hearts
  - Limits long-term survival, leading cause of mortality after 1 yr
  - Immune-mediated atherosclerosis, form of chronic rejection
- Infections:
  - 1st mo:
    ○ Bacterial infections are most common cause of mortality during this high-risk time period
    ○ Pneumonia (*Pseudomonas*, *Legionella*, other gram-negative organisms)
    ○ Mediastinitis
    ○ Wound infection
    ○ Urinary tract infection
  - 1st yr:
    ○ Opportunistic and conventional infections
    ○ Cytomegalovirus (CMV)
    ○ Herpes simplex virus (HSV)
    ○ *Legionella*
    ○ Fungal infections
    ○ *Pneumocystis carinii*

- Medication toxicity:
  - Cyclosporine, Neoral (2nd-generation cyclosporine), tacrolimus:
    ○ Nephrotoxicity (30% incidence)
    ○ Hepatotoxicity
    ○ Neurotoxicity
    ○ Hyperlipidemia, diabetogenic
  - Azathioprine, mycophenolate mofetil:
    ○ Bone marrow suppression
    ○ Leukopenia
  - Sirolimus:
    ○ Hyperlipidemia
    ○ Wound healing
  - Steroids:
    ○ Osteoporosis
    ○ Cushing disease
- Malignancy:
  - Secondary to immunosuppression
  - 10–100 times more common vs. general population
  - Skin and lip cancer
  - Lymphomas
  - Kaposi sarcomas
  - Solid organ neoplasms

### Pediatric Considerations
- If the patient is not on steroids, bacteremia risk is similar to that in the general population.
- High incidence of pneumonia
- Patients on steroids may not show meningeal signs.

### Pregnancy Considerations
- Pregnancy after cardiac transplant is becoming more common. Between 1991–2006, 42 women received either heart or heart-lung transplants. They have reported 66 pregnancies, all progressing to live births.
- Most common complications include HTN, preeclampsia, and rejection.
- Physiologic changes that occur with pregnancy do not relate to increased rate of heart failure in transplant patients.
- Special attention should be paid to these patients regarding rejection and infection, given their immunosuppression.

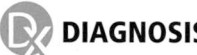 **DIAGNOSIS**

## SIGNS AND SYMPTOMS
- Acute rejection:
  - Nonspecific symptoms predominate because the heart is usually denervated:
    ○ Fatigue
    ○ Dyspnea
    ○ Low-grade fever
    ○ Nausea
    ○ Vomiting

- May be difficult to differentiate between infection
- Signs of heart failure:
  ○ Tachypnea
  ○ Rales
  ○ Hypoxia
  ○ S3
  ○ Murmur
  ○ Edema
- Allograft vasculopathy:
  - As early as 3 mo after transplantation (20–50% incidence by 5 yr)
  - Insidious onset:
    ○ Fatigue
    ○ Cough
    ○ Dyspnea
  - Acute onset:
    ○ Heart failure
    ○ Sudden death
    ○ Infarction
  - Denervated hearts do not present with typical angina.
  - Infection (opportunistic and conventional)
  - Fever
  - Skin lesions (zoster)
  - CMV:
    ○ Mild (flu-like illness)
  - Fever
  - Nausea
  - Malaise
  - Severe:
    ○ Pneumonitis (13–50% mortality)
    ○ Hepatitis
    ○ Gastroenteritis
    ○ Profound leucopenia

### Pediatric Considerations
- Higher risk for post-transplant lymphoproliferative disease with Epstein-Barr virus seroconversion
- Like adults, at risk for allograft vasculopathy and its associated cardiac ischemia

### History
- Comprehensive history is essential including specific and subtle symptoms.
- Contact information for coordinating transplant team if not at same center

## ESSENTIAL WORKUP
- Assess for signs of rejection, cardiac dysfunction, and infarction:
  - EKG
  - Cardiac enzymes
  - CXR
  - ECG
- Possible rejection requires biopsy: Consult transplant team.

### Pediatric Considerations
Normal fever workup plus chest radiograph and EKG; if on steroids, perform LP

## DIAGNOSTIC TESTS & INTERPRETATION
### Lab
- Electrolytes:
  - Cyclosporine effects:
    - Increased blood urea nitrogen, creatinine
    - Hyperkalemia
    - Metabolic acidosis
    - Hyponatremia
- CBC:
  - Relative eosinophilia may indicate rejection over infection.
- Blood and urine culture if febrile
- Lumbar puncture if seizures, altered mental status, or severe headache
- Consider:
  - BNP (expect baseline elevation)
  - CMV titers
  - Urine antigen test
  - Cyclosporine trough level

### Imaging
- EKG:
  - Tachycardia
  - 20% decrease in total voltage (nonsensitive)
  - Note that normal rhythm for denervated heart is sinus 90–110 bpm.
  - Depending on transplant surgical technique, may see 2 P waves (native and donor heart):
    - Native P waves do not correspond to quasi-random signal.
- CXR:
  - Cardiomegaly
  - Pulmonary edema
  - Pleural effusions
  - Compare with previous (healthy donor heart may appear large in small recipient)
- ECG:
  - Decreased mitral deceleration time
  - Initial diastolic dysfunction
  - Biventricular enlargement
  - Mitral/tricuspid regurgitation

## DIFFERENTIAL DIAGNOSIS
- Rejection
- Infection
- Ischemia
- CMV
- Viral illness
- Malignancy
- Cyclosporine toxicity

 TREATMENT

## INITIAL STABILIZATION/THERAPY
ABCs:
- IV access
- Oxygen
- Monitor
- Intubation
- Defibrillation/pacing
- Vasopressors as required
- Arrhythmias:
  - Advanced cardiac life support
  - Bradycardia does not respond to atropine; use isoproterenol

## ED TREATMENT/PROCEDURES
- Hemodynamically significant rejection:
  - Methylprednisolone
  - May also require OKT3 or other anti–T-cell antibody therapy
- Infarct/vasculopathy:
  - Aspirin
  - Heparin
  - Possible angioplasty
  - Likely need retransplantation
- CMV:
  - Empiric IV ganciclovir
- HSV:
  - Oral or IV acyclovir
- Gastroenteritis:
  - Search for CMV infection with culture, serology.
- Fever without a source:
  - Consult infectious disease or transplantation team.
- Headache:
  - Threshold for CT scan and lumbar puncture should be low (meningitis, abscess).
- Serious illness/trauma/operation:
  - Steroid burst
- Limit NSAID use because of risk for renal insufficiency from cyclosporine and tacrolimus.

## MEDICATION
- Acyclovir: 5–10 mg/kg IV q6h; genital herpes: 400 mg PO t.i.d. × 7–10 days; varicella: 20 mg/kg up to 800 mg PO q.i.d. for 5 days
- Ceftriaxone: 50 mg/kg IV
- Cyclosporine, CellCept, tacrolimus, sirolimus, Neoral, azathioprine, mycophenolate mofetil: Per transplantation team instructions
- Ganciclovir: 5 mg/kg b.i.d. for 2–3 wk (adjust for renal function)
- Isoproterenol 1–4 μg/min, titrate to effect; max. 10 μg/min
- Methylprednisolone: 1 g IV; peds: 10–20 mg/kg IV
- OKT3, daclizumab, or other antibody therapy: Per transplant team instructions

 FOLLOW-UP

## DISPOSITION
### Admission Criteria
- Hemodynamically significant rejection
- Vasculopathy/ischemia
- New dysrhythmia
- Poorly controlled HTN
- CHF
- Dyspnea
- Hypoxia
- Temperature >38°C in adult or child on steroids
- Suspected CMV (unexplained fever, gastroenteritis, or interstitial pneumonitis)
- Not tolerating oral medicines
- Syncope

### Discharge Criteria
- Mild rejection
- Only in consultation with transplantation team
- Fever in nontoxic child:
  - Do not give children stress-dose steroids.

## FOLLOW-UP RECOMMENDATIONS
All transplant patients should follow up with their coordinating transplant clinic after an ED visit.

## PEARLS AND PITFALLS
Cardiac allograft recipients are quite prone to develop coronary artery disease (CAD). This CAD is generally diffuse and quite different from "typical" atherosclerotic CAD.

## ADDITIONAL READING
- Chinnock R, Sherwin T, Robie S, et al. Emergency department presentation and management of pediatric heart transplant recipients. *Pediatr Emerg Care.* 1995;11(5):355–360.
- Deng MC. Cardiac transplantation. *Heart.* 2002;87:177–184.
- Massad MG. Current trends in heart transplantation. *Cardiology.* 2004;101:79–92.
- Mastrobattista JM, Gomez-Lobo V. Pregnancy after solid organ transplantation. *Obstet Gynecol.* 2008;112:919–932.
- Mill MR, Grady MS. Cardiac transplantation. In: Tintinalli JE, Kelen GD, Stapczynski JS, eds. *Emergency medicine: A comprehensive study guide,* 6th ed. San Francisco: McGraw-Hill, 2000:422–428.
- Miniati DN, Robbins RC, Reitz BA. In: Braunwald L, ed. *Heart disease: A textbook of cardiovascular medicine,* 6th ed. Philadelphia: WB Saunders, 2001:615–631.
- Mueller XM. Drug immunosuppression therapy for adult heart transplantation. *Ann Thorac Surg.* 2004;77:363–371.
- Poston RS, Griffith BP. Heart transplantation. *J Intensive Care Med.* 2004,19.3–12.

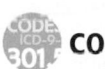 CODES

ICD9
996.83 Complications of transplanted heart

C

# CARDIOGENIC SHOCK
*Nadeem Al-Duaij*

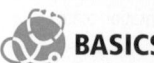 **BASICS**

## DESCRIPTION
- Persistent hypotension and tissue hypoperfusion due to cardiac dysfunction in the presence of adequate intravascular volume and left ventricular filling pressure
- Most common cause of death in hospitalized patients with acute MI (AMI)
- Underlying mechanisms in AMI:
  - Pump failure:
    - ≥40% left ventricle (LV) infarct
    - Infarct in pre-existing LV dysfunction
    - Reinfarction
  - Mechanical complications:
    - Acute mitral regurgitation
    - Ventricular septal defect
    - LV rupture
    - Pericardial tamponade
  - Right ventricular (RV) infarction
- 7% of patients with AMI develop cardiogenic shock.
- Role for a systemic inflammatory response syndrome via inducible nitric oxide in the pathophysiology of cardiogenic shock

## ETIOLOGY
- AMI
- Sepsis
- Myocarditis
- Myocardial contusion
- Valvular disease
- Cardiomyopathy
- Left atrial myxoma
- Drug toxicity:
  - β-Blocker
  - Calcium channel blocker
  - Adriamycin

## DIAGNOSIS

### SIGNS AND SYMPTOMS
- ABCs and vital signs:
  - Patent airway (early)
  - Labored breathing and tachypnea (early); respiratory failure (late)
  - Diffuse crackles or wheezing
  - Hypoxia
  - Hypotension:
    - Systolic BP <90 mm Hg
    - Decline by at least 30 mm Hg below baseline level
  - Tachycardia
  - Weak pulses

- General:
  - Cyanosis
  - Pallor
  - Diaphoresis
  - Dulled sensorium
  - Decrease in body temperature
  - Urine flow of <20 mL/h
- Neck:
  - Jugular venous distention
- Cardiac:
  - Ischemic chest pain
  - Systolic apical blowing murmur
  - Gallop rhythm:
    - S3 reflects severe myocardial dysfunction.
    - S4 is present in 80% patients in sinus rhythm with AMI.
  - Systolic click:
    - Suggests rupture of the chordae tendinea
- Abdominal:
  - Epigastric pain
  - Nausea and vomiting
- Neurologic:
  - Obtundation

### History
- Obtain history from patient, family, or EMS for clues to possible etiology.
- Medications history

### Physical Exam
- Perform rapid survey and stabilize ABCs.
- Distended neck veins and cool extremities distinguish cardiogenic shock from distributive and hypovolemic shock.
- Careful heart and lung exam

### ESSENTIAL WORKUP
Ancillary studies further define the type and degree of cardiac injury and determine the indications for emergent catheterization or surgical intervention.

### DIAGNOSTIC TESTS & INTERPRETATION
EKG:
- Normal EKG does not rule out AMI.
- Findings of AMI (ST-elevations in two or more contiguous leads)
- May occur in non-ST-elevation acute coronary syndrome
- Dysrhythmias
- LV hypertrophy

### Lab
- B-type natriuretic peptide (BNP):
  - Diagnostic and prognostic value
- Creatine kinase (CK), CK-MB, troponin
- Electrolytes and renal function:
  - Acute renal failure is a strong predictor of mortality.
- CBC:
  - Identify anemia or elevated WBC.
- Drug levels (eg, digoxin)

### Imaging
- CXR:
  - Pulmonary congestion
  - Pleural effusion
  - Cardiomegaly
  - Pneumonia
  - Pneumothorax
  - Pericardial effusion
- Emergent ECG:
  - Transthoracic echocardiography (TTE) with color Doppler
  - LV contractility looking for hypokinesis, akinesis or dyskinesis
  - Acute mitral regurgitation or septal defects
  - RV dilatation, tricuspid insufficiency, high pulmonary artery and RV pressures suggest pulmonary embolism
  - RV hypokinesis or akinesis, RV dilatation, normal pulmonary pressures suggest RV infarction
  - Pericardial effusion, right atrium or RV diastolic collapse suggest cardiac tamponade

### DIFFERENTIAL DIAGNOSIS
- Obstructive shock:
  - Tension pneumothorax
  - Cardiac tamponade
  - Pulmonary embolism
  - Spontaneous esophageal rupture
  - Air embolus
- Distributive shock:
  - Sepsis
  - Anaphylaxis
  - Addisonian crisis
  - Neurogenic shock
- Hypovolemic shock:
  - Hemorrhage
  - Gastrointestinal losses
  - Dehydration
  - Burns

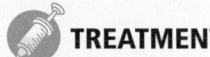 **TREATMENT**

### PRE-HOSPITAL
- ABCs, IV access, O$_2$, monitor
- Consider fluid bolus if no crackles.
- Aspirin
- Nitroglycerin or morphine sulfate for chest pain in absence of hypotension
- Transport AMI patients to facility with 24-hr cardiac revascularization capability.

### INITIAL STABILIZATION/THERAPY
- ABCs
- 2 large-bore peripheral IV lines
- Cardiac monitor
- Endotracheal intubation for airway compromise:
  - Consider etomidate for induction (minimal effect on BP)
- Fluid challenge (100–250 mL normal saline) in absence of pulmonary congestion
- Foley catheter to monitor urine output

### ED TREATMENT/PROCEDURES
- AMI:
  - Aspirin
  - Heparin
  - Thrombolysis if percutaneous coronary intervention or bypass surgery not available
  - GP IIb/IIIa inhibitors prior to percutaneous coronary intervention
- Hypotension:
  - Dopamine, 1st-line vasopressor
  - Norepinephrine may be used for hypotension unresponsive to dopamine or intra-aortic balloon pump (IABP), or for tachycardia.

- Normotensive patient:
  - Dobutamine may be used. It has additive effect when used with dopamine; combine with nitroprusside in acute mitral regurgitation
  - Milrinone may be considered in conjunction with dobutamine or dopamine.
- Pulmonary edema:
  - Nitroglycerin drip or furosemide in the normotensive patient
- Prompt cardiology consultation is crucial for the initiation of the following therapies:
  - IABP improves survival when combined with revascularization.
  - Early revascularization is the single most important life-saving measure.

### MEDICATION
- Dobutamine: 3–5 $\mu$g/kg/min, titrate to 20–50 $\mu$g/kg/min as needed IV
- Dopamine: 3–5 $\mu$g/kg/min, titrate to 20–50 $\mu$g/kg/min as needed IV
- Furosemide: 40–80 mg/d (peds: 1 mg/kg IV or IM, not to exceed 6 mg/kg) IV or IM
- Milrinone: 50 $\mu$g/kg loading dose, 0.375–0.75 $\mu$g/kg/min continuous infusion IV
- Nitroglycerin: 10–20 $\mu$g/min (pedis: 0.1–1 $\mu$g/kg/min) IV
- Nitroprusside: 0.3 $\mu$g/kg/min, titrate to a maximum of 10 $\mu$g/kg/min IV
- Norepinephrine: 2 $\mu$g/min, titrate up as needed IV

 **FOLLOW-UP**

### DISPOSITION
***Admission Criteria***
All patients in cardiogenic shock require admission to a critical care unit.

## PEARLS AND PITFALLS
- Cardiogenic shock is the leading cause of death in inpatient AMI.
- Early recognition of preshock states is essential.
- Early revascularization offers better outcomes.

## ADDITIONAL READING
- Hochman JS. Cardiogenic shock complicating acute myocardial infarction: Expanding the paradigm. *Circulation.* 2003;107:2998–3002.
- Peacock WF, Weber JE. Cardiogenic shock, in Tintinalli JE, Kelen GD, Stapczynski JS, eds: *Emergency Medicine: A Comprehensive Study Guide.* New York: McGraw-Hill, 2004:242.
- Topalian S, Ginsberg F, Parrillo JE. Cardiogenic shock. *Crit Care Med.* 2008;36:S66–S74.

**See Also (Topic, Algorithm, Electronic Media Element)**
Shock; MI

 **CODES**

ICD9
785.51 Cardiogenic shock

# CARDIOMYOPATHY

*Elizabeth Temin*
*James Feldman*

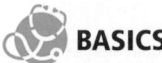 **BASICS**

## DESCRIPTION
Diseases of the myocardium associated with cardiac dysfunction:
- Dilated:
  – Idiopathic in 25% of all cases of heart failure
- Hypertrophic
- Restrictive
- Arrhythmogenic right ventricular (RV)
- Unclassified cardiomyopathy
- Specific cardiomyopathy:
  – Heart muscle disease associated with a systemic disease or condition

### Pediatric Considerations
- Genetic: 20–30%
- Acquired
- Idiopathic

### Pregnancy Considerations
See Cardiomyopathy, Peripartum.

## ETIOLOGY
- Dilated:
  – Idiopathic
  – Viral
  – Genetic/toxic
  – Immune
- Hypertrophic:
  – Familial disease with autosomal dominance
- Restrictive:
  – Idiopathic
  – Amyloid
- Arrhythmogenic RV:
  – Familial disease with dominant and recessive patterns
- Specific infectious:
  – Lyme disease
  – Viral
  – Chagas disease
  – HIV
- Toxic agents:
  – Alcohol
  – Chemotherapeutic agents
- Peripartum period
- Metabolic:
  – Hyperthyroidism
  – Pheochromocytoma
  – Takotsubo (stress catecholamine)
- General systems diseases:
  – Lupus
  – Scleroderma
  – Neuromuscular diseases
  – Amyloidosis

### Pediatric Considerations
- Idiopathic
- Genetic:
  – Inborn errors of metabolism
  – Malformation syndromes
  – Neuromuscular disease
  – Familial isolated cardiomyopathy disorders

- Acquired:
  – Vitamin and/or trace mineral deficiencies
  – Electrolyte disturbances
  – Endocrine disorders
  – Toxins
  – Collagen vascular disease
  – Immunologic disease
  – Malignancy
  – Morbid obesity
  – Myocarditis
  – Pulmonary disease
  – Kawasaki disease
  – Infection
  – Radiation
  – Congenital heart disease
  – Asphyxia

 **DIAGNOSIS**

## SIGNS AND SYMPTOMS
### History
- Antecedent illness or exposure:
  – Chemotherapy
  – HIV
  – Lyme disease
  – Viral
- Underlying systemic condition:
  – Hemochromatosis
  – Sarcoidosis
  – Pregnancy
- Family history:
  – Familial sudden death
- Exertional complaints (syncope, dyspnea)
- Dizziness
- Near syncope and syncope
- Palpitations
- Sudden death
- Ventricular arrhythmias
- CHF

### Pediatric Considerations
- Irritability
- Hepatomegaly
- Generalized muscle weakness
- Acute biochemical crisis
- Hypoglycemia
- Metabolic acidosis
- Hyperammonemia
- Cyanosis
- Encephalopathy
- Dysmorphic features

### Pregnancy Considerations
See Cardiomyopathy, Peripartum.

### Physical Exam
- Vital signs
- Cardiopulmonary exam
- Abdominal organomegaly
- Edema
- Other:
  – Rash
  – Goiter
  – Systemic illness

## DIAGNOSTIC TESTS & INTERPRETATION
### Lab
- CBC
- Electrolytes, BUN, creatinine, liver function tests
- Cardiac biomarkers
- Brain (B-type) natriuretic peptide: Level > 100 pg/mL
- Serologies: Not useful in the ED

### Imaging
- CXR:
  – Dilated cardiomyopathy:
    ○ Cardiomegaly
    ○ Pulmonary congestion
    ○ Pleural effusions
  – Hypertrophic cardiomyopathy:
    ○ See Cardiomyopathy, Hypertrophic.
  – Restrictive cardiomyopathy:
    ○ Normal cardiac silhouette
    ○ Pulmonary congestion
- Emergency transthoracic 2D ECG by emergency physician:
  – Depressed LV ejection fraction
  – Excludes pericardial tamponade
- Formal transthoracic ECG:
  – Study of choice
  – Identification of underlying disease
- Nuclear scintigraphy:
  – When ECG is indeterminate
  – Determination of the thickness of the septum and free wall
  – Alternative assessment to ECG
- CT and MRI distinguish between constrictive pericarditis and restrictive cardiomyopathy.
- MR comprehensive assessment of heart failure: Assess myocardial anatomy, regional and global function, and viability. Allows assessment of perfusion and acute tissue injury (edema and necrosis), and nonischemic heart failure, fibrosis, infiltration, and iron overload can be detected.

### Diagnostic Procedures/Surgery
EKG:
- Hypertrophic cardiomyopathy:
  – Left ventricle (LV) hypertrophy
  – Q waves in leads II, III, aVF, V5, and V6 in the early teenage years (most specific)
- Dilated, Lyme, Chagas, and toxic cardiomyopathies:
  – Atrial fibrillation
  – Heart block
  – Conduction abnormalities
  – Pseudoinfarct pattern with pathologic Q waves in anterior and inferior leads without coronary artery disease

### ALERT
Takotsubo (stress cardiomyopathy) can mimic STEMI (ST elevation MI).

- Cardiac catheterization:
  – Suspicion of ischemia
  – Treatable systemic disease
- Hypertrophic cardiomyopathy:
  – Assessment of hemodynamic abnormalities
  – Endomyocardial biopsy
  – Evaluation for myocarditis or define etiology
- Cardiac CT or MRI

*Pediatric Considerations*
- Electrolytes
- pH
- Glucose
- Ammonia level
- Cardiac output
- Dysmorphic evaluation
- EKG
- ECG:
  – Genetic workup; see individual causes

## DIFFERENTIAL DIAGNOSIS
- Other causes of dyspnea:
  – Chronic obstructive pulmonary disease
  – Anemia
  – Asthma
  – Interstitial lung disease
  – Pulmonary embolism
  – Pericardial tamponade:
    ○ Valvular heart disease
  – Ischemic heart disease
  – Hypothyroidism
  – Constrictive pericarditis, commonly confused with restrictive cardiomyopathy
- Other causes of syncope:
  – Hypovolemia
  – Heat disorder
  – Hypoglycemia

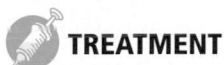 **TREATMENT**

### PRE-HOSPITAL
- Monitor
- Oxygen
- Hypertrophic cardiomyopathy, known or suspicion: Avoid or use a lower dose of nitroglycerine.
- LV heart failure:
  – Oxygen
  – Nitroglycerine spray
  – Furosemide

### INITIAL STABILIZATION/THERAPY
Airway, breathing, and circulation:
- Control airway as needed.
- Supplemental oxygen
- Continuous positive-airway pressure

### ED TREATMENT/PROCEDURES
- Anticoagulation:
  – Dilated cardiomyopathy
  – Standard treatment of atrial fibrillation
  – Systemic embolization
- Limited ED experience with agents effective in hypertrophic cardiomyopathy:
  – Disopyramide to reduce obstruction
  – Amiodarone to convert and maintain sinus rhythm
- Standard treatment of CHF
- Standard treatment of dysrhythmias

### ALERT
- Keep NPO until inborn errors of metabolism ruled out.
- IV fluids:
  – D10 should be given until defects in the protein or fatty acid metabolism pathways are ruled out.
  – IV fluids need to be given slowly to avoid rapid fluid shifts to the extravascular space.

### ALERT
Do not give any products with lactate to avoid worsening any metabolic acidosis or lactic acidemia:
- Antioxidants and vitamin cofactors
- l-Carnitine to increase mitochondrial energy metabolism
- Standard treatment of CHF
- Sodium dichloroacetate (DCA) acutely lowers acetic acid levels in patients with mitochondrial disorders.

### MEDICATION
- Amiodarone: 5 mg/kg over 10 min
- Carnitine: (peds: 50–300 mg/kg/d PO or IV)
- Digoxin: Start 0.125 mg IV
- Diltiazem IV: 0.25 mg/kg actual body weight over 2 min (average adult dose: 20 mg); repeat bolus dose (may be administered after 15 min if the response is inadequate): 0.35 mg/kg actual body weight over 2 min (average adult dose: 25 mg); continuous infusion 10 mg/hr; rate may be increased in 5 mg/hr increments up to 15 mg/hr as needed
- Disopyramide: 100–200 mg PO q6h
- Esmolol IV: Loading dose: 500 $\mu$g/kg over 1 min; follow with a 50 $\mu$g/kg/min infusion for 4 min; infusion may be continued at 50 $\mu$g/kg/min or, if the response is inadequate, titrated upward in 50 $\mu$g/kg/min increments (increased no more frequently than q4min) to a maximum of 200 $\mu$g/kg/min
- Furosemide: 20–40 mg IV to a maximum of 200 mg on subsequent doses (peds: 1 mg/kg IV q12–24h)
- Heparin: Load 80 IU/kg IV; then 18 IU/kg/hr
- Metoprolol IV: 2.5–5 mg q2–5min (maximum total dose: 15 mg over a 10–15-min period)
- Milrinone: Bolus 50 $\mu$g/kg IV over 10 min, then 0.375–0.75 $\mu$g/kg/min IV
- Nesiritide: Bolus 2 $\mu$g/kg IV, then 0.01 $\mu$g/kg/min IV with a maximum of 0.03 $\mu$g/kg/min
- Nitroglycerine: 5 $\mu$g/min IV titrate to SBP

*Geriatric Considerations*
Use caution in geriatric dosing.

 **FOLLOW-UP**

### DISPOSITION
*Admission Criteria*
- New or suspected cardiomyopathy
- Syncope in which dysrhythmias or HCM are possible etiologies
- Familial history of premature sudden death
- Cardiogenic shock

*Discharge Criteria*
- Diagnosed cardiomyopathy with mild CHF that improves with ED therapy
- Restrictive or hypertrophic cardiomyopathy
- Cardiology consultation for discharge planning

*Issues for Referral*
Patients with ejection fraction (EF) <35% may require referral for single-chamber implantable cardioverter defibrillator and resynchronization therapy with atrial-synchronized biventricular pacing.

### FOLLOW-UP RECOMMENDATIONS
- Primary care
- Cardiology
- Genetic testing may be indicated.

## PEARLS AND PITFALLS
- Diagnosing asthma without cardiac evaluation is a pitfall.
- Not obtaining a family history with syncope or cardiac complaint is a pitfall.

## ADDITIONAL READING
- Bybee KA, Prasad A. Stress-related cardiomyopathy syndromes. *Circulation*. 2008;118:397–409.
- Egan DJ, Bisanzo MC, Hutson HR. Emergency department evaluation and management of peripartum cardiomyopathy. *J Emerg Med*. 2009;36(2):141–147.
- Karamitsos TD, Francis JM, Myerson S, et al. The role of cardiovascular magnetic resonance imaging in heart failure. *J Am Coll Cardiol*. 2009;54:1407–1424.
- Nishimura RA, Holmes DR Jr. Hypertrophic obstructive cardiomyopathy. *N Engl J Med*. 2004;350:1320–1327.
- Schwartz ML, Cox GF, Lin AE, et al. Clinical approach to genetic cardiomyopathy in children. *Circulation*. 1996;94:2021–2038.

### See Also (Topic, Algorithm, Electronic Media Element)
- Cardiomyopathy, Hypertrophic
- Cardiomyopathy, Peripartum

 **CODES**

### ICD9
- 425.4 Other primary cardiomyopathies
- 425.5 Alcoholic cardiomyopathy
- 425.7 Nutritional and metabolic cardiomyopathy

# CARDIOMYOPATHY, HYPERTROPHIC

L. Kristian Arnold

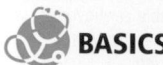 **BASICS**

## DESCRIPTION
- Hypertrophic cardiomyopathy (HCM):
  - Hypertrophied (regionally or globally), nondilated left ventricle (LV) in the absence of another cause of LV hypertrophy, such as hypertension or aortic stenosis
  - 2 general types:
    - Nonobstructive (HCM)—75% of patients. Estimated around 1% annual mortality.
    - Obstructive (HOCM)—25% of patients. More severe—Estimated 2% annual mortality—Includes older diagnosis of subaortic outflow track obstruction known as idiopathic hypertrophic subaortic stenosis, originally described in 1950s.
  - Now defined as primarily a genetic disorder affecting the sarcomere:
    - Many phenotypic variations
  - Predominant abnormality identified (1/3 of cases) in young (<35 yr old) athletes suffering sudden atraumatic death
  - Manifests in all ages, from neonate to elderly:
    - Average age of diagnosis is 30–40 yr old.
    - Usually more severe when diagnosed at younger age
    - Adolescence most common onset of hypertrophy
- Structural pathology:
  - Irregular, marked ventricular wall thickening with disarray of myofibrils in the thickened regions and fibrin deposition:
    - Affects higher pressure LV more than right and, in obstructive form, if obstruction removed, hypertrophy decreases.
    - Some evidence of progressive wall thinning with age associated with decreased death from arrhythmia
    - Some phenotypes with later age onset
  - Thickening usually asymmetric involving the septum to a greater extent than the free ventricular wall
  - Atrial dilatation secondary to diastolic filling stiffness

## RISK FACTORS
### Genetics
- 1st cardiac disorder for which genetic basis identified
- Autosomal-dominant inheritance:
  - >10 associated genes found:
    - Most encode proteins for sarcomere
    - >700 distinct mutations recognized
  - Variable penetrance
  - Variable phenotypic expression
  - Some genotypes significantly more lethal:
    - Routine screening impractical at present
    - Increasing complexity with more understanding of interplay between primary sarcomere abnormalities and other genetic and nongenetic factors
    - Some mutations affect cell wall pumps—thus, association with dysrhythmias.

- Prevalence ~1 in 500 general population:
  - Based on echocardiographic diagnosis

## ETIOLOGY
See "Genetics."

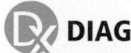 **DIAGNOSIS**

## SIGNS AND SYMPTOMS
### History
- Obstructive symptoms correlate with exertion, Valsalva maneuver, or suddenly assuming upright position—all activities that decrease venous return or ventricular filling.
  - Severity depends on the location and degree of ventricular wall thickening.
- Shortness of breath
- Dyspnea on exertion
- Exertional or postprandial angina
- Presyncope
- Syncope
- CHF
- Cardiovascular collapse
- Dysrhythmias:
  - Paroxysmal atrial fibrillation:
    - Often leads to significant, rapid clinical deterioration when present with CHF
  - Supraventricular tachycardia
  - Nonsustained ventricular tachycardia (VT) occurs in young adults.
  - Bradydysrhythmia less common
  - VT or ventricular fibrillation may lead to sudden death.
- Prior therapy for known HCM might include surgery or alcohol injection to reduce septal bulk:
  - Potential for conduction blocks
  - Potential septal rupture
- Known cases with higher risk of arrhythmia may have implanted defibrillators.

### Pediatric Considerations
Due to potential increasing severity in adolescence, any young child with syncope without clear cause, or in association with exercise, should have more extensive, focused history for familial sudden death (standard is 3 generations) and possible referral for evaluation.

### Physical Exam
- No or subtle physical findings
- Most findings in patients with outflow tract obstruction, variably:
  - Loud, left-sided S4
  - Double apical cardiac impulse at the mid to upper sternum
  - Murmur:
    - Crescendo-decrescendo midsystolic murmur at the left sternal edge
    - Radiation to aortic and mitral areas, not to neck or axilla

- Increasing in intensity with Valsalva maneuver or standing up
- Quieter with recumbency, squatting, or handgrips
- Frequent associated mitral regurgitation
  - With more severe obstruction, a more apparent murmur with radiation to the left sternal border
  - Radiation to the axilla if there is associated mitral insufficiency

## DIAGNOSTIC TESTS & INTERPRETATION
ECG findings:
- Normal in 15% of patients
- ST segment and T-wave abnormalities
- LV hypertrophy with strain, with quasi-random signal (QRS) complexes that are tallest in the midprecordial leads
- Large Q waves, particularly in inferolateral leads
- Left atrial enlargement
- Short pulse rate with slurred upstroke of QRS

### Lab
- Clinical laboratory testing is of no assistance.
- Genetic testing may help in outpatient workup, but not in ED.

### Imaging
- CXR:
  - Normal
  - Bulge along left heart border representing hypertrophy of free wall of LV
  - Right or left atrial enlargement
  - Pulmonary vascular redistribution
- Transthoracic cardiac echo/Doppler:
  - Establishes the diagnosis of HCM (standard >15-mm wall thickness in adults)
  - Demonstrates systolic outflow obstructions and diastolic filling abnormalities
- Nuclear MRI supplements indeterminate echocardiography and is a better definition of patchy hypertrophy.
- Stress thallium and PET evaluate ischemia.

### Diagnostic Procedures/Surgery
No ED-based procedures are of diagnostic utility.

## DIFFERENTIAL DIAGNOSIS
- Vagal and other causes of syncope and presyncope (if HCM is considered, it must be ruled out because it is much more likely to be fatal with repeat episodes)
- Aortic stenosis
- Pulmonic stenosis
- Ventricular septal defect
- Mitral regurgitation
- Mitral valve prolapse
- Arteriosclerotic coronary vascular disease
- Differentiate in patients presenting with CHF or angina:
  - More ominous in the setting of HCM

**TREATMENT**

### ALERT
Consider HCM in patients who decompensate during standard treatments for CHF, ischemia, or supraventricular tachycardia, and in young athletes who collapse during or just after exertion.

### INITIAL STABILIZATION/THERAPY
- ABCs
- IV catheterization
- Supplemental oxygen
- Cardiac monitor
- Pulse oximetry

### ED TREATMENT/PROCEDURES
- Depends on type of presentation: Dysrhythmia, cardiac failure, or ischemia
- Underlying principle to understand sensitivity to any situation that may impair cardiac filling:
  - Do *not* place in seated or Fowler position.
- Patient may need to remain supine.
- Standard CHF or anginal vasodilator therapy may lead to cardiovascular collapse; if this occurs, treat with fluid bolus.
- Attention to any hypovolemia as small degree may significantly impair cardiac output.
- Control HRT and improve diastolic filling (underlying principle in treating HCM-associated CHF and angina):
  - β-Blockers:
    - Mainstay of therapy
    - Decrease dysrhythmias and lower elevation of pressure gradient across the LV outflow tract
  - Calcium channel blockers:
    - Verapamil reduces obstruction by decreasing contractility and improving diastolic relaxation and filling.
    - Nifedipine relatively contraindicated due to vasodilatation
- Dysrhythmia management:
  - β-Blockers and calcium channel blockers 1st line for supraventricular dysrhythmias
  - Amiodarone:
    - Drug of choice for ventricular dysrhythmias
    - Used when β-blockers and calcium channel blockers fail
  - Disopyramide:
    - Effective for supraventricular and ventricular dysrhythmias
  - Electrical cardioversion:
    - Use early in HCM with new atrial fibrillation and CHF

### MEDICATION
- Most emergency presentations associated with this disorder requiring any ED treatment other than frank resuscitation are likely to be either tachydysrhythmias requiring or warranting electrical therapy or CHF.
- Amiodarone: 150 mg over 10 min, then 360 mg over 6 hr, then 540 mg over next 18 hr (peds: 5 mg/kg IV over 1 hr in 1 mg/kg bolus aliquots, off-label use per manufacturer, but class IIb for VT with a pulse and class indeterminate for VF and pulseless VT, per American Heart Association. Do not use in infants.)
- Diltiazem: 0.25 mg/kg (peds: Contraindicated <12 yr old) IV over 2 min; may repeat in 15 min at 0.35 mg/kg
- Propranolol: 1–3 mg (peds: 0.01–0.1 mg/kg slow IV push over 10 min; not to exceed dose 1 mg/dose) slow IV bolus
- Verapamil: 2.5 mg (peds: >1 yr: 0.1–0.2 mg/kg/dose over 2 min; repeat q10–30min as needed; not to exceed 5 mg/dose [1st dose] or 10 mg/dose [2nd dose]) IV bolus over 1–2 min, may repeat as 5.0 mg in 15–30 min

*First Line*
N/A

*Second Line*
N/A

 **FOLLOW-UP**

### DISPOSITION
*Admission Criteria*
- Consider for unexplained syncope, especially in younger adults.
- Telemetry admission for dysrhythmia
- ICU admission:
  - Syncopal episodes
  - CHF
  - Angina
  - Hemodynamically significant tachydysrhythmia

*Discharge Criteria*
When increased myocardial wall thickness is an incidental finding during the ED evaluation for another presentation with:
- No history of familial sudden death (proposed guidance—3 generations to rule out in face of suspicion) or personal history of syncope
- Need urgent follow-up with a cardiologist
- Counsel against any activities that may decrease diastolic filling pending follow-up.

*Issues for Referral*
See "Discharge Criteria."

### FOLLOW-UP RECOMMENDATIONS
See "Discharge Criteria."

## PEARLS AND PITFALLS

Increasing awareness of genetic and phenotypic variants with implications in definition of "normal variant":
- Some authors advocate cardiac ECHO screening for any youth participation in sports.

## ADDITIONAL READING

- Bos JM, Ommen SR, Ackerman MJ. Genetics of hypertrophic cardiomyopathy: One, two, or more diseases? *Curr Opin Cardiol*. 2007;22(3):193–199.
- Elliott P, McKenna WJ. Hypertrophic cardiomyopathy. *Lancet*. 2004;363(9424): 1881–1891.
- Maron BJ, McKenna WJ, Danielson GK, et al. American College of Cardiology/European European Society of Cardiology clinical expert consensus document on hypertrophic cardiomyopathy: A report of the American College of Cardiology Foundation Task Force on Clinical Expert Consensus Documents and the European of Cardiology Committee for Practice Guidelines. *J Am Coll Cardiol*. 2003;42(9): 1687–1713.
- Maron BJ, Seidman JG, Seidman CE. Proposal for contemporary screening strategies in families with hypertrophic cardiomyopathy. *J Am Coll Cardiol*. 2004;44(11):2125–2132.
- Roberts R, Sigwart U. Current concepts of the pathogenesis and treatment of hypertrophic cardiomyopathy. *Circulation* 2005;112(2); 293–296.
- Spirito P, Autore C. Management of hypertrophic cardiomyopathy. *BMJ*. 2006;332(7552): 1251–1255.

## CODES

ICD9
- 425.1 Hypertrophic obstructive cardiomyopathy
- 425.4 Other primary cardiomyopathies

**C**

# CARDIOMYOPATHY, PERIPARTUM
David W. Callaway

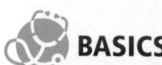 **BASICS**

## DESCRIPTION
- Cardiomyopathy occurring during the last month of pregnancy up to 5 mo following the delivery
- Diagnostic criteria (all required):
  - Onset of myocardial failure during last month of pregnancy or 1st 5 mo after delivery
  - Absence of a specific cause
  - Absence of prior cardiac disease
- Classified as a form of dilated cardiomyopathy
- Incidence: 1 in 3,000–15,000 live births
- ~50% of cases resolve spontaneously
- Mortality: 18–56%
- Risk factors:
  - Older women (>30 yr)
  - Multiparous women
  - Twin births
  - Prolonged tocolytic therapy
  - Obesity
  - Preeclampsia
  - African or Haitian origin
- Systemic and pulmonary embolism more frequent than with other forms of cardiomyopathy
- Factors indicating a poor prognosis:
  - Lower left ejection fraction at 6 mo postpartum
  - Onset >2 wk postpartum
  - Age >30 yr
  - African American descent
  - Multiparity

## ETIOLOGY
Various causes are suggested but remain unproved:
- Viral infection leading to myocarditis in presence of immunosuppression during pregnancy
- Immunologic response to an unknown maternal or fetal antigen
- Maladaptive response to the hemodynamic stresses of pregnancy
- Stress-activated cytokines
- Prolonged tocolysis
- Selenium deficiency

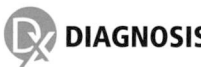 **DIAGNOSIS**

## SIGNS AND SYMPTOMS
- Dyspnea
- Chest pain
- Orthopnea
- Cough
- Paroxysmal nocturnal dyspnea
- Anorexia
- Fatigue

## History
- Onset and duration of symptoms
- Unexplained persistent cough
- Excessive weight gain:
  - ->2–4 lb/wk
- Prior cardiac disease
- Prior pregnancies and complications

## Physical Exam
- Palpitations
- Jugular venous distention
- Gallop rhythm
- Mitral regurgitation murmur
- Loud P2
- Pulmonary rales
- Peripheral edema (especially rapid onset)
- Hepatomegaly
- Hepatojugular reflux

## ESSENTIAL WORKUP
- CXR views:
  - Pulmonary venous congestion
  - Cardiomegaly
- EKG:
  - Nonspecific
  - Left ventricular hypertrophy
  - Left atrial enlargement
  - T-wave flattening or inversion
  - Arrhythmias
  - Ventricular ectopy (40%)
  - Atrial fibrillation (20%)

## DIAGNOSTIC TESTS & INTERPRETATION
### Lab
- Electrolytes:
  - Generally normal
- BUN, creatinine
- CBC:
  - Mild postpartum anemia may contribute to fatigue and dyspnea.
- Creatine kinase with muscle and brain fraction
- $\beta$-Natriuretic peptide (BNP):
  - Useful for distinguishing between heart failure due to diastolic and/or systolic dysfunction and a pulmonary cause of dyspnea
  - BNP >100 pg/mL diagnosed heart failure with a sensitivity of 90%, a specificity of 76%, and a predictive accuracy of 83%. BNP of ≤50 pg/mL has a high negative predictive value.

## Imaging
- CXR:
  - Cardiomegaly
  - Effusions (usually right-sided)
  - 3 phases of pulmonary findings:
    - Stage I: Pulmonary redistribution to upper lung fields (cephalization)
    - Stage II: Interstitial edema with Kerley B lines
    - Stage III: Alveolar edema
    - Bilateral confluent perihilar infiltrates leading to classic butterfly pattern
    - May be asymmetric and mistaken for pneumonia
- Echo:
  - Demonstrates chamber enlargement and decreased ejection fraction
  - Criteria for the diagnosis were established by Hibbard et al.:
    - Ejection fraction <45% or M-mode fractional shortening of <30%
    - End-diastolic dimension >2.72 cm/m$^2$
  - Exclude valvular pathology and cardiac tamponade.

## Diagnostic Procedures/Surgery
Endomyocardial biopsy:
- Indicated to assess for myocarditis and steroid therapy

## DIFFERENTIAL DIAGNOSIS
- Other causes of dilated cardiomyopathy:
  - Ischemia
  - Infarction
  - Valvular rupture or disease
  - Chronic HTN
  - Familial
  - Toxins:
    - Ethanol, anthracyclines, cocaine, drug allergy
  - Metabolic:
    - Thiamine
    - Selenium
    - Hypothyroidism
    - Thyrotoxicosis
    - Hypophosphatemia
  - Infectious:
    - Viral
    - Parasitic or rickettsial
    - Bacterial
    - Fungal
  - Systemic disorders:
    - Sarcoidosis
    - Scleroderma
    - Systemic lupus erythematosus
  - Eosinophilic myocarditis
  - Neuromuscular dystrophies
  - Mitochondrial cardiomyopathies

- Other causes of shortness of breath or edema:
  - Pulmonary embolism
  - Pneumonia
  - Asthma
  - Cardiac ischemia
  - Anemia
  - Hyperthyroidism
  - Constrictive pericarditis
  - Pericardial tamponade
  - Nephrotic syndrome
  - Cirrhosis

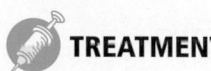 **TREATMENT**

### PRE-HOSPITAL
Differentiate pulmonary edema from acute reactive airway disease.

### INITIAL STABILIZATION/THERAPY
ABCs:
- Prompt evaluation of respiratory and hemodynamic status
- Control airway as needed.
- Supplemental oxygen
- Continuous positive airway pressure, as needed

### ED TREATMENT/PROCEDURES
- Prepartum therapy:
  - Amlodipine: A dihydropyridine calcium-channel blocker that has been shown to improve survival in nonischemic cardiomyopathy patients
  - Nitrates
  - Hydralazine
  - IV furosemide
  - Digoxin to control rate due to atrial fibrillation
- Postpartum therapy:
  - Consider adding ACE inhibitors (enalapril) or ARBs
  - Anticoagulation therapy often recommended:
    ○ 30% of cases complicated by systemic or pulmonary embolism
    ○ During pregnancy, use subcutaneous or IV heparin rather than warfarin, which causes birth defects.

- For severe symptoms or lack of response to standard therapy:
  - Dobutamine
  - Dopamine
  - Nitroprusside
  - Immunosuppressive therapy:
    ○ Advocated for patients who fail to improve within 2 wk of standard medical therapy
    ○ Prednisone with cyclosporine or azathioprine
    ○ Immunoglobulin therapy
    ○ Remains controversial

### MEDICATION
- Amlodipine: 2.5–10 mg/d PO
- Bumetanide: 0.5–2.0 mg IV
- Digoxin: 1 mg IV load over 1 day; 0.125–0.375 mg/d PO
- Milrinone: 50 $\mu$g/kg over 10 min
- Dobutamine: 2–10 $\mu$g/kg/min IV
- Dopamine: 2–20 $\mu$g/kg/min IV
- Enalapril: 0.625–1.25 mg IV; 2.5–20 mg/d PO
- Furosemide: 20–100 mg IV
- Metoprolol: 12.5 mg PO b.i.d.
- Morphine sulfate: 2–4 mg IV q5min
- Nitroglycerin: 0.4 mg sublingual; 1–2 inch of nitroglycerine paste; 5–20 $\mu$g per min IV, maximum of 100–200 $\mu$g/min IV
- Nitroprusside: 0.5–10 $\mu$g/kg/min IV

 **FOLLOW-UP**

### DISPOSITION
#### Admission Criteria
- Patients with pulmonary edema, cardiogenic shock, or evidence of ischemia should be admitted to ICU.
- All symptomatic patients with new onset of peripartum cardiomyopathy should be admitted.

#### Discharge Criteria
- Mild left ventricular dysfunction
- Established history of peripartum cardiomyopathy:
  - Mild fluid overload attributable to excessive salt intake
  - Complete resolution of symptoms following ED treatment
  - No evidence of cardiac ischemia
- Close follow-up arranged

*Issues for Referral*
Close follow-up with a cardiologist

### FOLLOW-UP RECOMMENDATIONS
- Drink 6–8 glasses of liquid each day.
- Avoid alcohol because it may worsen cardiomyopathy.
- Support socks may help decrease the swelling in legs and prevent clot formation.
- Daily weights:
  - Weight gain can be a sign of extra fluid in the body.
  - Call doctor if gain of >2 pounds in a day.
- Return for shortness of breath, feeling faint, palpitations.

## PEARLS AND PITFALLS

- Remember high rates of thromboembolism in pregnancy and peripartum cardiomyopathy.
- Utilize multidisciplinary approach with cardiology and obstetrics consultations.

## ADDITIONAL READING

- Brown CS. Peripartum cardiomyopathy: A comprehensive review. *Am J Obstet Gynecol*. 1998;178:409–414.
- Hibbard JU, Lindheimer M, Lang RM. A modified definition for peripartum cardiomyopathy and prognosis based on echocardiography. *Obstet Gynecol*. 1999;94(2):311–316.
- Murali S, Baldisseri MR. Peripartum cardiomyopathy. *Crit Care Med*. 2005;33:S340–S346.
- Pearson GD, Veille JC, Rahimtoola S, et al. Peripartum cardiomyopathy: National Heart, Lung, and Blood Institute and Office of Rare Diseases (National Institutes of Health) workshop recommendations and review. *JAMA*. 2000;283:1183–1188.
- Radhakrishnan R, Sorrell V. Peripartum cardiomyopathy: Causes, diagnosis, and treatment. *Clev Clin J. Med*. 2009;76(5):289–296.

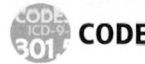 **CODES**

### ICD9
674.50 Peripartum cardiomyopathy, unspecified as to episode of care or not applicable

# CARPAL FRACTURES

Peter J. Chen
Wallace A. Carter

 **BASICS**

## DESCRIPTION
- Most commonly fractured carpals are the scaphoid (68%) and triquetrum (18%).
- Carpal bone fractures commonly occur with other wrist injuries:
  - Capitate fractures along with scaphoid (scaphocapitate syndrome) sometimes occur with perilunate dislocations.
  - Hamate fractures associated with injuries to 4th and 5th CMC and metacarpals

## ETIOLOGY
- Fall on outstretched hand (FOOSH) with a hyperextended wrist
- Direct blow
- Axial loading
- Chronic use injury

 **DIAGNOSIS**

## SIGNS AND SYMPTOMS
### History
- FOOSH or direct blow
- Hook of Hamate fractures:
  - Associated with a forceful swing of a racquet or club

### Physical Exam
- Pain, swelling, decreased range of motion
- Individual palpation of each carpal bone is possible with correct positioning of wrist.
- Scaphoid fractures:
  - Snuffbox tenderness is sensitive but not very specific.
  - Specificity improved with pronation and ulnar deviation of wrist
  - Scaphoid compression test (axial loading thumb causes pain) is also not very specific.
  - Tenderness of tubercle on palmar aspect at distal wrist crease with wrist in extension
  - More specific than snuffbox tenderness

## ESSENTIAL WORKUP
- A complete physical exam of the entire upper extremity and shoulder girdle:
  - Evaluate for associated injuries.
- Neurovascular exam is essential.
- Hamate fractures may be associated with ulnar nerve or artery injuries.

## DIAGNOSTIC TESTS & INTERPRETATION
### Imaging
- Anterior-posterior, lateral, oblique views of the hand and wrist
- Special views (eg, scaphoid views) may be obtained for most of the carpals if physical exam is suspicious.
- CT scan has superior sensitivity for fractures.
- MRI can diagnose ligamentous injuries.

## DIFFERENTIAL DIAGNOSIS
- Metacarpal base fractures
- Distal radius or ulna fractures
- Lunate or perilunate dislocations

### Pediatric Considerations
Be wary of epiphyseal injuries of the distal radius: Children rarely get simple sprains or fractures of the wrist.

 **TREATMENT**

## PRE-HOSPITAL
- Prevent contamination of any lacerations overlying the area.
- Patients with swelling or significant pain at the wrist or hand:
  - Elevate extremity and apply ice.
  - Remove jewelry, watches.
  - Immobilize extremity with padded board splints to reduce further injury.

## INITIAL STABILIZATION/THERAPY
As in any trauma, assess for other more serious injuries.

## ED TREATMENT/PROCEDURES
- Isolated carpal bone fractures can be initially managed with splinting.
- Thumb spica:
  - Scaphoid and trapezium fractures
  - Wrist held in slight extension
- Sugar tong splint:
  - Capitate and lunate fractures
  - Extends from MCP joint on dorsal side of hand, wrapping around the elbow, ending at midpalmar crease
  - Wrist neutral
- Volar splint:
  - Triquetrum, pisiform, trapezoid, hamate fractures
  - Extends from midpalmar crease to below the elbow
  - Wrist in slight extension
  - Splint suspected fractures (especially scaphoid) based on physical exam despite negative radiographs.

- Open carpal fractures:
  - Requires high-pressure irrigation
  - Parenteral antibiotics against *Staphylococcus aureus,* with gram-negative coverage in Grade III (involving significant soft tissue damage) open fractures
  - Tetanus prophylaxis
  - Immediate orthopedic consultation

## MEDICATION

- Mild oral analgesics, oral narcotics, NSAIDs for patient comfort
- Proper splinting will relieve most of the pain for these injuries.

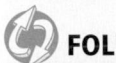

## FOLLOW-UP

### DISPOSITION

#### Admission Criteria

- Open fractures are admitted for early operative irrigation and debridement.
- Patients with injuries requiring surgical management (open reduction) sometimes are admitted for early intervention.

#### Discharge Criteria

Closed, nondisplaced carpal fractures treated with adequate splinting may be discharged to have orthopedic follow-up in 7–10 days.

## FOLLOW-UP RECOMMENDATIONS

- Confirmed fractures are referred to orthopedics for definitive casting and further management.
- Missed fractures can lead to long-term complications and disability:
  - Untreated scaphoid, capitate and lunate fractures lead to high rates of nonunion and avascular necrosis.
  - Immobilize any injury with significant pain and refer for repeat radiographs in 7–10 days or more advanced imaging (CT or MRI).

## PEARLS AND PITFALLS

- Carpal fractures may not be apparent on initial radiographs and may lead to long-term disability if not treated appropriately.
- Splint all suspected fractures and refer for repeat radiographs or consider CT scanning in ED or outpatient setting.
- Most (90%) scaphoid fractures are isolated injuries:
  - All other carpal fractures are more often associated with other wrist or hand injuries.
- Adequate treatment involves splinting in position of function and referral for definitive casting and management.

## ADDITIONAL READING

- Goddard N. Carpal fractures in children. *Clin Orthop Relat Res.* 2005;432:73–76.
- Papp S. Carpal bone fractures. *Orthop Clin North Am.* 2007;38(2):251–260.
- Phillips TG, Reibach AM, Slomiany WP. Diagnosis and management of scaphoid fractures. *Am Fam Physician.* 2004;70:879–884.
- Simon R, Sherman S, Koenigsknecht S, eds. Carpal fractures. In: *Emergency orthopedics: The extremities,* 1 + ed. New York: McGraw-Hill, 2007.
- Yaghoubian R, Goebel F, Musgrave DS, et al. Diagnosis and management of acute fracture dislocation of the carpus. *Ortho Clin N Am.* 2001;3(2):295–305.

 CODES

### ICD9

- 814.00 Closed fracture of carpal bone, unspecified
- 814.10 Open fracture of carpal bone, unspecified

# CARPAL TUNNEL SYNDROME

Matthew T. Spencer
Linda L. Spillane

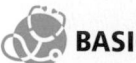 **BASICS**

## DESCRIPTION
- Carpal tunnel syndrome is caused by compression of the median nerve as it passes through the carpal tunnel.
- The carpal tunnel is the area bound by the carpal bones and the transverse carpal ligament.
- The median nerve, flexor digitorum profundus, flexor digitorum superficialis, and flexor pollicis longus are located in the carpal tunnel.
- Carpal tunnel syndrome can be classified as acute or chronic.

## ETIOLOGY
- Acute:
  - Trauma
  - Infection
  - Snakebite
  - Hemorrhage
  - High-pressure injection injury
- Chronic:
  - Occupational/overuse syndromes—high impact, repetitive motion
  - Pregnancy, birth control pills
  - Granulomatous disease: Tuberculosis, sarcoidosis
  - Mass lesions with median nerve compression
  - Osteophytes
  - Amyloid
  - Multiple myeloma
  - Rheumatoid arthritis
  - Endocrine disorders: Hypothyroidism, diabetes mellitus, acromegaly
  - Chronic hemodialysis
  - Idiopathic

### Pediatric Considerations
Idiopathic causes are rare in children; most cases have a correctable cause including:
- Trauma
- Mucolipidosis
- Hamartoma of the median nerve
- Anomalous flexor digitorum superficialis (FDS)
- Hemophilia with hematoma

## DIAGNOSIS

### SIGNS AND SYMPTOMS
*History*
- Acute or chronic onset
- Numbness/paresthesias in a median nerve distribution:
  - Thumb, index, middle, and radial aspect of ring finger
- Pain:
  - Location: Wrist or hand, sometimes radiating to elbow, forearm, or shoulder
  - Often worse at night—relieved by "shaking out" the hand
  - Exacerbated by repetitive wrist movement and by activities in which the wrist is flexed (eg, driving)

*Physical Exam*
- Weakness of the abductor pollicis brevis and opponens muscles:
  - Innervated by the recurrent branch of the median nerve
  - Patient may complain of dropping things or having decreased fine motor control.
  - Sensitivity of 29%; specificity of 80%, on average
- Loss of 2-point discrimination:
  - Late finding, highly specific
  - Sensitivity of 24%; specificity of 94%
- Atrophy of thenar muscles:
  - Late finding, highly specific
  - Sensitivity of 18%; specificity of 94%

### ESSENTIAL WORKUP
- History of characteristic nocturnal pain and paresthesias in the median nerve distribution.
- Muscle weakness and thenar wasting are later findings.
- Provocative testing:
  - Phalen test:
    - Wrist flexion for 60 sec produces numbness or tingling in the median nerve distribution.
    - Sensitivity of 68%; specificity of 73%
  - Tinel sign:
    - Gentle tapping over the median nerve at wrist produces tingling in the fingers in the median nerve distribution.
    - Sensitivity of 50%; specificity of 77%
  - Carpal compression test:
    - Direct pressure applied over the proximal carpal ligament for 30 sec produces tingling in the fingers in the median nerve distribution.
    - Sensitivity of 64%; specificity of 83%
  - Tourniquet test:
    - BP cuff inflated to just above the patient's systolic BP for 2 min produces paresthesias in the median nerve distribution.
    - Sensitivity of 59%; specificity of 61%

### DIAGNOSTIC TESTS & INTERPRETATION
*Lab*
- Not indicated in most cases
- Thyroid function studies; rheumatoid factor and immune panel if indicated by history and physical exam

*Imaging*
- Wrist radiograph if trauma or degenerative arthritis suspected
- CT in select cases (not routine):
  - May show encroachment of carpal tunnel
- MRI displays the soft tissues well but not recommended for routine diagnosis:
  - Findings: Palmar bowing of transcarpal ligament, flattened median nerve, median nerve or synovial swelling, fluid in carpal tunnel, signal abnormality of median nerve
- Ultrasound can be diagnostic:
  - Sensitivity of 44–95%; specificity of 57–100%
  - Findings: Median nerve swelling at proximal canal, median nerve flattening at distal canal, bowing of transcarpal ligament

*Diagnostic Procedures/Surgery*

Nerve conduction studies and electromyography are criterion standard tests.

## DIFFERENTIAL DIAGNOSIS

- Cervical nerve root compression:
  - Origin of median nerve is at the 6th and 7th cervical roots.
  - Symptoms are aggravated by erect posture and neck movement.
- Hand–arm vibration syndrome:
  - Characterized by Raynaud, numbness and tingling in ulnar and median nerve distributions when exposed to cold or vibration, weakened grip, and upper extremity myalgias
  - Associated with prolonged exposure to vibration
- Thoracic outlet obstruction
- Osteoarthritis of the 1st carpometacarpal joint
- Brachial plexitis
- Generalized neuropathy
- Syringomyelia

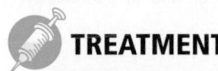 **TREATMENT**

### INITIAL STABILIZATION/THERAPY

None necessary

### ED TREATMENT/PROCEDURES

- Acute:
  - Hand surgery consultation for surgical release of transverse carpal ligament using either open or endoscopic technique
- Chronic:
  - Splint wrist in neutral position (0 degrees)
  - Aspirin or NSAIDs
  - Local corticosteroid injection
  - Avoidance of repetitive wrist movement
  - Wrist splint to be worn at night until follow-up
  - Referral to occupational medicine for ergometric testing if caused by repetitive motion, and tendon gliding or nerve gliding exercises
  - May need referral to a hand surgeon for consideration of surgical release of transverse carpal ligament using either open or endoscopic technique

## MEDICATION

- NSAIDs (there are many choices; a few are listed below):
  - Ibuprofen: 600 mg (peds: 5–10 mg/kg per dose) PO q8h
  - Naproxen: 250–500 mg (peds: 5–7 mg/kg/dose) PO q12h
  - Ketorolac: 30 mg IV or IM (peds: 0.5 mg/kg per dose) q6h or 10 mg PO q6h (peds: not approved for oral use in patients <17 yr of age)
- Local corticosteroid—transient relief in 2/3 of patients (many different regimens):
  - Hydrocortisone: 20 mg Methylprednisolone: 15–40 mg
  - Triamcinolone: 20 mg
  - Usually combined with 0.15–0.5 mL 2% lidocaine

 **FOLLOW-UP**

### DISPOSITION

*Admission Criteria*

Acute carpal tunnel syndrome requiring surgical decompression

*Discharge Criteria*

Chronic carpal tunnel syndrome after adequate pain control

### FOLLOW-UP RECOMMENDATIONS

Primary care physician or directly to a specialist in occupational medicine or hand surgery within 1–2 wk

## ADDITIONAL READING

- Boyer MI. Corticosteroid injection for carpal tunnel syndrome. *J Hand Surg Am.* 2008;33(8): 1414–1416.
- Cranford CS, Ho JY, Kalainov DM, et al. Carpal tunnel syndrome. *J Am Acad Orthop Surg.* 2007;15(9)L537–L548.
- Keith MW, Masear V, Chung K, et al. Diagnosis of carpal tunnel syndrome. *J Am Acad Orthop Surg.* 2009;17(6):389–396.
- Keith MW, Masear V, Chung K, et al. Treatment of carpal tunnel syndrome. *J Am Acad Orthop Surg.* 2009;17(6):397–405.
- MacDermid JC, Wessel J. Clinical diagnosis of carpal tunnel syndrome: A systematic review. *J Hand Ther.* 2004;17(2):309–319.
- Schnetzler KA. Acute carpal tunnel syndrome. *J Am Acad Orthop Surg.* 2008;16(5):276–282.
- Seror P. Sonography and electrodiagnosis in carpal tunnel syndrome diagnosis, an analysis of the literature. *Eur J Radiol.* 2008;67(1):146–152.

 **CODES**

### ICD9

354.0 Carpal tunnel syndrome

# CAUDA EQUINA SYNDROME

*Daniel Morris*
*Kyan J. Berger*

 **BASICS**

## DESCRIPTION
Compression of lumbar and sacral nerve fibers in cauda equina region:
- Nerve fibers below conus medullaris
- Fibers end at L1–L2 interspace.

## RISK FACTORS
- Neoplasm
- IV drug use
- Immunocompromised state

## ETIOLOGY
- Herniated disc most common:
  - L4–L5 discs > L5–S1 > L3–L4
  - Most common in 4th and 5th decades of life
- Mass effect from:
  - Myeloma, lymphoma, sarcoma, meningioma, neurofibroma, hematoma
  - Spine metastases (breast, lung, prostate, thyroid, renal)
  - Epidural abscess (especially in IV drug users)
- Blunt trauma
- Penetrating trauma
- Spinal anesthesia

**DIAGNOSIS**

## SIGNS AND SYMPTOMS
### History
- Low back pain
- Sciatica/radicular pain (unilateral or bilateral)
- Lower extremity numbness or weakness
- Difficulty ambulating owing to weakness or pain
- Bladder or rectal dysfunction:
  - Retention or incontinence

### Physical Exam
- Lumbosacral tenderness
- Lower extremity sensory or motor deficits:
  - May be asymmetric
- Decreased foot dorsiflexion strength
- Decreased quadriceps strength
- Decreased deep tendon reflexes
- Saddle hypalgesia or anesthesia
- Decreased anal sphincter tone

## ESSENTIAL WORKUP
- Neurologic exam most essential:
  - Straight-leg raise
  - Lasègue sign:
    - With patient supine, flex hip and dorsiflex foot.
    - Pain or spasm in posterior thigh indicates nerve irritation.
  - Perineal sensation
  - Rectal tone
  - Anal wink: Reflex contraction of external anal sphincter with gentle stroking of skin lateral to anus

- Postvoid residual volume:
  - Estimate by bladder catheterization or using US.
  - >50–100 mL is considered abnormal.
  - Residual increases with age.
  - Diagnosis unlikely if normal

## DIAGNOSTIC TESTS & INTERPRETATION
### Lab
- Based on differential diagnoses
- CBC, urinalysis, ESR, and C reactive protein (CRP)

### Imaging
- Radiographs of lumbosacral (LS) spine
- MRI of spine is definitive study.
- CT myelogram if MRI unavailable

## DIFFERENTIAL DIAGNOSIS
- Osteoarthritis, LS strain, sciatica
- Vertebral fracture (pathologic and nonpathologic)
- Osteomyelitis
- Spinal epidural abscess
- Conus medullaris or higher cord compression
- Ankylosing spondylitis, spinal stenosis
- Abdominal aortic aneurysm dissection
- Vascular claudication
- Hip pathology
- Acute transverse myelitis

C

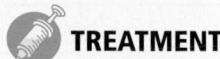 **TREATMENT**

**PRE-HOSPITAL**
- Manage airway and traumatic injuries as indicated.
- If evidence of trauma, patient should be transported with full spine immobilization.

**ALERT**
Even in nontrauma patient, consider spinal immobilization given possibility of unstable lesion.

**INITIAL STABILIZATION/THERAPY**
- Spine immobilization if trauma or unstable spine lesion suspected
- Analgesia
- NPO until evaluated by neurosurgery

**ED TREATMENT/PROCEDURES**
- Repeat neurologic exams to detect progression.
- For acute spinal cord trauma (<8 hr), begin high-dose methylprednisolone protocol.
- Immediate neurosurgical consultation in all cases
- Initiate antibiotics for epidural abscess in consultation with neurosurgery.
- Controversy exists regarding urgency of decompression:
  - Recommendations range from within 6 hr of onset to within 24 hr.

**MEDICATION**
- Methylprednisolone (high-dose steroid protocol): 30 mg/kg IV bolus, then 5.4 mg/kg/h infusion over next 23 hr
- Morphine sulfate: 2–4 mg (peds: 0.1 mg/kg per dose q5min PRN; max. 15 mg) IV/SC q5min PRN
- Ondansetron: 4–8 mg (peds: 0.15 mg/kg [up to 4 mg] IV q8h PRN nausea)
- Promethazine HCl: Adult: 25–50 mg IV q4h

 **FOLLOW-UP**

**DISPOSITION**
*Admission Criteria*
- All patients with acute cauda equina syndrome must be admitted to neurosurgical service.
- Patients have good prognosis with rapid surgical decompression.
- Treatment should not be delayed.
- Patients presenting late (>48 hr) also benefit from surgical decompression.

*Discharge Criteria*
Patients with established cauda equina syndrome with prior complete evaluation and no new neurologic deficits may be discharged with close follow-up with their neurosurgeon.

**PEARLS AND PITFALLS**

Ideally, diagnose patients in early phase before irreversible neurologic dysfunction:
- Back pain out of proportion
- Fever and back pain
- Back pain in high-risk groups; screen with ESR/CRP when infection suspected

**ADDITIONAL READING**

- Della-Giustina DA. Emergency department evaluation and treatment of back pain. *Emerg Med Clin North Am.* 1999;*27*:877–893.
- Fraser S, Roberts L, Murphy E. Cauda equina syndrome: A literature review of its definition and clinical presentation. *Arch Phys Med Rehabil.* 2009;90(11):1964–1968.
- Hussain SA, Gullan RW, Chitnavis BP. Cauda equina syndrome: Outcome and implications for management. *Br J Neurosurg.* 2003;17(2):164–167.
- Miller DW, et al. General methods of clinical exam. In: Youmans JR, et al., eds. *Neurological surgery,* 4th ed. Philadelphia: WB Saunders; 1996:40.
- Shapiro S. Medical realities of cauda equina syndrome secondary to lumbar disc herniation. *Spine.* 2000;25(3):348–352.

 **CODES**

**ICD9**
- 344.60 Cauda equina syndrome without mention of neurogenic bladder
- 344.61 Cauda equina syndrome with neurogenic bladder

# CAUSTIC INGESTION
*Paul Kolecki*

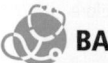 **BASICS**

## DESCRIPTION
- Alkalis:
  - Dissociate in the presence of $H_2O$ to produce hydroxy ($OH^-$) ions, which leads to liquefaction necrosis
  - Postingestion—mainly damages the esophagus:
    ○ Gastric damage can occur (see "Acids").
  - Esophageal damage (in the order of increasing damage) consists of:
    ○ Superficial hyperemia
    ○ Mucosal edema
    ○ Superficial blisters
    ○ Exudative ulcerations
    ○ Full-thickness necrosis
    ○ Perforation
    ○ Fibrosis with resulting esophageal strictures
  - Do *not* directly produce systemic complications.
- Acids:
  - Dissociate in the presence of $H_2O$ to produce hydrogen ($H^+$) ions, which leads to a coagulation necrosis with eschar formation
  - Postingestion—damages the stomach because of rapid transit time through esophagus:
    ○ Esophageal damage can occur (see "Alkalis").
  - Gastric damage (in the order of increasing damage) consists of:
    ○ Edema
    ○ Inflammation
    ○ Immediate or delayed hemorrhage
    ○ Full-thickness necrosis
    ○ Perforation
    ○ Fibrosis with resulting gastric outlet obstruction
  - Well-absorbed and can cause hemolysis of RBCs and a systemic metabolic acidosis

## ETIOLOGY
- Direct chemical injuries
- Injuries occur secondary to acid and alkali exposures.
- Many caustic agents (acids and alkalis) are found in common household and industrial products.
- Caustic substances:
  - Ammonia hydroxide
- Glass cleaners:
  - Formaldehyde:
    ○ Embalming agent
  - Hydrochloric acid:
    ○ Toilet bowel cleaners
  - Hydrofluoric acid:
    ○ Glass etching industry
    ○ Microchip industry
    ○ Rust removers

- Iodine:
  ○ Antiseptics
- Phenol:
  ○ Antiseptics
- Sodium hydroxide:
  ○ Drain cleaners
  ○ Drain openers
  ○ Oven cleaners
- Sodium borates, carbonates, phosphates, and silicates:
  ○ Detergents
  ○ Dishwasher preparations
  ○ Sodium hypochlorite
  ○ Bleaches
- Sulfuric acid:
  ○ Car batteries

 **DIAGNOSIS**

## SIGNS AND SYMPTOMS
- Oropharyngeal:
  - Pain
  - Erythema
  - Burns
  - Erosions
  - Ulcers
  - Drooling
  - Hoarseness
  - Stridor
  - Aphonia
  - Absence of visible lesions in the oropharynx does not exclude visceral injuries.
- Pulmonary:
  - Tachypnea
  - Cough
  - Pneumonitis if aspirated
- GI:
  - Pain
  - Emesis or hematemesis
  - Melena, dysphagia
  - Odynophagia
  - Esophageal or gastric perforation
  - Peritonitis owing to perforation
- Cardiovascular:
  - Tachycardia
  - Hypotension
  - Orthostatic changes
- Hematologic:
  - Acid ingestion can cause RBC hemolysis.
- Dermatologic:
  - Pain
  - Erythema
  - 1st-, 2nd-, or 3rd-degree burns

- Ocular:
  - Pain
  - Erythema
  - Injection
  - Corneal burns
  - Full-thickness corneal damage
- Metabolic:
  - Metabolic acidosis

## ESSENTIAL WORKUP
- History of or signs and symptoms of an exposure
- Absence of oropharyngeal lesions does *not* exclude visceral injury.

## DIAGNOSTIC TESTS & INTERPRETATION
### Lab
- CBC
- Electrolytes, BUN, creatinine, glucose
- Arterial blood gas
- Blood cultures:
  - If mediastinitis or peritonitis suspected
- Type and cross-match

### Imaging
Chest and abdominal radiographs for:
- Esophageal or gastric perforation

### Diagnostic Procedures/Surgery
- Esophageal and gastric endoscopy:
  - For symptomatic patients to determine the extent of injury
  - Perform within the 1st 12–24 hr after ingestion.
  - Not recommended in the presence of respiratory distress without proper airway management
  - Not recommended in the presence of severe pharyngeal damage
- Radiographic oral contrast imaging not recommended acutely:
  - May be used in follow-up for assessment for strictures

## DIFFERENTIAL DIAGNOSIS
- Chemical injuries from corrosives, acids, alkalis, desiccants, vesicants, and oxidizing and reducing agents
- Foreign body ingestion
- Upper airway infection or angioedema

**TREATMENT**

## PRE-HOSPITAL
- For oral burns or symptoms: Rinse mouth liberally with water or milk.
- Water or milk can be given to following patients:
  - Able to drink
  - Not complaining of significant abdominal pain
  - Do not have airway compromise or vomiting
- Copious irrigation for ocular or dermal exposure

## INITIAL STABILIZATION/THERAPY
- ABCs:
  - Prophylactic intubation if there is any evidence of respiratory compromise
  - Blind nasotracheal intubation contraindicated
- Treat hypotension with 0.9% NS IV fluid resuscitation.

## ED TREATMENT/PROCEDURES
- Decontamination:
  - Dermal or ocular exposure:
    - Immediate and thorough irrigation with water or 0.9% NS until physiologic pH attained
    - Alkalis typically require more irrigation than acids.
  - Ipecac, activated charcoal, gastroesophageal lavage, and a neutralizing acid or base are all contraindicated with caustic ingestions.
- Dilution:
  - Water or milk in the 1st 30 min of ingestion:
    - Especially useful for solid caustic alkali ingestions
    - Excessive intake may induce vomiting and worsen esophageal damage.
  - If respiratory distress, intubate before dilution.
  - Contraindicated if esophageal or gastric perforation suspected

- Keep patient NPO if oral exposure.
- Broad-spectrum antibiotics if mediastinitis or peritonitis suspected
- Antiemetics for nausea and vomiting
- Treat dermal exposures according to standard burn recommendations.
- Detailed examination for ocular exposures
- IV H$_2$ blockers for symptomatic relief
- Gastroenterology and surgical consultation
- Benefit of corticosteroids following esophageal damage is controversial:
  - May prevent the formation of esophageal stricture
  - May promote bacterial invasion, immune suppression, and tissue softening
  - The decision to initiate corticosteroids requires input from entire team caring for patient.
  - Initiate broad-spectrum antibiotics if corticosteroids are given.
- Laparoscopy or laparotomy for perforation and full-thickness necrosis
- Topical hydrofluoric acid exposure (options depend on severity and location):
  - IM injection of 5% calcium gluconate (0.5 mL/cm$^2$ of skin with 30-gauge needle)
  - Intra-arterial infusion of 10 mL of 10% calcium gluconate in 40 mL D$_5$W over 4 hr

## MEDICATION
- Methylprednisolone: 40 mg q8h IV (peds: 2 mg/kg/day IV); the course of therapy is 14–21 days followed by a corticosteroid taper.
- Prochlorperazine (Compazine): 5–10 mg IV (peds: 0.13 mg/kg per dose IM)
- Ranitidine (Zantac): 50 mg IV q6–8h

 **FOLLOW-UP**

## DISPOSITION
### Admission Criteria
- All symptomatic patients
- Nonaccidental ingestion

### Discharge Criteria
- Asymptomatic patients who accidentally ingested and are able to swallow without difficulty
- Minimal oropharyngeal pain with a corresponding visible lesion; no drooling; no respiratory compromise; no deep throat, chest, or abdominal pain; and able to swallow without difficulty

## FOLLOW-UP RECOMMENDATIONS
Psychiatric referral for intentional ingestion

## PEARLS AND PITFALLS

- Dilute with mild or water at home or in the ED within the 1st 30 min.
- Perform copious irrigation of ocular or dermal exposure:
  - Alkalis require more irrigation than acids.

## ADDITIONAL READING

- Nagi B, Kochar R, Thapa BR, et al. Radiological spectrum of late sequelae of corrosive injury to upper gastrointestinal tract. A pictorial review. *ACTA Radiologica*. 2004;1:712.
- Rao RB, Hoffman RS. Caustics and batteries. In: Goldfrank LR, Flomenbaum NE, Lewin NA, et al., eds. *Goldfrank's Toxicologic Emergencies*, 7th ed. New York: McGraw-Hill; 2002:1323–1340.
- Salzman M, O'Malley RN. Updates on the evaluation and management of caustic exposures. *Emerg Med Clin North A*. 2007;25(2):459–476.

**CODES**

ICD9
- 983.1 Toxic effect of acids
- 983.2 Toxic effect of caustic alkalis
- 983.9 Toxic effect of caustic, unspecified

# CAVERNOUS SINUS THROMBOSIS

*Tamara Espinoza*

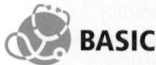 **BASICS**

## DESCRIPTION
- Thrombosis of a branch of the major intracerebral venous drainage system
- Most commonly infectious
- Spreads from odontogenic or sinus infectious source
- Less frequently occurs with hypercoagulable states

### Anatomy
3 primary sites of thrombosis:
- Cavernous sinus: Most common:
  - Drainage from superficial venous system
- Superolateral to the sphenoid sinus and surrounds the sella:
  - Cranial nerves (CN) III, IV, V1, and V2 traverse the lateral wall of the sinus.
  - CN VI and the internal carotid artery occupy the medial portion of the sinus.
- Can also involve transverse sinus and superficial sagittal sinus

## PATHOPHYSIOLOGY
- Hematogenous spread of facial, otic, or neck infection into venous drainage system
- Contiguous spread directly from infected sinus cavities (sphenoid, ethmoid, frontal)
- Bacterial overgrowth leads to inflammation and coagulation, resulting in thrombosis.
- Venous engorgement of cavernous sinus can affect adjacent structures:
  - Ophthalmoplegia from inflammation of CN III, IV, or VI
  - Pupillary fixation from CN III
  - Sensory deficits or paresthesias of forehead or cheek from CN V1 and V2

## ETIOLOGY
- Septic:
  - *S. aureus* is the most common infectious etiology followed by streptococcal species.
  - Cavernous sinus:
    - 30% mortality
    - Midface infection spreads into cavernous sinus
    - Maxillary dental infection and sphenoid sinusitis are most common.
  - Lateral:
    - 25% mortality
    - Primarily disease of young children
    - Spread from otogenic source
    - Otitis media or mastoiditis
  - Superior sagittal:
    - Extremely rare, with 80% mortality

- Aseptic:
  - Less common
  - Granulomatous conditions (tuberculosis [TB])
  - Inflammatory disorders
  - From mass effect (tumors at base of skull, aneurysms)
- Hypercoagulable states

### Pediatric Considerations
- Children may present with nonspecific symptoms such as decreased energy, vomiting, fever.
- Have high level of suspicion for any child with recent otitis or pharyngitis with worsening symptoms, declining mental status, or signs of increased intracranial pressure:
  - HTN, bradycardia, lethargy, vomiting, gait instability
- More common in the neonatal period, when diagnosis can be extremely difficult to make

 **DIAGNOSIS**

## SIGNS AND SYMPTOMS
- Signs:
  - Headache occurs in 90% of patients.
  - Fever if infectious cause
  - Ocular or retrobulbar pain
  - Facial swelling
  - Visual disturbance
  - Facial dysesthesias
  - Lethargy or altered mental status
- Symptoms:
  - Ptosis, proptosis
  - Chemosis with retinal vein engorgement
  - Facial or periorbital edema
  - Ophthalmoplegia
  - Cranial nerve palsies: Abducens nerve most commonly affected
  - Retinal hemorrhage or papilledema
  - Altered level of consciousness or coma
  - Seizures
  - Sepsis with cardiovascular instability or collapse

### History
High-risk historical factors include:
- A history of trauma
- Previous ENT or neurosurgical instrumentation
- Diabetes or immunocompromised state (HIV, steroid use, cancer)

## ESSENTIAL WORKUP
Clinical diagnosis based on:
- Symptoms of venous obstruction
- Ophthalmoplegia
- Sepsis or meningitis
- Symptoms that become unilateral and spread to become bilateral are diagnostic.

## DIAGNOSTIC TESTS & INTERPRETATION
### Lab
- Neither sensitive nor specific
- CBC:
  - Leukocytosis
- PT/PTT/INR
- Erythrocyte sedimentation rate (ESR) elevated in 50–60%
- Lumbar puncture/cerebrospinal fluid (CSF):
  - To evaluate fever and altered mental status
  - CSF with elevated protein and WBC

### Imaging
- CT scan:
  - Can be normal early in disease course
  - Findings include:
    - Nonspecific abnormalities
    - May identify original source of infection (eg, sinusitis)
    - Delayed filling of involved sinus
    - Filling defect of sinus owing to thrombosis
    - Dilated superior ophthalmic vein
    - Associated intracranial hemorrhage
    - Signs of increased intracranial pressure (ICP): Small ventricles, loss of sulci
- MRI with MR angiography (MRA)/MR venography (MRV):
  - Diagnostic modality of choice
  - Direct visualization of intracranial vessels and sinuses
  - Capable of visualizing thrombus at any stage

## DIFFERENTIAL DIAGNOSIS
- Meningitis/encephalitis
- Intracranial abscess
- Periorbital and orbital cellulitis
- Internal carotid artery aneurysm or fistula
- Pseudotumor cerebri
- Acute-angle closure glaucoma
- Intracranial hemorrhage
- Tolosa-Hunt syndrome:
  - Rare granulomatous inflammation of cavernous sinus

## ALERT
- This can be an extremely difficult diagnosis to make.
- Maintain a high level of suspicion in toxic-appearing patients with recent ear/nose/throat (ENT) infections, or in patients with refractory headache and risk factors for hypercoagulability or intracranial infection.

C

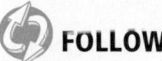

# TREATMENT

## PRE-HOSPITAL

### ALERT
- Patients can be altered and unstable.
- May require rapid assessment and stabilization of airway, breathing, and circulation (ABCs)

## INITIAL STABILIZATION/THERAPY
- Careful assessment of mental status with intubation for airway protection as needed
- Aggressive fluid resuscitation for cardiovascular instability

## ED TREATMENT/PROCEDURES
- Broad-spectrum antibiotics with multiple drug regimens:
  - Cover for gram-positives, gram-negatives, as well as anaerobes.
  - Nafcillin or vancomycin (for methicillin resistant *S. aureus* [MRSA]) plus ceftriaxone:
    - Add metronidazole or clindamycin in significant infections.
- Heparin:
  - Attenuates clot propagation and improves morbidity/mortality.
  - Controversial in transverse and sagittal thrombosis owing to higher risk of subsequent hemorrhage
  - Administer only after ruling out bleed on CT scan.
  - Questionable superiority of LMWH over IV heparin
- Systemic steroids:
  - Believed to be of benefit with concomitant pituitary insufficiency, and with infectious or inflammatory etiologies
- Appropriate management of increased ICP as needed
- Surgical consultation for drainage of primary site of infection (eg, dental abscess or sinusitis)

## MEDICATION
- Ceftriaxone: 2 g/d IV (peds: 80–100 mg/kg/d to q12h)
- Clindamycin: 300–900 mg IV q6–12h (neonates: 10–20 mg/kg/24 h IV divided q6–12h; peds: 25–40 mg/kg/24h divided q6–8h)
- Metronidazole: 500 mg IV q6h (neonates: 7.5–30 mg/kg/24 h IV divided q12–24h; peds: 30 mg/kg/24h IV divided q6h)

- Nafcillin: 1–2 g IV q4h (peds: 50–75 mg/kg/24 h IV divided q8–12h depending on age)
- Vancomycin: 1 g IV q12h (peds: 10–20 mg/kg IV q8–12h depending on age)

### First Line
- Broad-spectrum antibiotics
- Anticoagulation

### Second Line
- Dexamethasone is controversial.
- Endovascular thrombolytics in selected cases

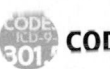

# FOLLOW-UP

## DISPOSITION
### Admission Criteria
- All patients with sinus thrombosis warrant admission to a monitored setting.
- Consider ICU admission.

### Discharge Criteria
None

## FOLLOW-UP RECOMMENDATIONS
Neurologic and neurosurgical consultation

## COMPLICATIONS
- Blindness can result from:
  Central retinal artery occlusion
  - Central retinal vein occlusion
  - Septic emboli
  - Arteritis
  - Ischemic optic neuritis
  - Glaucomatous optic atrophy
  - Corneal ulceration from loss of corneal reflex
- Hearing loss from otic invasion
- Local spread can cause meningitis or intracranial abscess.
- Seizures, especially in superior sagittal sinus thrombosis
- Pituitary necrosis and insufficiency from local invasion
- Sepsis can develop from systemic hematogenous seeding:
  - Septic emboli
  - Adult respiratory distress syndrome (ARDS)

# PEARLS AND PITFALLS
- Diagnosis is made on clinical evaluation and confirmatory laboratory evidence. Maintain a high index of suspicion.
- Noncontrast head CT is often negative or nonspecific. MRI/MRV is the diagnostic imaging modality of choice and should be pursued in high-risk individuals.
- Administer IV antibiotics early, especially in any ill-appearing patient with ENT or neurologic complaints.
- Hypercoagulable states result in *both* central and peripheral venous thrombosis. Workup and management decisions must include consideration of systemic thromboembolism.

# ADDITIONAL READING
- Cannon ML, Antonio BL, McCloskey JJ, et al. Cavernous sinus thrombosis complicating sinusitis. *Pediatr Crit Care Med*. 2004;5(1):86–88.
- Carvalho KS, Garg BP. Cerebral venous thrombosis and venous malformations in children. *Neurol Clin North Am*. 2002;20:1061–1077.
- Heilpern KL, Lorber B. Infectious disease emergencies: Focal intracranial infections. *Infect Dis Clin North Am*. 1996;10(4):879–898.
- Sztajnkrycer M, Jauch EC. The difficult diagnosis: Unusual headaches. *Emerg Med Clin North Am*. 1998;16(4):741–760.

## See Also (Topic, Algorithm, Electronic Media Element)
Headache

# CODES

ICD9
- 325 Phlebitis and thrombophlebitis of intracranial venous sinuses
- 437.6 Nonpyogenic thrombosis of intracranial venous sinus

# CELLULITIS

*John Mahoney*
*Dolores Gonthier*

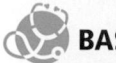

## BASICS

### DESCRIPTION
- Acute, spreading erythematous superficial infection of skin and subcutaneous tissues:
  - Variety of pathogens
  - Extension into deeper tissues can result in necrotizing soft tissue infection.
- Progressive spread of erythema, warmth, pain, and tenderness
- Predisposing factors:
  - Lymphedema
  - Tinea pedis
  - Open wounds
  - Pre-existing skin lesion (furuncle)
  - Prior trauma or surgery
  - Retained foreign body
  - Vascular or immune compromise
  - Injection drug use

### ETIOLOGY
- Simple cellulitis:
  - Group A streptococci
  - *Staphylococcus aureus*—including resistant strains such as community-acquired methicillin-resistant *S. aureus* (CA-MRSA; see below):
    - CA-MRSA risk factors include: Prior MRSA infection, household contact of CA-MRSA patient, daycare contact of MRSA patients, children, soldiers, incarcerated persons, athletes in contact sports, IV drug users, men who have sex with men
    - Different antibiotic susceptibility than nosocomial MRSA
    - Variable, rising local prevalence of CA-MRSA should be considered when starting empiric antibiotic therapy.
    - Suspect CA-MRSA in unresponsive infections.
- Extremity cellulitis after lymphatic disruption:
  - Nongroup A β-hemolytic streptococci (groups C, B, G)
- Cellulitis in diabetics:
  - Can be polymicrobial with *S. aureus*, streptococci, gram-negative bacteria, and anaerobes, especially when associated with skin ulcers
- Periorbital cellulitis:
  - *S. aureus*
  - Streptococcal species
- Buccal cellulitis:
  - *Haemophilus influenzae* type B
  - Anaerobic oral flora, associated with intraoral laceration or dental abscess
- Nosocomial MRSA:
  - Risk factors: Recent hospital or long-term care admission, surgery, injection drug use, vascular catheter, dialysis, recent antibiotic use, unresponsive infection
  - Resistant to most antibiotics (see "Treatment")

- Less common causes:
  - Clostridia
  - Anthrax
  - *Pasteurella multocida*—common after cat and dog bites
  - *Eikenella corrodens*—human bites
  - *Pseudomonas aeruginosa:*
    - Hot-tub folliculitis—self-limited
    - Foot puncture wound
    - Ecthyma gangrenosum in neutropenic patients
  - *Erysipelothrix* species—raw fish, poultry, meat, or hide handlers
  - *Aeromonas hydrophila*—freshwater swimming
  - *Vibrio* species—seawater or raw seafood

### Pediatric Considerations
- Facial cellulitis in children:
  - *Streptococcus pneumoniae*
  - *H. influenzae* type B, although incidence declining since introduction of HIB vaccine
- Perianal cellulitis:
  - Group A streptococci
  - Associated or antecedent pharyngitis or impetigo
- Neonates:
  - Group B streptococci

## DIAGNOSIS

### SIGNS AND SYMPTOMS
- Common to all syndromes:
  - Pain, tenderness, warmth
  - Erythema
  - Edema or induration
  - Fever/chills
  - Tender regional lymphadenopathy
  - Lymphangitis
  - Accompanying subcutaneous abscess possible
  - Suspect deep abscess especially if treatment failure on initial antibiotic
  - Superficial vesicles
- Buccal cellulitis:
  - Odontogenic cases more serious:
    - Toothache, sore throat, or facial swelling
    - Progressive extension into soft tissues of neck with fever, erythema, neck swelling, and dysphagia

### Pediatric Considerations
- Facial cellulitis in children:
  - Erythema and swelling of the cheek and eyelid
  - Rapidly progressive
  - Usually unilateral
  - Upper respiratory tract symptoms
  - Risk for cavernous sinus thrombosis and permanent optic nerve injury
- Perianal cellulitis:
  - Erythema and pruritus extending from the anus several centimeters onto adjacent skin
  - Pain on defecation
  - Blood-streaked stools

### History
Patients often incorrectly attribute CA-MRSA infection with spontaneous abscess to a spider bite.

### Physical Exam
In simple cellulitis, physical findings can suggest the etiology and help narrow empiric antibiotic coverage:
- Staph etiology: Focal abscess or pustule with any of: Fluctuance, yellow or white center, central point or "head", ordraining pus, indolent progression
- Strep etiology: Sharply demarcated borders, lymphangitis, pre-existing lymphedema, concomitant nausea from toxin

### ESSENTIAL WORKUP
- Cellulitis is a clinical diagnosis.
- Physical exam to reveal infection source

### DIAGNOSTIC TESTS & INTERPRETATION
#### Lab
- WBC count unnecessary
- Gram stain and culture to focus antimicrobial selection and reveal resistant pathogens (MRSA):
  - Aspirate point of maximal inflammation or punch biopsy if there is no wound to culture.
  - Perform in treatment failures and consider in admitted patients
- Blood culture:
  - Usually negative in uncomplicated cellulitis
  - May identify organism in patients with:
    - Lymphedema
    - Buccal or periorbital cellulitis
    - Salt water or freshwater source
    - Fever or chills

#### Imaging
- Plain radiographs may reveal abscess formation, subcutaneous gas, or foreign bodies:
  - Extension to bone (osteomyelitis) not visualized early on plain radiographs
- Extremity vascular imaging (Doppler US) can help rule out deep venous thrombosis.
- US useful for diagnosing abscess if physical exam is equivocal or if there is a broad area of cellulitis.
- CT or MRI can help rule out necrotizing fasciitis.

### DIFFERENTIAL DIAGNOSIS
- Necrotizing fasciitis
- Lymphangitis or lymphadenitis
- Thrombophlebitis or deep venous thrombosis:
  - Differentiation from cellulitis:
    - Absence of initial traumatic or infectious focus
    - No regional lymphadenopathy
    - Presence of risk factors for DVT
- Insect bite
- Allergic reaction
- Acute gout or pseudogout
- Ruptured Baker cyst
- Herpetic whitlow
- Neoplasm

- Phytophotodermatitis
- Erythema chronicum migrans lesion of Lyme disease
- Differential diagnosis of facial cellulitis:
  – Allergic angioedema
  – Conjunctivitis
  – Contusion

### Pediatric Considerations
Differential diagnosis of perianal cellulitis:

- Candida intertrigo
- Psoriasis
- Pinworm infection
- Child abuse
- Behavioral problem
- Inflammatory bowel disease

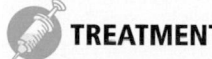 TREATMENT

### INITIAL STABILIZATION/THERAPY
Airway compromise possible with deep extension of facial or neck cellulitis

### ED TREATMENT/PROCEDURES
- General principles:
  – Consider local prevalence of MRSA and other resistant pathogens in addition to usual causes.
  – Usual outpatient treatment: 7–10 days
  – Cool compresses for comfort
  – Analgesics
  – Extremity elevation
  – Treat predisposing tinea pedis with topical antifungal such as clotrimazole.
- Simple cellulitis:
  – Outpatient:
    ○ Oral cephalexin plus TMP/SMX (to cover CA-MRSA)
    ○ Alternatives to cephalexin: Oral dicloxacillin, macrolide, or levofloxacin
    ○ Alternative to TMP/SMX: Clindamycin
  – Inpatient:
    ○ IV nafcillin or equivalent
- Extremity cellulitis after lymphatic disruption.
  – Same as simple cellulitis
- Cellulitis in diabetics:
  – Outpatient:
    ○ Amoxicillin/clavulanate or clindamycin
  – Inpatient:
    ○ IV ampicillin/sulbactam or imipenem cilastatin or equivalent
- Periorbital cellulitis in adults:
  – Outpatient: Oral dicloxacillin or azithromycin
  – Inpatient: IV vancomycin
- Buccal cellulitis in adults:
  – Outpatient: Oral amoxicillin/clavulanate
  – Inpatient: IV ceftriaxone
  – Odontogenic source:
    ○ Drainage essential
    ○ Coverage for anaerobes: Clindamycin
- Facial cellulitis in children:
  – IV ceftriaxone
- Perianal cellulitis:
  – Outpatient: Oral penicillin VK
  – Inpatient: IV penicillin G (aqueous)
- Animal or human bite:
  – Oral amoxicillin/clavulanate

- Foot puncture wound:
  – Oral or IV ciprofloxacin or IV ceftazidime
- MRSA:
  – Nosocomial MRSA: IV vancomycin or oral or IV linezolid
  – Severe CA-MRSA:
    ○ IV clindamycin or IV vancomycin

### MEDICATION
- Amoxicillin/clavulanate: 500–875 mg (peds: 45 mg/kg/24 h) PO b.i.d. or 250–500 mg (peds: 40 mg/kg/24 h) PO t.i.d.
- Ampicillin/sulbactam: 1.5–3 g (peds: 100–300 mg/kg/24 h up to 40 kg; over 40 kg give adult dose) IV q6h
- Azithromycin: (adults and peds) 10 mg/kg up to 500 mg PO on day 1, followed by 5 mg/kg up to 250 mg PO daily on days 2–5
- Ceftazidime: 500–1,000 mg (peds: 150 mg/kg/24 h; max., 6 g/24 h; use sodium formulation in peds) IV q8h
- Ceftriaxone: 1–2 g (peds: 50–75 mg/kg/24 h) IV daily
- Cephalexin: 500 mg (peds: 50–100 mg/kg/24 h) PO q.i.d.
- Ciprofloxacin: (adult only) 500–750 mg PO b.i.d. or 400 mg IV q8–12h
- Clindamycin: 450–900 mg (peds: 20–40 mg/kg/24 h) PO or IV q8h
- Dicloxacillin: 125–500 mg (peds: 12.5–25 mg/kg/24 h) PO q6h
- Erythromycin base: (adult) 250–500 mg PO q.i.d.
- Imipenem cilastatin: 500–1,000 mg (peds: 15–25 mg/kg) IV q6h; max. 4 g/24 h or 50 mg/kg/24 h, whichever is less
- Levofloxacin: (adult only) 500–750 mg PO or IV daily
- Linezolid: 600 mg PO or IV q12h (peds: 30 mg/kg/24 h div. q8h)
- Nafcillin: 1–2 g IV q4h (peds: 50–100 mg/kg/24 h divided q6h); max. 12 g/24 h
- Penicillin VK: 250–500 mg (peds: 25–50 mg/kg/24 h) PO q6h
- Penicillin G (aqueous): 4 mU (peds: 100,000–400,000 U/kg/24 h) IV q4h
- Trimethoprim/sulfamethoxazole (TMP/SMX): 2 DS tabs PO q12h (peds: 6–10 mg/kg/24 h TMP div. q12h)
- Vancomycin: 1 g IV q12h (peds: 10 mg/kg IV q6h; dosing adjustments required younger than age 5 yr); check serum levels

 FOLLOW-UP

### DISPOSITION
#### Admission Criteria
- Toxic appearing
- Tissue necrosis
- History of immune suppression
- Concurrent chronic medical illnesses
- Unable to take oral medications
- Unreliable patients

#### Discharge Criteria
- Mild infection in a nontoxic-appearing patient
- Able to take oral antibiotics
- No history of immune suppression or concurrent medical problems
- No hand or face involvement
- Has adequate follow-up within 24–48 hr

#### FOLLOW-UP RECOMMENDATIONS
- Follow-up within 24–48 hr
- Sooner if worsening symptoms, including new or worsening lymphangitis, increasing area of redness, worsening fever

## PEARLS AND PITFALLS
- Strep and staph are most common causes.
- CA-MRSA now significant cause of cellulitis, frequent enough to warrant including coverage in empiric treatment
- Clinicians not accurate at identifying MRSA at the bedside
- A deep abscess may be misclassified as cellulitis.
- Use clinical suspicion and ultrasound to avoid missing an abscess.

## ADDITIONAL READING
- Abrahamian FM, Talan DA, Moran GJ. Management of skin and soft-tissue infections in the emergency department. *Infect Dis Clin N Am.* 2008;22:89–116.
- Padmanabhan R, Fraser T. The emergence of methicillin-resistant *Staphylococcus aureus* in the community. *Cleve Clin J Med.* 2005;72:235–241.
- Pasternack MS, Swartz MN. Cellulitis, necrotizing fasciitis and subcutaneous tissue infections. In: Mandell GL, Bennett JE, Dolin R, eds. *Mandell, Douglas and Bennett's Principles and Practice of Infectious Diseases*, 7th ed. New York: Elsevier/Churchill Livingstone; 2010:1289–1312.
- Swartz MN. Cellulitis. *New Engl J Med.* 2004;350: 904–912.

### See Also (Topic, Algorithm, Electronic Media Element)
- Abscess, Skin/Soft Tissue
- Lymphadenitis
- Lymphangitis
- Necrotizing Fasciitis

## CODES

### ICD9
- 682.8 Cellulitis and abscess of other specified sites
- 682.9 Cellulitis and abscess of unspecified sites

# CENTRAL RETINAL ARTERY OCCLUSION

*Yasuharu Okuda*
*Braden J. Hexom*

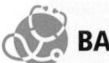 **BASICS**

## DESCRIPTION

- Obstruction of the central retinal artery associated with sudden painless loss of vision
- Usually occurs in persons 50–70 yr of age
- Ophthalmic artery is 1st branch of carotid.
- Risk factors include HTN, atherosclerotic disease, sickle cell disease, vasculitis, valvular heart disease, lupus, trauma, and coronary artery disease.
- Incidence of 1–10 per 100,000
- Often described as a "stroke of the eye"

## ETIOLOGY

- Embolic:
  - Occlusion by intravascular material from a proximal source:
    - Atherosclerotic disease (majority)
    - Carotid artery stenosis
    - Valvular heart disease (cardiogenic emboli)
    - Atrial myxoma
    - Dissection of the ophthalmic artery
    - Carotid artery dissection
- Thrombotic:
  - Obstruction of flow from the rupture of a pre-existing intravascular atherosclerotic plaque
  - Hypercoagulable states (sickle cell)
- Inflammatory:
  - Due to temporal arteritis, lupus, vasculitis
- Arterial spasm:
  - Associated with migraine headaches
- Decreased perfusion:
  - Low flow conditions such as in severe hypotension or high pressure situations seen in acute angle closure glaucoma or retrobulbar hemorrhage

 **DIAGNOSIS**

## SIGNS AND SYMPTOMS

### History
- Sudden, painless, monocular loss of vision
- Prior episodes of sudden visual loss:
  - May last a few seconds to minutes (amaurosis fugax)
  - Caused by transient embolic phenomena or decreased ocular blood flow

### Physical Exam
- Significantly decreased visual acuity
- Afferent pupillary defect usually present
- Retinal appearance:
  - Emboli visualized within vascular tree of the retina
  - Appears as glinting white or yellow flecks (Hollenhorst plaques) within the vessels
  - Ischemic edema visible within 15–20 min of occlusion
  - "Cherry-red spot" remains over the fovea (only area where there is very thin retina allowing the vascular choroids to show through).
  - Affected arteries empty or showing dark red stationary or barely pulsatile segmented rouleaux ("box-carring")
  - Within 1–2 hr opacification of the usually transparent infarcting retinal nerve layer occurs.
- Partial field deficits:
  - Occur if only if branch of central retinal artery involved

## ESSENTIAL WORKUP
- Visual acuity and visual field testing
- Funduscopic exam
- Intraocular pressure measurements
- Emergent ophthalmologic consultation

## DIAGNOSTIC TESTS & INTERPRETATION

### Lab
Directed towards evaluating underlying etiology of occlusion:

- CBC with differential and platelet count
- PT/PTT
- Electrolytes, BUN/creatinine, glucose
- Electronic spin resonance for giant cell arteritis (in patients >55 yr old)
- ANA, RF, CRP, ESR
- Rapid plasma regain (RPR)
- Hemoglobin electrophoresis
- Serum protein electrophoresis

### Imaging
Directed toward evaluating underlying etiology of occlusion:

- Carotid artery ultrasound/doppler
- Possibly echocardiography
- Fluorescein angiography or electroretinography to confirm the diagnosis

## DIFFERENTIAL DIAGNOSIS
- Acute angle closure glaucoma
- Central retinal vein occlusion
- Giant cell arteritis (temporal arteritis)
- Optic neuritis
- Retinal detachment

**TREATMENT**

### ALERT
Initiate treatment immediately because irreversible visual loss occurs at 90 min:
- Only immediate treatment may help to salvage or restore sight to the affected eye.
- Goals of therapy include dislodging or dissolving the embolus, arterial dilation to improve forward flow, and reduction of intra-ocular pressure to improve the profusion gradient.

### ED TREATMENT/PROCEDURES
- Immediate global massage in an attempt to dislodge the embolus:
  - Lay patient flat and apply digital global massage bolus.
  - On closed eyelid, apply constant pressure for 15 sec and remove for 15 sec. Repeat for 5 cycles.
- Increase $PCO_2$ to dilate retinal vessels:
  - Have patient breath into paper bag for 10 min each hour
  - May use inhaled carbogen (a mixture of carbon dioxide and oxygen gas)
- Administer IV acetazolamide to decrease intraocular pressure.
- Apply topical timolol maleate to reduce intraocular pressure.
- Administer aspirin and IV heparin for prevention of clot propagation.
- Obtain emergent ophthalmology consultation for:
  - Anterior chamber paracentesis to help reduce intraocular pressure
  - Possible intra-arterial fibrinolysis for clot lysis
- Administer high dose systemic steroids in suspected cases of inflammatory arteritis.

### MEDICATION
#### First Line
- Acetazolamide: 500 mg IV or PO
- Carbogen: Inhalation of 95% oxygen and 5% carbon dioxide mixture
- Heparin: 80 U/kg IV bolus then 18 U/kg/hr continuous infusions (rate adjusted based on PTT level)
- Timolol maleate 0.5% solution: 1 drop topically to affected eye

#### Second Line
- Methylprednisolone. 250 mg IV in suspected cases of inflammatory arteritis
- Aspirin: 325 mg PO
- Mannitol
- Sublingual nitroglycerin

 **FOLLOW-UP**

### DISPOSITION
#### Admission Criteria
Required for workup of proximal cause in acute cases (source of embolism, thrombosis, or inflammatory)

#### Discharge Criteria
Chronic retinal artery occlusion with no evidence of active disease can be worked up as an outpatient.

#### Issues for Referral
All suspected cases warrant emergent ophthalmology consultation.

### FOLLOW-UP RECOMMENDATIONS
Most cases will require carotid US to exclude atherosclerotic disease.

### PEARLS AND PITFALLS
- Amaurosis fugax (transient, possibly resolved retinal artery occlusion) is sentinel event and may lead to complete occlusion or stroke requiring further workup.
- Retinal artery occlusion is a medical emergency requiring immediate treatment to prevent loss of the eye.
- It is important to document a full eye exam including evaluation of the optic fundus.

### ADDITIONAL READING
- Arnold M, Koerner U, Remonda L, et al. Comparison of intra-arterial thrombolysis with conventional treatment in patients with acute central retinal artery occlusion. *J Neurol Neurosurg Psychiatry.* 2005;76(2):196–199.
- Fraser SG, Adams W. Interventions for acute non-arteritic central retinal artery occlusion. *Cochrane Database Syst Rev.* 2009;(1):CD001989.
- Hazin R, Daoud YJ, Khan F. Ocular ischemic syndrome: Recent trends in medical management. *Curr Opin Ophthalmol.* 2009;20:430–433.
- Morgan A, Hemphill R. Acute visual change. *Emerg Med Clin North Am.* 1998;16(4):825–843.

### See Also (Topic, Algorithm, Electronic Media Element)
- Central Retinal Venous Occlusion
- Visual Loss

**CODES**

#### ICD9
362.31 Central retinal artery occlusion

# CENTRAL RETINAL VEIN OCCLUSION

Lisa Jacobson
Yasuharu Okuda

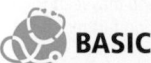 **BASICS**

## DESCRIPTION
Disease characterized by decreased visual acuity resulting from venous occlusion of any etiology

## ETIOLOGY
- Ischemic CRVO:
  - 20–25% of cases
  - Blocked venous return leads to backflow in capillaries, hemorrhage, and macular edema.
  - Limited space at lamina cribrosa predisposes to thrombosis due to slow flow and vessel wall changes
  - Theorize that arteriosclerotic changes in the adjacent artery may impinge upon the vein.
- Nonischemic CRVO:
  - Milder, incomplete occlusion

 **DIAGNOSIS**

## SIGNS AND SYMPTOMS
Classic description:
- Acute, unilateral, painless vision loss
- "Blood and thunder" appearance on funduscopy

## History
- Painless, unilateral vision loss
- If nonischemic, may be incomplete and intermittent vision loss

## Physical Exam
- Decreased visual acuity:
  - Usually worse than 20/200
- Afferent pupillary defect
- Dilated tortuous veins
- Retinal hemorrhages:
  - If central, findings in all 4 quadrants
  - Extensive hemorrhages give a dramatic look to fundus classically described as "blood and thunder appearance."
- Disk edema
- Cotton wool spots

## ESSENTIAL WORKUP
- BP
- Visual acuity:
  - Hand movements typically is all that is seen.
- Visual fields
- Funduscopy
- Tonometry:
  - Normal pressures are between 10 and 21 mm Hg.

## DIAGNOSTIC TESTS & INTERPRETATION
### Lab
- CBC
- PT/PTT
- ESR
- ANA
- Serum protein electrophoresis

## Imaging
Fluorescein angiography:
- Ophthalmologists use this to map areas of nonperfusion.
- Differentiates between ischemic and nonischemic

## Diagnostic Procedures/Surgery
Gonioscopy:
- Measure iris or angle neovascularization.

## DIFFERENTIAL DIAGNOSIS
- Amaurosis fugax/transient ischemic attack
- Cavernous sinus thrombosis
- DM
- HTN/hypertensive retinopathy
- Hyperviscosity syndromes:
  - Sickle cell, polycythemia, leukemia, multiple myeloma
- Hysterical blindness
- Ocular ischemia syndrome
- Papilledema
- Retinal artery occlusion
- Retinal detachment
- Severe anemia with thrombocytopenia
- Temporal arteritis
- Vitreal hemorrhage

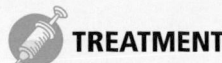

# TREATMENT

## PRE-HOSPITAL
No specific interventions need occur prior to arrival at the hospital in regards to the eye.

## INITIAL STABILIZATION/THERAPY
- Initiate steps to lower intraocular pressure if it is elevated.
- Treat underlying medical problems.

## ED TREATMENT/PROCEDURES
- Recognition and prompt ophthalmologic referral is the cornerstone of ED treatment.
- Though not proven, the following may be tried in consultation with an ophthalmologist:
  – Aspirin
  – Anti-inflammatory agents
  – Systemic steroids
  – Systemic anticoagulation
  – Fibrinolytics

## MEDICATION
There is no proven treatment for CRVO, ophthalmologists may treat with the following:
- Intravitreal triamcinolone
- Antivascular endothelial growth factor:
  – Bevacizumab

### Considerations in Prescribing
Use of oral contraceptives can increase the risk of CRVO.

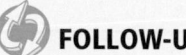

# FOLLOW-UP

## DISPOSITION
### Admission Criteria
Patients may be admitted for surgical intervention, depending upon the ophthalmologist.

### Discharge Criteria
Patients can be discharged from the ED as long as they have immediate follow-up with an ophthalmologist.

### Issues for Referral
- If no ophthalmologist is available, treatment should be initiated for concomitant conditions and patient transferred to nearest hospital with ophthalmologic consultation.
- Ophthalmologists often perform panretinal photocoagulation if neovascularization is found.

## FOLLOW-UP RECOMMENDATIONS
- Patients with ischemic CRVO need prolonged follow-up to catch neovascularization and glaucoma that typically develop.
- Patients with CRVO likely have other vascular diseases and need complete medical workups.
- Patients should also follow with an internist to manage comorbidities and risk factors.

## PEARLS AND PITFALLS
- Increased IOP resulting from neovascularization and edema can cause vascular insufficiency and with delayed treatment vision loss can be permanent.
- When patients present with bilateral CRVOs or CRVO at a young age, workup must search for hyperviscosity syndromes.

## ADDITIONAL READING
- Beran DI, Murphy-Lavoie H. Acute painless vision loss. *J La State Med Soc.* 2009;161(4):214–223.
- Di Capua, et al. Cardiovascular risk factors and outcome in patients with retinal vein occlusion. *J Thromb Thrombolysis.* 2009.
- Khare, et al. Common ophthalmologic emergencies. *Int J Clin Pract.* 2008;62(11):1776–1784.
- Marx JA, et al. *Rosen's Emergency Medicine: Concepts and Clinical Practice.* 6th ed. St. Louis, MO: Mosby; 2009.
- Turello M, et al. Retinal vein occlusion: Evaluation of "classic" and "emerging" risk factors and treatment. *J Thromb Thrombolysis.* 2009.
- Yanoff M, Duker J. *Ophthalmology.* 3rd Ed. St. Louis, MO: Mosby; 2008.

### See Also (Topic, Algorithm, Electronic Media Element)
- Central Retinal Artery Occlusion
- Visual Loss

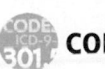 CODES

ICD9
362.35 Central retinal vein occlusion

# CEREBRAL ANEURYSM

*Veronique Au*
*Rebecca Smith-Coggins*

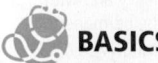 **BASICS**

## DESCRIPTION
- Abnormal, localized dilation or out-pouching of cerebral artery wall:
  - Occurs in 5–10% of population
- Rupture of saccular aneurysms account for 5–15% of strokes.
- Of those that rupture:
  - 40% occur at anterior communicating artery (ACA)
  - 30% at internal carotid (IC)
  - 20% in middle cerebral artery (MCA)
  - 5–10% in vertebrobasilar artery (VBA) system

## ETIOLOGY
- Asymptomatic in 2% of population
- "Congenital," saccular, or berry aneurysms most common (90%):
  - Develop at weak points in arterial wall and bifurcations of major cerebral arteries
  - Incidence increases with age.
  - Multiple in 20–30%
  - Increased incidence:
    - Polycystic kidney disease
    - Cerebral arteriovenous malformation
    - Type III collagen deficiency
    - Fibromuscular dysplasia
    - Ehlers-Danlos syndrome
    - Marfan syndrome
    - Pseudoxanthoma elasticum
    - Neurofibromatosis
    - Moyamoya disease
    - Coarctation of the aorta
    - Tuberous sclerosis
    - Sickle cell disease
    - Osler-Weber-Rendu syndrome
    - $\alpha$1-Antitrypsin deficiency
    - Systemic lupus erythematosus
    - Glucocorticoid remediable hyperaldosteronism
- Arteriosclerotic, fusiform or dolichoectatic (7%):
  - More common in peripheral arteries
- Inflammatory (mycotic):
  - 10% of patients with bacterial endocarditis
- Traumatic, associated with severe closed head injury
- Neoplastic, embolized tumor fragments
- Familial correlation: 1st-degree relative with history of aneurysm essentially doubles lifetime risk.

### Pediatric Considerations
- Although rare in children, more likely to be giant (>25 mm)
- Occur in the posterior circulation

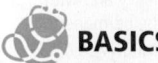 **DIAGNOSIS**

## SIGNS AND SYMPTOMS
- Commonly asymptomatic before rupture
- Sentinel headaches occur in 30–60% of patients before rupture:
  - Can be unilateral
- Seizures, syncope, or altered level of consciousness

### History
- Onset of headache
- Family history
- Altered mental status
- Focal neurologic deficits
- Rupture results in subarachnoid hemorrhage:
  - Headache: Severe ("worst headache ever") with sudden onset ("thunderclap")
    - Different from prior headaches
    - Classically without focal deficits
  - Nuchal rigidity (most common sign) secondary to blood in CSF

### Physical Exam
Compression of adjacent structures may cause neurologic symptoms:
- Anterior communicating artery aneurysms:
  - Optic tract: Altitudinal field cut or homonymous hemianopsia
  - Optic chiasm: Bitemporal hemianopsia
  - Optic nerve: Unilateral amblyopia
- Aneurysms at internal carotid–posterior communicating artery junction:
  - Oculomotor nerve: Fixed and dilated pupil, ptosis, diplopia, and temporal deviation of eye with inability to turn eye upward, inward, or downward
- Aneurysms in cerebral cortex may produce focal deficits including:
  - Hemiparesis
  - Hemisensory loss
  - Visual disturbances
  - Aphasia
  - Seizures

## ESSENTIAL WORKUP
- Complete neurologic examination
- Emergent noncontrast head CT scan will diagnose 90–95% of subarachnoid hemorrhages.
- Lumbar puncture with CSF analysis if CT scan is negative

## DIAGNOSTIC TESTS & INTERPRETATION
### Lab
- Coagulation studies
- Baseline CBC with platelets and differential
- Electrolytes
- Renal and liver function tests
- Arterial blood gas

### Imaging
- CXR for pulmonary edema
- 4-vessel cerebral angiography remains gold standard.
- MRA
- Helical CT scanning may be useful in detecting aneurysms >3 mm.
- Transcranial Doppler US may be useful in detecting vasospasm.

### Diagnostic Procedures/Surgery
Lumbar puncture if suspect aneurismal leak or rupture with normal head CT

## DIFFERENTIAL DIAGNOSIS
- Neoplasm
- Arteriovenous malformation
- Optic neuritis
- Migraine
- Meningitis
- Encephalitis
- Hypertensive encephalopathy
- Hyperglycemia or hypoglycemia
- Temporal arteritis
- Acute glaucoma
- Subdural hematoma
- Epidural hematoma
- Intracerebral hemorrhage
- Thromboembolic stroke
- Air embolism
- Sinusitis

**TREATMENT**

### PRE-HOSPITAL
- Cautions:
  - Neurologic examination in the field can be extremely helpful.
  - Assess:
    - Level of consciousness
    - Glasgow coma scale score
    - Gross motor deficits
    - Speech abnormalities
    - Gait disturbance
    - Facial asymmetry
    - Other focal deficits
- Patients with subarachnoid hemorrhage may need emergent intubation for rapidly deteriorating level of consciousness.
- Patients must be transported to a hospital with emergent CT scanning and intensive care unit–level treatment.

### INITIAL STABILIZATION/THERAPY
- ABCs:
  - Supplemental oxygen
  - Rapid-sequence intubation may be required for airway protection or for controlled ventilation.
  - Continuous cardiac monitoring and pulse oximetry
- For altered mental status:
  - Check blood glucose immediately, give $D_{50}$ (if glucose is low).
  - Naloxone
  - Thiamine
- Reversal of anticoagulation
- Prevention of acute increases in intracranial pressure from vomiting should be accomplished with antiemetics.
- Seizures should be managed acutely with IV benzodiazepines and fosphenytoin/phenytoin.
- Seizure prophylaxis is controversial and not recommended.

### ED TREATMENT/PROCEDURES
Following initial stabilization, the major goals of early treatment of ruptured or leaking aneurysms are to prevent re-rupture, cerebral vasospasm, and hydrocephalus (see "Subarachnoid Hemorrhage").

### SURGERY/OTHER PROCEDURES
- Optimal timing for angiography and surgery remain controversial, but trend is toward early surgery to decrease incidence of rebleeding and cerebral vasospasm.
- Early placement of ventriculostomy in appropriate patients may allow for direct intracranial pressure monitoring and often decreases systemic hypertension.

### Pediatric Considerations
Aneurysms in children have a high rate of hemorrhage and should be repaired early.

### MEDICATION
#### First Line
- Labetalol: 20–30 mg/min IV bolus, then 40–80 mg q10min max. 300 mg; follow with continuous infusion 0.5–2 mg/min
- Nimodipine: 60 mg PO/nasogastric q4h
- Ondansetron: 4 mg PO/SL/IV q4h PRN (peds: 0.1 mg/kg IV; max 4 mg/dose)
- Prochlorperazine: 5–10 g IV/IM q6–8h (peds: 0.2 mg/kg/day IM in 3 or 4 div. doses); max. 40 mg/day

#### Second Line
- Diazepam: 5–10 mg IV q10–15min max., 30 mg (peds: 0.2–0.3 mg/kg q5–10min max. 10 mg)
- Docusate sodium: 100 mg PO b.i.d.
- Fosphenytoin: 15–20 mg/kg phenytoin equivalents (PE) at rate of 100–150 mg/min IV/IM
- Hydralazine: 10–20 mg IV q30min
- Lorazepam: 2–4 mg IV q15min PRN (peds: 0.03–0.05 mg/kg per dose; max. 4 mg per dose)
- Nicardipine: 5 mg/h IV infusion, increase by 2.5 mg/h q5–15min max. 15 mg/hr (peds: Dosing unavailable)
- Phenytoin: 15–20 mg/kg IV load at max. 50 mg/min; max. 1.5 g (adult and peds); maintenance 4–6 mg/kg/day IV/IM

 **FOLLOW-UP**

### DISPOSITION
#### Admission Criteria
- Any patient with acute aneurismal subarachnoid hemorrhage should be admitted, preferably to ICU.
- Any patient with symptomatic unruptured aneurysm should receive admission and urgent neurosurgical consultation, given high rate of rupture.

#### Discharge Criteria
- Patients with incidentally discovered asymptomatic intracranial aneurysms may be discharged with close neurosurgical follow-up.
- Note that overall risk of rupture is 1–2% per year and that critical size at which risk for rupture outweighs risk for surgery is controversial (classically 10 mm, but probably in the 4–8-mm range).

### FOLLOW-UP RECOMMENDATIONS
- Neurosurgery
- Neurology
- Primary care

### PEARLS AND PITFALLS
- CT scan alone is not sufficient to exclude subarachnoid hemorrhage.
- Vasospasm is typically seen on day 3 after bleed or surgery.
- Nimodipine can prevent or treat vasospasm but should never be administered IV.
- Nitroprusside and nitroglycerine should be avoided due to tendency to increase cerebral blood volume and thereby intracranial pressure.

### ADDITIONAL READING
- Bederson JB, Connolly ES, Batjer HH, et al. Guidelines for management of aneurismal subarachnoid hemorrhage: A statement for healthcare professionals from a special writing group of the Stroke Council, American Heart Association. *Stroke.* 2009;40:994.
- Byyny RL, Mower WR, Shum N, et al. Sensitivity of noncontrast cranial computed tomography for the emergency department diagnosis of subarachnoid hemorrhage. *Ann Emerg Med.* 2008;51:697–703.
- Clarke G, Mendelow AD, Mitchell P. Predicting the risk of rupture of intracranial aneurysms based on anatomical location. *Acta Neurochir (Wien).* 2005;147(3):259–263.
- Edlow JA, Caplan LR. Avoiding the pitfalls in the diagnosis of subarachnoid hemorrhage. *New Engl J Med.* 2000;1:29–36.
- Naval NS, Stevens RD, Mirski MA, et al. Controversies in the management of aneurismal subarachnoid hemorrhage. *Crit Care Med.* 2006;34:511–524.
- Salary M, Quigley MR, Wilberger JE. Relation among aneurysm size, amount of subarachnoid blood, and clinical outcome. *J Neurosurg.* 2007;107(1):13–17.
- Swadron SP. Pitfalls in the management of headache in the emergency department. *Emerg Med Clin North Am.* 2010;28:127–147.

### See Also (Topic, Algorithm, Electronic Media Element)
Subarachnoid Hemorrhage

**CODES**

ICD9
- 430 Subarachnoid hemorrhage
- 437.3 Cerebral aneurysm, nonruptured

# CEREBRAL VASCULAR ACCIDENT

Veronique Au
Rebecca Smith-Coggins

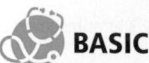

## BASICS

### DESCRIPTION
Interruption of blood flow to a specific brain region:
- Neurologic findings are determined by specific area affected.
- Onset may be sudden and complete, or stuttering and intermittent.

### RISK FACTORS
- Diabetes
- Smoking
- HTN
- Coronary artery disease
- Peripheral vascular disease
- Oral contraceptive use
- Polycythemia vera
- Sickle cell anemia
- Deficiencies of antithrombin III, protein C or S

### ETIOLOGY
- May be ischemic (thrombotic, embolic, or secondary to dissection/hypoperfusion) or hemorrhagic
- Thrombotic stroke is caused by occlusion of blood vessels:
  - Clot formation at an ulcerated atherosclerotic plaque is most common.
  - Sludging (sickle cell anemia, polycythemia vera, protein C deficiency)
- Embolic stroke is caused by acute blockage of a cerebral artery by a piece of foreign material from outside the brain, including:
  - Cardiac mural thrombi associated with mitral stenosis, atrial fibrillation, cardiomyopathy, CHF, or MI
  - Prosthetic or abnormal native valves
  - Atherosclerotic plaques in the aortic arch or carotid arteries
  - Atrial myxoma
  - Ventricular aneurysms with thrombi
- Arterial dissection:
  - Carotid artery dissection
  - Arteritis (giant cell, Takayasu)
  - Fibromuscular dysplasia
- Global ischemic or hypotensive stroke is caused by an overall decrease in systemic blood pressure: Sepsis, hemorrhage, shock
- Hemorrhagic stroke:
  - Intracranial hemorrhage
  - Subarachnoid hemorrhage

### Pediatric Considerations
Usually attributable to underlying disease process, such as sickle cell anemia, leukemia, or a blood dyscrasia

## DIAGNOSIS

### SIGNS AND SYMPTOMS
#### History
- Time of onset (or time last seen at baseline)
- Trauma/surgery
- Medications
- Altered mentation/confusion
- Headache
- Vertigo/dizzy
- Focal neurologic deficits

#### Physical Exam
- General:
  - Cheyne-Stokes breathing, apnea
  - HTN
  - Cardiac dysrhythmias, murmurs
- Anterior cerebral artery:
  - Contralateral hemiplegia (lower/upper)
  - Hemisensory loss
  - Apraxia
  - Confusion
  - Impaired judgment
- Middle cerebral artery:
  - Contralateral hemiplegia (upper/lower)
  - Hemisensory deficits
  - Homonymous hemianopsia
  - Dysphasia
  - Dysarthria
  - Agnosia
- Posterior cerebral artery:
  - Cortical blindness in half the visual field
  - Visual agnosia
  - Altered mental status
  - Impaired memory
  - 3rd-nerve palsy
  - Hemiballismus
- Vertebrobasilar system:
  - Impaired vision, visual field defects, nystagmus, diplopia
  - Vertigo, dizziness
  - Crossed deficits: Ipsilateral cranial nerve deficits with contralateral motor and sensory deficits
- Basilar system:
  - Quadriplegia
  - Locked-in syndrome
  - Coma
- Watershed area (boundary zone between anterior, middle, and posterior circulation):
  - Cortical blindness
  - Weakness of proximal upper and lower extremities with sparing of face, hands, and feet

### ESSENTIAL WORKUP
- Detailed neurologic exam; consider calculating National Institutes of Health stroke scale (NIHSS).
- Emergent noncontrast head CT scan to distinguish ischemic from hemorrhagic events:
  - May be normal in 1st 24–48 hr of ischemic stroke
- If CT is normal and subarachnoid hemorrhage is suspected, emergent lumbar puncture is indicated.
- EKG to evaluate for dysrhythmias and presence of MI
- Oxygen saturation measurement
- Rapid glucose determination

## DIAGNOSTIC TESTS & INTERPRETATION
### Lab
- Baseline CBC, electrolytes, renal function tests, liver function test, prothrombin time, partial thromboplastin time
- Urinalysis:
  - Hematuria can be seen in subacute bacterial endocarditis with embolic stroke.
- Sedimentation rate:
  - Elevated in subacute bacterial endocarditis, vasculitis, hyperviscosity syndromes
- Consider additional tests: Cardiac enzymes, urine pregnancy test, drug screen, alcohol level, ABG, and blood cultures.

### Imaging
- Noncontrast head CT
- MRI can detect ischemia <2 hr after onset.
- CXR
- ECG
- Carotid US

### Diagnostic Procedures/Surgery
- EKG to evaluate for arrhythmia
- Lumbar puncture if subarachnoid hemorrhage is suspected and head CT nondiagnostic

### DIFFERENTIAL DIAGNOSIS
- Intracranial bleeding
- Hypoglycemia
- Seizure disorder; Todd paralysis
- MI or CHF
- Panic attacks, depression, conversion reaction
- Transient global amnesia
- Meningoencephalitis
- Peripheral neuropathy
- Intracranial abscess
- Migraine
- Air embolism
- Transient ischemic attack
- Encephalopathy
- Neoplasm
- Subdural hematoma
- Giant cell/Takayasu arteritis
- Multiple sclerosis
- Compressive myelopathy
- Vestibulitis
- Medication effect/toxidrome

## TREATMENT

### PRE-HOSPITAL
- Patients may have difficulty moving or communicating after cerebral vascular accident.
- Neurologic exam in field is helpful:
  - Should include assessment of consciousness level, Glasgow coma scale score, gross motor deficits, speech abnormalities, gait disturbance, facial asymmetry, and other focal deficits
- Hyperglycemia may exacerbate an ischemic insult:
  - Perform rapid blood glucose testing before administration of glucose-containing fluids.

## INITIAL STABILIZATION/THERAPY

- Manage airway:
  - Supplemental oxygen 2–4 L via nasal cannula
  - Rapid-sequence intubation may be required for airway protection or controlled ventilation to decrease intracranial pressure.
  - IV access
  - Cardiac monitoring and pulse oximetry
- For altered mental status, give naloxone and thiamine and check blood glucose.

## ED TREATMENT/PROCEDURES

- Treat elevated BP with labetalol, nicardipine, nitroprusside, or hydralazine:
  - Systolic BP >220 mm Hg or diastolic BP >120 mm Hg on repeated measurements
  - If indicated for other concurrent problems (MI, aortic dissection, CHF, hypertensive encephalopathy)
  - Initial goal is systolic BP <180 mm Hg, diastolic <110 mm Hg.
- Control seizures with benzodiazepines, then phenytoin.
- Maintain euvolemia and normothermia.
- Thrombolytics:
  - Ischemic stroke only; administer within 4.5 hr of symptom onset
  - Contraindications:
    - Any history of intracranial hemorrhage
    - Recent stroke or head trauma <3 mo ago
    - Surgery <14 days ago
    - Systolic BP >185 mm Hg; diastolic BP >110 mm Hg
    - Bleeding diathesis
    - Noncompressible arterial puncture <7 days ago
    - MI <3 mo ago
    - Anticoagulation: INR >1.7, PT >15 sec, or prolonged PTT; use of heparin within 48 hr
    - Thrombocytopenia with platelets <100,000
    - Intracranial neoplasm
    - Seizure at stroke onset
    - Minor or rapidly improving symptoms
    - Pregnancy
    - Internal bleed (GI/GU) <3 wk ago
  - Avoid anticoagulants and antiplatelet drugs for 24 hr.
- Treat increased intracranial pressure and cerebral edema:
  - Elevate head of bed 30°
  - Controlled ventilation to keep partial pressure of carbon dioxide 35–40 mm Hg
  - Mannitol
- Urgent neurosurgical decompression may be required with brainstem compression in cases of vertebrobasilar stroke or hemorrhage.
- In patients with completed or minor strokes, aspirin may prevent recurrence.

- For focal embolic/thrombotic strokes:
  - Recannulation
  - US-enhanced thrombolysis
  - Intra-arterial thrombolysis

### ALERT

For patients presenting between 3 and 4.5 hr of onset, there are additional exclusion criteria:

- Age >80 yr
- Oral anticoagulant use (regardless of INR)
- NIH-SS >25 or >1/3 MCA territory involved
- History of previous stroke and diabetes

## MEDICATION

### First Line

- Alteplase (TPA): 0.9 mg/kg IV; max. 90 mg, with 10% of dose given as bolus and remainder infused over 60 min
- Aspirin: 81–325 mg PO daily
- Labetalol: 15–20 mg/min IV bolus, then 40–80 mg q10min max. 300 mg; follow with continuous infusion 0.5–2 mg/min

### Second Line

- Clopidogrel: 75 mg PO daily
- Diazepam: 5 mg IV q5–10 min max. 20 mg
- Enalapril: 0.675–1.25 mg IV
- Hydralazine: 10–20 mg IV q30min
- Mannitol (15–25% solution): 0.5–2 g/kg IV over 5–10 min, then 0.5–1 g/kg q4h–q6h
- Nicardipine: 5 mg/h IV infusion, increase by 2.5 mg/h q5–15min max. 15 mg/h
- Nitroprusside: 0.25–10 $\mu$g/kg/min
- Trimetaphan: 1–4 mg/min

## FOLLOW-UP

### DISPOSITION

#### Admission Criteria

- Patients with acute cerebral vascular accident should be admitted to hospital.
- Indications for ICU:
  - Severely decreased level of consciousness
  - Hemodynamic instability
  - Life-threatening cardiac dysrhythmias
  - Significantly increased intracranial pressure
  - Administration of alteplase

#### Discharge Criteria

- Patients who present with completed strokes that are days to weeks old may be discharged if they are able to function independently or have adequate social support.
- Patients with multiple prior strokes who experience relatively minor new episodes may also be treated on outpatient basis if similar criteria are met and stroke is completed.

### FOLLOW-UP RECOMMENDATIONS

- Neurology
- Primary care
- Speech therapy/occupational therapy

## PEARLS AND PITFALLS

- Always note pre-hospital observations.
- Timing of onset (new guidelines suggest TPA up to 4.5 hr after onset of symptoms):
  - Include additional exclusion criteria between 3 and 4.5 hr.
- Blood glucose testing
- Avoid aggressive blood pressure correction due to risk of hypoperfusion and extension of stroke.

## ADDITIONAL READING

- Adams HP, del Zoppo G, Alberts MJ, et al. Guidelines for the early management of adults with ischemic stroke: A guideline from the American Heart Association/American Stroke Association Stroke Council, Clinical Cardiology Council, Cardiovascular Radiology and Intervention Council, and the Atherosclerotic Peripheral Vascular Disease and Quality of Care Outcomes in Research Interdisciplinary Working Groups. Stroke. 2007;38(5):1655–1711.
- del Zoppo GJ, Saver JL, Jauch EC, et al. Expansion of the time window for treatment of acute ischemic stroke with IV/IV tissue plasminogen activator: A science advisory from the American Heart Association/American Stroke Association. Stroke. 2009;40:2945–2948.
- Fulgham JR, Ingall TJ, Stead LG, et al. Management of acute ischemic stroke. Mayo Clin Proc. 2004;11: 1459–1469.
- Hacke W, Kaste M, Bluhmki E, et al. Thrombolysis with alteplase 3 to 4.5 hours after acute ischemic stroke (ECASS III). N Engl J Med. 2008;359(13): 1317–1329.
- NINDS rt-PA Stroke Study Group. Tissue plasminogen activator for acute ischemic stroke. N Engl J Med. 1995;333:1581–1587.
- Williams M, Patil S, Toledo EG, et al. Management of acute ischemic stroke: Current status of pharmacological and mechanical endovascular methods. Neurol Res. 2009;31(8):807–815.
- www.ninds.nih.gov/doctors

### See Also (Topic, Algorithm, Electronic Media Element)

- Transient Ischemic Attack
- Intracranial Hemorrhage

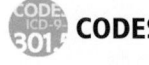 ## CODES

**ICD9**

434.91 Cerebral artery occlusion, unspecified with cerebral infarction

# CERVICAL ADENITIS

*Julie Zeller*

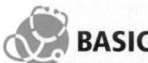 **BASICS**

## DESCRIPTION

- Cervical adenitis is an acute bacterial infection of a cervical lymph node, often arising after a prior bacterial infection of the head or neck area.
- Primarily a pediatric disease with 70–80% of patients falling in the 1–4-yr-old age group:
  - It is becoming more common in adults owing to immunocompromised disease states (HIV, cancer, transplant patients).
- Any cervical node can become infected:
  - >80% of childhood cervical lymphadenitis involves the submandibular or deep cervical nodes.
  - Jugulodigastric node located just below the angle of the mandible is very common site.
  - Cervical nodes act as the final common pathway for lymphatic drainage of all areas of the head and neck.
  - Initial lymphadenopathy results after bacterial invasion of regional areas of the head and neck.
  - Local lymph nodes swell secondary to hyperplasia of sinusoidal cells and infiltration of lymphocytes.
  - If the infection is not contained, the bacteria enter the lymph system and proliferate (lymphadenitis).
  - Pus forms when neutrophils are incited, and an abscess develops when host defenses are unable to clear infection.
  - Clinically manifests as warm, tender, swollen, erythematous node

## ETIOLOGY

- ~50–80% of cases are a result of group A β-hemolytic *Streptococcus* and *Staphylococcus aureus*.
- Infections secondary to community-acquired MRSA (CA-MRSA) have increased in frequency.
- Children have one of the highest rate of CA-MRSA colonization and invasive disease.
- Mycobacteria TB:
  - Scrofula or tuberculous lymphadenitis
  - Rarely seen
  - Usually a chronic lymphadenitis in the posterior cervical nodes
  - Purified protein derivative (PPD) is usually strongly reactive.
  - Treatment medical
- Atypical mycobacteria (nontuberculous) *Mycobacterium avium* complex:
  - More commonly seen
  - Usually a chronic lymphadenitis in the submandibular or anterior cervical nodes
  - PPD test results are unreliable.
  - Treatment is primarily surgical.

- *Bartonella henselae* (cat-scratch disease):
  - Subacute lymphadenitis
  - Fever and mild systemic symptoms occur in only ~3% of patients.
  - Has indolent course but usually spontaneously resolves after 4–6 wk
- Anaerobes:
  - Consider when associated with infections of the teeth or gingiva
- Rare organisms:
  - *Haemophilus influenzae*
  - *Yersinia pestis*
  - *Nocardia* species
  - *Francisella tularensis*
  - *Brucella melitensis*
  - *Mycoplasma pneumoniae*
  - *Treponema pallidum*
  - *Actinomyces israelii*

### Pediatric Considerations

- One of the most common causes of a neck mass in a child
- Overall, group A β-*Streptococcus* and *Staphylococcus aureus* most common causes
- In neonates, group B *Streptococcus* and *Staphylococcus aureus* most common
- Group B streptococcal cellulitis-adenitis syndrome:
  - Infants are usually 3–7 wk of age, male, febrile, with submandibular or facial cellulitis, and an ipsilateral otitis
  - 94% incidence of concurrent bacteremia
- *Staphylococcus aureus* associated with more indolent course and higher frequency of suppuration

### Geriatric Considerations

- Consider malignancy over infection in this population, especially in the absence of fever, leukocytosis, etc.
- Fixed, nontender, hard node most likely not cervical adenitis

## DIAGNOSIS

### SIGNS AND SYMPTOMS

- Enlarged, tender cervical lymph node
- Usually unilateral and solitary
- Warmth and erythema of overlying skin
- Early in course, node is firm but may become fluctuant later
- With or without fever
- Malaise
- Irritability in infants and children
- Usually a concurrent head and neck infection:
  - Pharyngitis, tonsillitis, peritonsillar abscess
  - Otitis media, otitis externa
  - Dental infection
  - Impetigo, scalp infection

### History

- Time of onset of symptoms
- Associated symptoms: Fever, weight loss, rash
- Exposures/travel history
- Comorbities/birth history for infants

### Physical Exam

Complete evaluation of head and neck with attention to airway and patient's clinical appearance

### ESSENTIAL WORKUP

- Cervical adenitis is a clinical diagnosis.
- Identify primary source of infection in head and neck area (eg, otitis media, tonsillitis).
- If no primary inflammatory source of infection in head and neck:
  - Address possible TB exposure with PPD.
  - Look for signs of systemic disease and viral illness.

### DIAGNOSTIC TESTS & INTERPRETATION

### Lab

- Unnecessary if a treatable primary source of infection confirmed
- Blood cultures for toxic-appearing patients
- Sepsis workup in neonates
- If cause unclear, the following lab tests may help to discern a nonbacterial cause (see "Differential Diagnosis"):
  - Leukocyte count with differential
  - Monospot
  - Throat cultures
  - Antibody titers (Epstein-Barr virus, CMV, toxoplasmosis)

### Imaging

- CXR study, lateral neck, or Panorex:
  - Helpful if source of infection unclear or to rule out a deep space infection
  - Chest radiograph study to screen for TB
- CT or MRI of neck:
  - Helpful in delineating embryonic developmental masses or ruling out deep-space infections
- US:
  - Can differentiate cystic from solid structures, but other findings nonspecific
  - Can identify deep-cavity abscess if not palpable on exam
- Excisional biopsy

### Diagnostic Procedures/Surgery

- Needle aspiration:
  - All fluctuant nodes should be aspirated.
  - Send for gram stain and acid-fast stains, aerobic and anaerobic cultures, mycobacteria, and fungi.
  - If any suspicion of tuberculous lymphadenitis, the node should not be aspirated owing to risk for sinus development and chronic drainage.
- Intradermal skin testing:
  - Mycobacteria, catscratch disease

## DIFFERENTIAL DIAGNOSIS

- Lymphadenopathy (inflammation of node but no bacterial infection) can be a sign of many systemic diseases; usually these nodes are multiple and bilateral.
- Viral infections are a common cause:
  - Respiratory viruses (adenoviruses, rhinoviruses, enteroviruses)
  - Epstein-Barr virus, herpes simplex virus, varicella-zoster virus, CMV
  - Mumps, rubella, rubeola
- Specific pediatric diseases with cervical adenitis in their diagnostic criteria:
  - Kawasaki disease
  - Kikuchi disease
  - Periodic fever, aphthous stomatitis, pharyngitis, and cervical adenitis known by mnemonic PFAPA (seen in preschool-aged children)
- Toxoplasmosis
- Congenital cysts:
  - Brachial cleft cysts, thyroglossal duct cysts, cystic hygromas
- Malignancies:
  - Leukemia, lymphoma, rhabdomyosarcoma, thyroid carcinoma
  - Rare cause of a nonspecific lump in children (<2% overall)
- Other systemic diseases:
  - Lupus, sarcoidosis

 **TREATMENT**

### INITIAL STABILIZATION/THERAPY

- Oxygen, monitor airway for any signs of compromise
- Universal precautions

### ED TREATMENT/PROCEDURES

- Treatment directed toward the primary source of infection in the head and neck:
  - If unsure of cause, treat for group A *Streptococcus* and *Staphylococcus aureus*.
  - Consider MRSA if symptoms not improving on standard antibiotic therapy
- Aspirate all fluctuant nodes.
- Many oral antibiotics are effective:
  - Cephalexin
  - Dicloxacillin
  - Amoxicillin/clavulanic acid
  - Erythromycin (not as effective against *Staphylococcus aureus*)
- Patients with suspected dental, periodontal, or anaerobic causes of illness:
  - Clindamycin
  - Penicillin V
  - Amoxicillin/clavulanic acid

- CA-MRSA:
  - Clindamycin (many isolates are now resistant)
  - Bactrim
  - Vancomycin if toxic and requiring inpatient care
- Treatment should be for at least 10 days, even if symptoms resolve sooner.
- Warm, moist compresses
- Analgesics, as needed

## MEDICATION

### First Line

- Dicloxacillin: 250–500 mg (peds: 25–50 mg/kg/24 h) PO q6h
- Cephalexin: 250–500 mg (peds: 25–50 mg/kg/24 h) PO q6h
- Penicillin VK: 250–500 mg (peds: 25–50 mg/kg/24 h) PO q6h
- Erythromycin: 250–500 mg (peds: 40 mg/kg/24 h) PO q6h **NOT effective against Staph aureus
- Amoxicillin/clavulanic acid: 250–500 mg (peds: 20–40 mg/kg/24 h) PO q8h
- Clindamycin: 300 mg (peds: 8–25 mg/kg/24 h) PO q6h
- TMP-SMX (Bactrim): DS (160/800) 2 tabs PO b.i.d. (peds: 40 mg/200 mg/10 kg) PO b.i.d. **MRSA

### Second Line

- Cefazolin: 1–2 g (peds: 25–50 mg/kg/24 h) IV q8h
- Nafcillin: 1–2 g (peds: 50–200 mg/kg/24 h) IV q4–6h
- Clindamycin: 600–900 mg (peds: 20–40 mg/kg/24 h) IV q8h
- Ampicillin-sulbactam: 1.5–3 g (peds: 200 mg/kg/day) q6h
- Vancomycin: 1 g (peds 40–60 mg/kg/day) q8h IV **MRSA

 **FOLLOW-UP**

### DISPOSITION

#### Admission Criteria

- Neonates
- Airway compromise
- Patient appears ill.
- Immunocompromised
- Inability to take PO
- Not improving on oral antibiotics

#### Discharge Criteria

- Most patients can be discharged on PO antibiotics.
- Close follow-up with a recheck in 2–3 days
- Ability to take PO antibiotics and fluids
- Return to the ED if:
  - Symptoms worsen
  - Abscess develops
  - Voice changes
  - Dyspnea develops
  - Systemic symptoms develop

### Issues for Referral

Clinical exam concerning for malignancy or congenital abnormality (brachial cleft/thyroglossal duct cyst)

### FOLLOW-UP RECOMMENDATIONS

- Mandatory recheck in 48 hr to ensure improvement
- Referral to dentist or ENT depending on source of infection

## PEARLS AND PITFALLS

Cervical adenitis is a clinical diagnosis:

- Unilateral warm, tender, swollen, erythematous lymph node
- Most common bacteria responsible for infection are group A *Strep* and *S. aureus*.
- Consider group B Strep in infants and MRSA for infections not improving on standard antibiotics.
- Disposition should be influenced by patient's clinical status.

## ADDITIONAL READING

- Dullin MF, Kennard TP, Leach L, et al. Management of cervical lymphadenitis in children. *Am Fam Physician.* 2008;78:1097–1098.
- Hay WW Jr, Levin MJ, Sondheimer JM, et al., eds. *CURRENT Diagnosis & Treatment: Pediatrics,* 19th ed. McGraw-Hill; 2009.
- Swanson D. Etiology and clinical manifestations of cervical lymphadenitis in children. *UpToDate.com/online*
- Shaikh U. Lymphadenitis. *Emedicine.* http://www.emedicine.com/ped/topic32.htm

### See Also (Topic, Algorithm, Electronic Media Element)

- Kawasaki Disease
- Lymphadenitis

 **CODES**

### ICD9

- 289.3 Lymphadenitis, unspecified, except mesenteric
- 683 Acute lymphadenitis

# CESAREAN SECTION, EMERGENCY

*James S. Walker*
*Jonathan B. Walker*

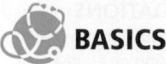

## BASICS

### ALERT
- The sole indication for ED physician to perform emergency perimortem cesarean section is a gravid female (>24 wk gestation) in cardiopulmonary arrest who has not responded to initial resuscitative measures, regardless of cause.
- The most important predictor of fetal survival is length of time between maternal cardiac arrest and cesarean delivery:
  – Cesarean section should begin within 4 min of maternal arrest.
  – Goal is delivering fetus within 1 min.
- Obtain immediate consultations from obstetrics, pediatrics (and surgery, if trauma related):
  – Do not defer or delay performing procedure until arrival of consultants.
- Do not perform emergent cesarean section if patient is <24 wk gestation.

### ETIOLOGY
- Trauma (penetrating or blunt):
  – Major cause of maternal mortality
- Pulmonary embolus:
  – Thromboembolism is number 1 cause of nontraumatic maternal mortality.
- Cerebral vascular accident
- Amniotic fluid embolism
- DIC
- Placenta previa
- Eclampsia
- Miscellaneous medical disorders:
  – Asthma
  – CHF
  – MI
  – Drug overdose

## DIAGNOSIS

### SIGNS AND SYMPTOMS
*History*
Gravid female (>24 wk gestation determined by uterine fundal height) who is in cardiopulmonary arrest.

*Physical Exam*
Patient is determined to be >24 wk gestation if uterus is at least 4 finger breadths above umbilicus

### ESSENTIAL WORKUP
- Physical examination for apnea and pulselessness in obviously gravid female:
  – Quickly evaluate for reversible causes of cardiopulmonary arrest:
    ○ Hypoxia
    ○ Hypovolemia
    ○ Hydrogen ion (acidosis)
    ○ Hypokalemia/hyperkalemia
    ○ Hypoglycemia
    ○ Hypothermia
    ○ Trauma
    ○ Thromboembolism
    ○ Toxins/poisons
    ○ Tension pneumothorax
    ○ Tamponade (pericardial)
  – Supine hypotension syndrome (compression of inferior vena cava by enlarged uterus)
- Assess gestational age by uterine fundal height.
- Distance from pubis to fundus in centimeters is roughly equivalent to gestational age in weeks.
- US is beneficial if *immediately* available to assess fetus.

### DIAGNOSTIC TESTS & INTERPRETATION
*Imaging*
- None necessary to establish cardiopulmonary arrest
- Do *not* use valuable time attempting to determine fetal heart tones.

### DIFFERENTIAL DIAGNOSIS
Cardiopulmonary arrest is final common pathway:
- Evaluate for underlying cause.

## TREATMENT

### PRE-HOSPITAL
Cautions:
- Minimal scene time, "scoop and run"
- Place the patient in the left lateral decubitus position to avoid compression of inferior vena cava (supine hypotension syndrome).
- Trauma patient requiring spinal immobilization:
  – Uterus can be manually displaced to left.
  – Backboard can be wedged to keep right hip elevated 45°.

### INITIAL STABILIZATION/THERAPY
- Standard resuscitation measures:
  – Emergency intubation
  – High-flow oxygen
  – Cardiac and BP monitoring
  – 2 large-bore peripheral IV lines:
    ○ Fluid resuscitation
    ○ O-negative blood if indicated
- Fetal survival correlates with maternal survival and adequacy of initial maternal resuscitation.
- If patient is at <24 wk gestation, use advanced cardiac life support and advanced trauma life support protocols directed at maternal resuscitation; do *not* perform emergent cesarean section.
- If patient is >24 wk gestation, use 4-min rule:
  – Perform advanced cardiac life support (ACLS) or advanced trauma life support for 4 min.
  – If no response, proceed to immediate emergency cesarean section.
  – Goal is to deliver fetus within 1 min.
  – If it is obvious there is no chance for maternal survival, begin perimortem cesarean section immediately.

### ED TREATMENT/PROCEDURES

- Call for immediate obstetric, surgical, and pediatric consultations:
  - Do *not* delay performing procedure while waiting for consultants.
- Ensure a Foley catheter has been inserted to decompress bladder, but do not delay procedure.
- Perform cesarean section:
  - Use linea nigra as landmark for vertical midline incision.
  - Incise abdominal wall from pubic hairline to 5 cm above umbilicus.
  - This incision should pass through fascial and peritoneal layers.
  - Retract urinary bladder inferiorly against pubic symphysis.
  - Make small vertical incision in lower uterine segment, just cephalad to urinary bladder.
  - Extend incision cephalad with scissors:
    - Insert your free hand into uterus.
    - Lift uterine wall away from fetus to avoid fetal injury.
  - Deliver fetus.
  - Clamp umbilical cord in 2 places and cut between the 2 clamps.
  - Manually deliver placenta.
  - Perform neonatal resuscitation, as indicated.
  - Immediately reassess maternal vital signs because occasionally spontaneous circulation may return.
  - Continue maternal resuscitation as appropriate.
  - Suture uterus with running lock stitch using no. 0 polyglactin suture.
  - Suture fascia and peritoneum with running stitch using no. 0 polyglactin suture.
  - Close the skin with staples or suture.
  - Administer broad-spectrum antibiotics.

### MEDICATION

#### First Line
Resuscitative measures/ACLS medications directed at mother:
- Treatment of underlying cause

#### Second Line
Neonatal resuscitation should be anticipated:
- Oral tracheal intubation

 **FOLLOW-UP**

### DISPOSITION

#### Admission Criteria
- The infant should be admitted to NICU.
- If maternal resuscitation is successful, patient should be admitted to appropriate ICU.

#### Discharge Criteria
Neither infant nor mother should be discharged from ED.

## PEARLS AND PITFALLS

- Only females >24 wk pregnant in cardiopulmonary arrest qualify for the procedure.
- Decision to perform perimortem cesarean section must be made quickly (within 4 min of maternal cardiopulmonary arrest). Procrastination can be fatal.
- Procedure must be done quickly (<1 min).

### ADDITIONAL READING

- Boyd R, Teece S. Towards evidence based emergency medicine: Best BETs from the Manchester Royal Infirmary. Perimortem caesarean section. *Emerg Med J*. 2002;19:324–325.
- Brown HL. Trauma in pregnancy. *Obstet Gynecol*. 2009;114:147–160.
- Cusick SS, Tibbles CD. Trauma in pregnancy. *Emerg Med Clin N Am*. 2007;25:861–872.
- Hill CC, Pickinpaugh J. Trauma and surgical emergencies in the obstetric patient. *Surg Clin N Am*. 2008;88:421–440.
- Muench MV, Canterino JC. Trauma in pregnancy. *Obstet Gynecol Clin N Am*. 2007;34:555–583.
- Roberts JR, Hedges JR, Chanmugan AS, et al., eds. *Clinical Procedures in Emergency Medicine*, 4th ed. Philadelphia: Saunders; 2004.
- Stallord TC, Burns B. Emergency delivery and perimortem C-section. *Emerg Med Clin North Am*. 2003;21:679–693.

 **CODES**

#### ICD9
- 669.70 Cesarean delivery, without mention of indication, unspecified as to episode of care
- 669.71 Cesarean delivery, without mention of indication, delivered, with or without mention of antepartum condition

# CHANCROID
*Norbert Elsner*

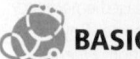 **BASICS**

## DESCRIPTION
- Sexually transmitted genital ulcerative disease:
  - Increased risk for HIV infection
- A common cause of genital ulceration in Africa, southeast Asia, and Latin America:
  - Uncommon in U.S. where HSV > syphilis >> chancroid, but likely underreported

## ETIOLOGY
Causative agent: Haemophilus ducreyi:
- Highly infectious bacterium

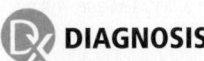 **DIAGNOSIS**

## SIGNS AND SYMPTOMS
- Begins as a single erythematous papule or pustule:
  - Quickly erodes into painful chancres (1–20 mm)
  - Soft and friable with ragged, irregular borders
- Primary ulcer usually excavated
- Moist, granulation tissue at base
- Purulent or hemorrhagic exudate
- Location:
  - Male:
    ○ Penile shaft, glans, internal surface of foreskin, anus
  - Female:
    ○ Cervix, vagina, vulva, perineum, anus

- Occurs 4–7 days (median) after exposure
- Incubation period 3–10 days (range 1–35 days)
- Inguinal adenopathy:
  - In ~50% of men; less common in women
  - Appears 3–14 days after initial ulcer
  - Unilateral (usually)
  - Painful
  - Suppurative large nodes (buboes)
  - May rupture and form chronic draining sinuses
- Dysuria, dyspareunia secondary to contact with lesions
- Variants:
  - Phagedenic:
    ○ Secondary superinfection (especially fusospirochetal) and rapid extensive tissue destruction
  - Giant chancroid:
    ○ Very large single ulcer
  - Serpiginous ulcer:
    ○ Rapidly spreading, indolent, shallow ulcers in groin or thigh
  - Follicular:
    ○ Multiple small ulcers with perifollicular distribution

## ESSENTIAL WORKUP
Clinical diagnosis based on appearance is often inaccurate, and lab tests difficult or unavailable, so consider:
- CDC case definitions:
  - Definite: Positive culture of *H ducreyi*
  - Probable: Typical signs, symptoms of chancroid PLUS negative darkfield exam for *T. pallidum* PLUS negative syphilis serology PLUS negative culture for HSV (or clinical exam atypical for herpes)

## DIAGNOSTIC TESTS & INTERPRETATION
*Lab*
- Gram stain unreliable (positive in 50–80%):
  - Gram-negative coccobacilli: Linear or "school-of-fish" pattern
- Culture extremely difficult (positive in 0–80%); requires complex media:
  - Obtain specimen from:
    ○ Base of ulcer
    ○ Needle aspiration of inguinal node by placing needle through normal skin (to avoid formation of fistula)
- Polymerase chain reaction (PCR) assay: Sensitive and specific, but not widely available
- RPR:
  - Coinfection with syphilis is common.
  - Part of CDC guidelines for probable clinical diagnosis of chancroid
- Herpes simplex virus (HSV) culture:
  - Part of CDC guidelines for probable clinical diagnosis of chancroid
- HIV testing

## DIFFERENTIAL DIAGNOSIS
- Infectious:
  - Syphilis (*T. pallidum*):
    ○ Chancre usually painless, indurated, clean
  - Herpes genitalis (*H. simplex):
    ○ Vesicular, multiple, recurrent
  - Granuloma inguinale (donovanosis) (*Klebsiella granulomatis*):
    ○ Ulcer margins elevated; + induration
  - Lymphogranuloma venereum (*C. trachomatis*):
    ○ Often single lesion; tender, fluctuant, unilateral lymphadenopathy
- Noninfectious:
  - Drug eruption
  - Less common:
    ○ Pyoderma gangrenosum; Behçet disease

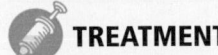 TREATMENT

### INITIAL STABILIZATION/THERAPY
Usual precautions for patient exam and handling of specimens

### ED TREATMENT/PROCEDURES
Antibiotics:

- Azithromycin: Single PO dose
- Ceftriaxone: Single IM dose (pregnancy: 1st line)
- Ciprofloxacin: PO × 3 days:
  – NOT for pregnant/lactating patients
- Erythromycin base: PO × 7 days:
  – Pregnancy: 2nd line
- Needle aspiration of suppurative nodes (>5 cm diameter):
  – To prevent chronic sinus drainage from spontaneous rupture
  – Use 18-gauge needle through lateral intact skin.
  – May require repetition
- Recommend concurrent HIV, syphilis, HSV testing *and* follow-up testing in 3 mo if initially negative.

### MEDICATION

**First Line**
- Azithromycin: 1 g PO × 1
- Ceftriaxone: 250 mg IM × 1

**Second Line**
- Ciprofloxacin: 500 mg PO b.i.d for 3 days
- Erythromycin base: 500 mg PO q.i.d. for 7 days

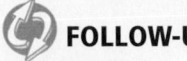 FOLLOW-UP

### DISPOSITION
**Discharge Criteria**
- Sexual abstinence or condom use until lesions healed
- Clinical course:
  – Symptoms improve within 2 days of treatment.
  – Ulcers improve within 3–7 days.
  – Possible delayed resolution in those HIV-positive or uncircumcised

### FOLLOW-UP RECOMMENDATIONS
Examine and treat sexual partners (regardless of presence/absence of symptoms) if contact within 10 days of symptom onset.

## PEARLS AND PITFALLS

- Initiate treatment if probable CDC case guidelines met. Do not wait for culture results.
- Higher risk of treatment failure in HIV-infected patients
- Presumptive treatment of sexual contacts.
- Treatment failure: Consider drug resistance, medication noncompliance, coinfection (syphilis).

## ADDITIONAL READING

- Centers for Disease Control and Prevention. Sexually Transmitted Diseases Treatment Guidelines 2006. Available at www.cdc.gov/std/treatment. Accessed March 15, 2010.
- Chancroid. *UpToDate Online*. 2008;v17.3. Available at www.uptodate.com
- Marx JA, Hockberger RS, Walls RM, et al. *Rosen's Emergency Medicine: Concepts and Clinical Practice*, 7th ed. St. Louis, MO: Mosby; 2009.

 CODES

### ICD9
099.0 Chancroid

# CHEMICAL WEAPONS POISONING

*Patrick M. Whiteley*

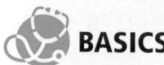

## BASICS

### DESCRIPTION
Chemical agents that affect CNS, pulmonary, cardiovascular, dermal, ocular, or GI systems when exposed to victims

### ETIOLOGY
- Blood agents: Cyanide:
  - Inhibition of cellular respiration by binding to ferric ion in cytochrome oxidase a-a3 and uncoupling oxidative phosphorylization
- Blister agents: Sulfur mustard, nitrogen mustard, lewisite, phosgene oxime:
  - Alkylation and cross-linking of purine bases of DNA and amino acids resulting in change in structure of nucleic acid, proteins, and cellular membranes
- Lacrimators and riot control agents: 1-chloroacetophenone (CN; Mace), o-chlorobenzylidene malononitrile (CS), oleoresin capsicin-pepper spray (OC), chloropicrin, adamsite (DM):
  - Mucous membrane irritators
- Pulmonary irritants (choking agents):
  - High water solubility: Ammonia:
    - Mucous membrane irritation of eyes and upper airway
  - Intermediate water solubility: Chlorine:
    - Forms hydrochloric acid, hydrochlorous acids, which form free radicals causing upper airway and pulmonary irritation
  - Low water solubility: Phosgene:
    - Mild irritant effects initially, then delayed pulmonary edema as late as 24 hr
    - Direct pulmonary damage after hydrolysis in lungs to hydrochloric acid
- Nerve agents:
  - Anticholinesterase inhibitors—causes cholinergic overstimulation at muscarinic, nicotinic, and CNS sites
- Incapacitating agents: 3-quinuclidinyl benzilate (BZ):
  - Anticholinergic (antimuscarinic)

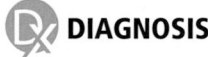

## DIAGNOSIS

### SIGNS AND SYMPTOMS
#### History
Multiple victims, house fire, known exposure (agent determines history findings)

#### Physical Exam
- Blood agents (cyanide and cyanogens):
  - Vital signs:
    - Tachypnea and hyperpnea (early); respiratory depression (late)
    - Hypertension and tachycardia (early); hypotension and bradycardia (late)
    - Death within seconds to minutes
  - CNS:
    - Headache
    - Mental status changes
    - Seizures

- Pulmonary:
  - Dyspnea
  - Noncardiogenic pulmonary edema
  - Cyanosis uncommon
- GI:
  - Odor of bitter almonds (sometimes)
  - Burning in mouth and throat
  - Nausea, vomiting
- Blister agents (mustards, lewisite):
  - General:
    - Mortality, 2–4%
  - Dermatologic:
    - Skin erythema, edema, pruritus can appear 2–24 hr after exposure.
    - Necrosis and vesiculation appear 2–18 hr after exposure.
  - Head, eyes, ears, nose, and throat (HEENT):
    - Airway occlusion from sloughing of debris
    - Laryngospasm, sore throat, sinusitis
    - Eye pain, photophobia, lacrimation, blurred vision, blepharospasm, periorbital edema, conjunctival edema, corneal ulceration
  - Pulmonary:
    - Bronchospasm, tracheobronchitis
    - Respiratory failure
    - Hacking cough
  - GI:
    - Nausea, vomiting
  - Hematologic:
    - Leukopenia
- Lacrimators and riot control agents (tear gases):
  - HEENT:
    - Eye pain
    - Lacrimation
    - Blepharospasm
    - Temporary blindness
  - Dermatologic:
    - Skin irritation
    - Papulovesicular dermatitis (tear gas)
    - Superficial burns
  - Pulmonary:
    - Cough
    - Chest tightness
    - Dry throat
    - Sensation of suffocation
    - Pulmonary edema when exposed to high concentrations without ventilation
- Pulmonary irritants (choking agents):
  - HEENT:
    - Eye pain, lacrimation, blepharospasm
    - Temporary blindness
  - Dermatologic:
    - Skin irritation, dry throat, nasal irritation
  - Pulmonary:
    - Shortness of breath, cough, bronchospasm
    - Chest pain
    - Pulmonary edema as late as 24 hr from exposure (phosgene)

- Nerve agents (sarin, tabun, soman, VX):
  - *SLUDGEBAM* syndrome:
    - *Salivation*
    - *Lacrimation*
    - *Urination*
    - *Defecation*
    - *GI cramps*
    - *Emesis*
    - *Bronchorrhea, bronchoconstriction, bradycardia (most life threatening)*
    - *Abdominal upset*
    - *Miosis*
  - HEENT:
    - Miosis
    - Hypersecretion by salivary, sweat, lacrimal, and bronchial glands
  - CNS:
    - Irritability, nervousness
    - Giddiness
    - Fatigue, lethargy, depression
    - Ataxia, convulsions, coma
  - Pulmonary:
    - Bronchoconstriction
    - Bronchorrhea
  - GI:
    - Nausea, vomiting, diarrhea
    - Crampy abdominal pains
    - Urinary and fecal incontinence
  - Musculoskeletal:
    - Fasciculations, skeletal muscle twitching
    - Weakness
    - Flaccid paralysis
- Incapacitating agents (BZ):
  - Anticholinergic (antimuscarinic) toxidrome:
    - Hot as a hare
    - Dry as a bone
    - Red as a beet
    - Blind as a bat
    - Mad as a hatter
    - Hypertension
    - Tachycardia
    - Hyperpyrexia
    - Urinary retention
    - Decreased bowel sounds

### ESSENTIAL WORKUP
- History and symptoms key to type of agent exposure
- Physical examination:
  - Cyanide (bitter almonds, comatose, hypotensive, metabolic acidosis)
  - Mustard (faint, sweet odor of mustard or garlic, blisters, sloughing of skin, dyspnea)
  - Check for SLUDGEBAM syndrome.
  - Lacrimators (eye irritation, lacrimation, blepharospasm)
  - Choking agents (dyspnea, bronchospasm)

## DIAGNOSTIC TESTS & INTERPRETATION
*Lab*
- Arterial blood gases:
  - Cyanide:
    - Decreased atrioventricular (AV) oxygen saturation gap
    - Lactic acidemia with high anion gap metabolic acidosis
    - Arterialization of venous blood
    - Cyanide levels cannot be performed in clinically relevant timeframe.
- CBC:
  - Leukopenia, thrombocytopenia, anemia with significant mustard exposure
- Electrolytes, BUN, creatinine, glucose
- Urinalysis
- Creatine phosphokinase (CPK)
- Lactate for cyanide
- Erythrocyte cholinesterase activity for nerve agents

*Imaging*
CXR for pulmonary edema

## DIFFERENTIAL DIAGNOSIS
- Asthma/COPD
- Stevens-Johnson syndrome
- Toxic epidermal necrolysis
- Pemphigus vulgaris
- Scalded skin syndrome
- Organophosphate or carbamate pesticide poisoning
- Botulism
- Radiation poisoning
- CHF
- Anaphylactoid reaction

 **TREATMENT**

### PRE-HOSPITAL
- Avoid contamination of environment and clinicians:
  - Use level A or level B personal protective equipment.
  - Decontamination:
    - Dermal wet decontamination primarily for nerve and blistering agents
    - Dry decontamination (removal of clothing and jewelry) for other agents
- Administer atropine even if patient is tachycardic because condition may result from hypoxia.

### INITIAL STABILIZATION/THERAPY
- ABCs
- Patient decontamination:
  - Brush off powder from chemical.
  - Irrigate skin and eyes with copious amounts of water or saline.
  - Remove and dispose of clothing in double bags.
- Protection for healthcare workers:
  - Level A or B personal protective suit
  - Chemical-resistant suit
  - Heavy rubber gloves and boots, neoprene gloves
- Administer oxygen, place on cardiac monitor, and measure pulse oximetry.
- Establish IV access with 0.9% NS.

## ED TREATMENT/PROCEDURES
- Decontamination: Reduce secondary exposure
- Blood agents:
  - High flow 100% NRB oxygen
  - Benzodiazepines for seizures
  - Hydroxocobalamin (1st line)
  - Cyanide antidote kit (2nd line), may be repeated.
- Blister agents:
  - Supportive care
  - Standard burn management
  - Atropine to relieve eye pain
  - Monitor fluids, electrolytes, complete blood chemistry.
  - Monitor CBC for nadir.
  - Supportive care for sepsis, anemia, hemorrhage
  - Granulocyte colony-stimulating factor (G-CSF) for neutropenia
- Choking agents, lacrimators, riot control agents:
  - Supportive care, bronchodilators
  - Eye irrigation
  - CXR and careful monitoring for respiratory complications
  - Phosgenes require monitoring for delayed pulmonary edema for 24 hr
- Nerve agents:
  - Supportive care:
    - 100% oxygen
    - Frequent airway suctioning
  - Atropine 2 mg IV q5min until reversal of bronchorrhea, bronchoconstriction, and hypoxemia:
    - Antagonizes muscarinic effects and some CNS but no effect on skeletal muscle weakness or respiratory failure
    - Pupillary response and heart rate are not useful measures of adequate atropinization.
    - Stop atropine after patient regains consciousness and spontaneous ventilation (may need for periodic relapses); give as much as it takes to reverse respiratory compromise.
  - Pralidoxime chloride (2-PAM or Protopam):
    - Regenerates cholinesterase by reversing phosphorylation (unless aging has occurred)
    - Reduces abnormal skeletal muscle movements, improves skeletal muscle weakness, and reverses flaccid paralysis
    - May repeat 1st dose or start on continuous infusion
    - If improvement from 1st dose, repeat 60–90 min later.
  - Diazepam: Administer for seizures.
- Incapacitating agents (BZ):
  - Supportive care
  - Aggressive IV fluid hydration
  - Benzodiazepines for agitation and increased muscular activity
  - Consider physostigmine in consultation with a poison center.

## MEDICATION
- Albuterol using nebulizer: 2.5 mg in 2.5 mL NS (peds: 0.1–0.15 mg/kg per dose)
- Atropine: 2 mg IM or IV (6 mg in severely intoxicated patients; peds: 0.02–0.08 mg/kg), then q5–10min titrate to clinical effect
- Diazepam: 5–10 mg IV over 3–5 min (peds: 0.2–0.4 mg/kg up to 10 mg over 2–3 min)

- Hydroxocobalamin: 5 g IV
- Cyanide antidote kit:
  - Inhale amyl nitrite ampule for 30 sec qmin until sodium nitrite given.
  - Sodium nitrite: 10 mL of 3% solution or 300 mg IV over 3–5 min (peds: 0.15–0.33 mL/kg):
    - Monitor methemoglobin levels to keep <30%.
  - Sodium thiosulfate: 50 mL IV of 25% solution or 12.5 g (peds: 1.65 mL/kg)
- Pralidoxime chloride (2-PAM, Protopam): 1–2 g IV over 20–30 min or 600 mg IM (diluted with water or saline to concentration of 300 mg/mL) given with 1st 3 atropine doses (peds: 25–50 mg/kg per dose IV), repeat in 2 hr if muscle weakness has not been relieved, and in 4- to 6-hr intervals if necessary. Continuous infusion of 500 mg/h has been used for organophosphate poisoning.

 **FOLLOW-UP**

### DISPOSITION
*Admission Criteria*
- ICU admission for symptomatic patients with significant exposure
- Hospital admission to monitor for developing complications for blister, choking, lacrimating agents, incapacitating agents

*Discharge Criteria*
Riot control exposures:
- Observe in ED for 6 hr and discharge if symptoms resolve.
- High/intermediate water solubility gas exposures can be discharged in 6 hr if asymptomatic.

### FOLLOW-UP RECOMMENDATIONS
Agent dependent. Long-term neurological symptoms possible.

## PEARLS AND PITFALLS
Inadequate decontamination

## ADDITIONAL READING
- Davis K, Aspera G. Exposure to liquid sulfur mustard. *Ann Emerg Med*. 2001;37:653–656.
- Ford M, Delaney K, Ling L, et al. *Clinical Toxicology*. Philadelphia: WB Saunders; 2001.
- Keyes DC. Chemical warfare agents. In: Dart RC, et al., eds. *Medical Toxicology*, 3rd ed. Philadelphia: Lippincott Williams & Wilkins; 2004:1777–1794.

 **CODES**

### ICD9
989.9 Toxic effect of unspecified substance, chiefly nonmedicinal as to source

# CHEST PAIN

*Edward Ullman*

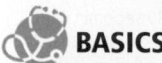 **BASICS**

## DESCRIPTION

- One of the most frequent chief complaints in the ED
- Often the presenting symptom of a high-risk etiology:
  - Acute coronary syndrome
  - Pulmonary embolism
  - Aortic dissection
- Assume life-threatening until proven otherwise.
- Categorization may suggest the underlying etiology, but the presentation of chest pain can be extremely variable and vague.
- Thoracic pain:
  - May involve the myocardium, pericardium, the ascending aorta, pulmonary artery, mediastinum, and esophagus
  - Pain is deep, visceral, and poorly localized.
  - Characteristics vary from severe and crushing to mild, burning, or indigestion.
- Epigastric pain:
  - May involve the descending aorta, diaphragmatic muscles, gallbladder, pancreas, duodenum, and stomach
  - Pain is generally referred to the xiphoid region and in the back.
- Pleuritic pain:
  - Inflammation or trauma to the ribs, cartilage, muscles, nerves, pleural or pericardial surface
  - Pain increased by breathing, laughing, coughing, sneezing
  - Tenderness to palpation may be present.
  - Diaphragmatic pleurisy:
    - ○ Sharp shooting pains in the epigastrium, lower retrosternal area, or shoulder intensified by thoracic movement
- Chest wall pain:
  - Inflammation of skin and subcutaneous structures of the chest wall
  - Pain is reproduced by:
    - ○ Palpation
    - ○ Horizontal flexion of the arms
    - ○ Extension of the neck
    - ○ Vertical pressure on the head

## ETIOLOGY

- Thoracic:
  - Acute coronary syndrome
  - Pericarditis
  - Myocarditis
  - Stress-induced cardiomyopathy
  - Cardiac syndrome X
  - Stimulant use
  - Thoracic aortic dissection
  - Esophagitis
  - Esophageal spasm
  - GERD
  - Esophageal hyperalgesia
  - Abnormal motility patterns and achalasia
  - Esophageal rupture and mediastinitis

- Epigastric:
  - Dissection of the descending aorta
  - Peptic ulcer disease
  - Pancreatitis
  - Cholecystitis
  - Splenic rupture
  - Hepatic injury
  - Subdiaphragmatic abscess
- Pleuritic pain:
  - Pulmonary embolism
  - Pneumothorax
  - Pneumonia
  - Costochondritis
- Diaphragmatic pleurisy:
  - Splenic rupture
  - Hepatic injury
  - Subdiaphragmatic abscess
- Esophageal rupture
- Intercostal myositis
- Intercostal neuralgia
- Pectoralis minor strain
- Pericarditis
- Pleuritis
- Pneumonitis
- Rib fractures
- Acute chest syndrome of sickle cell
- Chest-wall twinge syndrome:
  - Brief episodes of sharp anterior chest pain lasting 30 sec to 3 min, aggravated by deep breathing and relieved by shallow respirations
- Chest wall pain:
  - Chest wall hematoma
  - Chest wall laceration
  - Herpes zoster
  - Thrombophlebitis of the thoracoepigastric vein
  - Xiphisternal arthritis
  - Adiposis Dolorosa
  - Breast abscess, fibroadenosis, carcinoma

## DIAGNOSIS

### SIGNS AND SYMPTOMS

- Coronary artery disease:
  - Pressure
  - Squeezing pain
  - Radiation to arm, jaw
  - Shortness of breath
  - Diaphoresis
  - Nausea
  - Vomiting
  - Weakness
  - Fatigue especially in women or elderly
  - Signs of CHF
  - Anxiety

- Aortic dissection:
  - Sudden onset of pain with maximal intensity early
  - Tearing pain
  - Radiation to back and/or flank
  - HTN
  - Diastolic murmur of aortic insufficiency
  - Difference in upper extremity pulses
  - Syncope
  - Nausea
  - Vomiting
  - Associated neurological changes (ie, visual changes)
- Pulmonary embolism:
  - Pleuritic pain
  - Shortness of breath
  - Anxiety
  - Diaphoresis
  - Tachypnea
  - Tachycardia
  - Low-grade fever
  - Syncope
  - Localized rales
  - Wheezing
- Acute pericarditis:
  - Substernal pain
  - Varies with respiration
  - Increased with recumbency
  - Relieved by leaning forward
  - Anxiety
  - Anorexia
  - Fever
  - Pericardial friction rub

### History

- The history is the most important tool to distinguish between the various etiologies.
- Have the patient define the key features:
  - Duration
  - Location:
    - ○ Retrosternal
    - ○ Subxiphoid
    - ○ Diffuse
  - Frequency:
    - ○ Constant
    - ○ Intermittent
    - ○ Sudden vs. delayed onset
  - Precipitating factors:
    - ○ Exertion
    - ○ Stress
    - ○ Food
    - ○ Respiration
    - ○ Movement

– Timing:
  ○ Context of onset of pain (ie, at rest, exertional)
  ○ Duration of pain
– Quality:
  ○ Burning
  ○ Squeezing
  ○ Dull
  ○ Sharp
  ○ Tearing
  ○ Heavy
– Associated symptoms:
  ○ Shortness of breath
  ○ Diaphoresis
  ○ Nausea
  ○ Vomiting
  ○ Jaw pain
  ○ Back pain
  ○ Radiation
  ○ Palpitations
  ○ Syncope
  ○ Fever
  ○ Weakness: Generalized vs. focal
  ○ Fatigue

### Physical Exam
- Cardiac exam for murmurs, rub, decreased heart sounds, or extra heart sounds
- Chest exam for decreased breath sounds, rales, wheezing
- Extremity exam for decreased pulses, pulsus paradoxus
- Skin exam for lesions of herpes zoster
- Abdominal exam for tenderness, rebound, guarding

### DIAGNOSTIC TESTS & INTERPRETATION
EKG:
- Inexpensive and available
- Obtain and interpret within 10 min of arrival
- Serial EKG can be useful in patients with high concern for ACS and a negative initial EKG.
- See specific etiologies.

### Lab
- Lab testing should be individualized to the patient and the presentation, based on the risk of potential life threats.
- See "Cardiac Testing."
- D Dimer:
  – Sensitive but poor specificity for physical exam
  – Indicated for low-risk patient if there is an indication to rule out pulmonary embolus
  – Controversial use as a screening test for aortic dissection

### Imaging
- CXR:
  – Pneumothorax
  – Pneumonia
  – CHF
  – Aortic dissection:
    ○ Widened mediastinum seen in ~55–62% of patients

  ○ A pleural effusion is found in ~20% of patients.
  ○ Apical capping
  ○ Aortic knob obliteration
  ○ A normal chest radiograph is found in 12–15% of patients.
  – Acute pericarditis:
    ○ Usually normal unless massive effusion enlarges cardiac silhouette
  – Esophageal rupture:
    ○ Usually will show mediastinal air
    ○ May have left pleural effusion
- Helical CT scan:
  – Pulmonary embolism
  – Sensitive for aortic dissection
- Ventilation/perfusion scan:
  – Useful in pulmonary embolus
  – Must have normal CXR
- Angiography:
  – Pulmonary embolism; although rarely done
  – Useful in dissection, especially in stable patients
- US:
  – Test of choice for pericardial and valvular disease
  – Transesophageal ECG can be used in diagnosis of aortic dissection, especially in unstable patients and those unable to tolerate contrast.
  – Right ventricular dilation and hypokinesia is suggestive for pulmonary embolus.

### DIFFERENTIAL DIAGNOSIS
See "Etiology."

 TREATMENT

### PRE-HOSPITAL
- Therapeutic interventions should be guided by the patient's presentation, risk factors, and past history.
- If a cardiac life threat is suspected:
  – IV access
  – Cardiac monitoring
  – EKG
  – Oxygen
  – Baby aspirin
  – Pain control:
    ○ Nitrates
    ○ Morphine

### INITIAL STABILIZATION/THERAPY
As guided by the patient's presentation:
- ABCs
- IV
- Oxygen
- Cardiac monitoring

### ED TREATMENT/PROCEDURES
- IV, oxygen, and monitoring
- EKG
- Treatment varies based on suspected etiologies.

### MEDICATION
See "Etiology."

 FOLLOW-UP

### DISPOSITION
**Admission Criteria**
Dependent on the risk for life-threatening cardiopulmonary etiologies

**Discharge Criteria**
Very low risk for untoward event if discharge is planned

**Issues for Referral**
Follow-up with primary care physician on low-risk chest pain for outpatient assessment

### FOLLOW-UP RECOMMENDATIONS
Patient should be instructed to return if:
- Chest discomfort lasts >5 min
- Chest discomfort gets worse in any way
- History of angina, and discomfort not relieved by usual medicines
- Shortness of breath, sweats, dizziness, vomiting, or nausea with chest pain or chest discomfort
- Chest discomfort moves into your arm, neck, back, jaw, or stomach

## PEARLS AND PITFALLS
- Caution in only ordering a single biomarker
- Using response to medications as a diagnostic tool
- Not using serial EKG in patients with suspected ACS

## ADDITIONAL READING
- ACC/AHA Guidelines for the Management of Patients with unstable Angina and Non-ST-Segment Elevation MI: Executive Summary and Recommendations. *Circulation.* 2000;102:1193.
- Geraldine McMahon C, Yates DW, Hollis S. Unexpected mortality in patients discharged from the emergency department following an episode of nontraumatic chest pain. *Eur J Emerg Med.* 2008;15(1):3–8.
- Marcus GM, et al. The utility of gestures in patients with chest discomfort. *Am J Med.* 2007;120(1):83–89.
- Thoracic: Respiratory, cardiovascular, and lymphatic symptoms. In: LeBlond RF, DeGowin RL, Brown DD, et al., eds. *DeGowin's diagnostic examination*, 8th ed. New York: McGraw-Hill Professional, 2004.

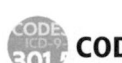 CODES

**ICD9**
786.50 Unspecified chest pain

# CHEST TRAUMA, BLUNT
*Lisa G. Lowe Hiller*

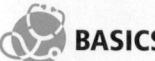

## BASICS

### DESCRIPTION
- Significant source of morbidity and mortality in the U.S.
- ~12 thoracic trauma victims per million population per day
- ~33% of these injuries require hospital admission.
- Directly responsible for 20–25% of all deaths attributed to trauma
- Contributing cause of death in 25% of patients who die from other traumatic injuries

### ETIOLOGY
- Common mechanisms of injury include:
  - Motor vehicle collisions (70–80%)
  - Motorcycle collisions
  - Pedestrians struck by a motor vehicle
  - Falls from great heights
  - Assaults
  - Blast injuries
  - Sports related injuries
- Injuries can result from direct blunt force to the chest or from forces related to rapid deceleration.

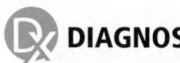

## DIAGNOSIS

### SIGNS AND SYMPTOMS
- Obvious contusion, wound, or other defect of the chest wall
- Paradoxical chest wall movement suggests flail chest segment.
- Usually occurs in combination with other injuries
- Hypotension
- Some patients with severe intrathoracic injuries, such as traumatic aortic disruption, may have *no* visible external signs of trauma.

### History
- Time of injury
- Mechanism of injury
- Estimates of motor vehicle accident (MVA) velocity and deceleration
- Loss of consciousness
- Chest pain
- Pain with deep inspiration or cough
- Dyspnea

### Physical Exam
- Unilaterally absent breath sounds
- Crepitus or subcutaneous air in the chest wall
- Decreased or absent breath sounds
- Tenderness to palpation on the chest wall
- Jugular venous distention
- Hyperresonance to percussion on involved side

## ESSENTIAL WORKUP
- Check airway, breathing, and circulation (ABCs) to determine the patient's stability
- Focused exam of the chest:
  - Respiratory effort and rate
  - Chest wall excursion
  - Crepitus
  - Subcutaneous air
  - Breath sounds and heart sounds
  - Presence of jugular venous distention
- Obtain a supine CXR immediately:
  - Avoid an upright CXR because of potential for other injuries (especially spinal injuries)
- EKG and monitor to detect myocardial ischemia or dysrhythmias
- Consider use of US for detecting small pneumothoraces, especially given the poor sensitivity of supine CXR in detecting such injuries.

## DIAGNOSTIC TESTS & INTERPRETATION
### Lab
- Baseline hemoglobin
- Pulse oximetry
- ABG
- Serum lactate
- Type and cross-match
- Coagulation profile
- Cardiac enzymes when indicated
- Periodic chemistry panel for patients receiving significant fluid resuscitation

### Imaging
- CXR is the initial radiologic study of choice:
  - If CXR reveals widened mediastinum and patient hemodynamically stable, repeat film in upright position.
- Chest CT is more specific for pneumothoraces and pulmonary contusions/occult injuries.
- Thoracic US can be efficiently used for detecting hemothoraces and pericardial injuries. The sensitivity, specificity, and overall accuracy in the ED setting for such injuries is >90%.
- Chest CT with contrast, or aortic angiogram, is useful in identifying aortic and large-vessel injuries.
- Esophagoscopy for direct endoscopic visualization if esophageal injury suspected
- Contrast esophagogram (with water and then barium) for possible esophageal injuries if esophagoscopy negative, but patient at risk for esophageal injury (eg, pneumomediastinum)
  - Combination of these 2 tests in sequence (each 80–90% sensitive individually) reaches close to 100% sensitivity
- EKG if sternal tenderness is present or abnormalities on cardiac monitor

### Diagnostic Procedures/Surgery
- If patient's condition is unstable, emergency thoracotomy may be necessary to repair a traumatic aortic disruption.
- If there are signs of cardiac tamponade, and patient is stable, perform an EKG urgently:
  - Pericardial effusions, wall motion defects, aortic injuries, valvular or other intracardiac pathology may also be identified.
- If there are signs of cardiac tamponade and the patient is unstable, consider emergent pericardiocentesis, followed by immediate transport to the OR for a pericardial window.
- Bronchoscopy for possible upper airway injuries (eg, large persistent air leak after chest tube)

### Pregnancy Considerations
- In pregnant patients, remember to use the least amount of radiation available and to shield the uterus during imaging when possible.
- Take note of the differences in anatomy of the thoracic cavity in pregnant patients, as well as differences in laboratory values, intravascular volume, and cardiovascular physiology.
- See Pregnancy, Trauma in, for details.

## DIFFERENTIAL DIAGNOSIS
- Simple pneumothorax
- Tension pneumothorax
- Open pneumothorax
- Hemothorax
- Rib fractures
- Flail chest
- Pulmonary contusion
- Myocardial contusion
- Myocardial rupture
- Cardiac (pericardial) tamponade
- Traumatic aortic disruption
- Esophageal injury
- Large vascular injury (subclavian artery, pulmonary artery)
- Tracheobronchial injury
- Diaphragmatic injury

### Pediatric Considerations
The rib cage is highly elastic in children and can withstand significant forces without overt signs of external trauma even in patients with major intrathoracic injuries.

### Geriatric Considerations
Elderly patients have been shown to have greater respiratory complications, including ARDS and pneumonia, than younger patients in the setting of blunt chest trauma. This is especially true in those >85 yr of age.

# TREATMENT

## PRE-HOSPITAL
- All patients with any signs of life in the field should be transported to a trauma center.
- Full spinal precautions should be employed.
- Needle decompression is indicated for tension pneumothorax:
  - Unilaterally absent breath sounds
  - Hypotension
  - Jugular venous distention
  - Hyperresonance to percussion
- If large, open pneumothorax exists, tape an occlusive dressing on 3 sides only to prevent causing a tension pneumothorax.
- Do not delay transport to hospital for IV access.

## INITIAL STABILIZATION/THERAPY
- ABCs management; intubate patient early if signs of respiratory insufficiency, shock, or altered mental status exist.
- Resuscitation attempts should be initiated only in patients who arrive in the ED with vital signs.
- Any patient who presents in blunt traumatic arrest is not likely to survive a thoracotomy in the ED, and it is therefore generally not indicated in this group.
- If the patient's condition is unstable and clinically shows signs of a tension pneumothorax, perform needle thoracostomy and place a chest tube immediately after.
- Do not wait to obtain a CXR.
- Place chest tube on the affected side or bilaterally if injury site is unclear.
- Deliver oxygen by nonrebreather face mask for stable patients.
- Obtain vascular access, preferably 2 large-bore IV lines (> 18 gauge).
- Maintain spinal immobilization.

## ED TREATMENT/PROCEDURES
- Tube thoracostomy if pneumothorax or hemothorax is identified:
  - 36-French chest tube in an adult
  - In children, use the largest tube that the intercostal space will accommodate.
- Provide resuscitation with isotonic fluids and blood products as necessary:
  - Aggressive fluid resuscitation may be harmful if severe pulmonary contusions exist.
- Workup for associated intra-abdominal injuries (eg, with diagnostic peritoneal lavage, abdominal US, abdominal CT scan):
  - Patients with chest trauma frequently have concomitant intra-abdominal injuries.

## MEDICATION
- Tetanus booster if indicated
- Consider methylprednisolone (for signs of spinal cord injury): 30 mg/kg IVI over 1 hr, followed by a continuous drip of 5.4 mg/kg/h for next 23 hr; this practice is currently under debate, so know your hospital's protocol.
- Judicious doses of short-acting analgesics (fentanyl 1–2 $\mu$g/kg IV, morphine 0.1 mg/kg IV) as needed for pain control

# FOLLOW-UP

## DISPOSITION
### Admission Criteria
- Patients with conduction blocks, frequent ectopy, or ischemic changes visible on EKG should be admitted to a monitored setting for possible myocardial contusion.
- Hemodynamically unstable patients should go to the OR on an emergency basis for thoracotomy or laparotomy.
- >1,000–1,500 mL of blood drawn out of the chest tube on initial insertion indicates need for thoracotomy/operative management.
- >200 mL of blood per hour from chest tube for several hours suggests the need for operative intervention.
- Patients with significant rib fractures should be admitted for pain control:
  - Consider epidural catheter for analgesia.
- Patients who lose vital signs in the ED should undergo rapid open thoracotomy.

### Discharge Criteria
Patients with clinically insignificant chest wall contusions and an initial negative upright CXR may be observed for 6 hr in the ED and often be discharged if a repeat radiograph at that time reveals no pneumothorax, hemothorax, or pulmonary contusion, the patient is able to breathe deeply and to cough, and has no other significant injuries.

### Issues for Referral
- Notify trauma surgeon promptly about patients with significant injuries requiring surgical intervention or admission.
- Indications for emergent surgical referral:
  - Traumatic thoracotomy with loss of chest wall integrity
  - Blunt diaphragmatic injuries
  - Massive air leak following chest tube insertion
  - Massive hemothorax or continued high rate of blood loss via the chest tube (ie, 1,500 mL on insertion of tube or continued loss of 200–300 mL/h)

- Radiographically or endoscopically confirmed tracheal, major bronchial, or esophageal injury
- GI tract contents recovered on chest tube placement
- Cardiac tamponade
- Radiographic confirmation of a great-vessel injury
- Embolism or missile into pulmonary artery, great vessel, or heart

## FOLLOW-UP RECOMMENDATIONS
- Patients should be closely followed by trauma or cardiothoracic surgeons after hospital discharge, as indicated, depending upon the injuries discovered and treatment rendered.
- Patients with thoracostomy tubes should have a CXR and routine wound care follow-up within 48 hr to remove the dressing and reassess clinical status.

# PEARLS AND PITFALLS
- Blunt chest trauma is responsible for up to 1/4 of all trauma-related deaths.
- Trauma patients arriving at a non-trauma center should be stabilized and transferred to facilities that can provide definitive care as soon as possible.
- Open thoracotomy in the ED has not been shown to improve survival in patients found in cardiopulmonary arrest after blunt trauma.
- The extent of injury is not always clinically obvious upon initial presentation.

# ADDITIONAL READING
- American Heart Association Guidelines for Cardiopulmonary Resuscitation and Emergency Cardiovascular. *Circulation*. 2005;112: IV-146–IV-149.
- Centers for Disease Control and Prevention. Accidents/unintentional injuries. Retrieved October 2008 from http://www.cdc.gov/nchs/FASTATS/acc-inj.htm
- Karmy-Jones R, Jurkovich GJ. Blunt chest trauma. *Curr Probl Surg*. 2004;41(3):211–380.
- Lotfipour S. Factors associated with complications in older adults with isolated blunt chest trauma. *West J Emerg Med*. 2009;10(2). Retrieved from http://escholarship.org/uc/item/9922n5
- Sartorelli KH, Vane DW. The diagnosis and management of children with blunt injury of the chest. *Semin Pediatr Surg*. 2004;13(2):98–105.

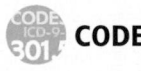 CODES

ICD9
862.8 Injury to multiple and unspecified intrathoracic organs without mention of open wound into cavity

# CHEST TRAUMA, PENETRATING

*Jean C.Y. Lo*

 **BASICS**

## ETIOLOGY
- Gunshot wounds or stab wounds most common
- Impalement on a sharp object from a fall can occur.

 **DIAGNOSIS**

## SIGNS AND SYMPTOMS
- Object impaled in the chest wall
- Obvious wound in the chest wall with or without bleeding
- Chest pain
- Dyspnea
- Respiratory distress
- Altered mental status from hypoxemia
- Absent or altered breath sounds on 1 or both sides
- Hypotension
- Jugular venous distention

## ESSENTIAL WORKUP
- Perform routine assessment of airway, breathing, and circulation.
- Rapid exam:
  - Respiratory effort and rate
  - Chest excursion
  - Crepitus
  - Subcutaneous air
  - Breath sounds and heart sounds
- Upright CXR is preferred for identifying a pneumothorax:
  - Supine CXR should be taken 1st if spinal precautions must be maintained.
- Baseline hemoglobin
- Pulse oximetry
- ABG
- Serum lactate
- Type and screen

## DIAGNOSTIC TESTS & INTERPRETATION
### Lab
- Perform EKG if signs of tamponade present or if wound is close to the heart:
  - In stab wound to precordium and pericardial sac, hemopericardium may decompress into hemothorax, thus not apparent on initial EKG:
    - Repeat pericardial US is recommended after tube thoracostomy decompression of the hemothorax.
    - Residual hemothorax represents pericardial injury or cardiac laceration.
- ECG

### Imaging
- With gunshot wounds, other areas (abdomen, pelvis) should be imaged:
  - Total number of wounds and bullets must be the same.
- Arteriogram of aortic arch, carotid arteries, or subclavian artery if great vessel injury is suspected
- Esophageal Gastrografin swallow or endoscopy to identify esophageal perforation
- Bronchoscopy to identify tracheobronchial injuries

## DIFFERENTIAL DIAGNOSIS
- Simple pneumothorax
- Tension pneumothorax
- Open pneumothorax
- Hemothorax
- Rib fractures
- Flail chest
- Pulmonary contusion
- Myocardial contusion
- Myocardial rupture
- Pericardial tamponade
- Traumatic aortic disruption
- Esophageal injury
- Large vessel injury
- Tracheobronchial injury
- Diaphragmatic injury
- Intra-abdominal injury
- Spinal cord injury

 **TREATMENT**

## PRE-HOSPITAL
- Cautions:
  - All patients with signs of life in the field according to reports from EMS personnel should be transported to a trauma center.
  - Full spinal immobilization if spinal injury suspected
  - Never remove objects impaled in the chest because exsanguination may follow.
  - Needle decompression may be necessary if tension pneumothorax suspected:
    - Unilaterally absent breath sounds, hypotension, jugular venous distention
  - If large open pneumothorax exists, occlusive dressing taped on 3 sides:
    - A totally occlusive dressing may produce a tension pneumothorax.
- Controversies:
  - Do not delay transport to hospital to obtain IV access:
  - IV access may be established en route.
  - Do not delay transport to hospital to apply full spinal immobilization to patients who do not have clear clinical signs of spinal injury.

## INITIAL STABILIZATION/THERAPY
- Airway, breathing, and circulation management:
  - Intubate for signs of serious chest injury, obvious respiratory distress, or hypotension.
- Oxygen by nonrebreather face mask for patients in stable condition
- Obtain vascular access, 2 peripheral large-bore IV lines (>18 gauge), and fluid resuscitation as needed:
  - 2-liter isotonic fluid bolus initially
  - In penetrating aortic trauma, permissive hypotension at systolic BP 90 mm Hg until definitive surgical control prevents further hemorrhage.
- For tension pneumothorax, perform a needle thoracostomy and place a chest tube immediately.
- Do not wait to get a CXR.
- For pericardial tamponade, perform an emergency pericardiocentesis:
  - Follow by rapid transport to the operating room for a pericardial window
- Maintain spinal immobilization if indicated.

## ED TREATMENT/PROCEDURES

- Notify trauma surgeon about patient's arrival.
- Tube thoracostomy if a pneumothorax or hemothorax is identified:
  - 36-gauge chest tube in an adult
  - In children, use largest tube intercostal space will accommodate.
- Fluid resuscitation as necessary:
  - Contused lung parenchyma will have leaky capillary beds, and aggressive crystalloid resuscitation may aggravate pulmonary dysfunction.
- Any wound with an entry or exit site below the nipple or the posterior tip of the scapula is concerning for an intra-abdominal injury:
  - Workup with a diagnostic peritoneal lavage (DPL), US, CT scan, exploratory laparotomy, or laparoscopy
  - DPL positive with 5,000 RBC
- Describe the nature of wounds accurately:
  - Retain any bullet fragments, clothes, or tissue removed from the wound.
- Probing a chest wound is contraindicated because it can create a pneumothorax or worsen hemorrhage.
- Impaled objects should be removed only in the operating room.
- Tetanus booster if indicated

## MEDICATION

- Methylprednisolone (for spinal cord injury): 30 mg/kg IV over 1 hr, followed by a continuous drip of 5.4 mg/kg/h for 23 hr
- Small doses of short-acting analgesics (fentanyl, 1–2 $\mu$g/kg IV, morphine 0.1 mg/kg IV) or sedatives (midazolam, 0.05 mg/kg IV) as needed for pain control and sedation
- Treat with IV antibiotics if wound grossly contaminated (eg, cephalexin 1 g IV).

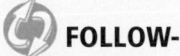 **FOLLOW-UP**

### DISPOSITION
#### Admission Criteria

- All patients with penetrating chest trauma should be admitted.
- A patient who has signs of life in the field but no BP on arrival in the ED should have an emergency thoracotomy performed by the most experienced person present:
  - If the source of bleeding is controlled and there are signs of cardiac activity, the patient should go to the operating room for formal operative repair.
- Hemodynamically unstable patients should go immediately to the operating room.
- Any patient with intrathoracic penetration should have a chest tube placed and should be admitted to a monitored setting.
- >1,000–1,500 mL of blood drawn out of the chest tube on initial insertion indicates the need for thoracotomy.
- >200 mL/hr of blood from a chest tube for several hours suggests the need for surgical intervention.
- Patients with large, persistent air leaks usually require surgery.
- Patients with significant rib fractures should be admitted and have an epidural catheter placed for pain control and pulmonary toilet.

#### Discharge Criteria

Patients with isolated minor chest wounds and a normal CXR can be observed for 3 hr in the ED and have a repeat radiographic study; if no intrathoracic penetration is suspected, the patient can be discharged:

- CT chest may be an alternative to CXR, if no intrathoracic penetration is suspected; patient can be discharged without repeat radiograph.

## ADDITIONAL READING

- Ball CG, Williams BH, Wyrzykowski AD, et al. A caveat to the performance of pericardial ultrasound in patients with penetrating cardiac wounds. *J Trauma.* 2009;67:1123–1124.
- Haut ER, Kalish BT, Efron DT, et al. Spinal immobilization in penetrating trauma: More harm than good. *J Trauma.* 2010;68:115–121.
- Ivatury RR, Cayten CG. *The textbook of penetrating trauma.* Baltimore: Williams & Wilkins, 1996.
- Magnotti LJ, Weinberg JA, Schroeppel TJ, et al. Initial chest CT obviates the need for repeat chest radiograph after penetrating thoracic trauma. *Am Surg.* 2007;73:569–572.
- Moloney HT, Fowler SJ, Chang W. Anesthetic management of thoracic trauma. *Curr Opin Anaesthesiol.* 2008;21:41–46.
- Seamon MJ, Medina CR, Pieri PG, et al. Follow-up after asymptomatic penetrating thoracic injury: 3 hours is enough. *J Trauma.* 2008;65:549–553.

 **CODES**

### ICD9
862.9 Injury to multiple and unspecified intrathoracic organs with open wound into cavity

C

# CHOLANGITIS

*Robert G. Buckley*

 **BASICS**

## DESCRIPTION
- Partial or complete obstruction of the common bile duct owing to gallstones, tumor, cyst, or stricture
- Increased intraluminal pressure in biliary tree
- Bacterial multiplication results in bacteremia and sepsis.
- Purulent infection of biliary tree, which may involve the liver and gallbladder
- Mirizzi syndrome is defined as common bile duct obstruction owing to extrinsic compression from gallbladder or cystic duct edema or stones.

## ETIOLOGY
- Bacterial sources of infection include:
  - Ascending duodenal source
  - Gallbladder infection
  - Portal venous seeding
  - Hematogenous spread with hepatic secretion
  - Lymphatic spread
- Bacterial organisms include:
  - Anaerobes (*Bacteroides* and *Clostridium* species)
  - Intestinal coliform (*Escherichia coli*)
  - Enterococcus
- AIDS sclerosing cholangitis characterized by:
  - Papillary stenosis
  - Sclerosing cholangitis
  - Extrahepatic biliary obstruction
  - Cytomegalovirus (CMV), *Cryptosporidium*, and microsporidia isolated, but causal role not established

 **DIAGNOSIS**

## SIGNS AND SYMPTOMS
### History
- Charcot's triad:
  - Classic presentation of fever and chills; right upper quadrant (RUQ) pain and jaundice found in only 50–70%
- Addition of shock and altered mental status denotes a more advanced form of biliary sepsis known as *Reynold's pentad*.
- Abdominal pain present in >70%— localizing to RUQ.
- AIDS sclerosing cholangitis presents with similar symptoms but with more chronic indolent course and near-normal serum bilirubin levels.

### Physical Exam
- Fever found in >90%
- Peritoneal findings found in 30%
- Clinically apparent jaundice may be absent in up to 40%.

## ESSENTIAL WORKUP
- ECG in patients at risk for coronary artery disease
- CBC
- LFT
- Amylase, lipase
- Urinalysis
- Blood cultures
- Gallbladder US or hepatoiminodiacetic acid (HIDA) scan

## DIAGNOSTIC TESTS & INTERPRETATION
### Lab
- CBC:
  - Leukocytosis with left shift unless immunocompromised or severe sepsis
- LFTs consistent with cholestasis:
  - Elevated direct bilirubin and alkaline phosphatase
- Minimal elevation of transaminases (<200 IU/mL)
- Changes may lag symptom onset by 24–48 hr.
- Amylase and lipase normal or mildly elevated
- Urinalysis positive for bilirubin

### Imaging
- US detects the level of ductal obstruction and the presence of gallstone etiology.
- Radionuclide scanning (HIDA):
  - Indicates obstruction when tracer not found in duodenum within 1 hr
  - More sensitive than US in detecting obstruction in the 1st 24–48 hr before ductal dilation occurs
- CT scan and CRX:
  - Useful to rule out intestinal obstruction, perforation, or pneumonia
  - 20% gallstones radiopaque

### Diagnostic Procedures/Surgery
Emergency invasive biliary imaging and drainage by endoscopic retrograde cholangiopancreatography [ERCP], (or surgical/percutaneous if not available), if no response to medical treatment in 12–24 hr

## DIFFERENTIAL DIAGNOSIS

- Acute cholecystitis
- Hepatitis or hepatic abscess
- Acute pancreatitis
- Right pyelonephritis
- Right lower lobe pneumonia or pulmonary embolism
- Perforated duodenal ulcer
- Appendicitis
- Sepsis with nonspecific elevation of LFTs
- Fitz-Hugh and Curtis syndrome

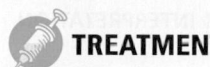 **TREATMENT**

### PRE-HOSPITAL
Stabilize septic shock.

### INITIAL STABILIZATION/THERAPY

- Immediate IV fluid resuscitation for dehydration, hemodynamic compromise, and sepsis
- Vasopressors (dopamine) for hypotension refractory to volume replacement

### ED TREATMENT/PROCEDURES

- Broad-spectrum antibiotics for coliforms, anaerobes, and enterococcus such as:
  - Ampicillin/sulbactam plus aminoglycoside (eg, gentamicin)
  - Piperacillin/tazobactam plus aminoglycoside (eg, gentamicin)
  - For penicillin allergy:
    o Adults—use levofloxacin (Levaquin) and metronidazole
    o Pediatrics—use clindamycin and metronidazole
  - Substitute aztreonam for aminoglycoside in renal insufficiency.

- NPO
- Nasogastric (NG) suctioning if protracted vomiting or ileus
- IV fluid (0.9% NS) replacement and maintenance
- Narcotic analgesia if hemodynamically stable and diagnosis reasonably established
- Immediate surgical consultation
- Emergency invasive biliary drainage procedure (surgical, percutaneous, or ERCP) if no response to medical treatment in 12–24 hr

### MEDICATION

- Ampicillin/sulbactam: 3.0 g (peds: 200 mg/kg/24 h) IV piggyback (IVPB) q6h
- Aztreonam: 2 g (peds: 120 mg/kg/24 h) IVPB q6h
- Clindamycin: 600–900 mg (peds: 25–40 mg/kg/24 h) IVPB q6–8h
- Dopamine: 2–20 $\mu$g/min IVPB; titrate to maintain BP
- Gentamicin: 1.5–2.0 mg/kg (peds: 6–7 mg/kg/24 h) IVPB q8h; follow levels
- Levaquin: 500 mg IVPB q24h; contraindicated in peds
- Hydromorphone: 0.5–2 mg IV, (0.01–0.02 mg/kg), titrated to pain relief. Metronidazole: 500 mg (peds: 30 mg/kg/24 h) IVPB q6h
- Piperacillin/tazobactam: 3.375 mg (peds: 300 mg/kg/24 h) IVPB q6h
- Ondansetron: 4–8 mg IV, (0.15—0.3 mg/kg) IV (not to exceed 8 mg/dose IV), q4h PRN vomiting

 **FOLLOW-UP**

### DISPOSITION

#### Admission Criteria

- All patients with acute cholangitis should be admitted with immediate surgical and gastroenterologic consultation.
- Admit patients with signs of septic shock to the ICU.

#### Discharge Criteria
None

#### Issues for Referral
Surgery/GI consultation

### FOLLOW-UP RECOMMENDATIONS
Admission to hospital for IV antibiotic and possible biliary drainage procedure.

## PEARLS AND PITFALLS

- Aggressively fluid resuscitate patients.
- Administer antibiotics.
- Obtain GI and surgical consultations.

## ADDITIONAL READING

- Chari RS, Shah SA. Biliary system. In: Townsend CM Jr, ed. *Sabiston textbook of surgery*, 18th ed. Philadelphia: WB Saunders; 2008:1547–1587.
- Hanau LH, Steigbigel NH. Cholangitis: Pathogenesis, diagnosis and treatment. *Curr Clin Top Infect Dis*. 1995;311:99–105.
- Lai EC, Mok FP, Tan ES, et al. Endoscopic biliary drainage for severe acute cholangitis. *N Engl J Med*. 1992;326;1582–1586.
- Mahajani RV, Uzer MF. Cholestasis. Cholangiopathy in HIV-infected patients. *Clin Liver Dis*. 1999;3: 669–684.
- Solomkin JS, Mazuski JE, Baron EJ, et al. Guidelines for the selection of anti-infective agents for complicated intra-abdominal infections. *Clin Infect Dis*. 2003;37:997–1005.

### See Also (Topic, Algorithm, Electronic Media Element)

- Cholecystitis
- Cholelithiasis

 **CODES**

ICD9
576.1 Cholangitis

# CHOLECYSTITIS
*Robert G. Buckley*

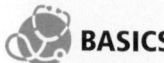 **BASICS**

## DESCRIPTION
Cholecystitis is defined as inflammation of the gallbladder.

## ETIOLOGY
- Acute calculous cholecystitis:
  - Owing to bile stasis secondary to prolonged obstruction by a gallstone (see "Cholelithiasis") in the gallbladder neck, cystic duct, or common bile duct
  - Leads to increased intraluminal pressure and mucosal damage
  - Release of inflammatory mediators results in distention, edema, and increased vascularity.
  - Coliforms and anaerobes lead to infection—primary causal role is controversial.
- Acalculous cholecystitis:
  - 10% of cases
  - Underlying critical illness leads to biliary stasis and mucosal ischemia.
  - Subsequent mucosal inflammation and infection

### Pediatric Considerations
- *Acute calculous cholecystitis* extremely rare in childhood (see "Cholelithiasis")
- *Acalculous cholecystitis* more common than calculous form in children:
  - Associated with systemic bacterial infections, scarlet fever, Kawasaki disease, and parasitic infections

 **DIAGNOSIS**

## SIGNS AND SYMPTOMS
### History
- Acute calculous cholecystitis:
  - Dull, aching, epigastric, or right upper quadrant (RUQ) pain
  - Radiation to tip of right scapula, acromion, or thoracic spine
  - Duration >6 hr more suggestive of cholecystitis than uncomplicated biliary colic
  - As inflammation progresses, parietal peritoneal irritation leads to sharp, localized pain.
  - Nausea, vomiting, fever, and chills often reported, but absent in most cases
  - Jaundice in 20%
  - History of prior attacks of biliary colic or known gallstones favors diagnosis.
- Acalculous cholecystitis:
  - Occurs in critically ill patients (burns, sepsis, trauma, or postoperative)
  - Localized pain and tenderness frequently absent
  - Often presents with symptoms of generalized sepsis of unknown source

### Physical Exam
- Localized parietal peritoneal signs:
  - Percussion tenderness
  - Rebound
  - Found as the disease progresses
- Murphy's sign:
  - Inspiratory arrest with gentle palpation of RUQ owing to increased pain
  - Found in most cases

## ESSENTIAL WORKUP
- ECG in patients at risk for coronary artery disease
- CBC
- LFT
- Amylase, lipase
- Urinalysis
- Human chorionic gonadotropin (hCG)
- Gallbladder US or HIDA scan

## DIAGNOSTIC TESTS & INTERPRETATION
### Lab
- CBC:
  - WBC >12,000 cells/mm$^3$ supports diagnosis, but may be normal in more than half of cases
- LFTs:
  - Transaminases, bilirubin, amylase, and lipase may be minimally elevated, but are generally normal.
  - Disproportionate elevation of direct bilirubin and alkaline phosphatase compared with transaminases suspicious for common duct obstruction or cholangitis

### Imaging
- US:
  - Generally the 1st-line imaging procedure
  - Positive findings include gallbladder wall thickening (>5 mm) or pericolic fluid—sensitivity, 90%; specificity, 80%.
  - Optimal if patient NPO >8 hr
- Radionuclide scanning (HIDA):
  - Most useful when clinical suspicion remains high despite equivocal findings on US or when acalculous cholecystitis suspected
  - Positive when tracer seen in small bowel but inflamed gallbladder fails to visualize
  - Sensitivity, >95%; specificity, 90%
  - False-positive results increase in nonfasting state.
- CT scanning:
  - Exclude intestinal perforation or obstruction
  - Air in the gallbladder wall consistent with emphysematous cholecystitis
  - Gallstones radiopaque in up to 20%

## DIFFERENTIAL DIAGNOSIS

- Biliary colic
- Hepatitis or hepatic abscess
- Cholangitis
- AIDS sclerosing cholangitis
- Pancreatitis
- Intestinal perforation
- Peptic ulcer disease
- Gastritis
- Duodenal perforation
- Right lower lobe pneumonia, pleurisy, or pulmonary infarction
- MI
- Abdominal aortic aneurysm
- Appendicitis
- Fitz-Hugh and Curtis syndrome
- Pyelonephritis

 TREATMENT

### PRE-HOSPITAL
Establish IV access for patients with vomiting or severe pain.

### INITIAL STABILIZATION/THERAPY
- IV, oxygen, cardiac monitoring until myocardial ischemic cause excluded
- Initiate IV fluid therapy for dehydration, hemodynamic compromise, or sepsis.

### ED TREATMENT/PROCEDURES
- Broad-spectrum antibiotics for coliforms, anaerobes, and enterococcus:
  - Ampicillin/sulbactam
  - Piperacillin/tazobactam
  - Add aminoglycoside if sepsis or cholangitis suspected (see "Cholangitis").
- Alternative antibiotics for penicillin allergic:
  - Adults: Levofloxacin ( Levaquin ) and metronidazole
  - Peds: Clindamycin with aminoglycoside
- NPO
- IV fluid replacement and maintenance
- Antiemetics (ondansetron) if vomiting
- Nasogastric (NG) suctioning if refractory vomiting or ileus

- Narcotic analgesics (hydromorphone) with antiemetic (ondansetron):
  - Administer for refractory pain once diagnosis is reasonably established.
  - Morphine sulfate may lead to spasm at sphincter of Oddi (clinical significance not well established).
- Anticholinergics (glycopyrrolate) of no proven benefit for acute biliary pain.
- Surgical consultation

### MEDICATION
- Ampicillin/sulbactam: 3 g (peds: 200 mg/kg/24 h) IV piggyback (IVPB) q6h
- Clindamycin: 600–900 mg (peds: 25–40 mg/kg/24 h) IVPB q6h to q8h
- Gentamicin: 1.5–2.0 mg/kg (peds: 6–7 mg/kg/24 h) IVPB q8h; follow levels
- Levaquin: 500 mg IVPB q24h; contraindicated in peds
- Hydromorphone: 0.5–2 mg IV (0.01–0.02 mg/kg), titrated to pain relief.
- Metronidazole: 500 mg (peds: 30 mg/kg/24 h) IVPB q6h
- Piperacillin/tazobactam: 3.375 mg (peds: 300 mg/kg/24 h) IVPB q6h
- Ondansetron: 4–8 mg IV (peds: 0.15–0.3 mg/kg) IV (not to exceed 8 mg/dose IV), q4h PRN vomiting

 FOLLOW-UP

### DISPOSITION
#### Admission Criteria
- All cases of cholecystitis should be admitted for parenteral antibiotics, analgesia, fluid replacement, and cholecystectomy in 24–72 hr.
- Unstable patients (gallbladder perforation or sepsis) require immediate surgery.

#### Discharge Criteria
None

#### Issues for Referral
General surgery consult for patients with cholecystitis

### FOLLOW-UP RECOMMENDATIONS
Inpatient admission for antibiotics and surgical evaluation

## PEARLS AND PITFALLS

- US is the 1st-line imaging procedure.
- Perform a radionuclide scanning (HIDA) when clinical suspicion is high with equivocal US or when acalculous cholecystitis suspected.

## ADDITIONAL READING

- Elwoood DR. Cholecystitis. *Surg Clin North Am.* 2008;88:1241–1252.
- Mahajani RV, Uzer MF. Cholestasis: Cholangiopathy in HIV-infected patients. *Clin Liver Dis.* 1999;3: 669–684.
- Silen W. Cholecystitis and other causes of acute pain in the right upper quadrant of the abdomen. In: Silen W, ed. *Cope's early diagnosis of the acute abdomen*, 20th ed. Oxford, UK: Oxford University Press; 2000:128–137.
- Singer AJ, McCracken G, Henry MC, et al. Correlation among clinical, laboratory, and hepatobiliary scanning findings in patients with suspected acute cholecystitis. *Ann Emerg Med.* 1996;28:267–272.
- Trowbridge RL, Rutkowski NK, Shojania KG. Does this patient have acute cholecystitis? *JAMA.* 2003;289:80–86.

### See Also (Topic, Algorithm, Electronic Media Element)
- Cholangitis
- Cholelithiasis

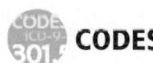 CODES

ICD9
575.10 Cholecystitis, unspecified

# CHOLELITHIASIS
*Robert G. Buckley*

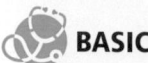 **BASICS**

## DESCRIPTION
- Symptoms arise when gallstones pass through the cystic or common bile ducts leading to impedance of normal bile flow and gallbladder spasm.
- Biliary dyskinesia produces symptoms identical to biliary colic in the absence of stones.

## ETIOLOGY
- Cholesterol stones:
  - Most common type of gallstone
  - Form when solubility exceeded
- Pigment stones:
  - 20%
  - Composed of calcium bilirubinate
  - Associated with clinical conditions such as hemolytic anemias that lead to increased concentration of unconjugated bilirubin
- Incidence increases with age and favors females to males 2:1.
- Gallstones are exceedingly rare in childhood and are most commonly associated with sickle cell disease, hereditary spherocytosis, or other hemolytic anemias that result in pigment stone formation.
- Biliary sludge:
  - Nonstone, crystalline, granular matrix
  - Associated with rapid weight loss, pregnancy, ceftriaxone or octreotide therapy, and organ transplantation
  - May develop symptoms identical to cholelithiasis and its complications

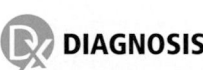 **DIAGNOSIS**

## SIGNS AND SYMPTOMS
### History
- Dull, aching epigastric or right upper quadrant (RUQ) pain:
  - Arising over 2–3 min, continuous (rather than colicky), and lasting from 30 min–6 hr before dissipating
  - May radiate to the tip of right scapula, acromion, or thoracic spine
  - Often correlated with ingestion of large, fatty meal
- Anorexia
- Nausea and vomiting
- Afebrile:
  - Fever and chills suggest cholecystitis or cholangitis

### Physical Exam
- Tenderness to deep palpation but without rebound
- Murphy sign (inspiratory arrest during deep palpation of the RUQ) may be present during the episode of colic, but should resolve when symptoms pass.

## ESSENTIAL WORKUP
- Obtain ECG on those whose pain may be owing to myocardial ischemia.
- CBC
- LFTs
- Amylase, lipase
- Urinalysis
- Human chorionic gonadotropin (hCG)

## DIAGNOSTIC TESTS & INTERPRETATION
### Lab
- CBC:
  - WBC count usually normal, but may elevate after vomiting
  - Leukocytosis suggestive of cholecystitis or cholangitis
- LFTs:
  - Usually normal
  - Elevation suggests common duct obstruction, cholangitis, cholecystitis, or hepatitis.
  - Amylase/lipase
  - Normal or minimally elevated with passage of gallstone
  - Elevation in context of severe persistent epigastric pain suggests pancreatitis.
- Urinalysis:
  - Exclude nephrolithiasis or pyelonephritis.
  - Bilirubinuria suggests common duct obstruction or hepatitis.

### Imaging
- US:
  - Detects gallstones with sensitivity and specificity >90%
  - Dilation of common bile duct >10 mm indicates obstruction, but may be normal with acute obstruction.
  - Gallbladder wall thickening >5 mm or pericolic fluid 90% sensitive and 80% specific for cholecystitis
  - Accuracy enhanced in fasting patient (>6 hr) with noncontracted gallbladder

- Radionuclide scanning (HIDA):
  - Cannot detect gallstones
  - Passage of tracer into small intestine without visualization of gallbladder highly diagnostic of cystic duct obstruction and cholecystitis:
    - Sensitivity and specificity roughly 95%
  - Failure of tracer to pass into duodenum suggests common bile duct obstruction.
- CT scanning:
  - Less sensitive than US to detect gallstones:
    - Only 20% radiopaque.
  - Most useful to exclude other causes of upper abdominal pain such as aortic aneurysm, perihepatic abscess, or pancreatic pseudocyst
  - Detects rare complications such as air in gallbladder wall in emphysematous cholecystitis or air-filled gallbladder in biliary-enteric fistula
- Plain radiographs:
  - Most useful for diagnosis of intestinal obstruction.

## DIFFERENTIAL DIAGNOSIS
- MI
- Abdominal aortic aneurysm
- Acute cholecystitis, cholangitis, or choledocholithiasis
- Renal colic or pyelonephritis
- Duodenal ulcer perforation
- Acute pancreatitis
- Intestinal obstruction
- Peptic ulcer disease, gastritis, or GERD
- Right lower lobe pneumonia, pleurisy, or pulmonary infarction
- Hepatitis or hepatic abscess
- Fitz-Hugh and Curtis syndrome

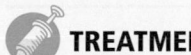 **TREATMENT**

### PRE-HOSPITAL
Initiate IV access for patients with nausea or vomiting.

### INITIAL STABILIZATION/THERAPY
IV fluid bolus if vomiting or hypotensive

### ED TREATMENT/PROCEDURES
- IV hydration with 0.9% NS if vomiting
- NPO
- Parenteral NSAIDs (ketorolac) may lessen biliary spasm, but may exacerbate peptic causes of pain.
- Narcotic analgesics (hydromorphone) with antiemetic (ondansetron):
  – Administer for refractory pain once diagnosis is reasonably established.
  – Morphine sulfate may lead to spasm at sphincter of Oddi (clinical significance not well established).
- Anticholinergics (glycopyrrolate) have no proven benefit in the treatment of acute biliary pain.

### MEDICATION
- Ketorolac: 60 mg IM or 30 mg (peds: Start 0.5 mg/kg for 1st dose up to 1 mg/kg/24 h) IV q6h. In elderly: 30 mg IM or 15 mg IV
- Hydromorphone: 0.5–2 mg IV (0.01–0.02 mg/kg), titrated to pain relief.
- Ondansetron: 4–8 mg IV (0.15–0.3 mg/kg) IV (not to exceed 8 mg/dose IV), q4h PRN vomiting.

 **FOLLOW-UP**

### DISPOSITION
#### Admission Criteria
Admission and surgical or gastroenterologic consultation for evidence of:
- Acute cholecystitis
- Acute cholangitis
- Common duct obstruction
- Gallstone pancreatitis

#### Discharge Criteria
- Lack of clinical, laboratory, or radiographic evidence of cholecystitis, cholangitis, common duct obstruction, or pancreatitis
- Resolution of all pain and tenderness
- Ability to tolerate oral fluids

#### Issues for Referral
General surgery referral for all cases of biliary colic with documented cholelithiasis

### FOLLOW-UP RECOMMENDATIONS
Surgical follow-up for patients with symptomatic gallstones

## PEARLS AND PITFALLS

- An ultrasound is more sensitive and specific for cholelithiasis.
- Radionuclide scanning (HIDA) is highly diagnostic of cystic duct obstruction and cholecystitis.
- CT scans may miss gallstones if the stones are not radiopaque.

## ADDITIONAL READING

- Antevil JL, Buckley RG, Johnson AS, et al. Treatment of suspected symptomatic cholelithiasis with glycopyrrolate: A prospective, randomized clinical trial. *Ann Emerg Med*. 2005;45:172–176.
- Chari RS, Shah SA. Biliary system. In: Townsend CM Jr, ed. *Sabiston textbook of surgery*, 18th ed. Philadelphia: WB Saunders; 2008:1547–1587.
- Silen W. The colics. In: Silen W, ed. *Cope's early diagnosis of the acute abdomen*, 20th ed. Oxford, UK: Oxford University Press; 2000:142–149.
- Trowbridge RL, Rutkowski NK, Shojania KG. Does this patient have acute cholecystitis? *JAMA* 2003;289:80–86.
- Vassiliou MC, Laycock WS. Biliary Dyskinesia. *Surg Clin North Am*. 2008;88(6):1253–1272.

### See Also (Topic, Algorithm, Electronic Media Element)
- Cholangitis
- Cholelithiasis

 **CODES**

### ICD9
- 574.00 Calculus of gallbladder with acute cholecystitis, without mention of obstruction
- 574.10 Calculus of gallbladder with other cholecystitis, without mention of obstruction
- 574.20 Calculus of gallbladder without mention of cholecystitis, without mention of obstruction

# CHRONIC OBSTRUCTIVE PULMONARY DISEASE

*Adam Z. Barkin*

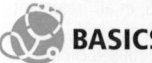

## BASICS

### DESCRIPTION
- A disease characterized by airflow obstruction due to several processes:
  - Emphysema: Irreversible alveolar destruction with loss of airway elastic recoil
  - Chronic bronchitis: Airway inflammation without alveolar destruction
  - Reactive airway disease: Reversible bronchospasm, mucous plugging, and mucosal edema
- COPD affects ~10% of the population and 50% of smokers.
- Increased incidence of hypertension, diabetes, heart failure, and cardiovascular disease in those with COPD

### RISK FACTORS
*Genetics*
$\alpha_1$-Antitrypsin deficiency

### ETIOLOGY
- Smoking is the overwhelming cause:
  - COPD develops in 15% of smokers.
- Air pollution
- Airway hyperresponsiveness
- $\alpha_1$-Antitrypsin deficiency
- Autoimmunity may play a role.
- Acute exacerbations:
  - Viral or bacterial infections
  - Pollutants

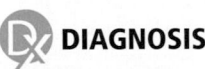

## DIAGNOSIS

### SIGNS AND SYMPTOMS
*History*
- Dyspnea on exertion
- Cough
- Sputum production
- Fatigue
- Wheezing
- Orthopnea
- Altered mental status

*Physical Exam*
- Wheezing
- Retractions
- Decreased air movement
- Cyanosis
- Prolonged expiratory phase
- Barrell chest
- Lower extremity edema
- Jugular venous distension
- S3 and S4 gallops
- Altered mental status secondary to carbon dioxide narcosis

### DIAGNOSTIC TESTS & INTERPRETATION
*Lab*
- CBC:
  - Elevated hematocrit may indicate chronic hypoxemia.
  - Increased neutrophils and elevated WBC may indicate infection.
- Arterial blood gas:
  - Retaining carbon dioxide
  - Acidosis
  - Oxygenation
- Beta natriuretic peptide:
  - Differentiate between COPD and CHF.
- Sputum sample
- Theophylline level as needed

*Imaging*
- CXR:
  - Pneumothorax, pneumonia, CHF, lobar collapse
- Chest CAT scan:
  - When needed to evaluate for pulmonary embolus or further characterize disease

*Diagnostic Procedures/Surgery*
- Pulse oximetry
- ECG
- Pulmonary function tests
- Echocardiography:
  - To diagnose left or right ventricular failure or strain

### DIFFERENTIAL DIAGNOSIS
- Pneumothorax
- CHF
- Pneumonia
- Pulmonary embolus
- Upper airway obstruction
- Asthma
- Restrictive lung disease
- ARDS
- Pleural effusions
- Acute coronary syndrome
- Pericardial effusion
- Metabolic derangement

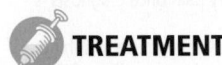

## TREATMENT

### PRE-HOSPITAL
Supplemental oxygenation:
- 100% via nonrebreather
- Do not withhold for fear of $CO_2$ retention.
- Initiate nebulized bronchodilator therapy.

### INITIAL STABILIZATION/THERAPY
- Oxygen therapy:
  - Maintain oxygen saturation >90–92%.
  - Patients at risk for $CO_2$ narcosis are those with slow respiratory rate.
  - Monitor closely for ventilation suppression.
- Noninvasive ventilation:
  - May prevent intubation
  - May help resolve hypercarbia
- Intubation for airway control:
  - Indicated if clinical tiring, altered mental status, or the inability to comply with emergent therapy
  - Ineffective ventilation
  - $CO_2$ narcosis

## ED TREATMENT/PROCEDURES

- Continuous ECG and pulse oximetry monitoring
- Bronchodilator therapy
- $\beta$-Agonists:
  - Albuterol
- Anticholinergics:
  - Ipratropium bromide
- Corticosteroids:
  - Anti-inflammatory effects
  - Reduce relapses
  - Methylprednisolone or prednisone
- Antibiotics:
  - Fever, increased sputum production, and/or dyspnea
- Methylxanthines
- Ventilator settings:
  - Allow sufficient expiratory time to minimize air trapping and subsequent barotrauma.
  - Permissive hypercapnia

## MEDICATION

- Albuterol: 2.5 mg nebulized q10–30min
- Azithromycin: 500 mg PO/IV once then 250 mg/day PO for 4 days
- Ceftriaxone: 1 g IV q24h
- Ipratropium bromide: 0.5 mg nebulized q6h
- Levofloxacin: 500 mg PO/IV q24h
- Methylprednisolone: 125 mg IV q6h
- Prednisone: 40–60 (1–2 mg/kg) mg PO per day for 5 days
- Terbutaline: 0.25 mg SC q30min

### First Line

- Albuterol
- Ipratropium bromide
- Prednisone or methylprednisolone

## FOLLOW-UP

### DISPOSITION

### Admission Criteria

- ICU admission:
  - Intubated patients
  - $CO_2$ narcosis with oxygen saturation <90%
  - Clinical tiring in the ED
  - Severe acidosis
  - Concomitant cardiac or pulmonary disease
  - Acute coronary syndrome
  - Arrhythmia
  - CHF
  - Pulmonary embolism
- Regular hospital bed:
  - COPD patients with an additional pulmonary insult:
    ○ Pneumonia
    ○ Lobar collapse
    ○ Increased work of breathing
- Exercise intolerance
- Failure to improve in ED
- Failed outpatient treatment
- 3 criteria can predict mortality at admission:
  - Age >70 yr
  - Number of clinical signs of severity:
    ○ Cyanosis, accessory muscle use, etc.
  - Dyspnea at baseline

### Discharge Criteria

- Mild flare
- Resolution in ED
- Ambulatory oxygen saturation >92%

### FOLLOW-UP RECOMMENDATIONS

- Smoking cessation
- Ensure vaccinations are up-to-date (influenza annually, pneumococcal at least once).
- Identify and avoid triggers (eg, cold air, perfumes).

## PEARLS AND PITFALLS

- Nebulized steroids may be used more for acute exacerbation of COPD in the future.
- Patients with COPD are at increased risk for diabetes, hypertension, and cardiovascular disease.
- Consider routine influenza and pneumococcal vaccinations for those with COPD.

## ADDITIONAL READING

- Celli BR. Update on management of COPD. *Chest.* 2008:133:1451–1462.
- Cosio MG, Saeta M, Agusti A. Immunologic aspects of chronic obstructive pulmonary disease. *NEJM.* 2009;360:2445–2454.
- Maclay JD, Rabinovich RA, MacNee W. Update in chronic obstructive pulmonary disease 2008. *Am J Respir Crit Care Med.* 2009;179:533–541.
- Marx JA, Hockberger RS, Walls RM, et al., eds. *Rosen's Emergency Medicine: Concepts and Clinical Practice,* 7th ed. St. Louis: Mosby; 2009.
- Sutherland ER, Cherniack RM. Management of chronic obstructive pulmonary disease. *NEJM.* 2004;350:2689–2697.

### See Also (Topic, Algorithm, Electronic Media Element)

- Asthma
- Congestive Heart Failure
- Dyspnea
- Pulmonary Embolism

## CODES

ICD9

- 491.21 Obstructive chronic bronchitis with (acute) exacerbation
- 496 Chronic airway obstruction, not elsewhere classified

C

# CIRRHOSIS

*Paul J. Allegretti*

 **BASICS**

## DESCRIPTION

- Progressive process of inflammation, cellular injury and necrosis, diffuse fibrosis, and formation of regenerative nodules
- Loss of lobular and vascular architecture
- Irreversible in advanced stages
- Intrahepatic portal hypertension owing to increased resistance at the sinusoid, compression of the central veins, and anastomosis between the arterial and portal systems
- Markedly reduced life expectancy
- 10th leading cause of death in the U.S.

## ETIOLOGY

- Chronic alcohol abuse (most common cause in U.S.)
- Chronic viral hepatitis, B or C (2nd most common cause in U.S.)
- Autoimmune hepatitis
- Biliary cirrhosis, primary (PBC) or secondary (sclerosing cholangitis)
- Metabolic:
  - Hereditary hemochromatosis
  - Wilson disease
  - Porphyria
- Drugs:
  - Acetaminophen
  - Methotrexate
  - Amiodarone
  - Methyldopa
- Hepatic congestion:
  - Right-sided heart failure
  - Pericarditis
  - Budd-Chiari syndrome (hepatic venous outflow obstruction)
- Infiltrative:
  - Sarcoidosis
  - Amyloidosis
  - Nonalcoholic steatohepatitis (NASH)
  - Hepatocellular carcinoma, diffusely infiltrating
- Infections:
  - Brucellosis
  - Echinococcosis
  - Tertiary syphilis
  - Schistosomiasis

### Pediatric Considerations

- Congenital
- Arteriohepatic dysplasia, biliary atresia, cystic fibrosis, $\alpha_1$-antitrypsin deficiency
- Metabolic
- Fructosemia, tyrosinemia, galactosemia, glycogen storage diseases
- Infectious
- Congenital hepatitis B

 **DIAGNOSIS**

## SIGNS AND SYMPTOMS

- May be silent
- Insidious onset with nonspecific findings:
  - Malaise
  - Fatigue
  - Anorexia
  - Nausea and vomiting
  - Weight loss
  - Pruritus
  - Hyperpigmentation
- Jaundice
- Fetor hepaticus
- Asterixis
- Hypotension
- Cruveilhier-Baumgartnen murmur
- Renal insufficiency
- Spider telangiectasias
- Palmar erythema
- Dupuytren contractures
- Parotid and lacrimal gland enlargement
- Nail changes
- Terry nails
- Muehrcke lines
- Clubbing
- Feminization:
  - Testicular atrophy
  - Impotence
  - Loss of libido
  - Gynecomastia
- Ascites
- Amenorrhea
- Abdominal collateral circulation including caput medusae
- Hepatomegaly
- Splenomegaly
- Abdominal discomfort or tenderness
- Fever
- Complications:
  - When complications develop, patient is considered to have decompensated disease.
  - Ascites
  - Spontaneous bacterial peritonitis (SBP)
  - Hepatic encephalopathy—may be precipitated by:
    ○ GI bleed
    ○ Infections
    ○ Increased dietary protein
    ○ Hypokalemia
    ○ Sedatives
    ○ Constipation
    ○ Azotemia
    ○ Alkalosis
  - Variceal hemorrhage:
    ○ 1/3 of patients with varicies bleed.
    ○ Each bleeding episode carries a 33% mortality rate.
    ○ Hepatic venous pressure gradient >12 mm Hg increases risk of bleed.

- Portal hypertensive gastropathy or peptic ulcer disease
- Hepatorenal failure:
  ○ Caused by decreased renal perfusion during severe decompensated cirrhosis
  ○ May be iatrogenic: Secondary to diuretics, NSAIDs, IV contrast, aminoglycosides, large-volume paracentesis
  ○ High mortality rate
- Hepatopulmonary syndrome:
  ○ Intrapulmonary vascular dilation and hypoxia
  ○ Results in increased alveolar-arterial gradient

## ESSENTIAL WORKUP

Detailed history and physical to search for clues to liver disease

## DIAGNOSTIC TESTS & INTERPRETATION
### Lab

- CBC:
  - Anemia
  - Macrocytosis
  - Leukopenia and neutropenia
  - Thrombocytopenia
- Impaired liver function:
  - High bilirubin
  - Low albumin
  - High globulins
  - Prolonged prothrombin time
  - Varying degrees of DIC
  - Hypoglycemia
- Increased liver enzymes:
  - Aspartate alanine aminotransferase (AST, SGOT), alanine aminotransferase (ALT, SGPT)—reflect injury
  - Ratio of AST:ALT $\geq$2.0 in alcoholic liver disease
  - Alkaline phosphatase and 5′-nucleotidase reflect cholestasis.
  - Gamma-glutamyltranspeptidase (GGT)
  - May be normal in inactive cirrhosis
- Electrolytes, BUN, and creatinine
- Hyponatremia:
  - Renal dysfunction and hepatorenal syndrome
- Arterial blood gases or pulse oximeter for:
  - Suspected pneumonia
  - CHF
  - Hepatopulmonary syndrome
- Search for cause:
  - Hepatitis B surface antigen
  - Hepatitis C antibody
  - Antinuclear antibody (ANA) and antismooth muscle antibody (autoimmune hepatitis)
  - Antimitochondrial antibody (primary biliary cirrhosis)
  - Serum iron, transferrin saturation, and ferritin (hemochromatosis)
  - Ceruloplasmin (Wilson disease)
  - $\alpha_1$-Antitrypsin deficiency
  - Serum immune electrophoresis (high IgM in PBC)
  - Cholesterol (chronic cholestasis)
  - Alpha fetoprotein (hepatocellular cancer)

### Imaging
- US for liver architecture, biliary obstruction, ascites, portal vein thrombosis, splenomegaly
- CT scan to explore abnormal finding on ultrasound
- CXR for pleural effusion, cardiomegaly, and CHF

### Diagnostic Procedures/Surgery
- Esophagogastroduodenoscopy (EGD) indicated for upper GI bleeding or variceal surveillance
- Variceal ligation or endoscopic sclerotherapy

## DIFFERENTIAL DIAGNOSIS
- Ascites:
  - Increased right heart pressure
  - Hepatic vein thrombosis
  - Peritoneal malignancy/infection
  - Pancreatic disease
  - Thyroid disease
  - Lymphatic obstruction
- Upper GI bleeding:
  - Peptic ulcer disease
  - Gastritis
- Encephalopathy:
  - Metabolic
  - Toxic
  - Intracranial process

## TREATMENT

### PRE-HOSPITAL
- Naloxone, dextrose (or Accucheck), and thiamine for altered mental status
- Reverse hypotension with IV fluids to prevent acute ischemic hepatic injury.

### INITIAL STABILIZATION/THERAPY
Treat complications such as GI bleeding or hepatic encephalopathy.

### ED TREATMENT/PROCEDURES
- For suspected variceal bleed:
  - IV proton pump inhibitors
  - IV octreotide—analog of somatostatin (splanchnic vasoconstrictor)
  - IV vasopressin with simultaneous nitroglycerin has been used, but has high complication rate:
    - Nitroglycerin decreases vasoconstriction of vasopressin.
  - Reverse coagulopathy:
    - Fresh-frozen plasma 1 IU/hr until bleeding is controlled
    - Desmopressin (DDAVP)—improves bleeding time and prolonged partial thromboplastin time
  - Balloon tamponade with Sengstaken-Blakemore tube or a variant for variceal compression (rarely used anymore, prophylactic intubation recommended)
  - Emergent endoscopic sclerotherapy
- Initiate broad-spectrum antibiotics in suspected sepsis or spontaneous bacterial peritonitis (SBP):
  - Cefotaxime
  - Ticarcillin-clavulanate
  - Piperacillin-tazobactam
  - Ampicillin-sulbactam
- Treat complicating conditions such as ascites, hepatic encephalopathy, SBP.

- Treat pruritus with:
  - Diphenhydramine 25–50 mg IM/IV q4h
  - Cholestyramine, ursodeoxycholic acid, or rifampin
  - Naloxone infusion 0.2 $\mu$g/kg/min for temporary relief for extreme cases
- For prolonged PT, administer vitamin K, 10 mg PO, or SC daily for 3 days. If bleeding, need FFP.
- Relieve biliary obstruction (eg, stricture) by endoscopic, radiologic, or surgical means.
- Provide nutritious diet; high in calories and adequate in protein (1 g/kg), unless there is complicating hepatic encephalopathy (HE)
- $\beta$-Blocker (propranolol) for esophageal varices:
  - Titrated to pulse rate of 60 or 25% reduction of resting pulse
  - With or without isosorbide dinitrate
  - Decreases rebleeding rate
  - May delay or prevent occurrence of 1st bleed
- Consult transplantation coordinator whenever post-liver transplantation patient presents to the ED with liver dysfunction, suspected sepsis, or possible treatment-related complication.

### SPECIAL THERAPY
- Hemochromatosis: Phlebotomy or deferoxamine (iron-chelating agent)
- Autoimmune hepatitis: Prednisone with or without azathioprine
- Chronic hepatitis B or C: Alpha interferon (avoid in decompensated cirrhosis)
- Primary biliary cirrhosis: Ursodeoxycholic acid
- Wilson disease: Penicillamine
- The only cure for most advanced cirrhosis is liver transplantation.

### MEDICATION
- Azathioprine: 1–2 mg/kg PO
- Cefotaxime: 1–2 g q6–8h (peds: 50–180 mg/kg/d q6h) IV
- Cholestyramine: 4 g PO 1–6 times per day
- Desmopressin (DDAVP): 0.3 $\mu$g/kg in 50-mL saline infused over 15–30 min
- Dextrose: $D_{50}W$ 1 amp (50 mL or 25 g; peds: $D_{25}W$ 2–4 mL/kg) IV
- Naloxone: 0.2–2 mg (peds: 0.1 mg/kg) IV or IM initial dose
- Lactulose: 15–30 mL t.i.d. aiming at 2–3 stools per day
- Octreotide: 25–50 $\mu$g IV bolus followed by 50 $\mu$g/hr IV infusion
- Piperacillin-tazobactam: 3.375 g IV q6h (peds: 100–400 mg/kg/d divided q6–8h; renal dosing required)
- Prednisone: 40 mg (peds: 1–2 mg/kg) PO daily
- Propranolol: 40 (initial) to 240 mg (peds: 1–5 mg/kg/d) PO t.i.d.
- Rifampin: 600 mg (peds: 10–20 mg/kg) PO daily
- Thiamine: 100 mg (peds: 50 mg) IV or IM
- Ursodeoxycholic acid: 8–10 mg/kg/d t.i.d.

## FOLLOW-UP

### DISPOSITION
**Admission Criteria**
- Acute decompensation or complicating conditions
- 1st presentation with clinically evident cirrhosis, unless close outpatient workup is possible
- Advanced grades hepatic encephalopathy, sepsis, active GI bleed, and hepatorenal and hepatopulmonary syndromes require ICU.

**Discharge Criteria**
Most patients with compensated cirrhosis can be treated as outpatients.

### FOLLOW-UP RECOMMENDATIONS
GI for all new cases

## PEARLS AND PITFALLS
- Prognosis is highly variable.
- Patients present with a wide variety of signs and symptoms related to end stage liver disease.
- New cases need full workup and GI consultation for management.
- Any complication puts patient in decompensated state.
- SBP symptoms are frequently vague:
  - Must have a high suspicion and low threshold for paracentesis when considering SBP

## ADDITIONAL READING
- Fauci A, Braunwald E, et al. Harrison's principles of internal medicine, 17th ed. New York: McGraw-Hill; 2008.
- Feldman M. Sleisenger and Fordtran's gastrointestinal and liver disease, 8th ed. Philadelphia: WB Saunders; 2006.
- Goldberg E. Diagnostic approach to the patient with cirrhosis. Wellesley, MA: UpToDate; 2009.
- Runyon BA. Management of adult patients with ascites due to cirrhosis. Hepatology. 2004;39(3): 841–856.

### See Also (Topic, Algorithm, Electronic Media Element)
- Ascites
- Hepatic Encephalopathy
- Hepatitis
- Spontaneous Bacterial Peritonitis
- Varices

## CODES

ICD9
- 571.2 Alcoholic cirrhosis of liver
- 571.5 Cirrhosis of liver without mention of alcohol
- 571.6 Biliary cirrhosis

# CLAVICLE FRACTURE

*Sean Patrick Nordt*
*Jeffrey A. Manko*

### Geriatric Considerations
Geriatric patients who sustain a clavicular fracture may have difficulty performing activities of daily living. The patient's social and living situations should be assessed to determine a safe discharge plan that may require additional assistance at home.

### Pregnancy Considerations
Clavicular fractures are the result of direct trauma. Patients who are pregnant should be appropriately worked up for other injuries but also should receive fetal monitoring to ensure the health of the fetus. Even minor injuries can result in trauma or harm to the fetus.

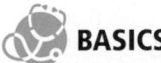 **BASICS**

## DESCRIPTION
- Clavicular fractures account for 5% of all fractures in all age groups.
- 80% of clavicular fractures involve the middle 3rd.
- 15% occur in the distal 3rd.
- 5% occur in the medial 3rd.

Classification.
- Group I: middle-3rd fractures
- Group II: distal-3rd fractures:
  - Type I: coracoclavicular ligaments are intact (nondisplaced).
  - Type II: severing of the coracoclavicular ligaments (conoid)
  - Type III: articular surface involvement of the acromioclavicular joint
- Group III: medial (proximal)-3rd fractures

## ETIOLOGY
Mechanism:
- Direct trauma to the clavicle
- Fall on the lateral shoulder
- Fall on the outstretched hand

### Pediatric Considerations
- Most common of all pediatric fractures
- May occur in newborns secondary to birth trauma

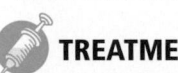 **DIAGNOSIS**

## SIGNS AND SYMPTOMS
### History
- Local pain, tenderness, and swelling over the fracture site
- Crepitus is often present owing to the clavicle's subcutaneous position
- Arm held in adduction against the chest wall with resistance to motion
- Shoulder displaced anteriorly and inferiorly

### Physical Exam
- Palpate the clavicle for tenderness, crepitus, and swelling.
- Examine the humerus and shoulder joint for other fractures, dislocations, or subluxations.
- Determine whether the fracture is open or closed.
- Evaluate for associated injuries (often serious and life threatening) that must be excluded:
  - Skeletal injuries:
    - 1st rib fracture with underlying aortic injury
    - Sternoclavicular joint separation/fracture-dislocation
    - Acromioclavicular joint separation/fracture-dislocation
    - Cervical spine injuries

## DIAGNOSTIC TESTS & INTERPRETATION
### Imaging
- AP radiographs of both clavicles are mandatory and must include:
- Upper 3rd of the humerus
- Shoulder girdle (rule out other fractures)
- Upper lung fields (rule out pneumothorax)
- Oblique and apical lordotic views:

- May be helpful, especially for medial and distal clavicle fractures that are not easily visualized on the AP view
- Stress views (weight-bearing) for distal clavicle fractures are no longer routinely recommended.
- Angiography:
  - Should be performed if there is any evidence or suspicion of vascular injuries (most commonly subclavian vessels)

## DIFFERENTIAL DIAGNOSIS
- Distal fractures: Consider acromioclavicular separation.
- Medial fractures: Consider sternoclavicular separation.
- Shoulder fracture-dislocation

**TREATMENT**

## PRE-HOSPITAL
- Ice packs to affected area
- Pain management using either narcotics or NSAIDs
- Immobilize affected side in a sling.

## INITIAL STABILIZATION/THERAPY
Airway management and resuscitate as indicated

## ED TREATMENT/PROCEDURES
- Open fracture: Uncommon occurrence, but usually requires open debridement and internal fixation (obtain immediate orthopedic referral)
- Closed fracture: If severely displaced, attempt closed reduction and immobilize depending on type of fracture:
  - Middle 3rd:
    - If nondisplaced, a sling or shoulder immobilizer is enough to provide support.

- Controversy exists as to whether closed reduction is necessary because the alignment is rarely maintained regardless of splinting technique.
- To perform a closed reduction, 1% lidocaine should be injected into the fracture hematoma. The shoulders are pulled upward, outward, and backward, and the fracture is then manipulated into place.
- Sedation may be given to alleviate pain or anxiety.
- A figure-of-eight splint or shoulder immobilizer is then applied.
- Ice should be applied for the 1st 24 hr.
- Analgesia (narcotics or NSAIDs) for pain
- Distal 3rd type I:
  - Ice for the 1st 24 hr.
  - Immobilization with a sling or shoulder immobilizer
  - Orthopedic referral
  - Analgesia (narcotics or NSAIDs) for pain
  - Early range of motion
- Distal 3rd type II:
  - Ice for the 1st 24 hr.
  - Immobilization with a sling or shoulder immobilizer
  - Orthopedic referral (may require operative repair)
  - Analgesia (narcotics or NSAIDs) for pain
- Distal 3rd type III: Same as type II
- Medial (proximal) 3rd:
  - Ice for the 1st 24 hr.
  - Immobilization in a sling or shoulder immobilizer for support
  - Analgesia (narcotics or NSAIDs) for pain
  - Orthopedic follow-up
- Reassess neurovascular status after all splints are applied.

### Pediatric Considerations
- Children who do not cooperate with the figure-of-eight splint should be referred to an orthopedic surgeon for possible shoulder spica placement.
- Most children will tolerate a shoulder immobilizer best.

### MEDICATION
- Acetaminophen: 500–1,000 mg PO q6h PRN (peds: 15–20 mg/kg PO q6h PRN)
- Ibuprofen: 600–800 mg PO q6h PRN with meals (peds: 5–10 mg/kg PO q6h PRN)

 FOLLOW-UP

### DISPOSITION
#### Admission Criteria
- Open fracture
- Associated injuries that are potentially life threatening

#### Discharge Criteria
- Isolated closed clavicle fracture without other injuries
- Appropriate support services at home (especially for elderly patients)
- Orthopedic follow-up
- Adequate pain management

#### Issues for Referral
Open fracture, complex injury, signs of neurovascular injury require immediate orthopedic referral.

### FOLLOW-UP RECOMMENDATIONS
Follow-up with an orthopedic surgeon:
- Seek medical care immediately with any changes in neurologic function, sensation, or motor strength.

## PEARLS AND PITFALLS

Always be wary of associated injuries that can be life-threatening including cervical spine injury, aortic injury, and other cardiopulmonary injuries:
- Always assess for any neurologic deficits associated with the fracture.

## ADDITIONAL READING

- Anderson K. Evaluation and treatment of distal clavicle fractures. *Clin Sports Med.* 2003;22:319–326.
- Eiff MP. Management of clavicle fractures. *Am Fam Physician.* 1997;55:12–128.
- Heckman J, Bucholz R. *Rockwood and Green's Fractures in Adults,* 5th ed. Philadelphia: Lippincott Williams & Wilkins, 2001.
- Post M. Current concepts in the treatment of fractures of the clavicle. *Clin Orthop.* 1989;245: 89–101.
- Judd DB, Pallis MP, Smith E, et al. Acute operative stabilization versus nonoperative management of clavicle fractures. *Am J Orthop.* 2009;38(7): 341–345.

 CODES

### ICD9
- 810.00 Closed fracture of clavicle, unspecified part
- 810.01 Closed fracture of sternal end of clavicle
- 810.02 Closed fracture of shaft of clavicle

# COCAINE POISONING
*Steven Aks*

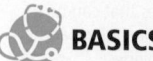 **BASICS**

## DESCRIPTION
- Sympathomimetic
- Inhibits neurotransmitter reuptake at the nerve terminal
- Metabolism:
  – Hepatic degradation
  – Nonenzymatic hydrolysis
  – Cholinesterase metabolism

## ETIOLOGY
- IV, nasal, oral administration of cocaine
- Oral ingestion:
  – Body stuffers:
    ○ Ingest hastily wrapped packets in attempt to evade police.
  – Body packers:
    ○ Ingest cocaine packets to smuggle the drug using couriers' oral, rectal, and vaginal cavities.
    ○ Cocaine is wrapped carefully in packets containing large amounts of drug.

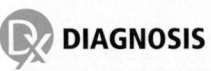 **DIAGNOSIS**

## SIGNS AND SYMPTOMS
- Sympathomimetic toxidrome
- Cardiovascular:
  – HTN
  – Tachycardia
  – Chest pain (angina)
- Respiratory:
  – Tachypnea
  – Pleuritic chest pain:
    ○ Pneumomediastinum
    ○ Pneumothorax
    ○ Bronchitis
    ○ Pulmonary infarction
  – Cough
- CNS:
  – Agitation
  – Tremulousness
  – Coma
  – Seizures
  – Stroke

- Miscellaneous:
  – Hyperthermia (poor prognosis)
  – Limb ischemia (inadvertent intra-arterial injection)
  – Corneal ulcerations (heavy crack smokers):
    ○ Owing to local chemical and thermal irritation that disrupts corneal epithelium
  – Rhabdomyolysis

### History
For body packers and stuffers:
- Time since ingestion
- Route of ingestion (oral, rectal, vaginal)
- Number of packets ingested
- Material and method of packing

### Physical Exam
Sympathomimetic toxidrome:
- HTN
- Tachycardia
- Tachypnea
- Hyperthermia
- Diaphoresis
- Mydriasis
- Neuromuscular hyperactivity

## ESSENTIAL WORKUP
- Recognition of the sympathomimetic toxidrome caused by cocaine:
  – Distinguish from anticholinergic toxidrome.
- Toxidrome recognition:
  – Sympathomimetic:
    ○ Heart rate (tachycardia)
    ○ BP (increased)
    ○ Moist skin
    ○ Bowel sounds present
    ○ Temperature (increased)
    ○ No urinary retention
  – Anticholinergic:
    ○ Heart rate (tachycardia)
    ○ BP (increased)
    ○ Dry skin
    ○ Bowel sounds diminished
    ○ Temperature (increased)
    ○ Urinary retention present

## DIAGNOSTIC TESTS & INTERPRETATION
### Lab
- CBC
- Electrolytes, BUN, creatinine, glucose
- Urinalysis dip for myoglobin
- Cardiac enzymes (troponin, creatine phosphokinase) for:
  – Anginal chest pain
  – Abnormal results on ECG
- Creatine phosphokinase (CPK) for evidence of myoglobinuria

### Imaging
- ECG:
  – For anginal chest pain
  – Consider possibility of myocardial infarction with cocaine-related chest pain.
- CXR:
  – For chest pain or shortness of breath
  – Check for pneumomediastinum, pneumothorax, aortic rupture.
- Abdominal radiograph:
  – For body packers/stuffers
  – Usually produces negative result for stuffers because drug is loosely packed in cellophane
  – Positive for packers because drug is densely packed and usually radiopaque
- CT of the abdomen with contrast:
  – When unreliable history of body packers/stuffers and nothing visualized on abdominal frontal radiograph
- CT brain scan:
  – For altered mental status or severe headache
  – Detects cerebral ischemia or hemorrhage

## DIFFERENTIAL DIAGNOSIS
- Other agents with sympathomimetic effects
- Theophylline
- Caffeine
- Amphetamines
- Albuterol
- Tricyclic antidepressants
- Antihistamines
- Phencyclidine (PCP)
- Thyrotoxicosis
- Neuroleptic malignant syndrome
- Hallucinogens

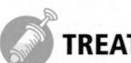 **TREATMENT**

## PRE-HOSPITAL
- Establish IV access
- Cardiac monitor:
  – Chest pain may be ischemic.
  – Benzodiazepine therapy to control agitation
- When drug is used as a "speedball" (combination of heroin and cocaine ), administer naloxone in increments to reverse coma.

## INITIAL STABILIZATION/THERAPY
- ABCs
- Establish IV access.
- Establish cardiac monitor.
- Provide therapy with naloxone (Narcan), thiamine, dextrose (or Accu-Check) for altered mental status

## ED TREATMENT/PROCEDURES
- Supportive care for mildly symptomatic patients
- Benzodiazepines:
  - For agitation and tremor
  - Initial agents for hypertension and tachycardia
- Cooling measures for hyperthermia.
  - Evaporative-convective method
- Treat rhabdomyolysis:
  - Hydrate with 0.9% NS
  - Alkalinization with IV bicarbonate in severe cases
- Cardiac chest pain:
  - Aspirin
  - Nitrates
  - Oxygen
  - Opiates
  - Avoid $\beta$-blockers because of unopposed $\alpha$-stimulation
  - Angiography/angioplasty/thrombolysis for acute myocardial infarction
- HTN/tachycardia:
  - Benzodiazepine initial agent
  - Use $\alpha$-blocking agent (phentolamine) as sole agent or combine with $\beta$-blocker (propranolol, esmolol) if unresponsive to benzodiazepine.
  - Use labetalol cautiously (does not have equal $\alpha$- and $\beta$-blocking properties).
  - IV nitroglycerin/nitroprusside for severe unresponsive hypertension
- Body packer/stuffers:
  - Treat asymptomatic or minimally symptomatic body packers and body stuffers:
    ○ Oral activated charcoal
    ○ Whole-bowel irrigation with polyethylene glycol-electrolyte lavage solution (efficacy unknown)
    ○ Most body stuffers if asymptomatic after 12–24 hr post ingestion
  - Consult with surgeons for symptomatic body packers and stuffers.
  - If toxicity is not easily managed with previously suggested pharmacologic therapy, remove the drug packets intraoperatively.

## MEDICATION
### First Line
- Diazepam: 5 mg incremental doses IV or
- Lorazepam: 2 mg incremental doses IV

### Second Line
- Activated charcoal slurry: 1–2 g/kg up to 90 g PO
- Dextrose: $D_{50}W$ 1 ampule (50 mL or 25 g) (peds: $D_{25}W$ 2–4 mL/kg) IV
- Esmolol: 50–200 $\mu$g/kg/min IV infusion titrated to effect
- Naloxone (Narcan): 2 mg (peds: 0.1 mg/kg up to 2 mg) IV or IM initial dose
- Nitroglycerin: 10–100 $\mu$g/min IV infusion
- Nitroprusside: 0.3 $\mu$g/kg/min IV (titrate to effect up to 10 $\mu$g/kg/min)
- Phentolamine: 5 mg IV q15–24min (titrate to clinical effect)
- Polyethylene glycol (GoLYTELY): 1–2 L PO per hour until packet passage (efficacy controversial)

 **FOLLOW-UP**

## DISPOSITION
### Admission Criteria
- Altered mental status
- Abnormal vital signs: Heart rate > 100 bpm, diastolic BP > 120 mm Hg, or hypotension
- Hyperthermia
- Cocaine-induced myocardial ischemia
- Body stuffers and body packers
- ICU admission for moderate to severe toxicity

### Discharge Criteria
- Mental status and vital signs normal after 6 hr of observation
- Body packers or stuffers with confirmed expulsion of packets and no clinical signs of toxicity
- Stuffers may be discharged if uncomplicated packets were ingested and if asymptomatic for 12–24 hr.

## PEARLS AND PITFALLS
- Benzodiazepines are the 1st line treatment for the sympathomimetic toxidrome from cocaine.
- Avoid $\beta$ blockers in the hyperdynamic cocaine intoxicated patient.
- Consider a broad differential in cocaine-associated chest pain.
- An abdominal flat plate radiograph will be of some value in a body packer, but of no value in imaging packets in a body stuffer.

## ADDITIONAL READING
- Hoffman RS. Cocaine. In: Goldfrank LR, ed. *Goldfrank's toxicologic emergencies,* 8th ed. Stamford, CT: Appleton & Lange; 2006:1133–1146.
- Jones JH, Weir WB. Cocaine-associated chest pain. *Emerg Med Clin N Am.* 2005;89:1323–1342.
- June R, Aks S, Keys N, et al. Medical outcome of cocaine bodystuffers. *J Emerg Med.* 2000;18: 221–224.
- Kalimullah FA, Bryant SM. Case files of the medical toxicology fellowship at the Toxikon Consortium in Chicago: Cocaine-associated wide-complex dysrhythmias and cardiac arrest-treatment nuances and controversies. *J Med Toxicol.* 2008;4:277–283.

 **CODES**

### ICD9
970.8 Poisoning by other specified central nervous system stimulants

# COLON TRAUMA
*Stephen R. Hayden*

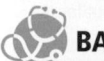 **BASICS**

## DESCRIPTION
- Trauma that perforates the colon inflames the cavity in which it lies.
- Peritoneal inflammation from hollow viscus perforation often requires hours to develop.
- Mesenteric tears from blunt trauma cause hemorrhage and bowel ischemia.
- Delayed perforation from ischemic or necrotic bowel may occur.
- Peritonitis and sepsis may develop from the extravasated intraluminal flora.
- Ascending and descending colon segments are retroperitoneal.
- The left colon has a higher bacterial load than the right.
- Morbidity and mortality increase if the diagnosis of colon injury is delayed.

## ETIOLOGY
- Penetrating abdominal trauma:
  - The colon is the second most commonly injured organ in penetrating trauma.
  - Gunshot wounds have the highest incidence.
  - Transverse colon is most commonly injured.
  - Often presents with peritonitis
- Blunt abdominal trauma:
  - Colon rarely injured in blunt trauma
  - Burst injury occurs from compression of a closed loop of bowel.
  - Intestine may be squeezed between a blunt object (lap belt) and vertebral column or bony pelvis.
  - Sudden deceleration may produce bowel-mesenteric disruption and consequent devascularization.
  - With deceleration, the sigmoid and transverse colon are most vulnerable.
- Transanal injury:
  - Iatrogenic endoscopic or barium enema injury
  - Foreign bodies used during sexual activities may reach and injure the colon.
  - Compressed air under high pressure such as at automobile repair facilities can perforate the colon even if the compressor nozzle is not fully inserted anally.
  - Swallowed sharp foreign bodies (toothpick) may penetrate the colon, particularly the cecum, appendix, and sigmoid:
    - Most foreign bodies pass without complications.

### Pediatric Considerations
Unlike adults, children have an equal frequency of blunt and penetrating colon injuries.

 **DIAGNOSIS**

## SIGNS AND SYMPTOMS
- Colon trauma is generally associated with other intra-abdominal and extra-abdominal injuries, commonly to the small intestine.
- Injuries of significant severity may have minimal early findings.
- It is uncommon to determine specific organ injury on physical exam.
- Assess on examination:
  - Abdomen for peritoneal signs
  - Ecchymosis or hematoma on lower abdomen from lap-belt compression
  - Ecchymosis on epigastric region from steering-wheel compression
  - Grey Turner sign (flank hematomas) resulting from retroperitoneal bleeding.
  - Foreign bodies or blood on digital rectal examination (particularly in the presence of pelvic fracture)
  - Note: Abdominal wall ecchymosis or hematoma is not always present despite existing injury.
  - Note: Bowel sounds are not helpful.

## ESSENTIAL WORKUP
- Serial abdominal examination because inflammation takes time to develop
- Abdominal CT with contrast is the best diagnostic study in stable patients.
- US and diagnostic peritoneal lavage (DPL) are helpful in the potentially unstable patient.

## DIAGNOSTIC TESTS & INTERPRETATION
- No individual test or combination of currently available diagnostic modalities is adequate to detect blunt colonic injury.
- Signs of peritoneal irritation owing to intestinal injury typically develop hours after the event.

### Lab
- Electrolytes
- Calcium, magnesium

### Imaging
- CT is more useful for detecting penetrating versus blunt colon injury.
- CT with triple contrast allows intraperitoneal and retroperitoneal visualization.
- Oral contrast is not essential in blunt abdominal trauma CT evaluation.
- Although CT may miss colon injuries, abnormal findings are typical.
- CT is only moderately sensitive at identifying hollow viscus injury.
- Hollow viscus injury associated CT findings include extraluminal gas or contrast, mesenteric fat streaking, and free fluid without solid organ injury.
- Water-soluble enema with fluoroscopy is useful if other test results are inconclusive.
- Plain abdominal radiographs can show indirect signs such as intraperitoneal and retroperitoneal free air.
- FAST US exam does not evaluate for enteric injury and retroperitoneal hemorrhage.
- See "Abdominal Trauma, Blunt"; "Abdominal Trauma, Imaging."

### Diagnostic Procedures/Surgery
- DPL or ultrasound in addition to CT will increase sensitivity.
- In blunt trauma, DPL will often not detect retroperitoneal injuries and enteric injury as intra-abdominal bleeding is limited.
- Fecal or vegetable material on DPL analysis indicates hollow viscus injury.
- Lavage white cell response may be negative secondary to delayed peritoneal inflammation.
- In hollow viscus injury, lavage WBC count: RBC ratio is higher than that seen with solid-organ injuries.

## DIFFERENTIAL DIAGNOSIS
- Other intra-abdominal injuries
- A fractured pelvis may present similarly to intraperitoneal injuries in children.

## TREATMENT

### PRE-HOSPITAL
- Cautions:
  - Follow standard prehospital guidelines for trauma treatment (ABCs).
  - Do not remove penetrating foreign bodies.
  - Do not attempt to replace eviscerated bowel; cover with moist saline dressings.
  - Obtain history regarding mechanism of injury, vehicular damage, and seat belt use.
- Controversies:
  - Use of intravenous crystalloid resuscitation is still considered the standard of care.

### INITIAL STABILIZATION/THERAPY
- Refer to topic on abdominal trauma.
- ABCs should precede abdominal evaluation.
- Aggressive management with intravenous crystalloid resuscitation and blood replacement as needed.

### ED TREATMENT/PROCEDURES
- Early surgical consultation; surgery is definitive treatment.
- Cover eviscerated bowel in moist saline gauze, in a nondependent position.
- Administer broad-spectrum antibiotics to cover gram-negative aerobic and anaerobic bacteria.
- The efficacy of multiple-agent and single-agent antibiotic regimens is similar.
- Ensure tetanus prophylaxis.

### MEDICATION
- Ampicillin: 2 g (peds: 50 mg/kg) IV q6h *plus* gentamicin 2 mg/kg (peds: 2.5 mg/kg) IV q8h *plus* metronidazole 500 mg IV q6h (peds: use clindamycin 25–40 mg/kg IV q24h div q6h–q8h)
- Aztreonam: 2 g IV q8h (peds: 90–120 mg/kg IV q24h div. q6h–q8h) *plus* clindamycin 900 mg IV q8h (peds: use clindamycin 25–40 mg/kg IV q24h div. q6h–q8h)
- Cefoxitin: 2 g IV q8h (peds: 40 mg/kg IV q6h)
- Piperacillin/tazobactam: 4.5 g (peds: 75 mg/kg) IV q8h

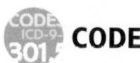

## FOLLOW-UP

### DISPOSITION

#### Admission Criteria
- Colon injuries require admission for surgical repair.
- All penetrating foreign bodies must be removed to prevent sepsis.
- Patients with abdominal ecchymosis require hospital admission and observation because of potential for undiagnosed hollow viscus injury.

#### Discharge Criteria
- Patients in whom serious abdominal injury is not suspected and with completely normal abdominal examination, normal hemodynamic status, and no other injury may be considered for discharge with appropriate precautions.
- If there is any doubt about the possibility of colon injury, the patient should be admitted and observed.

## PEARLS AND PITFALLS

Patients may initially present with paucity of symptoms:
- Observation for serial examination is indicated if mechanism suggests significant blunt abdominal trauma.

## ADDITIONAL READING
- Goldberg JE, Steele SR. Rectal foreign bodies. *Surg Clin North Am.* 2010;90(1):173–184.
- Cleary RK, Pomerantz RA, Lampman RM. Colon and rectal injuries. *Dis Colon Rectum.* 2006;49(8):1203–1222.
- ACEP Clinical Policies Committee and Clinical Policies Subcommittee on Acute Blunt Abdominal Trauma. Clinical policy: Critical issues in the evaluation of adult patients presenting to the emergency department with acute blunt abdominal trauma. *Ann Emerg Med.* 2004;43:278–290.
- Carrillo EH, Somberg LB, Ceballos CE, et al. Blunt traumatic injuries to the colon and rectum. *J Am Coll Surg.* 1996;183:548–552.
- Fealk M, Osipov R, Foster K, et al. The conundrum of traumatic colon injury. *Am J Surg.* 2004;188(6):663–670.
- Killeen KL, Shanmuganathanm K, Poletti PA, et al. Helical computed tomography of bowel and mesenteric injuries. *J Trauma.* 2001;51(1):26–36.
- Williams MD, Watts D, Fakhry S. Colon injury after blunt abdominal trauma: Results of the EAST Multi-Institutional Hollow Viscus Injury Study. *J Trauma.* 2003;55(5):906–912.
- Nelson R, Singer M. Primary repair for penetrating colon injuries. *Cochrane Database Syst Rev.* 2003;(3):CD002247.

## CODES

### ICD9
- 863.40 Injury to colon, unspecified site, without mention of open wound into cavity
- 863.50 Injury to colon, unspecified site, with open wound into cavity

C

# COMA

*Gregory D. Jay*
*Linda C. Cowell*

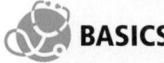 **BASICS**

## DESCRIPTION

- Light coma:
  - Responds to noxious stimuli
- Deep coma:
  - Does not respond to pain
- Unresponsiveness:
  - Loss of either arousability or cognition:
    - Loss of arousal
    - Arousal is primarily a brainstem function.
    - Impairment of the reticular activating system
    - Loss of cognition
    - Requires dysfunction of both cerebral hemispheres
  - Stupor:
    - Deep sleep, although not unconsciousness
    - Exhibits little or no spontaneous activity
    - Awaken with stimuli
    - Little motor or verbal activity once aroused
- Obtundation:
  - Mental blunting with mild or moderate reduction in alertness
  - Delirium:
    - Floridly abnormal mental status
    - Irritability
    - Motor restlessness
    - Transient hallucinations
    - Disorientation
    - Delusions
  - Clouding of consciousness:
    - Disturbance of consciousness
    - Impaired capacity to think clearly or perceive, respond to, and remember current stimuli

## ETIOLOGY

- Diffuse brain dysfunction (69%):
  - Lack of nutrients:
    - Hypoglycemia
    - Hypoxia
  - Poisoning:
    - Ethanol
    - Isopropyl alcohol
    - Ethylene glycol
    - Methanol
    - Salicylates
    - Sedative-hypnotics
    - Narcotics
    - Anticonvulsants
    - Isoniazid
    - Heavy metals
    - Opiates
    - Anticholinergics
    - Lithium
    - Phenylcyclidine
    - Cyanide
    - Carbon monoxide

- Infection:
  - Bacterial/tuberculous/syphilitic meningitis
  - Encephalitis
  - Falciparum meningitis
  - Typhoid fever
  - Rabies
- Endocrine disorders:
  - Myxedema coma
  - Thyrotoxicosis
  - Addison disease
  - Cushing disease
  - Pheochromocytoma
- Metabolic disorders:
  - Hepatic encephalopathy
  - Uremia
  - Porphyria
  - Wernicke encephalopathy
  - Aminoacidemia
  - Reye syndrome
  - Hypercapnia
- Electrolyte disorders:
  - Hypernatremia, hyponatremia
  - Hypercalcemia, hypocalcemia
  - Hypermagnesemia, hypomagnesemia
  - Hypophosphatemia
  - Acidosis, alkalosis
- Temperature regulation:
  - Hypothermia
  - Heat stroke
  - Neuroleptic malignant syndrome
  - Malignant hyperthermia
- Uremia
- Postictal state, status epilepticus
- Psychiatric
- Shock
- Fat embolism
- Hypertensive encephalopathy
- Supratentorial lesions (19%):
  - Hemorrhage (15%):
    - Intraparenchymal hemorrhage
    - Epidural hematoma
    - Subdural hematoma
    - Subarachnoid hemorrhage
  - Infarction (2%):
    - Thrombotic arterial occlusion
    - Embolic arterial occlusion
    - Venous occlusion
  - Tumor or abscess (2%):
    - Hydrocephalus
    - Herniation
    - Hemorrhage from erosion into adjacent blood vessels
- Subtentorial lesions (12%):
  - Infarction
  - Hemorrhage
  - Tumor
  - Basilar migraine
  - Brainstem demyelination

### Pregnancy Considerations
Eclampsia

 **DIAGNOSIS**

## SIGNS AND SYMPTOMS

### History
Ongoing disturbance of consciousness

### Physical Exam
- No spontaneous eye opening
- Lack of response to painful stimuli
- No motor activity
- Regular cardiorespiratory function
- Glasgow Coma Scale (GCS) scoring:
  - Eye opening (E):
    - Spontaneously 4
    - To verbal command 3
    - To pain 2
    - No response 1
  - Best motor response (M) to verbal command:
    - Obeys 6
  - Best motor response to painful stimulus:
    - Localizes to pain 5
    - Withdraws to pain 4
    - Flexion—abnormal 3
    - Extension—abnormal 2
    - No response 1
  - Best verbal response (V):
    - Oriented and converses 5
    - Disoriented and converses 4
    - Verbalizes 3
    - Vocalizes 2
    - No response 1
  - GCS = E + M + V
- Hypothermia:
  - Infection, hypoglycemia, myxedema coma, alcohol and sedative-hypnotic poisoning
- Fever:
  - Infection, thyrotoxicosis, anticholinergics, sympathomimetics, neuroleptic malignant syndrome, hypothalamic hemorrhage
- HTN
- Structural lesion, hypertensive encephalopathy
- Hypotension
- Mydriasis:
  - Organophosphates
- Miosis:
  - Narcotics
  - Anticholinergics
  - Pontine lesion
- Loss of pupillary reflexes or unequal pupils:
  - Structural lesions
- Evidence of head trauma
- Nuchal rigidity:
  - Meningitis
  - Subarachnoid hemorrhage
- Decorticate posturing:
  - Flexion of elbows and wrists
  - Adduction and internal rotation of shoulders
  - Supination of the forearms
  - Suggests severe damage above the midbrain

- Decerebrate posturing:
  - Extension of elbows and wrists
  - Adduction and internal rotation of shoulders
  - Pronation of the forearms
  - Suggests damage at the midbrain or diencephalon
- Asymmetric movements:
  - Structural lesions
  - Persistent twitching of an extremity:
    ○ Status epilepticus

## ESSENTIAL WORKUP
- Detect and treat reversible causes.
- Immediate exclusion of comalike states:
  - Noting resistance to passive opening of eyelids, fluttering of eyelids when stroked, abrupt eyelid closure, eye movements by saccadic jerks (rather than roving), or finding the eyes rolled back
  - Provocation of nystagmus with ice-water caloric testing
  - Before paralyzing a patient for intubation, an attempt should be made to detect a locked-in syndrome.
  - Demonstrating that the patient is able to blink on verbal command will establish this diagnosis.
  - Intubation is still indicated to prevent aspiration.

## DIAGNOSTIC TESTS & INTERPRETATION
### Lab
- Dextrostix
- CBC
- Electrolytes
- Blood and urine toxicologic screen

### Imaging
Head CT:
- Diagnosis of hemorrhage and midline shift
- CT angiography for suspected cerebrovascular accident

### Diagnostic Procedures/Surgery
- Lumbar puncture:
  - All patients with coma of unknown etiology, particularly if fever is present
  - Antibiotics may be administered for as long as 48 hr before lumbar puncture.
  - CT should be performed before lumbar puncture if there is evidence of increased intracranial pressure, a mass lesion, pre-existing trauma, or focal findings.
- Risk of tonsillar herniation in patients with a mass lesion is very small.
- Electroencephalography:
  - Performed to rule out suspected seizure activities
  - Little use in the emergency evaluation
  - Unlike electroencephalogram studies performed in a laboratory, lighting will cause artifacts.

## DIFFERENTIAL DIAGNOSIS
- Locked-in syndrome
- Psychogenic unresponsiveness
- Stupor
- Catatonia
- Akinetic mutism

## TREATMENT
### PRE-HOSPITAL
- Airway management if loss of airway patency
- Endotracheal intubation if no response to coma cocktail
- IV access
- Dextrose or Dextrostix
- Narcan
- Monitor
- Look for signs of an underlying cause:
  - Medical alert bracelets
  - GCS
  - Pupils
  - Extremity movements

### INITIAL STABILIZATION/THERAPY
- Airway management
- Empiric use of naloxone
- Empiric dextrose:
  - Administer if serum glucose cannot be measured at the bedside
  - Can safely be administered before thiamine
  - Does not worsen outcome in patients with stroke

### ED TREATMENT/PROCEDURES
- Specific therapy directed at underlying cause once identified
- Consider empiric use of antibiotics for coma of undetermined etiology:
  - Broad-spectrum with good cerebrospinal fluid penetration such as ceftriaxone
- Stop seizure activity with benzodiazepines, phenytoin, and phenobarbital.
- Empiric treatment for a toxic ingestion:
  - Activated charcoal
- Correct body temperature:
  - Aggressive rewarming for patients with core temperature between 32 and 35°C and invasive rewarming for <32°C
  - Ice packs and forced air movement over exposed wetted skin if severe hyperthermia

### MEDICATION
- Ceftriaxone: 100 mg/kg IV
- Dextrose: 1–2 mL/kg of $D_{50}$W IV; neonate 10 mL/kg $D_{10}$W IV; peds 4 mL/kg $D_{25}$W IV
- Diazepam: 0.1–0.3 mg/kg slow IV (max 10 mg/dose) q10–15min × 3 doses
- Flumazenil: 0.20 mg IV qmin × 1–5 doses
- Fomepizole: 15 mg/kg IV
- Lorazepam: 0.05–0.1 mg/kg IV (max 4 mg/dose q10–15min)
- Mannitol: 0.25–1.0 g/kg IV over 20 min
- Naloxone: 0.01 mg/kg IV/IM/SC/ET
- Narcan: 0.4–2.0 mg IV/IM/SQ
- Phenobarbital: 10–20 mg/kg IV
- Phenytoin: 18–20 mg/kg IV/IO or fosphenytoin 15–20 mg/kg IV/IO
- Physostigmine: 0.06–0.08 mg/kg IV
- Thiamine: 100 mg IM or 100 mg thiamine in 1,000 mL of IV fluid wide open

## FOLLOW-UP
### DISPOSITION
#### Admission Criteria
Patients who do not have a readily identifiable and completely reversible cause of coma should be admitted.

#### Discharge Criteria
Comatose patients with correctable hypoglycemia and opiate toxicity who respond completely to aggressive ED treatment can be discharged.

#### Issues for Referral
Further delineation or prevention of possible adverse medication reaction

### FOLLOW-UP RECOMMENDATIONS
- If discharged, urgent PCP F/U is needed.
- Consideration of adverse medication reaction
- Supervision for 24 hr post-discharge

## PEARLS AND PITFALLS
- Rapid medical stabilization
- Neuroimaging for structural lesions
- Metabolic and toxicologic assessment
- Identification of unusual causes of coma
- Dischargeable patients require period of ED observation.

## ADDITIONAL READING
- Glauser J. Coma: A systematic approach to patient evaluation and management 2008. Available at http://www.thefreelibrary.com/Coma.+A+Systematic +Approach+to+Patient+Evaluation+and +Management.-a0206595218
- Plum F, Posner J. The diagnosis of stupor and coma, 4th ed. Philadelphia: FA Davis, 2007.
- The Martin A. Samuels neurology review for primary care physicians. Available at http//www.cmeinfo. com/store_temp/The_Martin_A._ Samuels_Neurology_Review_for_Primary_Care_ Physicians.305.asp
- Weiner W, Shulman L. Emergent and urgent neurology, 2nd ed. Philadelphia: Lippincott, Williams & Williams, 1999.

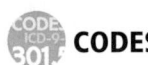 CODES

### ICD9
780.01 Coma

# COMPARTMENT SYNDROME

*Chet Shermer*

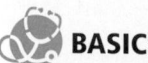 **BASICS**

## DESCRIPTION

- Elevated tissue pressure in closed spaces that compromises blood flow through capillaries
- Normal tissue pressure is <10 mm Hg.
- Capillary blood flow in a compartment is compromised at pressures >20 mm Hg.
- Muscles and nerves can develop ischemic necrosis at pressures >30 mm Hg.
- When distal pulses are diminished on exam, muscle necrosis is probably present.
- The four compartments of the leg are most frequently involved, but compartment syndrome can occur in the arm, forearm, hand, foot, shoulder, buttocks, and thigh.

## ETIOLOGY

- Decreased compartment size: Circumferential cast, burn eschar, or military antishock trousers (MAST)
- Increased compartment contents: Compression of the compartment from edema or hematoma caused by direct trauma, fracture, overexertion of muscles, postischemic time, or limb compression during prolonged recumbency

 **DIAGNOSIS**

### ALERT

- Keep the extremity at the level of the heart to promote arterial flow but not diminish venous return.
  - Do not use ice if compartment syndrome is suspected—it may compromise microcirculation.

## SIGNS AND SYMPTOMS

- Severe, constant pain over the compartment that is disproportionate to extent of injury
- Pain increases with active contraction and passive stretching.
- Muscle weakness
- Hypesthesia
- 6 *P's*: Pain, pressure, paresis, paresthesia, and pulses present

### History

- Elicit above symptoms.
- 6 *P's*

### Physical Exam

- Tenderness of muscle compartment
- Assess motor and neurologic function.

## DIAGNOSTIC TESTS & INTERPRETATION

### Imaging

Radiographs should be performed if fracture is suspected.

### Diagnostic Procedures/Surgery

- Measurement of compartment pressures with a system such as the Stryker IC pressure monitor system (Stryker Surgical, 420 East Alcott Street, Kalamazoo, MI 49001), using an 18-gauge needle or continuous pressure monitoring with the attachment for an indwelling catheter
- Technique is as follows:
  - Prep overlying skin with antiseptic solution.
  - Local anesthetic can be infiltrated into the *SC tissue only*, taking care not to inject intramuscularly.
  - The needle used for pressure measurements is advanced through the skin until a popping sensation is felt when the fascia is pierced.
  - 0.2 mL of saline is injected to clear the lumen of the needle, and the intracompartmental pressure measurement is then read.
  - To ascertain correct placement of the needle within the compartment, external pressure may be applied over the muscle compartment, or the muscles can be passively stretched to increase the intracompartmental pressure transiently; once these maneuvers are discontinued, the pressure should drop to baseline and stabilize.

## DIFFERENTIAL DIAGNOSIS

- Chronic compartment syndrome
- Fascial hernia
- Stress fracture
- Arterial occlusion
- Neurapraxia
- Deep venous thrombosis
- Cellulitis
- Osteomyelitis
- Tenosynovitis
- Synovitis

# TREATMENT

## INITIAL STABILIZATION/THERAPY

- Acutely injured extremities that are casted should have the cast univalved and spread and underlying cast padding should be cut.
- Keep the extremity at the level of the heart.

## ED TREATMENT/PROCEDURES

- Acute compartment syndrome is a surgical emergency.
- Mainstay of treatment is fasciotomy, particularly for compartment pressures >30–40 mm Hg.

## MEDICATION

- Medications are not helpful, including steroids or vasodilators, in the treatment of compartment syndrome.
- Pain medication is essential after diagnosis is made or consultant evaluation is begun.

### First Line

IV narcotic analgesics may provide some relief, although the pain is frequently so severe that only decompression in the OR can provide relief.

### Second Line

Oral narcotic analgesics and nonsteroidal agents are of very little benefit acutely.

# FOLLOW-UP

## DISPOSITION

### Admission Criteria

- Emergent orthopedic or surgical consultation for compartment pressures >30 mm Hg
- For compartment pressures >20 mm Hg but <30 mm Hg, surgical consultation should be sought and the patient admitted.
- For compartment pressures between 15 and 20 mm Hg, serial measurement of pressures should be taken; if the patient cannot be relied on to return for repeat measurements, the patient should be admitted.

### Discharge Criteria

Compartment pressure <10–15 mm Hg: Patients should be given symptomatic treatment and instructed to return for increased pain, swelling, development of paresthesias.

### Issues for Referral

If the clinician suspects chronic compartment syndrome, then prompt referral to orthopedic surgeon is necessary. Direct communication is best to express your concerns.

# PEARLS AND PITFALLS

- Must measure compartment pressures or arrange transfer to higher level of care if capability is lacking.
- Care must be taken when measuring compartment pressures to avoid injury to tendons, nerves, and blood vessels.
- Must consider concomitant rhabdomyolysis in crush-type injuries.

# ADDITIONAL READING

- Mabee JR. Compartment syndrome: A complication of acute extremity trauma. *J Emerg Med*. 1994;12(5):651–656.
- Farr D, Selesnick H. Chronic exertional compartment syndrome in a collegiate soccer player: A case report and literature review. *Am J Orthop*. 2008 July; 37(7):374–377.

- Naidu KS, Chin T, Harris C, et al. Bilateral peroneal compartment syndrome after horse riding. *Am J Emerg Med*. Sep 2009;27(7):901.e3–901.e5.
- Reis ND, Better OS. Mechanical muscle-crush injury and acute muscle-crush compartment syndrome. *J Bone Joint Surg Br*. 2005;87(4):450–453.

## See Also (Topic, Algorithm, Electronic Media Element)

- Compartment Syndrome, Extremity http://emedicine.medscape.com/article/828456-overview
- Compartment Syndromes of Extremities https://online.epocrates.com/u/2911502/Compartment+syndrome+of+extremities/Summary/Highlights?ICID=EMN0909

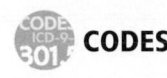

# CODES

### ICD9

- 958.8 Other early complications of trauma
- 958.90 Compartment syndrome, unspecified

**C**

# CONGENITAL HEART DISEASE, ACYANOTIC

*Lynne M. Palmisciano*
*William J. Lewander*

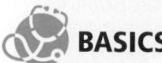 **BASICS**

## DESCRIPTION

Abnormality in the cardiocirculatory system that is present at birth but does not cause mixing of deoxygenated and oxygenated blood:

- L→R shunting lesions:
  - Ventricular septal defect (VSD)
  - Atrial septal defect (ASD)
  - Patent ductus arteriosus (PDA)
  - Endocardial cushion defects (AV canal)
- Ventricular outflow obstructions:
  - Coarctation of aorta (LV)
  - Aortic stenosis (LV)
  - Pulmonic stenosis (RV)
  - Hypoplastic left-heart syndrome (HLHS)
- Ductal dependent: Symptoms as DA closes:
  - Coarctation of aorta
  - Critical aortic stenosis
  - Critical pulmonic stenosis
  - Hypoplastic left-heart syndrome

## ETIOLOGY

For most forms, cause is unknown:

- Genetic: Down (AV canal), Turner (coarct)
- Environmental: Congenital rubella (PDA, AS)

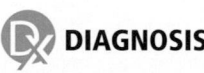 **DIAGNOSIS**

## SIGNS AND SYMPTOMS

### History

- Many asymptomatic
- Lethargy, poor feeding, and failure to thrive
- Dyspnea on exertion
- Recurrent respiratory infections

### Physical Exam

- VSD and AV canal:
  - Dusky color, hepatomegaly
  - Holosystolic and diastolic murmurs + thrill
  - Hyperdynamic precordium, displaced PMI
- ASD:
  - Fixed, split S2
  - Systolic ejection and diastolic murmurs
- PDA:
  - "Machine-like" murmur and bounding pulses
- Coarctation:
  - Differential cyanosis (pink only upper 1/2)
  - BP upper extremities > BP lower extremities
  - ↓ or absent lower extremity pulses
- AS:
  - Harsh systolic murmur, thrill, aortic click
- PS:
  - Systolic ejection murmur, thrill, pulmonic click
  - Widely split S2
  - Jugular venous a waves
- HLHS:
  - Dusky, listless, tachypneic, ↓ pulses
  - Single heart sound, systolic ejection murmur

## ESSENTIAL WORKUP

- Oxygen saturation (pre- and postductal)
- ABG, CBC, basic chemistries and glucose
- Sepsis evaluation
- CXR to assess pulmonary blood flow
- EKG (axis, hypertrophy, conduction delays)
- 4-extremity BPs
- Cardiology consult with ECG

## DIAGNOSTIC TESTS & INTERPRETATION

### Imaging

- CXR:
  - L→R shunting lesions all show cardiomegaly (specific chambers) and ↑ pulmonary markings
    - ASD (RA, RV), VSD (RV, LA), PDA (LA, LV)
    - AV canal (globular; all chambers enlarged)
- Obstructive lesions: Normal to cardiomegaly

### Diagnostic Procedures/Surgery

EKG:

- ASD: Right axis deviation:
  - RVH or right bundle branch block (RBBB)
- VSD–LAH, LVH (if large, also RVH):
  - Notched or peaked p waves (large VSD)
- PDA: Biventricular hypertrophy (large PDA)
- AV canal: Superior axis, LVH, RVH:
  - RBBB and prolonged PR interval
- AS: Normal to LVH (severe cases)
- PS: Normal to RVH, RAE (severe cases):
  - RBBB
- Coarctation of aorta: RVH or RBBB
- HLHS: RAE, RVH, peaked P waves

## DIFFERENTIAL DIAGNOSIS

- CHF
- Hypertrophic cardiomyopathy
- Cardiogenic shock
- Aortic dissection
- Myocarditis
- Bronchopulmonary dysplasia
- Pulmonary HTN
- Pneumonia/bronchiolitis
- Hypoglycemia
- Adrenal insufficiency, CAH
- Glycogen storage diseases
- Sepsis
- Shock

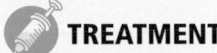 **TREATMENT**

### INITIAL STABILIZATION/THERAPY
- Maintain warmth and oxygenation.
- Treat hypoglycemia and acidosis.
- Establish IV access.
- Prepare for endotracheal intubation.

#### ALERT
High oxygen tensions promote ductal closure.

### ED TREATMENT/PROCEDURES
- Administer prostaglandin $E_1$ (PGE$_1$) to dilate or reopen the ductus arteriosus:
  - Continuous IV infusion 0.05–0.1 $\mu$g/kg/min
  - Complications include apnea, bradycardia, hypotension, and seizures.
- Evaluate and treat alternate causes cyanosis:
  - Septic workup and empiric antibiotics
  - Maintain normoglycemia
- Circulatory collapse from CHD:
  - Fluid resuscitation (increments of 10 mL/kg)
  - Inotropes
  - Aggressive treatment of acidosis
- CHF:
  - Digoxin and diuretics

### MEDICATION
- Ampicillin 50 mg/kg IV
- Digoxin dosing requires extreme caution:
  - Range 25–40 $\mu$g/kg IV
- Dobutamine: 5–20 $\mu$g/kg/min IV
- Dopamine: 2–20 $\mu$g/kg/min IV
- Epinephrine: 0.1–2 $\mu$g/kg/min IV
- Furosemide: 1 mg/kg IV
- Gentamicin: 4 mg/kg/d IV or 2.5 mg/kg/dose
- Milrinone 0.25–1 $\mu$g/kg/min
- Prostaglandin $E_1$: 0.05–0.1 $\mu$g/kg/min
- Sodium bicarbonate: 1–2 mEq/kg IV

 **FOLLOW-UP**

### DISPOSITION
#### Admission Criteria
- All newborns with suspected CHD:
  - Admit to pediatric ICU.
- CHD with acute worsening of cyanosis or CHF
- CHD with pneumonia or bronchiolitis

#### Discharge Criteria
Determine in consult with cardiologist

#### Issues for Referral
Primary care physician to coordinate care with cardiologist and cardiothoracic surgery

### FOLLOW-UP RECOMMENDATIONS
Plan for follow-up should be made in consult with the pediatric cardiologist.

## PEARLS AND PITFALLS
- Acyanotic lesions presenting at 2–12 wk:
  - Coarctation as DA closes
  - Septal defects as pulmonary vascular resistance drops
- Classic ECG in AV canal: Superior QRS axis
- Classic CXR in coarctation: Rib notching (late)

## ADDITIONAL READING
- Libby P, Bonow RO, Mann DL, et al., eds. Congenital heart disease. In: *Braunwald's heart disease*, 8th ed. Philadelphia: Saunders Elsevier, 2008: 1563–1623.
- Woods WA, McCulloch MA. Cardiovascular emergencies in the pediatric patient. *Emerg Med Clin N Am.* 2005;23:1233–1249.
- Yee L. Cardiac emergencies in the first year of life. *Emerg Med Clin N Am.* 2007;25:981–1008.

### See Also (Topic, Algorithm, Electronic Media Element)
- Congestive Heart Failure
- Failure to Thrive
- Neonatal Sepsis

 **CODES**

### ICD9
- 745.4 Ventricular septal defect
- 745.5 Ostium secundum type atrial septal defect
- 746.9 Unspecified congenital anomaly of heart

# CONGENITAL HEART DISEASE, CYANOTIC

Lynne M. Palmisciano
William J. Lewander

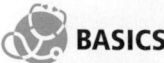

## BASICS

### DESCRIPTION
- Aberrant embryonic development results in mixing of deoxygenated and oxygenated blood returning to systemic circulation by 2 mechanisms:
  - Right-to-left intracardiac shunt
  - Anatomic defects of the aortic root
- Subtypes: 5 T's, 2 E's, single ventricle:
  - Tetralogy of Fallot (TOF):
    ○ Ventricular septal defect (VSD)
    ○ Right ventricular (RV) outflow obstruction
    ○ Overriding aorta
    ○ RV hypertrophy (RVH)
  - Transposition of the great arteries (TGA):
    ○ Aorta arises from RV and pulmonary artery from left ventricle (LV)
  - Tricuspid atresia:
    ○ No outlet from right atrium to RV
    ○ Obligatory atrial level connection
  - Truncus arteriosus:
    ○ Single arterial trunk for systemic, pulmonic and carotid circulations
  - Total anomalous pulmonary venous return (TAPVR):
    ○ Pulmonary veins drain into systemic venous circulation
    ○ Supracardiac, cardiac, infracardiac, or mixed
  - Ebstein anomaly of tricuspid valve:
    ○ Abnormal and displaced tricuspid valve divides RV resulting in poor RV function
  - Eisenmenger syndrome:
    ○ Complication in longstanding acyanotic heart disease with L→R shunts
    ○ Pulmonary vascular resistance reaches suprasystemic levels; R→L shunt
  - Single ventricle physiology:
    ○ Total mixing of systemic and venous return
- Subdivide by amount of pulmonary blood flow:
  - Decreased in TOF and tricuspid atresia
  - Increased in TGA, truncus, and TAPVR

### ETIOLOGY
For most forms, cause is unknown:
- Genetic cause: Chromosome 22 deletion in DiGeorge syndrome (conotruncal defects; TOF, truncus; also coarctation of aorta)
- Environmental/teratogenic: TGA seen more often in infants of diabetic mothers

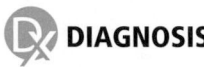

## DIAGNOSIS

- Most common initial ED presentations of cyanotic congenital heart disease (CHD):
  - Cyanosis
  - CHF
  - Circulatory collapse
- Physiologic stress triggers cyanosis in older patients with CHD:
  - Cardiac shunt obstruction
  - Pulmonary disease
  - Decreased systemic vascular resistance
  - Fever
  - Dehydration

### SIGNS AND SYMPTOMS
- Central cyanosis:
  - Visible in lips, nail beds, mucosa
  - Increases with cry or agitation
  - Minimal change with 100% $O_2$
- CHF:
  - Rales, gallop, hepatomegaly, scalp edema
- Hypercyanotic spells or "Tet spells":
  - Restless and hyperpneic then increased cyanosis then syncope
  - Follows reductions in already compromised pulmonary blood flow:
    ○ Wakening, feeding, vigorous cry, exercise
  - Older child may compensate by squatting.
  - Temporary reduction or absence of systolic ejection murmur during spell

### History
- Family history of CHD:
  - If parent or sibling: Increased risk of CHD
  - If 2 relatives: Risk of CHD triples
- Prenatal history:
  - Exposure to teratogens
  - Abnormal fetal ultrasound
- Tetralogy of Fallot:
  - Often asymptomatic at birth; symptoms develop as RV infundibulum hypertrophies
  - Severe RV outflow obstruction; neonatal cyanosis (duct dependent lesion)
  - Tet spells in toddlers
  - Older, uncorrected patients:
    ○ Dyspnea on exertion and growth delay
- Tricuspid atresia:
  - Usually cyanotic from birth
  - Feeding difficulties
  - Older patients show dyspnea on exertion and easy fatigability
- Ebstein anomaly:
  - Teens may present with dysrhythmias.
- Transposition of great arteries:
  - Presents in 1st hrs to days of life
- TAPVR:
  - Neonatal presentation; severely ill:
    ○ Cyanosis
    ○ Doesn't improve with mechanical ventilation
  - Infantile presentation; heart failure:
    ○ Mild cyanosis
  - If no obstruction to pulmonary venous return:
    ○ Asymptomatic or mild cyanosis
    ○ Frequent pneumonias
    ○ Growth problems
- Truncus arteriosus:
  - Mild cyanosis in newborn
  - Heart failure in older infants

### Physical Exam
- Tetralogy of Fallot:
  - Loud systolic murmur left sternal border (LSB)
  - Systolic thrill in 50%
  - +/− Continuous murmur of PDA
  - Loud, single 2nd heart sound (S2)
  - RV prominence/bulge
  - Older, uncorrected patients:
    ○ Dusky, blue skin
    ○ Clubbing of digits
    ○ Retinal engorgement

- Tricuspid atresia:
  - Tachypnea
  - Regurgitant murmur from VSD at LSB
  - +/− continuous PDA murmur
  - Single S2
  - Prominent LV impulse
- Ebstein anomaly:
  - Holosystolic murmur of tricuspid regurgitation
  - Many have diastolic murmur
  - Gallop
- Transposition of great arteries:
  - Single, loud S2
  - Severe hypoxemia
- TAPVR:
  - Neonatal; severe tachypnea and cyanosis
  - Infantile; heart failure:
    ○ Tachycardia
    ○ Systolic ejection murmur at LSB
    ○ Middiastolic murmur at lower LSB
    ○ Gallop
    ○ Fixed, split S2
    ○ Hepatomegaly
- Truncus arteriosus:
  - Newborn:
    ○ Mild cyanosis
    ○ Regurgitant systolic murmur at LSB
    ○ Single S2
  - Older infants; heart failure:
    ○ Hyperdynamic precordium
    ○ Bounding pulses
    ○ Wide pulse pressure
    ○ Loud, single S2
    ○ Systolic ejection murmur and thrill
    ○ Middiastolic murmur

### ESSENTIAL WORKUP
- Oxygen saturation
- ABG
- CBC, glucose
- Sepsis evaluation
- CXR to assess pulmonary blood flow
- EKG to assess for hypertrophy and QRS axis
- Cardiology consult and ECG

### DIAGNOSTIC TESTS & INTERPRETATION
#### Lab
- Decreased room air oxygen saturation
- Hyperoxia test:
  - ABG in room air and after several minutes 100% oxygen:
    ○ $PaO_2$ >150 in $O_2$; no intracardiac shunt
    ○ $PaO_2$ <100 in $O_2$; highly suspicious of cyanotic CHD
- CBC: Erythrocytosis with chronic cyanosis

#### Imaging
- CXR:
  - Decreased pulmonary blood flow:
    ○ Tetralogy of Fallot (enlarged RV)
    ○ Tricuspid atresia (enlarged LV)
    ○ Single ventricle physiology
  - Increased pulmonary flow:
    ○ Transposition of the great vessels (large RV)
    ○ TAPVR (large RV)
    ○ Truncus arteriosus (large LV and RV)

- Classic CXR descriptions:
  - Boot-shaped heart: TOF; large and upturned RV looks like toe of boot
  - Egg on a string: TGA; narrow mediastinum, great vessels anterior/posterior position
  - Snowman sign: Supracardiac TAPVR; upper portion formed by pulmonary veins
- ECG: In all new CHD cases to evaluate structure, function, and shunts

### Diagnostic Procedures/Surgery
EKG:

- Tetralogy of Fallot:
  - Right axis deviation (RAD)
  - Right ventricular hypertrophy (RVH)
- TAPVR:
  - RAD
  - RVH and right atrial enlargement (RAE)
- Transposition of the great vessels:
  - RAD
  - RVH
- Tricuspid atresia:
  - Superior axis
  - LVH, RAE, LAE
- Truncus arteriosus:
  - RVH, LVH
- Ebstein anomaly:
  - Right bundle branch block
  - Often Wolff-Parkinson-White

## DIFFERENTIAL DIAGNOSIS

- Pulmonary:
  - Pneumothorax/hemothorax
  - Bronchopulmonary dysplasia
  - Congenital lung hypoplasia/dysplasia
  - Pulmonary hemorrhage
  - Pulmonary embolus
  - Pulmonary HTN
  - Diaphragmatic hernia
  - Foreign body/anatomic obstruction
- Cardiac:
  - Cyanotic CHD
  - CHF
  - Cardiogenic shock
- Infectious:
  - Pneumonia, bronchiolitis
  - Sepsis
- Neurologic:
  - Seizure
  - Neuromuscular disease
  - Drug-induced respiratory depression
- Other:
  - Polycythemia
  - Methemoglobinemia
  - Dehydration
  - Hypoglycemia

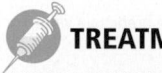 **TREATMENT**

### INITIAL STABILIZATION/THERAPY
- Maintain warmth (cold ↑ $O_2$ consumption).
- Treat hypoglycemia and acidosis.
- Maintain oxygenation.
- Establish IV access.
- Prepare for endotracheal intubation.

### ED TREATMENT/PROCEDURES
- Administer prostaglandin $E_1$ ($PGE_1$) to dilate or reopen the ductus arteriosus:
  - Continuous IV infusion 0.05–0.1 $\mu$g/kg/min
  - Complications include apnea, bradycardia, hypotension, and seizures:
    - Generally intubate prior to transport
  - Not effective for obstructed TAPVR:
    - May require ECMO awaiting surgery
  - Overall benefits far outweigh potential risks
- Evaluate and treat alternate causes of cyanosis:
  - Septic workup and empiric antibiotics
  - Fluid resuscitate (increments of 10 mL/kg)
  - Maintain normoglycemia
- Patients with Tet spells:
  - Provide a calming environment.
  - Place child in knee-chest position.
  - Supplemental $O_2$ if not agitating to patient
  - IV or IM morphine
  - For severe cases not responding to above:
    - IV bicarbonate to treat severe acidosis
    - IV phenylephrine to ↑systemic vascular resistance and reduce R→L shunt
    - IV propranolol for $\beta$-adrenergic blockade
- Cyanosis in the older patient with known CHD:
  - 10–20 mL/kg NS IV if dehydration likely
  - Supplemental $O_2$ if suspicious for pulmonary diseases
  - Antipyretics for fever
  - Antibiotics for pneumonia/infectious process
- Circulatory collapse from CHD:
  - Fluid resuscitation
  - Inotropes: Dobutamine, dopamine, milrinone
  - Aggressive treatment of acidosis

### MEDICATION
- Acetaminophen: 15 mg/kg PO or PR
- Ampicillin: 50 mg/kg IV
- Dobutamine: 5–20 $\mu$g/kg/min IV
- Dopamine: 5–20 $\mu$g/kg/min IV
- Gentamicin: 4 mg/kg/d IV or 2.5 mg/kg/dose
- Ibuprofen: 10 mg/kg PO (>6 mo)
- Milrinone: 0.25–1 $\mu$g/kg/min
- Morphine sulfate: 0.1 mg/kg SC, IM, or IV
- Phenylephrine: 0.5–5 $\mu$g/kg/min IV
- Propranolol: 0.1 mg/kg IV
- Prostaglandin $E_1$: 0.05–0.1 $\mu$g/kg/min
- Sodium bicarbonate: 1–2 mEq/kg IV

 **FOLLOW-UP**

### DISPOSITION
#### Admission Criteria
- All newborns with suspected CHD:
  - Admit to pediatric ICU.
- CHD with acute worsening of cyanosis or CHF
- CHD with symptomatic pneumonia or respiratory syncytial virus

#### Discharge Criteria
- Determine in consult with cardiologist
- Patients who respond to minimal intervention (ie, TOF patients treated noninvasively)
- Ensure close follow-up.

#### Issues for Referral
- Primary care physician to coordinate care
- Cardiologist for diagnosis, medical management, and ongoing monitoring
- Cardiothoracic evaluation for surgery

### FOLLOW-UP RECOMMENDATIONS
- Plan for follow-up should be determined in consult with the pediatric cardiologist.
- Clear instructions for return visits, as any physiologic stress may worsen condition.

## PEARLS AND PITFALLS

- Cyanotic heart disease: 5 "terrible" T's:
  - Tetralogy of Fallot
  - Transposition of the great arteries
  - Tricuspid atresia
  - Truncus arteriosus
  - TAPVR
- Visual appearance of cyanosis requires >3–5 mg/dL deoxygenated hemoglobin.
- Duct-dependent lesions:
  - Present at 2–3 wk of age
  - Sudden cyanosis or cardiovascular collapse
  - Treat with PGE1:
    - Beware apnea and hypotension

## ADDITIONAL READING

- Apitz C, Webb GD, Redington AN. Tetralogy of Fallot. Lancet. 2009;374:1462–1471.
- Fleisher GR, Ludwig S, Henretig FM, eds. Cardiac emergencies. In: Textbook of pediatric emergency medicine, 5th ed. Philadelphia: Lippincott, Williams, & Wilkins, 2006:717–758.
- Libby P, Bonow RO, Mann DL, et al., eds. Congenital heart disease. In: Braunwald's heart disease, 8th ed. Philadelphia: Saunders Elsevier, 2008:1563–1623.
- Woods WA, McCulloch MA. Cardiovascular emergencies in the pediatric patient. Emerg Med Clin N Am. 2005;23:1233–1249.
- Yee L. Cardiac emergencies in the first year of life. Emerg Med Clin N Am. 2007;25:981–1008.

### See Also (Topic, Algorithm, Electronic Media Element)
- Bronchiolitis
- Congestive Heart Failure
- Neonatal Sepsis

 **CODES**

#### ICD9
746.9 Unspecified congenital anomaly of heart

# CONGESTIVE HEART FAILURE

*Devin R. Sokolowski*
*Robert A. Partridge*

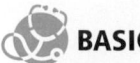 **BASICS**

## DESCRIPTION

- Inability of the ventricle to fill with (diastolic) or eject (systolic) blood. As a result, the heart fails to maintain adequate circulation.
- Low-output failure:
  - Decreased cardiac output secondary to myocardial muscle failure
- High-output failure:
  - Cardiac output is normal or high, but insufficient for metabolic needs:
    ○ Hyperthyroidism
    ○ Pregnancy
    ○ Anemia
    ○ A-V fistula
    ○ Beriberi
    ○ Paget disease
    ○ Severe anemia
- Acute CHF:
  - Rapidly progressive failure state (hours–days)
  - Usually caused by a precipitating event
  - The heart does not have the reserve to compensate for the added burden.
- Chronic CHF (weeks):
  - Slowly progressive failure state
- Left-sided failure:
  - Hemodynamic burden placed on left ventricle:
    ○ Resultant pulmonary congestion
- Right-sided failure:
  - Hemodynamic burden placed on right ventricle:
    ○ Hepatic enlargement, jugular venous distention (JVD), and dependent edema can occur.
- CHF affects ~5.7 million Americans.
- Estimated 2009 cost of CHF is $37.2 billion.
- Of all patients discharged for CHF from hospitals in 2006, 73% were ≥65.

## ETIOLOGY

- Decreased myocardial contractility:
  - Myocardial ischemia/infarction
  - Cardiomyopathy (including alcoholic and pregnancy-related cardiomyopathy)
  - Myocarditis
  - Dysrhythmias
  - Decreased contractile efficiency:
    ○ Drug related (negative inotropes)
    ○ Metabolic disorder
- Pressure overload states:
  - HTN
  - Valvular abnormalities
  - Congenital heart disease
  - Pulmonary embolism
- Restricted cardiac output:
  - Myocardial infiltrative disease
- Volume overload:
  - Dietary indiscretion (sodium overload)
  - Drugs leading to sodium retention (glucocorticoids, NSAIDs, nasal decongestants, vasodilators)
- Thyrotoxicosis
- Pregnancy
- Severe anemia

## Dx DIAGNOSIS

## SIGNS AND SYMPTOMS

- General:
  - Fatigue
  - Weakness
  - Anxiety
  - Shortness of breath
  - Cough
  - Malaise
  - Lightheadedness
- Left-heart failure:
  - Dyspnea
  - Orthopnea
  - Paroxysmal nocturnal dyspnea
  - Decreased exercise tolerance
  - Rales and/or wheezing ("cardiac asthma")
  - Pleural effusion (usually right sided)
  - Dullness at lung bases
  - S3 gallop (secondary to decreased left ventricle compliance)
  - S4 may be present
  - Laterally displaced apical impulse
- Right-heart failure:
  - Dyspnea on exertion
  - JVD
  - Hepatic enlargement/tenderness (may lead to right upper quadrant pain)
  - Nausea
  - A positive abdomino-jugular reflex
  - Ascites
  - Dependent edema
- Severe impairment:
  - Confusion
  - Tachypnea
  - Sinus tachycardia
  - Hypotension
  - Palpable dicrotic notch
  - Pulsus alternans
  - Frothy sputum
  - Cheyne-Stokes respirations

## ESSENTIAL WORKUP

- The CXR is important in confirming the diagnosis and assessing severity.
- 12-hr radiographic lag from onset of symptoms may occur.
- Radiographic findings may persist for several days despite clinical improvement.

## DIAGNOSTIC TESTS & INTERPRETATION

### Lab

- Electrolytes:
  - Obtained to establish baseline when initiating therapy with diuretics and/or ACE inhibitors
  - Hyperkalemia possible with severe low-output state
- CBC:
  - Anemia can be a cause or exacerbating factor.
- β-Natriuretic peptide (BNP) and creatinine:
  - Elevation in severe CHF
- Liver function tests:
  - May increase suggesting hepatic congestion
- Thyroid function tests:
  - Specifically in patients >65 yr old or patients in atrial fibrillation
- Cardiac enzymes:
  - May be useful if ischemia or infarction is presumed to be the underlying cause
- BNP:
  - Useful for distinguishing between heart failure and a primary pulmonary cause of dyspnea in patients without severe renal failure or pulmonary embolus
  - In the *Breathing Not Properly Study*, a BNP >100 pg/mL diagnosed heart failure with a sensitivity of 90% and a specificity of 73%.
  - BNP >500 pg/mL more consistent with CHF
  - BNP <100 pg/mL unlikely to be CHF
- NT-proBNP:
  - The prohormone proBNP is cleaved into BNP and the N-terminal fragment, NT-pro-BNP.
  - Similar test characteristics as BNP
  - NT-proBNP >1,000 pg/mL more consistent with CHF
  - NT-proBNP <300 pg/mL unlikely to be CHF

### Imaging

- CXR:
  - Cardiomegaly
  - Specific signs of CHF:
    ○ Cephalization (vascular prominence in the upper lung fields due to fluid overload)
    ○ Interstitial edema/Kerley B lines
    ○ Alveolar edema
  - Effusions (usually right-sided)
  - Bilateral confluent perihilar infiltrates leading to classic butterfly pattern:
    ○ May be asymmetric and mistaken for pneumonia
- EKG:
  - Underlying cardiac ischemia
  - Presence of dysrhythmias
  - Left-ventricular hypertrophy
  - Heart block
  - Normal EKG has high negative predictive value for systolic dysfunction.

- ECG:
  - Ejection fraction
  - Acute valvular pathology
  - Pericardial tamponade
  - Pericardial thickening in constrictive pericarditis
  - Ventricle size
  - Regional wall motion abnormalities

## DIFFERENTIAL DIAGNOSIS
- Left-sided CHF:
  - Acute exacerbation of chronic obstructive pulmonary disease
  - Asthma exacerbation
  - Acute respiratory distress syndrome
  - Pneumonia
  - Bronchitis
  - Constrictive pericarditis
  - Valvular disease
  - Pericardial tamponade
  - Coarctation of aorta
- Right-sided CHF:
  - Nephrotic syndrome
  - Cirrhosis
  - Left-side heart failure
  - Pulmonary embolism

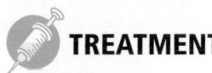 **TREATMENT**

### PRE-HOSPITAL
- IV access
- Supplemental oxygen
- Cardiac monitor
- Pulse oximetry
- EKG
- Sublingual nitrates for active chest pain without hypotension
- Furosemide
- Endotracheal intubation may be required.

### INITIAL STABILIZATION/THERAPY
- IV access
- Supplemental oxygen
- Elevate head of the bed with the patient's legs dependent to reduce venous return.
- Cardiac monitor
- Pulse oximetry
- Control airway as needed:
  - NIPPV (noninvasive positive pressure ventilation)
    - CPAP vs. BiPAP
    - Reduce work of breathing, improve oxygenation, decrease need for intubation, possible mortality benefit
    - Some studies with higher incidence of MI reported with BiPAP over CPAP in acute CHF; studies not conclusive
  - Endotracheal intubation for impending respiratory failure

### ED TREATMENT/PROCEDURES
- Normotensive or hypertensive patients:
  - Rapid-acting nitrates:
    - Sublingual nitroglycerin
    - Nitro paste
    - IV nitroglycerin
  - IV loop diuretics (furosemide, bumetanide)

- Severe persistent HTN:
  - IV nitroglycerin, nitroprusside, or nesiritide
  - Nesiritide:
    - Recombinant DNA form of human BNP
    - Vasodilation of arteries and veins, reducing preload and afterload
    - Promotes free water and sodium loss
- Hypotensive patients:
  - Avoid nitrates, morphine, and diuretics.
  - Agents that increase myocardial contractility:
    - Dobutamine
    - Dopamine
    - Inamrinone
    - Milrinone
- In less severe cases of low-output CHF:
  - ACE inhibitors improve hemodynamics and increase exercise capacity.
  - Use in conjunction with other diuretics.

### Pediatric Considerations
- Neonates (1st weeks of life):
  - Suspect ductal-dependant cardiac lesions if clinical CHF and no improvement with $O_2$:
    - Prostaglandin E1 infusion to maintain ductus
- Children:
  - IV furosemide, and IV dopamine or milrinone
  - IV nitroglycerin for pulmonary edema

### MEDICATION
- Aspirin: 325 mg PO/PR if acute MI is suspected
- Bumetanide (Burnex): 1–3 mg IV
- Dobutamine: 2–10 µg/kg/min IV, max. of 40 µg/kg/min
- Dopamine: 2–20 µg/kg/min IV, max. of 50 µg/kg/min
- Enalapril: 0.625–1.25 mg IV; 2.5–20 mg/d PO
- Furosemide (Lasix): No prior use—40 mg IVP; prior use—double 24-hr dose (80–180 mg IV); no effect in 30 min—redouble dose
- Inamrinone: 0.75 mg/kg IV load; 5–10 µg/kg/min IV
- Milrinone: 50 µg/kg IV load; 0.375 µg/kg/min–0.75 µg/kg/min IV
- Nesiritide: 2 µg/kg bolus, then infusion of 0.01 µg/kg per min
- Nitroglycerin: 0.4 mg sublingual; 1–2 inches of nitro paste; 5–20 µg/min IV, max. of 100–200 µg/min IV
- Nitroprusside: 0.3–10 µg/kg/min IV (starting dose), max. of 10 µg/kg/min

### Pregnancy Considerations
ACE inhibitors and ARBs should be held during pregnancy:
- Associated with multiple fetal abnormalities
- Oxygen
- Nitroglycerin
- Furosemide

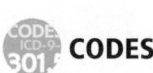 **FOLLOW-UP**

### DISPOSITION
**Admission Criteria**
- ICU:
  - Pulmonary edema
  - Cardiogenic shock
  - Concomitant MI or ischemia
- Medical wards:
  - New-onset CHF
  - Symptoms not relieved by aggressive ED therapy

**Discharge Criteria**
- Mild exacerbation of chronic CHF:
  - Responds to treatment
- Close follow-up should be arranged with continuation of diuretic, vasodilator, or ACE inhibitor therapy and patient lifestyle education.

**Issues for Referral**
ICD and/or biventricular pacer may be considered in advanced heart failure:
- Shown to decrease mortality and hospitalization rates in select patient groups

### FOLLOW-UP RECOMMENDATIONS
- Close follow-up with physician within 1 wk of discharge
- Medication and dietary compliance (strict salt restriction)
- Frequent home monitoring of body weight
- Monitor electrolytes and renal function during chronic diuretic therapy

## PEARLS AND PITFALLS
- In cases of diagnostic uncertainty, a BNP may help diagnose CHF.
- In severe CHF, NIPPV can improve impending respiratory compromise.
- Be vigilant in searching for and treating the underlying cause of the heart failure exacerbation (eg, MI, PE, acute valvular pathology).

## ADDITIONAL READING
- Heart Failure Society of America. Executive summary: HFSA 2006 Comprehensive Heart Failure Practice Guideline. *J Card Fail.* 2006;12(1):10–38.
- McCullough PA, Nowak RM, McCord J, et al. B-type natriuretic peptide and clinical judgment in emergency diagnosis of heart failure: Analysis from Breathing Not Properly (BNP) multinational study. *Circulation* 2002;106:416–422.
- Silvers S, et al. ACEP Clinical policy: Critical issues in the evaluation and management of adult patients presenting to the emergency department with acute heart failure syndromes. *Ann Emerg Med.* 2007;49(5):627–669.

**CODES**

### ICD9
428.0 Congestive heart failure, unspecified

# CONJUNCTIVITIS

*Jessica Freedman*

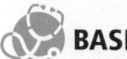

## BASICS

### DESCRIPTION
Inflammation of the conjunctiva arising from a broad group of etiologies

### ETIOLOGY
- Bacterial:
  - Staphylococcus aureus
  - Streptococcus pneumoniae
  - Haemophilus influenza
  - Gonococcal:
    - Ophthalmic emergency
  - Chlamydia:
    - Transmission occurs via autoinoculation from genital secretions.
    - Often occurs in newborns
- Viral:
  - Adenovirus most common
  - Epidemic keratoconjunctivitis (EKC) is caused by adenovirus subtypes.
  - Frequently associated with upper respiratory infections or exposure to someone with a red eye
  - Most commonly referred to as "pink eye"
  - Herpes simplex virus
  - Recurrent ocular infection occurs in 25% patients within 2 yr.
  - Use of steroids is *contraindicated*:
    - Allergic
  - Frequent history of allergy, atopy, nasal symptoms
  - Contact related
  - May be due to chemical irritation, hypersensitivity from preservatives, medications
  - *Pseudomonas* commonly implicated organism:
    - May be found in patients using saliva to clean contact lenses

## DIAGNOSIS

### SIGNS AND SYMPTOMS
General:
- Red eye (conjunctival irritation)
- Gritty, foreign body sensation
- Discharge
- Eyelid sticking (worse upon awakening)
- Conjunctival edema (chemosis) and eyelid edema
- Bacterial:
  - Mucopurulent or purulent discharge
- Gonococcal:
  - Hyperacute, copious purulent discharge:
    - Discharge starts 12 hr after inoculation.
  - Severe chemosis
  - Eyelid swelling
  - Preauricular lymphadenopathy typically absent
  - Invades intact conjunctiva and cornea within 24 hr and causes ulcerations, scarring, and perforations leading to blindness

- Chlamydia:
  - Lacrimation
  - Mucopurulent discharge
  - With or without photophobia
  - Concomitant genital infection (>50%)
  - Transmission occurs via autoinoculation from genital secretions
- Viral—general:
  - Preauricular adenopathy
- Viral syndrome:
  - Watery, mucous discharge, lacrimation
  - Gritty feeling or foreign body sensation in eye
  - Spreads to other eye in 24–48 hr
  - Pinpoint subconjunctival hemorrhages:
    - Tarsal conjunctiva may have a bumpy appearance.
- *Epidemic keratoconjunctivitis* (EKC):
  - Conjunctival hyperemia
  - Chemosis
  - Corneal infiltrates
  - Decreased vision
- Herpes simplex virus (HSV):
  - Acute follicular conjunctival reaction
  - Skin lesions or vesicles along eyelid margin or periocular skin
  - Corneal involvement—dendritic lesion
- Herpes zoster virus (HZV):
  - Associated with pain or paresthesias of the skin
  - Rash or vesicles involving the distribution of cranial nerve V1
  - Dendritic characters on cornea
  - Rarely vesicles or ulcers form on the conjunctiva.
- Allergic:
  - Hallmark: Itching
  - Red conjunctiva
  - Watery discharge
  - Papillary hypertrophy
  - Frequent history of allergy, atopy, nasal symptoms
- Contact related:
  - Acute symptoms result of corneal ulceration
  - Normal visual acuity and intraocular pressures

### ESSENTIAL WORKUP
- History for:
  - Onset of inflammation
  - Environmental or work-related exposure
  - Ill contacts
  - Sexual activity, discharge, rash
  - Use of over-the-counter medicines or cosmetics
  - Systemic diseases
- Careful physical examination including slit-lamp examination including fluorescein staining

## DIAGNOSTIC TESTS & INTERPRETATION
*Lab*
- Bacteriologic studies:
  - Not indicated in routine cases
  - Indications:
    - Ophthalmia neonatorum (except chemical)
    - Suspected gonococcal ophthalmia
    - Compromised host
    - Signs and symptoms of systemic disease
    - Refractory to treatment within 48–72 hr (with good compliance)
- Positive Gram stain for gram-negative intracellular diplococci:
  - Sufficient to initiate systemic and topical treatment for gonococcal disease
- Rapid plasma reagent (RPR):
  - For suspected cases of sexually transmitted disease

### DIFFERENTIAL DIAGNOSIS
- Acute angle-closure glaucoma (most serious cause)
- Allergies or hypersensitivity
- Anterior uveitis
- Corneal abrasion
- Dry eye
- Foreign body
- Keratitis
- Nasolacrimal obstruction
- Scleritis or episcleritis
- Subconjunctival hemorrhage

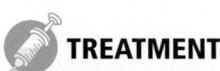

## TREATMENT

### INITIAL STABILIZATION/THERAPY
- Initiate empiric antibiotic therapy with broad-spectrum topical agent.
- Systemic therapy for gonococcal, chlamydial, and meningococcal conjunctivitis, ophthalmia neonatorum, and all severe infections regardless of cause
- Manage herpetic eye infections in consultation with an ophthalmologist.

### ED TREATMENT/PROCEDURES
- Remove discharge from the eye(s):
  - Contact lens wearers should discontinue use and throw away affected contact lenses.
  - Contact lens wearers should discontinue use until:
    - Eye is white.
    - Antibiotic therapy is completed.
    - No discharge for 24 hr
  - Frequent hand washing
  - No sharing of towels, tissues, cosmetics, linens
  - Frequent warm soaks until lashes and eyes free of debris

- Bacterial conjunctivitis:
  - Antibiotics—topical:
  - Can use ointment or drops
  - Continue therapy for 48 hr after clearing of symptoms.
  - Discontinue therapy and obtain cultures if no improvement in 48–72 hr (with good compliance).
- Antibiotics—systemic:
  - Parenteral therapy mandatory for gonococcal infection
  - Chlamydia requires systemic treatment of sexual partners and parents of neonates.
- Viral conjunctivitis:
  - No specific antiviral therapy
  - Limited use of topical antihistamine or decongestant
- EKC may require steroids and should be prescribed in consult with ophthalmology.
- Allergic conjunctivitis (there may be a lag time of up to 2 wk for improvement with these agents):
  - Antihistamine or decongestant drops (naphazoline [Naphcon-A])
  - Mast cell stabilizer/antihistamine or NSAID ophthalmic drops as 2nd line
- Noninfectious:
  - Eye lubricant drops or ointment
- Empiric treatment:
  - Topical antibiotic ointment or drops

## MEDICATION

- General:
  - All contact lens wearers require pseudomonal coverage.
  - Bacitracin ophthalmologic ointment (no pseudomonal coverage)
  - Ciprofloxacin: 0.35% 1 drop q1–6h (has antipseudomonal properties; may be used in children)
  - Erythromycin: 0.5% ointment
  - Gentamicin: 0.3% ointment q3–4h or drops q1–4h (has antipseudomonal coverage)
  - Sulfacetamide: 10% 1 drop q1–6h (lacks pseudomonal coverage)
  - Tobramycin ointment
- Chlamydia:
  - Doxycycline: 100 mg PO b.i.d. for 3 wk or
  - Erythromycin: 250–500 mg PO q.i.d. for 3 wk (peds: 50 mg/kg/d PO in 4 div. doses for 14 days) or
  - Sulfasoxazole 500–1,000 mg q.i.d. for 3 wk

- Gonococcal:
  - Adults:
    - Ceftriaxone: 1 g IV or IM daily for 3–5 days or PRN
    - Erythromycin: 500 mg PO q.i.d. for 2–3 wk or doxycycline 100 mg PO b.i.d. for 2–3 wk
    - *Plus* topical antibiotics as above
  - Neonates:
    - Penicillin G 100,000 IU/kg/d in 4 div. doses for 7 days or ceftriaxone 25–50 mg/kg/d IV for 7 days
- Viral:
  - Artificial tears
  - Naphcon-A or Visine AC 1 or 2 drops q.i.d. PRN for no more than 1 wk
- HSV or HZV:
  - Trifluorothymidine: 1% 5 times per day, *or*
  - Vidarabine: 3% ointment 5 times per day
- Allergic:
  - Naphazoline (Naphcon-A): 1 drop b.i.d.–q.i.d. or Visine AC
  - Acular: 1 or 2 drops b.i.d.
  - Cromolyn sodium 4% (Crolom): 1 drop q.i.d.
- Noninfectious and nonallergic:
  - Eye lubricant drops or ointment: Artificial tears or Lacri-Lube
- Empiric treatment:
  - Erythromycin ointment 0.5% (half inch q.i.d.)
  - Sulfacetamide 10% ophthalmic drops (1 or 2 drops q.i.d.) for 5–7 days

### Pediatric Considerations

- Often a manifestation of systemic disease in infants
- Conjunctivitis in the 1st 36 hr of life usually chemically induced caused by silver nitrate applied at birth.
- Neonates become infected during passage through the birth canal.
- Gonococcal, herpetic, chlamydial organisms most common
- Ophthalmia neonatorum is conjunctivitis within the 1st 4 wk of life.
- *Chlamydia trachomatis* is not eradicated by silver nitrate.
- Some newborns treated with erythromycin still develop conjunctivitis.
- Ointment is preferred over drops because of difficulty with administration of drops.

 **FOLLOW-UP**

### DISPOSITION

**Admission Criteria**

Known or suspected gonococcal infection (any age group)

**Discharge Criteria**

Close follow-up for all cases

**Issues for Referral**

Diagnosis of EKC and bacterial conjunctivitis requires ophthalmology referral.

### FOLLOW-UP RECOMMENDATIONS

All patients with bacterial conjunctivitis require ophthalmology follow up.

## PEARLS AND PITFALLS

- Be sure to disinfect slit lamp and chair used for patients to avoid contamination.
- Conjunctivitis is extremely contagious.
- Viral conjunctivitis contagious for up to 2 wk.
- EKC is especially contagious.
- Extreme caution should be taken when using corticosteroids, as they may worsen an underlying HSV infection.

## ADDITIONAL READING

- Alteveer JG, McCans KM. The red eye, the swollen eye, and acute vision loss. *Emerg Med Pract* 2002;4(6):27.
- Bertolini J, Pelucio M. The red eye. *Emerg Med Clin North Am.* 1995;13(3):561–579.
- Kunimoto D, Kanitkar K, Makar M. *The wills eye manual: Office and emergency room diagnosis and treatment of eye diseases*, 4th ed. Philadelphia: Lippincott Williams & Wilkins; 2004.
- Leibowitz HM. The red eye. *New Engl J Med.* 2000;343:345.
- Mueller JB, McStay C. Ocular infection and inflammation. *Emerg Med Clin North Am.* 2008;26(1).

### See Also (Topic, Algorithm, Electronic Media Element)

Red eye

 **CODES**

### ICD9

372.30 Conjunctivitis, unspecified

# CONSTIPATION

*Julia Sone*

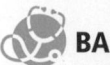 **BASICS**

## DESCRIPTION

**Rome Criteria** for the diagnosis of constipation requires 2 or more of the following for at least 3 mo:

- Straining more than 25% of the time
- Hard stools more than 25% of the time
- Incomplete evacuation more than 25% of the time
- 2 or fewer bowel movements per week

### Pediatric Considerations

- 3% of pediatric outpatient visits are because of defecation disorders.
- Children with cerebral palsy often develop functional constipation.
- Can be classified into subgroups:
  - Constipation with anatomical origins (anal stenosis/strictures, ectopic anus, imperforate anus, sacrococcygeal teratomas)
  - Colonic neuromuscular disease (Hirschsprung's disease)
  - Defecation disorders (functional constipation and nonretentive fecal soiling)
  - Function fecal retention
- Most common cause of fecal retention and soiling in children is functional fecal retention:
  - Caused by fears associated with defecation
  - Associated with irritability, abdominal cramps, decreased appetite, early satiety

## ETIOLOGY

- Metabolic and endocrine:
  - Diabetes
  - Uremia
  - Porphyria
  - Hypothyroidism
  - Hypercalcemia
  - Pheochromocytoma
  - Panhypopituitarism
  - Pregnancy
- Functional and idiopathic:
  - Colonic irritable bowel syndrome
  - Diverticular disease
  - Colonic inertia
  - Megacolon/megarectum
  - Pelvic intussusception
  - Nonrelaxing puborectalis
  - Rectocele/sigmoidocele
  - Posthysterectomy syndrome
  - Descending perineum

- Pharmacologic:
  - Analgesics
  - Anesthetics
  - Antacids
  - Anticholinergics
  - Anticonvulsants
  - Antidepressants
  - Antihypertensives
  - Calcium channel blockers
  - Diuretics
  - Ferrous compounds
  - Laxative abuse
  - MAOIs
  - Opiates
  - Paralytic agents
  - Parasympatholytics
  - Phenothiazines
  - Psychotropics
- Neurologic:
  - Central Parkinson disease
  - MS
  - Cerebrovascular accidents
  - Spinal cord lesions/injury
  - Peripheral Hirschsprung disease
  - Chagas disease
  - Neurofibromatosis
  - Autonomic neuropathy
- Mechanical obstruction:
  - Neoplasm
  - Stricture
  - Hernia
  - Volvulus

 **DIAGNOSIS**

## SIGNS AND SYMPTOMS

- Constipation is a symptom, not a disease.
- Passage of hard stool
- Straining/difficulty passing stool
- Infrequent bowel movements
- Abdominal distention/bloating
- Firm/hard stool on digital rectal exam:
  - May have empty rectal vault
- Diarrhea (liquid stool passes around firm feces)

## History

- Age of onset of symptoms
- Diet and exercise regimen
- Stool size, caliber, consistency, frequency, ease of defecation
- Medical and surgical history:
  - Medications that can slow colonic transit like $\beta$-blockers, high-dose calcium channel blockers, narcotics
- Use of enemas, laxatives, and digital manipulation to facilitate defecation
- Associated pelvic floor dysfunction:
  - Urinary symptoms
  - Rectocele

### Physical Exam

- Abdominal exam may reveal a mass due to stool
- Rectal examination to assess for outlet obstruction:
  - Ability to squeeze and relax the sphincter
  - Is there a rectocele or cystocele?
  - Assess firmness of stool

## ESSENTIAL WORKUP

Thorough history and physical exam:

- Medical, surgical, and psychiatric investigation and date of onset
- Note abdominal distention, hernias, tenderness, or masses
- Complete anorectal exam for anal stenosis, fissure, neoplasm, sphincter tone, perineal descent, tenderness, spasm

## DIAGNOSTIC TESTS & INTERPRETATION

### Lab

- Only necessary when considering metabolic/endocrine disorders
- CBC if inflammatory or neoplastic origin
- Electrolytes and calcium indicated if at risk of:
  - Hypokalemia
  - Hypocalcemia
- Thyroid function test if patient appears to be hypothyroid

## Imaging
- Rarely indicated unless an underlying process suspected
- Abdominal radiograph:
  - Large amount of feces in colon
  - Dilated colon that needs decompression
- CT scan of abdomen/pelvis to r/o perforation in elderly, constipated pt with abdominal pain/fever
- Barium/gastrografin enema study:
  - Diverticulosis
  - Megarectum
  - Megacolon
  - Hirschsprung disease
  - Stricture from inflammation or tumor

## DIFFERENTIAL DIAGNOSIS
- See "Etiology."
- Bowel obstruction

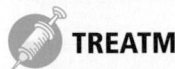 TREATMENT

### PRE-HOSPITAL
Establish IV access for patients with significant abdominal pain.

### INITIAL STABILIZATION/THERAPY
IV fluids for dehydrated/hypotensive patients

### ED TREATMENT/PROCEDURES
- Clean out colon:
  - Enemas, suppositories
  - Manual disimpaction of hard stool
  - Laxatives
- Maintain bowel regimen:
  - Increase noncaffeinated fluids (8–10 cups per day).
  - Increase dietary fiber intake (20 g/d).
  - Stool softeners
  - Exercise
  - Change medications causing constipation.

### MEDICATION
- Enemas:
  - Fleet: 120 mL (peds: 60–120 mL) per rectum (PR)
  - Mineral oil: 60–150 mL (peds: 5–11 yr old, 30–60 mL; older than 12 yr, 60–150 mL) PR daily
  - Tap water: 100–500 mL PR

- Fiber supplements:
  - Methylcellulose: 1 Tbs in cup water PO daily to t.i.d.
  - Psyllium: 1–2 tsp in cup of water/juice (peds: younger than 6 yr, 1/4–1/2 tsp in 2 oz water or juice; 6–11 yr, 1/2–1 tsp in 4 oz water or juice; older than 12 yr, 1–2 tsp in cup water or juice) PO daily to t.i.d.
- Laxatives (osmotic):
  - Lactulose: 15–30 mL (peds: 1 mL/kg) PO daily to b.i.d.
  - Polyethylene glycol: 17 g (peds: 0.8 g/kg/d dissolved in 4–8 oz of liquid) PO daily dissolved in liquid
- Laxatives (stimulant):
  - Bisacodyl: 10–15 mg PO daily (peds: Younger than 3 yr, 5 mg PR daily; 3–12 yr, 5–10 mg PO/PR daily; older than 12 yr, 5–15 mg PO daily or 10 mg PR daily)
  - Cascara sagrada: 5 mL (peds: Infants, 1.25 mL; 2–12 yr, 2.5 mL; older than 12 yr, 5 mL) PO at bedtime on an empty stomach
  - Castor oil: 15–60 mL (peds: 2–12 yr, 5–15 mL) PO daily; do not take at bedtime
  - Senna: 2–4 tabs PO daily to t.i.d. (peds: 2–6 yr, 1/2–1 tab PO daily to b.i.d.. 6–12 yr, 1–2 tabs PO daily to b.i.d.; older than 12 yr, 2–4 tabs PO daily to b.i.d.)
- Stool softeners:
  - Docusate sodium: 100 mg (peds: 3–5 mg/kg/d in divided doses) PO daily to b.i.d.
  - Mineral oil: 15–45 mL (peds: 5–15 mL) PO daily
- Suppositories:
  - Glycerin: 1 adult (peds: Infant, 1 infant suppository) PR PRN

 FOLLOW-UP

### DISPOSITION
#### Admission Criteria
- Patients with severe abdominal pain, nausea, and emesis
- Neurologically impaired, elderly, morbidly obese who cannot be cleaned out in the ED or home
- Bowel obstruction/peritonitis

#### Discharge Criteria
- No co-morbid illness requiring admission
- Pain free
- Adequately cleaned out

### Issues for Referral
GI follow-up for further evaluation and treatment

### FOLLOW-UP RECOMMENDATIONS
Primary care or GI follow-up for patients with longstanding constipation

## PEARLS AND PITFALLS
- Advise patients regarding appropriate dietary and lifestyle changes to decrease incidence of constipation.
- Perform thorough history and physical to exclude significant medical or surgical etiologies for constipation.

## ADDITIONAL READING
- Doody DP, Flores A, Rodriguez LA. Evaluation and management of intractable constipation in children. *Semin Colon Rectal Surg.* 2006;17(1):29–37.
- Talley N. Differentiating functional constipation from constipation-predominant irritable bowel syndrome: Management implications. *Rev Gastroenterol Disord.* 2005;5(1):1–9.
- Wexner SD, Pemberton JH, Beck DE, et al. eds. *The ASCRS Textbook of Colon and Rectal Surgery.* Springer; 2007.

### See Also (Topic, Algorithm, Electronic Media Element)
- Abdominal Pain
- Bowel Obstruction

 CODES

### ICD9
- 564.00 Constipation, unspecified
- 564.01 Slow transit constipation
- 564.02 Outlet dysfunction constipation

# CONTACT DERMATITIS

Gabrielle A. Jacquet
Jeffrey Druck

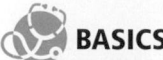 **BASICS**

## DESCRIPTION

- Irritant:
  - Immediate eczematous eruption (superficial inflammatory process primarily in epidermis)
  - Trigger substance itself directly damages the skin resulting in nonimmunologic inflammatory reaction with erythema, dryness, cracking, or fissuring.
  - May see vesicles
  - Usually owing to repeated exposure to mild irritant (eg, water, soaps, heat, friction)
  - Lesions itch or burn:
    ○ Usually gradual onset with indistinct borders
    ○ Most often seen on hands
- Allergic:
  - Delayed (type IV) hypersensitivity reaction (requires prior sensitization)
  - Allergen induced immune response
  - Local edema, vesicles, erythema, pruritus, or burning
  - Usually corresponds to exact distribution of contact (eg, watchband)
  - Onset usually within 12–48 hr with prior sensitization; may take 14–21 days for primary exposure
  - Common sources: Nickel, gold, neomycin, bacitracin
- Photocontact:
  - Interaction between an otherwise harmless substance on the skin and UV light

### Pediatric Considerations
- Allergic contact dermatitis is less frequent in children, especially infants, than in adults.
- Major sources of pediatric contact allergy:
  - Metals, shoes, preservatives, or fragrances in cosmetics, topical medications, and plants
  - Diaper dermatitis: Prototype for irritant contact dermatitis in children
- Circumoral dermatitis: Seen in infants and small children; may result from certain foods (irritant or allergic reaction)

## ETIOLOGY
- Irritant (80% of contact dermatitis), for example:
  - Soaps, solvents
  - Chemicals
  - Certain foods
  - Urine, feces
  - Diapers
  - Continuous or repeated exposure to moisture (hand washing)
  - Course paper, glass, wool fibers
  - Shoe dermatitis: Common; identify by lesions limited to distal dorsal surface of foot usually sparing the interdigital spaces

- Allergic:
  - Plants, poison ivy, oak, sumac (rhus dermatitis):
    ○ Most common form of allergic contact dermatitis in North America
    ○ Direct: Reaction to oleoresin urushiol from plant
    ○ Indirect: Contact with pet or clothes with oleoresin on surface or fur or in smoke from burning leaves
    ○ Lesions may appear up to 3 days after exposure with prior sensitization (12–21 days after primary exposure) and may persist up to 3 wk.
    ○ Fluid from vesicles is not contagious and does not produce new lesions.
    ○ Oleoresin on pets or clothes remains contagious until removed.
  - Cement (prolonged exposure may result in severe alkali burn)
  - Metals (especially nickel)
  - Solvents, epoxy
  - Chemicals in rubber (eg, elastic waistbands) or leather
  - Lotions, cosmetics
  - Topical medications (eg, neomycin, hydrocortisone, benzocaine, paraben)
  - Some foods
  - Ability to respond to certain antigens is probably genetically determined
- Photodermatitis:
  - Inflammatory reaction from exposure to irritant (frequently plant sap) and sunlight

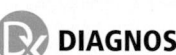 **DIAGNOSIS**

## SIGNS AND SYMPTOMS
### History
- Date of onset
- Time course
- Pattern of lesions
- Relationship to work
- Exposure to new products (eg, lotions, soaps, and cosmetics), foods, medications, and jewelry

### Physical Exam
- Special attention to character and distribution of rash
- *Acute lesions:* Skin erythema and pruritus:
  - May see edema, papules, vesicles, bullae, serous discharge, or crusting
- *Subacute:* Vesiculation less pronounced
- *Chronic lesions:* May see scaling, lichenification, pigmentation, or fissuring with little to no vesiculation; may have characteristic distribution pattern

## DIAGNOSTIC TESTS & INTERPRETATION
### Lab
No specific tests in ED are helpful.

### Imaging
No specific tests in ED are helpful.

### Diagnostic Procedures/Surgery
- Patch testing:
  - Generally not done in ED; refer to allergist/immunologist.
- When tinea is suspected, may use Wood lamp for fluorescence

## DIFFERENTIAL DIAGNOSIS
- Atopic dermatitis: Associated with family history of atopy
- Seborrheic dermatitis: Scaly or crusting "greasy" lesions
- Nummular dermatitis: Coin-like lesions
- Intertrigo: Dermatitis in which skin is in apposition
- Infectious eczematous dermatitis: Dermatitis with secondary bacterial infection, usually *Staphylococcus aureus*
- Cellulitis: Warm, blanching, painful lesion
- Impetigo: Yellow crusting
- Scabies: Intensely pruritic, frequently interdigital with tracks
- Psoriasis: Silvery adherent, scaling, lesions well delineated, affecting extensor surfaces, scalp, and genital region
- Herpes simplex: Groups of vesicles, painful, burning
- Herpes zoster: Painful, follows dermatomal pattern
- Bullous pemphigoid: Diffuse bullous lesions
- Tinea: Maximal involvement at margins, fluoresces under Wood lamp
- Pityriasis alba: Discrete, asymptomatic, hypopigmented lesions
- Urticaria: Pruritic raised lesions (wheal) frequently with surrounding erythema (flare)
- Acrodermatitis enteropathica: Vesiculobullous lesion of hands and feet, associated with failure to thrive, diarrhea, and alopecia
- Letterer-Siwe tumor (Langerhans cell histiocytosis): Associated with hepatosplenomegaly and adenopathy
- Dyshidrotic dermatitis (eczema)

## TREATMENT

### INITIAL STABILIZATION/THERAPY
Rarely required in absence of concomitant pathology

### ED TREATMENT/PROCEDURES
General:
- Primarily symptomatic
- Wash area with mild soap and water.
- Remove or avoid offending agent (including washing clothes).
- Cool, wet compresses; especially effective during acute blistering phase
- Antipruritic agents:
  - Topical:
    - Calamine lotion, corticosteroids (do not penetrate blisters); avoid benzocaine or hydrocortisone-containing products, which may further sensitize skin.
  - Systemic: Antihistamines, corticosteroids
- Aluminum acetate (Burrows) solution: Weeping surfaces

Irritant dermatitis:
- Remove offending agent
- Wash well with soap and warm water
- Decrease wet/dry cycles (hand washing)
- Bland emollient
- Topical steroids for severe cases (ointment preferred) medium to high potency (hands) b.i.d. for several weeks

Allergic dermatitis:
- Topical steroids (ointment preferred) b.i.d. for 2–3 wk:
  - Face: Low potency
  - Arms, legs, trunk: Medium potency
  - Hands and feet: High potency
- Oral steroids for severe cases

Rhus dermatitis:
- Follow general measures *plus*:
  - Wash all clothes and pets that have come in contact with the plant; oil persists and is contagious.
  - Oatmeal baths can provide soothing relief.
  - Aseptic aspiration of bullae may relieve discomfort.
  - Severe reaction (>10% TBSA): Systemic corticosteroids for 2–3 wk with gradual taper:
    - Premature termination of corticosteroid therapy may result in rapid rebound of symptoms.

Shoe dermatitis:
- Follow general measures *plus:*
  - Wear open-toe, canvas, or vinyl shoes.
  - Control perspiration: Change socks, use absorbent powder.

Diaper dermatitis:
- Follow general measures *plus:*
  - Topical zinc oxide, petrolatum ointment, or aquaphor
  - Change diapers after each soiling

### MEDICATION
Systemic:
- Antihistamine ($H_1$-receptor antagonist, 1st and 2nd generation):
  - Cetirizine: Adults and children >6 yr, 5–10 mg PO daily (peds: Age 2–6 yr, 2.5 mg PO daily/b.i.d.)
  - Diphenhydramine hydrochloride: 25–50 mg IV/IM/PO q6h PRN (peds: 5 mg/kg/24 h div. q6h PRN)
  - Fexofenadine: 60 mg PO b.i.d. or 180 mg PO daily (peds: Age 6–12, 30 mg PO b.i.d.)
  - Hydroxyzine hydrochloride: 25–50 mg PO IM up to q.i.d. PRN (peds: 2 mg/kg/24 h PO div q6h or 0.5 mg/kg IM q4–6h PRN)
  - Loratadine: 10 mg PO b.i.d.
  - For refractory pruritus: Doxepin: 75 mg PO daily may be effective.
- Corticosteroid:
  - Prednisone: 40–60 mg PO daily (peds: 1–2 mg/kg/24 h, max. 80 mg/24 h) div. daily/b.i.d.
- For refractory pruritus:
  - Doxepin: 75 mg PO daily may be effective.

Topical:
- Aluminum acetate (Burrows) solution: Apply topically for 30 min t.i.d. until skin is dry.
- Calamine lotion: q6h PRN
- Topical corticosteroid: Triamcinolone ointment 0.025, 0.1%; cream 0.025, 0.1%; lotion 0.025, 0.1% t.i.d. or q.i.d. daily

### First Line
- Topical steroids
- Oral antihistamines

### Second Line
Oral steroids

## FOLLOW-UP

### DISPOSITION
### Admission Criteria
Rarely indicated unless severe systemic reaction or significant secondary infection

### Discharge Criteria
- Symptomatic relief
- Adequate follow-up with primary care physician or dermatologic specialist

### FOLLOW-UP RECOMMENDATIONS
- Follow up with primary care physician in 2–3 days for recheck.
- Return to ED for: Facial swelling, difficulty breathing, mucosal involvement causing decreased PO intake.

## PEARLS AND PITFALLS

- Remove offending agent.
- Beware of progression to systemic anaphylaxis (eg, latex allergy).
- Rhus dermatitis wounds are no longer contagious after washed with soap and water:
  - Be sure to wash all clothes and animals that have come in contact with plant as oil remains contagious.

## ADDITIONAL READING

- Frosch PJ, Menne T, Lepoittevin J-P, eds. *Contact Dermatitis*, 4th ed. Germany: Springer; 2006.
- Marx JA, Hockberger RS, Walls RM, et al., eds. *Rosen's Emergency Medicine: Concepts and Clinical Practice*, 7th ed. St. Louis: Mosby, 2009.
- Rietschel RL, Fowler JF, eds. *Fisher's Contact Dermatitis*, 6th ed. Ontario: BC Decker; 2008.
- Saary J, Qureshi R, Palda V, et al. A systematic review of contact dermatitis treatment and prevention. *J Am Acad Dermatol*. 2005;53:845.

 CODES

ICD9
- 692.0 Contact dermatitis and other eczema due to detergents
- 692.1 Contact dermatitis and other eczema due to oils and greases
- 692.2 Contact dermatitis and other eczema due to solvents

# COR PULMONALE

E. Jedd Roe

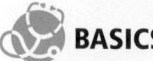 **BASICS**

## DESCRIPTION

- Ventricular failure confined to the right ventricle that occurs secondary to a pulmonary disorder:
  - Acute cor pulmonale is a right ventricular (RV) dilatation from an overload due to acute pulmonary HTN.
    - Most often caused by a massive pulmonary embolism
  - Chronic cor pulmonale occurs secondary to RV hypertrophy caused by an adaptive response to pulmonary HTN:
    - Predominately occurs as a result of alveolar hypoxia
- The pulmonary circulation is a low-resistance, low-pressure system:
  - The pulmonary arteries are thin walled and distensible.
  - Mean pulmonary arterial pressure is usually 12–15 mm Hg.
  - Normal left arterial pressure is 6–10 mm Hg.
  - The resulting pressure difference driving the pulmonary circulation is only 6–9 mm Hg.
- 3 factors affect pulmonary arterial pressure:
  - Cardiac output
  - Pulmonary venous pressure
  - Pulmonary vascular resistance
- Pulmonary HTN can arise through a number of mechanisms:
  - A marked increase in cardiac output
  - Left-to-right shunt secondary to congenital heart disease
  - Hypoxia:
    - The most common cause of increased pulmonary vascular resistance
    - The resulting hypercapnia and acidosis induces additional vasoconstriction.
    - Pulmonary venous pressure increases.
    - A compensatory rise in pressure is seen in the pulmonary arterial system, so flow is maintained across the pulmonary vascular bed.
  - Pulmonary embolus causes a similar change by increasing resistance to pulmonary blood flow.
  - LV failure achieves the same result by directly influencing pulmonary venous pressure.
  - Dramatic rises in blood viscosity or intrathoracic pressure also impede blood flow.

## EPIDEMIOLOGY

### Incidence

- ~86,000 patients die from COPD each year:
  - Associated RV failure is a significant factor in many of these cases, and accounts for 10–30% of heart failure admissions in the U.S.
- In patients >50 yr with COPD, 50% develop pulmonary HTN and are at risk of developing cor pulmonale.
- The course of cor pulmonale is generally related to the progression of the underlying disease process.
- Once cor pulmonale develops, patients have a 30% chance of surviving 5 yr.

## ETIOLOGY

- Chronic hypoxia:
  - COPD
  - Chronic hypoxia at high altitude
  - Sleep apnea:
    - Primary pulmonary HTN
- Cystic fibrosis
- Congenital heart disease:
  - Left-to-right shunts
- Severe anemia
- Pulmonary embolism
- Collagen vascular diseases
- Thoracic deformities:
  - Kyphoscoliosis
- Obesity
- Mitral stenosis
- Pulmonary venoocclusive disease
- Increased blood viscosity:
  - Polycythemia vera
  - Leukemia
- Increased intrathoracic pressure:
  - COPD
  - Mechanical ventilation with positive end-expiratory pressure
  - Idiopathic primary pulmonary HTN

 **DIAGNOSIS**

## SIGNS AND SYMPTOMS

- Exertional dyspnea
- Easy fatigability
- Weakness
- Syncope
- Cough
- Hemoptysis
- Wheezing
- Hoarseness
- Weight gain
- Jugular venous distention:
  - Prominent A and V waves
- Hepatomegaly
- Ascites
- Hepatojugular reflex
- Peripheral edema
- Left parasternal heave on cardiac palpation
- Pulmonic component of the 2nd heart sound increases in intensity.

### History

- Exercise intolerance
- Palpitations
- Chest pain
- Light-headedness
- Syncope
- Swelling of the lower extremites

### Physical Exam

- Increase in chest diameter
- Crackles and/or wheezes
- Splitting of the 2nd heart sound or murmurs of the pulmonary vasculature may be heard.
- Hepatojugular reflex and pulsatile liver
- Pitting edema of the lower extremities

## DIAGNOSTIC TESTS & INTERPRETATION

### Lab

- Pulse oximetry or ABG:
  - Resting $PO_2$ 40–60 mm Hg
  - Resting $PCO_2$ often 40–70 mm Hg
- Hematocrit:
  - Frequently elevated
- B-natriuretic peptide:
  - When elevated, is sensitive for moderate to severe pulmonary HTN, and may be an independent predictor of mortality
  - Elevated level alone is not enough to establish diagnosis of cor pulmonale.
- Other laboratory tests are not generally useful.

## Imaging

- CXR:
  - Signs of pulmonary HTN:
    - ○ Large pulmonary arteries (>16–18 mm)
    - ○ An enlarged RV silhouette
    - ○ Shows abnormalities in >90% of patients in the detection of cor pulmonale, but does not indicate the severity of disease
    - ○ Pleural effusions do not occur in the setting of cor pulmonale alone.
- EKG:
  - Right-axis deviation
  - Tall, peaked P waves (P pulmonale)
  - RV hypertrophy (specific not sensitive)
  - Transient changes due to hypoxia
  - Right precordial T-wave flattening
  - ST-segment depression in segments II, III, and arteriovenous fistula
- ECG: The noninvasive diagnostic method of choice:
  - RV dilation or hypertrophy in the setting of normal LV dimensions
  - Assessment of tricuspid regurgitation
  - Doppler quantization of pulmonary artery pressure, RV ejection fraction
- Chest CT, ventilation/perfusion scans, or pulmonary angiography:
  - Useful in the setting of acute cor pulmonale
- Right-heart catheterization:
  - The most precise estimate of pulmonary vascular hemodynamics
  - Gives accurate measurements of pulmonary arterial pressure and pulmonary capillary wedge pressure

## DIFFERENTIAL DIAGNOSIS

- Primary disease of the left side of the heart
- Congenital heart disease
- Hypothyroidism
- Cirrhosis

 **TREATMENT**

## PRE-HOSPITAL

- Supportive therapy:
  - Supplemental oxygen
- To an endpoint of 90% arterial saturation:
  - IV access
  - Cardiac monitoring
  - Pulse oximetry
- Treat bronchospasm from associated respiratory disease:
  - β-Agonist nebulizers

- Caution:
  - Vasodilators and diuretics do not have a role in the field.
  - Severely hypoxic patients may require endotracheal intubation.

## INITIAL STABILIZATION/THERAPY

ED therapy is directed at the underlying disease process and reducing pulmonary HTN.

## ED TREATMENT/PROCEDURES

- Supplemental oxygen sufficient to raise arterial saturation to 90%:
  - Improving oxygenation reduces pulmonary arterial vasoconstriction and RV afterload.
  - The improved cardiac output enhances diuresis of excess body water.
  - Care must be taken to monitor the patient's ventilatory status and $PCO_2$, as hypercapnia may reduce respiratory drive and cause acidosis.
- Diuretics, such as furosemide, may be added cautiously to reduce pulmonary artery pressure by contributing to the reduction of circulating blood volume:
  - Be wary of volume depletion and hypokalemia
- Patients should be maintained on salt and fluid restriction.
- There is no role for digoxin in the treatment of cor pulmonale.
- Bronchodilators:
  - Bronchodilator therapy is particularly helpful for those patients with COPD:
  - Selective β-adrenergic agents such as subcutaneous terbutaline 0.25 mg SC may be useful.
  - Bronchodilator affects and reduces ventricular afterload.
  - Theophylline may play a role to improve diaphragmatic contractility and reduce muscle fatigue.
  - Anticoagulation may be considered for those at high risk for thromboembolic disease.
- Acutely decompensated COPD patients:
  - Early steroid therapy
  - Antibiotic administration
- In general, improvement in the underlying respiratory disease results in improved RV function.

## MEDICATION

- Furosemide: 20–60 mg IV (peds: 1 mg/kg may increase by 1 mg/kg/q2h not to exceed 6 mg/kg)
- Terbutaline: 0.25 mg SC

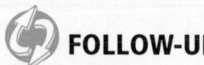 **FOLLOW-UP**

## DISPOSITION

### Admission Criteria
- New-onset hypoxia
- Anasarca
- Severe respiratory failure
- Admission criteria for the underlying disease process

### Discharge Criteria
Patients without hypoxia or a stable oxygen requirement

### Issues for Referral
- Close follow-up as long as the underlying etiology has responded to acute management
- The need for a sleep study to assess for sleep apnea should be coordinated by the patient's physician.

## FOLLOW-UP RECOMMENDATIONS
Ensure home oxygenation in patients with chronic hypoxia

## PEARLS AND PITFALLS

- The physical exam is unreliable for detecting cor pulmonale in patients with COPD, as hyperinflation of the chest obscures the classic findings.
- Vasodilator therapy should only be considered after conventional therapy and oxygenation have failed.

## ADDITIONAL READING

- Braunwald E. Heart failure and cor pulmonale. In: Kasper D, et al, eds., *Harrison's textbook of medicine*, 16th ed. New York: McGraw-Hill, 2005:1355–1359.
- Chaouat A, Naeije R, Weitzenblum E. Pulmonary hypertension in COPD. *Eur Respir J*. 2008;32: 1371–1385.
- Han MK, McLaughlin VV, Criner CJ, et al. Pulmonary diseases and the heart. *Circulation*. 2007;116: 2992–3005.
- Humbert M, Sitbon O, Simonneau G. Treatment of pulmonary arterial hypertension. *N Engl J Med*. 2004;351:14:1425–1436.
- Jardin F, Vieillard-Baron A. Acute cor pulmonale. *Curr Opin Crit Care*. 2009;15:67–70.
- Weitzenblum E. Chronic cor pulmonale. *Heart*. 2003;89:225–230.

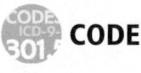 **CODES**

### ICD9
- 415.0 Acute cor pulmonale
- 416.9 Chronic pulmonary heart disease, unspecified

C

# CORNEAL ABRASION

*Denise S. Lawe*

 **BASICS**

## DESCRIPTION
- Any tear or defect in the corneal surface epithelium
- May be classified as traumatic, spontaneous, foreign body, or contact lens related

## ETIOLOGY
- Traumatic:
  - Human fingernail
  - Branches
  - Hairbrushes/combs
  - Sand/stones
  - Metallic object
  - Snow
  - Pens/pencils
  - Toys
  - Activated charcoal
  - Airbag deployment
  - Pepper spray
  - Paper/cardboard
  - Make-up applicator
  - Animal paws
  - Injury due to passage through the birth canal
- Foreign body related:
  - Wood
  - Glass
  - Metal
  - Rust
  - Plastic
  - Fiberglass
  - Vegetable matter
  - Eyelid foreign body
- Contact lens related:
  - Over-worn
  - Improperly fitting or cleaned
- Spontaneous:
  - Usually previous traumatic abrasion or an underlying defect in the corneal epithelium

**DIAGNOSIS**

## SIGNS AND SYMPTOMS
- Severe ocular pain
- Gritty (scratchy) discomfort
- Tearing
- Blepharospasm
- Foreign body sensation
- Photophobia (particularly if secondary traumatic iritis present)
- Conjunctival injection
- Diminished or blurred vision
- Headache

### History
- Any direct trauma to the globe
- Any known or potential foreign body
- Contact lens use
- Any history of previous corneal abrasion
- Ocular/periocular surgery
- Pre-existing visual impairment
- Time of onset
- Associated symptoms or concomitant injury
- Treatment before visit
- Use of safety glasses (pounding, drilling, grinding metal) or eyeglasses
- Systemic disease (diabetes, autoimmune disorders)
- Tetanus status

### Pediatric Considerations
- Signs and symptoms may differ:
  - Excessive crying
  - Conjunctival erythema
  - Tearing
  - Eye rubbing
  - Lid edema
- Younger than 12 mo:
  - Frequently no history of eye trauma
  - Often no eye signs may just be excessive crying
- Older than 12 mo:
  - More often will have history of minor eye trauma
  - Positive eye signs

### Physical Exam
- If indicated, evaluate for other life-threatening injuries with attention to the primary survey.
- Complete eye exam:
  - Gross visual inspection
  - Visual acuity
  - Penlight exam to evaluate for conjunctival injection, the pupil shape/reactivity, and for any evidence of corneal infiltrate or opacity
  - Evert upper lids to check for retained foreign body
  - Slit-lamp to evaluate anterior segment and depth of abrasion
  - Fluorescein to identify area of damaged corneal epithelium
  - Funduscopic examination

## DIAGNOSTIC TESTS & INTERPRETATION
### Pediatric Considerations
Handheld slit-lamp and Wood's lamp: Helpful in examination of pediatric eye

## DIFFERENTIAL DIAGNOSIS
- Conjunctivitis, viral, or bacterial
- Corneal dystrophy (inherited)
- Corneal ulcer
- Glaucoma
- Herpes zoster
- Keratitis, viral or bacterial, or ultraviolet induced
- Recurrent corneal erosion syndrome
- Uveitis
- More extensive pathology than corneal abrasion:
  - Laceration of cornea
  - Perforation of cornea
  - Hyphema
  - Iris prolapse
  - Lens disruption

C

 **TREATMENT**

### INITIAL STABILIZATION/THERAPY
- Instill topical anesthetic (proparacaine/tetracaine).
- Consider cycloplegic for intense pain owing to ciliary spasm (homatropine 5%).

### ED TREATMENT/PROCEDURES
- Removal of superficial foreign body:
  – A residual rust ring does not need emergent removal. It can be removed at 24–48 hr.
- Pain control (topical/oral):
  – Diclofenac (topical)
  – Ketorolac (topical)
  – Oral narcotics or NSAID
- Cycloplegic (optional):
  – Cyclopentolate (mydriasis 1–2 days)
  – Tropicamide (mydriasis 6 hr)
  – Homatropine 5%
- Topical antibiotic:
  – This practice has not been rigorously studied.
  – Concern is for superinfection
  – Ointment better than drops because also a lubricant
  – Discontinue antibiotics once symptom free for 24 hr
  – Contact lens wearers must be covered for *Pseudomonas:*
    ○ Ciprofloxacin
    ○ Erythromycin
    ○ Gentamicin
    ○ Sulfacetamide
    ○ Tobramycin/TobraDex
    ○ Polytrim
- Eye patch:
  – No patch required for small abrasions
  – Never patch contact lens related injury.
  – Never patch infection-prone injury (organic matter is at high risk).
  – More research needed to evaluate efficacy of patching in abrasions >10 mm

- Tetanus prophylaxis:
  – Routine tetanus not necessary
  – Update tetanus if abrasion caused by or contaminated with organic matter or dirt
- Emergent ophthalmologic consultation required for retained intraocular foreign body, penetrating injury to globe (or other more serious injury) and any patient with a corneal infiltrate, white spot or opacity

### MEDICATION
- Ciprofloxacin: 0.35% 1 drop q.i.d.
- Cyclopentolate: 0.5%, 1.0%, or 2.0% drops (mydriasis 1 or 2 drops t.i.d.)
- Diclofenac: 0.1% drops 1 drop q.i.d.
- Erythromycin: 0.5% ointment q.i.d.
- Gentamicin: 0.3% ointment q.i.d.
- Gentamicin: 0.3% 2 drops q6h
- Homatropine: 5% solution 2 drops b.i.d.
- Ketorolac: 0.5% drops 1 drop q.i.d.
- Proparacaine: 0.5% 1 drop once
- Sulfacetamide: 10% drops 2 drops q.i.d.
- Sulfacetamide: 10% ointment q.i.d.
- TobraDex: Suspension 0.1%/0.3% 2 drops q4–6h
- Tobramycin: 0.3% drops 2 drops q6h
- Tobramycin: 0.3% ointment q6h
- Tropicamide: 0.5%, 1.0% drops (mydriasis 6 hr) 1 drop q4h

 **FOLLOW-UP**

### DISPOSITION
*Admission Criteria*
Associated injuries requiring admission

*Discharge Criteria*
All simple corneal abrasions

*Issues for Referral*
All corneal abrasions require follow-up to ensure healing without infection or scarring.

### FOLLOW-UP RECOMMENDATIONS
- Follow-up with ophthalmologist for re-examination and ongoing care in 24 hr if contact lens wearer.
- Follow-up can be delayed to 48 hr if not a contact lens wearer and otherwise uncomplicated abrasion

## PEARLS AND PITFALLS
- Always diligently evaluate for penetrating trauma to the globe.
- Always diligently evaluate for evidence of infection.
- Do not discharge the patient with any topical anesthetic. It is toxic to the epithelium and retards healing.
- Do not use a mydriatic agent on a patient with a history of glaucoma.

## ADDITIONAL READING
- Calder LA, Fergusson D. Topical nonsteroidal anti-inflammatory drugs for corneal abrasions: Meta-analysis of randomized trials. *Acad Emerg Med.* 2005;12:467–473.
- Emedicine. Corneal abrasions, emergency medicine
- Marx JA, ed. *Rosen's Emergency Medicine: Concepts and Clinical Practice*, 7th ed. New York: Mosby; 2009.
- Turner A, Rabiu M. Patching for corneal abrasion. *Cochrane Database Syst Rev.* 2006;19(2).
- Upadhyay MP, Karmacharya PC, Koirala S, et al. The Bhaktapur eye study: Ocular trauma and antibiotic prophylaxis for the prevention of corneal abrasions in Nepal. *Br J Ophthalmol.* 2001;85:388–392.
- UpToDate. Corneal abrasions and corneal foreign bodies.
- Weavers CS, Terrell KM. Evidence based emergency medicine. Update: Do ophthalmic nonsteroidal anti-inflammatory drugs reduce the pain associated with simple corneal abrasions without delaying healing? *Ann Emerg Med.* 2003;41:134–140.

### See Also (Topic, Algorithm, Electronic Media Element)
- Conjunctivitis
- Corneal Burn
- Corneal Foreign Body
- Red Eye
- Ultraviolet Keratitis

**CODES**

### ICD9
- 371.82 Corneal disorder due to contact lens
- 930.0 Corneal foreign body
- 918.1 Superficial injury of cornea

# CORNEAL BURN
*Matthew A. Wheatley*

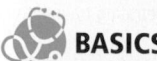 **BASICS**

## DESCRIPTION
- Inappropriate exposure of cornea to chemicals, heat, cold, electrical, or radiant energy causing damage to the cornea and often extending to adjacent structures
- Severity of injury related to duration of exposure, type of agent, anion concentration, pH level of solution
- Alkalis:
  - Cause immediate rise in pH level
  - Highly soluble in lipids, so rapidly penetrate the eye, causing severe corneal injury and continue to penetrate over time if no intervention undertaken
  - Penetration can occur in <1 min.
  - Exception: Calcium alkalis penetrate relatively poorly secondary to soap formation; can cause corneal opacification, so may appear worse but actually have better prognosis than other alkali burns.
- Acids:
  - Immediately coagulate proteins of corneal epithelium
  - Cause opacification
  - Coagulation produces barrier to deeper penetration.
  - Exception: Lipophilicity of hydrofluoric acid causes it to act similar to a base with more rapid penetration.
- Thermal burns:
  - Affect eyelids more than globe due to reflex blinking and Bell phenomenon (eyes roll up and outward)
  - Cause direct injury to cornea
  - Damage primarily depends on duration and intensity of heat.
- Electrical injury:
  - Occurs with current flow through head, with input at or near eye
- Radiation injury:
  - Due to ultraviolet light exposure to cornea

## ETIOLOGY
- Alkalis:
  - Ammonia:
    - Fertilizer, refrigerant, household ammonia, cleansing agents
  - Potassium hydroxide:
    - Caustic potash
  - Magnesium hydroxide:
    - Sparklers, flares, fireworks
  - Lye: NaOH:
    - Caustic soda, drain cleaners

  - Lime: $CaOH_2$:
    - Fresh lime, quicklime, calcium hydrate, slaked lime, hydrated lime, plaster, mortar, cement, whitewash
  - Nonspecific alkali:
    - Motor vehicle airbag on inflation releases alkali.
- Acids:
  - Sulfuric acid: $H_2SO_4$:
    - Car battery acid
  - Sulfurous acid: $H_2SO_3$:
    - Preservatives (fruit and vegetable)
- Bleach
- Refrigerants:
  - Hydrofluoric acid: HF:
    - Etching silicon/glass
    - Cleaning brick
    - Electropolishing metals
    - Control of fermentation in breweries
    - Commercial/household rust removal
- Thermal:
  - Hot liquids, molten metal
  - Flames
  - Hot smoke/gases
  - Flash burn
  - Steam
  - Cigarette burns
- Radiation:
  - Sun lamps
  - Tanning booths
  - High-altitude
  - Reflection off snow/water
  - Arc welding

### Pediatric Considerations
Consider child abuse or neglect.

 **DIAGNOSIS**

## SIGNS AND SYMPTOMS
- Severe ocular pain
- Photophobia
- Lacrimation
- Foreign body sensation
- Conjunctival injection
- Corneal edema
- Corneal opacification
- Impaired visual acuity
- Limbal blanching
- Lens opacification
- Vesicles clear fluid (hypothermal injury)
- Vesicles hemorrhagic fluid
- Necrosis of iris, ciliary body

## History
- Type of exposure:
  - Inspect any bottles accompanying the patient for active and inactive ingredients.
- Vehicle of exposure:
  - Aerosol: Common
  - Propellant: May result in intraocular foreign body/perforation
- Duration of exposure
- Time of onset
- Time irrigation initiated
- Pre-existing visual impairment
- Protective eyewear
- Contact lens use
- Treatment before arrival

## Physical Exam
Complete eye exam (after irrigation):
- Visual acuity
- Bright white light for visual inspection of cornea/conjunctivae/limbus
- Slit-lamp to evaluate anterior segment inflammation
- Fluorescein stain:
  - Corneal epithelial damage:
    - Punctate corneal lesions with discrete lower border from inferior lid seen in UV radiation burns
  - Perforation (Seidel's test)
- Check for lenticular clarity.
- Fundus exam
- Measure intraocular pressure (especially in delayed presentation).
- Lid/eyelash exam
- Check pH with acid/alkali burns with litmus paper or pH indicator on urine dipstick.

## DIAGNOSTIC TESTS & INTERPRETATION
### Diagnostic Procedures/Surgery
- Fluorescein stain
- Check pH

## DIFFERENTIAL DIAGNOSIS
- Infection:
  - Viral keratitis
  - Corneal ulcer
- Corneal erosion syndrome:
  - Corneal foreign body
  - Corneal abrasion
  - Hypothermal injury

### Pediatric Considerations
Handheld slit-lamp and Wood lamp helpful in examination of child's eye

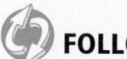

## TREATMENT

### PRE-HOSPITAL

- Irrigate at scene 15–30 min unless other coexisting life-threatening conditions require immediate transfer.
- Bring bottle of substance to hospital.
- Continuous irrigation en route to hospital with NS

### INITIAL STABILIZATION/THERAPY

- Chemical exposure:
  - Suspect acid or alkali in all exposures to unknown substances.
  - Irrigate with any available diluting substance but preferably water or NS.
- Thermal exposure:
  - Cool-moist dressing with overlying ice packs

### ED TREATMENT/PROCEDURES

- Chemical exposure: Alkalis/acids/mace:
  - Continuous irrigation to achieve pH 7.3–7.5 (1–2 L via a Morgan lens >30–60 min):
    ○ Measure pH with Nitrazine paper
    ○ Dip paper in inferior conjunctival fornix.
  - pH should be evaluated at 5 and 30 min after irrigation to ensure normalization of pH.
  - Evaluate fornices in detail and eye in full range of motion to ensure removal of all particulate chemical substance.
  - Topical anesthetic (proparacaine)
  - Antibiotic prophylaxis for *Staphylococcus/Pseudomonas* until epithelialization is complete:
    ○ Gentamicin ointment plus erythromycin or
    ○ Bacitracin
  - Cycloplegics to minimize posterior synechiae formation:
    ○ Cyclopentolate 1%
    ○ Atropine 1%
  - Oral analgesics
    If increased intraocular pressure:
    ○ Immediate ophthalmologic consultation
    ○ Administer acetazolamide 125 mg PO q.i.d. and timolol 0.5% drops b.i.d.
- Topical steroids to control anterior uveitis (consult ophthalmology)
- Eye patch (consult ophthalmology)
- May require surgical intervention if frank corneal penetration
- Ophthalmologic consultation by phone in mild injuries
- Immediate ophthalmologic consultation in all moderate to severe injuries; if unavailable at your hospital, arrange transfer to closest eye center

- Hydrofluoric acid:
  - Treat as above, plus 1% calcium gluconate eyedrops
  - Systemic analgesia for 24 hr
- Thermal exposure:
  - Frequent moist dressing changes
  - Antibiotics drop q.i.d.
  - Generous lubricant application
  - Moisture chamber when extensive injury to eyelid
  - Steroids (consult ophthalmologist; do not use for >1 wk)
  - Ophthalmology consultation for any 2nd- or 3rd-degree burn to eyelids
  - Cigarette ash and hot liquid splashes usually result in corneal epithelial injury:
    ○ Treat as corneal abrasion
- Electrical Injury:
  - Irrigation
  - Wound care
  - Antibiotic ointment
  - Cycloplegic (if anterior uveitis)
  - Analgesia
- Radiation injury:
  - Topical anesthetic
  - Short-acting cycloplegic
  - Antibiotic ointment
  - Consider oral opioids for pain control

### Pediatric Considerations

- Patching poorly tolerated
- May require systemic analgesia for complete examination

### MEDICATION

- Artificial tears
- Atropine: 0.5%, 1.0%, 2.0% drops (cycloplegia 5–10 days, mydriasis 7–14 days) 1 drop t.i.d.
- Bacitracin ointment: q.i.d.
- Ciprofloxacin: 0.35% 1 drop q.i.d.
- Cyclopentolate: 0.5%, 1.0%, 2.0% drops (cycloplegia 1–2 days, mydriasis 1–2 days) 1 drop t.i.d.
- Erythromycin: 0.5% ointment q.i.d.
- Gentamicin: 0.3% ointment q.i.d.
- Gentamicin: 0.3% drops 1 drop q6h
- Homatropine: 5% drops 1–2 drop b.i.d.–t.i.d.
- Proparacaine: 0.5% drops 1 drop
- Sulfacetamide: 10% ointment q.i.d.
- Sulfacetamide: 10% drops q.i.d.
- Tetracaine: 0.5% drops 1–2 drops
- Tobramycin: 0.3% ointment q6h
- Tobramycin: 0.3% drops q6h
- Tropicamide: 0.5%, 1.0% drops (cycloplegia none; mydriasis 6 hr) 1 drop

## FOLLOW-UP

### DISPOSITION

#### Admission Criteria

- Intractable pain
- Increased intraocular pressure
- Corneal penetration requiring immediate surgical intervention
- Hydrofluoric acid burn; admit for 24 hr of systemic analgesia
- Suspected child abuse

#### Discharge Criteria

All mild corneal burns

### FOLLOW-UP RECOMMENDATIONS

Mandatory follow-up with ophthalmologist in 12–24 hr; arrange before patient discharge

## PEARLS AND PITFALLS

- In chemical exposures, delay exam until eye has been irrigated.
- All patients with epithelial defects need 12–24-hr ophthalmology follow-up.
- Do not prescribe topical anesthetics for discharged patients.

## ADDITIONAL READING

- Keller G, Kuckelkorn R, Redbrake C, et al. Emergency treatment of chemical and thermal eye burns. *Acta Ophthalmologica Scandinavica.* 2002;80:4.
- Khaw PT, Shah P, Elkington AR. Injury to the eye. *Br Med J.* 2004;328:36–38.
- Naradzay J, Barish RA. Approach to ophthalmologic emergencies. *Med Clin N America.* 2006;90: 305–328.
- Marx J, Hockberger R, Walls R, eds. *Rosen's emergency medicine,* 7th ed. Elsevier, 2009.

### See Also (Topic, Algorithm, Electronic Media Element)

- Corneal Abrasion
- Red Eye

## CODES

### ICD9

- 940.2 Alkaline chemical burn of cornea and conjunctival sac
- 940.3 Acid chemical burn of cornea and conjunctival sac
- 940.4 Other burn of cornea and conjunctival sac

# CORNEAL FOREIGN BODY
*Carl G. Skinner*

 **BASICS**

## DESCRIPTION
- Foreign material on or in the corneal epithelium
- Corneal epithelium disrupted:
  - Abrasion if only epithelium disrupted
  - Scar if deeper layers of cornea involved

## ETIOLOGY
- Foreign material causes inflammatory reaction:
  - May develop conjunctivitis, corneal edema, iritis, necrosis
- Poorly tolerated:
  - Organic material (plant material, insect parts)
  - Inorganic material that oxidizes (iron, copper)
- Well tolerated:
  - Inert objects (paint, glass, plastic, fiberglass, nonoxidizing metals)

 **DIAGNOSIS**

## SIGNS AND SYMPTOMS
- Foreign body sensation
- Eye pain
- Conjunctiva and sclera injection
- Tearing
- Blurred or decreased vision
- Photophobia
- Visible foreign body or rust ring
- Iritis

### History
Common complaint: Something fell, flew, or otherwise landed in my eye:
- Hot, high-speed projectiles may not produce pain initially.

### Physical Exam
- Complete eye exam:
  - Visual acuity
  - Visual fields
  - Extraocular movements
  - Lids and lashes
  - Pupils
  - Sclera
  - Conjunctiva
  - Anterior chamber
  - Fundi:
    - Slit-lamp
    - Fluorescein exam
    - Perform Seidel test (visualization of flow of aqueous through corneal perforation during fluorescein slit-lamp examination)
    - Intraocular pressure if no evidence of perforation

## ESSENTIAL WORKUP
- Injury history to determine type of foreign body and likelihood of perforation
- Exclude intraocular foreign body:
  - Suspect intraocular foreign body with high-speed mechanisms, such as machine operated or hammering metal on metal, or positive Seidel test.

## DIAGNOSTIC TESTS & INTERPRETATION
### Imaging
- Orbital CT scan or B-mode US when suspect intraocular foreign body
- Orbital plain radiograph to screen for intraocular metallic foreign body

## ALERT
Avoid MRI for possible metallic foreign bodies.

## DIFFERENTIAL DIAGNOSIS
- Conjunctival foreign body
- Corneal abrasion
- Corneal perforation with or without intraocular foreign body
- Corneal ulcer
- Keratitis

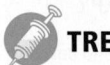 **TREATMENT**

### PRE-HOSPITAL
Place a Fox shield and position the patient upright.

### INITIAL STABILIZATION/THERAPY
Apply topical anesthetic to stop eye discomfort and assist in examination.

### ED TREATMENT/PROCEDURES
- Deep foreign bodies:
  - Refer those penetrating the Bowman membrane (next layer under epithelium) to an ophthalmologist, because permanent scarring may occur.
- Superficial foreign bodies:
  - Irrigation removal technique
- Apply topical anesthetic
- Try to wash foreign body off cornea by directing a stream of 0.9% NS at an oblique angle to cornea:
  - 25-gauge needle or foreign-body (FB) spud removal technique:
    - Using slit-lamp to immobilize patient's head and allow good visualization
    - Hold needle (bevel up) with thumb and forefinger, allowing other fingers to be stabilized on the patient's cheek.
    - Lift foreign body off cornea, keeping needle parallel to corneal surface.

- Rust rings removal:
  - Within 3 hr, iron-containing foreign bodies oxidize, leaving a rust stain on adjacent epithelial cells.
  - Removal recommended as rust rings delay healing and act as an irritant focus
  - Remove with needle or pothook burr either at same time as foreign body or delayed 24 hr
- Postremoval therapy:
  - Recheck Seidel test to exclude corneal perforation.
  - Treat resultant corneal abrasion with antibiotic drops or ointment.
  - Initiate cycloplegic agent when suspect presence of keratitis.
  - Update tetanus.
  - Initiate analgesia (nonsteroidal anti-inflammatory drug [NSAID] or acetaminophen with codeine).

### Pediatric Considerations
May require sedation to facilitate exam and foreign body removal

## MEDICATION
- Cycloplegics:
  - Cyclopentolate 1–2%: 1 drop t.i.d. (lasts up to 2 days)
  - Homatropine 2% or 5%: 1 drop daily (lasts up to 3 days)
- Topical antibiotics for 3 to 5 days: Often used but unproven benefit:
  - Erythromycin ointment: Thin strip q6h
  - Sulfacetamide 10%: 1 drop q6h
    Ciprofloxacin: 1 drop q6h
  - Ofloxacin: 1 drop q6h
  - Polymyxin/trimethoprim: 1 drop q6h
- Topical NSAIDs:
  - Ketorolac: 1 drop q6h
  - Diclofenac: 1 drop q6h

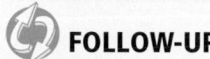 **FOLLOW-UP**

### DISPOSITION
### Admission Criteria
Globe penetration

### Discharge Criteria
All corneal foreign bodies

### Issues for Referral
- Consult ophthalmologist for:
  - Vegetative material removal owing to risk of ulceration
  - Any evidence of infection or ulceration
  - Multiple foreign bodies
  - Incomplete foreign body removal
- Ophthalmology follow-up in 24 hr for:
  - Abrasion in the visual field
  - Large abrasion
  - Abrasions that continue symptomatic or worsen the next day
  - Rust ring removal

### FOLLOW-UP RECOMMENDATIONS
Return or follow-up with a physician if symptoms continue or worsen in 1 or 2 days.

## PEARLS AND PITFALLS
- Consider intraocular foreign body, especially with history of high projectile objects.
- Clinical evidence does not support eye patching for pain or healing.
- After removal, most corneal foreign bodies can be treated as an abrasion and usually do well without further treatment.
- Topical anesthetics should not be prescribed for home use.

## ADDITIONAL READING
- Babineau MR, Sanchez LD. Ophthalmologic procedures in the emergency department. *Emerg Med Clin North Am.* 2008;26:17–34.
- Dargin JM, Lowenstein RA. The painful eye. *Emerg Med Clin North Am.* 2008;26:199–216.
- Khaw P, Shaw P, Elkington A. ABC of eyes. Injury to the eye. *Br Med J.* 2004;328:36–38.
- Knoop KJ, Dennis WR, Hedges JR. Ophthalmologic procedures. In: Roberts MD, Hedges JR, eds. *Clinical procedures in emergency medicine*, 5th ed. 2009:1153–1159.
- Turner A, Rabiu M. Patching for corneal abrasion. *Cochrane Database Syst Rev.* 2006;CD004764.

### See Also (Topic, Algorithm, Electronic Media Element)
- Corneal Abrasion
- Red Eye

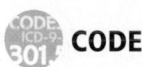 **CODES**

**ICD9**
930.0 Corneal foreign body

# COUGH

*Alison K. Sisitsky*

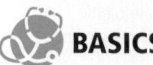 **BASICS**

## DESCRIPTION
- A sudden spasmodic contraction of the thoracic cavity resulting in violent release of air from the lungs and usually accompanied by a distinctive sound:
  - Deep inspiration
  - Glottis closes
  - Expiratory muscles contract
  - Intrapulmonary pressures increase
  - Glottis opens
  - Air expiration at high pressure
  - Secretion and foreign material excretion
  - Vocal cord vibration with tracheobronchial walls, lung parenchyma, and secretions
- Defense mechanism to clear the airway of foreign material and secretions:
  - Voluntary or involuntary
  - Involuntary coughing regulated by the vagal afferent nerves:
    - Voluntary coughing under cortical control allowing for inhibition or voluntary cough
    - Because of cortical control, placebos can have a profound effect on coughing.
  - Reflex involves respiratory tissue receptor activation of afferent neurons to the central cough center followed by efferent output to the respiratory muscles.
  - Mechanical receptors in larynx, trachea, and carina sense touch and displacement.
  - Chemical receptors in larynx and bronchi are sensitive to gases and fumes.
  - Activated by irritants, mucus, edema, pus, and thermal stimuli
- Complications of severe coughing:
  - Epistaxis
  - Subconjunctival hemorrhage
  - Syncope
  - Pneumothorax
  - Pneumomediastinum
  - Emesis
  - Hernia
  - Rectal prolapse
  - Incontinence
  - Seizures
  - Encephalitis
  - Intracranial hemorrhage
  - Spinal epidural hemorrhage
  - Clubbing
  - Pruriginous rash

## ETIOLOGY
- Acute (<3 wk):
  - Pneumonia
  - Left ventricular failure
  - Cough variant asthma
  - COPD exacerbation
  - Bronchiectasis
  - Pulmonary embolism
  - Upper respiratory tract infection
  - Acute bronchitis
  - Pertussis
  - Bacterial sinusitis
  - Upper airway cough syndrome:
    - Post nasal drip
    - GERD
    - Allergic rhinitis
    - Environmental irritant rhinitis
- Subacute (3–8 wk):
  - Postinfectious cough
  - Pertussis
  - Bronchitis
  - Bacterial sinusitis
  - Asthma
  - GERD
  - Pulmonary embolism
- Chronic (>8 wk):
  - Postnasal drip
  - Asthma
  - GERD
  - Chronic bronchitis
  - Tuberculosis
  - Bronchiectasis
  - Eosinophilic bronchitis
  - ACE inhibitor use
  - Bronchogenic carcinoma
  - Carcinomatosis
  - Sarcoidosis
  - Left ventricular failure
  - Aspiration syndrome
  - Psychogenic/habit

### Pediatric Considerations
- Most frequent causes:
  - Asthma
  - Sinusitis
  - GERD
- Less common causes:
  - Tracheobronchomalacia
  - Mediastinal tumor
  - Acyanotic congenital heart disease
  - Ventricular septal defect
  - Patent ductus arteriosus
  - Pulmonary stenosis
  - Tetralogy of Fallot
  - Lodged foreign body
  - Chronic aspiration of milk
  - Environmental exposure

- Consider:
  - Neonatal history
  - Feeding history
  - Growth and developmental history
  - Allergies
  - Eczema
  - Sleep disorders
- Indications for CXR:
  - Suspicion of foreign body ingestion
  - Suspect aspiration

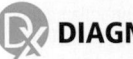 **DIAGNOSIS**

## SIGNS AND SYMPTOMS
- Sputum production:
  - Frothy (pulmonary edema)
  - Mucopurulent
  - Suggestive of bacterial pneumonia or bronchitis but also seen with viral infections
  - Rust colored (pneumococcal pneumonia)
  - "Currant jelly" (*Klebsiella* pneumonia)
  - Hemoptysis
- Posttussive syncope or emesis (suggests pertussis)
- Shortness of breath
- Chest pain
- Chills/fever
- Night sweats
- Wheezing
- GERD:
  - Heartburn
  - Dysphagia
  - Regurgitation
  - Belching
  - Early satiety
- Malignancy:
  - Weight loss
  - Poor appetite
  - Fatigue

### History
- Duration of cough to classify into acute, subacute, and chronic
- Description of sputum, if present, including hemoptysis
- Posttussive emesis or syncope and paroxysmal cough suggests pertussis.
- History of GI symptoms pointing to GERD
- Weight loss and night sweats suggestive of tuberculosis in chronic cough

C

### Physical Exam
- Vital signs
- Abnormal breath sounds:
  - Absence or decreased: Reduced airflow vs. overinflation
  - Rales (crackles): Popping or rattling when air opens closed alveoli:
    - Moist, dry, fine, coarse
  - Rhonchi: Snoring-like sounds when large airways are obstructed
  - Wheezes: High-pitched sounds produced by narrowed airways
  - Stridor: Upper airway obstruction
- Evidence of respiratory distress:
  - Use of accessory muscles
  - Abdominal breathing

### ESSENTIAL WORKUP
- Complete medical history:
  - Duration
  - Associated symptoms
  - Sick contacts
  - Smoking exposure
  - ACE inhibitor use
  - HIV/immunocompromised state
  - Potential exposure to tuberculosis
- EKG:
  - History of cardiac disease
  - Associated chest pain or abnormal vital signs
  - Lack of infectious symptoms

### DIAGNOSTIC TESTS & INTERPRETATION
#### Lab
Order according to presenting signs and symptoms:
- WBC count with differential
- Sputum gram stain, cultures, and sensitivities
- Acid fast bacilli (AFB) culture
- CD4 count
- Pertussis titers
- D-Dimer
- Flu swab (for high-risk patients or those to be admitted)

#### Imaging
- CXR:
  - For immunosuppressed patient
  - At least 1 of the following in healthy patients with acute cough and sputum production:
    - Heart rate >100 bpm
    - Respiratory rate >24 breaths/min
    - Oral body temperature of >38°C
    - Chest exam findings of focal consolidation, egophony, or fremitus
  - Ill appearing
  - Change in chronic cough
  - Continued cough after discontinuation of ACE inhibitor
- CT of chest:
  - Abnormal CXR
  - Assess for pulmonary embolism

#### Diagnostic Procedures/Surgery
- Peak flow
- Bronchoscopy:
  - For unknown mass on chest radiograph
  - Hemoptysis
  - Suspected cancer

### DIFFERENTIAL DIAGNOSIS
See "Etiology."

---

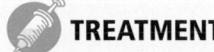

## TREATMENT

### INITIAL STABILIZATION/THERAPY
Assess airway, breathing, and circulation.

### ED TREATMENT/PROCEDURES
Specific treatment related to cause:
- Respiratory infection: Consider antibiotics, antivirals (flu), decongestants, and antitussives.
- Asthma: Inhaled $\beta_2$-agonist and steroids
- GERD: $H_2$-blockers, proton pump inhibitors, and antacids
- Suspicion of pertussis: Macrolide and 5 days isolation
- Exacerbation of chronic bronchitis: Inhaled $\beta_2$-agonist and steroids
- Malignancy: Supportive care

### MEDICATION
- Antibiotics:
  - Pick appropriate coverage for suspected bacteria.
- Antivirals:
  - Tamiflu: 75 mg (peds: 30–75 mg PO b.i.d. × 5 days) PO daily
- Antitussives:
  - Benzonatate (Tessalon Perles): 100–200 mg PO q6h
  - Codeine: 10–20 mg (peds: 1–1.5 mg/kg/d) PO q4h–q6h
  - Dextromethorphan: 10–20 mg (peds: 1 mg/kg/d) PO q6h–q8h
  - Hydrocodone: 5–10 mg (peds: 0.6 mg/kg/d q6h–q8h) PO q6h–q8h
- Bronchodilators:
  - Albuterol: 2.5 mg in 2.5 NS (peds: 0.1–0.15 mg/kg/dose q20min) q20min inhaled
  - Ipratropium: 0.5 mg in 3 mL NS (peds: Nebulizer 250–500 μg/dose q6h) q3h
- Decongestants:
  - Chlorpheniramine: 4–12 mg (peds: 2 mg PO q4h–6h) PO q4h–q12h
  - Phenylpropanolamine: 25–50 mg (peds: 6.25–12.5 mg PO q4h) PO q4h–q8h
- Mucolytics:
  - Guaifenesin: 5–20 mL (peds: 5–10 mL/dose if >6 yr; 2.5–5 mL/dose if <6 yr) PO q4h
- Steroids:
  - Dexamethasone: 2 sprays/nostril b.i.d.
  - Methylprednisolone: 60–125 mg IV (peds: 1–2 mg/kg/dose IV/PO q6h)
  - Prednisone: 40–60 mg (peds: 1–2 mg/kg/d q6h–q12h) PO

---

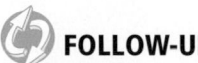

## FOLLOW-UP

### DISPOSITION
#### Admission Criteria
- Hypoxemia or critical illness
- Suspected tuberculosis with positive chest radiograph result
- Immunocompromised with fever
- Risk of bacteremia or sepsis

---

### Discharge Criteria
- Oxygenation at baseline for patient
- Oral medications
- Safe environment at home

### Issues for Referral
Close follow-up by primary care physician for outpatient management

### FOLLOW-UP RECOMMENDATIONS
- Stop smoking, avoid being around smokers or other harmful substances such as asbestos.
- Change diet.
  - Avoid coffee, tea, and soda.
  - Avoid eating for at least 4 hr prior to sleeping.
- Use pillows to keep head elevated at night.
- Seek care immediately with:
  - Chest pain
  - Coughing blood
  - Shortness of breath
  - Fainting

## PEARLS AND PITFALLS
- For patients fitting the clinical profile for cough due to GERD, it is recommended that treatment be initially started in lieu of testing.
- For patients with a presumed diagnosis of acute bronchitis, routine treatment with antibiotics is not justified and should not be offered.

## ADDITIONAL READING
- Irwin RS, Baumann MH, Bolser DC, et al. Diagnosis and management of cough executive summary: ACCP evidence based clinical practice guidelines. Chest. 2006;129:1S.
- Irwin RS. Unexplained cough in the adult. Otolaryngol Clin North Am. 2010;43(1):167–180, xi–xii.
- Schroeder K, Fahey T. Over-the-counter medications for acute cough in children and adults in ambulatory settings. Cochrane Database Syst Rev. 2004;18(4): CD001831.

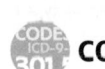 CODES

ICD9
786.2 Cough

---

# CROUP

*Dale W. Steele*

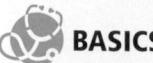 **BASICS**

## DESCRIPTION

- Viral infection of the upper and lower respiratory tract
- Most commonly presents in children 6 mo–3 yr:
  - Laryngotracheitis/laryngotracheo-bronchitis
  - Inspiratory stridor owing to extrathoracic airway obstruction
  - Expiratory wheeze suggests lower airway involvement.
  - Inflammatory edema of subglottic region
  - Narrowest part of pediatric airway
- May progress to respiratory failure
- Spasmodic croup:
  - Sudden onset at night without viral prodrome
  - Consistent response to mist or cool night air
  - Often recurrent
  - May represent allergic reaction to viral antigen

## ETIOLOGY

- Parainfluenza types 1, 2, and 3
- Influenza A and B
- Adenoviruses
- Respiratory syncytial virus
- Measles
- *Mycoplasma pneumoniae*
- Herpes simplex

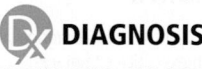 **DIAGNOSIS**

## SIGNS AND SYMPTOMS

### History

- Nonspecific upper respiratory prodrome with or without fever
- Duration of illness:
  - Prior airway manipulation
  - Possibility of foreign body aspiration
- Previous episodes
- History of wheeze
- Immunization status (*Haemophilus influenzae* type b [HIB]; diphtheria, pertussis, and tetanus [DPT])

### Physical Exam

- Toxic appearing?
- Cyanosis (not present in majority of patients. If present, suggests severe disease)
- Preferred position?
- Quality of cry/voice?
- Drooling/trismus/limited neck extension?
- Mental status
- Stridor at rest, increased work of breathing?
- Hydration status
- Westley croup score (maximum total points: 17):
  - Stridor (inspiratory or biphasic):
    - 0 = None
    - 1 = Audible with stethoscope at rest
    - 2 = Audible without stethoscope at rest
  - Retractions:
    - 0 = None
    - 1 = Mild
    - 2 = Moderate
    - 3 = Severe
  - Air entry:
    - 0 = Normal
    - 1 = Decreased
    - 2 = Severely decreased
  - Cyanosis:
    - 0 = None
    - 4 = With agitation
    - 5 = At rest
  - Level of consciousness:
    - 0 = Normal
    - 5 = Altered

## DIAGNOSTIC TESTS & INTERPRETATION

### Lab

- Continuous pulse oximetry
- Other tests are not routinely indicated.

### Imaging

Anteroposterior (AP) and lateral neck radiographs:

- Steeple sign indicates narrowing of subglottic trachea.
- Imaging not routinely indicated, unless atypical presentation or clinical course
- Subject to misinterpretation
- Should not delay definitive visualization and intubation in OR in child with concern for epiglottitis or bacterial tracheitis
- Monitor child during imaging, if done.

## DIFFERENTIAL DIAGNOSIS

- Infection:
  - Bacterial tracheitis
  - Retropharyngeal or parapharyngeal abscess
  - Epiglottitis
  - Peritonsillar abscess
  - Diphtheria
- Foreign body (airway or esophageal)
- Angioedema
- Vocal cord paralysis
- Congenital airway anomaly:
  - Laryngomalacia
- Acquired subglottic stenosis
- Thermal injury to upper airway
- Hemangioma
- Laryngeal papillomatosis
- Vocal cord dysfunction (VCD) (adolescents)

 **TREATMENT**

## PRE-HOSPITAL

- Allow child to maintain position of comfort.
- Defer interventions that may distress child such as:
  - IV access
  - IM injections
- If severe distress:
  - Immediate nebulized epinephrine with humidified oxygen

## INITIAL STABILIZATION/THERAPY

- Nebulized racemic epinephrine or l-epinephrine if distress or stridor at rest:
  - l-epinephrine containing only the active isomer; has been shown to be therapeutically equivalent to racemic epinephrine
- Oxygen (via blowby) for suspected or documented hypoxia suggesting severe disease
- Mist therapy often used, but no evidence for efficacy
- Dexamethasone:
  - Reduces need for intubation, shortens length of stay, and reduces admissions and return visits
  - Effective even in mild croup (Westley croup score ≤2)

C

- If poor response to nebulized racemic epinephrine or l-epinephrine:
  - Consider trial of heliox:
    o Heliox, when available, has been used to decrease the work of breathing in patients with an incomplete response to epinephrine.
- If impending or existing respiratory failure despite aforementioned therapy:
  - Tracheal intubation by most experienced person available
  - Use uncuffed endotracheal tube (ETT) $\leq 0.5 - <1.0$ mm usual size.
- If epiglottitis or foreign body suspected:
  - Ideally, to OR for inhalational anesthesia, direct laryngoscopy, and intubation
  - Surgeon standing by for emergent tracheostomy

## ED TREATMENT/PROCEDURES
See "Initial Stabilization."

## MEDICATION
- Racemic epinephrine 2.25%: 0.25–0.5 mL nebulized in 2.5 mL NS
- l-epinephrine 1:1,000: 5 mL (5 mg) nebulized
- Dexamethasone: Single dose of 0.6 mg/kg (max. 10 mg) PO (use crushed tablet with flavored syrup). Equally effective when given PO, IV, or IM
- Heliox (70% helium: 30% oxygen mixture administered via face mask or tent house)
- Antibiotics: Not indicated

 FOLLOW-UP

## DISPOSITION
### Admission Criteria
- Young infants, pre-existing upper airway obstruction
- Persistent or recurrent stridor at rest unresponsive to nebulized epinephrine, or recurring > 4 hours after dexamethasone given
- Pediatric intensive care unit:
  - Persistent severe obstruction
  - Need for frequent epinephrine treatments and/or heliox
  - Tracheal intubation with assisted ventilation

### Discharge Criteria
- Normal oxygenation in room air
- No stridor at rest after brief observation
- Children initially given epinephrine who no longer have stridor at rest should be observed for a minimum of 2–3 hr
- Reliable caretaker, communication, transport

### Issues for Referral
Concern for underlying anatomic abnormality

## FOLLOW-UP RECOMMENDATIONS
- Most children with croup do not require specific follow-up.
- Patients who have had prolonged stridor, or acute worsening of stridor should seek care with their primary care physician or return to the ED.

## PEARLS AND PITFALLS
- Beware young infants with stridor
- High incidence of congenital abnormalities

## ADDITIONAL READING
- Bjornson C, Johnson DW. Croup. Lancet. 2008; 371:329–339.
- Bjornson C, Klassen TP, Williamson J, et al. A randomized trial of a single dose of oral dexamethasone for mild croup. N Engl J Med. 2004;351:1306–1313.
- Castro-Rodríguez JA, Holberg CJ, Morgan WJ, et al. Relation of two different subtypes of croup before age three to wheezing, atopy, and pulmonary function during childhood. A prospective study. Pediatrics. 2001;170:512–518.
- Cherry J. Croup. NEJM. 2008;358:384–391.

- Kwong K, Hoa M, Coticchia JM. Recurrent croup presentation, diagnosis and management. Am J Otolaryngol. 2007;28:401–407.
- Ledwith CA, Shea LM, Mauro RD. Safety and efficacy of nebulized racemic epinephrine in conjunction with oral dexamethasone and mist in the outpatient treatment of croup. Ann Emerg Med. 1995;25:331–337.
- Rittichier KK, Ledwith CA. Outpatient treatment of moderate croup with dexamethasone: Intramuscular versus oral dosing. Pediatrics. 2000;106: 1344–1348.
- Scolnik D, Coates AL, Stephens D. Controlled delivery of high vs. low humidity vs. mist therapy for croup in emergency departments. JAMA. 2006;295: 1274–1280.
- Weber JE, Chudnofsky CR, Younger JG, et al. A randomized comparison of helium-oxygen mixture (heliox) and racemic epinephrine for the treatment of moderate to severe croup. Pediatrics. 2001; 107:e96.

## See Also (Topic, Algorithm, Electronic Media Element)
Guideline for the diagnosis and management of croup. Alberta, ON, Canada: Alberta Medical Association; 2003. Accessed December 29, 2009, http://www.topalbertadoctors.org/informed_practice/cpgs/croup.html

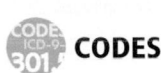 CODES

ICD9
464.4 Croup

# CUSHING SYNDROME

*Hugh A. Schuckman*
*Stephen L. Chesser*

 **BASICS**

## DESCRIPTION
- Cushing disease: Pituitary adenoma producing excess adrenocorticotropic hormone (ACTH)
- Cushing syndrome: Excessive glucocorticoid effects

## RISK FACTORS
### Genetics
- Multiple endocrine neoplasia type I
- Carney complex (pigmented lentigines, atrial myxoma, germ-cell tumors with Cushing disease)

## ETIOLOGY
- Most commonly exogenous administration of glucocorticoids either therapeutically or surreptitiously
- Pituitary adenoma secreting ACTH
- Adrenal production of cortisol from adenoma, carcinoma, or micronodular disease
- Tumor-producing ectopic ACTH:
  - Small cell lung carcinoma:
    - Most common
  - Uterine cervical carcinoma
  - Islet cell tumor of pancreas:
    - Multiple endocrine neoplasia (MEA) I-type syndrome
  - Medullary thyroid cancer
  - Pheochromocytoma
  - Ganglioneuroma
  - Melanoma prostate carcinoma
  - Carcinoid tumor:
    - Lung
    - Pancreas
    - GI tract
    - Thymus
    - Ovary

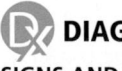 **DIAGNOSIS**

## SIGNS AND SYMPTOMS

### ALERT
- The most important aspect of Cushing syndrome in the ED is recognizing the potential for Addisonian (adrenal) crisis during periods of stress.
- Although nonemergent, the early recognition of Cushing syndrome may prevent morbidity and mortality.

### Pediatric Considerations
Suspect if increasing in obesity while failing to maintain height on the growth chart

### Pregnancy Considerations
Cushing syndrome rarely complicates pregnancy, but has been associated with severe pre-eclampsia and HELLP syndrome (*h*emolysis, *e*levated *l*iver function, and *l*ow *p*latelets).

### History
- Cushing disease previously diagnosed
- Prior use of corticosteroids
- Characteristic appearance should lead to questions concerning change in weight, facial appearance, hirsutism, or psychiatric symptoms.

### Physical Exam
- Diagnosis suggested by:
  - Abnormal fat deposition with moon facies
  - Buffalo hump
  - Central obesity with thin extremities
  - Supraclavicular fat deposition:
    - Above findings raise suspicion in a stressed patient of potentially developing Addisonian (adrenal) crisis
- Cardiovascular:
  - Uncontrolled hypertension
- Neurologic:
  - Atherosclerotic or embolic stroke
  - Pseudotumor cerebri (primarily with exogenous glucocorticoid administration):
    - Check fundi
  - Spinal lipomatosis with cord or nerve-root compression
- Gastroenterologic:
  - Peptic ulcers
  - GI hemorrhage
  - Pancreatitis (primarily with exogenous glucocorticoid administration)
  - Fatty liver
- Psychiatric:
  - Toxic psychosis
  - Mood disorders (40%)
  - Depression
  - Memory impairment
  - Euphoria

- Musculoskeletal:
  - Myopathy (proximal weakness)
  - Pathologic fractures
  - Osteoporosis
  - Aseptic necrosis humeral or femoral heads (primarily with exogenous glucocorticoid administration)
- Endocrine:
  - Glucose intolerance
  - Hyperlipidemia
  - Amenorrhea, female with male pattern balding, or hirsutism
- Hematologic:
  - Increased neutrophils
  - Decreased lymphocytes and eosinophils
  - Opportunistic infections
- Ophthalmologic:
  - Cataracts (primarily with exogenous glucocorticoid administration)
  - Glaucoma (primarily with exogenous glucocorticoid administration)
- Dermatologic:
  - Purple striae >1 cm in diameter
  - Hyperpigmentation—especially of buccal mucosa (from excess ACTH production)
  - Facial plethora
  - Thin skin
  - Impaired wound healing
  - Ecchymoses
  - Acne
  - Hyperhidrosis

## ESSENTIAL WORKUP
- Cannot confirm diagnosis in ED
- Anticipate impending Addisonian (adrenal) crisis:
  - Most frequent and common problem with Cushing syndrome is its recognition in patient with concurrent illness to prevent acute Addisonian crisis.
- Search for life-threatening conditions:
  - MI
  - Stroke
  - Sepsis
  - Pathologic fracture
  - Uncontrolled DM
  - Psychiatric emergency necessitating admission

## DIAGNOSTIC TESTS & INTERPRETATION
### Lab
- Electrolytes, BUN, creatinine, glucose:
  - Hypokalemia
  - 10% with metabolic alkalosis
  - Diminished glucose tolerance (75%)
  - 20% overt DM
- Urinalysis:
  - 50% have glycosuria.
- CBC:
  - Increased WBCs
  - Decreased eosinophils

### Imaging
- ECG for myocardial ischemia
- CXR for tumor-causing ectopic ACTH
- Plain films if suspect possible pathologic fractures:
  - Delayed bone age

### Diagnostic Procedures/Surgery
Nonemergent testing:
- MRI for pituitary tumor
- CT for adrenal carcinoma, adenoma, or hyperplasia
- Dexamethasone-suppression test (follow-up study with primary physician):
  - If suspicion of endogenous Cushing syndrome exists
  - Low-dose (screening test): 1 mg at 11:00 pm with an 8 am cortisol level drawn:
    - Low specificity
- False-positive results from alcohol, estrogens, spironolactone, phenytoin, barbiturates, and rifampin:
  - High-dose dexamethasone-suppression test needed to confirm the diagnosis:
    - 2 mg q.i.d. of dexamethasone with cortisol level 6 hr later
    - Compare day 2 urine-free cortisol and 17-hydroxyketosteroids with baseline levels.

## DIFFERENTIAL DIAGNOSIS
- Alcohol-induced pseudo–Cushing syndrome
- Obesity
- Psychiatric states:
  - Depression
  - Obsessive–compulsive disorder
  - Panic disorder
- Physiologic states:
  - Chronic stress
  - 3rd-trimester pregnancy
  - Chronic strenuous exercise

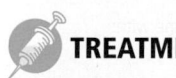 TREATMENT

## PRE-HOSPITAL
- Acute addisonian (adrenal) crisis under stress may develop with iatrogenic Cushing syndrome.
- Patients may have extremely labile behavior with violent behavior.
- Leading causes of death in untreated Cushing syndrome are:
  - Infection
  - Stroke
  - MI

## INITIAL STABILIZATION/THERAPY
- Anticipate Addisonian (adrenal) crisis.
- Initiate treatment for associated complications:
  - MI
  - Stroke
  - Psychiatric stabilization

## ED TREATMENT/PROCEDURES
- IV rehydration
- Glucose-lowering agents for hyperglycemia
- Appropriate cultures and antibiotics for suspected infection
- Antihypertensive agents for uncontrolled BP
- Administer steroids (hydrocortisone) with iatrogenic Cushing if patient under stress to prevent Addisonian crisis.
- Medications to lower cortisol levels (bromocriptine, ketoconazole, aminoglutethimide, metyrapone):
  - Used rarely with severe symptoms in patients awaiting surgery
  - Institute under the direction of an endocrinologist.

Definitive therapy:
- Iatrogenic:
  - Taper steroids as rapidly as possible
  - Calcium, vitamin D, and estrogen supplementation if possible
- Pituitary Cushing:
  - Transsphenoidal surgery
  - Radiation for surgical failures and a few select patients
- Adrenal adenoma/carcinoma:
  - Adrenal resection with medical therapy for metastatic lesions not resectable
- Ectopic ACTH:
  - Tumor resection (if possible) with medical therapy for metastatic lesions not resectable

## MEDICATION
### First Line
ONLY if in adrenal crisis: Hydrocortisone: 100 mg (peds: 1–2 mg/kg) IV q6h

### Second Line
- In consultation with an endocrinologist
- SYMPTOMATIC TREATMENT ONLY as adjunctive therapy in patients awaiting surgery or refractory to other treatment
- Steroidogenic inhibitors:
  - Ketoconazole 200 mg PO b.i.d.
  - Metyrapone 0.5–1 g/d PO in div. doses
  - Aminoglutethimide 250 mg PO q6h
- Adrenolytics:
  - Mitotane 500 mg PO daily
- ACTH release inhibitors:
  - Cyproheptadine 4 mg PO b.i.d.
  - Bromocriptine 2.5–30 mg/d
- Other:
  - Spironolactone for symptomatic relief of HTN or hypokalemia

 FOLLOW-UP

## DISPOSITION
### Admission Criteria
- Complications that require admission such as:
  - MI
  - Stroke
  - Sepsis
  - Pathologic fracture
  - Uncontrolled DM
  - Psychiatric emergency
- Impending Addisonian (adrenal) crisis

### Discharge Criteria
Well-appearing, stable patient without admission criteria

### Issues for Referral
- Any patient suspected of Cushing syndrome for further evaluation
- Conditions secondary to Cushing requiring treatment

## FOLLOW-UP RECOMMENDATIONS
Follow up testing to confirm diagnosis

## PEARLS AND PITFALLS
- Keep a high index of suspicion in the physiologically stressed patient by history or from body habitus for the need to prophylax against Addisonian crisis.
- The diagnosis of primary Cushing's disease may be life changing for the patient.
- Suspect Cushing's disease when there are supraclavicular fat pads.

## ADDITIONAL READING
- Goldman L, Bennett JC, eds. Cecil's Textbook of Medicine, 23rd ed. Philadelphia: Saunders-Elsevier; 2008.
- Guyton A, Hall J. Textbook of Medical Physiology. 11th ed. Philadelphia: Saunders-Elsevier; 2006
- Andreoli T, Carpenter C. Cecil Essentials of Medicine. 7th ed. Philadelphia: Saunders Elsevier; 2007.
- Wallach J, ed. Interpretation of Diagnostic Tests. 8th ed. Boston: Little, Brown and Company; 2007.

 CODES

ICD9
255.0 Cushing's syndrome

# CYANIDE POISONING
*Kirk L. Cumpston*

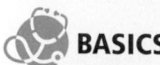 **BASICS**

## DESCRIPTION
- Toxicity through inhalation, dermal, or GI tract absorption
- Intracellular toxin that inhibits aerobic metabolism through interruption of oxidative phosphorylation:
  - Leads to decreased $O_2$ utilization and ATP production
- Detoxification:
  - Rhodanese: Hepatic mitochondrial enzyme responsible for the metabolism:
    - Combines cyanide (CN) with sulfur (rate-limiting step) covalently (irreversible) to form less toxic and water-soluble thiocyanate (T-CN)
    - Forms less toxic reversible cyanhemoglobin when combined with hemoglobin (Fe 3+)
    - Forms nontoxic cyanocobalamin (B12) when combined with hydroxocobalamin (B12a)
    - Rate of CN removal requires adequate bioavailability of sulfur compounds (thiosulfate [TS]).

## ETIOLOGY
- Fires:
  - Combustion by-product of natural and synthetic products
- Vehicle exhaust
- Industry:
  - Metal plating, microchip manufacturing
  - Chemical synthesis
  - Plastic manufacturing
  - Pesticides
- Solvents:
  - Artificial nail remover
  - Metal polishes
- By-product of nitroprusside metabolism (nonenzymatic)
- By-product of *Pseudomonas aeruginosa* and pyocyaneus infections
- Amygdalin (converted by intestinal flora to CN)-CN containing plants (apricot and peach pits, apple and pear seeds, and cassava)
- Jewelry making

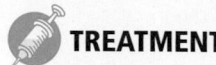 **DIAGNOSIS**

## SIGNS AND SYMPTOMS
- Dermal exposure: Standard decontamination
- Oral exposure: Can be caustic, 50 mg has caused death.
- Inhalational exposure:
  - 50 parts per min causes anxiety, palpitations, dyspnea, headache.
  - 100–135 ppm <1 hr is lethal.
- Heart and brain—most sensitive organs—1st to show manifestation of toxicity

- CNS:
  - Headache
  - Confusion
  - Syncope
  - Seizures
  - Coma
- Cardiovascular:
  - Dyspnea
  - Chest pain
  - Cardiorespiratory collapse and death
- Other:
  - Nausea/vomiting

## ESSENTIAL WORKUP
- History of exposure:
  - Smoke inhalation
  - Industrial exposure
  - Intentional suicide
  - Intentional homicide
- Clinical clues (frequently absent):
  - Peculiar odor of bitter almonds
  - Bright red (arterialization) retinal vessels
  - Abrupt onset and/or deteriorating toxic effects
  - Lactic acidosis
  - High venous $O_2$ saturation (secondary to blocked cellular $O_2$ consumption); arterialization of venous blood gases

## DIAGNOSTIC TESTS & INTERPRETATION
### Lab
- CBC
- Electrolytes, BUN, creatinine, glucose:
  - Anion gap acidosis
- Liver profile
- Creatine phosphokinase (CPK)
- Carboxyhemoglobin (CO) level
- Methemoglobin (MH) level
- CN level:
  - Send out lab that is not usually available in a clinically relevant time period.
  - Levels >0.5–1 mg/L: Toxic
  - Levels 2.5–3.0 mg/L: Fatal
- Blood gas determinations:
  - Increased arterial saturation gap (calculated direct [measure] $O_2$ saturation [cooximeter])
  - Elevated mixed venous $O_2$: $MvO_2$ (normal about 35–40)
  - Elevated mixed venous $O_2$ saturation (cooximeter): $SmvO_2$ (normal about 75%)
  - Decreased arteriovenous $O_2$ difference: $AVO_2D$ (normal about 3–4.8 mL/dL)
- Elevated lactate level >8 mmol/L:
  - An elevated lactate is a surrogate marker for the presence of cyanide with the appropriate history and physical examination.

### Imaging
CXR

## DIFFERENTIAL DIAGNOSIS
- Carbon monoxide
- Hydrogen sulfide
- MH
- Sulfhemoglobinemia
- Inert gases "asphyxiants"
- Other causes of high anion gap metabolic acidosis

**TREATMENT**

## PRE-HOSPITAL
- Remove source of CN.
- Prevent others from becoming contaminated.
- Remove and bag all contaminated clothing and wash affected areas copiously with soap and water. If vapor contamination, removal of clothing may be all that is necessary.

## INITIAL STABILIZATION/THERAPY
- ABCs:
  - Administer 100% oxygen:
    - Even in presence of normal $PaO_2$
    - Acts synergistically with antidotes
- Gastric decontamination for oral ingestions if within 1 hr:
  - Perform gastric lavage and administer activated charcoal (AC) if ingestion of CN or CN-containing products and no contraindications.
  - Do not induce emesis.

## ED TREATMENT/PROCEDURES
Hydroxocobalamin (B12a) Cyanokit®:
- Administer if manifesting significant CN toxicity with persistent high anion gap metabolic acidosis, with any syncope, seizures, and hypotension.
- Administration often instituted empirically; CN levels not immediately available
- Binds to CN:
  - Forms nontoxic cyanocobalamin (B12); renally excreted
- Advantages:
  - No methemoglobin induction
  - Does not cause hypotension
  - Intracellular distribution
- Limitations:
  - Cost

## ALERT
- Incompatible in the same IV line with:
  - Diazepam
  - Dobutamine
  - Dopamine
  - Fentanyl
  - Nitroglycerin
  - Pentobarbital
  - Propofol
  - Sodium thiosulfate
  - Sodium nitrite
  - Ascorbic acid
  - Blood products

- Side effects of hydroxocobalamin:
  - HTN
  - Red skin and all secretions
  - Interference of colorimetric assays of AST, ALT, total bilirubin, creatinine, Mg, iron
- Cyanide antidote kit:
  - Administer if manifesting significant CN toxicity with persistent high anion gap metabolic acidosis, with any syncope, seizures, and hypotension.
  - Administration often instituted empirically; CN levels not immediately available
  - Contents: Amyl nitrite pearls, sodium nitrite, and sodium thiosulfate
  - Nitrite action:
    - Induce a CN-scavenging MH by oxidizing hemoglobin ($Fe^{2+}$ to $Fe^{3+}$), which attracts extracellular CN away from the mitochondria-forming CN-MH, which is less toxic.
    - Do not administer empirically or prophylactically.
  - Sodium thiosulfate action:
    - Substrate for the enzyme rhodanase
    - Combines with CN to form a less toxic T-CN
- Hyperbaric oxygen therapy:
  - Can be used to treat CN exposures
  - Maximizes tissue oxygenation despite toxic MH level

## MEDICATION
Activated charcoal: 1 g/kg PO

### First Line
Hydroxocobalamin ($B_{12a}$):
- 70 mg/kg IV, max 5 g
- There are 22.5-g bottles with the drug in powder form in them
- Reconstitute the powder by gently rolling the bottle after filling with 100 mL of 0.9% NS
- Attach the bottle to an IV line and infuse over 7.5 min
- Both bottles are to be infused over 15 min

### Second Line
- Amyl nitrite, sodium nitrite, and sodium thiosulfate Cyanide Antidote Kit:
- Amyl nitrite pearls:
  - Crush 1 or 2 ampules in gauze and hold close to nose, in lip of face mask, or within Ambu bag.
  - Inhale for 30 sec–1 min until IV access obtained.
- Sodium nitrite ($NaNO_2$): 10 mL (300 mg) (peds: 0.15–0.33 mL/kg) IV as 3% solution over 5–20 min:
  - May repeat once at half dose within 30–60 min
  - Keep MH level <30%.
  - Dilute; infuse slowly if hypotensive.
- Sodium thiosulfate: 50 mL: 12.5 g (peds: 0.95–1.95 mL/kg) IV over 10–15 min of 25% solution:
  - 1/2 initial dose may be given after 30–60 min.

### Pregnancy Considerations
- Hydroxocobalamin is class C.
- Amyl nitrite is class X.
- Sodium nitrite is unknown.
- Sodium thiosulfate is class C.

### Geriatric Considerations
- ~50 known or suspected CN victims aged 65 or older received hydroxocobalamin and it had similar safety and efficacy as younger patients.
- Hydroxocobalamin is renally excreted unchanged in the urine so renal impairment could prolong the elimination half-life.
- The safety and effectiveness of hydroxocobalamin is unknown in hepatic impairment.
- Sodium thiosulfate is metabolized in the liver and excreted by the kidney. Impairment in either organ may prolong elimination.
- The nitrites are short acting impairment if hepatic and renal function may prolong elimination.

### Pediatric Considerations
The safety and effectiveness of hydroxocobalamin has not been established in children, but the 70 mg/kg dose has been used.

### ALERT
- Sodium nitrite has weight based dosing for children.
- Sodium nitrite dosing can be based on serum hemoglobin when the clinical scenario does **NOT** require life-saving administration of the antidote before lab testing:

| Hgb | Nitrite (mg/kg) | Nitrite (mL/kg) |
|-----|-----------------|-----------------|
| 7   | 5.8             | 0.19            |
| 8   | 6.6             | 0.22            |
| 9   | 7.5             | 0.25            |
| 10  | 8.3             | 0.27            |
| 11  | 9.1             | 0.30            |
| 12  | 10.0            | 0.33            |
| 13  | 10.8            | 0.36            |
| 14  | 11.6            | 0.39            |

 **FOLLOW-UP**

## DISPOSITION
### Admission Criteria
ICU admission of all symptomatic exposures

### Discharge Criteria
- Asymptomatic patients after at least 4 hr of observation
- Survival after 4 hr of acute exposure usually associated with complete recovery

### Issues for Referral
Psychiatry referral for intentional overdose and suicidal patients

## PEARLS AND PITFALLS
- In a patient with hypotension, high anion gap metabolic acidosis, seizures, syncope, altered mental status consider cyanide in the differential diagnosis and treat presumptively.
- Use serum lactate as a surrogate marker for cyanide exposure.
- Victims of smoke inhalation may have combination of:
  - CN toxicity
  - MH
  - CO toxicity
  - If the COHgb concentration is extremely elevated, considered a concomitant CN exposure as well
  - To avoid further reduction in oxygen transport; initially treat with hydroxocobalamin or sodium thiosulfate, without sodium nitrite to avoid methemoglobinemia.

## ADDITIONAL READING

- Baud F, Borron S, Megarbane B, et al. Lactic acidosis in cyanide poisoning: Pathophysiology and clinical considerations. *J Toxicol Clin Toxicol*. 2001;39:244.
- Fortin JL, Giocanti JP, Ruttimann M, et al. Prehospital administration of hydroxycobalamin for smoke inhalation-associated cyanide poisoning: 8 years of experience in the paris fire brigaide. *Clin Toxicol*. 2006;44:37–44.
- Borron SW, et al. Prospective study of hydroxycobalamin for acute cyanide poisoning in smoke inhalation. *Ann Emerg Med*. 2007;49(6): 794–801.
- Leikin J, Paloucek F. Cyanide, nitrites, sodium thiosulfate, sodium nitirite, hydrocobalamin. In. Leikin JB, Paloucek F, eds. *Leikin and Paloucek's Poisoning and Toxicology Handbook*, 4th ed. Boca Raton, FL: Lexi-Comp; 2000:701–702, 830, 991, 1,011.

 **CODES**

### ICD9
989.0 Toxic effect of hydrocyanic acid and cyanides

# CYANOSIS
*Michael S. Murphy*

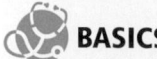 **BASICS**

## DESCRIPTION
- Caused by abnormal elevations of hemoglobin or hemoglobin derivatives:
  - Reduced hemoglobin >5 g/dL
  - Methemoglobin >1.5 g/dL
  - Sulfhemoglobin >0.5 g/dL
- The amount of oxyhemoglobin does not affect the blood's color.
- Cyanosis is more common in patients with polycythemia.
- Cyanosis is less common in patients with anemia.
- Methemoglobinemia cyanosis presents with normal PO$_2$ and chocolate-colored blood.

## ETIOLOGY
Central cyanosis/decreased saturation:
- Impaired pulmonary function:
  - Hypoventilation:
    - Pneumonia
    - Chronic obstructive pulmonary disease
    - Pulmonary edema
  - Ventilation/perfusion mismatch:
    - Asthma
    - Pulmonary embolus
  - Diffusion problems:
    - Interstitial lung disease
    - Anatomic shunts
  - Congenital cardiac causes:
    - Transposition
    - Tetralogy
  - Pulmonary arteriovenous fistula:
    - Hereditary hemorrhagic telangiectasia
  - High-altitude related, with decreased atmospheric pressure at 16,000 feet
- Low-oxygen affinity hemoglobin mutants:
  - Hb Kansas
  - Beth Israel
  - St. Mande

Central cyanosis/hemoglobin abnormalities:
- Methemoglobinemia:
  - Congenital:
    - Cytochrome *b*5 reductase deficiency
    - Hemoglobin M disease
  - Most cases are acquired:
    - Aniline dyes
    - Chloroquine, primaquine
    - Dapsone
    - Local anesthetic agents such as lidocaine
    - High doses of methylene blue
    - Naphthalene
    - Nitrites, nitroglycerine
    - Sulfonamides
    - Fava beans

- Sulfhemoglobin:
  - Generally benign
  - Irreversible alteration of hemoglobin
  - Caused by many medications
- Dimethyl sulfoxide
- Paint
- Phenacetin
- Phenazopyridine
- Phenylenediamine
- Phenylhydroxylamine
- Sulfanilamide
- Sulfapyridine
- Sulfathiazole
- Sulfur compounds
- Peripheral cyanosis
- Vasoconstriction to cold air or water
- Arterial obstruction seen in emboli or Raynaud
- Venous obstruction thrombophlebitis
- Decreased cardiac output compensatory vasoconstriction

Differential cyanosis:
- Lower extremities involved, but upper extremities spared
- Patent truncus arteriosus or pulmonary HTN:
  - Pediatric cyanosis
- Cardiac:
  - Cyanotic congenital defects:
    - Tetralogy of Fallot
    - Transposition of great vessels
    - Truncus arteriosus
    - Pulmonary and tricuspid atresia
    - Ebstein anomaly
  - Total anomalous pulmonary venous return

Pulmonary stenosis:
- Any right-to-left shunting
- Respiratory:
  - Upper airway disorders:
    - Croup
    - Bacterial tracheitis
    - Epiglottitis
    - Retropharyngeal abscess
    - Foreign body
    - Trauma
  - Lower airway disorders:
    - Asthma
    - Bronchiolitis
    - Pneumonia
    - Cystic fibrosis
    - Pulmonary edema/CHF
    - Pulmonary embolism
    - Chest wall injury
    - Pleural disorders such as pneumothorax or diaphragmatic hernia

- Neurologic:
  - CNS injury/lesions
  - Infection
  - Seizure
  - Toxins
  - Breath holding
  - Hemoglobinopathy

 **DIAGNOSIS**

## SIGNS AND SYMPTOMS
- A bluish discoloration of the skin and mucous membranes:
  - Chocolate color:
    - Methemoglobinemia
  - Slate gray color:
    - Methemoglobinemia or sulfhemoglobin
  - Varies based on skin thickness or pigment
- Central or generalized:
  - Visible in lips, nail beds, ears, or malar regions
  - Peripheral or local cyanosis:
    - Limited to extremities
- Differential cyanosis:
  - Lower extremities involved, but upper extremities spared
  - Clubbing
  - Dyspnea
  - Fatigue
  - Headache
  - Occupational exposure or use of certain chemicals or drugs
- Asymptomatic:
  - Suggests methemoglobinemia

## ESSENTIAL WORKUP
- Assess airway and ventilation as 1st priority:
  - Stabilize airway and provide adequate ventilation.
- Investigate hypoxemia causes:
  - Cardiac and respiratory most common
  - Consider methemoglobinemia.

## DIAGNOSTIC TESTS & INTERPRETATION
*Lab*
- Pulse oximetry:
  - Does not assess ventilation
  - Results inaccurate with:
    - Abnormal hemoglobins
    - Nail polish
    - Pigmented skin
    - Hypoperfusion
    - Used of vital dyes

- Arterial blood gas:
  - Oxygen tension
  - Measured hemoglobin saturation
  - Cyanosis in face of normal $PO_2$, think methemoglobinemia
  - Blood in methemoglobinemia is chocolate color.
  - Methemoglobin level
- Complete blood chemistry:
  - Check hemoglobin.
- Hyperoxia test for congenital cyanosis of newborn:
  - If $PO_2$ fails to increase to 100 mm Hg after 100% $O_2$, suspect congenital heart disease.

### *Imaging*
- CXR to investigate respiratory or cardiac pathology:
  - Inspiratory/expiratory views if foreign body
  - Expiratory view if occult pneumothorax suspected
- Radiograph of neck for upper airway disorders:
  - Foreign body
  - Steeple sign (croup)
  - Prevertebral swelling (retropharyngeal abscess)
  - Epiglottic swelling
- EKG:
  - Dysrhythmia, injury, or ischemia
- Echo:
  - Bubble study if septal defect/shunt suspected
  - Wall motion/valvular abnormalities
  - Pericardial fluid

### DIFFERENTIAL DIAGNOSIS
- Hyperpigmentation:
  - Drugs or metals
  - Chronic high-dose chlorpromazine
  - Minocycline
  - Argyria (silver deposits)
  - Tattoos
- Polycythemia

 **TREATMENT**

### PRE-HOSPITAL
- Assess and establish patent airway.
- Correct any airway obstruction.
- Recognize an incorrectly placed airway.
- 100% $O_2$ using a nonrebreathing device
- Ensure adequate ventilation.
- Recognize need to establish definitive airway.
- Protect cervical spine if trauma suspected.
- IV line, monitor, pulse oximetry
- Albuterol nebulizer for bronchospasm
- Racemic epinephrine nebulizer for severe croup
- Management of pulmonary edema per protocol

### INITIAL STABILIZATION/THERAPY
- Oxygen supplied through a 100% nonrebreathing device
- Immediately assess and address airway issues.

### TREATMENT-GENERAL-MEASURES
- Recognize and manage cardiopulmonary disorders.
- Methylene blue for methemoglobinemia exceeding 30%:
  - Do not use if patient has G6PD deficiency.

### MEDICATION
- Albuterol nebulized: 0.03 mL/kg (5 mg/mL)
- Dexamethasone: (for croup) 0.6 mg/kg IV/IM
- Furosemide: 1.0 mg/kg IV q6h
- Magnesium: 2.0 g IV over 10 min (40 mg/kg IV over 20 min)
- Methylene blue: 1–2 mg/kg IV of 1% solution over 5 min
- Methylprednisolone: 1–2 mg/kg IV q6h
- Morphine: 2–4 mg IV (0.05 0.1 mg/kg IV q2h PRN)
- Nitroglycerine: 0.4 mg sublingually or IV (0.5–5 $\mu$g/kg/min IV)
- Prostaglandin $E_1$: 0.05–0.1 $\mu$g/kg/min IV; max 0.4 $\mu$g/kg/min
- Racemic epinephrine nebulized: 0.05 mL/kg

 **FOLLOW-UP**

### DISPOSITION
#### *Admission Criteria*
- Most affected patients should be admitted to hospital.
- ICU admission is required for any instability or cyanosis.

#### *Discharge Criteria*
Reversible causes of hypoxia:
- Reactive airway disease responsive to $\beta$-agonists
- Pulmonary edema in patient with known CHF but no suspicion of myocardial injury and diuresis

### PEARLS AND PITFALLS
- Immediately assess airway and breathing and determine etiology of hypoxemia.
- Central cyanosis: Consider decreased saturation or hemoglobin abnormalities.
- Peripheral cyanosis: Vasoconstriction, environmental, obstruction or diminished inotropic function
- Chocolate-colored blood: Think methemoglobinemia.
- Beware of methemoglobinemia following excessive benzocaine.

### ADDITIONAL READING
- BheemReddy S., Messineo F, et al., Methemoglobinemia following transesophageal echocardiograph: A case report and review. *Echocardiography.* 2006;23(4):319–321.
- Braunwald E. Hypoxia, polycythemia, and cyanosis. In: *Harrison's principles of internal medicine,* 13th ed. New York: McGraw-Hill, 1994:178–183.
- Mansouri A, Lurie A. Concise review: Methemoglobinemia. *Am J Hematol.* 1993;42:7–12.
- Stack A. Cyanosis. In: *Synopsis of pediatric emergency medicine,* 4th ed. Philadelphia: Lippincott Williams & Wilkins; 2002:64–67.

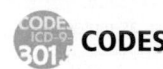 **CODES**

### ICD9
782.5 Cyanosis

# CYSTIC FIBROSIS

*Joseph Kahn*
*Roger M. Barkin*

## BASICS

### DESCRIPTION
- Defect of the cystic fibrosis transmembrane conductance regulator (CFTR)
- CFTR functions as an ATP-regulated chloride channel that regulates the activity of chloride and sodium channels on the cell surface:
  - Abnormal electrolyte transport in exocrine glands and secretory epithelia
  - Decreased exocrine pancreatic function with malabsorption
  - Thickened mucus, recurrent pulmonary infections, and progressive obstructive damage to the lungs
  - Recurrent sinus disease
- Occurs in 1:3,600 live births in white population, 1:29,000 in African American population; 1:6,500 in Hispanic population
- 30% of cases diagnosed by newborn screening
- Diagnosed in the 1st 2 yr of life in 75% of cases
- Approximately 30,000 children and young adults in U.S. have CF.
- Median life expectancy in the U.S. is about 37 yr.
- Approximately 40% of CF patients are older than 18 yr.
- 10 million Americans are unknown, asymptomatic carriers of the defective gene.
- CF is reason for 16% of lung transplants in U.S.

### RISK FACTORS
#### Genetics
Recessively inherited genetic disease, involving the CFTR gene on the long arm of chromosome 7:
- Different mutations produce variable phenotypes.
- Classic disease is homozygous for the DF508 mutation.
- CF is the most common lethal genetic disease in U.S.

### ETIOLOGY
Common organisms in patients with pneumonia; often multiple drug resistance:
- *Staphylococcus aureus:*
  - MSSA
  - MRSA
- *Pseudomonas aeruginosa:*
  - Prevalence increases with age; >70% of adults are chronically infected.
- *Haemophilus influenzae*
- *Stenotrophomonas maltophila*
- *Burkholderia cepacia:*
  - Prevalence 3%
  - Associated with rapid clinical deterioration
- Achromobacter xylosoxidans
- Mycobacteria (non-tuberculous):
  - M. avium complex
  - M. abscessus
- *Aspergillus*

## DIAGNOSIS

### SIGNS AND SYMPTOMS
- General:
  - Failure to thrive
  - Recurrent respiratory tract infections
  - Anasarca in infancy
  - Salty taste of skin
- Head, ears, eyes, nose, and throat (HEENT):
  - Nasal polyps
  - Severe headaches due to sinusitis
  - Otitis media
- Pulmonary:
  - Persistent cough:
    - Initially dry, then productive
  - Recurrent pneumonitis or bronchiolitis in 1st year of life
  - Wheezing
  - Hemoptysis
  - Pneumonia
  - Chronic bronchitis
  - Bronchiectasis
  - Respiratory distress
  - Pneumothorax
  - Pneumomediastinum
  - Most common cause of hospitalization in CF
- Cardiac:
  - CHF
  - Cor pulmonale
  - Pulmonary hypertension
- GI:
  - Abdominal pain
  - Meconium Ileus
  - Distal intestinal obstructive syndrome or "meconium ileus equivalent"
  - Gastro-esophageal reflux
  - Cholelithiasis
  - Pancreatitis/pancreatic insufficiency
  - Ileocecal intussusception
  - Foul smelling, fatty stools
  - Jaundice/cirrhosis
  - Rectal prolapse
  - Hematemesis
  - Small intestine bacterial overgrowth
- Extremities:
  - Bone pain
  - Edema/joint effusions
  - Decreased thickness of cortical bone
- Recurrent venous thrombosis
- Cardiorespiratory failure is most common cause of death.

### ESSENTIAL WORKUP
- Sweat chloride test
- DNA analysis if sweat test equivocal
- Nasal potential difference if DNA inconclusive

### DIAGNOSTIC TESTS & INTERPRETATION
#### Lab
- Sweat chloride test:
  - Chloride concentration >60 mEq/L
  - With classic signs and symptoms, a positive test result confirms the diagnosis.
- Stool sample:
  - Decreased elastase, trypsin, or chymotrypsin
  - Increased fat in 72-hour fecal fat excretion
- Immunoreactive trypsin (IRT):
  - Defines increased risk and/or diagnosis
  - May be falsely positive or negative
- DNA analysis:
  - Indicated if symptoms are highly suggestive, but sweat test result is negative
  - 90% of CF chromosomes identified
  - Positive if 2 abnormal genes present
  - Genotyping cannot establish the diagnosis.
  - 1,300 CTFR mutations listed
  - Ameliorating or neutralizing 2nd mutation may be present.
- CBC:
  - Thrombocytopenia
- Serum electrolytes:
  - Hyponatremic, hypochloremic alkalosis
- Serum glucose:
  - Hyperglycemia and new-onset diabetes in adolescents and adults; ketoacidosis is rare.
- Liver function tests and PT:
  - Obtain if hematemesis or hemoptysis or signs of liver failure
- ABG:
  - Hypoxemia
  - Metabolic alkalosis
- Sputum culture:
  - May have pseudomonal colonization.
- Studies indicated in high-risk patients with unclear diagnosis:
  - Nasal potential-difference measurements:
    - Complex and time-consuming study
  - Semen analysis:
    - Azoospermia

#### Imaging
- Chest radiograph:
  - Hyperaeration
  - Peribronchial thickening
  - Atelectasis
  - Hilar lymphadenopathy
  - Pneumothorax/pneumomediastinum
  - Bronchiectasis
  - Blebs
  - Chest CT identifies blebs/bronchiectasis
- Abdominal radiographs and/or CT:
  - Indicated if abdominal pain, vomiting, or abdominal distention
  - Distal intestinal obstruction syndrome
  - Intussusception
- Barium enema:
  - Indicated if suspicion of intussusception
- Sinus films:
  - Limited use because routine sinus films are always cloudy
  - CT scan is needed to assess sinuses.

#### Diagnostic Procedures/Surgery
Bronchoalveolar lavage:
- High percentage of neutrophils and absolute neutrophil count
- Unnecessary in patients with obvious pulmonary symptoms

## DIFFERENTIAL DIAGNOSIS

- Respiratory:
  - Asthma
  - Recurrent pneumonia
  - Bronchiectasis
  - Pertussis
  - Immunodeficiency
  - Foreign body aspiration
  - Alpha-1 antitrypsin deficiency
  - Ciliary agenesis
- GI:
  - Chronic diarrhea
  - Gastroenteritis
  - Milk allergy
- Elevated electrolyte levels in sweat:
  - Fucosidosis
  - Glycogen storage disease type I
  - Mucopolysaccharidosis
  - Hypothyroidism
  - Vasopressin-resistant diabetes insipidus
  - Adrenal insufficiency
  - Familial cholestasis
  - Familial hypoparathyroidism
  - Malnutrition
  - Ectodermal dysplasia
  - Atopic dermatitis
  - Infusion of prostaglandin E$_1$

## TREATMENT

### PRE-HOSPITAL

- Transcutaneous pacing for unstable type II 2nd- or 3rd-degree block
- Atropine:
  - Avoid with type II 2nd-degree block because it may precipitate 3rd-degree block.

### ED TREATMENT/PROCEDURES

- Stabilize airway, breathing, and circulation (ABCs):
  - Correct fluid, respiratory, electrolyte, and glucose abnormalities.
  - Consider bronchodilators/steroids if wheezing.
- Pneumothorax:
  - Observe if <5–10%.
  - Thoracostomy
- Consultation with the primary CF physician or pulmonary specialist
- Right heart failure:
  - Diuretics
- Hemoptysis:
  - Blood products as indicated (check INR)
  - Ventilatory support
- Distal intestinal obstructive syndrome:
  - Usually requires surgery
- Hematemesis:
  - Packed RBCs
  - Blood products for coagulation abnormalities
  - Early consultation with endoscopist
- Intussusception:
  - Correct with barium/air enema
  - May require surgery
- Rectal prolapse:
  - Manual reduction
  - Surgical consult if difficult case or recurrence
- Respiratory care:
  - Pulmonary toilet/physical therapy
  - Mucous thinning inhaled agents

- Antibiotics for pneumonia:
  - Based on culture and sensitivity
  - S. aureus (MSSA):
    - Cephalothin or Nafcillin
  - S. aureus (MRSA):
    - Vancomycin or linezolid
  - P. aeruginosa:
    - (Tobramycin or amikacin) plus (ticarcillin or ceftazidime or imipenem/cilastatin or meropenem)
  - S. aureus (MSSA) and P. aeruginosa:
    - (Ticarcillin/clavulanate or piperacillin/tazobactam or cefipime or imipenem/cilastatin or meropenem) plus (tobramycin or amikacin)
  - S. aureus (MRSA) and P. aeruginosa:
    - (Vancomycin or linezolid) plus coverage for Pseudomonas alone
  - B. cepacia:
    - Trimethoprim-sulfamethoxazole and/or meropenem and/or cipro and/or minocycline and/or chloramphenicol
  - H. influenzae:
    - Cefotaxime or ceftriaxone
  - Sinusitis
  - Antibiotics based on cultures and sensitivities
- Future directions:
  - Gene therapy: Compacted DNA
  - CFTR modulation:
    - Repair of protein function
  - Restore airway surface liquid:
    - Nebulized hypertonic saline
  - Mucous alteration:
    - DNase I to thin mucous in lungs
  - Anti-inflammatory:
    - High dose ibuprofen
  - Anti-infective agents:
    - Acute and chronic infections
  - Transplantation: Inhaled cyclosporine
  - Nutrition

### MEDICATION

- Amikacin: 5 mg/kg IV q8h
- Cefazolin: 30 mg/kg IV q8h
- Cefepime: 50 mg/kg IV q8h
- Ceftazidime: 50 mg/kg IV q8h
- Chloramphenicol: 15–20 mg/kg IV q6h
- Imipenem/cilastatin: 15–25 mg/kg IV q6h
- Meropenem: 40 mg/kg IV q8h
- Nafcillin: 25–50 mg/kg IV q6h
- Piperacillin: 100 mg/kg IV q6h
- Piper/tazo: 100 mg/kg IV q6h
- Ticarcillin: 100 mg/kg IV q6h
- Ticar/clav: 100 mg/kg IV q6h
- Tobramycin: 2.5–3.5 mg/kg IV q8h
- Tmp-Smx: 5–10 mg/kg IV q12h
- Vancomycin: 15 mg/kg q6h
- Note: Because many patients are undernourished, pharmacokinetics of antibiotics (especially aminoglycosides, penicillins, and cephalosporins) may be altered, requiring careful monitoring.

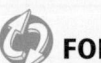

## FOLLOW-UP

### DISPOSITION

#### Admission Criteria

- Pulmonary exacerbation with significant deterioration from baseline, hypoxemia, resistant bacteria, failure of outpatient therapy
- Pneumothorax
- Hemoptysis
- Hematemesis
- Intussusception or unexplained abdominal pain or bowel obstruction
- Hyperglycemia

#### Discharge Criteria

- Close follow-up to verify the sensitivities of culture results and change therapy as needed
- Avoid hot weather.
- Oral salt supplements during times of profuse sweating
- Chloride sweat test of newly diagnosed child with CF

#### Issues for Referral

All patients with cystic fibrosis should be followed by a pediatric pulmonary center to ensure comprehensive management. Consultation is appropriate during acute exacerbations.

### FOLLOW-UP RECOMMENDATIONS

- Team approach of specialists
- Breathing treatments, chest PT, exercise programs, antibiotics, replacement of pancreatic enzymes

## PEARLS AND PITFALLS

- With CF patient in respiratory distress, always consider pneumothorax: Obtain CXR.
- For CF patients with abdominal pain/vomiting, always consider DIOS and intussusception: Consider imaging and surgical consult.

## ADDITIONAL READING

- Davies JC, Alton EW, Bush A. Cystic fibrosis. *BMJ*. 2007;335:1255–1259.
- Gibson RL, Burns JL, Ramsey BW. Pathophysiology and management of pulmonary infections in cystic fibrosis. *Am J Resp Crit Care Med*. 2003;168: 918–951.
- Moyer K, Balistreri W. Hepatobiliary disease in patients with cystic fibrosis. *Current Opinion in Gastroenterology*. 2009;25:272–278.
- Simon RH. Cystic fibrosis: Antibiotic therapy for lung disease. *UpToDate*; 2009; www.uptodate.com; accessed November 3, 2009.
- Cystic Fibrosis. *American Academy of Pediatrics: Pediatric Care Online* 2009.

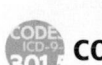 CODES

### ICD9

- 277.00 Cystic fibrosis without mention of meconium ileus
- 277.01 Cystic fibrosis with meconium ileus
- 277.02 Cystic fibrosis with pulmonary manifestations

# DACRYOCYSTITIS AND DACRYOADENITIS

*Shari Schabowski*

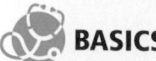 **BASICS**

## DESCRIPTION
- Dacryoadenitis and dacryocystitis are inflammatory conditions affecting the lacrimal system of the eye:
  - Dacryoadenitis is inflammation or infection of the lacrimal gland from which tears are secreted.
  - Dacryocystitis is an infection within the lacrimal drainage system.
- Dacryoadenitis may be a primarily inflammatory condition or an infectious process resulting from contiguous spread from a local source or systemic infection.
- Dacryocystitis is a suppurative infection involving an obstructed lacrimal duct and sac.

## EPIDEMIOLOGY
More commonly seen on the left:
- Acquired:
  - The majority of cases occur in woman over 40 yr with peak at 60–70 yr.
  - Rarely seen in African Americans
- Congenital risks

## Etiology—Dacryoadenitis
- Most commonly caused by systemic inflammatory conditions:
  - Autoimmune diseases
  - Sjögren syndrome
  - Sarcoidosis
  - Tumor
- Infectious causes may be primary or may occur secondary to contiguous spread from bacterial conjunctivitis or periorbital cellulites.
- Acute, suppurative:
  - Bacteria most common cause in adults:
    ○ Staphylococcus aureus
    ○ Streptococci
    ○ Chlamydia trachomatis
    ○ Neisseria gonorrhea
- Chronic dacryoadenitis:
  - Nasal flora > ocular flora

### *Pediatric Considerations*
- Viruses most common cause in children:
  - Mumps
  - Measles
  - Epstein-Barr virus
  - Cytomegalovirus
  - Coxsackie virus
  - Varicella-zoster virus
- Slowly enlarging mass may be dermoid.

## Etiology—Dacryocystitis
- Under normal conditions, tears drain via pumping action at the lacrimal duct, moving tears to lacrimal sac and then into middle turbinate/sinuses.

- Symptoms begin when duct to lacrimal sac becomes partially or completely obstructed:
  - In acquired form, chronic inflammation related to ethmoid sinusitis is a commonly implicated cause but many nasal and systemic inflammatory conditions have been correlated with this process:
    ○ May also occur secondary to trauma, a dacryolith, after nasal or sinus surgery or by any local process that might obstruct flow
  - Stasis in this conduit results in overgrowth of bacteria and infection.
  - Infection may be recurrent and may become chronic:
    ○ Most common bacteria: Sinus > ocular flora
    ○ *Staphylococcus aureus* is most common organism

### *Pediatric Considerations*
- In congenital form, presentation occurs in infancy.
- High morbidity and mortality associated with this form:
  - Caused by systemic spread of infectious process
- The most common organism is *Streptococcus pneumonia.*

 **DIAGNOSIS**

Both will present as a unilateral, red, painful eye.

## SIGNS AND SYMPTOMS
### *Dacryoadenitis*
May present as an acute or indolent swelling and erythema of upper eyelid
- Swelling and tenderness greatest in temporal aspect of upper lid under orbital rim:
  - S-shaped lid
- Mass may be palpable
- May be associated with:
  - Extensive cellulitis
  - Conjunctival injection and discharge
  - Increase or decrease in tear production
  - Ipsilateral conjunctival injection and chemosis
  - Ipsilateral preauricular adenopathy
- Normal visual acuity, slit-lamp, and funduscopic exams
- May cause pressure on the globe or globe displacement:
  - Visual distortion may occur.
- Chronic form: Slowly progressive, painless swelling

### ALERT
Promptly determine clinical probability of spread *from N gonorrhea* conjunctivitis:
- Morbidity very high:
  - Visual loss likely
  - Systemic illness probable
- Treatment differs significantly from other causes.

### *Dacryocystitis*
Presents as an acutely inflamed, circumscribed mass extending inferiorly and medially from inner canthus:
- Epiphora or excessive tearing—hallmark symptom:
  - Tear outflow is obstructed.
- Discharge from punctum:
  - Pressure on the inflamed mass may result in purulent material from the punctum.
  - This may be diagnostic.
- Cellulitis extending to lower lid may be present
- Low-grade fever may be present, but patient rarely appears toxic.

## ESSENTIAL WORKUP
Complete eye exam, including visual acuity, extraocular movements, slit-lamp, and funduscopic exam:
- Flip lids
- Examine nasal passages.

### *Pediatric Considerations*
Careful inspection for evidence of extension to orbital cellulitis or meningitis is essential.

## DIAGNOSTIC TESTS & INTERPRETATION
### *Lab*
- Tests of expressed material (used to help direct specific antibiotic treatment):
  - Gram stain
  - Culture and sensitivity
  - Chocolate agar plating if GC suspected
- CBC and blood cultures

### *Imaging*
CT of orbit/sinus to evaluate deep-tissue extension or possible underlying disorder in dacryoadenitis particularly with recurrent cases or in children at risk for orbital cellulitis extending from dacryocystitis.

## DIFFERENTIAL DIAGNOSIS
- Dacryoadenitis:
  - Autoimmune diseases
  - Lacrimal gland tumor
  - Hordeolum
  - Periorbital cellulitis
  - Severe blepharitis
  - Orbital cellulitis
  - Acute conjunctivitis
  - Insect bite
  - Traumatic injury
  - Orbital or lacrimal gland tumor
- Dacryocystitis:
  - Insect bite
  - Traumatic injury
  - Acute ethmoid sinusitis
  - Acute maxillary sinusitis
  - Periorbital cellulitis
  - Orbital cellulitis
  - Acute conjunctivitis
  - Acute blepharitis

**TREATMENT**

### ED TREATMENT/PROCEDURES
- Early diagnosis and initiation of treatment will reduce risk of extension of infection to adjacent structures and systemic infection.
- Topical antibiotics may be considered to treat or avoid conjunctivitis.

### *Dacryoadenitis*
- Cool compresses to decrease inflammation and nonsteroidal pain medication
- Viral etiology:
  – Typically self-limited inflammation
- Bacterial etiology:
  – Antibiotics
  – Oral for mild infection:
    ○ Cephalexin
    ○ Amoxicillin/clavulanate
  – IV for severe infection:
    ○ Cefazolin
    ○ Ticarcillin/clavulanate
- Tetanus toxoid if necessary
- Incision and drainage rarely necessary except in very severe cases:
  – Perform with consultation to facial surgery service or ophthalmology

### *Pediatric Considerations*
- Cool compresses
- Analgesics
- If cause unclear, treat with antibiotics as with adults

### *Dacryocystitis*
- Drainage of infected sac is essential:
  – Warm compresses and gentle massage to relieve obstruction
  – May facilitate outflow from obstructed tract with nasal introduction of vaso-constricting agent
  – Incision and drainage only in severe cases:
    ○ Typically done by ophthalmology
    ○ Avoid in ED when possible
    ○ May result in fistula formation
  – Duct instrumentation to facilitate drainage is not indicated in acute setting:
    ○ Reserve instrumentation for nonacute setting, if necessary at all
    ○ Manipulation while duct is inflamed may cause injury to duct and permanent obstruction from scarring and stenosis.
  – Topical ophthalmic antibiotic drops to prevent secondary conjunctivitis
- Systemic antibiotics to resolve infection and prevent spread to adjacent structures:
  – Oral for mild infection
  – Intravenous when febrile or severe infection
- Analgesics

### *Pediatric Considerations*
- Newborns respond well to massage and topical antibiotics in ~95% of cases.
- If no resolution in 1st yr of life, may require probing of duct by ophthalmologist

- Children <4 yr old who develop dacryocystitis:
  – At increased risk for *Haemophilus influenzae* infection, if not immunized:
    ○ Given typical age of presentation, complete immunization is unlikely at primary presentation.
    ○ Recommended schedule 2, 4, 6, and 12–15 mo
  – *Haemophilus influenzae* type B carries high risk for bacteremia, septicemia, and meningitis.
  – Treat afebrile, well-appearing children with responsible parent with oral cefaclor or amoxicillin/clavulanate.
  – Administer cefuroxime IV in acutely ill patients.

### MEDICATION
- Amoxicillin/clavulanate (Augmentin): 500 mg (peds: 20–40 mg of amoxicillin/kg/24 h) PO q8h
- Cefaclor: 500 mg (peds: 20–40 mg/kg/24 h) PO t.i.d.
- Cefazolin: 500–1,000 mg (peds: 50–100 mg/kg/24 h) IV q6–8h
- Cefuroxime: 750–1,500 (peds: 50–100 mg/kg/24 h) mg IV q8h
- Cephalexin: 500 mg (peds: 25–100 mg/kg/24 h) PO q.i.d.
- Cocaine hydrochloride: 4% topical solution single-dose nasal spray
- Erythromycin ophthalmic ointment: 2 drops q.i.d. to affected eye
- Tetracaine and phenylephrine topical solution single-dose nasal spray
- Ticarcillin/clavulanate: 3.2 g (peds: 200–300 mg of ticarcillin/kg/24 h) IV q4–6h
- Trimethoprim-polymyxin ointment: 2 drops q.i.d. to affected eye

 **FOLLOW-UP**

### DISPOSITION
### *Admission Criteria*
- Adults:
  – Febrile or toxic appearance
  – Concomitant medical problems including diabetes or immunosuppression
  – Extensive cellulitis
  – Suspicion of adjacent spread with deep tissue involvement or meningitis or *N meningitis*
- Children:
  – Acutely ill appearance
  – Concomitant medical problems
  – Extensive cellulitis
  – High risk for *Haemophilus influenzae*
  – If reliable follow-up within 24 hr cannot be arranged

### *Issues for Referral*
Dacryoadenitis and dacryocystitis should be referred promptly to ophthalmology:
- Patients with dacryocystitis require further evaluation to confirm complete drainage of sac and to assess need for further intervention to avoid recurrence.
- Availability of follow-up should be confirmed and ophthalmologic consultation should be completed prior to discharge.

### PEARLS AND PITFALLS
- In cases of red eye with lid swelling, specifically examine the lacrimal structures for evidence of involvement.
- Skin Incision and drainage of dacryocystitis should be avoided whenever possible to avoid fistula formation:
  – Intra-nasal vaso-constricting agents should be used primarily to facilitate drainage.

### ADDITIONAL READING
- Boruchoff SA, Boruchoff SE. Infections of the lacrimal system. *Infect Dis Clin North Am*. 1992;6:925–932.
- Brook I, Frazier EH. Aerobic and anaerobic microbiology of dacryoadenitis. *Am J Ophthalmol*. 1998;125:552–554.
- Kanski JJ. *Clinical ophthalmology*. Oxford, England: Butterworth-Heinemann; 1994:66–69.
- Lueder GT. Neonatal dacryocystitis associated with nasolacrimal duct cysts. *J Pediatr Ophthalmol Strabismus*. 1995;32:102–106.
- Rhee DJ, Pyfer MF, Rhee DM. *The Wills eye manual: Office and emergency room diagnosis and treatment of eye disease*. Philadelphia: Lippincott Williams & Wilkins; 1999.
- Rubin S, Hallagan L. Lids, lacrimals, and lashes. *Emerg Med Clin North Am*. 1995;13:631–648.
- Thompson CJ. Review of the diagnosis and management of acquired nasolacrimal duct obstruction. *Optometry*. 2001;72.103–111.

### See Also (Topic, Algorithm, Electronic Media Element)
- Conjunctivitis
- Hordeolum and Chalazion
- Periorbital and Orbital Cellulitis
- Red Eye

 **CODES**

#### ICD9
- 375.00 Dacryoadenitis, unspecified
- 375.01 Acute dacryoadenitis
- 375.02 Chronic dacryoadenitis

# DECOMPRESSION SICKNESS
*Peter J. Park*

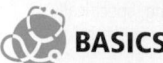

## BASICS

### DESCRIPTION
- Multisystemic disease process resulting from escape of nitrogen bubbles out of solution into body fluids and tissues
- Also known as "the bends" or caisson disease

### ETIOLOGY
Mechanism:
- Sequence of events:
  - Increases in ambient pressure cause increase in partial pressure of nitrogen inspired (per Henry's law, below).
  - Nitrogen accumulates in tissues in increasing concentrations the longer ambient pressures remain elevated.
  - Decompression sickness (DCS) results when ambient pressure keeping nitrogen in solution decreases too rapidly (on ascent), preventing gradual removal of excess body burden of nitrogen.
  - As the nitrogen removal gradient is overwhelmed, tissues become supersaturated and bubble formation occurs.
- Henry's law:
  - Amount of gas that will dissolve in a solution is directly proportional to partial pressure of that gas.
  - Increases in partial pressure result in larger amount of gas dissolved in tissue.
  - Decreases in partial pressure result in gas coming out of solution.
- Dalton's law:
  - Total pressure exerted by a mixture of gases is equal to the sum of the partial pressure of each of the component gases.
- Bubble location determines clinical effects:
  - Blood flow obstruction and tissue ischemia from intravascular bubbles
  - Tissue distention and compression from interstitial bubbles
  - Compression of arterioles, nerves, and lymphatics
  - Endothelial damage leading to stimulation of coagulation and clotting cascades
  - Bubbles sensed as foreign by host defenses, leading to release of chemotactic and other factors

- Risk factors for DCS:
  - Greater depth (increased ambient pressures), longer bottom time, and quicker rate of ascent
  - Proper use of dive tables and computers does *not* eliminate risk for DCS.
  - Increased incidence with age and weight (higher body fat), hypothermia, dehydration, exercise, multiple dives in a day
- Airplane flight following diving can precipitate DCS owing to lower cabin pressure.

## DIAGNOSIS

### SIGNS AND SYMPTOMS
- Cutaneous:
  - Scarlatiniform, erysipeloid, or mottled rash:
    - Cutis marmorata
  - Peau d'orange appearance owing to lymphatic obstruction
- Musculoskeletal:
  - Pain:
    - "The bends"
    - Dull, deep muscular aching
    - Often in a joint (elbow and shoulder most common)
    - Typically not exacerbated by movement or reproduced with palpation
  - No external physical signs of trauma
- GI:
  - Nausea and vomiting
  - Abdominal pain
- Pulmonary:
  - Shortness of breath
  - Chokes triad is thought to be owing to bubbles in pulmonary vascular tree:
    - Substernal pressure
    - Cough
    - Dyspnea
- CNS:
  - Weakness and fatigue
  - Numbness and paresthesia
  - Agitation
  - Headache
  - Dizziness
  - Vertigo
  - Convulsion
  - Bladder and/or bowel incontinence
  - Lethargy
  - Visual disturbances
  - The staggers:
    - Vestibular system and posterior column involvement

### History
Elicit time of symptom onset related to dive completion:
- Onset during ascent or immediately upon surfacing often due to arterial gas embolism or barotraumas.

### Physical Exam
Thorough physical exam including a detailed neurologic exam

### ESSENTIAL WORKUP
- Clinical diagnosis: Recognize risk factors and various clinical presentation.
- Careful neurologic exam to document possible waning symptoms
- Trial of pressure:
  - Rapid relief of symptoms upon recompression in a hyperbaric chamber may be only way to diagnose DCS conclusively.

### DIAGNOSTIC TESTS & INTERPRETATION
#### Lab
- CBC:
  - Increased hematocrit secondary to hemoconcentration
- Electrolytes, BUN, creatinine, glucose
- Urinalysis
- ABG and pulse oximetry:
  - Monitor oxygenation.

#### Imaging
- CXR:
  - Concomitant pulmonary barotrauma
  - Aspiration pneumonia
- Head CT when altered mental status or neurologic deficit

### DIFFERENTIAL DIAGNOSIS
- Musculoskeletal injury unrelated to bubble formation
- Inner or middle ear barotraumas
- Arterial gas embolism
- Cerebrovascular accident (CVA)

TREATMENT

## PRE-HOSPITAL
- Cautions:
  - Recognize DCS:
    - Post-dive extremity pain often attributed to muscle strain
    - Serious neurologic complaints often minimized because diver does not consider DCS
  - Time after surfacing to presentation of DCS:
    - 50%: Symptoms within 1 hr
    - 95%: Symptoms within 12 hr
    - 60% of neurologic DCS within 10 min
- Controversies:
  - In-water recompression:
    - Return injured diver/patient to depth where symptoms are ameliorated.
    - Extremely difficult
    - Need large amount of surface support
  - Corticosteroids and lidocaine:
    - No controlled studies demonstrating benefit

## INITIAL STABILIZATION/THERAPY
- Airway, breathing, and circulation management (ABCs)
- Provide normobaric (100%) oxygen via mask or endotracheal tube (ETT):
  - Increases inert gas (nitrogen) elimination from tissues, reducing gas bubble size
  - Increases oxygen delivery to injured tissue
- Early recompression in hyperbaric chamber

## ED TREATMENT/PROCEDURES
- IV rehydration with 0.9% normal saline (NS) to maintain goal urine output of 1–2 mL/kg/h:
  - Diver usually dehydrated owing to diuretic effect of pressure, exercise, breathing dry compressed air
  - Increased fluid assists with gas removal and dissolution of nitrogen

- Hyperbaric oxygen recompression therapy (see Hyperbaric Oxygen Therapy):
  - For all DCS except for cutaneous
  - Arrange transportation to nearest hyperbaric facility.
  - Aircraft capable of full pressurization maintaining barometric pressure below 1,000 feet best suited for transfers
  - Prophylactic chest tube for simple pneumothorax to prevent conversion to tension pneumothorax
  - Fill endotracheal and Foley catheter balloons with water or saline to avoid shrinkage/damage during recompression
- Divers Alert Network (DAN):
  - Based at Duke University Medical Center
  - Provides 24 hr emergency hotline for medical consultation on treatment of dive-related injuries and for referrals to hyperbaric chambers ([919] 684-8111)
- Analgesics

 FOLLOW-UP

## DISPOSITION
### Admission Criteria
Refer all patients with suspected or diagnosis DCS for hyperbaric therapy.

### Discharge Criteria
- Patients not requiring hyperbaric treatment
- Stable patients with mild symptoms may be discharged post–hyperbaric oxygen treatment.
- Air travel may exacerbate symptoms as ambient pressure decreases.

## FOLLOW-UP RECOMMENDATIONS
Hyperbaric referral

## PEARLS AND PITFALLS
- Difficult to distinguish musculoskeletal decompression sickness from musculoskeletal pain
- Avoid in-water recompression therapy.

## ADDITIONAL READING
- Bakker DJ. Treatment of the accidents induced by hyperbaric pressure. In: *7th European Consensus Conference on Hyperbaric Medicine*. 2004.
- Bartlett RD. Diving emergencies. In: *Critical decisions in emergency medicine*. Vol. 10, No. 10, Lesson 20. Dallas, TX: American College of Emergency Physicians; 1997.
- Kizer KW, van Hoesen KB. Diving medicine and decompression sickness. In: Auerbach PA, ed. *Wilderness medicine*, 5th ed. St. Louis: CV Mosby, 2007.
- Moon RE, Gorman DF. Treatment of decompression disorders. In: *The physiology and medicine of diving*, 5th ed. Philadelphia: WB Saunders, 2003.
- Newton HB. Neurologic complications of scuba diving. *Am Fam Physician*. 2001;63:2211–2218.
- Vann R, Denoble P, Uguccioni D, et al. DAN report on decompression illness, diving fatalities and project dive exploration. 2006 edition. Durham NC: Divers Alert Network, 2006.

### See Also (Topic, Algorithm, Electronic Media Element)
- Arterial Gas Embolism
- Barotrauma
- Hyperbaric Oxygen Therapy

 CODES

ICD9
993.3 Caisson disease

# DEEP VEIN THROMBOSIS
*Jonathan A. Edlow*

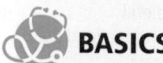

## BASICS

### DESCRIPTION
- A constant balance exists between intravascular clot formation and clot dissolution, clot forming when the former overpowers the latter.
- Clot can be superficial (to the fascia) or deep. The latter is called deep vein thrombosis (DVT).
- DVT can be upper or lower extremity and distal or proximal (to the popliteal vein).
- ~600,000–2,000,000 new cases present annually.
- Prevalence increases with advancing age in the general population.
- Diagnosis is more accurate using active surveillance rather than clinical suspicion.
- Common in both medical and surgical hospitalized patients
- Pulmonary embolism (PE) and DVT are different ends of the clinical spectrum of the same disease process.

### Pediatric Considerations
DVT in children is unusual, but when cases do occur, search for an underlying reason for hypercoagulability. Also, upper-extremity DVT is associated with central IV lines in children.

### ETIOLOGY
- 3 genetic factors promote clotting.
- Hypercoagulable states:
  – Cancer
  – Nephrotic syndrome
  – Sepsis
  – Inflammatory conditions:
    ○ Ulcerative colitis
  – Increased estrogen:
    ○ Pregnancy
    ○ Oral contraceptives
  – Antiphospholipid syndrome
  – Protein S, C, and antithrombin III deficiencies, factor V Leiden, prothrombin gene mutations, others
- Stasis:
  – Prolonged bed rest
  – Immobility (such as from a cast)
  – Long plane, car, or train ride
  – Neurologic disorders with paralysis
  – CHF
  – Obesity

- Vascular damage:
  – Trauma
  – Surgery
  – Central lines:
    ○ Especially with upper extremity DVT
- Multifactorial issues:
  – Advancing age:
    ○ Prior DVT or PE
- Genetics:
  – Important with respect to some of the risk factors; ask about family history of clotting.

### Pregnancy Considerations
Pregnancy is a risk factor for DVT, especially in the 3rd trimester and the 2 wk postpartum.

### Geriatric Considerations
Age in and of itself is a risk for DVT (and PE). As with many diseases, the presentation may be atypical in the elderly.

## DIAGNOSIS

### SIGNS AND SYMPTOMS
- Leg swelling:
  – >1 cm difference is usually significant.
- Leg warmth and redness
- Leg pain and tenderness
- Palpable cord
- In superficial thrombophlebitis, a red pipe-cleaner-like cord may be visible and palpable.
- Arm swelling, warmth, or tenderness:
  – Upper extremity or subclavian vein involved
- Phlegmasia cerulea dolens:
  – Cold, tender, swollen, and blue leg (secondary arterial insufficiency)
- In phlegmasia alba dolens:
  – Cold, tender, and white leg (secondary arterial insufficiency)

### ESSENTIAL WORKUP
- Determination of a patient's clinical (pretest) risk is a key step in a workup for DVT.
- A careful history and physical exam, interpreted in the context of the risk-factor profile, is the most important driver of subsequent diagnostic evaluation.

## DIAGNOSTIC TESTS & INTERPRETATION

### Lab
D-Dimer testing:
- D-Dimer, a byproduct of endogenous clot formation, is becoming increasingly used in evaluation of patients for DVT and PE.
- Only useful when the result is negative (to exclude DVT). Positive D-dimer does not make the diagnosis; it only mandates further testing.
- Methods of measuring D-dimer levels:
  – Latex agglutination (1st-generation tests) are not sufficiently sensitive and should not be used.
  – Microlatex agglutination tests (2nd-generation test) show some promise but remain insufficiently tested as compared with other methods.
  – Whole-blood latex agglutination (SimpliRED) is valuable if negative in low probability patients (using Well criteria).
  – Enzyme-linked immunosorbent assay testing gives a quantitative result and has been validated in large clinical studies in ED patients.

### Imaging
- Contrast venography:
  – Once the imaging test of choice; now rarely performed because it is invasive, is expensive, and has complications.
  – Involves injection of contrast medium into a leg vein, the inflammation from which can cause thrombophlebitis in several percent of patients undergoing the procedure.
  – Reactions to the contrast dye may also cause reaction.
- Radionuclide venography:
  – Radionuclide venous imaging is under investigation.
  – This test is not commonly used in routine clinical practice.
- Impedance plethysmography:
  – Another uncommonly used test, which can miss smaller distal clots
- Compression US:
  – Standard 1st-line diagnostic test
  – It examines the veins. Normal veins compress; those with clots do not.
  – Color Doppler can be useful for identifying the vein but does not add substantially to accuracy.
  – Duplex scanning refers to the combination of compression B-mode US and color Doppler.
  – Has a sensitivity in the high 90% range
  – Should be repeated (or followed up with contrast venography) in high-risk patients with negative USs.

## DIFFERENTIAL DIAGNOSIS

- Superficial thrombophlebitis
- Cellulitis
- Torn muscle and/or ligaments (including plantaris and gastrocnemius tears)
- Ruptured Baker cyst
- (Bilateral) edema secondary to heart, liver, or kidney disease
- (Unilateral) edema from abdominal mass (gravid uterus or tumor) or lymphedema
- Postphlebitic syndrome (from prior thrombophlebitis)

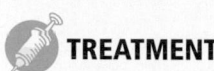 **TREATMENT**

### INITIAL STABILIZATION/THERAPY

In cases of phlegmasia cerulean, or alba dolens:

- IV access
- Supplemental oxygen
- Surgical or vascular consultation

### ED TREATMENT/PROCEDURES

- Systemic anticoagulation:
  - In patients without contraindications
  - Use either unfractionated heparin or low molecular-weight heparin (LMWH)
  - Carefully selected patients can be primarily treated with LMWH as outpatients
- Warfarin:
  - Started shortly after a heparin has been administered
  - Not before heparin because of the theoretic risk for inducing a transient hypercoagulable state
  - Ximelagatran, a direct oral thrombin inhibitor, is effective, but not FDA-approved at present because of concern about hepatotoxicity.
- Vena cava filters:
  - Indications:
    - ○ Contraindications to systemic anticoagulation
    - ○ New thromboembolic event while on adequate anticoagulation
  - Vena cava filters (or umbrellas) can be placed transcutaneously, usually by a vascular surgeon or radiologist.
  - Empiric filter placement may be useful in certain settings:
    - ○ Ongoing risk such as cancer
    - ○ Risk for a recurrent PE could be fatal because of poor cardiopulmonary reserve or a recent PE.
  - Randomized data suggest that filter placement is no more effective than anticoagulation.
  - Filters can also be deployed in the superior vena cava in the setting of upper-extremity DVT.
- Thrombolysis:
  - Rarely indicated
  - Roughly a 3-fold increase in bleeding complications
  - Catheter-administered lytic therapy is used more commonly in upper extremity DVT

- Thrombectomy:
  - Occasionally recommended for patients with extensive disease
  - Consult a vascular surgeon.
- Septic thrombophlebitis:
  - Surgical excision of the vein or IV antibiotics

### MEDICATION

- Enoxaparin: 1 mg/kg SC b.i.d. for outpatients (or inpatients); a dose of 1.5 mg/kg SC per day is FDA-approved for inpatients
- Heparin (unfractionated): 80 U/kg bolus followed by an 18 U/kg/hr drip, with the activated partial thromboplastin time (aPTT) titrated 2–2.5 times normal
- Tinzaparin: 175 IU/kg/d SC
- Warfarin: 5 mg/d with a prothrombin time being checked on the 3rd day

 **FOLLOW-UP**

### DISPOSITION

#### Admission Criteria

- Patients with DVT unable to receive LMWH as an outpatient
- Patients with concomitant PE or other serious diseases
- Patients thought to be at especially high bleeding risk
- Patients with phlegmasia

#### Discharge Criteria

- Outpatient treatment with a LMWH:
  - No serious concomitant disease that requires hospitalization
  - Patient has means of communication and transportation to return to the hospital if needed
  - Patient (or family member) is willing and able to inject the medication.
  - aPTT does not need to be checked.
  - Heparin-induced thrombocytopenia is less common with the LMWH but still occurs.
- Patients with superficial or distal thrombophlebitis can be discharged with close follow-up.

#### Issues for Referral

- Consult vascular surgery if there is any question about arterial insufficiency.
- Consider need for inferior vena cava filter in patients who have contraindications to full anticoagulation or form new clots on adequate anticoagulation.

### ALERT

When the clinical suspicion is high but the US is negative, remember to advise the patient to follow-up with his or her primary care physician, and to have a follow-up US in 5–10 days.

### FOLLOW-UP RECOMMENDATIONS

Outpatient treatment with a LMWH:

- Patient needs hematocrit, platelet count, and INR checked in 2–3 days.
- INR needs to be checked at about day 3.

## PEARLS AND PITFALLS

- Do not use a negative Homan's sign to exclude the diagnosis of DVT.
- Use some measure (whether it is clinical gestalt or a formal scoring system such as the Well's score) to determine pre-test probability for DVT.
- In high pre-test probability patients, do not rely on D-dimer testing; instead, perform venous imaging, usually compression US.
- In medium-risk patients with a negative D-dimer or negative US, strongly consider arranging or recommending a repeat study in 5–7 days.

## ADDITIONAL READING

- Brown DFM. Treatment options for DVT. *Emerg Med Clin North Am.* 2001;19:913–923.
- Hirsh J, Hoak J. Management of DVT and PE. *Circulation.* 1996;93:2212–2245.
- Kelly J, Hunt BJ. Role of D-dimers in diagnosis of venous thromboembolism. *Lancet.* 2002;359(9305): 456–458.
- Kyrle PA, Eichinger S. Deep venous thrombosis. *Lancet.* 2005;365(9465):1163–1174.
- Lawall H, Hoffmanns W, Hoffmanns P, et al. Prevalence of deep vein thrombosis (DVT) in non-surgical patients at hospital admission. *Thromb Haemost.* 2007;98(4):765–770.
- Tracy JA, Edlow JA. Ultrasound diagnosis of DVT. *Emerg Med Clin North Am.* 2004;22:775–796.

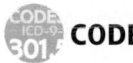 **CODES**

### ICD9

- 453.40 Acute venous embolism and thrombosis of unspecified deep vessels of lower extremity
- 453.41 Acute venous embolism and thrombosis of deep vessels of proximal lower extremity
- 453.42 Acute venous embolism and thrombosis of deep vessels of distal lower extremity

**D**

# DEFIBRILLATORS, IMPLANTABLE

*Robert Sidman*

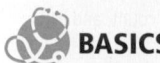 **BASICS**

## DESCRIPTION

- Small battery-powered electrical impulse generator implanted in patients at risk of cardiac arrest from cardiac arrhythmias
- The device is able to detect and convert ventricular and atrial arrhythmias into sinus rhythm with electric shocks defined as implantable cardiac device (ICD) therapy.
- Similar method of implantation as a pacemaker
- Recent devices no longer require cardiac leads reducing the risk of infection.
- 450,000 individuals experience sudden cardiac death yearly in the U.S.:
  - >100,000 devices implanted in U.S. each year
  - Implantable defibrillators have been shown to reduce mortality more effectively than antiarrhythmic drug therapy in patients with left ventricular dysfunction:
    - Absolute risk reduction of mortality of 7% in the 1st 2 yr
    - Benefit over antiarrhythmic drug therapy may be limited to patients with ejection fractions of <35%
  - Effective in reducing mortality in hypertrophic cardiomyopathy
  - Not more effective than antiarrhythmic drugs with nonischemic dilated cardiomyopathy
- The emergency physician is increasingly required to deal with ICD-related emergencies.
- Immediate post implant complications:
  - Pneumothorax
  - Vascular perforation
  - Acute lead dislodgement
- Appropriate shocks:
  - 5% a year for primary prevention
  - 20% a year for secondary prevention
- Electrical storm:
  - ≥2 appropriate shocks delivered within a 24-hr period
- Inappropriate shocks:
  - 10–20% of ICD recipients
  - Oversensing
  - Inappropriate classification of rapid supraventricular tachycardia
- Device infection:
  - 1–12% of patients
  - 31–66% mortality if the device is left in place
  - Infection may involve the skin, the generator, the defibrillation pocket, or the leads.
  - Coagulase-negative staphylococci (42%)
  - Methicillin-sensitive staphylococci (25%)
  - MRSA (4%)
  - Gram-negative bacilli (9%)
- Pocket hematoma
- Vascular occlusion

## ETIOLOGY

- Electrical storm:
  - Unknown
  - Decompensated heart failure
  - Acute ischemia
  - Metabolic disturbances
  - Drug proarrhythmia
  - Thyrotoxicosis
  - Fever with dilated cardiomyopathy
  - Brugada syndrome
  - Post cardiac surgery
  - ICD induced from left ventricular or T-wave pacing
- Inappropriate shocks:
  - Oversensing:
    - QRS, T wave, P wave, myopotential, electromagnetic interference
    - Frequent non sustained ventricular dysrhythmias
    - Lead fracture
    - Loose setscrew
    - Chatter between leads
    - Header problem
  - Inappropriate classification of rapid supraventricular tachycardia:
    - Atrial fibrillation
    - Sinus tachycardia
    - Atrial flutter
    - Other supraventricular tachycardias (SVT)
- Device/site related:
  - Wound infection:
    - *Staphylococcus aureus* (most aggressive and seen early)
    - *S. epidermidis* (more indolent and later)
    - *Escherichia coli*, *Pseudomonas* species, and *Streptococcal* species (less common)
  - Pocket hematomas
  - Vascular (venous thrombosis/embolism secondary to impedance of venous flow as a result of the ICD lead[s])

 **DIAGNOSIS**

## SIGNS AND SYMPTOMS

- Appropriate shocks:
  - Syncope or near syncope
  - Lightheadedness or dizziness
  - Shortness of breath
  - Palpitations (non-SVT)
  - Chest discomfort or pain
  - Diaphoresis
- Inappropriate shocks:
  - Palpitations (SVT)
  - Lead-related fractures, inappropriate sensing

- Device infection:
  - Fever
  - Chills
  - Malaise
  - Anorexia
  - Nausea
  - Diaphoresis
  - Hypotension
  - Heart murmur
  - Wound infection:
    - Pain
    - Erythema
    - Purulent drainage
    - Warmth
    - Fluctuance
    - Skin erosion
- Hematoma at the insertion site (pocket hematoma):
  - Pain (mild)
  - Swelling
- Vascular (thromboembolic phenomena):
  - Unilateral swelling in upper extremity
  - Superficial varicosities

### History

- Therapy-related:
  - Recent angina, heart failure
- Device-related:
  - Recent implant (<14 days)
  - Skin trauma to wound
  - Lead related:
    - Repetitive arm motions
    - "Twiddler's syndrome" (inadvertent manipulation of the device)
  - Vascular:
    - Recent implant
    - Multiple leads

### Physical Exam

- Vital signs
- Evidence of heart failure/acute coronary syndrome:
  - Displaced point of maximal impulse
  - Left ventricular heave
  - Presence of an S3 or S4
  - Presence of basilar rales
  - Dullness to percussion
  - Determination of jugular venous pressure
  - Hepato-jugular reflex
  - Peripheral edema
- Device/site-related:
  - Examination of wound/pocket:
    - Demarcation of pocket (erythema)
    - Purulent drainage
  - Examination of affected upper extremity

## ESSENTIAL WORKUP
- Following ICD therapy:
  - ICD interrogation will determine whether therapy was appropriate and can determine lead fracture if present.
  - EKG (transient ST-segment changes and elevations of the cardiac enzymes may be seen after shock delivery and do not necessarily indicate myocardial damage)
  - CXR may diagnose lead fracture.
- Device/site-related:
  - Signs and symptoms of local verses systemic infection
  - Upper extremity swelling suggests venous thrombosis.

## DIAGNOSTIC TESTS & INTERPRETATION
### Lab
- Therapy-related:
  - 12-lead EKG
  - Cardiac enzymes
- Device-related:
  - CBC with differential
  - Blood cultures
  - Do not aspirate pocket.

### Imaging
- PA and lateral chest radiograph:
  - Lead fractures
  - Lead dislodgment
- Vascular US of upper extremity
- MRI absolutely contraindicated:
  - Magnetic field may damage ICDs.

### Diagnostic Procedures/Surgery
- Therapy-related:
  - Device interrogation by electrophysiologist/cardiologist Application of magnet inhibits therapies.
- Device/site-related (pocket hematoma/infection): Referral to surgeon/electrophysiologist
  - Electrocautery should generally be avoided in patients with ICDs unless device is deactivated with programming or with magnet application.
- External defibrillation is safe, but avoid shock directly over ICD (see below).

## DIFFERENTIAL DIAGNOSIS
- Appropriate therapies.
  - Single shock following an episode of VT or VF
- Phantom shocks:
  - Patient awakened from sleep by a perceived shock

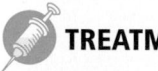 ## TREATMENT

### PRE-HOSPITAL
Following an ICD electrical discharge:
- IV access
- Continuous EKG monitoring
- Advanced cardiac life support (ACLS) protocols

## INITIAL STABILIZATION/THERAPY
- ACLS protocols
- Magnet application inhibits ICD therapies.
- Device-related:
  - Pain management
  - Elevation of affected extremity

## ED TREATMENT/PROCEDURES
- Patients with devices should receive treatment according to standard ACLS protocols.
- Electrical storm may require IV antiarrhythmic agents such as amiodarone.
- Inappropriate therapies:
  - Treatment of supraventricular dysrhythmia to prevent ICD shocks with β-blockers or calcium-channel blockers
- Lead-related problems may require further surgical intervention or device reprogramming; magnet application will inhibit therapies.
- Device infections:
  - Broad-spectrum antibiotics
  - Obtain blood cultures 1st

## MEDICATION
- Amiodarone 150 or 300 mg IVP followed by an infusion 1 mg/kg/hr for 6 hr, then reduce to 0.5 mg/kg/hr. Can rebolus (150 mg) as often as required
- Lopressor: 5 mg IV as needed to control heart rate
- Diltiazem: 5–20 mg IV, then a maintenance drip to control heart rate
- Cefazolin: 1 g IV q8h
- Vancomycin: 1 g IV q12h
- Cephalexin: 500 mg PO q.i.d.
- Warfarin for documented venous occlusion, INR 2–3 for 3 mo

 ## FOLLOW-UP

### DISPOSITION
#### Admission Criteria
- Therapy-related:
  - Ongoing/suspected cardiac ischemia or heart failure
  - Multiple ICD shocks and initiation of antiarrhythmic agents for VF/VT or other SVT
  - Treat underlying process and consult with electrophysiologist whether immediate interrogation is warranted.
- Device/site-related:
  - Skin erosion
  - Wound dehiscence
  - Systemic infection/endocarditis
  - Need for lead revision
  - Expanding pocket hematoma
  - Upper extremity thrombosis

### Discharge Criteria
- Therapy-related:
  - If patient is hemodynamically stable without evidence of active ischemia or heart failure, interrogation usually not required:
    - Single-shock therapy
    - Consult with electrophysiologist and arrange appropriate follow-up.
  - Device reprogrammed to avoid inappropriate therapy
- Device/site-related:
  - Localized infection
  - No signs of skin erosion
  - Pocket not expanding:
    - Prophylactic antibiotics are not indicated for pocket hematomas.
  - Wound stable

### Issues for Referral
Most ICD-related issues require follow-up with an electrophysiologist.

### FOLLOW-UP RECOMMENDATIONS
- Therapy-related:
  - Cardiologist or electrophysiologist
- Device-related:
  - Surgeon or cardiologist/electrophysiologist

## PEARLS AND PITFALLS
- Aspiration of device pocket is not recommended.
- Care should be taken not to deliver external shocks directly over the device, as it may shunt energy away from the heart.

## ADDITIONAL READING
- Dimarco JP. Implantable cardioverter-defibrillators. NEJM. 2003;349(19):1836–1847.
- Kowalski M, Huizar JF, Kaszala K, et al. Problems with implantable cardiac device therapy. Cardiol Clin. 2008;26:441–458.
- Maron BJ, Spirito P, Shen WK, et al. Implantable cardioverter-defibrillators and prevention of sudden cardiac death in hypertrophic cardiomyopathy. JAMA. 2007;298:405–412.
- Munter D. Assessment of implanted pacemaker/AICD devices. In: Roberts J, Hedges G, eds. Clinical procedures in emergency medicine, 4th ed. Philadelphia, PA: WB Saunders, 2003.
- Scher DL. Troubleshooting pacemakers and implantable cardioverter-defibrillators. Curr Opin Cardiol. 2004;19(1):36–46.

 ## CODES

### ICD9
V45.02 Automatic implantable cardiac defibrillator in situ

# DELIRIUM

*Arthur B. Sanders*
*Lori Stolz*

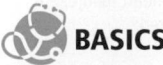 **BASICS**

## DESCRIPTION
- Delirium is a clinical syndrome characterized by acute changes in awareness, cognition, and perception with a waxing and waning course.
- Delirium is a syndrome secondary to an underlying medical condition.
- Pathophysiology unknown:
  - Diffuse cerebral dysfunction
  - Derangements of cerebral acetylcholine
  - CNS dopamine, $\gamma$-aminobutyric acid, and serotonin may be involved.
- Frequently missed by emergency medicine physicians

## ETIOLOGY
- Neurologic:
  - Meningitis or encephalitis
  - Seizure
  - Wernicke's encephalopathy
  - Hypoxia and hypoperfusion of the brain
  - Intracranial bleed or mass
- Pulmonary:
  - Pneumonia
  - Other pulmonary etiology of hypoxia
- Cardiovascular:
  - Hypertensive crisis
  - Acute coronary syndromes
  - Arrhythmia
- GI:
  - Hepatic encephalopathy
  - Dehydration
- Renal:
  - UTI
  - Acute renal failure
- Endocrine:
  - Hypoglycemia
  - Hyperglycemia
- Rheumatologic:
  - Collagen vascular disorder
- Toxicologic:
  - Environmental toxins
  - Medications
  - Withdrawal from barbiturates or alcohol
- Other:
  - Electrolyte abnormalities
  - Vitamin deficiencies
  - Hypothermia
  - Hyperthermia
  - Trauma

## Geriatric Considerations
- Common presentation in older ED patients
- Up to 10% of older ED patients may have delirium.
- Many patients will present with subtle symptoms and vague chief complaints:
  - Fall, dizzy, or not feeling well
- Waxing and waning symptoms
- Cause may be life-threatening condition.

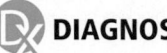 **DIAGNOSIS**

## SIGNS AND SYMPTOMS
- Disturbed consciousness:
  - Hyperalert:
    - Combative
    - Agitation
  - Hypoactive:
    - Lethargic
    - Stupor
    - Coma
  - Mixed hyperalert and hypoactive with rapid oscillations
- Cognitive changes:
  - Disorientation
  - Impaired memory
  - Disorganized thinking and speech
  - Misperceptions, illusions, delusions, and hallucinations
- Reduced awareness of environment
- Inattention:
  - Difficulties in focusing, shifting, and maintaining attention
  - Restlessness
  - Distractibility
  - Lability

## History
- History from caregivers is essential.
- Time course:
  - Hours to days
  - Fluctuating course
- Medications:
  - Prescribed and over-the-counter
  - Dosing
  - Recently added medications
  - Recently discontinued medications
- Associated signs and symptoms that would indicate underlying etiology

## Physical Exam
- Vital signs
- Complete neurologic examination:
  - Careful attention to changes in mental status
  - Orientation
  - Focal deficits
  - Hallucinations
- Psychiatric exam
- Use physical exam to determine possible underlying medical illness and to focus further workup.
- Several screening tools are available to evaluate for delirium:
  - Confusion assessment method consists of 4 key features:
    - 1: Acute onset or fluctuating course
    - 2: Inattention
    - 3: Disorganized thinking
    - 4: Altered level of consciousness
    - Diagnosis is made when features 1 and 2 are present with either 3 or 4
  - Mini-mental state exam:
    - Can be administered serially and will fluctuate

## ESSENTIAL WORKUP
- Awareness of delirium as syndrome is key.
- Workup should be broad to determine underlying organic disease.
- Ancillary studies as determined by history, physical, and initial workup

## DIAGNOSTIC TESTS & INTERPRETATION
### Lab
- Initial testing:
  - Electrolytes, calcium
  - Renal function
  - Hepatic function
  - Glucose
  - CBC
  - Urinalysis with culture and sensitivity
  - Toxicology screens
- Further studies based on signs and symptoms:
  - Arterial blood gas
  - Thyroid-stimulating hormone
  - Cardiac enzymes

### Imaging

- ECG
- Head CT scan
- CXR
- Other imaging based on history, physical, and possible etiologies

### Diagnostic Procedures/Surgery

- Lumbar puncture indicated for altered mental status with a fever
- EEG if indicated by potential seizure activity

## DIFFERENTIAL DIAGNOSIS

- Other disease processes that should be distinguished from delirium include:
  - Psychiatric illness:
    - Symptoms do not have fluctuating course that is typical of delirium.
    - Typically there are no changes in consciousness.
    - Delirium is classically associated with visual hallucinations, whereas psychiatric illness is more often auditory.
  - Dementia:
    - Delirium has rapid onset, while dementia has a slowly progressive, insidious course without fluctuation of symptoms.
    - Dementia is not associated with acute changes in consciousness.
- Once identified as delirium, the differential for the underlying cause is quite extensive.

 ## TREATMENT

### PRE-HOSPITAL

- IV access:
  - Pulse oximetry to monitor respiratory status:
    - Glucose measurement
    - ECG monitoring
- Naloxone if associated respiratory insufficiency
- Monitor patient:
  - Advanced life support (ALS) transport with all medications
- Look for signs of an underlying cause:
  - Medications
  - Medical alert bracelets
- Document basic neurologic examination:
  - Glasgow coma scale score
  - Pupils
  - Extremity movements

## ED TREATMENT/PROCEDURES

- Once delirium is identified, seek the underlying cause intensely.
- Treatment should be targeted at underlying medical condition.
- IV line access
- Oxygen if indicated by hypoxia
- Cardiac, pulse oximetry, and BP monitoring
- Thiamine should be administered to alcoholic and malnourished patients.
- For patients who are significantly agitated, chemical treatment of agitation may help facilitate ED workup.

## MEDICATION

- Treatment of delirium should be aimed at underlying condition.
- Benzodiazepines should be 1st-line for patients with alcohol or benzodiazepine withdrawal.
- Benzodiazepines should be avoided in patients with all other causes of delirium, if possible.

### First Line

- Haloperidol : 5–10 mg IV or IM:
  - Lower doses (0.5–2 mg) are appropriate for elderly patients.
- Recent studies show that atypical antipsychotics may be equally effective to typical antipsychotics.
- Thiamine: 100 mg IV, IM, or PO

### Second Line

- Alprazolam: 0.25–0.5 mg PO
- Lorazepam: 0.5–2 mg IV, IM, or PO

 ## FOLLOW-UP

### DISPOSITION

#### Admission Criteria

- When cause is unclear, admit.
- If delirium has not resolved, admit.

#### Discharge Criteria

Patient could be discharged if:

- Treatable cause is found and treated
- Mental status clears while in the ED
- Reliable caregivers are available
- Follow-up is ensured

## FOLLOW-UP RECOMMENDATIONS

- When cause is identified, follow-up is dependant upon underlying condition.
- When delirium has resolved within ED stay, close follow-up with primary care provider, preferably in <2 days.
- Patients and caregivers should be counseled carefully regarding return precautions:
  - Any recurrence of delirium should prompt a return to the ED.
  - Delirium can be a life-threatening condition.

## PEARLS AND PITFALLS

- Identify underlying cause
- Delirium is often missed by emergency physicians and maintaining an awareness of delirium as a syndrome is critical.

## ADDITIONAL READING

- Han JH, Zimmerman EE, Cutler N, et al. Delirium in older emergency department patients: Recognition, risk factors and psychomotor subtypes. *Acad Emerg Med.* 2009;16:193–200.
- Inouye SK. Delirium in older persons. *N Engl J Med.* 2006;354:1157–1165.
- Lonergan E, Luxenberg J, Areosa Sastre A. Benzodiazepines for delirium. *Cochrane Datab Syst Rev.* 2009;4(Art. No. CD006379).

 ## CODES

### ICD9

- 293.0 Delirium due to conditions classified elsewhere
- 293.1 Subacute delirium
- 780.09 Alteration of consciousness, other

# DELIVERY, UNCOMPLICATED

Jonathan B. Walker
James S. Walker

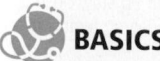 **BASICS**

## ETIOLOGY

- Delivery in ED is rare:
  - Incidence of ED deliveries in U.S. is not known.
  - Health care systems in which patients have little prenatal care tend to have greater incidence of ED deliveries.
- ED deliveries usually occur in 1 of following 3 scenarios:
  - Multiparous patient with history of prior rapid labor
  - Nulliparous patient who does not recognize symptoms of labor
  - Patients with lack of prenatal care, lack of transportation, or premature labor

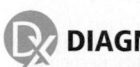 **DIAGNOSIS**

## SIGNS AND SYMPTOMS

- True labor presents as uterine contractions occurring at least every 5 min and lasting 30–60 sec.
- Significant vaginal bleeding with labor demands immediate assessment for placenta previa or abruption.

### History

- Last menstrual period and estimated gestational age (EGA)
- Recent infections
- Pregnancy history, complications
- Prior C-section
- Prenatal care
- Abdominal/pelvic cramping
- Ruptured membranes (amniotic sac)
- May report incontinence
- Urge to push or have a bowel movement
- Bloody show—loss of mucous plug

### Physical Exam

- Signs of imminent delivery:
  - Fully effaced and dilated cervix (~10 cm in term infant)
  - Palpable fetal parts
  - Bulging of perineum
  - Widening of vulvovaginal area
- Try to determine fetal position and presenting part by palpation of the uterus.

## ESSENTIAL WORKUP

- *Sterile* bimanual pelvic exam is most useful tool to assess presence of labor and possibility of imminent delivery:
  - Assess dilation, station, and effacement
  - No pushing until full dilation
  - Bimanual exam should *not* be done with vaginal bleeding until ultrasound (US) can rule out placenta previa.
- Fetal heart tones (FHTs) should be obtained by Doppler.

## DIAGNOSTIC TESTS & INTERPRETATION

### Lab

- If patient is in active labor, CBC, blood typing, and Rh screen should be sent:
  - Kleihauer-Betke testing should be ordered after delivery if Rh-negative mother gives birth to Rh-positive child.
  - Rh immunoglobulin can be administered to mother within 72 hr of delivery.
- Urinalysis if there is concern about urinary tract infection or pre-eclampsia

### Imaging

- Imaging studies are not needed for uncomplicated vaginal deliveries.
- 3rd-trimester vaginal bleeding should have emergent US to evaluate for placental abruption or placenta previa.
- If time permits, US can help locate the position and anatomy of the placenta.

## DIFFERENTIAL DIAGNOSIS

- Braxton Hicks contractions:
  - Irregular uterine contractions that do not result in cervical dilation or effacement
- Muscular low back pain
- Round uterine ligament pain
- Other causes of abdominal pain, such as torsion of the ovary, appendicitis, nephrolithiasis

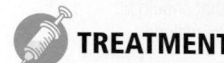 **TREATMENT**

## PRE-HOSPITAL

- Place patients in left lateral recumbent position.
- Emergency medical services (EMS) personnel should be adequately trained and have proper equipment available for delivery.
- EMS transportation of high-risk obstetric patients *before* delivery:
  - Lower neonatal morbidity and mortality
  - Faster and less expensive when compared with transportation of neonate *after* delivery
- Use of air transport for obstetric patients has been shown to be safe and effective:
  - If altitude during flight can result in hypoxia for fetus, pregnant patients should be placed on supplemental oxygen.

## INITIAL STABILIZATION/THERAPY

- Immediate sterile pelvic examination to assess for cervical dilation, effacement, station, or presenting parts (if no vaginal bleeding)
- Patients in active labor should be transferred to labor and delivery immediately unless delivery is imminent.
- If patient is completely dilated and fetal parts are on perineal verge, prepare for ED delivery.

## ED TREATMENT/PROCEDURES

- Obstetrician should be notified that delivery will be occurring in ED.
- Pediatrician or neonatologist and NICU should be notified.
- Begin IV saline or D5NS and supplemental oxygen, and place patient in lithotomy position.
- Assemble obstetric (OB) pack:
  - Bulb syringe
  - 2 sterile Kelly clamps
  - Sterile Mayo scissors
  - Umbilical clamp
- Neonatal resuscitative equipment should also be available.
- If time permits, sterilize vaginal area with povidone-iodine (Betadine).
- Uncomplicated vaginal delivery should occur as follows:
  - As crowning occurs, deliver head in controlled fashion, guiding it through introitus with each contraction.
  - Routine episiotomy is not necessary; however, if perineum is tearing, perform midline episiotomy by placing 2 fingers behind perineum and make straight incision toward (but not including) rectum with sterile Mayo scissors.
  - After fetal head is delivered, quickly suction nasopharynx, then feel around neck for nuchal cord:
    - If present, manually reduce over head.
    - If nuchal cord is too tight, double clamp, cut cord, and deliver infant immediately.
  - Apply gentle downward pressure on fetal head with uterine contractions:
    - Deliver anterior shoulder.
    - Posterior shoulder and remainder of infant will rapidly deliver.
  - After delivery, infant should be held at level of uterus and oropharynx suctioned again.
  - Double clamp cord with sterile Kelly clamps and cut between them.
  - Infant should be stimulated, warmed, and dried:
    - If cyanosis is present, infant should be given oxygen and resuscitated.
  - Place umbilical clamp.
  - Placenta will spontaneously deliver in 20–30 min:
    - Observe mother closely for postpartum hemorrhage.

- Uterine massage can aid in separation of placenta from uterus and limit uterine atony:
  - Avoid placing traction on umbilical cord because this can lead to inversion of uterus or rupture cord.
- If patient has severe bleeding and placenta is not passing spontaneously, patient should be taken immediately to operating room.
- After delivery of placenta, it should be examined for any irregular or torn areas suggestive of retained placental products.
- In uncomplicated delivery, use of drugs is not necessary:
  - Massage of uterus is all that is needed to facilitate cessation of bleeding after placenta has been delivered.
- Postpartum uterine bleeding is common:
  - Uterus, vagina, and perineum should be inspected for laceration.
  - If no laceration is found, assume uterine atony.
  - If uterus does not contract in response to uterine massage, administer oxytocin IV.
  - Continued massage of uterus may be helpful if bleeding still persists; then give methylergonovine maleate (Methergine) IM.
  - If bleeding is not responding to these measures, then carboprost tromethamine (Hemabate) can be administered IM.

## MEDICATION

- Carboprost tromethamine (Hemabate): 0.25 mg IM q15–60min (up to 2 doses)
- Methylergonovine maleate (Methergine): 0.2 mg IM
- Oxytocin : 20–40 IU in 1 L of crystalloid infused at 250–500 mL/hr IV

 **FOLLOW-UP**

## DISPOSITION

### Admission Criteria

- All women with uncomplicated deliveries and no significant postpartum bleeding should be admitted to labor and delivery or postpartum unit for care and monitoring.
- Obtain pediatric or neonatal consultation and admit to neonatal ICU:
  - All infants with respiratory distress
  - Gestational age <36 wk
  - Weight <5 lbs
  - Low Apgar scores

- Term infants with none of above complications may be admitted to the nursery or with mother to combined maternal–fetal unit.

### Discharge Criteria

- After adequate recovery from delivery, patient can be taken labor and delivery or postpartum unit.
- Patient should not be discharged home from ED.

## PEARLS AND PITFALLS

- Be ready for complications such as cord prolapse, shoulder dystocia, breech delivery.
- Be prepared to treat 2 patients after delivery—mother and infant.

## ADDITIONAL READING

- Enright K, Kidd A, Macleod A. Postpartum emergencies. *Emerg Med J*. 2009;26:310.
- Marx JA, Hockberger RS, Walls RM, et al. *Rosen's Emergency Medicine: Concepts and Practice*, 7th ed. St. Louis, MO: Mosby; 2009.
- Mirza FG, Gaddipati S. Obstetric emergencies. *Semin Perinatol*. 2009;33:97–103.
- Roberts JR, Hedges JR, Chanmugan AS, et al., eds. *Clinical Procedures in Emergency Medicine*, 4th ed. Philadelphia: Saunders; 2004.

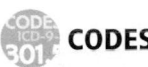 **CODES**

ICD9
650 Normal delivery

D

# DEMENTIA
*David A. Guss*

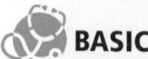 **BASICS**

## DESCRIPTION
- Progressive degenerative process of the CNS
- Prevalence 1% at age 60 yr to 30–50% by age 85 yr
- Pathophysiology varies, dependent on cause.
- Characterized by gradual decline in cognitive functioning:
  - Generally evolves over period of years
  - Course is highly variable, months to years in duration.
- Genetics:
  - Increased risk of Alzheimer's disease in 1st-degree relatives of patients with Alzheimer's

## ETIOLOGY
- Primary dementia:
  - Neurofibrillary tangles—Alzheimer's
  - Gliosis—Pick's disease
- Secondary dementia:
  - Ischemic—multiinfarct dementia
  - Subcortical degeneration—Parkinson's disease, Wilson's disease
  - Toxic, metabolic, nutritional derangements—vitamin $B_{12}$
  - Prions—Creutzfeldt-Jakob
  - Virus—HIV dementia
  - Bacterial—syphilis
  - Vasculitis—systemic lupus erythematosus (SLE), thrombotic thrombocytopenic purpura (TTP)
  - Binswanger
- Secondary dementia—see "Differential Diagnosis"

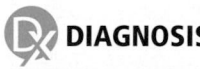 **DIAGNOSIS**

## SIGNS AND SYMPTOMS
Acquired loss of cognitive function leading to impairment of daily functioning, may be associated with the following:
- Loss of memory: Short followed by long term
- Impairment of abstract thinking
- Impaired judgment and impulse control
- Agnosia: Inability to recognize objects
- Aphasia: Language disorder
- Apraxia: Inability to perform motor functions
- Agitation
- Apathy
- Depression
- Inappropriate behavior
- Declining personal hygiene and appearance
- Urinary or fecal incontinence

## History
Full and complete history:
- Must include input from family and friends
- Complete list of medications
- Co-morbid diseases
- Prior history of similar behavior
- Onset and progression

## Physical Exam
Full and complete physical exam:
- Head-to-toe evaluation, all organ systems
- Meticulous neurologic examination:
  - Mental status evaluation
  - Cranial nerves
  - Reflexes
  - Motor, sensory, cerebellar, gait

## ESSENTIAL WORKUP
- Must eliminate acute reversible or exacerbating factors
- Extent of workup is related to history and course of illness:
  - Extensive evaluation for new diagnosis
  - Directed evaluation for sudden change of dementia
  - Limited evaluation for stable disease previously assessed

## DIAGNOSTIC TESTS & INTERPRETATION
### Lab
- Extent of evaluation dependent on patient condition and suspected cause
- New diagnosis or sudden deterioration:
  - CBC
  - ESR
  - C-reactive protein (CRP)
  - Glucose
  - Electrolytes
  - BUN, creatinine
  - Liver enzymes
  - Ammonia
  - Urinalysis
  - Toxicology screen
  - Thyroid-stimulating hormone
  - Vitamin $B_{12}$ level
  - Syphilis serology (RPR)
  - HIV
  - Blood cultures if fever present
  - Urine cultures if fever present
  - Antinuclear antibody if SLE suspected
- Established diagnosis with stable disease: No tests may be required.

## Imaging
- New diagnosis or sudden deterioration in established dementia:
  - CXR if infection considered
  - Head CT, without and with contrast
  - Electroencephalogram if suspicion of seizure disorder
  - Head MRI in selected cases
- Established diagnosis with stable disease: Studies may not be required.

## Diagnostic Procedures/Surgery
- Lumbar puncture and CSF analysis, syphilis serology
- EEG if seizure suspected

## DIFFERENTIAL DIAGNOSIS
- Toxic, metabolic, nutritional:
  - Narcotics, sedatives, hypnotics
  - Alcohol
  - Heavy metals
  - Dehydration
  - Hypothermia, hyperthermia
  - Hypoglycemia, hyperglycemia
  - Hyponatremia, hypernatremia
  - Hypercalcemia
  - Hepatic encephalopathy
  - Uremia
  - Thiamine deficiency
  - Vitamin $B_{12}$ deficiency
  - Niacin deficiency
- Infections:
  - UTI
  - Pneumonia
  - Sepsis
  - Meningitis, encephalitis
- Seizures–frontal lobe status
- Head trauma:
  - Bilateral chronic subdural hematomas
  - Pugilistic dementia
- Normal pressure hydrocephalus
- Stroke
- Tumor
- Vasculitis:
  - SLE
  - TTP
- Depression

**TREATMENT**

### PRE-HOSPITAL
- Obtain history from friends, family.
- Provide for patient and staff safety.
- Manage agitation.
- Attentiveness to co-morbid conditions
- Treat acute toxic and metabolic disorders:
  - Hypoglycemia
  - Hypothermia
  - Hyperthermia

### INITIAL STABILIZATION/THERAPY
- Ensure adequate airway.
- Administer $O_2$ if hypoxic.
- Ensure normal vital signs.
- Establish IV access if required.
- In agitated patients, provide for patient and staff safety.

### ED TREATMENT/PROCEDURES
- Evaluate for reversible causes of altered mental status.
- Consider full differential diagnosis—evaluate and treat appropriately:
  - Treat hypoglycemia with PO or IV dextrose.
  - Treat narcotic overdose or excess with naloxone.
  - Rewarm if hypothermic.
  - Antipyretic for hyperthermia
  - IV fluids for dehydration
  - Correct electrolyte abnormalities.
  - Administer antibiotics for infection:
    ○ UTI and pneumonia most common occult infections
  - Treat seizures:
    ○ Lorazepam for status epilepticus
    ○ Phenytoin for long-term management
- Sedation for agitation:
  - Start with low doses and increase as necessary to achieve clinical result.
  - Neuroleptics: Haloperidol, risperidone, ziprasidone
  - Benzodiazepines: Lorazepam, midazolam
- Soft restraints if chemical sedation ineffective
- Attempt to limit number of medications:
  - Reduced likelihood of toxicity
  - Reduced likelihood of drug–drug interaction
  - If agitation not an issue, eliminate all sedative-hypnotics
- Treat depression

### MEDICATION
- Alzheimer agents: Always start at lowest dose:
  - Donepezil: 5–10 mg PO at bedtime
  - Rivastigmine: 1.5–6 mg PO b.i.d.
  - Galantamine: 4–12 mg PO b.i.d.
  - Tacrine: 10–40 mg PO q.i.d.
  - Memantine: 5 mg PO q.i.d–10 mg PO b.i.d.
- Antidepressants: Start with lowest dose:
  - Oversedation a problem
  - May worsen dementia
  - Useful in patients who cannot sleep
  - Fluoxetine: 20–60 mg PO daily
  - Sedative agents: Always start with lowest dose
  - Droperidol: 0.625–2.5 mg IV—advantage, rapid onset; disadvantage, risk for QT prolongation, requires prolonged EKG monitoring
- Haloperidol: 0.5–2 mg PO b.i.d.; start with lowest dose 0.5–2.5 mg IM or IV if rapid onset required
- Lorazepam: 0.5–1 mg IV, 0.5–2 mg PO
- Midazolam: 0.5–2 mg IV slow push
- Naloxone: 0.4–2 mg IVP
- Risperidone: 0.5–2 mg PO b.i.d.; start with lowest dose
- Ziprasidone: 20–80 mg PO b.i.d., 10–20 mg IM q4h; start with lowest dose

 **FOLLOW-UP**

### DISPOSITION
#### Admission Criteria
- Unstable vital signs
- Significant comorbid condition requiring parenteral medications:
  - Pneumonia
  - UTI
  - Fluid and electrolyte disorder
- Uncertain diagnosis requiring evaluation and management that is not suitable for outpatients
- Inadequate home support coupled with inability to arrange suitable placement from ED

#### Discharge Criteria
- Stable vital signs
- No significant unstable co-morbid conditions
- Secure diagnosis or elimination of life-threatening organic disease
- Adequate home support
- Reliable access to follow-up care

### Issues for Referral
- Patients may need assistance with transportation, finances, etc.
- Patients with other comorbidities need referral to appropriate specialists.

### FOLLOW-UP RECOMMENDATIONS
- Primary care
- Geriatrician
- Psychiatrist
- Neurologist

## PEARLS AND PITFALLS
- Primary dementia is characterized by slow, steady progression:
  - Course is generally 5–10 yr from diagnosis to death.
- Can fluctuate as consequence of intervening illness and comorbid conditions
- Cholinesterase medications can improve functional status in patients with Alzheimer disease.
- Careful attention to medications, secondary illnesses, and prompt intervention for infections can improve quality of life and longevity.
- Death is generally consequence of infection, cardiovascular disease, or injury.

## ADDITIONAL READING
- Holsinger T, Deveau J, Boustani M, et al. Does this patient have dementia? *JAMA*. 2007;297: 2391–2404.
- Langa KM, Foster NL, Larson EB. Mixed dementia. *JAMA*. 2004;292:2901–2908.
- Mitchell SL, Teno JM, Kiely DK, et al. The clinical course of advanced dementia. *N Engl J Med*. 2009;361:1529–1538.
- Savva SM, Wharton SB, Ince PG, et al. Age, neuropathology, and dementia. *N Engl J Med*. 2009;360:2302–2309.

### See Also (Topic, Algorithm, Electronic Media Element)
- Altered Mental Status
- Delirium

**CODES**

### ICD9
- 290.0 Senile dementia, uncomplicated
- 290.10 Presenile dementia, uncomplicated
- 294.10 Dementia in conditions classified elsewhere without behavioral disturbance

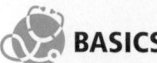 # DENGUE FEVER

*Jessica Freedman*

## BASICS

### DESCRIPTION

- Dengue fever occurs secondary to dengue viral infection.
- Poorly understood immunopathologic response causes dengue hemorrhagic fever (DHF) and dengue shock syndrome (DSS).
- DHF and DSS usually occur in patients with previous exposure to dengue virus.
- Hemorrhagic manifestations occur after defervescence of fever.
- Vascular permeability increases.
- Plasma extravasates into extravascular space, including pleural and abdominal cavities.
- Bleeding tendency
- Shock may ensue.
- Disseminated intravascular coagulation (DIC) may develop.
- Dengue fever, DHF, and DSS are all self-limited.
- World Health Organization—required criteria for diagnosis of DHF:
  - Fever
  - Bleeding evidenced by one of the following: Positive tourniquet test petechia, ecchymosis, purpura, GI tract bleeding, injection site bleeding
  - Increased vascular permeability and plasma leakage as evidenced by an elevated hematocrit (>20%), decreased hematocrit >20% after volume replacement or pleural effusions, ascites or hypoproteinemia
  - Thrombocytopenia (<100,000/mm$^3$)
- World Health Organization—required criteria for diagnosis of DSS:
  - All four criteria of DHF plus
  - Rapid and weak pulse
  - Narrow pulse pressure or hypotension for age
  - Cold, clammy skin
  - Restlessness

### ETIOLOGY

- Occurs in tropical and subtropical regions: Asia, Africa, Central and South America, and the Caribbean
- Caused by dengue virus serotypes 1–4
- Transmitted by mosquitoes: *Aedes aegypti* and *Aedes albopictus*
- Incubation period of 3–14 days

##  DIAGNOSIS

### SIGNS AND SYMPTOMS

- Fever:
  - Abrupt in onset rising to 39°C or higher
  - 2–7 days duration
  - Biphasic, returning to almost normal after 2–7 days
  - Associated with frontal or retro-orbital headache
- Rash:
  - Generalized maculopapular rash occurs with onset of fever.
  - After 3–4 days, rash becomes diffusely erythematous.
  - Faded areas appear.
  - Areas of desquamation may appear.
  - After defervescence of fever, scattered petechiae may develop over trunk, extensor surfaces of limbs, and axillae.
  - Palms and soles spared
- Musculoskeletal:
  - Arthralgias and myalgias after onset of fever
  - Severe lumbar back pain
- GI:
  - Anorexia
  - Nausea and vomiting
  - Abdominal pain (sometimes severe)
  - Altered taste
  - Hepatomegaly/ascites
  - GI bleeding

- Miscellaneous:
  - Epistaxis
  - Gingival bleeding
  - Hemoptysis
  - Hypotension
  - Narrowed pulse pressure (<20 mm Hg)

### ESSENTIAL WORKUP

- Primarily a clinical diagnosis
- Suspect in endemic areas
- Suspect in patients with history of travel

### DIAGNOSTIC TESTS & INTERPRETATION

#### Lab

- CBC:
  - Thrombocytopenia
  - Elevated hematocrit
- Electrolytes, BUN, creatinine:
  - Elevated BUN
  - Hyponatremia
- Liver function tests:
  - Elevated aspartate transaminase (AST; or serum glutamic-oxaloacetic transaminase [SGOT])
- Coagulation profiles:
  - Prolonged INR, prothrombin time (PT), and partial thromboplastin time (PTT)
  - Low fibrinogen:
    - D-Dimer
  - Virus isolation or detection of dengue virus–specific antibodies (available in only a few laboratories) through hemagglutination (HI) assay

#### Imaging

CXR:

- Pleural effusions

### Diagnostic Procedures/Surgery

Tourniquet test:

- Inflate BP cuff to median BP in patient's extremity.
- Test is positive when 3 or more petechiae appear per square centimeter.

## DIFFERENTIAL DIAGNOSIS

- Viral illness, nonspecific
- Influenza
- Rubella
- Measles
- Malaria
- Rocky Mountain Spotted fever
- Typhoid
- Kawasaki disease
- Scarlet fever
- Erythema infectiosum
- Mononucleosis
- Roseola infantum
- Secondary syphilis
- Enterovirus
- West Nile virus
- HIV
- Leptospirosis
- Chikungunya fever
- Toxic shock syndrome
- Hepatitis
- Appendicitis
- Meningitis

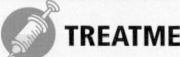

## TREATMENT

### INITIAL STABILIZATION/THERAPY

- IV access
- IV crystalloids for hypotension
- O$_2$ and monitor for unstable patients

### ED TREATMENT/PROCEDURES

- Treatment is supportive.
- IV fluids
- Acetaminophen (Tylenol) for fever
- Analgesics for pain
- Platelet transfusion for severe thrombocytopenia
- DIC therapy, if necessary

### Pediatric Considerations

- Neonatal dengue can occur by vertical transmission if mother infected 0–8 days before delivery:
  – Infants may develop DHF or DSS because of passive maternal immunity.
- DHF and DSS most common in children 7–12 yr of age

## FOLLOW-UP

### DISPOSITION

#### Admission Criteria

- ICU admission for the following:
  – Hypotension
  – DIC
  – Thrombocytopenia
  – Hemoconcentration
- Regular admission for the following:
  – 15 yr of age or younger
  – All patients with previous dengue exposure
  – Any patient where close follow-up is not available

### Discharge Criteria

- Close follow-up guaranteed
- Tolerating PO
- Pain controlled

## PEARLS AND PITFALLS

- Consider Dengue in patients presenting with fever and rash who recently traveled to endemic regions.
- Chikungunya fever is an emerging infectious disease also seen in travelers and must be considered in the differential:
  – Found in Asia and Africa

## ADDITIONAL READING

- Isturiz RE, Gubler DJ, del Castillo JB. Dengue and dengue hemorrhagic fever in Latin America and the Caribbean. *Infect Dis Clin North Am*. 2000;14(1): 121–140.
- Kautner I, Robinson MJ, Kuhnle U. Dengue virus infection: Epidemiology, pathogenesis, clinical presentation, diagnosis and prevention. *J Pediatr*. 1997;131(4):516–524.
- Mandell GL, Bennett JE, Dolin R. eds. *Principles and Practice of Infectious Diseases*, 6th ed. New York: Churchill Livingstone; 2004.
- Pincus LB, Grossman ME, Fox LP. The exanthema of dengue fever: Clinical features of two US tourists traveling abroad. *J Am Acad Dermatol* 2008;58(?): 308–316.

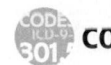 CODES

ICD9
- 061 Dengue
- 065.4 Mosquito-borne hemorrhagic fever

D

# DENTAL TRAUMA

*Brian N. Corwell*

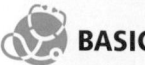

## BASICS

### DESCRIPTION
- Permanent teeth:
  - Begin to erupt at age 6
  - 32 total (4 central and 4 lateral incisors, 4 canines, 8 premolars, 12 molars)
  - Number from 1–32 starting with upper right 3rd molar (1) to upper left 3rd molar (16) and lower left 3rd molar (17) to lower right 3rd molar (32)
  - Better and often easier to describe the involved tooth anatomically
- Tooth fractures:
  - Fractures of the crown are classified as uncomplicated (involving only the enamel or both the enamel and dentin) or complicated (involving the neurovascular pulp)
  - May also classify by the depth of penetration using the *Ellis classification system*
  - Class I fracture: Uncomplicated fracture:
    - Involves only the superficial enamel
    - Fracture line appears chalky white.
    - Painless to temperature, air, percussion
  - Class II facture: Uncomplicated fracture:
    - Involves enamel and dentin
    - Fracture line will have ivory or pale-yellow appearance compared to whiter enamel.
    - Sensitive to temperature, air, percussion
  - Class III fracture: Complicated fracture:
    - True dental emergency
    - Involves enamel, dentin, and pulp
    - Pulp has pinkish, red, fleshy hue within surrounding dentin.
    - Frank bleeding or a pink blush after wiping tooth surface indicates pulp violation.
    - May be exquisitely painful or desensitized (with neurovascular disruption)
- Concussed teeth:
  - Tooth neither loose nor displaced
  - Sensitivity with chewing or percussion
- Subluxed teeth:
  - Tooth is loose but not displaced.
- Partial avulsion:
  - Partial displacement of a tooth from its socket
- Avulsed tooth:
  - Total displacement from the alveolar ridge
- Intrusion:
  - Tooth is driven into socket
- Extrusion:
  - Central dislocation of tooth from socket
- Lateral luxation:
  - Nonaxial displacement of the tooth
  - Associated with alveolar socket comminution or fracture
- Alveolar bone fractures:
  - Fractures of tooth-bearing portions of mandible, maxilla
  - Diagnosed clinically or radiographically
  - Bite malocclusion, painful bite, tooth mobility en bloc

### ETIOLOGY
- Age periods of greatest predilection:
  - Toddlers (falls and child abuse)
  - School-aged children and preteens (bicycle and playground accidents)
  - Adolescents (athletics, altercations, MVCs)
- Mouth guard use greatly reduces sport associated dental injury
- Assault, domestic violence, or multiple trauma
- Motor vehicle, motorcycle, bicycle accidents
- Laryngoscopy
- Certain predisposing anatomic factors increase risk:
  - Anterior overbite >4 mm increases risk for fracture 2–3 times
  - Short upper lip, mouth breathing, incompetent upper lip, physical disabilities

## DIAGNOSIS

### SIGNS AND SYMPTOMS
*History*
- Tooth mobility, avulsion or laxity
- Exacerbating factors (may indicate pulp exposure or inflammation):
  - Difficulty opening and closing jaw
  - Chewing
  - Drinking
  - Extremes of temperature
  - Pain on palpation
- Bite malocclusion:
  - Suggests displaced teeth or fracture of maxilla or mandible
- Mechanism:
  - Sufficient mechanism necessitates complete evaluation for multiple trauma and associated local injuries (eg, jaw fracture)
- Exact time of injury:
  - May affect treatment and prognosis

*Physical Exam*
- Examine all teeth for trauma or fracture.
- Examine all fractured teeth carefully for pulp exposure:
  - Dry the tooth with gauze, observe for frank bleeding or pink blush.
- Check for concomitant intraoral laceration.
- Inspect each tooth surface and percuss for mobility, sensitivity, or fracture.
- Assess for malocclusion and midface instability.
- Account for all missing teeth, tooth fragments, and prostheses (may have been swallowed, aspirated, embedded into adjacent soft tissue or impacted into alveolus).
- Inspect oral cavity carefully:
  - Adjacent soft tissue injuries
  - Fractures to alveolar bone, mandible, or maxilla
  - Suspect mandible fracture in those unable to open mouth >5 cm or with a positive tongue blade bite test.
  - Associated injuries:
    - Salivary glands, ducts, blood vessels
    - Nerves (test tooth sensitivity by tapping with tongue blade in addition to testing mental and infraorbital nerve function)

### ESSENTIAL WORKUP
- Thorough physical exam
- Imaging as necessary
- Stabilization and proper referral

### DIAGNOSTIC TESTS & INTERPRETATION
*Imaging*
- Plain dental radiograph:
  - To locate missing avulsed teeth
  - Ellis class III fractures
- Panorex:
  - Indicated for suspected or associated alveolar or mandibular fracture:
    - Foreign bodies
    - Displacement of teeth
- CT:
  - Indicated for suspected condyle fractures (may be missed by plain film)
- CXR:
  - Indicated for missing teeth or fragments
  - If the tooth is visualized below the diaphragm, it does not require retrieval.
- Bronchoscopy:
  - Indicated for removal in cases of dental aspiration located in bronchus or esophagus

### DIFFERENTIAL DIAGNOSIS
Rule out other significant concurrent facial or systemic injuries.

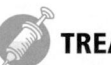

## TREATMENT

### PRE-HOSPITAL
- Maintain a patent airway.
- Avulsed teeth:
  - Rinse tooth with sterile saline or milk.
  - Immediate attempt to reimplant permanent tooth into socket by 1st capable person:
    - *Time is tooth:* Each minute tooth is out of socket reduces tooth viability by 1%.
    - Best chance of success if reimplant done in within 15 min
    - Poor tooth viability if avulsed for >1 hr
  - If unsuccessful, keep tooth hydrated
  - Place tooth in a transport solution (listed from most to least desirable):
  - Hanks balanced salt solution (HBSS)
    - Balanced pH culture media available commercially in the Save-a-Tooth kit
    - Works well even 30 min after avulsion or with dry tooth
  - Cold milk:
    - Best alternative storage medium
  - Saline
  - Saliva:
    - Place tooth in parent's mouth under tongue
    - In buccal pouch
    - In container of child's saliva
  - Sports drinks
  - Never use tap water or dry transport:
    - Causes cell damage

### INITIAL STABILIZATION/THERAPY
- Ensure patent airway.
- Have patient bite on gauze to control bleeding.
- Account for all teeth and tooth fragments.
- Reimplant avulsed tooth immediately.

## ED TREATMENT/PROCEDURES

- General considerations:
  - Splinting should occur before suturing any lacerations.
  - Occlusion is always the best guide to proper tooth position.
  - Dental fracture management:
    - Determined by patient age and extent of trauma
  - Tetanus prophylaxis:
    - Consider as a non-tetanus prone wound
    - Dirty wounds, deep lacerations, avulsed teeth, intrusion injuries, bone fracture
- Ellis Class I:
  - No emergency treatment indicated
  - File/smooth sharp edges with an emery board:
    - Prevents further injury to soft tissue
  - Dental referral for elective cosmetic repair
  - May restore normal tooth appearance later
- Ellis Class II:
  - Treatment goal is to prevent bacterial pulp contamination through exposed dentin.
  - Dry tooth surface prior to application.
  - Cover exposed surface with calcium hydroxide paste or similar barrier agent.
  - If no such agent exists, use Dermabond.
  - Next, cover and wrap tooth with dry foil to create protective barrier.
  - Prophylactic antibiotic coverage for 5–7 days
  - Pain control
  - Dental referral within 24–36 hr
  - In children <12 yr of age:
    - Protective dentin layer is thinner, placing pulp at greater risk of infection.
    - Dress in calcium paste and cover in foil.
    - Dental referral within 24 hr
    - Liquid diet until follow-up
- Ellis Class III:
  - Immediate dental referral
  - If dentist/oral surgeon is not available:
    - Place a piece of moist cotton over the exposed pulp.
    - Cover with dry tin foil.
  - If brisk bleeding, have patient bite into gauze soaked with topical anesthetic and epinephrine.
  - Prophylactic antibiotic coverage for 5–7 days
  - Children with primary teeth:
    - Nerve block, likely pulpotomy by dentist
  - Adults and older children:
    - Nerve block for significant pain
    - Dentist may provide root canal to avoid abscess formation.
- Concussed tooth:
  - No splinting required
  - Soft diet
  - Follow-up with dentist as needed
- Subluxed tooth:
  - Splinting only required for excess laxity
  - Soft diet for 1–2 wk
  - Follow-up with dentist
- Partial tooth avulsion:
  - Administer local anesthetic.
  - Carefully reduce to normal position.
- Lateral luxation:
  - Repositioning is a forceful and traumatic procedure.
  - Use 2-finger technique:
    - 1 finger guides the apex down and back.
    - 2nd finger repositions crown.
  - Soft diet for 1–2 wk
  - Follow-up with dentist
  - Splinting usually required for 10–14 days

- Intrusion:
  - Do not manipulate.
  - Palliative care
  - Dental follow-up within 24 hr
- Avulsed tooth:
  - Treatment based on age of patient:
    - Avulsed primary teeth are never replaced.
  - Handle the tooth only by the crown.
  - Remove debris by gentle rinsing in saline or tap water.
  - Do not scrub, curette, or attempt to disinfect tooth.
  - Administer local anesthesia if needed.
  - Gently suction clots with Frasier suction tip:
    - Use care not to damage socket walls.
  - Irrigate socket to remove clots if necessary. If extraoral time is <20 min:
    - Manually reimplant the tooth.
    - Should "click" into place
  - If pulp exposed, use bathing solution 1st:
    - Doxycycline 1 mg in 20 mL NaCl for 5 min
    - If tooth dry for >30 min outside mouth, soak in Hanks solution for 30 min before reimplanting.
  - Use firm but gentle pressure.
  - Splint usually required for 7–10 days
  - If tooth reimplanted pre-hospital:
    - Assure correct position and alignment.
  - Attempt reimplant regardless of time avulsed.
  - Once tooth inserted, have patient bite gently onto folded gauze pad to help maneuver tooth into proper position.
  - Stabilize with a splint or periodontal paste such as a Coe-Pak:
    - Mix resin and catalyst in even amounts to a firm consistency.
    - Apply to dried enamel and gingiva using gloves lubricated with water or jelly.
    - Apply to anterior or both anterior and posterior surfaces of the avulsed tooth and adjacent 2 teeth.
  - Prophylactic antibiotic coverage for 5–7 days
  - Tetanus immunization as necessary
  - Liquid diet until follow-up
  - Definitive stabilization by a dentist
- Alveolar bone fracture:
  - Pain control
  - Oral surgery/dental consultation for reduction and fixation (arch bar)
  - Prophylactic antibiotic coverage
  - Tetanus immunization
  - Liquid diet, advance to soft mechanical
  - Warm rinses t.i.d.
  - No straws

## MEDICATION

- Acetaminophen with codeine: 30–60 mg/dose 1–2 tabs PO q4h–q6h PRN (peds: Codeine: 0.5–1.0 mg/kg/dose [max. 30–60 mg] PO q4–6h)
- Acetaminophen with oxycodone: 1–2 tabs PO q4–6h PRN (peds: Oxycodone: 0.05–0.15 mg/kg/ dose [max. 5 mg/dose] PO q4–6h)
- Penicillin V: 250–500 mg PO q6h (peds: 25–50 mg/kg/24 h [max. 3 g] PO q6h)
- Erythromycin (use if penicillin allergic): Adult: 200–500 mg PO q6h (peds: 30–50 mg/kg/24 h [max. 2 g] PO q6h)
- Clindamycin (use if penicillin allergic): 150–300 mg PO q6h (peds: 10–25 mg/kg/24 h PO q6h)
- Tetanus prophylaxis: 0.5 mL IM

 FOLLOW-UP

### DISPOSITION

*Admission Criteria*

- Admission for other associated injuries
- Suspected child or elder abuse and those with no available safe environment

*Discharge Criteria*

All hemodynamically stable patients with dental injury without associated traumatic injury

*Issues for Referral*

- Ellis III injuries: Immediate dental referral
- Document recommendations and arrangements for dental follow-up care.

### FOLLOW-UP RECOMMENDATIONS

All patients with avulsions and Ellis II and III injuries should see dentist within 24 hr.

## PEARLS AND PITFALLS

- Avulsed teeth should never be transported dry or in tap water.
- Occlusion is best guide to proper tooth position after reimplantation
- Warn patients with dental trauma of risks of tooth resorption, color change, potential tooth loss, and/or need for future root canal.

## ADDITIONAL READING

- Layug ML, Barrett EJ, Kenny DJ. Interim storage of avulsed permanent teeth. *J Can Dent Assoc.* 1998;64:357–360.
- Nelson LP, Shusterman S. Emergency management of oral trauma in children. *Curr Opin Pediatr.* 1997;9:242–245.
- Wilson CF. Management of trauma to primary and developing teeth. *Dent Clin North Am.* 1995;39:133–167.
- Wolfson AB, Hendey GW, Ling LJ, et al., eds. *Harwood Nuss' Clinical Practice of Emergency Medicine,* 5th ed. Philadelphia: Lippincott, 2010.

### See Also (Topic, Algorithm, Electronic Media Element)

Tooth Pain

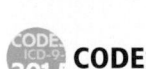 CODES

### ICD9

873.63 Open wound of internal structures of mouth, tooth (broken) (fractured) (due to trauma), uncomplicated

# DEPRESSION

Kathy M. Sanders
Felicia A. Smith

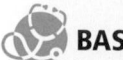 **BASICS**

## DESCRIPTION
Major depression:
- Psychiatric illness with depressed mood and neurovegetative signs and symptoms lasting ≥2 wk
- Significant associated morbidity and mortality
- Clinician should try to recognize this disorder in the medically ill.

## ETIOLOGY
- Major depression with suicidal ideation:
  - Biological illness associated with derangements in several neurotransmitter systems of the brain, including serotonin, norepinephrine, and dopamine
- Causes of neurobiological derangement include:
  - Genetic predisposition
  - Medical illness
  - Effects of medications
  - Chronic unremitting stressors in a predisposed individual
- Women are more likely to have major depression than men:
  - Men are more likely to complete suicide successfully (though women make more attempts)

### Pediatric Considerations
- Depressed children and adolescents are difficult to diagnose because the criteria are not as easily recognized.
- Indicators of major depression in children:
  - Irritability
  - Changes in school, home, and social functioning
  - Social withdrawal
  - Substance abuse
- Consultation with a child psychiatrist is crucial in further assessment and disposition.

 **DIAGNOSIS**

## SIGNS AND SYMPTOMS
- Criteria include depressed mood or loss of interest and pleasure for at least 2 wk and 5 (or more) of the following:
  - Loss of energy
  - Appetite disturbance
  - Sleep disturbance
  - Decreased attention span
  - Feeling of worthlessness
  - Recurrent thoughts of death
  - Psychomotor agitation or retardation
- Wide variety of presentations:
  - Quietly with somatic complaints, panic attacks, or psychosocial distress
  - More dramatic with suicidal ideation
- Associated somatic complaints:
  - Weakness, malaise
  - Weight loss
  - Headache
  - Back pain
- Diminished sense of self-esteem

### History
- Time course: Acute, episodic, chronic
- Collateral from family or outpatient providers
- Substance use
- Medications and medication adherence
- Family history
- History of self-injurious behavior or violence

### Physical Exam
- Vital signs
- Neurological exam:
  - Cognitive exam: Attention and orientation
  - Motor exam: Tone, abnormal movements

## ESSENTIAL WORKUP
- Eliciting the signs and symptoms of major depression is key to making the diagnosis (see "Signs and Symptoms" section for criteria).
- Use history and physical to guide further workup including labs and imaging.

## DIAGNOSTIC TESTS & INTERPRETATION
### Lab
- 1st line:
  - CBC
  - Electrolytes including calcium, blood urea nitrogen/creatinine, glucose
  - Urine and serum toxicology screen
  - Urinalysis
  - Liver function tests
  - Thyroid function tests
  - $B_{12}$ and folate
- 2nd line guided by history and physical findings:
  - HIV testing
  - Ceruloplasmin
  - Urine heavy metals
  - ESR/CRP/ANA
  - RPR/VDRL

### Imaging
- Overall yield low without focal neurological deficits but recommended for atypical presentation or focal findings
- MRI brain preferred over CT as screen: Higher yield for potentially clinically meaningful lesions:
  - White matter changes
  - Tumors or developmental anomalies
  - Cerebrovascular accident

## DIFFERENTIAL DIAGNOSIS
- Psychiatric illnesses:
  - Dysthymia
  - Adjustment reactions
  - Bipolar disorder
  - Substance induced mood disorders
  - Acute stress reactions
  - Schizophrenia

- Medical causes of depression:
  - Drug induced:
    - Antihypertensives
    - Oral contraceptives
    - Steroids
    - Sedative-hypnotics
    - Cocaine and amphetamine
    - β-Blockers
    - Metoclopramide
  - Endocrine disorders:
    - Hypothyroidism
    - Adrenal insufficiency
    - DM
  - Tumors:
    - Pancreatic
    - Lung
    - Brain
  - Neurologic disorders:
    - Dementia (early phase)
    - Epilepsy
    - Huntington disease
    - Multiple sclerosis
    - Parkinson disease
    - Stroke
    - Subdural hematoma
  - Infections:
    - Hepatitis
    - HIV
    - Mononucleosis
    - Neurosyphilis
  - Nutritional disorders:
    - Folate deficiency
    - Pellagra
    - Vitamin $B_{12}$ deficiency
  - Electrolyte disturbances
  - End-stage renal pulmonary and cardiovascular disease
  - Chronic pain syndromes

 **TREATMENT**

## PRE-HOSPITAL
- Ensure safety of patient and providers.
- Understand local laws for involuntary commitment to hospital.

## INITIAL STABILIZATION/THERAPY
ABCs of psychiatric assessment:
- Safety
- Evaluation
- Management:
  - 1-to-1 nursing and suicide precautions for suicidal patient safety
  - Work up potential medical causes.

## ED TREATMENT/PROCEDURES

- Psychological management:
  - Listen empathically to understand the stressors involved in the depression.
  - Emphasize that depression is a treatable condition to reassure, as well as to develop a treatment alliance.
- Initiate medications:
  - Use for diagnosed major depression
  - Decision to Initiate antidepressant medication should be for patients with established follow-up and only with enough medication given until the next appointment.
  - Low dose benzodiazepines or neuroleptics may be used for associated agitation, insomnia, or psychosis.
  - Usually takes weeks for antidepressant medications to resolve major depression.
- Choice of drug for the initiation of antidepressant therapy depends on:
  - Efficacy
  - Side-effect profile of the agent
  - Potential lethality if used to overdose
  - Compliance factors
- Selective serotonin reuptake inhibitors (SSRIs) (citalopram, escitalopram, fluoxetine, sertraline, paroxetine) SSRIs:
  - Well tolerated
  - Side effects include:
    ○ Mild nausea
    ○ Decreased appetite
    ○ Jitteriness
    ○ Somnolence
    ○ Sexual dysfunction
  - Weight gain:
    ○ Minimal overdose potential
- Serotonin norepinephrine reuptake inhibitors (SNRIs; venlafaxine, duloxetine):
  - Well-tolerated
  - Side effects similar to SSRIs
  - Minimal overdose potential
- Norepinephrine dopamine reuptake inhibitors (bupropion):
  - Agitation
  - Insomnia
  - Weight loss
  - Tremor
  - Decreased seizure threshold
- α₂-Receptor antagonist/agonist (mirtazapine):
  - Weight gain
  - Sedation
  - Orthostasis
  - Constipation
- Tricyclic antidepressants (amitriptyline, imipramine, nortriptyline, clomipramine):
  - Side effects include:
    ○ Anticholinergic effects
    ○ Weight gain
    ○ Postural hypotension
    ○ Sedation
    ○ Decreased seizure threshold
    ○ Overdoses of as little as 1 g of tricyclic antidepressant can be fatal
    ○ Nortriptyline is best tolerated and effective.

- Monoamine oxidase inhibitors (phenelzine, tranylcypromine, selegiline transdermal):
  - Dietary and other medication restrictions to avoid hypertensive crisis
  - Very dangerous in overdose
  - Best prescribed by psychiatrist

## MEDICATION

- Amitriptyline: Initial 25–50 mg/d PO
- Bupropion: 75–400 mg/d PO
- Citalopram: 20–40 mg/d PO
- Duloxetine: 30–120 mg/d PO
- Escitalopram: 10–20 mg/d PO
- Fluoxetine: 20–40 mg/d PO
- Imipramine: Initial 25–50 mg/d PO
- Mirtazapine: 15–45 mg/d PO
- Nortriptyline: Initial 25 mg/d PO
- Paroxetine: 20–40 mg/d PO
- Phenelzine: 15–60 mg/d PO
- Sertraline: 50–150 mg/d PO
- Tranylcypromine: 10–50 mg/d PO
- Venlafaxine: 75–300 mg/d PO

### First Line
- SSRIs, SNRIs, bupropion, mirtazapine
- Medication dosages for adults only
- Geriatric populations: Start at low dose range and titrate slowly.

### Second Line
- Tricyclics and monamine oxidase inhibitors
- Use with extreme caution in geriatric or medically ill populations.

 FOLLOW-UP

### DISPOSITION
#### Admission Criteria
- Patient is suicidal or at high risk for suicide:
  - See "Suicide, Risk Evaluation."
- Minimal or unreliable social supports
- Previous history of suicide or poor treatment response
- Symptoms so severe that continual observation or nursing supportive care is required
- Psychotic features
- Civil commitment for psychiatric hospitalization is necessary if the patient is refusing treatment and is suicidal or otherwise judged to be at-risk to harm self or others.

#### Discharge Criteria
- Low suicide risk
- Adequate social support
- Close follow-up available

#### Issues for Referral
- Insurance carrier determines inpatient disposition
- Options for any level of care are specified by the patient's insurance coverage.
- Outpatient follow-up appointments with mental health provider are important if discharging rather than admitting. Wait times for appointments may make this difficult.
- Case management or social services in ED is helpful for disposition issues.

## FOLLOW-UP RECOMMENDATIONS
Follow-up depends on severity of illness and risk of harm:
- If not being admitted, patients with significant symptomatology should be seen in follow-up in 1–2 wk.
- When medication is initiated, patient should be seen in follow-up in 1–2 wk.
- More stable patients or those with minor symptoms may be seen with less urgency.

## PEARLS AND PITFALLS
- Patients with depression experience significant morbidity and may present a risk of self-harm. Diagnosis is important.
- Consider medical, substance use, and neurological factors to presenting symptoms.
- Safety is key. Know hospitalization and involuntary commitment criteria in your area.

## ADDITIONAL READING
- Cassem NH, et al. Mood disordered patients. In: Stern TA, Fricchione GL, Cassem NH, et al., eds. *MGH Handbook of General Hospital Psychiatry*, 6th ed. St. Louis, MO: Mosby; 2010.
- Rosenbaum JF, Arana GW, Hyman SE, et al. Drugs for the treatment of depression. In: Rosenbaum JF, Arana GW, Hyman SE, et al., eds. *Handbook of Psychiatric Drug Therapy*, 5th ed. Philadelphia: Lippincott Williams & Wilkins; 2005:55–120.
- Stern TA, Herman JB, Slavin PL, eds. *MGH Guide to Primary Care Psychiatry*, 2nd ed. New York: McGraw Hill; 2004.
- Stern TA, Rosenbaum JF, Fava M, et al., eds. *MGH Comprehensive Clinical Psychiatry*. Philadelphia: Mosby; 2008.

### See Also (Topic, Algorithm, Electronic Media Element)
- Bipolar Disorder
- Psychosis, Acute
- Psychosis, Medical vs. Psychiatric
- Suicide, Risk Evaluation

 CODES

ICD9
- 296.20 Major depressive affective disorder, single episode, unspecified degree
- 296.30 Major depressive affective disorder, recurrent episode, unspecified degree
- 311 Depressive disorder, not elsewhere classified

# DERMATOMYOSITIS/POLYMYOSITIS
*Sean-Xavier Neath*

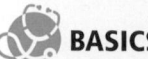 **BASICS**

## DESCRIPTION
- Dermatomyositis (DM) and polymyositis (PM) are systemic inflammatory myopathies, which represent the largest group of acquired and potentially treatable causes of skeletal muscle weakness.
- Patients experience a marked progression of muscle weakness over weeks to months.
- Can lead to respiratory insufficiency from respiratory muscle weakness
- Aspiration pneumonia can occur owing to a weak cough mechanism, pharyngeal muscle dysfunction, and esophageal dysmotility.
- Cardiac manifestations include myocarditis, conduction defects, cardiomyopathy and congestive heart failure (CHF).
- Arthralgias of the hands, wrists, knees, and shoulders
- Ocular muscles are not involved but facial muscle weakness may be seen in advanced cases.

## ETIOLOGY
- The exact cause is unknown, although autoimmune mechanisms are thought to be largely responsible.
- Incidence ~1:100,000 with a female preponderance
- Association with HLA-B8 and HLA-DR3
- There may be an association between PM and certain viral, bacterial, and parasitic infections.
- DM/PM occurs with collagen vascular disease about 20% of the time.
- In DM, humoral immune mechanisms are implicated, resulting in a microangiopathy and muscle ischemia.
- In PM, a mechanism of T cell–mediated cytotoxicity is posited. CD8 T cells, along with macrophages surround and destroy healthy, nonnecrotic muscle fibers that aberrantly express class I MHC molecules.
- Deposition of complement is the earliest and most specific lesion, followed by inflammation, ischemia, microinfarcts, necrosis, and destruction of the muscle fibers.

### Pediatric Considerations
- Although DM is seen in both children and adults, PM is rare in children.
- Similar to adult DM, juvenile DM (JDM) primarily affects the skin and skeletal muscles.
- Juvenile form may include vasculitis, ectopic calcifications (calcinosis cutis), and lipodystrophy.
- The juvenile form may be associated with coxsackievirus.

## DIAGNOSIS

### SIGNS AND SYMPTOMS
#### History
- Polymyositis (PM) is distinguished from dermatomyositis (DM) by the absence of rash.
- Patients with PM present with muscle pain and proximal muscle weakness.
- DM presents with skin rash, muscle pain, and weakness.
- Constitutional symptoms include weight loss, fever, anorexia, morning stiffness, myalgias, and arthralgias.
- Patients often note fatigue doing customary tasks:
  – Brushing hair, climbing stairs, reaching above the head, rising from a chair
  – May also complain of dysphagia, dyspnea, and cough
- Progressive weakness of the proximal limb and girdle muscles is seen early; distal muscle weakness can occur late in the disease.

#### Physical Exam
- General:
  – Fatigue
  – Fever
  – Weight loss
- Dysphagia
- Progressive muscle weakness:
  – Involves proximal muscles primarily
  – Symmetrical
- Skin findings of DM:
  – Skin rash occurs with or precedes muscle weakness.
  – Heliotrope rash (lilac discoloration) on the upper eyelids associated with edema
  – Gottron sign: Violaceous or erythematous papules over the extensor surfaces of the joints, particularly knuckles, knees, and elbows
  – Shawl sign: A V-shaped erythematous rash occurring on the back and shoulders
  – Periungual telangiectasias: Nail-bed capillary changes that include thickened irregular and distorted cuticles
  – "Machinist hands": Darkened horizontal lines across the lateral and palmar aspects of the fingers

### ESSENTIAL WORKUP
- Assess airway and breathing for any signs of aspiration or compromise.
- Assess for any signs of cardiac involvement and complications.

## DIAGNOSTIC TESTS & INTERPRETATION
### Lab
- Serum muscle enzymes:
  – Creatine phosphokinase (CPK) is elevated, other muscle enzymes such as aldolase, can also be elevated.
- Diagnostic criteria established in 1975 by Bohan and Peter:
  – Symmetric proximal muscle weakness with dysphagia and respiratory muscle weakness
  – Elevation of serum muscle enzymes
  – Electromyographic features of myopathy
  – Muscle biopsy showing features of inflammatory myopathy
  – Confidence limits for diagnosis (typical rash must be seen for diagnosis of DM):
    ○ Definite diagnosis: Three or four criteria
    ○ Probable diagnosis: Two criteria
    ○ Possible diagnosis: One criterion
- Newer diagnostic criteria using the immunohistological characterization (MHC/CD8) complex may prove to be more specific for this diagnosis.

### Imaging
- Chest radiograph may show interstitial lung disease, evidence of aspiration pneumonia, CHF, or cardiomyopathy.
- EM studies show myopathic potentials that are not specific for DM/PM.
- Increasing role for MRI in determining regions of inflammation best suited for biopsy

### Diagnostic Procedures/Surgery
- Muscle biopsy is the definitive test:
  – In PM, inflammatory infiltrates are often endomysial, although they may be perivascular.
  – In DM, inflammatory infiltrates are mostly perivascular and include a high percentage of B cells.
- Renal biopsies of patients may show focal proliferative glomerulonephritis.
- Pulmonary function tests are useful in following the progression of interstitial lung disease.

## DIFFERENTIAL DIAGNOSIS

- Collagen vascular diseases
- Muscular dystrophies
- Spinal muscular atrophy
- Myasthenia gravis
- Amyotrophic lateral sclerosis
- Poliomyelitis
- Guillain-Barré syndrome
- Hypothyroidism
- Hyperthyroidism
- Cushing syndrome
- Drug-induced:
  - Colchicine
  - Zidovudine (AZT)
  - Penicillamine
  - Ipecac
  - Ethanol
  - Chloroquine
  - Corticosteroids
- Infection:
  - Toxoplasmosis
  - Trichinosis
  - Coxsackievirus
  - HIV, influenza
  - Epstein-Barr virus
- Electrolyte disturbances:
  - Hypokalemia
  - Hypercalcemia
  - Hypomagnesemia
- Vasculitis
- Paraneoplastic neuromyopathy
- Hypereosinophilic myalgia syndrome

## TREATMENT

### PRE-HOSPITAL
- Assess ABCs
- Transport with elevation of head of bed

### INITIAL STABILIZATION/THERAPY
- Intubation and mechanical ventilation as required
- Nasogastric (NG) suction to prevent aspiration
- Pneumothorax has been described as a rare occurrence in childhood DM.

### ED TREATMENT/PROCEDURES
- Elevate head of the bed to prevent aspiration.
- Begin high-dose corticosteroids to suppress inflammation and improve muscle weakness.
- Avoid triamcinolone and dexamethasone because they may cause a drug-associated myopathy.
- Efficacy of prednisone determined by objective increase in muscle strength, not change in CK levels
- Immunosuppressive medications
- Azathioprine is limited by GI intolerance and bone marrow suppression.

- Cyclosporine has been used but with limited success.
- Methotrexate should be used immediately in children who do not respond to high dose steroids.
- Do not base treatment decisions solely upon CPK level.

### MEDICATION

#### First Line
Prednisone: 60 mg/d PO (peds: 1–2 mg/kg/d PO):
- Length of treatment and taper individualized to clinical response and normalization of CK

#### Second Line
- Methotrexate: 15–25 mg PO per week (peds: 0.5–1 PO mg/kg/wk—not to exceed adult dose)
- Azathioprine: 3 mg/kg/d PO for 4–6 mo
- Intravenous immunoglobulin (IVIG), mycophenolate, cyclosporine, cyclophosphamide are increasingly used by rheumatologists.

 FOLLOW-UP

### DISPOSITION

#### Admission Criteria
- Respiratory insufficiency
- Aspiration pneumonia
- Profound muscle weakness
- Weakened cough mechanisms
- Pharyngeal dysfunction
- CHF

#### Discharge Criteria
- Well-appearing patients with no respiratory dysfunction and no risk for aspiration
- Patients who can take oral corticosteroids and immunosuppressive agents as outpatients

#### Issues for Referral
Consultation with a rheumatologist should be made when the diagnosis is suspected for assistance with definitive diagnosis and further treatment.

### FOLLOW-UP RECOMMENDATIONS
- Compared to the general population, the incidence of malignant conditions appears to be increased in patients with DM (but not in those with PM).
- A complete annual physical examination with pelvic, breast, and rectal examinations, urinalysis; complete blood count; blood chemistry tests; and a chest film are often recommended for cancer surveillance in patients with a history of DM.

## PEARLS AND PITFALLS

- The diagnosis of an inflammatory myopathy is largely clinical supported by selected laboratory testing and muscle biopsy.
- Most patients improve with therapy, and many make a full functional recovery, which is often sustained with maintenance therapy.
- Up to 30% may be left with some residual muscle weakness.
- It is important to keep in mind that relapses may occur at any time despite successful response to therapy.

## ADDITIONAL READING

- Amato A, Barohn R. Evaluation and treatment of inflammatory myopathies. *J Neurol Neurosurg Psychiatry*. 2009;80:1060–1068.
- Caro I. Dermatomyositis as a systemic disease: Collagen vascular diseases. *Med Clin North Am*. 1989;73:1181–1191.
- Dalakas M. Polymyositis, dermatomyositis, and inclusion body myositis. In: Fauci AS, Braunwald E, Kasper DL, et al., eds. *Harrison's Principles of Internal Medicine*, 17th ed. New York, McGraw-Hill; 2008.
- Wedderburn L. Juvenile dermatomyositis: New developments in pathogenesis, assessment and treatment. *Best Pract Res Clin Rheum*. 2009;23: 665–678.

### See Also (Topic, Algorithm, Electronic Media Element)
- Hypokalemia
- Hypothyroidism
- Myasthenia Gravis
- Systemic Lupus Erythematosus

 CODES

#### ICD9
- 710.3 Dermatomyositis
- 710.4 Polymyositis

# DIABETES INSIPIDUS
*Melissa H. White*

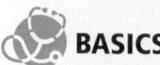 **BASICS**

## DESCRIPTION
- Disorder in which large volumes of dilute urine are excreted (polyuria) as an inappropriate response to arginine vasopressin (AVP)
- Often characterized by excessive fluid intake (polydipsia)
- 2 types:
  - Central diabetes insipidus (DI, CDI; failure or deficiency of AVP release):
    - 4 types:
      1. No AVP to release (loss or malfunction of posterior pituitary neurons)
      2. Defective osmoreceptors—release AVP only in response to severe dehydration
      3. Elevated threshold for AVP release
      4. Subnormal amount of AVP released
      5. Familial cases have been reported (autosomal dominant).
  - Nephrogenic DI (lack of renal response to AVP):
    - Differentiate from primary polydipsia.
    - Some cases are X-linked recessive in males.

## ETIOLOGY
- Central DI:
  - Any condition that disrupts the osmoreceptor-hypothalamus-hypophyseal axis:
    - Trauma (skull fractures, hemorrhage)
    - CNS neoplasm: DI can be considered a tumor marker.
    - Pituitary adenomas
    - Craniopharyngiomas
    - Germinomas
    - Pinealomas
    - Metastatic tumors
    - Leukemia
    - Histiocytosis X
    - Sarcoidosis
    - Congenital CNS defects
    - Pituitary or hypothalamic surgery
    - CNS infections (eg, meningitis, encephalitis)
    - Pregnancy (Sheehan syndrome)
    - Idiopathic (autoantibodies, occult tumor)
    - Wolfram syndrome (DI, DM, optic atrophy, deafness)

- Nephrogenic DI:
  - Any condition that disrupts the kidney:
    - Congenital renal disorders
    - Obstructive uropathy
    - Renal dysplasia
    - Polycystic kidney disease
    - Systemic disease with renal involvement
    - Sickle cell disease
    - Sarcoidosis
    - Amyloidosis
    - Drugs:
      - Amphotericin
      - Phenytoin
      - Lithium (persists past discontinuation of drug)
      - Aminoglycosides
      - Methoxyflurane
      - Demeclocycline
    - Electrolyte disorders:
      - Hypercalcemia
      - Hypokalemia

### Pregnancy Considerations
- Transient in the 2nd trimester:
  - Unclear etiology, but there is an increase of circulating vasopressinase.
  - Leads to a decrease in AVP and transient DI
  - Watch patient closely during anesthesia and periods of water restriction.
  - Typically clears after delivery
  - Desmopressin (DDAVP) resists this vasopressinase.
- Sheehan syndrome may cause DI.

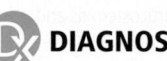 **DIAGNOSIS**

## SIGNS AND SYMPTOMS
### History
- Polyuria (up to 16–24 L/d of urine):
  - Note the voiding frequency.
- Polydipsia (often craves cold fluids):
  - Note the amount of PO fluid intake per day.
- Drug ingestion
- Signs and symptoms of hypothalamic tumors:
  - Headache
  - Visual disturbances
  - Growth disturbances
  - Obesity
  - Hyperpyrexia
  - Sleep disturbances
  - Sexual precocity
  - Emotional disturbances

### Physical Exam
- Dehydration
- Cachexia
- Head trauma
- Visual field defects
- Seizures

### Pediatric Considerations
- Polyuria and polydipsia may not be recognized by caregivers until symptoms of dehydration develop.
- In neonates:
  - Often present at birth
  - If unrecognized, dehydration and hypernatremia may cause permanent CNS damage.
- In infants:
  - Irritability
  - Poor feeding
  - Growth failure
  - Intermittent high fever
  - Abnormal behavior (hyperactivity, restlessness)
- In children:
  - Enuresis

## ESSENTIAL WORKUP
- Clinical diagnosis in the ED:
  - Elevated serum sodium concentration
  - Copious amounts of dilute urine
- History:
  - Usually an increased amount of PO fluid intake per day
  - Voiding frequency
  - Medication use history
- Physical exam
- Labs below

## DIAGNOSTIC TESTS & INTERPRETATION
### Lab
- Urinalysis:
  - Specific gravity will be low.
- Serum and urine osmolality:
  - High serum osmolality
  - Low urine osmolality
- Electrolytes, BUN, creatinine, and glucose:
  - Hypernatremia
  - Hypercalcemia
  - Hypokalemia
- CBC:
  - Anemia may be a sign of a neoplasm.
- Serum and urine AVP tests are expensive and unnecessary in the ED.

### Imaging
- As needed to evaluate for trauma or search for neoplasm
- CXR
- CT of brain
- MRI of pituitary axis is usually outpatient.

### Diagnostic Procedures/Surgery
Water deprivation test (dehydration test):
- Unnecessary in the emergency setting
- Can be dangerous in cases of hypotension or small children
- Performed as a confirmatory test for those receiving treatment

## DIFFERENTIAL DIAGNOSIS
- Primary water deficit:
  - Inadequate access to free water
  - Increased insensible water loss (eg, premature infants)
  - Inadequate breast-feeding
- Primary sodium excess:
  - Excessive sodium bicarbonate during resuscitation
  - Hypernatremic enemas
  - Ingestion of seawater
  - Hypertonic saline administration
  - Accidental substitution of salt (sodium chloride [NaCl]) for glucose in infant formulas
  - Intentional salt poisoning
  - High breast milk sodium
- Primary polydipsia (psychogenic polydipsia):
  - Solute-induced polyuria
  - Diuretic use
  - Resolving acute renal failure
  - Osmotic diuresis
  - Uncontrolled DM

 TREATMENT

### PRE-HOSPITAL
- ABCs
- Immobilize if trauma is suspected.
- Serum blood glucose
- IV access and fluids if signs of dehydration exist
- Control seizures according to medical direction guidelines.

### INITIAL STABILIZATION/THERAPY
- Manage ABCs.
- Manage traumatic injuries accordingly.
- High index of suspicion for head trauma

### ED TREATMENT/PROCEDURES
- Correction of hypotension:
  - Use of 0.9% NaCl is indicated for shock.
  - Intravascular losses represent only about 1/12 of total water losses.

- Central DI (vasopressin deficient):
  - Arginine vasopressin (aqueous vasopressin):
    - Half-life is too short.
    - May induce coronary vasospasm
    - Used only for dehydration test
  - Lysine vasopressin (lypressin):
    - Can be given intranasally
    - Frequent instillation needed
  - Desmopressin:
    - Drug of choice to control symptoms
    - Administer intranasally b.i.d. in dosage necessary to control polyuria or polydipsia. Also, PO form available
    - Caution in postoperative patients as cerebral edema may develop
  - Chlorpropamide (Diabinese):
    - Enhances effect of vasopressin at renal tubule
    - May stimulate AVP release
    - Useful only in partial CDI
    - Clofibrate stimulates the release of endogenous vasopressin.
- Nephrogenic DI:
  - Thiazide diuretics:
    - Induce natriuresis.
  - Dietary sodium restriction
  - Restrict solutes and avoid excessive drinking to prevent water intoxication.
  - Avoid alcohol (especially beer) intake
  - Check daily weights.
  - NSAIDs (indomethacin)
- Parenteral correction of initial water deficit in cases where PO is not an option:
  - Usually only in symptomatic hypernatremic cases
  - For fluid replacement, refer to "Hypernatremia."

## MEDICATION
- Aqueous arginine vasopressin: 5–10 U SC in the unconscious patient from head trauma or postoperative
- Chlorpropamide (Diabinese): 200–500 mg PO daily
- Clofibrate (Atromid-S): 500 mg PO q6h
- Desmopressin: 10–20 μg intranasally; 2–4 μg SC or IV; 0.1 mg PO
- Hydrochlorothiazide (HCTZ): 50 mg PO daily
- Lypressin nasal spray: 1–2 nasal spray t.i.d.–q.i.d. as needed

 FOLLOW-UP

### DISPOSITION
### Admission Criteria
- AMS
- Seizure
- Severe dehydration
- Electrolyte abnormalities
- Associated trauma
- Patients requiring DDAVP testing or a trial of water restriction

### Discharge Criteria
- Known diagnosis of DI
- Stable electrolytes
- Adequately hydrated

### FOLLOW-UP RECOMMENDATIONS
Referral to specialist depends on underlying etiology of DI.

## PEARLS AND PITFALLS
- Check urine osmolality and consider DI in polyuria.
- Central DI will typically respond to desmopressin.
- Nephrogenic DI will not respond to ADH:
  - Treat the underlying electrolyte abnormality, discontinue concerning drugs, and consult nephrology for further management.

## ADDITIONAL READING
- Behrman RE, ed. Nelson Textbook of Pediatrics, 16th ed. Philadelphia: WB Saunders, 2000.
- Braunwald E, et al. Diabetes insipidus. In: Braunwald E, ed. Harrison's Principles of Internal Medicine. New York: McGraw-Hill, 2002.
- Goroll AH, ed, Primary Care Medicine, 4th ed. Philadelphia: Lippincott Williams & Wilkins, 2000.
- Makaryus AN, et al. Diabetes insipidus: Diagnosis and treatment of a complex disease. Cleve Clin J Med. 2006; 73:65–71.
- Mavrakis AN, et al. Diabetes insipidus with deficient thirst: Report of a patient and review of the literature. Am J Kidney Dis. 2008;51:851.
- Rose BD. Diabetes insipidus. Wellesley, MA: 2005.
- Sainz Bueno JA, et al. Transient diabetes insipidus during pregnancy: A clinical case and review of the syndrome. Eur J Obstet Gynecol. 2005;118:251–254.
- Zink BJ. Traumatic brain injury outcome: Concepts for emergency care. Ann Emerg Med. 2001;37(3): 318–332.
- The author gratefully recognizes the contribution of Rahul Patwari for the previous edition of this chapter.

### See Also (Topic, Algorithm, Electronic Media Element)
- Head Trauma
- Hypernatremia

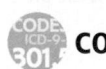 CODES

### ICD9
- 253.5 Diabetes insipidus
- 588.1 Nephrogenic diabetes insipidus

D

# DIABETES MELLITUS, JUVENILE
*Madeline M. Joseph*

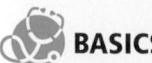

## BASICS

### DESCRIPTION
- Decrease in effective circulating insulin
- Increase in counter regulatory hormones including glucagon, catecholamines, cortisol, and growth hormone
- Hyperglycemia owing to:
  - Decreased peripheral glucose utilization
  - Increased hepatic gluconeogenesis
- Hyperosmolality and osmotic diuresis
- Ketoacidosis produced by increased lipolysis, with ketone body ($\beta$-hydroxybutyrate, acetoacetate) production, causes ketonemia and metabolic acidosis
- Potassium deficit:
  - Intracellular shifts into extracellular space owing to hydrogen ion exchange
  - Loss from osmotic diuresis

### ETIOLOGY
Mechanism:
- Immune-mediated pancreatic islet $\beta$-cell destruction
- Precipitating events leading to diabetic ketoacidosis (DKA):
  - Infection, often minor acute illness such as virus, group A strep pharyngitis or UTI
  - Stress
  - Endocrine: Pregnancy, puberty, hyperthyroidism
  - Psychiatric disorders, including eating disorders
  - Medication noncompliance, inappropriate interruption of insulin pump therapy, or treatment error
- Risk factors for cerebral edema:
  - Attenuated rise in measured serum sodium during DKA therapy (unrelated to the volume or sodium content of IV fluid or rate of change in serum glucose)
  - Bicarbonate treatment for acidosis correction
  - Hypocapnia
  - Increased serum urea nitrogen
  - No association with degree of hyperglycemia
  - Demographic factors that have been associated with an increase risk of cerebral edema include: Younger age, longer duration of symptoms, and new onset diabetes mellitus. These factors are also associated with increased risk of severe DKA.

## DIAGNOSIS

### SIGNS AND SYMPTOMS
- Polydipsia
- Polyuria (may have good urine output despite dehydration)
- Polyphagia
- Weight loss, unexplained
- Diabetic ketoacidosis (DKA):
  - Initial presentation in 20–40% of patients
  - Often associated with tachypnea (Kussmaul's respiration), tachycardia, orthostatic BP changes
  - Nausea
  - Vomiting
  - Abdominal pain, often resolving with reduction in ketosis/acidosis
  - Hyperpnea
  - Ketotic breath

#### Dehydration
- Mental status changes
- Shock
- Cerebral edema:
  - The incidence ranges from 0.87–1.1%.
  - Cerebral edema accounts for 57–87% of all DKA deaths.
  - It typically occurs 4–12 hr after treatment is initiated, but can be presenting (subclinical) before treatment has started.
  - Headache
  - Change in neurological status, such as drowsiness, irritability, or specific neurological deficit, such as pupillary responses or cranial nerve palsies
  - Inappropriate slowing in pulse rate
  - Increase in BP
- Hyperglycemic hyperosmolar nonketotic coma:
  - Glucose level of 800–1,200 mg/dL
  - Rare in children; more common in adults

### ESSENTIAL WORKUP
For DKA:
- Hourly vital signs and neurologic checks
- Frequent blood chemistries
- ECG monitoring (in severe DKA) to assess T waves for evidence of hyperkalemia/hypokalemia
- Accurate fluid input and output. Consider urinary catheterization in patients with impaired level of consciousness.

## DIAGNOSTIC TESTS & INTERPRETATION
### Lab
For DKA:
- Glucose, serum: Hyperglycemia
- Urinalysis:
  - Glycosuria
  - Ketonuria
  - Exclude UTI
- Blood chemistries every 2–4 hr until acidosis has resolved (more frequent as clinically indicated in the more severe cases)
- Electrolytes and venous pH
- Anion gap metabolic acidosis:
  - Potassium—high or normal (artifactual owing to extracellular shift)
  - Serum potassium rises 0.5 mEqL for each 0.1 decrease in pH
  - Sodium—low or normal (may be artifactual owing to hyperglycemia)
  - Corrected Na (mEq/L) = [measured serum Na (mEqL) + plasma glucose (mg/dL) − 100] × 0.016
  - Bicarbonate—low
- Serum ketones—elevated
- Serum osmolality
- CBC:
  - WBC often elevated owing to stress or infection
- Calcium
- Phosphate
- Cultures as indicated: Group A strep pharyngeal swab, urine
- Pregnancy test if indicated
- ECG if potassium markedly abnormal

### Imaging
CXR if any suggestion of pneumonia

### DIFFERENTIAL DIAGNOSIS
- Infection (may precipitate):
  - UTI
  - Gastroenteritis
  - Appendicitis
  - Sepsis
- Ingestion (salicylates, alcohols, glycols)
- Diabetes insipidus

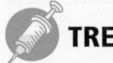

# TREATMENT

## PRE-HOSPITAL
For DKA:
- ABCs
- Airway protection
- Establish IV access and initiate fluid therapy.

## INITIAL STABILIZATION/THERAPY
For DKA:
- Oxygen
- Cardiac monitor
- IV access and volume resuscitation

## ED TREATMENT/PROCEDURES
For DKA:
- Fluid replacement:
  – Assume fluid deficit of 10% of body weight.
  – Initial volume expansion with 10–20 mL/kg of 0.9% NaCl; may repeat to achieve hemodynamic stability
  – Correct 50% of fluid deficit over 1st 8 hr, remainder over 24–48 hr.
  – Do not give >3 L/m² over 1st 24 hr.
- Begin IV insulin infusion after ketoacidosis confirmed:
  – Initial rate of continuous infusion (regular insulin) 0.1 U/kg/hr
  – Adjust rate to drop serum glucose maximum of 100 mg/dL/hr.
  – Add dextrose to infusion fluid when serum glucose <300 mg/dL.
  – Change to SC insulin when no longer significantly acidotic and able to eat.
- Some clinicians prefer IM route, commonly initially using regular insulin at a dose of 0.1–0.2 U/kg/hr.
- Replace potassium and phosphate losses:
  – Verify adequate urine output.
  – Add to fluids as KCl and K$_3$PO$_4$ in equal amounts. Large doses of K$^+$ may be necessary; guide therapy by frequent monitoring of K$^+$.
- Monitor serum sodium:
  – Risk for cerebral edema if Na$^+$ fails to rise as glucose falls
- Bicarbonate therapy:
  – Not recommended in most cases since generally it does not alter outcome and it increases risk for cerebral edema with its use
  – Use it with caution in patients with severe acidosis (pH <6.9) in whom peripheral vasodilation and decreased cardiac contractility may further impair tissue perfusion and in potentially life-threatening hyperkalemia.

- Cerebral edema:
  – Treat cerebral edema as soon as the condition is suspected due to its high mortality and morbidity rates: 21–25% and 10–26%, respectively.
  – Decrease fluid administration rate.
  – Mannitol (0.25–1.0 g/Kg over 20 min): No large studies to date demonstrate definitive beneficial or detrimental effects. Consider its use in patients with signs of cerebral edema before impeding respiratory failure. Dose can be repeated in 2 hr if there is no initial response.
  – Hypertonic saline (3%) 5–10 mL/kg over 30 min may be an alternative to mannitol
  – Endotracheal intubation and ventilation: Avoid aggressive hyperventilation since it has been associated with poor outcome in DKA-related cerebral edema (similar to that found in head trauma).

## MEDICATION
- Insulin drip: Start 0.1 U/kg/hr IV (some clinicians prefer the IM dosing and route).
- Mannitol: 0.25–1 g/kg IV

# FOLLOW-UP

## DISPOSITION
### Admission Criteria
For DKA:
- ICU:
  – Altered mental status
  – Shock or cardiac dysrhythmia
  – Initial glucose >700 mg/dL
  – Initial pH <7.0
- Inpatient unit:
  – Stable new-onset diabetic patients requiring intensive education
  – Patients with ketoacidosis not meeting requirements for ICU care
  – Compliance concerns or other social issues

### Discharge Criteria
- Known diabetic patients who respond well to therapy with normalization of glucose, pH, and ketosis
- Tolerating oral fluids
- Reliable parents
- Reliable follow-up within 24 hr including appropriate education

### Issues for Referral
- Critically ill
- Persistent abnormal mental status
- Poorly controlled diabetes

## FOLLOW-UP RECOMMENDATIONS
- Close follow-up with the primary care physician is important even after the resolution of DKA to ensure appropriate management of the patient's diabetes to prevent further occurrence of DKA.
- Many children with diabetes are followed at comprehensive diabetes centers in collaboration with primary care physician.

# PEARLS AND PITFALLS
Mortality from DKA is predominately related to the occurrence of cerebral edema. Therefore, early and appropriate treatment is of most importance in managing children with DKA.

# ADDITIONAL READING
- Dunger DB, et al. ESPE/LWPES consensus statement on diabetic ketoacidosis in children and adolescents. *Arch Dis Child*. 2004;89:188–194.
- Edge JA, et al. The risk and outcome of cerebral edema in children with diabetic ketoacidosis. *Arch Dis Child*. 2001;85:16–22.
- Glaser N, Barnett P, McCaslin I, et al. Risk factors for cerebral edema in children with diabetic ketoacidosis. *N Engl J Med*. 2001;344:264–269.
- Kamat P, et al. Use of hypertonic saline for the treatment of altered mental status associated with diabetic ketoacidosis. *Pediatr Crit Care Med*. 2003;4:239–242.
- Marcin JP, et al. Factors associated with adverse outcomes in children with diabetic ketoacidosis-related cerebral edema. *J Pediatr*. 2002;141:793–797.
- Rewers A, et al. Predictors of acute complications in children with type 1 diabetes. *JAMA*. 2002;287:2511–2518.
- Roberts JS, et al. Cerebral hyperemia and impaired cerebral autoregulation associated with diabetic ketoacidosis in critically ill children. *Crit Care Med*. 2006;34:2217–2223.
- Toledo JD, et al. Sodium concentration in rehydration fluids for children with ketoacidotic diabetes: Effect on serum sodium concentration. *J Pediatr*. 2009;154:895–900.
- Wolfsdorf J, Glaser N, Sperling MA. Diabetic ketoacidosis in infants, children and adolescents-a consensus statement from the American Diabetes Association. *Diabetes Care*. 2006;29:1150–1159.

# CODES

## ICD9
- 250.01 Diabetes mellitus without mention of complication, type I (juvenile type), not stated as uncontrolled
- 250.03 Diabetes mellitus without mention of complication, type I (juvenile type), uncontrolled
- 250.13 Diabetes mellitus with ketoacidosis, type I (juvenile type), uncontrolled

# DIABETIC KETOACIDOSIS

*Joseph M. Weber*

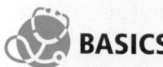 **BASICS**

## DESCRIPTION

Insulin deficiency and excess of counterregulatory hormones (catecholamines, glucagon, growth hormone, and cortisol) resulting in:

- Dehydration (osmotic, hyperglycemic, diuresis, and decreased oral intake)
- Acidosis (anion gap metabolic acidosis)
- Ketone formation (unrestrained lipolysis and ketogenesis)
- Hyperglycemia (unrestrained glycogenolysis and gluconeogenesis)
- Electrolyte disturbances (hypokalemia, hypo/hypernatremia, hypophosphatemia)

## ETIOLOGY

- Medication noncompliance (>50%)
- New-onset diabetes (type I or II)
- Underlying medical illness (increased counterregulatory hormones and insulin resistance):
  - Infectious process
  - MI
  - GI bleed
  - CNS event
- Pregnancy (relative insulin deficiency and counterregulatory hormone excess)
- Medications (protease inhibitors and atypical antipsychotics: Olanzapine, clozapine)
- Alcohol abuse

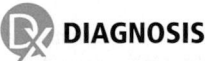 **DIAGNOSIS**

## SIGNS AND SYMPTOMS
### History
- Medication noncompliance
- Polyuria, polydipsia
- Weakness
- Abdominal pain, nausea, vomiting
- Altered mental status
- Chest pain
- Febrile illness

### Physical Exam
- Tachycardia
- Hypotension (dehydration, sepsis)
- Tachypnea (hyperpnea)
- Kussmaul respirations
- Hyperthermia/hypothermia (coexisting infection)
- Dehydration:
  - Poor skin turgor
  - Dry mucous membranes
- Odor of ketones on breath
- Diffuse abdominal tenderness

## ESSENTIAL WORKUP
- Diagnostic criteria:
  - pH <7.3, with ketonemia
  - Bicarbonate <15 mEq/L
  - Glucose >250 mg/dL
- Bedside glucose measurement
- Venous blood gas
- Urine dip for ketones
- Serum electrolytes, glucose, BUN/creatinine
- Search for precipitating cause

## DIAGNOSTIC TESTS & INTERPRETATION
### Lab
- Serum glucose measurement:
  - Confirm bedside test.
- Electrolyte measurement:
  - Increased anion gap metabolic acidosis: $[Na - (Cl + HCO_3)] > 12$
  - Sodium:
    - Pseudohyponatremia (from hyperglycemia) correction factor; add 1.6 mEq/L to the measured sodium for every 100 mg/dL of blood glucose >100 mg/dL.
  - Potassium:
    - Initial serum level may be normal to high owing to extracellular shift as compensation for acidosis.
    - Total body deficit usually 3–5 mEq/kg
    - As acidosis improves, for every 0.1 increase in the pH, serum potassium decreases 0.5 mEq/L.
    - Can drop precipitously with insulin and fluids
  - Bicarbonate:
    - Usually <15 mEq/L
    - May be higher owing to coexisting volume contraction alkalosis
- BUN/creatinine:
  - Usually shows prerenal azotemia owing to dehydration
- Serum ketones:
  - Must be present to make diagnosis of DKA.
  - $\beta$-Hydroxybutyrate is the predominant ketoacid, but acetoacetate and acetone are also present:
    - $\beta$-Hydroxybutyrate is not measured by most hospital serum and urine ketone tests (nitroprusside reaction measures only acetoacetate and acetone), thus there is a theoretical risk of missing the presence of ketones using these tests.
  - Urine ketone dip test (UKDT) is 97% sensitive for presence of serum ketones and a negative UKDT has a negative predictive value of 100% in ruling out the presence of DKA.
  - Point-of-care capillary testing for $\beta$-hydroxybutyrate is 98% sensitive for serum ketones:
    - May be used with capillary glucose testing in triage to detect DKA early in the ED course.

- Urinalysis:
  - Ketonuria, glucosuria
  - Pregnancy (UhCG)
- Venous blood gas:
  - Essential to assess patient's pH
  - pH correlates well with arterial pH.
  - Avoids need for repeated arterial sticks
  - ABG should be performed if oxygenation/ventilation need assessment.
- Serum osmolarity:
  - May be measured in the lab and calculated
  - Calculated: 2(Na) + glucose/18 + BUN/2.8 (normal 285–300 mOsm/L)
  - Significant hyperosmolarity >320
- CBC:
  - Leukocytosis may be present without infection.
  - If left shift in differential, suspect infection.
- Other lab tests:
  - Amylase: Elevation is nonspecific in DKA.
  - Lipase: Elevation specific for pancreatitis
  - Calcium, Mg, Phosphate: All usually decreased as is $K^+$

### Imaging
- CT head to rule out other causes of altered mental status.
- CXR if pneumonia suspected as precipitant or hypoxia present
- EKG to rule out ischemia as a precipitant, and look for signs of hyper/hypo $K^+$

## DIFFERENTIAL DIAGNOSIS
- Other causes of anion gap acidosis
- Use ACAT MUD PILES mnemonic:
  - **A**lcoholic ketoacidosis
  - **C**arbon monoxide/cyanide
  - **A**spirin
  - **T**oluene
  - **M**ethanol
  - **U**remia
  - **D**iabetic ketoacidosis
  - **P**araldehyde
  - **I**ron/isoniazid
  - **L**actic acidosis
  - **E**thylene glycol
  - **S**tarvation/sepsis
- Hyperglycemic hyperosmolar nonketotic syndrome

TREATMENT

### PRE-HOSPITAL
- Fluid bolus often initiated in field
- Quantify amount given by paramedics to guide further ED fluids.

### INITIAL STABILIZATION/THERAPY
- ABCs for patients with altered mental status
- Coma cocktail for AMS: Naloxone, thiamine, Accu-Chek
- 0.9% NS bolus for hypotension/tachycardia

### ED TREATMENT/PROCEDURES
- Cardiac monitor and pulse oximetry for patients with abnormal vitals
- Fluids:
  – Average adult water deficit is 100 mL/kg (5–10 L).
  – Initial 1–2 L bolus of 0.9% NS to restore intravascular volume over 1st hr.
  – If corrected serum sodium is low, continue with 0.9% NS, giving 1–2 more liters over the next 2–4 hr.
  – If corrected serum sodium is normal or elevated, use 0.45% NS giving 1–2 more liters over next 2–4 hr.
  – Be careful to avoid fluid overload in patients with cardiac disease.
  – Avoid precipitous falls in serum sodium/osmolality, as this may contribute to cerebral edema.
  – Total fluid replacement should take 24–36 hr.
- Insulin:
  – Reverses ketogenic state and downregulates counterregulatory hormones
  – Administered as continuous IV infusion of regular insulin at 0.1 units/kg/h:
    o Adjust infusion in response to changes in glucose and anion gap
  – Continue until pH >7.3 and resolution of anion gap
  – Serum glucose will fall sooner than resolution of acidosis and should be kept >250 mg/dL with glucose-containing fluids such as $D_5$45% NS.
- Potassium:
  – Administration is essential.
  – Total body deficit of 3–5 mEq/kg
  – Will drop precipitously with administration of fluid and insulin
  – Administer KCl, 10 mEq/h IV once renal function is established and $K^+$ is known to be <5.5 mEq/L.
  – May need to give up to 20–40 mEq/h IV in cases where initial $K^+$ is < 3.5 mEq/L
  – Some advocate checking $K^+$ before initiating insulin to avoid severe hypokalemia.
  – Should measure q1–2h during 1st 4–6 hr of therapy

- Bicarbonate:
  – No studies have shown clinical benefit in DKA, and its routine use is not advocated.
  – Complications include hypokalemia, alkalosis, cerebral acidosis, and edema.
  – Some advocate its use for pH <7.0 with cardiac instability.
- Phosphate:
  – Not routinely replaced during initial ED therapy
  – May supplement if <1.0 mg/dL
  – Administer as potassium phosphate.
- Magnesium:
  – May supplement if <1.2 mg/dL
  – Administer 2 g $MgSO_4$ IV over 1 hr.
- Identify and treat precipitating cause.

### Pediatric Considerations
- Fluids:
  – Average fluid deficit is 100 mL/kg.
  – Initial 10–20 mL/kg bolus of 0.9% NS to restore intravascular volume
  – May repeat once in severely dehydrated children
  – Should not exceed 40–50 mL/kg of fluid in 1st 4 hr of therapy
  – Replace remainder of deficit at 1.5–2.0 times maintenance over 24–36 hr.
  – Overzealous fluid administration is thought to contribute to cerebral edema.
- Cerebral edema:
  – Occurs in 1–2% of children with DKA
  – Causes 31% of deaths associated with DKA
  – Exact causes unclear
  – Suspect with coma, fluctuating mental status, bradycardia, HTN, severe headache, decreased urine output, or quickly falling corrected $Na^+$ or osmolality to below normal levels
  – Mannitol 0.25–1.0 g/kg IV over 30 min should be given immediately and can be repeated hourly.
  – Fluid rate should be decreased and other supportive measures instituted.

### MEDICATION
- $D_{50}$: 1 amp (25 g) of 50% dextrose IVP (peds: 2–4 mL/kg $D_{25}$)
- Insulin (100 units regular insulin in 100 mL NS) run at 0.1 U/kg/hr
- $MgSO_4$: 2 g of 20% solution

 FOLLOW-UP

### DISPOSITION
#### Admission Criteria
- ICU admission for pH <7.0, altered mental status, serious comorbid illness, and extremes of age (<2 yr or >60 yr)
- Monitored unit for moderate DKA (pH 7.01–7.24) with CHF or cardiac history
- General floor (nurses skilled with insulin infusions) for moderate DKA without comorbidities
- Observation unit (<23 hr admission) for mild DKA (pH 7.25–7.30) without precipitating illness

#### Discharge Criteria
- Resolution of anion gap acidosis
- Tolerating PO fluids
- No evidence of precipitating event
- Clear instructions on home insulin regimen
- Close primary care follow-up arranged

## PEARLS AND PITFALLS
- Decreasing or discontinuing insulin drip when glucose normalizes is a pitfall. Insulin should only be stopped when pH improves and anion gap normalizes.
- Failure to replete potassium is a pitfall.

## ADDITIONAL READING
- American Diabetes Association: Position statement: Hyperglycemic crises in diabetes. *Diabetes Care.* 2004;27(Suppl 1).
- Ma OJ, et al. Arterial blood gas results rarely influence emergency physician management of patients with suspected diabetic ketoacidosis. *Acad Emerg Med.* 2003;10(8):836–841.
- Naunheim R, et al. Point-of-care test identifies diabetic ketoacidosis at triage. *Acad Emerg Med.* 2006;13:683–685.
- White NH. Management of diabetic ketoacidosis. *Rev Endocr Metab Disord.* 2003;4:343–353.

### See Also (Topic, Algorithm, Electronic Media Element)
Hyperosmolar Syndrome

 CODES

### ICD9
- 250.13 Diabetes mellitus with ketoacidosis, type I (juvenile type), uncontrolled

D

# DIALYSIS COMPLICATIONS
Christopher B. Colwell

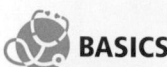 **BASICS**

## DESCRIPTION
Dialysis complications may be:
- Vascular access related (infection, bleeding)
- Nonvascular access related (hypotension, hyperkalemia)
- Peritoneal (abdominal pain)

## ETIOLOGY
- Vascular access–related:
  - Infections:
    ○ Infections (largely access related or peritonitis) are a major cause of death in dialysis patients.
    ○ Often caused by *Staphylococcus aureus*
    ○ Can present with signs of localized infection or systemic sepsis
    ○ Can also present with minimal findings
  - Thrombosis or stenosis:
    ○ Often presents with loss of bruit or thrill over access site
    ○ Must be addressed quickly (within 24 hr) to avoid loss of access site
  - Bleeding:
    ○ Can be life-threatening
- Nonvascular access–related:
  - Hypotension:
    ○ Most common complication of hemodialysis
    ○ After dialysis: Often owing to acute decrease in circulating blood volume
    ○ During dialysis: Hypovolemia (more commonly) or onset of cardiac tamponade owing to compensated effusion suddenly becoming symptomatic after correction of volume overload:
    ○ MI, sepsis, dysrhythmias, hypoxia
    ○ Hemorrhage secondary to anticoagulation, platelet dysfunction of renal failure
  - Shortness of breath:
    ○ Volume overload
    ○ Development of dyspnea *during* dialysis owing to: Tamponade, pericardial effusion, hemorrhage, anaphylaxis, pulmonary embolism, air embolism
  - Chest pain:
    ○ Ischemic:
      1. Dialysis patients are often at high risk for having atherosclerotic disease
      2. Dialysis is an acute physiologic stressor with transient hypotension and hypoxemia that increases myocardial oxygen demand.
    ○ Pleuritic:
      1. Pericarditis, pulmonary embolism
  - Neurologic dysfunction: Disequilibrium syndrome:
    ○ Rapid decrease in serum osmolality during dialysis leaves brain in comparatively hyperosmolal state.

- Peritoneal:
  - Peritonitis:
    ○ Owing to contamination of peritoneal dialysate or tubing during exchange
    ○ *S. aureus* or *S. epidermis* (70%)
  - Perforated viscus with abdominal pain that can be severe, fever, brown or fecal material in effluent, or localized tenderness
  - Fibrinous blockage of catheter resulting from infection or inflammation

 **DIAGNOSIS**

## SIGNS AND SYMPTOMS
- Vascular access–related:
  - Bleeding from puncture sites
  - Loss of bruit in graft
  - Local infection, cellulitis, fever
  - Decreased sensation and strength distal to access
- Nonvascular access–related:
  - Hypotension before, during, or after procedure
  - Palpitations
  - Syncope
  - Chest pain:
    ○ Ischemic
    ○ Pleuritic
  - Hemorrhage:
    ○ GI
    ○ Pleural
    ○ Retroperitoneal
  - Shortness of breath:
  - Neurologic symptoms (disequilibrium syndrome):
    ○ Headache
    ○ Malaise
    ○ Seizures
    ○ Coma
- Peritoneal:
  - Abdominal pain
  - Cloudy dialysis effluent
  - Nausea and vomiting
  - Exudates or inflammation at insertion site of Tenckhoff catheter

## ESSENTIAL WORKUP
- Careful physical exam:
  - Complete set of vital signs including auscultated BP, pulse, respiratory rate, accurate temperature, and pulse oximetry
  - Careful physical exam for occult infectious sources (odontogenic, perirectal abscess)
  - Auscultation of lungs for evidence of infection (rhonchi) or volume overload (rales)
  - Search for other evidence of volume overload (edema).
  - Careful cardiac exam including listening for murmurs or rubs
- EKG: Look for signs of electrolyte balance or conduction disturbances.
- Infection:
  - Blood and wound cultures
  - Cell count, Gram stain, culture of peritoneal fluid

- Bleeding:
  - CBC to evaluate anemia and platelet count
  - Coagulation studies
- Chest pain or shortness of breath:
  - EKG
  - Chest radiograph
  - ABG
  - Cardiac enzymes (if appropriate, based on history)
- Neurologic dysfunction: CT of brain for intracranial hemorrhage

## DIAGNOSTIC TESTS & INTERPRETATION
### Lab
- Electrolytes, BUN, and creatinine
- Glucose
- CBC

### Imaging
- ECG for suspected:
  - Hyperkalemia
  - Pericarditis
  - Effusion
  - Tamponade
- US of access for possible clotted graft or fistula
- Peritoneal catheterogram for catheter blockages
- CT scan for pulmonary embolism:
  - Dialysis patients are at risk for both bleeding and clotting problems.
  - Problematic in renal insufficiency owing to contrast dye load:
    ○ Can be done in renal failure, but contrast is then a fluid bolus and may need to be dialyzed off
    ○ Communicate contrast load to renal team, as dialysis may need to occur for longer-than-normal duration.

## DIFFERENTIAL DIAGNOSIS
- Hypotension:
  - Cardiogenic shock, acute MI, tamponade, primary dysrhythmias
  - Electrolyte abnormalities leading to dysrhythmias (hyperkalemia and hypokalemia)
  - Embolism: Air or pulmonary
  - Hypovolemia
  - Vascular instability: Autonomic neuropathy, drug-related, dialysate-related
- Neurologic complications:
  - Cerebrovascular accident
  - Disequilibrium syndrome
  - Hyperglycemia or hypoglycemia
  - Hypernatremia or hyponatremia
  - Hypoxemia
  - Intracranial bleed
  - Meningitis or abscess
  - Uremia
- Peritoneal complications:
  - Peritonitis
  - Hernia incarceration
  - Perforated viscus
  - Acute abdominal process: Appendicitis, cholecystitis

# TREATMENT

## PRE-HOSPITAL

### ALERT
- Do not perform IV access and BP measurement in extremity with functioning AV graft or fistula.
- Run IV fluids slowly and keep to minimum, if possible.
- Administer furosemide in pulmonary edema (anuric patients: Use high doses $\leq$200 mg).

### INITIAL STABILIZATION/THERAPY
- Check airway, breathing, and circulation.
- Vascular access–related:
  - Bleeding:
    - Firm pressure to site(s)
    - Do not totally occlude access; may cause clotting.
    - Will likely need pressure applied for at least 5–10 min to stop even minor bleeding
    - Document presence or absence of thrill after pressure was applied.
    - Apply Gelfoam.
- Nonvascular access–related:
  - Hypotension:
    - Search for underlying cause.
    - Vasopressors, fluids
  - Shortness of breath:
    - Preload and afterload reduction with nitrites and ACE inhibitors.
    - Attempt diuresis if fluid overload is suspected cause.
    - Arrange for dialysis.
  - Hyperkalemia:
    - Administer IV calcium, bicarbonate, insulin, and glucose when appropriate (see "Hyperkalemia").
    - Monitor cardiac rhythm.
    - Administer ion-exchange resin (Kayexalate).
    - Arrange for dialysis.
  - Neurologic complications:
    - Administer naloxone, thiamine, dextrose (or Accu-Chek) for altered mental status.
    - Control seizures with benzodiazepines.

### ED TREATMENT/PROCEDURES
- Vascular access–related:
  - Infection:
    - Initiate antistaphylococcal IV/IV antibiotics.
  - Clotted access:
    - Analgesia
    - Warm compresses
    - Vascular surgery consult
  - Hemorrhage:
    - Control bleeding.
    - Correct coagulopathies.
    - Administer IV fluids and blood products.
- Nonvascular access–related:
  - Electrolyte imbalances:
    - Treat hypercalcemia or hypermagnesemia with saline infusion if tolerated (dilution).
    - Diuresis with furosemide after preload and afterload reduction (nitroglycerin, enalapril)
    - Arrange for dialysis.

- Volume overload:
  - Attempt diuresis with nitrites and furosemide.
  - Arrange for dialysis.
- Pericardial effusion or tamponade:
  - Emergent pericardiocentesis may be necessary in unstable patient.
  - Arrange for dialysis.
- Acute MI:
  - Thrombolytics or angioplasty if patient is appropriate candidate
  - Nitrates to decrease myocardial workload
- Disequilibrium syndrome:
  - Rule out other causes of altered mental status.
  - Generally resolves over time
- Peritoneal:
  - Peritonitis: IV or intraperitoneal antibiotics
  - Culture catheter or tunnel infection, visible exudates:
    - Oral antibiotics (antistaphylococcal)
    - If recurrent or tunnel, may need to be unroofed
    - Meticulous site care
  - Perforated viscous:
    - IV antibiotics
    - Surgical consultation

## MEDICATION
- Calcium gluconate: 1 g slowly IV (cardioprotective in hyperkalemia with widened QRS complex)
- Cefazolin: 1 g IV or IM followed by 250 mg/2 L bag for 10 days (peritonitis)
- Captopril: 25 mg sublingually
- Dextrose $D_{50}W$: 01 amp: 50 mL or 25 g (peds: dextrose $D_{25}W$: 2–4 mL/kg) IV
- Dopamine: 2–20 $\mu$g/kg/min IV
- Enalapril: 1.25 mg IV
- Furosemide: 20–100 mg IV (may require doses of $\geq$30 mg to effect diuresis in chronic renal failure)
- Insulin: 5–10 U regular insulin IV (with $D_{50}$ for hyperkalemia)
- Naloxone (Narcan): 2 mg (peds: 0.1 mg/kg) IV or IM initial dose
- Nitroglycerin: 0.4 mg sublingually; 5–20 $\mu$g/min IV
- Sodium bicarbonate: 1 mEq/kg up to 50–100 mEq IV PRN
- Sodium polystyrene sulfonate (Kayexalate): 1 g/kg up to 15–60 g PO or 30–50 g retention enema q6h PRN (for hyperkalemia)
- Thiamine (vitamin $B_1$): 100 mg (peds: 50 mg) IV or IM
- Tobramycin: 1.7 mg/kg IV or IM followed by 10 mg/2 L bag for 10 days (peritonitis)
- Vancomycin: 1 g IV or IM followed by 50 mg/2 L bag for 10 days (peritonitis)

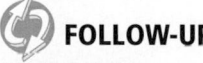

# FOLLOW-UP

## DISPOSITION
### Admission Criteria
- ICU admission:
  - Severe hyperkalemia
  - Pulmonary edema

- Volume overload
- Persistent hypotension
- Uncontrolled seizures
- Acute MI
- Cardiovascular accident
- Pericarditis
- Sepsis
- Peritonitis with toxic or systemic symptoms
- Regular admission:
  - Fever
  - Vomiting
  - Peritonitis without toxic or systemic symptoms
  - Non–life-threatening electrolyte disturbances
  - Inability to provide self-care for continuous ambulatory peritoneal dialysis with antibiotics

### Discharge Criteria
- Mild infections of access site
- Same-day surgery for some thrombectomy procedures
- Hemostasis at puncture sites

## FOLLOW-UP RECOMMENDATIONS
Most patients on dialysis are followed closely by their nephrologists.

## PEARLS AND PITFALLS
- Consider cardiac tamponade in dialysis patients, even when they don't exhibit classic symptoms.
- Always consider hyperkalemia in dialysis patients.
- Infections can have very subtle presentations in dialysis patients.

## ADDITIONAL READING
- Feldman HI, Held PJ, Hutchinson JT, et al. Hemodialysis vascular access morbidity in the United States. Kidney Int. 1993;43(Suppl 41): S1091–S1096.
- Kahn IH, Catto GRD. Long-term complications of dialysis: Infection. Kidney Int. 1993;43(Suppl 41): S143–S148.
- Wolfson AB. Renal failure. In: Marx JA, ed. Rosen's emergency medicine: Concepts and clinical practice, 7th ed. Philadelphia, PA: Mosby; 2010:1257–1281.

### See Also (Topic, Algorithm, Electronic Media Element)
- Renal Failure
- Hyperkalemia

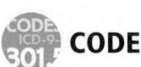 CODES

### ICD9
- 458.21 Hypotension of hemodialysis
- 998.11 Hemorrhage complicating a procedure
- 999.39 Infection following other infusion, injection, transfusion, or vaccination

# DIAPER RASH

Francesco Mannelli
Amy LePage
Kristine Thompson

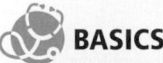 **BASICS**

## DESCRIPTION
- Very common dermatologic disorder of infancy
- Most common in 1st mo of life and again at 12–24 mo
- Incidence in adults unknown but common among incontinent patients
- Primary irritant/contact dermatitis:
  - Outer skin layers are broken down, leading to inflammation and loss of protective barrier function.
  - Increased skin moisture encourages growth of microorganisms on the surface of the skin.
  - Secondary fungal or bacterial infection can cause more severe forms of diaper dermatitis.
- Also known as irritant diaper dermatitis

## ETIOLOGY
- Irritants:
  - Moisture:
    ○ Prolonged overhydration owing to infrequent diaper changes, poorly absorbing diapers, or cloth diapers
  - Friction:
    ○ Diaper rubbing on skin or loose-fitting diaper
  - Chemicals:
    ○ Prolonged exposure to stool enzymes and urine
    ○ Scents or moisturizers in wipes or soap
    ○ Diaper material or adhesive used to hold diaper in place
- Infection:
  - *Candida albicans*:
    ○ Isolated in up to 80% of infants
    ○ Overgrowth common after systemic antibiotic use
  - Bacterial
  - Often complication of other causes of dermatitis:
    ○ *Staphylococcus aureus, Streptococcus, Escherichia coli* are common; *Peptostreptococcus* and *Bacteroides* may also be encountered.
- Seborrheic diaper dermatitis
- Atopic diaper dermatitis (contact dermatitis)
- Risk factors:
  - Oral thrush
  - Number of previous episodes of diaper rash
  - Duration of use of diapers
  - Diarrhea

 **DIAGNOSIS**

Diagnosis often empiric based on appearance of rash

## SIGNS AND SYMPTOMS
### History
Child may cry with diaper changes or wiping diaper area or may be irritable.

### Physical Exam
- Irritant
- Beefy-red confluent patches with distinct borders at diaper edges, typically sparing skin folds
- Infectious:
  - *Candida*—demarcated erythematous rash with satellite pustules or papules, typically involves skin folds
  - Bacterial—superficial erosions with yellow crust and occasionally bullae
- Seborrheic diaper dermatitis:
  - Lesions with erythematous base and greasy yellow or gray scale
  - Infant will likely have similar lesions on other body surfaces, especially scalp.
- Atopic diaper dermatitis:
  - Similar appearance to irritant dermatitis, but lesions also on other body surfaces such as the face.
- Variations include:
  - Jacquet form—erosive variant with ulcers or erosions with elevated margins usually seen with persistent diarrhea or adult urinary incontinence.
  - Psoriasiform—erythema, silvery surface scales and spared skin folds; also likely to have similar lesions on other body surfaces.
  - Granuloma gluteale infantum—violaceous papules and nodules on the buttocks and in the groin with a self-limited course, resolving in weeks or months, often with residual scarring.

## ESSENTIAL WORKUP
- Inquire about diaper-changing habits and urinary and fecal habits.
- Examine other body areas to identify associated rashes.
- Consider child abuse or neglect:
  - Child's overall hygiene
  - Burns or other trauma

## DIAGNOSTIC TESTS & INTERPRETATION
### Lab
- Laboratory evaluation usually not necessary for management of diaper dermatitis.
- Bacterial cultures usually not indicated except in complicated cases.
- Skin surface scrapings with KOH prep and/or culture may help distinguish between *Candida* and atypical seborrheic dermatitis:
  - Look for budding yeast and/or pseudohyphae.

## DIFFERENTIAL DIAGNOSIS
- Child abuse or neglect
- Infection:
  - Impetigo
  - Scabies
  - Herpes simplex
  - Varicella
  - Congenital syphilis
- Psoriasis
- Atopic dermatitis
- Seborrheic dermatitis
- Papular urticaria
- Bullous pemphigoid
- Epidermolysis bullosa
- Acrodermatitis enteropathica
- Acrodermatitis enteropathica-like eruption
- Langerhans cell histiocytosis

**TREATMENT**

### ED TREATMENT/PROCEDURES

- Environmental adjustments:
  - Education of parents and caregivers is essential:
    - Cleanse skin frequently using cotton balls and water.
    - Wet wipe and talcum powder are not recommended.
  - Frequent diaper changes, up to q1h for neonates and q3–q4h for infants and adults.
  - Gentle rinsing of affected area with warm water or saline.
  - Avoid harsh soaps or alcohol wipes.
  - Leave area uncovered as much as possible; allow time to air dry.
  - Highly absorbent diapers have less incidence of diaper rash than cloth diapers.
  - Cloth diapers are not recommended for patients with irritant diaper dermatitis.
  - New diapers that are "breathable" or contain top sheet of zinc oxide/petroleum and stearyl alcohol lining have been shown to decrease incidence.
- Barrier creams:
  - Many preparations available containing zinc oxide, petroleum, lanolin.
    Should be applied after each diaper change and continued after rash resolves to minimize recurrence
  - A substantial negative relationship exists between barrier cream use and number of previous episodes of diaper dermatitis.
  - If *Candidal* infection present, apply over antifungal medication.
- Corticosteroids:
  - For moderate to severe cases not responding to other therapy
  - Should not be stronger than 1% hydrocortisone: Anything stronger can cause serious side effects.
  - Discontinue after 3–5 days.

- Antifungals:
  - Nystatin cream, powder, or ointment:
    - Expect improvement in 1–2 days.
    - Ointment best tolerated on macerated skin.
  - Clotrimazole applied topically after diaper change.
  - Miconazole applied topically after diaper change.
  - Lotion is preferred in intertriginous areas.
  - Cream should be applied sparingly to avoid maceration effects.
  - Ciclopirox applied topically after diaper change.
  - Generally continue 1–2 days after clearing
  - Antifungal agent also found to have some antibacterial activity and anti-inflammatory properties.
  - Consider oral agent if concurrent cutaneous or oral candidiasis is present or in recalcitrant case because stool may be colonized with *C. albicans*.
- Antibacterials:
  - Typically concurrent with other therapies if suspicion of bacterial infection
  - Mupirocin (Bactroban ) applied after diaper changes
  - Systemic antibiotics rarely needed

### MEDICATION

- Ciclopirox 0.77% cream, gel, or suspension: Applied topically b.i.d. after diaper change
- Clotrimazole 1% cream: Applied topically b.i.d. after diaper change
- Hydrocortisone 0.5–1% topical cream: Applied b.i.d.
- Miconazole topical 2% cream: Applied b.i.d. after diaper change
- Miconazole nitrate 0.25% ointment: Apply after diaper change and bathing
- Mupirocin 2% ointment or cream (Bactroban): Applied topically 3–5 times daily after diaper changes (for infants >3 mo of age)
- Nystatin 100,000 U/g cream, powder, or ointment: Apply b.i.d. after diaper change

 **FOLLOW-UP**

### DISPOSITION
*Admission Criteria*
- Evidence of child abuse or neglect
- Evidence of sepsis

## ADDITIONAL READING

- Adalat S, Wall D, Goodyear H. Diaper dermatitis-frequency and contributory factors in hospital attending children. *Pediatr Dermatol*. 2007;24(5):483–488.
- Adam R. Skin care of the diaper area. *Pediatr Dermatol*. 2008;25(4):427–433.
- Gupta AK, Skinner AR. Management of diaper dermatitis. *Int Soc Derm*. 2004;43:830–834.
- Humphrey S, Bergman JN, Au S. Practical management strategies for diaper dermatitis. *Skin Therapy Lett*. 2006;11(7):1–6.
- Van L, Harting M, Rosen T. Jacquet erosive diaper dermatitis: A complication of adult urinary incontinence. *Cutis*. 2008;82(1):72–74.

**CODES**

### ICD9
- 112.3 Candidiasis of skin and nails
- 691.0 Diaper or napkin rash

# DIAPHRAGMATIC TRAUMA

*Jennifer Cullen*

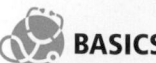 **BASICS**

## DESCRIPTION
- Penetrating injury:
  - Violation of the diaphragm by penetrating object (most commonly stab and gunshot wounds)
  - May involve any portion of diaphragm
- Blunt injury:
  - Increased intra-abdominal or intrathoracic pressure is transmitted to diaphragm, causing rupture.
  - Usually due to motor vehicle crashes
  - Injuries are more commonly left-sided:
    - Left hemidiaphragm has posterolateral embryologic point of weakness.
    - Right hemidiaphragm is protected by liver.
    - Injuries are larger than with penetrating injury (frequently between 5–15 cm in length).
- Diaphragmatic defects do not heal spontaneously because of pleuroperitoneal pressure gradient:
  - May exceed 100 cm $H_2O$ during maximal respiratory effort
  - Promotes herniation of abdominal contents through rent in diaphragm and into chest

## EPIDEMIOLOGY
### Incidence
Estimated to be 1–7% in substantial blunt trauma and 10–15% in penetrating injuries

## ETIOLOGY
- Lateral torso impact is 3 times more likely to result in ipsilateral diaphragmatic rupture than frontal impact.
- Suspect diaphragmatic injury:
  - Penetrating trauma to thoracoabdominal area
  - Injuries that cross plane of the diaphragm

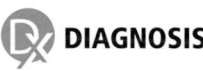 **DIAGNOSIS**

## ALERT
In acute phase, there may be no abdominal visceral herniation:
- This injury may even be missed on initial laparotomy or laparoscopy.

## SIGNS AND SYMPTOMS
- Vary depending on whether phase is acute, latent, or obstructive:
  - Acute:
    - Tachypnea
    - Hypotension
    - Absence of breath sounds
    - Abdominal distention
    - Bowel sounds in chest
  - Latent:
    - Abdominal discomfort from intermittent herniation of abdominal contents into thorax
    - Abdominal pain that is worse postprandially
    - Exacerbated by lying supine
    - Pain radiating to left shoulder
    - Nausea, vomiting, or belching
  - Obstructive:
    - Severe abdominal pain
    - Obstipation
    - Nausea, vomiting
    - Abdominal distention
- Strangulated abdominal organs may perforate and spill abdominal contents into chest.
- Respiratory compromise, sepsis, and death

## ESSENTIAL WORKUP
CXR may reveal herniated loops of bowel or other abdominal viscera in thorax:
- Pathognomonic finding is presence of nasogastric tube above diaphragm.
- Findings are often nonspecific:
  - Elevated hemidiaphragm
  - Irregular diaphragmatic contour
  - Mediastinal shift away from affected side
  - Unilateral pleural thickening or pleural effusion
  - Areas of atelectasis or consolidation at bases
  - Small hemothorax or pneumothorax
- 50% of initial CXRs may be normal.
- Diagnosis may be difficult in latent phase because of intermittent nature of herniation.
- Contrast studies of GI tract may be helpful.

## DIAGNOSTIC TESTS & INTERPRETATION
### Lab
- If diagnostic peritoneal lavage (DPL) is performed:
  - Red blood cell count of 1,000 $RBC/mm^3$ is considered positive for diaphragmatic injury after penetrating trauma.
  - May provide false-negative result in up to 40% of patients with isolated diaphragmatic injury
- No laboratory studies confirm or rule out presence of diaphragmatic injury.

### Imaging
- CXR is diagnostic in 90% of cases in which herniation is present, but sensitivity is limited in absence of acute hernia.
- GI contrast studies are the most useful in diagnosing chronic herniation of abdominal contents through diaphragm.
- US may be used, particularly on right side with accompanying hepatic herniation.
- Conventional CT is rarely diagnostic and has poor sensitivity.
- New multidetector CT (MDCT) has had much better success at diagnosing subtle diaphragmatic injuries.
- MRI is useful in its ability to visualize the diaphragm as a discrete structure, but is not practical in acute settings.

### Diagnostic Procedures/Surgery
- Diagnostic pneumoperitoneography:
  - Air is injected through DPL catheter.
  - Pneumothorax on subsequent CXR is diagnostic of diaphragmatic injury.
  - Poorly tolerated by unstable patients and may require chest tube placement.
- Thoracoscopy and laparoscopy are potentially valuable tools, both diagnostically and therapeutically:
  - Especially useful in penetrating trauma to left thoracoabdominal region, with its high prevalence of diaphragmatic injury

## DIFFERENTIAL DIAGNOSIS
- Atelectasis
- Hemothorax
- Pneumothorax
- Pulmonary contusion
- Gastric dilation, intra-abdominal fluid
- Traumatic pneumatocele
- Subdiaphragmatic abscess
- Intrathoracic cyst
- Empyema
- Congenital eventration of the diaphragm

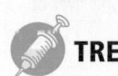 TREATMENT

### ALERT
Herniation of abdominal contents into chest wall may mimic hemothorax or tension pneumothorax:
- Bowel sounds in chest may help distinguish
- Be suspicious of diaphragmatic injury with lateral compression of chest:
  - Be cautious in placement of needle or tube thoracostomies.
- Fecal thorax has been reported with bowel rupture.

### INITIAL STABILIZATION/THERAPY
- Follow advanced trauma life support (ATLS) protocols.
- If respiratory distress is present, immediate placement of a nasogastric tube may decompress herniated abdominal contents.

### ED TREATMENT/PROCEDURES
- Palpate within the chest wall completely for visceral organs before placing chest tube.
- Patients with visceral perforations are septic and need aggressive resuscitation and antibiotic therapy.
- Early surgical intervention is paramount.
- Thoracoscopy or laparoscopy is useful in selected injuries and patients.
- Empiric broad-spectrum antibiotics are indicated in the case of perforated viscera.

### MEDICATION
- Gram-negative aerobes:
  - Gentamicin: Adults/peds: 2–5 mg/kg IV initial dose
- Gram-negative anaerobes:
  - Clindamycin: 900 mg (peds: 20–40 mg/kg/24 h) IV q8h
  - Metronidazole: 1 g (peds: 15 mg/kg) IV load, then 500 mg (peds: 7.5 mg/kg) IV q6h
- Both aerobic and anaerobic:
  - Ampicillin/sulbactam: 1.5–3 g (peds: 100–400 mg/kg/24 h) IV q6h
  - Cefotetan: 2 g (peds: 40–80 mg/kg/24 h) IV q12h
  - Cefoxitin: 2 g (peds: 80–160 mg/kg/24 h) IV q12h
  - Ticarcillin/clavulanate: 3.1 g (peds: 50 mg/kg per dose) IV q6h

 FOLLOW-UP

### DISPOSITION
#### Admission Criteria
- Patients with suspicion for diaphragmatic injury must be admitted to trauma surgery.
- Patients should be admitted to the monitored or ICU setting.

#### Discharge Criteria
Patients with diaphragmatic injury or any significant suspicion for it must not be discharged from ED.

### FOLLOW-UP RECOMMENDATIONS
Patients with diaphragmatic injuries s/p repair must be followed by trauma surgeon to monitor for recurrence.

#### Pediatric Considerations
- Pediatric anatomic differences predispose to diaphragmatic injury via less severe mechanisms:
  - Thinner abdominal wall
  - More horizontal orientation of diaphragm
  - Greater cartilaginous rib component
- Incidence of right- and left-sided injury is equal.
- More likely to be isolated injury

## PEARLS AND PITFALLS
- Overall mortality is 18–40% depending on mechanism.
- Highly associated with concomitant severe injuries to spleen and liver, and with pelvic fractures.
- Must have high index of suspicion for diaphragmatic injury with left-sided upper abdominal and lower thoracic penetrating trauma.
- Always obtain chest imaging.

## ADDITIONAL READING
- Blaivas M, Brannam L, Hawkins M, et al. Bedside emergency ultrasonographic diagnosis of diaphragmatic rupture in blunt abdominal trauma. *Am J Emerg Med*. 2004;22(7):601–604.
- Hanna WC, Ferri LE. Acute traumatic diaphragmatic injury. *Thorac Surg Clin*. 2009;19:485–489.
- Lewis JD, Starnes SL, Pandalai PK, et al. Traumatic diaphragmatic injury: Experience from a level I trauma center. *J Surgery*. 2009;146(4):578–584.
- Shah R, Sabanathan S, Mearns AJ, et al. Traumatic rupture of the diaphragm. *Ann Thorac Surg*. 1995;60(5):1444–1449.
- Shehata S, Shabaan BS. Diaphragmatic injuries in children after blunt abdominal trauma. *J Pediatr Surg*. 2006;41:1727–1731.
- Sliker CW. Imaging of diaphragm injuries. *Radiol Clin N Am*. 2006;44:199–211.

 CODES

### ICD9
002.0 Injury to diaphragm without mention of open wound into cavity

# DIARRHEA, ADULT
Isam F. Nasr

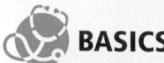

## BASICS

### DESCRIPTION
Bowel movements characterized as frequent (>3/day), loose and watery owing to an infectious or toxin exposure

### ETIOLOGY
- Viruses:
  - 50–70% of all cases
- Invasive bacteria:
  - Campylobacter:
    - Contaminated food or water, wilderness water, birds, and animals
    - Most common bacterial diarrhea
    - Gross or occult blood is found in 60–90%.
  - Salmonella:
    - Contaminated water, eggs, poultry, or dairy products
    - Typhoid fever (Salmonella typhi) characterized by unremitting fever, abdominal pain, rose spots, splenomegaly, and bradycardia
  - Shigella:
    - Fecal or oral route
  - Vibrio parahaemolyticus:
    - Raw and undercooked seafood
  - Yersinia:
    - Contaminated food (pork), water, and milk
    - May present as mesenteric adenitis or mimic appendicitis
- Bacterial toxin:
  - Escherichia coli:
    - Major cause of traveler's diarrhea
    - Ingestion of food or water contaminated by feces
  - Staphylococcus aureus:
    - Most common toxin-related disease
    - Symptoms 1–6 hr after ingesting food
  - Bacillus cereus:
    - Classic source—fried rice left on steam tables
    - Symptoms within 1–36 hr
  - Clostridium difficile:
    - Antibiotic-associated enteritis linked to pseudomembranous colitis
    - Incubation period within 10 days of exposure or initiation of antibiotics
  - Aeromonas hydrophila:
    - Aquatic sources primarily
    - Affects children <3 yr of age
    - Fecal leukocytes absent
  - Cholera:
    - Caused by enterotoxin produced by Vibrio cholerae
    - Profuse watery stools with mucus (classic appearance of rice-water stools)

- Protozoa:
  - Giardia lamblia:
    - Most common cause of parasite gastroenteritis in North America
    - High-risk groups: Travelers, children in day care centers, institutionalized people, homosexual men, and campers who drink untreated mountain water
  - Cryptosporidium parvum:
    - Commonly carried in patients with AIDS
  - Entamoeba histolytica (entamebiasis):
    - 5–10% extraintestinal manifestations (hepatic amebic abscess)

### Pediatric Considerations
- Most are viral in origin and self-limited.
- Rotavirus accounts for 50%.
- Shigella: Infections associated with seizures
- Focus evaluation on state of hydration.

## DIAGNOSIS

### SIGNS AND SYMPTOMS
#### History
- Loose, watery bowel movements
- Bloody stools with mucus
- Abdominal pain and cramps, tenesmus, flatulence
- Fever, headache, myalgias
- Nausea, vomiting
- Dehydration, lethargy, and stupor

#### Physical Exam
- Dry mucous membranes
- Abdominal tenderness
- Perianal inflammation, fissure, fistula

### ESSENTIAL WORKUP
- Digital rectal exam to determine presence of gross or occult blood
- Fecal leukocyte determination:
  - Present with invasive bacteria
  - Absent in protozoal infections, viral, toxin-induced food poisoning

## DIAGNOSTIC TESTS & INTERPRETATION
### Lab
- CBC—indications:
  - Significant blood loss
  - Systemic toxicity
- Electrolytes, glucose, BUN, creatinine—indications:
  - Lethargy, significant dehydration, toxicity, or altered mental status
  - Diuretic use, persistent diarrhea, chronic liver or renal disease
- Stool culture—indications:
  - Presence of fecal leukocytes
  - Historical markers: Immunocompromised, travel, homosexual
  - Public health: Food handler, day care or health care worker, institutionalized
- Blood cultures—indications:
  - Suspected bacteremia or systemic infections
  - Ill patients requiring admission
  - Immunocompromised
  - Elderly patients and infants

### Imaging
Abdominal radiographs:
- No value unless obstruction or toxic megacolon suspected

### DIFFERENTIAL DIAGNOSIS
- Ulcerative colitis
- Crohn disease
- Mesenteric ischemia
- Diverticulitis, anal fissures, hemorrhoids
- Irritable bowel syndrome
- Milk and food allergies
- Malrotation with midgut volvulus
- Meckel diverticulum
- Intussusception
- Appendicitis
- Drugs and toxins:
  - Mannitol
  - Sorbitol
  - Phenolphthalein
  - Magnesium-containing antacids
  - Quinidine
  - Colchicine
  - Mushrooms
  - Mercury poisoning

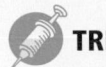 **TREATMENT**

**PRE-HOSPITAL**
- Difficult IV access with severe dehydration
- Avoid exposure to contaminated clothes or body substances.

**INITIAL STABILIZATION/THERAPY**
- ABCs
- IV fluid with 0.9% normal saline (NS) resuscitation for severely dehydrated

**ED TREATMENT/PROCEDURES**
- Oral fluids for mild dehydration (Gatorade/Pedialyte)
- IV fluids for:
  - Hypotension, nausea and vomiting, obtundation, metabolic acidosis, significant hypernatremia or hyponatremia
  - 0.9% NS bolus: 500 mL–1 L (peds: 20 mL/kg) for resuscitation, then 0.9% NS or D$_5$W 0.45% NS (peds: D$_5$W 0.25% NS) to maintain adequate urine output
- Bismuth subsalicylate (Pepto-Bismol):
  - Antisecretory agent
  - Effective clinical relief without adverse effects
- Kaolin-pectin (Kaopectate):
  - Reduces fluidity of stools
  - Does not influence course of disease
- Antimotility drugs: Diphenoxylate (Lomotil), loperamide (Imodium), paregoric, codeine:
  - Appropriate in noninfectious diarrhea
  - Initial use of sparse amounts to control symptoms in infectious diarrhea
  - Avoid prolonged use in infectious diarrhea—may increase duration of fever, diarrhea, and bacteremia and may precipitate toxic megacolon
- Antibiotics for infectious pathogens:
  - *Campylobacter*: Quinolone or erythromycin
  - *Salmonella*: Quinolone or trimethoprim-sulfamethoxazole (TMP-SMX)
  - Typhoid fever: Ceftriaxone
  - *Shigella*: Quinolone, TMP-SMX, or ampicillin
  - *Vibrio parahaemolyticus*: Tetracycline or doxycycline
  - *Clostridium difficile*: Vancomycin
  - *Escherichia coli*: Quinolone or TMP-SMX
  - *Giardia lamblia*: Metronidazole or quinacrine
  - *Entamoeba histolytica* (entamebiasis): Iodoquinol or metronidazole

**MEDICATION**
- Ampicillin: 500 mg (peds: 20 mg/kg/24 hr) PO or IV q6h
- TMP-SMX (Bactrim DS): 1 tab (peds: 8–10 mg TMP/40–50 mg SMX/kg/24 hr) PO or 4–5 mg/kg TMP IV b.i.d.
- Ceftriaxone: 1 g (peds: 50–75 mg/kg/12 hr) IM or IV q12h.
- Ciprofloxacin (quinolone): 500 mg PO or 400 mg IV q12hr (>18 yr)
- Doxycycline: 100 mg PO or 100 mg IV q12h
- Erythromycin: 500 mg (peds: 40–50 mg/kg/24 hr) PO q.i.d.
- Iodoquinol: 650 mg (peds: 30–40 mg/kg/24 hr) PO t.i.d.
- Metronidazole: 250 mg (peds: 35 mg/kg/24 hr) PO t.i.d. (>8 yr)
- Quinacrine: 100 mg (peds: 6 mg/kg/24 hr) PO t.i.d.
- Tetracycline: 500 mg PO or IV q6h
- Vancomycin: 500 mg (peds: 10–50 mg/kg/24 hr) IV q6h

 **FOLLOW-UP**

**DISPOSITION**
**Admission Criteria**
- Hypotension, unresponsive to IV fluids
- Significant bleeding
- Signs of sepsis or toxicity
- Intractable vomiting or abdominal pain
- Severe electrolyte imbalance or metabolic acidosis
- Altered mental status
- Children with >10–15% dehydration

**Discharge Criteria**
- Mild cases requiring oral hydration
- Dehydration responsive to IV fluids

**Issues for Referral**
Cases of prolonged diarrhea may be referred to a gastroenterologist for further workup.

**FOLLOW-UP RECOMMENDATIONS**
Since diarrhea is self-limiting, follow-up is optional.

**PEARLS AND PITFALLS**
- Avoid prolonged use of antimotility dugs in infectious diarrhea.
- TMP-SMX (Bactrim DS), ciprofloxacin, doxycycline and tetracycline are contraindicated in pregnancy. Metronidazole may be used in the third trimester.
- Health care providers and food handlers with documented infectious diarrhea may need clearance to return to work from their local health department.
- Infectious diarrhea with *C. difficile* is on the rise, especially in nursing home patients.

**ADDITIONAL READING**
- Chen L. Infectious diarrheal disease and dehydration. In: J Marx, Hockberger R, Walls S, eds. *Rosen's Emergency Medicine*, 7th ed. Philadelphia: Elsevier, 2009:2188–2199.
- Dupont HL. What's new in enteric infectious diseases at home and abroad. *Curr Opinion Infect Dis.* 2005;18:407–412.
- Hogan D. The emergency department approach to diarrhea. *Emerg Med Clin North Am.* 1996;14(4): 673–694.
- Leffler, DA, Lamont, JT. Treatment of Clostridium difficile–associated disease. *Gastroenterology.* 2009;136:1899.
- Reisdorff E, Pflug V. Infectious diarrhea: Beyond supportive care. *Emerg Med Rep.* 1996;17(14): 141–150.
- Surawicz CM. Infectious causes of chronic diarrhea. *Gastroenterol Clin North Am.* 2001;30(3):679–692.

**See Also (Topic, Algorithm, Electronic Media Element)**
Gastroenteritis

 **CODES**

**ICD9**
- 008.5 Bacterial enteritis, unspecified
- 008.8 Intestinal infection due to other organism, not elsewhere classified
- 787.91 Diarrhea

# DIARRHEA, PEDIATRIC

Richard Lichenstein
Rajender Gattu

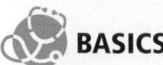

## BASICS

### DESCRIPTION
- One of the most common pediatric complaints; 2nd only to respiratory infections in overall disease frequency fo ED visits
- Leading cause of illness and death in children worldwide
- Acute infectious enteritis (AIE):
  - Vomiting and diarrhea
  - Children <5 yr in the U.S. typically have 2 episodes annually.
  - Responsible for ~10% of all pediatric ED visits and hospital admissions
- Acute change in the "normal" bowel pattern that leads to increased number or volume of stools and lasts <7 days; World Health Organization (WHO) defines case as 3 or more loose or watery stools per day.
  - Chronic if the diarrhea persists for >2 wk

### ETIOLOGY
- Acute enteritis:
  - Infectious:
    - Viruses: 70–80% of cases:
      - Rotavirus most common
      - Enteric adenovirus
      - Norovirus (food borne outbreaks)
    - Bacteria: 10–20%:
      - *E. coli*, Yersinia, *C. difficile*
      - Salmonella, Shigella, Campylobacter
      - Vibrio sp.
      - Aeromonas sp.
    - Parasites: 5%:
      - Cryptosporidiosis (water-borne)
      - *Giardia lambia*
  - Noninfectious:
    - Postinfectious
    - Food allergies and intolerance:
      - Cow's milk protein
      - Soy protein
      - Methyl xanthines
      - Lactose intolerance
    - Chemotherapy/radiation induced
    - Drug induced:
      - Antibiotics, laxatives, antacids
    - Ingestion of heavy metals-copper, zinc
    - Ingestion of plants-hyacinth, daffodils, amanita species
    - Vitamin deficiency: Niacin, folate
    - Vitamin toxicity: Vitamin C, B$_3$
  - Associated with other infections (parenteral):
    - Otitis media
    - UTI
- Chronic diarrhea:
  - Dietary factors: Excessive consumption of sorbitol or fructose from fruit juices
  - Enteric infections in immunocompromised
  - Malnutrition
  - Endocrine: Thyrotoxicosis, pheochromocytoma
  - Inflammatory bowel diseases: Crohn's disease, ulcerative colitis
  - Malabsorption syndromes (cystic fibrosis, celiac disease)
  - IBS

## DIAGNOSIS

### SIGNS AND SYMPTOMS
- Frequent, loose stools
- Signs of dehydration:
  - Watery
  - Bloody
  - Mucoid
  - Sometimes abdominal pain, fever, anorexia
  - Tenesmus
- Signs of dehydration reflect degree of loss of total-body water and vary with the degree of dehydration: Mild <5%, moderate 5–10%, severe >15%
- Severe dehydration:
  - Mental status change: Often depressed with significant dehydration associated with impaired muscle tone
  - Mucous membrane: Dry
  - Skin turgor: Decreased
  - Anterior fontanel: Depressed
  - Blood pressure: Decreased
  - Pulse: Tachycardia
  - Capillary refill: Prolonged (>2 sec)
  - Urine output: Decreased
  - Eyes: Sunken and absent tears
  - Thirst
- Patients with diabetes mellitus and DKA may be dehydrated in the face of increased thirst and ongoing urine output

### History
- Onset and duration
- Mental status and muscle tone
- Fever and associated symptoms, for example: Abdominal pain, emesis
- Stool frequency and character
- Urine output
- Feeding
- Recent antibiotics
- Recent travel
- Possible ingestions

### Physical Exam
- Abnormal capillary refill >2 sec
- Absent tears
- Dry mucus membranes
- General ill appearance. In several studies, appearance, degree of sunken eyes, dry mucus membranes, and tear production are associated with length of stay and need for IV fluids in children with acute gastroenteritis:
  - Clinical dehydration scales based on a combination of physical exam findings are better predictors than individual signs.

### ESSENTIAL WORKUP
Majority of children with acute diarrhea do not require any lab tests. Consider workup if:
- Temp >103°F
- Systemic illness
- Bloody diarrhea
- Prolonged course >2 wk

- Tenesmus
- Dehydration greater than mild, usually requiring parenteral therapy
- Diarrhea with blood or mucus suggests an enteroinvasive inflammatory or cytotoxin-mediated process (*Salmonella*, invasive *E. coli*).

### DIAGNOSTIC TESTS & INTERPRETATION
#### Lab
- CBC with differential, blood culture, urine culture, and UA—if any signs of systemic infection
- Basic metabolic panel including electrolytes, BUN, creatinine, bicarbonate, for any child treated with IV hydration for severe dehydration or with those patients with abnormal physical signs:
  - Recent evidence suggests that serum bicarbonate is particularly helpful in detecting moderate dehydration.
  - Stool pH <5.5 or positive stool-reducing substances are positive in lactose intolerance.
- Stool microscopy:
  - >5 fecal leucocytes per high-power field is suggestive of invasive bacterial infection:
    - Shigella
    - Salmonella
    - Campylobacter
    - Yersinia
    - Invasive *E. coli*
- Stool culture:
  - Unnecessary in most cases unless there is a high likelihood of identifying bacterial pathogens (positive guaiac and/or fecal leucocytes) for which the clinical course and period of contagion may be altered by antibiotic therapy
- Consider urine culture in febrile children ≤12 mo.

#### Imaging
Usually not indicated unless high clinical suspicion for other diagnoses based on history and physical exam

#### Diagnostic Procedures/Surgery
Usually not indicated unless high clinical suspicion for other diagnoses based on history and physical exam

### DIFFERENTIAL DIAGNOSIS
- *Giardia lamblia*
- Postinfectious:
  - Follows acute or bacterial or viral gastroenteritis; often associated with malabsorption, especially lactose
- *C. difficile* may follow use of antibiotics.
- Milk allergy
- Malrotation with midgut volvulus
- Inflammatory bowel disease
- Intussusception
- UTI
- Malabsorption syndromes

**TREATMENT**

## INITIAL STABILIZATION/THERAPY

- For severely dehydrated children in shock or near shock, IV or intraosseous access with 20 mL/kg 0.9% NS and 1 g/kg dextrose if hypoglycemic
- Pulse oximetry
- Endotracheal intubation may be required for children in shock.

## ED TREATMENT/PROCEDURES

- For mild to moderate dehydration, correct dehydration using oral rehydration therapy (ORT), 50 mL/kg and 100 mL/kg, respectively, over a 4-hr period:
  - Replace ongoing losses with 10 mL/kg of ORT for each stool.
  - Ideal ORT solution has a low osmolarity (210–250) and sodium content of 50–60 mmols/L.
- For moderate to severe dehydration, correct dehydration using parenteral fluids combining maintenance and deficit requirements.
- If diarrhea is not associated with dehydration, use 10 mL/kg of ORT for each stool alone.
- Antibiotics only for defined acute enteritis:
  - Erythromycin for *Campylobacter jejuni*
  - TMP-SMX for:
    - *Salmonella*—complicated (infant <6 mo old, disseminated, bacteremia, immunocompromised host, enteric fever)
    - *Shigella*
    - *Yersinia*
    - *E. coli*—enteroinvasive
  - Metronidazole or vancomycin for:
    - *C. difficile* (severe and or prolonged enteritis)
    - Neomycin for *E. coli*—enteroadherent
  - Furazolidone or metronidazole for G. lamblia
- Antidiarrheal agents *not* recommended
- Probiotics: *Lactobacillus GG* and *Saccharomyces boulardii* are an effective adjunct when treating the acute diarrhea in children in reducing the duration of symptoms.
- Post-ED diet:
  - While rehydrating, feed children with diarrhea age-appropriate diets.
  - Well-tolerated foods:
    - Rich in complex carbohydrates (rice, potatoes, bread)
    - Lean meats
    - Yogurt
    - Fruits
    - Vegetables
    - Full-strength milk and formula unless there is a strong suspicion of lactose intolerance
  - Avoid fatty foods and foods high in simple sugars.

## MEDICATION

- Ampicillin: 50–200 mg/kg/24 h IV/PO q6h
- Erythromycin: 40 mg/kg/24 h PO q6h; 10–20 mg/kg/24 h IV q6h
- Furazolidone: 6 mg/kg/24 h PO q6h
- Metronidazole: 30 mg/kg/24 h PO q.i.d. × 7 days
- Neomycin: 50–100 mg/kg/24 h PO q6–8h
- Nitazoxanide: 100 mg PO b.i.d. (age 1–3 yr); 200 mg PO b.i.d. for older
- TMP-SMX: 8–10 mg/kg/24 h as TMP PO b.i.d.
- Vancomycin: 40–50 mg/kg/24 h PO q6h
- Loperamide (not for use in children <6 yr old or in those with heme-positive stools): Age 6–8 yr, 2 mg PO b.i.d.; age 8–12 yr, 2 mg PO t.i.d.
- Cefixime: 8 mg/kg/d PO per day for 7–10 days
- Ceftriaxone: 50 mg/kg/d IV/IM for 7–10 days
- *Lactobacillus GG* and *Saccharomyces boulardii*: 5 billion doses/d
- Zinc: 10–20 mg/d for 10–14 days (children <5 yr)

### First Line
- TMP-SMX for *Salmonella* sp. and *Shigella* sp.
- Doxycycline for *V. cholera*
- Metronidazole for *C. difficile*

### Second Line
- Ceftriaxone and Cefotaxime for Salmonella and Shigella species
- Erythromycin for *V. cholera*.
- Vancomycin for resistant *C. difficile*

 **FOLLOW-UP**

## DISPOSITION

### Admission Criteria
- Surgical abdomen
- Inability to tolerate oral fluids
- 10% dehydration or greater
- Suspected complicated Salmonella enteritis
- Toxic-appearing child

### Discharge Criteria
- Improvement in the patient's condition
- Caregivers of child can follow through with appropriate ORT and diet.
- Caregivers able to report signs and symptoms of dehydration

### Issues for Referral
- Immunocompromised host
- Conditions associated with complications such as seizures
- Hypernatremic dehydration

## FOLLOW-UP RECOMMENDATIONS
Follow-up care depends on the length and severity of diarrhea, age of the child, and caregivers ability to comply with instructions:
- Uncomplicated diarrhea does not typically need follow-up.
- Neonates require strict follow-up care in a few days.

## PEARLS AND PITFALLS

- History and PE assists in differentiating uncomplicated diarrhea from other, often more serious conditions in children.
- Vast majority of children with acute diarrhea do not need extensive lab tests, which are unlikely to affect the management.
- Treatment with antidiarrheals and antibiotics has very limited role in childhood diarrhea.
- Diagnoses like appendicitis, intussusception, UTI, and sepsis may need to be considered.

## ADDITIONAL READING

- King CK, Glass R, Bresee JS, et al. Managing acute gastroenteritis among children: Oral rehydration, maintenance, and nutritional therapy. *MMWR Recomm Rep.* 2003;52(RR-16):1–16.
- Bellamare S, Harting L, Wiebe N. Oral rehydration versus intravenous hydration for treating dehydration due to gastroenteritis in children. A meta-analysis of randomized controlled trials. *BMC Med.* 2004;2:11.
- Canavan A, Arant BS Jr. Diagnosis and management of dehydration in children. *Am Fam Physician.* 2009;80(7):692–696.
- Allen SJ, Okoko B, Martinez E. Probiotics for treating infectious diarrhoea. *Cochrane Database Syst Rev.* 2004:CDC003048.
- Steiner MJ, DeWalt DA, Byerley JS. Is this child dehydrated? *JAMA.* 2004;291(22):2746–2754.
- Spandorfer PR, Alessandrini EA, Joffe MD, et al. Oral versus intravenous rehydration of moderately dehydrated children: A randomized controlled trial. *Pediatrics.* 2005;115:295–301.

### See Also (Topic, Algorithm, Electronic Media Element)
Vomiting, Pediatric

**CODES**

### ICD9
- 009.0 Infectious colitis, enteritis, and gastroenteritis
- 787.91 Diarrhea

# DIGOXIN, POISONING

*Kirk L. Cumpston*

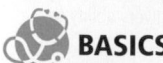

## BASICS

### DESCRIPTION
- Acute digitalis effects (elevated levels in children and intentional overdose):
  - Inhibits sodium-potassium ATPase pump in cell membranes
  - Allows more calcium ions to enter cell and cardiac cells to contract more strongly
  - Increases $K^+$ extracellularly
  - Increases vagal tone
  - Slows atrioventricular (AV) node conduction (vagotonic)
  - Increases automaticity and conduction system refractory period
  - Bradydysrhythmias
- Chronic digitalis effects (therapeutic to toxic levels in elderly patients):
  - Inhibits sodium-potassium ATPase pump in cell membranes
  - Increases intracellular calcium
  - Increases vagal tone
  - Increases automaticity
  - Usually hypokalemic secondary to diuretic use
  - Tachydysrhythmias

### ETIOLOGY
- Digoxin/digitoxin pharmaceuticals
- Plants and animals containing cardiac glycosides:
  - Foxglove
  - Oleander
  - Lily of the valley
  - Dogbane
  - Red squill
  - Cane toad, Colorado River toad

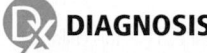

## DIAGNOSIS

### SIGNS AND SYMPTOMS
- Toxicity onset: 2 hr after PO ingestion and 15 min following IV
- Toxicity:
  - Occurs with normal digoxin levels (chronic)
  - May be absent with elevated digoxin levels (acute)
- Cardiovascular:
  - Dysrhythmias:
    - Paroxysmal atrial tachycardia (PAT) with AV block
    - Bidirectional ventricular tachycardia is pathognomonic
    - Premature ventricular contractions (PVCs) most common
    - Nonparoxysmal accelerated junctional tachycardia
    - Ventricular tachycardia (VT)
    - Atrial fibrillation
    - Bigeminy
    - Bradycardia
    - Nonparoxysmal atrial tachycardia
    - AV blocks
    - Sinus arrhythmia
    - Premature atrial contraction
  - CHF exacerbation
  - Hypotension
  - Shock
  - Cardiovascular collapse
  - Syncope
- CNS:
  - Mental status changes:
    - Agitation
    - Lethargy
    - Psychosis
- Visual perception:
  - Blurred
  - Scotoma
  - Green to yellow halo
  - Photophobia
  - Color perception changes
- GI:
  - Anorexia, nausea, vomiting, abdominal pain

### History
- Accidental adult or pediatric overdose of a known amount
- Intentional acute overdose in a patient not taking digoxin chronically
- Intentional acute on chronic overdose in a patient taking digoxin chronically
- Unintentional toxicity from chronic ingestion of digoxin in which renal clearance decreases or the dose chronically increases

### Physical Exam
- Altered mental status
- Bradycardia
- Tachycardia
- Irregular rhythm
- Hypotension

### ESSENTIAL WORKUP
- ECG:
  - For dysrhythmia
- Digoxin level:
  - Normal range: 0.5–2.0 ng/mL
  - Distribution after oral intake not complete until 6 hr; therefore, > 6-hr level is most accurate steady state concentration.
  - False elevations possible with spironolactone use, pregnancy, hyperbilirubinemia, chronic renal failure, liver failure, CHF
  - May be falsely elevated after digoxin-specific fab fragments given

## DIAGNOSTIC TESTS & INTERPRETATION
### Lab
- Electrolytes, BUN, creatinine, glucose:
  - Hypokalemia contributes to digitalis toxicity.
  - Hyperkalemia seen in acute toxicity and correlates with acute digitalis mortality better than digoxin serum levels.
  - Follow $K^+$ serially
- Calcium, magnesium

### ALERT
Serum digoxin concentration should not be obtained after digoxin-specific antibody Fab fragments have been administered because it will be inaccurate.

### DIFFERENTIAL DIAGNOSIS
- Overdoses:
  - Calcium channel blockers
  - $\beta$-Blockers
  - Quinidine, procainamide
  - Clonidine
  - Organophosphates
  - Antidysrhythmics
  - Other antihypertensives
- Primary cardiac dysrhythmias
- Acute gastroenteritis

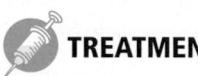

## TREATMENT

### PRE-HOSPITAL

### ALERT
If cardioversion is necessary for tachydysrhythmias, use low levels (50 J):
- May precipitate refractory tachydysrhythmias

### INITIAL STABILIZATION/THERAPY
ABCs:
- IV, oxygen, monitor:
  - IV fluid bolus if hypovolemic
- Administer naloxone, thiamine, dextrose, for altered mental status.

### ED TREATMENT/PROCEDURES
- Cardiac arrest resuscitation:
  - Defibrillate for ventricular fibrillation, pulseless VT.
  - Standard advanced cardiac life support (ACLS) protocol
  - Administer digoxin-specific antibody Fab fragments (Digibind), up to 5–20 vials IV push (IVP).
  - $MgSO_4$, 2 g IVP
  - Continue resuscitation for 30 min after digoxin-specific antibody Fab fragments.

- General measures:
  - Gastric lavage if <1 hr after acute ingestion and history of life-threatening ingestion, hemodynamically stable, and airway stabilization
  - Activated charcoal if acute ingestion
  - Replenish magnesium.
  - Treat hyperkalemia with insulin, dextrose, bicarbonate, sodium polystyrene sulfonate.

### ALERT
Calcium can probably be used to treat hyperkalemia, but because other safer alternatives exist it is not recommended. If the patient has hyperkalemia from digoxin toxicity treatment with digoxin-specific Fab fragments are indicated 1st.

Dysrhythmia management:

- 1st choice is digoxin-specific antibody Fab fragments. If these are not immediately available, initiate the following:
  - Lidocaine:
    - For ventricular dysrhythmias without AV block
    - Not harmful but not very effective
  - For bradydysrhythmias:
    - Atropine
  - Pacing for symptomatic bradydysrhythmia

### ALERT
IV pacemakers have been associated with greater mortality in digoxin poisoned patients

- MgSO$_4$ for ventricular dysrhythmias with torsades de pointes
- Quinidine, procainamide contraindicated

- Cardioversion is last resort for severe, life-threatening tachydysrhythmia:
  - Start at low energy 10–50 J, then increase to high levels if ineffective.
  - Safe if digoxin level <2.0 ng/mL
- Digoxin-specific antibody Fab fragments (Digibind, Digi Fab):
  - Indications:
    - Serum digoxin concentration ≥15 ng/mL at anytime or ≥10 ng/mL at steady state (6 hr)
    - Ingestion of >10 mg in adults or 0.2 mg/kg or 4 mg in children
    - Hyperkalemia >5.0–5.5 mEq/L
    - Hemodynamically unstable or life-threatening dysrhythmias
    - Ventricular tachycardia, ventricular fibrillation
    - Atrial tachycardia
    - Variable AV block
    - Bradycardia with no response to atropine
    - Hypotension

- Onset: 20–30 min
- Digoxin levels may increase, decrease, or stay in therapeutic range after therapy owing to Fab digoxin complexes.
- Renal clearance of drug–antibody complexes:
  - Too large to be removed by dialysis
- 2nd dose if rebound toxicity
- Complications:
  - Exacerbation of CHF
  - Hypokalemia
  - Atrial fibrillation with rapid ventricular response

### MEDICATION
- Activated charcoal slurry:
  - 1 mg/kg if within 1 hr
- Digoxin-specific antibody Fab fragments:
  - 40-mg vial neutralizes 0.6 mg of digoxin.
  - If amount ingested known:
    - Number of vials needed equals amount ingested mg/0.6.
  - If steady serum level known:
    - Number of vials needed equals serum digoxin level multiplied by patient's weight in kg/100.
  - If neither amount ingested or serum level known:
    - Acute toxicity: 5–10 vials adults or children
    - Chronic toxicity: 2–3 vials adults
  - Bolus for cardiac arrest
  - Additional doses as needed
- Standard treatment for hyperkalemia and bradycardia (calcium only if necessary)

#### Geriatric Considerations
- Dosage is based on weight and serum concentration. There is no change in the setting of renal or hepatic dysfunction.
- Recrudescence of toxicity has been reported in patients with concomitant renal failure. Redosing of digoxin-specific Fab fragments should be used again when indicated.

#### Pediatric Considerations
- Weight-based dosing for children is the same as it is for adults.
- On some occasions, accidental dose ingested by a child is known and the number of vials is indicated by the amount of digoxin bound by each vial. See dosing.

#### Pregnancy Considerations
Digoxin-specific Fab fragments are pregnancy class C.

 **FOLLOW-UP**

#### DISPOSITION
##### Admission Criteria
- ICU:
  - Unstable cardiovascular status in acute or chronic toxicity
- Telemetry:
  - Asymptomatic or mildly symptomatic dysrhythmia
  - High risk for developing toxicity

##### Discharge Criteria
Acute/chronic ingestion:
- Digoxin level <2.0 ng/mL
- Asymptomatic for 6 hr and no ECG abnormalities

#### FOLLOW-UP RECOMMENDATIONS
Psychiatric referral for stable patients who are suicidal

## PEARLS AND PITFALLS

When it is known that the patient is on digoxin and presents with cardiovascular instability, and/or hyperkalemia, treatment should begin with the antidote: Digoxin-specific Fab fragments.

## ADDITIONAL READING

- Bismuth C, Gaultier F, Conso Efthymiou ML. Hyperkalemia in acute digitalis poisoning: Prognostic significance and therapeutic implications. *J Toxicol Clin Toxicol.* 1973;6(2):153–162.
- Erickson CP, Olson KR. Case files of the medical toxicology fellowship of the California poison control system San Francisco-calcium plus digoxin more taboo than toxic? *J Med Toxicol.* 2008;4(1):33–39.

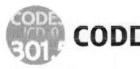 **CODES**

#### ICD9
972.1 Poisoning by cardiotonic glycosides and drugs of similar action

# DISSEMINATED INTRAVASCULAR COAGULATION

Steven H. Bowman
Rajan Parikh

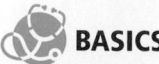 **BASICS**

## DESCRIPTION
- Normal coagulation: Series of local reactions among blood vessels, platelets, and clotting factors
- Disseminated intravascular coagulation (DIC) is systemic activation of coagulation and fibrinolysis by some other primary disease process.
- Coagulation system activation results in systemic circulation of thrombin and plasmin.
- Role of thrombin in DIC:
  - Thrombin circulates and converts fibrinogen to fibrin monomer.
  - Fibrin monomer polymerizes into fibrin (clot) in the circulation.
  - Clots cause microvascular and macrovascular thrombosis with resultant peripheral ischemia and end organ damage.
  - Platelets become trapped in clot with resultant thrombocytopenia.
- Role of plasmin in DIC:
  - Plasmin circulates systemically converting fibrinogen into fibrin degradation products (FDPs).
  - FDPs combine with fibrin monomers.
  - FDP–monomer complexes interfere with normal polymerization and impair hemostasis.
  - FDPs also interfere with platelet function.
- Acute DIC—uncompensated form:
  - Clotting factors used more rapidly than body can replace them
  - *Hemorrhage* predominant clinical feature, which overshadows ongoing thrombosis
- Chronic DIC—compensated form:
  - Body able to keep up with pace of clotting factor consumption
  - *Thrombosis* predominant clinical feature

## ETIOLOGY
- Precipitated by many disease states
- Complications of pregnancy:
  - Retained fetus
  - Amniotic fluid embolism
  - Placental abruption
  - Abortion
  - Eclampsia
  - HELLP syndrome
- Sepsis:
  - Gram-negative (endotoxin-mediated meningococcemia)
  - Gram-positive (mucopolysaccharide-mediated)
  - Other microorganisms (eg, viruses, parasites)

- Trauma:
  - Crush injury
  - Severe burns
  - Severe head injury
  - Fat embolism
- Malignancy:
  - Solid tumor or metastatic disease
  - Hematologic malignancy (eg, leukemia)
- Intravascular hemolysis:
  - Transfusion reactions
  - Massive transfusion
- Organ destruction:
  - Severe pancreatitis
  - Severe hepatic failure
- Vascular abnormalities:
  - Kasabach-Merritt syndrome
  - Large vascular aneurysm
- Thrombocytopenia:
  - Thrombotic thrombocytopenic purpura
  - Idiopathic thrombocytopenic purpura

 **DIAGNOSIS**

## SIGNS AND SYMPTOMS
- Excessive bleeding:
  - Petechiae
  - Purpura
  - Hemorrhagic bullae
  - Wound bleeding
  - Epistaxis
  - Hemoptysis
  - GI bleeding
- Excessive thrombosis:
  - Large vessels
  - Microvascular thrombosis and end organ dysfunction
  - Cardiac, pulmonary, renal, hepatic, CNS
  - Thrombophlebitis
  - Pulmonary embolus
  - Nonbacterial thrombotic endocarditis
  - Gangrene
  - Ischemic infarcts of kidney, liver, CNS, bowel
- Acute DIC:
  - Hemorrhagic complications predominate.
- Chronic DICL:
  - Thrombotic complications predominate.

## History
- Previous history of bleeding disorder
- Pregnancy/last menstrual period
- History of malignancy or immunocompromise

## Physical Exam
- Neuro:
  - Altered MS, confusion, lethargy
- Cardiovascular:
  - Hypotension, tachycardia
- Respiratory:
  - Tachypnea, rhonchi, rales
- GI:
  - Upper or lower GI bleeding, abdominal distension
- GU:
  - Oliguria, hematuria
- Skin:
  - Petechia, purpura, jaundice

## ESSENTIAL WORKUP
- Depends on precipitating illness
- Diagnosis generally not made in ED

## DIAGNOSTIC TESTS & INTERPRETATION
### Lab
- Platelet count:
  - Decreased
  - $<100,000/mm^3$
  - May be normal in chronic DIC
- Prothrombin time (PT)/partial thromboplastin time (PTT):
  - Increased
  - May be normal in chronic DIC
- Fibrinogen:
  - Decreased
  - $<150$ mg/dL in 70%
  - May be normal in chronic DIC
- FDPs:
  - Increased
  - $>40$ $\mu$g/mL
- D-dimer increased
- CBC/peripheral smear:
  - Red cell fragments
  - Low platelets
  - Peripheral smear confirms disease in chronic DIC
- Electrolytes, BUN, creatinine, glucose:
  - Elevated BUN, creatinine owing to renal insufficiency
- ABGs:
  - Oxygen, acid base status

### Imaging
- CXR for suspected pneumonia
- Head CT for altered mental status
- OB US in pregnant patients

## DIFFERENTIAL DIAGNOSIS
- Inherited coagulation disorders:
  - Factor deficiencies
- Other acquired coagulation disorders:
  - Anticoagulant therapy
  - Drugs
  - Hepatic disease
- Platelet dysfunction:
  - TTP/HUS
  - HIT
  - ITP

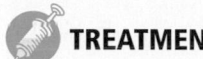 **TREATMENT**

### INITIAL STABILIZATION/THERAPY
- Airway management and resuscitation measures:
  - Control bleeding
  - Establish IV access
  - Restore and maintain circulating blood volume.
- Initiate therapy of precipitating disease:
  - Antibiotics in sepsis
  - Evacuate uterus of retained products of conception.
  - Chemotherapy in malignancy
  - Debridement of devitalized tissue in trauma

### ED TREATMENT/PROCEDURES
- Therapy of DIC is controversial and should be individualized based on:
  - Age
  - Hemodynamic status
  - Severity of hemorrhage
  - Severity of thrombosis
- Involve admitting service before initiating specific DIC therapy.
- Replace depleted blood components:
  - Fresh frozen plasma (FFP):
    - For prolonged PT
    - Provides clotting factors and volume replacement
    - Dose: 2 U or 10–15 mL/kg
  - Platelets:
    - If platelet count <20,000 or platelet count <50,000 with ongoing bleeding
    - Dose: 1 U/10 kg body weight
  - Cryoprecipitate:
    - Higher fibrinogen content than whole plasma
    - For severe hypofibrinogenemia (<50 mg/dL) or for active bleeding with fibrinogen <100 g/dL
    - Dose: 8 U
  - Washed packed cells
  - Albumin
  - Nonclotting volume expanders

- Inhibit intravascular clotting with heparin:
  - Use is controversial.
  - Consider when thrombosis predominates.
  - May be effective in mild to moderate DIC
  - Efficacy undetermined in severe DIC. Possible indications:
    - Purpura fulminans (gangrene of digits, extremities)
    - Acute promyelocytic leukemia
    - Dead fetus syndrome—several weeks after intrauterine fetal death
    - Thromboembolic complications of large vessels
    - Before surgery with metastatic carcinoma
  - Administer heparin, antithrombin concentrates alone or in combination (controversial):
  - Administer activated protein C (controversial):
    - Mortality benefit seen in severe sepsis complicated by DIC
- Inhibit fibrinolysis:
  - Block secondary compensatory fibrinolysis that accompanies DIC
  - Use complicated by severe thrombosis
  - Use only when DIC accompanied by primary fibrinolysis:
    - Promyelocytic leukemia
    - Giant hemangioma
    - Heat stroke
    - Amniotic fluid embolism
    - Metastatic carcinoma of prostate
  - Initiate in extreme cases only:
    - Profuse bleeding not responding to replacement therapy
    - Excessive fibrinolysis present (rapid whole blood lysis/short euglobulin lysis time)
    - ε-Aminocaproic acid (EACA)
    - Tranexamic acid

### MEDICATION
Specific DIC treatment is usually not initiated in the ED. Underlying precipitating diseases should be treated initially:

- Heparin:
  - Low-dose regimen: 5–10 U/kg/hr IV for chronic DIC
  - High-dose regimen: 10,000 U bolus followed by 1,000 U/h; 20,000–30,000 U q24h via constant infusion

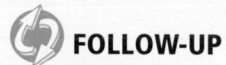 **FOLLOW-UP**

### DISPOSITION
**Admission Criteria**
Severe precipitating illness in combination with DIC requires ICU admission.

**Discharge Criteria**
None

### FOLLOW-UP RECOMMENDATIONS
Follow-up involves following platelets and coagulation factors.

## PEARLS AND PITFALLS
- Suspect DIC as a complicating factor in severe, life-threatening illness.
- Establish early clinical suspicion since the sequelae of DIC can be devastating.
- Remember to consider treating the underlying cause of DIC when the thromboembolic and bleeding complications of the process seem to be dominating the clinical picture.

## ADDITIONAL READING
- Bick RL. Disseminated intravascular coagulation: Current concepts of etiology, pathophysiology, diagnosis, and treatment. *Hematol Oncol Clin North Am.* 2003;17(1):149–176.
- Levi M. Disseminated intravascular coagulation. *Crit Care Med.* 2007;35:2191–2195.
- Rodgers GM. Acquired coagulation disorders. In: Greer I, et al., eds. *Wintrobe's Clinical Hematology.* 12th ed. Philadelphia: Lippincott Williams & Wilkins; 2009:1422–1455.
- Seligsohn U. Disseminated intravascular coagulation. In: Lichtman M, et al., eds. *Williams Hematology,* 7th ed. New York: McGraw-Hill; 2006;1959–1979.

### See Also (Topic, Algorithm, Electronic Media Element)
- Sepsis
- Idiopathic Thrombocytopenic Purpura
- Thrombotic Thrombocytopenic Purpura

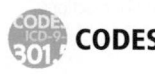 **CODES**

**ICD9**
286.6 Defibrination syndrome

# DISULFIRAM REACTION

Timothy J. Meehan
Sean M. Byrant

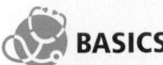 **BASICS**

## DESCRIPTION

- Inhibits various enzymes and its active metabolites exert additional effects.
- Disulfiram-ethanol reaction:
  - Usually occurs 8–12 hr after taking the drug; should not be observed >24 hr after dosing
  - Competitively and irreversibly inactivates aldehyde dehydrogenase
  - Ethanol metabolism is blocked, resulting in accumulation of acetaldehyde.
  - Acetaldehyde produces release of histamine resulting in vasodilation and hypotension.
  - Severe reactions may occur in drinkers with ethanol levels of 50–100 mg/dL.
  - Severity and duration of reaction is proportional to amount of ethanol ingested.
- Disulfiram blocks dopamine $\beta$-hydroxylase and limits synthesis of norepinephrine from dopamine:
  - Relative excess of dopamine may contribute to altered behavior.
  - Relative depletion of norepinephrine may contribute to hypotension.
- Disulfiram metabolite (carbon disulfide) interacts with pyridoxal 5-phosphate:
  - Diminishes concentration of pyridoxine available for formation of $\gamma$-aminobutyric acid (GABA) in CNS
  - Potentially lowers seizure threshold
  - Carbon disulfide is also cardiotoxic, hepatotoxic, and inhibits cytochrome P-450 (CYP2E1).
- Disulfiram metabolites may chelate important metals (copper, zinc, iron) essential in various enzyme systems.
- Disulfiram metabolites may cause peripheral neuropathies that are dose and duration dependent.

## ETIOLOGY

- Disulfiram is used as deterrent in treatment of chronic ethanol abuse.
- Many users of the medication wear medical alert bracelet.
- Other agents producing disulfiram-like reactions:
  - Antibiotics:
    - Cephalosporins
    - Nitrofurantoin
    - Metronidazole
  - Oral hypoglycemics:
    - Sulfonylureas
  - Industrial agents:
    - Carbon disulfide
    - Hydrogen sulfide
  - Mushrooms:
    - *Coprinus atramentarius*
    - *Clitocybe clavipes*

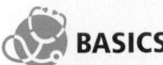 **DIAGNOSIS**

## SIGNS AND SYMPTOMS

- Disulfiram overdose:
  - Symptoms rare with <3 g ingested
  - 10–30 g may be lethal.
  - Tachycardia, hypotension, tachypnea
  - Abdominal pain, diarrhea, garlic, or rotten-egg breath
  - Agitation, irritability, ataxia
  - Dysarthria, hallucinations
  - Lethargy, coma, seizures, flaccidity
  - Parkinsonian syndrome
- Disulfiram–ethanol reaction:
  - Hypotension, tachycardia, tachypnea
  - Flushing of face, neck, torso
  - Pruritus, diaphoresis, sensation of warmth
  - Nausea, vomiting, abdominal pain, diarrhea
  - Headache, ataxia, confusion, anxiety, dizziness
  - Dyspnea, pulmonary edema, chest pain, dysrhythmias, myocardial infarction

## History

Ingestion of disulfiram or agents listed above may provide essential clues to diagnosis.

## Physical Exam

- Vital signs:
  - Hypotensive, tachycardic, tachypneic
- Cardiovascular:
  - Tachycardia, arrhythmias
- Pulmonary:
  - Pulmonary edema, dyspnea
- Abdominal:
  - Diffuse abdominal pain, nausea, vomiting
- Skin:
  - Flushed, diaphoretic
- Neurologic:
  - Dysphoric, confusion, signs of cerebellar dysfunction, seizures

## ESSENTIAL WORKUP

Suspect disulfiram–ethanol reaction with the following:

- Typical signs and symptoms are present.
- Treatment for chronic ethanol abuse in conjunction with recent ethanol ingestion, or exposure to ethanol-containing foods or medications, including mouthwash

## DIAGNOSTIC TESTS & INTERPRETATION
### Lab

- Ethanol level
- Electrolytes, BUN, creatinine, and glucose
- Liver function tests if hepatitis is suspected
- Creatine phosphokinase (CPK) if considering rhabdomyolysis in light of seizures or agitation
- Urinalysis (myoglobin)
- Serum levels of offending agent are NOT clinically useful.

### Imaging

- ECG to assess cardiac ischemia or dysrhythmia
- CT scan or MRI:
  - Indicated with altered mental status/seizure
  - Basal ganglia ischemia and infarction have been reported.
- EEG:
  - Diffuse slowing without focal abnormalities has been seen in cases of acute toxicity with coma.

## DIFFERENTIAL DIAGNOSIS

- Sepsis
- Meningitis, encephalitis
- Cardiogenic shock secondary to acute coronary syndrome
- Anaphylactoid/anaphylactic reaction
- Gastroenteritis/pancreatitis with dehydration
- Ethanol withdrawal

### Pediatric Considerations

- Acute poisonings yield mainly severe CNS toxicity.
- Ataxia, weakness, lethargy, seizures
- Reye syndrome-like encephalopathy in severe cases
- Adult symptoms may also be present.

**TREATMENT**

### PRE-HOSPITAL
- ABCs, IV access
- Begin resuscitation with IVF if no signs or symptoms of pulmonary edema.
- Rapid glucose determination (Accu-Chek)

### INITIAL STABILIZATION/THERAPY
- ABCs:
  - Airway protection if necessary
  - Supplemental oxygen
  - Mechanical ventilation as needed
  - Resuscitation with 0.9% NS IV for hypotension
- Pressor support with norepinephrine for refractory hypotension

### ED TREATMENT/PROCEDURES
- Management is primarily supportive with aggressive, appropriate care:
  - No specific antidote available
- GI decontamination:
  - Activated charcoal in cases of disulfiram overdose:
    - Caution if mental status depression
    - Caution if vomiting (potential for aspiration)
    - Do not intubate solely to give activated charcoal
  - Gastric lavage is unnecessary. Whole-bowel irrigation is not indicated.
- Alleviation of flushing:
  - Antihistamines ($H_1$ and $H_2$ antagonists)
  - Prostaglandin inhibitors (indomethacin, ketorolac)
- Antiemetics for intractable vomiting (ondansetron, metoclopramide)
- Seizures:
  - Benzodiazepines (diazepam, lorazepam)
  - Pyridoxine (vitamin $B_6$)
  - 4-Methylpyrazole:
    - Inhibits ethanol metabolism at alcohol dehydrogenase enzyme
    - Not indicated for disulfiram–ethanol reactions or disulfiram overdose
- Hemodialysis:
  - Consider after massive ingestion of disulfiram and ethanol with refractory hypotension.
  - No studies documenting beneficial effect

### MEDICATION
- Diazepam: 5–10 mg (peds: 0.2–0.5 mg/kg) IV
- Diphenhydramine: 25–50 mg (peds: 1–2 mg/kg) IV
- Indomethacin: 50 mg PO (peds: 0.6 mg/kg PO for age >14 yr)
- Lorazepam: 2–6 mg (peds: 0.03–0.05 mg/kg) IV
- Metoclopramide: 10 mg (peds: 1–2 mg/kg) IV
- Norepinephrine: 4 mL in 1,000 mL of $D_5W$, infused at 0.1–0.2 $\mu$g/kg/min
- Ondansetron: 4 mg (peds: 0.1 mg/kg for >2 yr old) IV
- Pyridoxine: 1 g (peds: 500 mg) IV, repeat PRN

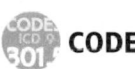 **FOLLOW-UP**

### DISPOSITION

#### Admission Criteria
- ICU admission for mechanical ventilation, coma, refractory hypotension requiring pressors, cardiac ischemia, refractory seizures, and severe agitation
- Persistent vomiting, abdominal pain, or flushing
- Elderly patients or those who have pre-existing cardiac disease

#### Discharge Criteria
- Mild reactions that resolve with supportive care after observation period of 8–12 hr:
  - Symptoms may recur on rechallenge with ethanol up to 7–10 days after last dose of disulfiram or agents that cause disulfiram-like reactions.
  - Abstain from ethanol use until at least 2 wk after last dose of such agents.
- Appropriate follow-up needed to assess development of hepatic or neurologic sequelae

### FOLLOW-UP RECOMMENDATIONS
- Psychiatry follow-up for intentional overdose with disulfiram
- Detox follow-up for patients with disulfiram–ethanol reactions

## PEARLS AND PITFALLS
- Educate patients who are prescribed medications with potential for disulfiram-like reactions to avoid ALL alcohol.
  - Includes: Mouthwash, alcohol-based hand gels, alcohol-based aftershaves, some cough syrups.
- Recommend abstinence for 3 days longer than the course of treatment to ensure low likelihood of reaction.

## ADDITIONAL READING
- Enghusen Poulsen H, Loft S, Anderson JR, et al. Disulfiram therapy adverse drug reactions and interactions. *Acta Psychiatr Scand*. 1992;86:59–66.
- Kuffner EK. Disulfiram and disulfiram-like reactions. In: Goldfrank LR. *Goldfrank's Toxicologic Emergencies*. McGraw-Hill; 2002;971–979.
- Johansson B. A review of the pharmacokinetics and pharmacodynamics of disulfiram and its metabolites. *Acta Psychiatr Scand*. 1992;86:15–26.
- Leikin J, Paloucek F. Disulfiram. In: *Poisoning and Toxicology Handbook*. Hudson, OH: Lexi-Comp; 2002;502–503.
- Park CW, Rissio S. Disulfiram ethanol induced delirium. *Ann Pharmacother*. 2001;35:32–35.
- Petersen EN. The pharmacology and toxicology of disulfiram and its metabolites. *Acta Psychiatr Scand*. 1992;86:7–13.
- Watson WA. Disulfiram. In: *Clinical Toxicology*. Philadelphia: WB Saunders; 2001;591–594.

### See Also (Topic, Algorithm, Electronic Media Element)
Alcohol Poisoning

## CODES

### ICD9
995.29 Unspecified adverse effect of other drug, medicinal and biological substance

# DIVERTICULITIS
*Ronald E. Kim*

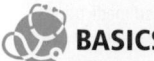

## BASICS

### DESCRIPTION
- Inflammation and/or perforation of diverticulum:
  - Microscopic or macroscopic
  - Uncomplicated vs. complicated
- Incidence increasing

### ETIOLOGY
- Fecal material in diverticulum hardens, forming fecalith.
- Fecalith abrades mucosa or compromises blood supply, causing inflammation.
- Inflammation causes microperforation of bowel wall:
  - Peridiverticulitis: Inflammation of wall not extending beyond serosa (uncomplicated diverticulitis)
  - Pericolic abscess: Serosal perforation, yet inflammation remains localized (complicated diverticulitis)
  - Peritonitis: Serosal perforation with generalized spread of inflammation (complicated diverticulitis)
- Uncomplicated diverticulitis:
  - Colonic wall thickening
  - Inflammatory changes (fat stranding on CT)
- Complicated diverticulitis:
  - Abscess
  - Bowel obstruction
  - Fistulas after recurrent attacks
  - Colovesical fistula (most common) presents with dysuria, frequency, urgency, pneumaturia, and fecaluria.

## DIAGNOSIS

### SIGNS AND SYMPTOMS
#### History
- Symptoms develop over hours to days
- Anorexia
- Nausea, vomiting
- Low-grade fever
- Malaise
- Abdominal pain:
  - Persistent
  - Initially vague
  - Becomes localized to left lower abdomen
- Abdominal distention
- Diarrhea (colon irritation) or constipation (inflammatory obstruction)
- Flatulence, heartburn
- Urinary frequency:
  - Owing to contact of inflamed colon against bladder

#### Physical Exam
- Tenderness at left lower quadrant with occasional mass palpated (phlegmon):
  - *Phlegmon*—inflamed bowel loops or abscess
- Bowel sounds normal, increased, or decreased
- Rectal tenderness with heme-positive stool:
  - Massive gross rectal bleeding (rare)
- Peritoneal signs if:
  - Perforation has occurred

- Unremarkable examination if:
  - Elderly
  - Immunocompromised
  - Taking corticosteroids

### ESSENTIAL WORKUP
- CBC:
  - Elevated WBC with left shift
  - Iron deficiency anemia suggests underlying carcinoma cause.
- CT of abdomen:
  - Preferred diagnostic modality
  - Better than contrast studies at diagnosing extraluminal processes (eg, diverticulitis)
  - Diagnostic criteria include:
    - Wall thickening >5 mm
    - Inflammation of pericolic fat
    - Pericolic abscess
  - Nondiagnostic criteria include:
    - Stricture
    - Diverticula
    - Fistula
  - Ability to diagnose nondiverticular causes of abdominal pain
  - CT-guided percutaneous needle aspiration of localized abscesses avoids further surgery.
  - Gastrografin PO/PR (per rectum) contrast may be used; avoid barium, especially when perforation is suspected.

### DIAGNOSTIC TESTS & INTERPRETATION
#### Lab
- UA:
  - WBC/RBC common
  - Colovesical fistula results in WBC, bacteria, or feces.
- Blood cultures:
  - If hospitalized with peritonitis

#### Imaging
- Abdominal (supine and upright) and chest radiographs:
  - Perforation indicated by free air
  - Obstruction indicated by air–fluid levels
- CT:
  - Perforation indicated by free air
  - Obstruction indicated by air–fluid levels
  - Accuracy enhanced with use of IV, PO, and PR contrast
- Endoscopy:
  - Not necessary to diagnose acute illness
  - Rigid sigmoidoscopy aids in diagnosing nondiverticular causes of abdominal pain (spasm, stricture, edema, pus, or peridiverticular erythema).
- US:
  - For diagnosing colonic wall thickening, inflammation, mass, abscess, or fistula
  - Greatly operator dependent
  - Not reliable in presence of intestinal gas
- Barium enema:
  - Indicated after resolution of acute illness to rule out fistula or other colonic pathology (eg, carcinoma)
- Avoid endoscopic procedures and barium contrast studies in acute cases so as not to cause perforation:
  - In select cases, water-soluble contrast may be safe alternative.

### DIFFERENTIAL DIAGNOSIS
- Colon carcinoma with perforation
- Ischemic colitis
- Bacterial colitis
- Appendicitis:
  - Left-sided pain if peritonitis from ruptured appendix
  - Right-sided diverticular pain with cecal diverticulum (rare) or redundant sigmoid colon
- Inflammatory bowel disease
- Irritable bowel syndrome
- Ruptured or torsed ovarian cyst
- Pancreatic disease
- Pelvic inflammatory disease
- Peptic ulcer disease
- Renal colic

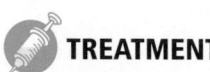

## TREATMENT

### PRE-HOSPITAL
Avoid opiates in abdominal pain when underlying cause is unclear.

### INITIAL STABILIZATION/THERAPY
- Rehydration with 0.9% normal saline (NS) to replace intravascular volume depletion
- Bowel rest:
  - NPO or liquid diet
  - Nasogastric tube (NG) tube if persistent vomiting or bowel obstruction present

### ED TREATMENT/PROCEDURES
- Uncomplicated diverticulitis:
  - Most respond to medical therapy.
- Complicated diverticulitis:
  - Most require percutaneous drainage or surgery.
- Analgesia:
  - Anticholinergics (dicyclomine):
    - Reduces colonic spasm
    - Does not mask underlying pathology
  - Opiates for more aggressive pain management (IV morphine or Demerol although morphine can theoretically increase intraluminal pressure, leading to perforation):
    - If hemodynamically stable
    - When not dependent on repeat abdominal examinations for diagnostic or therapeutic decisions
- Antibiotics to cover gram-negative aerobic and anaerobic bacteria:
  - Mild, uncomplicated cases (peridiverticulitis) for outpatient management:
    - Ciprofloxacin or Levaquin plus metronidazole or clindamycin
    - Trimethoprim/sulfamethoxazole (TMP/SMX) DS plus metronidazole
    - Amoxicillin/clavulanate
    - Duration of therapy is 7–10 days or until afebrile for 3–5 days.
  - Moderate uncomplicated and mild complicated cases for inpatient management:
    - Ceftriaxone or other 3rd-generation cephalosporin plus metronidazole or clindamycin

- ○ Ampicillin/sulbactam
- ○ Piperacillin/tazobactam
- ○ Ticarcillin/clavulanate
- ○ Ciprofloxacin or Levaquin plus metronidazole or clindamycin
- ○ Aztreonam
- – Complicated cases (with peritonitis from perforation):
  - ○ Imipenem/cilastatin
  - ○ Meropenem
  - ○ Aztreonam plus metronidazole or clindamycin
  - ○ Gentamicin plus metronidazole or clindamycin plus/minus ampicillin
  - ○ Trovafloxacin (alternative)
- Surgery:
  - – Emergent surgery:
    - ○ Indicated for generalized peritonitis from perforation
    - ○ Two-stage procedure with resection of diseased segment of colon and proximal colostomy followed later with reanastomosis
  - – Elective surgery:
    - ○ Indicated for: Multiple recurrent attacks (>2) without generalized peritonitis (controversial); fistula formation; intractable pain; unresolved obstruction; failure of medical therapy; single serious attack in patient <50 yr of age (controversial)
    - ○ One-stage procedure following resolution of inflammation from medical therapy
    - ○ Nonoperative management may be considered for complicated diverticulitis.
  - – Peridiverticular abscess drainage:
    - ○ Indicated if well circumscribed and easily accessible
    - ○ Accomplished by CT- or ultrasound-guided percutaneous needle aspiration
- Outpatient therapy:
  - Clear liquids with follow-up in 2–3 days
  - – When acute condition has resolved:
    - ○ High-fiber, low-fat diet to decrease recurrence of attacks

## MEDICATION

- Amoxicillin/clavulanate: 500/125 mg PO t.i.d. or 875/125 mg PO b.i.d.
- Ampicillin: 2.0 g IV q6h
- Ampicillin/sulbactam: 3.0 g IV q6h
- Cefotetan: 2.0 g IV q12h
- Cefoxitin: 2.0 g IV q8h
- Ciprofloxacin: 400 mg IV q12h or 500 mg PO b.i.d.
- Dicyclomine: 20 mg PO q.i.d. (up to 40 mg PO q.i.d.) or 20 mg IM q6h (*not* for IV use)
- Gentamicin: Multiple daily dose (MDD) regimen, 2.0 mg/kg load, then 1.7 mg/kg IV q8h, or once-daily dose (OD) regimen, 5.0–7.0 mg/kg IV q24h (assuming normal renal function)
- Imipenem/cilastatin: 500 mg IV q6h
- Meropenem: 1 g IV q8h
- Meperidine: 50–100 mg IM q3–4h PRN or 25–50 mg IV and titrate to clinical response
- Metronidazole: 1 g (15 mg/kg) IV load then 500 mg IV q8h or 500 mg PO q8h
- Morphine sulfate: 2–10 mg/70 kg body weight IV push slowly

- Piperacillin/tazobactam: 3.375 g IV q6h or 4.5 g IV q8h
- Ticarcillin/clavulanate: 3.1 g IV q6h
- Trimethoprim/sulfamethoxazole DS: 1 tablet PO b.i.d.
- Trovafloxacin: 300 mg IV for 1st dose, then 200 mg IV/PO daily

### First Line

- Uncomplicated diverticulitis (outpatient), 7 to 10 days:
  - – Trimethoprim/sulfamethoxazole DS one tablet PO b.i.d. and metronidazole 500 mg PO q6h or
  - – Ciprofloxacin 750 mg PO b.i.d. and metronidazole 500 mg PO q6h
  - – Amoxicillin/clavulanate extended release 1000/62.5 mg two tablets PO b.i.d.
- Mild to moderate infection (inpatient):
  - – Ticarcillin/clavulanate: 3.1 g IV q6h or
  - – Ampicillin/sulbactam: 3 g IV q6h or
  - – Ciprofloxacin 400 mg IV q12h and metronidazole 1 g IV q12h
- Severe infection (inpatient):
  - – Ampicillin: 2.0 g IV q6h and metronidazole 500 mg IV q6h and gentamicin 7 mg/kg q24h (or ciprofloxacin 400 mg q12h) or
  - – Imipenem 500 mg IV q6h

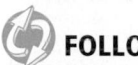 **FOLLOW-UP**

## DISPOSITION

### Admission Criteria

- Intractable pain
- High fever
- Peritonitis
- Failure to respond to outpatient management
- Severe disease on CT scan
- Immunocompromised or steroid-dependent patients
- Recurrent episodes
- Comorbidities: Renal insufficiency, liver dysfunction, COPD, diabetes with end-organ damage
- Extremes of age
- Uncertainty of diagnosis

### Discharge Criteria

- Mild cases (low-grade fever, mild discomfort) of known diverticular disease
- Minimal comorbidities

### Issues for Referral

GI or surgical consult

## FOLLOW-UP RECOMMENDATIONS

- Avoid NSAIDs
- Colonoscopy (or contrast enema x-ray with flexible sigmoidoscopy) should be obtained after resolution of initial episode.

## PEARLS AND PITFALLS

- CT scanning differentiates diverticulitis as complicated or uncomplicated:
  - – Surgery reserved for complicated cases, but nonoperative management becoming more prevalent
- Most cases of uncomplicated diverticulitis rarely progress to complicated disease:
  - – Multiple attacks do not seem to lead to increased complications.
- Diverticulitis does not seem to be a progressively worsening process:
  - – Acute episodes can present at any stage.
- Severe disease on initial CT scan:
  - – Increased risk of failure of medical therapy
  - – High risk of secondary complications

## ADDITIONAL READING

- Lorimer JW, Doumit G. Comorbidity is a major determinant of severity in acute diverticulitis. *Am J Surg.* 2007;193:681–685.
- Nelson RS, et al. Clinical outcomes of complicated diverticulitis managed nonoperatively. *Am J Surg.* 2008;196(6):969–974.
- Touzious IG, Dozois EJ. Diverticulosis and acute diverticulitis. *Gastroenterol Clin.* 2009;38(3):513–525.
- Töö PS, et al. Medical comorbidities predict the need for colectomy for complicated and recurrent diverticulitis. *Am J Surg.* 2008;196:710–714.

### See Also (Topic, Algorithm, Electronic Media Element)

Diverticulosis

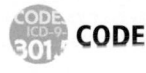 **CODES**

### ICD9

- 562.01 Diverticulitis of small intestine (without mention of hemorrhage)
- 562.03 Diverticulitis of small intestine with hemorrhage
- 562.11 Diverticulitis of colon (without mention of hemorrhage)

# DIVERTICULOSIS

*Ronald E. Kim*

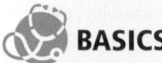 **BASICS**

## DESCRIPTION
- Single (diverticulum) or multiple (diverticula) colonic wall outpouchings from colonic muscle dysfunction, usually acquired
- Sequence:
  - Insufficient amounts of dietary fiber cause diminished stool bulk.
  - Increased colonic contractions to propel stool through colon cause increase in intraluminal pressure.
  - Increased pressure forces mucosa and submucosa to herniate through muscularis propria at its weakest point, where vasa recta penetrate.

## ETIOLOGY
- Occurs anywhere in GI tract, although generally a colonic disease:
  - Left-sided 95% (western countries)
  - Right-sided 70% (Asian countries)
  - Sigmoid colon most common site
- Pseudodiverticula:
  - Outpouchings of mucosa and submucosa only
  - Most common form of colonic diverticula
  - True congential diverticula (uncommon) contain all bowel wall layers.
- Incidence directly related to increase in age
- Common in western society, owing to refined diet and low intake of fiber
- Complications:
  - Massive arterial bleeding usually from right colon:
    - Fecalith (dry, hard stool) erodes through arterial branch.
  - Inflammation (diverticulitis)
  - Perforation
  - Abscess
  - Obstruction

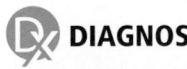 **DIAGNOSIS**

## SIGNS AND SYMPTOMS
### History
- Thorough history and physical examination essential to avoid excessive workup
- Clinical patterns:
  - Asymptomatic (70–85%)
  - Symptomatic (painful)
  - Hemorrhagic (5–15%)
- Chronic or intermittent left-lower-quadrant pain:
  - Often precipitated by eating
  - Sometimes relieved by flatulence or bowel movement

- Painless brisk hematochezia (maroon stools or bright red blood); often self-limiting
- Constipation (or diarrhea)
- Change in bowel pattern
- Dyspepsia
- Diverticulitis and diverticular bleeding are separate entities and rarely coexist.

### Physical Exam
- Abdominal palpation:
  - Tenderness in left lower quadrant
  - Firm sigmoid colon in left lower quadrant
- Rectal exam:
  - Predominantly reveals heme-negative stool
  - Bleeding typically mild
- Fever: Absent

## ESSENTIAL WORKUP
Thorough history and physical examination essential to avoid excessive workup

## DIAGNOSTIC TESTS & INTERPRETATION
### Lab
- Asymptomatic diverticulosis:
  - Requires no testing
- Uncomplicated painful disease (no peritoneal signs) with known history:
  - Requires no workup
- Uncomplicated painful disease (no peritoneal signs) without previous history:
  - Requires workup to rule out carcinoma (if weight loss, anorexia, heme-positive stool)
  - CBC for leukocytosis or anemia
  - Urinalysis to exclude hematuria or pyuria
- Hemorrhagic diverticulosis:
  - CBC
  - Electrolytes, BUN, creatinine, glucose, calcium
  - Type and cross for 4 units of packed RBCs
  - PT, PTT, INR
  - ECG

### Imaging
- Uncomplicated painful diverticulosis—outpatient options:
  - Flexible sigmoidoscopy, then barium enema:
    - Sigmoidoscopy: Rule out carcinoma (before barium studies for optimal visualization).
    - Barium enema: Search for classic diverticula and exclude carcinoma or polyps.
  - Colonoscopy

- Hemorrhagic diverticulosis:
  - Anoscopy:
    - If mild bleeding, to rule out hemorrhoids
  - Proctosigmoidoscopy:
    - If no blood in stool above rectum, assume rectal bleed.
  - Colonoscopy:
    - Cannot perform if bleeding excessive (difficult to visualize pathology)
    - Allows for therapeutic intervention
    - Usually done prior to radionuclide imaging or angiography
  - Radionuclide imaging:
    - Safe, no bowel prep needed
    - Poor localization of bleeding site
    - Ideal for detecting intermittent bleeding, owing to long half-life of radioisotope (24–36 hr)
    - No potential for therapeutic intervention
  - Angiography:
    - No bowel prep needed
    - Localizes site of bleeding (more exact after radionuclide scanning)
    - Allows for therapeutic intervention
    - Risk of intestinal infarction
  - Barium enema:
    - Rarely indicated, but most sensitive for diagnosis
    - Identifies diverticula but not bleeding (can hinder visualization of other imaging techniques)

## DIFFERENTIAL DIAGNOSIS
- Painful diverticulosis:
  - Irritable bowel syndrome (almost identical clinical presentation)
  - Diverticulitis
  - Colon carcinoma
  - Crohn disease
  - Urologic (renal colic)
  - Gynecologic (ruptured or torsed ovarian cyst)
- Hemorrhagic diverticulosis:
  - Hemorrhoids
  - Anal fissure
  - Proctitis
  - Colitis
  - Carcinoma
  - Polyps
  - Ischemic enteritis
  - Angiodysplasia
  - Amyloidosis
  - Vascular–enteric fistula
  - Upper GI source

**TREATMENT**

### PRE-HOSPITAL

- Avoid opiates in abdominal pain when underlying cause is uncertain.
- Establish 2 large-bore IV lines with 0.9% NS if significant rectal bleeding/hemodynamic instability.
- For hypotension:
  - 1–2 L (20 mL/kg) bolus 0.9% NS intravenously
  - Trendelenburg position

### INITIAL STABILIZATION/THERAPY

Hemorrhagic diverticulosis (massive):

- Airway control (100% $O_2$ or intubate if unresponsive)
- Intravenous access with at least 1 large-bore catheter or 2 if unstable
- 0.9% NS bolus 1–2 L (20 mL/kg) for hypotension
- Central catheter placement if unstable following initial fluid resuscitation for more efficient delivery of fluids and monitoring of central venous pressure
- Nasogastric tube to rule out upper GI bleed
- Bladder catheter to monitor urine output
- Transfuse O-negative RBCs immediately if arrest is impending.
- Consult surgeon (most diverticular bleeding stops spontaneously).

### ED TREATMENT/PROCEDURES

- Uncomplicated symptomatic diverticulosis:
  - High-fiber diet and/or hydrophilic bulk laxative (eg, psyllium)
  - Warm compresses to abdomen
  - Reassurance
  - Avoid cathartic laxatives.
  - No evidence to support use of antispasmodic (dicyclomine)
- Hemorrhagic diverticulosis (massive):
  - Initial stabilization (see above)
  - Monitor fluid status (input/output).
  - Radionuclide scan; sensitive and noninvasive, but requires active bleeding
  - Selective angiography with injection of vasopressin to control bleeding
  - Embolization controversial; may be considered before surgery
  - Surgical intervention for segmental colectomy

### MEDICATION

- Dicyclomine: 20 mg PO/IM q.i.d. (not for IV use)
- Propantheline: 15 mg PO 30 min ac/qhs

 **FOLLOW-UP**

### DISPOSITION

#### Admission Criteria

- ICU if unstable with massive hemorrhagic diverticulosis
- Mild or intermittent hemorrhagic diverticulosis that is otherwise stable so as to determine site of bleeding and evaluate need for definitive treatment

#### Discharge Criteria

- Uncomplicated, symptomatic diverticulosis
- Stable with trace heme-positive stool, negative gastric aspirate, no anemia, and no other complaints

#### Issues for Referral

GI follow-up for colonoscopy

### FOLLOW-UP RECOMMENDATIONS

- Colonoscopy within 48 hr of initial presentation for stable patients
- Discontinue aspirin and NSAIDs.
- Increase intake of dietary fiber.
- No evidence for avoidance of nuts, corn, popcorn

## PEARLS AND PITFALLS

- 15% with hematochezia have an upper GI source.
- Most cases (75–95%) resolve spontaneously or with conservative management.
- Massive blood loss seen in 9–19% of patients, especially those with comorbid diseases or advanced age.
- Colonoscopy is the initial diagnostic procedure of choice in stable patients.

## ADDITIONAL READING

- Bono MJ. Gastrointestinal emergencies. Part I: Lower gastrointestinal tract bleeding. *Emerg Med Clin North Am.* 1996;14(3):547–556.
- Kim YI, Marcon NEl. Injection therapy for colonic diverticular bleeding. A case study. *J Clin Gastroenterol.* 1993;17(1):46–48.
- Kohler L, Sauerland S, Neugebauer E. Diagnosis and treatment of diverticular disease: Results of a consensus development conference. The Scientific Committee of the European Association for Endoscopic Surgery. *Surg Endosc.* 1999;13(4): 430–436.
- McGuire IIII. Bleeding colonic diverticula: A reappraisal of natural history and management. *Ann Surg.* 1994;220(5):653–656.
- Touzious JG, Dozois EJ. Diverticulosis and acute diverticulitis. *Gastroent Clin.* 2009;38(3):513–525.
- Wilkins T, Baird C, Pearson AN, et al. Diverticular bleeding. *Am Fam Physician.* 2009;80(9):977–983.

### See Also (Topic, Algorithm, Electronic Media Element)

- Diverticulitis
- Gastrointestinal Bleeding

 **CODES**

### ICD9

- 562.00 Diverticulosis of small intestine (without mention of hemorrhage)
- 562.02 Diverticulosis of small intestine with hemorrhage
- 562.10 Diverticulosis of colon (without mention of hemorrhage)

# DIZZINESS
*Mitchell Adelstein*

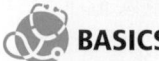

## BASICS

### DESCRIPTION
- Nonspecific feeling that may define a whirling sensation, a tendency to fall, feeling faint, weakness, or feeling confused
- May be caused by a number of problems:
  - Vertigo:
    - Vestibular dysfunction
    - Cerebellar disease
  - Disequilibrium:
    - Suggests a structural CNS disorder
    - Multiple sensory deficits
  - Near syncope/syncope:
    - Cardiovascular insufficiency
    - Faintness that is postural or paroxysmal suggests a cardiovascular disorder
  - Weakness
  - Psychiatric illness:
    - Constant, ill-defined dizziness unrelated to posture suggests a psychogenic etiology

### ETIOLOGY
- Peripheral vertigo (85%):
  - Benign paroxysmal positional (most common)
  - Acute labyrinthitis
  - Ménière disease
  - Vestibule neuritis
  - Acoustic neuroma
  - Ototoxic drugs:
    - Aminoglycosides
    - Antimalarials
    - Erythromycin
    - Furosemide
  - Otitis media and serous otitis with effusion
  - Foreign body in ear canal
- Central vertigo (15%):
  - Cerebellar hemorrhage
  - Vertebral basilar artery insufficiency
  - Cerebellar trauma
  - Cerebellopontine angle tumor
  - Temporal lobe epilepsy
  - Vertebral basilar migraines
  - Multiple sclerosis
  - Subclavian steal syndrome
  - Drugs suppressing the reticular activating system:
    - Sedative hypnotics
    - Anticonvulsants

- Disequilibrium:
  - Multiple sensory defects
  - Frontal lobe disorder:
    - Tumors: Meningioma, glioma, metastatic tumor
    - Anterior cerebral artery syndrome
    - Hydrocephalus
  - Subcortical disorders:
    - Multiple strokes
    - Ataxic hemiparesis
  - Brainstem disorders:
    - Stroke
    - Multiple sclerosis
  - Cerebellar disorders:
    - Cerebellar hemorrhage, infarct, tumor
    - Spinocerebellar degeneration
    - Alcoholism
    - Acute cerebellitis
- Cardiac and vascular insufficiency:
  - Hypovolemia
  - Orthostatic hypotension
  - Anemia
  - Myocardial ischemia
  - Structural cardiac or valvular disease
  - Cardiac dysrhythmias:
    - Preexcitation
    - Prolonged QT syndrome
    - Hypokalemia
    - Supraventricular tachycardia
    - Ventricular dysrhythmia
  - Pulmonary embolism:
  - Subarachnoid hemorrhage
  - Hypoglycemia
  - Hypoxia
  - Hypercarbia
  - Hyperventilation syndrome
  - Vasovagal episode
- Other:
  - Psychogenic:
    - Anxiety
    - Hyperventilation syndrome
    - Depression
  - Chronic fatigue syndrome
  - Familial periodic paralysis
  - Hypothyroidism

## DIAGNOSIS

### SIGNS AND SYMPTOMS
- Dizziness is used to describe a wide range of symptoms:
  - Abnormal sensation of motion
  - Feeling faint or fainting
  - Lightheadedness
  - Unsteadiness
- Classify dizziness into 1 of 4 categories by asking the patient to explain the sensation without using the word *dizzy*:
  - Vertigo:
    - Abnormal sensation of movement and position in space
    - Nystagmus
  - Nausea
  - Vomiting
  - Diaphoresis
- Disequilibrium:
  - Disorder of coordination and rhythm
  - Loss of equilibrium
  - May include sensory deficits such as peripheral neuropathy
- Near syncope/syncope:
  - Diaphoresis
  - Palpitations
  - Pallor during the episode
- Other:
  - Depression
  - Fatigue
  - Weakness
  - Hyperventilation

### ALERT
Vertical nystagmus is abnormal and should elicit concern for a central etiology.

### ESSENTIAL WORKUP
Must be tailored to each individual patient's signs and symptoms

## DIAGNOSTIC TESTS & INTERPRETATION
### Lab
- Hematocrit, if suspected anemia/blood loss
- Glucose in setting of DM
- Electrolytes in setting of volume depletion
- Toxicologic screen, if suspected exposure/ingestion

### Imaging
- CT scan if central vertigo or ataxia is present
- Magnetic resonance angiogram if vertebral basilar insufficiency is suspected

### Diagnostic Procedures/Surgery
EKG to detect cardiac causes of near syncope and weakness

## DIFFERENTIAL DIAGNOSIS
See "Etiology"

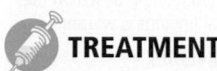

# TREATMENT

## INITIAL STABILIZATION/THERAPY
- Supplemental oxygen
- Stabilization should be determined by more specific classification of dizziness based on the history, physical exam, and ancillary studies.

## ED TREATMENT/PROCEDURES
Treatment should be determined by the underlying cause.

## MEDICATION
- Diazepam: 2.5–5 mg IV. q8h or 2–10 mg PO q8h
- Diphenhydramine: 25–50 mg IV, IM, or PO q6h
- Meclizine: 25 mg PO q6h PRN
- Promethazine: 12.5 mg IV q6h or 25–50 mg PO, IM, or PR q6h

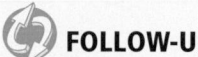

# FOLLOW-UP

## DISPOSITION
### Admission Criteria
Admission or discharge of patients with dizziness should be based on the underlying etiology or associated symptoms.

### Discharge Criteria
Admission or discharge of patients with dizziness should be based on the underlying etiology or associated symptoms.

### Issues for Referral
Refer for completion of workup as an outpatient to a primary care physician or a neurologist.

## FOLLOW-UP RECOMMENDATIONS
- The patient should be instructed:
  - Not to drive or operate machinery if he is feeling dizzy
  - To get up slowly after sitting or lying down
- He should return to the ED or see his doctor right away if:
  - Worsening headache
  - Stiff neck
  - Confusion, drowsiness, or any change in alertness
  - Loss of memory
  - Trouble moving arms or legs
  - Numbness anywhere
  - Abdominal (belly), back or chest pain.
  - Fever or shaking chills
  - Intractable vomiting
  - Blood in emesis or stools
  - Dark or black bowel movements
  - For women, bleeding or discharge from the vagina

## PEARLS AND PITFALLS
Although the current paradigm for evaluating the dizzy patient involves using symptom quality (vertigo vs. near-syncope, etc.), it may be more effective to use a system of timing and triggers to define temporal patterns of dizziness.

## ADDITIONAL READING
- Brown JJ. A systematic approach to the dizzy patient. *Neurol Clin.* 1990;8:209–24.
- Herr RD, Zun L, Mathews JJ. A directed approach to the dizzy patient. *Ann Emerg Med.* 1989;18:664.
- Kerber KA Vertigo and dizziness in the emergency - RCE > department. *Emerg Med Clin North Am.* 2009;27(1):39–50.
- Pigott DC, Rosco CJ. The dizzy patient: An evidence based diagnosis and treatment strategy. *Emerg Med Pract.* 2001;3(3):120.
- Walker JS, Barnes SB. Dizziness. *Emerg Med Clin North Am.* 1998;16(4):845–75.

### See Also (Topic, Algorithm, Electronic Media Element)
Vertigo

 CODES

**ICD9**
780.4 Dizziness and giddiness

# DOMESTIC VIOLENCE

*James Comes*

 **BASICS**

## DESCRIPTION

- Intimate partner violence and abuse is the infliction or the credible threat of physical harm against an intimate partner.
- Occurs in dating, married, cohabiting, or separated relationships
- Intimate partner violence and abuse is a pattern of assaultive and coercive behaviors that include physical, sexual, and psychologic attacks against the victim.
- The perpetrator uses these tactics to attain compliance from and to control the victim.
- Tactics used by perpetrators to gain power and control over their partners include:
  - Pushing
  - Shoving
  - Slapping
  - Punching
  - Kicking
  - Choking
  - Holding
  - Tying down
- Verbal abuse:
  - Threatening harm (including toward children or pets), intimidation, or destruction of property
  - Isolating the victim physically or socially
  - Degrading or humiliating behavior
  - Attempting to force or forcing the victim to perform sexual acts against his or her will or without protection against pregnancy
  - Causing physical harm during sex or assaulting genitalia

## ETIOLOGY

- Most victims are women, and most perpetrators are men.
- Partners in same-sex relationships and men may also be victims.
- Most rapes and assaults of women are by known assailants.

 **DIAGNOSIS**

Diagnosis and recognition in the ED, clinic, or office remains difficult and problematic.

## SIGNS AND SYMPTOMS

- Traumatic injuries:
  - Small subset of presenting complaints
  - Fractures
  - Contusions
  - Lacerations
  - Penetrating and blunt trauma to body
- Psychiatric:
  - Chronic pain syndromes
  - Physical symptoms related to stress
  - Anhedonia
  - Insomnia
  - Anorexia
  - Somatic complaints
  - Anxiety
  - Depression and suicidal ideation

## ALERT

Clinical clues:

- History not compatible with exam
- Repeat visits for the same chief complaint
- Delay in seeking care
- Any injury during pregnancy
- Interaction between woman and partner that suggests interpersonal problems
- Evidence of trauma not attributable to a motor vehicle accident
- Multiple symptoms without obvious physical findings

### History

- Short screening questions of a subset of female patients may be an effective means of identifying victims of domestic violence.
- Insufficient evidence to support universal screening
- Screening should be direct, nonjudgmental, supportive, and private.
- The Joint Commission requires hospitals to have policies and procedures in place for identifying and treating victims.

### Physical Exam

Document all signs of trauma.

## ESSENTIAL WORKUP

After identification, a directed workup based on the chief complaint and physical findings is warranted.

## DIFFERENTIAL DIAGNOSIS

- Partner violence may be the acute precipitant of the patient's reason for presenting to the ED, or it may be part of the patient's past or present social history.
- There is no traumatic or nontraumatic presentation that is pathognomonic for intimate partner violence.

 **TREATMENT**

## PRE-HOSPITAL

- Timely and appropriate medical attention
- Accurate description of events by EMS should be incorporated into the medical record.

## INITIAL STABILIZATION/THERAPY

- Provide timely and appropriate medical attention.
- Maintain advocacy by expressing messages of support and validating victim's dilemma.

## ED TREATMENT/PROCEDURES

- Document in the chart the victim's allegations in his or her own words.
- Diagram or photograph injuries (after consent) and incorporate them into the clinical record.
- Address the patient's safety in returning to the same home environment:
  - Important determinants in predicting future danger include violence that is increasing in frequency and severity, threats of homicide or suicide by the partner, or the availability of a lethal weapon
- With the aid of social services or domestic violence advocates, review the patient's options:
  Outpatient victim services
  - Emergency shelter information
  - Hotlines
  - Restraining order information
  - Legal services
- Mandatory reporting requirements vary among states:
  - Some states require the health care practitioner to make a verbal and written report if he or she suspects wound or physical injury results from assaultive and abusive conduct.
  - Determine how local authorities respond to reports of intimate partner violence and abuse from health care practitioners.
  - Recognize that mandatory reporting requirements may place the victim in more danger and create ethical dilemmas for the physician when the victim does not want the case reported to police or social service agencies.

## MEDICATION

- Acetaminophen: 650–975 mg PO
- Morphine sulfate: 0.1 mg/kg/dose IV or IM

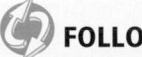 **FOLLOW-UP**

### DISPOSITION

#### Admission Criteria

- A victim whose life is in imminent danger and who cannot be safely discharged (to his or her home, family, friends, or shelter) may need to be admitted to the hospital (under an assumed name).
- Use appropriate admission guidelines depending on degree of trauma sustained.

#### Discharge Criteria

A victim whose safety is ensured and whose injuries can be managed as an outpatient may be discharged.

#### Issues for Referral

Availability of advocacy services varies considerably.

### FOLLOW-UP RECOMMENDATIONS

Provide information regarding outpatient services and emergency shelter information.

## PEARLS AND PITFALLS

- Failure to consider partner violence in the differential diagnosis of the patient's chief complaint
- Failure to inquire about patient's safety and provide referral options
- Mandatory reporting laws remain controversial and are of unclear benefit.

## ADDITIONAL READING

- Abbott J. Injuries and illnesses of domestic violence. *Ann Emerg Med.* 1997;29:781–785.
- Hyman A, Schillinger D, Lo B. Laws mandating reporting of domestic violence: Do they promote well-being? *JAMA.* 1995;273:1781–1787
- MacMillan HL, Wathen CN, Jamieson E, et al. Screening for intimate partner violence in health care settings. *JAMA.* 2009;302:493–501.
- Salber PR, Taliaferro F. Intimate partner violence and abuse. In: *Rosen's Emergency Medicine Concepts and Clinical Practice,* 5th ed. St. Louis, MO: Mosby; 2002:863–875.

### See Also (Topic, Algorithm, Electronic Media Element)

- Elder Abuse
- Trauma

 **CODES**

ICD9

- 995.80 Unspecified adult maltreatment
- V15.41 History of physical abuse

# DUODENAL TRAUMA

*Christanne M. Hoffman*

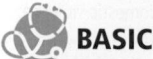

## BASICS

### DESCRIPTION
- Characteristics of duodenum:
  - 12 inches long
  - C-shaped
  - Divided into 4 sections:
    - Last 3 sections retroperitoneal along with distal portion of 1st section
  - Lies mostly over 1st 3 lumbar vertebrae
  - 2nd section is most commonly injured
- Types of injury:
  - Duodenal wall hematoma
  - Wall perforation
  - Hemorrhage, including retroperitoneal
  - Crush
- Incidence of duodenal injury is ~5% of all intra-abdominal injuries.
- Penetrating trauma accounts for ~75% of duodenal injuries:
  - Mortality ranges from 13–28%.
  - Associated with exsanguination
- Blunt duodenal trauma has a higher mortality due to greater force of injury and often delayed diagnosis due to retroperitoneal location:
  - If injury is diagnosed in <24 hr, mortality rate is about 11%.
  - If >24 hr, mortality rate approaches 40%.
  - Late mortality usually from sepsis

### Pediatric Considerations
- Majority secondary to recreational injuries (eg, bicycle handlebar injuries)
- Intramural duodenal hematomas may occur in nonaccidental trauma:
  - If suspected, prompt referral to appropriate child protective agency is required.
- In children, hematoma is most commonly seen in 1st portion of duodenum.

### Pregnancy Considerations
- Retroperitoneal hemorrhage more common due to increased pelvic and abdominal vascularity
- Large uterus serves as protection from bowel injury.
- Peritoneal irritation is blunted in the pregnant patient, therefore greater index of suspicion.

### ETIOLOGY
- Blunt trauma:
  - Shear strain: Abrupt acceleration/deceleration at point of attachment (most common retroperitoneal injury with rapid deceleration)
  - Tensile strain: Direct compression or stretching of tissue
- Penetrating trauma:
  - Creates cavitations, can lead to infection

## DIAGNOSIS

### SIGNS AND SYMPTOMS
- Complaints may be minimal with vague abdominal, flank, and back pain.
- High GI obstruction may be seen with duodenal hematomas.

### History
Penetrating or blunt abdominal trauma

### Physical Exam
- Retroperitoneal: Often subtle, RUQ pain, nausea, vomiting, tachycardia, fever
- Intraperitoneal: Peritonitis

### ESSENTIAL WORKUP
- Basic labs including amylase
- Acute abdominal series or CT
- DPL or Ex-lap if unstable, high suspicion

### DIAGNOSTIC TESTS & INTERPRETATION
#### Lab
- Laboratory tests are of little value.
- 50% of patients with duodenal injuries have elevated serum amylase.

### Imaging
- Upright chest and abdominal radiographs:
  - Intraperitoneal air
  - Retroperitoneal air
  - Air in biliary tree
  - Scoliosis to the right
  - Loss of psoas shadow
  - Air around right kidney
  - Injecting air into nasogastric tube may demonstrate retroperitoneal air more clearly.
  - Intramural hematomas without leakage may have coiled-spring appearance.
- CT with oral and IV contrast:
  - Perhaps best diagnostic test that shows small amounts of retroperitoneal gas and extravasated contrast material
  - Sausage-shaped mass in duodenal wall strongly suggests hematoma.

### Diagnostic Procedures/Surgery
- Ex lap is the ultimate diagnostic test when high suspicion remains, even after other diagnostic tests are negative.
- Diagnostic peritoneal lavage (DPL):
  - Often positive for blood, bile, or bowel content
  - Negative lavage does not exclude injury (65% false-negative rate).

### DIFFERENTIAL DIAGNOSIS
- Injury to hollow organs (stomach, small and large intestines)
- Liver and biliary tree injuries
- Vascular injuries (aortic and mesenteric arteries as well as venous injuries)
- Postoperative complications from prior duodenal surgery or injury repair, such as infection and suture line dehiscence

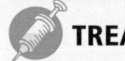 TREATMENT

### PRE-HOSPITAL
- Follow trauma protocols.
- Important to have prehospital personnel provide clear description of mechanism of injury and to transport to appropriate facility

### INITIAL STABILIZATION/THERAPY
- Airway management, resuscitation as needed
- Aggressive fluid therapy with warmed normal saline or lactated Ringer solution if patient hypotensive; transfuse as indicated
- Central line may be needed for unstable patients.
- Nasogastric decompression
- Early trauma surgical consultation

### ED TREATMENT/PROCEDURES
- Tetanus and antibiotic prophylaxis for penetrating wounds
- Definitive treatment involves laparotomy with exploration of duodenum for injuries.
- Broad-spectrum antibiotics to prevent sepsis in patients with perforation

### MEDICATION
- Cefoxitin: 2 g (peds: 40 mg/kg) IV *plus* gentamicin: 2 mg/kg IV loading dose (adult and peds) *or*
- Cefotetan: 2 g (peds: 20 mg/kg) IV *plus* gentamicin: 2 mg/kg IV loading dose (adult and peds) *or*
- Clindamycin: 600 mg IV (peds: 20–40 mg/kg/d IV in 3–4 div. doses) *plus* gentamicin: 2 mg/kg IV loading dose (adult and peds) *or*
- Ceftriaxone: 1–2 g IV (peds: 50–75 mg/kg/d in 2 div. doses, not to exceed 2 g) *plus* metronidazole: 15 mg/kg IV

 FOLLOW-UP

### DISPOSITION
#### Admission Criteria
- All patients with duodenal injuries need admission to trauma surgical service.
- Minor duodenal hematomas that do not require immediate surgery may require nasogastric decompression for obstruction (up to 7 days) and observation for possible expansion or rupture of the hematoma.

#### Discharge Criteria
- No patient with identified traumatic duodenal injury should be discharged from the ED.
- Complications: Intra-abdominal abscess, duodenal fistula, pancreatic fistula, sepsis

#### Issues for Referral
- Duodenal Organ Injury Scale (DIS) by American Association for the Surgery of Trauma:

| Grade | Duodenal Injury Description |
| --- | --- |
| I | Hematoma-single portion<br>Laceration-partial thickness, no perf |
| II | Hematoma: >1 portion<br>Lac. Disrupts <50% circumference |
| III | Lacerations only:<br>–Disrupts 50–75% circum D2<br>–Disrupts 50–100% circum D1, D3, D4 |
| IV | Lacerations only:<br>–Disrupts >75% circum D2<br>–Involves ampulla or CBD |
| V | Lac: Massive disruption pancreatico-duodenal complex<br>Vascular-devascularization |

- Majority injuries Grade II or III
- 80% primary repairs

### FOLLOW-UP RECOMMENDATIONS
- All patients with diagnosed duodenal injury should be admitted.
- If diagnostic studies are negative, recommend follow up with PMD within 24–48 hr.
- Diet: Clear liquids, advance as tolerated

## PEARLS AND PITFALLS
- Significant morbidity and mortality with delayed or missed diagnosis
- Physical exam can be misleading due to retroperitoneal location.
- If continued high suspicion despite negative diagnostic tests, get surgical consult.

## ADDITIONAL READING
- Degiannis E, Boffard K. Duodenal injuries. *Br J Surg.* 2000;87:1473–1479.
- Han J, et al. Multilevel duodenal injury after blunt trauma. *J Korean Surg Soc.* 2009;77:282–286.
- Linsenmaier U, et al. Diagnosis and classification of pancreatic and duodenal injuries in emergency radiology. *Radiographics.* 2008;28(6):1591–1602.
- Rickard M, et al. Pancreatic and duodenal injuries: Keep it simple. *Anz J Surg.* 2005;75(7):581–586.

### See Also (Topic, Algorithm, Electronic Media Element)
- Abdominal Trauma, Blunt
- Abdominal Trauma, Imaging
- Abdominal Trauma, Penetrating

 CODES

### ICD9
863.21 Injury to duodenum without open wound into cavity

D

# DYSFUNCTIONAL UTERINE BLEEDING

*Christy Rosa Mohler*

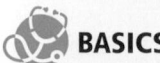 **BASICS**

## DESCRIPTION
- Excessive (>80 mL) or prolonged vaginal bleeding without demonstrable organic cause
- Also referred to as anovulatory bleeding
- Occurs secondary to anovulation or oligoovulation
- Typical blood loss during a normal menstrual cycle is 30 mL.
- Diagnosis of exclusion

## ETIOLOGY
- Unopposed estrogen stimulation of proliferative endometrium
- Anovulatory (most common):
  - Alteration of neuroendocrinologic function
  - Obesity
  - Very low calorie diets, rapid weight change, intense exercise
  - Psychologic stress
  - Most common in postmenarchal, premenopausal women
- Ovulatory:
  - Metrorrhagia:
    - Irregular bleeding between periods
  - Menorrhagia:
    - Regular periods with excess flow (>80 mL) or >7 days of bleeding
  - Oligomenorrhea:
    - Periods with intermenstrual cycles >35 days

### Pediatric Considerations
Anovulatory bleeding common in adolescence owing to immaturity of the hypothalamic-pituitary-ovarian axis

 **DIAGNOSIS**

## SIGNS AND SYMPTOMS
### History
- Abnormal uterine bleeding in the absence of systemic or structural disease
- Includes bleeding between normal menstrual cycles, change in normal pattern of menstrual cycle, and increased or decreased amount of menstrual bleeding
- Most common in postmenarchal, premenopausal women
- Typically painless

### Physical Exam
- Mild to moderate bleeding on pelvic exam
- Pallor, tachycardia, hypotension, orthostasis in severe cases
- Evaluate for trauma, foreign bodies

### ALERT
It is rare for women to be hemodynamically unstable simply from dysfunctional uterine bleeding; if such instability is present, concern is for ectopic pregnancy or other cause for hemorrhage.

## ESSENTIAL WORKUP
Pregnancy test

## DIAGNOSTIC TESTS & INTERPRETATION
### Lab
- CBC, PT/PTT, bleeding time
- May send iron studies, TSH, LH, FSH, prolactin level, cervical cultures for routine follow-up by primary medical doctor (PMD)/gynecology

### Imaging
Pelvic ultrasound may show uterine, tubal, or ovarian abnormality; may be needed to rule out other processes on differential diagnoses.

### Diagnostic Procedures/Surgery
- Dilation and curettage (D&C) may be required for heavy bleeding unresponsive to other interventions.
- Refer for endometrial biopsy if older than 35 yr of age

## DIFFERENTIAL DIAGNOSIS
- Pregnancy complications:
  - Threatened, incomplete, or spontaneous abortion; ectopic or molar pregnancy
- Infectious:
  - Vaginitis, cervicitis, pelvic inflammatory disease (PID)
- Coagulopathies:
  - Von Willebrand disease, idiopathic thrombocytopenic purpura, platelet defects, thalassemia
- Medications:
  - Warfarin, aspirin, oral contraceptives, tricyclic antidepressants, major tranquilizers
- Systemic illness:
  - Adrenal, hepatic, renal or thyroid dysfunction, diabetes mellitus, other endocrinopathies
- Anatomic lesions:
  - Fibroids, endometriosis, polyps, endometrial hyperplasia, neoplasm
- Intrauterine devices
- Trauma
- Anovulation:
  - Perimenarchal, perimenopausal
  - Prematory ovarian failure
  - Hyperprolactenmia
  - Hyperandrogenic
  - Hypothyroidism
  - Anorexia

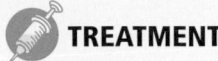 TREATMENT

### PRE-HOSPITAL
IV crystalloid boluses as needed for hypotension, tachycardia secondary to heavy bleeding

### INITIAL STABILIZATION/THERAPY
ABCs:
- Packed RBCs for significant bleeding unresponsive to crystalloids

### ED TREATMENT/PROCEDURES
- Observation usually adequate if bleeding mild
- IV crystalloid, packed RBCs for continued bleeding or hemodynamic instability
- Gynecology consultation if bleeding is severe and unresponsive to crystalloids, medications:
  - D&C may be necessary for hemodynamic instability.
  - Hysteroscopy or hysterectomy for continued heavy bleeding unresponsive to other measures

### MEDICATION
- Conjugated estrogen (Premarin) for heavy bleeding, hemodynamic instability:
  - 2.5 mg PO q.i.d.
    25 mg IV, repeat in 3 hr if needed
- Ibuprofen 400–800 mg PO q8h (reduces prostaglandin synthesis)
- IV dosing has not been shown to be superior to oral route:
  - Medroxyprogesterone acetate 5–10 mg/day PO is added when bleeding subsides.
- Oral contraceptive pills:
  - Ethinyl estradiol 35 $\mu$g and norethindrone 1 mg PO q.i.d. for 1 wk
- Medications may be deferred in mild cases with referral to gynecology
- Transdermal or long-acting estrogens are other options

 FOLLOW-UP

### DISPOSITION
#### Admission Criteria
- Significant blood loss
- Continued bleeding
- Hemodynamic instability requiring aggressive resuscitation and/or operative intervention

#### Discharge Criteria
Most patients can be discharged with gynecology referral once bleeding is controlled and patient is hemodynamically stable.

#### Issues for Referral
Endometrial biopsy if >35 yr old:
- Follow-up with either gynecologist or primary care physician is necessary for patients with dysfunctional uterine bleeding.
- Must evaluate for ongoing blood loss or potential malignancy as cause.

## PEARLS AND PITFALLS
- Dysfunctional uterine bleeding is a diagnosis of exclusion.
- Only 2% of endometrial carcinoma occur before age 40 yr.

## ADDITIONAL READING
- Berek JS, ed. *Berek & Novak's Gynecology*, 14th ed. Philadelphia: Lippincott Williams & Wilkins; 2007.
- Casablanca Y. Management of dysfunctional uterine bleeding. *Obstet Gynecol Clin North Am.* 2008;35: 219–234.
- Marx JA, Hockberger RS, Walls RM, et al., eds. *Rosen's Emergency Medicine: Concepts and Clinical Practice*, 7th ed. St. Louis, MO: Mosby; 2009.
- Pitkin, J. Dysfunctional uterine bleeding. *BMJ.* 2007;334:1110–1111.
- Tintinalli JE, Kelen GD, Stapczynski JS, eds. *Emergency: A Comprehensive Study Guide*, 6th ed. New York: McGraw-Hill; 2003.

### See Also (Topic, Algorithm, Electronic Media Element)
- Amenorrhea
- Vaginal Bleeding

 CODES

**ICD9**
626.8 Other disorders of menstruation and other abnormal bleeding from female genital tract

# DYSPHAGIA

*John Santoro*
*Kelvey R. Wilson*

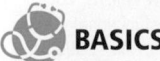 **BASICS**

## DESCRIPTION
- Difficulty swallowing
- Impaired passage of solids or liquids from the oral cavity to the stomach
- Can be neuromuscular or mechanical
- Frequency and severity increase with advancing age

## ETIOLOGY
- Oropharyngeal (transfer) dysphagia:
  - Difficulty transferring from the oropharynx to the proximal esophagus (difficulty initiating a swallow)
  - Easier to swallow solids vs. liquids
  - Immediate, within seconds of swallowing
  - Sensation of the bolus not passing below the cervical esophagus
  - Nasal or oral regurgitation
  - Coughing or choking (indicating aspiration)
  - Gurgling noise after swallowing (suggests Zenker diverticulum)
  - Vocal quality changes
  - Usually a neuromuscular disorder resulting in bulbar muscle weakness or impaired coordination
- Esophageal (transport) dysphagia:
  - Failure of normal transit through the esophagus
  - Retrosternal sticking sensation 10–15 sec after swallowing
  - Nocturnal regurgitation/aspiration
  - Drooling or regurgitation of undigested food and liquid (characteristic of esophageal obstruction)
  - Usually obstructive but consider motility disorders
- Functional dysphagia:
  - Diagnosis of exclusion
  - Full workup without evidence of mechanical or neuromuscular pathology
  - Symptoms >12 wk
- Odynophagia:
  - Pain with swallowing
  - Separate, but often related, entity
- Pain pattern:
  - Voluntary striated muscle in the upper 1/3 transitions to involuntary nonstriated muscle in the lower 2/3.
  - Somatic nerve fibers in the upper esophagus; excellent pain localization
  - Afferents, from the vagus nerve along with the cervical and thoracic sympathetic ganglia, innervate the lower esophagus; poor pain localization
  - Visceral pain from the lower esophagus may be difficult to distinguish from that of acute coronary syndrome.

## Pediatric Considerations
- Pediatric dysphagia:
  - Wide range of feeding and swallowing difficulties
  - Multifactorial pathophysiology:
    - Neuromuscular development
    - Anatomical changes from infancy to childhood
  - Esophageal disorders most common etiology
- Classification:
  - Oral phase:
    - Impaired ingestion/mastication and transfer to posterior pharynx
  - Pharyngeal phase:
    - Impaired swallow mechanism and transport of material through pharynx with appropriate airway closure (requires intact sensory and motor mechanisms to prevent aspiration)
  - Esophageal phase:
    - Impaired transport of material from esophagus to stomach

 **DIAGNOSIS**

## SIGNS AND SYMPTOMS
- Difficulty initiating swallowing
- Sensation of food stuck after swallowing
- Cough/choke after eating
- Impairment of gag reflex and ability to clear bolus
- Pocketing of food in mouth
- Voice change/dysphonia
- Drooling
- Dysarthria

## History
3 important questions:
- What causes symptoms?
  - Solids and liquids suggest a neuromuscular disorder.
  - Solids only or progression from solids to liquids suggests a mechanical abnormality.
- Are symptoms intermittent or progressive?
  - Intermittent symptoms suggest rings or webs.
  - Progressive symptoms suggest peptic or malignant strictures.
  - Motility disorders can be intermittent or progressive.
- Are there concomitant symptoms?
  - Odynophagia or chest pains
  - Chronic cough or nocturnal wheezing
  - Nasopharyngeal regurgitation
  - Weight loss
  - Chronic heartburn
  - Hematemesis
  - Recurrent pneumonia

## Physical Exam
- Often unremarkable
- Oropharyngeal inspection
- Pulmonary and cardiac auscultation
- Neurologic exam with emphasis on cranial nerves (esp. V, VII, IX, X, XII)
- Muscle strength, reflexes, coordination, gait and functional status

## ESSENTIAL WORKUP
- Adequate airway evaluation
- Thorough neurological exam

## DIAGNOSTIC TESTS & INTERPRETATION
EKG:
- Consider cardiac etiology for chest discomfort

## Lab
- No specific studies are indicated.
- Consider: CBC, TSH, vitamin $B_{12}$, creatine kinase (especially with neurogenic dysphagia)

## Imaging
- CXR:
  - Food dilating the esophagus
  - Aspiration pneumonitis
  - Extrinsic compressing mass
- Soft-tissue lateral neck radiograph
- Modified barium swallow (with solid bolus) or videofluoroscopy:
  - Defines esophageal anatomy
  - Assesses function
  - Do not perform if endoscopy anticipated
- CT/MRI of the head:
  - Indicated for new-onset neuromuscular dysphagia

## Diagnostic Procedures/Surgery
- Upper endoscopy:
  - Indicated to relieve obstruction and inspect the esophageal anatomy
  - Biopsy possible if indicated
- Esophageal manometry
- Fiberoptic nasopharyngeal laryngoscopy

## DIFFERENTIAL DIAGNOSIS
- Oropharyngeal:
  - Infectious:
    - Botulism
    - CNS infections
    - Dermatomyositis
    - Infectious pharyngitis
    - Lyme disease
    - Poliomyelitis

- Mechanical:
  - Congenital
  - Malignancy
  - Pharyngeal pouch
- Medications:
  - Aminoglycosides
  - Amiodarone
  - Anticholinergics
  - Aspirin and NSAIDs
  - Ferrous sulfate
  - HMG-CoA reductase inhibitors
  - Metoclopramide
  - Olanzapine
  - Penicillamine
  - Phenothiazines
  - Potassium
  - Procainamide
- Neuromuscular:
  - Amyotrophic lateral sclerosis
  - Cerebrovascular accident
  - Cranial nerve palsy
  - Cricopharyngeal spasm
  - Huntington chorea
  - Multiple sclerosis
  - Myasthenia gravis
  - Parkinson disease
  - Traumatic brain injury
- Psychological/behavioral
- Esophageal:
  - Mechanical:
    - Diverticula
    - Esophageal webs
    - Foreign body
    - Neoplasm
    - Peptic esophageal stricture
    - Postsurgical (laryngeal, spinal)
    - Radiation injury
    - Schatzki ring
  - Motor:
    - Achalasia
    - Chagas
    - Cushing syndrome
    - Diffuse esophageal spasm
    - Hyperthyroidism/hypothyroidism
    - Nonspecific motor disorders
    - Nutcracker esophagus
    - Scleroderma
    - Vitamin $R_{12}$ deficiency
  - Inflammatory:
    - Eosinophilic esophagitis
    - Pill esophagitis
  - Extrinsic:
    - Cardiovascular abnormalities (vascular rings, thoracic aneurysm, left atrial enlargement, aberrant subclavian artery)
    - Cervical osteophytes
    - Mediastinal mass

##  TREATMENT

### PRE-HOSPITAL
- Vigilant airway attention
- Position of comfort with suction available

### INITIAL STABILIZATION/THERAPY
- Vigilant airway attention
- Position of comfort with suction available
- NPO
- 0.9% NS 500 mL (peds: 20 mL/kg) IV fluid bolus for significant dehydration

### ED TREATMENT/PROCEDURES
- Nitroglycerin for esophageal spasm
- Glucagon for impacted foreign body
- Treat complications:
  - Airway obstruction
  - Aspiration, pneumonia, lung abscess
  - Dehydration, malnutrition
- Endoscopy
- Dietary modifications:
  - Thickened liquids for neuromuscular disorder
  - Thin liquids for mechanical disorders

### MEDICATION
#### First Line
- Glucagon: 1 mg IV followed by 2nd dose of 1 mg after 5 min if there is no improvement in symptoms (0.02–0.03 mg/kg in children, not to exceed 0.5 mg):
  - Success rates vary from 12–50%, which may not be better than spontaneous passage.
- Nitroglycerin: 0.4 mg SL q5min repeated up to 3 times:
  - Alert. Risk of significant hypotension

#### Second Line
- Diltiazem: Can aid in esophageal contractions and motility especially with nutcracker esophagus
- Isosorbide dinitrate in achalasia
- Cystine-depleting therapy with cysteamine if dysphagia is due to pretransplantation and posttransplantation cystinosis

##  FOLLOW-UP

### DISPOSITION
#### Admission Criteria
- Esophageal obstruction
- Compromised fluid or nutrition status
- Inability to protect airway
- Unable to tolerate own secretions
- Symptoms cannot be distinguished from cardiac ischemia.

#### Discharge Criteria
- Well-hydrated patient
- Urgent neurology, otolaryngology, or gastroenterology referral arranged for further evaluation and treatment

#### Issues for Referral
Next day follow-up with PCP or ENT

### FOLLOW-UP RECOMMENDATIONS
- Clear liquid diet prior to ENT follow-up
- Return if SOB, chest pain, or unable to tolerate own secretions.

## PEARLS AND PITFALLS
- Consider cardiac etiology.
- Dysphasia is a common presentation in stroke.
- Consider in patients with recurrent pneumonia.

## ADDITIONAL READING
- Al-Haddad M, Ward FM, Scolapio JS, et al. Glucagon for the relief of esophageal food impaction does it really work?. *Dig Dis Sci.* 2006;51(11):1930–1933.
- Fass R, Feldman M, Bonis P. *Approach to the patient with dysphagia.* Cited from UpToDate.com. 2009.
- Miller CK, Willging JP. Advances in the evaluation and management of pediatric dysphagia. *Cur Op in Otolaryn Head Neck Surg.* 2003;11(6):442–446.
- Paik N-J. *Dysphagia.* Cited from eMedicine.com, Inc., eMedicine Journal, 2008.
- Smith Hammond CA, Goldstein LB. Cough and aspiration of food and liquids due to oral-pharyngeal dysphagia; ACCP evidence-based clinical practice guidelines. *Chest.* 2006;129.1345.
- Varadarajulu S, Eloubeidi MA, Patel RS, et al. The yield and the predictors of esophageal pathology when upper endoscopy is used for the initial evaluation of dysphagia. *Gastrointest Endosc.* 2005; 61:804–808.

### See Also (Topic, Algorithm, Electronic Media Element)
Stroke

## 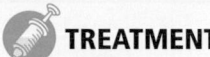 CODES

### ICD9
- 787.20 Dysphagia, unspecified
- 787.21 Dysphagia, oral phase
- 787.22 Dysphagia, oropharyngeal phase

# DYSPNEA
*Elizabeth L. Mitchell*

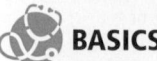 **BASICS**

## DESCRIPTION
- Inability to breath comfortably
- Usually an unconscious activity, dyspnea is the subjective sensation of breathing, from mild discomfort to feelings of suffocation.
- Dyspnea comes from the Greek word for "hard breathing."
- Often described as "shortness of breath"
- Common presenting complaint seen in 3.5% of ED visits
- Caused by difficulties in maintaining homeostasis with respect to gas exchange and acid–base status
- Dyspnea usually reflects an impairment in ventilation, perfusion, metabolic function, or CNS drive.
- Mechanisms that control breathing:
  - Control centers:
    - Brainstem and cerebral cortex affect both automatic and voluntary control of breathing.
  - Chemo, stretch, and irritant sensors:
    - $CO_2$ receptors located centrally and $PO_2$ receptors located peripherally
    - Mechanoreceptors lie in respiratory muscles and respond to stretch.
    - Intrapulmonary mechanoreceptors respond to chemical irritation, engorgement, and stretch.
  - Effectors of respiratory center output are in the respiratory muscles and respond to central stimulation to move air in and out of the thoracic cavity.
  - Motor-sensory control of the diaphragm and muscles of respiration are controlled by C3–C8 nerves and T1–T12 nerves.
- Derangements of any of these neurosensory pathways produces dyspnea:
  - Many etiologies for the sensation of dyspnea are due to the complex nature of mechanisms that control breathing.

## ETIOLOGY
- Upper airway:
  - Epiglottitis
  - Laryngeal obstruction
  - Tracheitis or tracheobronchitis
  - Angioedema
- Pulmonary:
  - Airway mass
  - Asthma
  - Bronchitis
  - Chest wall trauma
  - CHF

- Drug-induced conditions (eg, crack lung, aspirin overdose)
  - Effusion
  - Emphysema
  - Lung cancer
  - Metastatic disease
  - Pneumonia
  - Pneumothorax
  - Pulmonary embolism
  - Pulmonary HTN
  - Restrictive lung disease
- Cardiovascular:
  - Arrhythmia
  - Coronary artery disease
  - Intracardiac shunt
  - Left ventricular failure
  - Myxoma
  - Pericardial disease
  - Valvular disease
- Neuromuscular:
  - CNS disorders
  - Myopathy and neuropathy
  - Phrenic nerve and diaphragmatic disorders
  - Spinal cord disorders
  - Systemic neuromuscular disorders
- Metabolic acidosis:
  - Sepsis
  - DKA
  - AKA
  - Renal failure
  - Profound thiamine deficiency
- Toxic:
  - Methemoglobinemia
  - Salicylate poisoning
  - Cellular asphyxiants:
    - Carbon monoxide
    - Cyanide
    - Hydrogen sulfide
    - Sodium azide
  - Toxic alcohols
- Abdominal compression:
  - Ascites
  - Pregnancy
  - Massive obesity
- Psychogenic:
  - Hyperventilation
  - Anxiety
- Other:
  - Altitude
  - Anaphylaxis
  - Anemia

### Geriatric Considerations
Most common diagnoses in elderly patients presenting to the ED with dyspnea:
- Decompensated heart failure
- Pneumonia
- COPD
- Pulmonary embolism
- Asthma

### Pediatric Considerations
Unique conditions in differential diagnosis for age <2 yr:
- Croup
- Congenital anomalies of the airway
- Congenital heart disease
- Foreign-body aspiration
- Nasopharyngeal obstruction
- Shock

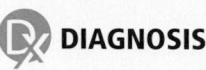 **DIAGNOSIS**

## SIGNS AND SYMPTOMS
- Difficult, labored, or uncomfortable breathing
- Upper airway:
  - Stridor
  - Upper-airway obstruction
- Pulmonary:
  - Tachypnea
  - Accessory muscle use
  - Wheezing
  - Rales
  - Asymmetric breath sounds
  - Poor air movement
- Cardiovascular:
  - S3 gallop
  - Murmur
  - Jugular venous distention
- CNS:
  - Altered levels of consciousness
- General:
  - Diaphoretic/cool versus hot/dry skin
  - Pallor
  - Upright patient position
  - Clubbing
  - Cyanosis
  - Edema
  - Ketotic breath odor

### History
- Time course, abruptness of onset, triggers, and severity
- History of stridor or wheezing
- Medication and compliance with these
- Exposure to allergens
- Past medical history
- Associated symptoms:
  - Chest pain
  - Fever
  - Cough
  - Hemoptysis

## Physical Exam
- Signs of acute distress
- Altered mental status
- Cyanosis
- Respiratory rate
- Retractions suggest severe dyspnea secondary to airway obstruction.
- Listen for abnormal lung sounds:
  - Stridor
  - Rales
  - Wheezing
  - Decreased breath sounds

## ESSENTIAL WORKUP
- Pulse oximetry:
  - May be falsely elevated due to increased ventilation or carbon monoxide
- CXR:
  - For diagnosis of pulmonary conditions
  - Assess heart size and evidence of CHF.
- ABG:
  - Oxygenation
  - Calculate arterial-alveolar gradient:
    - A-a (at sea level) $= 150 - (PO_2 - PCO_2)/0.8$
    - Normal $= 5-20$
  - Assess degree of acidosis.

## DIAGNOSTIC TESTS & INTERPRETATION
### Lab
- CBC:
  - Evaluation of anemia
  - Neutrophil count helpful in evaluation of infectious processes
- Electrolyte, BUN, creatinine, glucose:
  - Consider when specific metabolic derangements are suspected
  - B-natriuretic peptide may be elevated in CHF.
- Toxicology screen
- Methemoglobin/carboxyhemoglobin level
- Thyroid function tests
- D-Dimer (ELISA):
  - Useful for excluding pulmonary embolus if normal

### Imaging
- EKG for suspected myocardial ischemia, CHF
- Ventilation-perfusion scan or CT pulmonary angiogram for suspected pulmonary embolism
- Soft-tissue neck radiograph or fiberoptic visualization for suspected upper airway obstruction
- ECG for suspected pericardial effusion/tamponade
- Peak expiratory flow/spirometry to assess for reactive-airway disease
- Tensilon test for suspected myasthenia gravis

## DIFFERENTIAL DIAGNOSIS
- Adrenergic toxidrome
- Anticholinergic toxidrome
- Thyroid storm
- Munchausen syndrome

 **TREATMENT**

### PRE-HOSPITAL
- Place all patients on supplemental oxygen, pulse oximetry, and cardiac monitor.
- Initiate therapy for suspected cause of dyspnea when indicated:
  - Asthma
  - COPD
  - CHF
- Intubate patients in the face of impending respiratory failure.

### INITIAL STABILIZATION/THERAPY
- ABCs
- Immediate intubation for impending respiratory arrest:
  - Altered mental status
  - Unstable vital signs
- BiPAP in alert patients:
  - Contraindications:
    - Cardiac instability
    - Suspicion of upper airway obstruction
    - Inability to protect airway
    - Upper GI bleeding
    - Status epilepticus

### ED TREATMENT/PROCEDURES
- Based on underlying etiology
- Palliative care with opiates is indicated for the relief of dyspnea in terminal cancer patients.

 **FOLLOW-UP**

### DISPOSITION
#### Admission Criteria
- Assisted ventilation
- Hypoxia
- A-a gradient >40
- Medical condition requiring hospital therapy

#### Discharge Criteria
- Adequate oxygenation
- Stable medical illness that can be managed as outpatient

#### Issues for Referral
Based on suspected underlying etiology

### FOLLOW-UP RECOMMENDATIONS
- The patient should be told to not smoke while short of breath and to try to quit to help with some of the causes, as well as to prevent others from getting worse.
- The patient should return for any of the following problems:
  - No improvement or worsening in 24 hr
  - New chest pain, pressure, squeezing, or tightness
  - Shaking chills, or a fever >102°F
  - New or worsening cough or wheezing

- Abdominal (belly) pain, vomiting, severe headache
- Dizziness, confusion or change in behavior
- Any serious change in symptoms, or any new symptoms that are of concern

## PEARLS AND PITFALLS
- Altered mental status is an indication for immediate airway management in a patient with severe dyspnea.
- Dyspnea can and should be quantified.
- Dyspnea and tachypnea may occur without a respiratory etiology because of metabolic acidosis or a catastrophic CNS event.

## ADDITIONAL READING
- De Peuter S, Van Diest I, Lemaigre V, et al. Dyspnea: The role of psychological processes. *Clin Psychol Rev*. 2004;(5):557–581.
- Mahler DA, Selecky PA, Harrod CG, et al. American College of Chest Physicians consensus statement on the management of dyspnea in patients with advanced lung or heart disease. *Chest*. 2010;137(3):674–691.
- Manning HL, Mahler DA. Pathophysiology of dyspnea. *Monaldi Arch Chest Dis*. 2001;56(4): 325–330.
- Michelson E, Hollrah S. Evaluation of the patient with shortness of breath: An evidence based approach. *Emerg Med Clin North Am*. 1999;17(1): 221–237.
- Schwartzstein RM, Manning HL. Pathophysiology of dyspnea. *N Engl J Med*. 1995;12(3):1547–1552.
- Stenton C. The MRC breathless scale. *Occup Med*. 2009;58:226–227.
- Tobin MJ. Dyspnea: Pathophysiologic basis, clinical presentation, and management. *Arch Intern Med*. 1990;8:1604–1612.
- Weisman IM, Zeballos RJ. Clinical evaluation of unexplained dyspnea. *Cardiologia*. 1996;41(7): 621–634.

### See Also (Topic, Algorithm, Electronic Media Element)
Respiratory Distress

 **CODES**

### ICD9
786.09 Other dyspnea and respiratory abnormalities

# DYSTONIC REACTION
*Kenneth Jackimczyk*

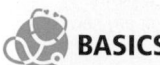 **BASICS**

## DESCRIPTION
- Normal pattern of CNS neurotransmission maintained by balance between dopaminergic and cholinergic receptors:
  - Certain drugs disrupt this balance, leading to involuntary muscle spasms.
- Although the spasms are uncomfortable and frightening, they are not life-threatening.
- Usually occurs within hours of ingestion:
  - Almost always within 1st wk after exposure to offending drug
- Age:
  - Twice as common in males
  - Uncommon in older patients
  - Children are more susceptible.

## ETIOLOGY
- Usually occur after patient has taken antipsychotic, antiemetic, or antidepressant drug
- Incidence of dystonic reactions in patients taking neuroleptics is 2–25%, depending on the agent.
- Neuroleptic agents:
  - Phenothiazine (Thorazine, Mellaril, Prolixin, Compazine, Stelazine, Phenergan)
  - Thioxanthenes (Navane)
  - Butyrophenones (Haldol, Droperidol)
  - Indole (Moban)
  - Dibenzoxipine (Loxitane)
- Antiemetic agents:
  - Metoclopramide (Reglan)
  - Trimethobenzamide (Tigan)

- Other agents:
  - Cyclic antidepressants
  - Antihistamines
  - Doxepin
  - Cimetidine
  - Prozac
  - Cocaine
  - Ketamine
  - Chloroquine
  - Lithium
  - Phencyclidine

### Pediatric Considerations
Children are particularly vulnerable to dystonic reactions when dehydrated or febrile.

 **DIAGNOSIS**

## SIGNS AND SYMPTOMS
### History
- Ingestion of antipsychotic, antiemetic, or other drug within week of symptom onset
- Difficulty with vocalization
- Completely alert and able to answer questions
- Involuntary muscle spasms usually involving the face, neck, and trunk (see "Physical Exam")

### Physical Exam
- Characteristic motor spasms occur.
- Oculogyric crisis:
  - Involves eye and periorbital muscles
  - Starts as blepharospasm
  - Evolves into painful upward or lateral deviation of eyes
- Buccolingual crisis:
  - Involves facial muscles and tongue
  - Bizarre grimacing
  - Trismus
  - Tongue protrusion
  - Dysphagia
  - Dysarthria
  - Rarely causes spasm of pharynx and larynx that can be severe enough to cause stridor

- Torticollic crisis:
  - Twisting of neck
- Tortipelvic crisis:
  - Abdominal wall muscle spasm
- Opisthotonos:
  - Involves muscles of trunk and back
  - Twisting and arching of spine

## ESSENTIAL WORKUP
- Clinical diagnosis is based on characteristic signs and symptoms with history of possible drug exposure.
- Diagnosis is confirmed by response to treatment.

## DIAGNOSTIC TESTS & INTERPRETATION
### Lab
No laboratory testing needed

### Imaging
No imaging studies needed

## DIFFERENTIAL DIAGNOSIS
- Tardive dyskinesia:
  - Complication of chronic antipsychotic therapy
  - Usually choreiform movements
- Akathisia:
  - Involuntary motor restlessness
  - May appear agitated
- Seizure:
  - History of prior seizures
  - Not responsive to verbal stimuli
  - Tonic-clonic-type motor movements rather than spasm
- Hysteria or pseudoseizure:
  - History of precipitating emotional event
  - Tonic-clonic motor activity rather than sustained spasm
- Tetanus
- Strychnine poisoning
- Chronic dystonias:
  - Cerebral palsy, familial choreas
  - Usually history of dystonia is associated with chronic neurologic process.
- Scorpion envenomation:
  - Oculogyric crisis and opisthotonos are common manifestations of scorpion envenomation.
  - Patient lacks history of drug exposure.
- Meningitis and encephalitis may present with atypical seizures that mimic dystonic reaction.

TREATMENT

### PRE-HOSPITAL
- Rarely life-threatening
- Direct attention toward spasm of larynx and tongue to be sure dystonic reaction is not causing respiratory compromise.
- Ask family and friends about ingestions of antipsychotic medications, antiemetics, and recreational drugs.
- Transport pill bottles.

### INITIAL STABILIZATION/THERAPY
Stabilize airway to prevent spasm of larynx or tongue from causing respiratory compromise.

### ED TREATMENT/PROCEDURES
- Administer diphenhydramine (Benadryl) or benztropine mesylate (Cogentin):
  - Rapid resolution of muscular spasm by restoring cholinergic-dopaminergic balance in CNS
  - IV administration is preferred route of treatment.
  - Onset of relief in 2–5 min
  - Complete resolution of symptoms in 15 min
  - IM administration is alternate route of treatment
  - Begins to work in 15–30 min
  - Continue oral administration for 3 days to prevent redevelopment of symptoms.
- Diazepam (Valium):
  - Administer in cases of dystonia unresponsive to adequate doses of anticholinergic medications.
  - Failure to respond to standard treatment should lead physician to consider other diagnoses.

### MEDICATION
- Benztropine mesylate (Cogentin): 1–2 mg either IV (over 2 min) or IM followed by 1–2 mg PO b.i.d. for 3 days:
  - Not to be used in children <3 yr old
  - For children >3 yr old: 0.02 mg/kg IV (over 2 min) or IM followed by 0.02 mg/kg PO b.i.d. for 3 days
- Diphenhydramine (Benadryl): 1–2 mg/kg up to 100 mg either IV (over 2 min) or IM followed by 25–50 mg (peds: 1–2 mg/kg) PO q6–8h for 3 days, or
- Diazepam: 5–10 mg IV followed by 5 mg PO q4–6h as necessary for 3 days

### First Line
Diphenhydramine (Benadryl)

### Second Line
Benztropine mesylate (Cogentin):
- Not to be used in children <3 yr old

 FOLLOW-UP

### DISPOSITION

#### Admission Criteria
Generally, patients are not admitted unless symptoms do not resolve with treatment, there are concerns about maintaining the airway, or the diagnosis is not certain.

#### Discharge Criteria
- Discharge after resolution of symptoms.
- Patient should not drive or perform tasks that require full alertness while taking sedating medications.

### FOLLOW-UP RECOMMENDATIONS
Patients should follow-up with the prescribing physician of the causative agent.

## PEARLS AND PITFALLS
- The diagnosis of acute dystonia is made based on the history of ingestion coupled with complete resolution of the symptoms after appropriate treatment.
- First-line of therapy is diphenhydramine.

## ADDITIONAL READING
- Sachdev PS. Neuroleptic-induced movement disorders: An overview. *Psychiatr Clin N Am.* 2005;28:255–274.
- Vena J, Dufel S, Paige T. Acute olanzapine-induced akathisia and dystonia in a patient discontinued from fluoxetine. *J Emerg Med.* 2006;30:311–317.
- Wolfson AB, Hendey GW, Ling LJ, et al., eds. *Harwood Nuss' Clinical Practice of Emergency Medicine,* 5th ed. Philadelphia: Lippincott, 2010.

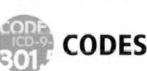 CODES

### ICD9
333.72 Acute dystonia due to drugs

# EATING DISORDER

David B. Herzog
Kathryn C. Eckstein
Kamryn T. Eddy

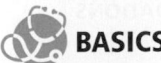 **BASICS**

## DESCRIPTION

### Anorexia Nervosa (AN)
- Refusal to maintain body weight at or above a minimally normal weight for age and height
- Failure to make expected weight gain during a period of growth
- Intense fear of gaining weight or becoming fat, even though underweight
- Severe body image disturbance
- Undue influence of body weight and shape on self-evaluation
- Denial of seriousness of low body weight
- In postmenarchal females, amenorrhea for 3 consecutive cycles
- Prevalence: 0.5% of females in U.S.

### Bulimia Nervosa (BN)
- Recurrent episodes of binge eating characterized by:
  - Eating a larger than usual amount of food in a discrete period of time
  - A sense of loss of control over eating during the episode
- Recurrent inappropriate compensatory behaviors used to prevent weight gain:
  - Self-induced vomiting
  - Misuse of laxatives
  - Diuretics
  - Enemas or other medications
  - Fasting
  - Excessive exercise
- Self-evaluation that is excessively influenced by weight or body shape
- Prevalence: 2% of females in U.S.

### Binge Eating Disorder (BED)
- Recurrent episodes of binge eating characterized by:
  - Eating a larger than usual amount of food in a discrete period of time
  - A sense of loss of control over eating during the episode
- Binge-eating episodes associated with 3 or more of the following:
  - Eating much more rapidly than normal
  - Eating until feeling uncomfortably full
  - Eating large amounts of food when not feeling physically hungry
  - Eating alone because of embarrassment about how much one is eating
  - Feeling disgusted with oneself, depressed, or very guilty after overeating
  - Marked distress regarding binge eating
- Prevalence: 3–5% of females and males in U.S. (3:2 ratio)

## ETIOLOGY
- Eating disorders result from a combination of genetic, neurochemical, developmental, psychological, and sociocultural factors.
- Typical age of onset for AN is bimodal at 13–14 yr and 17–18 yr.
- AN commonly onsets in a teenager whose initial dieting behavior escalates into an obsessive preoccupation with weight and thinness.
- BN and BED commonly onset in late adolescence or early adulthood.
- BN commonly onsets in an individual who:
  - Has attempted many diets and failed
  - May have learned purging behaviors from a friend or family member
- BED is associated with obesity, weight cycling, and dieting.

 **DIAGNOSIS**

## SIGNS AND SYMPTOMS
- Endocrine/metabolic complications:
  - Electrolyte imbalances
  - Hypothermia
  - Amenorrhea
  - Sleep disturbance
  - Growth retardation
  - Osteoporosis
  - Nutritionally based osteoporosis
- Cardiovascular problems:
  - Arrhythmias
  - Bradycardia
  - Hypotension
  - QTC prolongation
  - Ipecac cardiomyopathy
- Renal complications:
  - Hypokalemia
  - Edema
- Hematologic complications:
  - Anemia
  - Leukopenia
  - Thrombocytopenia
- GI complications:
  - Decreased motility
  - Intestinal dilatation
- Neurological complications:
  - Potentially irreversible structural brain changes
  - Peripheral neuropathy

## History
- Weight changes
- Restricting and bingeing behavior
- Purging (vomiting, laxatives, diuretics, enemas)
- Exercise patterns
- Medications, including over the counter (eg, stimulants, ipecac, diet pills)
- Menstrual history
- Family history of eating disorders and obesity
- Comorbid psychiatric disorder (eg, mood disorder, substance abuse, personality disorder)

## Physical Exam
- Weight, BMI (weight in kg/[height in meters]$^2$)
- Vital signs (including orthostatic BP and HR)
- Dry skin
- Lanugo:
  - A soft, downy body hair that develops on the chest and arms
- Breast atrophy
- Parotid swelling, submandibular swelling
- Hypercarotenemia
- Abnormal dentition
- Abrasions of dorsum of hand

## ESSENTIAL WORKUP
- Clinical diagnosis
- Medical evaluation
- Physical examination
- Nutritional assessment
- Psychiatric interview:
  - Concurrent psychiatric illness
  - Suicide risk assessment
  - Explore psychosocial context
- Family evaluation when patient lives with her or his family

## DIAGNOSTIC TESTS & INTERPRETATION
### Lab
- CBC
- Electrolytes, BUN, creatinine, glucose
- LFTs
- Calcium, magnesium, phosphorus
- UA including specific gravity
- Toxic screen
- Beta HCG
- Amylase
- Consider checking thyroid-stimulating hormone.

### Imaging
Specific tests may be useful in making differential diagnoses, eg, MRI (rule out brain tumor), abdominal CT (rule out obstruction)

### Diagnostic Procedures/Surgery
- ECG
- Consider cardiac ECHO if substantial weight loss

## DIFFERENTIAL DIAGNOSIS
- Borderline personality disorder
- Mood disorders
- Obsessive-compulsive disorder
- Substance abuse
- Medical conditions:
  – GI disease (eg, Crohn's disease, IBD, celiac disease)
  – Endocrine disorder (eg, DM, thyroid disorder, adrenal insufficiency)
  – Cancer

## TREATMENT

### INITIAL STABILIZATION/THERAPY
- ABCs
- IV 0.9% NS 1 L bolus (peds: 20 mL/kg) for severe dehydration
- Accu-Chek, correct hypoglycemia with dextrose
- Correct hypokalemia
- Warming blankets for severe hypothermia

### ED TREATMENT/PROCEDURES
Labs, physical examination, psychiatry consultation (including assessment of suicide risk), and medical stabilization

### MEDICATION
- Escitalopram (Lexapro): 10–20 mg PO daily for BN
- Fluoxetine (Prozac): 20–60 mg PO daily for BN and relapse prevention in AN
- Olanzapine (Zyprexa): 2.5–10 mg PO daily for AN
- Sertraline (Zoloft): 50–200 mg PO daily for BN

### First Line
- Only fluoxetine has a FDA indication for the treatment of BN.
- SSRIs are typically considered 1st line for BN and are the most commonly used medication for AN.

### Second Line
Olanzapine for AN

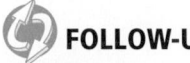

## FOLLOW-UP

### DISPOSITION
### Admission Criteria
- Medical risk:
  – Extremely low weight
  – Rapid weight loss
  – Serum electrolyte imbalance
  – Cardiac disturbance
  – Marked orthostatic hypotension
  – Bradycardia <40
  – Tachycardia >110
  – Hypothermia <97°F

- Psychiatric risk:
  – Severe depression
  – Suicidality
  – Severe denial
  – Severe impairment in functioning
  – Toxic family environment
  – Psychosis
  – Refractory symptoms

### Discharge Criteria
- Medically and psychologically safe enough to be managed on an outpatient basis
- Multimodal, multidisciplinary team in place to manage medical, nutritional, and psychological issues

### Issues for Referral
- Outpatient treatment requires a team approach composed of a:
  – Psychiatrist and/or psychologist
  – Nutritionist, preferably one who specializes in eating disorders
  – Pediatrician or internist
  – Family therapist
  – Group therapist
  – Dentist
- Prognosis:
  – AN and BN:
    ○ 20% chronic course
    ○ 30% improve
    ○ 50% recover
  – Mortality rate 5.6% per decade for AN
  – Outcomes improved with early diagnosis and treatment

### FOLLOW-UP RECOMMENDATIONS
- For outpatient treatment the team must establish modest goals and clear parameters, including expected weight gain for anorexic patients and compliance with follow-up appointments.
- Internist/pediatrician: Monitor vital signs, weight, BMI, electrolytes, and ECG.
- Nutritionist: Monitor diet, calorie intake, and exercise.
- Psychotherapy:
  – Cognitive behavioral therapy and interpersonal psychotherapy are the most effective forms of psychotherapy for BN.
  – Cognitive behavioral therapy, family therapy, and psychodynamic therapies are all useful for AN.
  – Family-based treatment is the preferred therapy for teenagers with AN and it is promising for teenagers with BN as well.

- Pharmacotherapy:
  – Only indicated within the context of psychotherapy, especially with comorbid psychopathology.
  – Antidepressant medications are shown to significantly reduce bingeing and purging behaviors:
    ○ Fluoxetine is the best studied.
  – No accepted pharmacologic treatment of AN.
  – Case studies suggest that 2nd-generation antipsychotics may be helpful in AN.
  – There is no clear evidence for specific treatment of osteoporosis in AN apart from weight restoration and nutritional calcium supplementation.

## PEARLS AND PITFALLS
- Eating disorders are associated with high medical risk and risk of suicide; prioritize safety assessment.
- Allow the control to reside with the patient as much as possible.
- Avoid trying to "out-obsess" the obsessional patient.
- Coordinate care with PCP and other members of a multidisciplinary team.

## ADDITIONAL READING
- American Psychiatric Association (APA). *Practice Guidelines for the Treatment of Patients with Eating Disorders*, 3rd ed. Washington, DC: Author; 2006.
- Katzman DK. Medical complications in adolescents with anorexia nervosa: A review of the literature. *Int J Eat Disord*. 2005;37:S52–S59.
- Le Grange D, Eddy KT, Herzog DB. Anorexia and Bulimia nervosa. In: Dulcan MK (Ed). *Textbook of Child and Adolescent Psychiatry*. Washington, DC: American Psychiatric Association; 2010:397–415.
- Mitchell JE, Crow S. Medical complications of anorexia nervosa and bulimia nervosa. *Curr Op in Psychiatry*. 2006;19(4):438–443.

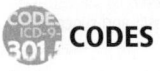

## CODES

### ICD9
- 307.1 Anorexia nervosa
- 307.50 Eating disorder, unspecified
- 307.59 Other disorders of eating

# ECTOPIC PREGNANCY

*Aviva Jacoby Zigman*

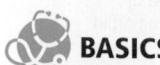 **BASICS**

## DESCRIPTION

- Implantation of fertilized ovum outside of uterus:
  – Most commonly fallopian tube
- Abdominal and peritoneal implantations:
  – Associated with higher morbidity
  – Difficulty in diagnosis
  – Tendency to bleed
- Occurs in 1.5–2.0% of pregnancies
- Accounts for 6% of all maternal deaths
- 60% of women with ectopic pregnancy are subsequently able to have a normal pregnancy.

## ETIOLOGY

- Risk factors include:
  – Woman >35 yr old
  – African American
  – Previous fallopian tube damage from infections, such as pelvic inflammatory disease (PID)
  – Previous tubal surgery (ie, tubal ligation)
  – Previous ectopic pregnancy
  – Intrauterine device (IUD) use:
    ○ 25–50% of pregnancies with IUD are ectopic.
  – Diethylstilbestrol (DES) exposure
  – In vitro fertilizations
- 43% of women with ectopic pregnancies have no risk factors.

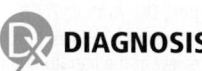 **DIAGNOSIS**

## SIGNS AND SYMPTOMS

Classic triad of amenorrhea, vaginal bleeding, and abdominal pain are present in only 15% of women with ectopic pregnancies:

- Amenorrhea (75–95%)
- Abdominal pain (80–100%):
  – Frequently unilateral
- Abnormal vaginal bleeding (50–80%)
- Symptoms of pregnancy (10–25%)
- Orthostatic hypotension, dizziness, and syncope (5–35%)
- Abdominal tenderness (55–95%)
- Adnexal tenderness (75–90%)
- Adnexal mass (35–50%)
- Cervical motion tenderness (43%)

### History

- Last menstrual period:
  – Majority of ectopics present 5–8 wk after LMP.
- Vaginal bleeding
- History of pelvic surgery, prior ectopic, IUD

### Physical Exam

- Evaluate for signs of peritoneal irritation.
- Pelvic exam:
  – Note uterine size.
  – Adnexal size
  – Adnexal tenderness
  – Presence of tissue in vaginal vault
  – Cervical OS open or closed

## ESSENTIAL WORKUP

- Pregnancy testing:
  – Women of potential childbearing age with vaginal bleeding or abdominal pain *must* have urine or serum pregnancy test.
  – Include testing of patients with history of recent elective or spontaneous abortion, tubal ligations, or IUD use.
  – Quantitative $\beta$-hCG in patients with positive qualitative test
- Vital signs unstable:
  – 2 large-bore IVs
  – Type and cross-match, hematocrit (Hct)
  – Bedside ultrasound (US), if immediately available, simultaneous with resuscitation
  – Consult gynecology and prepare for immediate surgical intervention.
- Vital signs stable:
  – Rapid hemoglobin determination
  – Type and Rh
  – US

## DIAGNOSTIC TESTS & INTERPRETATION

### Lab

- Urine pregnancy tests can detect $\beta$-human chorionic gonadotropin ($\beta$-hCG) levels of 25–50 mIU/L.
- Serum can detect $\beta$-hCG levels of 25 mIU/L.
- Quantitative serum $\beta$-hCG; for diagnosis and follow-up:
  – Doubles every 2 days in normal early pregnancy (early pregnancy <10,000 $\beta$-hCG mIU/L, 8 days to 7 wk)
  – $\beta$-hCG increases less in ectopic pregnancy.
  – Correlation with vaginal US increases predictive value.

### Imaging

- Ultrasonographic evidence of IUP makes ectopic pregnancy less likely:
  – Heterotopic pregnancies are possible.
- Positive IUP is indicated by double-ringed gestational sac, yolk sac, or fetal pole, and heartbeat seen in uterus.
- Transvaginal US; visualization of gestational sac at 5 wk, cardiac activity at 6.5 wk

- Transabdominal ultrasound; visualization of gestational sac at 5–6 wk, cardiac activity at 8 wk
- Complex adnexal mass and fluid in cul-de-sac seen in 22% of ectopics and has 94% positive predictive value when present.
- Positive pregnancy test with no confirmed IUP and fluid in pelvis; high risk for bleeding ectopic pregnancy

### Diagnostic Procedures/Surgery

- US in conjunction with quantitative $\beta$-hCG
- Patients with $\beta$-hCG levels >6,500 mIU/L and no intrauterine gestational sac seen on US have 100% chance of having ectopic pregnancy.
- Patients with $\beta$-hCG levels >6,500 mIU/L with intrauterine gestational sacs present have 94% chance of having normal pregnancy.
- Patients with $\beta$-hCG <2,000 mIU/L are too early to have gestational sac seen by abdominal ultrasound and thus cannot be ruled out for ectopic pregnancy.
- Patients with $\beta$-hCG >2,000 and <6,500 mIU/L should have IUP visualized on transvaginal US; suspect ectopic pregnancy if IUP is absent.
- Culdocentesis to evaluate for intraperitoneal blood if US is unavailable

## DIFFERENTIAL DIAGNOSIS

- Positive pregnancy test with vaginal bleeding:
  – Spontaneous abortion
  – Cervicitis
  – Trauma
- Positive pregnancy test with no evidence of IUP:
  – Completed spontaneous abortion
  – Early threatened abortion
- Positive pregnancy test with evidence of IUP, abdominal pain, or adnexal tenderness:
  – Septic abortion
  – Threatened abortion
  – Corpus luteal cyst
  – Ovarian torsion
  – UTI
  – Nephrolithiasis
  – Gastroenteritis
  – Appendicitis
  – Heterotopic pregnancy

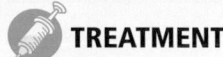 **TREATMENT**

### PRE-HOSPITAL
Cautions:

- Female patients of childbearing age presenting in shock may have unrecognized ruptured ectopic pregnancy.

### INITIAL STABILIZATION/THERAPY
- Vital signs unstable:
  - Airway management, resuscitate as needed
  - Fluid therapy with 2 large-bore IVs, oxygen, and monitor
  - Type specific, or O-negative blood if hypotensive after initial fluid bolus
  - Consult gynecology and transport to OR immediately for surgery.
- Vital signs stable:
  - Evidence of ectopic pregnancy on US:
    - Obstetric–gynecologic evaluation for surgery versus outpatient methotrexate treatment
    - For patients in whom future fertility is desired, methotrexate is the best option; otherwise surgery is the definitive treatment.
  - No evidence of ectopic pregnancy (early IUP vs. early ectopic):
    - Desired pregnancy: Serial $\beta$-HCG in stable, reliable patients and in conjunction with obstetrician
    - Undesired pregnancy: Dilation and curettage to evacuate uterus and confirm presence of products of conception

### ED TREATMENT/PROCEDURES
Methotrexate: Initiated only in conjunction with obstetric consultant and close follow-up:

- Reliable patients with unruptured ectopic pregnancies <4.0 cm
- $\beta$-HCG levels <6,000–15,000
- Contraindications:
  - Breast-feeding
  - Immunodeficiency
  - Pre-existing blood dyscrasia
  - Clinically significant anemia
  - Known sensitivity to methotrexate
  - Active pulmonary disease
  - Peptic ulcer disease
  - Hepatic dysfunction
  - Renal dysfunction

  - Alcoholism
  - Alcoholic liver disease
  - Ectopic mass >3.5 cm (relative contraindication)
  - Embryonic cardiac motion (relative contraindication)
- Most common dosing, single dose (50 mg/m²); serial $\beta$-hCG on days 2, 4, and 7. If <25% decline in $\beta$-hCG from day of 1st injection, 2nd dose is given.
- Multidose treatment is associated with less treatment failure.
- Common side effects:
  - Worsening abdominal pain
  - Nausea, vomiting, and diarrhea
- Worsening abdominal pain usually occurs 3–7 days after methotrexate initiation. These are usually tubal miscarriages; however, follow-up ultrasounds are essential to rule out ectopic rupture.
- Most common complication, tubal rupture in 4%
- Factors associated with methotrexate treatment failure:
  - Initial Hcg >5,000 mIU
  - Moderate to large free peritoneal fluid on US
  - Presence of fetal cardiac activity
  - Pretreatment increase in serum hCG level of more than 50% over a 48-hr period

### MEDICATION
- Methotrexate: 50 mg/m² IM/IV×1
- RhoGAM in Rh-negative women: 50 $\mu$g IM in women ≤12 wk pregnant; 300 $\mu$g IM in women >12 wk pregnant

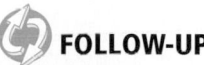 **FOLLOW-UP**

### DISPOSITION
#### Admission Criteria
- Any patient with confirmed ectopic pregnancy who is hemodynamically unstable
- Unreliable patients with increased risk factors, no available US, $\beta$-hCG >6,500 with no evidence of IUP should be admitted for observation and serial $\beta$-hCG tests.

#### Discharge Criteria
- Decision for outpatient management should be made in conjunction with obstetrician-gynecologist.
- Hemodynamically stable and reliable patients with workup that cannot rule out ectopic pregnancy:
  - Strict follow-up for serial $\beta$-hCG tests every 2 days
  - Patients should be recorded in logbook with phone numbers to ensure follow-up.

- *Ectopic precautions:* Patients should return to emergency room immediately for:
  - Increasing abdominal pain
  - Vaginal bleeding
  - Syncope or dizziness
  - Patients should not be left alone until diagnosis of ectopic pregnancy can be safely ruled out.
  - Family and friends should also be instructed on warning signs and symptoms of ruptured/bleeding ectopic pregnancies.

#### Issues for Referral
Phone consultation (at a minimum) with OB/GYN is essential when discharging a possible ectopic pregnancy.

### FOLLOW-UP RECOMMENDATIONS
All patients with positive pregnancy tests and unconfirmed IUP must be followed by an OB/GYN.

## PEARLS AND PITFALLS

- Always obtain a pregnancy test on women of childbearing age.
- Recognize the possibility of heterotopic pregnancies, especially in women undergoing fertility treatment.
- Secure close follow-up for any patient being evaluated and discharged for ectopic pregnancy.

## ADDITIONAL READING

- American College of Obstetricians and Gynecologists. *Practice Bulletin No. 94:* Medical management of ectopic pregnancies; June 2008.
- Barnhart KT. Ectopic pregnancy. *N Engl J Med* 2009;361:379–387.
- Marx JA, Hockberger RS, Walls RM, et al. *Rosen's Emergency Medicine: Concepts and Clinical Practice,* 7th ed. St. Louis, MO: Mosby, 2009.

### See Also (Topic, Algorithm, Electronic Media Element)
- Pregnancy, Uncomplicated
- Vaginal Bleeding

 **CODES**

### ICD9
- 633.00 Abdominal pregnancy without intrauterine pregnancy
- 633.10 Tubal pregnancy without intrauterine pregnancy
- 633.20 Ovarian pregnancy without intrauterine pregnancy

E

# ECZEMA/ATOPIC DERMATITIS

James A. Nelson

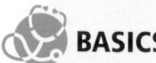 **BASICS**

## DESCRIPTION
- Pruritus is the hallmark.
- Chronic recurrent dermatitis characterized by signs of inflammation of the epidermis: Local redness, edema, crusting, and oozing
- Distribution tends to be in flexural areas such as the creases of elbows and knees.
- 90% of patients colonize with *Staphylococcus aureus*, and are prone to episodes of superinfection.

## RISK FACTORS
### Genetics
Family history of atopy (asthma, allergic rhinitis) in 30–70%

## ETIOLOGY
Thought to be a primary immunologic disease with secondary compromise of the epithelial barrier of the skin, causing dryness

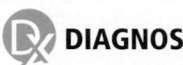 **DIAGNOSIS**

## SIGNS AND SYMPTOMS
### History
Diagnostic criteria suggest the patient must have itching and 3 of the 5 following:
- History of distribution at skin creases (flexural portions of extremities, head and neck)
- Atopic history (asthma or allergic rhinitis)
- History of dry skin
- Age at onset <2 yr
- Physical signs of flexural distribution

### Physical Exam
Dermatitis, characterized by:
- Inflammation: Redness, edema
- Epidermal compromise: Dry skin, weeping, oozing, then crusting
- Sequelae of scratching: Lichenification, cracking, excoriation, local bleeding

### Pediatric Considerations
- 45% of all cases start in the 1st 6 mo of life.
- 85% of all cases begin during the 1st 5 yr of life.

## ESSENTIAL WORKUP
History and physical exam

## DIAGNOSTIC TESTS & INTERPRETATION
### Lab
Remains a clinical diagnosis

### Diagnostic Procedures/Surgery
Generally reserved for settings outside of the ED:
- Radioallergosorbent test (RAST) sometimes used in severe cases to identify potential allergic triggers.
- Patch testing used if contact dermatitis is suspected.

## DIFFERENTIAL DIAGNOSIS
- Seborrheic dermatitis
- Neurodermatitis (lichen simplex chronicus)
- Allergic contact dermatitis
- Irritant dermatitis
- Psoriasis
- Dyshidrosis
- Ichthyosis
- Scabies

 **TREATMENT**

## PRE-HOSPITAL
No specific pre-hospital care necessary

## ED TREATMENT/PROCEDURES
- Mild disease or disease of the head and neck:
  - Low-potency corticosteroids such as hydrocortisone 1–2.5%
- Moderate or severe disease of the trunk and extremities:
  - Higher-potency corticosteroids such as triamcinolone 0.1% (moderate potency) or fluocinonide 0.05% ointment (high potency)
- Severe disease of the head and neck:
  - Topical calcineurin inhibitors such as pimecrolimus and tacrolimus
- First-generation antihistamines:
  - Diphenhydramine, hydroxyzine are used for relief of itching but are only weakly effective.
- Probiotics reduced symptoms in children by 56%.
- Behavioral interventions:
  - Avoid excessive bathing.
  - Use of tepid water and mild soaps
  - Frequent use of emollients (Eucerin cream, Aquaphor ointment)
- Bacterial superinfection: Cephalexin, cefazolin:
  - Consider MRSA

## MEDICATION
- Aquaphor ointment: Apply to affected areas b.i.d.
- Cefazolin: 1 g (peds: >1 mo 50–100 mg/kg/24 hr; <1 mo, see PDR) IV q8h
- Cephalexin: 500 mg (peds: 25–100 mg/kg/24 hr) PO q6h
- Cetirizine: 5–10 mg/d (peds: 2.5–5 mg/d) PO
- Diphenhydramine: 25–50 mg (peds: 5 mg/kg/24 h) PO or IV q6h
- Eucerin cream: Apply to affected areas b.i.d.
- Fexofenadine: 60 mg (peds: >12 yr) PO daily to b.i.d.
- Fluocinonide 0.05% ointment: Apply to affected areas of body b.i.d. for the duration of the flare (high potency).
- Hydrocortisone 2.5% ointment: Apply to affected areas of body/face b.i.d. for the duration of the flare (low potency).
- Hydroxyzine: 25–100 mg (peds: 2 mg/kg/24 hr) PO q4–6h
- Loratadine: 10 mg (peds: <30 kg: 5 mg) PO daily
- Pimecrolimus 1% cream: Apply to affected areas b.i.d. (peds: >2 yr of age) for the duration of the flare.
- Tacrolimus ointment: 0.1% (peds: >2 yr of age: 0.03%) apply to affected areas b.i.d. for the duration of the flare.
- Triamcinolone 0.1% ointment: Apply to affected areas of body b.i.d. for the duration of the flare (mid potency).

### First Line
- Hydrocortisone 2.5% ointment: Apply to affected areas of body/face b.i.d. for the duration of the flare (low potency).
- Triamcinolone 0.1% ointment: Apply to affected areas of body b.i.d. for the duration of the flare (mid potency). Avoid the face.
- Fluocinonide 0.05% ointment: Apply to affected areas of body b.i.d. for the duration of the flare (high potency). Avoid the face.
- Aquaphor ointment: Apply to affected areas b.i.d.

### Second Line
- Tacrolimus ointment: 0.1%: (peds: >2 yr of age: 0.03%) apply to affected areas b.i.d. for the duration of the flare. Can be used on the face.
- Pimecrolimus 1% cream: Apply to affected areas b.i.d. (peds: >2 yr of age) for the duration of the flare. Can be used on the face.

 FOLLOW-UP

## DISPOSITION
### Issues for Referral
Dermatology referral for problematic cases

## FOLLOW-UP RECOMMENDATIONS
- Patients should be warned of adverse consequences of treatment:
  - High-potency steroids can cause thinning of the skin.
  - Tacrolimus and pimecrolimus cause a stinging sensation for the 1st wk of therapy.

## PEARLS AND PITFALLS
- Consider secondary cellulitis, as 90% of patients with atopic dermatitis are eventually colonized with *Staphylococcus aureus*.
- Use tacrolimus and pimecrolimus for moderate to severe disease of the head and neck.
- Consider in any patient with a severely pruritic rash

## ADDITIONAL READING
- Bieber T. Mechanisms of disease: Atopic dermatitis. *N Engl J Med.* 2008;358:1483–1494.
- Buys LM. Treatment options for atopic dermatitis. *Am Fam Physician.* 2007;75:523–528.
- Wasserbauer N, Ballow M. Atopic dermatitis. *Am J Med.* 2009;122:121–125.
- Williams HC. Clinical practice: Atopic dermatitis. *N Engl J Med.* 2005;352:2314–2324.

## See Also (Topic, Algorithm, Electronic Media Element)
- Cellulitis
- CA-MRSA

 CODES

## ICD9
- 691.8 Other atopic dermatitis and related conditions
- 692.9 Contact dermatitis and other eczema, unspecified cause

E

# EDEMA

*Laura Macnow*

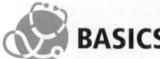 **BASICS**

## DESCRIPTION

- Clinically apparent accumulation of extravascular fluid due to a derangement in the balance of oncotic and hydrostatic forces:
  - Increase in venous hydrostatic pressure
- Systemically, as with CHF
- Locally, as with deep vein thrombosis:
  - Increase in lymphatic hydrostatic pressure
  - Decrease in oncotic pressure:
    ○ Systemically from hypoalbuminemia
    ○ Locally from increased capillary permeability
  - Increased venous hydrostatic pressure or decreased oncotic pressure results in pitting edema
  - Protein-rich extravasated fluid results in nonpitting edema
- Lymphedema
- Increased capillary permeability
- In certain disorders, there is no clear relation to Starling forces:
  - Myxedema
  - Idiopathic (cyclic) edema:
    ○ Worsened with heat
    ○ More common in women
    ○ Not necessarily related to menses

## ETIOLOGY

- Generalized:
  - Heart failure
  - Cor pulmonale
  - Cardiomyopathies
  - Constrictive pericarditis
  - Pulmonary HTN:
    ○ Sleep apnea
    ○ COPD
  - Acute glomerulonephritis
  - Renal failure
  - Medication related (often secondary to salt retention):
    ○ Steroids/estrogens/progestins
    ○ NSAIDs
    ○ Antihypertensives (especially vasodilators)
    ○ Lithium
    ○ Cyclosporine
    ○ Insulin
    ○ Thiazolidinediones (glitazones)
    ○ Growth hormone
    ○ Interleukin-2
    ○ MAOIs
    ○ Pramipexole
    ○ Docetaxel
    ○ Minoxidil
    ○ Acute withdrawal of diuretics

  - Idiopathic (cyclic) edema
  - Cirrhosis
  - Nephrotic syndrome
  - Protein-losing enteropathy
  - Starvation
  - Pregnancy
- Localized:
  - Deep vein thrombosis
  - Venous insufficiency
  - Thrombophlebitis
  - Chronic lymphangitis
  - Cellulitis
  - Baker cyst
  - Vasculitis
  - Angioedema:
    ○ Allergic
    ○ Acquired
  - Hypothyroidism (myxedema)
  - Mechanical trauma
  - Thermal injuries
  - Radiation injuries
  - Chemical burns
  - Hemiplegia
  - Reflex sympathetic dystrophy
  - Compressive or invasive tumor
  - Postsurgical resection of lymphatics
  - Postirradiation
  - Filariasis

 **DIAGNOSIS**

## SIGNS AND SYMPTOMS

- Weight gain of several kilograms
- Discomfort in the affected areas
- Swelling
- Tenderness
- Pitting edema:
  - Increased venous hydrostatic pressure or decreased oncotic pressure
- Nonpitting edema:
  - Protein-rich extravasated fluid
- Generalized edema (anasarca):
  - Edema is most prominent in dependent areas:
    ○ Feet
    ○ Sacrum
    ○ Bilateral lower extremities
    ○ Face/periorbital (especially in the morning)
  - Cardiac:
    ○ Dyspnea
    ○ Orthopnea
    ○ Paroxysmal nocturnal dyspnea
    ○ Increased jugular venous pressure
    ○ Rales
    ○ S3 gallop

  - Renal:
    ○ Anorexia
    ○ Puffy eyelids
    ○ Frothy urine
    ○ Oliguria
    ○ Dark urine
    ○ Hematuria
    ○ HTN
  - Hepatic:
    ○ Jaundice
    ○ Spider angiomas
    ○ Palmar erythema
    ○ Gynecomastia
    ○ Testicular atrophy
    ○ Ascites
- Localized:
  - Chronic venous insufficiency:
    ○ Chronic pitting
    ○ Skin discoloration (hemosiderin deposits)
    ○ Dermatitis/ulceration
    ○ Varicose veins
  - History of trauma:
    ○ Mechanical, thermal, radiation
  - Infectious/inflammatory:
    ○ Chills
    ○ Fever
    ○ Erythema
    ○ Increased warmth
  - Allergic:
    ○ Pruritus
    ○ Hives
    ○ Involvement of the lips and the oral mucosa
  - Myxedema:
    ○ Pretibial nonpitting edema
    ○ Dry waxy swelling of skin and subcutaneous tissues
    ○ Periorbital most common (puffy eyes)
    ○ Nondependent areas
    ○ Fatigue
    ○ Cold intolerance
    ○ Weight gain
    ○ Constipation
    ○ Slowed deep-tendon reflex relaxation
  - Idiopathic:
    ○ Diurnal weight gain/loss

### Pregnancy Considerations

- Common secondary to hormonally mediated fluid retention
- When involving hands and face, may be early sign of preeclampsia
- Dependent edema:
  - Usually in late pregnancy
  - From impedance of venous return
- Diuretics contraindicated

## ESSENTIAL WORKUP
Diagnostic studies should be directed by the underlying etiology suggested by the history and physical exam.

### DIAGNOSTIC TESTS & INTERPRETATION
*Lab*
- Cardiac etiology suspected:
  - BNP or NT-proBNP
- Deep vein thrombosis suspected:
  - D-Dimer (for patients with low clinical probability to rule out DVT)
- Renal etiology suspected:
  - Electrolytes
  - BUN and creatinine
  - Urinalysis
  - Urine electrolytes and protein
  - Serum lipids
- Hepatic etiology suspected:
  - Serum albumin
  - Liver function tests
  - Prothrombin time and partial thromboplastin time
- Myxedema suspected:
  - Thyroid function tests

*Imaging*
- Cardiac etiology suspected:
  - EKG
  - CXR
  - ECG
- Localized edema to an extremity:
  - US (duplex scanning) or contrast venography
- High suspicion for abdominal or pelvic malignancy:
  - Abdominal/pelvic CT

### DIFFERENTIAL DIAGNOSIS
- Cellulitis
- Contact dermatitis
- Diffuse subcutaneous infiltrative process
- Lymphedema
- Obesity

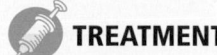 TREATMENT

### INITIAL STABILIZATION/THERAPY
See "ED Treatment."

### ED TREATMENT/PROCEDURES
- Treatment should be directed toward the underlying cause.
- Diuretics are usually indicated in cases of generalized edema but are not required emergently.
- Diuretics may be deleterious in patients with cirrhosis and ascites, as rapid fluid shifts may precipitate hepatorenal syndrome.

### MEDICATION
- Amiloride: 5–20 mg PO q.i.d.
- Captopril: 12.5–100 mg PO t.i.d. (max. 450 mg/d)
- Furosemide: 20–80 mg IV/PO q.i.d. (max. 600 mg/d)
- Hydrochlorothiazide: 25–200 mg PO q.i.d.
- Spironolactone: 25–200 mg PO q.i.d.

 FOLLOW-UP

### DISPOSITION
*Admission Criteria*
- Base the decision to admit the patient on the underlying etiology.
- Concomitant cardiovascular or pulmonary compromise
- Inability to ambulate without adequate home support
- Hypoxia

*Discharge Criteria*
- Patient should be advised to decrease salt intake.
- Elastic support stockings
- Elevation of involved limbs

*Issues for Referral*
- Patients >45 with chronic edema, or whose symptoms suggest a cardiopulmonary etiology require follow-up EKG.
- Patients with pulmonary HTN of unknown cause should be referred for a sleep study to evaluate for sleep apnea.
- A negative US in a patient at high-risk for DVT requires urgent repeat study in 5–7 days.

### FOLLOW-UP RECOMMENDATIONS
Patients with chronic edema may follow-up with primary care doctor for continued workup and treatment.

## PEARLS AND PITFALLS
- Classify edema as generalized vs. localized, pitting vs. nonpitting.
- Pitting edema is caused by "protein-poor" extravasated fluid (by increased hydrostatic pressure or decreased oncotic pressure).
- Nonpitting edema is caused by "protein-rich" extravasated fluids (lymphedema or increased capillary permeability).
- Generalized or bilateral leg edema necessitates workup of systemic disease.
- Acute unilateral leg edema requires evaluation for DVT.
- Consider preeclampsia in pregnant patients.

## ADDITIONAL READING
- Braunwald E, Loscalzo J. Edema. In: Fauci AS, et al., eds. *Harrison's Principles of Internal Medicine*, 17th ed. New York: McGraw-Hill, 2008.
- Ely JW, et al. Approach to leg edema of unclear etiology. *JABFM*. 2006;19:148–160.
- Mockler J, et al. What is the differential diagnosis of chronic leg edema in primary care?. *J Fam Pract*. 2008;57;188–189.
- Obrien JG, et al. Treatment of edema. *Am Fam Physician*. 2005;71:2111–2117.

### See Also (Topic, Algorithm, Electronic Media Element)
- Congestive Heart Failure
- Cor Pulmonale
- Deep Vein Thrombosis
- Angioedema
- Cirrhosis
- Venous Insufficiency
- Nephritic Syndrome
- Nephrotic Syndrome

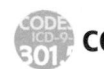 CODES

ICD9
782.3 Edema

E

# EHRLICHIOSIS

*Roger M. Barkin*
*Jonathan A. Edlow*

 **BASICS**

## DESCRIPTION
- Relatively recently described tick-borne human infection presenting as a nonspecific febrile illness
- Several forms of ehrlichiosis exist; 2 predominate in North America:
- Human monocytic ehrlichiosis (HME), 1st described in 1987:
  - Vector tick: *Amblyomma americanum* (lone star tick)
  - Geographic range: Central, southern, and mid-Atlantic states, with range expanding to parts of New England
- Human granulocytic ehrlichiosis or human granulocytic anaplasmosis (HGE or HGA), 1st described in 1994:
  - Vector tick: *Ixodes scapularis* (deer tick)
  - Geographic range: East Coast, mid-Central States, and Pacific Northwest (same areas as Lyme disease)
- A 3rd type may also be encountered, caused by *Ehrlichia ewingii,* which has the tick vector of the lone star tick.
- All are tick-borne but have different vectors and geographic ranges. Other species have been reported, but at present HME and HGE are the important ehrlichial human pathogens.

## ETIOLOGY
- 2 distinct species of obligate intracellular organisms
- The taxonomy of these pathogens has changed in recent years as more DNA and ribosomal RNA data become available.
- HME is caused by the organism *Ehrlichia chaffeensis.*
- HGE/HGA is caused by *Anaplasma phagocytophila* (a new name as of 2002).
- The vasculitis found in Rocky Mountain spotted fever (RMSF) is usually not present.
- Compared with RMSF, older individuals are usually affected, often those >40 yr of age.

## DIAGNOSIS

### SIGNS AND SYMPTOMS
- Signs and symptoms of HME and HGE/HGA are similar.
- Both of these are relatively newly recognized diseases:
  - Many patients who are infected undergo asymptomatic seroconversion.
  - The spectrum reported may overrepresent the more severely affected patients.
- With any tick-borne infection, patients can be coinfected by more than 1 pathogen from the same tick bite:
  - May have a complicated presentation of 2 different diseases
- Minority of children have severe disease.

### History
- The season and other epidemiologic factors are important in diagnosing tick-borne diseases:
  - Most commonly present from April–October
  - Variability is likely owing to changes in weather patterns from year to year and from region to region.
- Symptom onset from 1–2 wk (median 9–10 days) following the tick bite:
  - Bite of the larger lone star tick is more likely to be recalled by the patient than that of the smaller deer tick.
- Abrupt onset of:
  - Fever
  - Chills
  - Headache
  - Myalgias
  - Malaise
- Rash:
  - HME (35–60% of cases)
  - HGE or HGA (~5–10% of cases)
  - Often delayed and may be variable
- Symptoms may relate to complications of ehrlichiosis, such as:
  - ARDS
  - Renal failure
  - Hypotension and shock
  - Rhabdomyolysis
  - GI disturbances
  - CNS or peripheral nervous system (PNS) involvement, such as encephalopathy and meningitis
  - DIC
  - Immunocompromised patients have more severe complications.

### Physical Exam
- Fever
- Rash:
  - May be macular, maculopapular, or petechial
  - May be absent during 1st wk of illness
  - Usually involves trunk and spares hands and feet
- Lymphadenopathy
- Hepatosplenomegaly
- Neurologic findings:
  - Abnormal mental status
  - Meningismus
  - Nystagmus
- Pulmonary findings (rales, rhonchi) depending on pulmonary complications

### ALERT
- Ehrlichiosis is a potentially fatal tick-borne illness that is usually diagnosed clinically.
- Consider this diagnosis in all patients with nonspecific febrile illnesses, especially during the warm months of the year, and definitely if there is a history of tick bite.
- The Centers for Disease Control and Prevention (CDC) define the illness as fever with 1 or more of the following: Headache, myalgia, anemia, leukopenia, thrombocytopenia, or elevation of serum transaminase; plus serologic evidence of 4-fold change in IgG specific antibody by IFA or detection of specific target by PCR assay, demonstration of antigen on biopsy/autopsy sample, or isolation of organism in cell culture.

### DIAGNOSTIC TESTS & INTERPRETATION
*Lab*
- CBC:
  - Leukopenia
  - Thrombocytopenia
  - Anemia
- Hepatic transaminases:
  - Often elevated 2–6 times normal
- Indirect immunofluorescence antibody test:
  - Usual test available
  - Threshold for a positive test is usually made by the individual lab testing the serum.
  - 94–99% sensitive when 2nd sample obtained over 14 days from onset of illness

- Wright stain of peripheral blood:
  - Morula may be seen:
    - Small intracytoplasmic ehrlichial DNA inclusion bodies
    - Diagnostic
    - Sensitivity of seeing morulae depend on who is looking, for how long, and the immunologic competence of the patient.
    - Found more commonly in HGE/HGA (~50%) than in HME (~10–15%)
- Culture and PCR test:
  - Not routinely available
- Antibody titer tests:
  - Not available in real time

### Imaging
- Head CT for encephalopathy
- CXR for fever/dyspnea

### Other Studies
- CSF
- Pleocytosis with predominance of lymphocytes and increased total protein

## DIFFERENTIAL DIAGNOSIS
- Most tick-borne illnesses:
  - Rocky Mountain spotted fever
  - Lyme disease
  - Babesiosis
- Many viral and bacterial infections and numerous other infectious diseases, especially early in their course, can initially present with an undifferentiated febrile illness similar to ehrlichiosis.
- Mononucleosis
- Thrombotic thrombocytopenia purpura
- Hematologic malignancy
- Cholangitis
- Pneumonia

 **TREATMENT**

### INITIAL STABILIZATION/THERAPY
ABCs

### ED TREATMENT/PROCEDURES
- Initiate antibiotics:
  - Doxycycline:
    - Drug of choice
    - Children who are affected should also receive doxycycline. 14 days of treatment does not appear to cause significant discoloration of permanent teeth.
    - Treatment should be continued for at least 3 days past defervescence for a minimum total course of 7 days. Severe or complicated disease requires a longer course.

- Rifampin for:
  - Pregnant patients
  - Allergy to doxycycline
  - Mildly affected children <9 yr of age
  - Patients who are pregnant, allergic to doxycycline, or mildly affected can be given rifampin for 7–10 days.
- Initiate therapy for other tick-borne diseases that may have been cotransmitted.

### MEDICATION
Doxycycline:
- Adults: 100 mg IV/PO q12h
- Children (severely affected): 4 mg/kg q12h IV/PO up to maximum of adult dose; older children can be dosed as adult.

### Pediatric Considerations
Despite the fact that doxycycline is generally contraindicated in patients <9 yr old, it is the drug of choice in young children who are severely affected by ehrlichiosis. In less affected children, rifampin has been used successfully.

### Pregnancy Considerations
Rifampin can be used to treat pregnant women with ehrlichiosis.

 **FOLLOW-UP**

### DISPOSITION
### Admission Criteria
- Significant comorbidities/severely affected
- Cannot take PO antibiotics
- Immunosuppressed patients
- *E. chaffensis* (HME) has a case fatality rate up to 3%.

### Discharge Criteria
- Healthy appearing
- Symptoms typically last 1–2 wk; recovery occurring without sequelae.
- Long-term neurologic complications have been reported.

### Issues for Referral
Severe disease or presence of complications

## ADDITIONAL READING

- American Academy of Pediatrics. *2009 Report of the Committee on Infectious Diseases*. Elk Grove, IL: AAP, 2009.
- Edlow JA. *Bull's Eye: Unraveling the Medical Mystery of Lyme Disease*. New Haven, CT: Yale University Press, 2004.
- Olano JP, Walker DH. Human ehrlichioses. *Med Clin North Am*. 2002;86:375–392.
- Ramsey AH, Belongia EA, Gale CM, et al. Outcomes of treated HGE cases. *Emerg Infect Dis*. 2002;8(4):398–401.
- Schutze GE, Buckingham SC, et al. Human monocytic ehrlichiosis in children. *Pediatr Infect Dis*. 2007;26:475.
- Stone JH, Kerry D, Aram G, et al. Human monocytic ehrlichiosis. *JAMA*. 2004;292:2263–2270.
- www.cdc.gov/mmwr/pdf/rr/rr5504/pdf

### See Also (Topic, Algorithm, Electronic Media Element)
- Lyme Disease
- Rocky Mountain Spotted Fever
- Tick-Borne Diseases

 **CODES**

### ICD9
- 082.40 Unspecified ehrlichiosis
- 082.41 Ehrlichiosis chafeensis (e chafeensis)
- 082.49 Other ehrlichiosis

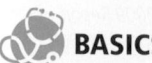 **BASICS**

## DESCRIPTION

### Bony Injuries

- Supracondylar fracture:
  - Most common in children
  - Peak ages 5–10 yr, rarely occurs >15 yr
  - Extension type (98%): FOOSH (*fall on outstretched hand*) with fully extended or hyperextended arm:
    - Type 1: Minimal or no displacement
    - Type 2: Slightly displaced fracture; posterior cortex intact
    - Type 3: Totally displaced fracture; posterior cortex broken
  - Flexion type: Blow directly to flexed elbow:
    - Type 1: Minimal or no displacement
    - Type 2: Slightly displaced fracture; anterior cortex intact
    - Type 3: Totally displaced fracture; anterior cortex broken
- Radial head fracture:
  - Usually indirect mechanism (eg, FOOSH)
  - Radial head driven into capitellum

### Soft Tissue Injuries

- Elbow dislocation:
  - Second only to shoulder as most dislocated joint
  - Most are posterior.
- Medial/lateral epicondylitis:
  - Overuse injuries usually related to rotary motion at elbow
  - Involving attachment points of hand and wrist flexor/extensor groups to elbow
  - Plumbers, carpenters, tennis players, golfers
  - Pain made worse by resisted contraction of particular muscle groups

### Pediatric Considerations

- Subluxed radial head (nursemaid's elbow)
- 20% of all upper extremity injuries in children
- Peak age 1–4 yr; occurs more frequently in females than males
- Sudden longitudinal pull on forearm with forearm pronated

## ETIOLOGY

- Mechanism aids in determining expected injury.
- Trauma predominates.
- Most elbow injuries caused by indirect trauma transmitted through bones of forearm (eg, FOOSH)
- Direct blows account for very few fractures or dislocations.

 **DIAGNOSIS**

## SIGNS AND SYMPTOMS

How patient carries arm may give clues to diagnosis.

### Bony Injuries

Supracondylar fracture:

- Flexion type:
  - Patient supports injured forearm with other arm and elbow in 90-degree flexion.
  - Loss of olecranon prominence
- Extension type:
  - Patient holds arm at side in S-type configuration.

### Soft Tissue Injuries

- Elbow dislocations:
  - Posterior: Abnormal prominence of olecranon
  - Anterior: Loss of olecranon prominence
- Radial head subluxation:
  - Elbow slightly flexed and forearm pronated, resists moving arm at elbow
- Medial/lateral epicondylitis:
  - Gradual onset of dull ache over inner/outer aspect of elbow referred to forearm
  - Pain increases with grasping and twisting motions.

## ESSENTIAL WORKUP

- Radiographs
- Assess wrist and shoulder for associated injury.
- Evaluate neurovascular status of limb.
- Assess skin integrity.
- Examine for compartment syndrome, which is more common in supracondylar fractures.

### ALERT

- Injuries to ipsilateral upper limb, particularly fractures to midshaft humerus and distal forearm, are common.
- Evaluate for associated neurovascular injuries (up to 20%).

## DIAGNOSTIC TESTS & INTERPRETATION

### Lab

None specific for elbow injuries

### Imaging

- Not usually necessary if overuse injury suspected
- Routine anteroposterior (AP) and lateral; add oblique for assessment of subtle injuries to radial head/distal humerus.

- Fat pad sign:
  - Seen with intra-articular injuries
  - Normally, anterior fat pad is narrow radiolucent strip anterior to humerus.
  - Posterior fat pad is normally *not* visible.
  - *Anterior fat pad sign* indicates joint effusion/injury when raised and becomes more perpendicular to anterior humeral cortex (sail sign).
  - *Posterior fat pad sign* indicates effusion/injury:
    - In adults, posterior fat pad sign without other obvious fracture implies radial head fracture.
    - In children, it implies supracondylar fracture.

### Pediatric Considerations

- Fractures in children often occur through unossified cartilage, making radiographic interpretation confusing.
- A line drawn down anterior surface of humerus should always bisect the capitellum in lateral view.
- If any bony relationships appear questionable on radiographs, obtain comparison view of uninvolved elbow.
- Suspect nonaccidental trauma if history does not fit injury.
- Ossification centers: 1st appear:
  - Capitellum: 3–6 mo
  - Radial head: 3–5 yr
  - Medial epicondyle: 5–7 yr
  - Trochlea: 9–10 yr
  - Olecranon: 9–10 yr
  - Lateral epicondyle: 9–13 yr

## DIFFERENTIAL DIAGNOSIS

- Sprain/strain
- Effusion
- Contusion
- Bursitis
- Arthritis

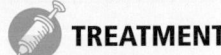 **TREATMENT**

**PRE-HOSPITAL**
Appropriate splinting

**INITIAL STABILIZATION/THERAPY**
Immobilization to prevent further injury before taking radiographs is essential.

**ED TREATMENT/PROCEDURES**
- Orthopedic consultation is recommended for all but nondisplaced, stable fractures, which can generally be splinted with 24–48-hr orthopedic follow up.
- Fractures generally requiring orthopedic consultation:
  – Transcondylar, intercondylar, condylar, epicondylar fractures
  – Fractures involving articular surfaces such as capitellum or trochlea
- Supracondylar fractures:
  – Type 1 can be handled by ED physician with 24–48-hr orthopedic follow-up.
  – Elbow may be flexed and splinted with posterior splint.
  – Types 2 and 3 require immediate orthopedic consult.
  – Reduce these in ED when fracture is associated with vascular compromise.
- Anterior dislocation:
  – Reduce immediately if vascular structures compromised.
  – Then flex to 90 degrees and place posterior splint.
- Posterior dislocation:
  – Reduce immediately if vascular structures compromised.
  – Then flex to 90 degrees and place posterior splint.
- Radial head fracture:
  – Minimally displaced fractures may be aspirated to remove hemarthrosis; instill bupivacaine (Marcaine) and immobilize.
  – Other types should have orthopedic consult.

- Radial head subluxation:
  – In one continuous motion, supinate and flex elbow while placing slight pressure on radial head.
  – Hyperpronation technique is possibly more effective—while grasping the patient's elbow the wrist is hyperpronated until a palpable click is felt.
  – Often will feel click with reduction
  – If exam suggests fracture but radiograph is negative, splint and have patient follow up in 24–48 hr for re-evaluation.
- Medial/lateral epicondylitis:
  – Severe cases can be splinted.
  – Rest, heat, anti-inflammatory agents

 **ALERT**
- Neurovascular injuries to numerous structures that pass about the elbow, including anterior interosseus nerve, ulnar and radial nerves, brachial artery
- Volkmann ischemic contracture is compartment syndrome of forearm.

**MEDICATION**
- Conscious sedation is often required to achieve reductions; see Conscious Sedation.
- Ibuprofen: 600–800 mg (peds: 5–10 mg/kg) PO t.i.d.
- Naprosyn: 250–500 mg (peds: 10–20 mg/kg) PO b.i.d.
- Tylenol with codeine no. 3. 1 or 2 tabs (peds: 0.5–1 mg/kg codeine) PO q4–6h
- Morphine sulfate: 0.1 mg/kg IV q2–6h

 **FOLLOW-UP**

**DISPOSITION**
*Admission Criteria*
- Vascular injuries, open fractures
- Fractures requiring operative reduction or internal fixation
- Admit all patients with extensive swelling or ecchymosis for overnight observation and elevation to monitor for and decrease risk for compartment syndrome.

*Discharge Criteria*
- Stable fractures or reduced dislocations with none of above features
- Splint and arrange orthopedic follow-up in 24–48 hr.
- Uncomplicated soft tissue injuries

**PEARLS AND PITFALLS**
- Failure to appreciate that a posterior fat pad sign is abnormal.
- Always educate parents of a child with a supracondylar fracture about the signs and symptoms of compartment syndrome.

**ADDITIONAL READING**
- Anderson BC. *Office Orthopedics for Primary Care: Diagnosis and Treatment*, 2nd ed. Philadelphia: Saunders; 1999.
- Carson S, Woolridge DP, Colletti J, et al. Pediatric upper extremity injuries. *Pediatr Clin North Am.* 2006;53(1):41–67, review.
- McCarty LP, Ring D, Jupiter JB. Management of distal humerus fractures. *Am J Orthop.* 2005;34(9):430–438.
- Macias CG, Bothner J, Wiebe R. A comparison of supination/flexion to hyperpronation in the reduction of radial head subluxations. *Pediatrics.* 1998;102(1):e10.
- Minkowitz B, et al. Supracondylar humerus fractures: Current trends and controversies. *Orthop Clin North Am.* 1994;25:4.
- Nicholson DA, et al. ABC of emergency radiology: The elbow. *Br Med J.* 1993;307:23.
- Simon R, Koenigsknecht S. *Emergency Orthopedics. The Extremities*, 4th ed. East Norwalk, CT: Appleton & Lange; 1996.

**CODES**

**ICD9**
- 726.31 Medial epicondylitis
- 812.41 Supracondylar fracture of humerus, closed
- 813.05 Fracture of head of radius, closed

# ELECTRICAL INJURY

*Marilyn M. Hallock*

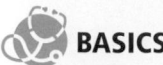 **BASICS**

## DESCRIPTION

- Electricity is the flow of electrons through a conductor, across a gradient, from high to low concentration.
- Nature and severity of electrical injuries depend on the voltage, current strength and type, resistance to flow, and duration of contact.
- Ohm's law: Voltage (V) = current (I) × resistance (R):
  - Voltage is directly proportional to current and is inversely proportional to resistance.
  - High-voltage (>600 V) and low-voltage injuries:
    - Telephone lines: 65 V
    - Household general circuit: 110 V
    - Electrical range or dryer: 220 V
    - Household power lines: 220 V
    - Subway 3rd rail: 600 V
    - Residential trunk line: 7,620 V
    - Industrial electrical power line: 100,000 V
  - Household devices can contain a transformer stepping up a seemingly low-voltage source to high voltage:
    - Microwave, television, computer
  - Resistance (R) is determined by the current's pathway through the body:
    - Nerves, muscles, blood vessels have low resistance and are better electrical conductors than are bone, tendon, fat.
    - Water and sweat on skin decrease resistance; calloused skin increases resistance.
    - More resistance means less flow, and more conversion to heat.
  - Current is measured in amperes (I) and is a measure of the amount of energy flowing through an object:
    - "Let go" current is the maximum current a person can grasp and release before muscle tetany inhibits letting go.
    - Household general circuit: 15–30 A
    - Tingling sensation/perception: 0.2–2 mA
    - Pain: 1–4 mA
    - Average child "let go" current: 3–5 mA
    - Adult "let go" current: 6–9 mA; higher for men than women
    - Skeletal muscle tetany current: 16–20 mA
    - Respiratory muscle paralysis: 20–50 mA
    - Ventricular fibrillation: 50–120 mA
- Alternating current (AC):
  - Electron flow rhythmically reverses direction:
    - Homes and offices in U.S. use standard 60 Hz
  - Can produce continuous tetanic muscle contraction, loss of voluntary control of muscles, prolongs contact
  - More dangerous than direct current (DC)
  - More likely to result in ventricular fibrillation at household current level:
    - Stimulation can continue through vulnerable T wave period of cardiac cycle.
- Direct current (DC):
  - Continuous electron flow in 1 direction
    - Defibrillators and pacemakers, industrial sources
  - Large, single muscle spasm tends to throw victim from source:
    - Increased risk of traumatic blunt injuries
    - Shorter duration of exposure
  - More likely to result in asystole
- Trimodal distribution of electrical injuries:
  - Toddlers (household outlets and cords)
  - Teenagers (risk-taking behavior)
  - Adults (work-related injuries)

## ETIOLOGY

Types of electrical injury:

- Direct contact causing tissue destruction:
  - Electrothermal burn may cause skin or deep tissue coagulation necrosis.
  - Minor visible injuries may be misleading for extensive deep tissue injury.
  - Location of damage is point of contact with source and point of contact with ground.
- Flame:
  - Burns from burning clothing or other substances
- Electrical arc indirect contact:
  - Burns from the heat of a high-voltage arc (a flashburn) that passes electricity through air
  - May cause thermal and flame burns
  - Flashburns usually result in superficial partial-thickness burns.
- Primary electrical phenomena:
  - Cardiac arrhythmias
  - Muscle contractions and tetany
- Secondary injury from trauma:
  - Supraphysiologic muscle contraction
  - Fall or being thrown

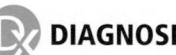 **DIAGNOSIS**

## SIGNS AND SYMPTOMS

- Head/neck/ENT:
  - Common entry site for high-voltage injuries:
    - Facial and corneal burns
    - Perforated tympanic membranes
    - Cataracts and optic nerve atrophy may present initially, or delayed 4–6 mo
    - Intraocular hemorrhage, uveitis
    - Cervical spine injury
- Cardiovascular:
  - Cardiac arrest, asystole, or ventricular fibrillation are leading causes of death.
  - Other arrhythmias and EKG findings: Sinus tachycardia, atrial fibrillation, premature ventricular contractions, transient ST elevation, reversible QT prolongation:
    - Sometimes delayed up to 12 hr
    - Usually resolve spontaneously
  - Myocardial damage occurs rarely:
    - Generally epicardial, not transmural
    - Damage does not follow distribution of coronary arteries.
    - EKG will not show standard injury patterns.

- Respiratory:
  - Brain injury causing respiratory center inhibition
  - Tetanic contraction/paralysis of chest wall/diaphragm muscles:
    - May cause respiratory arrest
  - Postcardiac arrest respiratory arrest
  - Traumatic lung injury
  - Lung tissue itself appears resistant to electrical injury, probably owing to air content.
- Neurologic:
  - Respiratory arrest
  - Amnesia, transient confusion
  - Loss of consciousness, altered mental status, seizures, coma
  - Spinal cord injury:
    - May result from blunt trauma or direct current effects (hand-to-hand flow)
    - Localized paresis up to/including quadriplegia
  - Long-term neurologic complications:
    - Seizures, peripheral nerve damage, spinal cord syndromes, psychiatric problems
- Vascular:
  - Muscle necrosis and compartment syndromes
  - Thrombosis in slow-moving venous system owing to coagulation
  - Intimal injury in fast-moving arterial system may lead to acute or delayed arterial malfunction.
- Renal failure secondary to myoglobinuria
- Skeletal system/orthopedics:
  - Supraphysiologic tetanic muscle contractions from electrostimulation
  - Classically described injuries:
    - Vertebral column fracture
    - Posterior shoulder dislocation
    - Femoral neck fracture
- Dermatologic:
  - Contact/ground wounds: Hands, feet, and head most common and most severe sites
  - "Kissing" burns from current exit and re-entry on flexor surfaces

### Pediatric Considerations

Mouth burn most common <4 yr; sucking/biting on household electrical cord:

- Cosmetic deformity risk if commissure involved
- Delayed bleeding (3–5 days) from labial artery when eschar separates
- Risk of damage to developing dentition

### Pregnancy Considerations

Fetus much less resistant to electrical shock than mother:

- Obstetric consult or referral for all pregnant patients regardless of symptoms
  - Risk of placental abruption or threatened miscarriage
  - Fetal monitoring if >20 wk gestation

## History
- Determine whether exposure was high- or low-voltage, the duration and location of contact, or concomitant trauma.
- If unwitnessed respiratory arrest or ventricular fibrillation in patient, consider electrical injury.

## Physical Exam
Search the skin for entry/exit wounds and kiss/arch wounds at flexor surfaces.

## ESSENTIAL WORKUP
- Urinalysis for myoglobin
- EKG and cardiac enzymes for high-voltage victims, and low voltage victims with cardiorespiratory complaints
- Cardiac monitoring indications:
  - Cardiac arrest
    Loss of consciousness
    Chest pain
  - Hypoxia
  - Abnormal EKG
  - Dysrhythmia in pre-hospital or ED setting
  - History of cardiac disease
  - Significant risk factors for coronary artery disease
  - Suspicion of conductive injury
  - Concomitant injury severe enough to warrant admission
- Prolonged monitoring is probably unnecessary in asymptomatic patients with normal EKG, no dysrhythmias, and exposure to <240 V

## DIAGNOSTIC TESTS & INTERPRETATION
### Lab
- For most exposures to household current, no testing is indicated:
  - Low-voltage burns can still cause dysrhythmias, seizures, and other complications if contact is near the chest or head.
- Urinalysis for myoglobinuria
- Creatinine kinase, electrolytes, BUN, creatinine:
  - Positive urine myoglobin and/or high-voltage exposure
  - Provides baseline renal function, possible presence of hyperkalemia and metabolic acidosis
- Cardiac markers in:
  - Abnormal EKG or dysrhythmia
  - High-voltage exposures or low-voltage victims with cardiorespiratory complaints

### Imaging
Dictated by clinical indications

## DIFFERENTIAL DIAGNOSIS
- Thermal burns from electrical arcing flash burn vs. deep electrothermal injury
- Instability owing to traumatic injuries vs. electrical burns

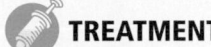 **TREATMENT**

### PRE-HOSPITAL
- Secure scene; turn off power source for high-voltage incident.
- Assume traumatic injury in unstable or unconscious patient:
  - Spinal immobilization
- Standard basic life support/advanced cardiac life support care
- Early CPR in post-electric shock arrest may allow time for heart to restart.
- Splint fractures and dislocations.
- Cover burns with clean, dry dressings.

### ALERT
Care must be exercised at scene to ensure that rescuers do not contact live electrical sources.

### INITIAL STABILIZATION/THERAPY
- ABCs
- Local wound care for thermal burns
- Immobilize/reduce fractures and dislocations

### ED TREATMENT/PROCEDURES
- IV fluid resuscitation:
  - Larger fluid volumes may be required owing to extensive 3rd spacing in injured muscle.
  - Rapid administration to reach urine output of 1 mL/kg/h
  - Foley catheter
- Evaluate for myoglobinuria and prevent renal failure:
  - Maintain good urine output.
  - IV sodium bicarbonate increases solubility of myoglobin in urine.
  - Consider furosemide/mannitol.
  - Monitor renal function.
- Tetanus prophylaxis
- Pain control as required

### MEDICATION
- Bicarbonate: 1 ampule IV, then 2 ampules added to 1 L of $D_5W$ to maintain urine pH >7.45
- Furosemide: 0.5 mg/kg IV
- Mannitol: 25 g (peds: 0.25–0.5 mg/kg) IV bolus, then 12.5 mg/kg/h IV titrated to urine flow >1 mL/kg/h

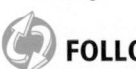 **FOLLOW-UP**

### DISPOSITION
#### Admission Criteria
- Documented loss of consciousness
- Dysrhythmias, abnormal EKG, or evidence of myocardial damage
- Suspicion of deep tissue damage
- Myoglobinuria or acidosis
- Burn criteria for admission or transfer to burn center
- Traumatic injuries requiring admission
- Pregnant patients >20 wk gestation

#### Discharge Criteria
- Minor, low-voltage injury (<240 V) with no associated injuries, normal physical exam, and asymptomatic
- Cutaneous burns or mild persistent symptoms with normal EKG and no urinary heme pigment
- Stable in ED after period of observation
- Discharge 1st-trimester patient with threatened miscarriage instructions.
- Pediatric patients with isolated oral burns and close adult care

### Issues for Referral
- Burn wound care
- Persistence of current symptoms or new delayed symptoms:
  - Neurology for delayed weakness, paresthesias
- Obstetrics for pregnant patients
- Dental or reconstructive surgery for pediatric oral burns

### FOLLOW-UP RECOMMENDATIONS
Ophthalmology for delayed cataracts in significant electrical current injuries

## PEARLS AND PITFALLS
- Prolonged cardiac monitoring is probably unnecessary in asymptomatic patients with normal EKG, no dysrhythmias, and exposure to <240 V.
- With significant electrical burn injuries, administer enough IV fluid to maintain adequate urine output and to stabilize the vital signs:
  - Extensive 3rd spacing may occur.

## ADDITIONAL READING

- Bailey B, Gaudreault P, Thivierge RL. Cardiac monitoring of high-risk patients after an electrical injury: A prospective multicentre study. *Emerg Med J.* 2007;24(5):348–352.
- Luz DP, Milan LS, Alessi MS, et al. Electrical burns: A retrospective analysis across a 5-year period. *Burns.* 1996;22(2):137–140.
- Price T, Cooper MA. Electrical and lightning injuries. In: Marx J, Hockberger R, Walls R. *Rosen's emergency medicine*, 5th ed. St. Louis: Mosby; 2002:2010–2020.
- Spies C, Trohman RG. Narrative review: Electrocution and life-threatening electrical injuries. *Ann Intern Med.* 2006;145(7):531–537.

### See Also (Topic, Algorithm, Electronic Media Element)
- Burns
- Lightning Injury
- Rhabdomyolysis

 **CODES**

### ICD9
994.8 Electrocution and nonfatal effects of electric current

# ENCEPHALITIS
*Arunchalam Einstein*

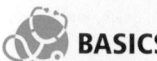 **BASICS**

## DESCRIPTION

- Acute infectious inflammation of the brain
- 20,000 cases in U.S. annually
- Mortality: 10%
- Inflammatory reaction occurs within brain parenchyma with destruction of neurons, parenchymal edema, and petechial hemorrhages.
- Route of CNS infection usually hematogenous; search for another site
- Neural migration occurs with rabies, herpes simplex virus (HSV), and varicella-zoster encephalitis.

## ETIOLOGY

- Viral is most common.
- 50% of cases have no identifiable cause.

### Specific Viruses

- HSV:
  - 10–20% of all encephalitides
  - Primary or reactivation
  - Early treatment improves prognosis.
- Arbovirus:
  - 10–15% of all encephalitides
  - Zoonotic transmission (mosquitoes, ticks) in warm months
  - Eastern equine causes fulminant encephalitis:
    ○ Tropism for the hippocampus
    ○ Abrupt onset of headache, fever, vomiting
  - Western equine occurs mostly in the western 2/3 of the U.S.:
    ○ Often preceded by nonspecific upper respiratory/GI tract symptoms
  - Japanese—most prevalent arboviral encephalitis worldwide:
    ○ Indolent course of fever, headache, myalgias, and fatigue followed by confusion, delirium, masklike facies, and parkinsonisms, seizures, brainstem dysfunction, coma, and death
- Flavivirus:
  - West Nile virus—increased incidence in North America:
    ○ Found in mosquitoes and birds
    ○ Febrile illness, often with rash
    ○ Headache
    ○ Lymphadenopathy
    ○ Polyarthropathy
    ○ Increased morbidity/mortality in elderly patients

- Enteroviral:
  - Occurs mainly in children <10 yr old
  - Relatively benign course with little or no long-term sequelae
- Measles encephalitis:
  - Occurs several days to 2–3 wk after primary infection and rash, or after years of latent infection
  - Abrupt onset and rapid progression to coma
  - Seizures common (50–60%)
  - Postimmunization incidence of 1 per 1 million vaccinated
- HIV encephalitis:
  - Lower CD4 counts predispose to encephalitis.
  - Typical features include motor spasticity and dementia.
  - Involvement of white matter with extensive neural degeneration
- Rhabdovirus: Rabies
- Nipah virus encephalitis, which appeared in Malaysia and Singapore, and is now present in Bangladesh, may be associated with exposure to pigs or bats.
- Hendra virus caused a disease affecting horses and humans in Australia in 1994 and 1995 and has since then caused sporadic encephalitis in humans.

### Nonviral

- *Mycoplasma pneumoniae*
- *Toxoplasma gondii*
- *Rickettsia rickettsii*
- *Mycobacterium tuberculosis*
- *Borrelia burgdorferi*
- *Coccidioides immitis*
- Leptospirosis

### Immunocompromised/HIV Patients

- Histoplasma
- *Cryptococcus neoformans*
- Varicella-zoster
- *Listeria monocytogenes*
- Cytomegalovirus
- *Toxoplasma gondii*
- Human herpesvirus type 6 (HHV-6)

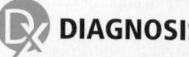 **DIAGNOSIS**

## SIGNS AND SYMPTOMS

- Often begins with a preceding flulike illness over a few days:
  - Mild headache, fever, sore throat, reduced appetite, myalgias
- Altered level of consciousness, drowsiness, coma
- Impaired cognitive ability and personality change, hallucinations, psychosis
- Restlessness, agitation, irritability, delirium
- Rash:
  - Lyme disease
  - Rocky Mountain spotted fever
  - Varicella
  - HSV
- Seizures
- Fever, headache, vomiting, possible meningismus
- Focal neurologic deficits, tremor, ataxia, cranial nerve palsies (more common than meningitis)
- Papilledema on funduscopy
- Clinical picture varies from mild headache and mild cognitive/emotional lability to severe agitation, seizures, coma, permanent neurologic sequelae, and death.
- Clinical course of symptoms may be slow moving or rapidly progressive.

## History

Arboviruses (eastern equine, western equine, St. Louis, Venezuelan equine encephalitis, and West Nile virus) cause disease when mosquitoes are active, whereas herpes simplex virus can occur at any time.

## Physical Exam

- Patients with encephalitis have an altered mental status ranging from subtle deficits to complete unresponsiveness.
- Other findings reflect neurological involvement.

## ESSENTIAL WORKUP
- Lumbar puncture—CSF analysis for
- Cell count/chemistry:
  - Elevated WBC, predominantly lymphocytes
  - Elevated protein
  - Glucose (normal in viral disease)
  - Gram stain with or without India ink for suspected/confirmed HIV
- Viral and bacterial cultures (fungi if indicated by history)
- Antigen assays for:
  - HSV
  - Cryptococcus
  - Toxoplasmosis
  - Other viral antigen and antibody assays if available (enterovirus, adenovirus, cytomegalovirus, mumps, varicella-zoster)

## DIAGNOSTIC TESTS & INTERPRETATION
### Lab
- CBC:
  - WBC usually elevated; however, a normal WBC does not exclude infection.
- Electrolytes, glucose, BUN, creatinine
- Bacterial and viral blood cultures
- Liver function tests, ammonia level if hepatic failure suspected
- Carboxyhemoglobin level if CO poisoning suspected
- Toxicology screen if ingestion suspected in differential
- Polymerase chain reaction (PCR):
  - Confirm viral nucleic acids in CSF
  - HSV, varicella, enteroviruses, others

### Imaging
- CT scan:
  - To rule out trauma, hemorrhagic conditions, and mass lesions
  - Cerebral edema may be the only finding consistent with encephalitis.
  - HSV may show parenchymal hemorrhagic areas of the frontal and temporal lobes, along with edema.
- MRI:
  - Hypodense temporal lobes in HSV

### Diagnostic Procedures/Surgery
EEG may be useful in presence proven or suspected seizures

## DIFFERENTIAL DIAGNOSIS
- Meningitis
- Brain abscess
- Sepsis
- Stroke (hemorrhagic or ischemic)
- Head injury
- Subarachnoid hemorrhage
- Encephalopathy (hepatic, uremic)
- Metabolic:
  - Electrolyte abnormalities ($Na^{2+}$, $K^+$, $Cl^-$, $Ca^{2+}$, $Mg^{2+}$, phosphate)
  - Hypoglycemia
  - Hyperglycemic nonketotic coma
- Neoplastic
- Drugs/toxins
- Carbon monoxide (CO) inhalation

 ## TREATMENT

### PRE-HOSPITAL
Stabilize. Treat seizures.

### INITIAL STABILIZATION/THERAPY
- ABCs:
  - Intubate patients who are obtunded/comatose/absent gag reflex.
- Naloxone, thiamine, glucose (or Accu-Chek) for altered mental status
- For signs of raised intracranial pressure on funduscopy or CT:
  - Hyperventilate to $PCO_2$ of 25–30 mm Hg
  - Administer mannitol
  - Neurosurgical consult for suspected hydrocephalus
- Run IV saline at KVO or half-maintenance to avoid cerebral edema.

### ED TREATMENT/PROCEDURES
- Seizure control:
  - Abort with lorazepam or diazepam.
  - Initiate antiseizure medication (Dilantin or phenobarbital) if more than 1 seizure has occurred.
- No specific treatment for most viral encephalitides:
  - Steroid use controversial
- Treat HSV encephalitis with acyclovir IV; initiate if considered likely based on clinical grounds, CT, and CSF findings.
- Initiate ganciclovir for suspected immunocompromised-related infections (cytomegalovirus [CMV], HHV-6).
- Administer antibiotic to cover for meningitis if diagnosis uncertain, especially when rash present (eg, meningococcemia, rickettsia).

### MEDICATION
- Acyclovir: 10 mg/kg IV q8h, max. 30 mg/kg/d
- Lorazepam: 2–4 mg per dose slow IV (peds: 0.05 to 0.1 mg/kg) per dose
- Diazepam: 5 mg IV per dose (peds: 0.1–0.2 mg/kg IV or 0.2–0.5 mg/kg per rectum)
- Dilantin: Loading dose 15 mg/kg IV to a max. 1 g
- Ganciclovir: 5 mg/kg IV q12h
- Mannitol: 0.5–1 g/kg of a 20% solution to run IV over 20–30 min
- Phenobarbital: Load 15–20 mg/kg to 300–800 mg IV at 25–50 mg/min

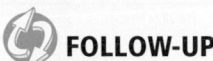 FOLLOW-UP

### DISPOSITION
*Admission Criteria*
All patients

## PEARLS AND PITFALLS
Empiric treatment for HSV-1 infection with acyclovir should always be initiated as soon as possible if the patient has encephalitis without apparent explanation.

## ADDITIONAL READING
- Kimberlin DW, Whitley RJ. Viral encephalitis. *Pediatr Rev.* 1999;20:192–198.
- Mandell G. *Mandell, Douglas, and Bennett's Principles and Practice of Infectious Diseases: Expert Consult Premium Edition*, 7th ed. New York: Churchill Livingstone; 2009.
- Reimann CA, Hayes EB, DiGuiseppi C, et al. Epidemiology of neuroinvasive arboviral disease in the United States, 1999–2007. *Am J Trop Med Hyg.* 2008;79(6):974–979.
- Tunkel AR, Whitley RJ. The management of encephalitis: Clinical practice guidelines by the Infectious Diseases Society of America. *Clin Infect Dis.* 2008;47(3):303–327.
- Solomon T. Flavivirus encephalitis. *New Engl J Med.* 2004;351:370–378.

### See Also (Topic, Algorithm, Electronic Media Element)
Meningitis

 CODES

### ICD9
- 049.9 Unspecified non-arthropod-borne viral diseases of central nervous system
- 323.9 Unspecified cause of encephalitis, myelitis, and encephalomyelitis

E

# ENDOCARDITIS

*Michael S. Murphy*

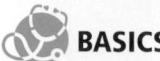 **BASICS**

## DESCRIPTION
- A microbial infection of the endothelial surface of the heart
- Characterized by the vegetation (a thrombus with superimposed microorganisms)
- Older population
- Frequently affects men
- Fewer patients at present demonstrate the classic signs once noted by Osler
- Risk factors:
  – Poor dental hygiene
  – IV drug abuse (IVDA):
    ○ Greater risk than rheumatic heart disease or prosthetic valves
    ○ Predilection for right-sided heart valves
- Risk factor for recurrent endocarditis:
  – Structural heart disease serves as common vegetative site due to altered intracardiac flow:
    ○ Mitral valve prolapse
    ○ Aortic valve dysfunction
  – Congenital heart disorders in the pediatric populations:
    ○ Tetralogy of Fallot
    ○ Aortic stenosis
    ○ Patent ductus arteriosus
    ○ Ventricular septal defects
    ○ Aortic coarctation
  – Prosthetic valves
  – Indwelling catheters
  – Any mechanical devices may serve as a portal of entry or attachment for microorganisms.

## ETIOLOGY
- Major categories:
  – Bacterial endocarditis
  – Prosthetic valve endocarditis
  – Nonbacterial thrombotic endocarditis:
    ○ Malignancy
    ○ Uremia
    ○ Burns
    ○ Systemic lupus erythematosus
- Common organisms:
  – *Streptococcus viridans*:
    ○ Found in oropharynx, common agent in native valve endocarditis
  – *S. bovis*:
    ○ Common association with colonic polyps or GI malignancy
  – *S. pneumoniae*:
    ○ Causes rapid valvular destruction, abscess, and CHF
    ○ Risk factor: Alcoholism

– *S. epidermidis*
– *S. aureus* (most common pathogen):
  ○ Seen in all populations, especially IVDA and toxic illness
  ○ Sometimes metastatic
– Enterococci:
  ○ Seen in young women and old men following instrumentation or infection
– *Candida* and *Aspergillus*:
  ○ Found in IVDA, prosthetic valves, or immunocompromised patients
– HACEK (*Haemophilus* sp.)
– Culture-negative endocarditis (Q fever, psittacosis, *Bartonella*, brucellosis)

 **DIAGNOSIS**

## SIGNS AND SYMPTOMS
- Fever:
  – Most common symptom
  – Often absent in certain settings:
    ○ Elderly
    ○ CHF
    ○ Severe debility
    ○ Chronic renal failure
    ○ Flulike illness
    ○ Chills
    ○ Sweats
    ○ Rigors
    ○ Malaise
- Head, eyes, ears, nose, and throat:
  – Retinal hemorrhages or Roth spots
- Respiratory:
  – Dyspnea
  – Cough
- Cardiac:
  – A new or changing murmur in 80–85% of patients
- Abdominal:
  – Abdominal or back pain
  – Splenomegaly (15–50%)
- Extremities:
  – Myalgias
  – Arthralgias
  – Digital clubbing
- Neurologic:
  – Septic embolization (stroke or mycotic aneurysm)
- Skin:
  – Cutaneous vasculitic lesions:
    ○ Mucosal and conjunctival petechiae
    ○ Splinter hemorrhages
    ○ Osler nodes: Erythematous, painful tender nodules
    ○ Janeway lesions: Erythematous or hemorrhagic, macular or nodular lesions, a few millimeters in diameter on the hands and feet

### History
- Fever duration and pattern
- Risk factors:
  – Prior cardiac disease
  – Source of bacteremia:
    ○ Indwelling intravascular catheters
    ○ IV drug use
    ○ Poor dental hygiene

### Physical Exam
- Heart and lung exam:
  – New cardiac regurgitant murmur
  – Heart failure
- Assess for splenomegaly.
- Assess for septic emboli:
  – Fundi, skin, nail beds
  – Careful neurologic exam for small focal deficits

## ESSENTIAL WORKUP
- Identify risk factors for endocarditis in patients with fever of unknown etiology.
- Blood cultures
- ECG is needed to confirm the diagnosis.

## DIAGNOSTIC TESTS & INTERPRETATION
### Lab
- CBC:
  – Anemia (sometimes hemolytic)
  – Leukocytosis (with granulocytosis and bandemia)
- Blood cultures:
  – Multiple sets (3 sets over a time period) should be obtained before antibiotic administration:
    ○ 5–10% with endocarditis have false-negative cultures
    ○ Consider culture of catheter device
- Elevated sedimentation rate and C-reactive protein (lacks specificity)
- Urinalysis:
  – Microscopic hematuria

### Imaging
- CXR:
  – CHF
  – Septic pulmonic emboli, which may be seen in right-sided endocarditis
- EKG:
  – Arrhythmia, new heart block
- ECG:
  – Acute valvular pathology
  – Abscess
  – Vegetations
  – Transesophageal ECG provides greater sensitivity.
  – CT may provide comprehensive information and valvular abnormalities

## DIFFERENTIAL DIAGNOSIS
- Rheumatic fever
- Atrial myxoma
- Acute pericarditis
- MI
- Aortic dissection with regurgitant valve
- Thrombotic thrombocytopenic purpura
- Systemic lupus erythematosus
- Occult neoplasm with metastasis
- Septicemia
- Cotton fever

 **TREATMENT**

### INITIAL STABILIZATION/THERAPY
- Monitor for signs of heart failure.
- Operative repair if:
  - Severe valvular dysfunction causing failure
  - Unstable prosthesis
  - Perivalvular extension with intracardiac abscess
  - Antimicrobial therapy failure
  - Large or fungal vegetations
- Antibiotic therapy:
  - IV, bactericidal, and empiric, pending culture results
  - Native valve or congenital abnormality:
    - Penicillin G + nafcillin + gentamicin
    - Vancomycin + gentamicin
  - Prosthetic valve or history of IVDA:
    - Vancomycin + gentamicin + rifampin
    - Nafcillin + gentamicin + rifampin (if methicillin-resistant S. aureus [MRSA] is not suspected)
    - If MRSA vancomycin failure/intolerant consider daptomycin or quinupristin-dalfopristin
    - Vancomycin-resistant Enterococcus faecium consider quinupristin-dalfopristin
    - Enterococcal: Penicillin G + gentamicin; vancomycin + gentamicin
    - Enterococcal (gentamicin resistant): Penicillin G + streptomycin
  - Fungal:
    - Amphotericin B
  - HACEK:
    - Ceftriaxone

## MEDICATION
- Amphotericin B:
  - Test dose 0.1 mg/kg up to 1 mg slow IV
  - Wait 2–4 hr.
  - If tolerated, begin 0.25 mg/kg IV and advance to 0.6 mg/kg IV q.i.d.
- Ceftriaxone: 2 g/d IV (peds: 100 mg/kg/24 hr)
- Daptomycin: 4 mg/kg/d IV
- Gentamicin: 1 mg/kg IV q8h (peds: 3 mg/kg/24 hr in 3 equally divided doses)
- Nafcillin: 2 g IV q4h
- Penicillin G: 4 million IU IV q4h (peds: 300,000 units/kg/d divided into 4 equal doses)
- Quinupristin-dalfopristin: 7.5 mg/kg IV q8h (peds: 7.5 mg/kg/12 hr)
- Rifampin: 600 mg PO q.i.d.
- Streptomycin: 15 mg/kg/24 hr IV/IM in 2 equally divided doses (peds: 20 mg/kg/24 hr IV in 2 equally divided doses)
- Vancomycin: 15 mg/kg IV q12h (peds: 40 mg/kg/24 hr in 2–3 equally divided doses)

 **FOLLOW-UP**

### DISPOSITION
#### Admission Criteria
- Patients with risk factors who exhibit pathologic criteria or clinical findings
- All IV drug users with fever
- Admit patients with cardiovascular instability to an intensive care unit/monitored setting.

#### Discharge Criteria
None

### FOLLOW-UP RECOMMENDATIONS
- Expected course:
  - Most patients will defervesce within 1 wk.
- Complications:
  - Cardiac: CHF, valve abscess, pericarditis, fistula
  - Neurologic: Embolic stroke, abscess, hemorrhage
  - Embolization: CNS, pulmonary, ischemic extremities
  - Mycotic aneurysms: Cerebral or systemic
  - Renal: Infarction, nephritis, abscess
  - Metastatic abscess: Kidney, spleen, tissue

## PEARLS AND PITFALLS
- Fever, new or changing murmur
- Recent health care exposure/device consider as risk factor
- S. aureus most common pathogen
- Common complications; watch for stroke, embolization, heart failure, intracardiac abscess
- Admit IV drug abusers presenting with fever to rule out endocarditis.
- Empiric therapy for acutely ill after 2–3 sets of blood cultures from separate venipuncture sites.

## ADDITIONAL READING
- Feuchtner G, Stolzmann P, et al. Multislice computed tomography in infectious endocarditis. J Am Coll Cardiol. 2009;53:436–444.
- Murdoch DF, Corey GR, et al. Clinical presentation, etiology and outcome of infective endocarditis in the 21st century: The International Collaboration on Endocarditis-Prospective Cohort Study. Arch Intern Med. 2009;169(5):463–473.
- Mylonakis E, Calderwood S. Infective endocarditis in adults. N Engl J Med. 2001;345(18):1318–1330.
- O'Gara PT. Infective endocarditis 2006: Indications for surgery. Trans Am Clin Climatol Assoc. 2007; 118:187–198.
- Saliman L, Prince A, et al. Pediatric infective endocarditis in the modern era. J Pediatr. 1993;122: 847–853.

 **CODES**

### ICD9
- 421.0 Acute and subacute bacterial endocarditis
- 421.9 Acute endocarditis, unspecified
- 424.90 Endocarditis, valve unspecified, unspecified cause

# ENDOMETRIOSIS

Christy Rosa Mohler

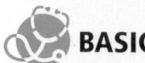 **BASICS**

## DESCRIPTION
- Ectopic endometrial tissue with cyclic hormonal responsiveness:
  - Primarily on pelvic peritoneum and ovaries
- Affects 5–10% of women of reproductive age
- Peritoneal endometriosis:
  - Endometriotic implants on surface of pelvic peritoneum and ovaries
- Endometrioma:
  - Endometrioid mucosal lining of ovarian cyst
- Rectovaginal endometriotic nodule:
  - Complex solid mass of endometriotic tissue, adipose, and fibromuscular tissue

## ETIOLOGY
- Unknown
- Theories include:
  - Retrograde menstruation
  - Immunologic factors
  - Metaplastic transformation
  - Toxins and/or oxidative stress

### Pediatric Considerations
Not seen before menarche

## RISK FACTORS
### Genetics
Familial disposition suggested by clinical, population, and twin studies

 **DIAGNOSIS**

## SIGNS AND SYMPTOMS
### History
- Pelvic or back pain, usually cyclic
- Dysmenorrhea may be severe.
- Dyspareunia
- Infertility

### Physical Exam
- Pelvic exam nonspecific:
  - Rarely immobile tender uterus or nodular masses are present.
- Abdominal exam typically benign unless ruptured endometrioma produces peritoneal signs.
- Endometriosis has been found in the lungs, brain, and many nonperitoneal sites; signs and symptoms can vary greatly depending on location of lesions.
- Catamenial pneumothorax occurs during menses due to endometriosis on the pleura.

## ESSENTIAL WORKUP
- Pregnancy test
- Rule out other, life-threatening diagnoses, as directed by history and physical exam.

## DIAGNOSTIC TESTS & INTERPRETATION
### Lab
- Pregnancy test
- Hematocrit if bleeding
- Type and screen if significant bleeding
- Other labs as needed to consider other disease processes on the differential diagnosis

### Imaging
- Pelvic US, CT, and MRI may show ovarian endometriomas, but rarely reveal implants.
- Not typically helpful in making the diagnosis

### Diagnostic Procedures/Surgery
Laparoscopy usually required for definitive diagnosis

## DIFFERENTIAL DIAGNOSIS
- Appendicitis
- Ectopic pregnancy
- Ovarian cysts
- Ovarian torsion
- Pelvic inflammatory disease/tubo-ovarian abscess
- Menstrual cramps/mittelschmerz
- Inflammatory bowel disease
- Irritable bowel disease
- Small bowel obstruction
- Diverticulitis
- Gastroenteritis

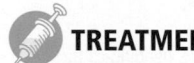 **TREATMENT**

## PRE-HOSPITAL
- Stabilize as needed.
- Pain control as necessary

## INITIAL STABILIZATION/THERAPY
- Manage hypotension initially with isotonic IV fluid.
- For severe bleeding not responsive to IV fluid, may need transfusion of packed red blood cells (PRBC)

## ED TREATMENT/PROCEDURES

- Analgesia
- Gynecology consultation for large or ruptured endometriomas
- Oral contraceptives, gonadotropin-releasing hormone agonists (eg, leuprolide [Lupron]), or other hormonal treatment may be started in consultation with the primary care physician or gynecologist.

### MEDICATION

- Acetaminophen: 650 mg–1,000 mg PO
- Ibuprofen: 400–800 mg PO
- Ketorolac: 15–30 mg IV or 30–60 mg IM
- Morphine: 4–8 mg IM/IV or equivalent analgesic

### First Line

- Ibuprofen: 400–800 mg PO
- Acetaminophen: 650–1,000 mg PO
- Ketorolac: 15–30 mg IV or 30–60 mg IM

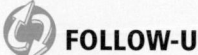 **FOLLOW-UP**

### DISPOSITION

### Admission Criteria

- Intractable pain
- Unclear diagnosis
- Need to follow serial exams or for further workup and treatment
- Ruptured endometrioma with peritoneal signs

### Discharge Criteria

Most patients with a clear exacerbation of endometriosis can be discharged with gynecology referral once pain is controlled.

### FOLLOW-UP RECOMMENDATIONS

Suspected cases of endometriosis should be referred to a gynecologist for evaluation and treatment.

## PEARLS AND PITFALLS

- Occurs in 5–10% of women of reproductive age
- Endometriosis often causes cyclical pelvic pain.

- Rule out other emergency medical conditions and treat symptoms as needed.
- Endometriosis is often a chronic condition that necessitates outpatient monitoring by a gynecologist or primary care physician.

## ADDITIONAL READING

- Berek JS, ed. *Berek & Novak's Gynecology*, 14th ed. New York: McGraw-Hill; 2007.
- Bulun SE. Endometriosis, *N Eng J Med*. 2009;360:268–279.
- Marx JA, Hockberger RS, Walls RM, et al, eds. *Rosen's Emergency Medicine: Concepts and Clinical Practice*, 7th ed. St. Louis: Mosby; 2009.
- Templeman C. Adolescent endometriosis. *Obstet Gyencol Clin North Am*. 2009;36:177–185.

 **CODES**

### ICD9

- 617.1 Endometriosis of ovary
- 617.2 Endometriosis of fallopian tube
- 617.3 Endometriosis of pelvic peritoneum

E

# EPIDIDYMITIS/ORCHITIS

Matthew D. Cook
Kevin R. Weaver

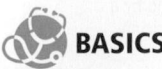 **BASICS**

## DESCRIPTION

### Epididymitis
- Definition: Inflammation or infection of the epididymis
- Rare in prepubertal boys
- Pathogenesis:
  - Initial stages:
    - Cellular inflammation begins in vas deferens
    - Descends to lower pole of epididymis
  - Acute phase:
    - Epididymis is swollen and indurated in upper and lower poles.
    - Spermatic cord thickened
  - Testis may become edematous owing to passive congestion or inflammation.
  - Resolution:
    - May be complete without sequelae
    - Peritubular fibrosis may develop, occluding ductules.
- Complications:
  - 2/3 of men have atrophy due to partial vascular thrombosis of testicular artery.
  - Abscess and infarction rare (5%)
  - Incidence of infertility with unilateral epididymitis unknown:
    - 50% with bilateral epididymitis

### Orchitis
- Definition: Inflammation or infection of the testicle:
  - Usually from direct extension of the same process within the epididymis
  - Isolated testicular infection is rare:
    - Can result from hematogenous spread of bacteria or following mumps infection
- Categories:
  - Pyogenic bacterial orchitis secondary to bacterial involvement of epididymis
  - Viral orchitis:
    - Most commonly due to mumps
    - Rare in prepubertal boys; occurs in 20–30% of postpubertal boys with mumps.
    - Occurs 4–6 days after parotitis but can occur without parotitis.
    - Unilateral in 70% of patients
    - Usually resolution in 6–10 days
    - 30–50% of testes involved have residual atrophy; rarely affects fertility
  - Granulomatous orchitis:
    - Syphilis
    - Mycobacterium and fungal diseases
    - Usually occurs in immunocompromised host

## ETIOLOGY

### Epididymitis
- Children:
  - Coliform or pseudomonal UTI
  - Sexually transmitted diseases rare in prepubertal males
  - Associated with predisposing abnormalities of lower urinary tract

- Young men, age <35 yr:
  - Usually sexually transmitted
  - *Chlamydia trachomaticum* (28–88%) with severe inflammation with minimal destruction
  - *Neisseria gonorrhoeae* (3–28%)
  - Coliform bacteria (7–24%):
    - Highly destructive with tendency for abscess
    - Coliform bacteria more common in insertive partners in anal intercourse
  - *Ureaplasma urealyticum* (sole organism in only 6% of cases)
- Older men, age >35 yr:
  - Commonly associated with underlying urologic pathology (benign prostatic hypertrophy, prostate cancer, strictures)
  - May have acute or chronic bacterial prostatitis
  - Coliform bacteria more common (23–67%), especially after instrumentation
  - Chlamydia trachomatis (8–80%)
  - Klebsiella and Pseudomonas species
  - Neisseria gonorrhoeae (15%)
  - Gram-positive cocci
- Drug related:
  - Amiodarone-induced epididymitis:
    - Usually with amiodarone levels > therapeutic levels
- Granulomatous:
  - Syphilis or mycobacterial and fungal causes:
    - May be presenting feature of *Mycobacterium tuberculosis* in high prevalence regions
    - Suspect in HIV patients
    - Urine cultures often negative for *M. tuberculosis*
- Vasculitis:
  - Polyarteritis nodosa
  - Behçet disease
  - Henoch-Schönlein purpura

### Orchitis
- Pyogenic bacterial orchitis:
  - Escherichia coli
  - Klebsiella pneumoniae
  - Pseudomonas aeruginosa
  - Staphylococci
  - Streptococci
- Viral orchitis:
  - Mumps:
    - 20% may develop epididymoorchitis.
    - Rarely associated with live-attenuated mumps vaccine
  - Coxsackie A and lymphocytic choriomeningitis virus
- Granulomatous orchitis: Syphilis and mycobacterial and fungal diseases:
  - Suspect in HIV patients
- Fungal orchitis:
  - Blastomycosis in endemic regions
  - Invasive candidal infections in immunosuppressed hosts
- Posttraumatic orchitis: Inflammation

 **DIAGNOSIS**

## SIGNS AND SYMPTOMS

### History
- Gradual onset of mild to moderate testicular or scrotal pain, usually unilateral
- Progressive scrotal swelling
- Dysuria (30%):
  - Recent UTI
  - History of abnormal bladder function
- Urethral discharge:
  - Of patients with gonococcal epididymitis, 21–30% did not complain of urethral discharge.
  - No demonstrable urethral discharge in 50%
- Fever (14–28%)
- Recent urethral instrumentation or catheterization

### Physical Exam
- Tenderness in groin, lower abdomen, or scrotum
- Scrotal skin commonly erythematous and warm (60%)
- Early:
  - May feel swollen, indurated epididymis
- Later:
  - May not be able to distinguish epididymis from testis
  - Spermatic cord may be edematous.
- Intact cremasteric reflex and Prehn sign:
  - Pain relief with testicular elevation
  - Commonly observed but not specific
- Coexistent prostatitis is rare (8%).
- Pyogenic bacterial orchitis:
  - Patients usually are acutely ill.
  - Fever
  - Intense discomfort
  - Swelling of testicle
  - Often reactive hydrocele

## ESSENTIAL WORKUP
- Must differentiate from testicular torsion
- Early consultation with urologist if strong suspicion of testicular torsion

## DIAGNOSTIC TESTS & INTERPRETATION

### Lab
- CBC:
  - Often leukocytosis in range of 10,000–30,000/mm$^3$
- Urinalysis and culture:
  - 15–50% of patients with epididymoorchitis have pyuria.
  - 24% of patients have positive urine bacterial cultures.
- Urethral swab (50–73% have demonstrable urethritis despite minority of symptoms)
  - Gram stain and culture or DNA amplification for *C. trachomatis/N. gonorrhoeae*
  - Avoid bladder emptying within 2 hr of tests (lowers sensitivity)
  - Especially for postpubertal and sexually active
- Blood culture if systemically ill

### Imaging

- US: Color Doppler imaging:
  - 82–100% sensitivity, 100% specificity in detecting testicular torsion or decreased blood flow
  - Epididymoorchitis:
    - Hyperemia
    - Increased vascularity and blood flow
  - Advantages:
    - Can evaluate for epididymitis or other causes of scrotal pain
    - 70% sensitivity, 88% specificity for epididymitis
  - Disadvantages:
    - Highly examiner dependent
    - Difficult in infants or children
- Testicular scintigraphy:
  - Radionuclide study to assess perfusion
  - 90–100% sensitivity, 89–97% specificity in detecting testicular torsion
  - Inflammatory processes have increased flow and uptake.
  - False-positive scans:
    - Large fluid collections in scrotum
    - Abscess
    - Hydrocele, hematocele
    - Bowel herniation
  - False-negative scans:
    - Early torsion
    - Spontaneous detorsion
    - Small children or infants

### Diagnostic Procedures/Surgery

Surgical exploration indications:

- Scrotal abscess
- If another scrotal problem, such as torsion, cannot be excluded
- Suspected or proved ischemia caused by severe epididymitis
- Patient with solitary testicle
- Scrotal fixation: Indicates severe inflammation and potential suppuration

### DIFFERENTIAL DIAGNOSIS

- Testicular torsion
- Testicular tumor
- Torsion of testicular appendages
- Trauma to scrotum
- Acute hernia
- Acute hydrocele

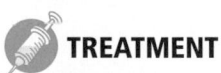 ## TREATMENT

### PRE-HOSPITAL

- IV access
- IV fluids, especially if systemically ill

### INITIAL STABILIZATION/THERAPY

- IV access
- IV fluids, especially if systemically ill

### ED TREATMENT/PROCEDURES

- Antibiotics:
  - Cover for chlamydial and gonococcal etiologies if adult or presumed sexually transmitted
  - Cover for coliform etiology:
    - Child, or adult >35 yr of age
    - Insertive partner in anal intercourse
    - Presumed nonsexually transmitted
  - Adjust according to culture and sensitivity
- Bed rest and scrotal support
- Ice packs
- Analgesics and anti-inflammatories

### MEDICATION

- Age <35 yr or sexually active postpubertal males:
  - Ceftriaxone 250 mg IM once, *plus* doxycycline 100 mg PO b.i.d. for 10 days:
    - May substitute azithromycin 1 g PO once for doxycycline if tetracycline allergy
    - Quinolone therapy no longer recommended if suspect STD due to *N. gonorrhoeae* resistance
- Age >35 yr or insertive partners in anal intercourse or negative culture/DNA amplification for *C. trachomatis/N. gonorrhoeae* or allergy to cephalosporins/tetracyclines:
  - Ofloxacin 300 mg PO b.i.d. *or* levofloxacin 500 mg/day PO for 10 days

### Pediatric Considerations

- Bacterial epididymitis is uncommon in prepubertal boys and antibiotic regimens are not well established.
- If concurrent UTI:
  - TMP-SMX 4 mg/kg TMP and 20 mg/kg SMX b.i.d. for 10 days
- Avoid quinolones and tetracyclines in children

 ## FOLLOW-UP

### DISPOSITION

#### Admission Criteria

- Surgical indications present
- Older age group if it is the only way to ensure appropriate workup:
  - Many will have underlying urologic pathology.
- Systemically ill, fever, nausea, vomiting
- Scrotal abscess
- Intractable pain

#### Discharge Criteria

- Fails to meet admission criteria
- Patient with good follow-up
- Able to take oral antibiotics

#### Issues for Referral

- Urologic consultation and follow-up
- Children need workup for urologic abnormalities:
  - Voiding cystourethrography
  - Renal US
- If bacteriuria present, examination of lower tract with cystoscopy after treatment completed

### FOLLOW-UP RECOMMENDATIONS

- Failure to improve within 3 days of commencing antibiotics warrants urologic evaluation.
- Persistence of symptoms after full antibiotic course warrants search for other causes of epididymitis:
  - Other considerations include TB or fungal epididymitis, scrotal abscess, tumor, infarction.
- Sexual partners of patients with suspected or confirmed *C. trachomatis/N. gonorrhoeae* should be tested/treated.
- Prepubertal boys need urology consult for evaluation of structural urogenital abnormalities.

## PEARLS AND PITFALLS

- Testicular torsion should be ruled out in all cases of new-onset testicular pain.
- Epididymitis usually due to STD in sexually active men <35 yr
- Epididymitis usually due to coliform bacteria in men >35 yr and prepubertal boys
- Antibiotic treatment is started immediately and empirically based on clinical picture.

## ADDITIONAL READING

- Brenner JS, Ojo A. Causes of scrotal pain in children and adolescents. *UpToDate*, at: www.uptodate.com. Accessed Nov 30, 2009.
- Centers for Disease Control and Prevention. Sexually transmitted diseases treatment guidelines; 2006. *Epididymitis*, at: www.cdc.gov/std/treatment/2006/epididymitis.htm. Accessed Nov 30, 2009.
- Marcozzi D, Suner S. The nontraumatic acute scrotum. *Emerg Med Clin North Am.* 2001;19: 547–568.
- Sabanegh ES, Ching CB. Epididymitis. *eMedicine* at: emedicine.medscape.com/article/436154-overview. Accessed Nov 30, 2009.
- Tracy CR, Steers WD, Costabile R. Diagnosis and management of epididymitis. *Urol Clin North Am.* 2008;35(1):101–108.
- Trojian TH, Lishnak TS, Heiman D. Epididymitis and orchitis: An overview. *Am Fam Physician.* 2009; 79(7):583–587.

### See Also (Topic, Algorithm, Electronic Media Element)

- Gonococcal Disease
- Prostatitis
- Testicular Torsion
- Urethritis

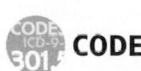 ## CODES

### ICD9

604.90 Orchitis and epididymitis, unspecified

# EPIDURAL ABSCESS

*Richard S. Krause*

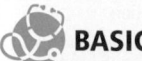

## BASICS

### DESCRIPTION
- A rare pyogenic infection of the spinal epidural space
- Most common in thoracic spine, followed by lumbar and cervical areas

### ETIOLOGY
- Focus of infection is present followed by either hematogenous spread (approximately 50%) or direct extension.
- Most common source is skin infection:
  – Any pyogenic infection may be source.
- *Staphylococcus aureus* accounts for >50% of cases:
  – Many are MRSA
  – *Streptococcus* is 2nd most common.
- *H. influenzae,* gram-negative bacilli, mycobacteria, anaerobic, and mixed infections also occur.
- May occur after lumbar puncture (usually follows multiple attempts)

#### Pediatric Considerations
- Children present similar to adults with back pain, fever, and neurologic signs as well as nonspecific systemic symptoms.
- Infants may exhibit only fever, irritability, and associated meningitis.
- Sphincter disturbance is frequently seen.
- Most cases are secondary to hematogenous spread.
- Location and bacteriology similar to adults

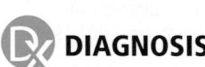

## DIAGNOSIS

### SIGNS AND SYMPTOMS
- Fever and severe back pain represent "red flag" for potentially serious condition:
  – If pain is radicular or there is neurologic disturbance, likelihood of epidural abscess is increased.

- Classic presentation:
  – Severe, progressive back pain (often radicular)
  – Fever
  – Neurologic deficit:
    ○ Weakness or paralysis
    ○ Sensory level
    ○ Sphincter disturbance
    ○ May present with signs and symptoms of sepsis without prominent back pain
- Occurs at all ages including infants:
  – Peak is at ages 60–70 yr
- Most patients have predisposing condition:
  – IV drug abuse (IVDA)
  – Diabetes
  – Malignancy
  – Chronic steroids
  – Chronic alcoholism
  – Instrumentation or spinal surgery
- May occur in absence of identifiable predisposing factors

### History
- Back pain
- Fever
- Neurologic deficit:
  – Weakness
  – Paresthesias
  – Incontinence

### Physical Exam
- Fever
- Localized spinal tenderness and/or erythema
- Neurologic deficit
- Evidence of IV drug use

### ESSENTIAL WORKUP
- History should include predisposing conditions when this diagnosis is suspected.
- Physical exam for source of infection, localized spinal tenderness, and neurologic findings:
  – Especially decreased sphincter tone
  – Saddle anesthesia
  – Lower extremity weakness

- Postvoid residual
- Younger adults should have <50 mL postvoid residual urine:
  – Older adults may have residual of 100 mL.
- Erythrocyte sedimentation rate (ESR) as below
- MRI with and without gadolinium contrast is the diagnostic test of choice:
  – When not available, obtain CT myelogram or CT with IV contrast (least sensitive).
  – Suspected epidural abscess is true neurosurgical emergency and requires emergent imaging.

### DIAGNOSTIC TESTS & INTERPRETATION
#### Lab
- ESR is almost always elevated (~100%), but is nonspecific:
  – Normal ESR makes diagnosis much less likely.
- C-reactive protein nearly always elevated.
- Blood cultures often positive (~60%).
- Leukocytosis with left shift is common (~70%).
- CSF often abnormal, but nondiagnostic; routine lumbar puncture should be avoided when epidural abscess is primarily suspected (may cause meningitis).

#### Imaging
- MRI is at least 90% sensitive:
  – Shows high-intensity lesion on T2 imaging
- Myelography and CT myelography are also sensitive, but risk dissemination.
- Plain films are often abnormal but nonspecific.

### DIFFERENTIAL DIAGNOSIS
- Diagnosis is difficult owing to rarity of condition and nonspecific symptoms:
  – Multiple physician encounters commonly precede diagnosis.
  – Most common initial diagnosis is benign musculoskeletal pathology: Muscular or ligamentous pain, degenerative arthritis, compression fracture, discogenic pain.

- Back pain with fever, systemic signs and symptoms:
  – Vertebral osteomyelitis
  – Spinal tumor (usually there is a known primary)
  – Meningitis (cervical epidural abscess may mimic, bacterial meningitis usually associated with abnormal mental status)
  – Discitis (usually post instrumentation)
  – Pyelonephritis
- Back pain with neurologic signs and symptoms:
  – Cord compression
  – Cord ischemia
  – Disc herniation

### Pediatric Considerations
Fever and back pain should be urgently investigated with MRI when epidural abscess is suspected.

 TREATMENT

### PRE-HOSPITAL
Spinal immobilization if trauma suspected or other cause of fracture suspected

### INITIAL STABILIZATION/THERAPY
Broad-spectrum parenteral antibiotics early for signs of sepsis:
- Must include coverage for *S. aureus*, streptococci, and gram-negative rods
- Vancomycin (for possible MRSA) and a 3rd-generation cephalosporin (for gram-negative coverage) are appropriate initial antibiotics.
- Cover *Pseudomonas* if IVDA

### ED TREATMENT/PROCEDURES
- Urgent imaging essential when diagnosis is considered
- Delay in treatment is associated with poorer outcome.
- If unable to localize lesion on physical exam, consider imaging entire spine.

- Urgent neurosurgical consultation or transfer for definitive therapy (surgical decompression) after diagnosis and antibiotic administration:
  – Conservative treatment (prolonged (6 wk) antibiotic therapy) may be successful in some cases.

### MEDICATION
- Ceftazidime: 2 g (peds: 50 mg/kg) q8h
- Ceftriaxone: 1–2 g IV q12h (peds: 100 mg/kg/d IM/IV q12–24h)
- Vancomycin: 1g IV q12h (peds: 10–15 mg/kg q6–8h)

### First Line
- Ceftriaxone
- Vancomycin
- Ceftazidime (if suspect *Pseudomonas*)

 FOLLOW-UP

### DISPOSITION

### Admission Criteria
Suspected epidural abscess should be admitted; MRI is needed emergently; transfer patient if necessary.

### Discharge Criteria
Patients with definite or suspected epidural abscess should not be discharged.

### Issues for Referral
Patients with spinal epidural abscess require admission to facility with neurosurgical capability:
- Transfer may be indicated if a neurosurgeon or MRI is unavailable:
  – Administer antibiotics and obtain blood cultures (positive in ~60%) prior to transfer.

## PEARLS AND PITFALLS
- Successfully treated epidural abscess may reoccur, especially in the setting of decreased immunity.
- Patients with Staphylococcal bacteremia and back pain or neurological signs/symptoms should be investigated for epidural abscess.

- Failure to order images that include the involved area:
  – Careful physical exam for areas of spinal tenderness and level of neurological deficit may help avoid this pitfall:
    ○ Consider both thoracic and lumbar imaging for a problem suspected in the mid back and cervical and thoracic imaging for upper back and neck pathology.
    ○ If unable to localize lesion on physical exam, consider imaging entire spine.

## ADDITIONAL READING

- Davis DP, Wold RM, Patel RJ. The clinical presentation and impact of diagnostic delays on emergency department patients with spinal epidural abscess. *J Emerg Med*. 2004;26:285–291.
- Siddiq F, Chowfin A, Tight R, et al. Medical vs surgical management of spinal epidural abscess. *Arch Int Med*. 2004;164:2409–2412.
- Soehle M, Wallenfang T. Spinal epidural abscesses: Clinical manifestations, prognostic factors, and outcomes. *Neurosurgery*. 2002;51:79–87.
- Karikari IO, Powers CJ, Reynolds RM, et al. Management of spontaneous spinal epidural abscess: A single-center 10-year experience. *Neurosurgery*. 2009;65:919–923.
- Darouiche RO. Spinal epidural abscess. *New Eng J Med*. 2006;355:2012–2020.
- Marx JA, Hockberger RS, Walls RM, et al. *Rosen's Emergency Medicine: Concepts and Clinical Practice*, 7th ed. St. Louis, MO: Mosby; 2009.

 CODES

### ICD9
- 324.1 Intraspinal abscess
- 324.9 Intracranial and intraspinal abscess of unspecified site

E

# EPIDURAL HEMATOMA
*Colleen Campbell*

 **BASICS**

## DESCRIPTION
- Direct skull trauma
- Inward bending of cavarum causes bleeding when dura separates from skull:
  – Middle meningeal artery is involved in bleed >50% of time.
  – Meningeal vein is involved in 1/3.
  – Diploic venous sinus bleed is seen in <10%.
- Skull fracture is associated in 75% of cases, less commonly in children.
- >50% have epidural hematoma (EDH) as isolated head injury:
  – Most commonly associated with subdural hematoma (SDH) and cerebral contusion
- Classic CT finding is lenticular, unilateral convexity, usually in temporal region.
- It usually does not cross suture lines, but may cross midline.

## ETIOLOGY
- Accounts for 1.5% of traumatic brain injury (TBI)
- Male/female incidence is 3:1.
- Peak incidence is 2nd–3rd decade of life.
- Motor vehicle accidents (MVAs), assault, and falls are most common causes:
  – Of all blunt mechanisms, assault has highest association with intracranial injury requiring neurosurgical intervention.
- Uncommon in very young (<5 yr) or elderly patients
- Mortality is 12% and is related to preoperative condition.

### Pediatric Considerations
- Head injury is the most common cause of death and acquired disability in childhood.
- Falls, pedestrian-struck bicycle accidents are most common causes:
  – Most severe head injuries in children are from MVA.
  – Always consider possibility of nonaccidental trauma.
- <50% have altered level of consciousness (LOC):
  – If EDH in differential diagnosis (DD), CT should be obtained.
- Bleeding is more likely to be venous.
- Good outcome in 95% of children <5 yr

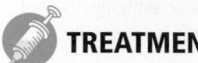 **DIAGNOSIS**

## SIGNS AND SYMPTOMS
### History
- Altered or deteriorating LOC
- LOC: 85% will have at some point in course:
  – Only 11–30% will have a lucid interval.
- Nausea and vomiting: 40%

### Pediatric Considerations
- Many times the only clinical sign is drop in hematocrit (Hct) of 40% in infants.
- Bulging fontanel with vomiting, seizures, or lethargy also suggest EDH in infants.
- Less than 50% of children have LOC at time of injury.
- Posterior fossa lesions are seen more commonly in children.

### Physical Exam
- Pupillary dilation: 20–40%:
  – Usually on same side as lesion (90%)
- Hemiparesis >1/3:
  – Usually on opposite side from lesion (80%)

## ESSENTIAL WORKUP
Head imaging, as below

## DIAGNOSTIC TESTS & INTERPRETATION
### Lab
- ABG, CBC, chemistry, PT/PTT
- Blood ETOH and drug screen as appropriate

### Imaging
- Noncontrast CT of head:
  – Admission perfusion CT may help predict prognosis.
  – Lenticular, biconvex hematoma with smooth borders may be seen.
  – Mixed density lesion may indicate active bleeding.
  – Most commonly seen in temporal parietal region
- Plain films may show skull fractures:
  – CT with bone windows is more often used.
- Spine series
- Further workup of trauma as indicated

### Pediatric Considerations
US may be used for diagnosis in infants with open fontanels.

## DIFFERENTIAL DIAGNOSIS
- History of recent head trauma lends itself to the diagnosis:
  – Trauma may be minor in infants and toddlers.
- Consider other diagnosis:
  – SDH
  – Cerebral concussion/contusion
  – Intracerebral bleed
  – Diffuse axonal injury
  – Subdural hygroma
  – Shaken baby syndrome
  – Toxic, metabolic, or infectious causes

# TREATMENT

## PRE-HOSPITAL
- Head-injured patients have 25% improved mortality when triaged to regional trauma centers.
- Spinal immobilization is essential.
- Ensure adequate oxygenation throughout transport:
  – Intubation and airway protection may be necessary.

## INITIAL STABILIZATION/THERAPY
- Prevent hypoxia and hypotension:
  – Rapid-sequence intubation for signs of deterioration or increased intracranial pressure (ICP)
  – Controlled ventilation to $PCO_2$ of 35–40 mm Hg
  – Avoid hyperventilation unless signs of brain herniation are present.
  – Avoid induction agents, which may increase ICP (eg, ketamine).
- Elevate head of bed 15–20% after adequate fluid resuscitation.
- Perform rapid neurologic assessment:
  – Glasgow coma scale (GCS) score:
- 14–15; minor head injury
- 9–13; moderate head injury
- Less than 8; severe:
  – Reflexes; pupils, corneal, gag, brainstem reflexes
- Secondary survey will reveal coexisting injury in >50%.

## ED TREATMENT/PROCEDURES

- Early surgical intervention (<4 hr) in comatose patients with EDH improves meaningful survival:
  - Burr hole is placed at fracture site or side with ipsilateral pupillary dilation.
  - Rapid craniectomy is occasionally performed if bleeding is not controlled at site of burr hole.
- Nonsurgical intervention in asymptomatic patients is associated with high rate of deterioration; >30% require surgical intervention.
- Maintain euvolemia with isotonic fluids.
- Continuous end tidal $CO_2$ monitoring:
  - Arterial line placement for close monitoring of MAP, $PO_2$, $PCO_2$
  - Foley catheter to monitor input/output (I/O) status
- Control ICP:
  - Prevent pain, posturing, and increased respiratory effort:
    ○ Sedation with benzodiazepines
    ○ Neuromuscular blockade with vecuronium or pancuronium in intubated patients
    ○ Etomidate is good induction agent.
    ○ Barbiturate coma should be initiated for refractory increased ICP in neurosurgical ICU.
  - Mannitol may be used once euvolemic:
    ○ Shown to increase MAP greater than coronary perfusion pressure (CPP) and cerebral blood flow (CBF), as well as decrease ICP
    ○ Keep osmolality between 295–310.
    ○ Use furosemide (Lasix) as adjunct only if no risk of hypovolemia.
- Treat HTN:
  - Labetalol or hydralazine
- Treat hyperglycemia if present:
  - Associated with increased lactic acidosis and mortality in patients with TBI
- Treat and prevent seizures:
  - Diazepam and Dilantin

- Not considered helpful:
  - Steroids
  - Antibiotic prophylaxis
  - Hyperventilation in absence of herniation
  - Fluid restriction
  - Calcium channel blockers
- Factors associated with poor outcome:
  - Age >40 yr
  - Increased admission base deficit
  - Large hematoma with rapid expansion
  - Increased midline shift
  - Lower admission GCS or unconsciousness at presentation
  - Postoperative ICP >3
  - Prolonged anisocoria
  - Associated brain injuries or concomitant trauma injuries

### Pediatric Considerations
Hemodynamically significant blood loss can result from scalp lacerations and subgaleal hematomas:

- Direct pressure and control of bleeding is indicated.

## MEDICATION

- Diazepam: 5–10 mg (peds: 0.1–0.2 mg/kg) IV
- Dilantin: Adult/peds: Load 18 mg/kg at 25–50 mg/min
- Etomidate: 0.3 mg/kg IV
- Fentanyl: 2–4 ug/kg IV
- Furosemide (Lasix): Adults/peds: 0.5 mg/kg IV
- Hydralazine: 10/mg/h IV (peds: Safety not established)
- Labetalol: 15–30 mg/h IV (peds: Safety not established)
- Lidocaine: As preinduction agent, 1.5 mg/kg IV
- Mannitol: Adults/peds: 0.25–1 g/kg IV q4h
- Pentobarbital: 1–5 mg IV q6h
- Rocuronium: 1 mg/kg IV
- Thiopental: As induction agent, 20 mg/kg IV
- Versed: 2–4 mg/h IV PRN (peds: 0.15 mg/kg IV)

### Pediatric Considerations
- Hypertonic saline has been shown to be beneficial in some pediatric studies (1.7–3%).
- NaCl 3%: 2–6 mL/kg IV. Infusion .1–1 mL/kg/hr

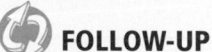

## FOLLOW-UP

### DISPOSITION

#### Admission Criteria
- All patients with CT abnormality or altered LOC should be admitted to ICU setting with frequent neurologic assessment.
- Patients should have repeated CT exam in 12–24 hr or if clinical deterioration occurs.
- Patients at increased risk of deterioration include those with rapid bleeds, associated skull fracture, or lower GCS or neurologic deficits.

#### Discharge Criteria
Admission is necessary for all patients with EDH.

## ADDITIONAL READING

- Bullock MR, et al. Surgical management of traumatic brain injury. *Neurosurgery*. 2006; 58(3 Suppl):S16–S24.
- Marion DM. Epidural hematoma. In: Bradley WG, ed. *Neurology in Clinical Practice*, 5th ed. Elsevier; 2008:54 A,B:1083–1114.
- Vincent JL, Berre J. Primer on medical management of severe brain injury. *Crit Care Med*. 2005;33(6): 1392–1399.
- Huh JW, Raghupathi R. New concepts of treatment in pediatric traumatic brain injury. *Anesth Clin*. 2009;27(2):213–240.
- Chestnut RM. Care of CNS Injuries. *Surg Clin N Am*. 2007;87(1):119–156, vii.
- Heegard W, Biros M. Traumatic brain injury. *Em Med Clin N Am*. 2007;25(3):655–678, viii.

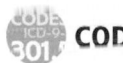

## CODES

### ICD9
852.40 Extradural hemorrhage following injury, without mention of open intracranial wound, with state of consciousness unspecified

# EPIGLOTTITIS, ADULT

Jonathan Fisher
Owen Lander

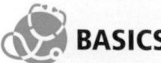 BASICS

## DESCRIPTION
- Rapidly progressive inflammation of the epiglottis and surrounding tissues leading to airway compromise
- May be more indolent in adults than pediatrics; rapid progression to total airway occlusion still seen in adults
- Although the incidence of pediatric epiglottitis has been decreasing, the incidence in adults is increasing.
- Inflammation of supraglottic structures:
  - Epiglottis:
    - Edema is primary airway concern.
    - May be primary or secondary from adjacent structures
  - Vallecula
  - Arytenoids
- Incidence is 1:100,000 adults per year
- More common in men: 3:1
- Adult mortality rate is 7% (<1% in children)
- Most common in 5th decade of life
- Immune-compromised patients may be particularly fulminant, with minimally associated symptoms and unusual pathogens, such as candida.
- Complications:
  - Total airway obstruction
  - Retropharyngeal abscess
  - Acute respiratory distress syndrome
  - Pneumonia
  - Empyema

## ETIOLOGY
- Infectious causes:
  - *Haemophilus influenzae B,* also type A and nontypeable strains
  - *Haemophilus parainfluenzae*
  - *Streptococcus pneumoniae*
  - *Staphylococcus aureus*
  - Group A strep
  - *Neisseria meningitis*
  - Herpes simplex
  - Cytomegalovirus
  - Numerous other uncommon agents
- Physical agents:
  - Chemical and thermal burns
  - Toxic or illicit drug inhalation
- Trauma, instrumentation

## DIAGNOSIS

### SIGNS AND SYMPTOMS
*History*
- General:
  - Fever
- Upper respiratory tract infection symptoms
- Prodrome absent in significant number of cases
- Head, eyes, ears, nose, throat:
  - Dysphagia
  - Muffled voice
  - Voice change:
    - "Hot potato" voice
    - Hoarseness
  - Foreign body sensation in throat
  - Drooling
  - Associated tonsillar, peritonsillar, uvular findings
- Respiratory:
  - Subjective sense of obstructed airway
  - Short of breath

*Physical Exam*
- General:
  - Fever
  - Toxic appearing
  - Sitting up in "tripod" stance
- Head, eyes, ears, nose, throat:
  - "Cherry red" epiglottis is classic, may be pale and edematous in up to 50%.
  - Hyoid/thyroid cartilage tender to gentle palpation
  - Tracheal rock: Pain with movement of the larynx from side to side.
  - Lymphadenopathy
- Respiratory:
  - Stridor
  - Sudden loss of airway
  - Respiratory distress with accessory muscle use

### ALERT
Patients with respiratory distress are at high risk for rapid progression to complete airway obstruction. Surgical airway management may be required.

### ESSENTIAL WORKUP
If significant respiratory distress:
- Avoid invasive diagnostic procedures
- Manage empirically with antibiotics and control of airway

### Pediatric Considerations
- Children with a high suspicion of epiglottitis are at risk of complete airway obstruction and should be quickly transferred to a setting where the airway can be definitively managed in a surgical setting.
- Staff capable of managing the airway should accompany the child until the airway has been secured.
- IV insertion, administration of antibiotics, and obtaining blood work should follow airway management.
- A needle cricothyrotomy may be required in extreme situations in young children.

### DIAGNOSTIC TESTS & INTERPRETATION
*Lab*
- CBC with differential
- Blood cultures
- Cultures of pharynx:
  - Only if no signs of respiratory distress

*Imaging*
- In patients with moderate to severe respiratory distress, the airway should be managed prior to imaging.
- Portable lateral soft-tissue x-ray:
  - Epiglottic "thumb" sign:
    - Thickening of the epiglottis
  - "Vallecula" sign:
    - The vallecula is normally well-delineated, deep, and roughly parallel to the pharyngotracheal air column.
    - Absence of a deep and well-defined vallecula, approaching the level of the hyoid bone
  - Swelling of the arytenoids and aryepiglottic folds
  - Prevertebral soft-tissue swelling
  - Significant false-negative with imaging
  - If suspected with negative film results, rule out with indirect visualization
- CT:
  - Indicated when a laryngoscopic evaluation cannot be performed or if coexistent soft-tissue complications are suspected

*Diagnostic Procedures/Surgery*
- Avoid prior to airway management if any signs of respiratory distress are present, including stridor
- Nasopharyngoscopy (mini-fiberoptic scope)
- Indirect laryngoscopy

## DIFFERENTIAL DIAGNOSIS

- Croup
- Airway foreign body
- Anaphylaxis
- Paradoxic vocal cord dysfunction
- Angioedema
- Laryngitis
- Pharyngitis
- Oropharyngeal abscess (peritonsillar or retropharyngeal)
- Bacterial tracheitis
- Congenital anomaly
- Meningitis

 **TREATMENT**

### PRE-HOSPITAL

- Transport patients in position of comfort.
- Supplemental oxygen as tolerated; avoid increasing anxiety
- Intubation indicated only if patient is in severe respiratory distress:
  - Likely difficult airway and significant chance of exacerbating compromise with laryngoscopy attempts
- Inhaled agents, racemic epinephrine, and $\beta$-agonists have no demonstrated value.

### INITIAL STABILIZATION/THERAPY

- ABCs
- Be prepared with all equipment on hand for definitive airway management, including a surgical airway, from presentation until diagnosis is ruled out or transport to intensive care setting.
- Examination of the airway can trigger airway obstruction.
- Orotracheal intubation in patients with signs of obstruction or significant respiratory distress:
  - Respiratory distress/airway failure may develop precipitously.
  - Consider ear-nose-throat/surgical consult if patient's condition permits for possible difficult/surgical airway.
- Needle jet insufflation may be a life-saving temporizing measure if a surgical airway is not immediately attainable with failed intubation.

## ED TREATMENT/PROCEDURES

- Humidified oxygen support
- IV access, hydration as indicated
- Begin antibiotic coverage empirically.
- Corticosteroids are controversial.

### MEDICATION

#### First Line

- Cefotaxime: 1–2 g IV initially, then 180 mg/kg/d in 4 divided doses
- Ceftriaxone: 1–2 g IV initially, then 100 mg/kg/d in 2 doses

#### Second Line

- Ampicillin/sulbactam: 3 g IV initially, then 200–300 mg/kg/d in 4 divided doses
- Trimethoprim-sulfamethoxazole: 320 mg IV initially, then 4–5 mg/kg IV q12h
- Consider adding increased coverage against *S. aureus*:
  - Nafcillin: 150–200 mg/kg IV per day in 4 divided doses
  - Vancomycin: 40–60 mg/kg IV per day in 3 divided doses if concern for MRSA
- Rifampin prophylaxis:
  - Adults: 600 mg/d PO for 4 days
  - >1 mo of age: 20 mg/kg/d PO for 4 days
  - <1 mo of age: 10 mg/kg/d PO for 4 days

 **FOLLOW-UP**

### DISPOSITION

#### Admission Criteria

Any patient with a suspected or confirmed diagnosis of epiglottitis should be admitted to an ICU setting for IV antibiotics and airway management.

#### Discharge Criteria

- Patients should not be discharged unless the diagnosis has been ruled out by visualization of the supraglottic structures by a physician familiar with physical appearance of the disease.
- Close contacts should receive prophylactic treatment with rifampin.

### Issues for Referral

ENT consultation should be obtained.

## PEARLS AND PITFALLS

- Failure to manage the airway in a timely manner is a pitfall.
- Avoid any unnecessary intervention until airway is secured.
- Mortality is 7% in adults with epiglottitis.

## ADDITIONAL READING

- Bowman JC. Epiglottitis, Adult. Emergency Medicine. Emedicine. Available at: http://emedicine.medscape.com/article/763612-overview. Accessed Jan 25, 2010.
- Ducic Y, Herbert PC, MacLachlan L, et al. Description and evaluation of the vallecula sign: A new radiologic sign in the diagnosis of adult epiglottitis. *Ann Emerg Med*. 1997;30:16.
- Guldfred LA, Lyhne D, Becker BC. Acute epiglottitis: Epidemiology, clinical presentation, management and outcome. *J Laryngol Otol*. 2008;122:818–823.
- Marx JA, Hockberger RS, Walls RM, et al. *Rosen's Emergency Medicine: Concepts and Clinical Practice*, 7th ed. St. Louis, MO: Mosby, 2009.
- Sobol SE, Zapata S, et al. Epiglottitis and croup. *Otolaryngol Clin North Am*. 2008;41:551–566.
- Woods CR. Epiglottitis. In: Rose BD, ed. *UpToDate*, Wellesley, MA: 2009.

 **CODES**

### ICD9

- 464.30 Acute epiglottitis without mention of obstruction
- 464.31 Acute epiglottitis with obstruction

**E**

# EPIGLOTTIS, PEDIATRIC

Beverly Bauman
Roger M. Barkin

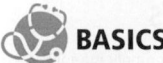 **BASICS**

## DESCRIPTION

- Inflammation of the epiglottis and surrounding supraglottic region, which is potentially life threatening owing to airway obstruction
- Children are at greater risk of upper airway obstruction owing to:
  - Decreased cross-sectional area of the upper airway (resistance is proportional to the inverse of the radius to the 4th power)
  - Loose attachment of mucosal surface and increased vascularity of mucosa allows for edema
  - Dynamic collapse of the airway
- A precipitous decline in the incidence of childhood epiglottitis since the introduction of the *Haemophilus influenzae* vaccination, although vaccine failure may result in rare cases among children who have been immunized
- In the post-Hib vaccine era, the mean age for this disease has increased, and it is now more commonly seen in adolescents and adults than in toddlers or young school-aged children.
- May occur throughout the year

### ALERT
All patients with suspected epiglottitis require intensive monitoring and intervention. Rapid progression of airway obstruction may occur.

## ETIOLOGY
- Infection:
  - *H. influenzae* type B
  - *S. pneumoniae*
  - Group A β-hemolytic *Streptococcus*
  - *Staphylococcus aureus*
  - Viruses
  - Less common infections include Klebsiella, Pseudomonas, Candida
- Caustic
- Thermal
- Traumatic
- Posttransplant lymphoproliferative disorder

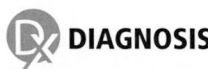 **DIAGNOSIS**

## SIGNS AND SYMPTOMS
### History
- Usually fulminant presentation without prodromal illness
- General:
  - Irritability, throat pain (often described as patient's worse sore throat), fever, noisy breathing
  - Progressive toxicity and respiratory distress

### Physical Exam
- General:
  - Toxic appearing
  - High fever is typical.
  - Rapid onset and progression
- Throat:
  - Drooling
  - Dysphagia
  - Muffled "hot potato" voice
  - Older patients often have very painful throat.
- Respiratory:
  - Rapidly progressive respiratory distress (dyspnea in only 1/3 of adults)
  - Children usually prefer to sit upright, leaning forward with open mouth ("tripod sniffing position") to maximize air entry.
  - Subtle stridor that may progress to severe stridor (stridor in only 10% of adults)
- Complications:
  - Airway obstruction is the most severe complication.
  - Epiglottic abscess
  - Associated pneumonia and atelectasis

## ESSENTIAL WORKUP
- Epiglottitis is a clinical diagnosis.
- Indirect laryngoscopy or any attempts to directly visualize the epiglottis are not indicated in children with suspected epiglottitis unless performed in a controlled environment. (In adolescents or adults, use of fiberoptic nasopharyngoscope may be indicated for patients without impending airway obstruction.)
- If infection is suspected, obtain cultures of the epiglottis during laryngoscopy after airway is secure.

## DIAGNOSTIC TESTS & INTERPRETATION
### Lab
- Avoid laboratory tests until airway is controlled.
- Throat cultures after control of airway
- Blood cultures after airway is secure:
  - Often positive if *H. influenzae* is the pathogen

### Imaging
- Radiographs of the soft tissue lateral neck:
  - Usually not necessary to make the diagnosis
  - Create additional risk by delaying stabilization of the airway, promoting airway obstruction by agitating the patient, and often removing the child from the ED to an uncontrolled environment. Children should never go unaccompanied to radiology. Personnel and equipment to control airway must always be available.
- Variable findings:
  - Normal
  - Swelling of the epiglottis ("thumbprint sign") and often supraglottic region
  - Ballooned hypopharynx
  - Obliteration of vallecula
  - EW/C3W (epiglottic width to 3rd cervical vertebral body width) ratio of >0.5

### Diagnostic Procedures/Surgery
Laryngoscopy:
- In a controlled environment whenever possible
- Cultures of the epiglottis during laryngoscopy after the airway is secured may help identify pathogens and direct treatment.
- Epiglottis will appear swollen, inflamed, reddened.

## DIFFERENTIAL DIAGNOSIS
- Other infectious processes:
  - Bacterial tracheitis
  - Mononucleosis
  - Diphtheria
  - Pertussis
  - Croup or laryngotracheobronchitis (primarily in younger children, but there is a significant overlap in the ages of presentation)
  - Ludwig's angina
  - Peritonsillar infection
  - Retropharyngeal abscess
- Anaphylactic reaction with angioedema
- Foreign body in upper airway
- Laryngeal trauma
- Laryngospasm
- Inhalation or aspiration of toxins (eg, hydrocarbons)
- Airway burns (have been related to crack cocaine)
- Hyperventilation
- CNS disorders

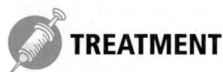 **TREATMENT**

## PRE-HOSPITAL
Degree and mode of intervention must reflect degree of obstruction, time and means of transport, capability of care providers, etc. Consult and notify receiving hospital.

## INITIAL STABILIZATION/THERAPY
- Airway management if patient is in extremis
- Bag-valve-mask ventilation with 100% $O_2$ with cricoid pressure often provides adequate ventilation and time to prepare for intubation and move to a controlled setting such as the operating room.
- Oral intubation:
  - Use an endotracheal tube (ETT) size that is 1 or 2 sizes smaller than indicated by age or length.
  - Direct compression of the anterior neck in the glottic region may help visualize air bubbles at the opening of the swollen glottis.
  - Instruments used for difficult airways may be adjunctive devices.
- If oral intubation fails:
  - Emergent cricothyrotomy or needle cricothyrotomy if age older than 10–12 yr
  - Needle cricothyrotomy if age younger than 10–12 yr

## ED TREATMENT/PROCEDURES

- 100% $O_2$ as tolerated by patient
- Allow child to remain in position of comfort and do not force child to lie down, which may worsen airway obstruction.
- Although not proven, racemic epinephrine or L-epinephrine by nebulizer may temporize symptoms while plans for a definitive airway are rapidly arranged. It must be done with caution to avoid agitating the child.
- Avoid procedures that agitate the child such as IV access and blood draws.
- Empiric invasive airway management may be indicated:
  - Patients with rapidly progressive respiratory difficulty, tachypnea, worsening throat pain, tachycardia, or hypoxemia
  - Patients at high risk of acute obstruction (eg, children with immunodeficiency disorders)
- Intubate in operating room or controlled environment by most skilled person.
- Use inhalational anesthesia before intubation.
- Have appropriate various diameters of endotracheal tubes available to accommodate the inflamed supraglottic region.
- Surgical backup is required in case intubation is not possible; then emergency tracheotomy or cricothyrotomy can be performed.
- Equipment for intubation and for a surgical airway or needle cricothyrotomy must be available at the bedside.
- Administer IV antibiotics: 2nd- or 3rd-generation cephalosporins are active against β-lactamase–producing *H. influenzae*.
- Steroids are controversial but frequently administered, particularly in patients with chemical or thermal epiglottitis.

## MEDICATION

### First Line
- Ampicillin/sulbactam: 100–200 mg/kg/24 h q6h IV
- Cefotaxime: 150 mg/kg/24 h q8h IV
- Ceftriaxone: 100 mg/kg/24 h q12h IV

### Second Line
- Ampicillin/sulbactam: 100–200 mg/kg/24 h q6h IV
- Ampicillin: 100–200 mg/kg/24 h q6h IV given with chloramphenicol
- Chloramphenicol: 75–100 mg/kg/24 h q6h IV
- Decadron: 0.6 mg/kg/d (max. 10 mg) IV
- Epinephrine, racemic: 0.05 mL/kg (max. 0.5 mL) q30min in 2.5 mL normal saline (NS) via nebulizer
- L-Epinephrine, 1:1,000: 0.5 mL/kg (max. 5 mL) q30min via nebulizer
- Rifampin for household contact prophylaxis: 20 mg/kg (max. 600 mg) daily for 4 days

 **FOLLOW-UP**

## DISPOSITION

### Admission Criteria
Patients with suspected or proven epiglottitis should be admitted to ICU after stabilization of airway and administration of antibiotics and fluids.

### Discharge Criteria
- Rifampin prophylaxis may be indicated for close contacts of *H. influenzae* epiglottitis. If the household has children younger than 12 mo of age or children who are unimmunized, incompletely immunized, or immunosuppressed, prophylaxis is indicated for nonpregnant household contacts. Child care center contacts should receive prophylaxis when 2 or more cases of Hib invasive disease have occurred within 60 days.
- All cases of invasive *H. influenzae* disease should be reported to the local or state public health department.

### Issues for Referral
Critical care or pulmonary consult on all patients

## PEARLS AND PITFALLS

True airway emergency. Patient must be monitored and accompanied at all times by someone with airway stabilization capabilities.

## ADDITIONAL READING

- American Academy of Pediatrics. *Red Book: 2009 Report of the Committee on Infectious Diseases*, 28th ed. Elk Grove Village, ILL: AAP; 2009.
- Faden H. The dramatic change in the epidemiology of pediatric epiglottitis. *Pediatr Emerg Care*. 2006;22:443–444.
- Rothrock S, et al. Radiologic diagnosis of epiglottitis: Objective criteria for all ages. *Ann Emerg Med*. 1990;19:978–982.
- Shah RK, Roberson DW, Jones DT. Epiglottitis in the *Hemophilus influenzae* type B era: Changing trends. *Laryngoscope*. 2004;114:557–560.
- Stroud RH, Friedman NR. An update on inflammatory disorders of the pediatric airway: Epiglottitis, croup and tracheitis. *Am J Otolaryngol*. 2001;22(4):268–275.

### See Also (Topic, Algorithm, Electronic Media Element)
- Bacterial Tracheitis
- Epiglottitis, Adult

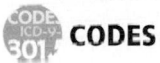 **CODES**

### ICD9
- 464.30 Acute epiglottitis without mention of obstruction
- 464.31 Acute epiglottitis with obstruction
- 476.1 Chronic laryngotracheitis

# EPIPHYSEAL INJURIES

*Neha Raukar*
*Daniel L. Savitt*

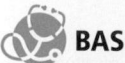 **BASICS**

## DESCRIPTION

Fractures through the physis accounts for 21–30% of pediatric long bone fractures with 30% of these leading to a growth disturbance:

- Most frequently seen in the distal radius and ulna, distal tibia and fibula, and the phalanges
- More common than ligamentous injury in children:
  - Tensile strength of pediatric bone is less than adjacent ligaments.
  - Physis is weakest part of pediatric bone.
  - Similar injury in an adult usually causes a sprain.
- Most common during peak growth:
  - Females: Age 9–12
  - Males: Age 12–15
  - Much less common in infancy and early childhood because epiphysis is not ossified and acts as a shock absorber
- Twice as common in males because female bones mature earlier
- Salter-Harris (SH) classification (introduced in 1963, simplest and most commonly used classification system):
  - Type I:
    - Fracture line confined to physis
    - Complete epiphyseal separation from metaphysis through the physis
    - If periosteum remains intact, epiphysis will not displace.
    - Clinical diagnosis made with focal tenderness over the physis
    - Most common example is SCFE.
    - Growth disturbance is rare.
  - Type II:
    - Accounts for ~80% of physeal fracture patterns
    - Fracture propagates along physis, and fragment from metaphysis accompanies the displaced epiphysis (Thurston Holland sign)
    - Periosteum torn opposite metaphyseal fragment
    - Growth is rarely disturbed.
  - Type III:
    - Rare
    - Fracture through a portion of physis extending through the epiphysis
    - Distal tibia most commonly affected
    - If displaced, requires reduction to maintain anatomic alignment
    - Growth disturbance may occur despite anatomic reduction because blood supply can be affected.

- Type IV:
  - Fracture originates at articular surface.
  - Extends through physis and into metaphysis
  - Distal humerus most commonly affected
  - Also has Thurston Holland fragment
  - Anatomic reduction essential and displaced fractures require ORIF
  - Growth arrest is common even with optimal treatment.
- Type V:
  - Results from severe crush injury to physis
  - No immediately visible radiographic alteration so almost impossible to diagnose initially
  - Compression forces lead to physeal injuries and inevitable growth disturbances.
  - Often found in retrospect
- Ogden modified the SH system to include injuries to the surrounding anatomy—periosteum, perichondrium, and Zone of Ranvier:
  - Ogden Type VI: Involves the peripheral perichondrium including the Zone of Ranvier
  - Ogden Type VII: Involves epiphysis only
- Peterson classification system, 1994:
  - Result of a 10 yr retrospective study
  - Showed that 16% of physeal injuries could not be classified by the SH system
  - Includes 2 different fracture patterns:
    - Peterson Type I—Transverse fracture through the metaphysis with 1 or more longitudinal extensions into the physis (this is similar to SH II except most of the energy is transmitted through the metaphysis, leading to a fracture, and not the physis so there is very little growth plate disturbance, this was actually the most common fracture pattern found)
    - Peterson Type VI—A part of the epiphysis, physis, and metaphysis are missing due to an open injury, classically by a lawnmower. Severe growth disturbance.

## ETIOLOGY

- Competitive and recreational injuries
- Traumatic injuries
- Child abuse
- Extreme cold
- Radiation injury
- Genetic, neurologic, and metabolic disease

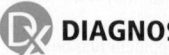 **DIAGNOSIS**

## SIGNS AND SYMPTOMS

### History

- Most commonly occurs after a fall
- Extreme cold and radiation can injure the physeal plate.

### Physical Exam

- Focal tenderness
- Swelling
- Limited mobility
- If lower extremity involved, patient may be non weight bearing
- Joint laxity:
  - Can be due to physeal injury and not ligamentous injury

## ESSENTIAL WORKUP

- Radiographs to classify the extent of the injury
- Assess pulses and capillary filling distal to injury.
- Evaluate distal motor and sensory function.
- Verify integrity of skin overlying injury.
- Address and manage coexisting injuries.

## DIAGNOSTIC TESTS & INTERPRETATION

### Imaging

- Plain radiography of injured extremity:
  - Type I fractures:
    - Usually normal
    - May appreciate a slightly separated physis or an associated joint effusion
    - Consider comparison views of contralateral joint to detect small defects.
    - Callus may be present on follow-up films.
  - Types II–IV: Films diagnostic of fracture
  - Types V:
    - Initial film often normal
    - Subsequent radiographs may reveal premature bone arrest.
- Ultrasound can be helpful in infants whose cartilage has not ossified.
- CT scan: Helpful in assessing orientation of comminuted fragments
- MRI:
  - Most accurate in the acute phase of injury
  - Can identify physeal arrest lines
  - Recommended if diagnosis remains equivocal and identification of a specific fracture would alter management

## DIFFERENTIAL DIAGNOSIS

- Strain
- Sprain
- Contusion

# TREATMENT

## PRE-HOSPITAL
- Immobilize limb in position found.
- Apply ice or cold packs to injury.
- Assess injured extremity for neurologic and vascular function.
- Consider concomitant injuries.

## INITIAL STABILIZATION/THERAPY
- Analgesia
- Apply sterile dressings to open wounds.
- Control bleeding of open wounds.

## ED TREATMENT/PROCEDURES
- Reduction/alignment required in displaced fractures:
  - Need to achieve anatomic alignment
- Vascular or neurologic compromise distal to injury requires immediate intervention.
- Immobilization of all suspected or radiographically confirmed physeal injuries:
  - Splint must immobilize joints proximal and distal to injury in anatomic alignment and neutral position.
  - Limit activity of the injured limb
- Open fractures:
  - IV antibiotics for *Staphylococcus aureus*, group A streptococcus, and potential anaerobes depending on mechanism and after cultures are obtained
  - Copious irrigation with saline
  - Sterile dressing
  - Orthopedic consultation
- Consultation:
  - Open fractures
  - Type II with displacement and types III and higher

## MEDICATION
### First Line
Pain management:
- Fentanyl: 2–3 $\mu$g/kg IV; transmucosal lollipops 5–15 $\mu$g/kg, max. 400 mg, contraindicated if <10 kg
- Morphine: 0.1 mg/kg IV/IM

### Second Line
If open:
- Cefazolin: 25–50 mg/kg/d IV/IM q6–8h
- Penicillin G: 100,000–300,000 U/kg/24 hr IM, or IV in 4–6 DD—has better strep and corny bacterium coverage
- Gentamycin: 5–7.5 mg/kg/day
- Flagyl: 15 mg/kg once then 7.5 mg/kg q6h—for contaminated wounds

# FOLLOW-UP

## DISPOSITION
### Admission Criteria
- Open fractures
- Open surgical reduction required
- Consider with Type III and IV fractures

### Discharge Criteria
- Low-grade fractures and fractures with higher grade if follow-up is definite
- Splint
- Analgesics
- Ice packs
- Elevation of affected limb
- Orthopedic follow-up within 1 wk

### Issues for Referral
All injuries involving the physis should follow-up with a musculoskeletal specialist.

## FOLLOW-UP RECOMMENDATIONS
Usually necessary, especially with higher grade injuries, to monitor limb length:
- Involves periodic physical exam and radiographic evaluation

# PEARLS AND PITFALLS
- Long-term complications:
  - Limb length discrepancy if entire growth plate affected
  - Angulation if only a part of the physis is affected
- In patients with suspected SH fracture and negative radiograph, immobilization with follow-up in a few days is appropriate.

# ADDITIONAL READING
- Rodriguez-Merchan EC. Pediatric skeletal trauma: A review and historical perspective. *Clin Orthop Relat Res.* 2005;432:8–13.
- Wilkins KE, Aroojis AJ. Incidence of fractures in children. In: Beaty JH, Kasser JR (Eds). *Rockwood & Wilkins' Fractures in Children*, 6th ed. Philadelphia: Lippincott Williams & Wilkins; 2006, p. 12.
- Rathjen KE, Birch JG. Physeal injuries and growth disturbances. In: Beaty JH, Kasser JR (Eds). *Rockwood & Wilkins' Fractures in Children*, 6th ed. Philadelphia: Lippincott Williams and Wilkins; 2006, p. 11
- Salter R, Harris W. Injuries involving the epiphyseal plate. *J Bone Joint Surg.* 1963;45A:587.

# CODES

## ICD9
- 813.42 Other closed fractures of distal end of radius (alone)
- 813.43 Fracture of distal end of ulna (alone), closed
- 813.44 Fracture of lower end of radius with ulna, closed

E

# EPISTAXIS

*Richard E. Wolfe*
*Christopher M. McCarthy, II*

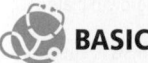 **BASICS**

## DESCRIPTION
- Nosebleeds are a common emergency presentation that is usually minor and self-limited but rarely may be life-threatening:
  - Lifetime incidence of ~60%:
    - The incidence decreases with age, with most cases seen in children <10 yr.
    - Male > Female
    - Severe bleeds requiring surgical intervention are more common in patients >50.
    - Occurs more frequently with low humidity during the winter, in northern climates, and at high altitude
- The nasal cavity is supplied with blood vessels originating from both the internal and external carotid arteries.
- Location of the hemorrhage determines therapy:
  - Anterior epistaxis (90% of cases):
    - Most commonly bleeding is located at Kiesselbach plexus, an anastomotic network of vessels on the anterior inferior nasal septum.
    - Rarely bleeding is found on the posterior floor of the nasal cavity or the nasal septum.
    - Presents as a unilateral bleed that can be visualized with a nasal speculum.
- Posterior epistaxis (10% of cases):
  - Posterolateral branch of sphenopalatine artery

## ETIOLOGY
- Idiopathic:
  - Dry nasal mucosa (low humidity)
- Nasal foreign body:
  - Children, mentally retarded patients, psychiatric patients
- Infection:
  - Rhinitis
  - Sinusitis
  - Nasal diphtheria
  - Nasal mucormycosis
- Allergic rhinitis
- Trauma:
  - Nose picking
  - Postoperative
  - Facial trauma
  - Barotrauma
- Environmental irritants:
  - Ammonia
  - Gasoline
  - Sulfuric acid
  - Glutaraldehyde

- Neoplasia:
  - Papilloma
  - Squamous cell carcinoma:
    - Most common nasal cancer
  - Hemangioma
  - Esthesioneuroblastoma
  - Melanoma
  - Adenocarcinoma
  - Juvenile nasal angiofibroma:
    - Uncommon tumor selectively affecting teenage boys
- Coagulopathy:
  - Hemophilia A or B
  - Von Willebrand disease
  - Thrombocytopenia
  - Liver disease
  - Leukemia
  - Chemotherapy
- Drug-induced:
  - Salicylates
  - NSAIDs
  - Heparin
  - Coumadin
- Hereditary hemorrhagic telangiectasia (Osler-Weber-Rendu disease)
- Atherosclerosis of nasal vasculature
- Endometriosis
- Renal failure
- Alcoholism

 **DIAGNOSIS**

## SIGNS AND SYMPTOMS
### History
- Laterality of the bleeding
- Intensity and amount of bleeding from the nares
- Recurrence of epistaxis and history of prior episodes
- Nasal obstruction and the duration of this symptom
- Complaints of vomiting or coughing blood
- Known tumors or coagulopathy
- Unusual bleeding or easy bruising suggests an underlying coagulopathy.
- Presence of systemic disease exacerbated by blood loss (coronary artery disease, chronic obstructive pulmonary disease)

### Physical Exam
- Careful exam for signs of coagulopathy:
  - Bruises
  - Petechiae and purpura
- Nasopharyngeal inspection:
  - Anesthetize nasopharynx prior to exam with cotton swab soaked in anesthetic and vasoactive agent.

- Attempt to identify bleeding source with nasal speculum (ie, Kiesselbach plexus vs. posterior source).
- Blood in mouth or oropharynx
- Tachycardia
- Hypotension

## ESSENTIAL WORKUP
- Assess stability: Airway compromise, hypovolemia.
- Determine source (anterior versus posterior).
- Consider underlying coagulopathy.

## DIAGNOSTIC TESTS & INTERPRETATION
### Lab
Consider for severe bleeding or suspected coagulopathy:
- Type and cross-match, hematocrit, PT, PTT, BUN

### Diagnostic Procedures/Surgery
Direct visualization of nasal mucosa with nasal speculum:
- Pretreat with topical vasoconstricting agent and anesthetic.
- Ensure adequate lighting (ie, headlamp) and suction.

## DIFFERENTIAL DIAGNOSIS
- Hematemesis
- Hemoptysis

### Pediatric Considerations
- Posterior epistaxis is rare in children; consider further workup for bleeding diatheses.
- Consider nasal foreign bodies or neoplasm, such as juvenile angiofibroma or papilloma.

 **TREATMENT**

## PRE-HOSPITAL
- Stable patients: Patient should bend forward at the waist, pinch nares closed, and spit out blood rather than swallow it.
- Unstable patients:
  - Intubation, if airway is compromised
  - IV access
  - Crystalloid resuscitation, if signs of hypovolemia

## INITIAL STABILIZATION/THERAPY
- Secure the airway in patients who are unconscious, have major facial trauma, or are otherwise at risk of obstruction or aspiration.
- Treat hypotension with crystalloids and blood products, if necessary, and ensure adequate IV access.

## ED TREATMENT/PROCEDURES

- Universal precautions against blood/fluid contamination
- Anterior source:
  - Instruct patient to bend forward at waist, pinch nares closed for 15 min, and spit out blood rather than swallow it.
  - If bleeding persists, use bayonet forceps to place cotton pledgets soaked in vasoconstricting and anesthetic agents into affected nares.
  - Visualize source of bleeding and cauterize limited area with silver nitrate or trichloroacetic acid.
  - Consider Gelfoam or Surgicel packing over cauterized site.
- Anterior nasal packing:
  - Indicated when cautery has failed to control bleeding
  - Associated with significant discomfort and infectious risk of sinusitis and toxic shock
  - Anterior nasal balloon:
    ○ Check the integrity of the balloons before insertion.
    ○ Cover with water-based lubricant or viscous lidocaine
    ○ Insert the device and inflate it slowly to avoid discomfort.
    ○ Use saline for the inflation if the balloon is to remain in place > a few hours.
  - Preformed nasal tampons:
    ○ Adequate anesthesia of the nasal passage should be ensured before placing the tampon.
    ○ Lubricate the tip of the Merocel tampon with antibiotic ointment.
    ○ Insert it at a 45 degree angle ~1–2 cm into the nasal cavity.
    ○ Rotate the long axis of the tampon into a horizontal plane and push it firmly back into the nasal cavity.
    ○ If the pack does not fully expand from the blood, then use saline to complete the expansion.
    ○ Secure the drawstring to the cheek.
  - Petroleum jelly-impregnated gauze:
    ○ Add an antibiotic ointment to the gauze.
    ○ Ensure that a free end remains outside the nose.
    ○ Place the gauze as far back as possible, starting on the floor of the nose.
    ○ Repeat while securing the placed gauze with the speculum until the nose is fully packed.
  - After anterior packing, persistent new bleeding may be a sign of inadequate packing or posterior source.
- Posterior source:
  - Posterior packing with balloon device such as Nasostat, Epistat; these are not left in for >3 days, with antibiotic prophylaxis for anterior packing.
  - If commercial packs are unavailable, a Foley catheter may be directed into posterior nasopharynx until the tip visible in mouth. The balloon is then inflated and the catheter retracted until the balloon is lodged in the posterior nasopharynx. The catheter is then held in place by umbilical clamp.

- Complications of posterior packing:
  - Pressure necrosis of posterior oropharynx (do not overfill balloon)
  - Nasal trauma
  - Vagal response
  - Aspiration
  - Infection
  - Hypoxia
  - Endoscopic cautery by otolaryngology is also useful and may obviate need for admission.

## MEDICATION

- Vasoactive solutions:
  - 4% cocaine
  - 1:1 mixture of 2% tetracaine and epinephrine (1:1,000)
  - 1:1 mixture of oxymetazoline 0.05% (Afrin) and lidocaine solution 4%
  - Phenylephrine (Neo-Synephrine)
- Amoxicillin-clavulanate potassium: 250 mg PO q8h
- Cephalexin: 250 mg PO q6h
- Clindamycin: 150 mg PO q6h
- Trimethoprim-sulfamethoxazole: 160/800 mg PO q12h

 FOLLOW-UP

### DISPOSITION

#### Admission Criteria

- Severe blood loss requiring transfusion
- Severe coagulopathy that places the patient at risk of further blood loss
- Posterior nasal packing: Otolaryngology consult and admission for supplemental oxygen, sedation, and observation; possible further surgical intervention (eg, arterial ligation or embolization)
- Patients with packing who cannot be relied upon to follow-up in a timely manner

#### Discharge Criteria

Stable patients:

- Use Afrin nasal spray for 2 days.
- Lubricate nares with an antibiotic ointment.
- Humidify air.
- Avoid nose picking.
- All patients with nasal packing in place should be prescribed an antistaphylococcal antibiotic (amoxicillin-clavulanate, cephalexin, trimethoprim-sulfamethoxazole) for the duration that the packing remains in place for prevention of both acute sinusitis and toxic shock syndrome.

#### Issues for Referral

- Refer all patients with packing to a specialist within 48 hr.
- Patients with nonvisualized source, suspicious-appearing lesions, recurrent same-side bleeding, or nasal obstruction should be referred to an ORL specialist for an exam to rule out a neoplastic etiology or a foreign body.

## FOLLOW-UP RECOMMENDATIONS

- Return to ED for bleeding not controlled by pressure, fever, difficulty breathing, or vomiting.
- Avoid any nose blowing for 12 hr after the bleeding stops.
- Avoid nose picking or putting anything into the nose.
- If the bleeding starts again, sit up and lean forward, pinch the soft part of the nose tightly for 10 min without letting go.
- Avoid lifting heavy objects or doing too much work right away.
- If there is no packing in the nose, put a small amount of petroleum jelly or antibiotic ointment inside the nostril 2 times a day for 4–5 days.
- Use a humidifier or vaporizer in the home.

## PEARLS AND PITFALLS

- Foreign bodies should be suspected in any unilateral nasal bleeding in small children, psychiatric patients, and patients with mental retardation.
- Avoid covering anterior nasal balloons with antibiotic ointment, as petroleum-based materials may cause a delayed rupture of the balloon.
- Avoid overinflating nasal balloons or placing a pack too tightly, as it can cause necrosis and eschars.

## ADDITIONAL READING

- Evans JA, Rothenhaus TC. Epistaxis. In: Wolfson AB et al., eds. *Harwood-Nuss' clinical practice of emergency medicine*, 4th ed. Philadelphia: Lippincott Williams & Wilkins, 2005:185–190.
- Frazee TA, Hauser MS. Nonsurgical management of epistaxis. *J Oral Maxillofac Surg* 2000;58:419–424.
- Gifford TO, Orlandi RR. Epistaxis. *Otolaryngol Clin N Am*. 2008;41:525–536.
- Kucik C, Klenny T. Management of epistaxis. *Am Fam Physician*. 2005;71:305–377.
- Middleton P. Epistaxis. *Emerg Med Australasia*. 2004;16:428–440.
- Pfaff JA, Moore GP. Otolaryngology. In: Marx J, Hockberger R, Walls R, eds. *Emergency medicine: Concepts and clinical practice*, 7th ed. St. Louis: Mosby, 2009:933–935.

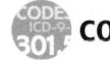 CODES

**ICD9**
784.7 Epistaxis

# ERYSIPELAS

*Irving Jacoby*

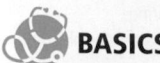

## BASICS

### DESCRIPTION
Superficial bacterial infection of the skin with prominent lymphatic involvement

### ETIOLOGY
- Group A β-hemolytic streptococcus is the causative organism (uncommonly, group C or G streptococci).
- Portals of entry are commonly skin ulcers, local trauma or abrasions, psoriatic or eczematous lesions, or fungal infections.

#### Pediatric Considerations
- *Haemophilus influenza* type b (HIB) causes facial cellulitis in children that may appear similar to erysipelas:
  - Should be considered in unimmunized children
  - Many will be bacteremic and require admission.
  - Cefuroxime or other appropriate *Haemophilus influenza* coverage is important.
  - *Haemophilus influenza* is much less common since widespread use of the HIB vaccine.
- Group B streptococci can cause erysipelas in the newborn.
- Can develop from infection of umbilical stump

## DIAGNOSIS

### SIGNS AND SYMPTOMS
- Most common sites of involvement are the face (5–20% of cases), lower legs (70–80% of cases), and ears.
- Skin has an intense fiery red color, hence the name "Saint Anthony's fire."
- Predilection for infants, children, and the elderly
- Systemic symptoms may include malaise, fever, chills, nausea, and vomiting.
- Traumatic portal of entry on skin is not always apparent.
- Rarely there may be an associated periorbital cellulitis or cavernous sinus involvement.

### History
- Facial erysipelas may follow an upper respiratory tract infection.
- Predilection for areas of lymphatic obstruction:
  - Particularly in the upper extremity following radical mastectomy
- May be a marker for previously undiagnosed lymphatic obstruction
- 30% recurrence rate within 3 yr, owing to lymphatic obstruction caused by an episode of erysipelas

### Physical Exam
- The involved skin is an edematous, indurated (peau d'orange), painful, well-circumscribed plaque with sharp, clearly demarcated edges.
- Classical butterfly rash on cheeks and across nose when affecting face
- Vesicles and bullae may be present in more serious infections.

### ESSENTIAL WORKUP
- The diagnosis is clinical:
  - Based on the characteristic skin findings and the clinical setting.
- Needle-aspirate wound cultures are seldom positive and not indicated.
- Positive blood cultures in 3–5%; leukocytosis is common; when complicating infected ulcers, cultures are positive in 30%.

### DIAGNOSTIC TESTS & INTERPRETATION
#### Lab
- Swabs of the skin are not indicated for culture, as they will show only skin organisms.
- CBC, differential, and blood cultures should be performed in diabetics and other high-risk populations, or in patients with hypotension and those who require admission:
  - Blood cultures more likely to be positive in patients with lymphedema.
- Check glucose in diabetics as infection may disrupt control.
- Urinalysis: To check for proteinuria, hematuria and red cell casts. This would suggest diagnosis of poststreptococcal glomerulonephritis (PSGN). If it occurs, is usually around 2 wk after onset of skin infection.

### Imaging
- There is no standard imaging for classical erysipelas. However, if deeper infection such as necrotizing fasciitis or myositis is suspected, plain films of an extremity can be taken to rule out the presence of gas.
- US may be useful to evaluate for abscess if this is a concern.

### DIFFERENTIAL DIAGNOSIS
- Abscess
- Allergic inflammation
- Cellulitis
- Contact dermatitis
- Deep vein thrombophlebitis (DVT)
- Diffuse inflammatory carcinoma of the breast
- Familial Mediterranean Fever
- Herpes zoster, second division of Cranial Nerve V
- Impetigo
- Inflammatory dermatophytosis
- Necrotizing fasciitis
- Periorbital cellulitis
- Systemic lupus erythematosus (SLE) with butterfly rash
- Streptococcal toxic shock syndrome
- Venous stasis dermatitis
- Viral exanthem

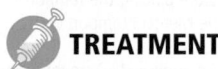

## TREATMENT

### PRE-HOSPITAL
Wearing gloves, followed by hand washing when managing patients, to decrease risk of transmission of streptococcal carriage

### INITIAL STABILIZATION/THERAPY
Patients may be toxic and in need of intravenous fluid resuscitation or pressure support.

### ED TREATMENT/PROCEDURES
- Appropriate antibiotic therapy; treatment should be for 10 days:
  - Patients with extensive involvement should be admitted for parenteral antibiotic treatment.
  - May switch to oral antibiotics when patient is stable and showing signs of response

- Mild cases: Patients can be discharged on oral therapy if nontoxic appearing, good compliance, and close follow-up can be ensured.
- Penicillin is the drug of choice when clearly the symptoms are consistent with erysipelas.
- If there is difficulty in distinguishing from cellulitis, staphylococcal coverage should be added:
  – Use penicillinase-resistant penicillin or first-generation cephalosporin
  – If in community with high incidence of methicillin-resistant *S. aureus* (MRSA), use vancomycin, or other anti-MRSA coverage. Reports of vancomycin-resistant Staphylococci are occurring.

## MEDICATION
- Cefuroxime: Peds: 50–100 mg/kg/d PO divided q8h
- Cephalexin: Adult: 500 mg PO q6h (peds: 40 mg/kg/d PO divided q8h) for 10 days
- Dicloxacillin: Adult: 500 mg PO q6h (peds: 30–50 mg/kg/d PO divided q6h) for 10 days
- Erythromycin: Adult: 250–500 mg PO q6h (peds: 40 mg/kg/d PO in divided doses q6h) for 10 days
- Penicillin G: Adult: 2 million U q4h IV (peds: 25,000 U/kg IV q6h)
- Penicillin G, procaine: 600,000 U q12h IM
- Penicillin V: Adult: 500 mg PO q6h (peds: 25–50 mg/kg/d div. q6h–q8h) for 10 days
- Clindamycin: 300 mg PO QID for 10 days; or 600 mg q6h or 900 mg q8h IV (peds: 20–40 mg/kg/d IV divided q6–8h; or 8–25 mg/kg/dsuspension PO divided TID or QID)
- Vancomycin: 1 g IV q12h given over 1.5–2 hr to decease risk of Red Man Syndrome (peds: 10–15 mg/kg IV q6h)

### First Line
- Oral or IV: Penicillin or first generation cephalosporin;
- Clindamycin for penicillin-allergic individuals

### Second Line
Oral: Erythromycin

 **FOLLOW-UP**

## DISPOSITION
### Admission Criteria
- Patients with extensive involvement, fever, toxic appearance, or those who live alone or are unable to take oral medications will require admission for IV antibiotics.
- Children more often require admission. Blood cultures, intravenous antibiotics, including coverage for *H. influenza,* should be initiated for patients who have not been immunized with HIB vaccine.

### Discharge Criteria
- Minimal facial involvement
- Nontoxic appearing
- Not immunosuppressed
- Able to tolerate and comply with oral therapy
- Adequate follow-up and supervision

### Issues for Referral
Refer to nephrologist for evaluation and treatment for poststreptococcal glomerulonephritis if hematuria, proteinuria and red cell casts are noted on UA, particularly in children between the ages of 3 and 15.

## FOLLOW-UP RECOMMENDATIONS
- Use of pressure stockings on the legs in the presence of lymphedema may reduce incidence of relapses.
- Following erysipelas of legs, use of topical antifungal cream or ointment to treat underlying tinea pedis when present

## PEARLS AND PITFALLS
- Failure to treat underlying dermatophyte infection of the feet and intradigital spaces associated with an episode of erysipelas of the leg may result in persistent breaks in the skin, and relapses.
- Treatment of underlying lymphedema is associated with reduced incidence of relapses.
- Failure to respond, or pain out of proportion to findings, might suggest deeper level of infection and require further work up to rule out necrotizing fasciitis, or mixed aerobic/anaerobic necrotizing cellulitis.
- Presence of micropustules would suggest Staphylococcal infection/cellulitis rather than erysipelas, and antibiotic coverage would need to be broader.
- Since infection is likely due to have entered skin through traumatic break in skin, should remember to check for tetanus immunization status and update if necessary.

## ADDITIONAL READING
- Bisno Al, Stevens DL. Streptococcal infections of skin and soft tissues. *N Engl J Med*. 1996;334:240–244.
- Damstra RJ, et al. Erysipelas as a sign of subclinical primary lymphoedema: A prospective quantitative scintigraphic study of 40 patients with unilateral erysipelas of the leg. *Br J Dermatol*. 2008;158: 1210–1215.
- Morris A. Cellulitis and erysipelas. *Clin Evid*. 2006;(15):2207–2211.

### See Also (Topic, Algorithm, Electronic Media Element)
- Abscess
- Cellulitis
- MRS, Community Acquired

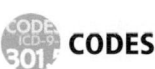 **CODES**

### ICD9
035 Erysipelas

# ERYTHEMA INFECTIOSUM

*Julie L. Story*
*Benjamin S. Heavrin*

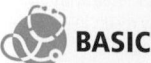 ## BASICS

### DESCRIPTION
- Characteristic viral exanthem also known as 5th disease:
  - 5th common childhood rash historically described
  - Measles (1st), scarlet fever (2nd), rubella (3rd), Duke's disease (4th), roseola (6th)
- Common symptoms: Viral prodrome followed by slapped-cheek rash and subsequent diffuse reticular rash +/− arthropathy
- Most common in school-aged children <14 yr
- Usually self-limited with lasting immunity
- Rare complications and chronic cases in patients with congenital anemias or immunosuppression
- Potential for severe complications to fetus if infection acquired during pregnancy
- Possible link to encephalopathy, epilepsy, meningitis, myocarditis, dilated cardiomyopathy, autoimmune hepatitis, HSP, ITP

### ETIOLOGY
- Caused by human parvovirus B19, small SS-DNA virus:
  - Infects human erythroid progenitor cells, suppressing erythropoiesis
- Most common in late winter and spring
- Transmitted via respiratory droplets and blood products as well as vertical maternal–fetal transmission
- Incubation period 4–21 days
- Most contagious during the week PRIOR to rash onset
- Majority of adults have serologic evidence of prior infection.

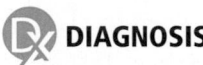 ## DIAGNOSIS

### SIGNS AND SYMPTOMS
- "Slapped-cheek" appearance most common in young children
- Fever
- Malaise
- Delayed symptoms 4–14 days later:
  - Diffuse, pruritic, lacy rash (absent in most adults), most pronounced in extremities
  - Symmetric polyarthropathy, most common in middle-aged women:
    - Small joints involved in adolescents and adults
    - Knees most commonly involved in children
    - Secondary to immune-complex deposition
  - However, most patients remain asymptomatic or only develop mild, nonspecific viral symptoms.

### History
- Mild constitutional symptoms (fever, headache, nasal congestion, nausea, sore throat)
- Contagious only until facial rash appears

### Physical Exam
- Stage 1:
  - "Slapped-cheek" rash of coalescent, warm, erythematous, edematous papules with circumoral pallor in young children
- Stage 2:
  - Nonspecific, diffuse, pruritic, maculopapular, reticular eruption
  - 4–21 days after facial rash, lasts up to 6 wk
  - More prominent on extremities
  - Usually spares palms and soles
- Stage 3:
  - Rash fades but recurs with exposure to sunlight, stress, exercise, and heat
- Usually complete resolution without scarring

### ESSENTIAL WORKUP
Clinical diagnosis based on characteristic signs and symptoms.

### DIAGNOSTIC TESTS & INTERPRETATION
- Usually not necessary
- CBC and reticulocyte count if concern for aplastic crisis
- Confirm diagnosis if immunocompromised or pregnant:
  - Viral DNA PCR now available
  - IgM antibody confirms acute infection and persists for 2–3 mo
  - IgG presence confers lasting immunity
- In pregnancy, ultrasound to detect hydrops fetalis

### DIFFERENTIAL DIAGNOSIS
- Allergic reaction
- Collagen vascular disease
- Coxsackie virus
- Drug eruptions
- Enterovirus
- Erysipelas
- Infectious mononucleosis
- Measles
- Nonspecific viral illness
- Rheumatoid arthritis
- Roseola
- Rubella
- Scarlet fever
- Sunburn

 ## TREATMENT

Erythema infectiosum is usually self-limited and does not require treatment.

### PRE-HOSPITAL
ABCs for severe cases and septic patients

### INITIAL STABILIZATION/THERAPY
- Supplemental oxygen if indicated
- Intubation with mechanical ventilation if patient in extremis
- IVF for hypotension with suspected dehydration
- Severe anemia may also cause hypotension and hypoxia, transfuse PRBCs as indicated.
- Pain control with acetaminophen, NSAIDs, or opiates as needed for severe arthropathy

### ED TREATMENT/PROCEDURES
- No specific antiviral treatment or vaccine is available.
- Send appropriate labs (CBC, reticulocytes, antibody testing) for severe cases.
- Symptomatic treatment as needed:
  - IVF for dehydration
  - NSAIDs for arthropathy if no underlying renal insufficiency
  - Consider diphenhydramine for prurutis, caution parents about possible AMS.
  - Antipyretics for fever
- PRBC transfusion for severe anemia
- ID consult: IVIG may have benefit for immunocompromised patients with chronic symptoms and red cell aplasia
- Hematology consult for severe cases
- Hospitalization and respiratory isolation for aplastic crisis

### MEDICATION
- Acetaminophen: 650 mg (peds: 15 mg/kg/dose) PO q6h PRN fever for up to 5 days
- Diphenhydramine: 25 mg (peds: 1–2 mg/kg/dose) PO q6h PRN itching for up to 5 days
- Ibuprofen: 400 mg (peds: 10 mg/kg/dose) PO q8h PRN pain for up to 5 days
- IVIG only in consultation with ID specialist

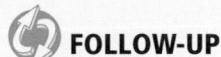

## FOLLOW-UP

### DISPOSITION

#### Admission Criteria

- Aplastic crisis or severe anemia
- Severely immunocompromised
- Hydrops fetalis
- Toxic appearance
- Severe arthritis

#### Discharge Criteria

- Nearly all patients
- Normal CBC, O2 sat, and BP
- Patients are no longer contagious following appearance of facial rash and may return to day care, school, or work.

#### Issues for Referral

- All patients without existing primary care physicians should be referred to a generalist for follow-up as needed.
- Patients with hereditary anemias should be referred to hematology for follow-up in 1–2 days.
- All immunocompromised patients require prompt subspecialty follow-up.
- Pregnant patients with new infection should have immediate follow-up with Ob/Gyn for further monitoring and ultrasound.

### FOLLOW-UP RECOMMENDATIONS

- Pregnant women with new Parvovirus B19 infection may need serial ultrasounds for 10–12 wk.
- Patients at risk for aplastic crisis should follow-up with the appropriate specialties 1–2 days after ED discharge for repeat CBC.

### PATIENT EDUCATION

Prevention:

- No vaccine available
- Frequent handwashing helps prevent spread.
- No current recommendations to keep children out of school, since most children are no longer contagious by the time the diagnosis is made.
- Pregnant women may choose to stay away from a workplace outbreak, but no current official recommendation exists.

## COMPLICATIONS

- Transient aplastic crisis in patients with anemias: Sickle cell disease, hereditary spherocytosis, thalassemia, iron-deficiency, or other conditions with shortened red cell lifespan:
  – Usually full recovery within 2 wk
- Persistent infection with severe anemia if immunocompromised and unable to mount antibody response, especially with HIV
- Arthritis or hypersensitivity dermatitis in adults:
  – May have transient rheumatoid factor positivity, but no true association with rheumatoid arthritis and no joint destruction
- Association with papular, purpuric gloves, and socks syndrome in adults:
  – Symmetric, painful progressive rash and edema of hands and feet
  – Erythema progresses to petechiae, purpura, and occasionally bullae
  – This syndrome is also associated with many other viruses and drugs.
- Rare hepatosplenomegaly, heart failure, CVA, thrombocytopenia, leukopenia

### Pregnancy Considerations

- Risk of hydrops fetalis in pregnancy
- 60% of pregnant women are susceptible to new infection.
- 30% risk of transplacental infection with new maternal infection
- Affects fetal liver (main site of erythropoiesis), leading to anemia, CHF, myocarditis, IUGR
- 2–6% risk of fetal loss, highest in 2nd trimester

## PEARLS AND PITFALLS

- Parvovirus B19 is usually a self-limited, mild illness.
- Common symptoms include "slapped-cheeks" rash with subsequent diffuse lacy rash and arthropathy.
- Patients are no longer contagious when the rash appears and aplastic crisis resolves.
- Evaluate all patients with history of hereditary or iron-deficiency anemia for aplastic crisis.
- Evaluate all patients with history of immunosuppression for chronic infection with persistent anemia.
- Confirm diagnosis in all pregnant patients. If no proven immunity, monitor for fetal complications and refer for follow-up.

## ADDITIONAL READING

- Servey JT, Reamy BV, Hodge J. Clinical presentations of parvovirus B19 infection. *Am Fam Physician*. 2007;75:373–377.
- Vafaie J, Schwartz RA. Erythema infectiosum. *J Cutan Med Surg*. 2005;9:159–161.
- Weir E. Parvovirus B19 infection: Fifth disease and more. *CMAJ*. 2005;172:743.

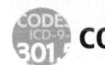 CODES

ICD9
057.0 Erythema infectiosum (fifth disease)

E

# ERYTHEMA MULTIFORME

Gregory W. Hendey
Thomas A. Utecht

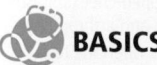 BASICS

## DESCRIPTION

- A rash caused by a hypersensitivity reaction:
  - May occur in response to various medications, infections, or other illness
- Divided into *major* and *minor* types:
  - Erythema multiforme major: Separate disease pattern that includes more severe disorders, such as Toxic Epidermal Necrolysis (TEN) and Stevens-Johnson syndrome (SJS).
  - Erythema multiforme minor is characterized by a benign, self-limited rash, generally not associated with acute, serious illness; simply referred to as *erythema multiforme*.
- Most often affects children and young adults (>50% younger than 20 yr)
- Males are affected more often than females.

## ETIOLOGY

- Hypersensitivity reaction, probably transient autoimmune defect
- Herpes simplex virus is the most common precipitant (>70%).
- Other causes include idiopathic, medications (antibiotics: Penicillin, sulfur-based, phenytoin, and others), malignancy, and *Mycoplasma* infections.

 DIAGNOSIS

## SIGNS AND SYMPTOMS

### History

- Prodrome: Infrequent systemic symptoms (mild fever/malaise), antecedent (within 3 wk) herpes simplex virus (HSV) in most cases
- Usually not associated with severe systemic illness

### Physical Exam

Characteristic rash:

- Lesions: Symmetric dull red macules and papules, evolving into round, well-demarcated target lesions with central clearing
- *Multiforme* refers to the evolution of the rash through various stages at different times.
- Distribution: Extremities, dorsal hands and feet, extensor surfaces, especially elbows and knees. **It is one of the few rashes that may involve palms and soles.**
- Spread: From extremities toward trunk
- Mucosal involvement: Often involves mild blistering or erosions on the lips or mouth
- Duration: Usually 1–4 wk, but may become chronic or recurrent

## ESSENTIAL WORKUP

Complete history and physical exam, with special attention to the skin, genitourinary system, recent infectious symptoms, and recent medications

## DIAGNOSTIC TESTS & INTERPRETATION

### Lab

No specific laboratory tests needed

### Imaging

No specific imaging is helpful.

### Diagnostic Procedures/Surgery

- Skin biopsy reveals mononuclear cell infiltrate around upper dermal blood vessels, without leukocytoclastic vasculitis and necrosis of epidermal keratinocytes.
- Biopsy is not necessary in most cases.

## DIFFERENTIAL DIAGNOSIS

- Systemic lupus erythematosus
- Fixed drug eruption
- Pityriasis rosea
- Secondary syphilis
- Erythema migrans
- Urticaria
- Stevens-Johnson syndrome
- Toxic epidermal necrolysis

**TREATMENT**

### PRE-HOSPITAL
Not contagious and does not require isolation or postexposure prophylaxis for exposed personnel

### INITIAL STABILIZATION/THERAPY
Generally benign and self-limited, requiring no initial stabilization

### ED TREATMENT/PROCEDURES
- Attempt to identify, treat, or remove underlying cause or precipitant
- Symptomatic: Cool compresses, antipruritics

### MEDICATION

#### First Line
Antiviral therapy:
- If HSV infection is present, see "Herpes" for specific treatment options.

#### Second Line
Antipruritic agents:
- Cetirizine (Zyrtec): 10 mg/day (peds: 2.5–5 mg) PO
- Diphenhydramine: 25–50 mg (peds: 5 mg/kg/24 hr) PO q6–8h
- Hydroxyzine: 25 mg PO q6–8h (peds: 2 mg/kg/24 hr div q6–8h)

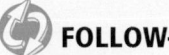 **FOLLOW-UP**

### DISPOSITION

#### Admission Criteria
Admission is not needed unless required for another concurrent disorder.

#### Discharge Criteria
Erythema multiforme is a benign disorder that does not require admission.

#### Issues for Referral
Patients should be referred to a dermatologist If the diagnosis is uncertain or the rash is atypical.

### FOLLOW-UP RECOMMENDATIONS
- Follow-up with primary care physician within 1 wk to assess:
  - Further evaluation of underlying conditions (HSV, medication reaction, malignancy, etc.)
  - Progression or resolution of rash
- Follow-up with a dermatologist within 1 wk if the diagnosis is uncertain.

## PEARLS AND PITFALLS

- In patients with severe systemic illness, a more serious diagnosis should be considered, such as SJS and TEN.
- Most patients with *E. multiforme* also have underlying HSV infection.

- Secondary syphilis may produce similar lesions on the palms and soles.
- Reassure patients that the rash of *E. multiforme* is benign and self-limited.

## ADDITIONAL READING

- Farthing P, Bagan JV, Scully C. Mucosal disease series. Number IV. Erythema multiforme. *Oral Dis*. 2005;11:261–267.
- Leaute-Labreze C, Lamireau T, Chawki D, et al. Diagnosis, classification, and management of erythema multiforme and Stevens-Johnson syndrome. *Arch Dis Chil*. 2000;83:347–352.
- Olufunmilayo O. Erythema multiforme. Available at www.emedicine.com, updated February 24, 2009.
- Scully C, Bagan J. Oral mucosal diseases: Erythema multiforme. *Br J Oral Maxillofac Surg*. 2008;46: 90–95.

### See Also (Topic, Algorithm, Electronic Media Element)
- Herpes
- Stevens-Johnson Syndrome
- Toxic Epidermal Necrolysis

 **CODES**

### ICD9
- 695.10 Erythema multiforme, unspecified
- 695.11 Erythema multiforme minor
- 695.12 Erythema multiforme major

E

# ERYTHEMA NODOSUM

*Herbert G. Bivins*
*Theresa Schwab*

## BASICS

### DESCRIPTION
- Erythema nodosum (EN) is characterized by multiple symmetric, nonulcerative tender nodules on the extensor surface of the lower extremities, typically in young adults.
- Peak incidence in 3rd decade, more common in women (4:1)
- Nodules are round with poorly demarcated edges and vary in size from 1–10 cm.
- Skin lesions are initially red, become progressively ecchymotic appearing as they resolve over 3–6 wk.
- Lesions are caused by inflammation of the septa between subcutaneous fat nodules (septal panniculitis).
- Spontaneous regression of lesions within 3–6 wk
- Major disease variants include:
  - EN migrans (usually mild unilateral disease with little or no systemic symptoms)
  - Chronic EN (lesions spread via extension, and associated systemic symptoms tend to be milder)

### ETIOLOGY
- Immune-mediated response; 30–50% of the time etiology is idiopathic.
- Often a marker for underlying disease; specific etiologies include:
  - Drug reactions (oral contraceptives, sulfonamides, penicillins)
  - Infections including streptococcal, mycobacterium tuberculosis (TB), atypical mycobacteria, and coccidioidomycosis, hepatitis, syphilis, chlamydia, *Rickettsia, Salmonella, Campylobacter, Yersinia*, parasites, and leprosy
  - Systemic diseases such as sarcoidosis, inflammatory bowel disease, Behçet, and connective tissue disorders
  - Malignancies such as lymphoma and leukemia
  - Cat-scratch disease
  - HIV infection
  - Rarely can be caused by vaccines for hepatitis and TB (BCG)

### Pediatric Considerations
Typically, EN begins 2–3 wk after onset of streptococcal pharyngitis.

## DIAGNOSIS

### SIGNS AND SYMPTOMS
- Tender erythematous nodules symmetrically distributed on extensor surface of lower legs
- Lesions occasionally occur on fingers, hands, arms, calves, and thighs.
- In bedridden patients, dependent areas may be involved.
- Fever, malaise, leukocytosis, arthralgias, arthritis, and unilateral or bilateral hilar adenopathy with any form of the disease

### History
- General symptoms may precede or accompany the rash:
  - Fever
  - General malaise
  - Polyarthralgias
- GI symptoms with EN may be a marker for:
  - Inflammatory bowel disease
  - Bacterial gastroenteritis
  - Pancreatitis
  - Behçet disease
  - A history of travel is important, as there are regional variations in etiology.

### Physical Exam
- A careful exam is important, as underlying etiology varies by region.
- Lesions are most common on the pretibial area but may occur on the thigh, upper extremities, neck and, rarely, the face.
- Absence of lesions on the lower extremities is atypical, as are ulcerated lesions.
- Lower-extremity edema may occur.
- Adenopathy should be evaluated.

## ESSENTIAL WORKUP
Careful history and physical exam directed at detecting precipitating cause

## DIAGNOSTIC TESTS & INTERPRETATION
### Lab
- CBC
- Throat culture/ASO titer
- ESR
- Appropriate chemistry tests
- Liver function tests
- Serologies for coccidioidomycosis in endemic regions
- TB skin testing in endemic regions

### Imaging
CXR: Hilar adenopathy may be evidence of sarcoidosis, coccidioidomycosis, tuberculosis, or other fungal infections.

### Diagnostic Procedures/Surgery
Definitive diagnosis made by deep elliptical biopsy and histopathologic evaluation (punch biopsy may be inadequate):
- Usually indicated for atypical cases or when TB is being considered

## DIFFERENTIAL DIAGNOSIS
- EN migrans and chronic EN
- Any type of panniculitis can resemble EN.
- Differences can be determined histopathologically.
- Other disorders include:
  - Periarteritis nodosum
  - Migratory thrombophlebitis
  - Superficial varicose thrombophlebitis
  - Scleroderma
  - Systemic lupus erythematosus
  - $\alpha_1$-Antitrypsin deficiency
  - Behçet syndrome
  - Lipodystrophies
  - Leukemic infiltration of fat
  - Panniculitis associated with steroid use, cold, and infection

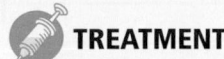 **TREATMENT**

### Pediatric Considerations
- Rare in children, streptococcal pharyngitis is the most likely etiology.
- Cat-scratch disease should be considered.

### PRE-HOSPITAL
Maintain universal precautions

### INITIAL STABILIZATION/THERAPY
Airway, breathing, and circulation (ABCs); IV, oxygen, monitoring as appropriate

### ED TREATMENT/PROCEDURES
- Treatment should be directed at underlying disease.
- Supportive therapies include rest and analgesics.
- Corticosteroids and potassium iodide may hasten resolution of symptoms.
- Systemic corticosteroids are contraindicated in presence of certain underlying infections such as TB or coccidioidomycosis, which may disseminate with their use.
- Potassium iodide is contraindicated in hyperthyroid states.

### MEDICATION
- Aspirin: 650 mg PO q4–6h PRN (peds: Contraindicated)
- Ibuprofen: 400–800 mg PO q8h (peds: 5–10 mg/kg PO q6h)
- Indomethacin: 25–50 mg PO q8h
- Potassium iodide/SSKI (used for resistant disease; contraindicated in hyperthyroidism): 900 mg PO daily for 3–4 wk
- Systemic corticosteroids (prednisone): 40 mg/d PO; duration determined by primary physician

### First Line
- Rest/supportive care
- NSAIDs
- Treatment of underlying disease

### Second Line
- Potassium iodide
- Steroids

 **FOLLOW-UP**

### DISPOSITION
### Admission Criteria
Dictated by the severity of symptoms and the etiologic agent

### Discharge Criteria
- Nontoxic patients, able to take PO fluids without difficulty
- Scheduled follow-up should be arranged.

### Issues for Referral
- EN is usually self-limited and resolves in 3–6 wk.
- Atypical cases may need excisional biopsy.
- Steroid and potassium therapy needs primary physician monitoring.

### FOLLOW-UP RECOMMENDATIONS
- Follow-up to assess for resolution with primary care physician or dermatologist.
- Evaluation of underlying etiology may require specialist referral.

## PEARLS AND PITFALLS
- EN is usually idiopathic but may be the 1st sign of systemic disease.
- Lesions may recur if underlying disease is not treated.
- Atypical and chronic lesions may indicate an alternative diagnosis and need biopsy.
- Patients taking potassium or steroids need close follow-up.

## ADDITIONAL READING
- Barbier SC, Faucher R. Erythema nodosum and adenopathy in a 15-year-old boy: Uncommon signs of cat scratch disease. *Arch Pediatr*. 2005;12: 295–297.
- Gonzalez-Gay MA. Erythema nodosum: A clinical approach. *Clin Exp Rheumatol*. 2001;19:365–368.
- James JD, Berger TG, Elston DM. *Andrew's Clinical Dermatology*, 10th ed. Philadelphia: WB Saunders, 2006.
- Kumbasar H. Erythema nodosum: An evaluation of 100 cases. *Clin Exp Rheumatol*. 2007;25:563–567.
- Schwartz RA. Erythema nodosum: A sign of systemic disease. *Am Fam Physician*. 2007;75:695–700.

 **CODES**

### ICD9
- 017.10 Erythema nodosum with hypersensitivity reaction in tuberculosis, unspecified examination
- 695.2 Erythema nodosum

E

# ESOPHAGEAL TRAUMA
*Susan Dufel*

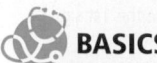 **BASICS**

## DESCRIPTION
- Adult esophagus is ~25–30 cm in length in close proximity to mediastinum with access to pleural space.
- It begins at hypopharynx posterior to larynx at level of cricoid cartilage.
- On either side of this slit are piriform recesses:
  - May be site for foreign body to lodge
- Sites of esophageal narrowing:
  - Cricopharyngeal muscle (upper esophageal sphincter)
  - Crossover of left main stem bronchus and aortic arch
  - Gastroesophageal junction (lower esophageal sphincter)
  - Areas of disease (cancer, webs, or Schatzki ring)
- Upper 3rd of esophagus is striated muscle:
  - Initiates swallowing
- Middle portion is mixture of striated and smooth.
- Distal portion is smooth muscle.
- It is fixed structure, but can become displaced by other organs:
  - Goiter
  - Enlarged atria
  - Mediastinal masses

## ETIOLOGY
### Mechanism
- External forces or agents (30%):
  - Penetrating: Leading to tears:
    ○ Stab wounds
    ○ Missile wounds
  - Perforation:
    ○ Foreign bodies via direct penetration
    ○ Pressure necrosis
    ○ Chemical necrosis
    ○ Radiation necrosis from selective tissue ablation
    ○ Instrumentation
  - Blunt: Motor vehicle accident
  - Caustic ingestions/burns:
    ○ Acid pH <2, alkali pH >12 accidental or intentional
    ○ Alkali: (42%) liquefaction necrosis causing burns, airway edema or compromise, perforation, chronic stricture, and cancer
    ○ Acid: (32%) coagulation necrosis, thermal injury, and dehydration causing perforation, ulceration, and infection, more likely to perforate than alkali
    ○ Chlorine bleach: (26%) mucosal edema, superficial erythema
  - Swallowed foreign bodies: Coins, bones, buttons, marbles, pins, button batteries
  - Food bolus impaction:
    ○ Most common type is meat.
    ○ In adults, often associated with prisoners, psychiatric patients, intoxicated patients, or edentulous patients

- Iatrogenic (55%):
  - Perforation secondary to instrumentation, endoscopy most common cause
  - Nasotracheal intubation/nasogastric tube most common cause in emergency department
- Increased gastric pressure (15%):
  - Large pressure differences between thorax and intra-abdominal cavity:
    ○ May lead to lacerations or perforation
  - Mallory–Weiss syndrome:
    ○ Longitudinal tears in distal esophageal mucosa with bleeding
  - Boerhaave syndrome:
    ○ Spontaneous esophageal rupture
    ○ Full-thickness rupture of distal esophagus
    ○ Classically after alcohol or large meals and vomiting

### Pediatric Considerations
- Foreign bodies
- Accounts for 75–80% of swallowed foreign bodies:
  - Typically in infants ages 18–48 mo
  - Entrapment usually at upper esophageal sphincter
  - Perforations
  - Commonly iatrogenic with NG insertion, stricture dilation and endotracheal intubation

 **DIAGNOSIS**

## SIGNS AND SYMPTOMS
- General:
  - Dysphagia: Difficulty swallowing
  - Odynophagia: Pain with swallowing
  - Chest pain: Anginalike, often pleuritic, severe, and unrelenting
  - Hoarseness
  - Dyspnea
- Tears or perforations:
  - Bleeding
  - Hematemesis
- Ingestions/foreign bodies:
  - Drooling or excessive salivation
  - Choking, gagging, vomiting, stridor, or wheezing
  - Inability of food or liquid to pass
- Caustic ingestions:
  - Oral pain
  - Abdominal pain
  - Vomiting
  - Drooling
- Esophagus injury scale:
  - I: Contusion/hematoma; partial thickness
  - II: Laceration ≤50% circumference
  - III: Laceration >50% circumference
  - IV: Segmental loss or devascularization <2 cm
  - V: Segmental loss or devascularization >2 cm

### History
- History of ingestions (type, time, amount)
- History of protracted vomiting
- History of inability to swallow after eating, foreign body sensation in throat
- History of penetrating trauma
- History of cancer therapy

### Physical Exam
- Tears or perforations:
  - SC air at base of neck
  - Hamman's crunch:
    ○ Systolic crunching sound secondary to air in mediastinum
  - Shock
  - Septicemia
  - Peritonitis
- Penetrating trauma:
  - Associated neck, chest, or abdominal injury with trauma:
    ○ Most commonly trachea
    ○ Associated with penetrating/blunt trauma
- Caustic ingestions:
  - Airway edema leading to stridor
  - Oral burns

## ESSENTIAL WORKUP
High level of suspicion and early diagnosis are key:
- Mortality <5% for perforation if repaired within 24 hr; 75% if delayed
- Early endoscopy for caustic ingestions
- Chest/lateral neck radiograph

## DIAGNOSTIC TESTS & INTERPRETATION
### Lab
- CBC in cases of gastrointestinal bleeding
- Type and cross for any extensive bleeding or if patient is OR candidate
- Coagulation studies
- Electrolytes for protracted vomiting or prolonged foreign body retention
- Arterial blood gas (ABG) for acid ingestions

### Imaging
- CXR for foreign body or perforation:
  - Pneumomediastinum
  - Widened mediastinum
  - Pneumothorax
  - Pleural effusion
- Lateral cervical spine films for foreign body or perforation:
  - Retropharyngeal air or fluid
  - Cervical emphysema
- Fiberoptic nasopharyngoscopy for foreign body removal
- Esophagram for foreign bodies or suspected perforation:
  - 10–25% false-negative rate
  - Current recommendations for water-soluble contrast (Gastrografin) 1st if perforation likely
  - Barium may limit visibility for later endoscopy:
    ○ More irritating if extravasates into mediastinum
  - Water-soluble contrast provides better visibility:
    ○ Less reaction if extravasates into mediastinum
    ○ May cause chemical pneumonitis if aspirated
  - Nonionic contrast may be safest, but is more expensive.
- Endoscopy for suspected perforation, caustic ingestions, and esophageal foreign body removal
- CT scanning with dilute oral contrast may be useful in diagnosis of perforations.

## DIFFERENTIAL DIAGNOSIS

- Pulmonary:
  - Tracheal injury
  - Pneumothorax
- Cardiovascular:
  - Myocardial infarction
  - Aortic dissection
  - Spontaneous pneumomediastinum
- Other esophageal emergencies:
  - Peptic stricture
  - Esophageal neoplasm
  - Schatzki ring
  - Diverticula
  - Achalasia
  - Diffuse esophageal spasm
  - Nutcracker esophagus
  - Gastroesophageal reflux
  - Esophagitis

 **TREATMENT**

### PRE-HOSPITAL

#### ALERT
- Chest pain should be presumed cardiac until proven otherwise.
- Airway protection, frequent suctioning
- Intravenous crystalloid if patient is hypotensive, vomiting, or if hematemesis is present
- Avoid neutralizing agents in caustic ingestions as that may worsen injury.
- Avoid copious amounts of oral fluids in caustic ingestions to prevent emesis.

### INITIAL STABILIZATION/THERAPY
- Manage airway and resuscitate as needed Intravenous access, monitoring
- Early intubation for penetrating neck and chest wounds
- Frequent suctioning of copious secretions
- Fluid replacement

### ED TREATMENT/PROCEDURES
- Foreign bodies/food impaction:
  - 80% pass, 20% need endoscopy, <1% need surgery
  - Glucagon may be tried: 1 mg IV and repeated in 20 min.
  - Nitroglycerin or nifedipine may be tried.
  - Carbonated beverages in combination with glucagon may be helpful.
  - Diazepam may be of benefit for foreign bodies in the upper (striated muscle) esophagus.
  - Gastrointestinal consultation and endoscopic extraction if not relieved

- Caustic ingestions:
  - Emesis/lavage contraindicated
  - Immediate decontamination with milk
  - Avoid neutralizing agents as they may cause exothermic reaction.
  - Gastrointestinal consultation for early endoscopy to provide prognostic information
- Tears/perforations:
  - Partial-thickness tears usually heal spontaneously.
  - Gastrointestinal consultation may be needed for diagnosis (endoscopy).
  - Perforation requires surgical consultation for thoracotomy and primary repair, some patients may be managed non-operatively.
  - Broad-spectrum parenteral antibiotics for perforation

### Pediatric Considerations
- Certain swallowed foreign bodies require gastrointestinal consultation and endoscopic removal:
  - Sharp objects: Fish bones, straight pins, razor blades, pencil
  - Caustic objects: Button batteries
- Other objects may pass on their own if below the lower esophageal sphincter and require follow-up only:
  - Coins, buttons, marbles
  - Open safety pins may pass spontaneously if blunt end forward.
- Consult pediatric gastrointestinal specialist.

### MEDICATION
- Foreign bodies/food impactions:
  - Glucagon: 1–2 mg (peds: 0.02–0.03 mg/kg) IV; may repeat once in 20 min
  - Nitroglycerin: 0.4 mg sublingually Diazepam: 3–10 mg (peds: 1–2 mg) IV
- Ingestions:
  - Antibiotics if perforated
- Perforation:
  - Cefoxitin: 1–2 g (peds: 100–160 mg/kg/24 hr) IV q6–8h
  - Gentamicin: 1.0–1.7 mg/kg (peds: 1.5–2.5 mg/kg/24 hr) IV q8h
  - Steroids not indicated in caustic ingestions

 **FOLLOW-UP**

### DISPOSITION
#### Admission Criteria
- Caustic ingestion
- Sharp foreign bodies
- Airway compromise
- Penetrating neck or chest trauma
- Evidence of sepsis, mediastinitis, or esophageal perforation
- Significant bleeding
- Inability to tolerate oral fluids

### Discharge Criteria
- Self-limited bleeding from partial-thickness tear
- Foreign body or food impaction that has passed lower esophageal sphincter

## PEARLS AND PITFALLS

Factors to predict outcomes in esophageal injuries:
- Time to diagnosis and definitive therapy: 24 hr decreases mortality by half.
- Location of injury: Cervical less than thoracic or abdominal
- Mechanism of injury: Spontaneous perforation has highest mortality 30–40%; iatrogenic 15–20% and direct trauma 5–10%.

## ADDITIONAL READING

- Poley JW, Steyerberg EW, et al. Ingestion of acid and alkaline agents: Outcome and prognostic value of early upper endoscopy. *Gastrointest Endosc.* 2004;60(3):372–377.
- Ghulam A, Schuchert M, et al. Contemporaneous management of esophageal perforation. *Surgery.* 2009;146(4):749–755.
- Gander JW, Berdon WE, et al. Iatrogenic esophageal perforation in children. *Pediatr Surg Int.* 2009;25(5):395–401.
- Plott E, Jones D. A state-of-the-art review of esophageal trauma: Where do we stand? *Dis Esoph.* 2007;20:279–289.

### See Also (Topic, Algorithm, Electronic Media Element)
- Boerhaave Syndrome
- Foreign Body, Caustic Ingestion, Esophageal
- Mallory-Weiss Syndrome

 **CODES**

### ICD9
- 862.22 Injury to esophagus without mention of open wound into cavity
- 862.32 Injury to esophagus with open wound into cavity
- 947.2 Burn of esophagus

# ETHYLENE GLYCOL POISONING

*Kirk L. Cumpston*

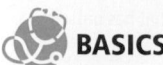 **BASICS**

## DESCRIPTION
- Peak levels in 1–4 hr
- Half-life, 2.5–4.5 hr
- <20% excreted unmetabolized by kidneys
- 3 stages (may overlap):
  - 1st stage: 1–12 hr after ingestion:
    - CNS depression
    - GI symptoms
    - Worsening acidosis
    - Coma
    - Convulsions
    - Cerebral edema
    - Tetany and myoclonus secondary to hypocalcemia
  - 2nd stage: 12–36 hr after ingestion:
    - Cardiopulmonary symptoms
    - When most deaths occur
  - 3rd stage: 36–72 hr after ingestion:
    - Oliguria
    - Flank pain
    - Acute renal failure
    - Bone marrow suppression and pancytopenia
- Pathophysiology:
  - Metabolized by hepatic alcohol dehydrogenase and aldehyde dehydrogenase ultimately to oxalic acid
  - Results in aldehyde and acid metabolites
  - Directly toxic to CNS, heart, lungs, and kidneys

## ETIOLOGY
- Ethylene glycol-containing products:
  - Antifreeze
  - Solvents
- Minimum reported lethal dose is 30 mL of 100% ethylene glycol.

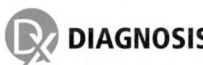 **DIAGNOSIS**

## SIGNS AND SYMPTOMS
- Cardiovascular:
  - Tachycardia/bradycardia/other dysrhythmias
  - Hypertension/hypotension
- CNS:
  - Inebriation/irritability
  - Ataxia
  - Obtundation
  - Coma
  - Cerebral edema
  - Convulsions
  - Peripheral nervous system
  - Cranial nerve abnormalities
- GI:
  - Nausea/vomiting
  - Abdominal pain
- Pulmonary:
  - Hyperventilation/tachypnea/Kussmaul respiration
  - Pulmonary edema
- Renal:
  - Acute renal failure
  - Costal-vertebral angle tenderness
  - Crystalluria

### History
- Intentional or unintentional ethylene glycol ingestion
- No history but a patient with an unexplained high anion gap metabolic acidosis
- Elevated unexplained osmol gap

### Physical Exam
- Tachypnea
- Altered mental status

## ESSENTIAL WORKUP
- History of all substances ingested
- Drawn simultaneously:
  - Arterial blood gas
  - Serum ethylene glycol, methanol, isopropyl alcohol, and ethanol levels
  - Electrolytes, BUN/creatinine, glucose
  - Measured serum osmolality (by freezing point depression)
  - Serum calcium, phosphorus, magnesium

## DIAGNOSTIC TESTS & INTERPRETATION
### Lab
- Determine the anion gap:
  - Anion gap $= (Na^+) - (Cl^- + HCO_3^-)$
  - Normal anion gap is 8–12.
- Determine osmol gap:
  - Osmol gap = measured osmolality – calculated osmolarity
  - Increased osmol gap: >10
  - Calculated osmolarity $= 2(Na^+) +$ glucose/18 + blood urea nitrogen/2.8 + ethanol (in mg/dL)/4.6
  - Calculated to screen for ethylene glycol ingestion because toxic alcohol levels are not commonly available in timely manner from most clinical laboratories
  - Most useful early in course of ethylene glycol poisoning or with concurrent ethanol ingestion
  - With concurrent ethanol ingestion, osmol gap tends to be larger and acidosis tends to be less severe because relatively less ethylene glycol has been converted to acid-producing metabolites.
  - Normal osmol gap does not rule out ethylene glycol ingestion.
  - Late presentation after ethylene glycol ingestion may manifest itself with only an elevated anion gap without a significant osmol gap.
- Ethylene glycol, methanol, isopropyl alcohol levels
- Ethanol level:
  - Measured to determine amount of ethanol bolus necessary to attain therapeutic level, and to determine coingestants
- Urinalysis:
  - Envelope-shaped oxalate crystals: Insensitive but specific finding.
  - Absence of urine calcium oxalate crystals does not rule out ethylene glycol exposure.
  - Ketones may be due to isopropyl alcohol ingestion, starvation, or diabetic ketoacidosis.

### Diagnostic Procedures/Surgery
Wood lamp inspection of urine or gastric contents:
- Detects presence of fluorescein, a common antifreeze additive
- Insensitive and not specific marker of antifreeze ingestion
- Absence of urinary fluorescence does not rule out ethylene glycol exposure.

## DIFFERENTIAL DIAGNOSIS
- Increased osmol gap:
  - **M**ethanol
  - **E**thanol
  - **D**iuretics (mannitol, glycerin, propylene glycol, sorbitol)
  - **I**sopropyl alcohol
  - **E**thylene glycol
  - **A**cetone, ammonia
  - **P**ropylene glycol
- Elevated anion gap metabolic acidosis: *A CAT MUDPILES*:
  - **A**lcoholic ketoacidosis
  - **C**yanide, CO, $H_2S$, others
  - **A**cetaminophen:
    - Rare in acute ingestion
    - Rare in chronic ingestion
    - Fulminant hepatic failure
  - **A**ntiretrovirals (NRTI)
  - **T**oluene
  - **M**ethanol, metformin
  - **U**remia
  - **D**iabetic ketoacidosis
  - **P**araldehyde, phenformin, propylene glycol
  - **I**ron, INH
  - **L**actic acidosis
  - **E**thylene glycol
  - **S**alicylate, acetylsalicylic acid (ASA; aspirin), starvation ketosis

 **TREATMENT**

## PRE-HOSPITAL
- Bring containers of all possible ingestants.
- Monitor airway and CNS depression.
- Dermal decontamination of an ethylene glycol chemical spill by removal of clothing and jewelry and irrigation with soap and water

## INITIAL STABILIZATION/THERAPY
- ABCs
- Supplemental oxygen, cardiac monitor, secured IV line with 0.9% NS
- $D_{50}W$ (or Accu-Chek), naloxone, and thiamine for altered mental status

## ED TREATMENT/PROCEDURES

- Prevent further ethylene glycol absorption:
  - Gastric lavage with nasogastric tube:
    - If <1 hr since ingestion, if patient is in coma, or if history of large ingestion
  - Ipecac contraindicated
  - Initial dose of activated charcoal for potential coingestants, but unlikely to help if only ethylene glycol:
    - Activated charcoal adsorbs ethylene glycol poorly.
- Prevent ethylene glycol conversion to toxic metabolites with fomepizole:
  - Fomepizole (4-MP, Antizol):
    - Initiate before ethylene glycol level returns, if accidental ingestion greater than a sip or intentional ingestion or altered mental status associated with unexplained osmol gap or elevated anion gap acidosis.
    - Competitive inhibitor of alcohol dehydrogenase
  - Disadvantage over ethanol:
    - Blurry vision
    - Transient elevation of LFTs
  - Advantages over ethanol:
    - Easy dosing
    - No need for continuous infusion
    - No inebriation/CNS depression
    - No hypoglycemia, hyponatremia, or hyperosmolality
    - Not necessary to check ethanol levels
    - Reduction in degree of nursing care and monitoring
- Ethanol therapy:
  - 2nd choice antidote if fomepizole is not available
  - Not FDA approved for treatment of ethylene glycol
  - Initiate before ethylene glycol level returns, if potentially toxic ingestion is suspected.
  - Ethanol: Greater affinity than ethylene glycol for alcohol dehydrogenase:
    - Slows conversion to toxic metabolites
  - Indications:
    - History of accidental ethylene glycol ingestion of greater than a sip or intentional ethylene glycol ingestion
    - Altered mental status associated with unexplained osmol gap or elevated anion gap metabolic acidosis
  - Goal: Serum ethanol level of 100–150 mg/dL
  - Continue ethanol therapy until ethylene glycol level is 0.
- Administer thiamine, pyridoxine, and magnesium:
  - Cofactors in metabolism of ethylene glycol that may promote conversion to nontoxic metabolites.
  - No human data supporting this theory
- Enhance elimination:
  - Hemodialysis:
    - Decreases elimination half-life of ethylene glycol and removes toxic metabolites
    - Indications: Severe acidosis or osmol gap; no ethylene glycol levels with metabolic acidosis, and clinical suspicion of significant ingestion; persistent electrolyte or metabolic acidosis; renal insufficiency; pulmonary edema; cerebral edema; serum ethylene glycol level >25–50 mg/dL
    - Continue hemodialysis until ethylene glycol level approaches 0.

- Correct secondary disorders:
  - Ensure adequate urine output via IV fluids.
  - Sodium bicarbonate therapy for acidemia with pH <7.1:
    - The goal is to maintain a serum pH in the normal range.
- Monitor/replace calcium:
  - Deposition of calcium into tissues can result in hypocalcemia.

### Pregnancy Considerations
- Fomepizole is class C in pregnancy.
- Ethanol is not recommended in pregnancy. Class D/X

### Pediatric Considerations
Ethanol can cause serious CNS depression and hypoglycemia when administered to children.

## MEDICATION

- Activated charcoal: 1 g/kg PO
- Dextrose: $D_{50}W$ 1 ampul: 50 mL or 25 g (peds: $D_{25}W$ 2–4 mL/kg) IV
- Ethanol:
  - PO: 50% ethanol solution (100-proof liquor) via nasogastric tube:
    - Loading dose: 1.5 mL/kg
    - Maintenance dose: 0.2–0.4 mL/kg/hr
    - Maintenance dose during hemodialysis: 0.4–0.7 mL/kg/hr
  - IV: 10% ethanol in $D_5W$:
    - Loading dose: 7.5 mL/kg over 30–60 min
    - Maintenance Infusion: 1–2 mL/kg/hr
    - Maintenance infusion during hemodialysis: 2–3.5 mL/kg/hr
- Fomepizole:
  - Loading dose: 15 mg/kg slow infusion over 30 min
  - Maintenance dose: 10 mg/kg q12h for 4 doses, then 15 mg/kg q12h until ethylene glycol levels are reduced to <20 mg/dL
  - Dosing related to hemodialysis:
    - Do not administer dose at beginning of dialysis if last dose was <6 hr previously.
    - Administer next dose if last dose was >6 hr previously.
    - Dose q4h during dialysis.
    - If time between last dose and end of dialysis was <1 hr from last dose, do not administer new dose.
    - If time between last dose and end of dialysis was 1–3 hr from last dose, administer 1/2 of next scheduled dose.
    - If time between last dose and end of dialysis was >3 hr from last dose, administer next scheduled dose.
- Magnesium: 25–50 mg/kg IV 1 dose up to 2 g
- Naloxone: 2 mg (peds: 0.1 mg/kg) IV or IM initial dose
- Pyridoxine: 100 mg/d for 2 days
- Sodium bicarbonate: 1–2 mEq/kg in $D_5W$ IV
- Thiamine: 100 mg (peds: 50 mg) IV or IM per day for 2 days

## FOLLOW-UP

### DISPOSITION
**Admission Criteria**
- All patients with significant ethylene glycol ingestion, even if initially asymptomatic
- ICU admission for seriously ill patients
- Transfer to another facility if hemodialysis or fomepizole is indicated but not readily available.

**Discharge Criteria**
Asymptomatic patient with isolated ethylene glycol ingestion, if serum ethylene glycol level is undetectable and no metabolic acidosis

### FOLLOW-UP RECOMMENDATIONS
Psychiatric referral for suicidal patients.

## PEARLS AND PITFALLS

- An osmol gap <10 mmol/L does not rule out an ethylene glycol exposure.
- Administer fomepizole immediately and confirm exposure with a serum concentration for patients with an elevated anion gap and ethylene glycol exposure in the differential diagnosis.
- If you cannot confirm an ethylene glycol exposure, or do not have hemodialysis capabilities 24/7, or no antidote, transfer the patient to a facility which has all of the above capabilities.
- Not all patients will have an elevated osmol and anion gap. Early presenters will have an osmol gap only, and late presenters may have an anion gap only.
- Do not use the absence of urine crystals or fluorescence of the urine to rule out an ethylene glycol exposure.

## ADDITIONAL READING

- Brent J, McMartin K, Phillips S, et al. Fomepizole for the treatment of ethylene glycol poisoning. *N Engl J Med.* 1999;340:832–838.
- Leikin J, Paloucek F. Ethylene glycol. Fomepizole. Alcohol. In: Leikin JB, Paloucek F, eds. *Leikin and Paloucek's Poisoning and Toxicology Handbook.* 4th ed. Boca Raton, FL: Lexi-Comp; 2008;989: 294–295, 794–795.
- Mycyk MB, Aks SE. A visual schematic for clarifying the temporal relationship between anion and osmol gaps in toxic alcohol poisoning. *Am J Emerg Med.* 2003;21(4):333–335.

## CODES

### ICD9
982.8 Toxic effect of other nonpetroleum-based solvents

# EXTERNAL EAR CHONDRITIS/ABSCESS

*Assaad J. Sayah*

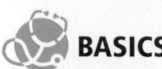 **BASICS**

## DESCRIPTION

Inflammation and infection of the pinna

## ETIOLOGY

- Mechanism:
  - Cartilage of the external ear is easily damaged due to:
    ○ Lack of overlying subcutaneous tissue
    ○ Relative avascularity
    ○ Exposed position
  - Chondritis:
    ○ Most commonly a secondary complication of otic trauma and burns
    ○ Onset is often insidious and may be delayed until apparent healing has occurred.
- Disfiguration of the pinna occurs without proper treatment:
  - Ranges from being a shriveled, cauliflower-like ear to complete loss of the external ear and possible stenosis of the auditory meatus.
- Causes:
  - Common causes of chondritis include:
    ○ Chemical or thermal burns
    ○ Frostbite
    ○ Hematoma formation
    ○ Mastoid surgery
    ○ Human bites
    ○ Deep abrasions
    ○ External otitis
    ○ High piercing of the ear lobe especially with poor technique, hygiene, and after-care.
  - Bacteria involved:
    ○ Pseudomonas aeruginosa
    ○ Staphylococcus
    ○ Proteus

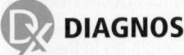 **DIAGNOSIS**

## SIGNS AND SYMPTOMS

- Initially a dull pain that increases in severity
- Fever
- Chills

### History

- Ear trauma
- Ear piercing

### Physical Exam

- Pinna:
  - Painful
  - Exquisite tenderness
  - Erythematous
  - Warmth
  - Loss of contours caused by edema often with sparing of the lobule.
- Increase of the auriculocephalic angle
- Fluctuant areas develop with eventual breakdown and suppuration.

## ESSENTIAL WORKUP

Clinical diagnosis:

- Typical physical findings in combination with aforementioned causes

## DIAGNOSTIC TESTS & INTERPRETATION
### Lab

Only if systemic signs of infection:

- CBC
- Blood cultures
- Local cultures for chondritis and abscess drainage

## DIFFERENTIAL DIAGNOSIS

- Allergic reaction
- Mastoiditis
- Dermatitis
- Hematoma

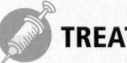 **TREATMENT**

## ED TREATMENT/PROCEDURES

General postinjury preventive measures:

- Prevention of chondritis is of the utmost importance:
  - Difficult management and disfiguring potential
- Avoid pressure to the injured ear.
- Minimize active débridement of eschars and crusts.
- Gentle washing twice daily with antibacterial soap and water followed by complete drying and application of topical antibiotics
- Keep hair away from the ear.
- Oral antibiotics for minor cases of early ear-lobe inflammation
- Parenteral antibiotics and early surgical drainage for patients with chondritis

## MEDICATION

- Ciprofloxacin: 500 mg PO b.i.d. (adult)
- Cephalexin: 500 mg (peds: 50 mg/kg/d) PO q.i.d.
- Dicloxacillin: 500 mg (peds: 25 mg/kg/d) PO q.i.d.
- IV antibiotics for severe infection
- Apply topical antibiotics when there's a break in skin barrier.

 **FOLLOW-UP**

## DISPOSITION

### Admission Criteria

- Edema, erythema, and significant ear tenderness
- Toxic patient with fever and chills
- Immunocompromised patient

### Discharge Criteria

Stable patient without systemic signs with close ear-nose-throat (ENT) follow-up

### Issues for Referral

ENT consult:

- For chondritis, abscess, and necrosis of the involved cartilage
- Early surgical drainage for chondritis and abscess

## PEARLS AND PITFALLS

Aggressive early management may prevent gross ear deformity:

- Antibiotic regimen should cover for pseudomonas.

## ADDITIONAL READING

- Fisher CG, Kacica MA, Bennett NM. Risk factors for cartilage infections of the ear. *Am J Prev Med*. 2005;29(3):204–209.
- Rowshan HH, Keith K, et al. Pseudomonas aeruginosa infection of the auricular cartilage caused by "high ear piercing" a case report and review of the literature. *J Oral Maxillofac Surg*. 2008;66(3):543–546.
- Van Wijk MP, Kummer JA, Kon M. Ear piercing techniques and their effect on cartilage, a histologic study. *J Plast Reconst Aesthet Surg* 2008;61 (Supp)1:104–109.

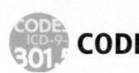 **CODES**

**ICD9**
380.03 Chondritis of pinna

# EXTREMITY TRAUMA, PENETRATING

*Gary M. Vilke*

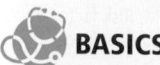 **BASICS**

## DESCRIPTION
Penetrating injury to extremity

## ETIOLOGY
- Stab or puncture
- Gunshot
- Laceration
- Bite
- High-pressure injection injury

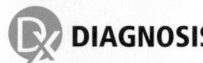 **DIAGNOSIS**

## SIGNS AND SYMPTOMS
- Entry and exit wound (if present), lacerations
- High-muzzle-velocity gunshot wounds:
  - Produce shock wave that results in significant tissue injury
  - Often exit wound demonstrates more tissue damage than entrance wound.
- Vascular injury:
  - Arterial injury:
    ○ Decreased or absent distal pulse
    ○ Distal ischemic changes
    ○ Expanding hematoma
    ○ Bruit or thrill over injury
  - Presence of distal pulse does not exclude proximal vascular injury.
- Neurologic injury:
  - Paresthesias
  - Decreased or absent motor function
  - Diminished sensation distal to injury
- Musculoskeletal injury:
  - Visible deformity
  - Ligamentous laxity in joints adjacent to injury suggests tendon injury.
  - Effusion in adjacent joint indicates fracture or ligamentous injury.
- Compartment syndrome:
  - Suggested by severe and constant pain over involved compartment
  - Pain on active and passive extension or flexion of distal extremity
  - Weakness, pain on palpation of compartment
  - Hypesthesia of nerves in compartment
  - Pulselessness and pallor are late findings.

## History
- Mechanism of injury
- Age of wound
- Circumstances of wounding:
  - Assault
  - Self-inflicted wound
  - Domestic violence
- Comorbid conditions:
  - Immunosuppression or diabetes
  - Valvular heart disease
  - Asplenia
  - Peripheral vascular disease

## Physical Exam
- Note location, length, depth, and shape of primary wound and exit wound, if present.
- Vascular injury:
  - Compare distal pulses by palpation and with Doppler study.
  - Assess capillary refill:
    ○ Abnormal if >2 sec
  - Ankle–brachial index (ABI):
    ○ Take BP in calf and arm (involved extremity).
    ○ Systolic pressure difference of >10 mm Hg suggests vascular injury.
  - Expanding hematoma, bruit, or thrill over injury also indicates vascular injury.
- Neurologic injury:
  - Assess distal motor function and sensory function:
    ○ 2-point discrimination
    ○ Light touch
    ○ Proprioception
- Musculoskeletal injury:
  - Note associated crush, tendon, or ligamentous injury and bony deformity.
  - Examine adjacent joints for range of motion.
  - Assess for compartment syndrome.
- Explore wound for foreign body.

## ESSENTIAL WORKUP
- Physical examination
- Imaging if findings suggestive of bony injury or possible foreign body

## DIAGNOSTIC TESTS & INTERPRETATION
### Lab
- Culture of acute wounds is not indicated.
- Wounds with signs of infection may be cultured to guide antibiotic choice.

### Imaging
- Radiograph to evaluate for radiopaque foreign body or underlying fracture:
  - Minimum AP and lateral views
- Radiolucent foreign bodies may be located by US, fluoroscopy, or CT.

### Diagnostic Procedures/Surgery
Arteriogram is indicated when vascular injury is suspected and immediate vascular surgery not required.

## DIFFERENTIAL DIAGNOSIS
Any medical condition that presents with findings consistent with extremity trauma or a wound

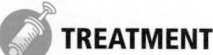 **TREATMENT**

## PRE-HOSPITAL
Cautions:
- Control hemorrhage with direct pressure over site.
- Elevate extremity.
- Evaluate neurovascular status.
- Leave impaled objects in place and stabilize in current position.
- Pain control

## INITIAL STABILIZATION/THERAPY
- Manage airway and resuscitate as indicated.
- Expose wound completely and remove constricting clothing or jewelry.
- Control hemorrhage with direct pressure.
- Blind clamping within wound and prolonged tourniquet use are not recommended.

## ED TREATMENT/PROCEDURES

- Pain control
- Complete neurologic assessment before local anesthesia
- Prolonged soaking of wounds, particularly with cytotoxic agents, is *not* recommended.
- Remove any visible debris and débride devitalized tissue.
- Most important is copious high-pressure irrigation with saline.
- Tetanus prophylaxis
- Stab wounds and gunshot wounds should receive single dose of cefazolin in ED.
- Immobilize extremity if there is suspicion of significant vascular injury, tendon injury, fracture, or joint violation.
- Loss of pulse or distal ischemia requires emergent surgery:
  - Do not delay surgical management for arteriogram.
- Lacerations may be closed if they have been adequately cleaned, have minimal tissue loss, and are seen within 6–8 hr of injury:
  - Delayed primary closure is alternative for older or contaminated wounds.
- Puncture or gunshot wounds should *not* be closed primarily.
- Special considerations:
  - Plantar puncture wounds:
    ○ Examine wound carefully under bright light.
    ○ Remove any foreign material.
    ○ Clean wound carefully.
  - Coring wound is controversial and should be reserved for removal of devitalized tissue or imbedded debris:
    ○ Probing or high-pressure irrigation of puncture wound will only force particulate matter further into wound.
    ○ Prophylactic antibiotics are not recommended (unless patient is diabetic or immunocompromised).
  - If not treated with aggressive debridement, can lead to osteomyelitis
  - High-pressure injuries of hand:
    ○ Orthopedic evaluation in ED is essential because wounds that appear trivial on surface may have product track up tendon sheaths into more proximal aspects of hand.
    ○ Some paints and other products are radiopaque, and plain radiographs may demonstrate extent of spread.

- Soft tissue foreign bodies (FB):
  ○ Small inert FB in wound, including bullets, not easily retrievable and not in close proximity to joint, tendon, vessel, or nerve can be left in place with close follow-up.
  ○ FB in hands and feet should be referred to specialist as they often migrate and become or remain symptomatic.
  ○ Organic materials (thorns, wood, spines, clothing) should be removed as they are very reactive.

## MEDICATION

- Tetanus prophylaxis: Td 0.5 mL IM
- Wounds >12 hr old, especially of hands and lower extremities, crush wounds with devitalized tissue, contaminated wounds:

### First Line

- Cefazolin: 1 g IV/IM (peds: 20–40 mg/kg IV/IM single dose in ED)
- Cephalexin: 500 mg PO (peds: 25–50 mg/kg/day) q.i.d. for 7 days *or*
  - Amoxicillin/clavulanate: 875/125 mg PO (peds: 25 mg/kg/day) b.i.d. for 7 days
- Erythromycin: 333 mg PO t.i.d. (peds: 40 mg/kg/day q6h for 7 days)
- Contaminated wounds in patients with pre-existing valvular heart disease:
  - Cefazolin: 1 g IV/IM, then cephalexin, 500 mg PO q.i.d. for 7 days

### Second Line

If penicillin-allergic:

- EES: 800 mg PO, then 400 mg PO q6h for 7 days *or*
- Clindamycin: 300 mg PO q6h for 7 days

 **FOLLOW-UP**

## DISPOSITION

### Admission Criteria

- Emergent surgical consultation and admission are required for any penetrating wounds with potential for vascular compromise, associated compartment syndrome, and joint penetration.
- High-muzzle-velocity penetrating gunshot wounds
- Diabetic or immunocompromised patients with contaminated wounds

### Discharge Criteria

Penetrating extremity injuries not requiring surgical intervention may be discharged after appropriate wound care with instructions to elevate extremity, keep wound clean, and to return for recheck in 24–48 hr or for any signs of infection.

### Issues for Referral

- Plantar puncture wounds: Close follow-up is necessary to assess for infection from unseen foreign body.
- Delayed primary closure is alternative for older or contaminated wounds.
- Wounds at high risk for infection should have close 1–2-day follow-up.

## FOLLOW-UP RECOMMENDATIONS

Return to the ED for increasing pain, numbness, tingling, redness, swelling drainage, fevers or other changes in clinical presentation.

## PEARLS AND PITFALLS

- Presence of distal pulse does not exclude proximal vascular injury.
- High-pressure injuries of hand may have wounds that appear trivial on surface but track up tendon sheaths into more proximal aspects of hand.

## ADDITIONAL READING

- American College of Emergency Physicians. Clinical policy for the initial approach to patients presenting with penetrating extremity trauma. *Ann Emerg Med.* 1999;33:612–636.
- Bekler H, Gokce A, Beyzadeoglu T, et al. The surgical treatment and outcomes of high-pressure injection injuries of the hand. *J Hand Surg Eur.* 2007;32(4):394–399.
- Chachad S, Kamat D. Management of plantar puncture wounds in children. *Clin Pediatr (Phila).* 2004;43(3):213–216.
- Manthey DE, Nicks. Penetrating trauma to the extremity. *J Emerg Med.* 2008;34(2):187–193.
- Newton EJ, Love J. Acute complications of extremity trauma. *Emerg Med Clin North Am.* 2007;25(3):751–761.
- Schnall SB, Mirzayan R. High pressure injuries to the hand. *Hand Clin.* 1999;15(2):245–248.

### See Also (Topic, Algorithm, Electronic Media Element)

- Bite, Animal
- Compartment Syndrome
- Ring/Constricting Band Removal

 **CODES**

ICD9

- 882.0 Open wound of hand except fingers alone, without mention of complication
- 884.0 Multiple and unspecified open wound of upper limb, without mention of complication
- 894.0 Multiple and unspecified open wound of lower limb, without mention of complication

E

# FACIAL FRACTURES

*David W. Munter*

## 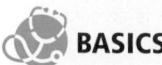 BASICS

### DESCRIPTION
- Typically due to blunt trauma from motor vehicle accidents, direct blows, or falls
- Consider physical assault and domestic violence, especially in women and children.
- Open fractures common
- Many facial fractures are complex and not easily classified.

### ETIOLOGY
- Le Fort fractures involve the maxilla and are classified as:
  - Le Fort I: Transverse fracture of maxilla below nose but above teeth through lateral wall of maxillary sinus to lateral pterygoid plate
  - Le Fort II: Pyramidal fracture from nasal and ethmoid bones through zygomaticomaxillary suture and maxilla, often involving maxillary sinuses and infraorbital rims
  - Le Fort III: Craniofacial disjunction with elongated, flattened face owing to fractures through frontozygomatic suture, orbit, base of nose, and ethmoid bone
  - Le Fort IV: Includes frontal bone in addition to Le Fort III
  - A patient may have different level Le Fort fractures on each side of the face.
- Zygomatic arch fractures often occur in two or three places and can involve the orbit and maxilla (tripod fracture).
- Inner plate frontal sinus fractures are associated with CSF leaks and ocular injuries.
- Orbital fractures most commonly involve the orbital floor (blowout fracture), and are commonly associated with ocular injuries.

### Pediatric Considerations
- Maxillofacial fractures rarely seen in children younger than 6 years; suspect nonaccidental trauma.
- Falls and motor vehicle accidents account for most cases.
- High incidence of associated head injury
- Fractures of the orbital roof are the most common facial fracture in children (excluding the nose).

## 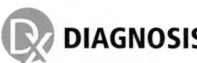 DIAGNOSIS

### SIGNS AND SYMPTOMS
- Most posttraumatic deformities of the face represent underlying fractures.
- Pain, swelling, ecchymosis, and deformity
- CSF rhinorrhea, facial hemorrhage, epistaxis, raccoon eyes
- Facial anesthesia with nerve entrapment or injury
- Associated injuries: Tooth, mandible, eye, tear duct, skull, and neck
- Bluish fluid-filled sac overlying nasal septum is a septal hematoma and is critical to detect.

### History
- Mechanism of injury
- Associated injuries

### Physical Exam
- Immediately assess airway.
- Most important:
  - Palpate entire face for tenderness, step-offs, depressions, and crepitus.
  - Check for mandibular injuries or malocclusion.
  - Nasal speculum exam for septal hematoma or CSF leak
  - Assess for areas of facial anesthesia.
  - Careful eye exam including funduscopic exam; obtain a visual acuity; assess for telecanthus (intercanthal width >30–35 mm), upward dysconjugate gaze (indicative of ocular muscle entrapment in an orbital floor blowout fracture).
- Le Fort fractures are assessed by placing thumb and index finger of one hand on the bridge of the nose and pulling upper teeth with other hand:
  - Le Fort I: Movement of hard palate and maxillary dentition only (your hand on the nose will not feel movement)
  - Le Fort II: Movement of hard palate, maxillary dentition, and nose (your hand on the nose will feel movement)
  - Le Fort III: Movement of entire midface

### Pediatric Considerations
Sedation with diazepam or midazolam may be needed to perform an adequate exam.

### ESSENTIAL WORKUP
- After airway is secured, other injuries take precedence.
- Radiologic studies are required in all cases of suspected facial fractures.

### DIAGNOSTIC TESTS & INTERPRETATION
#### Lab
Indicated for evaluation of associated injuries or if needed for pre-operative reasons

#### Imaging
- CT scanning with reconstructions is the imaging modality of choice for complex facial injuries.
- Obtain radiographs of any area of tenderness, crepitus, depression, or deformity, with the exception of isolated nasal injuries.
- A Waters view is a good screening exam; Caldwell and lateral facial films are less helpful:
  - May show fractures, asymmetry, or blood in the sinuses, or the classic teardrop opacity in the maxillary sinus representing an orbital floor blowout fracture
- Jug-handle views (submental vertex) may be needed to view zygomatic arch fractures.

### DIFFERENTIAL DIAGNOSIS
- Nasal fracture
- Zygoma fractures (arch or tripod fracture)
- Le Fort fracture
- Skull fractures including frontal sinus fractures and cribriform plate fractures
- Nasofrontoethmoid complex fractures
- Mandibular fractures
- Associated injuries to teeth, neck, brain
- Contusions or lacerations without underlying fractures

##  TREATMENT

### PRE-HOSPITAL

#### ALERT
- Airway control takes precedence:
  - Attempt chin lift, jaw thrust, and suctioning first.
  - Underlying injuries may make these attempts as well as use of bag-valve-mask (BVM) device unsuccessful.
  - Severe facial fractures may preclude oral intubation.
  - Nasotracheal intubation contraindicated in massive facial or nasal trauma.
  - Cricothyroidotomy performed if intubation using rapid sequence induction (RSI) cannot be performed.
- If associated injuries are present, protect cervical spine.

### INITIAL STABILIZATION/THERAPY
- Aggressively manage airway if not patent, patient requires airway protection, or ongoing swelling or bleeding threatens airway: RSI is initial airway management of choice in facial injuries; use etomidate or midazolam and vecuronium, rocuronium, or succinylcholine for rapid sequence induction.
- Surgical airway (cricothyroidotomy or needle cricothyroidotomy) may be required if RSI is unsuccessful.
- Nasotracheal intubation is contraindicated in most facial fractures.
- Protect cervical spine until clinically or radiographically cleared.
- Once airway is secure, other major injuries take precedence over facial injuries.
- Bleeding may be difficult to control and may require posterior packing if direct pressure does not work.

## ED TREATMENT/PROCEDURES

- Consult ENT specialist, plastic surgery, or oral surgery for complex fractures, including all Le Fort fractures and frontal sinus fractures involving the posterior table.
- Antibiotics (cefazolin or clindamycin in penicillin-allergic patients) for open fractures and CSF leak
- Tetanus prophylaxis
- Parenteral pain medication (morphine or fentanyl)
- A septal hematoma must be drained in the ED:
  – Anesthetize, aspirate with an 18- to 20-gauge needle, and pack both nares with Vaseline gauze.
  – Discharge on amoxicillin or erythromycin with recheck in 24 hr by ENT specialist.
- Patients with nondisplaced zygomatic fractures can be discharged with analgesics (acetaminophen or ibuprofen); refer displaced zygoma and tripod fractures that are otherwise stable for outpatient reduction in 2–3 days, after swelling is reduced.
- Overlying lacerations with simple fractures can be sutured in the emergency department; if patient is discharged, treat with amoxicillin or erythromycin.

### Pediatric Considerations

- Surgical cricothyroidotomy should not be performed in children <8 yr:
  – Needle cricothyroidotomy with jet ventilation may be performed.
- Children are at high risk of associated injuries.
- Repair of facial fractures should not be delayed more than 3–4 days (owing to rapid healing of facial fractures and the risk of malunion and cosmetic deformity).

## MEDICATION

- Acetaminophen: 650 mg (peds: 10–15 mg/kg) PO q4h
- Amoxicillin: 250 mg (peds: 40–80 mg/kg/24 hr) PO q8h
- Cefazolin: 1 g (peds: 50–100 mg/kg/24 hr) IV or IM
- Clindamycin: 600–900 mg (peds: 25–40 mg/kg/24 hr) PO q8h
- Diazepam: 5–10 mg (peds: 0.1–0.2 mg/kg) IV
- Erythromycin: 500 mg (peds: 30–50 mg/kg/24 hr) PO q.i.d.
- Etomidate: 0.2–0.3 mg/kg (peds: 0.2–0.3 mg/kg) IV
- Fentanyl: 2–10 bcg/kg (peds: 2–3 bcg/kg) IV
- Ibuprofen: 600–800 mg (peds: 20–40 mg/kg/24 hr) PO t.i.d.–q.i.d.
- Ketamine: 1–2 mg/kg (peds: 1–2 mg/kg) IV
- Midazolam: 2–5 mg (peds: Safety not established, but 0.02–0.05 mg/kg per dose has been used) IV
- Morphine sulfate: 0.1–0.2 mg/kg (peds: 0.1–0.2 mg/kg) IV q1h–q4h titrated
- Rocuronium: 0.6–1.2 mg/kg (peds: 0.6 mg/kg) IV
- Succinylcholine: 1–1.5 mg/kg (peds: 1–2 mg/kg) IV
- Vecuronium: 0.1–0.3 mg/kg (peds: 0.1–0.3 mg/kg) IV

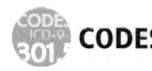 **FOLLOW-UP**

## DISPOSITION

### Admission Criteria

- Significant associated trauma
- Airway compromise
- Le Fort II and III fractures
- CSF leak
- Posterior table frontal sinus fractures
- Most open fractures excluding simple nasal fractures with lacerations

### Discharge Criteria

- No evidence of significant head, neck, or other injuries
- Closed fractures of the zygoma or anterior table of the frontal sinus with appropriate follow-up in 24–36 hr
- Septal hematomas that have been drained in the emergency department require follow-up in 24 hr.
- Refer displaced zygoma and tripod fractures that are otherwise stable for outpatient reduction in 2–3 days after swelling is reduced.

### Issues for Referral

ENT, plastic surgery, or neurosurgery may all handle facial fractures, actual referral depends on practice patterns at your institution. If there is no CSF leak or involvement of the posterior table of the frontal sinus, it is reasonable to initially consult ENT.

## PEARLS AND PITFALLS

Facial fractures and injuries can be very dramatic in appearance:

- Airway management always takes precedence
- After the airway is secured as necessary, evaluation of other injuries takes precedence—do not miss life-threatening injuries:
  – Cervical spine
  – Pulmonary or thoracic
  – Intra-abdominal injuries

## ADDITIONAL READING

- Chapman VM, Ellis E, Scott K. Assessment of patients. Fenton LZ, Gao D, Strain JD. Facial fractures in children: Unique patterns of injury observed by computed tomography. *J Comput Assist Tomogr.* 2009;33(1)70–72.
- Cole P, Kaufman Y, Hollier L. Principles of facial trauma: Orbital fracture management. *J Craniofac Surg.* 2009;20(1):101–104.
- Ellis E, Scott K. Assessment of patients with facial fractures. *Emerg Med Clin North Am.* 2000;18:411–447.
- Fraioli RE, Branstetter BF, Deleyiannis FW. Facial fractures: Beyond Le Fort. *Otolaryngol Clin North Am.* 2008;41(1):51–76.
- Kelley P, Hopper R, Gruss J. Evaluation and treatment or zygomatic fractures. *Plast Reconstruct Surg.* 2007;120:5S–15S.
- Mandolis S, Hollier LH Jr. Management of frontal sinus fractures. *Plast Reconstr Surg.* 2007;120:32S–48S.

### See Also (Topic, Algorithm, Electronic Media Element)

- Blowout Fracture
- Mandibular Fracture
- Nasal Fracture
- Rapid Sequence Intubation

## CODES

### ICD9

- 802.4 Closed fracture of malar and maxillary bones
- 802.6 Closed fracture of orbital floor (blowout)
- 802.8 Closed fracture of other facial bones

F

# FAILURE TO THRIVE

*David A. Listman*

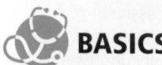 **BASICS**

## DESCRIPTION
- Not a single disease, but a description of a group of symptoms
- Inadequate physical growth:
  - Usually diagnosed earlier than age 2 yr
- Broadly divided into:
  - Organic (underlying medical condition)
  - Nonorganic (no underlying medical condition)
- Found in all socioeconomic groups
- Poverty increases risk of failure to thrive (FTT).
- May result in long-term growth, behavioral, and developmental difficulties, particularly in children who fail to thrive in the first few months of life

## ETIOLOGY
Many diseases with unique causes resulting in 1 or more of:
- Inadequate caloric intake
- Inadequate caloric absorption
- Excessive caloric expenditure

## DIAGNOSIS

### SIGNS AND SYMPTOMS
- No universally accepted diagnosis
- Failure to achieve or maintain a growth rate appropriate for age
- Weight less than 2 standard deviations below normal for age (corrected for prematurity)
- Weight that crosses downward through 2 major percentiles (major percentiles are 5th, 10th, 25th, 50th, 75th, and 90th percentiles) on standard growth chart (see References below)
- There is an associated change in the velocity of growth of 1 or more growth parameters. Any of the 3 routinely monitored growth parameters may be impaired initially:
  - Weight loss initially followed by impaired growth in length/height and finally head circumference usually caused with caloric inadequacy.
  - Primary length/height fall-off often associated with endocrinology problem while impairment in growth of head circumference commonly caused by CNS primary condition.

- Can manifest as:
  - Reduced muscle mass
  - Loss of subcutaneous fat
  - Alopecia
  - Dermatitis
  - Chronic disease
  - Marasmus
  - Kwashiorkor
  - Associated endocrinologic findings
  - Abnormal neurologic exam and development

### History
- Detailed feeding history:
  - Breast-feeding:
    - Prior breast-feeding experience
    - Frequency of feedings
    - Length of feedings
    - Family support for breast-feeding
  - Formula:
    - Type of formula (milk, soy, elemental, premie)
    - How formula is prepared (ready to feed, powder, liquid concentrate)
    - Frequency of feedings
    - Volume per feeding
  - Solid foods
  - Vomiting associated with feeds
  - Urine and stool output:
    - Blood in stool
- Gestational history:
  - Maternal medical complications
  - Drug or alcohol use
- Birth history:
  - Complications
  - Birth weight
- Developmental history:
  - Achievement of appropriate milestones
  - Child's perceived temperament
- Psychosocial history:
  - Family composition
  - Family/social support
  - Stresses
  - Maternal depression
  - Abuse or neglect

### Physical Exam
- Weight, length/height, head circumference:
  - Plotted on appropriate growth chart:
    - Include as many prior growth points as possible.
- Dysmorphic features:
  - Cardiac disorders
  - Pulmonary disorders
  - GI disorders
- Skin exam to include signs of child abuse

### ESSENTIAL WORKUP
- Detailed history and physical exam
- Growth parameters plotted on appropriate growth charts
- Observation of family–child interaction
- Direct observation of feeding
- CBC, CRP, electrolytes, urinalysis and urine culture, and if indicated, lead level

### DIAGNOSTIC TESTS & INTERPRETATION
#### Lab
- CBC:
  - Anemia
  - Infection
  - Leukemia/malignancy
  - Lead level
  - Lead poisoning
- Chemistry panel (electrolytes, BUN, creatinine, glucose, liver function, protein, albumin, calcium, phosphate, magnesium):
  - Hydration and acidosis
  - Metabolic and endocrinologic disorders including thyroid disease. Often checking the routine newborn screening (NBS) is useful.
  - Diabetes mellitus
  - Renal disease
  - Blood gas analysis
  - Renal tubular acidosis
  - Inborn errors of metabolism
- Urinalysis with culture:
  - Renal disease
  - Infection
- HIV

*Imaging*

CXR:

- TB
- Pneumonia
- Cardiomegaly

*Diagnostic Procedures/Surgery*

- pH probe:
  - Gastroesophageal reflux
- Sweat chloride test:
  - Cystic fibrosis (may be part of NBS)
- Tuberculin skin testing

## DIFFERENTIAL DIAGNOSIS

- Organic causes:
  - GI:
    - Malabsorption syndromes
    - Celiac disease
    - Cystic fibrosis
    - Food allergy
    - Inflammatory bowel disease
    - Hepatobiliary disease
    - Hepatitis
    - Cirrhosis
    - Biliary atresia
    - Obstructive disease
    - Pyloric stenosis
    - Malrotation
    - Hirschsprung disease
    - Gastroesophageal reflux
    - Vitamin deficiencies
  - Cardiac:
    - Congenital heart disease
    - Cyanotic
    - Congestive
    - Acquired heart disease
  - Pulmonary:
    - Bronchopulmonary dysplasia
    - Obstructive sleep apnea
    - Chronic lung disease
    - Cystic fibrosis
  - Hematologic/oncologic:
    - Iron deficiency anemia
    - Thalassemia
    - Lead poisoning
    - Leukemia

  - Renal:
    - Chronic renal insufficiency
    - Renal tubular acidosis
    - Recurrent UTIs
  - Neurologic/CNS:
    - Hydrocephalus
    - Hypertonia/hypotonia
    - Generalized weakness (ie, spinal muscular atrophy)
  - Immunologic:
    - AIDS
  - Endocrine:
    - Diabetes mellitus
    - Thyroid/parathyroid disease
    - Adrenal disease
    - Growth hormone deficiency
    - Hypopituitarism
    - Hypophosphatemic rickets
  - Infectious:
    - TB
    - Parasite
    - UTI
  - Genetic/congenital:
    - Fetal alcohol syndrome
    - Smith-Lemli Opitz syndrome
    - Cleft lip/palate
    - Inborn errors of metabolism
    - Many genetic syndromes can contribute.
  - Toxic
- Nonorganic causes:
  - Parent–child dysfunction:
    - Mother–infant bonding problems
    - Maternal mental illness/substance abuse
    - Inexperienced mother
    - Breast-feeding difficulties
    - Improper formula preparation
    - Chaotic family environment
    - Child abuse or neglect
    - Munchhausen syndrome by proxy

 **TREATMENT**

## INITIAL STABILIZATION/THERAPY

- Check for hypoglycemia
- Fluid resuscitation when dehydrated
- Supportive/nonjudgmental environment

## ED TREATMENT/PROCEDURES

- Recognize/identify child with FTT
- Rule out organic abnormalities:
  - Organic causes may have specific treatments.
- Social services consult
- Breast-feeding consult:
  - Advise on appropriate feeding.

## MEDICATION

Dependent on underlying cause

 **FOLLOW-UP**

## DISPOSITION

*Admission Criteria*

- Organic cause requiring medical admission
- Nonorganic causes to observe caregiver–child interaction
- Nonorganic causes to observe weight while monitoring oral intake
- Suspected child abuse/neglect
- Severe dehydration, malnutrition, or electrolyte imbalance

*Discharge Criteria*

- Case appropriately managed by primary care physician
- Follow-up is ensured.

*Issues for Referral*

Subspecialty referral depending on cause

## ADDITIONAL READING

- Bithoney WG, Dubowitz H, Egan H. Failure to thrive/growth deficiency. *Pediatr Rev.* 1992;13: 453–460.
- Centers for Disease Control and Prevention, National Center for Health Statistics: Growth charts. Available at www.cdc.gov/growthcharts. Accessed April 23, 2005.
- Gahagan S, Holmes R. A stepwise approach to evaluation of undernutrition and failure to thrive. *Pediatr Clin North Am.* 1998;45(1):169–187.
- Maggioni A, Lifshitz F. Nutritional management of failure to thrive. *Pediatr Clin North Am.* 1995;42:791.
- Shah MD. Failure to thrive in children. *J Clin Gastroenterol.* 2002;35(5):371–374.

 **CODES**

ICD9

783.41 Failure to thrive

F

# FATIGUE
*Matthew B. Mostofi*

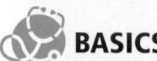 **BASICS**

## DESCRIPTION
- A subjective state of overwhelming, sustained exhaustion and decreased capacity for physical and mental work that is not relieved by rest
- Fatigue occurs with or without objective findings on physical exam.
- Fatigue is a common complaint in people with and without systemic disease, which makes this complaint a challenge to practicing physicians.

## ETIOLOGY
- The specific mechanisms of fatigue are unknown.
- Hematologic:
  - Anemia
  - Leukemia
- Endocrine:
  - Thyroid disorders
  - Adrenal insufficiency
  - Diabetes
  - Pregnancy
- Malignancy:
  - Paraneoplastic syndromes
- Psychiatric:
  - Chronic pain
  - Emotional distress
  - Depression
  - Eating disorders
  - Chemical dependency
  - Withdrawal syndromes
- Sleep disorders:
  - Insomnia
  - Sleep apnea
- Cardiac and pulmonary disorders
- Infections acute and chronic
- Rheumatic and autoimmune disorders
- Nutritional deficiencies including electrolyte abnormalities
- Physical inactivity and deconditioning
- Medications
- Chronic fatigue syndrome:
  - Symptom complex defined by the CDC
  - Severe fatigue lasting >6 mo
  - No definable organic disease
  - Presence of associated physical symptoms:
    - Headache
    - Arthralgias
    - Sleep disturbances
    - Lymphadenopathy
    - Exercise intolerance
    - Myalgias

## DIAGNOSIS

### SIGNS AND SYMPTOMS
- Fatigue is a subjective complaint of exhaustion or tired sensation that interferes with normal activities of life, and symptoms do not resolve with sleep.
- There are no specific signs of fatigue, but frequently physical signs may hint at the underlying cause of complaint.

### History
- Onset, pattern, duration of fatigue
- Associated symptoms: Fever, night sweats, weakness, dyspnea, weight loss/gain, sleep patterns
- Past medical and surgical history
- Psychiatric history: Emotional and mental stressors, depression
- Social history: Alcohol, drug use, major life events
- Medications
- Full review of systems

### Physical Exam
- A complete physical exam should be focused on trying to identify an underlying cause for patient's symptoms. No physical findings are specific to fatigue.
- A partial list of physical exam findings which may suggest an underlying cause include:
  - Vital signs: Abnormal vital signs should be investigated
  - HEENT:
    - Pupils for evidence of toxidrome
    - Sclera for icterus in liver disease
    - Conjunctiva pale in anemia
    - Thyroid for enlargement, pain or nodule that would suggest dysfunction
  - Heart: Murmurs or S3 may suggest LV dysfunction.
  - Lung: Abnormal AP diameter or breath sounds may suggest chronic or acute lung disease.
  - Abdomen: Tenderness or masses should be investigated.
  - Skin: Rash may suggest infectious or autoimmune disease, lack of turgor may suggest dehydration, hyperpigmentation in Addison disease.
  - Neurologic: True weakness or areflexia may suggest neuromuscular disorder, all new focal weakness should be investigated.
  - Musculoskeletal: Indwelling IV lines or dialysis catheters should prompt investigation of electrolyte abnormality or occult bacteremia.

### ESSENTIAL WORKUP
- Because fatigue is a subjective complaint, the essential workup is directed at identification of an underlying cause.
- Vital signs review, including pulse oximetry

### DIAGNOSTIC TESTS & INTERPRETATION
### Lab
- Lab evaluation should be directed by findings of history and physical exam.
- CBC:
  - Screen for anemia or leukemia.
- Serum glucose:
  - Both hyperglycemia and hypoglycemia can present with fatigue.
- Pregnancy test
- Electrolytes with blood urea nitrogen/creatinine
- Thyroid-stimulating hormone:
  - Screen for hypothyroidism.
- Urine drug screen

### Imaging
Imaging/special test: Special tests are reserved for evaluation of abnormal physical exam findings or history suggesting further evaluation.

### Diagnostic Procedures/Surgery
Any diagnostic procedures considered should be reserved for evaluation of abnormal physical exam findings or history suggesting further evaluation.

### DIFFERENTIAL DIAGNOSIS
- Infection:
  - Bacteremia
  - Urosepsis
  - Pneumonia
  - Viral syndromes
  - Abscess
  - Epstein-Barr virus, Monospot
  - Cytomegalovirus
  - HIV
  - Human herpes virus-6
- Immunologic/connective tissue:
  - Rheumatologic (rheumatoid arthritis, systemic lupus erythematosus, juvenile rheumatoid arthritis)
  - Osteoarthritis
  - Fibromyalgia
  - Myasthenia gravis
  - Lambert-Eaton syndrome
- Neoplastic:
  - Solid or hematologic cancers

- Metabolic:
  - Electrolyte abnormalities
  - Mitochondrial diseases
  - Bromism
- Hematologic:
  - Anemia
  - Hypovolemia
  - Hemoglobinopathy
- Endocrine:
  - Hyperthyroid or hypothyroid
  - Adrenal insufficiency
  - Diabetes
  - Hypoglycemia
- Neurologic:
  - Multiple sclerosis
  - Cerebrovascular accident
  - Amyotrophic lateral sclerosis
- Cardiovascular:
  - MI
  - Cardiomyopathy
  - CHF
- Pulmonary:
  - Pneumonia
  - Chronic obstructive pulmonary disease
  - Asthma
  - Sleep apnea
- GI:
  - Reflux
  - Peptic ulcer disease
  - Liver disease
- Autonomic dysfunction
- Lifestyle:
  - Excessive or insufficient exercise
  - Obesity
- Psychiatric:
  - Major depression
  - Anxiety
  - Grief
  - Stress
- Medication-related:
  - Drug interactions
  - Commonly caused by BP, cardiovascular, psychiatric, and narcotic medications
- Dehydration

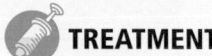 **TREATMENT**

### PRE-HOSPITAL
Evaluate vital signs:
- Collect relevant information that could help psychosocial evaluation.

### INITIAL STABILIZATION/THERAPY
- ABCs
- Administer supplemental oxygen for hypoxia.
- IV fluid bolus for signs of dehydration

### ED TREATMENT/PROCEDURES
- Treatment should be directed to correction of the underlying cause of fatigue:
  - Identify and treat any infectious process.
  - Correct metabolic and hematologic disturbances.
  - Diagnose progressive neurologic disease and acute psychiatric crisis.
  - Initiate workup for endocrine and neoplastic disease.
  - Stop any offending medications or toxins.
- Most cases will not have identifiable cause, so reassurance and close follow-up is required.
- Recommend appropriate diet, exercise regimen, and consistent sleep cycles.

### MEDICATION
*First Line*
Medication should be reserved for treatment of the underlying cause of symptoms.

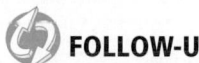 **FOLLOW-UP**

### DISPOSITION
*Admission Criteria*
- Underlying disease requiring IV medication or monitoring
- Failure to thrive as outpatient
- Unable to provide for self

*Discharge Criteria*
- Able to care for self
- Serious disturbances have been excluded.
- Adequate follow-up is arranged.

### *Issues for Referral*
Most patients who are evaluated for fatigue in the ED should be referred:
- When the cause of a patient's fatigue symptoms have been clearly identified, referral should be directed to the appropriate specialist.
- When the cause of a patient's fatigue symptoms are not clearly identified, a primary care referral is indicated.

## PEARLS AND PITFALLS
- Fatigue is a subjective symptom complex, and a complete history and physical are needed.
- Beware of patients with unreliable history and physical exam. The elderly, children, intoxicated, and those with decreased mental ability may all have life-threatening disease and present with a complaint of fatigue.

## ADDITIONAL READING
- Buchwald D, Wener MH, Pearlman T, et al. Markers of inflammation and immune activation in chronic fatigue and chronic fatigue syndrome. *J Rheumatol.* 1997;24(2):372–376.
- Dickinson CJ. Chronic fatigue syndrome etiological aspects. *Eur J Clin Invest.* 1997;27(4):257–267.
- Fukuda K. The chronic fatigue syndrome: A comprehensive approach to its definition and study International Chronic Fatigue Syndrome Study Group. *Ann Intern Med.* 1994;121(12):953–959.
- Manzullo EF, Escalante CP. Research into fatigue. *Hem/Onc Clinics of N Am.* 2002;16(3):619–628.
- Maul AC. Chronic fatigue syndrome. *Immunol Invest.* 1997;26(1–2):269–273.
- Morrison RE, Keating HJ. Fatigue in primary care. *Obstet Gynecol Clin.* 2001;28(2):225–240,v–vi.

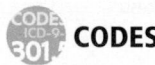 **CODES**

### ICD9
780.79 Other malaise and fatigue

F

# FEEDING PROBLEMS, PEDIATRIC

*Niels K. Rathlev*
*Richard Gabor*

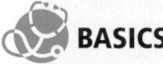 **BASICS**

## DESCRIPTION
- Problems may present in 1 or several of the components of "feeding:"
  - Getting food into oral cavity: Appetite, food-seeking behavior, ingestion
  - Swallowing food: Oral and pharyngeal phases
  - Ingestion and absorption: Esophageal swallowing, GI phase
- Acute feeding problems may be a component of acute systemic disease:
  - Infection, bowel obstruction
- Chronic feeding problems may result from underlying neuromuscular, cardiovascular, or behavioral issues:
  - Cerebral palsy, prematurity, congenital heart disease, chronic neglect
- Minor feeding difficulties reported in 25–50% of normal children:
  - Mainly colic, vomiting, slow feeding, and refusal to eat
- More severe problems observed in 40–70% of infants born prematurely or children with chronic medical conditions.

## ETIOLOGY
- Several distinct areas of pathology—but overlap is common
- Structural abnormalities:
  - Naso-oropharynx:
    - Cleft lip/palate
    - Choanal atresia
    - Micrognathia and/or Pierre Robin sequence
    - Macroglossia
    - Tonsillar hypertrophy
    - Retropharyngeal mass or abscess
  - Larynx and trachea:
    - Laryngeal cleft or cyst
    - Subglottic stenosis
    - Laryngeo or tracheo malacia
    - Tracheoesophageal fistula
  - Esophagus:
    - Esophageal strictures, stenosis, or web
    - Tracheoesophageal compression from vascular ring/sling
    - Esophageal mass or tumor
    - Foreign body
- Neurologic conditions:
  - Cerebral palsy
  - Muscular dystrophies
  - Mitochondrial disorders
  - Arnold-Chiari malformation
  - Myasthenia gravis
  - Brainstem injury
  - Pervasive developmental disorder (Autism Spectrum disorders)
  - Infant botulism
  - Brainstem glioma
  - Polymyositis/dermatomyositis

- Prematurity
- Immune disorders:
  - Allergy
  - Eosinophilic esophagitis
  - Celiac disease
- Congenital heart disease:
  - Precorrection: Fatigue, respiratory compromise, increased metabolic needs
  - Postcorrection: Any/all of above, recurrent laryngeal nerve injury
- Chronic aspiration
- Conditioned dysphagia:
  - Gastro-esophageal reflux (GER)
  - Prolonged tube or parenteral feeding early in life
- Metabolic disorders:
  - Hypothyroidism
  - Inborn errors of metabolism
- Acute illness or event:
  - Sepsis
  - Pharyngitis
  - Intussusception
  - Malrotation
  - Shaken baby syndrome
- Behavioral issues:
  - Poor environmental stimulation
  - Dysfunctional feeder–child interaction
  - Selective food refusal
  - Rumination
  - Phobias
  - Conditioned emotional reactions
  - Depression
  - Poverty (inadequate food available)

 **DIAGNOSIS**

## SIGNS AND SYMPTOMS
Common presentations:
- Caregiver concerns regarding feeding or postfeeding behavior
- Poor weight gain/failure to thrive
- Recurrent or chronic respiratory illness

### History
- Onset of problem
- Length of meals (often prolonged)
- Food refusal/oral aversion
- Independent feeding (if >8 mo):
  - Neuromuscular problems decrease ability to get food to the mouth
- Failure to thrive/poor weight gain
- Recurrent pneumonia/respiratory distress:
  - Most aspiration episodes are silent in infants
  - Recurrent pneumonia or wheezing may be primary symptoms of chronic aspiration
  - Chronic lung disease
- Recurrent vomiting or gagging:
  - If yes, when

- Diarrhea, rectal bleeding
- Onset of irritability or lethargy during feeding. Colic
- Duration of feeding highly variable, especially in breast fed infants—for all ages, feeding times >30 min on a regular basis is cause for concern:
  - Full-term healthy infant usually has 2–3 oz of formula every 2–3 hr.
  - Breast-fed baby eats 10–20 min on each breast every 2–3 hr.
  - As child gets older, duration and frequency may decrease.
  - 1-mo-old normally eats 4 oz every 4 hr.

### Physical Exam
- Vital signs, including oximetry
- Weight, length, head circumference:
  - Comparison with prior measurements is extremely helpful.
  - Slow velocity of growth
  - Impaired nutritional status. Severe cases may show emaciation, weakness, apathy.
  - Growth curve without prior data is harder to interpret.
- General physical exam—especially note:
  - Affect and social responsiveness
  - Dysmorphism (facial asymmetry, tongue and jaw size, etc.)
  - ENT—oropharyngeal inflammation, infection, or anatomic abnormality
  - Cardiovascular status (murmur, tachycardia, tachypnea, retractions)
  - Pulmonary—tachypnea, color change. Evidence of aspiration
  - Abdominal exam—bowel sounds, distension, tenderness, masses
  - Neurological—tone, coordination, alertness
  - Skin: Allergic rash or atopy:
    - Edema may occur with protein deficiency (kwashiorkor).
- Observation of feeding: Neuromuscular tone, posture, position; patient motivation; oral structure and function; efficiency of oral intake:
  - Ability to handle oral secretions
  - Pace of feeding
  - Noisy airway sounds after swallowing
  - Gagging, coughing, or emesis during feeding
  - Respiratory distress with feeding
  - Oximetry during feeding may be helpful
  - Onset of fatigue or irritability
  - Duration of feeding

## ESSENTIAL WORKUP
- A well-hydrated, comfortable child with a normal physical exam and recent history of good weight gain may not need any ED workup beyond assuring good follow-up.
- Children who show evidence of distress, dehydration, discomfort, respiratory distress, or poor weight gain require further evaluation.

## DIAGNOSTIC TESTS & INTERPRETATION

### Lab

- Initial assessment if child failing to thrive or appears malnourished:
  - CBC, urinalysis, electrolytes, BUN, glucose, erythrocyte sedimentation rate (ESR) and/or CRP, thyroid functions, LFT's, total protein and albumin
- Cultures of blood, urine, if concern of infection—CSF analysis and culture if concern for meningitis
- Serum NH3, urine for organic acids, and blood for inborn errors or metabolism if concern for metabolic disorders

### Imaging

- CXR film if suspected cardiopulmonary concerns
- EKG if cardiac disease suspected
- Referral or admission for ultrasound and other imaging studies as indicated. Fiberoptic or videofluoroscopic evaluation of swallowing may be needed.
- MRI if concerns for brainstem, skull base, or spinal problems

### Diagnostic Procedures/Surgery

- May need a multidisciplinary evaluation involving speech pathologist, pediatrician, and potentially an otolaryngologist.
- Surgical correction of specific pathology

## DIFFERENTIAL DIAGNOSIS

Feeding disorder encompasses symptoms observed as a final pathway for many disorders.
  Specific clues to the etiology may include:

- Prolonged feeding, fatigue:
  - Consider cardiac disease.
- Recurrent pneumonias:
  - Consider chronic aspiration.
- Stridor with feeds:
  - Consider glottic or subglottic anomalies.
- Suck-swallow-breathing coordination:
  - Consider nasal congestion, choanal atresia.
- Vomiting, diarrhea, abdominal pain, colic:
  - Consider allergy or GER.

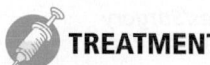 **TREATMENT**

### PRE-HOSPITAL

- Assess vital signs and hydration; resuscitate as necessary.
- Assess for and treat hypoglycemia.

### INITIAL STABILIZATION/THERAPY

- Cardiovascular/respiratory/fluid resuscitation as needed
- Assess for and treat hypoglycemia if suspected.

### ALERT

- Certain inborn errors of metabolism (glycogen storage diseases) can cause profound hypoglycemia if unable to take PO feeds—if known or suspected, IV dextrose should be started immediately.
- Bilious vomiting in a young infant may be a sign of malrotation with intestinal ischemia requiring emergent surgical consultation.

## ED TREATMENT/PROCEDURES

- Treat dehydration if present:
  - Oral rehydration if practical
  - IV if PO contraindicated, not tolerated or impractical
- Ondansetron for acute vomiting
- Treat respiratory distress if present:
  - Oxygen and other interventions as needed
- Treat infection if suspected.

### ALERT

Patients with severe malnutrition are at risk for sepsis AND may have blunted physiologic responses—a high index of suspicion for infection is warranted in severely malnourished patients.

### MEDICATION

Ondansetron: 0.1 mg/kg IV or PO q8h PRN nausea or vomiting—minimum oral dose 2 mg. Maximum dose 4 mg:

- For short-term use (2–3 doses) in patients >6 mo.

 **FOLLOW-UP**

### DISPOSITION

#### Admission Criteria

- Suspected systemic infection
- Inability to maintain hydration
- Sustained hypoxia during feeding
- Significant failure to thrive:
  - Particularly in infants <3 mo
- Decompensated cardiopulmonary disease
- Symptomatic anemia or endocrine dysfunction
- Negligent caretaker

#### Discharge Criteria

- Demonstrated ability to tolerate oral feedings
- Weight gain if failure to thrive
- Reliable caretaker and follow-up

#### Issues for Referral

- Specific referrals based on source of problem
- For complex or chronic feeding problems, a multidisciplinary approach is often needed.
- Chronic disease process may interfere with feeding AND increase caloric needs:
  - Nonoral nutrition such as PEG tubes are often needed to address these issues.

### FOLLOW-UP RECOMMENDATIONS

- When available, a primary provider is the most important resource for follow-up.
- In the case of complex problems, a multidisciplinary approach is often needed—the primary provider is often in the best position to coordinate this.

## PEARLS AND PITFALLS

- Successful feeding in infants requires coordinated, effective interaction of complex physiologic, developmental, and environmental factors.

- The factors are interdependent—disruption of 1 often leads to disruption of others:
  - Premature infant gavage fed for immature suck-swallow coordination, misses critical period for developing this reflex—develops aversion to oral stimulus because of recurrent noxious stimuli.
- Feeding problems of recent, acute onset are likely to have a single identifiable cause:
  - Gastroenteritis, pyloric stenosis, pharyngitis, sepsis
- More chronic, long-term problems are more likely to have multifactorial and/or subtle causes:
  - Feeding is an essential part of the parent–child interaction:
    - Dysfunctional interaction may be the cause of, or a response to a feeding problem.
  - Chronic feeding issues of medical origin may result in continued behavioral feeding difficulties even after the medical problem is corrected.
- Swallowing disorders and aspiration are frequently occult.

## ADDITIONAL READING

- Arvedson J. Assessment of pediatric dysphagia and feeding disorders. *Dev Disabil Res Rev.* 2008;14(2): 118–127.
- Bernard-Bonnin AC. Feeding problems of infants and toddlers. *Can Fam Physician.* 2006;52(10): 1247–1251.
- Rudolph CD, Link DT. Feeding disorders in children. *Pediatr Clin North Am.* 2002;49(1):97–112.

### See Also (Topic, Algorithm, Electronic Media Element)

- Failure to Thrive
- Feeding Tube Complications
- Inborn Errors of Metabolism
- Intussusception
- Irritable Infant
- Malrotation
- Pyloric Stenosis
- Vomiting, Pediatric

 **CODES**

### ICD9

- 779.31 Feeding problems in newborn
- 783.3 Feeding difficulties and mismanagement

# FEEDING TUBE COMPLICATIONS

Colleen N. Hickey
Jennifer L. Kolodchak

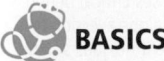 BASICS

## DESCRIPTION
- Extubation:
  - Accidental or intentional
  - More common with nasoenteric tubes compared with percutaneous endoscopic gastrostomy tubes (PEG), gastrostomy tubes (G tubes), or jejunostomy tubes (J tubes)
- Occlusion:
  - Small diameter:
    ○ Most common with nasoenteric tubes
  - Pill fragments
  - Inadequate flushing
  - Physical incompatibilities between formula and medications:
    ○ Adherence of formula residue to inner wall
  - Essential to rule out malposition, fracture, and dislodgment
- Peristomal wound infections:
  - Risk factors:
    ○ Malnutrition
    ○ Poor wound healing
    ○ Stomal leak
    ○ Local irritation
    ○ Poor wound care
    ○ Immunosuppression
    ○ Diabetes mellitus
    ○ Obesity
  - Excessive traction on tube:
    ○ Leads to delayed maturation of gastrocutaneous tract
    ○ Increases stomal leakage
- Stoma leak:
  - Problematic with distal obstruction (mechanical or dysmotility); more common with high gastric residual
  - Excessive tube motion
- Aspiration pneumonia:
  - At risk:
    ○ Impaired cough/gag reflex
    ○ Delayed gastric emptying from ileus
    ○ Obstruction
    ○ Gastroparesis
    ○ Gastroesophageal reflux (frequent with large nasoenteric tube)
- Diarrhea:
  - Medication induced:
    ○ Antibiotics
    ○ Promotility agents
  - Overgrowth of *Clostridium difficile*, other bacteria, or *Candida*
  - High-osmolar formula

- Feeding intolerance:
  - High residual suggests GI motility dysfunction
  - Delivery is too rapid.
  - High osmolarity formula
  - Lactose or fat intolerance
  - Low serum albumin
- Uncommon complications:
  - Abdominal wall hematoma
  - Fistulas:
    ○ Hepatogastric
    ○ Gastrocolic
    ○ Colocutaneous
  - Perforation (usually with placement)
  - Pressure sores/ulcerations

### Pediatric Considerations
Increased risk of aspiration:
- Delayed gastric emptying
- Immaturity of lower esophageal sphincter

 DIAGNOSIS

## SIGNS AND SYMPTOMS
- Extubation:
  - Tube removed from source
- Occlusion:
  - Unable to pass liquid through tube
- Tube migration:
  - Distal displacement of percutaneous endoscopic gastrostomy tube
  - Obstruction at or distal to pylorus
  - Dumping syndrome
  - Ischemia
  - Intussusception
  - Evidence of distal prolapse on external tube (if marked)
- Peristomal wound infections:
  - Cellulitis
  - Necrotizing fasciitis
  - Abscess formation
- Stoma leak:
  - Leakage of feedings/GI tract contents around stoma
- Aspiration pneumonia:
  - Cough
  - Dyspnea
  - Hypoxia
  - Food particulate in pulmonary secretions
  - Fever

- Misplacement of nasoenteric tube in pulmonary tree:
  - Pneumothorax
  - Hydrothorax
  - Pleural effusion
  - Bronchopleural fistula
  - Pneumonia
- Diarrhea:
  - Frequent loose stools
  - Dehydration
- Intolerance to enteral nutrition:
  - High residuals
  - Associated with increased risk of aspiration

## ESSENTIAL WORKUP
- Carefully examine the tube site and position of feeding tube within wound.
- For suspected tube migration, obtain a water soluble contrast radiography of the tube to establish the tube position within the abdomen/stomach/intestine.

## DIAGNOSTIC TESTS & INTERPRETATION
### Lab
- Peristomal wound infections:
  - CBC for significant infections
- Aspiration pneumonia:
  - Arterial blood gas or pulse oximetry
  - CBC
  - Electrolytes, BUN/creatinine, glucose
  - Blood and sputum culture
- Diarrhea:
  - Stool for white blood cells/culture/*C. difficile* toxin

### Imaging
- CXR:
  - Nasoenteric tube position
  - Aspiration pneumonia
- Water soluble contrast radiography for suspected tube migration

### Diagnostic Procedures/Surgery
Endoscopy to evaluate for tube migration

 TREATMENT

## PRE-HOSPITAL

### ALERT
If extubation of tube has occurred, transport tube with patient to facilitate easier replacement.

## INITIAL STABILIZATION/THERAPY
- ABCs
- IV fluid resuscitation for dehydration/sepsis

## ED TREATMENT/PROCEDURES

### Extubation
- Nasoenteric tube:
  – Replace in emergency department
  – Confirm position by radiograph before use.
- Percutaneous endoscopic gastrostomy (PEG) tube and gastrojejunal (G-J) tube:
  – Takes 4–6 wk for gastrocutaneous tract/fistula to mature
  – Improper or aggressive attempt at tube replacement could lead to disruption of gastrocutaneous tract and subsequent peritonitis.
  – PEG tube in place >4 wk:
    ○ Replace in emergency department (may use a Foley catheter of equivalent size)
    ○ Confirm by water soluble radiographic study.
    ○ Secure catheter to abdominal wall to prevent distal migration.
  – PEG tube in place <4 wk:
    ○ Do not replace in ED.
    ○ Risk of intraperitoneal placement
    ○ May need hospital admission and endoscopic tube replacement
  – Surgical G tube or J tube:
    ○ Management similar to that for PEG tube
    ○ Early dislodgment within first 3 days requires emergency surgical consult and antibiotic coverage for peritonitis.
    ○ May need endoscopic replacement if <4 wk old

### Occlusion
- Attempt gentle irrigation with NS, water, carbonated soda, pancreatic enzymes.
- If irrigation fails, replace tube.
- Do not use meat tenderizer.

### Tube Migration
- If retraction of tube is possible and well tolerated:
  – Secure tube externally.
  – Discharge home after brief trial of tube feeding.
- If feeding is not tolerated, or if there are signs of persistent obstruction or peritonitis:
  – Admit with consult to appropriate service (surgical/gastrointestinal).
- If external tube is cut (accidental or intentional) and the inner tube is within the abdomen:
  – Inner bumper usually passes through GI tract.
  – Cases of obstruction, subsequent perforation, and peritonitis have been reported, especially in children.

### Peristomal Wound Infections
- Local wound care
- Antibiotics:
  – 1st-generation cephalosporin (cefazolin or cephalexin)
  – Ampicillin/sulbactam
  – Amoxicillin/clavulanic acid
  – Clindamycin (penicillin-allergic)
- Outpatient management for milder cases
- More severe cases require surgical consult for possible drainage/débridement and inpatient care.
- Prophylactic use of antibiotic (cefazolin) before tube placement decreases wound infection.

### Peristomal Leak
- Change from intermittent to continuous delivery.
- Decrease rate of infusion.
- Optimize nutritional status.
- Relieve excess tension on tube.
- Administer prokinetic agents (eg, metoclopramide or erythromycin).
- Do NOT place larger tube.
- Local care:
  – Keep site clean and dry.
  – Barrier creams

### Aspiration Pneumonia
- Stop enteral feeding.
- Administer oxygen and broad-spectrum antibiotics.
- Endotracheal intubation with mechanical ventilation for respiratory failure and airway protection when indicated
- Prevent by:
  – Elevation of head of bed
  – Monitoring gastric residual
  – Use of continuous infusion at graduated rate
  – Use of prokinetic agent

### Diarrhea
- Manage cause
- Correct fluid and electrolyte imbalance.
- Try isotonic, hypotonic, or fat- or lactose-free formulas.
- High-fiber formula if above measures fail
- Antimotility agents:
  – Loperamide
  – Kaopectate
  – Cholestyramine

### Formula Intolerance
Prokinetic agents promote gastric emptying.

## MEDICATION
- Amoxicillin/clavulanic acid (Augmentin): 500–875 mg (peds: 25–45 mg/kg/24 h) PO q12h
- Ampicillin/sulbactam: 1.5–3 g (peds: 100–200 mg/kg/24 h) IV q6h
- Cefazolin (Ancef, Kefzol): 500 mg–1 g (peds: 25–100 mg/kg/24 h) IV q6h
- Cephalexin (Keflex): 250–500 mg (peds: 25–50 mg/kg/24 h) PO q6h
- Cholestyramine: 2–4 g (peds: >6 yr 80 mg/kg q8h) PO q6–12h
- Clindamycin: 150–400 mg (peds: 5–10 mg/kg) IV q6h
- Erythromycin: 50–100 mg (peds: 6–10 mg/kg/24 h) PO/IV q6–8h
- Kaopectate: 30 mL (peds: 3–6 yr old, 7.5 mL; 6–12 yr old, 15 mL) PO after each loose bowel movement up to 7 times per day
- Loperamide (Imodium): 4 mg initially, then 2 mg (peds: 1 mg q8h if 13–20 kg; 2 mg q12h if 20–30 kg; 2 mg q8h, if >30 kg) PO up to 16 mg/d
- Metoclopramide: 5–10 mg (peds: 0.1–0.2 mg/kg to max. 0.8 mg/kg/d) PO/IV/IM q6h (30 min before feeds and every night)

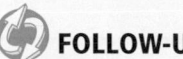

## FOLLOW-UP

### DISPOSITION

#### Admission Criteria
- Percutaneous endoscopic gastrostomy tube extubation within 1 wk of placement
- Surgical G tube or J tube extubation within 3 days of placement
- Significant peristomal wound infection
- Aspiration pneumonia
- Diarrhea associated with dehydration
- Peritonitis

#### Discharge Criteria
Successful replacement of extubated feeding tube

#### Issues for Referral
GI consult or surgical consult for feeding tube replacement when cannot be placed successfully in the emergency department

### FOLLOW-UP RECOMMENDATIONS
Primary care or GI follow-up for recurrent feeding tube complications

## PEARLS AND PITFALLS
- Radiography should be used to confirm placement of all feeding tubes.
- Do not attempt replacement of a newly placed PEG tube, G tube, or J tube in the ED.

## ADDITIONAL READING
- Lopez-Herce J. Gastrointestinal complications in critically ill patients: What differs between adults and children?. *Curr Opinion in Clin Nut and Met Care.* 2009;12.180–185.
- Metheny NA, Meert KL, Clouse RE. Complications related to feeding tube placement. *Curr Opinion in Gastroentrology.* 2007;23:178–182.
- Niv E, Fireman Z, Vaisman N. Post-pyloric feeding. *World J Gastroenterol.* 2009;15(11):1281–1288.
- Schrag SP, Sharma R, Jaik NP, et al. Complications related to percutaneous endoscopic gastrostomy (PEG) tubes: A comprehensive clinical review. *J Gastrointestin Liver Dis.* 2007;16(4):407–418.

F

# FEMUR FRACTURE

Alexander D. Miller
Colleen J. Buono

 **BASICS**

## DESCRIPTION
Fractures classified according to:
- Location:
  - Proximal 3rd (subtrochanteric region)
  - Middle 3rd
  - Distal 3rd (distal metaphyseal-diaphyseal junction)
- Geometry:
  - Spiral
  - Transverse
  - Oblique
  - Segmental
- Extent of soft tissue injury:
  - Open
  - Closed
- Degree of comminution: Winquist and Hansen classification:
  - Grade I: Fracture with small fragment <25% width of femoral shaft; stable lengthwise and rotationally
  - Grade II: Fracture with 25–50% width of femoral shaft; stable lengthwise; may or may not have rotational stability
  - Grade III: Fracture with >50% width of femoral shaft; unstable lengthwise and rotationally
  - Grade IV: Circumferential loss of cortex; unstable lengthwise and rotationally

## ETIOLOGY
- Usually requires major, high-energy trauma
- Patients are mostly young adults with high-energy injuries (motor vehicle accidents [MVAs], gunshot wounds [GSWs], falls):
  - Spiral fractures with falls from height
- Consider pathologic fracture if minor mechanism
- Can occasionally be due to stress fracture from repetitive activity
- Complications include compartment syndrome, fat embolism, adult respiratory distress syndrome (ARDS), hemorrhage.

### Pediatric Considerations
- 70% of femoral fractures in children <3 yr old are the result of nonaccidental trauma (NAT).
- Spiral fractures of the femur strongly suggest NAT.

 **DIAGNOSIS**

## SIGNS AND SYMPTOMS
### History
- Thigh pain, deformity, swelling, shortening
- Patient unable to move hip or knee
- Commonly presents as multitrauma:
  - Chest, abdominal, pelvic, hip, knee injury, including dislocation

### Physical Exam
- Rarely, open fracture unless injury is due to penetrating trauma
- Patient may be hypotensive due to hemorrhage into the thigh.
- Patient may have impaired circulation in the foot due to vascular compromise, compartment syndrome.

## ESSENTIAL WORKUP
- Radiographs (see Imaging)
- Assess distal pulses, palpate compartments, evaluate sensation and motor function.
- If pulses are not equal or palpable, bedside Doppler or angiography may be necessary.
- Search for associated injuries with multisystem trauma.
- In suspected NAT, obtain skeletal survey or bone scan.

## DIAGNOSTIC TESTS & INTERPRETATION
### Lab
CBC, type and cross-match
### Imaging
- AP pelvis, true lateral of the hip, AP and lateral views of the femur, complete knee series
- Baseline CXR, other films as indicated by trauma protocols

## DIFFERENTIAL DIAGNOSIS
- Hip fracture or dislocation
- Knee fracture or dislocation
- Thigh contusion or hematoma

 **TREATMENT**

## PRE-HOSPITAL
- Immobilization of the extremity and application of a traction splint can be important for tamponade of further blood loss into the thigh:
  - Backboard immobilization, rigid splinting, support of extremity for position of comfort
- Contraindications to traction:
  - Fractures close to the knee
  - Fracture or dislocation of the ipsilateral hip
  - Fractures of the pelvis
  - Fractures of the lower leg
- Do not attempt to reduce open fractures in the field; cover open wounds with sterile dressings.
- Monitor closely for development of hemorrhagic shock, as thigh can contain 4–6 units of blood.

## INITIAL STABILIZATION/THERAPY
- Airway, chest, abdominal injuries take precedence.
- Monitor BP continuously for signs of hemorrhagic shock.

## ED TREATMENT/PROCEDURES
- Maintain lower extremity stability.
- Remove splint and clothing.
- Pain control:
  - Isolated femur injuries: Parenteral analgesia
  - Multitrauma or pediatric patients: Femoral nerve block
- Orthopedic consultation necessary for all femur fractures:
  - Emergent if neurovascular compromise
  - Open fractures must go directly to the OR for irrigation and débridement.

- Antibiotics:
  - Fractures requiring surgery: Cefazolin if open fracture with laceration, extensive soft-tissue damage, contamination: Add gentamicin/tobramycin, tetanus.
  - If highly contaminated wound: Add penicillin G to cover clostridial species.
- Femur fractures with diminished or absent distal pulses, an expanding hematoma, or a palpable pulsatile mass require immediate angiography or femoral artery exploration.
- Skeletal traction should be applied if the patient will not go to the OR immediately.

## MEDICATION

- Antibiotics:
  - Cefazolin: 1 g IM/IV q6–8h (peds: 25–50 mg/kg IM/IV divided q6–8h max. 1 g)
  - Gentamicin/tobramycin: 3–5 mg/kg/d IV/IM divided 18h (peds: 2–2.5 mg/kg q8h)
  - Penicillin G: 2 million IU IV q4h (peds: 100,000–400,000 IU/kg/d IV divided q4–6h to max. 24 million IU in 24 h)
- Moderate sedation:
  - Etomidate: 0.1–0.3 mg/kg IV once (not recommended for <12 yr)
  - Fentanyl: 50–100 $\mu$g IV over 1–2 min once (peds: >6 mo 1–2 $\mu$g/kg IV once)
  - Ketamine: Caution in adults due to potential for emergence reaction (peds: 1.0–2 mg/kg IV, 4 mg/kg IM once)
  - Methohexital: 1–1.5 mg/kg IV once (peds: Not recommended)
  - Midazolam: 0.07 mg/kg IM or 1 mg slowly q2–3min up to 5 mg max. (peds: 0.25–1.0 mg/kg PO once to a max. of 20 mg) PO; 6 mo–5 yr: 0.05–0.1 mg/kg IV titrate to max. of 0.6 mg/kg; 6–12 yr: 0.025–0.05 mg/kg IV titrate to max. of 0.4 mg/kg
  - Propofol: 40 mg IV q10sec until induction; 5–60 $\mu$g/kg/min IV continuous infusion

- Pain control:
  - Hydromorphone: 0.5–2.0 mg IM/SC/slow IV q4–6h PRN; titrate for pain control (peds: 0.015 mg/kg per dose IV q4–6h PRN)
  - Morphine: 2–10 mg IV q4h; titrate for pain control (peds: 0.1 mg/kg IV q4h; titrate for pain control to max. 15 mg/dose)

### *Pediatric Considerations*

- Assess markers for NAT:
  - Delay in presentation
  - History of mechanism inconsistent with the injury
  - Isolated trauma to the thigh, associated burns, bruises, or linear abrasions
- Assess for dislocation of the femoral capital epiphysis.
- Depending on the age of the patient and the fracture type, pediatric femoral fractures may not require operative treatment.

 FOLLOW-UP

## DISPOSITION

### *Admission Criteria*

- All femur fractures must be admitted except as noted below in Discharge Criteria.
- Any suspicion of NAT in children

### *Discharge Criteria*

In certain rare circumstances of pathologic fracture or femur fractures in patients who are not ambulatory and would not undergo operative fixation, discharge can be considered in consultation with orthopedics if adequate pain control can be achieved and proper follow-up ensured.

## ADDITIONAL READING

- Abarbanell N. Prehospital midthigh trauma and traction splint use: Recommendations for treatment protocols. *Am J Emerg Med.* 2001;19:137–140.
- Buckley S. Current trends in the treatment of femoral shaft fractures in children and adolescents. *Clin Orthop.* 1997;338:60–73.
- Fractures of the femoral shaft. In: *Rockwood and Green's fractures in adults and children.* Philadelphia: Lippincott-Raven Publishers, 1991: Chapter 19.
- Kanlic E, Cruz M. Current concepts in pediatric femur fracture treatment. *Orthopedics.* 2007;30(12): 1015–1019.
- Rudman N, McIlmail D. Emergency department evaluation and treatment of hip and thigh injuries. *Emerg Med Clin North Am.* 2000;18:29–66.
- *Tarascon pocket pharmacopoeia,* 2006 edition. Lompoc, CA: Tarascon Publishing; 2006.
- *The Harriet Lane handbook,* 15th ed. Saint Louis, MO: Mosby; 2000.
- Ward K, Yealy D. Systemic analgesia and sedation in managing orthopedic emergencies. *Emerg Med Clin North Am.* 2000;18:141–166.

### See Also (Topic, Algorithm, Electronic Media Element)

Hip Injury

 CODES

### ICD9

- 821.00 Fracture of unspecified part of femur, closed
- 821.01 Fracture of shaft of femur, closed
- 821.20 Fracture of lower end of femur, unspecified part, closed

F

# FEVER, ADULT
*Richard E. Wolfe*

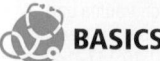

## BASICS

### DESCRIPTION
- Fever represents an elevation in the body's set thermoregulatory point.
- Core temperature is regulated by the anterior hypothalamus at 37°C ± 2°C.
- Fever is caused by increased prostaglandin E2 (PGE2) synthesis in the hypothalamus.
- Autonomic discharge from hypothalamus raises core temperature through shivering and dermal vasoconstriction.
- Normal circadian variation in core temperature occurs with nadir in early morning and peaks in late afternoon.
- Both exogenous and endogenous factors can raise the body's set thermoregulatory point:
  - Endogenous factors include IL-1 and IL-6, tumor necrosis factor, and IFN-γ.
  - Exogenous factors include endotoxin (lipopolysaccharide) and other toxins and metabolites produced by infectious organisms.
- Fever of unknown origin (FUO):
  - Fever >38.3°C for at least 3 wk as an outpatient and 3 days of inpatient evaluation or 3 outpatient visits without determining etiology.

### ETIOLOGY
- Any infectious process
- Iatrogenic infections (indwelling catheters, prostheses)
- Neoplastic
- Drug fever:
  - Most drugs can cause fever by a wide variety of mechanisms
  - Hypersensitivity:
    - Allergic reaction
    - Serum sickness
  - Jarisch-Herxheimer reaction
  - Local phlebitis from irritant drugs
- Severe withdrawal:
  - Alcohol, benzodiazepines
- Systemic inflammation:
  - Sarcoidosis
  - Inflammatory bowel disease
  - Rheumatoid arthritis
  - Takayasu's arteritis
  - Systemic lupus erythematosus
  - Polymyalgia rheumatica
  - Temporal arteritis
  - Periarteritis nodosa
- Endocrine:
  - Hyperthyroidism, pheochromocytoma
- Miscellaneous:
  - Alcoholic cirrhosis
  - Acute inhalation exposures:
    - Metal fume fever
  - Sickle cell disease
  - Hemolytic anemia
  - Pulmonary embolus
  - Familial Mediterranean fever
  - CNS lesions
  - Cotton fever:
    - Benign febrile reaction from an injected contaminant when IV drug abusers strain drug through cotton

- Common causes of FUO:
  - Infectious:
    - Cardiac (endocarditis, pericarditis)
    - TB (miliary, renal, or meningitic)
    - Abdominal and pelvic abscesses
    - Typhoid enteric fevers
    - Epstein Barr virus
    - Cat scratch disease
    - Cytomegalovirus
    - Visceral leishmaniasis
  - Neoplastic:
    - Lymphoma
    - Hypernephromas
    - Hepatomas/liver metastases
    - Myeloproliferative disorders
    - Preleukemias
    - Colon carcinomas
  - Inflammatory disorders

## DIAGNOSIS

### SIGNS AND SYMPTOMS
#### History
- Chills, shivering, and rigors:
  - Rigors suggest bacteremia
- Weight loss:
  - Suggestive of neoplastic, chronic infectious, or endocrine disorders
- Night sweats:
  - Suggestive of lymphoma, solid tumor, chronic inflammatory disease, or TB
- Specific fever patterns:
  - Daily morning temperature spikes:
    - Miliary TB, typhoid fever, periarteritis nodosum
  - Relapsing fevers: Febrile episode with alternating afebrile intervals:
    - Seen in malaria, *Borrelia* infections, rat-bite fever, and lymphoma (Pel Ebstein fevers)
  - Remittent fever: Temperature falls daily but does not return to normal:
    - Seen in TB and viral diseases
  - Intermittent fevers: Exaggerated circadian rhythm:
    - Seen in systemic infections, malignancy, and drug fever
  - Double quotidian fever:
    - Common pattern of 2 temperature spikes in 24 hr
    - In FUO, consider miliary tuberculosis, visceral leishmaniasis, and mixed malarial infections
- Risk factors:
  - s/p Splenectomy
  - Recent chemotherapy
  - IV drug use

#### Physical Exam
- Elevated core temperature:
  - Temperature >38°C (100.4°F) rectally or 37.5°C (99.5°F) orally
  - Lower thresholds in patients older than 65 yr, as the febrile response is not as strong
- Diaphoresis:
  - Absence of diaphoresis with severe hyperthermia suggests anticholinergic poisoning or heat stroke.

- Tachycardia:
  - For each degree of elevation in temperature in Fahrenheit, there should be a 10 bpm increase in pulse.
  - Relative bradycardia:
    - Useful finding in adults with temperature >102°F with normal cardiac response
    - Malaria, typhoid fever, CNS disorders, lymphoma, drug fever, brucellosis, psittacosis, leptospirosis, Legionnaire disease, Lyme disease, and factitious fevers
- Muscle rigidity:
  - Found in patients with neuroleptic malignant syndrome or serotonin syndrome
- Changes in mental status:
  - Can range from irritability to frank delirium and obtundation
- Rash:
  - Type of lesions and distribution can offer important clues to diagnosis.
  - Petechial rashes concerning for meningococcemia and Rocky Mountain spotted fever
- Signs of hyperthyroidism:
  - Goiter
  - Exophthalmos

### ESSENTIAL WORKUP
- Core temperature is most acutely measured rectally.
- Careful history and physical exam (PE) necessary to determine need for further diagnostic testing:
  - History should elicit any sick contacts, previous infections, recent travel, medications, animal or tick exposure, and immunization status.

### DIAGNOSTIC TESTS & INTERPRETATION
#### Lab
- CBC:
  - Commonly performed, but rarely helpful in management of fever in the ED
  - Important in determining neutropenia in patients with risk factors
  - Differential WBC count is unreliable but may give clues to certain etiologies.
  - Neutrophilia and bandemia suggestive of bacterial infection
  - Lymphocytosis suggestive of typhoid, TB, brucellosis, and viral disease
  - Atypical lymphocytosis seen in mononucleosis, cytomegalovirus, HIV, rubella, varicella, measles, and viral hepatitis
  - Monocytosis suggestive of TB, brucellosis, viral illness, and lymphoma
  - Platelet count <150,000 may be predictor of sepsis.
- Erythrocyte sedimentation rate is generally not useful in ED diagnosis of fever:
  - Very high values suggestive of endocarditis, temporal arteritis, TB, and polymyalgia rheumatica

- Urinalysis and urine culture
- Blood cultures:
  - Obtain for patients with signs of sepsis or altered mental status and ill-appearing patients
- Mono spot:
  - Consider if prolonged febrile illness and abnormal differential on the CBC

### Geriatric Considerations
- Certain infections will be prevalent in elderly patients in long-term care facilities.
- UTI, pneumonia, soft-tissue infection, gastroenteritis, prosthetic device associated infections
- High risk of methicillin-resistant *Staphylococcus aureus* and vancomycin-resistant *Enterococcus* species

### Imaging
- CXR:
  - In patients with PE finding of cardiopulmonary disease and patients with unclear fever source
- CT scanning, MRI, or may be indicated based on history, physical, and lab findings

## DIFFERENTIAL DIAGNOSIS
- Failure of thermoregulatory systems:
  - Core temperatures >41°C (105°F) more common in these states
  - Toxidromes:
    ○ Adrenergic (eg, cocaine)
    ○ Anticholinergic (eg, tricyclics)
  - Neuroleptic malignant syndrome
  - Malignant hyperthermia
  - Serotonin syndrome
  - Heat stroke
- Factitious fever

 TREATMENT

### PRE-HOSPITAL
- No specific field interventions required
- Monitoring and IV access should be obtained in the field for unstable patients or patients with altered mental status.

### INITIAL STABILIZATION/THERAPY
- Immediate treatment rarely required
- ABCs for unstable patients
- Initiate broad-spectrum antibiotic treatment immediately for immunocompromised patients and patients with unstable vital signs or profound mental status changes.

### ED TREATMENT/PROCEDURES
- Antipyretics:
  - Acetaminophen, NSAIDs, or salicylates:
    ○ Inhibit the cyclooxygenase enzyme, thereby blocking synthesis of prostaglandins.
  - Most febrile patients do not require antipyretic medication other than for comfort.
  - Selected patients require more aggressive antipyretic interventions:
    ○ Pregnant women
    ○ Patients with history of seizure disorders
    ○ Patients with significant cardiac disease
    ○ Hemodynamically unstable patients
    ○ Patients with altered mental status

- Glucocorticoids:
  - Inhibit phospholipase $A_2$ blocking prostaglandin synthesis
- Empiric antibiotics for neutropenic patients:
  - Combination therapy:
    ○ Extended spectrum $\beta$-lactam (ceftazidime, piperacillin) with an aminoglycoside
  - Monotherapy:
    ○ Cefepime
    ○ Ceftazidime
    ○ Imipenem
- Empiric antibiotics for asplenic patients:
  - Ceftazidime *or* Ceftriaxone
- External cooling mechanism rarely indicated

## MEDICATION
- Antipyretics:
  - Acetaminophen (B): 650–1,000 mg PO/PR q4–6h
  - Aspirin (D): 650 mg PO q4h
  - Ibuprofen (B): 800 mg PO q6h
- Antibiotics:
  - Cefepime: 2 g IV q12
  - Ceftazidime: 2 g IV q8
  - Gentamicin (D) or tobramycin (D): 2 mg/kg IV load then 1.7 mg/kg q8h plus piperacillin/tazobactam (B) 3.375 g IV q4h or ticarcillin/clavulanate (B) 3.1 g IV q4h
  - Imipenem/cilastatin (C): 500–1,000 mg IV q8h
  - Meropenem (B): 1 g IV q8h
  - Ciprofloxacin (C): 750 mg PO b.i.d. plus amoxicillin/clavulanate (B) 875 mg PO b.i.d.

 FOLLOW-UP

### DISPOSITION
#### Admission Criteria
- Patients with unstable vital signs require ICU admission.
- When identified, the underlying source of the fever usually determines the disposition.
- Certain high-risk groups who have fever without an identifiable source:
  - Neutropenic patients
  - Immunosuppressed or immunocompromised patients
  - Asplenic patients
  - IV drug abusers (high risk of endocarditis)
- Lower thresholds for admission in patients older than 60 yr and diabetics

#### Discharge Criteria
Immunocompetent patients with stable vital signs and an identified source of fever or a high suspicion of a nonthreatening viral infection may be safely discharged.

#### Issues for Referral
The suspected etiology of the fever determines the referral to a primary care physician or a specialist.

### FOLLOW-UP RECOMMENDATIONS
Appropriate outpatient treatment and follow-up for further outpatient assessment of the suspected etiology.

## PEARLS AND PITFALLS
- Empiric antibiotics immediately if fever and purpura
- IV drug abusers with fever need admission to rule out endocarditis.

## ADDITIONAL READING
- Cunha BA. Fever of unknown origin: Focused diagnostic approach based on clinical clues from the history, physical examination, and laboratory tests. *Infect Dis Clin North Am.* 2007;21:1137–1187.
- Kamal A, Kauffman CA. Fever of unknown origin. *Postgrad Med.* 2003;114(3):69–75.
- Knockaert DC, Vanderschueren S, Blockmans D. Fever of unknown origin in adults: 40 years on. *J Intern Med.* 2003;253:263–275.
- Mackowiak PA. Concepts of fever. *Arch Intern Med.* 1998;158:1870–1881.
- Plaisance KI, Mackowiak PA. Antipyretic therapy. *Arch Intern Med.* 2000;160:449–456.

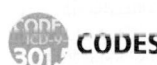 CODES

### ICD9
- 780.60 Fever, unspecified
- 780.61 Fever presenting with conditions classified elsewhere

# FEVER, PEDIATRIC

Nathan Mick
David A. Peak

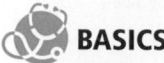 **BASICS**

## DESCRIPTION

- Fever is defined as a temperature of 38°C (100.4°F) rectally:
  - Oral and tympanic temperatures are generally 0.6–1.0°C lower.
- Tympanic temperatures are not accurate in children younger than 6 mo.
- Axillary temperatures are generally unreliable.
- Children who are afebrile but have a reliable history of documented fever should be considered to be febrile to the degree reported.

## ETIOLOGY

- Bacteremia (*Haemophilus influenzae* type B , *Streptococcus pneumoniae)*, viral illness, often accompanied by exanthem (varicella, roseola, rubella), coxsackievirus (hand-foot-mouth disease), abscess:
  - Haemophilus influenzae type B and Streptococcus pneumoniae vaccines have reduced incidence of Haemophilus and pneumococcal disease
- CNS: Meningitis, encephalitis
- Head, eyes, ears, neck and throat (HEENT): Otitis media, facial cellulitis, orbital/periorbital cellulitis, pharyngitis (group A *β*-hemolytic streptococcus, herpangina, adenovirus pharyngoconjunctival fever), viral gingivostomatitis (herpes and coxsackievirus), cervical adenitis, sinusitis, mastoiditis, conjunctivitis, peritonsillar/retropharyngeal abscess
- Respiratory: Croup (paramyxovirus), epiglottitis, bronchiolitis (respiratory syncytial virus [RSV]), pneumonia, empyema, influenza
- Cardiovascular: Purulent pericarditis, endocarditis, myocarditis
- Genitourinary (GU): Cystitis, pyelonephritis
- GI: Bacterial diarrhea, intussusception, appendicitis, hepatitis
- Extremity: Osteomyelitis, septic arthritis, cellulitis
- Miscellaneous: Herpes simplex virus infection in the neonate, Kawasaki disease, vaccine (DPT) reaction, heat exhaustion/stroke, factitious, familial dysautonomia, thyrotoxicosis, collagen vascular disease, vasculitis, rheumatic fever, malignancy, drug induced, overbundling (uncommon recheck 15 min after unbundling)

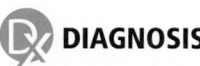 **DIAGNOSIS**

## SIGNS AND SYMPTOMS

- Clinical appearance must be evaluated. Airway, breathing, and circulation (especially dehydration with impaired perfusion/color) need specific evaluation.
- Toxicity associated with lethargy, poor perfusion, hypoventilation/hyperventilation, weak cry, decreased PO intake; purpuric or petechial rash, and/or hypotonia. Initial observation is crucial in this evaluation.

- Tachycardia or tachypnea may be the only finding in children with serious underlying condition.
- Fever with a temperature >38°C can raise a child's heart rate by 10 bpm for each degree Fahrenheit.
- Temperature >40°C have been associated with an elevated bacteremia rate in children <24 mo.
- Altered mental status:
  - Lethargy presenting with decreased level of consciousness
  - Irritability
  - Impaired interaction with environment, parents, physician, toys
- Physical exam (PE) to search for underlying condition.
- Tachypnea and low oximetry are the most sensitive signs for pneumonia. Also useful are rales, hypoxemia, cough >10 days, and fever >5 days.
- Risk factors for occult UTI include female sex, uncircumcised boys, fever without source and fever >39°C.
- Febrile seizures
- Temperatures >42°C often have a noninfectious cause.
- Serious infection may occur in the absence of fever.
- Antipyretics may change findings without impacting underlying disease. This may be useful in evaluation of patient.
- ~20% of children will have fever without definable source after history and physical.

## ESSENTIAL WORKUP

- Oxygen saturation as mandatory 5th vital sign
- Resuscitate as appropriate.
- Determine duration of illness, degree, pattern and height of fever, use of antipyretics, past medical history, drug allergies, vaccination status, recent medications/antibiotics, birth history if younger than 6 mo of age, exposures, feeding, activity, urine/bowel habits, travel history, and relevant review of systems.
- Search for underlying condition.
- Initiate antipyretic therapy.

## DIAGNOSTIC TESTS & INTERPRETATION
### Lab

- CBC with differential
- Urinalysis and culture in all male infants younger than 6 mo, uncircumcised infants younger than 12 mo, and females younger than 2 yr. Urines for culture should generally be obtained by catheterization or suprapubic techniques.
- Blood culture:
  - The development of automated blood culture systems has led to more rapid detection of bacterial pathogens.
- CSF for cell counts/culture for children toxic or 0–28/30 days of age; consider for nontoxic-appearing children 28–90 days of age as well as older in whom meningitis must be excluded.

- Stool for WBCs and culture when diarrhea present and suggestion of bacterial process
- C-reactive protein (CRP) elevation is commonly found and provides confirmatory data related to the presence of infection. The sedimentation rate (ESR) is also an adjunctive measure.
- Procalcitonin is being used in some settings as additional confirmatory information.

### Imaging

- CXR to exclude pneumonia if patient tachypneic or hypoxic
- Lumbar puncture as indicated
- Other studies as indicated to evaluate for specific underlying infection

## DIFFERENTIAL DIAGNOSIS
See "Etiology."

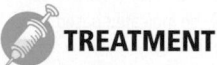 **TREATMENT**

## PRE-HOSPITAL

- Resuscitate as appropriate.
- Begin cooling with antipyretics or tepid towels.

## INITIAL STABILIZATION/THERAPY

- Treat any life-threatening conditions.
- Antipyretic therapy
- Evaporative cooling techniques, such as sponge bath, have minimal role.

## ED TREATMENT/PROCEDURES

- Focal infections require evaluation and treatment.
- Toxic children require prompt septic workup and appropriate antibiotics.
- All potential life-threatening conditions must be excluded before treating a minor acute illness, which is more common.
- Infants 0–28/30 days old need a full sepsis workup: CBC, urinalysis (UA), cultures (blood, urine, CSF), lumbar puncture. A CXR should be obtained if there is any evidence of respiratory illness:
  - Antibiotics: Cefotaxime or gentamicin and ampicillin; consider acyclovir for infants at risk for HSV
  - Admit
- Nontoxic infants 28/30–90 days old need workup, selective antibiotic use (ceftriaxone), and re-evaluation within 24 hr of admission:
  - *H. influenzae* type B and *S. pneumoniae* incidence has declined significantly with widespread vaccination.

– It is currently reasonable to perform blood culture and urine culture with selective lumbar puncture, coupled with ceftriaxone IM in low-risk patients (see definition under Disposition) if re-evaluation in 24 hr is ensured. Well-appearing infants 60–90 days of age may be managed without LP or antibiotics selectively.

– Lumbar puncture is optional in this setting, but should generally be considered if empiric antibiotics (ceftriaxone) are given to ensure that subsequent re-evaluation is not compromised.

– Presence of respiratory syncytial virus or influenza in this age group decreases but does not eliminate the risk of bacteremia and meningitis, but the rate of UTI is still appreciable.

- **Children 3 mo–3 yr of age** are evaluated selectively; those with recognizable viral syndrome (croup, stomatitis, varicella, bronchiolitis) generally do not require workup unless there is marked toxicity; antibiotic use is individualized for specific identifiable infections and pending appropriate cultures:

– Nontoxic children with temperatures >39°C and no identifiable infection should receive urinalysis/culture, chest radiograph, and CBC/blood culture as indicated, and selective empiric antibiotics.

– Children 3–6 mo of age who are incompletely immunized and have WBC >15,000/mm$^3$ and no identifiable infection may benefit from empiric antibiotics until preliminary blood cultures are available because of the risk of bacteremia.

– Widespread immunization for pneumococcus and *H. influenzae* have decreased the incidence of invasive infections by these bacteria.

- Immunocompromised children need aggressive evaluation, as do children with fever and petechiae/purpura or sickle cell disease.
- If methicillin resistant *S. aureus* is considered, clindamycin or trimethoprim-sulfamethoxazole may be useful.
- Those with underlying malignancy, central venous catheters, or ventricular-peritoneal shunts may have few findings others than fever.

## MEDICATION
### First Line
- Cefotaxime: 100–150 mg/kg/d IV q8h
- Ceftriaxone: 50–100 mg/kg/d IV/IM q12h
- Vancomycin: 40–60 mg/kg/d IV q6–8h if *S. pneumoniae* suspected until sensitivities defined
- Ampicillin: 150 mg/kg/d IV q4–q6h
- Gentamicin: 5 mg/kg/day IV divided q8

### Second Line
- Acetaminophen: 15 mg/kg per dose PO/PR (per rectum) q4–6h
- Ibuprofen: 10 mg/kg per dose PO q6–8h
- Specific antibiotics for identified or specific conditions

# FOLLOW-UP
## DISPOSITION
### Admission Criteria
- All toxic patients
- Infants 0–28/30 days of age with temperature >38°C
- Nontoxic infants 28/30–90 days of age with temperature >38°C who do not meet low-risk criteria (see definition under Discharge Criteria)
- Patients with fever and petechiae/purpura are generally admitted unless there is a specific nonlife-threatening cause.
- Immunocompromised children
- Poor compliance or follow-up

### Discharge Criteria
- Infants 28/30–90 days of age meeting low-risk criteria:
  – No prior hospitalizations, chronic illness, antibiotic therapy, prematurity
  – Reliable, mature parents with home phone, available transport, thermometer, and living in relative proximity to ED
  – No evidence of focal infection (except otitis media); nontoxic appearing; normal activity, perfusion, and hydration with age-appropriate vital signs
  – Normal WBC (5–15,000/mm$^3$), urine (negative Gram stain of unspun urine or leukocyte esterase or <5 WBC/high power field [HPF]), stool (<5 WBC/HPF) if performed, and CSF (<8 WBC/mm$^3$ and negative Gram stain) if performed
- Infants 3–36 mo of age who are nontoxic and previously healthy with good follow-up:
  – Antipyretics
  – Consider ceftriaxone and close follow-up.
- Follow-up by phone in 12–24 hr and re-evaluate in 24–48 hr with parental instructions to return if concerns develop or patient worsens.

## FOLLOW-UP RECOMMENDATIONS
Patients discharged with fever require close follow-up, usually by their primary care provider and guidelines of when to return with any change or worsening of signs or symptoms.

## PEARLS AND PITFALLS
- Fever is the most common presenting complaint in children. It may reflect a life-threatening condition.
- Children under 28/30 days of age are generally treated empirically, pending culture results.
- Older children need close follow-up and specific discharge instructions.
- Subtle findings such as tachycardia, tachypnea, or altered mental status may be indicative of significant underlying infection.

## ADDITIONAL READING
- Abramson JS, Baker CJ, Fisher MC. American Academy of Pediatrics. Committee on infectious diseases. Technical report. Prevention of pneumococcal infections, including the use of pneumococcal conjugate and polysaccharide vaccines and antibiotic prophylaxis. *Pediatrics*. 2000;106:367–376.
- American Academy of Pediatrics. *Red Book 2009 Report of the Committee on Infectious Diseases*. Elk Grove, IL: AAP; 2009.
- Baraff LJ. Management of fever without source in infants and children. *Ann Emerg Med*. 2000;36: 602–614.
- Claudius I, Baraff LJ. Pediatric emergencies associated with fever. *Emerg Med Clin North Am*. 2010;28:67–84.
- Hsiao AL, Baker MD. Fever in the new millennium: A review of recent studies of markers of serious bacterial infection in febrile children. *Curr Opin Pediatr*. 2005;17:56–61.
- Ishimine P. The evolving approach to the young child who has fever and no obvious source. *Emerg Med Clin North Am*. 2007;25:1087–1115.
- Krief WI, Levine DA, Platt SL, et al. Influenza virus infection and the risk of serious bacterial infections in young febrile infants. *Pediatrics*. 2009;124: 30–39.
- Levine DA, Platt SL, Dayan PS, et al. Risk of serious bacterial infection in young febrile infants with respiratory syncytial virus infections. *Pediatrics*. 2004;113:1728–1734.
- Oray-Schron P, Phoenix C, St. Martin D. Sepsis workup in febrile infants 0–90 days of age with respiratory syncytial virus infection. *Pediatr Emerg Care*. 2003;195:314–319.

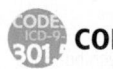

# CODES

**ICD9**
- 780.60 Fever, unspecified
- 780.61 Fever presenting with conditions classified elsewhere

# FIBROCYSTIC BREAST DISEASE

Michael W. Nielsen

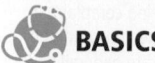 **BASICS**

## DESCRIPTION

- Generalized term for benign breast changes that are poorly defined
- Fibrocystic breast changes include:
  - Benign cysts
  - Cyclic and noncyclical mastalgia
  - Diffuse and focal nodularity
  - Fibroadenomas
  - Nipple discharge
- Term fibrocystic breast disease is considered synonymous with fibrocystic change.
- Fibrocystic breast changes:
  - Increased number of cysts or fibrous tissue in a normal breast
  - Most common of all benign breast conditions
  - Occurs in ~60% of women
  - Palpable thickening or lumpiness in the breast
  - Often associated with pain and tenderness
  - Symptoms are more prominent during the premenstrual phase and tend to improve with the onset of menses.
  - Often becomes progressively worse until menopause
  - Breast pain is most likely caused by rapid expansion of a simple cyst.
  - Breast pain alone is a rare symptom of cancer and accounts for only 0.2–2% of cases.
  - There are 3 indistinct clinical stages with significant overlap:
    ○ Termed *mazoplasia, adenosis,* and *cystic*
    ○ Each stage has predominant histological findings.
  - Synonym(s): Adenosis; benign breast disease; cystic mastitis; cystic disease of the breast; fibroadenosis; fibrocystic disease; mammary dysplasia

## ETIOLOGY

- Mechanism of development not well understood
- Considered a nonpathologic process because it is found in the majority of healthy breasts
- Enhanced or exaggerated reaction by breast tissue to cyclic levels of ovarian hormones:
  - May be caused by imbalance of the ratio of estrogen to progesterone
  - May occur secondary to increased daily prolactin production
- Most common in women 30–50 yr old
- May be carried into menopausal age with hormone replacement therapy
- Decreased incidence in women taking birth control pills
- Risk factors are controversial and may include:
  - Family history
  - Diet, including high fat intake
  - Methylxanthine-containing substances such as coffee, tea, cola, and chocolate

 **DIAGNOSIS**

## SIGNS AND SYMPTOMS
### History
- Breast pain (mastodynia) and tenderness:
  - Persistent or intermittent
  - Especially occurs during premenstrual phase of normal menstrual cycle
  - Pain is usually bilateral.
  - Pain may radiate to shoulders and upper arms.
- Lumpiness, nodularity:
  - May be localized or generalized
- Increased engorgement and breast density:
  - Breasts described as being dull and heavy
  - Fluctuations in the size of the cystic areas
- Spontaneous or expressible nipple discharge
- Nipple sensation changes, itching
- Family history of cysts is common.

### Physical Exam
- Palpate the 4 breast quadrants while patient is sitting and then while lying down.
- Identify discrete, mobile breast masses, rounded with smooth borders
- Examine for regional nodes.
- Fibrocystic changes feel doughy with vague nodularity.
- Usually more marked in the upper outer quadrants
- Small groups of cysts often described as palpating a "plate full of peas"
- Larger cysts have consistency of a balloon filled with water.
- Breast examination most sensitive 7–9 days after 1st day of menses when breasts are least congested.

## DIAGNOSTIC TESTS & INTERPRETATION
### Lab
- Prolactin and thyroid-stimulating hormone if galactorrhea is present
- Cyst aspiration cytology or biopsy of mass

### Imaging
- Diagnostic mammography if >30 yr old
- US if <30 yr old
- US:
  - Can differentiate cystic from solid breast masses
  - Useful in masses that appear on mammography
  - Benign cystic masses typically have uniform outer margin without asymmetry or irregular thickness of the cyst wall.
  - There are no echoes centrally, and posterior wall enhancement is noted.
  - Can assist in aspiration of deep cysts and nonpalpable cysts
  - Can be used to conservatively follow cyst size

- Mammography:
  - Mammographic findings of benign processes of the breast can appear as malignant.
  - Mammograms can be difficult to interpret in women <30 yr due to breast tissue density.
  - To avoid artifacts, should be performed either before aspiration or 7–10 days after aspiration.

### Diagnostic Procedures/Surgery
- Fine needle aspiration:
  - Usually done by specialist
  - Should completely evacuate cyst
  - Can be done for symptomatic or large masses
  - Allows differentiation between cystic and solid masses
  - Cells sent for cytology can diagnose cancer.
- Excisional biopsy:
  - Performed by surgeon
  - Indicated for solid lumps that are not proven benign

## DIFFERENTIAL DIAGNOSIS
- Benign breast masses:
  - Breast abscess
  - Duct ectasia
  - Mastitis
  - Simple fibroadenomas
  - Solitary papillomas
- Malignant breast masses:
  - Atypical hyperplasia
  - Complex fibroadenomas
  - Diffuse papillomatosis
  - Ductal hyperplasia without atypia
  - Sclerosing adenosis

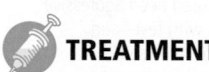 **TREATMENT**

## ED TREATMENT/PROCEDURES
- Not considered a disease process
- Majority of women will not require any medical treatment
- Conservative therapy:
  - Support bra:
    ○ Reduces tension on supporting ligaments of breast
    ○ May reduce inflammatory response and edema
  - Mild diuretic for 2–3 days before onset of menses
  - NSAIDs

- Dietary changes considered controversial:
  - Restricting dietary fat (to 25% of total calories) and eliminating caffeine
  - Increasing vitamin E and vitamin B6
  - Herbal preparations such as primrose oil
- Hormonal therapy:
  - Should be prescribed by primary care physician to enable follow-up during course of treatment
  - Oral contraceptives can decrease symptoms, particularly after 1 yr of use.
  - Danazol (synthetic androgen) and tamoxifen (partial estrogen antagonist):
    - To treat severe cyclical mastalgia
    - Shown to be equally effective
  - Bromocriptine (inhibits prolactin productions):
    - High incidence of side effects reported
- Surgical intervention:
  - If a nodule in a breast remains, excision is recommended regardless of mammographic or ultrasound findings.
  - If a large cyst recurs after aspiration on 2 occasions, it should be excised and sent for pathology.
  - Refer to general surgeon.

## MEDICATION

- Bromocriptine: 2.5–5 mg/d b.i.d.
- Danazol: 100–400 mg/d b.i.d. for 6 mo
- Tamoxifen: 10–20 mg/d
- Combined oral contraceptive pills

## FOLLOW-UP

### DISPOSITION
#### Discharge Criteria
- Patients may be discharged if the diagnosis is fibrocystic changes.
- Encourage patient to keep a breast pain record to determine whether pain is cyclic.
- It is important for patient satisfaction, as well as patient health and disease prevention, to ensure follow-up for all patients with breast masses.
- Encourage regular breast self-examination, annual physical exams, and annual mammograms, if appropriate.

#### Issues for Referral
- Lumps that persist throughout menses and are not cyclical should be further investigated with imaging and a fine needle biopsy.
- Referral to a general surgeon should be provided to diagnostically eliminate possibility of cancer.

## PEARLS AND PITFALLS

- Breast cancer may coexist with benign breast disease and fibrocystic changes:
  - Consider all cancer risk factors.
  - Confirm follow-up plan.

- Mastitis in a nonlactating patient should be treated as inflammatory carcinoma until proven otherwise.
- Fibrocystic change is usually bilateral; unilateral changes are suspicious for cancer.
- Fear of breast cancer is high in all patients:
  - Give reassurance that fibrocystic breast changes are not cancerous.
  - Low threshold for referral to specialists

## ADDITIONAL READING

- Institute for Clinical Systems Improvement (ICSI). *Diagnosis of breast disease.* Bloomington, MN: Institute for Clinical Systems Improvement; 2005.
- Marchant DJ. Benign breast disease. *Obstet Gynecol Clin North Am.* 2002;29:1–20.
- Parikh JR, Evans WP, Bassett L, et al. *Expert panel on women's imaging—Breast. Palpable breast masses.* American College of Radiology (ACR); 2005.
- Parikh JR. ACR appropriateness criteria on palpable breast masses. *J Am Coll Radiol.* 2007;4:285–288.
- Rastelli A. Breast pain, fibrocystic changes, and breast cysts. *Probl Gen Surg.* 2003;20:17–26.
- Santen RJ, Mansel R. Benign breast disorders. *N Engl J Med.* 2005;353:275–285.

## CODES

### ICD9
610.1 Diffuse cystic mastopathy

F

# FIBROMYALGIA
*Michael P. Wilson*

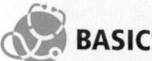

## BASICS

### DESCRIPTION
- Nonarticular, noninflammatory form of muscular and joint pain more common in females:
  - Widespread pain from stimuli that do not normally cause pain (allodynia)
  - >11 diffuse tender points
  - Fatigue
  - Sleep disturbance
  - Muscle stiffness
  - Difficulties with attention, memory
  - Limited physical findings
- Not diagnosis of exclusion, may occur with other rheumatic diseases

### ETIOLOGY
- Mechanism:
  - Painful symptoms believed to result from greater activation of pro nociceptive (pain-causing) system relative to antinociceptive (pain-dampening) system in brain and spinal cord.
- Abnormalities identified as possible mechanism:
  - Increased substance P (facilitates pro nociception)
  - Decreased biogenic amines (NE, serotonin, dopamine), which facilitate antinociception
  - Decreased gray matter in brain
  - Genetics: 1/3 of patients with fibromyalgia have close relative who is affected:
    - Candidate genes include 5-HT2A, serotonin transporter, D4 receptor, others
  - Like many complex diseases, psychologic factors play a role, with high incidence of psychiatric disorders.
  - In genetically predisposed individuals, likely starts as initial insult from age, trauma, illness, inflammation, etc.

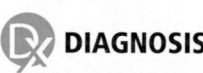

## DIAGNOSIS

### SIGNS AND SYMPTOMS
Widespread pain reported above the waist, below the waist, on the left side of the body, and on the right side of the body along with axial skeleton pain:
- Pain reported for >3 mo

### History
- Generalized musculoskeletal pain and morning stiffness
- Weakness and fatigue
- Sleep disturbance
- Muscle spasms
- Persistent fatigue not relieved with rest (consider chronic fatigue syndrome)
- Numbness or tingling in the arms or legs
- Impaired concentration or memory
- Nausea, vomiting
- Abdominal pain or discomfort relieved with bowel movements (consider irritable bowel syndrome)
- Ear pain
- Sinus pressure (consider sinusitis)
- Jaw or face pain (consider TMJ disorder)
- Temple pain (consider temporal arteritis)
- Pelvic or bladder discomfort
- Tension or migraine headaches (consider causes of chronic headache)
- Irritation or itching at introitus (consider vulvodynia)

### Physical Exam
Exam findings usually limited

### ESSENTIAL WORKUP
- History is key to diagnosis.
- In the ED, necessary only to distinguish between acute pain from trauma, injury, or new-onset medical conditions and chronic pain, which will require ongoing care and treatment.
- If a diagnosis of fibromyalgia is required, use classification criteria established by American College of Rheumatology (ACR) for fibromyalgia:
  - *Widespread* pain present for at least 3 mo defined as pain on both left and right side of body, above and below waist, and axial skeletal pain (cervical or anterior chest or thoracic spine or low back pain).
  - 11 of 18 specific tender points on digital palpation with force of <4 kg/cm (amount of pressure required to blanch thumbnail)
  - The 9 *paired* (bilateral) tender points are located at the:
    - Occiput: Suboccipital muscle insertions
    - Low cervical: Anterior aspects of C5–C7 intertransverse spaces
    - Trapezius: Midpoint of upper border
    - Supraspinatus: Above medial border of scapular spine
    - 2nd rib: 2nd costochondral junction just lateral to the junctions on upper surfaces
    - Lateral epicondyle: ~2 cm distal to epicondyles
    - Gluteal: Upper outer quadrant of buttocks
    - Greater trochanter: Posterior to trochanteric prominence
    - Knee: Medial fat pad proximal to joint line

## DIAGNOSTIC TESTS & INTERPRETATION
### Lab
- Required only for evaluation of alternative diagnoses or acute pain:
  - CBC
  - Blood chemistries
  - ESR
  - Muscle enzymes
  - Thyroid function tests
  - Urinalysis
- No specific laboratory abnormalities are characteristic of fibromyalgia.

### Imaging
No specific radiographic abnormalities are characteristic.

### Diagnostic Procedures/Surgery
Required only to evaluate causes of acute pain

### DIFFERENTIAL DIAGNOSIS
- Myofascial pain syndrome (*trigger points* present, not *tender points*)
- Chronic fatigue syndrome
- Major depression
- Polymyalgia rheumatica
- Lyme disease
- Hypothyroidism
- Collagen vascular disease
- Electrolyte imbalance
- Myopathies (metabolic and drug-induced)
- Osteomalacia
- Psychogenic rheumatism
- Eosinophilia-myalgia syndrome
- Urinary tract infection

## TREATMENT

### ED TREATMENT/PROCEDURES

- Patient education and reassurance:
  - Emphasize that fibromyalgia is not life-threatening and does not reduce life expectancy.
  - Disorder is chronic but not crippling or deforming.
  - Goal is to manage pain and improve functional disability.
- Patients will require ongoing care and should be referred to a primary physician or pain specialist.
- Pharmacologic therapy:
  - Pharmacotherapy for improving pain, relaxing muscles, and improving sleep quality has been most successful with CNS agents such as pregabalin or gabapentin.
  - Opioids are not indicated for chronic pain and may actually worsen a patient's long-term pain by acting as NDMA receptor agonists.
  - Combinations of medications (eg, amitriptyline and fluoxetine or amitriptyline and cyclobenzaprine) may be more beneficial than either medication alone.
  - Tricyclic antidepressants (TCAs; amitriptyline, nortriptyline) likely superior to SSRIs.
  - Serotonin norepinephrine reuptake inhibitors (duloxetine, milnacipran) may be more effective than SSRIs and better tolerated than TCAs.
  - Tramadol is an adjunctive agent.
  - Benzodiazepines (clonazepam) are of no benefit other than their role in sleep disturbances.
  - NSAIDs and corticosteroids have not been shown to be effective.
  - Steroids or local anesthetic (lidocaine) injection into tender points is controversial:
    - No studies available to prove efficacy

### MEDICATION

- Acetaminophen: 650 mg PO q4h
- Amitriptyline: 25–50 mg PO at bedtime
- Cyclobenzaprine: 5–10 mg PO t.i.d.
- Duloxetine: 60 mg PO daily or b.i.d.
- Gabapentin: Start 300 mg PO t.i.d., titrate upward to max of 1200 mg PO t.i.d. as tolerated
- Milnacipran: Start at 12.5 mg/d, then titrate upward to max of 50–100 mg PO b.i.d.
- Pregabalin: Start 50 mg PO t.i.d., titrate upward to max 450 mg/d PO in divided doses
- Tramadol: 300–400 mg/d PO

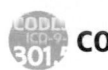

## FOLLOW-UP

### DISPOSITION

#### Admission Criteria

- Patients with serious underlying disease, intractable pain, or immunocompromised
- Patients with suicidal ideation

#### Discharge Criteria

Patients with uncomplicated fibromyalgia can be managed as outpatients.

### FOLLOW-UP RECOMMENDATIONS

Lifestyle modifications:

- Physical exercise should be encouraged:
  - Exercise program should be gradual to avoid overexertion and discouragement.
  - Aerobic exercise is more beneficial than simple stretching.
  - Efficacy not maintained if exercise stops
- Good sleep pattern should also be discussed:
  - Establishing nightly ritual in preparation for sleep
  - Avoiding caffeine-containing beverages or foods in afternoon or evenings

- Encourage stress management and coping strategies.
- Participation in educational programs (eg, cognitive-behavioral therapy):
  - Improvement is often sustained for months.

## PEARLS AND PITFALLS

As fibromyalgia patients can develop acute symptoms, distinguishing between acute and chronic pain is critical.

## ADDITIONAL READING

- Ablin JN, Buskila D, Clauw DJ. Biomarkers in fibromyalgia. *Curr Pain Headache Rep.* 2009;13(5): 343–349.
- Hansen GR. Management of chronic pain in the acute care setting. *Emerg Med Clin N Am.* 2005;23:307–338.
- Mease PJ, Choy EH. Pharmacotherapy of fibromyalgia. *Rheum Dis Clin N Am.* 2009;35: 359–372.
- Russell IJ, Larson AA. Neuropathogenesis of fibromyalgia syndrome: A unified hypothesis. *Rheum Dis Clin N Am.* 2009;35:421–435.
- Williams DA, Schilling S. Advances in the assessment of fibromyalgia. *Rheum Dis Clin N Am.* 2009;35:339–357.
- Wolfe F, Smythe HA, Yunus MB, et al. The American College of Rheumatology 1990 criteria for the classification of fibromyalgia. *Arthritis Rheum.* 1990;33(2):160–172.

## CODES

### ICD9
729.1 Myalgia and myositis, unspecified

F

# FLAIL CHEST
*Stephen L. Thornton*

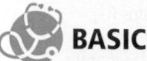 **BASICS**

## DESCRIPTION
- Free-floating segment of chest wall:
  - 3 or more adjacent ribs are fractured in 2 or more places.
  - Rib fractures in conjunction with sternal fractures or costochondral separations
- The free-floating segment of chest wall paradoxically moves inward during inspiration and outward during expiration.
- The principal pathology associated with flail chest is the *associated pulmonary contusion:*
  - There is no alteration in ventilatory mechanics owing to the free-floating segment.

## ETIOLOGY
- Blunt thoracic trauma
- Fall from a height
- Motor vehicle accident
- Assault
- Missile injury
- Ribs usually break at the point of impact or posterior angle:
  - Ribs 4–9 most prone to fracture.
  - Weakest point of ribs is 60-degree rotation from sternum.
- Transfer of kinetic energy to the lung parenchyma adjacent to the injury:
  - Disruption of the alveolocapillary membrane and development of pulmonary contusion
  - Arteriovenous shunting
  - Ventilation/perfusion mismatch
  - Hypoxemia
  - Respiratory failure may result.

### Pediatric Considerations
- Relatively elastic chest wall makes rib fractures less common in children.
- Presence of rib fractures implies much higher energy absorption.

### Geriatric Considerations
Much more susceptible to rib fractures:
- Described with low-energy mechanisms
- Complicated by osteoporosis

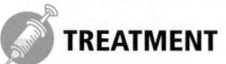 **DIAGNOSIS**

## SIGNS AND SYMPTOMS
### History
- Blunt thoracic trauma by any mechanism
- Mechanism as described by patient, parent, or prehospital personnel:
  - Seat belt usage
  - Steering wheel damage
  - Air bag deployment
- Localized chest wall pain increases with deep inspiration, coughing, moving
- Pleuritic chest pain
- Dyspnea
- Hemoptysis

### Physical Exam
- Flail chest paradoxically moves inward during inspiration and outward during expiration:
  - Initially this may not be seen because of muscle spasm and splinting respirations.
  - Inspection under tangential light may magnify paradoxical motion of the chest wall.
- Multiple rib fractures:
  - Bony step-offs
  - Ecchymosis
  - Crepitus
  - Edema
  - Erythema and tenderness associated with:
    - Splinting respirations
    - Intercostal muscle spasm
    - Dyspnea, tachypnea
  - Onset may be insidious, increasing over time.
- Cyanosis, tachycardia, hypotension
- Auscultation with initially normal breath sounds progressing to wet rales or absent breath sounds

## ESSENTIAL WORKUP
Diagnosis is initially made on clinical grounds and then supported by radiographs.

## DIAGNOSTIC TESTS & INTERPRETATION
### Lab
Arterial blood gas analysis:
- May reveal hypoxemia
- Elevated alveolar–arterial gradient

### Imaging
- Chest radiograph aids diagnosis and prognosis:
  - May reveal associated intrathoracic pathology:
    - Pneumothorax, hemothorax
    - Pneumomediastinum
    - Pulmonary contusion
    - Widened mediastinal silhouette
  - Pulmonary contusion appears within 6–12 hr after injury:
    - Ranges from patchy alveolar infiltrates to frank consolidation
- Thoracic CT is useful in detecting associated intrathoracic injuries not identified on chest radiograph:
  - Thoracic CT found to show on average of 3 additional rib fractures compared with plain chest radiographs.

## DIFFERENTIAL DIAGNOSIS
- Chest wall contusion or intercostal muscle strain
- Costochondral separation
- Sternal fracture and dislocation
- Radiographic differential diagnosis includes:
  - ARDS
  - Pulmonary laceration, infarction, or embolism
  - CHF
  - Pneumonia, abscess, other infectious process
  - Noncardiogenic causes of pulmonary edema

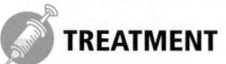 **TREATMENT**

## PRE-HOSPITAL
- Positioning the patient with the injured side down can stabilize the involved chest wall:
  - Improve ventilation in noninjured hemithorax.
- Thoracic trauma with significant mechanism or combined with pre-existing pulmonary disease should be routed to the nearest trauma center.

## INITIAL STABILIZATION/THERAPY
- Manage airway and resuscitate as indicated.
- IV line, $O_2$, continuous cardiac monitoring and pulse oximetry
- Control airway:
  - Endotracheal intubation
  - Indicated for patients with severe hypoxemia ($PaO_2$ <60 mm Hg on room air, <80 mm Hg on 100% $O_2$)
  - Significant underlying lung disease
  - Impending respiratory failure

## ED TREATMENT/PROCEDURES

- Maintain adequate oxygenation and ventilation.
- Monitor $O_2$ saturation and respiratory rate.
- In conscious and alert patients, $O_2$ administration via face mask is first-line therapy.
- If patient cannot maintain a $PaO_2$ >80 mm Hg on high-flow oxygen, consider continuous positive airway pressure via mask or nasal bilevel positive airway pressure.
- Early endotracheal intubation and mechanical ventilation if above fails:
  − Physiologic internal fixation of the flail segment
- External fixation or stabilization of the flail segment is not indicated.
- Adequate pain control is critical to maintaining adequate pulmonary function:
  − Avoid splinting, atelectasis, and pneumonia.
- Search for associated injuries and treat exacerbation of underlying lung disease.
- Intercostal nerve blocks with 0.5% bupivacaine are safe and effective when performed properly:
  − Provides 6–12 hr of pain relief
  − Perform intercostal nerve block posteriorly 2–3 fingerbreadths from the vertebral midline
  − Inject 0.5–1 mL just under the inferior surface of the rib where the neurovascular bundle is located.
  − Aspirate 1st to be certain the intercostal vessels have not been punctured.
- Prophylactic antibiotics are not indicated.

### ALERT

Avoid overhydration:

- In the setting of pulmonary contusion, the need for IV crystalloid resuscitation must be weighed against the risk of increasing interstitial pulmonary edema.

## MEDICATION

- Multiple acetaminophen/narcotic analgesic combinations are available; see alert below.
- Acetaminophen: 300 mg/codeine 30 mg (peds: 0.5–1 mg/kg codeine) PO q4–6h
- Acetaminophen: 500 mg/hydrocodone 5 mg PO q4–6h
- Acetaminophen: 750 mg/hydrocodone 7.5 mg PO q4h–q6h
- Acetaminophen: 325 mg/hydrocodone 10 mg PO q4–6h
- Acetaminophen: 325 mg/oxycodone 5 mg PO q6h
- Bupivacaine: 0.5% 0.5–1 mL per injection for intercostal nerve blocks
- Hydromorphone: 2–8 mg (peds: 0.03–0.08 mg/kg) PO q4–6h
- Hydromorphone: 1–4 mg (peds: 0.015 mg/kg) IV/IM/SC q4–6h
- Morphine sulfate: 0.05–0.1 mg/kg IV/IM/SC q2–6h
- Patient-controlled analgesia using hydromorphone or morphine sulfate is effective.

### ALERT

- Consider thoracic epidural analgesia for patients with intractable pain, oversedation, or hypoventilation secondary to narcotic analgesics.
- Avoid NSAIDs owing to the risk of gastrointestinal bleeding.
- The dose of acetaminophen/narcotic analgesic combinations is limited by the hepatic toxicity of acetaminophen.
- The maximum acetaminophen dose is 1 g per dose and 4 g/day (peds: 15 mg/kg per dose).

 **FOLLOW-UP**

## DISPOSITION

### Admission Criteria

All patients with flail chest are admitted to a critical care setting for close monitoring and adequate pain control.

### Discharge Criteria

Patients found to have flail chest, with or without pulmonary contusion, should not be discharged.

## PEARLS AND PITFALLS

- Early pain control is key.
- Beware of concomitant injuries such as pulmonary contusion and pneumothorax.
- Elderly patients have significantly poorer outcomes.

## ADDITIONAL READING

- Livingston D, Shogan B, John P, et al. Diagnosis of rib fractures and the prediction of acute respiratory failure. *J Trauma*. 2008;64:905–911.
- Wanek S, Mayberry JC. Blunt thoracic trauma: Flail chest, pulmonary contusion, and blast injury. *Crit Care Clin*. 2004;20(1):71–81.
- Ullman E, Donley L, Brady W. Pulmonary trauma: Emergency department evaluation and management. *Emerg Med Clin North Am*. 2003;21:291–313.
- Eckstein M, Henderson S. Thoracic trauma. In: Marx J, Hockberger R, Walls R, eds. *Rosen's Emergency Medicine: Concepts and Clinical Practice*, 7th ed. St. Louis: Mosby; 2009.

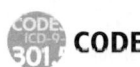 **CODES**

### ICD9

807.4 Flail chest

F

# FOOT FRACTURE
*Colleen Campbell*

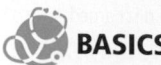 **BASICS**

## DESCRIPTION
Injury to tarsal bones or metatarsals including calcaneus, talus, navicular, cuboid, cuneiform, and metatarsals

## ETIOLOGY
- Most common foot injuries are of the metatarsals and phalanges.
- The calcaneus is the most commonly fractured of the tarsal bones.
- Calcaneus fractures: Compression injury from sudden high-velocity impact to heel:
  - 75% are intra-articular; 50% have associated injuries:
    - 10% spine fractures
    - 25% with associated lower extremity trauma
    - 9% bilateral, 5% open
- Metatarsal fractures: Divided into stress fractures, twisting injuries, or direct trauma:
  - 1st metatarsal: Direct applied force
  - 2nd and 3rd metatarsals are most often involved in stress fractures and twisting injuries.
  - 5th metatarsal: Avulsion fracture (dancer's fracture) of proximal apophysis is most common injury.
  - Jones fracture: Transverse fracture of the metaphyseal-diaphyseal junction of 5th metatarsal; results from twisting while foot inverted.
- Talus: Caused by dorsiflexion with axial load, common snowboarder's injury
- Navicular: Results from axial compression or stress fractures

- Cuboid and cuneiform fractures are rare and occur in conjunction with other injuries, often with tarsal-metatarsal injuries.
- Tarsal-metatarsal injuries (Lisfranc injuries) are high-energy injuries:
  - Axial load on plantar-flexed foot, or hindfoot fixed with forced foot eversion
  - Unstable forefoot on hindfoot
  - 20% go undiagnosed on initial visit.
  - 3 types: Convergent, divergent, and incongruent

### Pediatric Considerations
- Metatarsal fractures account for 90% of foot fractures in children, usually from direct trauma:
  - Lesser metatarsal fractures (2–4) most common followed by base of 5th then base of 1st metatarsal.
  - Physeal injury may occur with proximal 1st metatarsal fractures.
- Other common injuries include phalangeal fractures (17%) and navicular fractures (5%).
- Fractures of talus or calcaneus occur with distal tibia or fibula fractures (8%).
- Calcaneus fractures are less likely intra-articular. Less common to have associated spine fractures.

 **DIAGNOSIS**

## SIGNS AND SYMPTOMS
### History
- History of preceding trauma most common
- Stress fractures may present with increasing pain in setting of repetitive activities.

### Physical Exam
- Ecchymosis, pain, swelling, or deformity of foot
- Pain with weight bearing
- Joint instability

## ESSENTIAL WORKUP
- Physical exam of extremity is necessary to assess neurovascular status, skin integrity, gross swelling, deformity, or loss of function.
- Examination of spine is also essential in suspected calcaneus fractures, as there is a 10% incidence of coexistent injury.
- Anterior-posterior/lateral and oblique views are necessary for all foot fractures.
- Complications:
  - Compartment syndrome most commonly presents as severe pain in a swollen foot:
    - Pressures >35 mm Hg require opening of all major foot compartments.
    - May have hypesthesia of plantar foot
    - Weak toe flexion
    - Late findings include claw toe deformity.
  - Nonunion and avascular necrosis are common complications with talar neck fractures owing to distal blood supply.
  - Calcaneus fractures may be accompanied by sural nerve injury; test sensation along lateral aspect of foot.

## DIAGNOSTIC TESTS & INTERPRETATION
### Imaging
Special views may be needed for some fractures:
- Lisfranc fractures may require stress views with weight bearing. They may require MRI to evaluate ligamentous stability.
- Talar fractures may require a 45-degree internal oblique view. May require CT.
- Midfoot fractures may require an external oblique foot view.

- Calcaneus fractures require an axial view and may require CT:
  - Boehler angle <20 degrees suggests a compression fracture of calcaneus.
  - Lumbosacral spine films are necessary in all patients with calcaneus fractures.
- Stress fractures may require 2 wk to appear on plain films; bone scan or CT may be used to elucidate suspected fractures.

## DIFFERENTIAL DIAGNOSIS

- Anterior effects of calcaneus and talar dome fractures can be misdiagnosed as ankle sprains.
- Foot contusions
- Freiberg's disease: Osteochondrosis of 2nd metatarsal head may be mistaken for stress fracture.

 TREATMENT

### PRE-HOSPITAL

- Ice bag should be placed on affected foot and foot and ankle immobilized.
- All patients suspected of calcaneus fracture should have spinal immobilization; often, mechanism is fall from height >6 feet

### INITIAL STABILIZATION/THERAPY
Manage coexisting trauma as indicated.

### ED TREATMENT/PROCEDURES

- Airway, breathing, and circulation management
- Assess for neurovascular compromise distal to fracture site.
- Dislocations must be reduced as quickly as possible with assessment of neurovascular status before and after procedure:
  - Procedural sedation usually required

- Immobilize, ice, and elevate in a bulky splint:
  - Application of circumferential cast should be delayed until swelling subsides.
- Crutches
- Pain management:
  - If large amount of swelling and pain with toe movement, suspect compartment syndrome.
- Orthopedic consult indicated early for displaced fractures:
  - Many injuries require repair within 6 hr of injury to prevent delay of open reduction with internal fixation for 6–10 days owing to swelling.

### MEDICATION

- Cefazolin: 1 g IV/IM (peds: 25 mg/kg IV/IM)
- Diprivan: 40 mg IV q10s until sedation
- Etomidate: 0.1–0.2 mg/kg IV
- Fentanyl: 50–250 $\mu$g IV titrated (peds: 2 $\mu$g/kg IV)
- Hydromorphone 0.5 – 2 mg IV q2h (peds: 015 mg/kg IV q4–6h)
- Ibuprofen: 800 mg PO (peds: 10 mg/kg PO)
- Meperidine: 25–100 mg IV/IM titrated (peds: 1–1.75 mg/kg IV/IM)
- Methohexital: 1.0–1.5 mg/kg IV
- Morphine: 2–10 mg IV/IM titrated (peds: 0.1 mg/kg IV)

 FOLLOW-UP

### DISPOSITION
#### Admission Criteria

- Open fracture
- Evidence of compartment syndrome or neurovascular injury
- Open reduction internal fixation required immediately

### Discharge Criteria
Most patients with metatarsal fractures can be discharged with orthopedic follow-up.

### Issues for Referral
All open fractures, as well as all midfoot/Lisfranc injuries and displaced fractures that are not successfully reduced, should be seen in ED by an orthopedic specialist.

## ADDITIONAL READING

- Banarjee R, Nickishch F, Easley ME, et al. Foot fractures. *Browner Skeletal Trauma*, 4th ed. (Vol. 2, Chapter 61). Philadelphia: Saunders; 2008.
- Desmond EA, Chou LP. Current concepts review: Lisfranc injuries. *Foot Ankle Int.* 2006;8:653–660.
- Green NE, Swiontkowski M. *Skeletal Trauma in Children: Foot Fractures,* 4th ed. (Chapter 16). Philadelphia: Saunders; 2008.
- Newton EJ, Love L. Emergency department management of selected orthopedic injuries. *Emerg Med Clin N Am.* 2007;3:763–793.

 CODES

### ICD9

- 825.20 Fracture of unspecified bone(s) of foot (except toes), closed
- 825.21 Fracture of astragalus, closed
- 825.22 Fracture of navicular (scaphoid) bone of foot, closed

F

# FOREARM FRACTURE, SHAFT/DISTAL

Trevor J. Mills
Peter DeBlieux

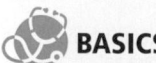 **BASICS**

## DESCRIPTION

- Forearm shaft fractures (single or paired) are often displaced by contraction of arm muscles; sometimes associated with concurrent dislocations:
  - *Galeazzi* fracture:
    - Distal radius fracture with distal radioulnar dislocation
  - *Monteggia* fracture:
    - Proximal ulnar fracture with dislocation of radial head
- Distal fractures include extension, flexion, and intra-articular classifications:
  - *Colles* fracture:
    - Hyperextension fracture of distal radius
    - Distal fragment displaced dorsally
    - Radial deviation
    - May also involve ulnar styloid and distal radioulnar joint
  - *Smith* fracture:
    - Hyperflexion fracture of distal radius
    - Distal fragment displaced volarly
  - *Barton* fracture:
    - Intra-articular fracture of dorsal rim of distal radius
    - Often associated with dislocation of carpal bones
  - *Hutchinson* fracture:
    - Intra-articular fracture of radial styloid

### Pediatric Considerations

- Shaft fractures:
  - *Torus* fracture:
    - Compression (buckling) of cortex on 1 or both sides
  - *Greenstick* fracture:
    - Distraction of 1 side of cortex with opposite side intact
  - Plastic deformity:
    - Bowing of radius or ulna without apparent disruption of cortex
    - Multiple microfractures
- Distal fractures:
  - *Salter-Harris*–type fractures (see Salter-Harris classification)

## ETIOLOGY

- Direct blow to forearm
- Longitudinal compression load:
  - Fall on outstretched hand (FOOSH)
  - Horizontal force
- Excessive pronation, supination, hyperextension, or hyperflexion

 **DIAGNOSIS**

## SIGNS AND SYMPTOMS

- Deformity
- Pain, edema, erythema

### History

- Associated events and concurrent injuries
- Past history of bone disease or old fractures
- History of repetitive stress of forearm movement
- Occupation
- Hand dominance

### Physical Exam

- Physical exam with special attention to skin integrity, deformity, and neurovascular status
- Forearm pain, crepitus, tenderness to palpation, deformity, shortening of forearm
- Forearm edema, ecchymosis, elbow or wrist joint effusions
- Abnormal mobility or loss of function at elbow/wrist/hand
- Neurologic abnormalities
- Vascular compromise

### ALERT
Impending compartment syndrome

## ESSENTIAL WORKUP
Suspected forearm fractures require anteroposterior (AP) and lateral radiographs, including joint above and joint below injury: Hand, wrist, and elbow.

## DIAGNOSTIC TESTS & INTERPRETATION
### Lab
Preoperative labs as warranted

### Imaging
Some intra-articular fractures may require CT imaging.

### Diagnostic Procedures/Surgery
Compartment pressures should be measured for suspected compartment syndrome.

## DIFFERENTIAL DIAGNOSIS

- Upper extremity muscle, ligamentous injury
- Elbow or wrist dislocations, including pediatric nursemaid's elbow
- Forearm contusions, hematomas
- Cellulitis, abscesses, soft tissue masses
- Forearm osteogenic tumors
- Osteomyelitis
- Upper extremity vascular or neurologic injuries
- Elbow or wrist arthritis, joint effusions
- Pediatric growth plates, nutrient vessels may be mistaken for fractures

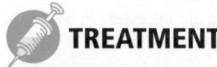 **TREATMENT**

## PRE-HOSPITAL

- All suspected forearm fractures should be elevated, splinted, and immobilized, including elbow and wrist joints.
- All open fractures should be wrapped with sterile dressing before immobilization:
  - Do not reduce open fractures back under skin in the field.
  - In patients with isolated extremity trauma, analgesia may be administered.

## ED TREATMENT/PROCEDURES

- Shaft fractures, nondisplaced:
  - Long-arm splint
  - Orthopedic referral
- Shaft fractures, displaced:
  - Orthopedic consultation
  - Often require open reduction, internal fixation
- Distal fractures, nondisplaced:
  - Forearm sugar-tong or AP splint
  - Orthopedic referral
- Distal fractures: *Colles/Smith:*
  - Simple, noncomminuted, extra-articular Colles and Smith fractures may be reduced in ED:
    - Splint (long-arm sugar-tong splint)
    - Sling
    - Referred to orthopedics
  - Complicated Colles and Smith fractures require orthopedic consultation.
- Distal fractures: *Barton/Hutchinson:*
  - Uncomplicated Barton and Hutchinson fractures
    - Splint (AP or sugar-tong splint)
    - Place in sling
    - Referred to orthopedics
  - Complicated fractures require orthopedic consultation.
- Open fractures:
  - Cover with sterile dressings.
  - IM/IV antibiotics
  - Tetanus immunization (if indicated)
  - Splint
  - Immediate orthopedic consultation
- Forearm fractures associated with compartment syndrome or neurovascular compromise require immediate orthopedic consultation.

### Pediatric Considerations
- *Torus* and *Greenstick* fractures with <10° of angulation may be treated with long-arm splint, sling, and orthopedic referral.
- *Plastic deformities* require orthopedic consultation:
  - Some minimally displaced plastic deformities may be placed in long-arm splint and sling.
- *Salter-Harris*–type fractures require orthopedic consultation.

## MEDICATION
- Acetaminophen: 325–1,000 mg PO q4h (peds: 10–15 mg/kg q4h PO)
- Antibiotics:
  - Open fractures require IM/IV antibiotics.
  - Cefazolin: 1–2 g IM/IV or equivalent 1st-generation cephalosporin; if contaminated, add an aminoglycoside
- Codeine: 15–60 mg PO/IM q4h (peds: >2 yr, 0.5–1.0 mg/kg q4h PO/IM)
- Hydrocodone: 5–10 mg PO q4h
- Ibuprofen: 200–800 mg q4–8h (peds >6 mo, 5–10 mg/kg per dose q6h)
- Morphine sulfate: 2–10 mg IV/IM; titrate to pain (peds: 0.1 mg/kg per dose IV/IM)
- Tetanus (Td): 0.5 mL IM every 10 yr

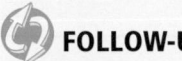 **FOLLOW-UP**

## DISPOSITION
### Admission Criteria
- Open fractures
- Fractures with compartment syndrome or neurovascular compromise
- Fractures needing immediate operative management or general anesthesia for reduction
- Suspected child abuse

### Discharge Criteria
- Appropriate reduction and immobilization
- Arranged orthopedic follow-up
- Adequate pain control measures
- Cast/splint care discharge instructions provided and understood by patient
- Documentation of intact neurovascular function after ED treatment

### Issues for Referral
All fractures (or suspected fractures) discharged from ED should be referred to orthopedic surgeon for close follow-up.

## FOLLOW-UP RECOMMENDATIONS
All patients should be referred to an orthopedic surgeon or hand surgeon.

## PEARLS AND PITFALLS
- Missed 2nd fracture
- Missed concurrent dislocation or subluxation
- Impending compartment syndrome

## ADDITIONAL READING
- Dicke TE, Nunley JA. Distal forearm fractures in children: Complications and surgical indications. *Orthop Clin North Am*. 1993;24(2):333.
- Handoll HH, Pearce P. Interventions for isolated diaphyseal fractures of the ulna in adults. *Cochrane Database Syst Rev*. 2009;(3):CD000523.
- Perron AD. Evaluation and management of the high-risk orthopedic emergency. *Emerg Med Clin North Am*. 2003;21(1):159–204.
- Szabo RM. Extra-articular fractures of the distal radius. *Orthop Clin North Am*. 1993;24(2):229.

 **CODES**

### ICD9
- 813.40 Closed fracture of lower end of forearm, unspecified
- 813.42 Other closed fractures of distal end of radius (alone)
- 813.43 Fracture of distal end of ulna (alone), closed

F

# FOREIGN BODY, EAR

Kathleen Nasci
Charles V. Pollack, Jr.

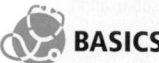 **BASICS**

## DESCRIPTION
- Foreign bodies lodged in the external auditory canal
- The external auditory canal:
  - Cartilaginous and bony passage lined with periosteum and skin
  - The periosteum is extremely sensitive, making removal a very painful procedure:
    - In small children general anesthesia may be required to remove the object.
  - Foreign bodies usually impact at the junction of the inner end of the cartilaginous portion of the canal or at the isthmus.
- Inanimate foreign objects are often associated with delayed presentations:
  - Children often delay reporting because of fear of punishment.
  - Often the foreign body is an incidental finding in children during an ear exam.
- Children and psychiatric patients may insert anything sufficiently small to enter the external auditory canal.
- Ear foreign bodies are most common in children <8 yr.
- Complications:
  - Canal laceration:
    - Usually caused by repeated attempts to remove a nongraspable object
  - Perforation of tympanic membrane:
    - More likely to result from removal procedure than the foreign body
  - Otitis externa
  - Malocclusion from erosion into the temporomandibular joint
  - Parapharyngeal abscess
  - Mastoiditis
  - Meningitis
  - Brain abscess
- Symptoms usually resolve within a few days after foreign body removal

## ETIOLOGY
- Children:
  - Stones
  - Small beads
  - Paper
  - Toys
  - Seeds and popcorn kernels
  - Beans and other food and organic materials
  - Button batteries:
    - High risk of tissue necrosis compared with other foreign bodies
- Competent adults:
  - Cotton-swab tips
  - Earplugs
  - Insects:
    - Cockroach most common in U.S.
  - Hidden illicit drugs

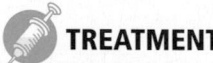 **DIAGNOSIS**

## SIGNS AND SYMPTOMS
- Decreased hearing
- Excessive crying in infants
- Unilateral ear pain
- Fullness
- Loud noises
- Buzzing sound (with live insects)
- Nausea
- Dizziness
- Ipsilateral tearing
- Purulent discharge from the external ear
- Itching
- Bleeding

### History
- Travel or camping history or poor living conditions suggests insects in the external ear canal.
- Inquire about previous attempts to remove the foreign body and any trauma associated with these attempts.

### Physical Exam
Otoscopic exam should be performed before and after removal of the foreign body:
- Identify type of foreign body to determine removal procedure:
  - Button battery
  - Live insect
  - Vegetable
  - Inanimate object
  - Size
  - Risk of swelling when exposed to water
- Perform a bilateral exam; especially important in children and psychiatric patients, and prevents overlooking a quiescent foreign body in the contralateral ear.
- Attempt to visualize tympanic membrane to assess for rupture.
- Assess for otitis externa.
- Assess for retained fragments after the removal.

## ESSENTIAL WORKUP
Careful otoscopic exam:
- Minimize pain.
- Gain the patient's trust.
- Identify the foreign body before attempting removal.

## DIAGNOSTIC TESTS & INTERPRETATION
### Lab
None indicated

### Imaging
CT scan if infectious or erosive sequelae are suspected

### Diagnostic Procedures/Surgery
Otomicroscope microscope:
- May be used when standard ED techniques fail or the equipment is available to emergency medical staff

## DIFFERENTIAL DIAGNOSIS
- Cerumen impaction
- Granuloma
- Hematoma
- Injury
- Otitis externa
- Perforated tympanic membrane
- Residual otitis externa after self-extraction of the foreign body
- Tumor

## TREATMENT

### PRE-HOSPITAL
- Cautions:
  - Severe ear pain, sensation of movement, and loud, buzzing sound:
    - Typical signs of a live insect in external auditory canal
    - Instill warm lidocaine or mineral oil into affected ear to kill insect
- Controversies:
  - Attempts at removal in the field are not indicated:
    - Lack of appropriate equipment
    - Prior failed attempts may make future attempts more difficult.

### INITIAL STABILIZATION/THERAPY
For a patient in distress because of a live insect:
- Drown or immobilize insect before any removal attempts
- Instill warm solution into the external auditory canal:
  - 2% lidocaine solution
  - Ether
  - Alcohol
  - Mineral oil
- Cold fluids should not be used so as to avoid a caloric response.

### ED TREATMENT/PROCEDURES
- Prepare the equipment and the patient:
  - Strong light source
  - Otoscope or operating microscope
  - Achieve proper head immobilization
  - Retract the pinna of the ear in a posterosuperior direction to straighten the canal

- Analgesia:
  - Lidocaine instillation for topical anesthesia:
    - Liquid 1–2% solution is preferred to viscous lidocaine.
    - Lidocaine injection of the 4 quadrants of the canal using a tuberculin syringe through the otoscope
    - 1–2% lidocaine, with or without epinephrine
- Procedural sedation:
  - Indicated for children and uncooperative adults
  - Use before attempts, as unsuccessful efforts may produce bleeding, edema, or injury to the tympanic membrane
  - Ketamine for children
  - Benzodiazepines for older patients
  - Consider fentanyl if analgesia is indicated during removal.
- Options for removal:
  - Water irrigation:
    - Perform careful visualization.
    - Place an Angiocath catheter adjacent to, or preferably distal to, the foreign body.
    - Inject warm water or sterile saline through catheter via a syringe.
    - Backwash the foreign body out.
    - Never attempt removal by irrigation when the foreign body is a button battery.
  - Use of instruments to dislodge the foreign body:
    - Alligator forceps removal
    - Cupped forceps: Numbers 3, 5, and 7 suction tips, preferably with Frazier suction cups
    - Cerumen loops
    - Right-angle blunt hooks
  - Suction catheters:
    - Best used for small objects
    Fogarty catheter:
    - Carefully pass beyond the foreign body and inflate and withdraw; this approach puts the tympanic membrane at particular risk of inadvertent injury.
  - Cyanoacrylate glue on the tip of a blunt probe:
    - Place on the foreign body for 10 seconds, and then pull.
    - May contaminate the ear with glue, and this technique has been associated with tympanic membrane rupture.
  - Acetone:
    - Used to dissolve Styrofoam foreign bodies or loosen superglue
  - Otomicroscopy:
    - Usually performed in the OR although reports of use in the ED have been positive
- Vegetable matter:
  - Avoid irrigation of foreign bodies that will swell when exposed to water.
  - Attempt removal with instrument.
  - Forceps usually work with graspable objects.
  - Be certain to delineate clearly between foreign body and inflamed external auditory canal tissue.

- Nonvegetable inanimate foreign body removal:
  - If easily grasped, attempt removal with forceps.
  - If not accessible, attempt removal with irrigation.
- Polished or smooth object extraction:
  - Visualize.
  - Direct suction
  - Blunt right-angled probe: Pass beyond the foreign body; rotate 90 degrees; remove it with the foreign body.
  - Fogarty catheter
  - Cyanoacrylate glue
- Insect removal:
  - Kill insect by rapidly instilling alcohol, 2% lidocaine (Xylocaine), or mineral oil into the ear.
  - Once killed, remove with forceps or by irrigation.
  - Reexamine to ensure that all insect parts are removed.
- Sharp objects:
  - Remove with operating microscope. Consider otolaryngologic referral if there is evidence of trauma or if patient is uncooperative.

## MEDICATION

### First Line

- Fentanyl. 1 μg/kg
- Ketamine: 1–2 mg/kg IV or 4 mg/kg IM
- Midazolam: 1 mg IV slowly q2–3min up to 5 mg (peds: 6 mo–5 yr, .05–.1 mg/kg, titrate to maximum of .6 mg/kg; 6–12 yr, .025–.05 mg/kg, titrate to max of .4 mg/kg)

### Second Line
- Cortisporin Otic: 4 gtt in ear q.i.d.
- Amoxicillin: 500 mg PO t.i.d. (peds: 80–90 mg/kg/24 h) PO b.i.d. for 7–10 days.
- Augmentin: 875 mg (peds: 90 mg/kg/24 h) PO b.i.d. for 7–10 days

 **FOLLOW-UP**

### DISPOSITION
### Admission Criteria
Hospital admission if the foreign body is a button battery that cannot be removed

### Discharge Criteria
- Foreign body removed
- Inability to remove a foreign body that will not cause rapid tissue necrosis
- Oral antibiotics (amoxicillin or Augmentin) should be initiated in cases with tympanic membrane perforation.

### Issues for Referral
Follow-up with ENT specialist as an outpatient:
- Inability to remove a foreign body
- Immunocompromised patients with signs of otitis externa

## FOLLOW-UP RECOMMENDATIONS
- Patient should be instructed not to place any objects in ear.
- A short course of analgesics after traumatic foreign body removal
- Otitis externa:
  - Topical antimicrobial such as Cortisporin suspension
- Immunocompromised patients may require oral antibiotics.
- Perforated tympanic membrane:
  - Prophylaxis with antibiotics
  - Follow-up with ENT specialist
- Avoid submersion in water until follow-up if trauma or infection present.

## PEARLS AND PITFALLS
- Use procedural sedation with uncooperative patients or when a difficult removal is anticipated.
- Irrigation in patients with button batteries in the ear should never be performed as the electrical current or battery contents can cause liquefaction tissue necrosis.

## ADDITIONAL READING
- Brown L, Denmark TK, Wittlake WA, et al. Procedural sedation use in the ED: Management of pediatric ear and nose foreign bodies. *Am J Emerg Med.* 2004;22(4):310–314.
- Cederberg CA, Kerschner JE. Otomicroscope in the emergency department management of pediatric ear foreign bodies. *Int J Pediatr Otorhinolaryngol.* 2009;73(4):589–591.
- Davies PH, Benger JR. Foreign bodies in the nose and ear: A review of techniques for removal in the emergency department. *J Accid Emerg Med.* 2000;17:91–94.
- Heim SW, Maughan KL. Foreign bodies in the ear, nose, and throat. *Am Fam Physician* 2007;76(8): 1185–1189.
- Kumar S, Kumar M, Lesser T, et al. Foreign bodies in the ear: A simple technique for removal analysed in vitro. *Emerg Med J.* 2005;22(4):266–268.

### See Also (Topic, Algorithm, Electronic Media Element)
- Tympanic Membrane Perforation
- Procedural Sedation

## CODES

### ICD9
931 Foreign body in ear

# FOREIGN BODY, ESOPHAGEAL

*Jason J. Prystowsky*

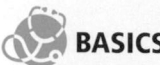

## BASICS

### DESCRIPTION
- Esophageal foreign bodies (FBs) typically lodge at 3 sites of physiologic constriction:
  - Cricopharyngeal muscle—63%, most common (C6)
  - Gastroesophageal junction—20% (T11)
  - Aortic arch—10% (T4)
- 90% of ingested FBs pass spontaneously.
- 10–20% are removed endoscopically, and 1% or less require surgery.

### ETIOLOGY
- Most common adult and adolescent FBs are food boluses and bones:
  - 88–97% of adults with food bolus impaction have underlying pathology.
  - Esophageal stricture, esophageal spasm, achalasia, esophageal motor disorder, tight fundoplication wraps, webs, extrinsic compression, esophageal cancer, eosinophilic esophagitis
  - Benign esophageal stenosis caused by Schatzki B-rings or peptic strictures are most common.
- Increased risk:
  - Edentulous adults
  - Intoxicated patients
  - Patients with underlying esophageal disease

### *Pediatric Considerations*
- 80% of foreign body (FB) ingestions occur in pediatric age group, peak ages 6 mo to 6 yr, particularly younger than 2 yr.
- Coins:
  - Most common: 80% of esophageal FBs
- Predisposing factor: Esophageal strictures

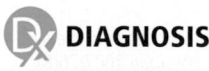

## DIAGNOSIS

### SIGNS AND SYMPTOMS
- Acute ingestion:
  - Dysphagia
  - Odynophagia
  - Drooling
  - Vomiting
  - Choking
  - Gagging
  - Blood-stained saliva
- Chronically retained FB:
  - Respiratory symptoms predominate (paraesophageal tissue swelling compromises adjacent trachea):
    - Cough
    - Stridor
    - Hoarseness
- Chest pain
- Site of FB sensation usually corresponds to esophageal level of FB
- Esophageal perforation (15–35% if ingest sharp object):
  - Redness
  - Swelling
  - Crepitus in the neck
  - Peritonitis
- <20% asymptomatic

### *Pediatric Considerations*
Infants: Signs/symptoms:
- Refusal to eat
- Stridor
- Upper respiratory tract infection
- Neck/throat pain

### *History*
- Adults:
  - Dysphagia, odynophagia, chest discomfort, drooling, retching (often self induced), stridor, choking, coughing:
    - 80% present within first 24 hr
    - 5% will present with airway obstruction (café coronary)
  - Children:
    - 50% asymptomatic
    - Drooling, refusal to eat, unexplained gagging, cough, wheeze, choking
    - More likely than adults to have respiratory symptoms

### ESSENTIAL WORKUP
- History about object ingested: Type, when, and how
- Physical exam focused by degree of distress exhibited:
  - Esophagus for:
    - Obstruction
    - Perforation
    - Hemorrhage
  - Oropharynx:
    - Red, irritated throat
    - Palatal abrasions
  - Lung:
    - Stridor and wheezing
  - Abdomen:
    - Peritonitis or bowel obstruction
- Direct or indirect laryngoscopy can be useful.

## DIAGNOSTIC TESTS & INTERPRETATION
### *Imaging*
- Biplane chest radiograph including all of neck for FB localization:
  - Need for additional radiographs dictated by clinical situation
  - Those with food bolus need no radiographs usually.
  - Esophageal FBs usually align themselves in coronal plane.
  - Esophageal perforation is noted by air in retropharyngeal space, in soft tissues of neck, or by pneumomediastinum.
- Esophageal contrast studies for nonradiopaque FBs:
  - Radiolucent objects (small pieces of glass, bone fragments, aluminum, plastic, pieces of wood)
  - Thin barium esophagogram: Changes in contour of barium column localize FB.
  - Passage of contrast solution into stomach: Partial versus complete obstruction
  - Contraindicated if evidence of perforation
  - Cautions:
    - Oral contrast in high-grade esophageal obstructions can increase risk of aspiration, and barium may coat mucosa, limiting subsequent endoscopy.
    - Traditional water-soluble contrast can cause severe tissue reaction in perforations because of its hyperosmolality.
- Commercially available metal detectors have been used in localizing ingested metal, particularly coins in pediatric population with 98–100% sensitivity.
- Endoscopy:
  - Method of choice for localizing and managing most esophageal FBs
  - Ability to inspect surrounding esophageal mucosa for pathology
  - Both diagnostic and therapeutic
- CT can often detect FBs not identified by other means, especially if use 3D reconstruction and can detect complications of perforation, fistula, or abscess

## DIFFERENTIAL DIAGNOSIS
- Globus hystericus phenomenon ("lump in throat")
- Esophagitis
- Croup
- Epiglottitis
- Upper respiratory tract infection
- Retropharyngeal abscess

## TREATMENT

### PRE-HOSPITAL
Cautions:
- Airway maintenance and prevention of aspiration paramount
- Oxygen for patients in distress
- Place patient in whatever position gives most comfort.
- Ipecac and cathartics contraindicated

### INITIAL STABILIZATION/THERAPY
- Airway, breathing, and circulation management 1st priority
- Prevent aspiration

### ED TREATMENT/PROCEDURES
- FBs lodged in upper or mid-esophagus:
  - Extraction required
- Asymptomatic patients with coins or smooth objects (not button batteries) in distal esophagus:
  - Observe up to 24 hr after ingestion to see whether it will pass into stomach.
    Danger of perforation increases after 24 hr.
- Impacted food bolus obstructing esophagus:
  - Emergent removal indicated
  - Digestion with proteolytic enzymes (papain) not recommended because of serious morbidity including esophageal perforation, hypernatremia, and aspiration
- Extricate sharp or pointed esophageal FBs regardless of their location:
  Perforation incidence ranges from 15–35%
  - Objects most commonly associated with complications are:
    - Chicken and fish bones
    - Straightened paper clips
    - Toothpicks
    - Needles
    - Bread bag clips
    - Dental bridgework
  - Direct laryngoscopy can be performed if above cricopharyngeus.
  - Objects that reach stomach and are shorter than 5 cm and <2 cm in diameter usually pass through GI tract without difficulty, but daily radiographs are still recommended.
- Button batteries:
  - Extract emergently wherever they lodge in esophagus
  - Batteries frequently leak: Potassium hydroxide and mercuric oxide are most toxic constituents.
  - Alkali produced from external flow of current can cause liquefaction necrosis.
  - Full-thickness mucosal burns can occur within 4–6 hr (combination of chemical, electrical, pressure injuries).
  - Battery in stomach will usually pass without difficulty:
    - Batteries remaining in stomach for >3–4 days should be removed.
    - Large-diameter batteries (>20 mm) should be removed from stomach after 48 hr.
  - Once past duodenal sweep, 85% are passed within 72 hr.

- Narcotic/amphetamine packets:
  - Body packing seen in regions of high drug traffic
  - Packets usually seen on radiographs
  - Rupture or leakage of contents can be fatal.
- Removal techniques:
  - Fluoroscopically guided Foley catheter extraction:
    - Successful and safe in experienced hands
    - Foley catheter (10–16 French) placed nasally, passed into esophagus, tip and balloon pushed beyond FB under fluoroscopic control
    - Foley balloon inflated with contrast and catheter slowly withdrawn
    - Contraindicated in chronic ingestions, uncooperative patients, sharp-pointed objects
  - Foley catheters may also be used to push distal FB into stomach
- Endoscopy:
  - Preferred method to remove acute or chronic FBs
  - 98% effective
  - Always used with impactions of long duration (>2–4 days) because of associated esophageal irritation/edema
  - General endotracheal anesthesia needed in difficult cases: Infants, psychiatric patients, difficult FB
  - Risk of complications increases after 24 hr, ideal to be done within 6–12 hr
  - Bougienage: Using dilator to push FB into stomach
  - Has been shown to be effective in experienced hands if endoscopy is unavailable
- IV glucagon:
  - Decreases lower esophageal sphincter tone without interfering with esophageal contractions
  - Falling out of favor for endoscopy
    Less effective if underlying Schatzki ring or stricture
  - Permits distal food boluses to pass into the stomach
  - For impactions <24-hr duration
  - Contraindicated if known insulinoma, pheochromocytoma, Zollinger-Ellison syndrome
- Gas-forming agents:
  - Useful in patients with esophageal food impactions <24 hr
  - Combining intravenous glucagon followed by oral gas-forming agents has also been successful.
  - Method has been occasionally associated with perforation.
- Surgical intervention:
  - Reserved for patients in whom FB cannot be removed by other methods
  - ~1–2% of all patients
  - Toothpicks and bones common objects

### MEDICATION
- E-Z Gas: 30 mL solution (NaHCO₃, citric acid, and simethicone) orally
- Glucagon: 1–2 mg IV push after test dose to determine hypersensitivity

## FOLLOW-UP

### DISPOSITION
#### Admission Criteria
- Seriously ill patients and those with complications such as esophageal perforation, migration of FB through esophageal wall, significant bleeding
- Airway compromise
- Symptomatic patients in whom attempts to remove FB are unsuccessful

#### Discharge Criteria
- Asymptomatic patients in whom FB has been removed or passed distal to esophagus
- Asymptomatic patients with distal esophageal smooth FBs need re-examination within 12–24 hr to ascertain whether spontaneous passage into stomach has occurred.

#### Issues for Referral
GI consult for sharp or pointed esophageal FBs, those obstructed in upper or mid esophagus and battery button FBs.

### FOLLOW-UP RECOMMENDATIONS
GI referral for patients with suspected underlying etiology for esophageal obstruction

## PEARLS AND PITFALLS
- Perform radiographs to locate radio-opaque FBs.
- Maintain a high suspicion for esophageal perforation.

## ADDITIONAL READING
- Eisen GM, Baron TH, Dominitz JA, et al. Guideline for the management of ingested foreign bodies. *Gastrointest Endosc.* 2002;55:802–806.
- Mosca S, Manes G, Martion R, et al. Endoscopic management of foreign bodies in the upper gastrointestinal tract: Report on a series of 414 adult patients. *Endoscopy* 2001;33:692–696.
- Ruben C, Liacouras C. Evaluation and management of foreign bodies in the upper gastrointestinal tract. *Pediatr Case Rev.* 2003;3:150–156.
- Smith M, Wong R. Foreign bodies. *Gastrointest Endosc Clin North Am.* 2007;17:361–382.
- Soprano JV, Mandl KD. Four strategies for the management of esophageal coins in children. *Pediatrics.* 2000;105:1497–1501.

## CODES

### ICD9
935.1 Foreign body in esophagus

F

# FOREIGN BODY, NASAL

*Richard E. Wolfe*
*Paul Blackburn*

 **BASICS**

## DESCRIPTION
- Object impacted in the nasal cavity
- Most common site of foreign body insertion in children
- Type of foreign body limited only by nostril size
- Population at risk:
  - Children between 2–6 yr most common
  - Mental retardation
  - Psychiatric illness
- Causes of worsening impaction and difficulties with removal:
  - Organic material may expand if moistened
  - Mucosal swelling over time
- Complications:
  - Sinusitis is the most common complication.
  - Foreign bodies may migrate into the sinuses.
  - Septal perforation
  - Bronchial aspiration
  - High risk of complications with button batteries:
    - Ischemic mucosa
    - Turbinate or septal damage
    - Saddle-nose deformity

## ETIOLOGY
- Food
- Sponge pieces
- Beans
- Seeds
- Vegetable matter
- Paper
- Pieces of toys
- Beads
- Rocks
- Insects and live worms
- Button batteries:
  - High risk of complications compared with other foreign bodies (tissue necrosis, septal perforation, saddle nose); require rapid removal
  - Magnets:
    - Used to simulate nasal piercing
    - Often imbedded in tissue, leading to difficult removal
    - May cause intestinal perforation if swallowed
- Traumatic:
  - Glass fragments

 **DIAGNOSIS**

## SIGNS AND SYMPTOMS
- Most nasal foreign bodies are asymptomatic.
- Unilateral nasal obstruction
- Nasal pain
- Difficulties with nasal breathing
- Nasal discharge:
  - Acute or chronic
  - Unilateral
  - Foul smelling
  - Halitosis
- Sinus discomfort
- Persistent epistaxis
- Local inflammation
- Septal perforation
- Ingestion or aspiration of foreign body

### History
- Someone witnesses child putting object into nose.
- Foreign body noticed by parent or caretaker.
- Many children are reluctant to admit to placing a foreign body for fear of adult disapproval.
- Delayed presentation:
  - When placement of the object is unwitnessed, the child may present weeks after with nasal discharge and bleeding.
  - Often misdiagnosed at this stage as sinusitis

## ESSENTIAL WORKUP
Visualization of the foreign body in the nostril:
- Always check both nostrils.

## DIAGNOSTIC TESTS & INTERPRETATION
### Imaging
- Fiberoptic visualization if foreign body cannot be visualized on rhinoscopy
- Sinus films if present for extended period:
  - Symptom persistence despite removal of the foreign body and antibiotics

## DIFFERENTIAL DIAGNOSIS
- Sinusitis
- Swollen inferior turbinate:
  - May be mistaken for a pink bead
- Rhinitis
- Nasal polyp
- Benign tumors:
  - Hemangioma most common

- Malignant tumors:
  - Lymphoma
  - Rhabdomyosarcoma
  - Nasopharyngeal carcinoma
  - Esthesioneuroblastoma
- Congenital masses:
  - Dermoid
  - Encephalocele
  - Glioma
  - Teratoma
- Retropharyngeal abscess
- Traumatic dislocation of nasal bones or septum
- Nasal deformity:
  - Usually associated with cleft palate
- Nasopharyngeal stenosis
- Rhinitis medicamentosa:
  - Rebound nasal mucosal edema

**TREATMENT**

## PRE-HOSPITAL
- Cautions:
  - Transport in sitting position:
    - Avoid posterior displacement, possible aspiration of foreign body.
- Avoid interventions that upset the child.

## ED TREATMENT/PROCEDURES
- Topical vasoconstrictors:
  - Presence of mucosal edema, or bleeding secondary to removal attempts
  - Nebulized epinephrine
  - Cocaine: 4%
  - Oxymetazoline: 0.05%
  - Phenylephrine: 0.125–0.5%
- Positive pressure:
  - Occlude contralateral nostril.
  - Positive pressure applied to mouth only
  - Deliver brisk puff as child begins to inhale.
  - Parent may tell the child he or she will be given a "big kiss."
  - Placement of 4 × 4 gauze pads on caregiver's cheek
  - Foreign body dislodges onto cheek of the provider or into room

- Repeated as necessary
- Alternatively, deliver puff with a bag-mask over the mouth and O$_2$ at 10–15 L/min.
- Alternatively, into contralateral nostril male-male adapter on oxygen tubing, deliver wall oxygen at 10–15 L/min.
  - Risk of barotrauma with sustained, unmodulated positive pressure
- Nasal wash with 7 mL saline via bulb syringe contralateral nostril described; controversial; aspiration risk?
- Hooked probe, alligator forceps:
  - Anterior foreign bodies that are easily grasped
  - Headlamp, nasal speculum facilitate use
  - Risk of further posterior displacement
- Suction catheter:
  - Best for round, smooth objects
  - Optimal retrieval with suction catheter
  - Suction tip placed against the object
  - Suction turned up to 100–140 mm Hg
  - Catheter and object withdrawn
- Cyanoacrylate tissue glue:
  - Film of glue applied to cut end of hollow plastic swab handle
  - Apply against object for 60 sec, then withdraw.
  - Caution with nontissue cyanoacrylate glues; tissue irritation
- Balloon catheters:
  - Used primarily when instrumentation fails
  - 5F or 6F Foley or Fogarty balloon catheter lubricated with 2% lidocaine jelly
  - Advance catheter past object.
  - Following inflation with 2–3 mL of air, gently withdraw catheter.
- Magnet for removal of metal foreign body described; limited experience

## MEDICATION

- Cocaine: 4% solution, 2 drops affected nares
- Lidocaine: 4% solution, 2 drops affected nares
- Oxymetazoline: 0.05%, 2–3 drops/sprays affected nares
- Phenylephrine: 0.125–0.5%, 2–3 sprays affected nares
- Procedural sedation may be of immense importance.

##  FOLLOW-UP

### DISPOSITION
#### Admission Criteria
Referral for ambulatory surgical removal:
- Foreign body cannot be recovered in ED.
- Removal under general anesthesia is required.

#### Discharge Criteria
- Ensure that all foreign bodies are removed from both nares.
- Return if bleeding, infection (nasal discharge)
- If a button battery was removed, monitor for delayed sequelae:
  - Ischemic mucosa
  - Turbinate or septal damage
  - Saddle-nose deformity

#### Issues for Referral
Follow-up with otolaryngologist if removal is successful in the ED.

### FOLLOW-UP RECOMMENDATIONS
- Return to the ED immediately if:
  - Coughing, wheezing, noisy or difficult breathing
  - Vomiting, gagging, choking, drooling, neck or throat pain, or inability to swallow
- Parents should be instructed to seek medical care for the following:
  - Fever
  - Headache or facial pain
  - Persistent epistaxis
  - Persistent drainage of nasal fluid

## PEARLS AND PITFALLS
- Consider nasal foreign bodies in children 2–6 years presenting with what appears to be sinusitis.
- Parents are best suited to perform positive-pressure removal to avoid frightening the child.

## ADDITIONAL READING
- Backlin SA. Positive-pressure technique for nasal foreign body removal in children. *Ann Emerg Med.* 1995;25(4):554–555.
- Chan TC, Ufberg J, Harrigan RA, et al. Nasal foreign body removal. *J Emerg Med.* 2004;26(4):441–445.
- Douglas SA, Mirza S, Stafford FW. Magnetic removal of a nasal foreign body. *Int J Pediatr Otorhinolaryngol.* 2002;62(2):165–167.
- Heim SW. Foreign bodies in the ear, nose, and throat. *Am Fam Physician.* 2007;76(8):1185–1189.
- Hills RW, Brown JC, Brownstein D. Barotrauma: A complication of positive pressure for nasal foreign body removal in a pediatric patient. *Ann Emerg Med.* 2008;52(6):623–625.
- Kadish HA, Corneli HM. Removal of nasal foreign bodies in the pediatric population. *Am J Emerg Med.* 1997;15(1):54–56.
- Lichenstein R, Guidice EL. Nasal wash technique for nasal foreign body removal. *Pediatr Emerg Care.* 2000;16(1):59–60.
- Lin VY, Daniel SJ, Papsin BC. Button batteries in the ear, nose, and upper aerodigestive tract. *Int J Pediatr Otorhinolaryngol.* 2004;68(4):473–479.
- Myer CM 3rd, Cotton RT. Nasal obstruction in the pediatric patient. *Pediatrics.* 1983;72(6):766–777.

## 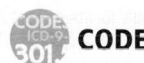 CODES

ICD9
932 Foreign body in nose

# FOREIGN BODY, RECTAL

*Jason J. Prystowsky*

 **BASICS**

## DESCRIPTION
- Self-insertion (autoeroticism):
  - Phallic substitutes inserted by patient or partner
  - Usually men age 20–40 yr, with male to female ratio 20:1
- Ingested objects lodged in rectum:
  - Chicken bones
  - Fish bones
  - Toothpick
- Iatrogenic accidental:
  - Thermometer
  - Enema tips
  - Foreign bodies (FBs) used to aid in removal of feces
- Assault:
  - Knife or pipe forcibly inserted
  - Incidence of perforation is very high.
- Concealment:
  - Body packing, "mules" illegally transporting drugs

 **DIAGNOSIS**

## SIGNS AND SYMPTOMS
- Complaint of rectal foreign body (FB)
- Rectal fullness
- Rectal pain
- Perirectal abscess (with imbedded bones/toothpick)
- FB on rectal examination:
  - High-lying foreign bodies are located proximal to rectosigmoid junction and are not palpable on rectal exam.
  - Low-lying foreign bodies are usually located in rectal ampulla and are palpable on rectal exam.
- Some patients may not be forthcoming with history:
  - Men will only admit to rectal FB if directly asked about it.
- Can present with vague symptoms of abdominal pain or obstruction
- Can present as bowel perforation with full peritonitis
- Often late presentation hours or days after placement, following repeated failed attempts at removal

- Rectal Organ Injury Scale (proposed by American Association for the Surgery of Trauma):
  - Grade I—Hematoma: Contusion or hematoma without devascularization:
    - Most injuries due to rectal FB are Grade I
  - Grade II—Laceration 50% circumference
  - Grade III—Laceration >50% circumference
  - Grade IV—Full-thickness laceration with extension into perineum
  - Grade V—Devascularized segment

## ESSENTIAL WORKUP
- Identify number, type, and duration of FBs and mechanism of insertion.
- Physical exam with emphasis on abdominal and rectal exam
- Biplane radiographic films to confirm number and size of FBs
- For assaulted patients, workup as for blunt trauma to abdomen.

## DIAGNOSTIC TESTS & INTERPRETATION
### Lab
- CBC:
  - For bleeding or peritonitis
- Urinalysis:
  - For urethral/bladder injuries

### Imaging
- Plain radiograph:
  - Consider doing kidneys, ureters, and bladder (KUB) radiograph prior to rectal exam to rule out objects harmful to examiner.
  - Define and locate FB.
  - Assess for complications of retained FB including bowel perforation and obstruction.
  - May be used serially to follow descent of FB
- CT scan of abdomen/pelvis:
  - To exclude perforation or abscess formation

## DIFFERENTIAL DIAGNOSIS
- Pseudo-FB:
  - Patients insist there is FB when radiograph, rectal exams, and proctoscopy results are normal.
- Perirectal abscess
- Hemorrhoid

 **TREATMENT**

## PRE-HOSPITAL
Cautions:
- Patient has usually tried to remove FB and failed.
- Further attempts at extraction will not work and could cause perforation.

## INITIAL STABILIZATION/THERAPY
- Perforation with peritonitis and sepsis:
  - 0.9% NS IV fluid 500 mL bolus
  - Broad-spectrum antibiotics (anaerobic and gram-negative aerobes):
    - Cefoxitin, cefotetan, ticarcillin-clavulanate, ampicillin-sulbactam, imipenem, meropenem, ertapenem, *or*
    - Metronidazole/clindamycin plus aminoglycoside/3rd-generation cephalosporin/fluoroquinolone/aztreonam
  - Urgent surgical consult
- Advanced trauma life support (ATLS) with evidence of other trauma

## ED TREATMENT/PROCEDURES
- Use appropriate sedation and analgesia.
- Avoid enemas or suppositories.
- Low-lying small rectal FBs that are not fragile or sharp:
  - Can be removed transanally if object can be firmly held
  - Remove with gentle but firm continuous traction to overcome anal sphincter.
- Colonic mucosa tightly adherent to distal end of FB creates vacuum and impedes withdrawal of object:
  - Passage of Foley catheter beyond object with insufflation of air breaks vacuum and permits retrieval.
- Awake and cooperative patients can facilitate transanal extraction with Valsalva.
- May use instruments to assist with extraction: Obstetrical forceps, tenaculum, ring forceps, vacuum extractor
- Can attempt bimanual manipulation if low-lying FB

- 60% of rectal FBs may be removed transanally in the ED under proper sedation.
- Following extraction, anorectum must be thoroughly evaluated to rule out occult injury.
- High-lying rectal FBs:
  - Not immediately accessible through rectum
  - Usually require surgical or GI consult
  - Attempt may be made to position object into low-lying position.
  - Direct visualization with large operating anoscope (after blockage of sphincter and pudendal nerve with local anesthesia)
  - Bimanual manipulation
  - Admission and observation for spontaneous descent (with serial radiographs)
  - Laparotomy may be necessary as last resort if other methods fail, or if patient has evidence of perforation.
- Consider surgical or GI consult for other complicated rectal FBs:
  - Larger objects
  - Objects that have remained >24 hr with resulting edema
  - Objects with sharp edges
  - Proctoscopy/sigmoidoscopy after extraction to examine colonic mucosa
- Body packers:
  - Ruptured packets of concealed illicit drugs can cause systemic toxicity, bowel necrosis, and death.
  - Sharp instruments should not be used for retrieval, and other instruments should be used with extreme caution.

## MEDICATION

- Ampicillin-sulbactam (Unasyn): 3g IV q6h (peds: 100–200 mg/kg/d div. q6h)
- Aztreonam (Azactam): 0.5–2g IV q8–12h (peds: 30 mg/kg IV q6–8h, max 120 mg/kg/d)
- Cefoxitin (Mefoxin): 1–2 g (peds: 30–40 mg/kg) IV q6h
- Cefotetan (Cefotan): 1–2 g (peds: 20–40 mg/kg) IV q12h
- Ceftriaxone (Rocephin): 1–2 g IV q12h (peds: 50–75 mg/kg IV daily)

- Ciprofloxacin (Cipro): 400 mg IV q8–12h
- Clindamycin: 600–900 mg (peds: 20–40 mg/kg/24 h) IV q8h
- Ertapenem (Invanz): 1 g IV q24h
- Gentamicin: 1 mg/kg (peds: 2–2.5 mg/kg) IV q8h
- Imipenem (Primaxin): 0.5–1 g (peds: 15–25 mg/kg) IV q6h
- Levofloxacin (Levoquin): 500 mg IV q24h
- Meropenem (Merrem): 1 g (peds: 60 mg/kg/d) IV q8h
- Metronidazole: 15 mg/kg IV once, then 7.5 mg/kg IV q6h
- Piperacillin-tazobactam (Zosyn): 3.75 g IV q6h or 4.5 g IV q8h (peds: 240–400 mg/kg/d div. q6–8h)
- Ticarcillin-clavulanate (Timentin): 3.1 g (peds: 200–300 mg/kg/d) IV q4–6h

### Pediatric Considerations

- Removal under general anesthesia for children who are too young to cooperate
- It is probably child abuse if FB other than enema tips or thermometer is present.

 **FOLLOW-UP**

### DISPOSITION

#### Admission Criteria

- Failed extraction in ED requires surgical removal in OR.
- Evidence of mucosal tear on proctoscopy should be observed for 24 hr (no antibiotic indicated).
- Symptom of rectal pain associated with removal of sharp FB indicates possibility of small perforation with developing abscess and requires examination under anesthesia.
- Any invasive procedure with analgesia and sedation requires inpatient observation for 24 hr.

#### Discharge Criteria

- Reliable patient with atraumatic insertion and removal of rectal FB
- Instruct to return for rectal pain, abdominal pain, fever, or massive rectal bleeding.

#### Issues for Referral

GI or surgery consult if unable to remove FB in ED

## FOLLOW-UP RECOMMENDATIONS

Flexible sigmoidoscopy or rigid proctoscopy to evaluate for mucosal injury following retrieval of rectal FB regardless of method used is recommended.

## PEARLS AND PITFALLS

- Passage of Foley catheter beyond object with insufflation of air breaks vacuum and permits retrieval.
- Provide adequate sedation/analgesia when attempting foreign body removal in the ED.

## ADDITIONAL READING

- Abcarian H. Colorectal foreign bodies. In: Mazier PW, et al., eds. *Surgery of the Colon, Rectum, and Anus*. Philadelphia: WB Saunders; 1995.
- Clarke DL, Buccumazza I, Anderson FA, et al. Colorectal foreign bodies. *Colorectal Dis*. 2005;7:98.
- Eftaiha M, Hambrick E, Abcarian H. Principles and management of colorectal foreign bodies. *Dis Colon Rectum*. 1977;112:691–695.
- Hellinger M. Anal trauma and foreign bodies. *Surg Clin North Am*. 2002;1253–1260.
- Janicke DM, Pundt MR. Anorectal disorders. *Emerg Clin North Am*. 1996;14:757–788.
- Smith M, Wong R. Foreign bodies. *Gastrointest Endosc Clin North Am*. 2007;17:361–382.
- Rodriguez-Hermosa JI, Codina-Cazador A, Ruiz B, et al. Management of foreign bodies in the rectum. *Colorectal Dis*. 2007;9:543.

### See Also (Topic, Algorithm, Electronic Media Element)

Rectal trauma

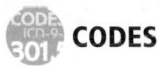 **CODES**

### ICD9

937 Foreign body in anus and rectum

**F**

# FOURNIER GANGRENE

*Gary M. Vilke*

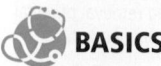 **BASICS**

## DESCRIPTION

- Inadequate hygiene leads to scrotal skin maceration and excoriation:
  - Portal of entry for bacteria in tissue
- Once skin barrier is broken, polymicrobial flora spread along *fascial planes* of perineum.
- Colles fascia fuses with urogenital diaphragm, slowing propagation posteriorly and laterally.
- Anteriorly, buck, and scarpa fascia are continuous, allowing rapid extension to anterior abdominal wall and laterally along fascia lata.
- Testes and urethra are usually spared.
- 3 anatomic origins account for most cases:
  - Lower urinary tract (40%): Urethral strictures, indwelling catheters
  - Penile or scrotal (30%): Condom catheters, hydradenitis, balanitis
  - Anorectal (30%): Fistulas, perirectal infections, hemorrhoids
- Rarely, intra-abdominal sources such as perforating appendicitis, diverticulitis, or pancreatitis have produced Fournier gangrene by dependent contiguous spread.

## ETIOLOGY

- Infection by polymicrobial flora (mixed aerobic and anaerobic organisms)
- Mixed bacteria exert synergistic tissue-destructive effect.
- End arterial thrombosis in subcutaneous tissues produces anaerobic environment.
- Bacterial toxins and tissue necrosis factors may contribute to clinical presentation.
- Risk factors:
  - Trauma
  - Diabetes
  - Alcoholism
  - Other immunocompromised states
  - Morbid obesity
  - Abdominal surgery

 **DIAGNOSIS**

## SIGNS AND SYMPTOMS

- Rapidly progressive necrotizing infection of *perineum* involving subcutaneous and fascial tissues and often muscle layers:
  - Usually seen in diabetics or immunocompromised patients
- Sources of infection may be flora from genitourinary, rectal, or penile/scrotal regions.

### Pediatric Considerations

- Though unusual in children, >50 cases have been described.
- Most often are complications of burns, circumcision, balanitis, severe diaper rashes, or insect bites
- Organisms are more frequently *Staphylococcus* or *Streptococcus*.
- Pediatric patients have more local disease and are less toxic.

### History

- Duration of symptoms:
  - Fevers or chills
  - Pain is out of proportion to examination in early phases, but eventually dead tissue becomes insensate.
  - Nausea and vomiting
  - Urinary infection symptoms
- Rapidity with which symptoms are progressing
- Identify if diabetic or immunocompromised
- Lethargy and inappropriate indifference to the illness are common.

### Physical Exam

- Patients are often toxic in appearance with nausea, vomiting, fever, chills, and pain.
- Careful examination of the genitalia and perirectal region
- Assess for skin findings:
  - Bronze or violaceous discoloration of skin
  - Thin brown watery discharge
  - Ulceration, bullous vesicles
  - Crepitance, SC air
  - Frank necrosis and eschar formation

## ESSENTIAL WORKUP

- Fournier gangrene is a clinical diagnosis.
- History and physical exam with special attention to perineum
- Evaluate for signs of sepsis.
- Early surgical consultation for emergent débridement is essential.
- Other workup directed toward relevant co-morbid factors such as diabetes or immunocompromised status

## DIAGNOSTIC TESTS & INTERPRETATION

### Lab

- Other than Gram stain of tissue and associated drainage, there are no specific laboratory tests that are diagnostic of Fournier gangrene.
- Urinalysis should be performed.
- Leukocytosis, anemia, electrolyte imbalances, acidosis, and renal failure are common.
- Disseminated intravascular coagulation (DIC) may be present; PT, PTT, fibrin-split products, and fibrinogen levels help identify.
- If patient is suspected of or known to have diabetes, glucose, electrolytes, and serum ketones to evaluate for diabetes and diabetic ketoacidosis (DKA)
- Culture of blood, urine, and tissue (when available)

### Imaging

- Plain films of the pelvis may reveal subcutaneous emphysema and ileus.
- CT scanning helps if intra-abdominal or ischiorectal source is suspected.
- US may be useful in differentiating from other causes of acute scrotum.

### Diagnostic Procedures/Surgery

Retrograde urethrography, anoscopy, proctosigmoidoscopy, and barium enemas may be helpful to localize anatomic sources of infection.

## DIFFERENTIAL DIAGNOSIS

- Epididymitis/orchitis
- Insect and human bites
- Perirectal infections
- Scrotal abscess/inguinal abscess
- Scrotal cellulitis
- Testicular torsion
- Tinea cruris

**TREATMENT**

### PRE-HOSPITAL
Patients may be hypotensive from septic shock and require aggressive fluid resuscitation and pressor support.

### INITIAL STABILIZATION/THERAPY
- Manage airway and resuscitate as indicated.
- Central venous access, aggressive fluid resuscitation, and pressure support as indicated:
  - Avoid femoral access, femoral venipuncture, and lower extremity venous access
- Early goal-directed therapy if septic
- Foley catheter placement or suprapubic access if indicated

### ED TREATMENT/PROCEDURES
- Empiric broad-spectrum antibiotics
- Early emergent aggressive surgical débridement
- Adjunctive hyperbaric oxygen therapy coordinated with surgical care
- Treat dehydration and correct electrolytes.
- Blood products as needed for DIC or anemia; oxygen debt can be minimized by keeping hematocrit >30%.
- Tetanus prophylaxis as indicated

### Pediatric Considerations
- More conservative surgical approach
- Adequate staphylococcal coverage

### MEDICATION
- Antibiotic regimens:
  - Multidrug regimen:
    - Ampicillin: 2 g IV q6h (peds: 50 mg/kg) *and*
    - Clindamycin: 900 mg IV q8h (peds: 10 mg/kg) *and*
    - Gentamicin: 5 mg/kg daily load IV q8h
    - Ciprofloxacin: 500 mg IV *and*
    - Clindamycin: 900mg IV initial ED dose

- Single-drug regimens (peds: Safety not established)
  - Ampicillin/sulbactam: 3 g IV initial ED dose
  - Imipenem: 1 g IV initial ED dose
  - Piperacillin/tazobactam: 3.375 g IV initial ED dose
  - Ticarcillin/clavulanate: 3.1 g IV initial ED dose
- Cover for possible MRSA with Vancomycin 1 g IV initial ED dose
- Blood products as indicated
- Dopamine or dobutamine IV drips starting at 5 μg/kg/min titrating to effect if hypotensive after aggressive hydration
- Insulin adjusted to control glucose and acidosis

 **FOLLOW-UP**

### DISPOSITION

#### Admission Criteria
- *All* patients with Fournier gangrene require admission and surgical ICU care.
- Mortality estimates of 3–38% emphasize need for early aggressive care.
- Consider early transfer to facility capable of providing adjunctive hyperbaric oxygen therapy if stable for transport.

#### Discharge Criteria
No patients with Fournier gangrene should be discharged.

## PEARLS AND PITFALLS
- Failure to perform a careful genital examination, particularly in a pediatric patient
- Failure to initiate antibiotics in a timely manner

## ADDITIONAL READING

- Burch DM, Barreiro TJ, Vanek VW. Fournier's gangrene: Be alert for this medical emergency. *JAAPA*. 2007;20(11):44–47.
- Jallali N, Withy S, Butler PE. Hyperbaric oxygen as adjuvant therapy in the management of necrotizing fasciitis. *Am J Surg*. 2005;189:462–466.
- Levenson RB, Singh AK, Novelline RA. Fournier gangrene: Role of imaging. *Radiographics*. 2008;28(2):519–528.
- Marynowski MT, Aronson AA. Fournier's gangrene. Emedicine: http://emedicine.medscape.com/article/778866-overview
- Morpurrgo E, Galandiuk S. Fournier's gangrene. *Surg Clin N Am*. 2002;82:1213–1224.

### See Also (Topic, Algorithm, Electronic Media Element)
- Cellulitis
- Urinary Tract Infection, Adult

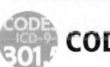 **CODES**

**ICD9**
608.83 Vascular disorders of male genital organs

F

# FRACTURE, OPEN
*Christy Rosa Mohler*

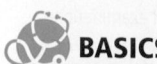

## BASICS

### DESCRIPTION
- Continuity between skin violation and fracture site, ranging from a puncture wound to grossly exposed bone
- Surgical emergency, as delays in care increase risk of infection and rate of complications
- Predisposition to complications in certain patients:
  – Massive soft tissue damage
  – Severe wound contamination
  – Compromised vascularity
  – Fracture instability
  – Compromised host (diabetes, vascular disease)

### ETIOLOGY
Open fractures typically result from significant blunt force or penetrating trauma.

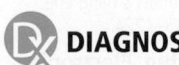

## DIAGNOSIS

### SIGNS AND SYMPTOMS
- Deformity with nearby violation in skin integrity
- Neurovascular compromise may occur.
- Additional traumatic injuries are frequently present.

### History
Significant trauma

### Physical Exam
- Complete neurologic and vascular exam
- Examine thoroughly for other traumatic injuries.

### ESSENTIAL WORKUP
- Plain radiographs including joints above and below the affected area
- Guided workup based on mechanism and evidence of other traumatic injuries

### DIAGNOSTIC TESTS & INTERPRETATION
#### Lab
- CBC, chemistry panel, coagulation studies for large-bone (femur, pelvis) fractures or multiple-trauma victims
- Type and screen or type and cross-match for potential of significant blood loss.
- Predebridement and postdebridement cultures have limited value and are not recommended.

#### Imaging
Doppler or angiography if vascular damage is suspected:
- Posterior knee dislocation
- Ischemic extremity
- Massive soft tissue injury in high-risk areas

#### Diagnostic Procedures/Surgery
- Measurement of compartment pressures if concern for compartment syndrome
- Consider arthrogram by intra-articular injection of saline or methylene blue if joint involvement is suspected.
- Angiography if noninvasive techniques are inadequate for ruling out vascular compromise

### DIFFERENTIAL DIAGNOSIS
Noncontinuous laceration/abrasion

## TREATMENT

### PRE-HOSPITAL
- Moist, sterile dressings over open wounds
- Immobilize joints above and below fracture.
- Control bleeding with local compression.
- Consider tourniquet for traumatic amputations or uncontrollable hemorrhage.
- Longitudinal traction of involved extremity if distal pulses absent

### INITIAL STABILIZATION/THERAPY
- Management of ABCs.
- Gentle reduction and immobilization of fracture

### ED TREATMENT/PROCEDURES
- Intravenous access
- Keep patient NPO
- Tetanus vaccination, if needed
- Antibiotics reduce the incidence of early infection in open fractures and should be given early in the ED course.
- Minimize number of times dressing is removed to avoid secondary contamination:
  – Redressing the wound increases the infection rate by a factor of 3–4.

- Examine limb regularly for compartment syndrome and neurovascular status.
- Early orthopedic consultation for formal irrigation, debridement, and operative fixation (if needed):
  – Irrigation and debridement are optimally performed within 6 hr to reduce likelihood of infection.
- Vascular surgery consultation for injuries with potential vascular damage

## MEDICATION

- Cefazolin: 1–2 g (peds: 20 mg/kg IM/IV)
- Add gentamicin: 3–6 mg/kg IV for more extensive injuries and highly contaminated wounds (peds: 2.5 mg/kg IV)
- Add penicillin G: 4–5 million U IV in farmyard injuries, vascular injuries, and in wounds at risk of contamination with Clostridium (peds: 50,000 U/kg IV)
- Tetanus booster: 0.5 mL IM
- Tetanus immunoglobulin: 250 IU IM if not previously immunized against tetanus
- Morphine sulfate: 2–10 mg (peds: 0.05–0.1 mg/kg per dose IV or equivalent analgesic)

### Pediatric Considerations

DTaP booster for children < 7 yr of age

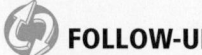

## FOLLOW-UP

### DISPOSITION

#### Admission Criteria

Most patients will be admitted for irrigation and IV antibiotics and possibly debridement or operative fixation.

#### Discharge Criteria

Simple open fractures may be washed out and immobilized in the ED after consultation with an orthopedic surgeon. The patient should be discharged with oral antibiotics.

#### Issues for Referral

Most open fractures will require emergent orthopedic consultation and may require trauma team evaluation for other injuries.

### FOLLOW-UP RECOMMENDATIONS

Patients discharged from the emergency department should be followed-up with an orthopedic surgeon in 1–2 days.

## PEARLS AND PITFALLS

- Open fractures are surgical emergencies requiring prompt orthopedic consultation.
- 40%–70% of patients with open fractures have other traumatic injuries.
- Prompt and thorough ED assessment and treatment can significantly decrease morbidity in patients with open fractures.

## ADDITIONAL READING

- Browner BD, Jupiter JB, Levine AM, et al., eds. *Skeletal Trauma*, 4th ed. Philadelphia: Saunders; 2008.
- Canale ST, Beaty JH, eds. *Campbell's Operative Orthopaedics*, 11th ed. Philadelphia: Mosby Elsevier; 2007.
- Gosselin RA. Antibiotics for preventing infection in open limb fractures. *Cochrane Database Syst Rev*, 2004;(1):CD003764.
- Marx JA, Hockberger RB, Walls RM, eds. *Rosen's Emergency Medicine*, 7th ed. Philadelphia: Mosby–Year Book, 2009.

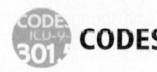 CODES

### ICD9

829.1 Fracture of unspecified bone, open

F

# FRACTURES, PEDIATRIC
*Adam Z. Barkin*

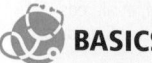 **BASICS**

## DESCRIPTION
- Anatomy:
  - Diaphysis: Physis to physis; bone shaft
  - Epiphysis: Cartilaginous center at or near end of bone that is site of bone growth
  - Physis (growth plate): Radiolucent line between epiphysis and metaphysis; cartilaginous
  - Metaphysis: Region of rapidly growing trabecular bone underlying base of cartilaginous growth plate; between diaphysis and epiphysis
- Bones are highly resilient, elastic, and springy
- Allow for fractures not seen in adults:
  - Greenstick fracture:
    ○ Incomplete fracture through cortex on opposite side of impact
  - Torus (buckle) fracture:
    ○ Usually at junction of metaphysis and diaphysis
    ○ Compression of bone of 1 cortex
  - Plastic deformity:
    ○ Bowing without disruption of cortex
  - Fractures involving the physis
- Cartilaginous growth plates are potential areas of injury.
- Ligaments more resistant to injury than growth plates
- Salter-Harris classification:
  - Risk of growth disturbance increases from type I to type V.
  - Type I:
    ○ Separation of epiphysis from metaphysis without displacement or injury to the growth plate
    ○ Tenderness and pain at point of growth plate
    ○ Radiograph typically normal
    ○ Growth disturbance is rare.
  - Type II:
    ○ Metaphyseal fracture extending to physis
    ○ Most common
    ○ Growth disturbance is rare.
  - Type III:
    ○ Intra-articular fracture extending through the epiphysis into the physis
    ○ Most common site is distal tibial epiphysis.
    ○ Growth disturbance possible
  - Type IV:
    ○ Epiphyseal, physeal, and metaphyseal fracture
    ○ Lateral condyle of humerus is most common site.
    ○ Growth disturbance highly likely
  - Type V:
    ○ Crush injury to epiphyseal plate, producing growth arrest
    ○ Usually occurs in joints that move in only 1 plane such as knee
- Fractures often accompany dislocations.
- Nonaccidental trauma (NAT) if history inconsistent with findings

## ETIOLOGY
- Mechanism is useful in defining the potential and type of injury:
  - Falls, motor vehicle accidents, blunt trauma, NAT
- Obesity and rapid growth spurts are risk factors.
- Common fractures include lower forearm, clavicle, tibia or fibula, supracondylar fracture of humerus.
- Nonaccidental trauma (NAT):
  - Any fracture in a child younger than 1 yr of age in whom history is not consistent with injury
  - Metaphyseal "corner" fractures are pathognomonic.
  - Posterior rib fractures
  - Spiral femur fracture
  - Fractures at different stages of healing
  - Skull fractures crossing suture lines, especially in children younger than 1 yr
  - Unusual behavior in child or parent

 **DIAGNOSIS**

## SIGNS AND SYMPTOMS
- Decreased limb movement, unwilling to use
- Swelling
- Tenderness
- Deformity
- Ecchymosis
- Crepitus
- Limp
- Abnormal neurovascular status of extremity
- Compartment syndrome:
  - Severe pain, especially in forearm, calf, foot
  - Pain with passive stretching of fingers or toes
  - Sensory deficit in the distal extremity
  - Cool extremity
  - Pulseless extremity
- Open fracture may be obvious or subtle (collection of blood with fat globules under skin)

### History
- Mechanism of injury:
  - Velocity of car, bike, etc.
  - Height of fall
- Neurologic compromise
- Events surrounding injury
- Other injuries

### Physical Exam
- Thorough secondary survey looking for deformities, bruising, other injuries
- Assess neurovascular status:
  - Motor/sensation
  - Distal pulses
  - Capillary refill
- Range of motion of all joints involved
- Exclude concurrent injuries
- Ensure that history consistent with injury

## ESSENTIAL WORKUP
- Prompt immobilization
- Imaging as below

## DIAGNOSTIC TESTS & INTERPRETATION
### Lab
- Required only if concomitant injuries, surgery anticipated, or multiple/major bone involvement
- CBC, ESR if infection suspected

### Imaging
- Anteroposterior (AP), lateral, and oblique radiographs as necessary, including the joint above and below the fracture
- Comparison views may be useful if growth plates involved.
- Follow-up radiographs at 7–10 days may be required to exclude avascular necrosis or Salter I fractures.
- Bone scan/CT/MRI may be useful to exclude fractures if plain radiographs are unhelpful or to evaluate for infection.

### Diagnostic Procedures/Surgery
Arthrocentesis if infection is suspected

## DIFFERENTIAL DIAGNOSIS
- Sprain or strain
- Contusion
- Infection
- Tumor
- Neurologic deficits
- Subtle dislocations such as radial head subluxation (nursemaid's elbow)
- NAT

 **TREATMENT**

## PRE-HOSPITAL
Immobilization

## INITIAL STABILIZATION/THERAPY
- Resuscitation for concurrent injuries
- Immobilization

## ED TREATMENT/PROCEDURES
- Management of life-threatening concurrent injuries
- Pain control
- Dislocations require immediate assessment and attention to neurovascular compromise:
  - Mechanism helps in understanding the direction of the force required to reduce.
- Alignment is essential, particularly when fracture involves a joint surface.
- Appropriate reporting of NAT

### Salter-Harris Fractures

- Type I and type II fractures require immobilization and orthopedic follow-up.
- Type II distal femur fractures, type III, and type IV require urgent orthopedic consultation for anatomic reduction.
- Type V fractures require immobilization and consultation.
- Anatomic reduction does not eliminate possibility of growth disturbance.

### Clavicle Fracture

- Figure-of-8 splint or sling for comfort
- Distal 3rd clavicle fractures should be referred with initial sling and swathe or shoulder immobilizer.

### Supracondylar Humerus Fracture

- May present with only posterior effusion on lateral radiograph
- Orthopedic consultation because of potential neurovascular complications
- Brachial artery injury, median nerve injury possible
- Volar compartment syndrome of forearm (results in Volkmann contracture)
- Epiphyseal injury with long-term growth abnormalities

### Distal Radius and Ulna Fractures

- Rotational deformities must be eliminated.
- Reduce angulated fractures >15°
- Immobilize for 4–6 wk.
- Colles fracture:
  - Reduce by traction in the line of deformity to disimpact the fragments, followed by pressure on the dorsal aspect of the distal fragment and volar aspect of the proximal fragment.
  - Correct radial deviation.
  - Immobilize the hand in ulnar deviation, wrist in neutral, and forearm in full pronation.
  - Orthopedic consultation
- Torus fracture (incomplete fracture; buckling or angulation on the compression side of the bone only):
  - Most often in distal forearm
- Greenstick fracture (incomplete fracture of diaphysis of long bone with fracture on tension side of cortex):
  - Immobilize.
  - Reduction if angulation >30° in infants, >15° in children

### Tibia or Fibula Fracture

- Isolated fibular fractures: Short-leg walking cast
- Nondisplaced tibial fracture: Long-leg posterior splint, non–weight bearing
- Displaced tibial fracture and complex fractures require consultation.
- Toddler's fractures:
  - Nondisplaced, oblique, distal tibia fracture
  - May need tangential view radiograph or bone scan to diagnose
  - Splint if suspect and repeat radiograph in 7–10 days.

### Radial Head Subluxation (Nursemaid's Elbow)

- Infant or preschooler
- Longitudinal traction on wrist or hand
- Radiograph if bony tenderness
- Reduction:
  - Supination of wrist and elbow flexion
  - Hyperpronation of wrist while cradling elbow with other hand
- Follow-up in 24–72 hr.

### Slipped Capital Femoral Epiphysis

- Disruption though capital femoral epiphysis
- Overweight adolescent boys
- May have referred pain to knee, thigh, or groin
- Non–weight bearing with prompt orthopedic follow-up
- Prophylactic treatment of contralateral hip remains controversial.

### Femur Fracture

- Most common long bone fracture

### Stress Fractures

- Increasingly common
- Insidious onset
- Vague, achy pain
- Usually associated with rigorous activity
- Treatment:
  - Selective bracing
  - Activity modification

### Open Fractures

- True orthopedic emergency
- Irrigate and dress with moist saline gauze
- Immobilize
- Cefazolin if only small laceration and minimal contamination
- Gentamicin if moderate contamination, high-energy injury, or significant soft tissue injury
- Consider penicillin if concern for clostridia infection (farm injury, fecal or soil contamination)

### MEDICATION

- Acetaminophen: 10–15 mg/kg PO/PR (per rectum) q4–6h
- Cefazolin: 25—100 mg/kg daily IM/IV q8h
- Gentamicin: 2.5 mg/kg IV/IM q8h or 6.5–7.5 mg/kg IV/IM q24h
- Hematoma block: 1% lidocaine without epinephrine (max. 3–5 mg/kg)
- Ibuprofen: 10 mg/kg PO q6–8h (first-line treatment)
- Morphine: 0.05–0.2 mg/kg SC/IM/IV q2–4h

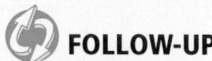

## FOLLOW-UP

### DISPOSITION

#### Admission Criteria

- NAT (or per social services)
- Open fracture
- Potential neurovascular compromise/compartment syndrome:
  - Condylar or supracondylar humerus fracture
  - Femoral shaft

#### Discharge Criteria

- Uncomplicated fracture: No concurrent injury or neurovascular/compartment compromise
- Follow-up arranged and parents understand injury and management

#### Issues for Referral

All Salter-Harris fractures should have orthopedic follow-up.

## PEARLS AND PITFALLS

- History is essential in evaluation of nonaccidental trauma.
- Have a low threshold to splint and/or consult orthopedist.
- Pain control is essential and often under-dosed.

## ADDITIONAL READING

- Heyworth BE, Green DW. Lower extremity stress fractures in pediatric and adolescent athletes. *Curr Opin Pediatr*. 2008;20:58–61.
- Kim Y, Noonan KJ. What's new in pediatric orthopaedics. *J Bone Joint Surg Am*. 2009;91: 743–751.
- Rodriguez-Merchan EC. Pediatric skeletal trauma: A review and historical perspective. *Clin Orthop Relat Res*. 2005;432:8–13.
- Wolfson AB, Hendey GW, Ling LJ, et al., eds. *Harwood Nuss' Clinical Practice of Emergency Medicine*, 5th ed. Philadelphia: Lippincott; 2010.

### See Also (Topic, Algorithm, Electronic Media Element)

- Conscious Sedation
- C-spine Fractures, Pediatric
- Fractures, Epiphyseal
- Fractures, Open
- Nursemaid's Elbow
- Shoulder Dislocation
- Slipped Capital Femoral Epiphysis

F

# FROSTBITE

*Joseph M. Weber*

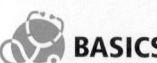 **BASICS**

## DESCRIPTION
- Tissue damage caused by cold temperature exposure
- Mechanism:
  - Tissue damage results from:
    - Direct cell damage: Intracellular ice crystal formation
    - Indirect cell damage: Extracellular ice crystal formation leads to intracellular dehydration and enzymatic disruption.
    - Reperfusion injury: Occurs upon rewarming. Fluid rich in inflammatory mediators (prostaglandin and thromboxane) extravasates through damaged endothelium promoting vasoconstriction and platelet aggregation.
    - Clear blisters form from extracellular exudation of fluid.
    - Hemorrhagic blisters occur when deeper subdermal vessels are disrupted, indicating more severe tissue injury.
    - The end result is arterial thrombosis, ischemia, and ultimately, necrosis.
  - Devitalized tissue demarcates as the injury evolves over weeks to months, hence the phrase "frostbite in January, amputate in July."

## ETIOLOGY
- Cold exposure: Duration of exposure, wind chill, humidity, and wet skin and clothing all increase the likelihood of frostbite.
- Predisposing factors:
  - Extremes of age
  - Altered mental status (intoxication or psychiatric illness)
  - Poor circulatory status

## DIAGNOSIS

### SIGNS AND SYMPTOMS
- Extremities (fingers, toes) and head (ears, nose) most commonly affected.
- After rewarming frostbite can be classified, however, initial classification often fails to provide an accurate prognosis and does not alter initial management.
- Superficial frostbite:
  - Only skin structures involved. Usually no tissue loss.
  - 1st degree: Erythema and edema with stinging, burning, and throbbing. No blisters or necrosis.
  - 2nd degree: Significant edema, clear blister formation. Numbness common.

- Deep frostbite:
  - Tissue loss inevitable.
  - 3rd degree: Involves subcutaneous tissue. Hemorrhagic blister formation due to subdermal venous plexus injury:
    - Initially insensate, injuries develop severe pain/burning on rewarming.
  - 4th degree: Involves muscle, tendon, and bone. Initially mottled, deep red or cyanotic.
  - Unfavorable prognostic indicators include: Hemorrhagic blisters, persistent cyanosis, mottling, anesthesia, and reduced mobility after rewarming.
  - Devitalized tissue demarcates as the injury evolves over weeks to months forming skin necrosis and dry black eschar.

### ESSENTIAL WORKUP
- Diagnosis is based on the clinical presentation. Wound description should include skin color and temperature, blister formation and color, and soft tissue consistency.
- A neurologic and vascular exam should include pulses (by Doppler if necessary), cap refill, and 2-point discrimination.
- Look for underlying factors contributing to cold exposure and co-morbid conditions requiring emergency management:
  - Hypothermia
  - Trauma
  - Hypoglycemia
  - Cardiac or neurologic problems
  - Intoxication/overdose
  - Compartment syndrome

### DIAGNOSTIC TESTS & INTERPRETATION
#### Lab
- None indicated in mild cases
- For deep frostbite:
  - CBC
  - Electrolytes, BUN/creatinine, glucose
  - Urinalysis/CK for evidence for myoglobinuria
- Cultures and gram stains from open areas when infection suspected

#### Imaging
Technetium-99 scintigraphy or MRA:
- May be helpful in early identification of salvageable versus unsalvageable tissue
- Permits earlier decision about amputation

### Diagnostic Procedures/Surgery
Method to create a warm water bath in the ED:
- Whirlpool hydrotherapy ideal, however, most ED's do not have
- Mix hot and cold tap water from a standard hospital sink in a large basin
- Use a thermometer to keep temperature between 40–42°C.
- The water will cool quickly: Intermittently add warm water or replace the water to keep the temperature in the proper range.
- Warmer temperatures can cause thermal injury while cooler temperatures delay thawing and decrease tissue survival.

### DIFFERENTIAL DIAGNOSIS
- Frostnip:
  - Superficial, reversible ice crystal formation without tissue destruction
  - Transient numbness and paresthesia resolve after dry rewarming.
- Trench (Immersion) foot:
  - Exposure to wet cold for prolonged periods
  - Neurovascular damage without ice crystal formation
  - Pallor, mottling, paresthesias, pulselessness, paralysis, and numbness
  - May be difficult to distinguish from post-thaw phase of frostbite
  - Hyperemia with dry rewarming may last up to 6 wk.
- Chilblains:
  - Chronic repeated exposure to dry cold
  - Localized erythema, cyanosis, plaques, and vesicles
  - Recurrent episodes common in patients with underlying vasculitis
  - Symptomatic treatment, dry rewarming

# TREATMENT

## PRE-HOSPITAL
- Protect and immobilize frostbitten area during transport
- Remove restrictive or wet garments
- Avoid dry rewarming of the frostbitten limb if there is a likelihood of refreezing injury during transport.
- If evacuation will be delayed and suitable facilities are available, field rewarming in warm (40–42°C) water can be attempted.
- Rubbing, manipulating the limb, or applying snow while it is still frozen is contraindicated.

### ALERT
Hypothermia:
- Common in frostbite victims
- In the severely hypothermic patient, avoid rough handling to minimize risk of cardiac dysrhythmias.

## INITIAL STABILIZATION/THERAPY
- ABCs management
- Identify and correct hypothermia.
- IV fluid volume expansion with 0.9% NS for severe frostbite
- Protect frostbitten areas from excessive handling during resuscitation.

## ED TREATMENT/PROCEDURES
- If the injury is <24 hr old and has not yet been rewarmed:
  - Initiate rapid rewarming of the frostbitten extremity in a 40–42°C water bath for 15–30 min.
  - Stop treatment when the limb is warm, red, and pliable.
  - Monitor water temperature closely to prevent thermal injury.
- Analgesia: IV morphine
- NSAIDs (eg, ibuprofen) to combat the effects of prostaglandins on skin necrosis.
- Aloe vera topical cream:
  - Recommended for all intact blisters
  - Combats the arachidonic acid cascade
  - Avoid preparations containing alcohol, scent, salicylates, all of which interfere with aloe effectiveness.

- Blister débridement or aspiration:
  - Indicated for clear blebs:
    - Removes thromboxane and prostaglandins
  - Contraindicated for hemorrhagic blebs:
    - Exposes deeper structures to dehydration and infection
- Tetanus prophylaxis
- Antibacterial prophylaxis:
  - Consider during the hyperemic recovery phase (at least 2–3 days) in severely frostbitten areas
  - Against *Streptococci*, *Staphylococci*, and *Pseudomonas* species (cephalosporin, penicillinase-resistant penicillin, quinolone)
  - Topical antibacterial agents interfere with the use of aloe vera cream and should be considered a 2nd-line approach.
- Elevation and splinting of frostbitten area
- Change dressing 2–4 times daily.
- Avoid vasoconstrictive agents (including tobacco).
- Adjunctive/controversial treatments include:
  - Thrombolytic therapy:
    - Both intra-arterial and systemic tPA may improve tissue salvage rates.
  - Pentoxifylline
  - Hyperbaric oxygen
  - Sympathectomy
  - Early débridement and free tissue transfer

## MEDICATION
- Aloe vera: Topical cream (70% concentration) q6h
- Cephalexin (cephalosporin): 500 mg (peds: 25–50 mg/kg/24 h q6h) PO q.i.d.
- Ciprofloxacin (quinolone): 500 mg PO b.i.d.
- Dicloxacillin (penicillinase-resistant penicillin): 500 mg (peds: 12.5–25 mg/kg/24 h q6h) PO q.i.d.
- Ibuprofen (NSAID): 800 mg (peds: 40 mg/kg/24 h q6–8h) PO t.i.d.
- Morphine sulfate: 0.1–0.2 mg/kg (peds: 0.1 mg/kg) IV or IM PRN (titrate to patient response)

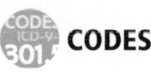 FOLLOW-UP

## DISPOSITION
### Admission Criteria
- All but the most superficial cases should be admitted.
- Lower admission threshold where risk of refreezing exists.
- Immersion (trench) foot patients may be discharged only if an environment that allows for proper treatment can be provided.

### Discharge Criteria
Minimal superficial injury, all others should be admitted.

### Issues for Referral
General, burn, or hand surgeon should be consulted in all but the most superficial of cases.

### FOLLOW-UP RECOMMENDATIONS
All discharged patients should be referred to a general, burn, or hand surgeon.

## PEARLS AND PITFALLS

Pitfalls:
- Allowing freeze, thaw, refreeze cycle to occur
- Failure to keep warm water bath between 40°C and 42°C during rewarming
- Failure to address hypothermia or other systemic illness
- Failure to consider compartment syndrome in a pulseless frostbitten extremity

## ADDITIONAL READING

- Biem J, et al. Out of the cold: Management of hypothermia and frostbite. *Can Med Assoc J*. 2003;168(3):305–311.
- Bruen K, et al. Treatment of digital frostbite: Current concepts. *J Hand Surg Am*. 2009;34(3):553–554.
- Murphy JV, et al. Frostbite: Pathogenesis and treatment. *J Trauma*. 2000;48(1):171–178.
- Wolfson AB, et al., eds. *Harwood-Nuss' Emergency Medicine*, 5th ed. Philadelphia: Lippincott Williams & Wilkins; 2010:1599–1603.

## See Also (Topic, Algorithm, Electronic Media Element)
Hypothermia

## CODES

ICD9
- 991.0 Frostbite of face
- 991.1 Frostbite of hand
- 991.2 Frostbite of foot

F

# GALLSTONE ILEUS
*Tamara Espinoza*

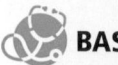 **BASICS**

## DESCRIPTION
- Mechanical intestinal obstruction secondary to impaction of a gallstone within bowel lumen
- Stone is usually >2.5 cm
- 1–3% of all intestinal obstructions
- Most cases occur in patients >65:
  - 25% of bowel obstructions in patients >65 yr
- Female > Male (5:1)
- Mortality 15–18%

## ETIOLOGY
- Chronic gallbladder inflammation causes adhesions between gallbladder and adjacent bowel wall.
- Cholecystenteric fistula develops, permitting stone passage into intestine:
  - Duodenum is most common site of fistula formation, followed by colon.
  - Gastric fistulas are rare.
- Site of impaction:
  - Terminal ileum most common (54–65%):
    - Narrowest part of small intestine.
  - Jejunum (27%)
  - Duodenum (1–3%):
    - Gastric outlet obstruction caused by duodenal impaction referred to as *Bouveret syndrome*.
  - Colonic obstruction is rare.
- Stones spilled intraperitoneally during cholecystectomy—open or laparoscopic—may also lead to bowel obstruction:
  - Can have recurrent obstruction from subsequent gallstones.

# DIAGNOSIS

## SIGNS AND SYMPTOMS
- "Tumbling" abdominal discomfort:
  - Episodic abdominal pain as stone lodges and dislodges throughout the intestines.
  - Complete impaction leads to severe, often acute abdominal pain.
- Nausea
- Vomiting:
  - Can be bilious or feculent
- Obstipation
- Abdominal distention and tympany
- Abdominal tenderness:
  - Peritoneal findings develop late in the course of disease
- Abnormal bowel sounds
- Occasional jaundice

### History
- Only 50–60% of patients have history of biliary colic or disease.
- Gallstone ileus has been associated with cardiovascular disease, diabetes, and obesity.

### Physical Exam
- Abdominal exam for:
  - Abdominal distension/tenderness
- Jaundice may occur

## ESSENTIAL WORKUP
Evaluate for intestinal obstruction.

## DIAGNOSTIC TESTS & INTERPRETATION
### Lab
- Electrolytes, BUN/creatinine, glucose since decreased oral intake and vomiting leads to:
  - Hypochloremia
  - Hypokalemia
  - Hyponatremia
  - Alkalosis
  - Prerenal azotemia
- Liver function panel and bilirubin may be elevated.
- Amylase:
  - Elevated in late obstructions
- CBC/hematocrit:
  - Hemoconcentration secondary to dehydration
- Elevated WBC nonspecific

### Imaging
- Flat and upright abdominal radiographs:
  - Multiple air fluid levels and distended bowel consistent with bowel obstruction
  - Rigler triad: 2 of 3 pathognomonic (present in 30–50%):
    - Air in the biliary tree (pneumobilia)
    - Partial or complete bowel obstruction
    - Ectopic stone visualized within the intestinal tract
- CXR:
  - Evaluate for pneumoperitoneum
- Abdominal CT scan:
  - Increasing use in evaluating small-bowel obstruction
  - Can directly visualize and localize stone within intestinal lumen
- Abdominal US:
  - Can identify pneumobilia and gallstones, but lower yield in locating obstructing stone

## DIFFERENTIAL DIAGNOSIS
- Paralytic ileus
- Extrinsic bowel obstruction:
  – Adhesions
  – Volvulus
  – Hernia
  – Intussusception
- GI malignancy
- Diverticulitis
- Bezoar
- Inflammatory bowel disease
- Pseudo-obstruction
- Cholecystitis
- Ascending cholangitis
- Pancreatitis

 **TREATMENT**

### PRE-HOSPITAL
Establish IV access.

### INITIAL STABILIZATION/THERAPY
IV fluid resuscitation

### ED TREATMENT/PROCEDURES
- Nasogastric suction to decompress the stomach and intestine
- Nothing PO
- Electrolyte replacement.
- Monitor urine output.
- Analgesics
- Broad-spectrum antibiotics to cover bowel flora:
  – Piperacillin/tazobactam.
  – Ampicillin/sulbactam.
  – Ticarcillin/clavulanate.
  – Alternatives include Imipenem, meropenem, 3rd-generation cephalosporins plus metronidazole.
- Surgical consultation

### MEDICATION
- Ampicillin/sulbactam: 3 g IV q6h (peds: 100–200 mg/kg/24 h)
- Piperacillin/tazobactam: 3.375 g IV q6h (peds: 240–400 mg/kg/24 h)
- Ticarcillin/clavulanate: 3.1 g IV q4–6h

 **FOLLOW-UP**

### DISPOSITION
**Admission Criteria**
- Admit all patients with gallstone ileus.
- Surgical evaluation for emergent operative intervention

**Discharge Criteria**
None

### FOLLOW-UP RECOMMENDATIONS
Surgical consultation in ED for evaluation and operative intervention

## PEARLS AND PITFALLS
- Gallstone ileus is a mechanical intestinal obstruction rather than a true ileus. Emergent surgical consultation is required for definitive management.
- High mortality rates stem from delay in diagnosis and patient comorbidities.
- Suspect gallstone ileus in all elderly patients, especially women, with signs/symptoms of bowel obstruction and no previous surgical history.

- Only 10% of ectopic gallstones can be visualized on plain radiographs. CT imaging is more sensitive and specific for detecting intraluminal stones.
- Only 1/2 of the patients have a previous history of biliary colic or gallstone disease.

## ADDITIONAL READING
- Bennett G, Balthazar E. Ultrasound and CT evaluation of emergent gallbladder pathology. *Radiol Clin North Am.* 2003;41:1203–1216.
- Chou JW, Hsu CH, Laio HC, et al. Gallstone ileus: Report of two cases and review of the literature. *World J Gastroenterol.* 2007;13:1295–1298.
- Lobo D, Jobling J, et al. Gallstone ileus: Diagnostic pitfalls and therapeutic successes. *J Clin Gastroenterol.* 2000;30(1):72–76.
- Rosenberg M, Parsiak K. Vomiting gravel. *Am J Emerg Med.* 2004;22(2):131–132.
- Zaliekas J, Munson JL. Complications of gallstones: The Mirizzi syndrome, gallstone ileus, gallstone pancreatitis, complications of "lost" gallstones. *Surg Clin North Am.* 2008;88:1345–1368.

### See Also (Topic, Algorithm, Electronic Media Element)
- Cholecystitis
- Cholelithiasis

 **CODES**

**ICD9**
560.31 Gallstone ileus

G

# GANGRENE

Karen B. Van Hoesen
Stephen R. Hayden

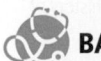 **BASICS**

## DESCRIPTION
- Gas gangrene or clostridial myonecrosis
- An acute, rapidly progressive, gas-forming necrotizing infection of muscle and subcutaneous tissue
- Can be seen in posttraumatic or postoperative situations
- Progressive invasion and destruction of healthy muscle tissue

## ETIOLOGY
- Clostridial organisms:
  - Facultative anaerobic, spore-forming, gram-positive bacillus
  - Produces a number of toxins; the most prevalent and lethal is $\alpha$-toxin.
- *Clostridium perfringens* is the most common bacterium; found in 80–90% of wounds.
- Other clostridial bacteria include *Clostridium novyi, Clostridium septicum, Clostridium histolyticum, Clostridium bifermentans,* and *Clostridium fallax.*
- 2 distinct mechanisms for introduction of clostridial organisms:
  - Traumatic and postoperative
  - Nontraumatic associated with diabetes mellitus, peripheral vascular disease, alcoholism, IV drug abuse, and malignancies

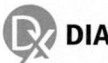 **DIAGNOSIS**

## SIGNS AND SYMPTOMS
- Sudden severe pain of extremity or involved area
- Low-grade fever
- Tachycardia out of proportion to fever
- Bronzing of the skin over involved area; later can turn purple or red
- Crepitus
- Formation of blebs and bullae
- Thin, serosanguineous exudate and sweet odor
- Rapid local extension
- Obtunded sensorium
- Systemic toxicity

## ESSENTIAL WORKUP
- History and physical exam with special attention to clinical evidence of crepitus in soft tissue
- Soft tissue x-rays of involved area to detect gas dissecting along fascial planes:
  - The absence of gas does not exclude significant disease.
- Stat Gram's stain of wound exudate for gram-positive bacillus with paucity of leukocytes

## DIAGNOSTIC TESTS & INTERPRETATION
### Lab
- CBC with differential, electrolytes, BUN, and creatinine
- Coagulation studies
- Evaluate for hemolysis
- Stat Gram's stain of wound exudates
- Anaerobic cultures of wound or tissue biopsy

### Imaging
- Radiographs may reveal soft tissue gas.
- CT if area involves abdomen or flank.

### Diagnostic Procedures/Surgery
All patients with gas gangrene must undergo surgical debridement.

## DIFFERENTIAL DIAGNOSIS
- Cellulitis
- Necrotizing fasciitis
- Nonclostridial myositis and myonecrosis
- Other causes of gas in tissues, as from dissection from respiratory or GI tracts

 **TREATMENT**

## PRE-HOSPITAL
Establish IV and infuse isotonic fluids

## INITIAL STABILIZATION/THERAPY
Manage airway and resuscitate as indicated:
- Rapid sequence intubation as needed.
- Supplemental oxygen:
  - Cardiac and oxygen saturation monitors should be placed.
- IV access; Consider central venous pressure monitoring.
- Aggressive volume expansion, including crystalloid, plasma, packed RBCs, and albumin if there is septic shock.

## ED TREATMENT/PROCEDURES
- Parenteral antibiotic therapy:
  - Initial empiric therapy should cover *Clostridium* species and group A *Streptococcus* as well as mixed aerobes and anaerobes
  - Primary definitive therapy: penicillin G plus clindamycin
  - Alternative: ceftriaxone or erythromycin
  - If mixed infection: penicillin plus clindamycin, metronidazole, or vancomycin and gram-negative coverage with gentamicin
  - Follow local sepsis protocols

- Surgical consultation:
  - Debridement, amputation, or fasciotomy is required.
- Hyperbaric oxygen (HBO) as adjunctive therapy:
  - Early transfer to hyperbaric facility may be lifesaving.
  - Lack of randomized trials with HBO but nonrandomized studies suggest benefit
- Tetanus prophylaxis
- Observe for major complications including ARDS, renal failure, myocardial irritability, and DIC.
- Polyvalent antitoxin is not made in the U.S. and studies have not demonstrated efficacy:
  - Because of the unacceptable hypersensitivity reactions, it is not routinely recommended.

## MEDICATION

- Ceftriaxone: 2.0 g (peds: 100 mg/kg/24 hr max. 4 g) IV q24h
- Clindamycin: 600–900 mg (peds: 40 mg/kg/day q6h) IV q8h.
- Gentamicin: 2.0 mg/kg (peds: 2.0 mg/kg IV q8h) IV q8h
- Metronidazole: 500 mg (peds: safety not established) IV q8h
- Penicillin G: 24 million IU/24 hr (peds: 250,000 IU/kg/24 hr) IV q4–6h
- Tetanus immune globulin: 500 IU IM
- Tetanus toxoid: 0.5 mg IM

### First Line
Primary definitive therapy for clostridial species; combination of penicillin G and clindamycin

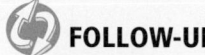 **FOLLOW-UP**

## DISPOSITION
### Admission Criteria
- All patients with gas gangrene and evidence of myonecrosis *must be admitted* for surgical débridement and IV antibiotics.
- Use of HBO therapy is an important adjunct.

### Discharge Criteria
No patient with acute gangrene should be discharged.

### Issues for Referral
After stabilization with antibiotics and surgical debridement, consider referral for hyperbaric oxygen treatment as an adjunct.

## PEARLS AND PITFALLS

- Bacteremia occurs in about 15% and can progress quickly to intravascular hemolysis.
- Hyperbaric oxygen as adjunctive therapy to surgical debridement and early antibiotics if patient is hemodynamically stable

## ADDITIONAL READING

- Kaide CG, Khandelwal S. Hyperbaric oxygen: Applications in infectious disease. *Emerg Med Clin North Am.* 2008;26(2):571–595.
- Brook I. Microbiology and management of soft tissue and muscle infections. *Int J Surg.* 2008;6(4):328–338. Epub July 15, 2007.
- Brook I. Microbiology and management of myositis. *Int Orthop.* 2004;28(5):257–260.
- Clark LA, Moon RE. Hyperbaric oxygen in the treatment of life-threatening soft-tissue infection. *Respir Care Clin North Am.* 1999;5(2):203–219.
- Headley AJ. Necrotizing soft tissue infections: A primary care review. *Am Fam Physician.* 2003;68(2):323–328.
- Langhan M, Arnold L. Clostridial myonecrosis in an adolescent male. *Pediatrics.* 2005;116(5):e735–e737.
- Perry BN, Floyd WE 3rd. Gas gangrene and necrotizing fasciitis in the upper extremity. *J Surg Orthop Adv.* 2004;13(2):57–68.

 **CODES**

### ICD9
- 040.0 Gas gangrene
- 785.4 Gangrene

G

# GASTRIC OUTLET OBSTRUCTION

*Jenny J. Lu*

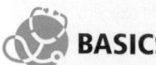

## BASICS

### DESCRIPTION
- Mechanical obstruction that impedes gastric emptying, resulting from any disease process
- Not limited to gastric pathology and may involve duodenal or extraluminal cause
- Benign and malignant causes:
  – Edema, scarring, stricture, or hyperplasia of pylorus or duodenum
  – Intrinsic or extrinsic mass, causing compression at pylorus or at proximal duodenum

### ETIOLOGY
- Neoplasms (pancreatic, gastric lymphoma, duodenal, gallbladder)
- Peptic ulcer disease (PUD) (no longer most common cause, with H2 blocker and Helicobacter Pylori treatment)
- Pyloric stenosis (most common in pediatric population)
- Inflammation/edema (chronic pancreatitis)
- Strictures/webs
- Caustic injury
- Gallstone obstruction

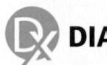

## DIAGNOSIS

### SIGNS AND SYMPTOMS
*History*
- Intermittent symptoms until obstruction becomes complete
- Vomiting, usually nonbilious
- Abdominal pain, variable
- Early satiety and epigastric fullness
- Epigastric discomfort relieved with emesis

*Physical Exam*
- Vital signs:
  – Often normal
  – Tachycardia, hypotension with significant volume depletion
- Abdominal examination:
  – Variable epigastric distention
  – Tympany
  – Succession splash >4 hr after eating
- Malnutrition in chronic or late obstruction
- Weight loss when chronic and with malignancy

*Geriatric Considerations*
- Abdominal pain, nausea/vomiting: Also common in elderly patients with acute myocardial infarctions:
  – Obtain EKG in persons at risk of acute coronary syndrome

*Pediatric Considerations*
- Pyloric stenosis:
  – Most common cause in pediatric population
  – As early as 1st wk up to age 3 mo
- Initially occasional nonprojectile postprandial vomiting, progressing to projectile (nonbilious) vomiting
- Midepigastric peristaltic wave prior to vomiting may be seen.
- Epigastric "olive" mass palpable in 80–90% of patients

### ESSENTIAL WORKUP
- Careful history and physical exam
- Abdominal US in pediatric patients:
  – Reveals elongated hypertrophic pyloric sphincter

### DIAGNOSTIC TESTS & INTERPRETATION
*Lab*
- CBC:
  – Anemia if blood loss from ulcer
  – High hematocrit indicates hemoconcentration.
- Electrolytes, BUN/creatinine, glucose:
  – Hypokalemia
  – Hypochloremic metabolic alkalosis
  – Hypoglycemia
  – Prerenal azotemia
- Urinalysis
- Amylase/lipase
- Liver function tests, if malignancy suspected
- Helicobacter pylori, if PUD suspected

*Imaging*
- Plain abdominal radiographs (obstructive series):
  – Dilated stomach
  – Absence of air in bowel distally
- Abdominal CT for detecting neoplastic, luminal, and extraluminal causes of obstruction

*Diagnostic Procedures/Surgery*
- Upper GI:
  – To demonstrate site of obstruction
- Upper endoscopy:
  – To visualize gastric outlet

### DIFFERENTIAL DIAGNOSIS
- Proximal bowel obstruction
- Exacerbation of peptic ulcer disease
- Gastroenteritis
- Cholelithiasis
- Cholecystitis
- Acute pancreatitis
- Diabetic gastroparesis
- Psychogenic vomiting

# TREATMENT

## PRE-HOSPITAL
IV fluid resuscitation if dehydrated or with history of recent vomiting.

## INITIAL STABILIZATION/THERAPY
- 0.9% NS IV fluid resuscitation for prolonged obstruction and significant volume depletion:
  - Adults: 1 L bolus
  - Peds: 20 ml/kg bolus
- Correct electrolyte abnormalities, especially hypokalemia.

## ED TREATMENT/PROCEDURES
- Nasogastric tube (NGT)
- Foley catheter to monitor urine output
- Surgical consultation/intervention:
  - Balloon dilatation of benign strictures
  - Enteral stent placement (malignant causes)
  - Gastrojejunostomy (malignant causes)
  - Vagotomy and antrectomy or pyloroplasty or gastrojejunostomy or other variation (benign causes)

## MEDICATION
- Famotidine: Adults: 20 mg (peds: 0.6–0.8 mg/kg/24 h div. q6–8h) IV q12h *or*
- Ranitidine: Adults: 50 mg (peds: 2–4 mg/kg/24 h div. q6–8h) IV q8h
- Pantoprazole: Adults: 40 mg IV daily (also H. *pylori* treatment as needed)

# FOLLOW-UP

## DISPOSITION
### Admission Criteria
All patients with gastric outlet obstruction require admission for fluid resuscitation, electrolyte repletion, gastroenterological, and surgical evaluation.

### Discharge Criteria
In the rare case, patients with previously diagnosed gastric outlet obstruction and planned intervention:
- Abdominal pain, vomiting have resolved completely
- Evaluated by surgeon or gastroenterologist during presentation
- Laboratory parameters and patient's volume status are normal

### Issues for Referral
Gastroenterology/surgery consultation.

## FOLLOW-UP RECOMMENDATIONS
Any discharged patient requires definite follow-up evaluation with surgeon or gastroenterologist:
- Specific instructions to return if symptoms recur

# PEARLS AND PITFALLS
- Misdiagnosing gastric outlet obstruction as gastroenteritis
- Failure to consider gastric outlet obstruction and malignancy in patient with epigastric pain and vomiting
- Failure to adequately replete electrolytes and fluids, especially in the elderly or pediatric patient

# ADDITIONAL READING
- Cherian PT, Cherian S, Singh P. Long-term follow-up of patients with gastric outlet obstruction related to peptic ulcer disease treated with endoscopic balloon dilatation and drug therapy. *Gastrointest Endosc.* 2007;66(3):491–497.
- Chowdhury A, Dhali GK, Banerjee PK. Etiology of gastric outlet obstruction. *Am J. Gastroenterol.* 1996;91:1679.
- Ozcan C, Ergun O, Sen T, et al. Gastric outlet obstruction secondary to acid ingestion in children. *J Pediatr Surg.* 2004;39(11):1651–1653.
- Shone DN, Nikoomanesh P, Smith-Meek MM, et al. Malignancy is the most common cause of gastric outlet obstruction in the era of H2 blockers. *Am J Gastroenterology.* 1995;90:1769–1770.
- Yusuf TE, Brugge WR. Endoscopic therapy of benign pyloric stenosis and gastric outlet obstruction. *Curr Opin Gastroenterol.* 2006;22(5):570–573.

## See Also (Topic, Algorithm, Electronic Media Element)
- Abdominal pain
- Bowel obstruction
- Pyloric stenosis
- Vomiting

# CODES

## ICD9
537.0 Acquired hypertrophic pyloric stenosis

G

# GASTRITIS
Yanina A. Purim-Shem-Tov

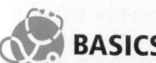 **BASICS**

## DESCRIPTION
- Inflammatory response of gastric mucosa to injury—"gastritis"
- 3 lines of defense of gastric mucosa:
  - Mucous layer that forms protective pH gradient
  - Surface epithelial cells that can repair small defects
  - Postepithelial barrier that neutralizes any acid that has traversed 1st 2 layers
- No definite link between histologic gastritis and dyspeptic symptoms
- Epithelial cell damage with no associated inflammation—"gastropathy"

## ETIOLOGY
- Common causes of gastritis: Infectious, autoimmune, drugs, hypersensitivity, stress.
- Common causes of gastropathy:Endogenous or exogenous irritants, such as bile reflux, alcohol, or aspirin and NSAIDs, ischemia, stress, chronic congestion.
- Acute gastritis:
  - Stress (sepsis, burns, trauma):
    - Decrease in splanchnic blood flow leading to decreased mucus production, bicarbonate secretion, and prostaglandin synthesis
    - Results in mucosal erosions and hemorrhage
  - Alcohol:
    - Induces production of leukotrienes that cause microvascular stasis, engorgement, and increased vascular permeability
    - Leads to hemorrhage
  - NSAIDs, including aspirin:
    - Interfere with prostaglandin synthesis, leading to similar cascade as induced by alcohol
    - Results in mucosal erosions
  - Steroids
- Chronic gastritis:
  - Produced by *Helicobacter pylori*
  - Mechanism of *H. pylori* unclear:
    - Gram-negative spiral bacteria found in gastric mucous layer
    - Contains enzyme urease that allows it to change pH level (alkaline) of its microenvironment

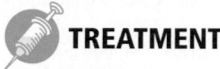 **DIAGNOSIS**

## SIGNS AND SYMPTOMS
- Dyspepsia
- Bloating
- Nausea/vomiting
- Anorexia
- Epigastric tenderness
- Heartburn

### History
- Dyspepsia
- Epigastric pain or discomfort (episodic and chronic)
- Bloating, indigestion, eructation, flatulence, and heartburn
- Anorexia, nausea/vomiting
- Dehydration, tachycardia, and electrolyte disturbances (with vomiting)
- Hematemesis, melena, pallor, and signs of volume depletion (hemorrhagic gastritis)

### Physical Exam
- Careful physical exam including stool Hemoccult testing and vital signs with orthostatics
- Nasogastric tube (NGT) when history of hematemesis or unstable vital signs
- Abdominal exam nonspecific

## ESSENTIAL WORKUP
- ABCs
- Hematocrit determination
- Evaluation for dehydration/shock

## DIAGNOSTIC TESTS & INTERPRETATION
### Lab
- Normal laboratory values in uncomplicated gastritis
- CBC:
  - Anemia with acute hemorrhagic gastritis
  - Leukocytosis: Infection
- Electrolytes, BUN, creatinine, glucose
- Amylase/lipase for pancreatitis in differential
- Urinalysis:
  - Assess dehydration/ketosis (starvation)
  - Bilirubin present with hepatitis

### Diagnostic Procedures/Surgery
- ECG:
  - For elderly patients
  - Myocardial ischemia in differential
- Endoscopy:
  - Outpatient unless significant hemorrhage
  - Allows for visualization of bleeding sites, histologic confirmation of mucosal inflammation, and detection of *H. pylori*

- Noninvasive *H. pylori* testing:
  - $^{13}$C and $^{14}$C urea breath tests
  - Stool antigen test
  - Serology to detect antibodies to *H. pylori*
  - Serum pepsinogen isoenzymes
    - The ratio of pepsinogen isozymes I and II in serum correlates with presence of metaplastic atrophic gastritis (principally autoimmune metaplastic atrophic gastritis and pernicious anemia)

## DIFFERENTIAL DIAGNOSIS
- Peptic ulcer disease (PUD)
- Nonulcer dyspepsia (symptoms without ulcer on endoscopy)
- Gastroesophageal reflux
- Biliary colic
- Cholecystitis
- Pancreatitis
- Hepatitis
- Abdominal aortic aneurysm
- Aortic dissection
- Myocardial infarction

**TREATMENT**

## PRE-HOSPITAL
- ABCs
- IV fluid resuscitation

## INITIAL STABILIZATION/THERAPY
- ABCs with acute erosive or hemorrhagic gastritis that presents with hemodynamic instability
- IV fluid resuscitation with lactated Ringer solution or 0.9% normal saline (NS) via 2 large-bore catheters
- NGT for gastric decompression and lavage
- Foley catheterization to assess volume replacement

## ED TREATMENT/PROCEDURES
- Pain control with:
  - Antacids
  - GI cocktail:
    - 30 mL antacids plus 10–20 mL viscous lidocaine
  - $H_2$ antagonists
  - Proton pump inhibitors (PPIs)
  - Sucralfate
  - Avoid narcotics—may mask serious illness
- Acute hemorrhagic gastritis:
  - IV fluid resuscitation
  - Blood transfusion if low hematocrit
  - Reverse causes (alcohol, sepsis, NSAIDs, or trauma)
  - Prevent *acute* or *erosive* gastritis in critically ill:
    - Antacids hourly or IV PPI or $H_2$ antagonists
    - Goal is to keep pH level at >4.

- Chronic gastritis—*H. pylori* therapy:
  - Treatment of *H. pylori* infection:
    - Invasive or noninvasive testing to confirm infection
    - Oral (PO) eradication antibiotic therapy options:
  - Most common therapies for *H. pylori* infection:
    - PPI (omeprazole 20 mg or lansoprazole 30 mg), clarithromycin 500 mg BID for 2 wk, amoxicillin 1 g BID for 2 wk.
    - For penicillin-allergic patients: PPI plus clarithromycin 500 mg BID plus metronidazole 500 mg BID for 14 days
    - 4 drug therapy: $H_2$ blocker, bismuth subsalicylate (Pepto-Bismol) plus either amoxicillin 1,000 mg BID or tetracycline 500 mg QID in combination with either metronidazole 250 mg QID or clarithromycin 500 mg BID for 14 days
  - Drug resistance:
    - Metronidazole: 30–48%
    - Clarithromycin: >10%
    - Amoxicillin: uncommon
    - Bismuth: none
  - Treatment controversial for asymptomatic or nonulcer dyspepsia gastritis
- Vitamin $B_{12}$ supplementation for *atrophic gastritis*

## MEDICATION

- Bismuth subsalicylate: 525-mg tabs 2 PO QID
- Cimetidine ($H_2$-blocker): 800 mg PO at bedtime nightly (peds: 20–40 mg/kg/24 h) for 6–8 wk
- Famotidine ($H_2$-blocker): 40 mg PO at bedtime nightly (peds: 0.5–0.6 mg/kg q12h) for 6–8 wk
- Lansoprazole (PPI): 30 mg PO BID for 2 weeks
- Maalox Plus: 2–4 tablets PO QID
- Misoprostol: 100–200 $\mu$g PO QID
- Mylanta II: 2–4 tablets PO QID
- Nizatidine ($H_2$ blocker): 300 mg PO at bedtime nightly for 6–8 wk
- Omeprazole (PPI): 20 mg PO BID (peds: 0.6–0.7 mg/kg q12h–q24h) for 2 weeks
- Pantoprazole (PPI): 40 mg PO/IV daily for 2 wk
- Ranitidine ($H_2$-blocker): 300 mg PO at bedtime nightly (peds: 5–10 mg/kg/24 h given q12h) for 6–8 wk
- Sucralfate: 1 g PO QID for 6–8 wk

### First Line
Triple therapy using a PPI with clarithromycin and amoxicillin or metronidazole given twice daily remains the recommended 1st choice treatment.

### Second Line
- Bismuth-based quadruple therapies remain the best 2nd choice treatment.
- The rescue treatment should be based on antimicrobial susceptibility testing.

 **FOLLOW-UP**

### DISPOSITION
#### Admission Criteria
- Acute hemorrhagic or erosive gastritis that presents with upper GI tract bleeding, tachycardia, and hypotension
- Uncontrolled pain or vomiting
- Coagulopathy from medication or liver disease

#### Discharge Criteria
- Unremarkable physical exam with normal CBC and heme-negative stools
- If heme-positive stools, discharge if stable vital signs, normal hematocrit, and negative NGT aspiration for upper GI tract hemorrhage:
  - Outpatient evaluation for endoscopy

#### Issues for Referral
- Outpatient referral for endoscopy and *H. pylori* testing
- Biopsy for gastric dysplasia and malignancy

### FOLLOW-UP RECOMMENDATIONS
Close follow up with gastroenterologist for endoscopy with biopsy for diagnostic reasons.

## PEARLS AND PITFALLS

- Gastritis/gastropathy is a common presentation to ED.
- Symptoms typically are dyspepsia, nausea, and vomiting.
- ED management depends on patient's clinical symptoms, but should include diagnostic and therapeutic components.
- Therapeutic management usually involves treatment of *H. pylori*.
- Drug resistance of *H. pylori* to antibiotics is increasing.
- Close follow up with gastroenterologist recommended for biopsy and to detect gastric cancers.

## ADDITIONAL READING

- Czinn SJ. *Helicobacter pylori* infection: detection, investigation, and management. *J Pediatr.* 2005;146:S21–26.
- Eswaran S, Roy MA. Medical management of acid-peptic disorders of the stomach. *Surg Clin North Am.* 2005;85:895–906.
- Leung WK, et al. Ulcer and gastritis. *Prim Care.* 2001;28(3):487–503.
- Smoot DT, Go MF, Cryer B. Peptic ulcer disease. *Prim Care.* 2001;33(1):8–15.
- Malfertheiner P, et al. Current concepts in the management of Helicobacter pylori infection: The Maastricht III Consensus Report. *Gut.* 2007;56(6): 772–781.
- Oishi Y, Kiyohara Y, Kubo M, et al. The serum pepsinogen test as a predictor of gastric cancer: The Hisayama study. *Am J Epidemiol* 2006;163:629.
- Ricci C, Vakil N, Rugge M, et al. Serological markers for gastric atrophy in asymptomatic patients infected with Helicobacter pylori. *Am J Gastroenterol* 2004;99:1910.
- Haj Sheykholeslami A, Rakhshani N, Amirzargar A, et al. Serum pepsinogen I, pepsinogen II, and gastrin 17 in relatives of gastric cancer patients: Comparative study with type and severity of gastritis. *Clin Gastroenterol Hepatol* 2008;6:174.

### See Also (Topic, Algorithm, Electronic Media Element)
- Gastrointestinal Bleeding
- Gastroesophageal Reflux Disease
- Peptic Ulcer Disease

G

 **CODES**

### ICD9
- 535.50 Unspecified gastritis and gastroduodenitis (without mention of hemorrhage)
- 535.51 Unspecified gastritis and gastroduodenitis with hemorrhage
- 537.9 Unspecified disorder of stomach and duodenum

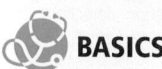

# GASTROENTERITIS
*Isam F. Nasr*

## BASICS

### DESCRIPTION
Inflammation of stomach and intestines associated with diarrhea and vomiting; often the result of infectious or toxin exposure.

### ETIOLOGY
#### Infectious
- Viruses:
  - 50–70% of all cases
- Invasive bacteria:
  - *Campylobacter*: Contaminated food or water, wilderness water, birds and animals:
    - Most common cause
    - Gross or occult blood is found in 60–90%.
  - *Salmonella*: Contaminated water, eggs, poultry, or dairy products:
    - *Typhoid fever (Salmonella typhi)* characterized by unremitting fever, abdominal pain, rose spots, splenomegaly, and bradycardia
    - Immunocompromised susceptible
  - *Shigella*: Fecal–oral route
  - *Vibrio parahaemolyticus*: raw and undercooked seafood
  - *Yersinia*: Contaminated food (pork), water, and milk:
    - May present as mesenteric adenitis or mimic appendicitis
  - Specific food-borne disease (food poisoning):
    - Staphylococcus aureus:
    - Most common toxin-related disease
    - Symptoms 1–6 hr after ingesting food
  - *Bacillus cereus*:
    - Classic source is fried rice left on steam tables.
    - Symptoms within 1–36 hr
  - Cholera: profuse watery stools with mucous (rice-water stools)
  - Ciguatera:
    - Fish intoxication
    - Onset 5 min to 30 hr (average 6 hr) after ingestion
    - Paresthesias, hypotension, peripheral muscle weakness
    - Amitriptyline may be therapeutic.
  - Scombroid:
    - Caused by blood fish: tuna, albacore, mackerel, and mahi mahi
    - Flushing, headache, erythema, dizziness, blurred vision, and generalized burning sensation
    - Symptoms last <6 hr.
    - Treatment includes antihistamines.
- Protozoa:
  - *Giardia lamblia*;
    - High-risk groups: travelers, day care children, homosexual men, and campers who drink untreated mountain water

#### Noninfectious Causes
- Toxins:
  - Zinc, copper, cadmium
  - Organic chemicals: Polyvinyl chlorides
  - Pesticides: Organophosphates
  - Radioactive substances
  - Alkyl mercury
- Altered host response to food substance
- (tyramine, monosodium glutamate, tryptamine)

#### Pediatric Considerations
- Focus evaluation on state of hydration.
- Most of viral origin and self-limited
- Rotavirus accounts for up to 50%.
- *Shigella* infections associated with seizures

## DIAGNOSIS

### SIGNS AND SYMPTOMS
#### History
- Nausea, vomiting, diarrhea
- Bloody/mucous diarrhea
- Abdominal cramps or pain
- Fever
- Malaise, myalgias, headache, anorexia
- Hypotension, lethargy, and dehydration (severe cases)

#### Physical Exam
- Dry mucous membranes
- Tachycardia
- Abdominal tenderness
- Perianal inflammation, fissure, fistula

### ESSENTIAL WORKUP
- Digital rectal examination to determine presence of gross or occult blood
- Fecal leukocyte determination:
  - Present with invasive bacteria
  - Absent in protozoal infections, viral, toxin-induced food poisoning

### DIAGNOSTIC TESTS & INTERPRETATION
#### Lab
- CBC indications:
  - Significant blood loss
  - Systemic toxicity
- Electrolytes, glucose, BUN, creatinine—indications:
  - Lethargy, significant dehydration, toxicity, or altered mental status
  - Diuretic use, persistent diarrhea, chronic liver or renal disease

- Stool culture indications:
  - Presence of fecal leukocytes
  - Historical markers (immunocompromised, travel, homosexual)
  - Public health (food handler, day/health care worker)
- Blood cultures indications:
  - Suspected bacteremia or systemic infections
  - Ill patients requiring admission
  - Immunocompromised
  - Elderly patients and infants

#### Imaging
Abdominal radiographs have no value unless obstruction or toxic megacolon suspected.

#### Pediatric Considerations
- Laboratory studies not required in most cases
- Rotazyme assay detects rotavirus:
  - Rarely indicated in managing outpatients
  - Helpful to cohort and avoid cross-contamination among inpatients
- Stool cultures indication:
  - Fecal leukocytes
  - Toxic
  - Infants
  - Immunocompromised

### DIFFERENTIAL DIAGNOSIS
- Gastritis/peptic ulcer disease
- Milk and food allergies
- Appendicitis
- Irritable bowel syndrome
- Ulcerative colitis/Crohn disease
- Malrotation with midgut volvulus
- Meckel diverticulum
- Drugs and toxins:
  - Mannitol
  - Sorbitol
  - Phenolphthalein
  - Magnesium-containing antacids
  - Quinidine
  - Colchicine
  - Mushrooms
  - Mercury poisoning

**TREATMENT**

**PRE-HOSPITAL**
- Difficult IV access with severe dehydration.
- Avoid exposure to contaminated clothes or body substances.

**INITIAL STABILIZATION/THERAPY**
- Management of ABCs
- IV fluid with 0.9% NS resuscitation for severely dehydrated

**ED TREATMENT/PROCEDURES**
- Oral fluids for mild dehydration (Gatorade/Pedialyte)
- IV fluids for:
  - Hypotension, nausea and vomiting, obtundation, metabolic acidosis, significant hypernatremia or hyponatremia
  - 0.9% NS bolus (adults: 500 mL–1 L, peds: 20 mL/kg) for resuscitation, then 0.9% NS or $D_5$ 0.45% peds: NS (peds: $D_5$ 0.25% NS) to maintain adequate urine output
- Bismuth subsalicylate (Pepto-Bismol):
  - Antisecretory agent
  - Effective clinical relief without adverse effects
- Kaolin–pectin (Kaopectate):
  - Reduces fluidity of stools
  - Does not influence course of disease
- Antimotility drugs (diphenoxylate [Lomotil], loperamide [Imodium], paregoric, and codeine):
  - Appropriate in noninfectious diarrhea
  - Initial use of sparse amounts to control symptoms in infectious diarrhea
  - Avoid prolonged use in infectious diarrhea—may increase duration of fever, diarrhea, and bacteremia and may precipitate toxic megacolon.
- Antibiotics for infectious pathogens:
  - *Campylobacter*: quinolones or erythromycin
  - *Salmonella*: quinolones or trimethoprim–sulfamethoxazole (TMP–SMX)
  - Typhoid fever: ceftriaxone
  - *Shigella*: quinolone, TMP–SMX, or ampicillin
  - *Vibrio parahaemolyticus*:tetracycline or doxycycline
  - *Clostridium difficile*:vancomycin
  - *Escherichia coli*: quinolones or TMP–SMX
  - *Giardia lamblia*:metronidazole
- Antiemetics for nausea/vomiting:
  - Prochlorperazine
  - Promethazine

**MEDICATION**
- Ampicillin: 500 mg (peds: 20 mg/kg/24 h) PO or IV q6h
- TMP–SMX; Bactrim DS: one tab (peds: 8–10 mg TMP/40–50 mg SMX/kg/24 hr) PO b.i.d.
- Ceftriaxone: 1 g (peds: 50–75 mg/kg/12 hr) IM or IV q12h
- Ciprofloxacin (quinolone): 500 mg PO or 400 mg IV b.i.d. (>18 yr)
- Doxycycline: 100 mg PO or 400 mg IV b.i.d.
- Erythromycin: 500 mg (peds: 40–50 mg/kg/24 h) PO q.i.d.
- Iodoquinol: 650 mg (peds: 30–40 mg/kg/24 h) PO t.i.d.
- Metronidazole: 250 mg (peds: 35 mg/kg/24 hr) PO t.i.d. (>8 yr)
- Prochlorperazine (Compazine): 5–10 mg IV q3–4h; 10 mg PO q8h; 25 mg per rectum (PR) q12h
- Promethazine (Phenergan): 25 mg IM/IV q4h; 25 mg PO/PR (peds: 0.25–1 mg/kg PO/PR/IM)
- Tetracycline: 500 mg PO or IV q.i.d.

 **FOLLOW-UP**

**DISPOSITION**

*Admission Criteria*
- Hypotension unresponsive to IV fluids
- Significant bleeding
- Signs of sepsis/toxicity
- Intractable vomiting or abdominal pain
- Severe electrolyte imbalance
- Metabolic acidosis
- Altered mental status
- Children with >10–15% dehydration

*Discharge Criteria*
- Mild cases requiring oral hydration
- Dehydration responsive to IV fluids

*Issues for Referral*
Cases of prolonged symptoms may be referred to a gastroenterologist for further work up.

**FOLLOW-UP RECOMMENDATIONS**
Most cases are self-limiting; therefore, follow-up is optional.

## PEARLS AND PITFALLS

- Viruses account for over 50% of cases
- Avoid antimotility drugs in cases due to infectious pathogens.
- Trimethoprim–sulfamethoxazole (TMP–SMX; Bactrim DS) ciprofloxacin, doxycycline, and tetracycline are contraindicated in pregnancy.Metronidazole may be used during the third trimester.

## ADDITIONAL READING

- Blacklow NR, Greenberg HB. Viral gastroenteritis. *N Engl J Med*. 1991;325:252.
- Craig SA, Zich DK. Gastroenteritis. In: Marx JA, Hockberger RB, Walls RM, eds. *Rosen's Emergency Medicine*, 7th ed. Philadelphia: Elsevier, 2009:1200–1227.
- Dupont HL. What's new in enteric infectious diseases at home and abroad. *Curr Opinion Infect Dis*. 2005;18:407–412.
- Hill, DR, Ericsson, CD, Pearson, RD, et al. The practice of travel medicine:Guidelines by the Infectious Diseases Society of America. *Clin Infect Dis*. 2006;43:1499.

**See Also (Topic, Algorithm, Electronic Media Element)**
- Diarrhea, Adult
- Diarrhea, Pediatric

 **CODES**

**ICD9**
- 005.9 Food poisoning, unspecified
- 008.5 Bacterial enteritis, unspecified
- 008.8 Intestinal infection due to other organism, not elsewhere classified

G

# GASTROESOPHAGEAL REFLUX DISEASE
Yanina A. Purim-Shem-Tov

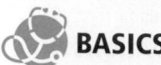 **BASICS**

## DESCRIPTION
- Spectrum of pathology in which gastric reflux causes symptoms and damage to esophageal mucosa
- Reflux esophagitis versus nonerosive reflux disease
- c40% of general population experience symptoms monthly.

## ETIOLOGY
- Incompetent reflux barrier allowing increase in frequency and duration of gastric contents into esophagus
- Transient lower esophageal sphincter relaxations (TLESRs):
  - Occur with higher frequency in gastroesophageal reflux disease (GERD) patients
  - Exposed esophageal mucosa becomes acidified and with time necroses.
  - Main antireflux barrier
- Lower esophageal sphincter (LES):
  - Crural diaphragm attachment (diaphragmatic sphincter)
  - Contributes to pressure barrier at gastroesophageal junction
  - Esophageal acid clearance via peristalsis and esophageal mucosal resistance are additional barriers.
  - Most healthy individuals have brief episodes
  - f reflux without symptoms.
- Decreased LES tone:
  - Smoking
  - Foods: alcohol, chocolate, onion, coffee, tea
  - Drugs: calcium channel blockers, morphine,
  - meperidine, barbiturates, theophylline, nitrates
- Delayed gastric emptying, increased body mass, and gastric distention contribute to reflux.
- Hiatal hernias associated with GERD:
  - Significance varies in any given individual
  - Most persons with hiatal hernias do not have clinically evident reflux disease.
- Acid secretion is same in those with or without GERD.
- Associated medical conditions: pregnancy, chronic hiccups, cerebral palsy, Down syndrome, autoimmune diseases, diabetes mellitus (DM), hypothyroidism.

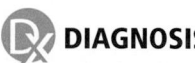 **DIAGNOSIS**

## SIGNS AND SYMPTOMS
- Esophageal manifestations
  - Heartburn (or pyrosis)
  - Regurgitation
  - Dysphagia.
- Extraesophageal manifestations
  - Bronchospasm
  - Laryngitis
  - Chronic cough

## History
- Typical signs and symptoms:
  - Heartburn (pyrosis):
    ○ Retrosternal burning pain
    ○ Radiates from epigastrium through chest to neck and throat
  - Dysphagia:
    ○ Dysphagia suggests esophageal spasm or stricture.
  - Odynophagia:
    ○ Odynophagia suggests ulcerative esophagitis.
  - Regurgitation
  - Water brash
  - Belching
  - Esophageal strictures, bleeding
  - Barrett esophagus (esophageal carcinoma)
  - Early satiety, nausea, anorexia, weight loss
  - Symptoms worse with recumbence or bending over
  - Symptoms usually relieved with antacids, although temporarily
- Atypical signs and symptoms:
  - Noncardiac chest pain
  - Asthma
  - Persistent cough, hiccups
  - Hoarseness
  - Pharyngeal/laryngeal ulcers and carcinoma
  - Frequent throat clearing
  - Recurrent pneumonitis
  - Nocturnal choking
  - Upper GI tract bleeding

## Physical Exam
- Nonspecific, may have some epigastric tenderness.
- Symptoms worsen with placing patient flat on the bed or Trendelenburg position

## Pediatric Considerations
- Regurgitation is common in infants:
  - Incidence decreases from twice daily in 50% of those age 2 mo to 1% of 1-yr-olds.
- Signs:
  - Frequent vomiting, irritability, cough, crying, and malaise
  - Arching the body (hyperextension) at feeding and refusals of feedings
- Failure to thrive
- Formula intolerance
- Sepsis

## ESSENTIAL WORKUP
- Differentiate GERD from more emergent conditions such as ischemic heart pain, esophageal perforation, or aortic pathology.
- History: Typical
- Thorough physical exam: Vital signs, head, ears, eyes, nose, throat (HEENT), chest and abdominal exams

## DIAGNOSTIC TESTS & INTERPRETATION
- No gold standard

### Lab
- CBC:
  - Chronic anemia from esophagitis
- Stool testing for occult bleeding

### Imaging
- No routine Imaging
- Chest radiograph:
  - Evidence of esophageal perforation, hiatal hernia, aortic disease

### Diagnostic Procedures/Surgery
- Diagnostic trial of antacid:
  - Those with persistent symptoms should be referred for endoscopy.
  - 90% of GERD patients respond to proton pump inhibitor (PPI) therapy.
- Barium esophagram for prominent dysphagia
- Esophageal pH monitoring:
  - Correlate symptoms to acid reflux,
- Esophageal manometry (poor sensitivity):
  - Evaluate LES resting pressure and esophageal peristaltic contractions.
- Esophagogastroduodenoscopy (EGD)—detects reflux esophagitis and complications (Barrett's esophagus, hiatal hernia, stricture, ulcers, malignancy)

## DIFFERENTIAL DIAGNOSIS
- Ischemic heart disease
- Asthma
- Peptic ulcer disease
- Gastritis
- Hepatitis/pancreatitis
- Esophageal perforation
- Esophageal foreign body
- Esophageal infection
- Cholecystitis/cholelithiasis
- Mesenteric ischemia

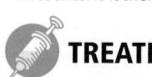 **TREATMENT**

## PRE-HOSPITAL
- Esophageal pain may mimic angina.
- Airway may need active control secondary to vomiting.

## INITIAL STABILIZATION/THERAPY
- ABCs need to be evaluated.
- IV fluid resuscitation for blood loss or shock

## ED TREATMENT/PROCEDURES
- Symptomatic relief:
  - Antacids
  - Antacids with viscous lidocaine
  - Sublingual nitroglycerine for esophageal spasm
  - Analgesics

- Lifestyle modifications:
  - Avoid late-night or heavy/fatty meals.
  - Minimize time in supine position after eating.
  - Elevation of head of bed
  - Weight loss
  - Eliminate smoking and alcohol intake.
- Avoid direct esophageal irritants such as citric juices and coffee
- Avoid foods that decrease LES pressures such as fatty foods, chocolate, and coffee.
- Avoid drugs that lower LES tone.
- Antacids (Maalox, Mylanta, etc.):
  - Treatment of mild and infrequent reflux symptoms
  - Not effective for healing esophagitis
  - Alginic acid slurry floats on surface of gastric contents, providing mechanical barrier
- Sucralfate:
  - Binds to exposed proteins on surface of injured mucosa to form protective barrier
  - May also directly stimulate mucosal repair
- Metoclopramide (prokinetic drug):
  - Improves peristalsis
  - Accelerates gastric emptying
  - Increases LES pressure
- $H_2$-blockers:
  - Effective for mild to moderate disease
  - Severe disease requires greater dosage than that used for peptic ulcer disease
- Proton pump inhibitors:
  - More potent long-acting inhibitors of gastric acid secretion
  - Faster healing than other drug therapies
  - More efficacious in severe GERD and frank esophagitis
- Endoscopic therapy:
  - Suturing (plication), thermal injury, chemical injection
- Antireflux surgery (goal: increase LES pressure):
  - Chronic reflux, younger patients, nonhealing ulceration, severe bleeding
  - Fundoplication can be more effective than medical therapy in selected cases

### Pregnancy Considerations

- Pyrosis present in 30–50% of pregnancies
- Increased intra-abdominal pressure, hormonal fluctuations lead to increased TLESRs.
- EGD reserved for severe presentations
- $H_2$-blockers—first-line therapy (longer safety record)
- PPIs—limited safety history in pregnancy

## MEDICATION

- Antacids: 30 mL plus viscous lidocaine, 10 mL, PO q6h
- Cimetidine: 400 mg PO b.i.d., 300 mg IM/IV q6h–q8h
- Esomeprazole: 20–40 mg PO daily
- Famotidine: 20 mg PO/IV BID (peds: 0.5–1.0 mg/kg/d div. q8h–q12h, max. 40 mg/d)
- Lansoprazole: 15–30 mg daily
- Metoclopramide: 10–15 mg PO/IV/IM q6h before meals and nightly at bedtime

- Nizatidine: 150 mg PO BID
- Omeprazole: 20–40 mg PO daily
- Pantoprazole: 40 mg PO/IV daily
- Rabeprazole: 20 mg PO daily
- Ranitidine: 150 mg (peds: 5–10 mg/kg q12h) PO BID or 300 mg PO nightly at bedtime
- Sucralfate: 1 g PO 1 hr before meals and nightly at bedtime

### First Line

- Life style modifications:
  - Head of bed elevation
  - Dietary modification
  - Refraining from assuming a supine position after meals
  - Avoidance of tight fitting garments
  - Promotion of salivation by either chewing gum
  - Restriction of alcohol use
  - Reduction of obesity
- Acid-suppressive medications:
  - $H_2$ blocker or a proton pump inhibitor
- Treatment of H-pylori infections

### Second Line

- Prokinetic drugs (bethanechol, metoclopramide)
- Drugs that inhibit transient LES relaxations (baclofen)

 FOLLOW-UP

## DISPOSITION

### Admission Criteria

- Seriously ill patients
- Significant esophageal bleeding
- Uncontrolled reactive asthma
- Dehydration
- Starvation and failure to thrive

### Discharge Criteria

Uncomplicated GERD: Refer to patient's primary care physician (PCP) or gastroenterologist for further evaluation.

### Issues for Referral

Extraesophageal manifestations (asthma, laryngitis, etc.)

## FOLLOW-UP RECOMMENDATIONS

Gastroenterologist for endoscopy in patients who require continuous maintenance medical therapy to rule out Barrett's esophagus

## PEARLS AND PITFALLS

- GERD therapy should include lifestyle changes
- In patients with worse than mild and intermittent GERD symptoms—acid-suppressive therapy
- In patients with GERD and moderate to severe esophagitis, provide acid suppression with a PPI rather than an $H_2$ blockers
- Endoscopy for patients who fail chronic therapy (at least 8 wk)

- Antireflux surgery for patients on high doses of PPIs, specially in young patients who may require lifelong therapy
- Complications of GERD
  - Esophagitis
  - Peptic stricture and Barrett's metaplasia
  - Extraesophageal manifestations of reflux: asthma, laryngitis, and cough.

## ADDITIONAL READING

- Cappell MS. Clinical presentation, diagnosis, and management of gastroesophageal reflux disease. *Med Clin North Am.* 2005;89(2):243–291.
- Spechler SJ, Lee E, Ahnen D, et al. Long-term outcome of medical and surgical therapies for gastroesophageal reflux disease. *JAMA.* 2001;205: 2331–2338.
- DeVault KR, Castell DO. American College of Gastroenterology. Updated guidelines for the diagnosis and treatment of gastroesophageal reflux disease. *Am J Gastroenterol* 2005;100:190.
- Diav-Citrin O, Arnon J, Shechtman S, et al. The safety of proton pump inhibitors in pregnancy: a multicentre prospective controlled study. *Aliment Pharmacol Ther* 2005;21:269
- Kaltenbach T, Crockett S, Gerson LB. Are lifestyle measures effective in patients with gastroesophageal reflux disease? An evidence-based approach. *Arch Intern Med* 2006;166:965.
- Kahrilas PJ, Shaheen NJ, Vaezi MF. American Gastroenterological Association Institute technical review on the management of gastroesophageal reflux disease. *Gastroenterology* 2008;135:1392.

### See Also (Topic, Algorithm, Electronic Media Element)

- Gastritis
- Peptic Ulcer Disease

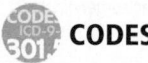 CODES

### ICD9

- 530.11 Reflux esophagitis
- 530.81 Esophageal reflux

G

# GASTROINTESTINAL BLEEDING

*Samantha Foy*
*Leon D. Sanchez*

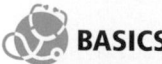 **BASICS**

## DESCRIPTION
- Bleeding from the GI tract:
  - Upper GI tract:
    - Proximal to the ligament of Treitz
    - Male > Female (2:1)
  - Lower GI tract:
    - Distal to the ligament of Treitz
    - Female > Male
- Mortality rate of GI bleed (GIB):
  - 10% overall with <5% in children to as high as 25% in adults >70

## ETIOLOGY
### Upper GIB (UGIB):
- Ulcerative disease of upper GI tract:
  - Peptic ulcer disease (40%):
    - *Helicobacter pylori* infection
    - Drug-induced (NSAIDs, aspirin, K supplements, Fe supplements)
    - Alcohol abuse
    - Cushing ulcers from severe damage to the CNS
  - Gastric or esophageal erosions (25%):
    - Reflux esophagitis
    - Infectious esophagitis (*Candida*, HSV, CMV)
    - Pill-induced esophagitis:
  - Gastritis and stress ulcerations:
    - Toxic agents (NSAIDs, alcohol, bile)
    - Mucosal hypoxia (trauma, burns, sepsis)
    - Chemotherapy
    - Esophageal foreign body
- Portal HTN:
  - Esophageal or gastric varices (20%)
  - Portal hypertensive gastropathy
- Arteriovenous malformations:
  - Aortoenteric fistula (s/p aortoiliac surgery)
  - Idiopathic angiomas
  - Osler-Weber-Rendu syndrome
  - Dieulafoy vascular malformations
  - Watermelon stomach (idiopathic)
  - Gastric antral vascular ectasia
- Mallory-Weiss tear (5%)
- Gastric and esophageal tumors
- Hemorrhage from a pancreatic source
- Hemobilia

### Lower GIB (LGIB):
- Diverticulosis (33%)
- Cancer or polyps (19%)
- Colitis (18%):
  - Ischemic, inflammatory, or infectious
- Vascular:
  - Angiodysplasia (8%)
  - Radiation telangiectasia
  - Aortocolonic fistula
- Inflammatory bowel disease:
  - Crohn disease or ulcerative colitis
- Postpolypectomy
- Anorectal (4%):
  - Internal or external hemorrhoids
  - Anal fissures
  - Rectal ulcer

### Pediatric Considerations
Meckel diverticulum and intussusception are the most common causes of LGIB in children.

 **DIAGNOSIS**

## SIGNS AND SYMPTOMS
- Both UGIB and LGIB may present with signs/symptoms of hypovolemia
- Classic presentation of UGIB:
  - Hematemesis or coffee ground emesis
  - Melena: Black tarry stool
- Classic presentation of LGIB:
  - Hematochezia: Bright red or maroon stool

### ALERT
Hematochezia classically signals a LGIB, but can be seen with a brisk UGIB as well.

### History
- Hematemesis and melena most common
- Coffee ground emesis
- Black, melanotic stools
- Bright red blood per rectum
- Abdominal pain
- Fatigue
- Weakness or lightheadedness
- Dyspnea
- Confusion or agitation

### Physical Exam
- Tachycardia
- Hypotension
- Orthostasis
- Pale appearance of conjunctiva/nail beds
- Altered mental status
- Melanotic, bloody, or heme positive stools
- Dry mucous membranes

### ESSENTIAL WORKUP
- Distinguish between hemoptysis and GIB:
  - Pulmonary source:
    - Bright red blood or frothy in appearance
    - Sputum mixed with blood is likely pulmonary.
    - pH >7
  - GI source:
    - Dark red/brown blood, +/− gastric contents
    - Associated with nausea/vomiting
    - pH <7
- CBC, coagulation studies, electrolytes
- Nasogastric aspiration and lavage for UGIB:
  - False negative rate is 25% if bleeding from duodenal source.
  - Presence of bile in aspirate is helpful in lowering false negative rate.
  - Lavage at least 500 cc of normal saline or until clear.
  - Iced lavage is not useful to stop bleeding and can cause hypothermia.

- Rectal exam:
  - Inspect for external hemorrhoids or anal fissure
  - Examine stool for black, red, maroon, or normal color.
  - False-positive Hemoccult result:
    - Raw red meat
    - Some iron preparations
    - Fruits: Cantaloupe, grapefruit, figs
    - Raw broccoli, cauliflower, radish
    - Methylene blue, chlorophyll
    - Iodide, bromide
  - False-negative Hemoccult result:
    - Bile
    - Mg containing antacids
    - Ascorbic acid
  - Agents causing black stools but negative Hemoccult:
    - Iron
    - Charcoal
    - Bismuth (ie, Pepto-Bismol)
    - Food dyes
    - Beets

### Pediatric Considerations
Bloody stool in newborns may be caused by the infant swallowing maternal blood.

### DIAGNOSTIC TESTS & INTERPRETATION
#### Lab
- CBC:
  - Anemia
  - Low mean corpuscular volume associated with chronic blood loss
  - Thrombocytopenia
- Electrolytes, BUN, creatinine, glucose
- Coagulation profile (PT/PTT/INR)
- LFTs, if upper GI bleeding suspected
- Type and screen/cross for active bleeding or unstable vital signs
- Lactate if mesenteric ischemia suspected

### ALERT
A drop in hematocrit may not be seen immediately and can remain normal for a period of time after acute blood loss.

#### Imaging
- Upright CXR if concern for aspiration
- Upright abdominal radiograph if concern for perforation, obstruction, or signs of peritonitis
- Multidetector helical CT emerging as a diagnostic imaging tool
- Angiography/arterial embolization:
  - Effective if large, active bleeding, LGIB > UGIB
- Radionucleotide scans:
  - Effective for identifying slow, active bleeding

### Diagnostic Procedures/Surgery
- Anoscopy:
  - For suspected internal hemorrhoids
- Esophagogastroduodenoscopy (EGD):
  - Diagnostic and possibly therapeutic
- Colonoscopy:
  - Diagnostic only
  - Best if done after adequate bowel preparation
- Bowel resection:
  - Reserved for refractory bleeding, usually in an unstable patient

## DIFFERENTIAL DIAGNOSIS
- Hemoptysis
- Oral/pharyngeal bleeding/epistaxis
- Hematuria
- Vaginal bleeding
- Acute abdomen
- Visceral trauma

## TREATMENT

### PRE-HOSPITAL
- Stabilize the airway/breathing:
  - Place the patient on 100% oxygen via mask
  - Intubate for massive upper GI bleed if not protecting airway
- Insert at least 1 large-bore IV line (16–18 g):
  - Administer crystalloid to keep SBP >90 mm Hg
  - Attempt 2nd IV line en route to hospital.

### INITIAL STABILIZATION/THERAPY
- Assess airway, breathing, and circulation.
- Control airway in patients with massive GI bleeding who are unstable or unable to protect airway.
- Administer 100% oxygen, apply cardiac monitor and pulse oximeter.
- Initiate 2 large-bore (16-g) IV lines:
  - Administer 1 L NS bolus (peds: 20 cc/kg) and repeat once if necessary.
  - Transfuse packed RBCs if still unstable after NS boluses or Hct <10 mg/dL:
    - Cross-matched or type-specific blood if available. Otherwise, use O negative for premenopausal women, O positive for others.
    - Administer fresh frozen plasma (FFP) and vitamin K if coagulopathic.
    - Consider platelets and FFP if large volumes of RBCs are being transfused.

### ED TREATMENT/PROCEDURES
- Consult gastroenterology for any significant GI bleeding.
- Consider surgical consult and/or interventional radiology (if available) for massive ongoing bleeding, unstable patient, or evidence of perforation.
- Place Foley catheter to monitor urine output.
- Place nasogastric tube (NGT), as above.
- Blood transfusion for:
  - Unstable vital signs despite crystalloid bolus
  - Ongoing chest pain/ischemic EKG changes
  - Significant anemia

- Treatment for UGIB:
  - IV proton pump inhibitor (PPI) (ie, pantoprazole)
  - Octreotide for suspected variceal bleeding
  - Consider vasopressin for variceal bleeding:
    - Administer concurrently with IV nitroglycerin to prevent tissue necrosis/myocardial ischemia.
  - Emergent endoscopy
  - Any 2 of these 3 factors indicates high risk for active bleeding
    - Bright bleeding from NGT
    - Hemoglobin <8 g/dL
    - WBC >12,000/uL
  - Hemodynamic instability may also require urgent endoscopy
  - Therapeutic options:
    - Cauterization of bleeding ulcers/vessels
    - Injection sclerosis of visible vessels
    - Endoscopic sclerotherapy for varices
  - Balloon tamponade for varices with Blakemore tube is a last resort.
- Treatment for lower GI bleeding:
  - Consider angiography for massive, active bleeding with directed vasopressin infusion.
  - Consider bowel resection for massive active bleeding that is refractory to medical management.

## MEDICATION

### First Line
- Pantoprazole: 80 mg (peds: Dosing not approved) IV bolus followed by an infusion of 8 mg/h for 72 hr
- Octreotide: 50 $\mu$g (peds: 1–2 $\mu$g/kg) bolus, then 50 $\mu$g/hr (peds: 1–2 $\mu$g/kg/hr) IV
- Vasopressin: 0.2–0.4 IU/min (peds: 0.002–0.005 IU/kg/min) IV, titrate up as needed. When no bleeding for 12 hr, taper over 24–48 hr.

### Second Line
- Nitroglycerin: 5–50 $\mu$g/min (peds: Not established) IV
- Somatostatin: 250 $\mu$g (peds: Not established) IV bolus and 250–500 $\mu$g/h for 2–5 days
- Terlipressin: 2 mg (peds: Not established) IV q4–6h for 48 hr
- Vitamin K: 10 mg (peds: 1–5 mg) PO/SC/IV q24h.

 FOLLOW-UP

## DISPOSITION

### Admission Criteria
- Unstable vital signs at any time
- Decreased hematocrit with recent GI bleeding
- Coagulopathy
- Age >65 or comorbid conditions
- Active bleeding

### Discharge Criteria
- Resolution of UGIB with negative nasogastric lavage and EGD
- Minor or resolved LGIB
- Stable vital signs
- Stable hematocrit >30 or hemoglobin >10 g/dL
- Normal coagulation
- Otherwise healthy patient, no ascites/portal HTN

### Issues for Referral
Consider referral to gastroenterologist for outpatient colonoscopy and/or EGD.

### FOLLOW-UP RECOMMENDATIONS
- Patients discharged from the ED should have close follow-up within 24–36 hr.
- Strict discharge instruction to return if further bleeding or concerning symptoms (lightheadedness, dyspnea, chest pain, etc.) occurs.
- Those with UGIB should be discharged on a PPI, liquid antacids, and advised to avoid caffeine, alcohol, tobacco, NSAIDs, and aspirin.

## PEARLS AND PITFALLS
- 10–15% of patients with UGIB can present with hematochezia.
- Common pitfall is failure to adequately resuscitate with crystalloid and blood products.
- Consider GIB in patients presenting with signs of hypovolemia or hypovolemic shock.

### Geriatric Considerations
PUD is the predominant cause of GIB in the elderly (68% of patients >60 and 27% of patients >80) with a higher mortality in this age group.

## ADDITIONAL READING
- Das AM, Sood N, Hodgin K, et al. Development of a triage protocol for patients presenting with gastrointestinal hemorrhage: A prospective cohort study. Crit Care. 2008;12:R57.
- Gralnek IM, Barkun AN, Bardou M. Management of acute bleeding from a peptic ulcer. N Engl J Med 2008;359(9):928–937.
- Hoedema RE, Luchtefeld MA. The management of lower gastrointestinal hemorrhage. Dis Colon Rectum. 2005;48:2010–2024.
- Marx J, Hockberger R, Walls R, eds. Rosen's Emergency Medicine, 7th ed. Philadelphia: Mosby/Elsevier, 2009.
- Wolfson AB, et al., eds. Harwood-Nuss' Clinical Practice of Emergency Medicine, 4th ed. Philadelphia: Lippincott, Williams, & Wilkins, 2005.

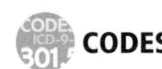 CODES

### ICD9
578.9 Hemorrhage of gastrointestinal tract, unspecified

G

# GHB, POISONING

*Mark B. Mycyk*
*Amy V. Kontrick*

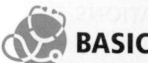 **BASICS**

## DESCRIPTION
- Naturally occurring analog of b3-aminobutyric acid (GABA)
- Used medically for narcolepsy
- Nonmedical uses:
  – Bodybuilding agent
  – Euphoric agent
  – Date-rape/predatory agent
- Onset of activity: 15–30 min after ingestion
- Duration of effect: 2–6 hr

## ETIOLOGY
Deliberate or accidental ingestion of γ-hydroxybutyrate (GHB)

 **DIAGNOSIS**

## SIGNS AND SYMPTOMS
- CNS:
  – CNS depression
  – Ataxia/dizziness
  – Impaired judgment
  – Aggressive behavior
  – Clonic movements of the extremities
  – Coma
  – Seizures
- Pulmonary:
  – Respiratory depression
  – Apnea
  – Laryngospasm (rare)
- GI:
  – Nausea
  – Vomiting
- Cardiovascular:
  – Bradycardia
  – Atrioventricular block
  – Hypotension
- Other:
  – Nystagmus
  – Hypothermia
- Withdrawal symptoms:
  – HTN
  – Tachycardia
  – Hyperthermia
  – Agitation
  – Diaphoresis
  – Tremors
  – Nausea, vomiting, and abdominal cramping
  – Hallucinations, delusions, and psychosis

## ESSENTIAL WORKUP
- Diagnosis based on clinical presentation and an accurate history
- Exclude coingestants if signs and symptoms inconsistent with GHB intoxication.

## DIAGNOSTIC TESTS & INTERPRETATION
### Lab
- Confirmatory GHB screen is typically a send-out lab and does not change ED management.
- Urine toxicology screen to exclude coingestants
- Serum alcohol level
- Urinalysis and creatine kinase (CPK) if suspected rhabdomyolysis from prolonged immobilization or agitation

### Imaging
- ECG:
  – Sinus bradycardia
  – Atrioventricular block
- CXR:
  – Aspiration pneumonia
- Head CT if suspected occult head trauma

## DIFFERENTIAL DIAGNOSIS
- Alcohol intoxication
- Barbiturate overdose
- Benzodiazepine overdose
- Neuroleptic overdose
- Opiate overdose
- Withdrawal:
  – Alcohol withdrawal
  – Sedative-hypnotic withdrawal

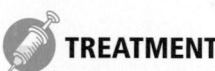 **TREATMENT**

## PRE-HOSPITAL
- Transport all pills/bottles and drug paraphernalia involved in overdose for identification in ED.
- γ-Hydroxybutyrate (GHB) precursors (γ-butyrolactone [GBL], 1,4 butanediol [1,4-BD], GHV [γ-hydroxyvalerate], and GVL) have same effects as γ-hydroxybutyrate.

## INITIAL STABILIZATION/THERAPY
- ABCs:
  – Airway control essential
  – Administer supplemental oxygen.
  – Intubate if indicated.
- Administer thiamine, dextrose (or Accu-Chek), and naloxone for depressed mental status.

### ED TREATMENT/PROCEDURES

- Supportive care
- Bradycardia:
  - Atropine
  - Temporary pacing
- Hypotension:
  - 0.9% NS IV fluid bolus
  - Trendelenburg
  - Dopamine titrated to pressure
- Seizures:
  - Treat initially with benzodiazepine.
  - Treat refractory seizures with phenobarbital.
- Withdrawal:
  - Treat aggressively with benzodiazepine.
  - Treat with phenobarbital or propofol if large doses of benzodiazepines unsuccessful.

### MEDICATION

- Dextrose: 50–100 mL $D_{50}$ (peds: 2 mL/kg of $D_{25}$ over 1 min) IV; repeat if necessary
- Diazepam: 5–10 mg (peds: 0.2–0.5 mg/kg) IV q10–15min
- Dopamine: 2–20 $\mu$g/kg/min with titration to effect
- Lorazepam: 2–4 mg (peds: 0.03–0.05 mg/kg) IV q10–15min
- Naloxone: 0.4–2 mg (peds: 0.1 mg/kg; neonatal: 10–30 $\mu$g/kg) IV or IM
- Phenobarbital: 10–20 mg/kg IV (loading dose)
- Propofol: 0.5–1.0 mg/kg IV (loading dose), then 5–50 $\mu$g/kg/min (maintenance dose)
- Thiamine (vitamin $B_1$): 100 mg (peds: 50 mg) IV or IM

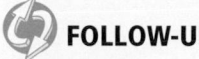 **FOLLOW-UP**

### DISPOSITION

#### Admission Criteria

- Intubated patient
- Patient with hypothermia or other hemodynamic instability
- Coingestion prolonging duration of intoxication

#### Discharge Criteria

- Asymptomatic after 6 hr of observation
- No clinical evidence of withdrawal syndrome

> **ALERT**
> Withdrawal from GHB is life-threatening and appears similar to alcohol withdrawal. Prolonged inpatient treatment may be indicated.

### FOLLOW-UP RECOMMENDATIONS

- Substance abuse referral for patients with recreational drug abuse.
- Patients with unintentional (accidental) poisoning require poison prevention counseling.
- Patients with intentional (eg, suicide) poisoning require psychiatric evaluation.

## PEARLS AND PITFALLS

- Consider nontoxicologic causes for persistent altered mental status
- Routine hospital drug testing will not confirm GHB or other common recreational drugs of abuse

## ADDITIONAL READING

- Caldicott DG, Chow FY, Burns BJ, et al. Fatalities associated with the use of gamma- hydroxybutyrate and its analogues in Australasia. *Med J Aust.* 2004;181(6):310–313.
- Dyer JE, Roth B, Hyma BA. Gamma-hydroxybutyrate withdrawal syndrome. *Ann Emerg Med.* 2001;37:147–153.
- Gahlinger PM. Club drugs: MDMA, gamma-hydroxybutyrate (GHB), Rohypnol, and ketamine. *Am Fam Physician.* 2004,69(11):2619–2926.
- Liechti ME, Kunz I, Greminger P, et al. Clinical features of gamma-hydroxybutyrate and gamma-butyrolactone toxicity and concomitant drug and alcohol use. *Drug Alcohol Depend.* 2006;81(3): 323–326.
- Shannon M, Quang LS. Gamma-hydroxybutyrate, gamma-butyrolactone, and 1,4-butanediol: A case report and review of the literature. *Pediatr Emerg Care.* 2000;16:435–440.
- Van Noorden MS, Van Dongen LC, Zitman FG, et al. Gamma-hydroxybutyrate withdrawal syndrome: Dangerous but not well known. *Gen Hosp Psychiatry.* 2009;31(4):394–396.

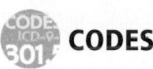 **CODES**

### ICD9

968.4 Poisoning by other and unspecified general anesthetics

G

# GIANT CELL ARTERITIS

*Donald J. Lefkowits*

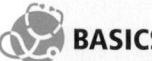 **BASICS**

## DESCRIPTION

- Chronic vasculitis of large- and medium-size vessels that occurs among individuals >50 yr of age
- Most common vasculitis in adults
- Most commonly causes inflammation of arteries originating from the arch of the aorta.
- Other vessels, including veins, are sometimes involved.
- Often referred to as temporal arteritis because of frequent involvement of temporal artery:
  - Most significant complication is monocular blindness
  - Ischemic optic neuritis
  - Usually several months after onset of symptoms
- Takayasu arteritis—involvement of aortic arch:
  - Usually young woman with nonspecific constitutional symptoms
  - Evidence of large vessel occlusion occurs months to years later
  - CVA, myocardial ischemia, extremity ischemia
  - Aortic aneurysm may result:
    o Thoracic aneurysm is 17 times higher than those without GCA
    o Abdominal aortic aneurysm is twice a common
- Inflammation of arteries supplying the muscles of mastication results in jaw claudication
- Pathologic specimens feature patchy mononuclear granulomatous inflammation resulting in a markedly thickened intima and occlusion of the vessel lumen.
- Age is the greatest risk factor:
  - Rare in patients <50 yr old
  - >90% are >60 yr old
- Increased prevalence in Northern latitude
- 2–4 times more common in women
- Rare in African American patients, common in whites
- Frequently associated with polymyalgia rheumatica (50%)

## RISK FACTORS

### Genetics

Genetic predisposition is linked to HLA-DR4—60% prevalence.

## ETIOLOGY

Autoimmune disease but etiology is not known

## DIAGNOSIS

- Difficult to diagnose Takaysu arteritis in the ED
- Temporal arteritis: Presence of any 3 or more of the following in patients with vasculitis:
  - Erythrocyte sedimentation rate >50
  - Age >50 yr
  - New onset of localized headache.
  - Tenderness or decreased pulsation of temporal artery
  - Biopsy revealing necrotizing arteritis.
- Up to 30% may not present with the classic features of headache, scalp tenderness, visual changes, or jaw claudication.

## SIGNS AND SYMPTOMS

### History

- May present with acute, subacute, or chronic symptoms:
  - Headache is the single most frequent symptom (70%):
    o Often localized, boring, or lancing in quality
    o Often described as unilateral over a temple
- Visual findings:
  - Findings are usually in 1 eye.
  - May develop weeks to months after the onset of other symptoms
  - May fluctuate, but visual impairment does not usually improve over time, even with treatment
  - Amaurosis fugax
  - Blindness
  - Diplopia
  - Ptosis
  - Extraocular muscle weakness
  - Scotoma
  - Blurred vision
- Tongue or jaw claudication upon mastication are common symptoms (50%).
- Constitutional symptoms:
  - Fatigue
  - Malaise
  - Anorexia
  - Weight loss
  - Weakness
  - Arthralgias
  - Low-grade fever
- Neurologic symptoms:
  - Neuropathy
  - Symptoms of TIA/CVA

- Polymyalgia rheumatica (up to 50%):
  - Stiffness
  - Aching pain in the proximal muscles
  - Worse in the morning and decreasing with exercise
- Rare symptoms:
  - Chest pain compatible with ischemia
  - Symptoms of CHF
  - Respiratory symptoms

### Physical Exam

- General:
  - Low-grade fever
  - Muscle tenderness to palpation (PMR)
  - Jaw claudication
- Skin:
  - Temporal artery may be erythematous, tender, and/or nodular
  - Pulsations over temporal artery:
    o Increased in early disease
    o Decreased in late disease
- Ophthamalogic:
  - Monocular vision loss
  - Decreased visual acuity
  - Visual field deficit
  - Funduscopy:
    o Often normal initially
    o Iritis and fine vitreous opacities may be early findings
    o Optic nerve edema
    o Swollen, pale disc with blurred margins
    o Pallor
    o Hemorrhage
    o Scattered cotton-wool spots
    o Vessel engorgement and exudates are seen later.
- Cardiovascular:
  - Extremity ischemia
  - Signs of CHF
  - Bruits or decreased pulses over large arteries
  - Raynaud phenomena
- Neurologic:
  - Evidence of CVA
  - Neuropathy
- Rare:
  - Tongue infarction

## ESSENTIAL WORKUP

Focused physical examination with emphasis on:

- Temporal artery and scalp abnormalities
- Complete neurologic examination
- Ophthalmic examination
- Any pulse differences in the extremities or bruits over large arteries should be noted.

## DIAGNOSTIC TESTS & INTERPRETATION
### Lab
- Elevated ESR, often >100 mm/h. ESR <40 is rare.
- Elevated C-reactive protein
- CBC:
  - Mild normochromic anemia is typical
  - Platelets tend to be elevated
  - White blood cell count can be normal or slightly elevated and differential is usually normal.
- LFTs and PTT may be elevated
- Creatine phosphokinase, renal function, and urinalysis are generally normal.
- Elevation in interleukin-6 (IL-6) is seen during flares.

### Imaging
- Doppler US:
  - Decreased blood flow in temporal, facial, and ophthalmic arteries
  - Presence of a halo is highly suggestive of active temporal arteritis.
- Angiogram:
  - Smooth, tapered occlusions or stenosis
- MRI or CT angiogram:
  - Indicated for examination of large arteries

### Diagnostic Procedures/Surgery
- Temporal artery biopsy.
  - Multiple sections should be done in 24–48 hr and no longer than 96 hr after initiation of steroids.
  - Gold standard for diagnosis

## DIFFERENTIAL DIAGNOSIS
- Vasculitides:
  - Polyarteritis nodosa
  - Hypersensitivity vasculitis
  - Systemic lupus erythematosus
  - Wegener granulomatosis
- Thrombosis of retinal, ophthalmic, or temporal arteries
- Lyme disease

 **TREATMENT**

## PRE-HOSPITAL
- Acute symptoms may be confused with stroke.
- Initiate appropriate monitoring and oxygen.
- Patients may be hypotensive from 1 of the rare sequelae (aortic dissection, abdominal aortic aneurysm, or myocardial infarction).

## INITIAL STABILIZATION/THERAPY
- Although rare, patients may present with vascular catastrophe such as aortic dissection or myocardial infarction and need appropriate aggressive early management.

## ED TREATMENT/PROCEDURES
- Steroids:
  - Strong clinical indications should be present if started before temporal artery biopsy.
  - Early, aggressive treatment can significantly reduce the incidence of blindness.
  - Steroids effectively control systemic and local symptoms within days to weeks.
  - Treatment with prednisone may continue for years—usual disease length is 3–4 yr.
- Symptomatic pain management with NSAIDs, salicylates, and/or narcotics as indicated.

## MEDICATION
### First Line
- Prednisone: 60–100 mg PO per day for at least 2 wk before considering tapering.
- Pain management with NSAID and/or narcotics

### Second Line
- For acute onset visual symptoms, consider 1,000 mg methylprednisolone IV pulse therapy for the 1st 1–3 days.
- Low dose aspirin to reduce thrombotic risk

 **FOLLOW-UP**

## DISPOSITION
### Admission Criteria
- Patients with impending vascular complications or acute focal neurologic findings.
- Patients with associated acute visual loss

### Discharge Criteria
- Less symptomatic patients without evidence of end-organ involvement
- Able to be seen in follow-up within 1–2 days

### Issues for Referral
- Rheumatology
- Ophthalmology if associated with visual symptoms
- Neurology with acute focal neurologic findings
- Cardiology, cardiothoracic surgery, and/or vascular surgery for involvement of aorta

## FOLLOW-UP RECOMMENDATIONS
- Rheumatology for steroid management and search for associated connective tissue disorders
- Ophthalmology and neurology for visual disturbance and/or focal neurologic findings.

## PEARLS AND PITFALLS
- Permanent visual loss is the most feared complication of temporal arteritis.
- Do not delay initiation of steroid therapy to await biopsy if strong clinical suspicion for GCA exists or if visual changes are reported:
  - Biopsy should be performed within 48 hr of initiation of steroid therapy.
- Jaw claudication and amaurosis fugax, while often dramatic, are symptoms patients often neglect to report. Query directly and specifically about them if GCA is being considered.
- 25–50% of patients who present with acute loss of vision in 1 eye who go untreated will develop bilateral blindness.

## ADDITIONAL READING
- Firestein GS, Budd RC, Harris Jr FD, et al., eds. Kelley's Textbook of Rheumatology, 8th ed. WB Saunders; 2008.
- Klig JE. Ophthalmologic complications of systemic disease. Emerg Med Clin North Am. 2008;26: 217–231.
- Nordberg E, Nordberg C. Giant cell arteritis: Strategies in diagnosis and treatment. Curr Opin Rheumatol. 2004;16:25–30.
- Salvarani C, Cimino F, Hunder GG. Polymyalgia rheumatica and giant-cell arteritis. Lancet. 2008;372:234–245.
- Unwin B, Williams CM, Gilliland W. Polymyalgia rheumatica and giant cell arteritis. Am Fam Physician. 2006;74:1547–1554.

 **CODES**

### ICD9
446.5 Giant cell arteritis

G

# GIARDIASIS

*Ann P. Nguyen*

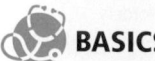 **BASICS**

## DESCRIPTION
- Noninvasive diarrhea
- Found worldwide:
  - 2–15% prevalence in developed nations
  - 20–40% prevalence in developing nations
- 5% of all travelers' diarrhea
- Most common intestinal parasite in the U.S.:
  - Highest incidence in summer months
  - Highest incidence in children aged 1–9 yr and adults aged 30–39 yr
- Fecal-oral transmission:
  - Humans are major reservoir.
  - Zoonotic reservoir in both domestic and wild mammals
  - Reservoir in contaminated surface water
- Populations at risk:
  - Travelers to endemic areas (developing countries, wilderness areas of U.S.)
  - Children in day care centers and their close contacts
  - Institutionalized persons
  - Practitioners of anal sexual activity

## ETIOLOGY
- *Giardia lamblia:*
  - A protozoan flagellate
- Also called *Giardia intestinalis* or *Giardiaduodenalis*
- Ingested Giardia attach to intestinal villi
- Alters the intestinal brush-border enzymes, impairing digestion of lactose, and other saccharides
- No toxin produced

## DIAGNOSIS

### SIGNS AND SYMPTOMS
#### History
- Onset 1–2 wk postexposure
- Infection may be asymptomatic (most common).
- Diarrhea of acute onset (90% of symptomatic patients):
  - Foul-smelling stools
  - Steatorrhea
  - Nonbloody
  - Self-limiting within 2–4 wk
  - More severe in immunocompromised patients and patients with underlying bowel disease
- Flatulence and bloating (70–75%)
- Abdominal cramping (70%)
- Nausea (70%)
- Vomiting (30%)
- Malaise (86%)

- Anorexia (66%)
- Weight loss (60–70%)
- Fever is rare (15%).
- 30–50% of acute cases progress to chronic giardiasis (>4 wk):
  - Fat malabsorption
  - Severe macrocytic anemia secondary to folate deficiency
  - Secondary lactase deficiency (in 20–40% of patients)
- Infection is more severe and harder to eradicate in immunosuppressed patients.

#### Pediatric Considerations
- Acute infection:
  - Severe dehydration
- Chronic infection:
  - Failure to thrive
  - Growth retardation and cognitive impairment owing to nutrient malabsorption

#### Physical Exam
- Abdominal exam is benign.
- Extraintestinal manifestations (10% of patients):
  - Polyarthritis
  - Urticaria
  - Aphthous ulcers
  - Maculopapular rash
  - Biliary tract disease

### ESSENTIAL WORKUP
- History:
  - Possible sources of exposure
  - Membership in high-risk group
- Physical exam:
  - If gross or occult blood on digital rectal exam, unlikely to be *Giardia*

### DIAGNOSTIC TESTS & INTERPRETATION
#### Lab
- Stool sample for microscopy (ova and parasites):
  - 50–70% sensitive if 1 sample
  - 85–90% sensitive if 3 samples taken at 2-day intervals (ideal)
  - 100% specific
  - Ability to detect other parasites as well
- Stool enzyme-linked immunosorbent assay (ELISA) or immunofluorescent antibody (IFA) assay for *Giardia* antigen:
  - 95% sensitive, 95–100% specific
  - Unlike microscopy, cannot rule out other parasites
- Stool polymerase chain reaction (PCR):
  - 100% sensitive and 100% specific
- Fecal leukocytes and stool culture unnecessary unless enteroinvasive organisms suspected (fever, bloody stool)

- Serology for anti-Giardia antibodies not helpful in the ED setting
- Electrolytes, BUN/Cr, glucose:
  - If prolonged diarrhea or evidence of dehydration
- CBC:
  - Macrocytic anemia in chronic giardiasis
  - Nondiagnostic in acute giardiasis

#### Imaging
Abdominal CT or ultrasound may show bowel wall thickening and flattened duodenal folds (nonspecific findings)

#### Diagnostic Procedures/Surgery
- Duodenal sampling:
  - Entero-Test (patient swallows a weighted string, which is later retrieved and examined for *Giardia* using microscopy)
- Endoscopy:
  - Duodenal aspiration
  - Endoscopic duodenal biopsy

### DIFFERENTIAL DIAGNOSIS
- Viral gastroenteritis:
  - Norwalk virus
  - Rotavirus
  - Hepatitis A
- Bacterial infections:
  - Staphylococcus
  - *E. coli*
  - *Shigella*
  - *Salmonella*
  - *Yersinia*
  - *Campylobacter*
  - *Clostridium difficile*
  - *Vibrio cholerae*
- Other protozoa:
  - *Cryptosporidium*
  - Microsporidia
  - *Cyclospora*
  - *Isospora*
  - *Entamoeba*
- Inflammatory bowel disease
- Irritable bowel syndrome
- Lactase deficiency
- Tropical sprue
- Drugs and toxins:
  - Antibiotics
  - Calcium channel blockers
  - Magnesium antacids
  - Caffeine
  - Alcohol
  - Sorbitol
  - Laxative abuse
  - Quinidine
  - Colchicine
  - Mercury poisoning

- Endocrine:
  - Addison disease
  - Thyroid disorders
- Malignancy:
  - Colorectal carcinoma
  - Medullary carcinoma of the thyroid

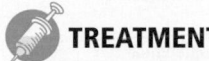

# TREATMENT

## INITIAL STABILIZATION/THERAPY
- ABCs: airway, breathing, circulation
- IV 0.9 NS if signs of significant dehydration

### Pediatric Considerations
- For severe dehydration (>10%):
  - IV bolus with 0.9% NS at 20 mL/kg
  - Cardiac monitor
  - Blood glucose determination

## ED TREATMENT/PROCEDURES
- Oral fluids for mild dehydration
- Correct any serum electrolyte imbalances.
- Stool sample for microscopy
- If stool sample is positive for *Giardia:*
  - Metronidazole or tinidazole are the treatment of choice:
    - 90% cure rate for each
  - Albendazole (78–90% efficacy), quinacrine (90% efficacy), or nitazoxanide (75% efficacy) if first-line therapy fails
- If stool sample negative for *Giardia:*
  - Refer to gastroenterologist for further specialized testing.
  - Consider empiric course of metronidazole if high suspicion for *Giardia.*
- Immunocompromised patients at risk for disease that is refractory to standard drug regimens:
  - Try drug of a different class/mechanism or metronidazole plus quinacrine for at least 2 wk

### Pediatric Considerations
- Metronidazole is first-line therapy (80–95% efficacy)
- Alternatives:
  - Furazolidone (80–85% efficacy)
  - Nitazoxanide (60–80% efficacy)
  - Paromomycin (55–90% efficacy)

### Pregnancy Considerations
- Metronidazole contraindicated in 1st trimester
- Albendazole, quinacrine, and tinidazole are contraindicated throughout pregnancy
- Use nitazoxanide instead
- If mild symptoms only, consider deferring treatment until late pregnancy or postpartum

## MEDICATION

### First Line
- Metronidazole: 250–500 mg (peds: 15 mg/kg/24 h) PO q8h for 5–10 days
- Tinidazole: 2 g (peds: 50 mg/kg) PO once

### Pregnancy Considerations
Metronidazole only (contraindicated in 1st trimester)

### Second Line
- Albendazole: 400 mg (peds: 10–15 mg/kg/24 h) PO daily for 5–7 days
- Furazolidone: 100 mg (peds: 6–8 mg/kg/24 h) PO q6h for 7–10 days
- Nitazoxanide: 500 mg (peds: 100 mg for ages 2–3 yr, 200 mg for ages 4–11 years) PO b.i.d. for 3 days
- Paromomycin: 500 mg (peds: 25–30 mg/kg/24 h) PO q8h for 5–10 days
- Quinacrine: 100 mg (peds: 6 mg/kg/24 h) PO q8h for 5–7 days

### Pediatric Considerations
Furazolidone, nitazoxanide, or paromomycin

### Pregnancy Considerations
Nitazoxanide

### ALERT
- Use furazolidone in older children only:
  - Causes hemolytic anemia in infants
  - Causes hemolytic anemia in persons with G6PD deficiency
- Avoid quinacrine in G6PD deficiency (causes hemolytic anemia)
- Avoid paromomycin in renal failure

# FOLLOW-UP

## DISPOSITION

### Admission Criteria
- Hypotension or tachycardia unresponsive to IV fluids
- Severe electrolyte imbalance
- Children with >10% dehydration
- Signs of sepsis/toxicity (rare in isolated giardiasis)
- Patients unable to maintain adequate oral hydration:
  - Extremes of age, cognitive impairment, significant co-morbid illness

### Discharge Criteria
- Able to maintain adequate oral hydration
- Dehydration responsive to IV fluids

## FOLLOW-UP RECOMMENDATIONS
Gastroenterology referral for diagnostic endoscopy if symptoms persist for >4 wk despite drug therapy

## PEARLS AND PITFALLS

Diagnosis is the greatest challenge in this disease:
- Include giardiasis in the differential diagnosis of all patients with diarrhea:
  - Giardia occasionally reported in domestic water supply
  - Patients may not present with the classic history and risk factors to have giardiasis

## ADDITIONAL READING

- Escobedo AA, Almirall P, Alfonso M, et al. Treatment of intestinal protozoan infections in children. *Arch Dis Child.* 2009;94:478–482.
- Escobedo AA, Alvarez G, Gonzalez ME, et al. The treatment of giardiasis in children: Single-dose tinidazole compared with 3 days of nitazoxanide. *Ann Trop Med Parasitol.* 2008;102:199–207.
- Escobedo AA, Cimerman S. Giardiasis: A pharmacotherapy review. *Expert Opin Pharmacother.* 2007;8:1885–1902.
- Huang DB, White AC. An updated review on cryptosporidium and giardia. *Gastroenterol Clin North Am.* 2006;35:291–314.
- Kiser JD, Paulson CP, Nichols W. What's the most effective treatment for giardiasis? *J Fam Pract.* 2008;57(4).

### See Also (Topic, Algorithm, Electronic Media Element)
- Amebiasis
- Diarrhea, Adult

# CODES

ICD9
007.1 Giardiasis

G

# GLAUCOMA

*Yasuharu Okuda*
*Lisa Jacobson*

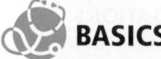 **BASICS**

## DESCRIPTION
Disease characterized by elevation of intraocular pressure, optic neuropathy, and progressive loss of vision

## ETIOLOGY
- Primary glaucoma:
  - Open-angle glaucoma:
    - Normal anterior chamber angle
    - Insidious onset with persistent rise in intraocular pressure
    - Most common type accounting for 90% of glaucomas in U.S.
    - Leading cause of blindness in African Americans
    - Risk factors include: African American, age >40 yr, family history, myopia, diabetes, and HTN
  - Acute angle-closure glaucoma:
    - Narrowing or closing of anterior chamber angle precluding natural flow of aqueous humor from posterior to anterior chamber of eye and through its filtering portion of trabecular meshwork
    - Usually abrupt onset with sudden increase in intraocular pressure
    - Risk factors include: Asians and Eskimos, hyperopia, family history, increased age, and female gender
- Secondary glaucoma occurs from other diseases, including diseases of eye, trauma, and drugs:
  - Can be either open or closed angle
  - Drugs: Steroids
  - Diseases: Neurofibromatosis, uveitis, neovascularization, and intraocular tumors
  - Trauma
  - Rapid correction of hyperglycemia

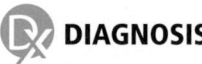 **DIAGNOSIS**

## SIGNS AND SYMPTOMS
Classic descriptions:
- Open angle:
  - Painless and gradual loss of vision
- Closed angle:
  - Painful loss of vision with fixed midsized pupil

## History
- Primary open-angle glaucoma:
  - Gradual reduction in peripheral vision or night blindness
  - Typically bilateral
  - Painless
- Primary angle-closure glaucoma:
  - Severe deep eye pain and ipsilateral headache often associated with nausea and vomiting
  - Decrease in visual acuity often described as visual clouding with halos surrounding light sources
  - Associated abdominal pain, which may misdirect diagnosis
  - Concurrent exposure to dimly lit environment such as movie theater
  - Use of precipitating medications:
    - Mydriatic agents: Scopolamine, atropine
    - Sympathomimetics: Pseudoephedrine, albuterol
    - Antihistamines: Benadryl, Antivert
    - Antipsychotics: Haldol
    - Phenothiazines: Compazine, Phenergan
    - Tricyclic antidepressants: Elavil
    - Sulfonamides: Topiramate

## Physical Exam
- Primary open-angle glaucoma:
  - Decreased visual acuity
- Primary angle-closure glaucoma:
  - Decreased visual acuity
  - Pupil is mid-dilated and nonreactive.
  - Corneal edema with hazy appearance
  - Conjunctival injection, ciliary flush
  - Firm globe to palpation

## ESSENTIAL WORKUP
- Detailed ocular examination
- Visual acuity:
  - Hand movements typically all that is seen
- Tonometry:
  - Normal pressures are 10–21 mm Hg.
  - Primary open-angle glaucoma:
    - Degree of elevation can vary, but 25–30% of patients may have normal intraocular pressures.
  - Primary angle-closure glaucoma:
    - Any elevation is abnormal, but usually seen in ranges >40 mm Hg.
- Slit-lamp exam:
  - Evaluation of anterior chamber angle
  - Used to eliminate other possibilities in differential including corneal abrasion and foreign body

## DIAGNOSTIC TESTS & INTERPRETATION
*Lab*
Directed toward workup of differential

*Imaging*
Directed toward workup of differential

*Diagnostic Procedures/Surgery*
Gonioscopy:
- This is direct measurement of the angle of closure

## DIFFERENTIAL DIAGNOSIS
- Cavernous sinus thrombosis
- Acute Iritis and uveitis
- Retinal artery or vein occlusion
- Temporal arteritis
- Retinal detachment
- Conjunctivitis
- Corneal abrasion

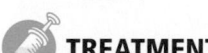 **TREATMENT**

## PRE-HOSPITAL
- No specific interventions need occur prior to arrival at the hospital in regards to the eye:
  - Pain control may be necessary
  - In traumatic etiologies, stabilize other injuries

## INITIAL STABILIZATION/THERAPY
- Initiate steps to lower intraocular pressure in acute closed-angle glaucoma:
  - Address other effects of trauma if this was the etiology
  - Discontinue inciting medication when involved

## ED TREATMENT/PROCEDURES
- Primary open-angle glaucoma:
  - Recognition and prompt ophthalmologic referral
  - Patients maintained on topical $\beta$-blockers or prostaglandin analogs to decreased IOP
- Primary angle-closure glaucoma (ophthalmologic emergency):
  - Intraocular pressure reduction:
    - Topical $\beta$-blocker, timolol maleate, to decrease aqueous humor production
    - Topical $\alpha_2$-agonist, apraclonidine, to decrease aqueous humor production
    - Carbonic anhydrase inhibitor, acetazolamide, for reduction of formation of aqueous humor
    - Hyperosmotic agent, mannitol, to draw aqueous humor from vitreous cavity into blood. (Indicated for severe attacks)

– Movement of iris away from trabecular meshwork:
  ○ Topical parasympathomimetic, pilocarpine hydrochloride, to constrict pupil once intraocular pressure is <40 mm Hg
– Reduction of inflammation:
  ○ Topical corticosteroid, prednisolone acetate
– Emergent ophthalmology consultation for possible definitive surgical treatment, laser iridectomy, if no improvement with medical management
– Adequate narcotic analgesia and antiemetics as needed

## MEDICATION
- Acetazolamide: 500 mg IV or PO
- Mannitol 20%: 1–2 g/kg IV over 30–60 min
- Pilocarpine hydrochloride 1–2% solution: 1 drop q15–30min until pupillary constriction occurs, then 1 drop q2–3h
- Prednisolone acetate 1% solution: 1 drop q15–30min for total of 4 doses

### First Line
- β-agonists:
  – Timolol maleate 0.25% or 0.5%:
    ○ 1 drop to affected eye b.i.d.
  – Levobunolol 0.25% or 0.5%:
    ○ 1 drop to affected eye b.i.d.
  – Carteolol HCL 1%:
    ○ 1 drop to affected eye b.i.d.
  – Betaxolol 0.25% or 0.5%:
    ○ 1–2 drop(s) to affected eye b.i.d.

### Second Line
- Adrenergic agonists:
  – Apraclonidine 0.5%, 1%:
    ○ 1–2 drop(s) to affected eye b.i.d.
  – Brimonidine:
    ○ 1 drop to affected eye t.i.d.
- Carbonic anhydrase inhibitors:
  – Acetazolamide:
    ○ 125–250 mg PO q.i.d.
  – Methazolamide:
    ○ 50–100 mg PO b.i.d.
  – Dorzolamide HCl 2%:
    ○ 1 drop in affected eye t.i.d.
  – Brinzolamide:
    ○ 1 drop to affected eye t.i.d.

- Prostaglandin analogs:
  – Latanoprost:
    ○ 1 drop in affected eye QHS
  – Bimatoprost 0.03%:
    ○ 1 drop in affected eye QHS
  – Travoprost:
    ○ 1 drop in affected eye QHS
  – Unoprostone:
    ○ 1 drop to affected eye b.i.d.

### Considerations in Prescribing
- Prostaglandin analogs have become standard of care for open-angle glaucoma due to an improved side effect profile
- Due to cost, topical β-blockers are often still used primarily

## FOLLOW-UP

### DISPOSITION
#### Admission Criteria
- Severe pain, nausea, or vomiting
- Patients receiving parenteral medications should be observed for side effects.
- Patients without improvement of symptoms or intraocular pressures should be admitted for continued monitoring of intraocular pressure, medical treatment, and possible definitive surgical management:
  – Laser intervention is more likely than operative

#### Discharge Criteria
Patients with minor symptoms and significant improvement of intraocular pressure may be safely discharged once seen by ophthalmology and with close, <24-hour follow-up.

#### Issues for Referral
If no ophthalmologist is available, treatment should be initiated and patient transferred to nearest hospital with ophthalmologic consultation.

### FOLLOW-UP RECOMMENDATIONS
- Open-angle glaucoma patients need urgent ophthalmology follow-up to optimize medical management
- Closed-angle glaucoma patients need immediate intervention

## PEARLS AND PITFALLS
- Increased IOP can cause vascular insufficiency and with delayed treatment vision loss can be permanent
- Eye pain/headache can be associated with severe abdominal pain—don't ignore the eye and miss the diagnosis
- Patients maintained on topical β-blockers for open-angle glaucoma may present with systemic side effects including orthostatic hypotension, bradycardia, or syncope

## ADDITIONAL READING
- Berkoff D, Sanchez L. An uncommon presentation of acute angle closure glaucoma. *J Emerg Med.* 2005;29(1):43–44.
- Dargin JM, Lowenstein RA. The painful eye. *Emerg Med Clin North Am.* 2008;26(1):199–216.
- Marx JA, et al. *Rosen's Emergency Medicine: Concepts and Clinical Practice*, 6th ed. St. Louis, MO: Mosby; 2009.
- Morgan A, Hemphill R. Acute visual change. *Emerg Med Clin North Am.* 1998;16:825–843.
- Muskens RP, et al. Topical beta-blockers and mortality. *Opthalmology.* 2008;115(11): 2037–2043.
- Tripathi R, Tripathi B, Haggerty C. Drug-induced glaucomas: Mechanism and management. *Drug Saf.* 2003;26:749–767.

### See Also (Topic, Algorithm, Electronic Media Element)
- Red Eye
- Visual Loss

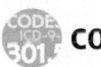

## CODES

### ICD9
- 365.9 Unspecified glaucoma
- 365.10 Open-angle glaucoma, unspecified
- 365.20 Primary angle-closure glaucoma, unspecified

G

# GLOBE RUPTURE

*Alexander T. Limkakeng, Jr.*
*Jeffrey J. Schaider*

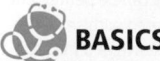 **BASICS**

## DESCRIPTION
- A full-thickness corneal or scleral injury owing to trauma
- Blunt trauma:
  - Causes an abrupt rise in intraocular pressure diffusely
  - Subsequent rupture of the eye either opposite the point of impact or at the weakest points:
    ○ Extraocular muscle insertion
    ○ Corneoscleral junction
- Penetrating injury:
  - Occurs with sharp objects or projectiles injuring the sclera or anterior eye directly
  - Most commonly anterior—the bony orbit protects the globe laterally and posteriorly
  - Posterior injury can occur with fracture of the bony orbit or with penetrating injuries of the eyelid or eyebrow.
- Prognosis worse with:
  - Larger lacerations
  - Injury posterior to the rectus insertion
  - Blunt injury
  - Intraocular foreign body, especially if made of organic material
  - Vitreous extrusion
  - Lens damage
  - Hyphema
  - Retinal detachment
  - Poor visual acuity at presentation
  - Afferent pupillary defect
  - Increased time to OR

## ETIOLOGY
- Falls, impact injuries
- Sport-related injuries (eg, elbow, ball impacts, arrows, etc.)
- Indirect concussive injuries (explosions)
- Sharp instrument/stabbing injuries, accidental or intentional
- Projectile injuries (industrial, firearms, BB pellets, blast explosion shrapnel—glass, etc.)

## DIAGNOSIS

### SIGNS AND SYMPTOMS
- Pain
- Localized ecchymosis and swelling
- Scleral or corneal laceration
- Extrusion of intraocular contents
- Markedly decreased visual acuity
- Limited extraocular motion
- Hyphema
- Severe subconjunctival hemorrhage and edema, especially if circumferential bloody chemosis
- Abnormally deep or shallow anterior chamber
- Low intraocular pressure:
  - Note: Do not perform tonometry if there is obvious rupture.
- Irregular pupil (points toward lesion)
- Subluxed lens
- Commotio retinae—gray-white discoloration of the retina

### History
- Mechanism of injury:
  - Assess for possibility of retained intraocular foreign body
- History of previous eye surgery
- Preinjury visual acuity
- Assess tetanus status
- Ascertain time of last PO intake

### Physical Exam
- Penlight or slit-lamp examination observing for signs of globe rupture
- If the diagnosis of ruptured globe is made, defer further ocular examination until the time of surgical repair:
  - Prevents placing any undue pressure on the eye and risking extrusion of the intraocular contents
- If no evidence of globe rupture on initial survey, proceed with thorough ophthalmologic examination:
  - Visual acuity
  - Slit-lamp examination

- Cornea
- Anterior chamber
- Iris
- Sclera:
  - Fluorescein
- Seidel test: Observe if fluorescein moves away as contents (which appear yellow-green) leak out at site of rupture:
  - Visualize fundus/retina.
  - Measure intraocular pressure
- Perform only if globe rupture is definitely *not* present.

### ESSENTIAL WORKUP
Perform thorough ocular examination as outlined above:
- Once diagnosis of globe rupture is suspected or made, defer further exam until time of repair.

### DIAGNOSTIC TESTS & INTERPRETATION
#### Lab
Preoperative labs:
- CBC
- Electrolytes
- Coagulation studies

#### Imaging
- Orbital radiograph (anteroposterior/lateral) for metallic intraocular foreign body
- CT scan of the orbits (axial and coronal views)
- MRI scan of the orbits after retained metallic foreign body is ruled out
- B-scan US of the eye

#### Diagnostic Procedures/Surgery
- Slit-lamp
- Fluorescein

### DIFFERENTIAL DIAGNOSIS
- Intraocular foreign body
- Hyphema
- Severe subconjunctival hemorrhage and chemosis
- Partial corneal laceration
- Partial scleral laceration

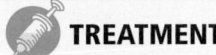 **TREATMENT**

### PRE-HOSPITAL
- Place a shield (not patch) over eye with no pressure on the globe.
- Use a Styrofoam cup if no shield available.

### INITIAL STABILIZATION/THERAPY
- Keep manipulation of the eye to a minimum If ruptured globe is suspected.
- Try to prevent any activity that will cause an increase in intraocular pressure such as straining, coughing, or vomiting.

### ED TREATMENT/PROCEDURES
- Emergent ophthalmologic consultation
- Bed rest
- No food or drink (NPO)
- Administer antiemetic for nausea/vomiting:
  – Prochlorperazine (Compazine)
- Update tetanus status.
- Administer prophylactic antibiotics IV:
  – Cefazolin (Ancef)
  – Gentamicin or clindamycin
- Succinylcholine is relatively contraindicated. However, with a defasciculating dose of a nondepolarizing agent and sufficient anesthesia, it may be used.

### *Pregnancy Considerations*
- Because of risk of extrusion of intraocular contents, straining should be avoided.
- If necessary, delivery by cesarean section or tocolysis should be considered in conjunction with obstetric consultation.

## MEDICATION
- Cefazolin (Ancef): 1 g (peds: 25–50 mg/kg/24 h) IV q6–q8h
- Clindamycin: 450 mg (peds: 25–40 mg/kg/24 h div. q6–q8h) IV q8h
- Gentamicin: 1 mg/kg (peds: 2–2.5 mg/kg) IV q8h
- Prochlorperazine (Compazine): 5–10 mg IV/IM

 **FOLLOW-UP**

### DISPOSITION
#### *Admission Criteria*
- All patients with globe rupture/penetrating eye injuries
- Early enucleation for severe injury

#### *Discharge Criteria*
Globe penetration excluded

#### *Issues for Referral*
- Emergent ophthalmologic consultation in the ER may be needed to definitively rule out globe rupture owing to difficulty with exam and the desire to minimize manipulation of the eye.
- Speed is of the essence since the risk of infection increases with prolonged time to operative repair.
- If appropriate, patient should be counseled on use of protective eyewear to prevent recurrence.

### FOLLOW-UP RECOMMENDATIONS
Postoperative ophthalmology follow-up

## PEARLS AND PITFALLS
- Do not manipulate the eye if you suspect or confirm a ruptured globe:
  – Place eye shield over affected eye.
- Administer antiemetic for patients with nausea and vomiting to prevent extrusion of globe contents.

## ADDITIONAL READING
- Anesthesia. In: Miller RD, ed. *Anesthetic Agents*. Philadelphia: Churchill Livingstone; 2000:473.
- Dunya IM, Rubin PAD, Shore JW. Penetrating orbital trauma. *Int Ophthalmol Clin*. 1994;34:25–36.
- Klystra JA, Lamkin JC, Runyan DR. Clinical predictors of scleral rupture after blunt ocular trauma. *Am J Ophthalmol*. 1993;115(4):530–535.
- Linden JA, Renner GS. Trauma to the globe. *Emerg Med Clin North Am*. 1995;13(3):581–605.
- Navon SE. Management of the ruptured globe. *Int Ophthalmol Clin*. 1994;34:71–91.
- Sabaci G, Bayer A, Mutlu M, et al. Endophthalmitis after deadly-weapon-related open-globe injuries. *Am J Ophthalmol*. 2002;133:62–69.

### See Also (Topic, Algorithm, Electronic Media Element)
- Blowout Fracture
- Corneal Abrasion
- Corneal Foreign Body
- Hyphema
- Retinal Detachment
- Visual Loss

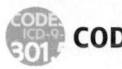 **CODES**

### ICD9
871.0 Ocular laceration without prolapse of intraocular tissue

G

# GLOMERULONEPHRITIS
*Melissa H. White*

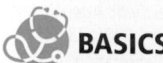 **BASICS**

## DESCRIPTION
- Syndrome characterized by:
  - Hematuria
  - Red blood cell casts
  - Proteinuria
  - Hypertension
  - Renal insufficiency
- Common pathway of multiple diseases resulting in intraglomerular inflammation and cellular proliferation
- Contributing factors:
  - Genetics
  - Antibody deposition:
    ○ Antibody attaches to glomerular antigen (native or implanted).
    ○ Circulating antigen-antibody complex deposited
  - Influx and activation of inflammatory mediators:
    ○ Leukocytes, complement, cytokines
    ○ Cell-mediated immune mechanisms
- Results in glomerular dysfunction
- Persistent inflammation can lead to scarring and permanent damage.
- Most common cause of chronic renal failure (CRF)

## ETIOLOGY
- Postinfectious:
  - Poststreptococcal glomerulonephritis (PSGN):
    ○ Occurs 7–21 days after *Streptococcal pharyngitis* or skin infection
    ○ Most common in children and men
    ○ Ranges from asymptomatic hematuria to oliguric renal failure
  - Can follow other bacterial, fungal, viral, or parasitic infections
- IgA nephropathy (Berger's disease):
  - Most common in men in the 3rd and 4th decades of life
  - Possibly related to increased production of IgA after infection
- Rapidly progressive glomerulonephritis (RPGN):
  - Can destroy renal function in days
  - Crescentic deposits in glomeruli destroy function.
  - Pauci-immune (small vessel vasculitides):
    ○ Often antineutrophil cytoplasmic antibody (ANCA)-positive
    ○ Can involve other areas (ie, lungs, skin)
    ○ Wegener granulomatosis
    ○ Microscopic polyangiitis
  - Immune complex deposits:
    ○ Postinfectious
    ○ Systemic disease (ie, systemic lupus erythematosus [SLE], Henoch-Schönlein purpura [HSP])
  - Antiglomerular basement membrane deposits:
    ○ Goodpasture disease with pulmonary involvement

- Membranoproliferative glomerulonephritis (MPGN):
  - Complement deposits in basement membrane
  - Hepatitis C

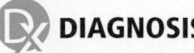 **DIAGNOSIS**

## SIGNS AND SYMPTOMS
- Cardinal signs:
  - Hematuria
  - Proteinuria
- Edema:
  - Owing to renal salt and water retention
  - Periorbital
  - Ascites
  - Pleural effusion
- HTN
- Oliguria
- Azotemia
- CHF
- Renal failure
- Nonspecific manifestations:
  - Fatigue
  - Weight loss
  - Abdominal pain
  - Nausea/vomiting
- Autoimmune disorders:
  - Arthralgias
  - Arthritis
  - Rash
  - Fever

### Geriatric Considerations
- Pauci-immune RPGN is common in this population (hematuria, proteinuria, and elevated CR)
- Urgent diagnosis and biopsy are indicated as this may progress to ESRD.
- Consult nephrology to discuss steroids, cyclophosphamide, and plasma exchange.

## ESSENTIAL WORKUP
Urinalysis for:
- Hematuria, proteinuria, and RBC casts

## DIAGNOSTIC TESTS & INTERPRETATION
### Lab
- Electrolytes, BUN, Cr, GFR:
  - Renal function
  - Hyperkalemia
- Albumin, total protein:
  - Varying degrees of hypoalbuminemia depending on clinical process

- CBC:
  - Anemia secondary to chronic renal disease, neoplasm, Goodpasture disease
  - With or without elevated WBC in infections
- PT, PTT:
  - Coagulation factors consumed in certain types of GN
- Labs to be considered for consultants:
  - Cultures—throat, skin, blood
  - 24-hr urine collection—protein, urine electrolytes
  - Streptozyme or antistreptolysin O titer
  - Complement levels (C1, C3, C4, $CH_{50}$)—reduced in PSGN, MPGN, SLE
  - ANA, rheumatoid factor—connective tissue diseases
  - Anti—glomerular basement membrane (GBM)—Goodpasture
  - cANCA—Wegener; pANCA-pauciimmune
  - Anti-DNA antibodies (SLE)
  - Hepatitis B and C serologies

### Imaging
- Renal ultrasound (if GFR is decreased):
  - Kidney size predictor of potential reversibility of disease, alternative diagnosis (ie, neoplasm, stone)
- Chest radiograph (CXR): Heart size, pulmonary edema, or hemorrhage

### Diagnostic Procedures/Surgery
Renal biopsy: Discern primary glomerulopathies vs. other causes.

## DIFFERENTIAL DIAGNOSIS
- Hematologic:
  - Sickle cell disease
  - Coagulopathy
- Renal:
  - Infectious
  - Malformation
  - Neoplasm
  - Ischemic
  - Trauma
  - Vasculitis
- Postrenal:
  - Mechanical (ie, stones, reflux, obstruction, catheterization)
  - Inflammatory (ie, cystitis, prostatitis, epididymitis, endometriosis, periurethritis)
  - Neoplasm
- Factitious:
  - Food
  - Drugs
  - Pigmenturia (ie, myoglobin, porphyria, hemoglobin)
  - Vaginal bleeding

TREATMENT

### PRE-HOSPITAL
- Supportive
- ABCs and fluid restriction in stable patients with significant edema.

### INITIAL STABILIZATION/THERAPY
ABCs: airway, breathing, circulation

### ED TREATMENT/PROCEDURES
- Treatment mainly supportive care:
  - BP control:
    - Loop diuretics
    - ACE inhibitor for maintenance
    - Treat hypertensive emergencies.
  - Dialysis:
    - Fluid overload
    - Hyperkalemia
    - Uremia
- PSGN:
  - Usually resolves spontaneously
  - No benefit to antibiotics
- IgA nephropathy:
  - Supportive care
  - Immunosuppressives if inflammation on biopsy
  - Variable course, but most recover
- RPGN:
  - Can irreversibly destroy renal function in days
  - Emergently consult nephrologist to discuss starting potentially toxic therapies.
  - Immunosuppressives and high-dose steroids:
    - Methylprednisolone and prednisone
    - Cyclophosphamide
    - Plasmapheresis for anti-GBM antibody
- MPGN:
  - Treat underlying disease if known. May include plasma exchange, cyclophosphamide, and/or steroids

### MEDICATION
- Benazepril: 5–40 mg PO daily (or any other ACE inhibitor)
- Cyclophosphamide: Dose in conjunction with nephrology
- Diazoxide: 1–3 mg/kg IV, max. 150 mg, repeat q15min
- Furosemide: 20–80 mg IV; max. 2 mg/kg/d
- Methylprednisolone: 30 mg/kg IV on alternative days for 3 doses, followed by oral prednisone (dose in conjunction with nephrology)
- Nitroprusside: 0.3–10 μg/kg/min IV
- Prednisone: 0.5–2 mg/kg/d

 FOLLOW-UP

### DISPOSITION
#### Admission Criteria
- Unstable vital signs
- Oliguria, anuria
- Uremia
- Acute renal failure
- Electrolyte abnormality
- Hypertensive emergency
- CHF
- Infectious cause of GN

#### Discharge Criteria
Healthy patients with no comorbid illness who present with mild hematuria and proteinuria with:
- Stable vital signs
- No signs of infection
- Otherwise normal lab work
- Close follow-up recommended

### FOLLOW-UP RECOMMENDATIONS
All patients with glomerulonephritis should follow-up with nephrology

## PEARLS AND PITFALLS
- Discussion with nephrology if management with immunosuppressives is sought.
- The finding of proteinuria or hematuria should always prompt follow-up to ensure that the patient is not progressing to GN.

## ADDITIONAL READING
- Beck LH, et al. Glomerular and tubulointerstitial diseases. *Prim Care*. 2008;35(2):265–96vi.
- Glassock RJ. Glomerular disease in the elderly. *Clin Geriatr Med*. 2009;25(3):413–422.
- Glassock RJ. Management of rapidly progressive glomerulonephritis. *Hosp Pract*. 2000;35(2): 59–62,65–66,69–70.
- Madaio MP, Harrington JT. The diagnosis of glomerular diseases: Acute glomerulonephritis and the nephrotic syndrome. *Arch Intern Med*. 2001;161(1):25–34.
- Vinen CS, Oliveira DB. Acute glomerulonephritis. *Postgrad Med J*. 2003;79:206–213.
- The author gratefully acknowledges the contribution of Scott A. Miller for the previous edition of this chapter.

### See Also (Topic, Algorithm, Electronic Media Element)
- Nephritic Syndrome
- Nephrotic Syndrome
- Renal Failure

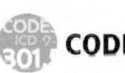 CODES

### ICD9
- 580.0 Acute glomerulonephritis with lesion of proliferative glomerulonephritis
- 583.4 Nephritis and nephropathy, not specified as acute or chronic, with lesion of rapidly progressive glomerulonephritis
- 583.9 Nephritis and nephropathy, not specified as acute or chronic, with unspecified pathological lesion in kidney

G

# GONOCOCCAL DISEASE

*JiWon E. Lee*

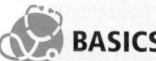 **BASICS**

## DESCRIPTION

- 2nd most frequently reported STD in U.S.:
  - Estimated 700,000 new cases per year
  - 50% reported
  - Increasing incidence in men who have sex with men (MSM):
    - Prevalence differs by HIV status (21% in HIV positive, 12% in HIV negative)
  - Humans only known host
- Concurrent infection with *Chlamydia trachomatis* is common
- Affects the urethra, rectum, cervical canal, pharynx, upper female genital tract, and conjunctiva
- Urethritis most common presentation in men
- Often asymptomatic in women

## ETIOLOGY

*Neisseria gonorrhoeae:*

- Gram-negative aerobic diplococci

 **DIAGNOSIS**

## SIGNS AND SYMPTOMS

- Cervicitis:
  - Defined as:
    - Mucopurulent endocervical discharge OR
    - Easily induced endocervical bleeding
  - Most common site of infection
  - 50% asymptomatic
  - Most symptoms nonspecific:
    - Vaginal discharge
    - Menorrhagia
    - Pelvic pain
    - Dyspareunia
    - Frequency and dysuria
- Pelvic inflammatory disease (PID):
  - 10–40% of untreated cases
  - Lower abdominal pain—most common presenting symptom
  - Other common signs and symptoms:
    - Dyspareunia, abnormal bleeding, abnormal cervical or vaginal discharge
  - Symptoms often occur at onset of menses.
  - Fever (50%)
  - 2/3 have mild, vague symptoms, may go unrecognized
  - Fitz-Hugh Curtis syndrome: (Perihepatitis):
    - 10% occurrence rate
    - Right upper quadrant pain/tenderness
- Bartholin's Abscess
- Urethritis:
  - Incubation period 3–7 days
  - Symptoms occur in 10–14 days:
    - Dysuria
    - Penile discharge

- Prostatitis—can occur in untreated urethritis
- Epididymitis:
  - Acute, unilateral testicular pain and swelling:
- Proctitis:
  - Often asymptomatic
  - Only site of infection in 40% of MSM
  - Rectal infection occurs in 35–50% of women with endocervical infection
  - 3-fold increase in HIV infection risk
  - Symptoms:
    - Perianal pruritis, mucopurulent discharge, mild rectal bleeding, severe rectal pain, tenesmus, and constipation
- Pharyngitis:
  - Sore throat, exudative tonsillitis
- Disseminated gonococcal infections (DGI):
  - Gonococcal bacteremia
  - Arthritis: Dermatitis syndrome:
    - 0.5–3% of untreated mucosal infections
    - Triad of tenosynovitis, dermatitis, and polyarthralgia
    - Fever, chills, malaise
  - Dermatitis:
    - Tender necrotic pustules on an erythematous base, few lesions, begin distally
  - Acute monoarticular or oligoarticular arthritis:
    - Knee most common
    - Warm, erythematous joint with effusion and pain with range of motion
  - Female > Male, 3:1:
    - Risk factors: Recent menstruation or recent pregnancy
  - Rare manifestations:
    - Hepatitis
    - Myocarditis
    - Endocarditis
    - Meningitis

## Physical Exam

- Cervicitis:
  - Cervical edema, congestion, friability:
- PID:
  - Uterine tenderness, bilateral adnexal, or cervical motion tenderness
- Urethritis:
  - Yellow-white thick discharge, urethral meatal erythema

## ESSENTIAL WORKUP

- Clinical diagnosis in male gonorrhea:
  - Gram stain 95% sensitive
- Cervical culture in female gonorrhea
- Also test for chlamydia and syphilis

## DIAGNOSTIC TESTS & INTERPRETATION

### Lab

- Cultures (gold standard):
  - Thayer-Martin medium:
    - Mainstay for blood and synovial fluid
- Gram stain:
  - Intracellular gram-negative diplococci:
    - 60% sensitive in symptomatic women
    - 95% sensitive in symptomatic men
- Nucleic acid amplification tests (NAATs):
  - DNA or RNA sequences using polymerase chain reaction (PCR)
  - Many also test for chlamydia
  - Useful in urethral, cervical, and urine specimens
- Pharyngeal/rectal cultures for local symptoms in high-risk individuals
- Disseminated gonococcal infection (DGI):
  - Synovial fluid analysis:
    - Neutrophilic leukocytosis, >50,000 cells/mm$^3$
    - Positive cultures when >80,000 cells/mm$^3$
  - 2 or more sets of blood cultures
  - Synovial, skin, urethral or cervical, and rectal cultures:
    - Thayer-Martin media
- PID/lower abdominal pain in female:
  - CBC
  - Urinalysis
  - Pregnancy test
- Rapid plasma reagin (RPR): For associated syphilis

## DIFFERENTIAL DIAGNOSIS

- Urethritis:
  - Chlamydia
  - Trichomonas
  - UTI
  - Syphilis
- DGI:
  - Bacterial arthritis:
    - Meningococcus (rash)
  - Hepatitis B
  - Connective tissue disease:
    - Reiter syndrome
    - Rheumatoid arthritis
    - Psoriatic arthritis
  - Acute rheumatic fever:
    - Poststreptococcal arthritis
  - Infective endocarditis
  - Others:
    - HIV
    - Secondary syphilis
    - Viral infection
    - Lyme disease (rash)
    - Gout (arthritis)

# TREATMENT

## ED TREATMENT/PROCEDURES
- Hydration (0.9% NS) for nausea/vomiting
- Generally treat sexual partner.
- Patient with gonorrhea should often be presumptively treated for chlamydial infection.
- Cervical, urethral, and anorectal infection:
  - Ceftriaxone: 125 or 250 mg IM once OR
  - Cefixime: 400 mg PO once OR
  - Spectinomycin: 2 g IM
  - Also treat for chlamydia:
    ○ Azithromycin: 1 g PO once OR
    ○ Doxycycline: 100 mg PO b.i.d. for 7 days
- Salpingitis/PID:
  - Outpatient:
    ○ Ceftriaxone: 250 mg IM once or cefoxitin 2 g IM and probenecid 1 g PO once or another 3rd-generation cephalosporin (ceftizoxime or cefotaxime) *plus* doxycycline 100 mg b.i.d. for 14 days with or without Metronidazole 500 mg PO b.i.d. for 14 days
  - Inpatient:
    ○ Cefoxitin 2 g IV q6h or cefotetan 2 g IV q12h *plus* doxycycline 100 mg PO or IV q12 h
    ○ Clindamycin 900 mg IV q8h plus gentamicin loading dose (2 mg/kg) followed by (1.5 mg/kg) q8h
    ○ Ampicillin/sulbactam: 3 g IV q6h plus doxycycline 100 mg PO or IV q12h
- Pharyngitis:
  - Ceftriaxone 125 or 250 mg IM single dose plus treatment for chlamydia if not ruled out
  - Spectinomycin if cephalosporin allergic
  - Pharyngeal culture 3–5 days post treatment to ensure eradication
- Epididymitis:
  - Ceftriaxone 250 mg IM once plus doxycycline 100 mg b.i.d. for 10 days
  - For negative NAAT or gonococcal culture or if enteric organisms most likely cause:
    ○ Ofloxacin 300 mg PO b.i.d. for 10 days OR
    ○ Levofloxacin 500 mg PO once a day for 10 days
- Treat sexual partner
- DGI:
  - Ceftriaxone: 1 g IV/IM daily (recommended)
  - Cefotaxime: 1 g IV q8h OR
  - Ceftizoxime: 1 g IV q8h OR
  - Spectinomycin: 2 g IM q12h (penicillin allergic)
  - After 24–48 hr of above therapy, additional 7 days with:
    ○ Cefixime: 400 mg PO b.i.d. OR
    ○ Cefpodoxime: 400 mg PO b.i.d.
- Conjunctivitis:
  - Adults:
    ○ Ceftriaxone 1 g IM once
  - Ophthalmia neonatorum:
    ○ Penicillin G 100,000 IU/kg/24 h IV q6h
    ○ Ceftriaxone 25–50 mg/kg/24 h IM/IV daily
    ○ Ceftriaxone 125 mg IM/IV

- Meningitis/endocarditis:
  - Ceftriaxone 1–2 g IV q12h:
    ○ 10–14 days for meningitis
    ○ 4 wk for endocarditis
- Severe cephalosporin allergy:
  - Consult infectious disease
  - Cephalosporin use post desensitization best alternative
  - Azithromycin 2 g PO for uncomplicated gonococcal infection:
    ○ Limit use to prevent resistance

### Pediatric Considerations
- Gonococcal ophthalmia neonatorum:
  - Mother with genital tract infection
  - Sight threatening infection
  - Bilateral conjunctivitis 2–5 days postpartum:
    ○ If untreated, leads to globe perforation

### Pregnancy Considerations
- Gonorrhea: Ceftriaxone/spectinomycin
- Chlamydia: Erythromycin

# FOLLOW-UP

## DISPOSITION
### Admission Criteria
PID—CDC recommendations
- Severely ill (eg, nausea, vomiting, and high fever)
- Pregnant
- Does not respond to or cannot take oral medication
- Tubo-ovarian abscess
- Other emergency surgical condition possible (eg, appendicitis)

### Discharge Criteria
Uncomplicated genital, pharyngeal, or conjunctival infection

### Issues for Referral
- Infertility
- Recurrent infection despite multiple therapy

# PEARLS AND PITFALLS

- Epididymitis—rule out torsion
- DGI—strongly consider in young sexually active patient with acute nontraumatic oligoarthritis or tenosynovitis

# ADDITIONAL READING

- CDC. Fact Sheet Gonorrhea: CS115145, Content updated December 2007. Centers for Disease Control and Prevention. U.S., Department of Health and Human Services, Atlanta. http://www.cdc.gov/std/gonorrhea/gonorrhea-fact-sheet.pdf. Accessed October 29, 2009.
- Updated recommended treatment regimens for gonococcal infections and associated conditions — United States, April 2007.CDC/NCHHSTP/DSTDP, Centers for Disease Control and Prevention. U.S., Department of Health and Human Services, Atlanta.http://www.cdc.gov/STD/treatment/2006/GonUpdateApril2007.pdf.1. Accessed October 29, 2009.
- Committee on Infectious Diseases, American Academy of Pediatrics. "Gonococcal Infections." Red Book(r): 2009 Report of the Committee on Infectious Diseases-28th Edition (2009).Editor: Larry K. Pickering, MD, FAAP. Printed in the United States of America. Stat!REF Online Electronic Medical Library-http://aapredbook.aappublications.org/cgi/content/full/2009/1/3.45 or http://online.statref.com/document.aspx?.fxid=76&docid=51. Accessed October 29, 2009.
- Pelvic Inflammatory Disease. Marx: Rosen's Emergency Medicine, 7th ed. 2009 Mosby, An Imprint of Elsevier. Chapter 96- Sexually Transmitted Diseases: Disorders Characterized By Genital Dischargehttp://www.mdconsult.com/book/player/book.do?.method=display&type=bookPage&decorator=header&eid=4-u1.0-B978-0-323-05472-0..00096 7-s0140&uniq=168081379&isbn=978 0-323-05472-0&sid=910003838. Accessed October 29, 2009
- Marx. Gonorrhea: Rosen's Emergency Medicine, 7th ed. 2009 Mosby, An Imprint of Elsevier. Chapter 96-Sexually Transmitted Diseases: Disorders Characterized By Genital Dischargehttp://www.mdconsult.com/book/player/book.do?.method=display&type=bookPage&decorator=header&eid=4-u1.0-B978-0-323-05472-0..00096-7-s0105&uniq=168081379&isbn=978-0-323-05472-0&sid=910009290. Accessed October 29, 2009.
- Marrazzo JM, Hoffman J. Infections Due to Neisseria. Chapter 18. Infectious Diseases: The Clinicians Guide to Diagnosis, Treatment, and Prevention. (c)2007 WebMD Inc. http://online.statref.com/titleinfo/fxid-65.html. Accessed October 29, 2009.

## See Also (Topic, Algorithm, Electronic Media Element)
- Chlamydia
- Urethritis

# CODES

### ICD9
- 098.0 Gonococcal infection (acute) of lower genitourinary tract
- 098.6 Gonococcal infection of pharynx
- 098.15 Gonococcal cervicitis (acute)

# GOUT/PSEUDOGOUT

*Delaram Ghadishah*

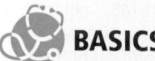
## BASICS

### DESCRIPTION
- Uric acid deposition into tissues, affecting mainly middle-aged men and postmenopausal women:
  - Most common crystalline diseases
  - Four phases:
    - Asymptomatic hyperuricemia (serum urate >7 mg/dL)
    - Acute gout
    - Intercritical gout: Quiet intervening periods
    - Tophaceous gout (up to 45% of cases)
  - Risk factors:
    - Age >40
    - Male/female ratio 2:1–6:1 <65 yr old; 1:1 ≥65 yr old
    - Hypertension
    - Use of loop or thiazide diuretics
    - High intake of alcohol, meat, seafood, and fructose-sweetened beverages
    - Obesity
  - Urologic deposition of uric acid calculi may cause renal dysfunction.
  - Associated with avascular necrosis and deforming arthritis
  - Most frequent in previously damaged joints, tissues:
    - Synovium
    - Subchondral bone
    - Bursae (olecranon, infrapatellar, prepatellar)
    - Achilles' tendon
    - Extensor surface of the forearms, toes, fingers, ear
    - Rarely CNS or cardiac (valves)
- Pseudogout: A disorder caused by calcium pyrophosphate crystal deposition:
  - Most common cause of acute monarthritis >60 yr of age
  - Risk factors:
    - Hypercalcemia (eg, hyperparathyroidism, familial)
    - Hemochromatosis; hemosiderosis
    - Hypothyroidism and hyperthyroidism
    - Hypophosphatemia, hypomagnesemia
    - Amyloidosis
    - Gout

### ETIOLOGY
- Deposition of monosodium urate crystals in tissues from supersaturated extracellular fluid owing to:
  - Underexcretion (most commonly) or excessive production of uric acid
  - Any rapid change in uric acid levels
    - Initiation or cessation of diuretics
    - Alcohol, salicylates, niacin
    - Cyclosporine
    - Lead acetate poisoning
    - Uricosurics or allopurinol
- Pseudogout occurs secondary to excess synovial accumulation of calcium pyrophosphate crystals
- Precipitants for both gout and pseudogout include minor trauma and acute illnesses:
  - Surgery, ischemic heart disease

## DIAGNOSIS

### SIGNS AND SYMPTOMS
- Gout and pseudogout both present as acute monoarticular or polyarticular arthritis:
  - Increased warmth, erythema, and joint swelling are present.
  - Early attacks subside spontaneously within 3–21 days, even without treatment.
  - Later attacks may last longer, cluster, be more severe, and be polyarticular.
- Gout:
  - Symptoms present maximally within 12–24 hr.
  - Tophi and joint desquamation may be present.
  - Women predominantly present after menopause and have polyarticular predominance (up to 70%).
  - Less dramatic presentations in immunosuppressed and elderly
  - Most common: 1st metatarsophalangeal joint (75%) > ankle; tarsal area; knee > hand; wrist
- Pseudogout:
  - Typically involves larger joints than with gout
  - Most common: knee > wrist > metacarpals; shoulder; elbow; ankle > hip; tarsal joints
  - Monoarticular (25%)
  - Asymptomatic (25%)
  - Pseudo-osteoarthritis (45%): Progressive degeneration, often symmetric
  - Pseudorheumatoid arthritis (in elderly)
- Polyarticular variant with fever and confusion

### ESSENTIAL WORKUP
- Arthrocentesis and aspiration of tophi:
  - Examine aspirant for crystals, Gram stain, cultures, leukocyte count, and differential
  - Fluid is typically thick pasty white:
    - Gout: 20,000–100,000 WBC/mm$^3$; poor string and mucin clot; no bacteria
    - Pseudogout: Up to 50,000 WBC/mm$^3$; no bacteria
- Microscopic examination of crystals under polarized light:
  - Gout:
    - Needle shaped
    - Strong birefringence
    - Negative elongation
  - Pseudogout:
    - Rhomboid
    - Weak birefringence
    - Positive elongation

## DIAGNOSTIC TESTS & INTERPRETATION
### Lab
- CBC often shows leukocytosis.
- Chemistry panel to assess for renal impairment
- Magnesium and calcium, thyroid-stimulating hormone (TSH), and serum iron
- Uric acid level has limited value.
- If infectious arthritis is suspected:
  - Blood and urine cultures
  - Urethral, cervical, rectal, or pharyngeal gonococcal cultures

### Imaging
- Plain radiographs to assess the presence of:
  - Effusion
  - Joint space narrowing
  - Baseline status of joint
  - Contiguous osteomyelitis
  - Fractures or foreign body
- Acute gout: Soft tissue swelling; normal mineralization; joint space preservation
- Chronic gout: Calcified tophi; asymmetric bony erosions; overhanging edges; bony shaft tapering
- Pseudogout: Chondrocalcinosis; subchondral sclerosis or cysts (wrist); radiopaque calcification of cartilage, tendons, and ligaments; radiopaque osteophytes
- Dual energy CT to assess for kidney stones or soft tissue urate crystals

### Diagnostic Procedures/Surgery
- Arthrocentesis
- Aspiration of tophi

### DIFFERENTIAL DIAGNOSIS
- Infectious arthritis
- Trauma
- Osteoarthritis
- Reactive arthritis
- Miscellaneous crystalline arthritis
- Aseptic necrosis
- Rheumatoid arthritis
- Systemic lupus erythematosus
- Sickle cell
- Osteomyelitis
- Psoriatic arthritis

**TREATMENT**

### INITIAL STABILIZATION/THERAPY
- Relieve pain.
- Rule out infectious cause.

### ED TREATMENT/PROCEDURES
- NSAIDs are first-line treatment.
- If NSAIDS ineffective or contraindicated:
  - Steroids (oral, intravascular, intramuscular, intra-articular)
  - Colchicine (limited by toxicity)
- Joint aspiration
- Avoid aspirin.
- Reduction of hyperuricemia and long-term management of gout and pseudogout are not within the usual scope of ED care:
  - Careful withdrawal of gout-producing agent
  - Uricosurics (eg, probenecid, sulfinpyrazone)
  - Allopurinol to reduce uric acid synthesis
  - Increased fluid intake and urine alkalization to prevent renal stones
  - Long-term colchicine or NSAIDs prophylactically

### MEDICATION
- Anakinra: 100 mg SQ qd:
  Off label use for chronic, treatment refractory gout or pseudogout and with renal failure
- Allopurinol: 100 mg PO qd, increased weekly to max 800 mg qd:
  - Start 1–2 wk after attack has resolved
  - Adjust for kidney disease.
  - Discontinue with rash or fever.
  - Treatment of choice with uric acid kidney stones
- Colchicine: 0.5 mg/hr PO up to pain relief, 8 mg total, or GI toxicity:
  - Can cause bone marrow suppression at high doses
  - Not dialyzable
  - Long-term use may cause myopathy.
  - Adjust dose for liver or kidney disease.
  - Does not prevent monosodium urate deposition or joint damage of chronic gout
- Corticosteroids:
  - Corticotropin: 40 units IM, q8h, up to 3 doses
  - Methylprednisolone: 40 mg (peds: 1–2 mg/kg) IM or IV qd for 3–4 days
  - Prednisone: 40 mg (peds: 1–2 mg/kg) PO qd for 3–4 days; taper over 7–14 days
  - Triamcinolone: 10–40 mg plus dexamethasone 2–10 mg intra-articularly

- Febuxostat: 40–80 mg qd:
  - Give with NSAID or colchicine when 1st started
- NSAIDs in maximal doses initially for 3 days, then taper over 4 days:
  - Ibuprofen: 800 mg (peds: 10 mg/kg) PO q.i.d.
  - Indomethacin: 25–50 mg PO t.i.d.–q.i.d. (peds: 2 mg/kg/d t.i.d.–q.i.d.; *not* for children <14 yr old)
  - Ketorolac: 15–30 mg IM/IV in ED, may repeat for 1 dose (peds: 1 mg/kg to max 30 mg IM or 0.5 mg/kg to max 15 mg IV) IM:
    - Naproxen: 500 mg PO t.i.d. (peds: 5 mg/kg PO h i d )
    - Sulindac: 200 mg PO t.i.d.
- Probenecid: 250–500 mg PO t.i.d., max. 3 g qd:
  - Not effective or less effective with renal disease or aspirin or diuretic use
  - Relatively contraindicated with presence of uric acid kidney stones
- Sulfinpyrazone: 50 mg t.i.d., max 800 mg qd

### Geriatric Considerations
NSAIDs may worsen renal function, fluid retention, gastropathy, hepatotoxicity, and cognitive function, particularly in the elderly.

### Pediatric Considerations
Gout not usually seen in children, although possible during chemotherapy treatment for cancer.

 **FOLLOW-UP**

### DISPOSITION
#### Admission Criteria
- Suspected infectious arthritis
- Acute renal failure
- Intractable pain

#### Discharge Criteria
- No evidence of infection
- Adequate pain relief

#### Issues for Referral
- Septic arthritis
- Renal failure

### FOLLOW-UP RECOMMENDATIONS
- Rheumatology follow-up in severe or difficult to control cases
- Renal follow-up if renal insufficiency is present
- Urology follow-up if uric acid stones are present
- Orthopedic follow-up in cases of septic arthritis or significant joint damage
- Advise patient to follow a low-purine diet.

## PEARLS AND PITFALLS
- Septic arthritis can occur simultaneously with an acute gout attack.
- NSAIDs are first-line treatment if tolerated.
- Attacks generally tend to be self-limited.
- Gout and pseudogout can lead to bony and cartilaginous damage.

## ADDITIONAL READING
- Agudelo CA, Wise CM. Crystal-associated arthritis in the elderly. *Rheum Dis Clin North Am.* 2000;26(3): 527–546.
- Laubscher T, et al. Taking the stress out of managing gout. *Can Fam Physician.* 2009;55:1209 1212.
- Terkeltaub R. Update on Gout: New therapeutic options and strategies. *Nat Rev Rheumatol.* 2010;6:30–38.
- Wiesner T, Fried I. Gouty tophi. *N Engl J Med.* 2009;361:21.
- Yanai H, et al. Clinical, radiological, and biochemical characteristics in patients with diseases mimicking polymyalgia rheumatica. *Clin Intervent Aging.* 2009;4:391–395.

### See Also (Topic, Algorithm, Electronic Media Element)
- www.Epocrates.com

## CODES

### ICD9
- 274.00 Gouty arthropathy, unspecified
- 274.03 Chronic gouty arthropathy with tophus (tophi)
- 712.20 Chondrocalcinosis, due to pyrophosphate crystals, involving unspecified site

# GRANULOCYTOPENIA

*Richard E. Wolfe*
*Elicia Sinor Kennedy*

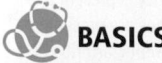 **BASICS**

## DESCRIPTION

- A significant decrease in the number of granulocytes
- 3 classes of granulocytes:
  - Neutrophils or polymorphonuclear cells (PMN) and bands
  - Eosinophils
  - Basophils
- As PMNs predominate, the terms neutropenia is often used interchangeably with granulocytopenia, as almost all granulocytopenic patients are neutropenic.
- Granulocytes are a key component of the nonspecific infection-fighting immune system.
- The clinical risks resulting from granulocytopenia are best defined by the level of the Absolute Neutrophil Count (ANC):
  - $ANC = WBC \times$ percentage (PMN + Bands)
- Neutropenia: ANC <1,500 cells/mm$^3$:
  - Mild: Between 1,000 and 1,500
  - Moderate: Between 500–1,000
  - Severe: <500; also incorrectly called agranulocytosis as there is usually a small number of granulocytes still present.
  - Patients with a count <1,000 that has recently or rapidly fallen are at greater risk for infection than those with a count <500 but rising.
  - Patients with myelodysplastic syndromes should be considered granulocytopenic with higher counts because of defective neutrophils.
- 4 basic mechanisms cause granulocytopenia:
  - Decreased production
  - Ineffective granulopoiesis
  - Shift of circulating PMNs to vascular endothelium
  - Enhanced peripheral destruction.
- Mortality of fever and neutropenia is as high as 50% if untreated:
  - Mortality correlates with the duration and severity of the neutropenia and the time elapsed until the 1st dose of antibiotics.
- 21% of patients with cancer and neutropenic fever develop serious complications.

### Pediatric Considerations

- Newborn infants have a physiologically elevated ANC in the 1st few days of life and may be granulocytopenic with levels >1,500/$\mu$L.
- Children >3 mo without underlying immunodeficiency or a central venous catheter unexpectedly found to have isolated moderate neutropenia are not at high risk of serious bacterial infection.

## ETIOLOGY

- Most common in patients undergoing myelosuppressive drug therapy or radiation treatment for neoplasms
- Adverse reaction to drugs
- 2nd most common cause:
  - Excludes cytotoxic drugs and requires at least 4 wk of administration prior to the onset of granulocytopenia
  - Discontinuation usually results with correction within 30 days.
  - Drugs with the highest risk:
    - Antipsychotic: Clozapine
    - Antibiotic: Sulfasalazine
    - Antithyroid: Thioamides
  - Antiplatelet agents
  - Antiepileptic drugs
  - NSAIDs
- Drugs that suppress the bone marrow:
  - Methotrexate
  - Cyclophosphamide
  - Colchicine
  - Azathioprine
  - Ganciclovir
- Chemicals
- Bacterial infections:
  - Typhoid
  - Shigella enteritis
  - Brucellosis
  - Tularemia
  - Tuberculosis
- Rickettsial infections:
  - Rickettsialpox
  - Ehrlichiosis
  - Rocky Mountain spotted fever
- Viral Infections
- Postinfectious neutropenia:
  - Most severe and protracted following HIV, hepatitis B, and Epstein-Barr viral infections
- Immune-related:
  - Primary immune neutropenia:
    - Due to antineutrophil antibodies
  - Bone marrow infiltration
- Transfusion reaction:
- Vitamin deficiency (B$_{12}$/folate)
- Chronic idiopathic neutropenia
- Pure white cell aplasia

### Pediatric Considerations

- Congenital neutropenia:
  - Neutropenia with abnormal immunoglobulins
  - Reticular dysgenesis
  - Severe congenital neutropenia or Kostmann syndrome
  - Cyclic neutropenia
- Chronic benign neutropenia
- Neonatal isoimmune neutropenia
- Shwachman-Diamond syndrome
- Cartilage-hair hypoplasia
- Dyskeratosis congenital
- Barth syndrome
- Chédiak-Higashi syndrome
- Myelokathexis
- Lazy leukocyte syndrome

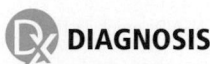 **DIAGNOSIS**

## SIGNS AND SYMPTOMS

- Signs of infection:
  - Fever
  - Localized erythema or fluctuance
- Signs of pancytopenia:
  - Fatigue
  - Pallor
  - Petechiae
  - Epistaxis and other spontaneous bleeding

### History

- Medical list should be reviewed for causative drugs.
- Family history of granulocytopenia in neonates and children
- Records of past ANC levels to assess for chronicity
- Question the patient carefully about fever, chills, dizziness, and vomiting as indicators of an underlying serious infection.
- Ask about localizing signs of infection such as cough; shortness of breath; chest pain; dysuria; urinary retention, urgency, or frequency; abdominal pain; and rectal pain.

## Physical Exam
Focus on finding signs of infection:

- Oral exam: Thrush, ulcers, periodontal disease
- Lungs: Rales, Rhonchi
- Skin: Rashes, ulcers, abscesses
- Perirectal: Although the rectal exam is relatively contraindicated until antibiotics are started, check for abscesses and mucosal lesions.

## ESSENTIAL WORKUP
Complete physical exam:

- Detailed exam of oral mucosa and perianal area
- Palpation of skin
- Location of fluctuance or tenderness
- Careful lung exam
- Rectal exam if symptoms suggest perirectal abscess

## DIAGNOSTIC TESTS & INTERPRETATION
### Lab
- CBC with differential:
  - Absolute neutrophil count = WBC (cells/$\mu$L) $\times$ percent (polymorphonuclears + bands)
- Blood culture from 2 different sites, with 1 from IV catheter site if present
- Urinalysis and urine culture:
  - Urinalysis may be normal

### Imaging
- CXR even in absence of lung findings
- Cerebrospinal fluid analysis for altered mental status/signs of meningitis

## DIFFERENTIAL DIAGNOSIS
- Lab error
- African Americans may have a lower but normal ANC value of 1,000 cells/mm$^3$

 TREATMENT

## INITIAL STABILIZATION/THERAPY
For patients presenting in shock:

- Administer 1 L 0.9% NS IV fluid bolus (peds: 20 cc/kg).
- Initiate pressors as needed to stabilize BP if no response to IV fluids.
- Consider starting goal-directed therapy.

## ED TREATMENT/PROCEDURES
- Strict isolation in a negative airflow room if possible
- Administer broad-spectrum combination antibiotics after cultures for suspected or documented infection:
  - Imipenem/cilastatin or fluoroquinolone
  - Ceftazidime alone or with aminoglycoside (amikacin, tobramycin, gentamicin)
- Cefepime alone
- Aminoglycoside plus antipseudomonal $\beta$-lactam (mezlocillin, piperacillin, or ticarcillin)
- Vancomycin if patient is at risk to be carrier of Staphylococcus aureus or has history of previous staphylococcal infections

## MEDICATION
- Amikacin: 15 mg/kg/24 hr (peds: 15–30 mg/kg/24 hr) divided q8–12h IV
- Cefepime: 0.5–2 g q12h
- Ceftazidime: 1–2 g (peds: 30–50 mg/kg q8h) q8–12h IV
- Gentamicin: 1 mg/kg (peds: 2–2.5 mg/kg) q8h or 5 mg/kg q24h
- Imipenem/cilastatin: 250–1,000 mg q6–8h
- Levofloxacin: 500 mg IV q.i.d.
- Mezlocillin: 3 g q4h over 30 min
- Piperacillin: 3 g q4h over 30 min
- Ticarcillin: 3 g (peds: 200–300 mg/kg per 24 hr) q4h over 30 min
- Tobramycin: 1 mg/kg q8h IV (peds: 2–2.5 mg/kg q8h IV)
- Vancomycin: 1–2 mg/kg q8–12h IV

 FOLLOW-UP

## DISPOSITION
### Admission Criteria
- Signs of infection
- Unreliable patient
- Close follow-up unavailable

### Discharge Criteria
- Previously diagnosed granulocytopenia
- Completely asymptomatic
- Close follow-up ensured
- Reliable patient

## Issues for Referral
All patients with granulocytopenia should be referred to their physician or a hematologist.

### FOLLOW-UP RECOMMENDATIONS
- Patient should return immediately to the ED with fever.
- Follow-up within 48 hr with the patient's physician

## PEARLS AND PITFALLS
- Usual signs of infection may be masked because of the impaired immune response in patients with granulocytopenia.
- Rectal exams are relatively contraindicated in neutropenic patients but should be performed once antibiotics are started to avoid missing a perirectal abscess.
- Antipyretic drugs should be avoided if there is a need to detect a fever to determine management.
- Patients with fever and an ANC <500 requires immediate and aggressive therapy with broad-spectrum antibiotics and IV fluids.

## ADDITIONAL READING
- Andres E, Noel E, Kurtz JE. Life-threatening idiosyncratic drug-induced agranulocytosis in elderly patients. Drugs Aging. 2004;21(7):427–435.
- Avery RK, Longworth DL. Evolving concepts in the management of patients with neutropenia and fever. Cleve Clin J Med. 1999;66:173–180.
- Bagby GC. Disorders of neutrophil production. In: Bennett JC, et al., eds. Cecil's Textbook of Medicine. Philadelphia: WB Saunders; 1996:908–915.
- Bozing K, Klein C. Novel genetic etiologies of severe congenital neutropenia. Curr Opin Immunol. 2009;21(5):472–480.
- Kaufman DW, Kelly JP, Levy M, et al. The Drug Etiologies of Agranulocytosis and Aplastic Anemia. New York: Oxford University Press, 1991.
- Melendez E, Harper MB. Risk of serious bacterial infection in isolated and unsuspected neutropenia. Acad Emerg Med. 2010;17:1–5.

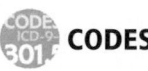 CODES

### ICD9
- 288.00 Neutropenia, unspecified
- 288.09 Other neutropenia

**G**

# GUILLAIN-BARRÉ SYNDROME

*John E. Houghland*
*Jeffrey Druck*

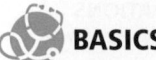 **BASICS**

## DESCRIPTION
- Group of autoimmune conditions involving demyelination and acute axonal degeneration of peripheral nerves:
  - Humoral and cellular immune mediated
- Usually preceded by triggering event, for example, respiratory or GI infection in 75%
- Leading cause of acute, flaccid paralysis in western countries
- All ages, but rare in infancy
- Weakness reaches nadir at 2–4 wk.
- Spontaneous resolution occurs over weeks to months.
- Acute inflammatory demyelinating polyradiculoneuropathy (AIDP):
  - Most common form of Guillain-Barré syndrome (GBS; 90%); formerly synonymous with GBS
  - Triggered by antecedent bacterial/viral infection
  - Demyelination sometimes accompanied by axonal loss
  - Usually complete recovery:
    - 85% with full recovery in 1 yr
    - 20% unable to walk at 6 mo
    - 10% mortality rate (from complications such as PE, infection, cardiac)
- Other forms of GBS:
  - Acute motor axonal neuropathy (AMAN):
    - Pure motor axonal involvement
    - 67% seropositive for *campylobacter*
    - Recovery often rapid
    - Often pediatric patients
  - Acute motor sensory axonal neuropathy (AMSAN):
    - Degeneration of myelinated motor and sensory nerves, but without significant inflammation or demyelination
    - Similar to AMAN, but also involves sensory nerves
  - Acute panautonomic neuropathy:
    - Very rare
    - Involves sympathetic and parasympathetic nerves
    - Postural hypotension, dysrhythmias, tachycardia, hypertension
    - Blurry vision, dry eyes, anhydrosis
    - Recovery gradual, often incomplete
  - Miller-Fisher syndrome:
    - Rare
    - Rapidly evolving ataxia, areflexia, ophthalmoplegia, no weakness
    - Demyelination and inflammation of cranial nerves II and VI, spinal ganglia, and peripheral nerves
    - Resolves in 1–3 mo

## ETIOLOGY
- Postinfectious:
  - 2/3 with antecedent illness, usually respiratory or GI
  - 1–3 wk between prodromal illness and neurologic symptoms
  - *Campylobacter jejuni* most common antecedent infection
  - Cytomegalovirus most common viral infection
  - Epstein Barr virus
  - Mycoplasma
  - Human immunodeficiency virus
- Relationship to vaccines is questionable

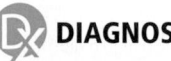 **DIAGNOSIS**

## SIGNS AND SYMPTOMS
### History
- Rapidly evolving, symmetric, ascending paralysis
- Absent or mild sensory symptoms (e.g., paresthesias of fingertips or toes)
- Pain, commonly of pelvis, shoulder girdles, posterior thighs
- Cranial nerve involvement may affect swallowing, facial muscles, eye movements.
- Preceding bacterial or viral infection

### Physical Exam
- Ascending symmetric weakness; proximal muscles, legs more affected than arms
- Loss of deep tendon reflexes
- Look for cranial nerve involvement.
- Normal sensory exam:
  - Autonomic dysfunction:
    - Hypertension
    - Orthostatic hypotension
    - Ileus
    - Dysrhythmias
    - Urinary retention
  - Miller-Fisher syndrome:
    - Ataxia, areflexia, ophthalmoplegia, mild limb weakness
- Other subtypes described above
- Features that suggest alternative diagnosis:
  - Fever
  - Normal reflexes
  - Upper motor neuron signs
  - Asymmetric neurologic deficits
  - Sharply demarcated sensory level

## DIAGNOSTIC TESTS & INTERPRETATION
- Diagnosis is generally made on clinical grounds
- Laboratory and imaging tests can assist with diagnosis and rule out other causes of symptoms

### Lab
- Electrolytes (some patients have SIADH)
- Lumbar puncture:
  - Increased protein (55–250), may be present only after 7–10 days as disease and blood–brain barrier dysfunction progress
  - Few or no WBCs (WBCs >10–50 suggests other etiology)
  - Normal opening pressure

### Imaging
CT or MRI to rule out cord compression

### Diagnostic Procedures/Surgery
Electrophysiologic studies will be abnormal (nerve conduction confirmatory)

## DIFFERENTIAL DIAGNOSIS
- Cord compression
- Hypokalemia
- Lyme disease
- Chagas disease
- Leprosy
- Sarcoidosis
- Vasculitides
- Tick paralysis
- Transverse myelitis
- Neuromyelitis optica
- Botulism
- Myasthenia gravis
- Neoplastic meningitis
- Acute periodic paralysis
- Poliomyelitis
- Diphtheria
- Eaton-Lambert syndrome
- Acute intermittent porphyria
- Chronic heavy metal poisoning
- Tetrodotoxin poisoning
- Psychogenic, malingering

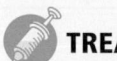 **TREATMENT**

**PRE-HOSPITAL**
Attention to airway management

**INITIAL STABILIZATION/THERAPY**
Airway assessment and management:
- Progression to respiratory failure can be rapid.

**ED TREATMENT/PROCEDURES**
- Airway management:
  – ~30% will need ventilatory support.
  – May need intubation within 24–28 hr of onset
  – Frequent monitoring of respiratory parameters:
    ○ Forced vital capacity (FVC) or negative inspiratory flow (NIF) helpful
    ○ ICU admission if FVC <20 mL/kg or NIF <30 cm H2O
    ○ Intubation recommended if FVC <15 mL/kg
- Watch for autonomic dysfunction.
- Supportive therapy
- Early neurology consult

**MEDICATION**
- Plasmapheresis or IV immunoglobulin (IVIG), in conjunction with neurologic consultation:
  – Unclear benefit for Miller Fischer or mild GBS
- IVIG: 400 mg/kg/d for 5 days
- Pain control:
  – Acetaminophen: 325–1,000 mg PO q6h
  – Ibuprofen: 400–800 mg PO q8h
  – Gabapentin: Start 300 mg PO per day
- Steroids not beneficial for pain or deficits:
  – Oral steroids delay recovery
  – IV steroids with no benefit

 **FOLLOW-UP**

**DISPOSITION**
*Admission Criteria*
- All patients with GBS or suspected GBS warrant admission for close observation
- ICU admission for those with signs of respiratory compromise or autonomic dysfunction

*Discharge Criteria*
Patients should be considered for discharge only after consultation with neurologist

**FOLLOW-UP RECOMMENDATIONS**
- Follow-up determined by neurologist
- Poor outcome associated with:
  – Older age
  – Longer time to nadir
  – Necessity for ventilator support
  – Preceding diarrheal illness, *C. jejuni*

## PEARLS AND PITFALLS

- Pearls:
  – Check FVC and/or NIF frequently to anticipate airway compromise
  – Consider other etiologies if CSF WBC count >10–50
- Pitfalls:
  – Failure to obtain appropriate imaging of the brain and spinal cord to rule out other potential causes
  – Failure to consult neurology and admit or observe all patients with suspected GBS

## ADDITIONAL READING

- Brettschneider J, Petzold A, Sussmuth S, et al. Cerebrospinal fluid biomarkers in Guillain-Barre syndrome—Where do we stand? *J Neurol*. 2009;256:3–12.
- Lunn MT, Willison HJ. Diagnosis and treatment in inflammatory neuropathies. *Postgrad Med. J* 2009;85;437–46.
- Pandey CK, Raza M, Tripathi M, et al. The comparative evaluation of gabapentin and carbamazepine for pain management in Guillain-Barre syndrome patients in the intensive care unit. *Anesth Analg*. 2005;101:220–5.
- Vucic S, Kiernan MC, Cornblath DR. Guillain-Barre syndrome: An update. *J Clin Neurosci*. 2009;16: 733–741.
- Winer JB. Guillain-Barre syndrome. *BMJ*. 2008;337:a671.

**See Also (Topic, Algorithm, Electronic Media Element)**
- Myasthenia Gravis
- Spinal Cord Syndromes
- Spine Injury
- Tick Bites

 **CODES**

**ICD9**
357.0 Acute infective polyneuritis

G

# HALLUCINOGEN POISONING

*Joanne C. Witsil*

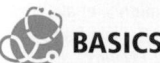

## BASICS

### DESCRIPTION
- Predominantly alters perception, cognition, and mood
- All hallucinogens potentiate neurotransmitter release or bind directly to receptors:
  - Serotonin (5-hydroxytryptamine; 5-HT): Many hallucinogens are agonists or antagonists at 5-HT receptor subtypes.
  - Norepinephrine, N-methyl-D-aspartate (NMDA), dopamine

### ETIOLOGY
- Most exposures are intentional.
- Common hallucinogens:
  - Indoleamine:
    - Lysergic acid diethylamide (LSD) (duration 6–12 hr)
    - Morning glory (*Ipomoea* spp.)
  - Tryptamines:
    - Psilocybin (*Psilocybe* mushrooms); frequently adulterated with LSD
    - N,N-dimethyltryptamine (DMT); 5-MeO-DMT (cfoxy-methoxyd), and other tryptamine congeners
  - Phenylethylamines (hallucinogenic amphetamines):
    - Methylenedioxyamphetamine (MDA)
    - Methylenedioxymethamphetamine (MDEA)
    - Methylenedioxymethamphetamine (MDMA; "ecstasy"; duration 8–12 hr)
    - Paramethoxyamphetamine
    - Dimethoxyamphetamine
    - Mescaline (peyote cactus); frequently adulterated with LSD (duration 6–12 hr)
  - Arylcycloalkylamines:
    - Phencyclidine (PCP), (duration is variable 11–96 hr in 1 report)
    - Ketamine, (duration depends on route of administration 30–120 min)
  - Anticholinergic:
    - Deadly nightshade (*Atropa belladonna*)
    - Jimsonweed (*Datura stramonium*)
  - Other:
    - Piperazines: Benzyl piperazine (BZP) and trifluoromethyl phenylpiperazine (TFMPP)
    - Dextromethorphan (DXM), (duration 3–6 hr)
    - Marijuana

## DIAGNOSIS

### SIGNS AND SYMPTOMS
- Considerable individual variation; effects may last 4–12 hr and ≤96 hr depending on agent/dose.
- Symptoms characterized by sympathetic arousal
- Usually oriented and able to give history of exposure even while having delusions
- Initial symptoms:
  - Nausea, flushing, chills, tremor
- Neurologic symptoms:
  - Restlessness and dizziness early after ingestion
  - Affective lability
  - Desire to laugh (especially with *Psilocybe* mushrooms)
  - Anxiety, despair, helplessness, dread
  - Intensified perceptions, visual distortions/intensification
  - Tactile distortions (especially with mescaline)
  - Synesthesia (blending of sensory modalities, eg, seeing sounds)
  - Religious or mystical experiences
  - Sleep disruption
- Neurologic signs:
  - Unusual/bizarre behavior
  - Speech disruption
  - Mydriasis
  - Piloerection
  - Hyperreflexia
  - Coma with massive exposure
  - Convulsions:
    - Hallucinogenic amphetamines
    - Children who become hyperpyrexic after *Psilocybe* mushroom ingestion
- Pulmonary:
  - Mild tachypnea
  - Respiratory arrest (with massive exposure)
- Cardiovascular:
  - Tachycardia
  - HTN (with hallucinogenic amphetamines)
  - Dysrhythmia (with hallucinogenic amphetamines)
  - Intracerebral hemorrhage (with hallucinogenic amphetamines)
- Gastrointestinal:
  - Nausea/vomiting (especially with mescaline)
- Metabolic:
  - Hyperpyrexia:
    - Especially with MDMA use at "rave" clubs
    - Hepatic failure, renal failure, and disseminated intravascular coagulopathy may follow.
    - May be lethal
  - Hyponatremia: Has been reported with MDMA use
- Hematopoietic:
  - Coagulopathies and hemorrhage at high doses owing to disruption of platelet serotonin function

### History
Identity of agent or agents used including:
- Method of usage
- Quantity
- Time of exposure
- Knowledge of place of exposure

### Physical Exam
- Obtain accurate vital signs including temperature.
- Perform detailed neurologic and psychiatric examination

### ESSENTIAL WORKUP
- Core temperature measurement and other vital signs
- ECG monitoring
- Determination of risk of rhabdomyolysis:
  - Creatine kinase level
  - Urine dip or myoglobin level

### DIAGNOSTIC TESTS & INTERPRETATION
### Lab
- Electrolytes, BUN, creatinine, glucose levels, coagulation screen, arterial or venous blood gas
- Urine toxicology screen:
  - Rarely indicated
  - Distinguishing between hallucinogens is of little value.
  - Most hallucinogenic substances are not tested for on routine drug screens.
  - Amphetamine screen is frequently negative for hallucinogenic amphetamines (eg, MDMA).

### Imaging
- Consider chest x-ray if looking for aortic dissection, pulmonary aspiration, or trauma-related injury
- Consider abdominal x-ray if there is suspicion of ingested packets

### DIFFERENTIAL DIAGNOSIS
- Meningitis
- Intracranial bleeds or lesions
- Withdrawal (ethanol, sedative–hypnotic, baclofen)
- Serotonin syndrome (especially with concomitant serotonergic agents involved)
- Psychiatric illnesses:
  - LSD associated with prolonged psychoses resembling schizoaffective disorders
  - Chronic amphetamine/cocaine abuse
  - Steroids
- Infectious/febrile seizures in hyperpyretic child

### Pediatric Considerations
Assess parent-child relationships for possibility of neglect or abuse.

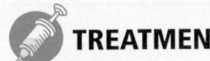 **TREATMENT**

### PRE-HOSPITAL

- Controversies:
  - Sedation with benzodiazepines versus haloperidol versus physical restraints:
    - Benzodiazepines are generally preferred.
    - Sedation masks symptoms and may limit history.
- Cautions:
  - Sedate or restrain patient to ensure safe transport.
  - For hyperthermic patient:
    - Use sedation rather than physical restraint.
    - Begin cooling measures.

### INITIAL STABILIZATION/THERAPY

- Management of ABCs
- Aggressive cooling if hyperthermic
- IV access/rehydration with isotonic fluids for significant fluid loss or evidence of rhabdomyolysis
- Naloxone, Accu-Chek, dextrose, and thiamine if patient has altered mental status

### ED TREATMENT/PROCEDURES

- Cooling measures:
  - Cool mist and fans
  - Benzodiazepines if agitated
  - Paralytics with intubation if needed (generally not succinylcholine)
- Sedate for agitation or autonomic signs:
  - Benzodiazepines
  - Rarely neuroleptics:
    - May intensify hallucinogenic experience
    - Possibly lower seizure threshold
- Activated charcoal (AC) is not expected to be helpful for most agents owing to rapid absorption and delayed patient presentation:
  - Consider AC for oral ingestions within 2–3 hr in patients with intact protective airway reflexes; especially for anticholinergics or seeds owing to delayed GI motility/absorption.
- Place in a quiet, calm environment.
- Maintain urine output of 2–3 mL/kg/hr and consider urine alkalinization for treatment of rhabdomyolysis.

### MEDICATION

- Dextrose D$_{50}$W for hypoglycemia: 1 ampule: 25 g/50 mL (peds: D$_{25}$W, 0.5–1 g/kg or 2–4 mL/kg) IV
- Benzodiazepines (diazepam): 5–10 mg IV (peds: 0.2–0.5 mg/kg) IV or lorazepam: 1–4 mg IV/IM (peds: 0.02–0.05 mg/kg) IV/IM
- Haloperidol (Haldol): 2.5–5 mg IV or IM; not recommended for children
- Naloxone (Narcan): initial dose: 2 mg (peds: 0.01–0.1 mg/kg) IV or IM
- Sodium bicarbonate drip for rhabdomyolysis: 3 ampules in 1 L of D$_5$W; infuse at 1.5–2 times maintenance rates (keep urine pH >7.5)
- Thiamine (vitamin B$_1$): 100 mg (peds: 25 mg) IV or IM

 **FOLLOW-UP**

### DISPOSITION

#### Admission Criteria

- Severely intoxicated
- Atypical presentation
- Prolonged symptoms (>12 hr after exposure)
- Prolonged periods of agitation and hyperthermia:
  - Risk of rhabdomyolysis or organ damage

#### Discharge Criteria

After receiving supportive therapy and observation, most patients can be discharged once they are asymptomatic.

#### Issues for Referral
#### Pediatric Considerations

Suspected cases of child abuse or neglect require referral to child protective services.

### FOLLOW-UP RECOMMENDATIONS

- Upon discharge, patients should receive follow-up care from their PCP, psychiatrist, or drug counseling facility.

### PEARLS AND PITFALLS

- Do not delay in the diagnosis and treatment of hyperthermia. Once hyperthermia is identified, aggressively lower body temperature.
- Use appropriate physical and chemical restraints to control violent and agitated patients to protect the patient and staff from physical injury.
- Conduct serial examinations and vital signs (especially temperature). Do not assume once a violently agitated patient is calm that the patient is recovering. The patient may be progressing to serious illness.

### ADDITIONAL READING

- Acute reactions to drugs of abuse. *Med Lett Drugs Ther*. 2002;44:21–24.
- Graeme KA. New drugs of abuse. *Emerg Med Clin North Am*. 2000;18:625–636.
- Greene SL. Review article: Amphetamines and related drugs of abuse. *Emerg Med Australas*. 2008;20(5):391–402.
- Hall AP, Henry JA. Acute toxic effects of "ecstasy" (MDMA) and related compounds: Overview of pathophysiology and clinical management. *Br J Anaesth*. 2006;96:678–685.
- Liechti ME, Kunz I, Kupferschmidt H. Acute medical problems due to Ecstasy use. *Swiss Med Wkly*. 2005;135:652–657.

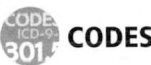 **CODES**

### ICD9

969.6 Poisoning by psychodysleptics (hallucinogens)

H

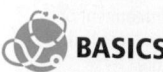

# HAND INFECTION
*Chet Shermer*

##  BASICS

### DESCRIPTION
- Hand infections are commonly seen in the ED.
- The range of pathology is broad and may include acute *and* chronic conditions.

### ALERT
- Serious hand infections are potential liability issues and must be handled with extreme caution.
- Referral to hand surgeon is almost always indicated.

### ETIOLOGY
- Bacterial infection of the hand is associated with skin pathogens:
  – *Staphylococcus* or *Streptococcus* spp.
  – History of a puncture wound
- Anaerobes are identified in 75% of paronychia in children owing to thumb sucking and nail biting.
- Chronic paronychia may be caused by *Candida albicans*.
- Herpetic whitlow is caused by type 1–2 herpes simplex virus.
- Clenched fist injuries involve a variety of pathogens, including anaerobic *Streptococcus* and *Eikenella* spp.

##  DIAGNOSIS

### SIGNS AND SYMPTOMS
- Paronychia:
  – Localized edema, erythema, and pain in proximal portion of lateral nail fold
  – Fluctuance may be present and may extend beneath the nail margin.
  – Systemic signs and symptoms are usually not present.
- Felon:
  – Erythema and tense swelling of the distal pulp space that does *not* extend proximal to the proximal interphalangeal (PIP) joint
  – Aching pain early, severe throbbing pain late
  – Systemic signs are usually not present.
- Herpetic whitlow:
  – Distal pulp space is swollen, but remains soft.
  – Lateral nail folds may be affected.
  – Throbbing pain of the distal pulp space
  – Vesicles containing nonpurulent fluid are present and may form bullae.
  – Systemic symptoms may be present:
    ○ Fever
    ○ Lymphadenopathy
    ○ Constitutional symptoms

- Flexor tenosynovitis:
  – Kanavel signs:
    ○ Severe pain and symmetric edema of the digit
    ○ Tenderness over the course of tendon sheath
    ○ Flexed position of the finger at rest
    ○ Pain on passive extension of the finger—may be the only finding in early infection
- Clenched fist injury:
  – Laceration over the metacarpophalangeal (MCP) joint from striking an object with a clenched fist
  – Any laceration over the MCP must be assumed to be a *human bite wound* until proven otherwise.
- Web space abscess:
  – Pain and edema of the affected web space and adjacent palm
  – Fingers are held abducted.
- Palmar space infections:
  – Thenar space infection:
    ○ Pain, tenderness, tense edema of thenar eminence
    ○ Dorsal edema without tenderness
    ○ Thumb is held abducted and flexed, and passive adduction is painful.
  – Midpalmar space infection:
    ○ Pain, edema, and tenderness of the midpalmar space
    ○ Dorsal edema without tenderness
    ○ Motion of middle and ring fingers is painful.
  – Hypothenar space infection:
    ○ Pain and fullness over hypothenar eminence
    ○ No limitation of finger movement

### History
See Signs and Symptoms.

### Physical Exam
See Signs and Symptoms.

### ESSENTIAL WORKUP
Most hand infections are diagnosed by history and physical examination with special attention to neurovascular status.

### DIAGNOSTIC TESTS & INTERPRETATION
#### Lab
- Although usually not necessary, herpetic whitlow may be confirmed by Tzanck test.
- Gram's stain and culture may guide antibiotic choice in felons.
- Blood cultures, CBC are not routinely indicated.

#### Imaging
- Radiographs are usually not helpful unless there has been trauma or a suspected foreign body.
- With felon, flexor tenosynovitis, and palmar space infection, radiograph may identify osteomyelitis or foreign body.
- Radiographs in clenched fist injury may reveal a fracture.

### DIFFERENTIAL DIAGNOSIS
- Paronychia should be differentiated from herpetic whitlow and felon.
- The differential for palmar space infection includes flexor tenosynovitis, cellulitis, and web space infection.

## TREATMENT

### PRE-HOSPITAL
Hand immobilization as appropriate

### ED TREATMENT/PROCEDURES
- Paronychia:
  – Early paronychia/simple cellulitis without purulence present may be managed with oral antibiotics and rest:
    ○ Cephalexin, dicloxacillin
    ○ Clindamycin or erythromycin if associated with nail biting or oral contact
  – Superficial infections are drained by inserting a No. 11 blade between nail and eponychium and lifting the eponychium from the nail.
  – If necessary, the lateral nail fold may be incised tangential to the curvature of the nail.
  – When pus is present under the adjacent nail, 1/4 of the nail should be removed.
  – When pus is present under the dorsal roof of the proximal nail, remove 1/3 of the proximal nail.
- Felon:
  – A lateral incision avoiding the neurovascular bundle is preferred.
  – More extensive felons are drained through a unilateral longitudinal incision that does not cross the distal interphalangeal (DIP) flexor crease.
  – Disruption of fibrous septa is no longer recommended:
    ○ Results in an unstable fingertip
    ○ Loculations may need to be broken up.
  – Give oral antibiotics to cover skin pathogens, place a drain, and recheck in 48 hr:
    ○ Cephalexin, dicloxacillin

- Herpetic whitlow:
  - Usually self-limited; do not incise and drain.
  - Oral acyclovir may be given to patients with systemic involvement.
- Flexor tenosynovitis, web space abscess, palmar space infection:
  - Elevation, IV antibiotics, and pain control:
    - Ampicillin/sulbactam, cefoxitin, ticarcillin/clavulanate
  - All of these infections require immediate consultation with a hand surgeon.
- Clenched fist injury:
  - Elevation, IV antibiotics, tetanus prophylaxis, and pain control in the ED:
    - Ampicillin/sulbactam, cefoxitin, ticarcillin/clavulanate
  - All bite wounds with evidence of infection or joint involvement require emergent consultation with a hand surgeon.
  - If there are no signs of infection and no joint penetration, patients may be considered for outpatient treatment with oral antibiotics after appropriate irrigation and wound care:
    - Ampicillin/clavulanate or penicillin V plus cephalexin or dicloxacillin
    - Do *not* primarily close lacerations associated with a human bite; delayed primary closure or healing by secondary intention is appropriate.

### MEDICATION

- Acyclovir: 400 mg PO t.i.d. for 10 days (peds: Not recommended for herpetic whitlow)
- Ampicillin/clavulanate: 875/125 mg PO b.i.d. (peds: 40 mg/kg/d PO div. q6h)
- Ampicillin/sulbactam: 1.5–3.0 g IV q6h (peds: Safety not established)
- Cefoxitin: 2 g IV q8h (peds: 80–160 mg/kg/day IV or IM div. q6h)
- Cephalexin: 500 g PO q.i.d. for 7 days (peds: 40 mg/kg/day PO div. q6h)

- Clindamycin: 300 mg PO q.i.d. for 7 days (peds: 20–40 mg/kg/day div. q6h PO IV or IM)
- Dicloxacillin: 500 mg PO q.i.d. for 7 days (peds: 12.5–50 mg/kg/day PO div. q6h)
- Erythromycin: 500 mg PO q.i.d. for 7 days (peds: 40 mg/kg/day div. q6h PO)
- Penicillin V: 250 mg PO q.i.d. (peds: 40 mg/kg/d PO div. q6h)
- Ticarcillin/clavulanate: 3.1 g IV q4–q6h (peds: Safety not established)

### First Line
Tailor to etiology

### Second Line
Tailor to etiology

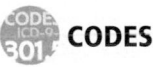

## FOLLOW-UP

### DISPOSITION

#### Admission Criteria
- Flexor tenosynovitis, web space abscess, palmar space infections:
  - All these infections require admission for IV antibiotics and drainage.
- Clenched fist injury with signs of infection:
  - Requires admission for surgical debridement and IV antimicrobials

#### Discharge Criteria
- Paronychia and felons:
  - Patients with uncomplicated paronychia or felon may be discharged from the ED with a recheck and drain removal in 48 hr.
- Herpetic whitlow:
  - Patients with herpetic whitlow may be discharged from the ED with appropriate follow-up.
- Clenched fist injury without infection:
  - May be discharged on oral antibiotics with follow-up in 24 hr

### Issues for Referral
Immediate consultation in emergency department is indicated

### FOLLOW-UP RECOMMENDATIONS
Usually arranged by admitting physician after operative therapy

## PEARLS AND PITFALLS

- Missed or delay in diagnosis
- Failure to obtain history of clenched fist injury
- Failure to consult surgeon promptly

## ADDITIONAL READING

- Antosia RE, Lyn E. The hand. In: Rosen P, et al., eds. *Emergency Medicine: Concepts and Clinical Practice*. 4th ed. St. Louis: Mosby, 1997;1998:625–668.
- Ong YS, Levin LS. Hand infections. *Plast Reconstr Surg*. 2009;124(4):225e–233e.
- Bach HG, Steffin B, Chhadia AM, et al. Community-associated methicillin-resistant Staphylococcus aureus hand infectieons in an urban setting. *J Hand Surg [Am]*. 2007;32(3):380–383.

### See Also (Topic, Algorithm, Electronic Media Element)
- Hand Infections http://emedicine.medscape.com/article/783011-overview

## CODES

### ICD0
- 681.02 Onychia and paronychia of finger
- 682.4 Cellulitis and abscess of hand, except fingers and thumb
- 686.9 Unspecified local infection of skin and subcutaneous tissue

H

# HAZMAT

*Moses S. Lee*

## 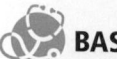 BASICS

### DESCRIPTION
- Hazmat refers to exposure to hazardous materials causing local or systemic toxicity.
- Pathophysiology:
  - Acids cause coagulation necrosis with eschar, usually limiting penetration to deeper tissue.
  - Alkalis cause liquefaction necrosis and soluble complexes that penetrate into deep tissues.
  - Damage also occurs through oxidation, protein denaturation, cellular dehydration, local ischemia, and by metabolic competition/inhibition.

### ETIOLOGY
- Hazardous materials are encountered in household, industry, agriculture, and transportation accidents and in criminal/terrorist activities.
- The toxicity of the materials relates to the particular substances and their effects.

## 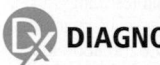 DIAGNOSIS

### SIGNS AND SYMPTOMS
- Skin:
  - Chemical burns; may appear deceptively mild at 1st
  - Visible liquid or powder on skin
  - Absorption through skin may cause systemic toxicity.
- Mucous membranes (eyes, nasopharynx; see "Corneal Burn"):
  - Ranges from subjective irritation to serious mucosal burns
  - Potential airway compromise
- Pulmonary:
  - Cough
  - Pleuritic chest pain
  - Bronchospasm
  - Dyspnea
  - Pulmonary edema (immediate or delayed)
- Systemic (after skin or pulmonary absorption):
  - Altered mental status
  - Seizures
  - Tachy/brady dysrhythmias
  - Hypotension/HTN
  - GI symptoms
  - Electrolyte disturbances
  - Carboxyhemoglobinemias and methemoglobinemias
  - Cyanide toxicity
  - Cholinergic syndrome (see "Chemical Weapons Poisoning, Nerve Agents")

### History
Elicit type, circumstances, and duration of exposure

### ESSENTIAL WORKUP
- Attempt to identify substance using prehospital providers, Material Safety Data Sheet, and Chemtrec (*Chemical Transportation Emergency Center*).
- Material Safety Data Sheet (MSDS):
  - Identifies chemicals
  - Differentiates vapor versus skin hazard
  - Determines need for decontamination
  - Limited treatment data
- Determine route and duration of exposure.
- Inhalation injury more likely in an enclosed space
- Determine toxicity using poison control; computerized databases, such as POISINDEX or TOXNET; or standard toxicology text.
- Observe as needed for systemic toxicity.

### DIAGNOSTIC TESTS & INTERPRETATION
#### Lab
- Depends on substance
- Electrolytes, BUN, creatinine, and glucose levels
- LFTs
- Calcium level
- Magnesium level
- Phosphorus level
- Arterial blood gases:
  - Metabolic acidosis
  - Carboxyhemoglobinemias and methemoglobinemias
  - Respiratory failure

#### Imaging
Chest radiograph for pulmonary edema

### DIFFERENTIAL DIAGNOSIS
- Skin:
  - Hypersensitivity reaction
  - Thermal burns
- Pulmonary:
  - Pneumonia
  - Pulmonary embolism
  - Anaphylaxis
- Systemic:
  - Status epilepticus
  - Overdose
  - Psychiatric illness
  - Myocardial infarction

## TREATMENT

### PRE-HOSPITAL
- Recognize a hazmat situation:
  - Accident at industrial/agricultural site
  - Accident involving transport of hazardous materials
  - Suspected terrorist mass casualty incident
  - Cholinergic syndrome
  - Irritant mucous membrane symptoms
  - Chemical burns
- Protect yourself:
  - Approach from upwind.
  - Do not enter scene until safety of material is determined.
  - Use level A protective gear if safety not established
  - Anyone able to walk and talk is minimally contaminated.
- Personal chemical protective equipment:
  - Level A: Positive-pressure self-contained breathing apparatus (SCBA), fully encapsulated chemical-resistant suit, double chemical-resistant gloves, chemical-resistant boots, and airtight seals between suit, gloves, boots
  - Level B: SCBA, nonencapsulated chemical suit, double gloves, boots
  - Level C: Air-purification device, suit, gloves, boots
  - Level D: Common work clothes
  - Identify substance:
    ○ Department of Transportation (DOT) placard, MSDS, shipping papers, hazard labels
    ○ If unsuccessful, call Chemical Transportation Emergency Center (Chemtrec: 1[800] 424-9300) to determine substance and toxicity.
    ○ Hazmat teams can do chemical testing.
- Determine toxicity and need for decontamination:
  - Poison control (1[800] 222-1222)
  - Chemtrec
- Decontaminate:
  - Hazmat team
- Treat:
  - Provide basic life support and advanced life support care as indicated.
  - Generally basic list support only in a "hot zone"
  - Irrigate skin and ocular burns immediately and continue until arrival at hospital.

## INITIAL STABILIZATION/THERAPY

- Protect ED personnel:
  - Secondary contamination can occur from dermal contact or through inhalation of volatile gases/particles.
- Keep patients outside in designated hot zones until decontaminated.
- When in doubt, decontaminate.
- Expect contaminated patients to arrive via emergency medical services or private vehicle.
- If treatment is required before/during decontamination:
  - Use minimum necessary staff in appropriate personal protection gear.
  - Focus on life- and limb-saving care only.
- Decontamination:
  - Security to enforce hot zone
  - Remove, label, and double-bag clothing (including contact lens).
  - Copious irrigation with soap and water for 10–15 min with special attention to obviously contaminated areas, wounds, and exposed eyes
  - Recapture water to prevent contamination of the sewer and downstream areas:
    - In an emergency or mass casualty situation, it is acceptable to let water drain into sewer.
  - Hydrotherapy:
    - Mainstay of therapy for chemical burns
    - Contraindicated only for elemental metals (sodium and potassium)
  - Allow patient to decontaminate himself or herself or use trained decontamination team.
  - Decontaminate children, dependent elderly, mentally/physically challenged and their appliances (eg, wheelchairs) with caregivers
  - Gloves, masks, goggles, and disposable gowns provide some protection
  - Remove/replace bandages, tourniquets, airway adjuncts, IV sets
  - Retriage after decontamination.

## ED TREATMENT/PROCEDURES

- Provide supportive care as needed.
- Determine if antidotal treatment would be effective and available.
- Hazmat incidents provoke extreme fear:
  - Expect casualties suffering from collective hysteria.
  - Knowledge of toxicologic profile can exclude contamination in these patients.
- ED staff may become symptomatic even if chemical concentrations in the air are below toxic levels and may need to be escorted to fresh air.

- Chemical burns:
  - Irrigation should be started as soon as possible and, if owing to a strong alkali, may need to be continued for hours.
  - Aggressive fluid resuscitation 2–4 mL/kg lactated Ringer solution per total burn surface area (TBSA) percent over 24 hr with 1/2 given over the 1st 8 hr
  - Pain control
- Pulmonary symptoms:
  - Bronchodilators, oxygen, intubation, and mechanical ventilation
- Selected special treatments:
  - Hydrofluoric acid burns:
    - Calcium gluconate via topical cutaneous gel, subcutaneous, or intra-arterial
    - For systemic toxicity: IV calcium gluconate and magnesium
  - Phenol burns:
    - Remove phenol from skin with polyethylene glycol 300 or 400 or with isopropyl alcohol.
  - Nitrates:
    - Ingested or extensive burns may cause methemoglobinemia.
    - Treat levels >30% with high-flow oxygen and IV methylene blue.
  - Elemental metals (sodium/potassium):
    - Water lavage is contraindicated and dangerous
    - Cover with oil until substance can be débrided from skin.
  - Cyanide toxicity:
    - Hydroxocobalamin administration
  - Organophosphates/carbamate insecticides (see: Chemical Weapons Poisoning)

## MEDICATION

- Albuterol: 2.5–5.0 mg nebulized
- Calcium gluconate: 10 mL of 10% solution
- Magnesium: 2 g IV over 20 min
- Methylene blue: 1–2 mg/kg slow IV (peds: *not* recommended for <6 yr old; >6 yr old: 1 mg/kg IV/IM over 5 min)
- Hydroxocobalamin: 5 mg IV over 5 min, repeat × 1

 **FOLLOW-UP**

### DISPOSITION

#### Admission Criteria

- Airway compromise, respiratory difficulty (hypoxia)
- Significant systemic symptoms
- Admit patients with chemical burns to burn center.

### Discharge Criteria

- Patients who are well after a period of observation and consultation with poison control
- Superficial chemical burns owing to a toxin without potential for systemic toxicity (weak acid/alkali)

## FOLLOW-UP RECOMMENDATIONS

Psychiatric or social work referral for victims of chemical terrorist attacks.

## PEARLS AND PITFALLS

- Decontaminate stable victims on site when possible.
- Protect medical providers (prehospital and ED) with appropriate personal protective equipment.
- Provide specific antidotes for exposures when indicated.
- Victims who can walk and talk are minimally contaminated.

## ADDITIONAL READING

- Clarke SFJ, Chilcott RP, Wilson JC, et al. Decontamination of multiple casualties who are chemically contaminated: A challenge for acute hospitals. *Prehosp Disast Med.* 2008;23(2): 175–181.
- Freyberg CW, Arquilla B, Fertel BS, et al. Disaster preparedness: Hospital decontamination and the pediatric patient—Guidelines for hospitals and emergency planners. *Prehosp Disast Med.* 2008;23(2):166–172.
- Goldfrank LR, Flomenbaum NE, Howland MA, et al. *Goldrank's Toxicologic Emergencies.* 8th ed. New York: McGraw-Hill; 2006;1764–1774.
- Hick JL, Penn P, Hanfling D, et al. Establishing and training health care facility decontamination teams. *Ann Emerg Med.* 2003;42:381–390.

### See Also (Topic, Algorithm, Electronic Media Element)

- Chemical Weapons Poisoning
- Cyanide Poisoning
- Radiation Injury

 **CODES**

### ICD9

989.9 Toxic effect of unspecified substance, chiefly nonmedicinal as to source

# HEAD TRAUMA, BLUNT

*Gary M. Vilke*

 **BASICS**

## DESCRIPTION

Blunt trauma to head resulting in a variety of injuries ranging from closed head injury to death

## ETIOLOGY

Blunt trauma to head may cause several types of closed head injuries:

- Concussion: Transient loss of consciousness or amnesia with normal head CT
- Subdural hematoma: Tearing of subdural bridging veins and bleeding into the subdural space
- Epidural hematoma: Dural arterial injury, especially the middle meningeal artery often associated with a skull fracture:
  - Classically, transient loss of consciousness followed by a lucid interval, then rapid demise
- Subarachnoid hemorrhage: Bleeding into the subarachnoid space following trauma
- Cerebral contusion: Focal injuries to the brain characterized as coup (beneath area of impact) or contrecoup (area remote from impact)
- Intracerebral hemorrhage: Mass intracranial lesion with bleeding into the brain parenchyma
- Diffuse axonal injury: Microscopic injuries scattered throughout the brain in a patient in deep coma

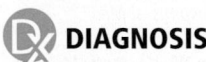 **DIAGNOSIS**

## SIGNS AND SYMPTOMS

- Evidence of trauma to head includes:
  - Scalp laceration, cephalohematoma, or ecchymosis
  - Raccoon eyes: Bilateral ecchymosis of orbits associated with basilar skull fractures
  - Battle sign: Ecchymosis behind the ear at mastoid process associated with basilar skull fracture
  - Hemotympanum
  - Cerebral spinal fluid rhinorrhea or otorrhea
- Evidence of increasing intracranial pressure includes:
  - Decreasing level of consciousness, falling score on Glasgow Coma Scale
  - Cushing response, bradycardia, HTN, and diminished respiratory rate
  - Dilated pupils associated with decorticate or decerebrate posturing

## History

- Mechanism
- Loss of consciousness (LOC) or amnesia for event
- Use of anticoagulants
- Headache, visual changes, or hearing loss
- Focal neurologic complaints
- Associated neck pain

## Physical Exam

- Evaluation of head for hematoma, Battle sign, Raccoon's eyes
- Complete neurologic examination
- Examination of neck/cervical spine

## ESSENTIAL WORKUP

- Imaging indicated for patients with any of the following:
  - LOC or amnesia of events
  - Progressive headache
  - Alcohol or drug intoxication
  - Unreliable history or dangerous mechanism
  - Posttraumatic seizure
  - Repeated vomiting
  - Signs of basilar skull fracture
  - Possible skull penetration or depressed skull fracture
  - Glasgow Coma Scale score <15
  - Focal neurologic findings
- Patients on coumarin or heparin or those with a history of bleeding dyscrasias must undergo imaging.
- Alcoholics have an increased risk for bleeding, low threshold for imaging

## Geriatric Considerations

- Older patients (>60–65 yr of age ) are at higher risk of intracranial hemorrhage
- Have a low threshold for obtaining CT scan

## DIAGNOSTIC TESTS & INTERPRETATION
### Lab

- Rapid check of blood glucose level
- CBC, platelet count, and coagulation parameters
- Type and cross-match for surgical candidates.
- Baseline electrolytes, BUN, and creatinine levels
- Blood alcohol level if indicated

## Imaging

- CT or MRI of head as indicated
- Cervical spine radiographs or helical CT when indicated

## Diagnostic Procedures/Surgery

Lumbar puncture if question of subarachnoid blood on head CT

## DIFFERENTIAL DIAGNOSIS

- Penetrating head trauma
- Any condition that alters mental status that may have produced a fall and caused external evidence of head trauma (eg, hypoglycemic episode, seizure)

 **TREATMENT**

## PRE-HOSPITAL

- Blunt head trauma patients with risk for intracranial lesion must go to a trauma center:
  - High-risk patients include those with depressed consciousness, focal neurologic signs, multiple trauma, or palpable depressed skull fractures.
- Moderate-risk patients should go to a hospital with availability of prompt neurosurgical consultation:
  - Moderate-risk patients include those with progressive headache, alcohol or drug intoxication, unreliable history, posttraumatic seizure, repeated vomiting, posttraumatic amnesia, signs of basilar skull fracture.
- Protect and manage the airway, including intubation:
  - Routine hyperventilation without signs of cerebral herniation should be avoided.
- If evidence of cerebral herniation (see "Signs and Symptoms") or progressive neurologic deterioration in a normotensive patient, initiate measures to decrease intracranial pressure:
  - Mild hyperventilation to keep ETCO$_2$ about 30–35 mm Hg:
    - 20 breaths per minute in adults
    - 25 breaths per minute in children
    - 30 breaths per minute in infants <1 yr
  - Elevating head of bed 20–30 degrees
- Cervical spine precautions must be maintained in all patients.
- Cautions:
  - Avoid hypotension (systolic BP <90 mm Hg); use IV crystalloid solutions to maintain BP.
  - Avoid hypoxia (oxygen saturation <90%); administer 100% oxygen.
  - Check blood glucose level.

## INITIAL STABILIZATION/THERAPY
Management of ABCs:

- Control airway as needed:
  - Rapid sequence intubation if Glasgow Coma Scale score <8, unable to protect airway, or evidence of hypoxia
  - Normalize Pco$_2$, avoid hyperventilation and hypoventilation.
- Treatment with etomidate or fentanyl as induction agent, succinylcholine (pretreat with minidose paralytic), rocuronium, or vecuronium; morphine for ongoing sedation
- Caution with fentanyl in hemodynamically labile patients
- IV catheter placement with crystalloid solution as needed to avoid hypotension (keep systolic BP >90 mm Hg)
- Cervical spine precautions

## ED TREATMENT/PROCEDURES

- Early neurosurgical consultation
- If patient has evidence of cerebral herniation (see "Signs and Symptoms"), initiate measures to decrease intracranial pressure:
  - *Mild* hyperventilation: 20 breaths per min in adults, 25 breaths per MIN in children, and 30 breaths per min in infants <1 YR to keep ETCO$_2$ about 30–35.
  - Elevate head of bed 20–30 degrees
  - Mannitol boluses IV: Do not administer mannitol unless systolic BP >100 mm Hg and patient is adequately fluid-resuscitated
- Phenytoin to prevent *early* posttraumatic seizures
- Reverse hypocoagulable states
- The use of glucocorticoids is *not* recommended to lower intracranial pressure in head trauma patients.
- Barbiturates are *not* recommended in the initial ED treatment of head-injured patients.
- If definitive neurosurgical care is not immediately available, a single burr hole may preserve life until neurosurgical intervention can be obtained:
  - Perform only in comatose patients with decerebrate or decorticate posturing on the side of a known mass lesion who have not responded to hyperventilation and mannitol.
- Transfuse as needed to keep hematocrit >30%.
- Avoid hypothermia, which will increase risks of coagulopathy during surgery.
- Maintain NPO status.
- Surgery:
  - Surgical procedure based on findings of CT scan and neurosurgical consultation

## MEDICATION

For RSI intubation, increased ICP, seizures, and pain control

### First Line

- Etomidate: 0.2–0.3 mg/kg IV
- Fentanyl: 3–5 bcg/kg IV if systolic BP >100 mm Hg
- Mannitol: 0.25–1 g/kg IV bolus
- Morphine sulfate: 2–20 mg IV (peds: 0.1 mg/kg IV up to adult doses)
- Phenytoin: 15–20 mg/kg IV up to 1,000 mg
- Rocuronium: 0.6 mg/kg IV
- Succinylcholine: 1–2 mg/kg IV
- Vecuronium bromide: 0.1 mg/kg IV; minidose pretreatment: 0.01 mg/kg IV

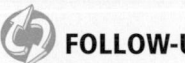 FOLLOW-UP

### DISPOSITION

#### Admission Criteria

- Patients with mass lesion associated with head trauma must be admitted to the ICU or undergo surgery.
- Patients with subarachnoid hemorrhage and diffuse axonal injury should be initially admitted to the ICU.
- Patients with ongoing symptoms including repetitive questioning, anterograde amnesia, or disorientation should be admitted to a monitored unit for neurologic evaluation.

#### Discharge Criteria

- Patients with resolved symptoms, negative findings on head CT, and no other comorbid factors (eg, intoxication, additional trauma needing treatment) may be discharged.
- Patients with minor head trauma, no loss of consciousness or amnesia, and normal neurologic exam findings may be discharged home with a friend or family member and head injury instructions.

#### Pediatric Considerations

Cases of suspected nonaccidental trauma must be reported to the appropriate legal agency.

#### Issues for Referral

If there are symptoms of concussion, patient will need follow-up with PMD, sports medicine physician, or neurologist to determine return to sports will be safe.

### FOLLOW-UP RECOMMENDATIONS

Return if worsening headache, visual changes, confusion, focal neurological changes, or other changes in clinical status.

## PEARLS AND PITFALLS

- Failure to query about anticoagulant use and image appropriately
- Failure to aggressively reverse hypocoagulable states
- Failure to counsel patient with a concussion for no contact sports until cleared by PMD, sports medicine physician, or neurologist.

## ADDITIONAL READING

- Badjatia N, Carney N, Crocco TJ, et al. Brain Trauma Foundation. *Guidelines for Prehospital Management of Traumatic Brain Injury*, 2nd ed. *Prehosp Emerg Care*. 2008;12(Suppl 1):S1–S52.
- Bernhardt DT. Concussion: emedicine: http://emedicine.medscape.com/article/92095-overview
- Bratton SL, Chestnut RM, Ghajar J. Guidelines for the management of severe traumatic brain injury. Brain Trauma Foundation; American Association of Neurological Surgeons, Congress of Neurological Surgeons; Joint Section on Neurotrauma and Critical Care, AANS/CNS. *J Neurotrauma*. 2007;24 (Suppl 1):S1–S95.
- Committee on Trauma. *Head trauma: Advanced Trauma Life Support*. 8th ed. Chicago: American College of Surgeons, 2008.
- Espinosa-Aguilar A, Reyes-Morales H, Huerta-Posada CE, et al. Design and validation of a critical pathway for hospital management of patients with severe traumatic brain injury. *J Trauma*. 2008;64(5):1327–1341.
- Warner KJ, Cuschieri J, Copass MK, et al. The impact of prehospital ventilation on outcome after severe traumatic brain injury. *J Trauma*. 2007;62(6): 1330–1336.

### See Also (Topic, Algorithm, Electronic Media Element)

- Head Trauma, Penetrating
- Spine Injury: Cervical, Adult

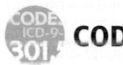 CODES

### ICD9

- 850.5 Concussion with loss of consciousness of unspecified duration
- 854.00 Intracranial injury of other and unspecified nature, without mention of open intracranial wound, with state of consciousness unspecified
- 959.01 Other and unspecified injury to head

H

# HEAD TRAUMA, PENETRATING

*Gary M. Vilke*

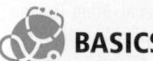 **BASICS**

## DESCRIPTION
Penetrating injury to intracranial contents:
- High-velocity penetration: Usually bullets, which cause trauma directly to brain tissue but also have a "shock wave" injury to local surrounding brain
- Low-velocity penetration: Usually knives, picks, or other sharp objects, with direct local trauma to brain tissue

## ETIOLOGY
- Direct penetration of the skull into the intracranial cavity by foreign object:
  - Direct or local damage to brain tissue
  - Intracranial hemorrhage, including subdural, epidural, and intraparenchymal bleeds
- A bullet that hits the skull, ricochets off, and does not fracture the skull can still cause significant trauma to the underlying brain tissue.

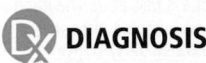 **DIAGNOSIS**

## SIGNS AND SYMPTOMS
- Alteration in level of consciousness and neurologic exam varies based on object and location.
- Evidence of increasing intracranial pressure:
  - Decreasing level of consciousness
  - Falling Glasgow Coma Scale score
  - Cushing response: Bradycardia, hypertension, and diminished respiratory rate
  - Blown pupil associated with decorticate or decerebrate posturing
- Evidence of penetrating injury to head or basilar skull fracture, or object still remaining in head:
  - Raccoon eyes: Bilateral ecchymosis of orbits associated with basilar skull fractures
  - Battle sign: Ecchymosis behind the ear at mastoid process associated with basilar skull fracture
  - Hemotympanum
  - CSF rhinorrhea or otorrhea

## History
- Determine the weapon type or caliber of weapon at scene.
- Loss of consciousness (LOC) or amnesia for event
- Use of anticoagulants
- Headache, visual changes, or hearing loss
- Focal neurologic complaints

## Physical Exam
- Evaluation of head evidence of penetrating injury and if a projectile, for multiple sites
- Complete neurologic examination
- Alteration in level of consciousness and neurologic exam varies based on object and location.
- Evidence of penetrating injury to head

## ESSENTIAL WORKUP
- Thorough history and exam to assess extent of injuries
- Imaging study

## DIAGNOSTIC TESTS & INTERPRETATION
### Lab
- CBC
- Platelet count
- Coagulation perimeters
- Type and cross-match
- Electrolytes, BUN, and creatinine baseline levels

### Imaging
- CT of head depicts location of lesion and extent of damage.
- Skull radiographs may reveal depth of impalement, location of bone fragments, and presence of fragments within the cranium.
- Cervical spine evaluation (when indicated):
  - Helical CT scanning or anteroposterior, lateral, and odontoid views plain radiographs

## DIFFERENTIAL DIAGNOSIS
- Blunt head trauma
- Basilar skull fracture
- Any condition that alters mental status that may have induced a fall and caused secondary penetrating trauma

 **TREATMENT**

## PRE-HOSPITAL
- Stabilize but do not remove foreign object (eg, knife).
- Determine the weapon type or caliber of weapon at scene.
- Protect and manage the airway to avoid hypoxemia.
- Avoid hyperventilation.
- Maintain cervical spine precautions.
- Transport to trauma center.
- Avoid hypoxia (oxygen saturation <90%):
  - 100% oxygen
- Avoid hypotension (systolic BP <90 mm Hg):
  - Administer IV crystalloid solutions

## INITIAL STABILIZATION/THERAPY
- Management of ABCs
- Rapid sequence intubation:
  - For Glasgow Coma Scale score <8, inability to protect airway, hypoxia, or cerebral herniation
  - Medications include etomidate or fentanyl as induction agent, succinylcholine (pretreat with minidose paralytic), rocuronium, or vecuronium; and morphine sulfate for ongoing sedation
  - Caution with fentanyl in the hemodynamically labile patient
  - Normalize $Pco_2$. Avoid hyperventilation or hypoventilation.
- IV catheter placement
- Crystalloid solution to maintain systolic BP >90 mm Hg
- Address other sources of associated trauma.
- Cervical spine precautions should be maintained.

### ED TREATMENT/PROCEDURES

- Early neurosurgical consultation
- If patient has evidence of cerebral herniation (see "Signs and Symptoms"), initiate measures to decrease intracranial pressure:
  - *Mild* hyperventilation: 20 breaths per minute in adults, 25 breaths per minute in children, and 30 breaths per minute in infants <1 yr to keep $ETCO_2$ about 30–35 mm Hg.
  - Elevate head of bed 20–30 degrees.
  - Mannitol boluses IV: Do not administer mannitol unless systolic BP >100 mm Hg and patient is adequately fluid-resuscitated.
- Phenytoin intravenously to prevent *early* posttraumatic seizures
- Reverse hypocoagulable states
- Glucocorticoids are *not* recommended to lower intracranial pressure in head trauma patients.
- Barbiturates are *not* recommended in the initial ED treatment.
- Transfuse as needed to keep hematocrit >30%.
- If definitive neurosurgical care is not immediately available, a single burr hole may preserve life until neurosurgical intervention can be attained:
  - Perform only in comatose patients with decerebrate or decorticate posturing who have not responded to initial treatment on the side of a known mass lesion/hematoma.
- Avoid hypothermia, which will increase risks of coagulopathy during surgery.
- Maintain NPO status.
- Surgery:
  - Based on clinical and radiologic findings and neurosurgical consultation

### MEDICATION

For RSI intubation, increased ICP, seizures, and pain control

#### First Line

- Etomidate: 0.2–0.3 mg/kg IV
- Fentanyl: 3–5 µg/kg IV.
  - If systolic BP >100 mm Hg
- Mannitol: 0.25–1 g/kg IV bolus
- Morphine sulfate: 2–20 mg IV (peds: 0.1 mg/kg up to adult doses)
- Phenytoin: 15–20 mg/kg IV up to 1,000 mg
- Rocuronium: 0.6 mg/kg IV
- Succinylcholine: 1–2 mg/kg IV
- Vecuronium bromide: 0.1 mg/kg IV:
  - Pretreatment minidose: 0.01 mg/kg IV

## FOLLOW-UP

### DISPOSITION

#### Admission Criteria

Admit all patients to ICU or transport directly to surgery.

#### Discharge Criteria

Do not discharge.

### FOLLOW-UP RECOMMENDATIONS

All patients with penetrating skull injuries should have been admitted.

## PEARLS AND PITFALLS

- Failure to query about anticoagulant use and image appropriately
- Failure to aggressively reverse hypocoagulable states

### ADDITIONAL READING

- Badjatia N, Carney N, Crocco TJ, et al. Brain Trauma Foundation. *Guidelines for Prehospital Management of Traumatic Brain Injury,* 2nd ed. *Prehosp Emerg Care.* 2008;12(Suppl 1):S1–S52.
- Bratton SL, Chestnut RM, Ghajar J. Guidelines for the management of severe traumatic brain injury. Brain Trauma Foundation; American Association of Neurological Surgeons; Congress of Neurological Surgeons; Joint Section on Neurotrauma and Critical Care, AANS/CNS. *J Neurotrauma.* 2007;24 (Suppl 1):S1–S95.
- Committee on Trauma. *Head Trauma: Advanced Trauma Life Support.* 8th ed. Chicago: American College of Surgeons, 2008.
- Espinosa-Aguilar A, Reyes-Morales H, Huerta-Posada CE, et al. Design and validation of a critical pathway for hospital management of patients with severe traumatic brain injury. *J Trauma.* 2008;64(5):1327–1341.
- Warner KJ, Cuschieri J, Copass MK, et al. The impact of prehospital ventilation on outcome after severe traumatic brain injury. *J Trauma.* 2007;62(6): 1330–1336.

### See Also (Topic, Algorithm, Electronic Media Element)

- Head Trauma, Blunt
- Spine Injury: Cervical, Adult

## CODES

### ICD9

- 801.50 Open fracture of base of skull without mention of intracranial injury, with state of consciousness unspecified
- 853.10 Other and unspecified intracranial hemorrhage following injury, with open intracranial wound, with state of consciousness unspecified
- 873.8 Other and unspecified open wound of head without mention of complication

H

# HEADACHE

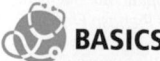

*Richard E. Wolfe*
*Jonathan A. Edlow*

 **BASICS**

## DESCRIPTION
- Prolonged pain in the cranial vault, orbits, or nape of the neck
- Intracranial and extracranial pain-sensitive structures project pain to the cranial surface:
  - Intracranial:
    ○ Arteries, veins, dura, meninges
  - Extracranial:
    ○ Skin, scalp, fascia, muscles
    ○ Mucosal linings of the sinuses
    ○ Arteries
    ○ Temporomandibular joints, teeth
- Pain is transmitted via the 5th cranial nerve.
- Pain may be caused by a number of mechanisms:
  - Nerve irritation
  - Traction on pain-sensitive vessels
  - Vasodilatation of pain-sensitive vessels
    ○ Hypoxia, hypercapnia, fever, histamine injection, nitroglycerin ingestion
- 2–4% of all ED visits have a chief complaint of headache:
  - 95% have a benign etiology (this number is somewhat lower in patients >50)
  - Life-threatening etiologies are rare but are sometimes difficult to diagnose and can be missed.

## ETIOLOGY
- Vascular:
  - Intra/extracranial vasodilatation and constriction of pain-sensitive blood vessels
  - Throbbing headache
- Tension:
  - Requires ≥10 attacks of a specific nature
  - Unknown etiology (possibly serotonin imbalance, decreased endorphins)
  - Most common type of recurring headache
  - Secondary to sustained contraction of head and neck muscles
  - Triggered by poor posture, stress, anxiety, depression, cervical osteoarthritis
  - Bilateral, nonpulsatile, band-like
  - Mild to moderate intensity
  - 4–13-hr duration
- Cluster headaches:
  - Triggered by alcohol, certain foods, altered sleep habits, strong emotions
- Intracranial (traction):
  - Mass lesions
- Extracranial:
  - Pathology causing pain in a peripheral nerve of the head and neck
- Unassociated with a structural lesion:
  - Idiopathic stabbing headache
  - Cold stimulus headache
  - Benign cough headache
  - Benign exertional headache

### Pediatric Considerations
Serious causes of headache in children are unusual but those who come to the ED for this complaint should all have follow-up with a pediatrician.

### Geriatric Considerations
Older patients with new-onset of headache have a higher likelihood of having a serious cause for their headache and, in general, should undergo a more thorough evaluation.

### Pregnancy Considerations
In addition to all other usual causes of headache, pregnant women (and those in the early postpartum period) are at increased risk for cerebral venous sinus thrombosis, eclampsia, and a related problem called PRES (posterior reversible leukoencephalopathy syndrome).

## DIAGNOSIS

### SIGNS AND SYMPTOMS
*History*
- Attributes of the pain—PQRST:
  - Provocative and palliative features:
    ○ Position of the head, effect of coughing, straining (increase suggests elevated ICP), and movement
  - Quality:
    ○ Throbbing or continuous
    ○ Deep or superficial
    ○ Change compared with any prior headaches
  - Region
  - Severity
  - Is this the worst headache of life?
  - Timing
  - Is the onset sudden or gradual?
- Associated findings:
  - Visual symptoms, dizziness, nausea, vomiting
- Historical factors indicating testing beyond the history and physical exam:
  - New onset:
    ○ >50
    ○ HIV or cancer patient?
  - Severe headache or "worst headache of my life"
  - Persistent vomiting
  - Any new focal neurological or visual symptoms
- Risk factors for cerebral sinus thrombosis:
  - Malignancy
  - Pregnancy (or postpartum)
  - Protein S or protein C deficiency
  - Oral contraceptive
  - Ulcerative colitis
  - Behçet's syndrome

*Physical Exam*
- Complete neuro exam including cranial nerves, motor, sensation, deep tendon reflexes, gait
- Examine for papilledema.
- Evaluate skin for rashes:
  - Zoster
  - Purpura
- Palpate temporal arteries

## ESSENTIAL WORKUP
- Detailed history and CNS, HEENT, and neck exam
- Depends on the clinical differential diagnosis
- Factors indicating testing beyond the history and physical exam:
  - Abnormal vital signs:
    ○ Severely elevated diastolic BP
    ○ Fever
  - Altered level of consciousness
  - Papilledema
  - Abnormal neurologic findings or meningismus

## DIAGNOSTIC TESTS & INTERPRETATION
*Lab*
- Lab tests are only useful in selected cases when the history or physical exam suggests etiologies placing the patient at risk of death or functional impairment.
- ESR:
  - If temporal arteritis or other inflammatory disorders suspected:
    ○ See Giant Cell Arteritis

*Imaging*
- Head CT scan:
  - Indications:
    ○ Unclear diagnosis based on history and physical exam (leaving open the possibility of serious causes)
    ○ Signs of increased ICP
    ○ "First or worst" headache
    ○ Abrupt onset
    ○ New focal neurologic abnormalities
    ○ Papilledema
    ○ Recurrent morning headache
    ○ Persistent vomiting
    ○ Headache associated with fever, rash, and nausea without systemic illness
    ○ Head trauma with loss of consciousness (LOC), focal neurologic findings, or lethargy
    ○ Altered mental status, meningismus
  - >95% sensitive for subarachnoid hemorrhage (SAH) <24 hr (but sensitivity falls rapidly with time and is 50% at 7 days out)
  - Must do lumbar puncture (LP) if SAH suspected and CT is negative.
- Sinus imaging is occasionally helpful for acute bacterial sinusitis; chronic mucosal thickening rarely is the cause of an acute headache.
- Vascular assessment with angiogram or MR angiography:
  - May be indicated if nonmigrainous vascular cause suspected
- MRI:
  - Indicated to assess for etiologies that are missed by CT scan and LP:
    ○ Posterior fossa lesion (not imaged well on CT)
    ○ Pituitary apoplexy (this may be visualized with newer-generation CT scanners)
    ○ Cerebral sinus thrombosis
- MRA:
  - Indicated if subarachnoid hemorrhage suspected, CT is negative, and unable to perform lumbar puncture
  - Also for suspicion of carotid or vertebral dissection

## *Diagnostic Procedures/Surgery*

Lumbar puncture:

- Perform CT 1st if:
  - New focal neurological finding
  - Papilledema
  - Abnormal mental status
  - HIV positive
- Detect intracranial and meningeal infections
- Detect blood not evident on CT scan:
  - Note that there is no specific threshold number of red cells below which SAH is excluded and that the RBC count is a function of time from onset of headache.
- Measure opening pressure to help diagnose pseudotumor cerebri and cerebral venous thrombosis and to help distinguish traumatic tap vs. true hemorrhage.
- Xanthochromia:
  - Should be visible by spectrometry 12 hr after onset of a subarachnoid hemorrhage
  - Spectrophotometry (although more sensitive) has a high false-positive rate.
  - Visual inspection is the most commonly used method in North America.

## DIFFERENTIAL DIAGNOSIS

- Note: There can be significant overlap in these temporal groupings.
- Acute single headache:
  - Single episode presenting within hours of onset
  - SAH
  - Meningitis
  - Vascular:
    - Acute intracerebral hemorrhage
    - Hypertensive encephalopathy
    - Cranial artery dissection
    - Cerebral venous sinus thrombosis
  - Ocular:
    - Acute narrow-angle glaucoma
    - Pituitary apoplexy
    - Temporal neuritis
  - Traumatic
  - Acute sinusitis
  - Toxic/Metabolic:
    - Fever
    - Hypoglycemia
    - High-altitude disease
    - Carbon monoxide poisoning
  - Narcotic, alcohol, or benzodiazepine withdrawal
- Acute recurrent headache:
  - Presenting within days to weeks of onset
  - Cerebral sinus thrombosis
  - Pseudotumor cerebri
  - Temporal arteritis
  - SAH (rebleed)
  - Migraine, cluster, tension
  - Hypoxic
  - Trigeminal neuralgia
  - Postherpetic neuralgia
  - Coital and exertional headache
- Subacute headache:
  - Presenting within weeks to months of onset
  - Chronic subdural hematoma
  - Brain tumor
  - Brain abscess
  - Chronic sinusitis
  - Temporomandibular joint syndrome
  - Chronic posttraumatic headache
  - Pseudotumor cerebri (Idiopathic intracranial HTN)
  - Temporal arteritis
  - HIV

- Chronic headache:
  - Presenting within months to years of onset
  - Chronic tension headache
  - Transformational migraine
  - Analgesic abuse/rebound
  - Depression
  - Extracranial:
    - Trigeminal neuralgia: Transient, shock like facial pain
    - Temporal arteritis: Elderly, severe, scalp artery tenderness/swelling
    - Metabolic: Severe anemia
    - Acute glaucoma: Nausea/vomiting, eye pain, conjunctival injection, increased IOP
    - Cervical: Spondylosis, trauma, arthritis
    - Temporomandibular joint syndrome

 **TREATMENT**

 **FOLLOW-UP**

## DISPOSITION

### *Initial Stabilization*

- ABCs if altered mental status
- Empiric antibiotics if bacterial meningitis is suspected

### *Admission Criteria*

- Headache secondary to suspected organic disease
- Pain refractory to outpatient management
- Intractable vomiting and dehydration
- Intracranial infection
- Intracranial hemorrhage
- Consider ICU admission:
  - Suspected symptomatic aneurysm
  - Acute subdural hematoma
  - SAH
  - Stroke
  - Increased ICP
  - Intracranial infection

### *Discharge Criteria*

- Most migraine, cluster, and tension headaches after pain relief
- Local or minor systemic infections

### *Issues for Referral*

Patients with recurrent headaches should have follow-up with a neurologist or PCP.

## ED TREATMENT/PROCEDURES

- Migraine (See Headache, Migraine)
- Tension:
  - Aspirin
  - Acetaminophen
  - NSAID
  - Nonpharmacologic (meditation, massage, biofeedback)
- Cluster (See Headache, Cluster)
- Temporal arteritis (See Giant Cell Arteritis)
- Intracranial infection (See Meningitis)
- Intracranial hemorrhage (See Subarachnoid Hemorrhage)

## MEDICATION

- Chlorpromazine: 25–50 mg IM/IV (peds: 0.5–1 mg/kg/dose IM/IV/PO) q4–6h
- Dihydroergotamine: 1 mg IM/IV, repeat q1h; max dose 3 mg
- Ergotamine: 2 mg PO/SL at onset, then 1 mg PO q 30 min; max dose 10 mg/wk
- Ketorolac: 30–60 mg IM; 15–30 mg IV once, then 15–30 mg q6h (peds 1 mg/kg IV q6h)
- Lidocaine 4%: 1 mL intranasal on same side as symptoms
- Metoclopramide: 5–10 mg IM/IV/PO q6–8h
- Morphine: 2.5–20 mg (peds: 0.1–0.2 mg/kg/dose) IM/IV/SQ q2–6h
- Prochlorperazine: 5–10 mg IM/IM/PO t.i.d.–q.i.d.; max 40 mg/day
- Sumatriptan: 6 mg SQ, repeat in 1 hr, up to 12 mg/24 hr

### ALERT

DO NOT use the response of any medication to indicate a benign cause of a headache; any of the above medications can relieve the pain from serious, life-threatening causes.

## PEARLS AND PITFALLS

- Consider cerebral venous thrombosis in those with risk factors.
- The sensitivity for detecting SAH on CT scan falls rapidly after 24 hr.

## ADDITIONAL READING

- Edlow JA, Panagos PD, Godwin SA, et al. Clinical policy: Critical issues in the evaluation and management of adult patients presenting to the Emergency Department with acute headache. *Ann Emerg Med*. 2008;52:407–436.
- Edlow JA, Malek A, Ogilvy CS. Aneurysmal subarachnoid hemorrhage: Update for emergency physicians. *J Emerg Med*. 2008;34: 237–251.
- Pope JV, Edlow JA. Favorable response to analgesics does not predict a benign etiology of headache. *Headache*. 2008;48:944–950.
- Savitz SI, Levitan S, Wears, et al. Pooled analysis of patients with thunderclap headache evaluated by CT and LP: Is angiography necessary in patients with negative evaluations? *J Neurol Sci*. 2009;276: 123–125.
- Wolfson AB, Hendey GW, Ling LJ, et al., eds. *Harwood Nuss' Clinical Practice of Emergency Medicine*, 5th ed. Philadelphia: Lippincott Williams & Wilkins; 2010.

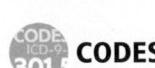 **CODES**

### ICD9

- 307.81 Tension headache
- 339.00 Cluster headache syndrome, unspecified
- 784.0 Headache

# HEADACHE, CLUSTER

*Gary A. Johnson*

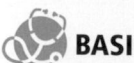 **BASICS**

## DESCRIPTION

- Rare headache and infrequent cause of ED visit
- Often has abated by time of presentation
  - 75% last <60 min
  - Rarely last >3 hr
- More common in men
- Onset usually between 20 and 40 yr of age
- Headaches occur in clusters lasting weeks to months followed by remission >1 mo
- Commonly occur 1–3 times per day during cluster period that lasts 2–3 mo
- Often occur during the same time of day and year
- Highest incidence in spring and fall
- Chronic cluster headache:
  - Remission <1 mo
  - Do not experience remission
  - 10% of patients
- Not clearly understood, but may be result of vasoactive substances released from mast cells
- May have many clinical and pathophysiologic similarities with migraine and variants
- Often follows a trigeminal nerve dermatome
- Pain is so severe it may lead to suicide

## ETIOLOGY

- Cause is unclear at present.
- Affects 0.1% of the population

 **DIAGNOSIS**

## SIGNS AND SYMPTOMS

### History

- Headache:
- Unliateral (usually does not change sides between headaches)
- Sharp, stabbing, boring
- Acute onset and builds in intensity quickly with climax at 5–15 min
- Pain stops abruptly
- Often exhausted after episode
  - Location:
    - Eye
    - Temple
  - Radiation to:
    - Ear
    - Cheek
    - Jaw
    - Teeth (often have had extensive dental workup for pain in the past
    - Nose
    - Ipsilateral neck
- Episodes are often nocturnal
- Attacks are more likely after ingestion of alcohol, nitroglycerine, or histamine-containing compounds.
- More likely in times of stress, prolonged strain, overwork, and upsetting emotional experiences
- No prodrome or aura

### Physical Exam

- Agitated, restless
- Prefer to stand and move around
  - Versus patients with migraines who prefer to lie quietly in a dark room
- Complete neurologic exam
- Accompanying autonomic symptoms:
  - Criteria for diagnosis
  - Ipsilateral to headache
    - Nasal congestion
    - Lacrimation
    - Rhinorrhea
    - Conjunctival injection
    - Facial flushing
    - Eyelid edema
    - Ptosis
    - Miosis
    - Sweating of face/forehead
- Horner syndrome may be seen.

## ESSENTIAL WORKUP

- An accurate history and physical examination should confirm the diagnosis.
- Life-threatening alternatives need to be ruled out.
- Relieve the acute attack and cluster

## DIAGNOSTIC TESTS & INTERPRETATION

### Lab

- Lumbar puncture (if meningitis or subarachnoid hemorrhage is suspected)
- Erythrocyte sedimentation rate (ESR; if temporal arteritis is suspected)

### Imaging

CT scan/MRI (to rule out hemorrhage, tumor)

## DIFFERENTIAL DIAGNOSIS

- Migraine headache
- Trigeminal neuralgia
- Meningitis
- Temporal arteritis
- Intracerebral mass lesion
- Herpes zoster
- Intracerebral bleed
- Dental causes
- Orbital/ocular disease (acute glaucoma)
- Temporal mandibular joint syndrome

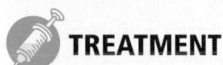 **TREATMENT**

### PRE-HOSPITAL
- Recognize more severe life-threatening causes of headache.
- Administration of oxygen by face mask may alleviate symptoms.

### INITIAL STABILIZATION/THERAPY
- Rule out life-threatening causes of headache.
- Administration of supplemental oxygen.

### MEDICATION
- Ergots: DHE 0.5–1 mg IV; repeat in 1 hr if necessary
- Fentanyl: 2–3 $\mu$g/kg IV
- Morphine: 2–4 mg IV or IM, may repeat q10min
- NSAIDs; Ketorolac 15–30 mg IM or IV
- Oxygen: 100% via face mask
- Prochlorperazine: 10 mg IM or IV
- Somatostatin: 100 $\mu$g SQ
- Sumatriptan: 6 mg SC, may repeat in 1 hr (max. of 2 doses in 24 hr)

### First Line
- Oxygen: 7–10 L/min via nonrebreather mask for 15 min:
  – May increase to 15 L/min if refractory headache
- Sumatriptan
- DHE

### Second Line
- Narcotics
- Corticosteroids
- Verapamil (prophylaxis)

 **FOLLOW-UP**

### DISPOSITION
#### Admission Criteria
- Persistent headache unresponsive to usual measures.
- Unclear headache diagnosis.

#### Discharge Criteria
- Patients with moderate to complete pain relief, a normal neurologic exam, and with a confident diagnosis of cluster headache.
- Consider prescribing oxygen and or subcutaneous sumatriptan for management at home

#### Issues for Referral
Follow-up with a neurologist should be arranged

## PEARLS AND PITFALLS

- History is essential to diagnose cluster headache as pain may be improved upon presentation
- 100% oxygen should be the first treatment initiated
- Cluster headaches may be so severe that they lead to suicide
  – Follow-up is essential to manage clusters which may last months

## ADDITIONAL READING

- Adams SM, Standridge JB. Practical strategy for detecting and relieving cluster headaches. *J Fam Pract*. 2005;54:1035–1040.
- Friedman BW, Grosberg BM. Diagnosis and management of the primary headache disorders in the emergency department setting. *Emerg Med Clin N Am*. 2009;27:71–87.
- McGeeney BE. Cluster Headache Pharmacotherapy. *Am J Ther*. 2005;12:351–358.

### See Also (Topic, Algorithm, Electronic Media Element)
- Headache
- Headache, migraine

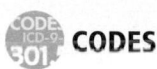 **CODES**

### ICD9
- 339.00 Cluster headache syndrome, unspecified
- 339.01 Episodic cluster headache
- 339.02 Chronic cluster headache

H

# HEADACHE, MIGRAINE

*Gary A. Johnson*

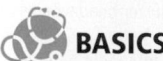

## BASICS

### DESCRIPTION
- Chronic and recurrent
- Often unilateral, throbbing, pulsating
- Often exacerbated by physical activity
- Bilateral in 40%
- Side of headache may vary
- Poorly understood:
  - May involve vasoconstriction, cortical excitation, or both
  - May originate in brainstem
  - Trigeminal nerve activation may account for some headaches.
- 1 million ED visits per year
- Usually begin in 2nd decade of life
- Common migraine:
  - 80% of migraines
  - Do not occur with aura
- Criteria for common migraine:
  - A. 5 attacks fulfilling criteria B, C, D, E
  - B. Attack lasts 4–72 hr
  - C. Headache has 2 of the following:
    - 1. Unilateral location
    - 2. Pulsating
    - 3. Moderate to severe pain
    - 4. Aggravation by or avoidance of physical activity
  - D. During headache, nausea/vomiting and/or photophobia/phonophobia
  - E. Not attributable to other cause
- Classic migraine:
  - Less common
  - Reversible neurologic symptoms that preceded headache (aura or prodrome)
- Criteria for classic migraines:
  - A. 2 attacks that fulfill B
  - B. At least 3 out of 4 of the following:
    - 1. 1 or more fully reversible aura symptoms
    - 2. At least 1 aura developing gradually over >4 min or 2 or more symptoms occurring in succession
    - 3. No single aura lasting >60 min
    - 4. Headache begins during or after aura with symptom free interval <60 min (may begin before aura)
  - C. Not attributable to other cause

### *Pediatric Considerations*
Migraines do present in the pediatric age group, but are less common.

### ETIOLOGY
- May be precipitated by chocolate, cheese, nuts, alcohol, sulfites, monosodium glutamate (MSG), stress, or puberty.
- Family history of migraines in 60% of cases
- Affects 5–15% of the population:
  - Women 3 times more than men
  - 15% of women have correlation with menses

## DIAGNOSIS

### SIGNS AND SYMPTOMS
#### History
- Worst headache of life
- Neurologic symptoms
- Usually gradual onset
- Usually lasts 4–72 hr
- Some patients have depression, memory problems, mania, anger
- Common migraine:
  - Headache is recurrent, throbbing, and frequently unilateral.
  - Usually associated with photophobia, phonophobia, nausea, and vomiting
- Classic migraine:
  - Similar to common migraine except it is preceded by a prodrome; often visual symptoms such as bright lights, selective field defects, or jagged lines
- Complex migraine:
  - Migraine headache with associated focal neurologic symptoms such as numbness, weakness, paralysis, or aphasia

#### *Physical Exam*
Thorough physical exam including detailed neurologic exam for any focal deficits:
- Ophthalmoplegic migraine:
  - Paresis of ocular nerve
  - Usually 3rd nerve
  - Must rule out other causes
- Hemiparetic migraine:
  - Episodic hemiparesis as an aura
  - Typically lasts 30–60 min
- Basilar type migraine may include:
  - Blindness
  - Dysarthria
  - Vertigo
  - Paresthesisas
  - Paresis
  - Altered mental status

### ESSENTIAL WORKUP
- An accurate history and physical exam should confirm the diagnosis.
- Patients with new onset of headache syndrome need an objective evaluation to rule out more serious causes of severe headaches:
  - Complete neurologic examination
  - Imaging may be appropriate in ED

### DIAGNOSTIC TESTS & INTERPRETATION
#### *Lab*
- Not needed for classic migraine or established migraines with typical symptoms
- LP if meningitis, subarachnoid hemorrhage, or pseudotumor cerebri is suspected
- ESR if temporal arteritis is suspected
- Carbon monoxide (CO) level if there is history or suspicion of CO exposure
- Intraocular pressure measurements if suspect glaucoma

#### *Imaging*
CT or MRI of the head when indicated

#### *Diagnostic Procedures/Surgery*
LP when indicated

### DIFFERENTIAL DIAGNOSIS
- Meningitis/encephalitis
- Subarachnoid/intracranial hemorrhage
- Cerebral ischemia (if complex migraine)
- HTN
- Brain tumor
- CO poisoning
- Temporal mandibular joint (TMJ) syndrome
- Glaucoma
- Pseudotumor cerebri
- Giant cell arteritis

**TREATMENT**

### PRE-HOSPITAL
- It is important to recognize life-threatening causes of headache and transport rapidly:
  - Sudden onset of symptoms, altered mental status, neck stiffness, fever, or neurologic deficit is a useful sign that suggests a more serious cause of headache.
  - Prior history of similar headache, absence of above symptoms, or strong family history is more suggestive of migraine.
- Allow patients with migraine headache to be in a calm, dark environment.

### INITIAL STABILIZATION/THERAPY
Patients with convincing evidence of increased intracranial pressure may need rapid-sequence intubation and controlled ventilation.

### ED TREATMENT/PROCEDURES
- Abortive therapy and pain management are the primary issues for patients in whom life-threatening causes of headache have been ruled out.
- Generally, abortive therapy options should be attempted 1st.
- Narcotic pain medications may be administered as rescue therapy.
- IV saline hydration is often a helpful adjunct for migraine headaches.
- Triptans and dihydroergotamine (DHE) should not be used within 24 hr of use of ergotamine or DHE

### Pregnancy Considerations
DHE is contraindicated in pregnancy and breastfeeding

### MEDICATION
- Abortive therapy in ED:
  - NSAIDs:
    - Ibuprofen: 400–800 mg PO q8h
    - Acetaminophen: 325–1,000 mg PO q6h
    - Ketorolac: 30–60 mg IM; 15–30 mg IV
  - Triptans:
    - Sumatriptan: 6 mg SC or nasally; may repeat in 1 hr (max. 2 doses per 24 hr); 25–100 mg PO
    - Zolmitriptan: 2.5–5 mg PO
    - Almotriptan: 25 mg PO

  - Ergot alkaloids:
    - Dihydroergotamine: 1 mg IM or IV, then repeat in 1 hr if necessary.
    - Droperidol (if ECG normal): 0.625–2.5 mg IM/IV
    - Metoclopramide: 10 mg IV
    - Prochlorperazine: 10 mg IV
    - Valproic acid: 250–1,000 mg IV
- Rescue pain medication:
  - Hydromorphone: 1–2 mg IM/IV per dose
  - Morphine: 2–10 mg IM/IV per dose
  - NSAIDs: ketorolac 15–30 mg IM/IV, indomethacin 25 mg PO/PR
- Prophylactic therapy:
  - $\beta$-Blockers: Propranolol 40 mg PO b.i.d.
  - $Ca^{2+}$ channel blockers: Verapamil 40 mg PO t.i.d.
  - Cyclic antidepressants: Amitriptyline 25 mg PO t.i.d.
  - Topiramate: 50–200 mg PO daily

### First Line
Abortive therapy with NSAIDs, triptans, DHE, and neuroleptic agents

### Second Line
- Narcotic pain medication
- Steroids:
  - Used in refractory attacks

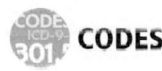 **FOLLOW-UP**

### DISPOSITION
#### Admission Criteria
- Severe intractable headache pain
- Intractable vomiting, electrolyte imbalance, or inability to take oral food or fluid
- Unresolved complex migraines

#### Discharge Criteria
Patients with moderate to complete pain relief, a normal neurologic exam, and a confident diagnosis of migraine.

### Issues for Referral
Rapidly evolving therapeutic options suggest neurologic follow-up is important.

### FOLLOW-UP RECOMMENDATIONS
- Patients with migraines should work to identify and avoid triggers
- Primary care or neurologic evaluation is indicated for those with recurrent migraines.

## PEARLS AND PITFALLS
- Narcotics are not first-line treatment for migraines
- Must exclude other potential serious causes of headaches
- Include CO poisoning on differential diagnosis

## ADDITIONAL READING
- Charles A. Advances in the basic and clinical science of migraine. *Ann Neurol.* 2009;65:491–498.
- Colman I, Rothney A, Wright SC, et al. Use of narcotic analgesics in the emergency department treatment of migraine headache. *Neurology.* 2004;62:1695–1700.
- Marx JA, Hockberger RS, Walls RM, et al. *Rosen's Emergency Medicine: Concepts and Clinical Practice*, 7th ed. St. Louis, MO: Mosby; 2009.
- Mett, A, Tfelt-Hansen P. Acute migraine therapy: Recent evidence from randomized comparative trials. *Curr Opin Neurol.* 2008;21:331–337.

## CODES

### ICD9
346.90 Migraine, unspecified, without mention of intractable migraine without mention of status migrainosus

H

# HEART MURMUR

*Leon D. Sanchez*
*Francis J. O'Connell*

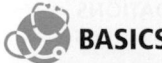 **BASICS**

## DESCRIPTION

- Sounds created by physiologic processes or functional and structural anomalies of the heart.
- Stenotic lesions:
  - Pressure overload in the chamber preceding the valve, leading to hypertrophy of the chamber in an attempt to overcome the increased resistance
- Regurgitant lesions:
  - Volume overload of the chamber preceding the valve, leading to chamber dilatation in an attempt to accommodate the regurgitant blood volume.
- Genetic abnormalities:
  - Congenital defects because of abnormal cardiac blood flow

## ETIOLOGY

- Aortic stenosis:
  - Rheumatic heart disease
  - Congenital bicuspid valve
  - Calcification of valve from aging
  - Prosthetic valve
- Aortic regurgitation:
  - Rheumatic heart disease
  - Endocarditis
  - Aortic dissection
  - Prosthetic valve
- Mitral stenosis:
  - Rheumatic heart disease
  - Rheumatologic disorders (systemic lupus erythematosus)
  - Calcification
  - Cardiac tumors (atrial myxoma)
  - Congenital
  - Prosthetic valve
- Mitral regurgitation, acute:
  - Endocarditis
  - Papillary muscle dysfunction
  - Rupture of papillary muscle
  - Rupture of chordae tendineae
  - Prosthetic valve
- Mitral regurgitation, chronic:
  - Rheumatic heart disease
  - Mitral valve prolapse
  - Connective tissue disease (Marfan disease)
- Mitral valve prolapse:
  - Congenital
  - Connective tissue disease
- Tricuspid stenosis:
  - Rheumatic heart disease
- Tricuspid regurgitation:
  - Rheumatic heart disease
  - Endocarditis
  - Pulmonary HTN
- Pericardial friction rub:
  - Pericarditis
  - Pericardial effusion

## *Pediatric Considerations*

- Pulmonic stenosis:
  - Congenital
  - Maternal–fetal rubella exposure
  - Rheumatic heart disease
- Pulmonic regurgitation:
  - Congenital
  - Rheumatic heart disease
  - Pulmonary HTN
- Atrial septal defect:
  - Congenital
  - Several different types of defects
  - Genetic predisposition in some cases
- Ventricular septal defect:
  - Congenital
- Patent ductus arteriosus:
  - Congenital
  - Prematurity
  - Maternal–fetal rubella exposure
- Coarctation of the aorta:
  - Congenital
  - Turner syndrome
- Idiopathic hypertrophic subaortic stenosis (HCM):
  - Congenital
  - Genetic predisposition

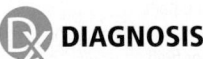 **DIAGNOSIS**

## SIGNS AND SYMPTOMS

- Aortic stenosis:
  - Systolic crescendo-decrescendo murmur radiating to carotids
  - Carotid pulse is described as parvus and tardus (diminished intensity and late upstroke).
  - Angina
  - Dyspnea on exertion
  - Exertional syncope
- Aortic regurgitation:
  - Diastolic blowing murmur at left sternal border
  - Austin Flint murmur is a diastolic rumble from exposure of the mitral valve to the aortic regurgitant flow.
  - Pulmonary edema
  - Dyspnea
  - Tachycardia
  - Chest pain
  - Pulse pressure may be widened.
  - Corrigan pulse or water hammer pulse; a rapid upstroke and downstroke of the carotid pulse
  - Quincke pulse, pulsations seen at the nail beds
  - Musse sign: Bobbing with carotid pulse

- Mitral stenosis:
  - Diastolic, rumbling murmur heard at the apex
  - Loud $S_1$ with an opening snap
  - Dyspnea
  - Orthopnea
  - Hemoptysis
  - Pulmonary edema
  - Emboli to systemic circulation
  - Atrial fibrillation
- Mitral regurgitation, acute:
  - Systolic, harsh, crescendo-decrescendo murmur heard at the base
  - Pulmonary edema
- Mitral regurgitation, chronic:
  - Holosystolic murmur heard at the apex radiating to the axilla
  - Dyspnea on exertion
  - Fatigue
  - Atrial fibrillation is common.
- Mitral valve prolapse:
  - Early to midsystolic click often followed by systolic murmur
  - Palpitations
  - Chest pain
- Tricuspid stenosis:
  - Diastolic, high-pitched murmur
  - Peripheral edema
  - Hepatosplenomegaly
  - Ascites
  - Fatigue
  - Atrial fibrillation is common.
  - Large A wave in the jugular venous pulse
- Tricuspid regurgitation:
  - Holosystolic, blowing murmur best heard along the left sternal margin
  - Peripheral edema
  - Hepatosplenomegaly
  - Ascites
  - Atrial fibrillation is common.
  - Large V wave in the jugular venous pulse
- Patent ductus arteriosus:
  - Continuous machinery murmur
  - CHF
- Pericardial friction rub:
  - Intermittent murmur
  - May have systolic and/or diastolic component
  - Symptoms owing to pericarditis or pericardial effusion

## Pediatric Considerations

- Pulmonic stenosis:
  - Systolic crescendo-decrescendo ejection murmur in the left upper sternal border
  - Severe lesions may have a thrill
  - Widely split $S_2$
  - Dyspnea with exertion in serious cases
  - May have signs of right heart failure
- Pulmonic regurgitation:
  - High-pitched early decrescendo diastolic murmur
  - Widely split $S_2$
  - Associated with Graham Steell murmur of pulmonary HTN
  - May have signs of right-heart failure
- Atrial septal defect:
  - No murmur in PFO
  - Systolic ejection murmur in secundum defect
  - Wide fixed $S_2$
  - Secundum associated with pulmonary HTN
- Ventricular septal defect:
  - Harsh, holosystolic murmur is loudest along the lower left sternal border
- Patent ductus arteriosus:
  - Continuous or machinery murmur at upper left sternal border with systolic thrill
  - Cyanosis
  - Bounding peripheral pulses
  - Tachypnea
- Coarctation of the aorta:
  - Continuous/late systolic murmur
  - May aortic click related to bicuspid valve
  - Difference between upper and lower extremity pulses
- Idiopathic hypertrophic subaortic stenosis (HCM):
  - Systolic, harsh, crescendo-decrescendo murmur heard at left sternal border
  - Increases in volume of the left ventricle at end diastole will decrease the intensity of the murmur.
  - Dyspnea
  - Chest pain
  - Exertional syncope
  - Sudden death

## Physical Exam

- Auscultation of heart and lung sounds
- Evaluation of pulses, peripheral perfusion, and edema

## ESSENTIAL WORKUP

For more details, see Valvular Heart Disease, Mitral Valve Prolapse, Congenital Heart Disease, Patent Ductus Arteriosus, Pericarditis, and Pericardial Effusion/Tamponade.

## DIAGNOSTIC TESTS & INTERPRETATION

### Imaging

- EKG
- CXR
- ECG:
  - Evaluate valves, chambers, flow.
- CT:
  - Rule out aortic dissection.

### Diagnostic Procedures/Surgery

Acute regurgitant lesions:

- Cardiac catheterization

## DIFFERENTIAL DIAGNOSIS

See "Etiology."

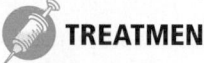 **TREATMENT**

### PRE-HOSPITAL

- IV fluids:
  - Patients with critical aortic stenosis are very sensitive to fluid shifts.
- Oxygen as appropriate

### INITIAL STABILIZATION/THERAPY

- Oxygen
- IV access
- Cardiac monitor
- Treat symptoms (CHF, dysrhythmias).
- Exercise care with fluids and medications in aortic stenosis

### ED TREATMENT/PROCEDURES

For more details, see Endocarditis, Valvular Heart Disease, Mitral Valve Prolapse, Congenital Heart Disease, Patent Ductus Arteriosus, Pericarditis, and Pericardial Effusion/Tamponade.

### MEDICATION

- Digoxin: 0.5 mg IV, then 0.25 mg IV 6 and 12 hr later
- Diltiazem (Cardizem):
  - 0.25 mg/kg (17.5 mg for 70 kg person) IV over 2 min
  - May rebolus after 15 min with 0.35 mg/kg IV
  - Start drip at 5–15 mg/hr.
- Furosemide (Lasix):
  - 20–80 mg IV, may increase dose if necessary
  - Max. of 600 mg per 24 hr
- Heparin:
  - 80-U/kg bolus IV, then drip at 18 U/kg/hr
  - Monitor partial thromboplastin time.
- Metoprolol (Lopressor): 5 mg IV q5–15 min for 3 doses, as tolerated
- Nitroglycerin:
  - 10–20 $\mu$g/min IV
  - Titrate to effect.
  - Max. 300 $\mu$g/min
- Nitroprusside:
  - 0.3 $\mu$g/kg/min IV
  - Titrate to effect
  - Max. 10 $\mu$g/kg/min
  - Protect bag from light
  - Thiocyanate toxicity from prolonged use
- Propranolol (Inderal): 1 mg IV q2min

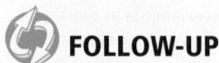 **FOLLOW-UP**

### DISPOSITION

#### Admission Criteria

- Signs of cardiac ischemia
- Syncope or near syncope
- Pulmonary edema
- Hemodynamic instability
- Endocarditis
- Arrhythmia

#### Discharge Criteria

- Asymptomatic
- Hemodynamically stable

#### Issues for Referral

Patients with new murmurs should be referred to their caregiver or a cardiologist.

### FOLLOW-UP RECOMMENDATIONS

- Patients should always inform their medical and dental caregivers that they have a heart murmur.
- To avoid an infection of the lining of the heart, antibiotics may be needed before procedures such as teeth cleaning.

## PEARLS AND PITFALLS

Patients with new heart murmurs and fever need to be assessed for endocarditis.

## ADDITIONAL READING

- Bonow RO, Carabello BA, Chatterjee K, et al. ACC/AHA 2006 guidelines for the management of patients with valvular heart disease. *Circulation.* 2006;114:e84–e231.
- Frommelt MA. Differential diagnosis and approach to heart murmur in term infants. *Pediatr Clin N Am.* 2004;51:1023–1032.
- http://sprojects.mmip.mcgill.ca/mvs/mvsteth.htm
- Nishimura RA, Carabello BA, Faxon DP, et al. ACC/AHA 2008 Guideline update on valvular heart disease: Focused update on infective endocarditis. *Circulation.* 2008;118:887–896.
- www.blaufuss.org/tutorial/

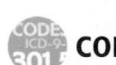 **CODES**

### ICD9

785.2 Undiagnosed cardiac murmurs

H

# HELLP SYNDROME
*Michael J. Bono*

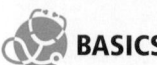 **BASICS**

## DESCRIPTION
- HELLP syndrome: *H*emolysis *E*levated *L*iver enzymes
- Continuum with severe preeclampsia as most patients will be hypertensive and *Low Platelets*
- Liver involvement is hallmark:
  - Other organs may be involved (eg, brain, kidneys).
- HELLP syndrome divided into 3 groups, representing severity of the disease; severity is directly related to the platelet count:
  - Class 1: Most severe form; platelet nadir <50,000 cells/$\mu$L
  - Class 2: Less severe; platelet nadir between 50,000 and 100,000 cells/$\mu$L
  - Class 3: Least severe; platelet nadir between 100,000 and 150,000 cells/$\mu$L
- Most maternal deaths occur with class 1.
- Increased mortality rate is associated with hemorrhage hepatic or CNS or vascular insult to the cardiopulmonary or renal systems.
- Incidence: 0.3% of all pregnancies
- 12–18% have normal BP
- Occurs in 20% of pregnancies with severe preeclampsia
- At diagnosis:
  - 52% preterm
  - 18% term
  - 32% postpartum

## RISK FACTORS
Frequently white, multiparous, older

### Pediatric Considerations
Infant mortality is greater in women with HELLP.

## ETIOLOGY
- Unclear, but vasospasm is the basis:
  - Vascular constriction causes resistance to blood flow and HTN.
  - Vasospasm probably damages vessels directly.
  - Angiotensin II causes endothelial cells to contract.
  - Endothelial cell is damaged and interendothelial cell leaks are the result.
- Small-vessel leaks:
  - Platelets and fibrinogen get deposited subendothelially.
  - Fibrin deposition develops in severe cases.
- Vascular changes and local tissue hypoxia lead to hemorrhage, necrosis, and end organ damage.

 **DIAGNOSIS**

## SIGNS AND SYMPTOMS
### History
- History and physical exam with attention to symptoms of abdominal pain, nausea, vomiting, and headache
- Obstetric history:
  - Parity
  - Deliveries
  - History of hypertensive disorder during pregnancy
  - Estimated gestational age
  - Prenatal care
- May present with flulike symptoms, such as fatigue or malaise
- Nausea, usually with vomiting
- Right upper quadrant or epigastic pain:
  - Pain increases with severity of disease
- Headache, often with visual changes
- Symptoms which carry higher morbidity:
  - Dyspnea and/or fluid overload to suggest cardiogenic/noncardiogenic pulmonary edema
  - Dyspnea associated with pulmonary embolus
  - Chest pain suggestive of myocardial ischemia
  - Altered mental status, seizures of focal neurologic deficit:
    - Hypertensive encephalopathy
    - Cerebral edema
    - Hemorrhagic cerebrovascular accident
  - Peripheral edema
  - Ascites
  - Hematuria
  - Low urine output

### ALERT
Determination of gestational age and fetal viability is critical in HELLP.

### Physical Exam
- Vital signs with attention to BP
- May not have systolic or diastolic HTN
- Many patients will have right upper quadrant pain
- Evidence of fluid overload
- Careful neurologic exam
- Fetal heart tones

## ESSENTIAL WORKUP
- Immediate CBC with platelet count and smear, BUN, creatinine, LFTs, coagulation profile, and magnesium level
- Urinalysis for protein; screen for UTI.
- Weigh patient to determine recent weight gain.

## DIAGNOSTIC TESTS & INTERPRETATION
### Lab
- CBC:
  - Anemia
  - Thrombocytopenia
  - Peripheral smear demonstrates microangiopathic hemolytic anemia (burr cells or schistocytes).
  - Other hemolysis markers are elevated lactate dehydrogenase (LDH) levels, increased reticulocyte count, and elevated bilirubin levels.
- Platelet count and smear:
  - Less than 100,000 cells per $\mu$L
- Disseminated intravascular coagulation screen
- Coagulation profile:
  - PT
  - PTT
- BUN, creatinine, and magnesium levels
- LFTs to assess hemolysis markers and hepatic dysfunction:
  - Elevated aspartate aminotransferase level: >40 IU/L
  - Elevated alanine aminotransferase level: >40 IU/L
  - Elevated lactate dehydrogenase: >600 IU/L

### Imaging
- CXR:
  - Suspected pulmonary edema
- CT of head:
  - Mental status changes or focal neurologic deficit
- US of the pelvis (transabdominal or transvaginal):
  - Image fetus and placenta

## DIFFERENTIAL DIAGNOSIS
- GI:
  - Cholecystitis
  - Cholelithiasis
  - Biliary colic
  - Pancreatitis
  - Hepatitis
  - Ulcer disease
  - Acute fatty liver of pregnancy
  - Acute gastritis
  - Hiatal hernia
  - Severe gastroesophageal reflux
- Hematologic:
  - Preeclampsia-associated thrombocytopenia
  - Gestational thrombocytopenia
  - Idiopathic thrombocytopenic purpura
  - Thrombotic thrombocytopenic purpura
  - Hemolytic uremic syndrome
- Neurologic:
  - Epilepsy
  - Encephalitis
  - Meningitis
  - Encephalopathy
  - Brain tumor
  - Intracranial hemorrhage

- Other:
  - Drug abuse
  - Pyelonephritis
  - Sepsis

## TREATMENT

### PRE-HOSPITAL
Cautions:

- Transport patient in left lateral decubitus position to prevent inferior vena cava syndrome.
- Venous access for anticipated seizure activity
- Routine seizure management (preferably with magnesium sulfate) if the patient seizes

### ALERT
Transport to a facility capable of providing high-risk obstetric care.

### INITIAL STABILIZATION/THERAPY
- ABC management
- Left lateral decubitus position to prevent inferior vena cava syndrome
- High flow oxygen via face mask
- Maternal monitoring:
  - Cardiac
  - Pulse oximetry
  - Tocography
- Fetal monitoring

### ED TREATMENT/PROCEDURES
- Control HTN with antihypertensives (see "Medication"):
  - Avoid ACE inhibitors because of fetal side effects.
- Heparin should be avoided because of bleeding complications.
- Treat preeclampsia or eclampsia with IV magnesium sulfate.
  - Magnesium sulfate is not given to treat HTN.
- Order type and screen for possible transfusion.
- Call for emergent obstetric consult, consider neonatology consult:
  - Consider emergent delivery.
  - Early plasma exchange therapy has shown promise in postpartum patients with severe disease.
- Discuss administration of glucocorticoid with consultant:
  - Helps fetal lung maturity
  - IV dexamethasone more effective than IM betamethasone
  - Depends on gestational age of fetus
  - Does not reduce disease severity or duration
- Limit IV fluid administration unless clinical evidence of dehydration:
  - Excess fluids promote further capillary leak
  - Lactated Ringers or NS at 60 mL/hr (no more than 125 mL/hr)
  - Monitor urine output with Foley catheter.

### TREATMENT-GENERAL-MEASURES
Activity: Bed rest
Blood products:

- Correct thrombocytopenia by platelet transfusion in women with platelet counts <20,000 cells/$\mu$L, even without active bleeding, as risk of postpartum bleeding is significantly increased.
- Platelet counts >40,000 cells/$\mu$L are safe for vaginal delivery.
- Correct thrombocytopenia to platelet counts >50,000 cells/$\mu$L if cesarean delivery planned.
- If coagulation dysfunction is present, transfusion with fresh frozen plasma and packed RBCs in consultation with obstetrics
- Transfusion with packed RBCs for hemoglobin <10 g/dL

### MEDICATION
#### First Line
- Hydralazine: 2.5 mg IV, then 5–10 mg q15–20min:
  - Up to 40 mg total dose, to keep diastolic BP <110 mm Hg
  - IV drip 5–10 mg/hr titrated
- Labetalol: 10 mg IV, then 20–80 mg IV q10min:
  - Up to 300 mg total dose
  - IV drip 1–2 mg/min titrated

#### Second Line
- Nitroprusside: 0.25 $\mu$g/kg/min as a drip:
  - Increase 0.25 $\mu$g/kg/min q5min
  - Use only if no response to hydralazine or labetalol
- Magnesium sulfate: 4–6 g in 100 mL IV over 15–20 min as loading dose:
  - Maintenance drip starting at 2 g/hr
  - Titrate to clinical effect
  - Watch for toxicity (antidote is calcium gluconate 10%, 10 mL IV over 3 min).
  - Measure magnesium sulfate level at 4–6 hr; adjust drip to achieve levels between 4 and 7 mEq/L.

## FOLLOW-UP

### DISPOSITION
#### Admission Criteria
- Admit all patients to obstetric service for continuous monitoring of mother and fetus.
- ICU admission:
  - Pulmonary edema
  - Respiratory failure
  - Cerebral edema
  - GI bleeding with hemodynamic instability

#### Discharge Criteria
Patients with HELLP syndrome should always be admitted. Discharge should be a decision of the OB Consultant

#### Issues for Referral
After stabilization in the ED, transfer to facility capable of managing high-risk obstetric conditions unless delivery is imminent.

### FOLLOW-UP RECOMMENDATIONS
Patients should be followed closely by OB:

- May develop HELLP after delivery, usually within 48 hr

## PEARLS AND PITFALLS

- Hypertensive pregnant women with abdominal pain, elevated LFTs, and decreased platelets need emergent treatment and OB consultation
- Patients with HELLP syndrome may have a normal BP
- Transport to a facility capable of caring for these patients after stabilization is essential

## ADDITIONAL READING

- Haram K, Svendsen E, Abildgaard U. The HELLP Syndrome: Clinical issues and management: A review. *BMC Pregnancy Childbirth*. 2009;9:8.
- Leeman L, Fontaine P. Hypertensive disorders of pregnancy. *Am Fam Physician*. 2008;78:93–100.
- Martin JN Jr, Rose CH, Briery CM. Understanding and managing HELLP syndrome: The integral role of aggressive glucocorticoids for mother and child. *Am J Obstet Gynecol*. 2006;195(4):914–934.
- Martin JN, Thigpen BD, Moore RC, et al. Stroke and severe preeclampsia and eclampsia: A paradigm shift focusing on systolic blood pressure. *Obstet Gynecol*. 2005;105:237–238.
- Yoder SR, Thornburg LL, Bisognano JD. Hypertension in pregnancy and women of childbearing age. *Am J Med*. 2009;122:890–895.

## See Also (Topic, Algorithm, Electronic Media Element)
- Preeclampsia

## CODES

### ICD9
642.50 Severe pre-eclampsia, unspecified as to episode of care

H

# HEMATURIA/PROTEINURIA

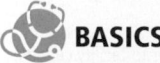

*Edward Ullman*
*Jonathan S. Anderson*

## 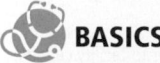 BASICS

### DESCRIPTION
- Microscopic hematuria: ≥T3 red blood cells per high-power field in 2 of 3 properly collected urine specimens
- Gross hematuria: Visible blood in properly collected urine specimen
- Proteinuria: Urinary protein excretion of >150 mg/d
- Risk factors for disease in asymptomatic proteinuria:
  – Diabetes
  – HTN
  – NSAID abuse
  – Heroin use
- Risk factors for disease in asymptomatic hematuria:
  – Tobacco use
  – Occupational exposure to benzenes, aromatic amines, and dyes
  – History of gross hematuria
  – Age >40 yr old
  – History of urologic disorder or disease
  – History of painful voiding
  – History of urinary tract infections (UTI)
  – Analgesic abuse
  – History of pelvic irradiation

### ETIOLOGY
- Proteinuria:
  – Glomerular:
    ○ Nephritic (postinfectious, IgA, lupus, vasculitis)
    ○ Nephrotic (minimal change, diabetes, preeclampsia)
  – Tubular
  – Overflow (hemolysis, rhabdo, multiple myeloma)
- Hematuria:
  – UTI
  – Stones (renal, bladder)
  – BPH
  – Cancer (bladder, renal, prostate)
  – Transient unexplained
  – Acute glomerulonephritis

##  DIAGNOSIS

### SIGNS AND SYMPTOMS
- Dysuria
- Blood in urine
- Fever
- Flank pain
- Flank ecchymosis
- Initial hematuria (anterior urethral lesion)
- Terminal hematuria (posterior urethra, bladder, neck, trigone)
- Cyclic hematuria (endometriosis or urinary tract)
- Previous upper respiratory tract infection (10–21 days prior)
- Previous skin infection (10–21 days prior)

- Deafness (Alport syndrome)
- Peripheral edema
- CHF
- Hemoptysis (Goodpasture disease)
- Concurrent menstruation
- Testicular, epididymal, and prostatic tenderness or trauma
- Terminal urethral lesion
- Enlarged prostate
- Penile/scrotal hematoma
- Atrial fibrillation:
  – Renal artery embolus or thrombus
- Organomegaly, flank mass
- Pregnancy consideration
- Headache
- HTN (>140/90 mm Hg)
- Right upper quadrant pain

### History
- Characteristics of complaint (onset, duration)
- Associated symptoms (recent illness)
- Past medical history (DM, HTN, pregnancy)
- Medications (nephrotoxic, anticoagulation)

### Physical Exam
- Complete physical exam, special attention to:
  – Edema, including periorbital
  – Thorough GU exam, including prostate
  – Rashes
  – Flank (ecchymosis, tenderness)

### ESSENTIAL WORKUP
- Urine dipstick
- Urinalysis with microscopic analysis
- Consider urine culture.
- BUN level
- Serum creatinine level
- CBC
- Pregnancy consideration
- Liver function test
- Platelet count
- Consider coagulation panel.

### DIAGNOSTIC TESTS & INTERPRETATION
#### Lab
- Urine:
  – Culture
  – Cytology
  – 24-hr urine protein and creatinine levels
  – Spot ratio of urine protein to creatinine
  – Spot ratio of urine protein to osmolality
  – Protein electrophoresis
- Serum:
  – Coagulation studies
  – Protein electrophoresis

### Imaging
- Helical CT scan
- Renal US

### Diagnostic Procedures/Surgery
- Cystourethroscopy
- Urethrogram
- Cystogram
- Retrograde pyelogram
- IV pyelogram

### DIFFERENTIAL DIAGNOSIS
- Glomerular hematuria:
  – IgA nephropathy (Berger disease)
  – Postinfectious glomerulonephritis
  – Membranoproliferative glomerulonephritis
  – Focal glomerular sclerosis
  – Lupus nephritis
  – Wegener granulomatosis
  – Polyarteritis nodosa
  – Henoch-Schönlein syndrome
- Thrombotic thrombocytopenic purpura:
  – Hemolytic uremic syndrome
  – Alport syndrome
  – Goodpasture disease
- Nonglomerular hematuria:
  – Infection (pyelonephritis, tuberculosis, schistosomiasis)
  – Inflammation (drug-induced, radiation induced)
  – Renal and extrarenal tumor
  – Interstitial nephritis
  – Papillary necrosis
  – Polycystic kidney disease
  – Medullary sponge disease
  – Renal artery embolism/thrombosis
  – Renal vein thrombosis
  – Sickle cell disease
  – Malignant HTN
  – Hypercalcuria
  – Hyperuricosuria
  – Urolithiasis
  – Strictures
  – Endometriosis
  – Foreign bodies
  – Benign prostatic hypertrophy
  – Coagulopathy/bleeding disorders
  – Trauma (renal pedicle injuries, urethral disruptions, bladder rupture)
  – Recent instrumentation
  – Frequent or interrupted coitus
  – Factitious
- Glomerular proteinuria (>2 g per day):
  – Minimal-change disease
  – Membranous glomerulonephritis
  – Focal segmental glomerulonephritis
  – Membranoproliferative glomerulonephritis
  – DM
  – Collagen vascular diseases
  – Amyloidosis
  – Preeclampsia
  – Infection (HIV, hepatitis B, hepatitis C, poststreptococcal infection, syphilis)

- Lymphoma
- Chronic renal transplant rejection
- Heroin use
- Penicillamine
- Tubular proteinuria:
  - Hypertensive nephrosclerosis
  - Uric acid nephropathy
  - Acute hypersensitivity interstitial nephritis
  - Fanconi syndrome
  - Sickle cell disease
- Overflow proteinuria:
  - Monoclonal gammopathy
  - Leukemia
- Proteinuria, other:
  - Dehydration
  - Stress
  - Fever
  - Heat injury
  - Inflammatory process
  - Orthostatic proteinuria

 TREATMENT

### PRE-HOSPITAL
- Airway, breathing, and circulation management
- Control other trauma, if present.

### INITIAL STABILIZATION/THERAPY
- Airway, breathing, and circulation management
- Treat hemodynamically unstable injuries 1st, if present.
- Obtain initial labs (urinalysis with microscopic analysis, BUN, serum creatinine).

#### Pregnancy Considerations
If considering preeclampsia:
- Aggressive BP control
- Magnesium if indicated
- Prompt OB/GYN consultation

### ED TREATMENT/PROCEDURES
- Uncomplicated UTIs:
  - Antibiotics
- Pyelonephritis:
  - Antibiotics
  - Analgesics
  - Antipyretics
- Rapidly progressing glomerulonephropathy:
  - Steroid therapy
  - Urologic/nephrology consultation
- Acute renal failure:
  - Hemodialysis
  - Renal US
  - Urine electrolytes
  - Nephrology consultation
- Renal colic:
  - IV fluids
  - Analgesics
  - If initial presentation, noncontrast helical CT scan
- Gross hematuria:
  - Insertion of 3-way Foley catheter with bladder irrigation to clear blood clots that may cause urinary retention from bladder obstruction

### MEDICATION
- Uncomplicated UTI:
  - 3–5-day treatment:
  - Trimethoprim/sulfamethoxazole as first-line therapy:
    - Ciprofloxacin or levofloxacin when the patient is allergic to sulfa or after failure of trimethoprim/sulfamethoxazole
    - Ciprofloxacin: 250 mg PO b.i.d. (do not use in pediatric/pregnant patients)
    - Levofloxacin: 250 mg PO daily (do not use in pediatric and pregnant patients)
    - Nitrofurantoin: 2 mg/kg/d PO
    - Trimethoprim/sulfamethoxazole DS: PO b.i.d. for 3 days (peds: 2 mg trimethoprim/10 mg sulfamethoxazole per kilogram PO daily)
    - Cefpodoxime: 100 mg b.i.d. for 7 days
    - Amoxicillin-clavulanate: 500 mg b.i.d. or 250 mg 3 t.i.d. for 7 days
    - Cefdinir: (peds) 14 mg/kg/d PO divided in 2 doses
    - Amoxicillin: (peds) 30–50 mg/kg PO t.i.d. for 7–10 days
- Outpatient pyelonephritis:
  Outpatient treatment with 7 days of ciprofloxacin or levofloxacin or 14 days of amoxicillin/clavulanate:
    - Amoxicillin/clavulanate: 500/125 mg PO t.i.d. for 14 days
    - Ciprofloxacin: 500 mg PO b.i.d. for 7 days
    - Levofloxacin: 250 mg PO daily for 7 days
    - Trimethoprim/sulfamethoxazole DS: PO b.i.d. for 14 days

#### Pediatric Considerations
In children, a 3rd-generation cephalosporin is preferable; amoxicillin-clavulanate or TMX sulfa are alternatives.

#### Pregnancy Considerations
In pregnant patients, the preferable antibiotics are nitrofurantoin, cefpodoxime, and amoxicillin-clavulanate.

 FOLLOW-UP

### DISPOSITION
#### Admission Criteria
- Intractable pain
- Intolerance of PO fluids and medications
- Hemodynamic instability
- Hematuria with traumatic injuries
- Obstructing ureteral stones with evidence of systemic infection or renal failure
- Hypertensive emergency
- Acute renal failure:
  - Azotemia/uremia/hyperkalemia
- Oliguria/anuria
- Pregnant with preeclampsia, pyelonephritis, obstructing nephrolithiasis

#### Discharge Criteria
- Hemodynamically stable without life-threatening issues
- Infected ureteral stones without renal failure or obstruction
- Mild hematuria or proteinuria without renal failure
- Hematuria:
  - Gross hematuria, except in young women with proven UTIs, needs urology follow-up.
  - Microscopic hematuria needs repeated U/As and PCP follow-up, and may need urology/nephrology in the future.
  - Pregnant patients with possible infections should have close follow-up to ensure treatment success.
- Proteinuria:
  - Mild cases should be referred to their primary care physician for further workup in an outpatient setting.
  - Large amounts of proteinuria should be referred to a nephrologists without delay.

## PEARLS AND PITFALLS
- Missing acute glomerulonephritis in children, either by misdiagnosing as a UTI based on the U/A, or by failing to consider it in the differential is a pitfall.
- Periorbital edema can be a sign of nephritic syndrome, not just allergic reaction.
- Failing to ensure follow-up for asymptomatic hematuria, especially in patients >40 is a pitfall.

## ADDITIONAL READING
- Ahmed Z, Lee J. Asymptomatic urinary abnormalities. *Med Clin North Am.* 1997;81: 641–652.
- Rao PK, Jones JS. How to evaluate 'dipstick hematuria': What to do before you refer. *Cleve Clin J Med.* 2008;75:227–233.
- Sokolosky MC. Hematuria. *Emerg Med Clin North Am.* 2001;19:621–632.
- Wolfson AB, et al., eds. *Harwood-Nuss' clinical practice of emergency medicine,* 4th ed. Philadelphia: J.B. Lippincott Publishers, 2005.

### See Also (Topic, Algorithm, Electronic Media Element)
- Urinary Tract Infection, Adult
- Urinary Tract Infection, Pediatric
- Preeclampsia/Eclampsia
- Renal Failure
- Renal Calculus

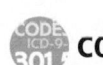 CODES

### ICD9
- 599.70 Hematuria, unspecified
- 599.71 Gross hematuria
- 599.72 Microscopic hematuria

# HEMOPHILIA

Steven H. Bowman
Theresa Gandor

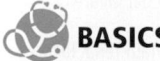 **BASICS**

## DESCRIPTION
- Caused by deficiency of factor VIII or factor IX
- Absence of factors causes partial inactivation of coagulation cascade and impaired hemostasis.
- 2 types:
  - Hemophilia A: Factor VIII deficiency
  - Hemophilia B (Christmas disease): Factor IX deficiency
- Severity varies among different individuals reflecting available natural factor activity:
  - 70% type A hemophiliacs are severe.
- Symptoms dependent on factor activity:
  - 5–30% factor activity (mild hemophilia):
    ○ Bleeding almost exclusively with major trauma/surgery/dental extractions
    ○ Rarely has bleeds
  - 1–5% factor activity (moderate hemophilia):
    ○ Occasional spontaneous hemorrhages
    ○ Bleeding into joints and muscles after minor injuries
    ○ May bleed as often as 1 time per month
  - <1% factor activity (severe):
    ○ Frequent spontaneous hemorrhages into joints and muscles
    ○ Internal bleeding after trauma/surgery
    ○ May bleed as often as 1–2 times per week
- Complications of the disorder:
  - Death from hemorrhage
  - Patients with recurrent joint bleeding leads to chronic arthropathy, pain, loss of function
- Complications related to treatment:
  - Transfusions-transmitted infections (risk reduced with purification of concentrates)
  - Development of IgG antibodies (inhibitors) to factors that prevent hemostasis

## ETIOLOGY
### Genetics
- X-linked recessive
- Rare disease:
  - Hemophilia A: 1 in 10,000 males.
  - Hemophilia B: 1 in 30,000 males
- Prevalence of inhibitors: 20–30% of severe hemophilia A and <5% of severe hemophilia B patients

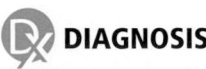 **DIAGNOSIS**

## SIGNS AND SYMPTOMS
- Bleeding:
  - Hemarthrosis (most common):
    ○ Knee (most common) > elbow > ankle > shoulder > wrist (least common)
  - Muscle hemorrhage
  - Bleeding from soft tissue lacerations
  - Postextraction or oral mucosal bleeding
  - Epistaxis (only in severe disease)
  - Hematuria
  - Intracranial hemorrhage
  - GI bleeding
  - Pseudotumors (blood cysts)

## ESSENTIAL WORKUP
Thorough history and physical examination

## DIAGNOSTIC TESTS & INTERPRETATION
### Lab
- CBC: Platelet count normal
- PT: Normal
- PTT: Increased
- Bleeding time: Normal
- Urinalysis: Asymptomatic hematuria (often)
- Specific factor assays:
  - Factor VIII: Ag (measures factor VIII quantity): Decreased
  - Factor VIII: c (measures factor VIII activity): Decreased
  - vWF (measures von Willebrand factor activity): Normal
  - vWF: Ag (measures von Willebrand factor quantity): Normal

### Imaging
Radiographic studies may be required in certain circumstances:
- Head CT to evaluate or exclude intracranial bleed
- Renal US/IV pyelograph to evaluate excessive hematuria or renal trauma
- Abdominal CT to evaluate or exclude retroperitoneal bleeding

## DIFFERENTIAL DIAGNOSIS
- Von Willebrand disease
- Anticoagulant drugs
- Antiplatelet agents
- Thrombocytopenia
- Hepatic dysfunction

 **TREATMENT**

## INITIAL STABILIZATION/THERAPY
- Control bleeding/type and screen.
- Establish IV access.
- Consider ordering pRBCs for transfusion.

## ED TREATMENT/PROCEDURES
### General
- Abort current bleeding episode by raising factor level.
- Coordinate ED care with hematologist
- Patients generally understand their disease and know doses/type of factor they have had in the past and if they have inhibitors or not.
- Determine desired factor level based on risk of bleeding and location/system:
  - 1 Unit in 1 mL of normal plasma is considered 100% clotting factor activity
  - Normal individuals have a factor VIII and factor IX level somewhere between 60–150%
  - Calculate factor VIII level of activity desired:
    ○ Factor VIII required (in units) = wt (kg) × 0.5 × (% factor activity desired).
    ○ 1 IU factor VIII/kg raises activity by 2%.
  - Calculate factor IX level of activity required:
    ○ Factor IX required (in units) = wt (kg) × 1.0 × (% factor activity desired).
    ○ 1 IU factor IX/kg raises activity by 1%.

### Approach to Factor Replacement
- Factor replacement given IV push over 1–2 min
- Low to moderate level of bleeding:
  - Soft tissue injury/lacerations
  - Joint or muscle bleeding (except iliopsoas)
  - Desired level of clotting-factor activity: 30–50%
    ○ Factor VIII dose: 25 IU/kg
    ○ Factor IX dose: 40–50 IU/kg
- Moderate to severe level of bleeding:
  - GI or genitourinary (GU) bleeding
  - Major muscle bleeds (Iliopsoas)
  - Desired level of clotting-factor activity: 50–100%
    ○ Factor VIII dose: 25–50 IU/kg
    ○ Factor IX dose: 50–100 IU/kg
- Severe level of bleeding (life-threatening):
  - CNS injury/intracranial bleed
  - Bleeding from major trauma/postsurgical
  - Intra-abdominal/retroperitoneal bleeding
  - Throat/neck bleeds compromising airway
  - Desired level of clotting-factor activity: 100%
    ○ Factor VIII dose: 50 IU/kg
    ○ Factor IX dose: 100–120 IU/kg

### Specific Management Considerations
- Hemarthrosis:
  - Splint, ace, ice
  - Arthrocentesis rarely indicated
- Muscle hemorrhage:
  - Forearm/calf—consider compartment syndrome.
  - Psoas hematoma—groin pain, femoral nerve paresthesias
- Postextraction or oral mucosal bleeding:
  - Treat locally with Avitene or other microfibrillar collagen hemostatic agent.
  - Replace factor if severe.
  - Amicar and Cyklokapron may be useful.
- Hematuria (generally mild):
  - Hydrate
  - Avoid Amicar and cryoprecipitate.
- Intracranial hemorrhage:
  - All head injuries should be considered significant, especially in children.
  - Do not delay therapy for CT head.
  - Replace factor to 100%.
- GI bleeding:
  - Secondary to ulcers, polyps, hemorrhoids
  - Replace factor promptly (50–100%).
  - Replace factor prior to endoscopy.

## MEDICATION
To calculate doses for recombinant and plasma-derived factor VIII and factor IX concentrates refer to section "Approach to Factor Replacement" above.

### First Line
- Patient without inhibitors:
  - Recombinant factor VIII for hemophilia A
    ○ Examples: Recombinate, Kogenate, ReFacto, Advate
  - Recombinant factor IX for hemophilia B:
    ○ Examples: BeneFIX

- Patient with inhibitors:
  - Recombinant factor VIIa (NovoSeven):
    - 90–120 $\mu$g/kg every 2–3 hr
    - Higher doses of up to 300 $\mu$g/kg may promote thrombin formation and stabilize fibrin clot in the case of inefficient hemostasis
    - Bypasses the coagulation cascade
    - Very efficacious, strong safety profile, minimal risk of inhibitor development, expensive

### Second Line
- Patient without inhibitors:
  - Plasma-derived factor VIII high-purity concentrates (for hemophilia A)
    - Examples: Monoclate-P, Hemofil-M, Monarc-M
    - Next best option if recombinant factor VIII is not available
    - Purification/viral inactivation by affinity chromatography, with monoclonal antibody
  - Plasma-derived factor VIII intermediate-purity concentrates (for hemophilia A):
    - Examples: Humate, Alphanate, Koate-HS, Profilate-HT
    - Purification/viral inactivation by heating in dry state or aqueous solution or solvent/detergent method
    - Only use when recombinant factor VIII or high-purity plasma VIII concentrates not available.
  - Plasma-derived factor IX high-purity concentrates (for hemophilia B)
    - Examples: AlphaNine, mononine
    - Next best option after recombinant factor IX
  - Cryoprecipitate (useful only in hemophilia A):
    - Obtained from FFP after thawing at 4°C
    - Contains factor VIII, vWF, fibrinogen
    - Estimated 80–100 units of factor VIII in 1 unit of cryo
    - Give 10 bags initially, peds dose 1 bag/6 kg
    - Not recommended if factor VIII concentrates available
  - FFP (contains factor VIII and IX):
    - 1 unit of FFP contains about 200–300 units each of both factor VIII and factor IX
    - 1 unit of FFP will raise factor level 5–10% in 60 kg person
    - Readily available in most EDs; useful in life-threatening bleeds when access to specific factor treatment might be delayed
  - Adjunct to factor therapy: DDAVP
    - Raises factor VIII level 2–4 times (only use in patients with mild hemophilia with mild bleeds)
    - Not useful in patients with hemophilia B
    - Side effects: Mild flushing, headache, tachycardia, hypotension, hyponatremia
    - Dose 0.3 $\mu$g/kg of DDAVP diluted in 50 mL 0.9% NS given over 15–30 min given IV or SC (intranasal "Stimate" 1 spray each nostril if >50 kg)
    - Should not be used in children <1 yr old
  - Adjunct to factor therapy: Antifibrinolytic agents (for mild bleeds):
    - Inhibit plasmin activity, prevents clot lysis
    - Only for mucosa/oral/dental bleeding
    - Do not use in children.
    - Examples: Amicar (aminocaproic acid) 75 mg/kg every 6 hr up to 4 g and Cyklokapron (tranexamic acid) 25 mg/kg every 8 hr

- Adjunct to factor therapy: Topical thrombin:
  - Useful for control of localized bleeding from lacerated superficial tissues
- Patient with inhibitors:
  - Activated prothrombin complex concentrates (APCCs):
    - Examples: FEIBA and Autoplex-T
    - Dose: 75–100 IU/kg every 8–12 hr
    - Contains VIIa, IXa, and Xa
    - Bypasses coagulation cascade
    - Thromboemolic events occur with higher doses: DVT, PF, acute MI, DIC
  - High dose recombinant or plasma-derived factor concentrates (2–3 times normal range):
    - For patients that have low-titer antibodies and do not have increasing titers when exposed to factor infusions (low-responders)
  - Porcine factor VIII:
    - Examples: Hyate: C
    - Dose: 50–200 IU/kg every 6–12 hr
    - Useful in patients with inhibitors; should not substitute for recombinant factor VII
    - Risk of transient thrombocytopenia

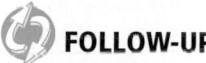 **ALERT**
- Avoid all IM injections of factor concentrates
- Avoid aspirin and aspirin-containing products
- For patients who necessitate an invasive procedure (arterial blood draw, central line, lumbar puncture, arthrocentesis), factor replacement therapy should be given beforehand

## FOLLOW-UP
### DISPOSITION
#### Admission Criteria
- Low threshold for admission
- All joint/muscle bleeds, internal bleeding, severe bleeds
- Bleeding that may require multiple infusions
- Severe complications or any head trauma

### Discharge Criteria
Minor soft tissue bleeding, superficial lacerations with resolution/control of bleeding

### Issues for Referral
Hematology for all bleeds

### FOLLOW-UP RECOMMENDATIONS
- Hematologist as outpatient
- Return to ER for recurrent bleeding episodes

## PEARLS AND PITFALLS
- Do not wait for a head CT before treatment in the setting of head trauma
- In a suspected bleeding emergency in a patient with unknown clotting factor level, assume the level to be 0 and treat as a severe bleed
- Be familiar with different factor replacement therapies for patients with and without inhibitors
- Consult hematologist for appropriate dosing in ER/length of treatment/inhibitor vs. noninhibitor treatment and have low threshold for admission

## ADDITIONAL READING

- Astermark J. Treatment of the bleeding inhibitor patient. *Semin ThrombHemost/*. 2003;29;77–85.
- Bolton-Maggs P. Haemophilias A and B. *Lancet*. 2003;361:1801–1809.
- Cohen AJ, Kessler CM. Treatment of inherited coagulation disorders. *Am J Med*. 1995;99:675.
- DiMichele D. Hemophilia 1996: New approach to an old disease. *Pediatr Clin North Am*. 1996;43:709.
- Friedman K, et al. Inherited coagulation disorders. In: Lee G, et al., eds. *Wintrobe's Clinical Hematology*, 11th ed. Philadelphia: Lippincott Williams & Wilkins; 2004:1619–1667.
- Furie B, Limentani SA, Rosenfield C. A practical guide to the evaluation and treatment of hemophilia. *Blood*. 1994;843.
- Kempton C, et al. How we treat a hemophilia A patient with a factor VIII inhibitor. *Blood*. 2009;113.11–17.
- Key N, et al. Coagulation factor concentrates: Past, present, future. *Lancet*. 2007;370.439–448.
- National Hemophilia Foundation. *Guidelines for emergency dept management of individuals with hemophilia*. MASAC document 175. www.hemophilia.org.
- Pipe S. Recombinant clotting factors. *Thromb Haemost*. 2008;99:840–850.
- Roberts HR, et al. Hemophilia A and Hemophilia B. In: Beutler E, et al., eds. *Williams' Hematology*, 6th ed. New York: McGraw-Hill; 2001:1639–1657.
- Singleton T, et al. Emergency Dept Care for patients with hemophilia and von Willibrand disease. *J Emerg Med*. 2008

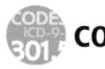 **CODES**

### ICD9
- 286.0 Congenital factor viii disorder
- 286.1 Congenital factor ix disorder

**H**

# HEMOPTYSIS

*Navneet Cheema*
*Peter S. Pang*

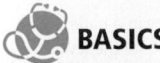 **BASICS**

## DESCRIPTION
- Expectoration of blood, originating from the tracheobronchial tree
- Source of bleeding is typically from bronchial arteries (95%) or pulmonary arteries (5%):
  - Lesions to the bronchial arteries usually produce profuse bleeding, whereas bleeding from the pulmonary arteries generates only small amounts.
- Threshold of massive hemoptysis defined has been defined from 100 mL–1L/24 h:
  - >8 mL/kg/d in children
  - Most common definition is >399 mL/24 hr
- Mortality:
  - Massive hemoptysis (>500 mL/24 hr): 38%
  - Trivial to moderate hemoptysis (<500 mL/24): 4.5%
  - Malignancy and coagulopathy increase the risk of mortality.

## ETIOLOGY
- Infectious (most common cause):
  - Acute or chronic bronchitis
  - Pneumonia
  - Tuberculosis
  - Viral (influenza, varicella)
  - Fungal (*Aspergillus, Coccidioides, Histoplasma, Blastomyces*)
  - Parasitic (*Ascariasis, Amebiasis, Paragonimiasis, Echinococcus*)
- Neoplastic:
  - Squamous cell, small cell, carcinoid
  - Bronchial adenoma
  - Metastatic disease
- Pulmonary:
  - Bronchiectasis
  - Pulmonary embolism
  - Pulmonary infarction
  - Cystic fibrosis
  - Bronchopleural fistula
- Cardiac:
  - Mitral stenosis
  - Tricuspid endocarditis
  - Heart failure
- Systemic disease:
  - Goodpasture syndrome
  - Systemic lupus erythematosus
  - Vasculitis (Wegener granulomatosis, Henoch-Schönlein purpura, Behçet disease)
- Hematologic:
  - Coagulopathy
  - Thrombocytopenia
  - Platelet dysfunction
  - DIC
- Vascular:
  - Pulmonary HTN
  - Arteriovenous malformation
  - Aortic aneurysm
  - Pulmonary artery aneurysm
  - Aortobronchial fistula

- Drugs/toxins:
  - Aspirin/antiplatelet therapy
  - Anticoagulants
  - Penicillamine, amiodarone, propylthiouracil
  - Cocaine ("crack") lung
  - Solvents (organic solvents, trimellitic anhydride)
- Trauma:
  - Tracheobronchial rupture
  - Pulmonary contusion
- Iatrogenic:
  - Bronchoscopy/lung biopsy
  - Pulmonary artery or central venous catheterization
  - Transtracheal aspirate
- Miscellaneous:
  - Foreign-body aspiration
  - Catamenial hemoptysis (pulmonary endometriosis)
  - Amyloidosis
  - Idiopathic or cryptogenic (between 5–30%, depending on patient population)

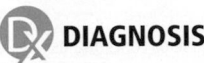 **DIAGNOSIS**

## SIGNS AND SYMPTOMS
- Chest pain
- Dyspnea
- Fever
- Weakness
- Fatigue
- Night sweats
- Weight loss

### History
- Inquire about prior lung, renal, or valvular heart disease
- History of cigarette smoking
- Chemical, asbestos, or infectious exposure
- Travel history (consider parasitic or fungal infectious etiology)
- Aspirin, NSAID, or anticoagulant use
- Consider Goodpasture syndrome if a history of hematuria is present.
- Recurrent or chronic hemoptysis raises suspicion of arteriovenous malformations, bronchiectasis, and cystic fibrosis.

### Physical Exam
- Clubbing of the fingers (chronic inflammatory lung diseases)
- Cutaneous ecchymosis (blood dyscrasia or anticoagulants)
- Aphthous ulcers (Behçet disease)
- Nasal septal perforation (Wegener granulomatosis)
- Hematuria (Goodpasture syndrome)
- Unilateral lower extremity edema may indicate DVT.
- Suggestive of pseudohemoptysis:
  - Sinusitis, epistaxis, rhinorrhea, pharyngitis, upper respiratory infection, aspiration

### Pediatric Considerations
- Thorough head, eyes, ears, nose, and throat exam to exclude nonpulmonary source of bleeding
- Pulmonary exam is often normal.
- Wheezing may suggest obstruction (eg, foreign body).
- Crackles may indicate an underlying pulmonary etiology (eg, pneumonia, hemothorax, heart failure).
- Telangiectasias or hemangiomas raise suspicion of arteriovenous malformations.

## ESSENTIAL WORKUP
- Differentiate between hemoptysis and pseudohemoptysis:
  - Note any precipitating factors, duration of symptoms, quantity, and quality of blood.
  - Pulmonary source:
    - Bright red blood
    - Frothy in appearance
    - Sputum mixed with blood is likely pulmonary
    - pH >7
  - GI source:
    - Dark red or brown blood
    - Accompanied by gastric contents
    - Worsens in setting of nausea/vomiting
    - pH <7
    - Gastric lavage may be used to rule out GI source of bleeding; however, nasal or other trauma may cause further bleeding.

## DIAGNOSTIC TESTS & INTERPRETATION
### Lab
- CBC with differential
- Basic metabolic panel
- PT/INR, PTT
- Urinalysis (eg, hematuria suggests Goodpasture or pulmonary-renal syndrome)
- Febrile patient or suspected infectious etiology:
  - Blood cultures
  - Sputum culture and gram/acid-fast/potassium hydroxide stain with cytology
- Hypotensive patient (criteria for massive hemoptysis):
  - Type and cross
  - Complete metabolic (liver and renal function) panel
  - Coagulation profile:
    - Fibrin and fibrinogen degradation products (FDP) or antithrombin III if disseminated IV coagulation suspected
- Pediatric patient:
  - Consider sweat-chloride test if cystic fibrosis is suspected.

### Imaging
- CXR:
  - Characterizes pathology (eg, tumor, cavity, effusion, infiltrate, pneumothorax)
  - Early pulmonary hemorrhage may present as infiltrate.
  - ~20% will be normal.

- CT:
  - High-resolution CT has become gold standard for diagnosing bronchiectasis.
  - Ideal study for stable patients with hemoptysis and a normal CXR
  - Can predict active TB by detecting cavitary lesions and acinar nodules
  - Higher sensitivity for peripheral tumors that may not be apparent on bronchoscopy
- Ventilation-perfusion or pulmonary arteriography if PE is suspected. VQ scan has limited utility if x-ray is abnormal.

### Diagnostic Procedures/Surgery
Bronchoscopy:

- Allows direct visualization of tumors, foreign bodies, granulomas, and infiltration
- Valuable for collecting bronchial secretions for cytology and histology
- Limited diagnostic yield in lesions outside the bronchial wall, distal to bronchial stenosis or occlusion, or peripheral lesions.

## DIFFERENTIAL DIAGNOSIS
Pseudohemoptysis:

- Epistaxis
- Pharyngeal bleeding
- GI bleeding

# TREATMENT

## PRE-HOSPITAL
- Respiratory and contact precautions
- Airway management:
  - Oxygen
  - Suctioning as needed
  - Endotracheal Intubation if airway compromised, severe respiratory distress, or hypoxemia
- Dual large-bore IV access
- Volume resuscitation as needed
- Continuous pulse oximetry, close hemodynamic and cardiac monitoring

## INITIAL STABILIZATION/THERAPY
- Airway and breathing:
  - Endotracheal intubation for impending respiratory failure
  - >8 Fr endotracheal tube to facilitate suctioning and subsequent bronchoscopy
  - Selective intubation of nonbleeding lung with single- or double-lumen endotracheal tubes may be required.
  - Supplemental oxygen as needed
  - Continuous pulse oximetry and cardiac monitoring
- Massive hemoptysis:
  - Principal risk to life is asphyxiation, not exsanguination
  - Maintain dual large-bore IV access.
  - Volume resuscitation with crystalloid or type specific blood as needed

## ED TREATMENT/PROCEDURES
- Antibiotic therapy if infiltrate present on CXR
- Correct hypoxemia and/or coagulopathy.
- If massive hemoptysis:
  - Large-bore IV or central access with volume resuscitation and blood products as needed
  - Early involvement of pulmonary, anesthesiology, interventional radiology and/or thoracic surgery
  - Patient should be positioned upright, or with side of hemorrhage in most dependent position.
  - Intubation for airway protection, impending respiratory failure, or to facilitate bronchoscopic evaluation
  - Endobronchial tamponade with Foley or Fogarty (<4 Fr) catheter, or double-lumen endotracheal tube (temporary measures)
  - Bronchial artery embolization (success rates reported as high as 98%); rebleeding presents in 20% of cases
  - Surgery:
    ○ Lobectomy or pneumonectomy if unsuccessful embolization or in presence of thoracic aneurysm, trauma, or arteriovenous malformation
    ○ Surgical resection is most effective for patients with localized lesions and adequate cardiopulmonary reserve.

## MEDICATION
Refer to specific etiology

# FOLLOW-UP

## DISPOSITION
### Admission Criteria
- ICU:
  - Intubation
  - Massive hemoptysis Hemodynamic instability
  - Hypovolemic shock
  - Severe or refractory hypoxemia
  - Impending respiratory failure
  - Impending airway compromise
- General ward:
  - Mild hemoptysis
  - TB (isolation)
  - Stable foreign body
  - Lung abscess
  - Cavitary lung disease

### Discharge Criteria
- Hemodynamically stable
- Mild hemoptysis
- No coagulopathy
- No supplemental oxygen requirement
- History of chronic stable hemoptysis
- Discharge with cough suppressants (benzonatate, codeine)
- Close follow-up

### Issues for Referral
- PCP within 7–10 days
- Specialist if etiology warrants referral

## FOLLOW-UP RECOMMENDATIONS
- Council patient not to smoke.
- The patient should avoid herbal medicines that may increase the risk of bleeding such as garlic, gingko, or ginseng.
- The patient should seek care immediately for:
  - Shortness of breath
  - Chest pain
  - Severe dizziness on standing
  - Fainting

# PEARLS AND PITFALLS

- Consider early airway management as clinical picture warrants.
- If severe unilateral hemorrhage with hypoxemia, place patient "bad lung" down
- Bronchial artery embolization can be very effective. Discuss case early with IR.

# ADDITIONAL READING

- Bidwell J, Pachner R. Hemoptysis: Diagnosis and management. *Am Fam Physician*. 2005;72(7): 1253–1260.
- Cahill B, Inghar D. Massive hemoptysis: Assessment and management. *Clin Chest Med*. 1994;15(1): 147–167.
- Coss-Bu JA, Sachdeva RC. Hemoptysis: A 10-year retrospective study. *Pediatrics*. 1997;100(3):7e–7.
- Jean-Baptiste E. Clinical assessment and management of massive hemoptysis. *Crit Care Med*. 2000;28:1642–1647.
- Hirschberg B, Biran I, et al. Hemoptysis: Etiology, evaluation, and outcome in a tertiary referral hospital. *Chest*.1997;112:440–444.
- Sirajuddin A, Mohammed TL. A 44-year-old man with hemoptysis: A review of pertinent imaging studies and radiographic interventions. *Cleve Clin J Med*. 2008;75(8):601–607.

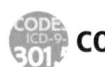 CODES

ICD9
786.3 Hemoptysis

# HEMORRHAGIC FEVERS

*David A. Tanen*

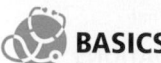

## BASICS

### DESCRIPTION
Hemorrhagic fevers are a group of illnesses that are caused by several distinct families of viruses. Viral hemorrhagic fever is used to describe a severe multisystem syndrome.

### RISK FACTORS
- Travel in endemic region
- Biologic warfare
- Exposure to pathogens via animal or insect bite or ingestion

### PATHOPHYSIOLOGY
- Viral hemorrhagic fevers cause endothelial damage and increase vascular permeability, hemorrhage, and hypovolemic shock.
- Disseminated intravascular coagulation (DIC) appears to be regular feature of Marburg and Crimean-Congo hemorrhagic fever but is less frequent with *Arenavirus* infections.
- Dengue hemorrhagic fever is thought to be immune mediated and is usually the result of secondary infection.

### ETIOLOGY
- Infection with RNA viruses that have zoonotic life cycles in specific geographic areas
- Short incubation period (<10–21 days)
- Examples of viral hemorrhagic fevers include the following:
  - Filoviruses: Fruit bat reservoir, unclear mode of transmission:
    ○ Ebola
    ○ Marburg
  - Arenaviruses: Rodent reservoir, transmitted via inhalation of aerosolized virus in rodent excreta:
    ○ Lassa
    ○ South American hemorrhagic fevers
  - Flaviviruses: Human reservoir, transmitted via mosquito:
    ○ Dengue hemorrhagic fever
    ○ Yellow fever
  - Bunyaviridae: Small mammal reservoir, transmitted via mosquitoes or ticks:
    ○ Rift Valley fever
    ○ Crimean-Congo hemorrhagic fever
  - Hantavirus: Rodent reservoir, transmitted via inhalation of aerosolized virus in rodent excreta:
    ○ Hemorrhagic fever with renal syndrome

### ALERT
- These viruses represent a potential biowarfare threat:
  - Highly infectious by aerosol (with exception of dengue)
  - Associated with high morbidity and in some cases high mortality
  - Replicate well in cell culture, which permits weaponization

## DIAGNOSIS

### SIGNS AND SYMPTOMS
- Most common (>50%) symptoms:
  - Acute febrile illness
  - Malaise
  - Headache
  - Nausea/vomiting
  - Flushing
  - Diarrhea (nonbloody)
  - Abdominal pain
  - Myalgias
- Less common (<30%) symptoms:
  - Gingival hemorrhage
  - Conjunctival injection/hemorrhage
  - Petechia
  - Hematemesis
  - Melena
  - Epistaxis
- Delayed presentations (>3 days into disease):
  - As above with hemorrhagic symptoms becoming more prominent
- Bleeding from gums, nose, lungs, GI tract, or uterus:
  - Exanthems
- Marburg and Ebola: Nonpruritic centripetal, papular, erythematous eruption appearing between days 5 and 7, which then coalesce into well-demarcated macules that may be hemorrhagic
- Yellow fever: Jaundice
- Dengue: Bright maculopapular truncal erythroderma that blanches dramatically under light pressure:
  - Shock
  - Seizures
  - Coma

### History
- Travel to endemic regions
- Sick contacts
- Unusual spread or numbers of a rare disease should raise concerns of a bioweapon attack

### Physical Exam
- Protection of health care workers:
  - Universal blood and body precautions
- Hemorrhage:
  - Conjunctival or gingival
  - Petechiae
  - Hematemesis
  - Melena
  - Epistaxis
- Exanthems:
  - Marburg and Ebola: Nonpruritic centripetal, papular
- Yellow fever: Jaundice
- Dengue: Bright maculopapular truncal erythroderma that blanches dramatically under light pressure

## ESSENTIAL WORKUP
- Focus on differentiating from other acute febrile illnesses, especially in the traveler.
- Recognize possible biologic attack when unusual number of patients present with similar and/or unusual findings.
- History to identify potential pathogen:
  - Include recent travel, illnesses, or other sources of exposure.

### DIAGNOSTIC TESTS & INTERPRETATION
*Lab*
- CBC:
  - May see leukocytosis or leukopenia, thrombocytopenia
- Electrolytes, BUN, creatinine, and glucose levels:
  - Look for renal failure
- Liver function tests:
  - Hepatic involvement is common, but jaundice occurs mainly with Yellow fever.
- Prothrombin time, partial thromboplastin time, and d-dimer tests:
  - Look for coagulopathy and DIC (seen in Crimean-Congo hemorrhagic fever, Ebola, and Marburg)
- Special lab test:
  - In specialized laboratories (biohazard level 4), definitive diagnosis can be made by viral isolation, real-time reverse transcriptase polymerase chain reaction (RT-PCR), and immunohistochemistry techniques:
    ○ Coordinated with CDC
    ○ Thick and thin smears to help differentiate from malaria

*Imaging*
CXR, head, and abdominal CT scanning:
- Rule out pneumonia
- Intracranial and intra-abdominal bleeding

*Diagnostic Procedures/Surgery*
Serum and saliva can be analyzed by RT-PCR in specialized laboratories.

### DIFFERENTIAL DIAGNOSIS
- Malaria:
  - A concern for traveler with fever
- Dengue fever:
  - Common source of fever in traveler
- Rickettsial:
  - Rocky Mountain spotted fever
  - Typhus
- Bacterial:
  - Meningococcemia
  - Sepsis
- Systemic disease:
  - Leukemia
  - Thrombotic thrombocytopenic purpura
- Pit viper envenomation

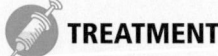

## TREATMENT

### PRE-HOSPITAL

#### ALERT
- Any place in the world can now be reached within significantly shorter time than incubation period of almost all infectious diseases.
- Early detection of viral hemorrhagic fever, natural, or biologic attack is key to control an outbreak.
- Most cases will derive from patients who traveled to or had contact with persons from parts of the world where the viruses are endemic.

### INITIAL STABILIZATION/THERAPY
Protection of health care workers:
- Universal blood and body precautions
- Isolation of patient
- Use of protective clothing plus HEPA-filtered respirators to minimize exposure to aerosols for those involved in procedures such as suctioning, catheter placement, and wound dressing

### ED TREATMENT/PROCEDURES
- Supportive therapy
- Empiric therapy with antimalarial regimens until definitive diagnosis is obtained
- Aggressive treatment of secondary infections
- Bleeding is usually mild, and life-threatening loss of blood is rare:
  – If indicated, hemorrhage can be managed by replacement of blood, platelets, and clotting factors.
- Aggressive support for shock:
  – Patients are often hypovolemic because of 3rd spacing and hemorrhage, but may readily develop pulmonary edema with crystalloid infusion.
- Ribavirin—a synthetic nucleoside:
  Useful for Lassa, South American hemorrhagic fever, Crimean-Congo hemorrhagic fever, and hemorrhagic fever with renal syndrome; ineffective against filoviruses
  – Causes a reversible hemolytic anemia
- Transfusion of immune plasma (convalescent plasma therapy) for South American hemorrhagic fever within 1st week of symptoms

### MEDICATION
- Ribavirin:
  – IV loading dose of 33 mg/kg followed by 16 mg/kg q6h for 4 days, then 8 mg/kg q8h for 3 days
  – Prophylactic 500 mg by mouth q6h for 7 days
- Vaccines:
  – Yellow fever is widely available.
  – South American hemorrhagic fever, Rift Valley fever, Hantavirus, Dengue, and Ebola/Marburg are under development.
- Other medications under investigation:
  – Nucleoside analog inhibitors of S-adenosylhomocysteine hydrolase inhibit Ebola replication in mice.
  – Zidampidine—a derivative of AZT—increases survival of mice infected with Lassa virus

#### First Line
- Ribavirin
- Antimalarials

#### Second Line
Contact the CDC about experimental vaccines and antivirals for postexposure prophylaxis (770) 488-7100 or (800) 311-3435 for all suspected cases.

## FOLLOW-UP

### DISPOSITION

#### Admission Criteria
Suspected cases of viral hemorrhagic fever:
- Isolation precautions
- ICU for signs of shock or multiorgan system failure

#### Discharge Criteria
None—if you suspect viral hemorrhagic fever, the patient needs to be isolated and the CDC notified

### FOLLOW-UP RECOMMENDATIONS
Consider experimental postexposure prohylaxis for staff and patient contacts that may include antivirals and vaccines. Coordinate with the CDC at (770) 488-7100 or (800) 311-3435.

## PEARLS AND PITFALLS
- Consider hemorrhagic viruses in your differential diagnosis when caring for a sick patient returning from endemic regions of the world
- Employ universal precautions and isolation to minimize the spread of the disease
- Contact the CDC at (770) 488-7100 or (800) 311-3435 for all suspected cases.

## ADDITIONAL READING
- Jeffs B. A clinical guide to viral hemorrhagic fevers: Ebola, Marburg and Lassa. *Trop Doct.* 2006;36:1–4.
- Pigott DC. Hemorrhagic fever viruses. *Crit Care Clin.* 2005;21:765–783.
- Mahanty S, Bray M. Pathogenesis of filoviral haemorrhagic fevers. *Lancet Infect Dis.* 2004;4:487–498.
- Franz DR, Jahrling PB, Friedlander AM, et al. Clinical recognition and management of patients exposed to biological warfare agents. *JAMA.* 1997;278: 399–411.

### See Also (Topic, Algorithm, Electronic Media Element)
- Dengue Fever
- Disseminated Intravascular Coagulation
- Hemorrhagic Shock
- Malaria
- Meningococcemia

## CODES

ICD9
- 065.4 Mosquito-borne hemorrhagic fever
- 065.9 Arthropod-borne hemorrhagic fever, unspecified
- 078.7 Arenaviral hemorrhagic fever

H

# HEMORRHAGIC SHOCK
*Theodore C. Chan*

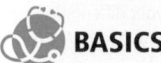 **BASICS**

## DESCRIPTION
- Loss of effective circulating blood volume resulting in inadequate organ perfusion
- Blood loss exceeds ability to compensate and tissue and organ perfusion decrease. At the tissue level, hypoperfusion leads to inadequate oxygenation, anaerobic metabolism, cell death.
- Compensated shock:
  - Patient's physiologic reserve prevents significant alteration in vital signs.
- Decompensated shock:
  - Loss of circulating volume overcomes patient's physiologic reserve, resulting in signification alteration in vital signs.
- Blood loss estimate:
  - Total blood volume ~7% of ideal body weight (4,900 mL in 70 kg adult) or 70 mL/kg
  - Multiply 70 mL/kg times body weight (kg) times percentage loss as determined by class of hemorrhage.

## RISK FACTORS
- Trauma
- Chronic or acute illness
- Physical anomalies
- Medications (anticoagulants)
- Genetics:
  - Arteriovenous malformations
  - Bleeding disorders
  - Other genetic anomalies

## ETIOLOGY
- Trauma—penetrating and blunt:
  - Abdominal:
    - Splenic injury (40% of abdominal hemorrhage)
    - Liver injury (20% of abdominal hemorrhage)
  - Chest:
    - Hemothorax
    - Aorta or great vessel injury
  - Pelvis:
    - Pelvic fracture with vascular injury
- Vascular malformations:
  - May lead to thoracic, intraperitoneal, or retroperitoneal bleeding
  - Aneurysms:
    - Abdominal aortic aneurysm most common
    - Mycotic aneurysm secondary to endocarditis
  - Aortogastric fistula
  - Arteriovenous malformations
- Abortion: Complete, partial, or inevitable
- Ectopic pregnancy
- Epistaxis
- Fractures (especially pelvis and long bones)
- GI bleeding
- Hemoptysis
- Malignancies
- Mallory-Weiss tear
- Placenta previa
- Postpartum hemorrhage
- Retroperitoneal bleeds
- Splenic rupture
- Vascular injuries

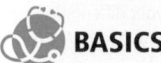 **DIAGNOSIS**

## SIGNS AND SYMPTOMS
- Class I hemorrhage: Loss of up to 15% of blood volume (up to 750 mL in 70-kg adult):
  - HR <100
  - BP normal
  - Respiratory rate (RR) 14–20
  - Increased or normal pulse pressure
  - Slight anxiety
- Class II hemorrhage: Loss of 15–30% of blood volume (750–1,500 mL):
  - Tachycardia: HR >100
  - BP normal, or slightly low systolic BP
  - Tachypnea: RR 20–30
  - Narrowed pulse pressure
  - Mild anxiety
  - Small decrease in urine output
- Class III hemorrhage: Loss of 30–40% of blood volume (1,500–2,000 mL):
  - Marked Tachycardia: HR >120
  - Hypotension: BP decreased
  - Marked Tachypnea: RR 30–40
  - Marked narrowing of pulse pressure
  - Significant change in mental status: Confusion
  - Delayed capillary refill
  - Marked decrease in urine output
- Class IV hemorrhage: Loss of >40% of blood volume (>2,000 mL):
  - HR >140
  - Marked hypotension: BP decreased
  - RR >35
  - Very narrow pulse pressure
  - Depressed mental status: Confusion, lethargy, loss of consciousness
  - Negligible urine output
  - Cold and pale skin

### Pediatric Considerations
- Children often have greater physiologic reserve than adults and can preserve normal vital signs longer.
- Systemic responses to blood loss in the pediatric patient include:
  - Volume loss <25%: Weak, thready pulse and tachycardia; lethargy, irritability, and confusion; cool, clammy skin; decreased urine output/increased urine specific gravity
  - Volume loss 25–40%: Tachycardia; marked change in consciousness; dulled response to pain; cyanotic, cold extremities with decreased capillary refill; minimal urine output
  - Volume loss >40%: Hypotension, tachycardia, or bradycardia; comatose; pale, cold skin; no urine output

### Pregnancy Considerations
Physiologic maternal hypervolemia requires greater blood loss to manifest maternal perfusion abnormalities which may result in decreased fetal perfusion.

### Geriatric Considerations
Underlying disease and medications may alter responses to hemorrhage and blood loss.

### History
Thorough health and past medical history:
- Underlying disease, risk factors, age
- Medications
- Trauma

### Physical Exam
- Complete physical exam to determine shock class category and assess for hemorrhage source
- Vital signs including HR, RR, BP
- Temperature
- Mental status (anxiety, confusion, lethargy, obtundation, coma)
- Capillary refill and skin perfusion
- Pulse pressure
- Abdominal examination
- Pelvic/rectal exam for bleeding as indicated

## ESSENTIAL WORKUP
- Thorough history and physical examination
- IV access for resuscitation
- Hemoglobin and hematocrit levels
- Blood type and cross-match

## DIAGNOSTIC TESTS & INTERPRETATION
### Lab
- CBC
- Blood type and cross-match
- Coagulation studies:
  - PT, PTT
  - International normalized ratio
- Other measures of tissue hypoperfusion:
  - Arterial blood gas
  - Base deficit
  - Serum lactate level
  - Serum electrolytes
- Pregnancy test/b-HCG

### Imaging
- CXR:
  - Hemothorax:
    - Blunt chest injuries
    - Thoracic arteriovenous malformation
- Pelvic radiograph for possible occult fracture
- Focused Abdominal Sonography for Trauma (FAST exam):
  - Abdominal trauma
  - Possible abdominal aortic aneurysm
  - Nontraumatic intraperitoneal hemorrhage
  - Fluid in Morrison's pouch implies significant hemorrhage or ascites.
  - Negative findings do not rule out intraperitoneal hemorrhage.
- Endovaginal US:
  - Positive pregnancy test
  - Fluid in the cul-de-sac
  - Ectopic pregnancy
- Abdominal CT scan (once patient stable):
  - Detects both intraperitoneal and retroperitoneal hemorrhage
  - Abdominal aortic aneurysm

### Diagnostic Procedures/Surgery
* Insert Foley catheter:
  - Monitor urine output.
* Nasogastric tube:
  - For undifferentiated hypovolemic shock to rule out GI hemorrhage
* Diagnostic peritoneal lavage:
  - For unstable trauma patients when US fails to show intraperitoneal hemorrhage
* Endoscopy:
  - In the setting of upper or lower GI bleeding
* Angiography:
  - Pelvic fracture
  - Retroperitoneal hemorrhage
  - Lower GI bleeding
  - Embolization therapy for bleeding from arterial sources can be performed.

## DIFFERENTIAL DIAGNOSIS
* Cardiac tamponade
* Tension pneumothorax
* Cardiogenic shock
* Sepsis
* Adrenal insufficiency
* Neurogenic shock

 TREATMENT

* The goal is to restore organ perfusion with fluids and to control source of hemorrhage. Controversy exists as to whether aggressive fluid resuscitation can increase bleeding risk
* Approach is to balance goal of organ perfusion and risks of rebleeding and may vary with type of patient:
  - In blunt trauma patients, maintenance of BP may take precedence to reduce risk of traumatic brain injury
  - In penetrating trauma patients with hemorrhage, delayed aggressive fluid resuscitation until definitive control may reduce bleeding risk

## PRE-HOSPITAL
* Rapid assessment and transport to appropriate care center
* IV access and fluid resuscitation are standard, though delaying aggressive fluid resuscitation may be warranted in cases of penetrating trauma with hemorrhage.

## INITIAL STABILIZATION/THERAPY
* Airway and breathing:
  - Intubation as indicated by patient's respiratory and mental status
  - 100% oxygen via face mask should be administered.
* Circulation:
  - 2 large-bore peripheral IV lines (16-gauge or larger)
  - Central venous line or venous cutdown (saphenous) may be necessary.
  - Intraosseous route may be considered
  - Aggressive crystalloid resuscitation
  - 1-to-1 rule: For 1 unit volume of blood loss, give 3 volumes of crystalloid.

* Early transfusion class III or IV hemorrhage:
  - Type-specific and cross-matched blood is preferred when time permits, often 1 hr.
  - Type-specific blood is usually available within 10–15 min.
* Type O blood can be used in immediate, life-threatening situations (type O Rh-negative blood only for women of child-bearing age).

## ED TREATMENT/PROCEDURES
* Place patient on continuous monitor.
* NPO status, strict bed rest
* Control hemorrhage (direct pressure, pelvic fixation/stabilization, etc.).
* Central venous access may be indicated for CVP monitoring, but placement of such lines should not interfere with resuscitation measures.
* Continually reassess patient for clinical response/deterioration:
  - Vital signs, mental status, and urine output.
  - Follow serial blood gas, lactate level, and hemoglobin/hematocrit measurements.
  - Maintain urine output at 50 mL/hr.
* Response to initial fluid resuscitation is the key to determining subsequent therapy:
  - Rapid response to fluid indicates minimal (<20%) blood loss.
  - Transient response to volume resuscitation indicates ongoing hemorrhage or inadequate resuscitation; continue fluid and blood administration and rapidly obtain necessary studies and consultations.
  - Minimal or no response to volume resuscitation indicates ongoing severe blood loss; immediate angiography or surgical intervention is warranted.
* Use fluids warmed (~39°C [102.2°F]) by microwave ovens, fluid warmers.
* Transfuse platelets and coagulation factors as indicated.
* Consider autotransfusion devices with tube thoracostomy treatment and decompression of large hemothoraces.
* Specialty consultation and additional procedures (surgery) as indicated by cause and source of hemorrhagic shock

### Pediatric Considerations
* Access may be obtained by intraosseous route after 1 or 2 unsuccessful attempts at peripheral access.
* Maintain urine output at 1 mL/kg/hr for children and 2 mL/kg/hr for infants.

### Pregnancy Considerations
Optimizing perfusion and treatment of the mother is treatment of choice for fetus.

## MEDICATION
### First Line
* IV Fluids:
  - Crystalloids: NS or lactated Ringer
  - Adults: 1- to 2-L bolus
  - Pediatric: 20 mL/kg bolus:
    ○ Reassess for clinical response/deterioration.

* Blood products: Cross-matched, type-specific, O-positive, or O-negative:
  - O-negative should be reserved for women of child-bearing age
  - Adult: Initiate with 4–6 units of packed RBCs.
  - Pediatric: 10 mL/kg of packed RBCs

### Second Line
* Other blood products:
  - Platelets
  - Coagulation factors, such as fresh frozen plasma and cryoprecipitate
* Individual coagulation factors (factor VII), Antifibrinolytic agents, Hemoglobin-based oxygen carriers, Perfluorocarbons:
  - Under study, but of no proven benefit

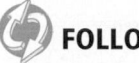 FOLLOW-UP

### DISPOSITION
#### Admission Criteria
All patients with hemorrhage should be admitted to the appropriate service.

#### Discharge Criteria
N/A.

#### Issues for Referral
N/A

## PEARLS AND PITFALLS
* Severity of hemorrhagic shock class and volume loss can be determined by vitals signs and careful physical examination.
* Fluid resuscitation should balance goal of restoring organ perfusion and potential risk of exacerbating bleeding before definitive control.
* Response to fluid resuscitation should guide subsequent therapy.

## ADDITIONAL READING
* American College of Surgeons, Committee on Trauma. *Advanced Trauma Life Support for Doctors*, 8th ed. Chicago: American College of Surgeons; 2008.
* Angele MK, Schneider CP, Chaudry IH. Bench-to-bedside review: Latest results in hemorrhagic shock. *Critical Care.* 2008;12:218–231.
* Cocchi MN, Kimlin E, Walsh M, et al. Identification and resuscitation of the trauma patient in shock. *Emerg Med Clin North Am.* 2007;25:623–642.
* Kortbeek JB, Al Turki SA, Ali J, et al. Advanced trauma life support, 8th edition, the evidence for change. *J Trauma.* 2008;64:1638–1650.

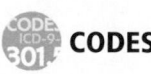 CODES

### ICD9
* 785.59 Other shock without mention of trauma
* 958.4 Traumatic shock
* 998.0 Postoperative shock, not elsewhere classified

H

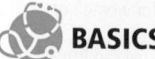
# HEMORRHOID
*Julia H. Sone*

## BASICS

### DESCRIPTION
- General:
  - Normal venous sinusoids of the distal rectum and proximal anal canal
  - Normal vascular cushions of anal canal that contribute to anal continence
  - Arteriovenous shunt system exists at the level of the internal hemorrhoids that accounts for the bright red blood per rectum
- When the hemorrhoids become symptomatic, hemorrhoid disease develops.
- Do not cause pain unless thrombosed or strangulated
- Discrete masses of thick submucosa contain:
  - Blood vessels
  - Smooth muscle
  - Elastic and connective tissue
- Sliding down of part of anal canal lining
- External hemorrhoids:
  - Vessels situated below dentate line
  - Covered by skin/anoderm
  - Drain to internal iliac veins
- Internal hemorrhoids:
  - Submucosal vessels above dentate lines
  - Drain to portal system
  - Usually at left lateral, right posterolateral, and right anterolateral positions
  - Grade 1: Painless, bleeding
  - Grade 2: Prolapse with bowel movement (BM), spontaneously reduce
  - Grade 3: Prolapse with BM, require manual reduction
  - Grade 4: Chronically prolapsed, not reducible

## ETIOLOGY
- Exact cause unknown
- Gravitational forces and abdominal pressure cause distention of the sinusoids
- Associated with straining and irregular bowel habits:
  - Hard, bulky stools or diarrhea cause tenesmus/straining.
  - Push anal cushions out of anal canal
  - Weaken submucosal tissue leading to prolapse
- Higher resting anal pressures:
  - Erect posture
- Heredity:
  - Absence of valves in veins
- Increased intra-abdominal pressure:
  - Ascites
  - Pregnancy
- Portal hypertension

##  DIAGNOSIS

### SIGNS AND SYMPTOMS
- Painless, rectal bleeding with defecation
- Blood on stool or toilet paper
- Bright red blood drips into toilet bowel
- Rectal discomfort or pressure
- Severe pain if:
  - Internal hemorrhoids prolapse and strangulate.
  - External hemorrhoids thrombose
- Pruritus ani
- May also have fissure

### History
- Length of bleeding:
  - Pain?
  - Duration?
- Any new lumps or masses by rectum?
- What is the stool consistency: Hard or liquid
- Is this a recurring problem?
- Are the stools pencil thin?

## Physical Exam
- Examination of perianal area:
  - Gently spread buttocks.
  - Discrete, dark blue, tender mass covered with skin: Thrombosed external hemorrhoid:
    - Can have internal component
  - Purplish, tender mucosal covered mass: Prolapsed, strangulated internal hemorrhoid:
    - Usually associated with enlarged, thrombosed external hemorrhoid
  - Have patient bear down to check for prolapsing hemorrhoids.
  - Digital rectal exam mandatory to rule out cancer
- Anoscopy to visualize anal canal:
  - Identify bleeding internal hemorrhoids.

### ESSENTIAL WORKUP
Detailed history with thorough anorectal examination

### DIAGNOSTIC TESTS & INTERPRETATION
#### Lab
- CBC if history of significant blood loss:
  - Hemoglobin/hematocrit
- Platelet count
- PT/PTT/INR if patient on anticoagulants or severe co-morbid condition

### DIFFERENTIAL DIAGNOSIS
- Rectal prolapse
- Anal fissure
- Perirectal abscess/fistula
- Condyloma acuminate
- Carcinoma

## 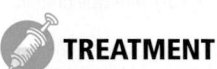 TREATMENT

### PRE-HOSPITAL
Establish IV access if sever bleeding

### INITIAL STABILIZATION/THERAPY
Direct digital pressure to control bleeding

## ED TREATMENT/PROCEDURES
- Conservative therapy for all patients:
  - Hot sitz baths for 15 min t.i.d. and after each bowel movement
  - High-fiber diet—30 g/d:
    ○ Eat more fresh fruits and vegetables.
    ○ Increase bran intake.
  - 10–12 glasses of water per day
  - Stool softeners
  - Bulk-forming laxatives
- NSAIDS: Analgesic and anti-inflammatory effects
- Excise thrombosed external hemorrhoid if severe pain, <5 days old and clot not resolving:
  - Follow with conservative therapy.
  - Place patient in prone jackknife position or left lateral decubitus and tape buttocks apart
  - Infiltrate surrounding skin and underneath clot using 27-gauge needle with lidocaine-containing epinephrine.
  - Make an elliptical incision to excise clot/skin.
  - May need silver nitrate sticks for hemostasis
  - Place a small piece of Gelfoam and/or gauze onto the wound and tape.
  - Remove dressing at time of 1st sitz bath in about 6 hr
  - Give analgesics:
    ○ Nonsteroidal anti-inflammatory drugs (NSAIDs)
    ○ Acetaminophen
    ○ Lidocaine 5% ointment to anus: Topical anesthetic for pain relief
    ○ 0.2% topical nitroglycerin ointment to anus—decreases pain by inhibiting sphincter spasm
- Manually reduce nonthrombosed, prolapsed internal hemorrhoids:
  - Follow with conservative therapy. May need topical anesthetic or anal sphincter block with local anesthesia
  - Can sclerose bleeding internal hemorrhoids with 2.5% sodium morrhuate or 3% hypertonic saline
  - Can rubber band ligate 1 or 2 internal hemorrhoids:
    ○ Avoid in immunocompromised patients due to perineal sepsis
- Nonreducible internal hemorrhoids:
  - Nonstrangulated: Conservative management and surgical referral
  - Strangulated: Immediate surgical referral for excision

### Pregnancy Considerations
Usually become symptomatic in the 3rd trimester and can be treated conservatively.
Do not use analpram-HC (class C)

## MEDICATION
- Acetaminophen: 325–650 mg (peds: 15 mg/kg) with codeine 15–30 mg (peds: 0.5 mg/kg) PO q4h PRN
- Bran/fiber: 20 g PO daily
- Docusate sodium (Colace): 50–200 mg (peds: <3 yr, 10–40 mg/d; 3–6 yr, 20–60 mg/d; >6–12 yr, 40–150 mg/d) PO q12h
- ELA-Max 5 (5% lidocaine anorectal cream): Apply to perianal area q4h PRN pain (peds: not for <12 yr of age).
- Hydrocortisone/pramoxine topical (Analpram-HC) 1%/1% cream; 2.5%/1% cream/lotion (peds: Same dosing) apply to area t.i.d.–q.i.d.
- Hydrocortisone/lidocaine topical (AnaMantle HC) 0.5%/3% cream; 2.5%/3% gel (peds: Not indicated) apply to anal canal b.i.d..
- Ibuprofen (Motrin): 400–600 mg (peds: 10 mg/kg/d) PO q6h
- Nitroglycerin 0.2% ointment: Apply to area t.i.d. with cotton-tipped applicator
- Psyllium seeds: 1–2 tsp (peds: 0.25–1 tsp/d) PO q24h

 **FOLLOW-UP**

## DISPOSITION
### Admission Criteria
- Strangulated grade 4 hemorrhoids:
  - Surgical consult for prolapsed, thrombosed internal hemorrhoids
- Severe anemia with bleeding hemorrhoids
- Severe bleeding hemorrhoid in pt on anticoagulation or with portal hypertension

### Discharge Criteria
Most patients will go home
### Issues for Referral
Surgical referral for:
- Grade 3 or 4 internal hemorrhoids
- Suspected anorectal or colonic tumors, inflammatory bowel disease, coagulopathy, pregnancy, or immunocompromised

## FOLLOW-UP RECOMMENDATIONS
- Colorectal follow up for grade 3 or 4 internal hemorrhoids or suspected tumor
- Primary care follow-up for uncomplicated hemorrhoids.

### ALERT
All patients with bright red blood per rectum should be referred to GI or Colorectal surgery to r/o malignancy

## PEARLS AND PITFALLS
Hemorrhoids are not the only cause of anorectal pain and bleeding. Investigate for other etiologies when indicated.

## ADDITIONAL READING
- Sack J. Pathophysiology of hemorrhoidal disease. *Semin Colon Rectal Surg.* 2003;14(2):93–99.
- Wexner SD, Pemberton JH, Beck DE, et al., eds. *The ASCRS Textbook of Colon and Rectal Surgery.* New York: Springer; 2007.

### See Also (Topic, Algorithm, Electronic Media Element)
- Anal Fissure

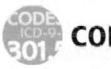 **CODES**

### ICD9
455.6 Unspecified hemorrhoids without mention of complication

# HEMOTHORAX

*Anthony C. Salazar*

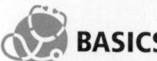 **BASICS**

## DESCRIPTION

- Accumulation of blood in the intrapleural space after blunt/penetrating chest trauma or other nontraumatic etiology. Bleeding is usually a result of disruption of the tissues/vessels of the chest wall, pleura, or intrathoracic structures:
  - Results in decreased vital capacity, hypoxia, and respiratory compromise.
  - Loss of large intravascular volume results in hemodynamic instability and hemorrhagic shock.
  - Massive hemothorax can cause increased intrathoracic pressure, resulting in compromised venous return and decreased cardiac output.
- Rarely a solitary finding in blunt trauma:
  - Commonly associated with pneumothorax (25% of cases), extrathoracic injuries (73% of cases), and pulmonary contusion.
- Large hemothoraces cause the release of substances that can act as anticoagulants and contribute to continued intrathoracic bleeding.
- If left untreated, can lead to empyema and fibrothorax (lung trapping due to adhesions).

## ETIOLOGY

- Traumatic injuries (including iatrogenic) to major blood vessels:
  - Common vessels, including intercostal artery, internal mammary artery, pulmonary artery, pulmonary vein, aorta, vena cava, and heart are associated with hemorrhage into the thoracic cavity.
- Traumatic lung parenchymal injuries:
  - Often stops spontaneously as a result of low pulmonary pressures and high concentrations of thromboplastin in the lung.
  - Often associated with pneumothorax.
- Nontraumatic or spontaneous hemothoraces:
  - Very rare.
  - Consider coagulation disorder, malignancy, primary vascular event (such as aortic dissection, ruptured aneurysm), PE with infarction, infection (TB), bullous emphysema, pulmonary AV malformation, lobar sequestration.
- Torn pleural adhesions as a complication of spontaneous pneumothorax or tube thoracostomy

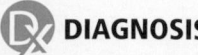 **DIAGNOSIS**

## SIGNS AND SYMPTOMS

- Small amount of blood in thorax (<400 mL): Little or no change in patient's appearance, vital signs, or physical findings
- Large amount of blood (>1,000 mL): Restlessness, anxiety, pallor, pleuritic chest pain, hemoptysis, dyspnea, or air hunger:
  - Signs of shock with loss of blood volume $\geq$30% (1,500–2,000 mL).
  - Tachycardia, tachypnea, hypotension.
- With insidious onset (ie, malignancy): Dyspnea is most common presenting sign since blood loss is usually not acute enough to produce a visible hemodynamic response.

### History

- Acute blunt or penetrating trauma to chest
- Recent rib fracture or flail chest
- Delayed hemothorax can occur hours to days later without initial evidence of intrathoracic pathology on CXR; may be related to rupture of chest wall hematoma or disruption of intercostal vessels by rib fracture edges during movement
- Malignancy or metastatic disease
- Recent surgical procedure: Thoracentesis, thoracostomy, etc.

### Physical Exam

- Vitals signs: Depending on severity and time course, hypoxia, tachypnea, tachycardia, and hypotension maybe seen.
- Neck: JVD if increased intrathoracic pressure, tracheal deviation
- Chest inspection: Asymmetric expansion, gross deformity, paradoxical wall movement, abrasion, hematoma, and contusion
- Chest wall palpation: Tenderness or crepitus over ribs, clavicles, scapulae, or the sternum; subcutaneous emphysema, dullness to percussion
- Auscultation: Decreased or absent breath sounds over ipsilateral side (best appreciated in the upright patient)

## ESSENTIAL WORKUP

CXR is the ideal diagnostic tool:

- In the hemodynamically stable patient, upright posteroanterior (PA) projection at full inspiration is optimal:
  - Fluid collections >200–300 mL can usually be seen on upright or decubitus CXR.
  - In a normal unscarred pleural space, fluid will be noted as a meniscus/fluid level blunting the costophrenic angle.
- In the supine anteroposterior (AP) radiograph (ie, portable), up to 1,000 mL of blood may not be readily apparent:
  - Only a slight hazy infiltrate over the involved hemithorax maybe seen.
- Look for associated injuries (pneumothorax, rib fractures, pulmonary contusion, widened mediastinum, etc.) when reading chest radiography.

## DIAGNOSTIC TESTS & INTERPRETATION

### Lab

- Hematocrit may be helpful if it shows a drop or changes on serial evaluations.
- Type and cross-match.
- Pulse oximetry, ABG
- Pleural fluid removed should reveal a hematocrit >50% of the blood hematocrit.

### Imaging

- US diagnostic imaging is a valuable tool in the evaluation of intrapleural fluid collection:
  - An extended FAST scan can diagnose hemothorax with a higher sensitivity than a portable CXR in trained hands.
- CT is useful in detecting small amounts of intrapleural fluid not visible on the chest radiograph.

## DIFFERENTIAL DIAGNOSIS

- Hemopneumothorax
- Pneumothorax
- Pulmonary contusion
- Pleural effusion
- Empyema/pneumonia

## TREATMENT

### PRE-HOSPITAL
- Assess vital signs and pulse oximetry; administer oxygen and obtain IV access.
- Fluid resuscitation as needed for hypotension
- Cautions:
  - Difficult to differentiate hemothoraces from pneumothoraces clinically:
    - All may present with dyspnea, pleuritic chest pain, decreased breath sounds, and hemodynamic instability.
    - Certain clues aid in making the diagnosis, such as subcutaneous emphysema for pneumothorax and dullness to percussion for hemothorax.
  - Perform needle thoracostomy for potential tension pneumothorax if the patient is hemodynamically unstable.

### INITIAL STABILIZATION/THERAPY
- Manage airway, breathing, circulation:
  - Control airway as needed; endotracheal intubation for patients with impending respiratory failure
  - Supplemental oxygen
  - 2 large-bore IV access sites and fluid bolus to restore circulating blood volume
    Needle thoracostomy should be performed in patients with hemodynamic instability unless chest tube kit is immediately available.
- Patient should be positioned to sit upright unless contraindicated.

### ED TREATMENT/PROCEDURES
- Obtain upright CXR as quickly as possible, but if patient unstable do not wait to administer definitive therapy.
- Hemothorax is treated by evacuating accumulated blood in the intrapleural space.
- Tube thoracostomy evacuates blood; allows for reexpansion of the lung, as well as constant monitoring of blood loss.
- Tube thoracostomy:
  - Use a large-bore chest tube (36–40 French).
  - Insert in the 4th-5th intercostal space at the mid-axillary line aiming posteriorly and superiorly.
    Tube is then connected to underwater seal drainage and suction (20–30 mL $H_2O$).
  - Correct placement and adequate drainage is confirmed via CXR.
- Autotransfusion should be used if available to replace blood loss.

- Indications for OR thoracotomy:
  - Initial tube drainage >20 mL/kg of blood (or 1,000 mL of blood for adults from the pleural cavity)
  - Persistent bleeding at a rate >7 mL/kg/h (or 200 mL/h for 4 hr)
  - Increasing hemothorax seen on chest radiography
  - Patient remains hypotensive despite adequate blood replacement and other sites of blood loss have been ruled out
  - Patient decompensates after initial response to resuscitation
- Indications for ED thoracotomy:
  - Penetrating trauma:
    - Traumatic arrest in the ED or within 10 min of ED arrival.
    - Severe shock with clinical signs of cardiac tamponade
  - Blunt trauma: Traumatic arrest in the ED at a trauma center or with surgeon available within 10 min

### MEDICATION
- Local anesthetics for cutaneous anesthesia prior to tube thoracostomy in awake, conscious patients
- Procedural sedation (midazolam) and analgesia (fentanyl) may be used for stable, awake patients prior to tube thoracostomy:
  - Fentanyl: Adult/peds: 2–5 $\mu$g/kg per dose
  - Midazolam: Adult/peds: 0.02–0.04 mg/kg per dose
  - Other sedative agents may be considered.

## FOLLOW-UP

### DISPOSITION
#### Admission Criteria
Patients with hemothoraces requiring tube thoracostomies should be admitted for monitoring and thoracostomy tube management to the trauma, cardiothoracic, or general surgery service. The admitting unit should be experienced in managing chest tube equipment.

#### Discharge Criteria
- Patients with isolated small hemothoraces (detected incidentally on US or CT imaging) may be considered for discharge after 4–6 hr of observation if there is no evidence of continued bleeding, the patient is not hypoxic, and is asymptomatic.
- Patients with asymptomatic blunt chest trauma and normal initial chest radiographs do not require repeat films prior to discharge.

## PEARLS AND PITFALLS
- Because the pleural cavity of an average 70 kg man can hold over 4 L of blood, an exsanguinating hemorrhage can occur without any evidence of external blood loss.
- Auscultation and percussion of a supine trauma patient with substantial hemothorax may produce equivocal findings due to distribution of blood along the entire posterior aspect of pleural space.
- Without a clear history of trauma, CXR may be incorrectly read as pneumonia.
- If there is a concurrent diaphragmatic injury, a hemothorax may have an intraabdominal origin.
- Prepare for autotransfusion early, as most blood loss occurs on initial chest tube insertion.
- In the supine trauma patient, a common error in chest tube insertion is placement too anterior and superior, making complete drainage difficult.
- Be sure all chest tube fenestrations are within the thoracic cavity.
- Prophylactic antibiotics administered with chest tube insertion do not decrease the risk of pneumonia or empyema.

## ADDITIONAL READING
- Ali HA, Lippmann M, Mundathaje U, et al. Spontaneous hemothorax: A comprehensive review. *Chest.* 2008;124(5):1056–1065.
- McEwan K, Thompson P. Ultrasound to detect haemothorax after chest injury. *Emerg Med J.* 2007;24(8):581–582.
- Parry GW, Morgan WE, Salama FD, Management of haemothorax. *Ann R Coll Surg Engl.* 1996;78(4):325–326.
- Vukich DJ, Markovchick V. Thoracic trauma. In: Rosen P, et al., eds. *Emergency Medicine: Concepts and Clinical Practice,* 6th ed. St. Louis, MO: Mosby; 2006:391–392.

## CODES

### ICD9
- 511.81 Malignant pleural effusion
- 511.89 Other specified forms of effusion, except tuberculous

H

# HENOCH SCHÖNLEIN PURPURA

*Mark A. Hostetler*

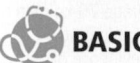 **BASICS**

## DESCRIPTION
Vasculitis

## ETIOLOGY
Mechanism:

- Increased serum IgA:
  - Circulating IgA complexes
  - Glomerular mesangial deposition of IgA
- Although cause is undefined, there are many associated conditions:
  - Infections
  - Group A strep
  - Mycoplasma
  - Viral: Varicella, Epstein-Barr (EB)
  - Drugs: Penicillin, tetracycline, aspirin, sulfonamides, erythromycin
  - Allergens: Insect bites, chocolate, milk, wheat
- Peak incidence: School-aged children and young adults
- More common in whites
- Males > Females
- Occurs more often in winter/spring
- Multisystem involvement can lead to life-threatening or long-term complications:
  - Intussusception
  - Proliferative glomerulonephritis
  - Chronic renal failure:
  - More common in older children and adults (13–14%)
  - Intracranial hemorrhage

## DIAGNOSIS

## SIGNS AND SYMPTOMS
- General:
  - Well-appearing child, despite nature and extent of rash
  - Recent or current upper respiratory tract infection
  - Malaise
  - Low-grade fever
  - Hypertension, if associated renal failure
  - Children <3 mo may have only skin manifestations.
- Skin:
  - Purpuric rash:
    - Presenting sign in 50% of patients
    - 100% of patients develop purpura
    - 1st appears as pink rounded papules that blanch
    - Progresses to 2–3 cm circular palpable purpura within 24 hr; may be discrete or confluent
    - Rash begins in gravity-dependent areas of legs and buttocks.
    - Symmetric distribution
    - May involve lower back
    - Rarely involves the face
    - Rash recurs in up to 40% of patients (within 6 wk).

- Abdominal:
  - Abdominal pain:
    - 70–80% of cases
    - Colicky to severe
    - Abdominal findings may precede the rash by 4 wk.
  - GI bleeding:
    - 75% of cases
    - Occult to severe blood loss
    - Intussusception (ileo-ileal or ileocolic)
- Renal-genitourinary:
  - Asymptomatic hematuria:
    - Occurs in 80% of cases
  - Scrotal pain
  - Testicular swelling
  - Renal failure
- Extremities:
  - Arthritis:
    - 70–80% of cases
    - Migratory periarticular pain
    - Most frequent in knees and ankles
    - Angioedema
- Neurologic:
  - Headache
  - Seizure
  - Focal deficits

### History
- Constitutional symptoms:
  - Fever
- Rash:
  - Location, timing, duration, and progression of rash
- Associated symptoms:
  - Abdominal pain, vomiting
  - Timing, duration, and progression of symptoms
- Progression of symptoms:
  - Timing, duration, and progression of symptoms

### Physical Exam
- General appearance:
  - Level of responsiveness, vital signs
- Cardiovascular:
  - Quality of heart tones
  - Perfusion (pulses, capillary refill)
- GI:
  - Abdominal distention, tenderness, palpable masses
- Genitourinary:
  - Testicular swelling, tenderness
- Skin:
  - Location
  - Blanching versus nonblanching
  - Raised (purpura) versus macular (petechia)
- Neurologic:
  - Level of consciousness
  - Presence of focal deficits

## ESSENTIAL WORKUP
Exclude life-threatening causes of purpura, severe abdominal pain, hematuria, and CNS findings, if appropriate.

## DIAGNOSTIC TESTS & INTERPRETATION
### Lab
- CBC:
  - Platelet count normal
  - WBC often elevated
- PT, PTT (if bleeding or in shock; or if unsure of diagnosis and concerned about possibility of coagulopathy)
- Electrolytes (if hypertension or urinalysis abnormal)
- BUN, creatinine (if hypertension or urinalysis abnormal):
  - May be elevated in cases with serious renal complications
- Urinalysis:
  - Hematuria is common
  - Proteinuria is suggestive of glomerulonephritis
- Cultures to exclude common infections

### Imaging
- Abdominal imaging studies:
  - Indicated if abdominal pain or GI bleeding
  - Flat and upright abdominal films of limited use
  - Abdominal US, barium enema, or CT scan may be necessary to rule out intussusception.
- Testicular US:
  - Indicated in patients with testicular pain and swelling
- Head CT:
  - Indicated if CNS findings to exclude bleed

### Diagnostic Procedures/Surgery
Lumbar puncture, as clinically indicated

## DIFFERENTIAL DIAGNOSIS
- Abdominal pain:
  - Gastroenteritis
  - Appendicitis
  - Inflammatory bowel disease
  - Intussusception
  - Meckel diverticulum
- Arthralgias:
  - Acute rheumatic fever
  - Polyarthritis nodosa
  - Juvenile rheumatoid arthritis
  - Systemic lupus erythematosus

- Rash:
  - Infection:
    - Meningococcemia
    - Bacterial sepsis: *Streptococcal* or *staphylococcal*
    - Rocky Mountain spotted fever
    - Infectious mononucleosis
    - Bacterial endocarditis
    - Viral exanthem
  - Trauma/child abuse
  - Functional platelet disorders
  - Thrombocytopenia
  - Vasculitis
  - Erythema nodosum
  - Drugs/toxins
- Renal disease:
  - Acute glomerulonephritis
- Testicular swelling:
  - Incarcerated hernia
  - Orchitis
  - Testicular torsion

 TREATMENT

**PRE-HOSPITAL**
Stabilize as clinically indicated

**INITIAL STABILIZATION/THERAPY**
- IV fluids for shock
- Packed RBCs for massive GI hemorrhage

**ED TREATMENT/PROCEDURES**
- Emergent intervention for life-threatening conditions, if any
- NSAIDs (ibuprofen):
  - Arthralgias
- Prednisone:
  - Severe abdominal pain once life-threatening pathology excluded
  - Painful subcutaneous edema or arthritis
  - Renal disease (high-dose pulse therapy required)
  - CNS involvement
- Polyclonal immunoglobulin therapy:
  - Severe, life-threatening disease (controversial)

**MEDICATION**

**First Line**
Ibuprofen: 600 mg (peds: 5–10 mg/kg per dose) PO q6h

**Second Line**
Prednisone: 60 mg (peds: 1–2 mg/kg/24h) PO daily for 5–7 days

 FOLLOW-UP

**DISPOSITION**
**Admission Criteria**
- Severe abdominal pain
- CNS findings
- GI bleeding
- Intussusception
- Evidence of renal failure

**Discharge Criteria**
- Normal platelet count
- Normal renal function
- Minimal or no abdominal pain
- If steroids started, follow up within 24 hr.

**Issues for Referral**
- GI:
  - Severe abdominal pain
- Renal:
  - Evidence of renal failure or insufficiency

**FOLLOW-UP RECOMMENDATIONS**
Primary care physician:
- Recheck CBC, urinalysis as clinically indicated

## PEARLS AND PITFALLS

- Exclude life-threatening causes
- NSAIDs are usually adequate
- Most patients do not require systemic corticosteroids

## ADDITIONAL READING

- Chang W, Yang Y, Wang L, et al. Renal manifestations in Henoch-Schoenlein purpura: A 10-year clinical study. *Pediat Nephrol*. 2005;20:1269–1272.
- Rostoker G. Schonlein-Henoch purpura in children and adults. Diagnosis, pathophysiology and management. *Biodrug*. 2001;15:99–138.
- Saulsbury FT. Clinical update: Henoch-Schoenlein purpura. *Lancet*. 2007;369:976–978.
- Weiss PF, Feinstein JA, Luan X, et al. Effects of corticosteroid on Henoch-Schoenlein purpura: A systemic review. *Pediatrics*. 2007;120:1079.

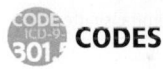 CODES

**ICD9**
287.0 Allergic purpura

H

# HEPATIC ENCEPHALOPATHY

Matthew N. Graber
Eduardo J. Menjivar

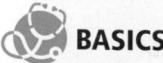

## BASICS

### DESCRIPTION

Hepatic encephalopathy (HE) is characterized by changes in behavior, consciousness, and motor disturbances, associated with hepatic insufficiency and the accumulation of substances normally metabolized by the liver. HE may result from a combination of:

- Accumulation of ammonia from:
  – Protein degradation by colonic bacteria
  – Deamination of glutamine in small bowel
  – Accumulated ammonia crosses the blood–brain barrier. The astrocyte uptakes this ammonia and metabolizes it into glutamine which causes cellular swelling. Ultimately leading to cerebral edema.
- Accumulation of other neurotoxins:
  – Short-chain fatty acids
  – Manganese toxicity
  – Neurosteroid
  – Phenols
  – Mercaptans
  – Amino acids such as tryptophan
- Increased levels of inhibitory neurotransmitters:
  – Benzodiazepines
  – $\gamma$-Aminobutyric acid (GABA)
  – Serotonin
- Decreased levels of excitatory neurotransmitters:
  – Glutamate
  – Dopamine
  – Aspartate
  – Catecholamines
- Other contributing factors to HE:
  – Decreased cerebral blood flow and oxygen
  – Increased glucose consumption and possible hypoglycemia
  – Zinc deficiency
- Genetics:
  – Inherited errors of the urea cycle

### ETIOLOGY

- Classification based on the 11th World congress of Gastroenterology:
  – Type A: HE associated with acute liver failure.
  – Type B: HE associated with portosystemic bypass and no intrinsic liver disease.
  – Type C: HE associated with cirrhosis and portal hypertension.
- Precipitating events:
  – GI bleeding (more common in elderly)
  – Hypokalemia
  – Alkalosis
  – Sepsis (eg, spontaneous bacterial peritonitis)
  – Constipation
  – Noncompliance with treatment regimen in chronic liver failure
  – High-protein diet
  – Hypoglycemia
  – Hypovolemia (eg, post-large-volume paracentesis)
  – Azotemia (eg, diuretic induced)
  – Narcotics or sedatives, including alcohol

– Zinc deficiency as multiple urea cycle enzymes are zinc dependent
– Hepatocellular injury
– Viral- or drug-induced hepatitis
– Post portosystemic shunt placement
– Recurrent encephalopathy can occur without precipitating factors.

## DIAGNOSIS

### SIGNS AND SYMPTOMS

- Type A: Rapidly progresses to seizures, decerebrate rigidity, coma, and frequently death.
- Type B and C are chronic conditions that may manifest as minimal or overt HE. Overt HE may be classified as episodic or persistent:
  – Minimal HE: Characterized by impaired psychomotor speed, visual perception, attention and concentration; slow mental processing; and memory loss. Only detected by psychometric testing.
  – Overt HE: Slow monotonous speech pattern, loss of fine motor skills, hyperreflexia, clonus, hyperventilation, extrapyramidal type movement disorder, seizures, confusion, coma, decerebrate/decorticate posturing.
  – Overt HE episodic: Characterized by short period of changes in consciousness over hours to days that usually return to a normal mental state with treatment. In persistent HE, patients do not return to a normal mental state.
- Grading (West Haven Criteria):
  – Stage 0:
    ○ No apparent clinical changes
    ○ Abnormal neurophysiologic and neuropsychologic tests
    ○ No asterixis
  – Stage I:
    ○ Personality changes, irritability, depression, or euphoria
    ○ Reversal of normal sleep pattern
    ○ Impairment of writing, drawing, addition, subtraction
    ○ Asterixis may be present
  – Stage II:
    ○ Significant behavioral changes, often inappropriate
    ○ Lethargy
    ○ Slow responses
    ○ Asterixis
    ○ Slurred speech
    ○ Ataxia
  – Stage III:
    ○ Disorientation to time and place
    ○ Amnesia
    ○ Paranoia
    ○ Nystagmus
    ○ Hypoactive reflexes
    ○ Positive Babinski reflex
    ○ Semi stupor to stupor
  – Stage IV:
    ○ Dilated pupils
    ○ Stupor or coma

### ESSENTIAL WORKUP

- Elicit history of liver disease and prior episodes of HE.
- Search for precipitating cause (particularly GI bleeding and infection).
- Check for electrolyte abnormalities:
  – Even minimal abnormalities may manifest as significant clinical changes.

### DIAGNOSTIC TESTS & INTERPRETATION

*Lab*

- Blood ammonia level:
  – Level correlates poorly with the degree of HE or the presence of cerebral edema.
  – CSF glutamine levels correlate closely with degree of HE.
  – Helpful in detecting HE in cases of altered mental status of unknown cause
  – Normal ammonia level with suspected HE warrants search for other causes of altered mental status.
- Hemoccult testing and nasogastric lavage to rule out GI bleeding
- CBC to search for anemia
- Electrolytes, BUN, creatinine, glucose
- PT/INR with elevations suggesting significant liver failure
- Liver profile/liver enzymes
- Urinalysis for possible infection
- Culture urine and ascitic fluid to search for infectious cause
- Toxicology screen for alternate cause of altered level of consciousness:
  – Acetaminophen and alcohol level as necessary
- Additional labs as clinical scenario dictates:
  – TSH
  – Blood gases
  – Magnesium
  – Viral serology

*Imaging*

- CXR for pneumonia and signs of CHF
- Head CT scan: For new-onset altered mental status, focal neurologic deficit, suspected cerebral edema, or trauma.
- MRI of the brain is especially helpful in diagnosing HE in patients with portosystemic shunts but no intrinsic liver disease.

*Diagnostic Procedures/Surgery*

- ECG for arrhythmia and electrolyte imbalance
- CSF examination:
  – For new-onset or unexplained worsening of HE
  – CSF glutamine level correlates with severity of HE.
- Paracentesis for spontaneous bacterial peritonitis (SBP) workup and culture of ascitic fluid
- EEG is usually abnormal, most commonly with generalized slowing and other nonspecific changes.

## DIFFERENTIAL DIAGNOSIS

- Alcohol withdrawal syndromes including delirium tremens
- Cerebrovascular accident
- CHF
- $CO_2$ narcosis
- Head trauma with concussion or intracranial bleed
- Hypocalcemia and hypercalcemia
- Hypoglycemia
- Hypokalemia
- Meningitis or encephalitis
- Metabolic encephalopathy
- Neuropsychiatric disorders
- Toxic confusional states secondary to:
  - Sedative overdose
  - Alcohol intoxication
  - Illicit drugs
  - Medications
- Uremia

### Pediatric Considerations

- Consider Reye syndrome early (most common cause of fulminate hepatic failure in children) even if PT is only mildly prolonged.
- Consider fatty acid $\beta$-oxidation disorder:
  - Freeze serum and urine sample for subsequent testing.

 ## TREATMENT

### INITIAL STABILIZATION/THERAPY

- Oxygen
- Airway protection:
  Patients with grade 3 or 4 HE may require intubation for airway protection. Propofol is the preferred agent for sedation.
- Cardiac monitor
- Fluid resuscitation
- Initial altered mental status treatment:
  - Naloxone
  - $D_{50}W$ (or bedside glucose)
  - Thiamine

### ED TREATMENT/PROCEDURES

Identification and removal of precipitating factors is key and may improve clinical picture alone.

#### ALERT

- Liver failure predisposes patients to both hypoglycemia and HE, and these can be additive to the clinical picture; therefore, frequent glucose checks are of absolute importance.
- Identification of early cerebral edema is important as brain perfusion must be preserved and herniation prevented (associated but not limited to grade 3 and 4 HE)

- Treatment of complicating conditions:
  - Acute GI bleeding
  - Sepsis
  - Electrolyte abnormalities
  - Coagulopathy
  - Renal and electrolyte disturbances
- Avoid sedative/narcotics if possible:
  - If necessary, use agents not metabolized by the liver.

- Increase ammonia elimination:
  - Bowel cleansing with laxatives and nonabsorbable sugars (ie, lactulose [mainstay of treatment], sorbitol PO or per rectum [PR])
- Decrease ammonia-producing intestinal flora (in combination with lactulose):
  - Neomycin (nephrotoxic and ototoxic)
  - Metronidazole
  - Vancomycin (PO)
  - Rifaximin: Recommended for the lactulose resistant HE. Current data suggests is as effective as lactulose and neomycin and has a favorable safety and tolerability profile, although more expensive.
- Treat associated cerebral edema if present.
- Correct zinc deficiency with zinc acetate or sulfate.
- Short-term restriction of protein intake in diet
- Flumazenil in patients who have received benzodiazepines may provide moderate, short-term improvement.
  - Avoid flumazenil unless you are sure that the patient is not a chronic alcoholic or benzodiazepine user as resultant seizures may occur.
- Precautions to prevent bodily harm to the confused patient with HE
- Liver transplantation provides cure for severe, spontaneous, or recurrent HE.
- Possibly of benefit:
  - L-carnitine
  - Albumin dialysis
  - Bromocriptine
  - Broad-spectrum antibiotic coverage
  - N-acetylcysteine
  - *Lactobacillus acidophilus* supplementation
    Ornithine aspartate
  - Benzoate
  - Branched-chain amino-acid supplementation
  - Chelation of manganese with edetate calcium disodium

### MEDICATION

- Dextrose: 1 Amp (25 g) of 50% dextrose (child: 2 mL/kg $D_{25}W$) IV
- Lactulose: 30 mL (peds: 0.3 mL/kg) PO or via nasogastric (NG) tube q6h titrated to produce 2 or 3 soft stools per day and stool pH <5
- Metronidazole: 250 mg (peds: 10–30 mg/kg/d) q8h for 2 wk
- Narcan: 2 mg (peds: 0.1 mg/kg) IV/IM initial dose
- Neomycin: 1–3 g (peds: 50–100 mg/kg/d) PO q6h
- Rifaximin: 1,200 mg/d q8h. (safety not established for children <12 yr)
- Mannitol: 0.5 –1 g/Kg IV
- Thiamine (vitamin $B_1$): 100 mg (peds: 50 mg) IV/IM
- Zinc acetate or sulfate: 220 mg PO q8h

 ## FOLLOW-UP

### DISPOSITION

#### Admission Criteria

- HE grade II, III, or IV or inadequate social support
- Type A HE (any grade) and type B or C (grade II or above) should be admitted to the ICU with urgent GI consult
- Associated complicating condition (GI bleeding and sepsis)
- Uncertainty about cause of altered mental status

#### Discharge Criteria

- Known chronic or intermittent HE
- Grades 0 or I with remediable cause
- Adequate supervision at home
- Close follow-up
- Those appropriate for discharge should go home with:
  - Low-protein diet
  - Lactulose prescription

#### Issues for Referral

- Refer to primary physician or GI for consideration of medication or diet changes if recurrent early stage HE episodes.
- For any grade of type A HE, consider transfer to a liver transplant facility.

### FOLLOW-UP RECOMMENDATIONS

- Dietary consultation if possible cause of exacerbation
- Alcohol counseling if a concern

## PEARLS AND PITFALLS

- Consider rifaximin for the lactulose-resistant HE
- Hypoglycemia is common in HE patients.
- Avoid sedatives and narcotics as is possible in HE patients. If necessary, use medications not metabolized by liver.

## ADDITIONAL READING

- Eroglu Y, Byrne WJ. Hepatic encephalopathy. *Emerg Med Clin North Am.* 2009;27(3):401–414.
- Riordan SM, Williams R. Treatment of hepatic encephalopathy. *New Engl J Med.* 1997;337(7):473–479.
- Sundaram V, Shaikh OS. Hepatic encephalopathy: Pathophysiology and emerging therapies. *Med Clin North Am.* 2009;93(4):819–836, vii.

### See Also (Topic, Algorithm, Electronic Media Element)

- Hypoglycemia

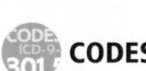 ## CODES

ICD9
572.2 Hepatic encephalopathy

H

# HEPATIC INJURY
*Todd Baumbacher*

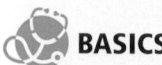 **BASICS**

## DESCRIPTION
- The size and location of the liver places it at significant risk for injury:
  - The liver is the solid organ most frequently injured in penetrating trauma.
  - The liver is the 2nd most commonly injured in blunt abdominal trauma, 2nd to the spleen.
  - Highly susceptible to blunt injuries, by direct blow or deceleration forces
- Mechanism of injury and description of forces are important factors in evaluating patients for possible hepatic injury:
  - Blunt trauma:
    ○ Obtain information about the forces and direction (horizontal or vertical) of any deceleration or compressive forces.
  - Penetrating trauma:
    ○ Type and caliber of the weapon
    ○ Distance from the weapon
    ○ Variety and length of knife or impaling object
- Hepatic injuries are graded by severity, ranging from subcapsular hematoma and lacerations to severe hepatic fragmentation.
- Associated conditions include rib fractures and injuries to the spleen, diaphragm, kidney, lung, gallbladder, pancreas, and blood vessels.
- Overall mortality of hepatic injury is reported at 8–10%.
- More often nonoperative management is becoming more common in isolated blunt hepatic trauma.

### Pediatric Considerations
Poorly developed musculature and relatively smaller anteroposterior diameter increase the vulnerability of liver to compressive forces in children.

## ETIOLOGY
Trauma:
- Blunt mechanism:
  - Deceleration
  - Acceleration
  - Compression
- Penetrating mechanism:
  - Stab wound
  - Gunshot wound
  - Impaled object

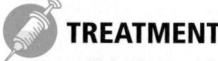 **DIAGNOSIS**

## SIGNS AND SYMPTOMS
Physical exam and history can be variable.

### History
History of trauma usually available from patient or prehospital providers

### Physical Exam
- Neither sensitive nor specific for hepatic injury
- Systemic signs related to acute blood loss:
  - May present with dizziness and weakness
  - Signs of shock including tachycardia and hypotension
- Local signs:
  - Right upper quadrant tenderness
  - Guarding
  - Abdominal distention
  - Rigidity
  - Rebound
  - Tenderness
  - Contusions/abrasions
  - Penetrating wounds to the right chest, flank, or abdomen

## ESSENTIAL WORKUP
- Physical exam is unreliable.
- Objective evaluation includes imaging of the abdomen or surgical exploration.

## DIAGNOSTIC TESTS & INTERPRETATION
### Lab
- No hematologic laboratory studies are specific for diagnosis of injury to the liver.
- Obtain baseline hemoglobin level.
- Liver function tests are not helpful in the acute setting.
- Consider type and cross if active hemorrhage is suspected.

### Imaging
- Consider imaging based on mechanism and physical exam.
- Plain abdominal radiographs:
  - Little value
- Bedside US:
  - Screening tool for both blunt and penetrating abdominal trauma
  - Procedure of choice in unstable patient
  - May identify intraabdominal fluid in the hepatorenal (Morison) pouch or parenchymal injuries
  - Suggests intraabdominal hemorrhage in patient with blunt, multiple-organ trauma

- CT scan with IV contrast:
  - Best depicts extent of hepatic injury and injuries to adjacent organs
  - Requires patient to be hemodynamically stable
  - Extravasation of IV contrast during arterial phase of CT injection indicative of vascular or high-grade liver injury requiring surgical intervention

### Diagnostic Procedures/Surgery
- Diagnostic peritoneal lavage (DPL):
  - Usually done in conjunction with trauma surgeon
  - Sensitive for presence of hemoperitoneum
  - Nonspecific for source of bleeding
  - Surgery and exploratory laparotomy if positive
  - Operative management may be necessary for unstable patients and those with high-grade lesions.
- Lower-grade injuries have been increasingly managed successfully without surgery.

## DIFFERENTIAL DIAGNOSIS
- Other causes of intraperitoneal injury
- Retroperitoneal injury
- Thoracic injury
- Diaphragmatic injury
- Splenic injury
- Vascular Injury

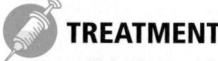 **TREATMENT**

## PRE-HOSPITAL
- Obtain details of mechanism of injury.
- Initiate large-bore IV access:
  - Hemorrhage may be rapid and life-threatening.
- Moist saline dressings over penetrating wounds or evisceration
- Direct pressure to control active bleeding
- Full spinal immobilization except in isolated penetrating trauma

## INITIAL STABILIZATION/THERAPY
ABCs:
- Control airway as needed; may have associated injuries including head injury.
- Supplemental oxygen, cardiac monitor, pulse oximetry
- Adequate IV access, including central line, intraosseous line, and cutdown as dictated by the patient's status
- Fluid resuscitation, initially with 2 L of crystalloid (normal saline or Ringer lactate), followed by blood products such as packed red blood cells. Consider fresh frozen plasma (FFP) as needed.

## ED TREATMENT/PROCEDURES

- Immediate laparotomy may be appropriate in the acutely injured patient with the following conditions:
  - Hemodynamic instability
  - Gunshot wounds to the anterior abdomen
  - Frank signs of intraperitoneal hemorrhage
  - Indications based on diagnostic procedures, such as diagnostic peritoneal lavage
  - Failure of nonoperative management
- Stab wounds can be managed by local wound exploration followed by US or DPL when intraperitoneal penetration is not demonstrated or equivocal.
- Consider nonoperative management for the following patients:
  - Hemodynamically stable with normal mental status
  - No evidence of other intraabdominal injury
  - Isolated low-grade (1–3) hepatic injury confirmed by imaging study
  - Transfusion requirements $\leq 2$ units of packed red blood cells
- High-grade liver injuries (4 and 5) have less successful nonoperative rates.
- Diet: Nothing per mouth (NPO)
- Activity: Strict bedrest
- Special therapy:
  - Angiography with embolization: Selective use in patients with persistent bleeding may decrease the need for operative management and blood transfusions
  - Factor VIIa has been used as an adjunct in nonoperative management to control bleeding.

## MEDICATION

- Crystalloid IV fluids: NS or lactated Ringers
- Packed red blood cells
- Fresh frozen plasma
- Recombinant factor VIIa

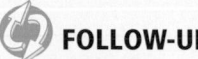

## FOLLOW-UP

### DISPOSITION

#### Admission Criteria

- All patients with hepatic injury require hospitalization for definitive laparotomy or close hemodynamic observation with serial exams or CT scans, as well as hematocrit measurements.
- ICU admission is often indicated in the 1st 48 hr after injury.

#### Discharge Criteria

Patients with proven or suspected hepatic injuries should not be discharged.

#### Issues for Referral

Report all gunshot and stab wounds to appropriate local authorities.

### FOLLOW-UP RECOMMENDATIONS

Follow-up US, physical exam, and hematocrits are crucial in noting changes in initially benign presentations.

## PEARLS AND PITFALLS

- Obtain early surgical consultation in unstable patients.
- Failing to obtain appropriate and adequate imaging studies is a pitfall.
- Do not rely on negative US to rule out hepatic injury.
- Failing to adequately resuscitate with IV fluids and blood products is a pitfall.
- If hepatic injury is confirmed, ensure no trauma to surrounding organ systems.
- Check for pregnancy in women

## ADDITIONAL READING

- Jacobs IA. Nonoperative management of blunt splenic and hepatic trauma in the pediatric population. *Am Surg*. 2001;67:149–154.
- Leone RT Jr. Nonoperative management of pediatric blunt hepatic trauma. *Am Surg*. 2001;67:138–142.
- Malhotra AK, Fabian TC, Croce MA, et al. Hepatic injury: A paradigm shift from operative to nonoperative management in the 1990s. *Ann Surg*. 2000;231:804–813.

- Marx J. Abdominal trauma. In: Marx J, Hockberger R, Walls R, et al., eds. *Emergency Medicine: Concepts and Clinical Practice*, 7th ed. St. Louis, MO: Mosby, 2010:415–434.
- Ochsner MG, Jaffin JH, Golocovsky M, et al. Major hepatic trauma. *Surg Clin North Am*. 1993;73:337–352.
- Townsend CM. Abdominal trauma. In: Townsend CM, Beauchamp DR, Evers MB, et al., eds. *Sabiston Textbook of Surgery*, 17th ed. Philadelphia: WB Saunders, 2004:521–523.
- Trunkey DD. Hepatic trauma: Contemporary management. *Surg Clin North Am*. 2004;84: 437–450.
- Vick LR, Islam S. Recombinant factor VIIa as an adjunct in nonoperative management of solid organ injuries in children. *J Pediatr Surg*. 2008;43: 195–199.
- Wolfson AB. Blunt abdominal trauma. In: *Clinical Practice of Emergency Medicine*, 5th ed. Philadelphia: Lippincott Williams and Wilkins, 2010:227–232.

## See Also (Topic, Algorithm, Electronic Media Element)

- Abdominal Trauma, Blunt
- Abdominal Trauma, Penetrating
- Abdominal Trauma, Imaging
- Colon Trauma
- Diaphragmatic Trauma
- Pancreatic Trauma
- Renal Injury
- Small Bowel Injury
- Trauma, Multiple

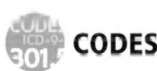

## CODES

### ICD9

864.00 Unspecified injury to liver without mention of open wound into cavity

H

# HEPATITIS

*Michael Schmidt*
*Lucas C. Rosiere*

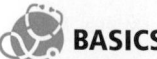 **BASICS**

## DESCRIPTION
- Inflammation of the liver owing to infectious, toxic, and autoimmune disorders
- Infectious causes are the most common:
  - Of infectious causes, hepatitis A is the cause of 30%, hepatitis B 50%, hepatitis C 20%

## ETIOLOGY
- Hepatitis A (HAV):
  - Transmission: Enteric > sexual > close contact
  - Mean incubation: 1 mo
  - Fulminant hepatic failure (FHF) in 0.1%
  - No chronic disease
- Hepatitis B (HBV):
  - Transmission: Mucous membrane or percutaneous exposure to bodily fluids > perinatal
  - Mean incubation: 75 days
  - FHF in 1%
  - 10% progress to chronic disease:
    ◦ Risk increases with earlier age of initial infection
    ◦ Risk of cirrhosis, hepatocellular carcinoma
- Hepatitis C (HCV):
  - Transmission: Blood > sexual > perinatal
  - Mean incubation: 1.5 mo
  - FHF extremely rare
  - 80% progress to chronic disease
  - Risk of cirrhosis, hepatocellular carcinoma
- Hepatitis D (HDV):
  - Superinfection of HBV, augments all pathologic actions of HBV
  - Same transmission as HBV
  - Mean incubation: 1 mo
  - FHF in 3%
  - 5% progress to chronic disease
- Hepatitis E (HEV):
  - Endemic to developing countries only
  - Transmission: Enteric > blood > perinatal > zoonotic
  - Mean incubation: 1.5 mo
  - FHF in 10%
- Abscess-induced hepatitis:
  - Entamoeba histolytica, pyogenic
- Secondary hepatitis viruses:
  - CMV, EBV, HSV, HIV
- Toxin-induced:
  - Acetaminophen (most common), EtOH, ecstasy (MDMA), industrial solvents and cleaning solutions, iron (hemochromatosis)

- Medication-induced:
  - Acetaminophen
  - Amiodarone
  - Aspirin
  - Carbamazepine
  - Isoflurane
  - Isoniazid
  - Ketoconazole
  - Labetalol
  - Methotrexate
  - Nicotinic acid
  - Phenytoin
  - Propylthiouracil
  - Pyrazinamide
  - Rifampin
  - Sulfonamides
  - Tetracycline
  - Valproic acid
- Autoimmune hepatitis:
  - Display concurrent stigmata of autoimmune disease

### Pediatric Considerations
- Vast majority of cases are caused by HAV.
- Perinatal HBV infection develops into chronic disease 90% of the time.

### Pregnancy Considerations
- 20% case-fatality for HEV during pregnancy.
- Acute fatty liver of pregnancy (AFLP):
  - May progress to DIC
- HELLP syndrome (*H*emolysis, *E*levated *L*iver enzymes, and *L*ow *P*latelets)
- All forms of immunoprophylaxis are safe during pregnancy.

 **DIAGNOSIS**

## SIGNS AND SYMPTOMS
- Often asymptomatic
- Preicteric phase:
  - Often misdiagnosed as a nonspecific viral syndrome or gastroenteritis
- Icteric phase:
  - Present in 70% of HAV, 30% of HBV, and 20% of HCV
- FHF:
  - Coagulopathy
  - Encephalopathy
  - Cerebral edema

### History
- Preicteric phase:
  - Fever, chills
  - Malaise
  - Nausea, vomiting, anorexia
  - Arthralgia
  - Aversion to smoking
- Icteric phase:
  - Jaundice
  - Dark Urine
  - Light Stools
  - Pruritus
  - Rash
  - Right upper quadrant pain
- FHF:
  - Bleeding
  - Altered mental status

### Physical Exam
- Preicteric phase:
  - Fever
  - Arthritis
  - Dehydration
- Icteric phase:
  - Fever
  - Icterus of skin, sclerae, mucous membranes, and tympanic membranes
  - Nonspecific maculopapular or urticarial rash
  - Dehydration
  - Tender hepatomegaly
- FHF:
  - Bruising
  - Disorientation
  - Asterixis

## ESSENTIAL WORKUP
- Detailed history for risk factors for hepatitis, including toxic exposure and drug use
- Viral serologies are the mainstay of diagnosis of viral causes.

## DIAGNOSTIC TESTS & INTERPRETATION
### Lab
- CBC with differential
- Basic metabolic panel (Chem7):
  - Azotemia with hepatorenal syndrome in FHF
  - Hypoglycemia with severe liver damage
- LFTs:
  - Elevation in transaminases reflects injury
  - Degree of elevation does not correlate with severity
  - If Alkaline phosphatase more than twice normal, consider primary cholestatic process rather than viral hepatitis.
  - Mild to moderate elevation of conjugated bilirubin due to decreased excretion

- Amylase, lipase may indicate pancreatic or biliary etiology
- PT/PTT/INR:
  - Prolonged PT/INR reflects more severe injury.
- Ammonia level:
  - For patients with altered mental status
- Viral serologies:
  - HAV:
    ○ Anti-HAV IgM: Acute infection
    ○ Anti-HAV IgG: Previous exposure, immunity
  - HBV:
    ○ HBsAg: Acute infection (appears before symptoms), chronic infection
    ○ Anti-HBs: Acute infection (may appear after HBsAg gone), past infection, immunization
    ○ Anti-HBc IgM: Acute infection
    ○ Anti-HBs IgG: Past infection, chronic infection
    ○ HBeAg: Acute infection, chronic infection
    ○ HBeAb: Acute infection, chronic infection
  - HCV:
    ○ Anti-HCV: Acute infection, chronic infections, first-line test
    ○ HCV RNA: Acute infection, chronic infections; confirmatory
  - HDV: Anti-HDV or viral RNA, not routine
  - HEV: Anti-HEV or viral RNA, not routine
- α-fetoprotein:
  - For chronic HBV or HCV to evaluate for hepatocellular carcinoma
- Monospot: For EBV
- Urinalysis for bilirubin

### Imaging
- Head CT to evaluate hepatic encephalopathy
- RUQ US to evaluate for biliary obstruction

### DIFFERENTIAL DIAGNOSIS
- Alcohol hepatitis
- Autoimmune hepatitis
- Nonalcoholic fatty liver disease
- Hemochromatosis
- Cholecystitis
- Cholangitis
- Liver abscess
- Wilson disease
- Infectious mononucleosis
- Heat stroke
- Fitz-Hugh and Curtis syndrome
- Biliary pathology

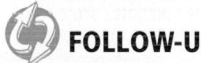 **TREATMENT**

### INITIAL STABILIZATION/THERAPY
ABCs for FHF and severe hepatic encephalopathy.

### ED TREATMENT/PROCEDURES
- Treat hypovolemia aggressively with isotonic fluids.
- Correct electrolyte imbalance.
- Treat vomiting with metoclopramide.
- Avoid hepatotoxic agents: Acetaminophen, alcohol, phenothiazines.
- Correct coagulopathy if active bleeding.
- Ursodeoxycholic acid or cholestyramine for cholestasis-induced itching
- Evaluate for the differential diagnoses and treat accordingly
- Postexposure prophylaxis (PEP):
  - HAV:
    ○ HAV IG 0.02 mL/kg IM within 2 wk of exposure
    ○ HAV vaccine 1 mL (peds: 0.5 mL) IM
  - HBV:
    ○ HBV IG 0.06 mL/kg IM within 7 days of exposure
    ○ HBV vaccine 1 mL (peds: 0.5 mL) IM
  - No effective immunoprophylaxis for HCV, HDV, or HEV

### MEDICATION
- Cholestyramine: 4 g PO 2–4 times per day for pruritus
- Dextrose $D_{50}W$: 1 amp or 25 g (peds: $D_{25}W$ 2–4 mL/kg) IV
- Metoclopramide: 10 mg IV/IM q6–8h, 10–30 mg PO q.i.d.
- Naloxone: 2 mg (peds: 0.1 mg/kg) IV/IM
- Thiamine: 100 mg (peds: 50 mg) IV/IM:
  - Prior to glucose if malnutritioned
- Ursodeoxycholic acid: 3 mg/kg t.i.d.

 **FOLLOW-UP**

### DISPOSITION
#### Admission Criteria
- Intractable vomiting, dehydration, or electrolyte imbalance not responding to ED treatment
- Acute hepatitis with evidence of significant liver dysfunction:
  - PT >3 sec above control or INR >1.5
  - Bilirubin >20 mg/dL
  - Hypoglycemia
  - Albumin <2.5 g/dL
- ICU admission for FHF
- Hepatic encephalopathy
- Pregnancy
- Immunocompromised host
- Possibility of toxic hepatitis
- Age >50

#### Discharge Criteria
- Normalized electrolytes
- PO tolerance
- Mild hepatic impairment

#### Issues for Referral
Most patients may be discharged home with gastroenterology or infectious disease follow up for further serologic diagnosis and definitive treatment.

### FOLLOW-UP RECOMMENDATIONS
- Strict personal hygiene instructions
- Avoid acetaminophen and alcohol.
- Avoid prolonged physical exertion.

## PEARLS AND PITFALLS
- Acute hepatitis is often misdiagnosed as a nonspecific viral syndrome—screen with urinalysis or serum LFTs
- ED treatment is primarily supportive
- Maintain high index of suspicion for AFLP and HELLP in pregnant patients with compatible symptoms

## ADDITIONAL READING
- Buggs AM. Hepatitis. www.emedicine.com. Accessed November 15, 2009.
- Emerson SU, Purcell RH. Running like water—the omnipresence of hepatitis E. *N Engl J Med*. 2004;351:23–67.
- Furbee RB, Barlotta KS, Allen MK, et al. Hepatotoxicity associated with herbal products. *Clin Lab Med*. 2006;26(1):227–241.
- Guntupalli SR, Steingrub J. Hepatic disease and pregnancy: An overview of diagnosis and management. *Crit Care Med*. 2005;33(10 Suppl): S332–S339.

### See Also (Topic, Algorithm, Electronic Media Element)
- Cholecystitis
- Cirrhosis
- Coma
- HELLP Syndrome
- Hepatic Injury
- Jaundice
- Mononucleosis
- Reye Syndrome

## CODES

### ICD9
- 070.1 Viral hepatitis a without mention of hepatic coma
- 070.30 Viral hepatitis b without mention of hepatic coma, acute or unspecified, without mention of hepatitis delta
- 573.3 Hepatitis, unspecified

**H**

# HEPATORENAL SYNDROME

*Matthew T. Keadey*

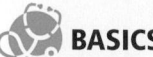 **BASICS**

## DESCRIPTION

- Renal failure (RF) in patients with acute or chronic liver disease with no other identifiable cause of renal pathology.
- Hepatorenal syndrome (HRS) represents significant decline in renal perfusion due to severe liver disease:
  - Type I hepatorenal syndrome:
    - Acute form with spontaneous RF in patients with liver disease
    - Rapidly progressive
    - Decrease in creatinine clearance (CrCl) by 50% or doubling of Cr in 2 wk (>2.5)
    - 90% mortality within 3 mo
    - Seen with acute liver failure or alcoholic hepatitis
    - Oliguric or anuric
  - Type II hepatorenal syndrome:
    - Slow course of RF
    - Seen in patients with diuretic resistant ascites
    - Lower mortality rate than type I HRS
- Hallmarks of HRS:
  - Prerenal disease
  - Reversible renal vasoconstriction and mild systemic hypotension
  - Kidneys have normal histology and structure.
  - Lack of improvement in renal function after volume expansion
- Liver disease causes systemic vasodilation with decrease in arterial blood volume:
  - Reflex activation of sympathetic nervous system
  - Activation of renin-angiotensin–aldosterone system (RAAS)
  - Stimulation of numerous vasoactive substances:
    - Nitric oxide
    - Prostacyclin
    - Atrial natriuretic peptide (ANP)
    - Arachidonic acid metabolites
    - Platelet-activating factor
    - Endothelins
    - Catecholamines
    - Angiotensin II
    - Thromboxane
- Action of vasoconstrictors prevails over vasodilator effects:
  - Renal hypoperfusion ensues due to renal cortical vasoconstriction.
  - Decrease in renal blood flow and glomerular filtration rates
- Decreased urine sodium excretion (U Na <10 mEq/d)
- Incidence of HRS:
  - 18% at 1st year, 39% at 5 yr
- Hyponatremia and high plasma renin levels are risk factors.

## ETIOLOGY

- Chronic liver disease, especially alcohol related (cirrhosis, severe alcoholic hepatitis)
- Fulminate hepatic failure
- Precipitating factors:
  - Decreased effective blood volume:
    - GI bleeding
    - Vigorous diuresis
    - Large-volume paracentesis
  - Use of nephrotoxic agent:
    - NSAIDs
    - Aminoglycoside
  - Sepsis:
    - Spontaneous bacterial peritonitis (SBP) leads to a 33% chance of developing renal failure during that year
    - Prophylaxis of SBP reduces the chance of developing acute renal failure

 **DIAGNOSIS**

## SIGNS AND SYMPTOMS

Signs of acute or chronic liver disease:

- Signs of portal hypertension
- Ascites, often tense
- Progressive oliguria
- Jaundice or hepatic encephalopathy
- Coagulopathy
- Tachycardia
- Hypotension
- Dyspnea, tachypnea due to tense ascites

### History

Acute or chronic hepatic disease with advanced hepatic failure and portal hypertension:

- Worsening liver function often predates acute renal dysfunction

### Physical Exam

- Consistent with severe hepatic disease
- Vital signs may show:
  - Fever in signs of sepsis
  - Hypotension in sepsis, intestinal bleeding, or even a low baseline intrinsic to liver disease

## DIAGNOSTIC TESTS & INTERPRETATION

### Lab

- CBC:
  - Anemia due to GI bleed
- Electrolytes:
  - Hyperkalemia
  - Acidosis

- Glucose
- Elevated BUN, creatinine (Cr):
  - Normal Cr found with low glomerular filtration rate (GFR) in association with muscle wasting, poor nutrition, and ascites.
  - Cr increased by some medications (cimetidine, trimethoprim, and spironolactone) due to inhibition of tubular secretion of creatinine.
  - Hyperbilirubinemia can artifactually lower serum creatinine.
- PT, PTT
- Urinalysis:
  - Absence of casts distinguishes HRS from acute tubular necrosis (ATN).
  - Check for UTI.
- Spot urine sodium and creatinine, and serum and urine osmolality:
  - Spot urine $Na^+$ <10 mEq/L
  - Fractional excretion of $Na^+$ <1%
  - Urine/plasma creatinine >30:1
  - Hyperosmolar urine > plasma osmolarity
- 24-hr urine output (low in absence of diuretics)
- 24-hr urine creatinine clearance:
  - Accurately assess GFR
- Blood, ascitic fluid, and urine culture as indicated
- Urinary excretion of $\beta_2$-microglobulin—useful marker of acute tubular damage

### Imaging

- CXR for signs of CHF or fluid overload
- Renal US: Rule out obstructive uropathy:
  - Duplex Doppler US can be used to assess degree of renal vasoconstriction.

### Diagnostic Procedures/Surgery

- ECG for dysrhythmia or signs of hyperkalemia
- Foley catheter placement to assess for urine output and exclude urinary retention as cause of renal failure
- Central venous pressure (CVP) measurements may help assess volume status:
  - Differentiates prerenal (low) from HRS (elevated)

## DIFFERENTIAL DIAGNOSIS

- HRS is diagnosis of exclusion
- Glomerulopathy:
  - Hepatitis B can lead to glomerulonephritis
  - Hepatitis C can cause intrinsic renal damage due to cryoglobulinemia
- ATN:
  - Urine sodium >30 mEq/L
  - Urine osmolality equals plasma osmolality
  - Urine casts and cellular debris
- Prerenal azotemia:
  - Overdiuresis
  - GI bleeding
  - Urine output improves following correction of hypovolemia
- Obstructive uropathy
- Infections or sepsis
- Medications—NSAID's
- Interstitial nephritis
- Postliver transplant renal dysfunction due to:
  - HRS due to failure of transplanted liver
  - Medications (eg, cyclosporine)
  - Pre-existing renal disease
  - Perioperative hypovolemia

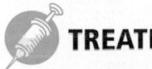 TREATMENT

### PRE-HOSPITAL
Attention to ABCs:

- Airway control may be a concern in severe encephalopathy.
- Respiratory failure seen with tense ascites as well as volume overload
- Correction of hypotension and ensure adequate IV access

### INITIAL STABILIZATION/THERAPY

- ABCs
- Aggressive correction of hypovolemia with:
  - 0.9% NS IV fluid
  - Colloid volume expanders: 100 g albumin in 500 mL of NS
  - Closely monitor clinical status including use of CVP
  - Urine output should improve with correction of prerenal azotemia
- Manage life-threatening emergencies of renal failure:
  - Hyperkalemia
  - Severe acidosis
  - Hypoxemia
  - Uremic pericarditis

## ED TREATMENT/PROCEDURES

- Exclude reversible or treatable causes of HRS.
- Supportive care until hepatic function recovers
- *Do no harm*—discontinue potentially nephrotoxic agents:
  - NSAIDs
  - Aminoglycosides
  - Demeclocycline
- Treat primary disease
- Search for and treat coexisting renal disease
- Correct electrolyte imbalances
- Treat any associated cardiopulmonary disorder and hypoxia
- Initiate broad-spectrum antibiotics if sepsis suspected
- Correct liver-associated complications:
  - Obstructive jaundice
  - Hepatic encephalopathy
  - Hypoglycemia
  - Peritonitis
- Consider large-volume paracentesis with IV albumin replacement (to relieve tense ascites):
  - Increases renal blood flow
  - May briefly improve HRS
- Transhepatic Intrahepatic Portosystemic Shunt:
  - Promising results, but small studies
  - Those who survived the procedure had 40% survival at 12 mo compared to 90% at 3 mo.
- Dialysis:
  - Useful in correcting fluid, electrolytes, acid–base imbalances, pulmonary edema
  - Indicated for patients who have likelihood of hepatic regeneration, hepatic recovery, or liver transplantation
- Liver transplant:
  - Is currently the only definitive therapy

## MEDICATION

- No medications are first line and should only be considered after other causes of renal dysfunction excluded
- Dopamine (renal dose): 2–5 $\mu$g/kg/min:
  - May improve renal function
  - Not curative
- Midodrine (7.5–12.5 mg PO t.i.d.) and octreotide (100–200 $\mu$g SC t.i.d.):
  - Octreotide is analog of somatostatin
  - Midodrine is sympathomimetic drug
- Misoprostol: 0.4 mg PO q.i.d.:
  - Synthetic analog of prostaglandin $E_1$
- Ornipressin: 2-hr infusion at 6 IU/h:
  - Vasopressin analog
  - Increases renal perfusion pressure and function
  - Not available in U.S.
- Terlipressin: 2 mg/d for 2 days:
  - Synthetic analog of vasopressin
  - Intrinsic vasoconstrictor activity
  - Not available in U.S.

 FOLLOW-UP

### DISPOSITION
*Admission Criteria*

- All suspected HRS with GI and nephrology consults
- ICU admission for associated cardiopulmonary disease, hepatic encephalopathy, marked electrolyte imbalances

*Discharge Criteria*
None

## PEARLS AND PITFALLS

Any degree of renal dysfunction needs to be evaluated very seriously in patients with liver disease.

## ADDITIONAL READING

- Arroyo V, Guevara M, Gines P. Hepatorenal syndrome in cirrhosis. *Gastroenterology*. 2002;122:1658–1676.
- Dagher L, Moore K. The hepatorenal syndrome. *Gut*. 2001;49:729–737.
- Gentilini P, Vizzutti F, et al. Ascites and hepatorenal syndrome. *Eur J Gastroenterol Hepatol*. 2001;13: 313–316.
- Gines P, Guevara M, Arroyo V, et al. Hepatorenal syndrome. *Lancet*. 2003;362:1819–1827.
- Roberts LR, Kamath PS. Ascites and hepatorenal syndrome: Pathophysiology and management. *Mayo Clin Proc*. 1996;71:874.
- Senzolo M, Cholangitas E, Tibballs J, et al. Transjugular intrahepatic portosystemic shunt in the management of ascites and hepatorenal syndrome. *Eur J Gastroenterol Hepatol*. 2008;18:1143–1150.
- Wong F, Blendis L. New challenge of hepatorenal syndrome: Prevention and treatment. *Hepatology*. 2001;34:1242–1251.

### See Also (Topic, Algorithm, Electronic Media Element)

- Hepatic Encephalopathy
- Hepatitis

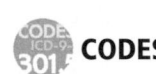 CODES

### ICD9
572.4 Hepatorenal syndrome

**H**

# HERNIA
*Jenny J. Lu*

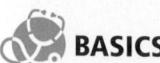 **BASICS**

## DESCRIPTION
- Weakness or disruption of fibromuscular layer of abdominal wall
- Hernia repair is most common general surgical procedure
- Incarceration of hernia:
  - Contents of hernia cannot be manipulated back into abdomen
- Strangulation of hernia:
  - Vascular compromise of entrapped bowel contained within hernia leading to ischemia and gangrene
  - Signs and symptoms of bowel obstruction or ischemia may occur (nausea/vomiting, fever, leukocytosis)

## ETIOLOGY
- Indirect inguinal hernia:
  - Results from persistent process vaginalis
  - Peritoneal contents herniates through internal ring
  - Right side more common than left
  - 27% lifetime risk of repair for men; 3% for women
- Direct inguinal hernia:
  - Due to weakness or defect in transversalis area in Hesselbach triangle:
    - Inguinal ligament inferiorly
    - Inferior epigastric vessels laterally
    - Lateral border of rectus abdominus medially
- Incisional hernia:
  - Resultant breakdown of previous surgical fascial closure
- Femoral hernia:
  - Peritoneum herniates into femoral canal beneath inguinal ligament.
  - Incarceration frequent due to protrusion through small orifice
- Obturator hernia:
  - Passes through obturator membrane and exits beneath pectineal muscle
- Umbilical hernia:
  - Congenital failure of umbilical ring to close
  - Protrusion through fibromuscular umbilical ring/umbilicus
  - 20–45% recurrence rate

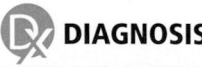 **DIAGNOSIS**

## SIGNS AND SYMPTOMS
### History
- Pain and swelling:
  - Localized to region of hernia
- Constant pain, vomiting, fever may indicate:
  - Incarceration
  - Strangulation
  - Bowel obstruction

### Physical Exam
- Vital signs:
  - Frequently normal
  - Tachycardia with pain, dehydration, infection
  - Hypotension with dehydration, strangulation, infection/sepsis
  - Fever with infection/sepsis
- Inguinal hernia:
  - Pain:
    - Localized to inguinal region
    - Exacerbated by straining/positional changes
    - Relieved by rest
  - Swelling:
    - Males: Intermittent bulge in scrotum
    - Females: Bulge immediately inferior to inguinal ligament or in labia
  - Swelling of spermatic cord, scrotum, or testes
  - Valsalva maneuver performed with finger directed towards internal ring—may allow hernia sac to descend against finger
- Femoral hernia:
  - Pain/swelling:
    - Localized to femoral orifice inferior to inguinal ligament
- Incisional Hernia:
  - Pain/swelling:
    - Localized to previous incision/scar
- Obturator hernia:
  - Nonspecific abdominal pain
  - Intermittent intestinal obstruction
  - Weight loss
  - Pain:
    - Owing to pressure on obturator nerve from hernia (Howship-Romberg sign)
    - Along medial thigh
    - Radiating to hip
    - Relieved with thigh flexion
    - Exacerbated by hip extension, adduction, or external rotation
- Spigelian hernia:
  - Abdominal pain/mass along anterior abdominal wall
  - Increased pain with maneuvers increasing intra-abdominal pressure
  - Intermittent bowel obstruction
  - Palpable mass along spigelian line:
    - Convex line extending from costal arch to pubic tubercle along lateral edge of rectus muscle

### Pediatric Considerations
- Diagnosis often difficult:
  - Parents describe bulge in inguinal area often no longer present at time of exam.
  - Incarcerated hernias may present with irritability, abdominal pain, or intermittent vomiting.
- Incidence of incarceration/strangulation is 10–20%:
  - >50% in patients younger than 6 mo of age
  - Incidence of incarceration higher in girls than boys
- Umbilical hernias:
  - Strangulation and incarceration rare
  - Most close spontaneously
  - Most surgeons will delay closure until 4 yr of age.
- Inguinal hernias (consider hydrocele):
  - If hydrocele, neck narrows at external inguinal canal without extension into inguinal canal

### Pregnancy Considerations
- Hernias uncommon during pregnancy, manifesting before or during
- Inguinal hernia: 1:1,000–3,000 incidence, 75% occurring in multiparas
- Recognition of emergent situations (incarceration, strangulation) may be a diagnostic and management challenge
- No consensus exists regarding treatment of unreducible hernia during pregnancy; complications during pregnancy may outweigh elective hernioplasty and emergent surgical consultation recommended

### Geriatric Considerations
- Higher risk of bowel resection if older than 65 yr with incarcerated hernias
- Higher postoperative pulmonary and cardiovascular complications

## ESSENTIAL WORKUP
Careful history and physical exam:
- Palpate inguinal/femoral area for tenderness/masses.
- Attempt examination with the patient standing or straining (Valsalva maneuver) if hernia not obvious.
- Pelvic exam in women to evaluate gynecological etiologies of groin pain

## DIAGNOSTIC TESTS & INTERPRETATION

### Lab
- CBC:
  - Leukocytosis with strangulation
- Electrolytes, BUN/creatinine, glucose:
  - If vomiting/dehydration
- Urinalysis:
  - Genitourinary causes of groin pain

### Imaging
- Plain abdominal radiographs:
  - Obstructive bowel pattern with incarceration or strangulation
- US:
  - For identifying masses in groin or abdominal wall
  - May be difficult in obese patients
- CT:
  - To diagnose obturator or spigelian hernia
  - Consider in symptomatic patients in whom body habitus precludes adequate physical exam or US study

## DIFFERENTIAL DIAGNOSIS
- Hydrocele
- Varicocele
- Lymphadenitis
- Testicular torsion
- Testicular tumor
- Undescended testis
- Renal calculi
- UTI
- Ovarian torsion
- Lymphogranuloma venereum

# TREATMENT

## INITIAL STABILIZATION/THERAPY
0.9% NS IV fluid resuscitation for dehydration, bowel strangulation, obstruction, or sepsis:
- Adults: 1 L bolus
- Peds: 20 mL/kg bolus

## ED TREATMENT/PROCEDURES
- Incarcerated or strangulated hernias:
  - IVFs
    Nasogastric tube (NGT)
  - Surgical consultation
  - Preoperative broad spectrum antibiotics for strangulated hernia
- Hernia reduction procedure:
  - IV sedation (benzodiazepines) and analgesia (opiates) if necessary
  - Place patient in Trendelenburg position.
  - For spontaneous reduction, allow 20–30 min

- For manual reduction:
  - Place constant, gentle pressure on hernia.
  - For inguinal hernias, achieve reduction by putting fingers of 1 hand on internal ring while gently pulling then pressing on hernia distal to external ring.
- Obtain surgical consultation if reduction is unsuccessful after 1 or 2 attempts.
- Contraindications to reduction include:
  - Fever
  - Leukocytosis
  - Signs of strangulation
- Complications:
  - Introduction of strangulated bowel into abdomen
  - Further ischemia/necrosis occurs with no clinical improvement.
- Reduction in girls may be more difficult if ovary encased within hernia.

## MEDICATION
- Antibiotics (perioperative/controversial):
  - Cefazolin: 1–1.5 g (peds: 25–50 mg/kg/d div. q6–8h) IV q6–8h
  - Cefoxitin: 1–2 g (peds: 0–7 days: 40 mg/kg/24 h q12h; >7 days: 80–160 mg/kg/24 h div. q4–6h) IV q6–8 h
- Analgesics:
  - Morphine sulfate: 2–10 mg per dose (peds: 0.1–0.2 mg/kg IV/IM/SC q2–4h) IV/IM/SC q2–6h PRN
  - Fentanyl: 1–4 µg/kg (peds: 1–4 µg/kg IV PRN) IV PRN
- Sedatives:
  - Lorazepam: 1–2 mg
  - Midazolam: 2.5–5 mg (peds: 0.07 mg/kg) IV PRN

# FOLLOW-UP

## DISPOSITION

### Admission Criteria
- Strangulated hernias require immediate surgical intervention.
- Incarcerated hernias require admission for urgent surgical intervention.
- Intestinal obstruction
- Peritonitis
- Vomiting/dehydration
- Severe pain

### Discharge Criteria
- After successful reduction has been achieved
- Scheduled re-evaluation in 24 hr and referral to surgery

### Issues for Referral
As above

## FOLLOW-UP RECOMMENDATIONS
General surgery referral for surgical repair, if patient discharged:
- For large, recurrent, and/or symptomatic hernias

## PEARLS AND PITFALLS
- Failure to recognize signs and symptoms of an incarcerated or strangulated hernia
- Forcing reduction of incarcerated hernia
- Reintroducing strangulated bowel back into abdominal cavity

## ADDITIONAL READING
- Augustin G, Matosevic P, Kekez T, et al. Abdominal hernias in pregnancy. *J Obstet Gynaecol Res*. 2009;35(2):203–211.
- Brooks DC. Abdominal wall hernias. Available at www.uptodate.com. Accessed January 2010.
- Derici H, Unalp HR, Bozdag AD, et al. Factors affecting morbidity and mortality in incarcerated abdominal wall hernias. *Hernia*. 2007;11(4): 341–346.
- Lau ST, Lee YH, Caty MG. Current management of hernias and hydroceles. *Semin Pediatr Surg*. 2007; 16(1):50–57.
- Mensching JJ, Musielewicz AI. Abdominal wall hernias. *Emerg Med Clin North Am*. 1996;14(4): 739–756.
- Nicks BA. Hernias: Treatment & Medication. Available at http://emedicine.medscape. com/article/775630-treatment. Accessed January 2010.
- Ramsook C, Endom LL. Overview of inguinal hernia in children. Available at www.uptodate.com. Accessed January 2010.
- Sanchez-Manuel FJ. Antibiotic prophylaxis for hernia repair. *Cochrane Database Syst Rev*. 2007;18(3): CD003769.

## See Also (Topic, Algorithm, Electronic Media Element)
Abdominal Pain

# CODES

### ICD9
- 553.00 Unilateral or unspecified femoral hernia without mention of obstruction of gangrene
- 553.1 Umbilical hernia without mention of obstruction or gangrene
- 553.21 Incisional hernia without mention of obstruction or gangrene

H

# HERPES, GENITAL

Wender Hwang
Mark Richmond
Seth M. Oskie

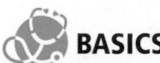 **BASICS**

## DESCRIPTION

- Genital herpes is a lifelong recurrent infection.
- ~1 in 4 Americans older than age 30 are seropositive for HSV-2:
  - Most are asymptomatic.
- 1st episode/primary HSV infection:
  - 2–12-day incubation
  - Symptoms peak 8–10 days after onset.
  - Lesions heal in 3 wk.
  - Primary infection may have more prominent clinical syndrome and complications (eg, encephalitis, meningitis, hepatitis).
  - Primary infection may also go unnoticed:
    ○ >50% of 1st recognized signs and symptoms are not primary infection.
- Recurrent HSV infection:
  - Average patient has 3 or 4 recurrences per year.
  - Virus reactivated from dorsal root ganglia
  - Triggered by local trauma, emotional stress, fever, sunlight, cold or heat, menstruation, or infection
  - Milder clinical syndrome and fewer lesions that usually heal within 10 days
- Asymptomatic HSV infection:
  - Virus is shed intermittently and often transmitted by persons who are without lesions or symptoms.

## ETIOLOGY

- 70–90% caused by a DNA virus herpes simplex virus, type 2 (HSV-2):
  - Remainder caused by herpes simplex virus type 1 (HSV-1)
- Increasing prevalence of genital HSV-1 infection:
  - Higher rates of oral sex
  - Falling incidence of childhood (nonsexual) transmission owing to improved social conditions resulting in a larger pool of susceptible adolescents and adults
- Primary genital infection by HSV-1 is similar to HSV-2 in symptoms and duration, but recurs much less frequently.
- Acquisition of HSV-2 in patients with pre-existing HSV-1 infection is less commonly associated with systemic symptoms:
  - Acquisition of HSV-1 in persons with pre-existing HSV-2 infection is rare.
- HSV vaccines currently in early clinical trials
- High association with HIV and other STDs

### ALERT

- Contact isolation and universal precautions should be maintained.
- Patients with HIV coinfection have higher HIV viral levels in the blood and skin lesions during HSV recurrence.

 **DIAGNOSIS**

## SIGNS AND SYMPTOMS

- Local pain and itching
- Herpetic cervicitis, vaginitis, or urethritis may present with dysuria, urinary hesitance or retention, vaginal discharge, or pelvic pain.
- Herpetic pharyngitis or gingivostomatitis may occur with oral acquisition.
- Systemic symptoms like fever, headache, malaise, photophobia, anorexia, myalgias, and lymphadenopathy are more common with primary infection.

### History

- 1–2-day prodrome of local tingling, burning, itching, or pain prior to eruption (can mimic sciatica)
- Classically, lesions are noted on day 2 as macules and papules, then progress to vesicles, pustules, and then ulcerate by day 5.
- Skin lesions crust over; mucosal membrane lesions heal without crusting.

### Physical Exam

- Lesions on vulva, vagina, cervix, perineum, buttocks; penile shaft or glans
- Grouped vesicles on an erythematous base
- On moist mucosal surfaces, ulcers may predominate.
- Atypical features may include localized edema, erythema, crusts, or fissures.

### Pediatric Considerations

- Neonatal infections are often disseminated or involve the CNS with high morbidity and mortality.
- Congenital HSV in the neonate without vesicles may mimic rubella, cytomegalovirus (CMV), or toxoplasmosis.
- Consider sexual abuse in children with genital HSV; culture lesions and test for other STDs in suspected cases.

## ESSENTIAL WORKUP

- Diagnosis based on history and physical examination

## DIAGNOSTIC TESTS & INTERPRETATION
### Lab

- Viral load in lesions of primary infection >> recurrence
- Tzanck preparation and staining of fluid from lesions is insensitive and nonspecific.

- Viral culture of vesicle fluid or ulcer base positive in 80–95% of cases, decreasing sensitivity as lesions crust and heal:
  - 3–10 days for result
- PCR 1.5–4 times more sensitive than viral culture; test of choice for CSF analysis in suspected CNS infection
- Serologic tests not helpful in acute disease:
  - Highly sensitive and specific; detect anti-gG1 and anti-gG2 antibodies
  - Require from 2 wk to >3 mo to detect seroconversion
  - Cannot distinguish acute from chronic disease
  - HerpeSelect HSV-1/HSV-2 enzyme-linked immunosorbent assay (ELISA):
    ○ Takes hour to days in lab
  - POCkit HSV2, bedside results in 10 min

### Imaging
No imaging generally indicated

## DIFFERENTIAL DIAGNOSIS

- Syphilis (*T. pallidum*)
- Chancroid (*H. ducreyi*)
- Lymphogranuloma venereum (LGV)
- Granuloma inguinale (*C. granulomatis*)
- Candidiasis
- Behçet syndrome

 **TREATMENT**

## PRE-HOSPITAL
Universal precautions should be maintained

## INITIAL STABILIZATION/THERAPY
Rarely required unless associated with systemic symptoms requiring hospitalization:

- Disseminated infection
- Hepatitis
- Pneumonitis
- Meningoencephalitis

## ED TREATMENT/PROCEDURES

- Treatment partially controls symptoms and lesions; does not eradicate latent virus nor affect recurrences after drug is discontinued.
- Episodic treatment of recurrences may shorten duration of lesions or ameliorate recurrences.
- Daily suppressive therapy in patients with frequent recurrences (6 or more per year) reduces frequency of recurrences by 75%.
- Acyclovir interferes with viral DNA polymerase; equally effective medications with less frequent dosing regimens are famciclovir and valacyclovir.
- Resistance to acyclovir in immunocompromised individuals is 5–10%:
  - Foscarnet 40 mg/kg IV t.i.d. may be effective.
- Consider testing for concomitant STDs.

### Pregnancy Considerations

- Women with primary HSV infection during pregnancy should receive antiviral therapy:
  - High rates of neonatal morbidity in both symptomatic and asymptomatic patients
- Asymptomatic antiviral therapy after 36 wk associated with decreased incidence of lesions at delivery:
  - Decreased cesarean delivery rates
  - Unknown effect on transmission because neither control nor therapy arms had cases of neonatal herpes

## MEDICATION

- Systemic or severe infection requiring hospitalization:
  - Acyclovir: 5–10 mg/kg IV t.i.d. until clinical improvement:
    o Neonate: 20 mg/kg IV t.i.d.

- 1st episode (7–10-day therapy; extend if not healed in 10 days):
  - Acyclovir: 400 mg PO t.i.d. or 200 mg PO 5 times per day:
    o Peds: 20 mg/kg PO t.i.d. or 5 mg/kg IV t.i.d.
  - Famciclovir: 250 mg PO t.i.d.
  - Valacyclovir: 1,000 mg PO b.i.d.
- Recurrent infection (5-day therapy):
  - Must start within 1 day of appearance of lesion or during prodrome
  - Acyclovir: 800 mg PO b.i.d. or 400 mg PO t.i.d. or 200 mg PO 5 times per day
  - Famciclovir: 125 mg PO b.i.d.
  - Valacyclovir: 500–1,000 mg PO b.i.d.
- Suppressive therapy (daily):
  - Acyclovir: 400 mg PO b.i.d.
  - Famciclovir: 250 mg PO b.i.d.
  - Valacyclovir: 500–1,000 mg PO daily
- Treatment of patients with HIV coinfection:
  - Recurrent infection. Use the non-HIV 1st-episode regimen above.
  - Suppressive therapy: Use the non-HIV recurrent-infection regimen.

 **FOLLOW-UP**

## DISPOSITION

### Admission Criteria

- Systemic involvement (encephalitis, meningitis), significant dissemination
- Severe local symptoms (pain, urinary retention)
- Severely immunocompromised patient

### Discharge Criteria

- Immunocompetent patient without systemic involvement
- Discharge counseling:
  - Avoid sexual contact during prodrome until healed
  - Practice safe sex techniques even if there are no lesions.

- Expect future recurrences; consider suppressive therapy if frequent.
- Analgesics and antipruritics as needed
- Dysuria and urinary retention may be relieved with sitz baths or pouring warm water over lesions during urination.

### Issues for Referral

- Neonatal herpes infection
- Sexual abuse in children
- Herpes infection during pregnancy

## PEARLS AND PITFALLS

- Treat primary infections
- Consider sexual abuse in children with genital herpes
- Herpes is a lifelong infection

## ADDITIONAL READING

- Cernik C, Gallina K, Brodell RT. The treatment of herpes simplex infections: An evidence based review. *Arch Intern Med.* 2008;168:1137–1144.
- Kimberlin DW, Rouse DJ. Clinical practice: Genital herpes. *N Engl J Med.* 2004;350:1970–1977.
- Moll HK. Management of oral and genital herpes in the emergency department. *Emerg Med Clin North Am.* 2008;26:475–473.
- Sexually transmitted diseases treatment guidelines 2006. Centers for Disease Control and Prevention. Available at: http://www.cdc.gov/std/treatment/2006/genital-ulcers.htm#genulc3

### See Also (Topic, Algorithm, Electronic Media Element)

- Herpes Simplex

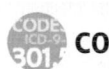 **CODES**

### ICD9

054.10 Genital herpes, unspecified

H

# HERPES SIMPLEX

Michael Homeyer
Mark Richmond

 **BASICS**

## DESCRIPTION
- Viral disease characterized by recurrent painful vesicular lesions of mucocutaneous areas
- Lips, genitalia, rectum, hands, and eyes most commonly involved
- Characterized by latency in sensory ganglia and reactivation
- Incubation period is approximately 4 days from exposure.
- Viral shedding occurs from 7–10 days (up to 23 days) in primary infection and 3–4 days in recurrent infections.
- Neonatal infections can occur in utero, intrapartum (most common), or postnatal; occur in 1/3,500 births per year in the U.S.
- Human-to-human transmission; 60–90% of population is infected with herpes simplex type 1 (HSV-1) or type 2 (HSV-2).
- More common in blacks than whites in ages <40 yr
- Females affected more than males

## ETIOLOGY
- HSV-1 or HSV-2 are DNA viruses of the Herpesviridae family.
- Viral transmission occurs through mucosa or abraded skin by direct contact with infected secretions:
  – Recurrent mucosal shedding of HSV may transmit the virus.
- Both viruses infect oral or genital mucosa:
  – Most common for HSV-1 to cause genital infections and HSV-2 to cause orofacial infections

 **DIAGNOSIS**

## SIGNS AND SYMPTOMS
- Primary infection may be unrecognized.
- Classically presents with grouped 1- to 2-mm vesicles on an erythematous base
- Vesicles may be filled with clear or cloudy fluid or may appear as frank pustules.

**Orofacial infection:**
- Primary infection:
  – Gingivostomatitis or pharyngitis:
    ○ Ulcerative exanthem involving gingival and mucous membranes
    ○ Fever, malaise, irritability, headache, myalgias, cervical adenopathy.
    ○ Primary infection symptoms typically last 10–14 days.
    ○ Inability to eat owing to pain is a risk for dehydration

- Recurrent infection (recrudescence):
  – Usually involves lips, specifically the vermillion border
  – Commonly incited by sunlight, heat, stress, trauma, or immunosuppression
  – Prodrome of itching, tingling, throbbing, or burning followed by erythema, papule/vesicle, ulcer, crust, and healing
  – Transmission can occur in absence of recognizable lesions
  – Fewer constitutional symptoms

**Skin infection:**
- History of exposure to HSV-1 or HSV-2
- Abrupt onset of fever, edema, erythema, and localized tenderness
- Herpetic whitlow:
  – HSV-2 more common than HSV-1
  – Infection of pulp and lateral aspect of finger with single or multiple vesicles
  – May occur from autoinoculation with primary oral or genital infection or from direct inoculation from occupational exposure
  – Can last 3–4 wk
  – Recurrence possible
- Traumatic herpes:
  – Can occur following cosmetic procedures of face, surgical and dental interventions, sun exposure, or burns
- Herpes gladiatorum:
  – Mucocutaneous infection of chest, face, and hands in wrestlers transmitted through traumatized skin
- Eczema herpeticum:
  – HSV-1 more command than HSV-2
  – Occurs in children and young adults with atopic dermatitis
  – Higher risk if on steroids or infected with HIV
  – Varicelliform eruption with spread to surrounding skin
  – Fever, headache, and fatigue
- HSV-associated erythema multiforme:
  – Usually presents on palms and soles
  – Lasts 2–3 wk

**Eye:**
- Most common cause of corneal blindness
- Caused by extension of facial lesions or direct inoculation
- Acute onset of pain and photophobia
- Periauricular adenopathy, blurry vision, chemosis, and conjunctivitis
- May be unilateral or bilateral
- Dendritic lesions of cornea noted on fluorescein exam
- Different from herpes varicella zoster as dermatome not involved

- Hutchinson's sign:
  – Vesicles on tip of nose may indicate ocular disease
  – Involvement of nasociliary nerve

**CNS/encephalitis:**
- Most common cause of severe sporadic encephalitis in the western world
- Usually from HSV-1 reactivation disease

### History
May or may not have known history of exposure to HSV-1 or HSV-2.

### Physical Exam
Vesiculoulcerative lesions in orofacial or genital area

### Pediatric Considerations
- Up to 60–80% of babies who develop neonatal HSV are born to mothers without history of genital herpes.
- Vesicular skin lesions may or may not be present on initial exam.
- Primary genital disease of the mother increases risk of transmitting virus to fetus.
- Most primary infections occur during childhood; symptomatic in only 5–10% of children
- Orofacial disease is most likely to present as gingivostomatitis in children younger than 5 yr of age.
- Whitlow may be caused by thumb-sucking children with oral herpes.

## ESSENTIAL WORKUP
- Herpes encephalitis:
  – Lumbar puncture if herpes encephalitis is considered.
- Herpes ophthalmicus:
  – Fluorescein exam if ocular herpes is a concern.

## DIAGNOSTIC TESTS & INTERPRETATION
- Orofacial:
  – Presumptive diagnosis made by history and exam
  – If definitive diagnosis is necessary (eg, systemic disease, child abuse):
    ○ Viral culture or polymerase chain reaction testing of swabs from vesicles
    ○ Fluorescent antibody detection of antigen; serum antibody studies
    ○ Scrapings for Tzanck smear or Papanicolaou stain
    ○ Skin biopsy if hyperkeratotic or lichenoid lesions
- Eye:
  – Dendritic corneal lesions by fluorescein exam
  – Swab of affected area for viral culture or fluorescent antibody detection
- CNS/encephalitis:
  – Lumbar puncture with CSF pleocytosis and negative bacterial antigens
  – CSF polymerase chain reaction (PCR) test
  – MRI/CT
  – EEG diagnostic if spike and waves in temporal region

### Lab

- Lesion scrapings can be sent for culture or PCR testing
- Tzanck smear demonstrating multinucleated giant cells, atypical keratinocytes, and large nuclei
- Serum testing has limited ED use.
- Enzyme-linked immunosorbent assay (ELISA) testing may demonstrate HSV antibodies, determining past exposure only.
- Requires from 2 wk to >3 mo to detect seroconversion

## DIFFERENTIAL DIAGNOSIS

- Orofacial and skin:
  - Bacterial pharyngitis
  - Mycoplasma pneumoniae pharyngitis
  - Stevens-Johnson syndrome
  - Herpes zoster
  - Varicella
  - Pemphigus
  - Contact or chemical dermatitis
  - Impetigo
- Eye:
  - Conjunctivitis: Viral, bacterial, or allergic
  - Herpes zoster ophthalmicus
  - Scleritis/episcleritis
  - Angle-closure glaucoma
  - Corneal abrasion

 TREATMENT

### PRE-HOSPITAL

- Maintain universal precautions.
- Pain control

### INITIAL STABILIZATION/THERAPY

Protect airway in comatose or obtunded patients with suspected CNS disease.

### ED TREATMENT/PROCEDURES

- Orofacial/gingivostomatitis:
  - Primary disease in healthy children is generally not treated.
  - Primary disease in normal host with mild disease requires only supportive treatment with hydration and analgesia.
  - Severe disease or immunocompromised patients: IV or oral acyclovir, valacyclovir, or famciclovir
  - Oral acyclovir is first-line medication
  - If recurrent disease, oral antivirals are most helpful if started with prodrome or at 1st sign of lesion:
    - Reduces lesions and symptoms by 1–2 day
  - Consider prophylaxis in patients with more than 6 episodes per year; history of herpes associated erythema multiforme or herpes gladiatorum; upcoming intense sun exposure or stress; perioral/intraoral surgery; cosmetic facial procedures:
    - Prophylaxis reduces frequency and severity of herpes labialis and may help decrease asymptomatic shedding, leading to decreased transmission
    - Does not cure or terminate the disease
    - When prophylaxis is stopped, most patients have recurrences

- Skin (other than orofacial or genital):
  - May be treated with oral acyclovir
  - Antibiotics if secondary bacterial infection
  - *Do not incise and drain*: May lead to spread of infection.
- Eye:
  - Oral acyclovir and topical antiviral therapy with trifluridine or vidarabine
  - Vidarabine ointment for children
  - *Do not treat with steroids*: May cause increased viral replication
  - Ophthalmology consult

### Pregnancy Considerations

Acyclovir has been used to suppress genital herpes near end of pregnancy and appears safe, but is not FDA approved

## MEDICATION

- Acyclovir:
  - Orofacial and skin: 400 mg PO t.i.d. for 7–10 days or 5–10 mg/kg IV (5–10 mg/kg) q8h for 7–14 days
  - Pediatric mucocutaneous primary infection: 1,200 mg/24 h divided q8h for 7–10 days max 80 mg/kg/24 hr or 15 mg/kg/24 hrs divided q8h for 7 days.
  - Eyes for suppression therapy: 400 mg PO b.i.d.
  - Encephalitis: 60 mg/kg/24 hrs IV divided q8h for 14–21 days
- Famciclovir:
  - Primary Orofacial: 250 mg PO t.i.d. for 7–10 days (immunocompetent), 500 mg PO b.i.d. for 7–10 days (immunocompromised).
- Trifluridine:
  - Adults and peds older than 6 yr: 1 drop of 1% ophthalmic ointment to eye q2h while awake (max. 9 drops per day) for at least 10 days and then taper under ophthalmology consultation.
- Valacyclovir:
  - Adults primary mucocutaneous: 1,000 mg PO b.i.d. for 7 days
  - Adult recurrent mucocutaneous (nongenital): 500 mg PO b.i.d. for 1 day
- Vidarabine:
  - Adults or peds older than 2 yr: topical 0.5-inch ribbon of 3% ophthalmic ointment to eye 5 times per day.
- Recurrent mucocutaneous herpes:
  - Acyclovir: 400 mg PO t.i.d. for 5 days
  - Famciclovir: 1,000 mg PO b.i.d. for 1 day
  - Valacyclovir: 500 mg PO b.i.d. for 3 days
- Long-term prophylaxis:
  - Acyclovir: 400 mg PO b.i.d.
  - Valacyclovir: 500 mg PO daily
  - Famciclovir: 250 mg PO b.i.d.

### ALERT

- Antiviral dosing may need adjustment for renal failure.
- Topical antivirals are available but have not been shown to reduce the length of symptoms or decrease recurrence.

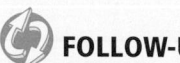 FOLLOW-UP

### DISPOSITION

#### Admission Criteria

- Encephalitis, disseminated disease, dehydration
- Severe local or disseminated disease in immunocompromised host
- Neonatal HSV
- ICU versus ward based on toxicity and need for airway support
- Ophthalmology consult versus admission for ocular involvement

#### Discharge Criteria

Uncomplicated local disease

#### Issues for Referral

- Suppressive treatment options
- Herpes infection during pregnancy

### FOLLOW-UP RECOMMENDATIONS

Skin/genital infection:

- Follow-up with the patient's primary doctor to discuss risks and benefits of suppressive therapy.

## PEARLS AND PITFALLS

- Failure to consider herpes simplex encephalitis in patients whom you have a concern for meningitis/encephalitis.
- Failure to consider ocular herpes in patients presenting with eye pain, decreased vision, and or lesions on nose.
- Failure to warn patients about the risk of transmission to others especially during outbreaks and for 1–2 wk thereafter.
- Failure to warn patients to avoid touching the lesions during outbreaks to prevent spread of the lesions to other body areas.

## ADDITIONAL READING

- Cernik C, Gallina K, Brodell R. The treatment of herpes simplex infections: An evidence based review. *Arch Intern Med*. 2008;168:1137–1144.
- Chayavichitsilp P, Buckwalter JV, Krakowski AC, et al. Herpes simplex. *Pediatr Rev*. 2009;30: 119–130.
- Mell HK. Management of oral and genital herpes in the emergency department. *Emerg Med Clin North Am*. 2008;26:457–473.

### See Also (Topic, Algorithm, Electronic Media Element)

- Genital Herpes
- Varicella
- Zoster

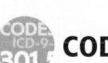 CODES

### ICD9

- 054.2 Herpetic gingivostomatitis
- 054.3 Herpetic meningoencephalitis
- 054.10 Genital herpes, unspecified

H

# HERPES ZOSTER

*Jeremy B. Hammel*
*Mark Richmond*

 **BASICS**

## DESCRIPTION
- Commonly known as shingles or dermatomal zoster
- Most common in patients with decreased cell-mediated immunity:
  – Older than 50 yr of age
  – Neoplastic diseases (lymphoproliferative cancers)
  – Immunosuppressive drugs
- Disseminates rarely in normal hosts and frequently in immunocompromised hosts
- *Ramsay Hunt syndrome* is characterized by zoster oticus, peripheral facial palsy, regional adenopathy, vertigo, and anesthesia of anterior 2/3 of hemitongue:
  – From 7th and 8th cranial nerve involvement
- Postherpetic neuralgia (PHN) is a complication of zoster:
  – Described as pain that persists at site of zoster lesions for >3 mo after cutaneous disease has healed
  – 10–70% of patients will have pain after resolution of lesions.
  – Incidence increases with age older than 50 yr, severe rash, and severe pain.
- Syndrome of herpes zoster occurring without rash is called *zoster sine herpete*.

## ETIOLOGY
- Caused by varicella-zoster virus (VZV), a DNA virus in the Herpesviridae family
- Mostly in individuals who previously had chickenpox and very rarely in vaccinated individuals
- Reactivation of a virus that lies dormant in dorsal root ganglia

### Pregnancy Considerations
Low rate of fetal complications

### Pediatric Considerations
Childhood zoster is most common when varicella occurred in utero or within 6 mo of life.

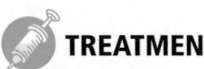 **DIAGNOSIS**

## SIGNS AND SYMPTOMS
- Prodrome of pain and paresthesias in dermatomal distribution:
  – Character of pain may be sharp, dull, tingling, burning, or intense pruritus.
  – Pain precedes rash by 1–10 days.
  – Prodrome less likely in young patients
  – Classical rash is grouped vesicles on erythematous base.
  – Initially are patches of erythema and then vesicles
  – Progress to scab and crust formation over 10–12 days
  – Crusts fall off in 2–3 wk.
  – Lesions evolve synchronously.
  – One dermatome typically affected, rarely crosses midline
  – Most common nerve distributions are thoracic and lumbar, followed by trigeminal and cervical.
- Ocular involvement occurs in half of cases involving ophthalmic division of trigeminal nerve:
  – Closely associated with disease occurring at tip of nose (Hutchinson sign)
  – Corneal involvement begins as punctate keratitis, which may coalesce to form pseudodendritic or stellate pattern.
- Disseminated disease may cause signs and symptoms of meningoencephalitis, myelitis, peripheral neuropathy, hepatitis, and pneumonitis.
- Immunosuppressed patients are more likely to have severe disease and visceral involvement.

## ESSENTIAL WORKUP
- Clinical presentation is sufficient for diagnosis in most patients.
- Herpes zoster ophthalmicus (HZO) is diagnosed by slit-lamp exam:
  – The pseudodendrites of HZO are elevated and plaquelike, sitting on top of epithelium, and stain brighter with rose bengal.
  – Is less ulcerative than HSV and stains less brightly with fluorescein

## DIAGNOSTIC TESTS & INTERPRETATION
*Lab*
- Cell yields are highest if base of vesicular lesions are scraped.
- Numerous rapid immunofluorescence assays exist to detect VZV in vesicular fluid and are preferred method:
  – Can distinguish between HSV and VZV
- Tzanck smear demonstrates giant cells and intranuclear inclusions.
- IgM and IgG are most commonly measured by ELISA:
  – Antibody titers rise 2 wk after acute infection.
- PCR may be useful in CSF analysis or verrucous lesions in which cultures are otherwise negative.

## DIFFERENTIAL DIAGNOSIS
- Zosteriform herpes simplex
- Varicella
- Herpes simplex (HSV)
- Nonherpetic conjunctivitis
- Enteroviral infections (eg, hand-foot-and-mouth disease)
- Insect bites
- Bullous impetigo
- Molluscum contagiosum

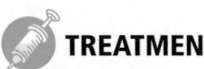 **TREATMENT**

## PRE-HOSPITAL
- Zoster is potentially contagious and may cause varicella in nonimmune health care workers:
  – Lesions should be covered.
- Maintain universal precautions.

## INITIAL STABILIZATION/THERAPY
- Rarely necessary
- IV access to administer fluids and antiviral therapy
- Disseminated disease to CNS or lungs may require airway support.

## ED TREATMENT/PROCEDURES

- Goal of treatment is to treat acute viral infection, decrease pain, and prevent postherpetic neuralgia (PHN).
- Acyclovir, valacyclovir, or famciclovir is recommended:
  - Should be started within 72 hr of rash formation, but some experts recommend to start later if new vesicles are still appearing
  - Speeds acute healing and resolution of acute pain
  - Does not decrease the rate of PHN
- Foscarnet recommended for acyclovir-resistant VZV in immunocompromised patients
- Ocular involvement:
  - Necessitates ophthalmologic consultation
  - Oral (normal host) or intravenous (immunocompromised host) acyclovir is best started within 72 hr; may be beneficial up to 1 wk after symptom onset.
- Oral corticosteroids in acute zoster are controversial:
  - Several studies showed modest improvement in cutaneous healing and acute neuritis
  - Do not help prevent PHN
  - If not contraindicated, recommended in patients >50 yr old, severe disease (>21 lesions), or severe pain
- Long-acting narcotics and topical lidocaine patches are recommended for moderate to severe pain.
- OTC analgesia for mild pain
- PHN is difficult to manage:
  - Topical lidocaine and prilocaine cream provide short-term relief.
  - Topical capsaicin is controversial and should not be initiated in ED.
  - Sustained-release oxycodone or other long-acting narcotics are useful for analgesia
    Gabapentin and pregabalin are safe and effective.

### Pediatric Considerations

Aspirin should be avoided because of risk of Reye syndrome.

## MEDICATION

### First Line

- Antivirals:
  - Acyclovir:
    - Immunocompetent: 800 mg PO 5x/d for 7 days (peds: <12 yo: 30 mg/kg/d or 1,500 m$^2$/d PO div q8h for 7–10 days; >12 yr of age: 4,000 mg/d PO div 5x/d for 5–7 days or 30 mg/kg/d or 1,500 m$^2$/d PO div q8h for 7–10 days)
    - Immunocompromised: 10 mg/kg IV q8h (peds: <12 yr of age: 60 mg/kg/d IV div q8h for 7–10 days; >12 yr of age: 30 mg/kg/d IV div q8h for 7–10 days)
    - Herpes zoster ophthalmicus: 800 mg PO 5x/d for 7 days or 10 mg/kg IV q8h
  - Famciclovir: Adults: 500 mg PO t.i.d. for 7 days
  - Valacyclovir: 1,000 mg PO t.i.d. for 7 days
- Pain medication as needed

### Second Line

- Foscarnet: 40 mg/kg IV q8h for 14–26 days
- Gabapentin: 100–300 mg nightly at bedtime increasing 100–300 mg every 3 days until adequate response or max. 3,600 mg/d div q8h
- Lidocaine patch 5%: apply up to 3 patches for <12 hr within a 24-hr period.
- Prednisone: 30 mg PO b.i.d. days 1–7, 15 mg PO b.i.d. days 8–14, and 7.5 mg b.i.d. days 15–21
- Pregabalin: Start 50 mg PO t.i.d. or 75 mg PO b.i.d. increase to 100 mg t.i.d. within 1 wk
- Varicella-zoster immunoglobulin (VZIG): Adults and peds: Specialized dosing

 ## FOLLOW-UP

### DISPOSITION

#### Admission Criteria

- Disseminated disease
- Immunocompromised patients with any of the following:
  - Involvement of trigeminal nerve
  - Herpes zoster ophthalmicus
  - Ramsay Hunt syndrome
  - Involvement of >2 dermatomes
  - Visceral involvement
  - Intractable pain
- ICU vs. ward depends on severity of disease.

#### Pediatric Considerations

Zoster in the neonate requires admission and treatment with IV acyclovir.

#### Discharge Criteria

- Most are managed as outpatients.
- Patients should be instructed that lesions may heal with scarring or leave depigmented areas.
- Recommend isolation from steroid-dependent, pregnant, or immunocompromised persons until lesions are crusted:
  - VZIG recommended within 72 hr for exposed immunocompromised contacts

- Neonates born to seronegative mothers exposed to zoster should receive VZIG within 24 hr.
- Recommend referral of patients older than 60 yr to primary care physician for vaccination therapy:
  - Recent published data support Oka/Merck VZV vaccine; was found to be beneficial in reducing incidence of herpes zoster as well as PHN.
- PHN may require long-term follow-up; referral to pain specialist may be required.

## PEARLS AND PITFALLS

- Pearls:
  - Remember to look for ocular involvement if rash is in V1 branch of trigeminal nerve
  - Start antivirals, pain meds on all patients:
    - Strongly consider steroids
  - Warn all patient about the risk for postherpetic neuralgia
- Pitfalls:
  - Failure to consider the diagnosis in the absence of rash
  - Failure to evaluate for ocular involvement with rash to face

## ADDITIONAL READING

- Liesegang TJ. Herpes zoster ophthalmicus. natural history, risk factors, clinical presentation, and morbidity. *Ophthalmology.* 2008;115:S3–S12.
- Opstelten W, Eekhof J, Neven AK, et al. Treatment of herpes zoster. *Can Fam Physician.* 2008;54: 373–377.
- Sampathkumar P, Drage I A, Martin DP. Herpes zoster (shingles) and postherpetic neuralgia. *Mayo Clin Proc.* 2009;84:274–280.
- Whitley RJ. A 70-year-old woman with shingles. A review of herpes zoster. *JAMA.* 2009;302:73–80.

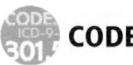 ## CODES

### ICD9

053.9 Herpes zoster without mention of complication

H

# HICCUPS

*Carrie Tibbles*
*James L. Smith, Jr.*

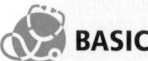 **BASICS**

## DESCRIPTION

- Sudden, involuntary, contraction of the diaphragm (usually unilateral) and other inspiratory muscles terminated by abrupt closure of the glottis
- Medical terminology: Singultus
- Usually occur with a frequency of 4–60/min
- Occurs as a result of stimulation of the hiccup reflex arc:
  - Irritation of the vagus and phrenic nerves
  - The "hiccup center" is located in the upper spinal cord or brainstem
- Classification:
- Hiccup bout: <48 hr
- Persistent hiccups: 48 hr–1 mo
- Intractable hiccups: >1 mo
- Male > Female (4:1)

## ETIOLOGY

- GI:
  - Gastric distention*, overeating, eating too fast
  - Esophageal: Gastroesophageal reflux*, achalasia, candida esophagitis, cancer
  - Gastric: Ulcers, cancer
  - Hepatic: Hepatitis, hepatoma
  - Pancreatic: Pancreatitis, pseudocyst, cancer
  - Bowel obstruction
  - Inflammatory bowel disease
  - Cholelithiasis, cholecystitis
  - Appendicitis
  - Abdominal aortic aneurysm
  - Postoperative, abdominal procedure
- Diaphragmatic irritation:
  - Hiatal hernia
  - Intraabdominal mass
  - Pericarditis
  - Eventration
  - Splenomegaly, hepatomegaly
  - Peritonitis
- CNS:
  - Vascular lesions: Ischemic/hemorrhagic stroke*, head trauma*, arteriovenous malformations,
  - Infectious: Encephalitis, meningitis, abscess
  - Structural: Cancer, Parkinson disease, Multiple sclerosis, hydrocephalus
  - Ventriculoperitoneal shunt

- Thoracic:
  - Infectious: Pneumonia, TB
  - Cardiac: MI, pericarditis
  - Aortic aneurysm
  - Cancer
  - Mediastinal lymphadenopathy*
- Head and neck:
  - Otic foreign body irritating the tympanic membrane
  - Pharyngitis
  - Laryngitis
  - Goiter
  - Retropharyngeal/peritonsillar abscess
  - Neck mass
- Metabolic:
  - Uremia
  - Hyponatremia
  - Hypocalcemia
  - Gout
  - DM
- Toxic/drug-induced:
  - Alcohol*
  - Tobacco
  - $\alpha$-Methyldopa
  - Benzodiazepines
  - Steroids
  - Barbiturates
  - Narcotics
  - Chemotherapeutic agents
  - Antibiotics
  - General anesthesia
- Psychogenic causes:
  - Stress/excitement
  - Grief
  - Malingering
  - Conversion disorder
- Idiopathic
  * More common causes

 **DIAGNOSIS**

## SIGNS AND SYMPTOMS

- Characteristic sound abruptly ending an inspiratory effort
- Attacks usually occur at brief intervals and last only a few seconds or minutes.
- Attacks lasting >48 hr or persisting during sleep suggest an organic etiology.

### History

- Targeted history and review of systems to determine likelihood of potential underlying etiology:
  - Severity and duration of current episode
  - History of previous episodes and treatment attempts

### Physical Exam

- Careful physical exam in search of an underlying cause, with exam focused on:
  - Head and neck
  - Chest
  - Abdomen
  - Neurologic

## ESSENTIAL WORKUP

For persistent or intractable hiccups, a thorough history and physical exam dictate further diagnostic testing.

## DIAGNOSTIC TESTS & INTERPRETATION

### Lab

- CBC with differential
- Electrolytes, BUN, creatinine

### Imaging

- CXR
- Further imaging may be indicated depending on clinical suspicion of a particular etiology; this can often be performed on an outpatient basis.

## DIFFERENTIAL DIAGNOSIS

Eructation

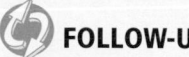 **TREATMENT**

### ED TREATMENT/PROCEDURES

- Treat specific causes when identified:
  - Remove foreign bodies from the ear.
  - Relieve gastric distention with a nasogastric tube.
- Nonpharmacologic maneuvers:
  - Catheter stimulation of the posterior pharynx
  - Direct stimulation of the uvula with a cotton swab
  - Supraorbital pressure
  - Carotid sinus massage
  - Digital rectal massage
- Pharmacologic treatment:
  - First-line, only FDA approved medication for hiccups:
  - Chlorpromazine
- Additional medications:
  - Gabapentin
  - Metoclopramide
  - Baclofen
  - Haloperidol
  - Nebulized lidocaine
  - Amitriptyline
  - Phenytoin

### MEDICATION

- Amitriptyline: 10 mg PO t.i.d.
- Baclofen: 10 mg PO t.i.d.
- Chlorpromazine: 25–50 mg IV/IM, 25–50 mg PO t.i.d–q.i.d.
- Gabapentin: 100 mg PO t.i.d–q.i.d.
- Haloperidol: 2–5 mg IM
- Lidocaine (4%): 3 mL nebulized, repeat if necessary
- Metoclopramide: 10 mg IV/IM, 10–20 mg PO q.i.d.
- Phenytoin: 200 mg IV

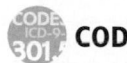 **FOLLOW-UP**

### DISPOSITION

#### Admission Criteria
For cases of hiccups that interfere with daily activities and could lead to decreased nutritional or fluid intake, aspirations, insomnia, wound dehiscence

#### Discharge Criteria
- If hiccups last <48 hr
- Workup inconsistent with underlying organic etiology

#### Issues for Referral
Referral in cases of intractable hiccups for investigation into underlying cause and more definitive therapeutic measures:

- Phrenic nerve block, crush, or transection
- Hypnosis
- Behavioral modification
- Acupuncture
- Psychiatric interventions

### FOLLOW-UP RECOMMENDATIONS
Home remedies in case of recurrence:

- Swallowing a spoonful of sugar
- Sucking on a hard candy or swallowing peanut butter
- Breath holding/Valsalva maneuver
- Biting a lemon
- Tongue traction
- Lifting the uvula with a cold spoon
- Drinking from the far side of a glass
- Fright
- Noxious stimuli
- Rebreathing into a paper bag

## PEARLS AND PITFALLS

Protracted hiccups are strongly suggestive of underlying organic disease.

## ADDITIONAL READING

- Kolodzik PW, Eilers MA. Hiccups (singultus): Review and approach to management. *Ann Emerg Med.* 1991;20:565–573.
- Launois S. Hiccup in adults: An overview. *Eur Respir J.* 1993;6(4):563–575.
- Lewis JH. Hiccups: Reasons and remedies. In: Lewis JH, ed. *A pharmacologic approach to gastrointestinal disorders.* Baltimore: Williams & Wilkins; 1994:116.
- Marinella MA. Diagnosis and management of hiccups in the patient with advanced cancer. *J Supportive Oncol.* 2009;7:122–227.
- Rosseau P. Hiccups. *South Med J.* 1995;88(2):175–181.
- Schuchmann JA, Browne BA. Persistent hiccups during rehabilitation hospitalization. *Am J Physical Med Rehabil.* 2007;86:1013–1018.

**CODES**

**ICD9**
786.8 Hiccough

# HIGH ALTITUDE ILLNESS

*Christopher B. Colwell*

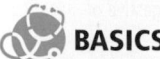

## BASICS

### DESCRIPTION
- Incidence dependent on:
  - Rate of ascent
  - Final altitude
  - Sleeping altitude
  - Duration at altitude
- Acute mountain sickness (AMS) incidence:
  - Up to 67% incidence with rapid ascent (1–2 days) to >14,000 ft
  - 22% incidence for skiers visiting resorts and sleeping at 7,000–9,000 ft, 40% at 10,000 ft
- AMS risk factors:
  - Previous history of high-altitude illness
  - Exertion
  - Younger persons (<50)
  - Physical fitness not protective
- High-altitude pulmonary edema (HAPE) incidence:
  - <1–2%
  - Varies with rate of ascent
- High-altitude cerebral edema (HACE) incidence <1%

### Pregnancy Considerations
- Relationship between pregnancy and high-altitude illness is not clearly established.
- Pregnancy-induced hypertension, proteinuria, and peripheral edema are more common at high altitude, which may be related to maternal hypoxemia.
- No evidence of increase in spontaneous abortions, placental abruption, or placenta previa at high altitudes
- Travel by pregnant women with normal pregnancies to moderate altitudes appears safe, although caution should be exercised when traveling >13,000 ft and for women with complicated pregnancies.

### Geriatric Considerations
Although elderly persons are more likely to have underlying health problems that may be affected by altitude, such as HTN, COPD, and coronary artery disease, the risk of development of AMS is less in those older than age 55 than in other age groups.

### ETIOLOGY
- Rapid ascent >8,000 ft without proper acclimatization is the most common cause of high-altitude–related illness.
- Rapidity of ascent, final altitude reached, sleeping altitude, and individual susceptibility all play a role in development of high-altitude illness as well.

## DIAGNOSIS

### SIGNS AND SYMPTOMS
#### History
- Acute Mountain Sickness (AMS):
  - Headache plus at least 1 of the following:
    - Nausea/vomiting
    - Fatigue/lassitude
    - Dizziness
    - Difficulty sleeping
  - Onset 4–12 hr after ascent
  - Generally benign and self-limited
  - Symptoms may become debilitating.
- High-altitude pulmonary edema (HAPE):
  - Onset 2–4 days after ascent, most commonly on 2nd night
  - Cough (dry at 1st, then productive)
  - Dyspnea at rest
- High-altitude cerebral edema (HACE):
  - Life threatening
  - Occurs in presence of HAPE and/or AMS:
    - Seen rarely as isolated entity
  - Onset:
    - May occur 12 hr after onset of AMS
    - Usually requires 2–4 days for development
  - Altered mental status
  - Severe or increasing headache
  - Nausea/vomiting

#### Pediatric Considerations
- AMS in infants and young children manifested by:
  - Increased fussiness
  - Decreased playfulness
  - Decreased appetite
  - Vomiting
  - Sleep disturbances
- Incidence of HAPE greater in younger individuals (<20 yr) than adults
- No cases of HAPE or HACE reported in children <4 yr old

#### Physical Exam
- AMS:
  - Without presence of high-altitude pulmonary or cerebral edema, the physical exam will often be normal:
    - More mild stages of AMS are often misdiagnosed as viral syndromes or hangovers from alcohol ingestions
- HAPE:
  - Tachypnea
  - Rales
  - Cyanosis
  - Fever may be present.
  - Severe respiratory distress and death may occur.

- HACE:
  - Ataxia
  - Papilledema, retinal hemorrhages
  - Altered mental status/global encephalopathy:
    - Focal neurologic deficit less common
    - Seizure (rare)
    - Coma

### ESSENTIAL WORKUP
- Clinical diagnosis in setting of recent altitude gain
- AMS:
  - Diagnosis made with history of headache plus at least 1 of the following:
    - Nausea/vomiting
    - Lassitude/fatigue
    - Dizziness
    - Insomnia
  - No diagnostic laboratory or imaging studies
- HAPE:
  - Dyspnea on exertion—universal finding at altitude
  - Dyspnea at rest—symptom of HAPE, worse at night
  - Rales, cyanosis, or cough support diagnosis.
  - Tachycardia, tachypnea correlate with severity.
- HACE:
  - Cerebellar ataxia with or without other symptoms of AMS
  - Papilledema, retinal hemorrhages are associated findings.

### DIAGNOSTIC TESTS & INTERPRETATION
#### Lab
Arterial blood gas (ABG) for HAPE:
- Reveals hypoxemia ($pO_2$ 30–50) and respiratory alkalosis, *not* acidosis

#### Imaging
- CXR in HAPE:
  - Reveals patchy alveolar infiltrates with areas of clearing between patches
  - Unilateral or bilateral infiltrates (right midlung field being most common)
  - Cardiomegaly, "batwing" distribution of infiltrates, and Kerley B lines (typical of cardiogenic pulmonary edema)—absent in HAPE
- CT and MRI scans in HACE:
  - Vasogenic edema of white matter

#### Diagnostic Procedures/Surgery
ECG in HAPE:
- Tachycardia
- Evidence of right-heart strain

## DIFFERENTIAL DIAGNOSIS

- AMS:
  - Alcohol hangover
  - Carbon monoxide poisoning
  - Encephalitis
  - Exhaustion
  - Meningitis
  - Viral syndrome
- HAPE:
  - High-altitude bronchitis and pharyngitis
  - Pneumonia
  - Pulmonary embolism:
    - More rapid onset
    - Pleuritic chest pain
- HACE:
  - Cerebrovascular accidents/transient ischemic attacks:
    - Focal neurologic signs suggest vascular lesion.

 TREATMENT

### PRE-HOSPITAL

- Severe cases require immediate evacuation to lower altitude.
- Do not proceed to higher altitude in presence of symptoms.
- Oxygen delivery or simulated descent in portable hyperbaric chamber (Gamow bag) can be lifesaving temporary measure making self-rescue possible.

### INITIAL STABILIZATION/THERAPY

- HAPE and HACE:
  - ABCs:
    - Endotracheal intubation for impending respiratory failure, hyperventilation, or airway protection
  - Establish IV access.
    Supplemental oxygen and monitoring
  - CPAP for HAPE

### ED TREATMENT/PROCEDURES

- AMS:
  - Mild cases usually self-limited:
    - Symptomatic treatment
    - Halt ascent until symptoms resolve
  - Acetazolamide for moderate to severe symptoms
  - Ibuprofen or acetaminophen for headache
  - Promethazine for nausea
  - Supplemental oxygen in severe cases
  - Descent for severe or persistent symptoms
  - Acetazolamide for AMS prophylaxis:
    - In high-risk individual with planned rapid ascent

- HAPE:
  - Immediate descent for moderate/severe symptoms
  - Mild cases may be managed without descent if:
    - Adequate oxygen supplies available
    - Serial medical examinations possible
    - Immediate descent for any deterioration in clinical status
  - Bed rest to avoid exercise-induced pulmonary HTN
  - Supplemental oxygen:
    - High flow rates (6–8 L/min) until improvement, then continue with lower flow rates
  - Nifedipine when other interventions are unavailable
  - β-agonist inhalers may be helpful.
  - Hyperbaric therapy is available and immediate descent is not possible.
- HACE:
  - Immediate evacuation to lower altitude
  - Oxygen
  - Dexamethasone
  - Bed rest with elevation of head at 30°, and in severe cases, aggressive management of elevated intracranial pressure

### MEDICATION

- Acetazolamide:
  - AMS treatment: 250–500 mg (peds: 5 mg/kg) PO b.i.d.
  - AMS prophylaxis: 250 mg PO b.i.d. (peds: 5 mg/kg) PO b.i.d.; start 24 hr before ascent
- Dexamethasone: 8 mg IV, then 4 mg PO/IV q.i.d.
- Ibuprofen: 800 mg (peds: 5–10 mg/kg) PO t.i.d.
- Nifedipine: 10 mg PO, then 30 mg sustained release (SR) PO b.i.d.
- Promethazine: 12.5–25 mg (peds: 0.25–1 mg/kg) PO/PR (per rectum)/IM q4–6h

### First Line

- Acetazolamide (AMS)
- Nifedipine (HAPE)

### Second Line

Dexamethasone

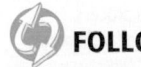 FOLLOW-UP

### DISPOSITION

Descent to a lower altitude mandatory in severe cases

### Admission Criteria

- Persistent symptoms after observation in lower altitude ED require admission.
- HAPE
- HACE

### Discharge Criteria

Once clinical improvement seen and oxygen saturation >95% on room air

### Issues for Referral

Offer prophylactic therapy for future ascents in patients with recurrent AMS (acetazolamide) or HAPE (nifedipine).

## PEARLS AND PITFALLS

- The symptoms of high-altitude illness can resemble mild viral syndromes.
- Failure to consider high-altitude illness is a common pitfall.
- When managing altitude illness, once symptoms have developed and until they resolve, further ascent is contraindicated.
- Ataxia and dyspnea at rest are potentially early indicators of HACE and HAPE, respectively.
- Hyperbaric oxygen and adjunctive medications should be considered when descent is not possible.

## ADDITIONAL READING

- Grissom CK, Roach RC, Sarnquist FH, et al. Acetazolamide in the treatment of acute mountain sickness: Clinical efficacy and effect on gas exchange. *Ann Intern Med*. 1992;116(6):461–465.
- Hackett PH, Roach RC. High-altitude illness. *N Engl J Med*. 2001;345:107–114.
- Roach RC, et al. How well do older persons tolerate moderate altitude? *West J Med*. 1995;162:32–36.
- Spaulding SC, Markovchick VJ. High-altitude illness. In: Wolfson AB, ed. *Harwood-Nuss' Clinical Practice of Emergency Medicine*, 5th ed. Philadelphia: Lippincott Williams & Wilkins; 2010:1605–1608.
- Yaron M, Honigman B. High altitude medicine. In: Marx JA, ed. *Rosen's Emergency Medicine: Concepts and Clinical Practice*, 7th ed. Philadelphia, PA: Mosby; 2010:1917–1928.

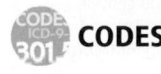 CODES

ICD9
993.2 Other and unspecified effects of high altitude

H

# HIP INJURY

*Siobhan Gray*
*Colleen Buono*

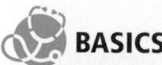 **BASICS**

## DESCRIPTION
- Hip injury includes hip fractures and dislocations of the proximal femur due to minor or major trauma or overuse.
- Hip fracture: Fracture of proximal femur. Classified as intracapsular or extracapsular:
  - Intracapsular fracture: Femoral head or neck; often associated with disruption of femoral neck vessels; significant morbidity due to AVN:
    - Femoral head fracture: Usually associated with hip dislocation (anterior > posterior).
    - Femoral neck fracture: Usually older adults with minor trauma, or young patient with major trauma; symptoms vary. Patient may or may not be ambulatory. Often site of stress fracture in runners/military recruits.
  - Extracapsular fractures: Below acetabular capsule. Normally do not disrupt blood flow. Morbidity typically due to patient immobilization: DVT, PE:
    - Trochanteric fractures: Greater trochanter usually fractured by avulsions at insertion in gluteus medius. Lesser trochanter usually avulsion due to forceful contraction of iliopsoas, seen in young athletes and children.
    - Intertrochanteric fracture: Defined as occurring in line between greater and lesser trochanters. Common in elderly, osteoporosis patients often due to fall. Marked external rotation and shortening. Can be stable or unstable. Nonambulatory.
    - Subtrochanteric fracture: Usually due to direct, significant trauma in younger patients or lesser trauma in elderly. Common site of pathologic fracture. Can be site of significant blood loss and shock.
- Hip dislocation: Disarticulation of femoral head. Classified as posterior, anterior, and central:
  - Posterior dislocation (most common):
    - Often from motor vehicle accident (MVA) in which knees strike dashboard
    - 10% associated with sciatic nerve injury
  - Anterior dislocation: 10% hip dislocations:
    - Often due to trauma with sudden abduction of thigh
    - Associated femoral head fractures, femoral nerve injury
    - Can be anterior superior, or anterior inferior
  - Central dislocation with acetabular fracture:
    - Usually from direct impact to greater trochanter
    - Associated significant blood loss, sciatic nerve injury

### Pediatric Considerations
- Hip dislocation: Uncommon; often spontaneously reduced at time of injury. Concern for tissue trapped in joint space:
  - Trivial force required for posterior hip locations in children <10 yr old
- Proximal femoral physeal fracture: Fracture at growth plate; great risk for osseous necrosis
- Slipped capital femoral epiphysis: Minimal trauma, decreased ROM.

- Femoral neck fractures: Relatively common; stress fractures young athletes
- Intertrochanteric fractures: Rare.
- Must suspect nonaccidental trauma (NAT)
- Consider pathologic fracture with minor trauma.

## ETIOLOGY
See individual injuries above.

 **DIAGNOSIS**

## SIGNS AND SYMPTOMS
### History
- Groin, hip, thigh, medial knee pain, pain with ambulation/weight-bearing in the setting of trauma
- Minor trauma in the elderly due to osteoporosis; high-impact trauma in young adults
- Rarely overuse injury, stress fracture.

### Physical Exam
- Obvious signs of trauma:
  - Deformity or angulation, swelling, open fracture, or missile entrance wound
  - Lower extremity held in position of comfort
- Hip fracture: Flexion, abduction, external rotation
- Posterior hip dislocation: Flexion, *adduction, internal rotation* of hip, flexion of knee, hip immobile
- Anterior hip dislocation: Flexion, *abduction, external rotation* of hip, thigh shortening, hip immobile

### Pediatric Considerations
- Pediatric fracture patterns different due to developing cartilaginous components:
  - Assess for dislocation of the femoral capital epiphysis.
- Fracture classification and management are also different.
- Suspect NAT without obvious mechanism of injury.
- Consider hip pain due to a separate process (limb-length discrepancy, neuromuscular disorders, neoplastic invasion of bone).

## ESSENTIAL WORKUP
- Assess distal pulses, palpate compartments, evaluate sensation and motor function.
- If pulses are not equal or palpable, bedside Doppler or angiography may be necessary.
- Search for associated injuries:
  - Neurologic deficits
  - Vascular injury
  - Pelvic fractures (include acetabular fractures)
  - Spinal fractures
  - Blunt abdominal trauma
- Radiographs as outlined below:
  - Remove splints and clothing when taking films.
  - Positive exam plus negative standard films indicates hip fracture until proven otherwise; further imaging (CT or MRI scan) is indicated.
  - Hip dislocations are orthopedic emergencies and require prompt reduction (<6 hr) with limited attempts.

### Pediatric Considerations
- In suspected child abuse, obtain appropriate radiographs to evaluate for other injuries.
- Assess markers for nonaccidental trauma:
  - Delay in presentation; history of mechanism inconsistent with injury
  - Isolated trauma to the thigh, associated burns, bruises, linear abrasions

## DIAGNOSTIC TESTS & INTERPRETATION
### Lab
CBC, type and crossmatch

### Imaging
- Standard films: AP pelvis and true lateral of hip, oblique view.
- Femoral neck fracture: AP pelvis with hip internally rotated 15–20 degrees
- Pubic rami and acetabular fractures: Pelvic inlet and outlet views
- Acetabular fractures: Judet views (oblique views of hip)
- High suspicion with negative plain films: CT, MRI, or bone scan
- Must get postreduction x-ray and/or CT scan.

### Diagnostic Procedures/Surgery
- Joint aspiration with or without arthrogram under fluoroscope if suspect a septic joint, foreign body, or hemarthrosis, especially in gunshot wounds to hip
- Operative repair or wash out

## DIFFERENTIAL DIAGNOSIS
- Pubic ramus fracture
- Acetabular fracture
- Septic joint
- Thigh, knee, ankle, or foot injury
- Trochanteric bursitis
- Iliotibial band tendinitis
- Hip contusion

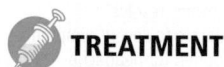 **TREATMENT**

## PRE-HOSPITAL
- Neurovascular exam is essential.
- Immobilize extremity in position of comfort for patient.

## INITIAL STABILIZATION/THERAPY
- Airway, head, chest, or abdominal injuries take precedence in multiple trauma.
- Maintain pelvis and hip stability.
- Monitor BP continuously.
- Cautions:
  - DO NOT apply traction.
  - Monitor closely for development of hemorrhagic shock as thigh can contain 4–6 units of blood.

## ED TREATMENT/PROCEDURES

- Maintain pelvis and hip stability.
- Remove splint and clothing.
- Pain control:
  - Isolated hip injuries: Parenteral analgesia
  - Multitrauma or pediatric patients: Femoral nerve block
- Orthopedic consultation:
  - Necessary for all hip fractures and dislocations
  - Emergent if neurovascular compromise
  - Open fractures must go directly to the OR for irrigation and debridement.
  - May need reduction in OR after 1–2 quick ED attempts to reduce.
- Fractures requiring surgery:
  - Cefazolin IV
- Open fractures with lacerations, extensive soft-tissue damage, or contamination:
  - Add gentamicin/tobramycin, tetanus.
- If highly contaminated wound: Add penicillin G to cover clostridial species.
- Gunshot wounds:
  - Culture missile track, iodine dressing
- Hip dislocation:
  - A true orthopedic emergency
  - Incidence of avascular necrosis and degenerative joint disease increases linearly with time to reduction:
    - Perform reduction in ED, ideally <6 hr from onset.
    - Allis or Stimson maneuvers
    - Also described: With patient in lateral decubitus position, move hip from flexed and adducted position to full external rotation with tibia perpendicular to floor.
  - Procedural sedation with etomidate, ketamine, or methohexital plus midazolam, propofol plus fentanyl
  - Look for fractures on postreduction imaging (plain film, CT).
  - Patients with prior hip arthroplasty may be reduced in the ED with procedural sedation and appropriate monitoring.

## MEDICATION

- Antibiotics
  - Cefazolin: 1 g IM/IV q6–8h (peds: 25–50 mg/kg IM/IV div q6–8h max. 1 g)
  - Gentamicin/tobramycin: 3–5 mg/kg/d IV/IM div q8h (peds: 2–2.5 mg/kg q8h)
  - Penicillin G: 2 million IU IV q4h (peds: 100,000–400,000 IU/kg/d IV div q4–6h to max. 24 million IU in 24 hr)
- Moderate sedation:
  - Etomidate: 0.1–0.3 mg/kg IV once (not recommended for <12 yr)
  - Fentanyl: 50–100 $\mu$g IV over 1–2 min once (peds: >6 mo 1–2 $\mu$g/kg IV once)
  - Ketamine: Not recommended in adults owing to emergence reaction (peds: 1.0–2 mg/kg IV, 4 mg/kg IM once)
  - Methohexital: 1–1.5 mg/kg IV once (peds: Not recommended)

- Midazolam: 0.07 mg/kg IM or 1 mg slowly q2–3min up to 5 mg max. (peds: 0.25–1.0 mg/kg PO once to a max. of 20 mg PO; 6 mo–5 yr: 0.05–0.1 mg/kg IV titrate to max. 0.6 mg/kg; 6–12 yr: 0.025–0.05 mg/kg IV titrate to max. 0.4 mg/kg
- Propofol: 40 mg IV q10sec until induction; 5–10 $\mu$g/kg/min IV continuous infusion
- Pain control:
  - Hydromorphone: 0.5–2.0 mg IM/SC/slow IV q4–6h PRN; titrate for pain control (peds: 0.015 mg/kg/min per dose IV q4–6h PRN)
  - Morphine: 2–10 mg IV q4h, titrate for pain control (peds: 0.1 mg/kg IV q4h, titrate for pain control to max. 15 mg/dose)

### First Line

- Antibiotics: Cefazolin IV
- Pain: Morphine
- Sedation: User dependent. Etomidate adults, ketamine children.

### Second Line

- Antibiotics: Ceftriaxone plus gentamicin
- Pain: Hydromorphone, fentanyl, nerve block
- Sedation: methohexital, midazolam, propofol

 **FOLLOW-UP**

## DISPOSITION

### Admission Criteria

- All hip fractures
- Septic joint
- Suspicion of occult fracture
- Suspicion of nonaccidental trauma in children
- All pediatric hip fractures and dislocations
- Most dislocations of hip

### Discharge Criteria

- Hip pain attributable to other cause
- Fracture ruled out (negative radiographs *plus* negative clinical exam)
- Patient with successful reduction of dislocated hip arthroplasty may be considered for discharge in consultation with orthopedics and with appropriate follow-up.
- Stress fracture, crutches follow-up with bone scan or repeat x-rays.

### Issues for Referral

- Chronic pain may need primary physician and pain specialist.
- Pediatric patients and elderly may need physical therapy.

## FOLLOW-UP RECOMMENDATIONS

- Discharged patients with hip pain not due to fracture/dislocation are referred to appropriate primary doctor.
- Stress fracture, non–weight-bearing: Follow-up orthopedics 2–3 days

## PEARLS AND PITFALLS

- Location of fracture determines risk factors for morbidity such as AVN and bleeding.
- Hip dislocations are orthopedic emergencies and require prompt reduction and few attempts.
- Be suspicious of occult fractures, as x-ray may miss 10% fractures. Follow-up study needed (CT or MRI) and possible admission.

## ADDITIONAL READING

- Dominguez S, Liu P, Roberts C, et al. Prevalence of traumatic hip and pelvic fractures in patients with suspected hip fracture and negative initial standard radiographs—a study of ED patients. *Acad Emerg Med*. 2005;12:366–369.
- Liporace FA, Egol KA, Tejwani N, et al. What's new in hip fractures? (Current concepts). *Am J Orthop*. 2005;34:66–74.
- Parker M, Johansen A. Hip fracture. *BMJ*. 2006;333:27–30.
- Quick TJ, Eastwood DM. Pediatric fractures and dislocations of the hip and pelvis. *Clin Orthop Relat Res*. 2005;432:87–96.
- Rudman N, McIlmail D. Emergency department evaluation and treatment of hip and thigh injuries. *Emerg Med Clin North Am*. 2000;18:29–66.
- *Tarascon pocket pharmacopoeia*, 2006 Edition. Lompoc, CA: Tarascon Publishing.
- Ward K, Yealy D. Systemic analgesia and sedation in managing orthopedic emergencies. *Emerg Med Clin North Am*. 2000;18:141–166.

### See Also (Topic, Algorithm, Electronic Media Element)

- Femur Fracture
- Pelvic Fracture

 **CODES**

### ICD9

- 820.8 Fracture of unspecified part of neck of femur, closed
- 835.00 Closed dislocation of hip, unspecified site
- 959.6 Other and unspecified injury to hip and thigh

H

# HIRSCHSPRUNG DISEASE

*Andrea Bracikowski*
*Sally Santen*

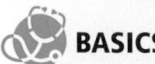 **BASICS**

## DESCRIPTION

- Congenital aganglionosis megacolon
- 1:5,000 live births
- Genetics:
  - Mutations of the *ret* proto-oncogene found in both familial and sporadic forms
  - Male-to-female ratio 4:1
  - 10% have positive family history; 5–12% of siblings.
  - Associated chromosomal abnormality (12%); most commonly Down's syndrome
  - Children with Down's Syndrome and Hirschsprung's often have more co-morbidities resulting in more complicated medical and surgical management
  - 20% of infants have other congenital anomalies (GI, cardiac, craniofacial, cleft palate)

## ETIOLOGY

- Absence of enteric ganglia in the distal colon
- Creates functional obstruction to passage of stool
- Failure of neural crest cells to migrate into parasympathetic Meissner (submucosal) and Auerbach (myenteric) ganglions
- Begins at the internal anal sphincter and involves the rectosigmoid colon (75% of cases)
- May extend entire length of GI tract (often fatal)
- Aganglionic segment chronically contracts, forming an obstruction to the passage of stool.
- Proximal colon distends to hold stool that has not passed.
- Stimulation of the anus allows passage of stool.
- Toxic megacolon may develop.

 **DIAGNOSIS**

## SIGNS AND SYMPTOMS

- 3 presentations, varying with age:
  - Neonatal:
    - Abdominal distention
    - Delayed passage of meconium in 1st 48 hr
    - Vomiting
    - Neonatal enterocolitis
    - Sepsis
  - Infancy:
    - Severe constipation
    - Chronic abdominal distention
    - Vomiting
    - Failure to thrive
  - Later childhood and adulthood:
    - Chronic constipation with obstruction
    - Enterocolitis at any age
    - Fever
    - Lethargy or toxic-appearing child
    - Abdominal distention
    - Bloody, foul-smelling diarrhea
    - Malnutrition
    - Reversible UTI (hydronephrosis, hydroureter, recurrent UTIs)
    - Acute appendicitis
    - Septicemia

### History

- Bowel movements frequently require rectal stimulation or enemas.
- Narrow caliber stools
- Encopresis and diarrhea are uncommon.
- Absence of inciting factors associated with functional constipation (ie, fissures, toilet training, diet)

### Physical Exam

- Possible palpable colon on the left
- Occult blood possibly owing to enterocolitis or anal fissures (constipation)

## ESSENTIAL WORKUP

Abdominal radiographs:

- Distended small bowel and proximal colon with an empty rectum are common findings.
- Transition zone into a narrowed rectosigmoid segment
- In neonates, films will commonly show a distal obstructive pattern.
- In children, with chronic constipation films may show only large amounts of stool.
- In children with enterocolitis, bowel wall edema or pneumatosis intestinalis may be present.
- Consider genetics consultation
- Look for other co-morbidities

## DIAGNOSTIC TESTS & INTERPRETATION

### Lab

- CBC, electrolytes, glucose, BUN, Cr,
- Urinalysis
- Blood culture if toxic
- PT, PTT, INR

### Imaging

Barium enema:

- Obtain after stabilization.
- Dilated colon proximal to the contracted aganglionic colon with uncoordinated peristalsis
- Delayed barium evacuation

## Diagnostic Procedures/Surgery
- Rectal manometry may assist in diagnosis, but is often abnormal in long-standing constipation.
- Full-thickness rectal biopsy confirms diagnosis by the lack of ganglion cells.

## DIFFERENTIAL DIAGNOSIS
- Infants:
  - Meconium ileus or meconium plug from cystic fibrosis
  - Intestinal or anal atresia or hypoplasia
  - Malrotation or duplication with volvulus
  - Necrotizing enterocolitis
  - Functional constipation
  - Sepsis
- Children:
  - Functional constipation
- Toxic:
  - Opiates, anticholinergics
- Infectious:
  - Botulism
  - *Trypanosoma cruzi*
- Acquired aganglionic colon
- Metabolic or endocrine:
  - Hypothyroid/parathyroid, adrenal insufficiency, electrolyte abnormality
- Structural
- Spinal cord defects, abdominal masses

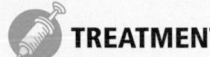 

# TREATMENT

## PRE-HOSPITAL
Rapid transport of infant with acute abdomen/septic appearing

## INITIAL STABILIZATION/THERAPY
- Ill-appearing children
- ABCs with monitoring
- Initial bolus 0.9% IV fluids (20 mL/kg) for shock, dehydration, sepsis

## ED TREATMENT/PROCEDURES
- Infants should be managed for bowel obstruction.
- Consultation with a pediatric surgeon and pediatric gastroenterology
- Unstable patient may require decompression by loop colostomy; stoma must contain normal bowel.
- Stable children:
  - Workup may be done as outpatient.
- Definitive treatment is resection of the aganglionic section of bowel; staging unnecessary in relatively well child:
  - Return to normal bowel function is the usual result.
  - Ultimate surgical goal is to place normal ganglion containing bowel within 1 cm of the anal opening.
- Enterocolitis may occur at any time.

## MEDICATION
- When a child is toxic or has enterocolitis, administer broad-spectrum antibiotics.
- IVF and replace electrolyte deficits

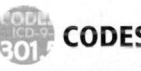

# FOLLOW-UP

## DISPOSITION

### Admission Criteria
- Infants and neonates presenting with bowel obstruction
- Enterocolitis
- Ill-appearing infants should be admitted to a PICU/NICU.
- If pediatric surgery is not available, transfer to a pediatric tertiary care center.

### Discharge Criteria
- Older children with constipation
- Well hydrated and taking oral fluid
- Responsible parents
- Close follow-up with primary care provider, surgeon, and gastroenterologist

### Issues for Referral
Care should be supervised by pediatric gastroenterologist/pediatric surgeon.

## ADDITIONAL READING

- Amiel J, Lyonnet S. Hirschsprung disease, associated syndromes, and genetics: A review. *J Med Genet*. 2001;38:729–739.
- Hackam DJ, Reblock K, Barsdale EM, et al. The influence of Down's syndrome on the management and outcome of children with Hirschsprung's disease. *J Pediatr Surg*. 2003;38(6):946–949.
- Rudolph C, Benaroch L. Hirschsprung disease. *Pediatr Rev*. 1995;16:5–11.

# CODES

## ICD9
751.3 Hirschsprung's disease and other congenital functional disorders of colon

H

# HIV/AIDS

Colleen Gibson
Mercedes Torres

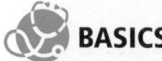 **BASICS**

## DESCRIPTION
- AIDS: Defined as lab evidence of HIV with CD4 <200 or AIDS defining illness—infection (eg, cryptosporidium), malignancy (eg, Karposi's, cervical cancer), or other (eg, HIV wasting disease, HIV encephalopathy)
- Opportunistic diseases:
  - CD <500 cells/mm$^3$:
    ○ Oroesophageal candidiasis
    ○ Pneumococcal infection
    ○ Hairy leukoplakia
    ○ Immune thrombocytopenic purpura
  - CD4 <200 cells/mm$^3$:
    ○ Pneumocystis jiroveci pneumonia (PCP)
    ○ Cryptococcal infection
    ○ Disseminated tuberculosis
    ○ Cryptosporidiosis
    ○ Isosporiasis
    ○ Toxoplasmosis
    ○ Histoplasmosis
  - CD4 <50 cells/mm$^3$:
    ○ CNS lymphoma
    ○ Mycobacterium avium complex (MAC)
    ○ TB pericarditis or meningitis
    ○ Cytomegalovirus (CMV)
    ○ Cholangiopathy: Most common cause cryptosporidium parvum

 **DIAGNOSIS**

## SIGNS AND SYMPTOMS
- Primary HIV infection: 2–6 wk after exposure:
  - Fever and malaise
  - Rash on face and trunk
  - Flu-like syndrome with lymphadenopathy and hepatosplenomegaly
  - Pharyngitis
  - Diarrhea
- Advanced HIV disease (CD4 <200):
  - Fatigue
  - Fevers and night sweats
  - Weight loss/wasting
  - Alopecia
  - Chronic diarrhea
  - Cough
  - Dyspnea
  - Hemoptysis
  - Chronic low-grade headache
  - Altered mental status
  - Seizures
  - Dementia
  - Neuropathy
  - Painless visual loss
  - Skin lesions

### History
- Risk factors:
  - Sexual promiscuity, multiple sexual partners
  - IV drug abuse
  - Men who have sex with men
  - Blood transfusions prior to 1985
  - Unprotected sex with at-risk partners

- Most recent CD4 count and viral load, lowest CD4 count
- History of or current use of antiretroviral medications
- Medication compliance
- Length of diagnosis/illness
- History of opportunistic infections
- Previous hospitalizations or ICU admissions

## ESSENTIAL WORKUP
- HIV serologic tests as noted below:
  - There is a window of 24 wk between primary infection and seroconversion, during which tests may be negative.
- Respiratory symptoms:
  - Chest radiograph
  - Arterial blood gas (ABG)
  - Sputum for gram stain, AFB, and culture
  - Serum LDH—elevated in PCP
  - Blood cultures
- Cardiac symptoms:
  - Serum cardiac markers, electrolytes
  - CXR
  - EKG
  - ECG in cases of suspected pericarditis, effusion, or tamponade
  - Blood cultures if endocarditis is suspected
  - Drug screen for cocaine and amphetamines
- Neurologic symptoms:
  - Head CT with and without contrast
  - Lumbar puncture with opening pressure
  - CSF for glucose, protein, Gram stain and culture, cell count with differential, AFB smear, India ink stain, herpes simplex and cryptococcus antigen, and VDRL
- GI symptoms:
  - Stool for ova and parasites, Gram stain, culture, and *Clostridium difficile* assay
  - Urine analysis
  - For women: Urine pregnancy test, pelvic exam with wet mount, and gonorrhea/chlamydia testing
  - Liver functions tests, amylase, and lipase
  - Hepatitis serologies
  - Low threshold for CT abdomen/pelvis
  - US if biliary symptoms present
  - Low threshold for surgical consult, as HIV patients may not present with classic acute abdomen
- Fever workup:
  - Include aerobic/anaerobic, fungal, AFB, and MAC blood cultures
- Ocular symptoms:
  - Fluorescein staining with slit lamp examination

## DIAGNOSTIC TESTS & INTERPRETATION
### Lab
- ELISA:
  - Detects IgG antibody against HIV
  - Sensitivity and specificity ~99%
  - Can be negative during the window period
- Western blot:
  - Detects IgG antibody against HIV proteins p24, gp 120, gp 41
  - Used to confirm a positive ELISA
  - Able to detect HIV during the 6-mo seroconversion period

- Rapid HIV testing:
  - Results available in 5–20 min
  - 4 types of tests currently available
  - Samples include oral swabs, whole blood, serum, or plasma
  - All reactive tests require confirmatory testing with western blot or ELISA
  - >99% specific and sensitive
- Absolute lymphocyte count (ALC):
  - Multiply WBC × percent lymphocytes
  - If ALC >2,000, likely CD4 >200, if ALC <1,000, likely CD4 <200

### Imaging
- CXR:
  - Bilateral interstitial infiltrates: PCP
  - Reticulonodular infiltrates: TB, KS, or fungal pneumonia
  - Hilar lymphadenopathy with infiltrate: TB, cryptococcosis, histoplasmosis, neoplasm
  - Lobar consolidation: Bacterial pneumonia
  - Cavitation: TB, necrotizing bacterial pneumonia, coccidioidomycosis
  - Normal x-ray does not rule out PCP or TB
- Head CT with and without IV contrast:
  - Multiple ring-enhancing lesions with edema in basal ganglia or cortex: Toxoplasmosis or CNS lymphoma
  - Subcortical nonenhancing lesions: PML
- Abdominal/pelvic CT:
  - Splenomegaly: CMV, TB
  - Intestinal perforation or bowel obstruction: CMV colitis, lymphoma, histoplasmosis, MAC, appendicitis, ulcer disease, KS
  - Cholecystitis or cholangitis: Cryptosporidium, Microsporidium, CMV
  - Pancreatitis: Medication-related, neoplasm, infectious

## DIFFERENTIAL DIAGNOSIS
- For pulmonary symptoms with HIV:
  - Pulmonary emboli
  - Pulmonary HTN
  - TB
  - Pneumonia: Bacterial, fungal, viral
  - Pulmonary malignancies
  - Lymphocytic interstitial pneumonitis
- For CNS symptoms with HIV:
  - Neurosyphilis
  - CMV or HSV encephalitis
  - Toxoplasmosis
  - CNS lymphoma
  - Meningitis (bacterial, coccidioidal, etc)
  - Subarachnoid hemorrhage
  - Cerebral infarction
  - HIV or metabolic encephalitis
  - Progressive multifocal leukoencephalopathy
- Cardiac symptoms with HIV:
  - Cardiomyopathy
  - Pericarditis/myocarditis
  - Endocarditis
  - Acute coronary syndrome
  - Pericardial effusion

- Oral symptoms with HIV:
  – Fungal infection (ie, candidiasis)
  – Viral lesions (HSV, CMV, hairy leukoplakia)
  – Bacterial lesions (TB, periodontal disease)
  – Autoimmune (salivary gland disease, aphthous ulcers)
  – Neoplasm (KS, lymphoma)
- Esophageal symptoms with HIV:
  – Infectious esophagitis (candida, CMV, HSV)
  – Reflux esophagitis
- Diarrhea with HIV:
  – Medication side effect
  – Parasites (cryptosporidium, Giardia, Isospora)
  – Bacteria
  – Viral (CMV, HSV, HIV)
  – Fungi (histoplasmosis, cryptococcus)
- Hepatomegaly with HIV:
  – Hepatitis
  – Opportunistic infection (CMV, MAC, TB)
- Renal disease with HIV:
  – Drug nephrotoxicity
  – HIV nephropathy
  – Vasculitis
  – Obstruction

 **TREATMENT**

### ED TREATMENT/PROCEDURES

- Patients who appear to have bacterial infections, appear toxic, or have rapidly progressive symptoms should receive their 1st dose of antibiotics in the ED.
- Begin HIV treatment if: Low CD4 (<350) or high viral load, pregnancy, AIDS defining illness or HIV-assoc nephropathy
- Triple therapy (HAART):
  – 1 nonnucleoside reverse transcriptase inhibitors (NNRTI) and 2 nucleoside reverse transcriptase inhibitors (NRTI)
  – 1 PI and 2 NRTIs
  – Triple NRTI
- Postexposure prophylaxis:
  – Start therapy within 2 hr if possible and continue for 4 wk
  – 2-drug regimen for most exposures:
    ○ Zidovudine + lamivudine
    ○ Lamivudine + stavudine
    ○ Stavudine + didanosine
  – 3-drug regimen for very high-risk exposure
- Toxoplasmosis: Pyrimethamine:
  – Sulfadiazine
  – Leucovorin
  – Steroids for cerebral edema
  – Treat for at least 6 wk
- Cryptococcal meningitis:
  – Amphotericin B
  – Flucytosine
  – Treat with above for 2 wk, then fluconazole for 8 wk
- CMV Retinitis: Ganciclovir
- Esophageal candidiasis:
  – Fluconazole for 14–21 days
- MAC: Clarithromycin:
  – Ethambutol
  – May add rifabutin if severe immunosuppression

- PCP:
  – Trimethoprim/sulfamethoxazole
  – Pentamidine or dapsone for sulfa-allergic patients
  – If PaO$_2$ <70 mm Hg or A-a gradient >35 mm Hg, add prednisone 40 mg PO b.i.d. for 5 days, then taper
- Oral candidiasis: Clotrimazole troches
- HIV acute demyelinating polyneuropathy: Plasmapheresis

### MEDICATION

- Common medication complications:
  – Hypersensitivity reaction: Abacavir
  – Pancreatitis:
    ○ Dideoxyinosine
    ○ Dideoxycytidine
    ○ Didanosine
    ○ Lamivudine
    ○ Cotrimoxazole
    ○ Pentamidine
    ○ Ritonavir
    ○ Stavudine
    ○ Zalcitabine
  – Peripheral neuropathy:
    ○ Didanosine
    ○ Isoniazid
    ○ Linezolid
    ○ Stavudine
    ○ Zalcitabine
  – Kidney stones: Indinavir and Atazanavir
  – Hepatotoxicity: All agents to some degree:
    ○ Nevirapine
    ○ Didanosine
    ○ Stavudine
  – Lactic Acidosis: Stavudine:
    ○ Didanosine
  – Stevens-Johnson syndrome:
    ○ Nevirapine
    ○ Atazanavir
    ○ Delavirdine
    ○ Efavirenz
    ○ Cotrimoxazole
    ○ Bactrim
  – Hemolytic anemia:
    ○ Dapsone (used for treatment of TB)
    ○ Zidovudine with ribavirin
  – Psychosis: Efavirenz
  – Hypoglycemia: Pentamidine
  – Postural hypotension: Maraviroc
  – Hyperlipidemia, truncal obesity, and atherosclerosis: Stavudine:
    ○ Protease inhibitors
  – Dilated cardiomyopathy: Zidovudine
  – Benign increase in unconjugated bilirubin: Atazanavir and indinavir
  – Macrocytic anemia: Zidovudine
  – Many cause some hematologic effects, GI upset, and rash

 **FOLLOW-UP**

### DISPOSITION

**Admission Criteria**

- Unexplained fever with CNS involvement or suspected endocarditis
- Neutropenic fever
- Hypoxemia (PaO$_2$ <70 mm Hg)
- Cardiac symptoms suggestive of ACS

- Pericardial effusion
- Suspected bacterial pneumonia or TB
- A change in neurologic status
- New-onset seizures
- Hemodynamic instability
- Inability to ambulate or tolerate oral intake
- Intractable diarrhea with dehydration

**Discharge Criteria**

The patient can maintain adequate oral intake, provide self-care, and ambulate.

**Issues for Referral**

- Patient should be referred to a primary HIV care provider for initiation of HAART therapy regimen and ongoing care.
- Be alert for signs of depression and refer for counseling or psychiatric treatment as this may inhibit treatment compliance.
- HIV patients are at higher risk for many malignancies—refer those with concerning symptoms for follow-up.

## PEARLS AND PITFALLS

- Immune Reconstitution Inflammatory Syndrome usually manifests within 8 wk of initiation of HAART as symptoms of opportunistic or autoimmune disease.
- For occupation exposures, there is a low risk of seroconversion (0.3% for significant percutaneous exposure and 0.09% for mucocutaneous).
- HIV patients on HAART should be considered at higher risk for acute coronary syndrome and insulin resistance.
- Measure oxygen saturation after walking in patients with a normal CXR and symptoms of pneumonia to help diagnose PCP
- HIV is an independent risk factor for COPD, pulmonary hypertension, CVA, venous thromboembolic disease, TTP, osteoporosis, and osteonecrosis of the hip.

## ADDITIONAL READING

- Bartlett J, Gallant J. *Medical management of HIV infection.* Baltimore, MD: Johns Hopkins Medicine Health Publishing B Group; 2007.
- Belleza WG, Browne B. Pulmonary considerations in the immunocompromised patient. *Emerg Med Clin North Am.* 2003;21(2):499–531.
- Church JA. Pediatric HIV in the emergency department. *Clin Ped Emerg Med.* 2007;8:117–122.
- Marco C, Rothman, R. HIV infection and complications in emergency medicine. *Emerg Med Clin North Am.* 2008;26:367–387.
- Venkat A, et al. Care of the HIV-positive patient in the emergency department in the era of HAART. *Ann Emerg Med.* 2008;52:274–285.

 **CODES**

### ICD9

- 042 Human immunodeficiency virus (hiv) disease
- V08 Asymptomatic human immunodeficiency virus (hiv) infection status

H

# HORDEOLUM AND CHALAZION

*Shari Schabowski*

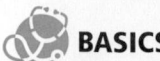 **BASICS**

## DESCRIPTION

- Result from inflammatory processes involving the glands of the eyelid along the lash line:
  - Hordeolum—acute glandular obstruction resulting in inflammation and abscess formation
  - Chalazion—end result of inspissations of glandular contents and chronic granulomatous inflammation
- Hordeolum:
  - Develops owing to outflow obstruction in 1 or more of the glands of the eyelid
  - Obstructed glands may become secondarily infected.
  - May progress to localized abscess formation or be complicated by periorbital cellulitis
- Chalazion:
  - Chronic granulomatous inflammation in the meibomian gland:
    - Originates from inspissated secretions
    - Blockage of the gland's duct at the eyelid margin may result in release of the contents of the gland into the surrounding eyelid soft tissue.
    - A lipogranulomatous reaction ensues
    - Occasionally, chalazia become secondarily infected.
    - May evolve from incompletely drained internal hordeolum

## ETIOLOGY

Hordeolum:

- May become secondarily infected:
  - Staphylococcus most common
- Predisposing conditions:
  - Meibomian gland dysfunction
  - Blepharitis
  - Rosacea
  - Previous hordeolum

 **DIAGNOSIS**

## SIGNS AND SYMPTOMS

- Hordeolum:
  - Develops acutely when glandular outflow is obstructed
  - Red, tender, painful, swollen mass along the eyelid margin
  - Typically solitary, rarely may be multiple
  - May be recurrent
  - Well localized inflammation
  - Presentation depends on which gland is affected:
    - External hordeolum (stye):
    - Originates from obstruction of the superficial sebaceous or sweat glands whose ducts are located between the eye lashes
    - Exquisitely tender small mass that typically points anteriorly
    - Internal hordeolum:
    - Originates from obstruction of the sebaceous glands whose ducts are located on the inner aspect of the lid margin
    - Painful small mass that is palpable through the eyelid
    - May cause a foreign body sensation in the eye and visual disturbance
    - Typically more inflamed, larger, and more painful
    - May point internally or through skin
  - Nonsystemic process
  - May be complicated by:
    - Conjunctivitis
    - Periorbital cellulitis
- Chalazion:
  - Firm, circumscribed, nontender, or minimally tender nodule:
    - Typically long-standing
  - Noninflamed
  - Symptoms most commonly owing to physical properties:
    - Disrupts natural contour of eye
    - Obstructs visual field/peripheral vision
    - Pressure on globe
    - Corneal desiccation or injury due to exposure
  - Nonacute, nonemergent process, which requires no urgent or emergent intervention unless secondary corneal or significant globe pressure is present.

## History

Hordeolum—sudden, well localized, painful mass along the margin of eyelid:

- No systemic symptoms

### Physical Exam

Focal, tender, inflammation of an external or internal gland of the eyelid:

- Minimal surrounding edema may be seen
- Abscess may point within lash line, from palpebral conjunctiva or externally via skin of the lid

## ESSENTIAL WORKUP

- Complete ophthalmologic examination including slit lamp exam and corneal evaluation
- Evaluation for evidence of associated cellulitis and/or systemic findings
- Hordeolum:
  - Identify the origin of the abscess
- Chalazion:
  - Determine whether physical properties of chalazion result in corneal exposure and injury.

## DIAGNOSTIC TESTS & INTERPRETATION

### Lab

Cultures of any drainage rarely aids in management

## DIFFERENTIAL DIAGNOSIS

- Blepharitis
- Dacryocystitis
- Dacryoadenitis
- Pyogenic granuloma
- Sebaceous cell carcinoma
- Basal cell carcinoma
- Squamous cell carcinoma

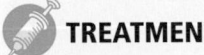 **TREATMENT**

**ED TREATMENT/PROCEDURES**
- Hordeolum—relieve obstruction and prevent abscess formation
  - Warm compresses for 15 min 4–6 times per day
  - Gently massage the nodule to express obstructed material
  - Rarely, in severe cases, incision and drainage of internal hordeolum may be necessary:
    ○ Typically done by ophthalmologist
    ○ If pointed toward the conjunctiva, vertical incision is made to avoid injury to the meibomian glands and reduce corneal injury from inadvertent scarring.
    ○ External skin incision is very rarely indicated.
  - When necessary, horizontal incision is used
  - Removing single involved eyelash may be helpful in rare more severe cases of external hordeolum
- Chalazion—complaints typically reflect nonemergent aesthetic and cumbersome physical properties of the mass:
  - Referral to ophthalmology for incision and curettage or steroid injection
  - Lubricating eye drops may provide symptomatic relief

**MEDICATION**
Ophthalmologic moisturizing drops as needed for comfort.

 **FOLLOW-UP**

**DISPOSITION**
**Discharge Criteria**
No indication for admission unless secondary complication is present (i.e., marked periorbital cellulitis with systemic symptoms)

**Issues for Referral**
- Urgent consultation with ophthalmologist should be considered if incision and drainage of internal hordeolum is deemed indicated.
- Chalazia should be referred to ophthalmologist for definitive treatment options.

**FOLLOW-UP RECOMMENDATIONS**
- Follow-up with ophthalmology in 1–2 days to evaluate response to conservative management.
- Symptoms should complete resolve in 1–2 wk

**PEARLS AND PITFALLS**

- Conservative treatment of hordeola with warm compresses and gentle massage is the standard:
  - Majority of cases respond without further intervention
    Emergent incision and drainage is rarely indicated and should only be considered in extreme cases
  - Incision and drainage may result in long-term complications including corneal injury, fistula formation, and aesthetic complications
  - Consult ophthalmology for incision and drainage if possible
- Chalazia do not require emergent intervention:
  - Referral is the standard management

**ADDITIONAL READING**

- Cullom R. *The Will's Eye Manual: Office and Emergency Room Diagnosis and Treatment of Eye Disease*. Philadelphia: Lippincott-Raven; 1998.
- Hassan AS, Nelson CC. Benign eyelid tumors and skin diseases. *Int Ophthalmol Clin*. 2002;42(2):135–149.
- Kanski JJ. *Clinical Ophthalmology*. London: Butterworth-Heinemann; 1994:24.
- Lederman C, Miller M. Disorders of the lacrimal system apparatus. Hordeola and chalazia. *Pediatr Rev*. 1999;20(8):283–284.
- Prochazka MD, MSc, Allan V. Diagnosis and treatment of red eye. *Primary Care Case Rev*. 2001;4(1)23–31.
- Rubin S, Hallagan L. Lids, lacrimals and lashes. *Emerg Clin North Am*. 1995;13(3):631–647.

**See Also (Topic, Algorithm, Electronic Media Element)**
- Dacryoadenitis
- Dacryocystitis
- Red Eye

 **CODES**

**ICD9**
- 373.2 Chalazion
- 373.11 Hordeolum externum

# HORNER SYNDROME
*Richard S. Krause*

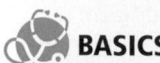 **BASICS**

## DESCRIPTION
Unilateral sympathetic denervation of the eye produces signs of Horner syndrome:
- Relaxation of retracting muscles in upper and lower lids:
  - *Ptosis* (drooping of the lids)
- Loss of pupillary dilator innervation:
  - *Miosis* (unopposed pupillary constriction)
- Loss of sympathetic stimulation of sweat glands:
  - Anhidrosis

## ETIOLOGY
- 40% unknown (in 1 large series)
- Tumors of lung or metastases to cervical nodes:
  - May interrupt preganglionic sympathetic fibers (between thoracic sympathetic trunk and superior cervical ganglion)
- Trauma: Penetrating neck wounds directly injure sympathetic fibers
- Pneumothorax:
  - Tension pneumothorax may cause traction on sympathetic fibers owing to shift of mediastinal structures.
- Infiltration or infection of cervical nodes:
  - Sarcoidosis, tuberculosis
- Vascular disorders:
  - Migraine or cluster headaches
  - Carotid artery dissection
- Lateral medullary infarction produces Horner syndrome as part of the Wallenberg syndrome:
  - Presents with vertigo and ataxia, which may overshadow the Horner syndrome.
- Cavernous sinus thrombosis may present with some of the features of Horner syndrome:
  - The condition typically causes headache and/or eye pain.
  - Ocular signs include ocular palsies, pain, chemosis, and proptosis.

## Pediatric Considerations
- Hereditary Horner syndrome:
  - Blue iris (or irregular coloration) on affected side
  - Brown on unaffected side (heterochromia iridis)
- Birth trauma:
  - May cause damage to sympathetic chain
- New Horner syndrome in a child should prompt workup for tumor (neuroblastoma).

 **DIAGNOSIS**

## SIGNS AND SYMPTOMS
- Horner syndrome is characterized by:
  - *Ptosis:* Drooping of eyelid on affected side, usually slight
  - *Miosis:* Decrease in pupillary size on involved side (pupillary asymmetry ≥1 mm)
  - *Anhidrosis:* Lack of sweating on involved side of face
- The importance of Horner syndrome is its association with certain disease states.

## History
Focus on pre-existing conditions that predispose to Horner syndrome or are risk factors for these conditions:
- Tumors, vascular disease, trauma:
  - Minor trauma often precedes carotid dissection.
- Cardiovascular risks
- Exposures:
  - For pseudo-Horner
- Pain:
  - Suggests carotid dissection

## ALERT
- Acute Horner syndrome with neck or facial pain:
  - Presume carotid dissection until proven otherwise:
    - c50% of internal carotid artery dissections present with a painful Horner syndrome.

## Physical Exam
Concentrate on a focused neurologic exam looking to confirm Horner syndrome and exclude other neurologic deficits:
- General physical should focus on identifying signs of other suspected conditions, such as tumor.

## ESSENTIAL WORKUP
- History and physical exam focused on neurologic findings
- CXR to screen for tumor or pneumothorax

## DIAGNOSTIC TESTS & INTERPRETATION
Provocative testing:
- Pharmacologic (cocaine) testing confirms diagnosis of sympathetic ocular lesion:
  - 1 drop of 5% ocular cocaine solution is instilled into each eye.
  - Failure of pupil on involved side to dilate as much as other pupil (increase in amount of anisocoria) in 1 hr is confirmatory (positive test).

## Lab
Not useful for Horner per se:
- Often needed as part of the workup of causative or associated conditions.

## Imaging
- CXR is usually indicated because of the association of chest pathology and Horner syndrome.
- CT or MRI of head, neck, or chest may be indicated depending on signs and symptoms.
- For suspected carotid dissection:
  - MRI/MRA or CTA of the neck compares favorably with contrast angiography:
    - Either test is appropriate.
    - The lesion is expected to be ipsilateral to the Horner syndrome.
- Choice of neuroimaging in suspected stroke depends heavily on local protocols and resources.
  - At a minimum, if stroke is suspected CT of the brain is indicated to rule out hemorrhagic stroke.

*Diagnostic Procedures/Surgery*

Ocular tonometry is indicated if acute glaucoma is suspected.

## DIFFERENTIAL DIAGNOSIS

- Increased intracranial pressure (ICP):
  - Almost always associated with altered level of consciousness (LOC), headache
- *Simple anisocoria (pseudo-Horner syndrome):*
  - 15–20% of the population has anisocoria and 3–4% also has miosis and ptosis.
  - Cocaine test is negative (both pupils dilate equally)
  - Inspect photo ID for pre-existing anisocoria.
- Topical medications or exposures are a common cause of miosis.
- Migraine or cluster headache
- Glaucoma, inflammatory ocular diseases, or ocular trauma

# TREATMENT

## PRE-HOSPITAL

Cautions:

- The importance of Horner syndrome is its association with more serious underlying conditions.
- Patients with increased ICP or tension pneumothorax must be recognized and treated as soon as possible.

## INITIAL STABILIZATION/THERAPY

- If increased ICP is suspected, initiate measures to control ICP:
  - Intubation, osmotic diuretics
- Tension pneumothorax:
  - Needle thoracostomy followed by chest tube

## ED TREATMENT/PROCEDURES

Horner syndrome per se requires no ED treatment:

- Causative or associated conditions may require treatment.

## MEDICATION

Cocaine: 5% (adult), 2.5% (peds) ophthalmic solution: 1 drop in each eye is diagnostic.

# FOLLOW-UP

## DISPOSITION

### Admission Criteria

Admission for isolated Horner syndrome is not needed:

- Admission may be needed for underlying condition.

### Discharge Criteria

- Stable patients with isolated Horner syndrome may be discharged with appropriate follow-up arranged for continued workup as outpatient:
  - When Horner syndrome is suspected, emergencies such as carotid dissection or stroke should be ruled out prior to discharge.

## FOLLOW-UP RECOMMENDATIONS

Neurologists and ophthalmologists must often be involved in the workup of Horner syndrome.

# PEARLS AND PITFALLS

Must search for underlying etiology

## ADDITIONAL READING

- Debette S, Leys D. Cervical-artery dissections: Predisposing factors, diagnosis, and outcome. *Lancet Neurol.* 2009;8(7):668–678.
- Arcasoy S, Jett J. Current concepts: Superior pulmonary sulcus tumors and Pancoast's syndrome. *N Engl J Med.* 1997;337:1370–1376.
- Fields C, Barker F. Review of Horner's syndrome and a case report. *Optom Vis Sci.* 1992;69(6):481–485.
- Maloney WF, Younge BR, Moyer NJ. Evaluation of the causes and accuracy of pharmacologic localization in Horner's syndrome. *Am J Ophthalmol.* 1980;90(3):394–402.
- Thanvi B, et al. Carotid and vertebral artery dissection syndromes. *Postgrad Med.* 2005;81:383–388.
- Wilheim H, et al. Horner's syndrome: A retrospective analysis of 90 cases and recommendations for clinical handling. *Ger J Ophthalmol.* 1992;1(2):96–102.

 CODES

### ICD9

- 337.9 Unspecified disorder of autonomic nervous system
- 954.0 Injury to cervical sympathetic nerve, excluding shoulder and pelvic girdles

H

# HUMERUS FRACTURE

G. Richard Bruno

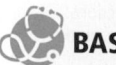 **BASICS**

## DESCRIPTION
- Proximal humeral fractures:
  - Typically described as nondisplaced, displaced, and/or fracture/dislocation
  - Account for 5% of all fractures
  - Increased incidence with age
  - Vast majority of patients are >60 yr old
  - **Neer classification**: A system that identifies the number of fragments and their location:
    - Fractures consist of 2–4-part fractures; the locations include the anatomic neck, surgical neck, greater tuberosity, and lesser tuberosity.
    - Fracture/dislocations also part of the Neer classification
- Humeral shaft fractures:
  - Account for <3% of fractures
  - May be spiral, oblique, or transverse
  - Humeral shaft fractures (AO classification):
    - Simple
    - Wedge
    - Comminuted (complex)

## ETIOLOGY
- Proximal humerus fractures:
  - Most often a history of a fall
  - Most common is fall on outstretched hand
  - Less common is violent muscle contraction from shock or seizure
- Humeral shaft fractures:
  - High-energy direct trauma (penetrating or blunt) or bending force
  - Less common from fall
  - Stress fractures from throwing injury

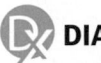 **DIAGNOSIS**

## SIGNS AND SYMPTOMS
- Pain, swelling, and tenderness
- Difficulty in initiating active motion
- Arm often closely held against chest
- Shortening of the extremity
- Crepitus may be present
- Ecchymosis
- Neurovascular compromise

### History
- Mechanism of injury
- Contributory comorbid factors (age, fall risk, malignancy)
- Associated injuries

### Physical Exam
- Complete exam of the affected extremity:
  - Inspect shoulder and humerus for obvious deformity, shortening, and open injuries
  - Assess ROM at shoulder, elbow
  - Neurovascular exam

## ESSENTIAL WORKUP
- Assess individual nerves:
  - Radial (special attention in midshaft humeral fractures)
  - Median
  - Ulnar
  - Axillary (sensation to the lateral aspect of the shoulder)
  - Musculocutaneous nerve (sensation to the extensor aspect of the forearm)
- Assess vascular supply:
  - Presence of radial, ulnar, and brachial pulses
  - Good capillary refill in all digits
- Radiology exams to define injury

### Pediatric Considerations
- Most common in age <3 or >12 yr
- Neonatal fractures from delivery trauma:
  - Most common in neonates >4.5 kg and breech births
  - May see pseudoparalysis
- Older children: Same injury mechanisms as adults
- Periosteum thicker in children and limits displacement of humeral shaft fractures
- Proximal humerals fractures:
  - Salter I fractures should be considered when films of proximal humerus are normal but significant pain is present
  - Salter II most common in younger children
- Consider abuse (especially <3 yr):
  - Injury patterns:
    - Transverse (direct blow)
    - Oblique/spiral (traction and humeral rotation)
    - Metaphyseal fractures (bucket-handle fractures)

## DIAGNOSTIC TESTS & INTERPRETATION
### Imaging
- Plain films:
  - Proximal humeral fractures:
    - Anteroposterior (AP), lateral views, axillary
    - Axillary view to assess tuberosity displacement, glenoid articular surface, and relationship of the humeral head to glenoid
  - Humeral shaft fractures:
    - AP and lateral views of entire humerus are mandatory.
    - Include shoulder and elbow views to exclude associated joint involvement.
- CT scan:
  - Helpful in proximal humeral fractures to define complex/comminuted injures and plan surgery
  - Help define relationship of humeral head to glenoid fossa in suspected fracture/dislocations

### Diagnostic Procedures/Surgery
Not applicable

## DIFFERENTIAL DIAGNOSIS
- Acute hemorrhagic bursitis
- Traumatic rotator cuff tear
- Dislocation
- Acromioclavicular separation
- Calcific tendinitis
- Contusion
- Tendon rupture
- Neurapraxia
- Pathologic fracture

 **TREATMENT**

## PRE-HOSPITAL
Cautions:
- Avoid excessive movement of the arm, which may produce further neurovascular injury.
- Immobilize with sling and swath and transport.
- Rapid transport in presence of neurologic or vascular deficits

## INITIAL STABILIZATION/THERAPY
- Primary and secondary survey for associated injuries
- Immobilization:
  - For comfort
  - Prevent fracture displacement
  - Prevent neurovascular injury
- Axillary pad may also be used for comfort.
- Pain control
- Application of ice to limit swelling
- Open fractures:
  - Cover with a sterile dressing
  - Tetanus prophylaxis
  - Parenteral antibiotics

## ED TREATMENT/PROCEDURES
- Patient should receive adequate analgesia during diagnosis and treatment of injury:
  - Narcotics PO/IM/IV are first-line therapy
- Proximal humeral fractures:
  - Single-part proximal humeral fractures:
    - >80% of proximal humeral fractures
    - Can be treated nonoperatively
    - Treatment is sling and swath
    - Early ROM exercises often employed
  - Displaced, multipart proximal humeral fractures:
    - Use Neer classification to describe
    - >1 cm separation or >45 degrees are considered displaced
    - Orthopedic review and referral is appropriate for 2-part or higher fractures
    - Many 2-part fractures can be reduced and managed nonoperatively

- 3- and 4-part fractures may need ORIF/hemiarthroplasty
  - Surgical options depend not only on type of fracture, but also patient's age, comorbities, and patient's functional expectations of the extremity
- Indications for emergent orthopedic consult for proximal humeral fractures:
  - Open fracture
  - Fracture/dislocation that cannot be reduced in ED
  - Vascular compromise
- Humeral shaft fractures:
  - Most humeral shaft fractures can be managed nonoperatively and do not require reduction
  - 20 degrees of anterior angulation and 30 degrees of varus angulation are well tolerated by the musculature around the humerus.
  - Humerus can tolerate up to 3 cm of shortening with little functional deficit
- Nondisplaced humeral shaft fractures:
  - ED can treat with a coaptation splint
  - Except transverse fractures
  - Functional brace may be utilized by orthopedist
- Transverse fractures:
  - ED treatment should be sling and swath
  - Higher incidence of nonunion
- Displaced humeral shaft fractures:
  - Orthopedist may utilize hanging cast to treat and reduce displaced or shortened fractures.
- Indications for emergent orthopedic consult for humeral shaft fractures:
  - Neurovascular compromise
  - Segmental fractures
  - Fractures extending into articular surface
  - Open fractures
  - "Floating elbow" (fractures with concurrent ipsilateral forearm fractures)

### Pediatric Considerations
In children nearing skeletal maturity, it is essential to determine the degree of displacement or separation of the proximal humeral epiphysis, as exact reduction is important to prevent later disturbance of growth.

### MEDICATION
- Pain medications:
  - Narcotics (first line)
  - NSAIDS (second line)
- Conscious sedation with closed reductions (see "Conscious Sedation")

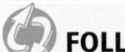 FOLLOW-UP

### DISPOSITION
#### Admission Criteria
- Open fractures for operative management and parenteral antibiotic therapy
- Fractures associated with vascular compromise
- Displaced fractures that cannot be treated adequately through closed reduction
- Significant associated injuries that require admission and observation

#### Discharge Criteria
- Nondisplaced fracture
- Fracture that is treated with closed reduction
- Most closed humeral shaft fractures without other injuries
- More complicated proximal humeral fractures, (ie, proximal humeral fracture of Neer 3 and 4 type), that may require nonemergent surgery. Discharge should be done in consultation with orthopedist.

#### Pediatric Considerations
- Pediatric patients are often less compliant with immobilization and less able to verbalize complaints; they may benefit from admission.
- Assess safety of environment in cases suspicious of NAT.

#### Issues for Referral
- Most humeral fractures should have outpatient orthopedic referral.
- Complicated proximal humeral fractures (Neer classification 2–4) should be reviewed with orthopedist to develop outpatient plan and possible nonemergent intervention.
- Some single-part nondisplaced proximal humeral fractures may be managed by the PCP.
- Displaced humeral shaft fractures require orthopedic referral for definitive care (functional bracing, hanging cast, ORIF, etc.).

### FOLLOW-UP RECOMMENDATIONS
- Most patient should be seen in close follow-up for repeat exam of the injured extremity, to verify adequate pain control, and to review treatment plan soon after ED visit.
- Proximal humeral fractures that are stable should be evaluated for early ROM therapy to minimize risk of adhesive capsulitis.

## PEARLS AND PITFALLS
- All humeral fractures should have diligent neurovascular exams:
  - Neurovascular exam should be repeated after manipulation.
  - Radial nerve injuries are the most common deficits seen in humeral shaft fractures.
  - Most radial nerve deficits will resolve spontaneously over time (months).
- Avascular necrosis is a risk in proximal humeral fractures that involve the surgical neck or articular surface.
- Patients with multiple-part proximal humeral fractures (Neer 2 or higher) may often be discharged from the ED, but a plan must be developed with the orthopedist because surgical intervention and/or hemiarthroplasty are possible.

## ADDITIONAL READING
- Burton DJ, Watters AT. Management of proximal humeral fractures. *Curr Orthop.* 2006;20:222–233.
- Caviglia H, Garrido CP, et al. Pediatric fractures of the humerus. *Clin Orthop Rel Res.* 2005;432:49–56.
- Green A, Norris TR. Proximal humerus fractures and glenohumeral dislocations. In: Browner, ed. *Skeletal Trauma: Basic Science, Management, and Reconstruction,* 4th ed. Saunders–Elsevier; 2008.
- Neer CS. Displaced proximal humeral fractures: I. Classification and evaluation. *J Bone Joint Surg.* 1970;52A:1077–1089.
- Schemitsch E, Bhandari M, Talbot M. Fractures of the humeral shaft. In: Browner, ed. *Skeletal Trauma: Basic Science, Management, and Reconstruction,* 4th ed. Saunders–Elsevier; 2008.

### See Also (Topic, Algorithm, Electronic Media Element)
- Conscious Sedation
- Elbow Fracture
- Shoulder Dislocation

 CODES

#### ICD9
- 812.00 Fracture of unspecified part of upper end of humerus, closed
- 812.21 Fracture of shaft of humerus, closed
- 812.40 Fracture of unspecified part of lower end of humerus, closed

# HYDATIDIFORM MOLE

*Emi Latham*

 **BASICS**

## DESCRIPTION

- Noninvasive localized tumors arising from trophoblastic tissue
- Can be associated with malignancy
- Twinning with normal pregnancy possible:
  - Higher risk for maternal persistent disease and metastasis
  - Possible to have normal infant
- Complete mole:
  - Fetal tissue not present
  - Diffuse chorionic villi swelling
  - Diffuse trophoblastic hyperplasia
  - Malignancy associated in 15–20%, usually lung
  - Genetics:
    ○ Karotype: 46,XX (90%); 46,XY (10%)
    ○ Paternal DNA expressed
    ○ Enucleate egg fertilized by 2 sperm or by a haploid sperm that duplicates
- Partial mole:
  - Fetal or embryonic tissue often present
  - Focal chorionic villi swelling
  - Focal trophoblastic hyperplasia
  - Malignancy associated in 4–12%
  - Genetics:
    ○ Karyotype: Triploid 69XXX (90%); 69XXY (10%)
    ○ Maternal and paternal DNA
    ○ Haploid ovum duplicates and is fertilized by normal sperm, or haploid ovum fertilized by 2 sperm.

## ETIOLOGY

- Largely unknown
- Advanced maternal age is the best estimated risk factor:
  - >40 yr old carries 5–10-fold risk
  - Disease has also been seen in <20 yr old
- Frequency multiple times greater in Asian countries:
  - 1 per 1,200 live births in the U.S. and Western Europe
  - Reported up to 1 per 100 live births in other countries (but maybe due to methodologies used to detect)
- Deficiency in animal fat and vitamin A
- Smoking
- Previous molar pregnancy carries 1–2% risk in future pregnancies
- Finding in 1 of 600 therapeutic abortions

 **DIAGNOSIS**

## SIGNS AND SYMPTOMS

- Usually exaggerated subjective symptoms of pregnancy
- Complete mole:
  - Vaginal bleeding, most common (97%):
    ○ Late 1st trimester
    ○ Usually painless and like "prune juice"
  - May also have vaginal tissue passage:
    ○ Often described as grapelike vesicles
    ○ Usually occurs in 2nd trimester <20 wk
  - Preeclampsia (27%):
    ○ Visual changes
    ○ HTN
    ○ Proteinuria
    ○ Hyperreflexia
    ○ Possibly convulsions
  - Hyperthyroidism (7%):
    ○ Marked tachycardia, tremor
    ○ Due to $\beta$-hCG stimulating thyrotropin receptors
  - Acute respiratory distress (2%):
    ○ Tachypnea, diffuse rales, tachycardia, mental status changes
    ○ Possibly embolism of trophoblastic tissue
    ○ May also be due to cardiopulmonary changes from preeclampsia, hyperthyroidism, or iatrogenic fluid replacement
- Partial mole:
  - Usually does not exhibit dramatic clinical features of complete mole
  - Frequently presents with symptoms similar to patients with threatened or spontaneous abortion:
    ○ Vaginal bleeding
    ○ May have fetal heart tones
  - Often presents at more advanced gestational age

## History

Similar to that of pregnancy:
- Missed menstrual periods
- Positive pregnancy test
- Nausea, vomiting, vaginal bleeding

## Physical Exam

- Uterine size/date discrepancy (50–66%):
  - Complete mole usually larger than dates would indicate
  - Partial mole can be smaller than dating suggests
- Ovarian masses:
  - Multiple bilateral theca lutein cysts due to high levels of $\beta$-hCG
  - Present in complete moles, rarely in partials

## ESSENTIAL WORKUP

- hCG
  - Complete mole:
    ○ Usually $\beta$-hCG >100,000 mIU/mL, but can be normal
  - Partial mole: Usually lower than that seen with normal pregnancy
  - $\beta$-hCG >40,000 mIU/mL carries poor prognosis
- US:
  - Original technology most accurate in 2nd trimester
  - Complete mole:
    ○ Characteristic "snowstorm" vesicular pattern
    ○ Absence of fetal tissue and swelling of chorionic villi with anechoic spaces
    ○ No amniotic fluid
  - Partial mole:
    ○ Produces "swiss-cheese" appearance
    ○ From cystic changes in placenta with scalloping of villa and in shape of gestational sac
    ○ Fetus may be present
  - Newer high-resolution US allows for diagnosis within the 1st trimester:
    ○ Complex intrauterine mass with many small cysts
  - Theca lutein cysts:
    ○ More commonly seen in complete moles
    ○ Bilateral, multiloculated
    ○ Large at 6–12 cm

## DIAGNOSTIC TESTS & INTERPRETATION

### Lab

- $\beta$-hCG
- Blood type, Rh and crossmatch
- CBC to assess for anemia and thrombocytopenia
- Coagulation profile to assess for disseminated intravascular coagulation
- Electrolytes with BUN and creatinine
- LFTs
- TSH and thyroxin (free T4) if hyperthyroidism suspected
- Urinanalysis to evaluate for protein if preeclampsia suspected

### Imaging

- US:
  - May be performed at bedside
- CXR:
  - To assess for pulmonary edema in acute respiratory distress
  - To check for metastatic disease
  - For baseline study

## Diagnostic Procedures/Surgery

Pathology/histology:

- All conception products should be evaluated
- Products may be the only way to diagnose a partial molar pregnancy
- Complete mole:
  - Edematous chorionic villi
  - Hyperplasia of trophoblasts
- Partial mole:
  - Fetal tissue and vessels
  - Amnion
  - Edematous chorionic villi

## DIFFERENTIAL DIAGNOSIS

- Threatened abortion
- Missed abortion
- Incomplete abortion
- Ectopic pregnancy
- Hyperthyroidism
- Hyperemesis gravidarum
- HTN
- Preeclampsia

 TREATMENT

### PRE-HOSPITAL

- Ensure patent airway, provide oxygen.
- IV access
- Treat convulsions appropriately with benzodiazepine
- Save passed tissue for histological evaluation

### INITIAL STABILIZATION/THERAPY

- IV access
- Cardiac monitoring
- Type and cross-match for blood, especially if patient requires uterine extraction

### ED TREATMENT/PROCEDURES

- Acute respiratory distress:
  Intubation and mechanical ventilation
  - CXR
- Hyperthyroidism:
  - β-adrenergic blockers:
    ○ Administer before molar evacuation
    ○ Stress of anesthesia or surgery may precipitate thyroid storm
- Preeclampsia/eclampsia:
  - Convulsions
    ○ Administer benzodiazepine (diazepam)
    ○ Administer magnesium sulfate
  - HTN:
    ○ Administer hydralazine or labetalol

- Coagulopathy:
  - Transfuse with blood products as needed
  - Human anti-D immunoglobulin (RhoGAM):
    ○ Although fetal blood not present in complete mole, maybe delay in distinguishing partial vs. complete
- Suction curettage:
  - Done by obstetrician, possibly in ED
  - Curative in 80% of cases
  - Method of choice in women wishing to preserve fertility
  - Oxytocin infusion to induce myometrial tone, may require other uterotonic formulations
- Chemoprophylaxis:
  - Very controversial
  - Prescribed by obstetrician only for patients with follow-up
  - Usually used in high-risk complete mole or if hormonal monitoring is unavailable
- Hysterectomy:
  - Patients in older age group
  - Patients not interested in keeping fertility
  - High-risk disease
  - Does not prevent possible metastasis

## MEDICATION

- Diazepam: 0.2–0.4 mg/kg IV, or 0.3–0.5 mg PR, up to 5–10 mg, for max. 30 mg
- Hydralazine: 5–10 mg IV q20m, up to 60 mg
- Labetalol: 20 mg IV with doubled dosing q10m for max. 300 mg
- Magnesium sulfate: 4–6 g IV over 15–20 min then maintenance 1–2 g/h
- Oxytocin: Postpartum bleeding, 10 units IM
- Propranolol: 1 mg IV increments q2m
- RhoGAM: 300 mcg within 72 hr

 FOLLOW-UP

### DISPOSITION

#### Admission Criteria

- Enlargement of uterus beyond 16 wk of gestation size:
  - The larger the uterus, the greater the risk for uterine perforation during suction curettage, hemorrhage, and pulmonary complications due to embolism
- Clinical evidence of preeclampsia, hyperthyroidism, respiratory distress
- Hysterectomy
- Partial molar pregnancy
- Hemodynamic instability

#### Discharge Criteria

- Uncomplicated dilation and curettage of low-risk and small-size mole in reliable patient
- Stress importance of follow-up
- Pelvic rest for 4–6 wk after uterine evacuation
- Recommend no pregnancies for 12 mo
- Future pregnancies should have early sonographic evaluation due to increased risk in future pregnancies.

### FOLLOW-UP RECOMMENDATIONS

- Close follow-up and monitoring by OB-Gyn
- Serial hCG levels:
  - Obtained weekly for at least 4 wk, then monthly intervals
  - Levels should consistently drop and never increase
  - If increase is noted, evaluation for metastatic disease should ensue
- Use contraception
- US:
  - Early in all future pregnancies
  - Increased risk for future molar pregnancies (1–1.5% with 2nd, 20% after 2 moles)

## PEARLS AND PITFALLS

- Missed diagnosis in conjunction with:
  - Normal pregnancy
  - Preeclampsia, especially <24 wk gestation
  - Hyperemesis with normal pregnancy
- The importance of follow-up must be stressed:
  - If hCG is not followed, may lead to undiagnosed metastatic disease.
  - 20% can develop malignancy

## ADDITIONAL READING

- Hydatidiform Mole. Emedicine. Available at: http://emedicine.medscape.com/article/254657-overview
- Sebire MJ, Seckl MJ. Gestational trophoblastic disease: Current management of hydatidiform mole. *BMJ.* 2008;337:a2076.
- Soper JT, et al. Diagnosis and treatment of gestational trophoblastic disease: ACOG practice bulletin #53. *Gynecol Oncol.* 2004;93:575–585.

### See Also (Topic, Algorithm, Electronic Media Element)

- Preeclampsia/Eclampsia
- Pregnancy

 CODES

### ICD9

630 Hydatidiform mole

H

# HYDROCARBON POISONING

Seth M. Oskie
James W. Rhee

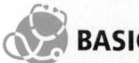 **BASICS**

## DESCRIPTION

- Main complication from hydrocarbon exposure is aspiration:
  - Hydrocarbon aspiration primarily affects central nervous and respiratory systems.
- Physical properties determine type and extent of toxicity:
  - Viscosity (resistance to flow):
    - Higher aspiration risk from products with lower viscosity
  - Volatility (ability of a substance to vaporize):
    - Hypoxia from aromatic hydrocarbons displacing alveolar air
  - Surface tension (ability to adhere to itself at liquid's surface):
    - Low surface tension allows easy spread from oropharynx to trachea, promoting aspiration (eg, mineral oil, seal oil).
- Volatile substance abuse:
  - Common solvents abused:
    - Typewriter correction fluid
    - Adhesive
    - Gasoline
    - Cigarette-lighter fluid
  - *Sniffing:* Product inhaled directly from container
  - *Huffing:* Product inhaled through a soaked rag held to face
  - *Bagging:* Product poured into bag and multiple inhalations taken from bag
- Major classes of hydrocarbons:
  - Aliphatics:
    - Include kerosene, mineral oil, seal oil, gasoline, solvents, and paint thinners
    - Pulmonary toxicity via aspiration
    - Asphyxiation from gaseous methane and butane by displacement of alveolar oxygen
  - Halogenated hydrocarbons:
    - Include carbon tetrachloride and trichloroethane
    - Found in industrial settings as solvents
    - Well absorbed by lungs and gut
    - High toxicity
    - Liver and renal failure associated with ingestion
  - Cyclics or aromatic compounds include toluene and xylene:
    - Highly volatile and well absorbed from gut
    - Death from benzene reported with 15-mL ingestion
  - Terpenes or wood distillates include turpentine and pine oil:
    - Significant GI tract absorption
    - Significant CNS depression

## ETIOLOGY

- Accidental exposures typical in young children
- Inhalation abuse of volatile hydrocarbons
- Suicide attempts in adolescents and adults

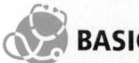 **DIAGNOSIS**

## SIGNS AND SYMPTOMS

- Often asymptomatic at presentation
- Odor of hydrocarbons on breath
- Early: Euphoria:
  - Disinhibition
- Late: Dysphoria:
  - Ataxia
  - Confusion
  - Hallucination
- Sudden sniffing death:
  - Cardiac arrest in volatile substance abusers secondary to hypersensitization of myocardium leading to malignant dysrhythmias on adrenergic stimulation
- Pulmonary:
  - Mild to severe respiratory distress
  - Cyanosis
  - Aspiration (primary complication)
- CNS:
  - Intoxication
  - Euphoria
  - Slurred speech
  - Lethargy
  - Coma
- GI tract:
  - Local mucosal irritation
  - Gastritis
  - Diarrhea
- Cardiac:
  - Tachycardia
  - Dysrhythmias (volatile substance abuse)
- Dermal:
  - Local erythema
  - Maculopapular or vesicular eruptions
  - Defatting dermatitis from chronic skin exposure
  - Huffer face rash in chronic abusers

## History

- Route, type, quantity, and time of exposure:
  - Determine intentionality and coingestions
- Symptoms:
  - Vomiting, respiratory distress, mental status change or pain
- Bystander actions or prehospital interventions

## Physical Exam

- Evaluate for airway compromise in patients with decreased level of consciousness and vomiting
- Respiratory symptoms generally occur within 30 min but are frequently delayed several hours
- Monitor for hypoxia, hypotension and cardiac dysrrhythmias
- Cyanosis and hypoxia suggest respiratory failure but may result from methemoglobinemia
- Temperature may be elevated at presentation following aspiration and indicates pneumonitis:
  - Fever after 48 hr suggests bacterial super-infection

## ESSENTIAL WORKUP

Obtain information on the following:

- Product: exact name on label, manufacturer, and ingredients
- Nature of ingestion or exposure: accidental or intentional
- Estimated amount ingested
- In industrial settings, Material Safety Data Sheets (MSDSs)

## DIAGNOSTIC TESTS & INTERPRETATION

ECG for intoxicated volatile substance abusers

### Lab

- Pulse oximetry:
  - If abnormal, follow with arterial blood gases.
- Electrolytes; BUN, creatinine, and glucose levels; and liver function tests:
  - For halogenated and aromatic hydrocarbon exposure
  - Metabolic acidosis
  - Hypokalemia
- Carboxyhemoglobin levels for methylene chloride exposure:
  - Methylene chloride metabolized to carbon monoxide in vivo

### Imaging

CXR:

- Abnormalities visible 20 min to 24 hr after exposure (usually by 6 hr)
- Increased bronchovascular marking and bibasilar and perihilar infiltrates (typical)
- Lobar consolidation (uncommon)
- Pneumothorax, pneumomediastinum, and pleural effusion (rare)
- Pneumatoceles resolve over weeks
- Repeat chest radiograph if worsening respiratory symptoms

## DIFFERENTIAL DIAGNOSIS

- Caustic, pesticide, or toxic alcohol ingestions
- Accidental vs. intentional:
  - Psychiatric evaluation for all intentional ingestions
- Child neglect:
  - Poor supervision or unsafe home environment

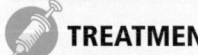 **TREATMENT**

## PRE-HOSPITAL
- Decontaminate clothes, skin, and hair of any hydrocarbon exposure
- Do not induce emesis.
- Ipecac contraindicated owing to increased risk of aspiration
- Keep volatile-substance abusers calm and avoid interventions that cause anxiety or distress.
- Management of *accidental* hydrocarbon exposures at home controversial:
  - <1% require physician intervention.
  - For asymptomatic or quickly asymptomatic after ingestion with reliable observer available
  - Applies only when exact product and its components are known and there is no indication for gastric decontamination or possibility for delayed organ toxicity

## INITIAL STABILIZATION/THERAPY
- ABCs
- IV access and fluid resuscitation if hypotensive or ongoing fluid losses
- Oxygen
- Cardiac monitor
- Naloxone, thiamine, $D_{50}W$ (or Accu-Chek) if altered mental status

## ED TREATMENT/PROCEDURES
- Supportive care
- Treat respiratory symptoms:
  - Oxygen
  - Nebulized $\beta_2$-agonist for bronchospasm (albuterol)
  - Endotracheal intubation and mechanical ventilation for respiratory failure
  - Steroids not indicated for bronchospasm
  - Avoid using epinephrine in volatile substance abusers as it may precipitate dysrhythmias
- Gastric evacuation not indicated for vast majority of hydrocarbon ingestions:
  - Aspiration risk higher than risk of systemic absorption for aliphatic hydrocarbon mixtures, which account for most ingestions
  - Contraindicated if spontaneous emesis has occurred
  - Small-bore nasogastric tube aspiration of stomach contents may be indicated for some hydrocarbon (CHAMP) ingestions that have systemic toxicity:
    - CHAMP: *c*amphor, *h*alogenated hydrocarbons, *a*romatic hydrocarbons, *m*etals (eg, lead, mercury), *p*esticides
    - Only for very recent ingestions (60 min)
    - Benefit of doing this procedure needs to be weighed heavily against risk of aspiration and subsequent pneumonitis.
    - Cuffed-tube endotracheal intubation for airway protection during lavage if no gag reflex or altered mental status

- Activated charcoal not indicated except for significant coingestants
- Cathartics not indicated:
  - Diarrhea common with hydrocarbon

## MEDICATION
- Dextrose: $D_{50}W$ 1 ample of 50 mL or 25 g (peds: $D_{25}W$ 2–4 mL/kg) IV
- Naloxone (Narcan): 2 mg (peds: 0.1 mg/kg) IV or IM initial dose
- Thiamine (vitamin $B_1$): 100 mg (peds: 50 mg) IV or IM
- Bronchospasm:
  - Albuterol 2.5–5 mg NEB (peds: 0.15–0.3 mg/kg)

 **FOLLOW-UP**

## DISPOSITION
### Admission Criteria
- Symptomatic patients
- Patients with potential delayed organ toxicity (carbon tetrachloride or other toxic additives)

### Discharge Criteria
- Observe for 6 hr then discharge:
  - Asymptomatic patients with normal chest radiograph and pulse oximetry findings
  - Asymptomatic patients with abnormal CXR and normal oxygenation and respiratory rate may be discharged if reliable follow-up is ensured.
  - Symptomatic patients on presentation who quickly become asymptomatic
- Observe volatile-substance abusers until mental status clears.

### Issues for Referral
Psychiatry consult as needed

### FOLLOW-UP RECOMMENDATIONS
- Follow up in 24 hr for patients who remain asymptomatic after a minimum of 6 hr observation
- Asymptomatic patients with an abnormal CXR should have a repeat study in 24 hr

## PEARLS AND PITFALLS
- Main complication from hydrocarbon exposure is aspiration:
  - Aspiration risk inversely related to viscosity and surface tension and directly related to volatility
- Provide external decontamination
- Gastric decontamination is rarely indicated

- Avoid induced emesis and cathartics
- Observe patients a minimum of 6 hr post ingestion for evidence of toxicity
- Admit symptomatic patients to hospital:
  - Admit when there is potential for delayed organ toxicity:
    - CHAMP: *C*amphor, *h*alogenated hydrocarbons, *a*romatic hydrocarbons, *m*etals (eg, lead, mercury), *p*esticides

## ADDITIONAL READING
- Anas N, Namasonthi V, Ginsburg C. Criteria for hospitalizing children who have ingested products containing hydrocarbons. *JAMA.* 1981;246: 840–843.
- Dice WH, Ward G, Kelly J, et al. Pulmonary toxicity following gastrointestinal ingestion of kerosene. *Ann Emerg Med.* 1982;11:138–142.
- Esmail A, Meyer L, Pottier A, et al. Deaths from volatile substance abuse in those under 18 years: Results from a national epidemiological study. *Arch Dis Child.* 1993;69:356–360.
- Hydrocarbons. In *Poisindex®System [internet database].* Greenwood Village, Colo: Thomson Reuters (Healthcare) Inc. Updated periodically.
- Klein BL, Simon JE. Hydrocarbon poisonings. *Pediatr Clin North Am.* 1986;33:411.
- Machado B, Cross K, Snodgrass WR. Accidental hydrocarbon ingestion cases telephoned to a regional poison center. *Ann Emerg Med.* 1988;17: 804–807.

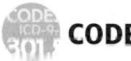 **CODES**

ICD9
987.0 Toxic effect of liquefied petroleum gases

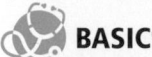

## BASICS

### DESCRIPTION
- Most common cause of painless scrotal swelling.
- Classified as congenital or acquired:
  - Congenital result from a patent process vaginalis and communication between tunica vaginalis and peritoneal cavity:
    - Normally occurs spontaneously and most are closed by 2 yr of age
  - Acquired occur secondary to interscrotal infection, neoplasm, inguinal or scrotal surgery, or regional or systemic disease.
- Communicating hydrocele:
  - Patent processus vaginalis
  - Scrotum fills and empties with peritoneal fluid depending on body position.
- *Noncommunicating hydrocele* is owing to production of serous fluid by a disease process

### ETIOLOGY
- Imbalance between production and resorption of fluid within space between tunica vaginalis and tunica albuginea.
- Disease processes causing adult noncommunicating hydrocele include:
  - Epididymitis
  - Hypoalbuminemia
  - TB
  - Trauma
  - Mumps
  - Spermatic vein ligation
  - In 3rd World, hydrocele is primarily caused by infections such as *Wuchereria bancrofti* or *Loa Loa*.
  - Rarely malignancy (1st-degree testicular neoplasm or lymphoma)

- Rare etiology is the abdominoscrotal hydrocele that may cause hydroureter or unilateral limb edema owing to compression:
  - US reveals single sac extending from scrotum into abdominal cavity via the deep inguinal ring.

### Pediatric Considerations
- Congenital in 6% of newborn boys
- Usually diagnosed in newborn nursery
- Caused by patent processus vaginalis, a structure that remains patent in 85% of newborns
- May vary in size owing to position or crying:
  - Patients may present with history of scrotal mass that has resolved.
- Most close by age of 2 yr

## DIAGNOSIS

### SIGNS AND SYMPTOMS
Painless scrotal swelling with a sensation of pulling or dragging.

### History
History and examination with special attention to identifying torsion of testicle.

### Physical Exam
- Mass may be soft and doughy or firm depending on the amount of fluid present.
- Initial diagnostic test is transillumination of affected side:
  - This is rapidly being replaced as diagnostic test of choice by bedside US.

### ESSENTIAL WORKUP
- Bedside US:
  - Allows visualization of hydrocele as well as of testicle
  - Especially in cases of massive fluid collection, bedside US should be diagnostic test of choice.
- Because of possibility in adults that a hydrocele may be owing to a primary neoplasm, the testicle must be palpated in its entirety.

### DIAGNOSTIC TESTS & INTERPRETATION
#### Lab
No specific laboratory testing is indicated unless underlying cause demands it.

#### Imaging
US is diagnostic and allows visualization of testicular anatomy:
- Appears as large anechoic fluid-filled space surrounding the anterolateral testicle

### DIFFERENTIAL DIAGNOSIS
- Epididymitis
- Indirect inguinal hernia
- Orchitis
- Testicular neoplasm
- Testicular torsion

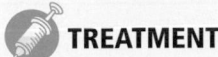 **TREATMENT**

**INITIAL STABILIZATION/THERAPY**
Stabilization should focus on underlying cause (eg, trauma).

**ED TREATMENT/PROCEDURES**
Appropriate examination of testicle to exclude primary neoplasm and referral.

**MEDICATION**
Treat underlying cause.

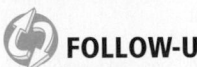 **FOLLOW-UP**

**DISPOSITION**
*Admission Criteria*
Patients with secondary hydrocele may need admission for further evaluation of underlying pathology (eg, neoplasm, trauma).

*Discharge Criteria*
- Otherwise healthy patients without co-morbid illness may be referred for further evaluation to urologist.
- Hydrocele is usually repaired if cosmesis is a factor or in cases where it causes discomfort.
- Repair can be:
  – Surgical:
    ○ Aspiration or sclerotherapy are alternatives to open hydrocelectomy.
  – Medical:
    ○ Aspiration of hydrocele contents and sclerotherapy to prevent recurrence.

*Pediatric Considerations*
- Most hydroceles in infant population will spontaneously resolve by 12 mo of age:
  – Referral and observation are appropriate once diagnosis is made.
- After age of 12–18 mo, refer for surgical repair as communicating hydroceles usually have hernia that needs repair.

**FOLLOW-UP RECOMMENDATIONS**
Patients should be referred to Urology.

**PEARLS AND PITFALLS**

The mass may fail to transilluminate due to thickening of the tunica vaginalis.
- Bedside US should visualize both the fluid filled mass and the testicle.

**ADDITIONAL READING**

- Akin EA, Khati NJ, Hill MC. Ultrasound of the scrotum. *Ultrasound Q.* 2004;20:181–200.
- Hoerauf A. Filiariasis: New drugs and new opportunities for lymphatic filiariasis and onchocerciasis. *Curr Opin Infect Dis.* 2008;21: 673–681.
- Rabinowitz R, Hulbert WC. Acute scrotal swelling. *Urol Clin North Am.* 1995;22:101–105.
- Rubenstein RA, Dogra VS, Seftel AD, et al. Benign intrascrotal lesions. *J Urol.* 2004;171:1765–1772.

**See Also (Topic, Algorithm, Electronic Media Element)**
- Epididymitis/Orchitis
- Hernia
- Testicular Torsion

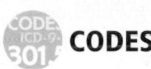 **CODES**

ICD9
603.9 Hydrocele, unspecified

H

# HYDROCEPHALUS
*Richard S. Krause*

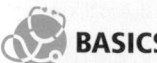 **BASICS**

## DESCRIPTION
- Increased CSF in cranial cavity:
- Cerebral atrophy also leads to increased CSF in the cranial vault but CSF pressure is not increased
- *Obstructive hydrocephalus* is most common form:
  - Obstruction is within ventricular system or in subarachnoid space.
- Acute obstructive hydrocephalus may cause rapid rise in intracranial pressure (ICP), rapidly leading to death or permanent cerebral damage.
- *Nonobstructive hydrocephalus* causes subacute symptoms and is a potentially treatable form of dementia
- Also described as "communicating" and "noncommunicating":
- Communicating hydrocephalus: Flow of CSF is blocked after it exits the ventricles (ventricles still "communicate")
- Noncommunicating hydrocephalus: Flow of CSF blocked along one or more of the passages connecting the ventricles (ventricles do not "communicate")

## ETIOLOGY
- Obstructive hydrocephalus:
  - Obstruction of:
    - Aqueduct of Sylvius (most common, both lateral ventricles and third ventricle dilated, 4th ventricle is spared)
    - Foramen of Monro (lateral ventricle dilated)
    - Foramina of Luschka and Magendie (fourth ventricle blocked followed by third and lateral ventricles)
    - Subarachnoid space around brainstem (postinfectious or postsubarachnoid hemorrhage [post-SAH] entire system dilated)
  - Acute presentations usually secondary to CSF shunt blockage, SAH, or severe head trauma
- Nonobstructive hydrocephalus:
  - Normal pressure hydrocephalus:
    - Increased intracranial volume of CSF without intracranial hypertension
    - Increased ventricular size on CT (without volume loss as in atrophy)
    - Sometimes called "chronic hydrocephalus"
- Pediatric hydrocephalus:
  - Congenital hydrocephalus owing to neonatal hemorrhages, congenital malformations, or acquired postmeningitis secondary to subarachnoid scarring around brainstem

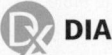 **DIAGNOSIS**

## SIGNS AND SYMPTOMS
- Obstructive hydrocephalus:
  - Headache
  - Nausea and vomiting
  - Decreased level of consciousness
  - Urinary incontinence
  - Ocular palsies
  - Papilledema, decreased vision
  - Pupillary dilation
  - Cushing response:
    - Raised systolic pressure and bradycardia secondary to increased ICP
  - Pediatric patients:
    - Full fontanelle, irritability, and lethargy
  - May present like nonobstructive hydrocephalus if obstruction develops slowly
- Nonobstructive hydrocephalus:
  - Progressive dementia, somnolence
  - Gait disturbance
  - Urinary incontinence
  - Impaired upward gaze
  - Generalized weakness and lethargy
  - Dementia is often insidious with subacute onset of progressive intellectual deterioration.
  - No headache or papilledema

### Pediatric Considerations
- Pediatric patients increase CSF volume slowly:
  - Craniomegaly
  - Retardation
  - Prominent scalp veins
  - Impaired upward gaze (setting sun sign)

### History
- Onset of symptoms
- History of CSF shunt
- Nausea/vomiting
- Headache
- Weakness
- Confusion
- Visual changes
- Incontinence

### Physical Exam
- Thorough neurologic exam:
  - Motor
  - Sensation
  - Deep tendon reflexes
  - Gait
  - Cranial nerve exam
  - Papilledema may be seen
- Confusion
- Decreased mental status
- Palpate CSF shunt if present
- Full anterior fontanelle in children:
  - Other findings as noted in "Signs and Symptoms"

## ESSENTIAL WORKUP
CT scan of the head will allow assessment of ventricular size and symmetry:
- Aid in diagnosis of cerebral edema, mass lesions, and hemorrhage

## DIAGNOSTIC TESTS & INTERPRETATION
### Lab
Lumbar puncture (LP) is typically performed after head CT (for nonobstructive causes):
- Opening pressure on LP will reflect increased ICP in nonobstructive hydrocephalus.
- CSF should be sent for routine tests if infection is suspected.
  - Gram stain, culture, protein, and glucose, cell count

### Imaging
MRI of brain reveals ventricular size and symmetry and may allow for better visualization of masses than CT.

### Diagnostic Procedures/Surgery
Lumbar puncture may be indicated

## DIFFERENTIAL DIAGNOSIS
- Acute cerebral infarction or hemorrhage
- Intracranial infection
- Mass effect from fast-growing tumor or hematoma
- Dementia or delirium of other cause
- Toxic or metabolic encephalopathies

### Pediatric Considerations
- Suspect hydrocephalus in infant whose head circumference is increasing excessively, has progressive lethargy, persistent vomiting, impaired upward gaze, etc.
- Congenital anomalies:
  - Dandy-Walker malformation
  - Arnold-Chiari malformation
  - Meningomyelocele
  - Choroid plexus papilloma
  - Hypoplasia/dysfunction of arachnoid villi

- Infections:
  - Rubella
  - Cytomegalovirus (CMV)
  - Toxoplasmosis
  - Syphilis
  - Bacterial meningitis
  - Reye's syndrome
- Tumors, especially posterior fossa tumors:
  - Medulloblastoma
  - Astrocytoma
  - Ependymoma
- Hemorrhage:
  - Intraventricular
  - Subarachnoid

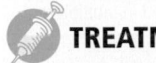 **TREATMENT**

### PRE-HOSPITAL
Cautions:

- Elevated ICP/hydrocephalus cannot be definitively diagnosed in the field.
- When it is suspected, supplemental $O_2$ and airway management (if needed) are indicated.
- Patients should be transported with head elevated at ~30°.

### INITIAL STABILIZATION/THERAPY
- Signs of impending herniation:
  - Rapid-sequence intubation (RSI)
    - Thiopental or etomidate for induction
    - Paralytic choice is controversial.
    - Depolarizing agents (succinylcholine) may increase ICP, although this effect may not be clinically significant.
    - Nondepolarizing agents (rocuronium, vecuronium) may be preferable.
  - Controlled ventilation to maintain $PaCO_2$ at ~35 mm Hg
  - Maintain systolic blood pressure (BP) >100 mm Hg (adult) with fluids or pressors.
  - Mannitol
- If a CSF shunt is present and there are signs of impending herniation:
  - Forced pumping of shunt chamber:
    - Flush device with 1 mL saline to remove distal obstruction.
    - Slow drainage of CSF from reservoir to achieve pressure <20 cm $H_2O$.
    - IV mannitol to lower ICP

### ED TREATMENT/PROCEDURES
- When signs of impending herniation or acute shunt malfunction are absent, hydrocephalus does not require ED treatment.
- Definitive treatment involves either placement (or revision) of shunting device or treatment of underlying cause (eg, tumor).
- Neurological symptoms (gait disturbance) or severe headache associated with normal pressure hydrocephalus may respond to removal of CSF by LP (20–30 mL).
- If intraventricular hemorrhage (usually from trauma or SAH) causes acute obstructing hydrocephalus a ventriculostomy may be placed in the lateral ventricle

### MEDICATION
- Atropine: 0.02 mg/kg IV (max. 0.1 mg)
- Etomidate: 0.2–0.3 mg/kg
- Lidocaine: 1 mg/kg IV
- Mannitol: 0.5–1 mg/kg
- Rocuronium: 0.6 mg/kg IV
- Succinylcholine: 1–1.5 mg/kg IV
- Vecuronium: 0.1 mg/kg

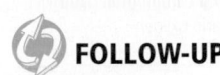 **FOLLOW-UP**

### DISPOSITION
#### Admission Criteria
Evidence of increased ICP or shunt malfunction requires admission.

#### Discharge Criteria
Patients with presumed normal pressure hydrocephalus may be discharged for follow-up.

#### Issues for Referral
Involvement of a neurosurgeon may be needed in acute obstructive hydrocephalus or for acute shunt malfunction

- Consider transfer if a neurosurgeon is not available at presenting hospital
- Airway management prior to transfer should be considered in acute cases

### FOLLOW-UP RECOMMENDATIONS
If patient is stable for discharge, follow-up with neurologist and/or neurosurgeon is essential.

## PEARLS AND PITFALLS

- LP should not be performed in obstructive hydrocephalus (risk of herniation)
- Suspect hydrocephalus in children whose head circumference is growing rapidly
- Consider hydrocephalus in patients with CSF shunts and any neurologic complaint

## ADDITIONAL READING

- Graff-Radford NR. Normal Pressure hydrocephalus. *Neurol Clin.* 2007;25:809–832.
- Mayer S, Chong J. Critical care management of increased intracranial pressure. *J Intensive Care Med.* 2002;17:55–67.
- Newman JP, Segal R. Images in clinical medicine: Communicating Hydrocephalus. *N Engl J Med.* 2004;351:e13
- Rekate HL. A contemporary definition and classification of hydrocephalus. *Semin Pediatr Neurol.* 2009;6:9–15.

### See Also (Topic, Algorithm, Electronic Media Element)
Ventricular Peritoneal Shunts

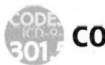 **CODES**

### ICD9
- 331.3 Communicating hydrocephalus
- 331.4 Obstructive hydrocephalus
- 331.5 Idiopathic normal pressure hydrocephalus (INPH)

H

# HYPERBARIC OXYGEN THERAPY

*Trevonne M. Thompson*

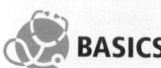 **BASICS**

## DESCRIPTION

- Administration of 100% oxygen at >1 atmospheric pressure (typically 2–3 atm)
- Mechanisms of action:
  - Increases oxygen availability at the cellular level:
    - Breathing 100% oxygen at 3 atm supplies enough dissolved oxygen to support life without hemoglobin.
  - Compresses formed gas bubbles (in cases of air embolism or decompression sickness)
- 2 types of hyperbaric oxygen chambers:
  - Monoplace:
    - Accommodates one supine patient
    - Technician outside the chamber for monitoring
    - Compressed with 100% oxygen
  - Multiplace:
    - Holds multiple patients
    - Holds attendants who "dive" with the patients
    - Airlocks available for medication/equipment transfer outside of the chamber
    - Compressed with air—patients breath oxygen by face mask, endotracheal tube, or face hood.

# DIAGNOSIS

## SIGNS AND SYMPTOMS

Indications for hyperbaric oxygen therapy:

- Arterial gas embolism
- Decompression sickness
- Carbon monoxide toxicity
- Soft tissue infections:
  - Clostridial myonecrosis
  - Necrotizing fasciitis
  - Refractory osteomyelitis
  - Chronic nonhealing wounds
- Wound care:
  - Radiation-induced tissue injury
  - Crush injuries
  - Thermal burns
  - Compromised skin grafts and flaps

## ALERT

The ED physician should focus on arterial embolism, decompression sickness, and carbon monoxide toxicity as uses for hyperbaric oxygen.

## ESSENTIAL WORKUP

- Determine need for hyperbaric oxygen therapy as described above.
- Perform a comprehensive physical examination to screen for contraindications to therapy and to establish a pretreatment baseline examination.
- Contraindications to therapy:
  - Untreated pneumothorax is the absolute contraindication:
    - May convert to a tension pneumothorax
  - Cardiovascular instability:
    - Unstable patient cannot be treated in a monoplace chamber.
    - Such a patient may be treated in multiplace chamber if benefit outweighs risk.

## DIAGNOSTIC TESTS & INTERPRETATION

### Lab

Arterial blood gas:

- To evaluate for hypoxia in appropriate cases

### Imaging

Chest radiography:

- To evaluate for occult pneumothorax

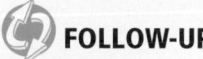 TREATMENT

### INITIAL STABILIZATION/THERAPY
- Manage ABCs
- Establish IV access.
- 100% oxygen
- Cardiac monitor (when appropriate)

### ED TREATMENT/PROCEDURES
- Determine need for hyperbaric oxygen therapy.
- Fill any devices with balloons (Foley catheters, endotracheal tubes) with fluid to avoid rupture during therapy.
- Pretreat patients with any sinus complaints with decongestants.
- Place myringotomy tubes in obtunded or mechanically ventilated patients or in patients with middle ear pathology (eg, otitis media).

### ALERT
Complications of hyperbaric oxygen therapy:
- Sinus/ear pain
- Barotrauma:
  - Ruptured tympanic membranes
  - Tension pneumothorax
- Seizures:
  - May be a result of oxygen toxicity
- Decompression sickness:
  - When decompression is too rapid
    - Inability to access an unstable patient when using a monoplace chamber

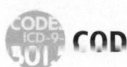 FOLLOW-UP

### DISPOSITION
#### Admission Criteria
- Arterial gas embolism
- Decompression sickness
- Significant carbon monoxide toxicity

#### Discharge Criteria
Stable patient with resolved symptoms

#### Issues for Referral
- May need to transfer to a facility that has a hyperbaric oxygen chamber
- Evaluate risks and benefits when considering the transfer of a potentially unstable patient.
- Divers Alert Network:
  - 24-hr emergency hotline for consultation of dive-related injuries
  - Referral source for hyperbaric oxygen chambers
  - Telephone numbers:
    - 919-684-9111
  - Website:
    - www.diversalertnetwork.org

### FOLLOW-UP RECOMMENDATIONS
Hyperbaric follow up for repeat recompression therapy.

## PEARLS AND PITFALLS
- Fill any devices with balloons (Foley catheters, endotracheal tubes) with fluid to avoid rupture during therapy.
- Check for occult pneumothorax.

## ADDITIONAL READING
- Sheridan RL, Shank ES. Hyperbaric oxygen treatment: A brief overview of a controversial topic. *J Trauma*. 1999;47(2):426–435.
- Tibbles PM, Edelsberg JS. Hyperbaric-oxygen therapy. *N Engl J Med*. 1996;334(20):1642–1648.
- Weaver LK. Carbon monoxide poisoning. *N Engl J Med*. 2009;360:1217–1225.

### See Also (Topic, Algorithm, Electronic Media Element)
- Carbon Monoxide Toxicity
- Decompression Sickness

## CODES

### ICD9
- 958.0 Air embolism as an early complication of trauma
- 986 Toxic effect of carbon monoxide
- 993.3 Caisson disease

H

# HYPERCALCEMIA

*Matthew A. Wheatley*

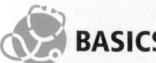 **BASICS**

## DESCRIPTION
- Severity depends on serum calcium level and rate of increase
- 0.1–1% of patients on routine screening
- Most cases mild (<12 mg/dL) and asymptomatic
- Hypercalcemic crisis, usually >14 mg/dL, causes serious signs and symptoms
- Calcium in bloodstream in 3 forms:
  - Ionized: 45%
  - Bound to protein (primarily albumin): 40%
  - Bound to other anions: 15%
- Ionized calcium—only physiologically active form

## ETIOLOGY
- Primary hyperparathyroidism
- Malignancy
- Miscellaneous

 **DIAGNOSIS**

## SIGNS AND SYMPTOMS
### History
- Neurologic:
  - Headache
  - Fatigue
  - Weakness, lethargy
  - Difficulty concentrating
  - Confusion
- Renal:
  - Polyuria, polydipsia
  - Complaints related to oliguric renal failure
  - Chronic, complaints related to:
    - Renal calculi
    - Nephrocalcinosis
    - Interstitial nephritis
- GI:
  - Anorexia
  - Nausea
  - Vomiting
  - Abdominal pain
  - Constipation
  - Chronic, complaints related to:
    - Peptic ulcer disease
    - Pancreatitis
- Dermatologic:
  - Pruritus

### Pediatric Considerations
- Failure to thrive
- Slow development
- Mental retardation may ensue

## Physical Exam
- Neurologic:
  - Irritability
  - Lethargy
  - Stupor
  - Coma
  - Hyporeflexia
- Cardiovascular:
  - Hypotension, if severely volume depleted, or HTN
  - Sinus bradycardia
  - Cardiac arrest with severe hypercalcemia (rare)
- Renal:
  - Signs of dehydration
- Dermatologic:
  - Band keratopathy
  - Ectopic calcification

### Pediatric Considerations
- Characteristic facies: Pug nose, fat nasal bridge, "cupid's bow" upper lip
- Hypotonia

## ESSENTIAL WORKUP
- Ionized and total serum calcium levels, albumin levels:
  - Normal total calcium level is <10.5 mg/dL
  - Must correct for calcium that is protein bound, primarily to albumin
  - Corrected total calcium (mg/dL) = measured total calcium (mg/dL) + 0.8 × [4.0 − albumin concentration (g/dL)]
- Electrolytes, BUN/creatinine, glucose
  - Possible oliguric renal failure
- ECG:
  - Shortening of QT interval
  - Prolongation of PR interval
  - QRS widening
  - Accentuated side effects of digoxin
  - Sinus bradycardia, bundle branch block, AV block, cardiac arrest with severe hypercalcemia (rare)
  - Can cause Osborn J wave at end of QRS complex that is usually associated with hypothermia

## DIAGNOSTIC TESTS & INTERPRETATION
### Lab
- Phosphate
- Protein
- Urinalysis
- Parathyroid hormone level:
  - If elevated or high normal, likely primary hyperparathyroidism.
  - If <20 pg/mL, consider testing PTH-related peptide and vitamin D metabolites.

- Vitamin D metabolites, if suspected
  - 25-hydroxy vitamin D (calcidiol):
    - If elevated, consider exogenous source (i.e., meds, vitamins, supplements).
  - 1,25-dihydroxyvitamin D (calcitriol):
    - If elevated, consider lymphoma or sarcoid
- Digoxin level, if taking
- Thyroid function tests

### Imaging
- CT head for altered mental status
- Chest x-ray and workup for occult malignancy, if no other cause for hypercalcemia

### Diagnostic Procedures/Surgery
Parathyroidectomy:
- For primary hyperparathyroidism resulting in symptomatic or severe hypercalcemia
- Some patients require urgent parathyroidectomy.

## DIFFERENTIAL DIAGNOSIS
- Primary hyperparathyroidism:
  - Most common cause among outpatients
  - Parathyroid adenoma 80%; hyperplasia 15%; carcinoma 5%
  - Usually mild, <11.2 mg/dL
  - Patients can be asymptomatic or have chronically elevated calcium
  - Increased bone resorption, relative decrease in calcium excretion, increased intestinal calcium absorption
- Malignancy:
  - Most common cause in hospitalized patients
  - Usually a rapid rise in serum calcium
  - Patients are more often symptomatic
  - Higher serum calcium concentrations
  - Most common paraneoplastic complication of cancer
  - Common tumors causing hypercalcemia: Breast, lung, colon, stomach, cervix, uterus, ovary, kidney, bladder, head and neck, multiple myeloma, and lymphoma
  - Most commonly from production of parathyroid hormone-related protein with similar actions
  - May result from production of other bone-resorbing substances by tumor
  - May result from local effects of osteolytic skeletal metastasis

- Miscellaneous:
  - Hypercalcemia associated with granulomatous diseases
  - Excessive calcium supplements
  - Thiazide diuretics causing increased renal reabsorption.
  - Granulomatous disorders may lead to activation of vitamin D.
  - Acute vitamin A intoxication
  - Increased exogenous vitamin D intake
  - Milk-alkali syndrome from excessive ingestion of calcium and nonabsorbable antacids, such as milk or calcium carbonate
  - Long-term lithium therapy
  - Renal transplantation
  - Hyperthyroidism
  - Acute tubular necrosis

### Pediatric Considerations
Differential diagnosis: Differences from adults:

- Primary hyperparathyroidism:
  - Less common than in adults
- Infantile hypercalcemia:
  - Uncertain cause
    Possibly hypersensitivity and in utero excessive exposure to vitamin D
- Immobilization hypercalcemia:
  - Typically adolescent who is growing rapidly
  - Prolonged immobilization, especially in traction, leads to hypercalciuria and then hypercalcemia.
  - Presumably from increased bone resorption with decreased or arrested bone mineralization

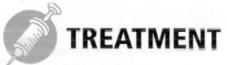 **TREATMENT**

**PRE-HOSPITAL**
Routine stabilization techniques

#### INITIAL STABILIZATION/THERAPY
- ABCs, IV access, oxygen, cardiac monitor
- 0.9% NS 1 L bolus (20 mL/kg) for hypotension or severe dehydration
- Naloxone, thiamine, $D_{50}W$ (or stat serum glucose measurement) for altered mental status

#### ED TREATMENT/PROCEDURES
- General:
  - Immediate therapy for severe hypercalcemia (corrected total >14 mg/dL) regardless of symptoms, or for symptomatic hypercalcemia
  - Asymptomatic, mild hypercalcemia does not require emergency treatment.

- Restoration of intravascular volume:
  - Isotonic saline:
    - 200–300 mL/hr adjusted to maintain urine output 100–150 mL/hr
  - Often need 2–5 L/d
  - Bedside vigilance necessary to prevent fluid overload
  - Correct other electrolyte abnormalities.
  - Cardiovascular status of patient may necessitate central venous pressure monitoring to adjust fluid administration rates.
- Renal elimination:
  - After volume expansion and if needed to avoid overload, administer loop diuretics (furosemide).
  - Avoid thiazide diuretics.
  - May need peritoneal or hemodialysis against a low calcium dialysate in renal failure
- Inhibition of osteoclastic activity:
  - Reduce mobilization of calcium from bone
  - Administer drug therapy when corrected calcium level >14 mg/dL or signs or symptoms
  - First-line drug therapy:
    - Bisphosphonates: Pamidronate (more potent and possibly less toxic), etidronate
    - Calcitonin: Rapid onset but modest decrease in levels
  - Other potential drug therapy:
    - Plicamycin: Efficacious but numerous side effects
    - Hydrocortisone: Especially useful with malignancies, granulomatous disorders, or vitamin D intoxication
  - Encourage ambulation in appropriate patients.
- Treat underlying disorder:
  - Parathyroidectomy for primary hyperparathyroidism resulting in symptomatic or severe hypercalcemia
  - Discontinue medication if cause.

### MEDICATION
#### First Line
- Calcitonin: 4 IU/kg IM/SC q12h
- Etidronate: 7.5 mg/kg over 4 hr daily for 3–7 days IV
- Furosemide: 10–40 mg q6–8h (peds: 1–2 mg/kg) IV
- Pamidronate: Single 24-hr infusion of 60–90 mg IV (peds: consult pediatrician)

#### Second Line
- Gallium nitrate: Continuous infusion of 200 mg/m²/d for 5 days IV
- Hydrocortisone: 200–400 mg/d IV for 3–5 days (peds: Consult pediatrician)
- Plicamycin: 25 $\mu$g/kg/d over 4–6 hr IV for 3–8 doses

 **FOLLOW-UP**

#### DISPOSITION
##### Admission Criteria
- Corrected total calcium level >13.0 mg/dL
- Signs or symptoms attributed to hypercalcemia, especially EKG changes.
- Monitored bed or ICU for corrected level >14 or serious signs and symptoms

##### Discharge Criteria
Corrected calcium level <13.0 mg/dL and no signs or symptoms of hypercalcemia

##### Issues for Referral
- Rapid follow-up arranged to determine cause and long-term therapy
- Consultation with endocrinologist should be considered.

#### FOLLOW-UP RECOMMENDATIONS
- Fluid hydration
- Watch for mental status changes

### PEARLS AND PITFALLS
- Make decisions based on symptoms or corrected Ca levels
- All patients with serum Ca >14 mg/dL require treatment regardless of symptoms
- Pay careful attention to EKG changes
- Careful monitoring is required for patients receiving intravascular volume repletion:
  - They often require a large volume of fluid but care must be taken to avoid volume overload

### ADDITIONAL READING
- Ariyan EA, Sosa JA. Assessent and management of patients with abnormal calcium. *Crit Care Med.* 2004;32(4 Suppl):S146–S154.
- Carroll ME, Schaide DS. A practical approach to hypercalcemia. *Am Fam Physician.* 2003;67: 1959–1966.
- Inzucci SE. Management of hypercalcemia. *Postgrad Med.* 2004;115:27–36.
- Marx JA, Hockberger RS, Walls RM, eds. *Rosen's Emergency Medicine.* Philadelphia: Elsevier; 2009.

#### See Also (Topic, Algorithm, Electronic Media Element)
- Hyperparathyroidism
- Hypocalcemia
- Hypoparathyroidism

 **CODES**

**ICD9**
275.42 Hypercalcemia

H

# HYPEREMESIS GRAVIDARUM

David Della-Giustina
Bradley N. Younggren

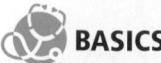

## BASICS

### DESCRIPTION

- Hyperemesis gravidarum is the most severe form along the continuum of nausea and vomiting of pregnancy.
- Also known as pernicious vomiting of pregnancy
- Characterized by unexplained intractable vomiting and dehydration.
- Occurs in 0.3–2% of pregnancies.

### ETIOLOGY

- Exact cause unknown
- Possible causes include the following:
  - Elevated gestational hormone levels of human chorionic gonadotropin (hCG) and/or estradiol
  - Thyrotoxicosis
  - Upper GI motility dysfunction
  - Hepatic abnormalities
  - Autonomic nervous system dysfunction
  - Psychologic factors
  - *Helicobacter pylori* infection
  - Genetic predisposition

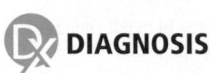

## DIAGNOSIS

### SIGNS AND SYMPTOMS

- Nausea and vomiting during pregnancy affects between 50% and 90%.
- Onset of symptoms by the 4th–10th wk of pregnancy with resolution by the 20th:
  - Symptoms after the 20th wk should raise one's suspicion of another process.
- Hyperemesis gravidarum is a clinical diagnosis defined by the following:
  - Persistent and severe nausea and vomiting
  - Dehydration
  - Weight loss of >5% of total body weight
  - Laboratory findings: Increased urine specific gravity, ketonuria, electrolyte disturbances, ketonemia

### History

- Onset of vomiting
- Gestational history:
  - Similar symptoms in prior pregnancies
- Last menstrual period
- Oral intake
- Urine output
- Bloody or bilious vomiting
- Abdominal pain
- Risk factors include the following:
  - History of motion sickness
  - Younger age
  - Migraine headaches
  - Symptoms earlier in the day
  - Low prepregnancy body mass index
  - More common in nulliparous women
  - 15% recurrence rate if manifested in previous pregnancy

### Physical Exam

- Observe for signs of dehydration
- Abdominal tenderness

### ESSENTIAL WORKUP

- History and physical examination with special attention to state of hydration and abdominal exam for other diagnoses associated with vomiting (appendicitis, cholecystitis, etc.)
- Obtain an uncontaminated urinalysis.
- If patient has unremitting vomiting for >24 hr, obtain a CBC, electrolytes, renal function, liver enzymes, bilirubin, and lipase.
- The PUQE score is a validated scoring system to determine severity of symptoms and the presence of hyperemesis gravidarum.

### DIAGNOSTIC TESTS & INTERPRETATION

#### Lab

- Urinalysis:
  - Increased specific gravity and ketonuria
  - Presence of glucose mandates checking serum glucose to rule out diabetes.
  - Presence of bilirubin mandates a search to rule out hepatobiliary cause for the vomiting.
- CBC:
  - May have an elevated hematocrit owing to dehydration
  - WBC is usually normal.
- Electrolytes:
  - Elevated BUN indicating volume depletion; elevated creatinine if renal failure present
  - Hyponatremia, hypokalemia, hypochloremia, and metabolic alkalosis from loss of HCl in emesis
- Liver function tests:
  - Mild increases in bilirubin may occur, but should be <4 mg/dL.
  - AST and ALT may also be mildly elevated, but not >100 IU/L
- Amylase/lipase:
  - In 1 study, amylase was elevated in 24% of patients with hyperemesis gravidarum; however, the amylase was salivary in origin; use lipase rather than amylase to evaluate for pancreatitis.

### Imaging

- US to rule-out molar pregnancy when routine 1st-trimester US imaging is not performed:
  - Not a mandated study

### DIFFERENTIAL DIAGNOSIS

- Pyelonephritis; most commonly missed
- Gastroenteritis; gastroparesis; intestinal obstruction; Mallory Weiss Tear
- Hepatobiliary disease; hepatitis, cholecystitis, fatty liver of pregnancy, achalasia
- Pancreatitis
- Appendicitis
- Diabetic ketoacidosis
- Hyperthyroidism; hyperparathyroidism
- Uremia; persistent nausea and vomiting are seen with severe renal dysfunction.
- Pseudotumor cerebri

**TREATMENT**

### PRE-HOSPITAL
- IV, monitor if signs of significant volume depletion
- IV hydration

### INITIAL STABILIZATION/THERAPY
IV hydration using a crystalloid with dextrose ($D_5LR$ or $D_5NS$)

### ED TREATMENT/PROCEDURES
- IV hydration using up to 3 L of $D_5LR$ or $D_5NS$
- Dextrose is added to help break cycle of ketosis
- Treat until patient is no longer symptomatic from hypovolemia
- Antiemetics administered IV are given to break the vomiting cycle
- Most commonly used medications:
  - Metoclopramide:
    ○ FDA category B
  - Promethazine and prochlorperazine:
    ○ Both FDA category C
    ○ Recent FDA warning regarding complications of IV promethazine administration
  - Selective 5HT3 receptor antagonist (ondansetron):
    ○ FDA category B with increasing use but recommended as a second-line agent
  - These medications have been used extensively in pregnancy, and there is little or no evidence that these antiemetics are associated with an increased risk of congenital anomalies.
  - Antiemetics are preferable to the risk of prolonged ketosis and hypovolemia
- Oral rehydration in the ED after the initial fluid resuscitation and antiemetics
- Thiamine 100 mg IV/IM/PO in the patient who requires IV rehydration:
  - There are case reports of patients developing Wernicke encephalopathy owing to hyperemesis gravidarum.
- Methylprednisolone may be effective for patients with hyperemesis gravidarum:
  - 2 studies demonstrated relief in symptoms and decreased need for admission for hyperemesis.
  - Antihistamines have been shown to be effective

### MEDICATION
*First Line*
- Metoclopramide (category B): 10–20 mg IV
- Ondansetron (category B): 4–8 mg IV
- Prochlorperazine (category C): 5–10 mg IV not to exceed 40 mg/d
- Promethazine (category C): 12.5–25 mg IM
- Discharge outpatient medications:
  - Meclizine (category B): 25 mg PO q6h PRN nausea
  - Metoclopramide (category B): 10 mg PO q6–8h PRN
  - Ondansetron (category B): 4 mg PO or ODT q8h
  - Prochlorperazine (category C): 5–10 mg PO q6h or 25 mg PR q12h PRN
  - Promethazine (category C): 12.5–25 mg PO or PR q4–6h PRN
  - Pyridoxine (vitamin $B_6$; category A): 25 mg PO t.i.d. (OTC)
  - Ginger (zingiber officinale): 500–1,500 mg divided b.i.d./t.i.d.
  - Doxylamine (Unisom—OTC) 12.5 mg PO q6–8h
  - Vitamin $B_6$ 25 mg PO t.i.d.–q.i.d.
  - Thiamine: 50 mg PO per day for symptoms >3 wk

*Second Line*
Methylprednisolone (category C): 16 mg IV or PO q8h × 3 days and then taper. Should be prescribed in consultation with obstetrician.

 **FOLLOW-UP**

### DISPOSITION
*Admission Criteria*
- Inability to tolerate oral intake after treatment
- Inability to control the emesis despite treatment
- Severe electrolyte or metabolic disturbances
- At highest risk <8 wk gestation

*Discharge Criteria*
- Most patients can be discharged as long as they are able to tolerate oral intake and have adequate follow-up.
- Correction of dehydration and associated symptoms
- Decreased ketonuria
- Patients should be reassured that their symptoms are common and almost always self-limited.
- Patients should be counseled that frequent, small meals may be helpful:
  - Meals should contain simple carbohydrates and be low in fats.
  - Avoid irritant or spicy foods.
- Home IV therapy can be arranged if indicated.

### FOLLOW-UP RECOMMENDATIONS
- All patients with diagnosis should take at least 3 mg thiamine/day to help prevent Wernicke's; a supplement of 50 mg/d PO is recommended
- Risk for 1st-trimester fetal loss is less in women with hyperemesis

## PEARLS AND PITFALLS
- Other diagnoses should be explored in patients presenting after 9 wk gestation with 1st symptoms
- The use of PICC lines has been shown to carry a significantly increased risk or maternal morbidity when compared to patients managed with either NG tube or medications alone.
- Be aware of the risk for central pontine myelinosis in hyponatremia patients when replacing sodium
- Wernicke's encephalopathy is the most devastating maternal complication:
  - Patients may not have the classic triad of ataxia, nystagmus, and dementia. Be concerned for any evidence of apathy or confusion.
  - Be sure to give patients thiamine 100 mg IV for any patient who presents with apathy or confusion

## ADDITIONAL READING
- Bottomley C, Bourne T. Management strategies in hyperemesis. *Best Prac Res Clin Obstet Gynaecol.* 2009;23:549–564.
- Einarson A, Maltepe C, et al. The safety of ondansetron for nausea and vomiting of pregnancy: A prospective comparative study. *Br J Obstet Gynaecol.* 2004;111(9):940–943.
- Goodwin T. Hyperemesis gravidarum. *Clin Obstet Gynecol.* 2008;35(3):401–417.
- Koren G, Boskovic R, Maltepe C, et al. Motherrisk-PUQE scoring system for nausea and vomiting of pregnancy. *Am J Obstet Gynecol.* 2002;186:S228–231.

**CODES**

### ICD9
- 643.00 Mild hyperemesis gravidarum, unspecified as to episode of care
- 643.10 Hyperemesis gravidarum with metabolic disturbance, unspecified as to episode of care
- 643.20 Late vomiting of pregnancy, unspecified as to episode of care

H

# HYPERKALEMIA

*Christopher B. Colwell*

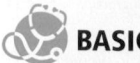 **BASICS**

## DESCRIPTION
- Potassium distribution:
  - Extracellular space: 2%
  - Intracellular space: 98%
- Potassium excretion:
  - Renal: 90%
  - GI: 10%
- Renal and extrarenal mechanisms maintain normal plasma concentration between 3.5 and 5.0 mmol/L.
- Renal excretion of potassium affected by:
  - Dietary intake
  - Distal renal tubular function
  - Acid–base balance
  - Mineralocorticoids
- Regulation between intracellular and extracellular potassium balance affected by:
  - Acid–base balance
  - Insulin
  - Mineralocorticoids
  - Catecholamines
  - Osmolarity
  - Drugs

## ETIOLOGY
- Decreased potassium excretion:
  - Most common cause: Renal failure (acute or chronic)
  - Distal tubular diseases:
    - Acute interstitial nephritis
    - Renal transplant rejection
    - Sickle cell nephropathy
    - Renal tubular acidosis (diabetes)
  - Mineralocorticoid deficiency:
    - Addison disease
    - Hypoaldosteronism
  - Drugs:
    - ACE inhibitors/angiotensin receptor blockers
    - $\beta$-blockers
    - Potassium-sparing diuretics
    - NSAIDs
    - Cyclosporine
    - High-dose trimethoprim
    - Lithium toxicity
- Intracellular to extracellular potassium shifts:
  - Metabolic acidosis:
    - Serum $K^+$ rises 0.2–1.7 mmol/L for each 0.1 unit fall in arterial pH.
  - Hyperosmolar states
  - Insulin deficiency
  - Cell necrosis
  - Rhabdomyolysis
  - Hemolysis
  - Chemotherapy
  - Drugs:
    - Digitalis toxicity
    - Depolarizing muscle relaxants (eg, succinylcholine)
    - $\beta$-Blockers
    - $\alpha$-Agonists
  - Hyperkalemic periodic paralysis
- Excess exogenous potassium load:
  - Cellular breakdown:
    - Trauma
    - Tumor lysis
  - Salt substitutes
  - Oral potassium
  - Potassium penicillin G
  - Rapid transfusions of banked blood
- Pseudohyperkalemia:
  - Traumatic venipuncture with hemolysis
  - Postvenipuncture release of potassium can occur in setting of:
    - Thrombocytosis (platelets >800,000/mm$^3$)
    - Extreme leukocytosis (WBC >100,000/mm$^3$)
  - Prolonged tourniquet time

 **DIAGNOSIS**

## SIGNS AND SYMPTOMS
### History
- Hyperkalemia is often asymptomatic, even at high levels.
- Neuromuscular symptoms, predominantly weakness, which can progress to paralysis.
- Dyspnea owing to respiratory muscle weakness.
- Cardiac dysrhythmias may be the initial manifestation, so patients could also present with chest pain, palpitations, or syncope.

### Physical Exam
- Muscular weakness (rare except in severe cases)
- Cardiac dysrhythmias (see ECG Changes)

## ESSENTIAL WORKUP
- Serum potassium >5.0 mmol/L
- Collect in heparinized tube if pseudohyperkalemia suspected.

## DIAGNOSTIC TESTS & INTERPRETATION
### Lab
- Electrolytes, BUN, creatinine, glucose:
  - Elevated BUN, creatinine in renal failure
  - Hyponatremia with mineralocorticoid deficiency
  - Mild metabolic acidosis with type IV renal tubular acidosis
- Arterial blood gases:
  - Assess acid–base status
- Creatinine kinase:
  - Rhabdomyolysis can lead to renal insufficiency and result in hyperkalemia
- $Ca^{2+}$
- For hyperkalemia in face of normal renal function, calculate transtubular potassium gradient (TTKG):
  - TTKG = urine K × Posm/Plasma K × Uosm
  - Posm, plasma osmolality; Uosm, urine osmolality
  - TTKG >8 suggests extrarenal cause; TTKG <6 indicates renal excretory defect.

### Diagnostic Procedures/Surgery
- ECG: Changes correlate with degree of hyperkalemia:
  - >5.0–6.5: peaking of T waves; shortening of $QT_c$ interval
  - >6.5–8.0: PR prolongation; loss of P waves; widening of QRS complexes
  - >8.0: Intraventricular blocks; bundle branch blocks; QRS axis shifts; sine wave complex
- Serum potassium cannot be reliably predicted by ECG:
  - Some patients (particularly those with chronic renal failure) will tolerate higher potassium levels than others.
  - Potassium effects (as seen on ECG) are more important than potassium level

## DIFFERENTIAL DIAGNOSIS
Pseudohyperkalemia

### ALERT
Most common cause of hyperkalemia reported by lab is pseudohyperkalemia owing to hemolysis.

**TREATMENT**

### PRE-HOSPITAL
- Treatment of hyperkalemic-induced dysrhythmias/cardiac arrest involves different drugs from usual advanced cardiac life support (ACLS) measures (see Treatment, below):
  - Inhaled albuterol can lower potassium temporarily by 1 mmol/L.
  - Sodium bicarbonate can be effective.
  - Calcium chloride or gluconate is available in some prehospital systems and should be considered in the unstable patient when hyperkalemia is suspected.
- Diagnosis suggested by prehospital rhythm strip or in at-risk populations (renal failure)

### INITIAL STABILIZATION/THERAPY
- ABCs
- IV access
- Cardiac monitor

### ED TREATMENT/PROCEDURES
- Hyperkalemia with ECG changes (widened QRS complexes): Antagonize potassium-mediated cardiotoxicity:
  - Administer calcium gluconate (in awake patient) or calcium chloride (in patient without pulse):
    - Onset 1–3 min
    - 30–60-min duration
    - No effect on total serum potassium levels
- Severe (>7.0) or Moderate (6.0–7.0) with ECG Changes (Heightened T waves or loss of P wave): Shift potassium intracellularly:
  - Administer combination of insulin and glucose:
    - Onset 20–30 min
    - 2–4-hr duration
  - IV sodium bicarbonate:
    - Much more effective in patient who is acidotic
    - Onset 20 min
    - 2-hr duration
    - Caution in patients at risk for volume overload
    - Worsens concomitant hypocalcemia
  - Inhaled albuterol:
    - Onset within 30 mins
    - 2–4-hr duration
  - Calcium should be administered if the patient is unstable
- Enhanced excretion for $K^+$ >6.0 without ECG changes:
  - Administer cation exchange resin:
    - Calcium or sodium polystyrene sulfonate PO or per rectum (PR)
    - Avoid in patients with suspected ileus or bowel obstruction.
- All patients:
  - Limit exogenous potassium and potassium-sparing drugs.
  - Treat underlying cause.

### Special Situations
- Renal failure:
  - Hemodialysis immediately effective at removing potassium
  - Furosemide:
    - Effective in absence of oliguric renal failure
    - Causes potassium-losing diuresis
- Cardiac arrest:
  - Administer $CaCl_2$ and $NaHCO_3$ with known or suspected hyperkalemia.
- Digoxin toxicity:
  - Avoid calcium:
  - When necessary, administer small doses very slowly.
  - Consider Digibind for $K^+$ >5.5 mmol/L.
- Mineralocorticoid deficiency:
  - Administer hydrocortisone

### MEDICATION
- Albuterol: 10–20 mg (peds: 2.5 mg if <25 kg; 5.0 mg if ≥25 kg) nebulized over 10 min
- Calcium chloride 10%: 10-mL amp (peds: 0.2 mL/kg per dose) IV over 2–5 min
- Calcium gluconate 10%: 20-mL amp (peds: 0.6–1.0 mL/kg) IV over 2–5 min
- Furosemide: 40–80 mg (peds: 1.0 mg/kg) IV—modify dose to achieve appropriate diuresis
- Hydrocortisone: 100 mg (peds: 1–2 mg/kg) IV
- Insulin and glucose: 10 IU (peds: 0.1 IU/kg) regular insulin plus 50 mL 50% (peds: 0.5–1 g/kg) dextrose IV
- Sodium bicarbonate: 1–3 amps (44 mEq per amp) IV over 20–30 min (peds: 1.0–2.0 mEq/kg per dose)
- Sodium polystyrene sulfonate (Kayexalate) or calcium polystyrene sulfonate (preferred with volume overload):
  - Oral: 15 g mixed with water or 50 mL of sorbitol q2h to total of 5 doses
  - Rectal enema: 50 g in 200 mL of sorbitol q4–6h
  - Peds: 1.0 g/kg orally or rectally

### First Line
- Calcium (under appropriate situations)
- Insulin and glucose

### Second Line
- Sodium bicarbonate
- Kayexalate
- Albuterol

 **FOLLOW-UP**

### DISPOSITION
#### Admission Criteria
Admit most cases:
- Process of potassium removal is relatively slow.
- Most potassium is intracellular and, therefore, not measured on serum electrolytes.
- Significant changes in levels will take time.
- Levels may continue to rise.

#### Discharge Criteria
Mild hyperkalemia (<5.5 mmol/L) provided that:
- Response to treatment has been demonstrated
- Known correctable cause
- Further rises in serum potassium not anticipated
- Early follow-up possible

#### Issues for Referral
Follow-up to address the underlying cause is important. In many cases, the underlying cause is renal insufficiency and the potassium will become elevated again if this is not addressed. Often this will mean regular hemodialysis.

#### FOLLOW-UP RECOMMENDATIONS
Many patients with hyperkalemia will be admitted. For those who are not, close follow-up and in many cases access to hemodialysis will be important.

## PEARLS AND PITFALLS
- Potassium effect is more important than absolute potassium level. The ECG is the most important determinate of need to treat acutely.
- Do not wait for confirmation of the potassium level to treat when the ECG indicates a hyperkalemic emergency
- Hyperkalemia is often asymptomatic until late: Obtain an ECG early in patients at risk.
- Sodium bicarbonate administration can easily lead to volume overload if not careful.

## ADDITIONAL READING
- Freeman K, et al. Effects of presentation and electrocardiogram on time to treatment of hyperkalemia. *Acad Emerg Med*. 2008;15(3):239.
- Halperin M, Kamel K. Potassium. *Lancet*. 1998;352:135–140.
- Mattu A, Brady W, Robinson D. Electrocardiographic manifestations of hyperkalemia. *Am J Emerg Med*. 2000;18:721–728.
- Rastegar A, Soleimani M. Hypokalaemia and hyperkalaemia. *Postgrad Med J*. 2001;77:759–764.
- Rodriguez-Soriano J. Potassium homeostasis and its disturbances in children. *Pediatr Nephrol*. 1995;9(3):364–374.
- Weisberg LS. Management of severe hyperkalemia. *Crit Care Med*. 2008;36(12):3246.

### See Also (Topic, Algorithm, Electronic Media Element)
- Dialysis Complications
- Renal Failure

**CODES**

ICD9
276.7 Hyperpotassemia

H

# HYPERNATREMIA

*Linda Mueller*

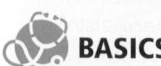 **BASICS**

## DESCRIPTION

Hypernatremia definition: Sodium >145 mEq/L:

- Mild hypernatremia: Serum sodium 146–155 mEq/L
- Severe hypernatremia: Serum sodium >155 mEq/L

## ETIOLOGY

Divided into 3 categories

### Hypovolemic Hypernatremia

- Most common
- Loss or deficiency of water and sodium with water losses being greater than sodium losses
- Examples:
  – Diuretics
  – Glucosuria
  – Mannitol
  – Renal failure
  – High-protein feedings
  – Lactulose
  – Excess sweating
  – Respiratory loss
  – Defective thirst mechanism
  – Lack of access to water
  – Diarrhea/vomiting
  – Burn victims
  – Intubated patients

### Isovolemic Hypernatremia

- Water deficiency without sodium loss; free water loss
- Examples:
  – Fever
  – Hypothalamic diabetes insipidus:
    ○ Head trauma
    ○ Tumor
    ○ Congenital
    ○ Infection (TB, syphilis, mycoses, toxoplasmosis, encephalitis)
    ○ Granulomatous disease (sarcoid, Wegner)
    ○ Cerebrovascular accident
    ○ Aneurysm
  – Nephrogenic diabetes insipidus:
    ○ Congenital
    ○ Drugs (lithium, amphotericin B, foscarnet, demeclocycline)
    ○ Obstructive uropathy
    ○ Chronic tubulointerstitial disease (sickle cell nephropathy, multiple myeloma, amyloidosis, sarcoidosis, systemic lupus erythematosus, polycystic kidney)
    ○ Electrolyte disorders (hypercalcemia, potassium depletion)

### Hypervolemic Hypernatremia

- Gain of water and sodium, with sodium gain greater than water gain.
- Examples:
  – Iatrogenic—most common cause:
    ○ Sodium bicarbonate administration
    ○ NaCl tablets
    ○ Hypertonic parenteral hyperaliment
    ○ Hypertonic IV fluid (IVF)
    ○ Hypertonic dialysis
  – Hypertonic medicine preparations such as ticarcillin and carbenicillin
  – Cushing disease
  – Adrenal hyperplasia
  – Primary aldosteronism
  – Sea water drownings

### Pediatric Considerations

- More prone to iatrogenic causes
- More likely to die or to have permanent neurologic sequela
- Morbidity ranges from 25–50%.
- May present with high-pitched cry, lethargy, irritability, muscle weakness
- Poor breast feeding and inappropriate formula preparations are a potential cause in neonates
- If hypernatremia is due to DKA, follow pediatric DKA protocols for fluid resuscitation
- DDAVP dose for 3 mo—12 yr is 5–30 mcg/day intranasally

### Geriatric Considerations

- Most commonly affected group due to impaired renal concentrating ability and reduced thirst mechanism
- Consider neglect if underlying etiology is dehydration alone

### Pregnancy Considerations

- May encounter transient DI of pregnancy
- Vasopressin and desmopressin are category B drugs in pregnancy
- Hydration status much more difficult to evaluate accurately by exam

 **DIAGNOSIS**

## SIGNS AND SYMPTOMS

- Most symptoms attributed to underlying cause (eg, dehydration)
- More marked with acute changes
- Death likely to occur with sodium of ≥185 mEq/L
- May see the following symptoms, usually at levels ≥160 mEq/L:
  – Neurologic:
    ○ Headache
    ○ Tremulousness
    ○ Irritability
    ○ Ataxia
    ○ Mental confusion
    ○ Delirium
    ○ Seizures
    ○ Coma
    ○ Hyperreflexia
    ○ Asterixis
    ○ Chorea
    ○ Subarachnoid, intracerebral, and subdural hemorrhages
    ○ Dural sinus thrombosis
  – Musculoskeletal:
    ○ Spasticity
    ○ Muscle weakness
    ○ Muscle twitching
  – Other:
    ○ Anorexia
    ○ Tachypnea
    ○ Poor skin turgor
    ○ Nausea/vomiting

### Hypovolemic Hypernatremia

- Tachycardia
- Orthostasis
- Dry mucous membranes
- Oliguria
- Azotemia

### Hypervolemic Hypernatremia

- Pulmonary edema
- Peripheral edema

### Physical Exam
- Evaluate for hydration status
- Look at mucous membranes, neck veins, and skin turgor
- Perform a complete neurologic exam and repeat throughout ED stay
- Obtain orthostatic vital signs

### ESSENTIAL WORKUP
Serum $Na^+$ level

### DIAGNOSTIC TESTS & INTERPRETATION
*Lab*
- Electrolytes, BUN/creatinine, glucose
- CBC
- Urinalysis:
  - Specific gravity
  - Urine/serum osmolality
  - Urine $Na^+$

*Imaging*
- CXR:
  - For infection/aspiration
  - Pulmonary edema with hypervolemic hypernatremia
- CT brain:
  - For altered mental status
  - Venous sinus thrombosis
  - Subarachnoid hemorrhages
  - Subdural hematoma

### Diagnostic Procedures/Surgery
Consider Foley catheter to accurately monitor input and output

### DIFFERENTIAL DIAGNOSIS
- Diabetic ketoacidosis
- Hyperosmolar coma
- Primary CNS lesions

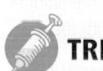

## TREATMENT

### PRE-HOSPITAL
Volume resuscitation if hypovolemic or evidence of hemodynamic compromise

### INITIAL STABILIZATION/THERAPY
- ABCs
- 0.9% NS IV bolus for severe hypotension
- Naloxone, thiamine, $D_{50}W$ (or Accu-Chek) for altered mental status

### ED TREATMENT/PROCEDURES
General:
- Calculate water deficit:
  - Water deficit = 0.6 (weight in kg) × (1- desired sodium/actual sodium)
- Do not rapidly correct hypertonicity to normal serum osmolality:
  - Rapid correction may cause seizures.
  - Reduce serum sodium level by <0.5–0.7 mEq/L/h.

### Hypovolemic Hypernatremia
- Replace volume contraction with 0.9% NS IV bolus.
- Change to $D_5W$ or hypotonic saline once volume replenished and hemodynamically stable.

### Isovolemic Hypernatremia
- Calculate water deficit.
- Correct water deficit with $D_5W$ or hypotonic saline:
  - Replace half of deficit in 1st 24 hr, then remainder over 1–2 days.

### Hypervolemic Hypernatremia
- Remove excess water with diuretics or dialysis.
- When euvolemic, replace water deficit with $D_5W$.
- Avoid hypotonic saline solutions because patient already has excess of total body sodium.

### Diabetes Insipidus (DI) Hypernatremia
- Sodium restriction
- Desmopressin:
  - Aqueous vasopressin (DDAVP)
  - Best therapeutic agent
- Chlorpropamide (Diabinese) enhances effect of vasopressin at renal tubule.
- Carbamazepine causes release of vasopressin.
- Hydrochlorothiazide enhances sodium excretion.
- Discontinue DI inducing drugs.

### MEDICATION
- Chlorpropamide (Diabinese): 100–500 mg/d
- Vasopressin (DDAVP): 1–2 μg IV/SC q12h or 5–20 μg intranasally

### First Line
Volume correction starting initially with NS

### Second Line
Correct the underlying cause.

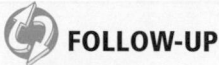

## FOLLOW-UP

### DISPOSITION
*Admission Criteria*
- Newly diagnosed sodium >150 mEq/L for monitoring and treatment
- Admit sodium >160 mEq/L or symptomatic patients to ICU.

*Discharge Criteria*
- Sodium <150 mEq/L in asymptomatic patient
- Sodium >150 mEq/L in patients with history of chronically elevated sodium who are at their baseline and asymptomatic

### FOLLOW-UP RECOMMENDATIONS
Repeat serum sodium levels with in a week.

## PEARLS AND PITFALLS

- Up to 30% of acute hypernatremia patients will have permanent neurologic sequelae, a complete and well-documented neurologic exam is a must.
- Patients at extreme ages and with chronic conditions are most susceptible to neurologic complications:
  - On going fluid losses may require recalculation of fluid needs
  - Repeat lab work to confirm controlled correction of sodium

## ADDITIONAL READING

- Adrogue HS, Madias NE. Hypernatremia. *N Engl J Med.* 2000;342:1493–1499.
- Ellison D, Disorders of sodium and water. *Am J Kidney Dis.* 2004;46(2):356–361.
- Fall P. Hyponatremia and hypernatremia. A systematic approach to causes and their correction. *Postgrad Med.* 2000;107(5):75–82.
- Fried LF, Palevsky PM. Hyponatremia and hypernatremia. *Med Clin North Am.* 1997;81(3): 585–609.
- Lin M, Lu S, Lim I. Disorders of water imbalance. *Emerg Med Clin North Am.* 2005;23:749–770, ix.
- Ranadive S, Rosenthal S. Pediatric disorders of water balance. *Endocrinol Metabol Clin.* 2009;38(4).

### See Also (Topic, Algorithm, Electronic Media Element)
- Diabetic Ketoacidosis
- Hyperosmolar Coma
- Hyponatremia

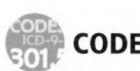

## CODES

**ICD9**
276.0 Hyperosmolality and/or hypernatremia

**H**

# HYPEROSMOLAR SYNDROME
*Matthew Robinson*

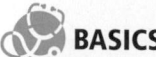 **BASICS**

## DESCRIPTION
- Results from a relative insulin deficiency in the undiagnosed or untreated diabetic
- Sustained hyperglycemia creates an osmotic diuresis and dehydration:
  - Extracellular space maintained by the osmotic gradient at the expense of the intracellular space
  - Eventually profound intracellular dehydration occurs.
- Total body deficits of $H_2O$, $Na^+$, $Cl^-$, $K^-$, $PO_4^-$, $Ca^{2+}$ and $Mg^{2+}$
- In contrast to diabetic ketoacidosis (DKA), significant ketoacidosis does not occur:
  - Circulating insulin levels are higher.
  - The elevation of insulin counterregulatory hormones is less marked.
  - The hyperosmolar state itself inhibits lipolysis (the release of free fatty acids) and subsequent generation of ketoacids

### Geriatric Considerations
- Most commonly seen in elderly type II diabetics who experience a stressful illness that precipitates worsening hyperglycemia and reduced renal function
- In the elderly, 30–40% of cases are associated with the initial presentation of diabetes.

### Pediatric Considerations
- Hyperosmolar hyperglycemic states (HHS) rare in pediatric patients

## ETIOLOGY
- Hyperosmolar state precipitated by factors that:
  - Impair peripheral insulin action
  - Increase endogenous or exogenous glucose
  - Decrease patient's ability to replace fluid loss
- Infection is most common precipitating factor in 32–60% of cases.
- Other precipitating causes include:
  - Inadequate diabetes therapy
  - Medication omission
  - Diet indiscretion
  - Infections
  - Pneumonia
  - UTI
  - Sepsis
  - Medications/drugs
  - Diuretics
  - $\beta$-blockers
  - Calcium channel blockers
  - Phenytoin
  - Cimetidine
  - Amphetamines
  - Ethanol
  - Myocardial infarction
  - Stroke
  - Renal failure
  - Heat stroke
  - Pancreatitis
  - Intestinal obstruction
  - Endocrine disorders
  - Burns
  - Heat stroke

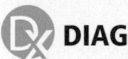 **DIAGNOSIS**

## SIGNS AND SYMPTOMS
### History
- Progression of signs and symptoms typically occur over days to weeks.
- Polyuria/polydipsia/weight loss
- Dizziness/weakness/fatigue
- Blurred vision
- Leg cramps

### Physical Exam
- Dehydration
- Tachycardia
- Sunken eyes
- Hypotension
- Orthostasis
- Dry mucous membranes
- Decreased skin turgor
- Collapsed neck veins
- Coma/lethargy/drowsiness
- Urinary output maintained until late
- Seizures/focal neurologic deficits
- Concurrent precipitating medical illness

## ESSENTIAL WORKUP
Diagnostic criteria:
- Serum glucose $\geq$600 mg/dL (usually >1,000 mg/dL)
- Minimal ketosis
- pH $\geq$7.30, $HCO_3$ $\geq$15 mEq/L
- Effective serum osmolality >320 mOsm/kg:
  - $= 2 \times Na^+ + glucose/18$
  - BUN not included because it is freely permeable between fluid compartments

## DIAGNOSTIC TESTS & INTERPRETATION
### Lab
- Broad testing indicated to evaluate hyperosmolar syndrome and for precipitating causes
- Electrolytes:
  - $K^+$ may be elevated even in presence of total body deficit owing to shift from intracellular space to extracellular space.
  - Mild anion gap metabolic acidosis owing to lactic acid, $\beta$-hydroxybutyric acid, or renal insufficiency
  - Increased sodium—Correct for hyperglycemia: Corrected $[Na^+] = [Na^+] + 1.6 \times [(glucose$ in mg/dL$) - 100]/100$

- BUN, creatinine:
  - Azotemia with elevated BUN/creatinine ratio owing to prerenal and intrarenal causes
- Venous blood gas (VBG) or arterial blood gas (ABG) to rapidly determine pH:
  - ABG necessary to evaluate mixed acid–base disorders
- Serum ketones, $\beta$-hydroxybutyrate, and lactate level if pH < 7.3 or significantly elevated anion gap to evaluate mixed acid–base disorder
- Serum osmolarity
- CBC:
  - Leukocytosis due to infection, stress, or hemoconcentration
  - Increased hemoglobin and hematocrit due to hemoconcentration
- Lipase and amylase:
  - Pancreatitis common
  - Elevated amylase and lipase with no evidence of pancreatitis common
  - May be due to increased salivary secretion, hemoconcentration, or decreased renal clearance
- Urinalysis:
  - Check for ketones/glucose.
  - Assess for UTI.
- Magnesium, calcium, phosphate
- Blood cultures in sepsis
- Creatine kinase for rhabdomyolysis:
  - Incidence as high as 17%
- Urine pregnancy test in females of childbearing years
- Cardiac enzymes and troponin for myocardial infarction

### Imaging
- CXR to evaluate for possible underlying pneumonia
- Head CT: When indicated for AMS or with focal neurologic deficit

### Diagnostic Procedures/Surgery
ECG:
- Evaluate for electrolyte abnormalities causing conduction impairment
- Evaluate for signs of ischemia as triggering event

## DIFFERENTIAL DIAGNOSIS
Differentiate from DKA:
- If acidosis or significant anion gap present, must determine cause (ie, ketosis, DKA, lactic acidosis, [hypoperfusion, sepsis, or postictal], or other cause of metabolic acidosis)
- Mixed disorder of HHS and DKA present in up to 33% of patients

# TREATMENT

## PRE-HOSPITAL
IV Fluid resuscitation and initial stabilization

## INITIAL STABILIZATION/THERAPY
ABCs:
- Secure airway in comatose patients.
- Cardiac monitor and 18-gauge IV
- Naloxone, thiamine, and blood glucose for coma of unknown cause
- Restore hemodynamic stability with IV fluids.
- 0.9% NS 1–2 L over the 1st hr
- Larger volumes of fluid may be needed to normalize the vital signs and establish urine output.

## ED TREATMENT/PROCEDURES
- General strategy:
  – Frequent reassessment of volume and mental status
  – Electrolyte assessment difficult:
    ○ Serum levels of $Na^+$, $K^+$, $PO_4^-$ do not accurately reflect the total body solute deficits or the intracellular environment.
    ○ Repeat electrolyte and glucose levels hourly.
  – Search for a precipitating illness.
- Fluids:
  – Begin resuscitation with 0.9% NS 1–2 L over 1–2 hr to restore intravascular volume and achieve hemodynamic stability.
  – Use 0.45% saline after initial resuscitation
  – Calculate total body water (TBW) deficit using corrected serum sodium:
    ○ TBW deficit $= 0.6 \times$ weight (Kg) $\times$ $(1 - 140/$corrected $Na^+)$
    Average fluid deficit is 9 L.
  – Replace 50% of the fluid deficit over the next 12 hr.
  – Add $D_5$ to IV fluids when serum glucose <300 mg/dL.
- Potassium:
  – Anticipate hypokalemia:
    ○ Total body deficit of ~5–10 mEq/kg body weight (replace over 3 days)
  – Begin potassium repletion after urine output is established. Do not start in anuric patients or if initial $K^+$ level is >5.0 mEq/L.
    ○ If the initial $K^+$ is normal (4.0–5.0 mEq/L), give 20–30 mEq KCl in the 1st L of fluids, then give 20 mEq/h.
    ○ If the initial $K^+$ is low (3.0–4.0 mEq/L), give 40 mEq in 1st L
    ○ If serum K+ is <3.0mEq/L hold insulin and give 10–20 mEq/h until K+ >3.3, then add 40 mEq to each lister
    ○ Follow repeat serum $K^+$ levels q1–2h and adjust treatment accordingly.

- Insulin:
  – No role in the early resuscitation
  – Earlier use of insulin may cause rapid correction of hyperglycemia with collapse of the intravascular space, hypotension, and shock or hypokalemia and dysrhythmias.
  – Some patients will not require insulin.
  – Use insulin as sole therapy in patients with fluid overload (ie, acute renal failure [ARF]).
  – Begin only after achieving hemodynamic stability and evaluating for hypokalemia:
    ○ Do not use unless serum $K^+$ > 3.3 mEq/L
  – SC or IM insulin not recommended due to erratic absorption
  – Titrate drip to decrease serum glucose by 50–100 mg/dL/h.
  – Decrease drip rate by 1/2 when serum glucose <250 mg/dL.
- Phosphate:
  – Routine replacement not recommended
  – If serum levels <1 mg/dL, give 20–30 mmol potassium phosphate over 24 hr
  – Monitor serum calcium levels closely
- Magnesium:
  – 0.35 mEq/kg magnesium in fluids for 1st 3–4 hr (2.5–3.0 g $MgSO_4$ in 70-kg patient)
  – Caution in ARF
- Anticoagulation:
  – Arterial thrombosis may complicate hyperosmolar state:
    ○ Consider SC heparin as prophylaxis.
  – Remain vigilant to detect thrombotic complications (eg, MI, pulmonary embolus, mesenteric ischemia).

## MEDICATION
- Insulin: Begin with 0.05–0.1 U/kg/h, modify after assessing clinical response.
- $MgSO_4$ (magnesium sulfate): 50% (5 g/10 ml; dilute to at least 20% before IV use)
- Naloxone: 2 mg (peds: 0.1 mg/kg) IV push (IVP)
- Potassium phosphate IV: Phosphates 3 mmol/mL and potassium 4.4 mEq/mL
- Potassium phosphate PO: Phosphorus 250 mg per tablet and potassium 1.1 mEq per tablet
- Thiamine: 100 mg (peds: 10–25 mg) IVP

# FOLLOW-UP

## DISPOSITION
### Admission Criteria
- All but the mildest cases should be admitted to ICU:
  – Frequent serial labs for the 1st 24 hr
  – Rapid shifts in fluids and electrolytes and the potential for deterioration in mental status and arrhythmias mandate close monitoring.
- Mild cases may be managed in an observation unit over 12–24 hr.

### Discharge Criteria
- Patients meeting the diagnostic criteria for hyperosmolar syndrome should not be discharged.
- Mild hyperglycemia patients with mild volume deficits and normal serum osmolarity can be discharged after hydration and correction of hyperglycemia.

### Issues for Referral
Patient should follow-up with endocrinology and with their primary physician within 1 wk postdischarge for long-term blood glucose monitoring and insulin therapy.

## PEARLS AND PITFALLS
- Failure to look for precipitating event or cause
- Too rapid correction of glucose—may lead to hypotension
- Continuing isotonic fluids after volume resuscitation—may lead to hypernatremia
- Continuing hypotonic fluids without frequent electrolytes—may lead to cellular edema, cerebral edema
- Failure to prevent hypokalemia: Respiratory depression, dysrhythmias
- Avoid Dilantin in the event of seizure activity:
  – Inhibits the endogenous release of insulin

## ADDITIONAL READING
- Chiasson JL, et al. Diagnosis and treatment of diabetic ketoacidosis and the hyperglycemic hyperosmolar state. *Can Med Assoc J.* 2003;168:859.
- Gaglia JL, et al. Acute hyperglycemic crisis in the elderly. *Med Clin N Am.* 2004;88:1063.
- Kitabchi AE, Nyenwe EA. Hyperglycemic crisis in diabetes mellitus: Diabetic ketoacidosis and hyperglycemic hyperosmolar state. *Endocrinol Metab Clin N Am.* 2006;35(4)725–751.

### See Also (Topic, Algorithm, Electronic Media Element)
- Diabetic Ketoacidosis

# CODES

## ICD9
- 250.20 Diabetes mellitus with hyperosmolarity, type ii or unspecified type, not stated as uncontrolled
- 250.21 Diabetes mellitus with hyperosmolarity, type I (juvenile type) not stated as uncontrolled
- 276.0 Hyperosmolality and/or hypernatremia

H

# HYPERPARATHYROIDISM

*Hugh A. Schuckman*
*Stephen L. Chesser*

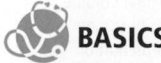
## BASICS

### DESCRIPTION
- Parathyroid hormone (PTH) excess with symptoms owing to PTH actions:
  - Decreases urinary $Ca^{2+}$ loss
  - Increases urinary $PO_4^{-2}$ loss
  - Stimulates vitamin D conversion from 25(OH)-D to 1,25(OH)-D in kidney
  - Liberates $Ca^{2+}$ and $PO_4^{-2}$ from bone
- Hypercalciuria produces increased magnesium losses in urine.
- Magnesium (negative feedback to prevent hypercalcemia):
  - Cofactor in production of PTH
  - Essential for action of PTH in target tissues
- Genetics:
  - Associated with multiple endocrine neoplasia type I:
    - Hyperparathyroidism
    - Pancreatic islet disease (secrete any combination of gastrin, insulin, pancreatic polypeptide, vasoactive polypeptide, or glucagons)
    - Pituitary disease: Hypersecretion of ACTH, prolactin, or growth hormone; foregut carcinoid tumor that may secrete corticotrophin-releasing hormone
- Associated with multiple endocrine neoplasia type 2a:
  - Hyperparathyroidism
  - Medullary carcinoma of the thyroid
  - Pheochromocytoma

### ETIOLOGY
- Excess secretion of PTH owing to:
  - Primary hyperparathyroidism (adenoma 85%, hyperplasia 14%, carcinoma <1%)
  - Secondary hyperparathyroidism (response to vitamin D deficiency or chronic renal failure with hyperphosphatemia):
    - Calcium is low or normal, but PTH levels are elevated.

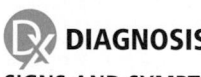
## DIAGNOSIS

### SIGNS AND SYMPTOMS
Stones, bones, abdominal groans, and psychic moans

#### ALERT
- Hypercalcemic crisis:
  - Anorexia, nausea, vomiting
  - Mental obtundation

### History
- Depend on the severity and rapidity of hypercalcemia
- Usually either an incidental finding or a secondary manifestation such as renal calculi, peptic ulcer disease, pancreatitis, pseudo gout, gout, and so on.

### Pediatric Considerations
- Neonate:
  - Hypotonia, weakness, and listlessness
  - Following delivery to hypoparathyroid mothers
- Hypercalcemic infants:
  - Broad forehead
  - Epicanthal folds
  - Underdeveloped nasal bridge
  - Prominent upper lip
  - Mental retardation
- Midteens—nonspecific symptoms of hypercalcemia

### Physical Exam
- Dehydration
- Cardiac:
  - Hypertension (even in the face of dehydration)
  - Cardiac conduction abnormalities (*not* proportional to degree of hypercalcemia)
  - Bradydysrhythmia
  - Bundle branch blocks
  - Complete heart block
  - Asystole
  - Short QT interval (shortening of ST segment)
  - Potentiation of digitalis effects (Hypercalcemia plus digoxin equals digitalis toxicity)
- Neurologic:
  - Headaches
  - Decreased reflexes
  - Proximal muscle weakness
  - Dementia
  - Lethargy
  - Coma
- Psychiatric:
  - Personality changes
  - Depression
  - Inability to concentrate
  - Anxiety
  - Psychosis
- GI:
  - Anorexia, nausea, vomiting
  - Constipation
  - Peptic ulcer disease
  - Pancreatitis
- General:
  - Fatigue
  - Weight loss
  - Polyuria and polydipsia
- Musculoskeletal:
  - Gout/pseudogout
  - Bone pain, bone cysts (osteitis cystica)
  - Arthralgias
  - Chondrocalcinosis
- Renal:
  - Kidney stones
  - Nephrocalcinosis
  - Decreased renal concentrating ability

### ESSENTIAL WORKUP
- Calcium level
- Albumin:
  - Elevated albumin—falsely elevated calcium level
  - Low albumin—falsely lowered calcium level
- Evaluate for symptoms of hypercalcemia, especially impending parathyroid storm (hypercalcemic crisis—anorexia, nausea, vomiting, obtundation progressing to coma).
- Review history for medication ingestion (see Differential Diagnosis below).
- No further ED workup if:
  - Asymptomatic
  - Normal ECG
  - Calcium level <14 mg/dL when corrected for albumin
- If symptomatic with $Ca^{2+}$ <14 mg/dL or any patient with $Ca^{2+} \geq 14$ mg/dL, check:
  - Ionized calcium
  - Chest radiograph (for CHF/malignancy)
  - Phosphorus
  - Electrolytes, BUN, creatinine
  - Sed rate
  - Alkaline phosphatase
  - Magnesium
  - Thyroid-stimulating hormone (TSH)
  - CBC

### DIAGNOSTIC TESTS & INTERPRETATION
#### Lab
- Calcium correction for albumin:
  - Corrected $Ca^{2+}$ (mg/dL) = measured $Ca^{2+}$ (mg/dL) + 0.8 [4.0 − albumin (g/dL)]
  - Acidosis:
    - Shifts binding to albumin—increases ionized (metabolically active) $Ca^{2+}$
    - Decrease of 0.1 pH unit increases the ionized $Ca^{2+}$ by 3–8%
- Phosphorus:
  - Low in primary hyperparathyroidism
  - Usually high in secondary hyperparathyroidism
  - Normal or high in malignancy-related hypercalcemia
- Chloride/$PO_4^{-2}$ ratio:
  - >33—hyperparathyroidism
  - <30—malignancy
- Alkaline phosphatase:
  - Increased in 50% of patients with hyperparathyroidism
  - Normal with vitamin D excess
- Erythrocyte sedimentation rate (ESR):
  - Normal in hyperparathyroidism
  - Elevated in malignancy or granulomatous diseases
- Anemia:
  - Present with malignancy or granulomatous disease
  - Absent in hyperparathyroidism

- Magnesium:
  – Low or low normal
- Parathyroid hormone (PTH):
  – Elevated in primary and secondary hyperparathyroidism
- PTH-related peptide:
  – Secreted by squamous cell carcinomas of lung, head, neck; renal carcinomas, bladder carcinomas, adenocarcinomas, and lymphomas

### Imaging
- Chest radiograph:
  – To assess CHF risk during IV hydration
  – Granulomatous disease or malignancy if cause of hypercalcemia is uncertain

### Diagnostic Procedures/Surgery
Definitive treatment is parathyroidectomy to treat and establish cause of hyperparathyroidism

## DIFFERENTIAL DIAGNOSIS
- PTH related:
  – Primary or secondary hyperparathyroidism
  – Familial hypocalciuric hypercalcemia
- Malignancy related:
  – PTH-related peptide or $Ca^{2+}$ release from osteolytic tumor
- Vitamin D-related excess vitamin D intake or vitamin D production by granulomas
- Immobilization—associated with Paget disease
- Drug induced:
  – Thiazide diuretics
    Lithium
  – Aluminum-containing antacids
  – Tamoxifen
  – Estrogens
  – Androgens
  – Vitamin A

 **TREATMENT**

### PRE-HOSPITAL
May present as a primarily psychiatric disorder

### INITIAL STABILIZATION/THERAPY
- Cardiac monitor if:
  – Symptomatic hypercalcemia
  – $Ca^{2+}$ level >14 mg/dL
- Hydrate with IV 0.9% NS.
- Correct acidosis.

### ED TREATMENT/PROCEDURES
- Treat hypercalcemia:
  – Vigorous hydration with 0.9% NS at minimum of 250 mL/h unless CHF:
    ○ Lowers calcium 1.5–2.0 mg/dL in 24 hr
    ○ Achieve urine output 100 mL/h
  – Administer furosemide or other loop diuretic (calciuric) after adequate volume replacement or in presence of CHF:
    ○ Common error: Administration of furosemide before adequate hydration
    ○ If urinary sodium losses exceed replacement sodium, then renal conservation measures retard calcium excretion.

– Avoid thiazide diuretics (retard calcium excretion).
– Consider glucocorticoid administration (decreases gut absorption and increases renal excretion of $Ca^{2+}$); most effective with vitamin D intoxication or granulomatous diseases.
– Start bisphosphonates (pamidronate or etidronate) in conjunction with primary physician (inhibits calcium mobilization from bone).
- Treat cardiac dysrhythmias in standard fashion:
  – Correct acidosis.
- Determine the cause of the hypercalcemia.
- Stop all medications that may contribute to hypercalcemia.
- Exercise extreme caution in use of digoxin.
- Anticipate CHF and electrolyte imbalance with frequent reassessment of patient and monitoring of serum electrolytes and magnesium levels.
- Calcitonin if unable to use hydration
- Emergent dialysis with renal failure

### MEDICATION
### First Line
- NS hydration: Initial 250–300 mL/hr depending on patient's propensity to CHF
- Calcitonin salmon 4 units/kg SC if saline hydration contraindicated (Intradermal test dose 0.1 mL of 10 unit/mL solution recommended)
- Furosemide: 40 mg IV q2–4h after assurance of adequate hydration
- Prednisone: 40–60 mg PO OR Hydrocortisone: 100 mg (peds: 1–2 mg/kg) IV

### Second Line
- IN CONSULTATION WITH ENDOCRINOLOGIST
- Calcitonin salmon: 4 units/kg SC q12h
- Pamidronate:
  – If albumin-corrected $Ca^{2+}$ level 12–13.5 mg/dL: 60 mg IV infused over 2 hr
  – If albumin-corrected $Ca^{2+}$ level > 13.5 mg/dL: 90 mg IV over 4 hr
  – Dosage should be reduced in renal impairment and infusion time may be extended to reduce nephrotoxic potential but no formal recommendations exist (pregnancy category C—used, but safety not established in peds).
- Zoledronic acid: 4 mg IV over 15–30 min (first-line agent due to efficacy and convenience, but less preferred due to lack of less expensive available generic)
- Cinalcet (Sensipar): 30 mg PO daily or b.i.d. (calcimimetic for secondary hyperparathyroidism or parathyroid carcinoma)

 **FOLLOW-UP**

### DISPOSITION
### Admission Criteria
- Corrected calcium >14 mg/dL
- Symptomatic hypercalcemia
- Evidence of abnormal cardiac rhythm or conduction

### Discharge Criteria
- Not meeting admission criteria
- Able to maintain adequate hydration

### Issues for Referral
If diagnosis is suspected, referral to check PTH levels and response to therapy

### FOLLOW-UP RECOMMENDATIONS
- If hyperparathyroidism is suspected arrange follow-up and send a PTH level.
- Patient needs to be instructed to maintain hydration and stop medications associated with hypercalcemia (see list in differential diagnosis)

## PEARLS AND PITFALLS
- The hypercalcemia of hyperparathyroidism is rarely symptomatic and $Ca^{2+}$ level rarely >14. (Higher levels are most frequently attributable to neoplastic disease)
- The importance of diagnosis is to prevent long-term complications.
- Be careful to correct the calcium level for the albumin level
- Administration of loop diuretics prior to adequate saline hydration will worsen hypercalcemia; some experts suggest that loop diuretics may be no longer warranted for this indication.

## ADDITIONAL READING
- Andreoli T, Carpenter C. *Cecil Essentials of Medicine*, 7th ed. Philadelphia: Saunders-Elsevier; 2007.
- Goldman L, Bennett JC, eds. *Cecil's Textbook of Medicine*, 23rd ed. Philadelphia: Saunders-Elsevier; 2008.
- Guyton A, Hall J. *Textbook of Medical Physiology*, 11th ed. Philadelphia: Saunders-Elsevier; 2006.
- Wallach J, ed. *Interpretation of Diagnostic Tests*, 8th ed. Boston: Little, Brown and Company; 2007.

### See Also (Topic, Algorithm, Electronic Media Element)
- Hypoparathyroidism

 **CODES**

### ICD9
- 252.00 Hyperparathyroidism, unspecified
- 252.01 Primary hyperparathyroidism
- 252.02 Secondary hyperparathyroidism, non-renal

**H**

# HYPERTENSIVE EMERGENCIES

David F. M. Brown
Katja Goldflam

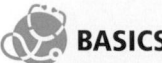

## BASICS

### DESCRIPTION
- 2/3 of hypertensive patients are poorly controlled
- Hypertensive urgency:
  - Severely elevated BP without end-organ damage
- Hypertensive emergency:
  - Uncontrolled HTN associated with acute end-organ damage
  - Generally > 180 mm Hg/120 mm Hg
  - Organs affected:
    - Heart (MI, aortic dissection, CHF)
    - Kidneys (acute renal failure)
    - Brain (encephalopathy, CVA, SAH)
    - Placenta (eclampsia)
- Loss of autoregulation of blood flow in hypertensive emergency:
  - Arterioles vasoconstrict to counter pressure.
  - High pressures overwhelm arterioles and endothelial damage occurs.
  - Lower BP slowly; hypotension below auto-regulatory zone may lead to ischemia.
- End-organ ischemia:
  - Prompts the renewed release of vasoconstrictors
  - Triggers a vicious cycle
- 1–2% of hypertensive patients will have a hypertensive emergency.
- Malignant HTN:
  - Classically in young African American men
  - Underlying renal disease
  - Flame-shaped hemorrhages, soft exudates, papilledema on funduscopic exam
- Hypertensive encephalopathy:
  - Sudden severe HTN
  - Cerebral edema with altered mental status
  - Papilledema
  - Posterior reversible encephalopathy syndrome (PRES) on MRI

### ETIOLOGY
- Primary hypertensive event:
  - Hypertensive encephalopathy
  - Accelerated malignant HTN
- CNS:
  - Subarachnoid hemorrhage
  - Intracranial hemorrhage
  - Cerebral infarction
  - Head trauma
  - Transient ischemic attacks
- Cardiovascular:
  - MIs
  - Unstable angina
  - Acute aortic dissection
  - Acute CHF
- Renal:
  - Acute renal insufficiency
  - Acute glomerulonephritis
  - Renal artery stenosis
- Excessive catecholamine states:
  - Pheochromocytoma
  - Adrenocortical tumors
  - Monoamine oxidase inhibitor (MAOI) interactions
- Antihypertensive medication withdrawal
- Pregnancy-related:
  - Pregnancy-induced HTN
  - Preeclampsia
- Autonomic dysfunction:
  - Guillain-Barré syndrome
  - Acute intermittent porphyria
- Drugs/toxins:
  - Cocaine
  - Amphetamines
  - Cold remedies
  - Oral contraceptives
  - Corticosteroids
  - Heavy metals

## DIAGNOSIS

### SIGNS AND SYMPTOMS
- Persistent elevation of BP
- Assess signs of end-organ damage:
  - Chest pain (myocardial ischemia)
  - Back pain (aortic dissection)
  - Dyspnea (CHF)
  - Headache
  - Altered mental status/confusion
  - Focal neurological symptoms
  - Seizures
  - Visual disturbance

### History
- Duration and severity of preexisting HTN
- Previous end-organ compromise:
  - Renal
  - Cerebrovascular
  - Cardiovascular
  - Great vessels
- Details of antihypertensive therapy:
  - Compliance
- Illicit drug use

### Physical Exam
- BP measured in both arms
  - Use proper cuff size
- Assess for end-organ compromise:
  - Neurologic:
    - Level of consciousness
    - Visual fields
    - Focal motor/sensory deficits
  - Ophthalmologic:
    - Funduscopic exam (retinal hemorrhages, papilledema)
- Cardiovascular:
  - Elevated JVP
  - Lung crackles
  - S3

### ESSENTIAL WORKUP
- 12-lead EKG:
  - Ischemic changes
  - Left ventricular hypertrophy
- Assess kidney function
  - Acute renal failure may be asymptomatic

## DIAGNOSTIC TESTS & INTERPRETATION

### Lab
- Standard hospital protocols for chest pain
- BUN, creatinine:
  - Acutely elevated in new renal failure
- Electrolytes
- Urinalysis:
  - Proteinuria and casts in renal injury
- Urine toxicology screen:
  - If illicit drugs are suspected
  - Cocaine, amphetamines
- HCG

### Imaging
Head CT:
- For headache, confusion, neurologic findings

### Diagnostic Procedures/Surgery
- Arterial line
- Lumbar puncture:
  - Exclude subarachnoid hemorrhage

### DIFFERENTIAL DIAGNOSIS
- Acute coronary syndrome (ACS)
- Acute pulmonary edema
- Aortic dissection
- Subarachnoid hemorrhage
- Intracerebral hemorrhage
- Cerebral infarction
- Preeclampsia/eclampsia
- Withdrawal syndromes:
  - β-Blockers
  - Clonidine (central α2-agonist)
- States of catecholamine excess:
  - Pheochromocytoma
  - Cocaine/sympathomimetic drug intoxication
  - Tyramine ingestion when on MAOIs

## TREATMENT

### PRE-HOSPITAL
- ABCs
- Consider gentle BP reduction as clinically indicated.

### INITIAL STABILIZATION/THERAPY
- ABCs
- Cardiac monitoring
- Pulse oximetry
- Oxygen administration
- IV access

### ED TREATMENT/PROCEDURES
- Treat end-organ damage, not absolute BP
- Hypertensive urgency:
  - No need to treat, but close follow-up
  - Oral agents only
  - Give any missed home dose
  - Can start HCTZ for diastolic > 100 mm Hg
- Reduce the mean arterial pressure by no more than 20–25% in the 1st hr
- Goal: Systolic ~160 mm Hg, diastolic ~100 mm Hg in 2–6 hr

- More gradual reduction recommended in:
  - Long history of poorly controlled HTN
  - Acute ongoing injury to CNS
- Ideal medication has rapid onset, rapid maximal effect, and rapid offset for easy titration.
- Labetalol:
  - Combined $\alpha$- and $\beta$-blocker
  - Rapid onset in 5–10 min
  - 3–6 hr duration, so bolus instead of drip
  - No reflex tachycardia due to $\beta$-blockade
  - Avoid in COPD, CHF, bradycardia
- Nitroprusside:
  - Short-acting arterial and venous dilator
  - Quick on/off:
    - Immediate onset
    - 2–3 min duration of action
  - Complications:
    - Reflex tachycardia
    - Cyanide toxicity after prolonged use
  - Contraindicated in pregnancy, renal failure (relative)
  - Avoid in ACS (decreases coronary perfusion) and aortic dissection (reflex tachycardia)
- Nitroglycerin:
  - Venous > arteriolar dilation
  - Perfuses coronaries, decreasing ischemia
  - Dilates cerebral capacitance vessels, increasing ICP
  - Similar pharmacokinetics as nitroprusside
  - Causes headache and reflex tachycardia
- Nicardipine:
  - Calcium channel blocker
  - Smooth onset, titration harder due to prolonged half-life
- Esmolol:
  - $\beta 1$-Blockade
  - Quick on/off, lasts ~30 min
- Enalaprilat:
  - ACE inhibitor
  - Onset peaks in 4 hr, may last up to 24 hr
  - Avoid in renal artery stenosis
  - Watch for hyperkalemia.
  - Contraindicated in pregnancy
- Hydralazine:
  - Arteriolar dilator
  - Effect in 30 min, duration 2–4 hr
  - Hypotensive effect may be less predictable.
  - Safe in pregnancy
- Fenoldopam:
  - Selective postsynaptic dopaminergic receptor agonist (DA1)
  - Quick on/off:
    - Onset 3–4 min
    - Duration 8–10 min
  - No reflex tachycardia
  - Maintains renal perfusion unlike most agents
  - Contraindicated in glaucoma, increases IOP
- Phentolamine:
  - $\alpha 1$-Blocker, peripheral vasodilator
  - first line for states of catecholamine excess
- Use caution with oral agents:
  - Difficult to reverse and titrate
- Accelerated malignant HTN:
  - Nitroprusside

- Cerebrovascular emergencies:
  - Ischemic:
    - $CPP = MAP - ICP$
    - Decreased CPP from hypotension (low MAP) or cerebral edema (high ICP) may extend infarct
    - Treat only SBP >220 mm Hg or DBP > 120
    - Lytic candidates should have BP lowered to <185/110 mm Hg
    - Labetalol or nicardipine are first line, due to minimal effect on cerebral vasculature
    - Avoid other calcium channel blockers that may increase ICP
  - Hemorrhagic CVA or SAH:
    - Stricter BP control, especially if aneurysmal
    - Goal MAP 110 mm Hg, BP 160/90 mm Hg
    - If ICP is high, keep CPP >60–80
    - Labetalol, nicardipine, esmolol are first line
    - Avoid dilating cerebral vessels with nitroglycerin or nitroprusside
- Cardiovascular emergencies:
  - ACS:
    - Nitroglycerin, reduces pre- and afterload
  - CHF:
    - Nitroglycerin paste or drip
    - Avoid $\beta$-blockers
    - Lasix PRN, not clear
  - Aortic dissection:
    - Reduce shear force (dP/dT) by reducing both BP and heart rate
    - Labetalol first line, decreases BP and HR
    - Avoid reflex tachycardia (eg, use nitroprusside only with $\beta$-blockade)
    - Goal: Rapid reduction to SBP <120 mm Hg
- Sympathomimetics (pheochromocytoma, cocaine, amphetamines):
  - Avoid pure $\beta$-blockade as $\alpha$ is left unopposed
  - Benzodiazepines
  - Phentolamine, pure $\alpha$-blockade
  - Nitroprusside

### Pregnancy Considerations

Preeclampsia:

- Frequently in primigravid women
- >20 wk gestation until 4 wk postpartum
- Headache, vision changes, peripheral edema, RUQ pain, proteinuria
- May progress to HELLP, eclampsia (seizures)
- Treatment:
  - Magnesium
  - Hydralazine
  - Diazoxide (second line)

### MEDICATION

- Enalaprilat: 1.25–5 mg q6hr IV bolus
- Esmolol: 500 $\mu$g/kg loading dose, then 25–300 $\mu$g/kg/min IV infusion
- Fenoldopam: 0.1–0.3 $\mu$g/kg/min IV infusion
- Hydralazine: 10–20 mg IV bolus
- Labetalol: 20–80 mg IV bolus q10min (total 300 mg); 0.5–2.0 mg/min IV infusion
- Nicardipine: 5–15 mg/hr IV infusion
- Nitroglycerin: 5–100 $\mu$g/min IV infusion
- Nitroprusside: 0.25–10 $\mu$g/kg/min IV infusion
- Phentolamine: 5–15 mg q5–15min IV bolus

## FOLLOW-UP

### DISPOSITION

**Admission Criteria**

- All patients with hypertensive emergencies
- Signs of end-organ damage
- ICU for cardiac and BP monitoring with arterial line

**Discharge Criteria**

Hypertensive urgency:

- Absence of cerebral, ocular, cardiac, or renal damage
- Likely to be compliant with primary care
- Known history of HTN
- Reversible precipitating cause (eg, medication noncompliance)
- Able to resume previous medication regimen
- Able to be seen in follow-up within 7 days
- Return with chest pain or headache

### FOLLOW-UP RECOMMENDATIONS

Initiation of a suitable medication regimen under care of a primary care provider

## PEARLS AND PITFALLS

- Avoid reflex tachycardia in aortic dissection.
- Avoid nitroprusside in renal failure (cyanide toxicity).
- Avoid unopposed $\alpha$ in states of catecholamine excess.

## ADDITIONAL READING

- Adams HP Jr., et al. AHA/ASA Guidelines for the early management of adults with ischemic stroke. *Stroke.* 2007;38(5):1655–1711.
- Broderick J, et al. AHA/ASA Guidelines for the management of spontaneous intracerebral hemorrhage in adults: 2007 update. *Stroke.* 2007;38(6):2001–2023.
- Marik PE, Varon J. Hypertensive crises: Challenges and management. *Chest.* 2007;131(6):1949–1962.

### See Also (Topic, Algorithm, Electronic Media Element)

- Acute Coronary Syndrome
- Acute Stroke
- Aortic Dissection
- Congestive Heart Failure
- Preeclampsia/Eclampsia
- Subarachnoid Hemorrhage

## CODES

ICD9

- 401.0 Malignant essential hypertension
- 401.1 Benign essential hypertension
- 401.9 Unspecified essential hypertension

**H**

# HYPERTHERMIA
*Michelle Sergel*

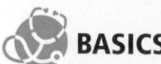 **BASICS**

## DESCRIPTION
- Hyperthermia is defined as elevation of core body temperature above the normal range of 36–37.5°C, due to failure of thermoregulation.
- Continuum of increasingly severe illnesses secondary to overwhelming heat stress.
- Begins with dehydration and electrolyte abnormalities and progresses to thermoregulatory dysfunction and multisystem organ failure
- Body temperature is maintained within a narrow range by balancing heat load with heat dissipation.
- Temperature elevation is accompanied by an increase in oxygen consumption and metabolic rate.
- Oxidative phosphorylation becomes uncoupled and a variety of enzymes cease to function >42°C (108°F).
- Prickly heat:
  - Blockage of sweat glands leading to rash
- Heat cramps:
  - Secondary to excessive sweating and sodium loss
- Heat exhaustion:
  - Core temp: <104°F (40°C)
  - Fluid and electrolyte depletion
  - Thermoregulatory function is maintained.
  - CNS function is preserved.
- Heat stroke:
  - Core body temp >105°F (40.5°C)
  - Loss of thermoregulatory function, severe CNS dysfunction, multisystem organ failure
  - Classic heat stroke (nonexertional):
    ○ Occurs in those with compromised thermoregulation or an inability to remove themselves from a hot environment (extremes of age, debilitated)
    ○ Develops over days to weeks
    ○ Severe dehydration, skin warm and dry
  - Exertional heat stroke:
    ○ Occurs in younger, athletic individuals with a combined environmental and exertional heat stress
    ○ Develops over hours
    ○ Internal heat production overwhelms dissipating mechanisms.
    ○ May be sweating

## ETIOLOGY
- Pre-existing conditions that hinder the body's ability to dissipate heat:
  - Age extremes
  - Dehydration
  - Cardiovascular disease
  - Obesity
  - Hyperthyroidism
  - Febrile illness
  - Skin diseases that hinder sweating (psoriasis, eczema)

- Pharmacologic contributors:
  - Sympathomimetics
  - LSD/PCP
  - MAO inhibitors
  - Anticholinergics
  - Antihistamines
  - β-blockers
  - Diuretics
  - Laxatives
  - Drug or alcohol withdrawal
- Physical/environmental factors:
  - Prolonged exertion
  - Lack of mobility
  - Lack of air conditioning
  - Excessive humidity
  - Lack of acclimatization

### Pediatric Considerations
Children are at increased risk of heat illness owing to increased body surface area to mass ratio.

### Geriatric Considerations
Debilitated elderly may be more susceptible to heat illness due to inability to remove themselves from a hot environment

 **DIAGNOSIS**

## SIGNS AND SYMPTOMS
- Prickly heat:
  - Pruritic maculopapular rash over clothed areas
- Heat edema:
  - Swelling of dependent areas of body
  - Resolves after acclimatization
- Heat tetany:
  - Carpal-pedal spasm—secondary to hyperventilation
- Heat cramps:
  - Cramps in heavily exercised muscles
  - During or after exercise
  - Primarily in lower extremities
- Heat exhaustion:
  - Core temp: <104°F (40°C)
  - CNS:
    ○ Headache
    ○ Fatigue
    ○ Malaise
    ○ Agitation
  - CV:
    ○ Mild tachycardia
    ○ Dehydration
  - Pulmonary:
    ○ Tachypnea
  - GI:
    ○ Nausea
    ○ Vomiting
  - Skin:
    ○ Perspiration present, often profuse

- Heat stroke:
  - Classic triad: Hyperthermia, CNS dysfunction, anhydrosis:
    ○ Perspiration is often present in early stages.
  - Core temp: >105°F (40.5°C)
  - CNS:
    ○ Severe confusion
    ○ Lethargy
    ○ Coma
    ○ Seizure
    ○ Ataxia
  - Cardiovascular (CV):
    ○ Tachycardia
    ○ Hypotension
    ○ Wide pulse pressure
    ○ Conduction disturbances
  - Pulmonary:
    ○ Tachypnea
    ○ Rales owing to noncardiac pulmonary edema
  - GI:
    ○ Nausea
    ○ Vomiting
    ○ Diarrhea
  - Skin:
    ○ Cutaneous vasodilation
    ○ Dry and hot if severe dehydration
    ○ Sweating may be present if patient is not dehydrated.
  - Acute oliguric renal failure owing to rhabdomyolysis, dehydration
  - Hepatic failure
  - Acute bleeding owing to disseminated intravascular coagulation (DIC)

## ESSENTIAL WORKUP
- Accurate core temperature
- History of heat exposure
- Heat exhaustion—diagnosis of exclusion
- Core temperature >105°F (40.5°C) and CNS dysfunction required to make diagnosis of heat stroke

## DIAGNOSTIC TESTS & INTERPRETATION
### Lab
- Heat stroke and heat exhaustion:
  - CBC:
    ○ Leukocytosis, hemoconcentration often present
  - Electrolytes, BUN, creatinine, glucose:
    ○ Hypernatremia with severe dehydration
    ○ Hyponatremia can occur if drinking copious free water.
    ○ Acute renal failure
  - Urinalysis (UA):
    ○ Myoglobin present in rhabdomyolysis
  - Blood and urine cultures to rule out infection
  - Toxicology screen
  - Serum creatinine kinase to rule out rhabdomyolysis

- Heat stroke:
  – Liver function tests:
    o Hepatic necrosis presents with elevated transaminases.
  – PT/PTT/DIC panel:
    o Coagulopathy, DIC
  – Consider lumbar puncture.

### Imaging
- ECG indicated in the elderly or those at cardiac risk
- CT head for altered mental status
- CXR for adult respiratory distress syndrome (ARDS), aspiration pneumonia

## DIFFERENTIAL DIAGNOSIS
- Febrile illness/sepsis
- Thyroid storm
- Pheochromocytoma
- Malignant hyperthermia
- Cocaine/PCP
- Anticholinergics
- MAO inhibitors
- Meningitis/encephalitis
- Cerebral falciparum malaria
- Delirium tremens
- Neuroleptic malignant syndrome

## TREATMENT
### PRE-HOSPITAL
Institute cooling measures for severe heat illness:
- Remove from heat stress
- Disrobe patient
- Cover body with wet sheet

### INITIAL STABILIZATION/THERAPY
- ABCs
- Continuous core temperature monitoring with a rectal or esophageal probe
- Immediate/rapid cooling if temperature >104°F (40°C)
- IV 0.9% NS 500 mL fluid bolus if hypotensive
- If altered mental status, administer glucose, thiamine, naloxone

## ED TREATMENT/PROCEDURES
- Cooling measures:
  – Initiate for body temperature >104°F (40°C).
  – Evaporative cooling:
    o Extremely effective (0.05–0.3°C/min)
    o Spray disrobed patient with fine mist of warm water (prevents shivering).
    o Airflow with fans blowing over patient
  – Conductive cooling:
    o Ice packs to groin/axilla—combine with evaporative cooling treatment above.
    o Cooling blankets
    o Cold oxygen administration
    o Iced or cold water immersion—effective but impractical
  – Iced peritoneal lavage, cold IV fluids, cold gastric lavage, and cardiopulmonary bypass for refractory cases
  – To avoid hypothermia, stop cooling therapy at 102°F (39°C)
  – Antipyretic agents are not helpful—underlying mechanism does not involve a change in the hypothalamus set point.
  – Avoid alcohol sponge baths—toxicity can occur owing to dilated cutaneous vessels.
- Supportive measures:
  – Rehydration for heat stroke/heat exhaustion:
    o Initial rehydration with 0.5–1.0 L 0.9% NS
    o Avoid overhydration—may contribute to development of ARDS
    o Peds: 20 mL/kg bolus
    o Place Foley catheter to monitor urine output for heat stroke victims.
  – Benzodiazepines for seizures or shivering
  – For heat cramps:
    o Administer analgesics and oral or IV hydration with electrolyte-containing fluid.
  – For hyperventilation heat tetany:
    o Provide reassurance/calming measures/rebreathing in closed system (bag or nonrebreather without oxygen).
  – For heat edema:
    o Lower extremity elevation
    o Remove from heat stress.

## MEDICATION
- Dextrose: 50–100 mL $D_{50}$ (peds: 2 mL/kg of $D_{25}W$ over 1 min) IV push (IVP)
- Diazepam: 5–10 mg (peds: 0.2–0.4 mg/kg) IVP
- Lorazepam: 1–2 mg (peds: 0.05–0.1 mg/kg) IVP
- Naloxone: 2 mg (peds: 0.1 mg/kg) IVP

 FOLLOW-UP

### DISPOSITION
#### Admission Criteria
- Heat stroke—admit to the ICU.
- Heat exhaustion—admit to general or monitored floor:
  – Severe electrolyte abnormalities
  – Renal failure/evidence of rhabdomyolysis
  – Elderly

#### Discharge Criteria
All patients except those with heat stroke or severe heat exhaustion may be discharged.

### FOLLOW-UP RECOMMENDATIONS
May require close follow-up if patient has compromised thermoregulation.

## PEARLS AND PITFALLS
- Management of heat stroke requires ensuring ABCs and initiation of rapid cooling.
- Continuous core temperature monitoring with a rectal or esophageal probe is mandatory.
- Evaporative cooling is the cooling modality of choice.

## ADDITIONAL READING
- Khosla R, Guntapalli KK. Heat-related illness. *Crit Care Clin.* 1999;15:251.
- Lee-Chiong TL, Stitt JT. Heat stroke and other heat-related illnesses. *Postgrad Med.* 1995;98(1):26–36.
- Walker JS, Barnes SB. Heat emergencies. In: Tintinalli JE, ed. *Emergency Medicine: A Comprehensive Study Guide.* 5th ed. New York: McGraw-Hill; 2000:1237–1242.

 CODES

### ICD9
- 780.60 Fever, unspecified
- 992.0 Heat stroke and sunstroke
- 992.2 Heat cramps

**H**

# HYPERTHYROIDISM

*Rita K. Cydulka*
*Kellie Kirkpatrick*

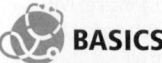 **BASICS**

## DESCRIPTION
- Excessive thyroid hormone production results in a continuum of disease caused by both the direct physiologic effect of thyroid hormones as well as increased catecholamine sensitivity:
  - Subclinical or mild hyperthyroidism
  - Thyrotoxicosis
  - Thyroid storm or thyrotoxic crisis with life-threatening manifestations:
    ○ 1–2% of patients with hyperthyroidism
- Regulation of thyroid hormone:
  - Thyrotropin-releasing hormone (TRH) from hypothalamus acts on the anterior pituitary.
  - Thyroid stimulating hormone (TSH) released by anterior pituitary gland and results in increased $T_3$ and $T_4$ from the thyroid gland:
    ○ Most of circulating thyroid hormone is $T_4$, which is peripherally converted to $T_3$.
    ○ $T_3$ is much more biologically active than $T_4$ although it has a shorter half-life.
- Genetics:
  - Interplay between genetics and environment.
  - Graves' disease is associated with HLA-B8 and HLA-DR3.
  - Autosomal dominant inheritance seen in some families with nontoxic goiter.

## ETIOLOGY
- Primary hyperthyroidism:
  - Toxic diffuse goiter (Graves' disease)
  - Toxic multinodular (Plummer's disease) or uninodular goiter
  - Excessive iodine intake (Jod-Basedow disease)
- Thyroiditis:
  - Postpartum thyroiditis
  - Radiation thyroiditis
  - Subacute thyroiditis (de Quervain's)
  - Chronic thyroiditis (Hashimoto's/lymphocytic)
- Metastatic thyroid cancer
- Ectopic thyroid tissue (struma ovarii)
- Pituitary adenoma
- Drug induced:
  - Amiodarone
  - Lithium
  - Iodine (radiographic contrast agents)
  - Excessive thyroid hormone (factitious thyrotoxicosis)

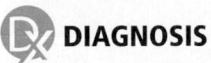 **DIAGNOSIS**

## ALERT
Thyroid storm is a life-threatening condition, which may be precipitated by:
- Infection
- Trauma
- Diabetic ketoacidosis
- Myocardial infarction
- Cerebrovascular accident
- Surgery
- Abrupt withdrawal of antithyroid medication or acute ingestion of thyroid medication

## SIGNS AND SYMPTOMS
- Signs and symptoms reflect end organ responsiveness to thyroid hormone:
  - Signs:
    ○ Fever
    ○ Tachycardia, wide pulse pressure
    ○ Diaphoresis/sweating
    ○ CHF
    ○ Shock
    ○ Tremor
    ○ Disorientation/psychosis
    ○ Goiter/thyromegaly
    ○ Thyrotoxic stare/exophthalmos/lid lag
    ○ Hyperreflexia
    ○ Pretibial myxedema
  - Symptoms:
    ○ Weight loss despite increased appetite
    ○ Dysphagia or dyspnea secondary to obstruction by a goiter
    ○ Rash/pruritus/hyperhidrosis
    ○ Palpitations/chest pain
    ○ Diarrhea
    ○ Myalgias and weakness
    ○ Nervousness/anxiety
    ○ Menstrual irregularities
    ○ Heat intolerance
    ○ Insomnia and fatigue
- Thyroid storms involves exaggerated signs and symptoms of thyrotoxicosis:
  - Extreme tachycardia/dysrhythmias
  - CHF
  - Shock
  - Disorientation and mental status changes including coma and seizure

### Geriatric Considerations
Apathetic hyperthyroidism:
- Owing to multinodular goiter, often have history of nontoxic goiter
- Subtle clinical findings that often reflect single-organ system dysfunction:
  - CHF
  - Atrial fibrillation resistant to standard therapy
  - Weight loss
  - Depression, emotional lability, flat affect
  - Tremor
  - Hyperactivity

### History
Gradual onset of aforementioned signs and symptoms

### Physical Exam
- Vital signs:
  - Fever
  - Tachycardia
  - Elevation of systolic blood pressure
  - Tachypnea/hypoxia
- Alopecia
- Exophthalmos or lid lag
- Thyromegaly or goiter, thyroid bruit
- Fine, thin, diaphoretic skin
- Irregularly irregular heartbeat

- Lung rales (CHF)
- Right upper quadrant tenderness/jaundice
- Muscular atrophy/weakness
- Tremor
- Mental status changes/coma

## ESSENTIAL WORKUP
- Find underlying cause/precipitating factors.
- Plasma TSH is the initial ED test of choice:
  - Normal level usually rules out hyperthyroidism:
    ○ TSH may be low with normal $T_4$. Get $T_3$ level to rule out $T_3$ thyrotoxicosis.
  - If TSH levels are not available, strong clinical picture should prompt initiation of therapy.

## DIAGNOSTIC TESTS & INTERPRETATION
### Lab
- Thyroid function tests for:
  - Symptoms of hyperthyroidism
  - Elderly patient with new-onset CHF
  - New atrial fibrillation/supraventricular tachycardia (AFib/SVT)
- TSH (usually decreased)
- Free $T_4$ (usually elevated):
  - If free $T_4$ is unavailable, total $T_4$ and resin $T_3$ uptake
  - 5% will have $T_3$ thyrotoxicosis, if low TSH with normal $T_4$, send $T_3$ to rule out.
- Lab studies are often not helpful/nonspecific, get as needed to look for underlying precipitants:
  - CBC to rule out anemia
  - Chemistry panel:
    ○ BUN, creatinine may be elevated secondary to dehydration
    ○ Hypokalemia, hyperglycemia
- Liver function tests (increased transaminases)
- Arterial blood gases for hypoxemia
- Cardiac markers

### Imaging
CXR (in CHF or sepsis)

### Diagnostic Procedures/Surgery
EKG:
- Most commonly sinus tachycardia.
- Rule out MI as precipitant of thyroid storm
- New onset atrial fibrillation

## DIFFERENTIAL DIAGNOSIS
- Pheochromocytoma
- Sepsis
- Sympathomimetic ingestion
- Psychosis
- Heat stroke
- Delirium tremens
- Malignant hyperthermia
- Neuroleptic malignant syndrome
- Hypothalamic stroke
- Hypothyroidism (may mimic apathetic hyperthyroidism)
- Factitious thyrotoxicosis

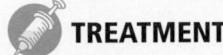 **TREATMENT**

## PRE-HOSPITAL
Stabilization and supportive care.

## INITIAL STABILIZATION/THERAPY
- Airway, breathing, and circulation management (ABCs)
- Cardiac monitor
- Supplemental oxygen
- IV fluids
- Initiate cooling measures:
  - Acetaminophen for fever:
    - Avoid aspirin (displaces thyroid hormone from thyroglobulin, elevates free $T_4$).
  - Cooling blanket

## ED TREATMENT/PROCEDURES
- Identify and treat the precipitating event.
- For thyroid storm, initiate treatment sequence outlined below based on clinical suspicion alone
- Inhibit hormone synthesis using thioamides:
  - Propylthiouracil (PTU):
    - Drug of choice
    - Decreases hormone synthesis and reduces peripheral conversion of $T_4$
  - Methimazole (MMI)
- Block hormone release using iodine *only after hormone synthesis is inhibited as above:*
  - Potassium iodide, *or*
  - Oral Lugol solution, *or*
  - Ipanoic acid (Telepaque)
  - Give iodine at least 1 hr after thioamides to prevent increased hormone production
  - Consider lithium in patient allergic to iodine
- Block peripheral effects of thyroid hormone:
  - $\beta$-blockade:
    - Propranolol is first line as it also inhibits $T_4$ conversion to $T_3$.
    - Esmolol. $\beta$-1 selective so may be used in patient with active CHF, asthma, etc.
  - Reserpine, guanethidine
- Dexamethasone/hydrocortisone:
  - Prevents peripheral $T_4$ to $T_3$ conversion
- Treatment of thyrotoxicosis, secondary thyroiditis:
  - $\beta$-blockade
    Anti-inflammatory medications
- General thyrotoxicosis support:
  - Acetaminophen for hyperpyrexia
  - Treat CHF with usual methods
  - Manage dehydration
  - Steroids

## MEDICATION
- Dexamethasone: 2 mg IV q6h (peds: 0.15 mg/kg q6h)
- Esmolol: 500 $\mu$g/kg IV over 1 min followed by maintenance dose of 50 $\mu$g/kg/min IV; titrate to effect
- Guanethidine: 30–40 mg PO q6h
- Hydrocortisone: 100 mg IV q8h

- Ipanoic acid: 1 g IV q8h for the 1st 24 h, then 500 mg IV b.i.d.
- Lithium carbonate: 800–1,200 mg PO per day (peds: 15–60 mg/kg/day div t.i.d.–q.i.d.)
- Lugol solutions: 8–10 drops PO q6h
- Methimazole: 40 mg (peds: 0.4 mg/kg) PO initially, then 25 mg (peds: 0.2 mg/kg/24 h) PO per day
- Potassium iodide (SSKI): 5 drops PO q6h
- Propranolol: 1–2 mg IV, repeated q10–15min PRN
- Propylthiouracil (PTU): 600–1,000 mg initially, then 200–250 mg PO q4h (peds: 5–7 mg/kg/24 h)
- Reserpine: 1–5 mg IM q4–6h, up to 15 mg/24 h

### First Line
- Propylthiouracil
- Propranolol
- Iodine therapy (1 hr after PTU)

### Second Line
- Methimazole
- Esmolol
- Lithium (only with iodine allergy)
- Guanethidine, reserpine

### Pregnancy Considerations
- Physiologic changes associated with pregnancy may resemble many symptoms of hyperthyroidism, thus causing a delay in diagnosis.
- Poorly controlled hyperthyroidism during pregnancy may result in:
  - Premature labor
  - Preeclampsia
  - Low birth weight
  - Spontaneous abortion
  - Stillbirth
- Thyroid storm often precipitated by stressors including infection, labor, birth
- Treatment:
  - Initial stabilization as in the nonpregnant patient (ABCs, supportive measures)
  - PTU considered safer than MMI. Both cross the placenta.
  - Propranolol may be safely used.
  - Radioactive iodine absolutely contraindicated during pregnancy or while nursing
  - Thyroidectomy only other option if unable to tolerate PTU while pregnant.
- Postpartum thyroiditis:
  - 5–10% of patients within 6 mo of delivery
  - May require antithyroid medications
  - Half of those affected become euthyroid within 1 yr
  - Transient hypothyroidism may follow

 **FOLLOW-UP**

## DISPOSITION
### Admission Criteria
- Thyroid storm
- Requiring IV medications to control heart rate
- Significantly symptomatic or unstable patients

### Discharge Criteria
Minimally symptomatic individuals who respond well to oral therapy

## FOLLOW-UP RECOMMENDATIONS
- Should have primary care physician follow-up within a few weeks depending on symptoms.
- May benefit from endocrinology referral.

## PEARLS AND PITFALLS
- Thyroid storm can be fatal. Diagnosis requires a high level of suspicion and treatment often needs to be started presumptively.
- Hyperthyroidism presents with a wide variety of signs and symptoms.
- Radioactive iodine is never a treatment option in the pregnant patient with hyperthyroidism.
- Never give iodine before blocking hormone synthesis with PTU or MMI in thyroid storm.

## ADDITIONAL READING
- Kronenberg H, et al. *Williams' Textbook of Endocrinology.* 11th ed. Philadelphia: WB Saunders; 2007.
- Mestman I. Hyperthyroidism in pregnancy. *Best Pract Res Clin Endocrinol Metab.* 2004;18:267–288.
- Nayak B, Burman K. Thyrotoxicosis and thyroid storm. *Endocrinol Metab Clin North Am.* 2006;35(4):663–686, vii.
- Wogan JM. Selected endocrine disorders. In: Marx J, et al. eds. *Rosen's Emergency Medicine: Concepts and Clinical Practice.* 5th ed. St. Louis, MO: Mosby; 2001.

### See Also (Topic, Algorithm, Electronic Media Element)
- Hypothyroidism

 **CODES**

### ICD9
- 242.90 Thyrotoxicosis without mention of goiter or other cause, and without mention of thyrotoxic crisis or storm
- 242.91 Thyrotoxicosis without mention of goiter or other cause, with mention of thyrotoxic crisis or storm

**H**

# HYPERVENTILATION

*Robert F. McCormack*

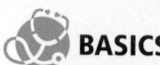 **BASICS**

## DESCRIPTION

- Hyperventilation describes a constellation of symptoms:
  - Most commonly: Dyspnea, chest pain, lightheadedness, and paresthesias
- Produced by a nonphysiologic increase in minute ventilation:
  - Minute ventilation may be increased by increasing respiratory rate or tidal volume (sighs).
- Pathologic or physiologic causes of hyperventilation must be excluded before the diagnosis of hyperventilation syndrome can be assigned.
- Prevalence:
  - 10–15% in the general population
  - More common in women (may be related to progesterone)

## ETIOLOGY

- Etiology of symptoms is unclear:
  - Usually a response to psychological stressors
- Controversy exists regarding underlying disorders that may contribute to hyperventilation:
  - Hypocapnia
  - Hypophosphatemia
  - Hypocalcemia

## DIAGNOSIS

### SIGNS AND SYMPTOMS

**History**
- Cardiac:
  - Chest pain
  - Dyspnea
  - "Air hunger"
  - Palpitations
- Neurologic:
  - Dizziness
  - Light-headedness
  - Syncope
  - Paresthesias
  - Headache
  - Carpopedal spasm
  - Tetany
- Psychiatric:
  - Intense fear, anxiety
  - Giddiness
  - Feeling of unreality
- General:
  - Fatigue
  - Weakness
  - Malaise

**Physical Exam**
- Clinical signs are rare and varied:
  - Tachypnea most common
  - However, tachypnea may not be present. Patient may increase tidal volume rather than respiratory rate.
- Carpopedal spasm:
  - May be dramatic
- Chvostek sign may be present

## ESSENTIAL WORKUP

- Diagnosis of exclusion:
  - Primary pathologic or physiologic causes of hyperventilation must be investigated and excluded.
- Clinical diagnosis based on the history and physical exam
- Vital signs including pulse oximetry
- Hyperventilation syndrome will not result in hypoxia.

## DIAGNOSTIC TESTS & INTERPRETATION

### Lab
- Consider an ABG in any hypoxic patient.
- Electrolytes, BUN, creatinine, and glucose levels for suspected acidosis/diabetic ketoacidosis
- EKG if chest pain present

### Imaging
CXR of any patient with hypoxia or focal findings on lung exam

### Diagnostic Procedures/Surgery
- Hyperventilation provocation test after resolution of symptoms:
  - Forced overbreathing for 3 min may be attempted to reproduce the symptoms.
  - Diagnostic accuracy is controversial.
  - Reproducibility of the symptoms may help the patient understand the role of overbreathing and help manage future attacks.

## DIFFERENTIAL DIAGNOSIS
- Pathologic
- Hypoxia:
  - Asthma
  - CHF
  - Pulmonary embolus
  - Pneumonia

- Severe pain
- CNS lesions
- Acidosis (DKA)
- Pulmonary HTN
- Pulmonary embolus
- Hypoglycemia
- Mild asthma
- Drugs:
  – Aspirin intoxication
  – Withdrawal syndrome (eg, alcohol, benzodiazepines)
- Physiologic
- Pregnancy
- Pyrexia
- Altitude

 **TREATMENT**

### PRE-HOSPITAL
- Patients with abnormal vital signs require IV access and pulse oximetry.
- Supplemental oxygen if hypoxic

### INITIAL STABILIZATION/THERAPY
- Patients with abnormal vital signs require IV access and pulse oximetry.
- Initiate therapy for pathologic or physiologic cause of hyperventilation.

### ED TREATMENT/PROCEDURES
- Initiate treatment of hyperventilation syndrome if initial workup does not support a pathologic or physiologic cause, and history and physical exam findings suggest the diagnosis of hyperventilation syndrome.
- Reassurance, calming, and explanation of the voluntary component of the patient's symptoms often have immediate dramatic results.

- Do not use paper bag rebreathing to increase the $PCO_2$. This has not been supported in the literature:
  – It may be dangerous in patients with hypoxia or a pathologic or physiologic cause for hyperventilation.
- Clarification of the psychologic stressors helps the patient avoid further attacks.
- Assess for need of psychiatric evaluation (ie, suicidal ideation).
- Anxiolytics:
  – Benzodiazepine if symptoms persist to break the cycle of anxiety and hyperventilation
  – Short course of anxiolytics may benefit patients with definable temporary stressors.

### MEDICATION
- Lorazepam: 1–2 mg PO or IV
- Diazepam: 2–5 mg PO or IV
- Outpatient treatment:
  – Buspirone: 5 mg PO t.i.d.
  – Diazepam: 2–5 mg PO b.i.d–q.i.d.

 **FOLLOW-UP**

### DISPOSITION
**Admission Criteria**
Hyperventilation syndrome does not require admission.

**Discharge Criteria**
- Exclusion or successful treatment of primary pathologic or physiologic causes of hyperventilation
- No acute psychiatric issues
- Adequate follow-up with a primary care physician

### FOLLOW-UP RECOMMENDATIONS
- Follow-up with primary care physician
- Assess the need for psychiatric follow-up.

### PEARLS AND PITFALLS
- Exclude pathologic or physiologic causes of hyperventilation.
- Hyperventilation syndrome will not result in hypoxia.

### ADDITIONAL READING
- Block M, Szidon P. Hyperventilation syndromes. *Compr Ther*. 1994;20:306–311.
- Callaham M. Hypoxic hazards of traditional paper bag rebreathing in hyperventilating patients. *Ann Emerg Med*. 1989;18:622–628.
- Gardner W. The pathophysiology of hyperventilation disorders. *Chest*. 1996;109:516–534.
- Nardi AE, Freire RC, Zin, WA. Panic disorder and control of breathing. *Resp Physiol Neurobiol*. 2009;167(1):133–143.
- Saisch S, Wessely S, William N. Patients with acute hyperventilation presenting to an inner–city emergency department. *Chest*. 1996;110(4): 952–957.

 **CODES**

ICD9
- 306.1 Respiratory malfunction arising from mental factors
- 786.01 Hyperventilation

H

# HYPERVISCOSITY SYNDROME

*Matthew B. Mostofi*

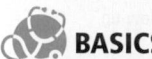 **BASICS**

## DESCRIPTION
- Hyperviscosity syndrome is the clinical consequences of increased blood viscosity.
- The classic clinical symptoms are the triad of mucosal bleeding, visual disturbances, and neurological signs.
- Viscosity is the resistance a material has to change in form.
- The higher the blood viscosity, the more internal resistance to blood flows.
- Increased cardiac output is required to provide adequate perfusion of hyper viscous blood.
- Oxygen delivery is impaired as transit through the microcirculatory system slows. This impaired microcirculatory oxygenation gives rise to the clinical symptoms of this syndrome.

## ETIOLOGY
- Hyperviscosity occurs when there is elevation of either the cellular or acellular components of circulating blood.
- Acellular (protein) hyperviscosity:
  - The most common cause (85–90%) of hyperviscosity is increased concentration of gamma globulins:
    ○ Monoclonal gammopathies: In malignant diseases like Waldenstrom macroglobulinemia and multiple myeloma
    ○ Polyclonal gammopathies: Usually rheumatic diseases (very rare)
- Cellular (blood cell) hyperviscosity:
  - Much less common (10–15%)
  - Increased numbers of RBC, as in polycythemia vera
  - Increased concentration (>100,000) of WBC, as in acute and chronic leukemia
  - Thrombocytosis

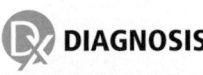 **DIAGNOSIS**

## SIGNS AND SYMPTOMS
- Classic triad:
  - Mucosal bleeding
  - Visual disturbances
  - Neurological
- Hematological:
  - Bleeding is the most common manifestation. Mechanism thought to be platelet dysfunction.
  - Epistaxis
  - Gingival, rectal, uterine bleeding
  - Prolonged postprocedural bleeding
  - Blood dyscrasias
  - Pruritus owing to red cell breakdown products
  - Splenic enlargement

- Ocular:
  - Change in visual acuity:
    ○ Blurring
    ○ Diplopia
    ○ Visual loss
  - Characteristic "link-sausage effect" on funduscopy
  - Alternating bulges and constrictions within the retinal veins
  - Retinal hemorrhage, detachment
  - Exudate, microaneurysm formation
  - Papilledema
- Renal:
  - Nephritic or nephrotic syndrome
  - Hematuria
  - Sterile pyuria
- Neurological:
  - Headache
  - Ataxia
  - Mental status changes/coma
  - Dizziness/vertigo
  - Nystagmus
  - Tinnitus, hearing loss
  - Paresthesia, peripheral neuropathy
  - Seizure
  - Intracranial hemorrhage
- Cardiovascular:
  - Angina or myocardial infarction
  - Dysrhythmias
  - CHF
- Dermatologic:
  - Raynaud phenomenon
  - Livedo reticularis
  - Palpable purpura
  - Eruptive spider nevus–like lesions
  - Digital infarcts
  - Peripheral gangrene

## History
Hyperviscosity syndrome should be considered in the following patient:
- Any patient presenting with the classic symptom triad of bleeding, visual disturbance, and neurological dysfunction.
- Any patient with an established immunoglobin-producing hematologic disease that presents with signs or symptoms of microvascular end organ damage or cardiac decompensation.
- Any patient with an established hypercellular hematologic disease that presents with signs or symptoms of microvascular end organ damage or cardiac decompensation.

## Physical Exam
There are no specific physical exam findings unique to hyperviscosity syndrome. However, patient will exhibit findings based on the affected end organs. Mucosal bleeding, petechial rash or bruising, focal neurologic findings, signs of decompensated heart failure, and funduscopic abnormalities have all been reported.

## ESSENTIAL WORKUP
- Evaluate end-organ ischemia and bleeding.
- Measure serum or whole blood viscosity.
- Suspect diagnosis if the laboratory evaluation is hampered by serum stasis and increased viscosity causing analyzer blockage

## DIAGNOSTIC TESTS & INTERPRETATION
### Lab
- CBC with WBC differential:
  - Anemia or erythrocytosis can be seen in hyperviscosity syndrome.
  - Anemia usually normocytic and normochromic
  - Rouleaux of erythrocytes on the peripheral smear important diagnostic clue
  - WBC for leukemia
- Electrolyte, BUN, creatinine, and glucose levels:
  - Renal dysfunction is commonly noted in hyperviscosity syndrome.
  - Hypercalcemia and pseudohyponatremia in multiple myeloma
- Urinalysis:
  - Proteinuria
  - Hematuria
  - Sterile pyuria
- Coagulation profile
- Serum and urine protein electrophoresis
- Measurement of serum viscosity (not routinely available in ED setting):
  - Ostwald viscosimeter
  - Normal range for the serum viscosity relative to water is 1.4–1.8.
  - Minimal viscosity at which symptoms develop is 4.0 centipoise (cp).
- Elevated leukocyte alkaline phosphatase, lactate dehydrogenase, and serum vitamin $B_{12}$ levels

### Imaging
One should consider CT of head in patients with signs or symptoms of central neurological dysfunction to exclude intracranial hemorrhage.

### DIFFERENTIAL DIAGNOSIS

- Bleeding and clotting disorders:
  - Platelet disorders (qualitative and quantitative)
  - Hereditary factor deficiencies
  - Acquired disorders (vitamin K deficiency, liver disease)
  - Disseminated intravascular coagulation

 TREATMENT

#### PRE-HOSPITAL
IV fluid resuscitation with hemorrhage

#### INITIAL STABILIZATION/THERAPY
- Rehydrate with 0.9% NS IV fluid.
- Bleeding or end-organ ischemia may not be controlled by any treatment except plasmapheresis.
- In patients with anemia and a leukemic picture, avoid blood transfusion until plasmapheresis is performed to avoid exacerbation of hyperviscosity syndrome.

#### ED TREATMENT/PROCEDURES
- Hydration, supportive care, and early hematologist consultation are initial ED management.
- Phlebotomy or emergent plasma exchange: This temporizing measure can be performed in a patient with HVS and severe neurological findings like coma or seizures:
  - Easily performed in the ED and is useful in acute severe cases if plasmapheresis not readily available
  - Simply draw off (100–200 mL) of whole blood and replace volume with isotonic saline. Should be performed in consultation with hematologist when possible.
  - Treatment of choice in patients with polycythemia vera.

- Plasmapheresis/leukapheresis: Definitive treatment for hyperviscosity syndrome.
- Should be performed in consultation with plasmapheresis team.
- ED physician can help in urgent situations by establishing or facilitating the establishment of large-bore central dialysis catheter, caution should be taken to avoid bleeding complications of this procedure:
  - In stable patients: 40 mL/kg of body weight
  - In critical patients: 60 mL/kg of body weight
  - Side effects include hypocalcemia with use of a citrate-containing anticoagulant and dysrhythmia (rare).
  - Many patients require more than 1 plasmapheresis.
  - Leukapheresis is reserved as the initial treatment in patients with hyperleukocytosis.

 FOLLOW-UP

#### DISPOSITION

##### Admission Criteria
- Patients with hyperviscosity and significant symptoms or any evidence of end-organ ischemia or hemorrhage should be admitted for treatment of the underlying hematological disorder.
- ICU admission for the following:
  - Hemorrhage
  - Altered mental status
  - Acute MI

##### Discharge Criteria
Discharge after definitive treatment of the underlying disorder.

##### Issues for Referral
All patients with hyperviscosity syndrome should be referred to hematologist.

### PEARLS AND PITFALLS
- Avoid diuretics in patients with hyperviscosity syndrome because they can increase blood viscosity.
- The classic triad of symptoms of hyperviscosity syndrome includes visual disturbances, bleeding, and neurologic manifestations.

### ADDITIONAL READING

- Adams B, Baker R, Lopez A. Myeloproliferative disorders and the hyperviscosity syndrome. *Emerg Clin N Am*. 2009;27:459–476.
- Forconi S, Pieragalli D, Guerrini M, et al. Primary and secondary blood hyperviscosity syndromes and syndromes associated with blood hyperviscosity. *Drug*. 1987;33(Suppl 2):19–26.
- Geraci JM, Hansen RM, Kueck BD. Plasma cell leukemia and hyperviscosity syndrome. *South Med J*. 1990;83:800–805.
- Gertz MA. Hyperviscosity syndrome. *J Intensive Care Med*. 1995;10:128–141.
- Pimentel L. Medical complications of oncologic disease. *Emerg Med Clin North Am*. 1993;22:407–419.
- Somer T, Meiselman HJ. Disorders of blood viscosity. *Ann Med*. 1993;25:31–39.
- Stolz JF, Donner M, Larcan A. Introduction to hemorheology: Theoretical aspects and hyperviscosity syndromes. *Int Angiol*. 1987;6:119–132.

#### See Also (Topic, Algorithm, Electronic Media Element)
Disseminated Intravascular Coagulation

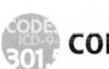 CODES

#### ICD9
273.3 Macroglobulinemia

# HYPHEMA

*Jamil D. Bayram*
*Sami H. Uwaydat*

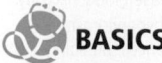 **BASICS**

## DESCRIPTION
- Blood in anterior chamber (AC) of the eye (between iris and cornea).
- Hyphema: Grossly visible layering of blood.
- Microhyphema: Suspended RBCs visible by slit-lamp only.
- Genetics:
  – Genetic predisposition is related to hereditary blood dyscrasias (see below).

## ETIOLOGY
- Blunt trauma: Most common (70–80%).
- Anteroposterior compression of the globe with simultaneous equatorial globe expansion causing rupture of iris stromal/ciliary body vessels
- Penetrating trauma: Direct injury to stromal vessels or sudden ocular decompression.
- Spontaneous: Less common, lower incidence of complications:
  – Tumors:
    ○ Melanoma
    ○ Retinoblastoma
    ○ Xanthogranuloma
    ○ Metastatic tumors
  – Blood dyscrasias:
    ○ Hemophilia
    ○ Leukemia
    ○ Thrombocytopenia
    ○ Von Willebrand disease
  – Blood thinners: Aspirin, Coumadin, heparin
  – Neovascularization of iris: In proliferative diabetic retinopathy, retinal vein occlusion, carotid stenosis.
  – Postsurgical: Cataract extraction, trabeculectomy, pars plana vitrectomy.

**ALERT**
In children with no history of trauma, suspect child abuse.

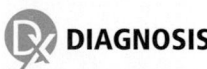 **DIAGNOSIS**

## SIGNS AND SYMPTOMS
- Photophobia
- Blurring of vision
- Decreased visual acuity
- Ocular pain
- Nausea/vomiting

## History
- Previous visual acuity
- Prior eye surgery
- Prior glaucoma treatment.
- Past medical history (blood disorders including sickle cell disease).
- Mechanism of trauma.
- Exact time of injury and of visual loss.
- History of excessive tearing after injury.

**ALERT**
History of excessive tearing may indicate open globe injury.

## Physical Exam
- General physical exam with emphasis on associated bodily injuries.
- Periorbital ecchymosis
- Eyelid lacerations
- Enophthalmos (depression of the globe within the orbit)
- Limited ocular movement with diplopia (may indicate orbital floor fracture)
- Proptosis (may indicate retro-orbital hemorrhage)
- Ocular exam:
  – Visual acuity
  – Rule out open globe (positive Seidel sign, corneal laceration, prolapse of intra-ocular structures)
  – Pupillary reaction to light (check for afferent pupillary defect prior to using dilating drops)
  – Tonometry for intraocular pressure (IOP) measurement

**ALERT**
Exclude globe perforation before measuring intraocular pressure (IOP); low pressure can indicate globe perforation.

- Slit-lamp exam; look for layer of blood in AC:
  – 4 grades of hyphema depending on percentage of anterior chamber occlusion by blood:
    ○ Grade I: <1/3
    ○ Grade II: 1/3–1/2
    ○ Grade III: >1/2
    ○ Grade IV: Total (called 8-ball hyphema; blood is dark and filling 100% of AC)
  – High-grade hyphemas are:
    ○ More likely to rebleed (25% of grade I compared with 67% of grade III)
    ○ More likely to develop glaucoma and corneal staining
    ○ Less likely to recover visual acuity
  – Dilated fundus exam (avoid pressure on globe)

## DIAGNOSTIC TESTS & INTERPRETATION
### Lab
- Laboratory tests should be individualized depending on the case.
- Platelet count, PT/PTT, bleeding time if bleeding disorder is suspected, or if the patient is on anticoagulants.
- BUN, creatinine, and pregnancy test if aminocaproic acid is to be used (see below)
- Factor VIII assay if family history of hemophilia
- Sickle cell screen especially in African Americans and Mediterranean descent

### Imaging
- CT orbits (1-mm cuts) if open globe injury, intraocular foreign body, or orbital wall fracture is suspected
- US biomicroscopy (B scan) if total hyphema and intraocular structures cannot be visualized.

**ALERT**
Do not perform B scan if open globe injury is suspected (pressure applied during this procedure may cause extrusion of intraocular contents).

## ESSENTIAL WORKUP
- Exam: Visual acuity, status of globe, intra-ocular pressure, associated ocular/bodily injuries
- Labs: Platelet count, PT/PTT, and sickle cell screen if indicated
- Imaging: B scan or CT orbits if indicated

## DIFFERENTIAL DIAGNOSIS
- Uveitis
- Endophthalmitis

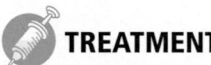 **TREATMENT**

## PRE-HOSPITAL
Place eye shield in case of corneal perforation.

## INITIAL STABILIZATION/THERAPY
- Keep head upright to allow blood in AC to settle down.
- Limit activity; avoid bending, straining, or exertion.
- Place metal or plastic shield over involved eye until integrity of globe is confirmed.
- Do not patch affected eye (if eye is patched, patient cannot notice sudden loss of vision).
- Note that metal and plastic shields have holes that let patient see through whereas patch completely blocks patient's vision.

## ED TREATMENT/PROCEDURES

- Mild analgesics (avoid NSAIDs because of antiplatelet effect)
- Antiemetics (associated N/V may worsen hyphema by increasing IOP)
- Cycloplegics decrease pain from iritis:
  - Atropine 1% eyedrops: b.i.d.–t.i.d. until hyphema resolves.
- Topical steroids may decrease inflammation from iritis:
  - Prednisolone acetate: 1% eyedrops (or equivalent) 4–8 times per day until hyphema resolves (usually 7–10 days).
- Aminocaproic acid (antifibrinolytic):
  - Use in consultation with ophthalmologist:
    - Not commonly used because of frequent systemic side effects.
  - Stabilizes fibrin clot in AC and decreases incidence of rebleed, but has no effect on final visual outcome.
  - 50 mg/kg PO q4h for total of 5 days (do not exceed 30 g/d). Dose should be adjusted in renal failure.
  - May cause postural hypotension, nausea, vomiting, diarrhea.
  - New topical form is not yet FDA approved.
  - Do not use in pregnant women or in patients prone to thrombosis. It can also cause acute renal failure in patients with hemophilia.
- Prednisone:
  - Indications:
    - Hemophilia
    - Uncooperative children
    - Total hyphema
    - History of thrombotic disease
  - Dose: 0.6–0.75 mg/kg/24 h in div. doses, up to 60 mg/d for 5 days
- For increased IOP:
  - For non–sickle cell patients, treat if IOP >30 mm Hg.
  - For sickle cell patients, treat if IOP >24 mm Hg.
  - Treat until IOP is controlled as indicated above.
  - Always start with 1 medication. Add another if unsuccessful in controlling pressure:
    - β-blockers—drug of choice: Timolol or Levobunolol 0.5% b.i.d.
    - α-agonist: Brimonidine 0.2% or apraclonidine 0.5% t.i.d.
    - Topical carbonic anhydrase inhibitors (CAI): Dorzolamide 2% or brinzolamide 1% t.i.d.
    - Oral CAI: Acetazolamide 500 mg PO q12h (peds: 8–30 mg/kg/24 h q6–8h) or methazolamide 50 mg q8h.
    - Mannitol (1–2 mg/kg IV over 45 min q24h) when all other eyedrops fail to lower IOP to acceptable level.
    - Avoid CAI and Mannitol in sickle cell patients, as they may cause acidosis and induce sickling.

- Allow 25–30 min for each eyedrop to work. If after using all the drops and mannitol, IOP is still high, then surgical evacuation of blood clot is warranted (AC tap or washout).
- Drugs to avoid:
  - Pilocarpine: Constricts pupil and prevents visualization of lens and retina
  - Prostaglandin eyedrops (eg, Latanoprost): Increase inflammatory response

### ALERT
Criteria for immediate consultation with ophthalmologist from the ED (If possible, consultation should be arranged within 24 hr.):
- Visual acuity worse than 20/200 at presentation.
- Sickle cell disease/trait with high IOP
- Large hyphema (filling >1/3 of AC).
- Medically uncontrolled IOP.

## MEDICATION
### First Line
- Atropine: 1% t.i.d.
- Prednisolone acetate: 1% q.i.d.

### Second Line
- Timolol 0.5% or levobunolol 0.5% b.i.d.
- Brimonidine 0.2 % or apraclonidine 0.5% t.i.d.
- Dorzolamide 2% or brinzolamide 1% t.i.d.
- Acetazolamide: 500 mg PO q12h.

 FOLLOW-UP

### DISPOSITION
- Discharge patient on atropine, prednisolone, and any appropriate IOP-lowering medications. Continue aminocaproic acid if decision was made to start it in ED.
- Antiemetics if needed.
- Stool softeners to minimize straining during bowel movements.

### Admission Criteria
- Hyphema size is not a criterion for discharge or admission; IOP control is the most important.
- Medically uncontrolled IOP requiring surgical intervention
- Ruptured globe
- Noncompliant patients
- Associated ocular or orbital injuries
- Children <7 yr of age:
  - Age group is usually at risk of amblyopia (also called lazy eye, which is irreversible visual loss secondary to visual deprivation in early childhood).
- Patients at risk of complications (sickle cell disease, hemophilia).

### Discharge Criteria
Absence of any admission criteria with IOP <30 mm Hg for non–sickle patients and <24 mm Hg for patients with sickle cell disease/trait.

### FOLLOW-UP RECOMMENDATIONS
Arrange for follow-up with ophthalmologist:
- Daily slit-lamp exam for 3 days after initial trauma, to monitor for rebleeding, corneal staining, and increased IOP.
- Follow-up exam will determine length of treatment with atropine, prednisone acetate, and IOP-lowering eyedrops.

## PEARLS AND PITFALLS

- Rule out ruptured globe prior to checking intraocular pressure and prior to initiating treatment.
- IOP control is not immediate. Allow at least 30 min for any treatment to take effect:
  - Always check for sickle cell disease in African Americans.

## ADDITIONAL READING

- Berke S. Post-traumatic glaucoma. In: Yanoff M, Duker J, eds. *Ophthalmology*, 2nd ed. St. Louis, MO: Mosby; 2004:1518–1521.
- Crouch ER Jr, Crouch FR. Management of traumatic hyphema: Therapeutic options. *J Pediatr Ophthalmol Strabismus*. 1999;35(5):238–250.
- Culom RD Jr, Chang B., eds. Hyphema and microhyphema. In: Rhee DJ, Pyfer MF, eds. *The Wills Eye Manual: Office and Emergency Room Diagnosis and Treatment of Eye Disease*. 3rd ed. Philadelphia: Lippincott Williams & Wilkins, 1999:32–37.
- Hamill MR. Current concepts in the treatment of traumatic injury to the anterior segment. *Ophthalmol Clin North Am*. 1999;12(3):457–464.
- Sankar PS, Chen TC, Grosskrentz CL. Traumatic hyphema. *Int Ophthalmol Clin*. 2002;42(3):57–68.
- Walton W, Von Hagen S, Grigorian R. Management of traumatic hyphema. *Survey Ophthalmol*. 2002;47(4):297–334.

### See Also (Topic, Algorithm, Electronic Media Element)
- Endophthalmitis
- Globe Rupture
- Uveitis
- Vitreous Hemorrhage

 CODES

### ICD9
- 364.41 Hyphema of iris and ciliary body
- 921.3 Contusion of eyeball

H

# HYPOCALCEMIA
*Michelle Sergel*

 **BASICS**

## DESCRIPTION
- Hypocalcemia is defined as a total plasma calcium level <8.7 mg/dL:
  - Ionized calcium may be normal and, therefore, have no clinical manifestations occurring.
- Normal total serum calcium concentrations are 8.7–10.5 mg/dL.

## ETIOLOGY
- Incidence in the general population is 0.6%.
- Mechanism:
  - From either increased loss of calcium from the circulation or decreased entry into the circulation
  - Intravascular calcium circulates in 3 forms:
    - Bound to proteins (mainly albumin): 45–50%
    - Bound to complexing ions (citrate, phosphate, carbonate): 5–10%
    - Ionized (free) calcium (physiologically active form): 45–50%
  - Serum levels of calcium are primarily controlled by 3 hormones:
    - Parathyroid hormone (PTH)
    - Decrease in calcium levels leads to an increase in PTH secretion (increasing bone resorption, renal absorption, intestinal absorption, urinary phosphate excretion).
  - Vitamin D (1,25-dihydroxyvitamin D):
    - Decrease in calcium level activates vitamin D (increasing bone resorption and intestinal absorption).
  - Calcitonin:
    - Causes a direct inhibition of bone resorption with increased calcium levels
- Hypoalbuminemia—the most common cause:
  - Each g/dL decrease in serum albumin decreases protein-bound serum calcium by 0.8 mg/dL.
  - Will not change ionized (free) calcium

### Pediatric Considerations
- Children have higher values of normal calcium (9.2–11 mg/dL).
- Neonatal hypocalcemia: Total serum calcium concentrations <7.0 mg/dL or serum-ionized calcium levels <4.4 mg/dL
- Symptoms of hypocalcemia in infancy:
  - Hyperactivity, jitteriness
  - Tachypnea
  - Apneic spells with cyanosis
  - Vomiting

 **DIAGNOSIS**

## SIGNS AND SYMPTOMS
- Occur when ionized calcium <3.2 mg/dL
- Depends on both the absolute and the rate of fall in calcium concentration
- Neuromuscular:
  - Paresthesias
  - Hyperreflexia
  - Muscle spasm
  - Tetany:
    - Neuromuscular irritability
    - Uncommon unless ionized calcium <4.3 mg/dL
  - Latent tetany (Chvostek and Trousseau signs)
  - Laryngeal stridor
  - Seizures
  - Choreoathetosis
- Cardiovascular:
  - Dysrhythmias:
    - Torsades de pointes
    - Heart block
  - Hypotension
  - Impaired contractility (CHF)
  - ECG changes:
    - Bradycardia
    - QT and ST prolongation
    - T-wave abnormalities
- Psychiatric:
  - Irritability/anxiety
  - Psychosis
  - Depression
  - Confusion
  - Delusions
  - Chorea
  - Parkinsonisms
- Ocular:
  - Papilledema
  - Cataracts
  - May occur in patients with acute onset hypocalcemia

## ESSENTIAL WORKUP
Serum-ionized calcium level confirms the diagnosis

## DIAGNOSTIC TESTS & INTERPRETATION
### Lab
- Arterial blood gas:
  - Change from normal pH of 0.1 units equals a reciprocal change in ionized calcium of approximately 1.7 mg/dL.
- Serum albumin
- Electrolytes, BUN/creatinine, glucose
- Magnesium
- Phosphate:
  - Increase in phosphate associated with hypoparathyroidism
  - Decrease in phosphate associated with vitamin D deficiency
- PTH:
  - Very high levels of PTH associated with pseudohypoparathyroidism
  - High levels of PTH associated with vitamin D deficiency
  - Low levels of PTH associated with hypoparathyroidism
- Serum calcidiol or calcitriol

### Diagnostic Procedures/Surgery
ECG:
- Prolonged QT interval
- Heart block

## DIFFERENTIAL DIAGNOSIS
- Impaired PTH action or secretion:
  - Parathyroid or thyroid surgery or radical neck surgery and/or irradiation for head and neck cancer
  - Autoimmune disease (typically presents in childhood)
  - Congenital hypoparathyroidism
  - Neonatal secondary to maternal hyperparathyroidism
  - Pseudohypoparathyroidism (resistance to PTH)
  - Infiltrative (amyloidosis, sarcoidosis, metastases, iron overload)
  - HIV infection
- Impaired vitamin D synthesis or action:
  - Nutritional malabsorption or poor intake
  - Renal disease
  - Pronounced hypophosphatemia
- Sepsis or severe burns:
  - Impaired secretion of PTH and calcitriol
  - End-organ resistance to the action of PTH
- Calcium complex formation or sequestration:
  - Hyperphosphatemia
  - Ethylene glycol, ethylenediaminetetraacetic acid (EDTA), citrate (from transfusion)
  - Pancreatitis, rhabdomyolysis
  - Alkalosis (ie, hyperventilation)
- Hypomagnesemia:
  - Causes end-organ PTH resistance
  - Decreased PTH secretion
  - Seen in chronic and/or critical illness
  - Must give magnesium to correct hypocalcemia

- Medications:
  – Mithramycin, plicamycin, phosphate, calcitonin, bisphosphonates
  – Phenobarbital, phenytoin
  – Cisplatin
  – Cadmium, colchicine
  – Fluoride, citrate
- Malignancies:
  – Prostate cancer
  – Breast cancer
  – Lung cancer
  – Chondrosarcoma
- "Hungry bone syndrome:"
  – After parathyroid removal
  – Rapid accretion of calcium as bone is remineralized

 **TREATMENT**

### INITIAL STABILIZATION/THERAPY
ABCs:
- Establish IV catheter access.
- Cardiac monitor

### ED TREATMENT/PROCEDURES
- Acute management:
  – Treat symptomatic hypocalcemia as a medical emergency with parenteral calcium administration.
  – Calcium IV bolus:
    ○ Calcium gluconate 1–2 g in 50 mL of 5% dextrose
    ○ Infuse over 10–20 min
    ○ Faster IV rates can cause cardiac dysrhythmias
    ○ Calcium salts are irritating to veins.
    ○ IM calcium gluceptate or calcium gluconate if IV access not available
    ○ Bolus dose increases ionized calcium for only 1–2 hr, therefore, must be followed by an infusion
  – Calcium infusion:
    ○ Calcium infusion rate: 0.5–1.5 mg/kg/h
    ○ Do not mix with bicarbonate or phosphate or precipitation of salts may form.
    ○ Administer cautiously in patients taking digitalis—may initiate and exacerbate digitalis toxicity
  – Response to therapy:
    ○ Individual responses vary.
    ○ Monitor calcium concentrations q1–4h during therapy.
    ○ Titrate treatment to symptoms or ECG changes.
    ○ Consider hypomagnesemia if the patient fails to respond to calcium therapy—correct hypomagnesemia with Mg 2 g IVPB 10% solution over 10 min
    ○ In the setting of acidosis, correct calcium 1st; alkalosis will further reduce ionized calcium.
    ○ Side effects of IV calcium include: Nausea, vomiting, hypotension, and dysrhythmias

- Chronic management:
  – Oral calcium supplementation
  – 1–4 g/d of elemental calcium in divided doses
  – Vitamin D:
    ○ Enhances intestinal absorption
    ○ Initiate with calcium supplementation—alone not sufficient to restore calcium levels.
    ○ 200 IU for ages 19–50 yr
    ○ 400 IU for ages 51–70 yr
    ○ 600–800 for ages >70 yr
    ○ Multivitamins contain 400 IU of vitamin D
  – Vitamin D preparations:
    ○ Ergocalciferol: 125 μg/d
    ○ Dihydrotachysterol: 100–400 μg/d
    ○ Calcifediol: 50–200 μg/d
    ○ Calcitriol: 0.25–0.2 μg/d:
    ○ Rapid onset (preferred)
    ○ Most active metabolite of vitamin D

### Pregnancy Considerations
Calcitriol requirements may double or triple toward the end of pregnancy.

### MEDICATION
- IV calcium:
  – Calcium chloride: 1 g in 10 mL (1 g = 360 mg [13.6 mEq] elemental calcium)
  – Calcium gluceptate (IV/IM): 1 g in 5 mL (1 g = 90 mg [4.5 mEq] elemental calcium)
  – Calcium gluconate: 1 g in 10 mL (1 g = 90 mg [4.5 mEq] elemental calcium)
- Oral calcium:
  – Calcium carbonate: 350- to 1,500-mg tablets (1 g = 400 mg)
  – Calcium citrate: 950-mg tablets (1 g = 211 mg elemental calcium)
  – Calcium glubionate: 18 g/5 mL of syrup (1 g = 65 mg elemental calcium)
  – Calcium gluconate: 500- to 1,000-mg tablets (1 g = 90 mg elemental calcium)
  – Calcium lactate: 350- to 1,000-mg tablets (1 g = 130 mg elemental calcium)

### Pediatric Considerations
- Initial calcium bolus with 10% calcium gluconate should be 9–18 mg of elemental calcium/kg or 1–2 mL/kg not to exceed 5 mL in premature infants or 10 mL in term infants.
- Calcitriol dose in children ranges from 0.1–3 μg/d.
- MISCELLANEOUS:
  – Calcium content of common foods:
    ○ Milk or yogurt, 8 oz = 300 mg
    ○ Cheddar cheese, 1 oz = 200 mg
    ○ Calcium-fortified cereal, 1 cup = 300 mg
    ○ Calcium-fortified orange juice, 1 cup = 270 mg
    ○ Shrimp, 3 oz = 50 mg
    ○ Peanuts = 130 mg
    ○ Orange = 50 mg

 **FOLLOW-UP**

### DISPOSITION
#### Admission Criteria
- Symptomatic or severe ionized hypocalcemia (<3.2 mg/dL)
- Continuous IV calcium preparations necessary to maintain calcium levels

#### Discharge Criteria
- Asymptomatic hypocalcemia
- Ionized calcium >3.2 mg/dL in healthy patients with no co-morbid illness

### FOLLOW-UP RECOMMENDATIONS
Close follow-up with an endocrinologist may be necessary for impaired PTH or vitamin D action or synthesis.

## PEARLS AND PITFALLS

- Hypocalcemia has many causes
- Treatment of hypocalcemia varies with its severity and underlying cause
- Patients that are severely symptomatic require rapid correction with IV calcium therapy
- To effectively treat hypocalcemia with concurrent magnesium deficiency, magnesium must first be normalized

## ADDITIONAL READING

- Horak HA, Poumand R. Endocrine myopathies. *Neurol Clin.* 2000;18(1):203–213.
- Kapoor M, Chan Z. Fluid and electrolyte abnormalities. *Crit Care Clin.* 2001;17(3):503–529.
- Riggs JE. Neurologic manifestations of electrolyte disturbances. *Neurol Clin.* 2002;20(1):227–239, vii.
- Thakker R. Hypocalcemia: Pathogenesis, differential diagnosis, and management. In Favus M, ed. *Primer on the Metabolic Bone Diseases and Disorders of Mineral Metabolism*, American Society of Bone and Mineral Research; 2006:6:213.
- Thomas MK, Demay MB. Vitamin D deficiency and disorders of vitamin D metabolism. *Endocrinol Metab Clin North Am.* 2000;29(3):611–627, viii.

### See Also (Topic, Algorithm, Electronic Media Element)
- Hypercalcemia
- Hyperparathyroidism
- Hypoparathyroidism

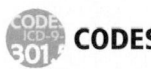 **CODES**

### ICD9
275.41 Hypocalcemia

H

# HYPOGLYCEMIA

*Matthew N. Graber*
*Brian V. Maneevese*

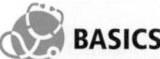 **BASICS**

## DESCRIPTION
- Deficiency in counterregulatory hormones (glucagon, epinephrine, cortisol, growth hormone) or excessive insulin response
- Serum glucose < 70 mg/dL

## RISK FACTORS
### Genetics
- Congenital metabolic and endocrine disorders that decrease gluconeogenic ability (eg, hereditary fructose intolerance)
- Congenital hyperinsulinism
- Neonatal diabetes mellitus (often a mutation effecting an ATP-dependent potassium channel)

## ETIOLOGY
- Increased insulin levels:
  - Overdose of oral hypoglycemic agent or insulin
  - Oral antihyperglycemics (ie, $\alpha$-glucosidase inhibitors, biguanides, and thiazolidinediones) do not cause hypoglycemia alone, but may enhance the risk when used with insulin or sulfonylureas.
  - Sepsis
  - Insulinoma
  - Autoimmune hypoglycemia
  - Alimentary hyperinsulinism
  - Renal failure (partially responsible for insulin metabolism)
  - Liver cirrhosis (responsible for significant insulin metabolism)
- Underproduction of glucose:
  - Alcohol (inhibitory effect on glycogen storage and gluconeogenesis)
  - Drugs
  - Salicylates
  - $\beta$-blockers (including eyedrops)
  - SSRIs
  - Some antibiotics (eg, sulfonylureas, pentamidine)
  - Adrenal insufficiency
  - Malnutrition
  - Dehydration
- Cerebral edema
- Extremes of age
- CHF
- Counterregulatory hormone deficiency
- Hypothyroidism or hyperthyroidism

### Pregnancy Considerations
- 3rd-trimester pregnant patients risk relative substrate deficiency–induced hypoglycemia.
- The fetus is less likely to become hypoglycemic during mother's hypoglycemic episode secondary to active glucose transport across placenta:
  - Oral hypoglycemic use in pregnancy may lead to profound and prolonged neonatal hypoglycemia.

### Pediatric Considerations
Most common cause of hypoglycemia in the 1st 3 mo of life is persistent hyperinsulinemic hypoglycemia of infancy (PHHI) in mothers with diabetes.

 **DIAGNOSIS**

## SIGNS AND SYMPTOMS
- Adrenergic caused by excessive counterregulatory hormones (ie, epinephrine):
  - Diaphoresis
  - Anxiety
  - Tachycardia
  - Hunger
- Neuroglycopenic:
  - Dizziness
  - Confusion
- Hyperactive or psychotic behavior:
  - Slurred speech
  - Cranial nerve palsies
  - Seizures
  - Hemiplegia
  - Decerebrate posturing
- Neonatal presentation:
  - Asymptomatic
  - Limp
  - Bradycardia
  - Irritable
  - Tremulous
  - Seizures
  - Poor feeding

### ALERT
Patients with "hypoglycemia unawareness" have reduced warning signals, do not recognize that their blood sugar is low, and instead may present with only late findings such as seizure, focal neurologic findings, altered mental status, and coma.

## History
- Underlying diseases or conditions: Diabetes, renal failure, liver failure, alcohol use.
- Certain medications—long acting insulin and oral agents—are more concerning.
- Possible insulin or oral hypoglycemia overdose.

### Physical Exam
See signs and symptoms

## ESSENTIAL WORKUP
- Diagnosis requires:
  - Demonstration of neuroglycopenic signs and symptoms as defined above
  - Lab evidence of hypoglycemia
  - Clearing of symptoms following glucose administration

## DIAGNOSTIC TESTS & INTERPRETATION
### Lab
- Blood glucose (initial and posttreatment)
- Electrolytes, BUN, creatinine
- Prothrombin time
- Urinalysis for possible infection
- Urine and other cultures as appropriate in evaluation for infection

### Imaging
CXR for:
- Possible aspiration during hypoglycemic episode
- Pneumonia as source of sepsis

### Diagnostic Procedures/Surgery
ECG if suspect MI/ischemia owing to hypoglycemia or as cause of hypoglycemia

## DIFFERENTIAL DIAGNOSIS
The differential diagnosis is extensive; see Altered Mental Status for a complete list. Major concerns include:
- Neurologic:
  - Cerebral vascular accident/transient ischemic attack (CVA/TIA)
  - Seizure disorder
- Drug or alcohol intoxication
- Hypoxia
- Sepsis
- Metabolic derangements
- Endocrine derangements
- Environmental stressors
- Psychosis, depression, or anxiety

### Pediatric Considerations
- Growth hormone deficiency
- Inborn errors of metabolism
- Ketotic hypoglycemia
- Reye syndrome
- Salicylate ingestion

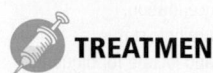 TREATMENT

### PRE-HOSPITAL
- Diagnosis with finger stick glucose
- IV dextrose preferred
- Oral glucose–containing fluids if unable to obtain IV.

### INITIAL STABILIZATION/THERAPY
- ABCs with aspiration and seizure precautions
- Glucose:
  - Dextrose IV push (IVP)—this should always be given if possible.
  - Oral glucose in awake patient (with no IV) without risk of aspiration
  - Glucagon IM if unable to establish IV access

### ED TREATMENT/PROCEDURES
- Administer $D_{50}W$ 50 mL for decreased level of consciousness:
  - 2nd or 3rd amp may be necessary.
  - Complications include volume overload and hypokalemia.
- Administer octreotide:
  - If hypoglycemia refractory to glucose administration
  - If hypoglycemia secondary to sulfonylureas
  - Initiate continuous IV infusion of 5–20% glucose solution for persistent mild hypoglycemia or if patient cannot eat.
- Administer glucagon:
  - If hypoglycemia refractory to glucose
  - If IV access delayed
  - Ineffective in alcohol induced hypoglycemia and significant liver disease
  - May repeat twice q20–30min
  - Administer hydrocortisone with glucagon for adrenal insufficiency.
  - Effective in 10–20 min

### Geriatric Considerations
Elderly patients often require significant time for resolution of symptoms, even after appropriate treatment of hypoglycemia.

### MEDICATION
#### First Line
$D_{50}W$: 1 amp (25 g) of 50% dextrose 1–2 mL/kg (child: 2 mL/kg $D_{25}W$; infants: 5 mL/kg $D_{10}W$) IVP

#### Second Line
- Octreotide: 50 $\mu$g q12h SC/IV or 50 uq IV then 50 $\mu$g IV/hr drip
- Glucagon: 0.5–2 mg IV/IM/SC:
  - Child: 0.03–0.1 mg/kg IV/IM/SC
  - Infant: 0.3 mg/kg IV/IM/SC; may repeat in 4 hr
- Hydrocortisone: 100 mg (peds: 1–2 mg/kg) IV
- Oral glucose: 20 g orally equals ~12-oz nondiet fruit juice, 14-oz nondiet cola, 2.5-oz chocolate

 FOLLOW-UP

### DISPOSITION
#### Admission Criteria
- Overdose of long-acting oral hypoglycemic agent (eg, sulfonylureas) or long-acting insulin mandate observation for at least 24 hr.
- Failure of neuroglycopenic symptoms to improve with glucose administration suggests neurologic injury, pre-existing neurologic condition, or another cause for these symptoms.
- Recurrent hypoglycemic state in ED
- Patients unable to tolerate oral fluids or food
- Suicidal intentions
- Older patients may require several days for complete recovery from severe or prolonged hypoglycemia.

#### Discharge Criteria
- Discharge mild unintentional insulin overusage or failure to take oral calories if blood glucose normal, symptoms resolved, tolerating oral intake, and can be observed.
- Families of patient with recurrent hypoglycemia should be instructed in IM glucagon administration.
- Monitor blood glucose for at least 3 hr prior to discharge.

### Issues for Referral
Refer to primary physician for consideration of medication or diet changes if recurrent hypoglycemic episodes.

### FOLLOW-UP RECOMMENDATIONS
PMD follow-up for medication re-evaluation within 48 hr

## PEARLS AND PITFALLS
- Administration of PO glucose or food may initially further decrease glucose level; therefore, IV dextrose always preferred if possible:
  - Multiple amps of $D_{50}W$ commonly required
  - Do not over rely on D10/D20 as even these concentrations contain relatively small amounts of glucose.
  - Hypoglycemia should be in the differential for all neurologic and psychiatric presentations.

## ADDITIONAL READING
- Guettier JM, Gorden P. Endocrinology and metabolism. *Clin North Am.* 2006;35:753–766.
- Service FJ. Hypoglycemia. *Med Clin North Am.* 1995;79(1):16.
- Service FJ. Medical progress: Hypoglycemic disorders. *N Engl J Med.* 1995;332:1144–1152.
- Stanley CA, Baker L. The causes of neonatal hypoglycemia. *N Engl J Med.* 1999;340:1200–1201.

### See Also (Topic, Algorithm, Electronic Media Element)
- Adrenal Insufficiency
- Altered Mental Status
- Cirrhosis
- Renal Failure

 CODES

### ICD9
- 250.80 Diabetes mellitus with other specified manifestations, type ii or unspecified type, not stated as uncontrolled
- 250.81 Diabetes mellitus with other specified manifestations, type I (juvenile type) not stated as uncontrolled
- 251.2 Hypoglycemia, unspecified

H

# HYPOGLYCEMIC AGENT POISONING

*Timothy J. Meehan*
*Mark B. Mycyk*

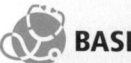 **BASICS**

## DESCRIPTION
- Oral or parenteral agents that may cause hypoglycemia or other metabolic imbalances.
- Hypoglycemic poisoning may be intentional or unintentional (accidental).

## ETIOLOGY
- Insulin:
  - Enhances glucose uptake into cells
  - Limits glucose availability to the brain (most sensitive to hypoglycemia)
  - Influences potassium redistribution (hypokalemia)
- Sulfonylurea agents:
  - Enhance insulin release from pancreatic $\beta$ cells, reduce hepatic glucose production, and increase peripheral insulin sensitivity
  - Hypoglycemic effect enhanced by:
    ○ Polypharmacy (drug interactions)
    ○ Alcohol use and hepatic dysfunction (poor nutritional stores)
    ○ Renal insufficiency (decreased clearance)
- Biguanide agents (metformin):
  - Antihyperglycemic agents:
    ○ Decrease elevated serum glucose concentrations
    ○ Generally do not cause hypoglycemia in isolation.
  - In the presence of insulin, biguanides do the following:
    ○ Increase glucose uptake into cells
    ○ Limit glucose availability to the brain (most sensitive to hypoglycemia)
    ○ Influence potassium redistribution (hypokalemia)
    ○ Decrease gastrointestinal glucose absorption
    ○ Decrease hepatic gluconeogenesis
    ○ Metabolize glucose to lactate in intestinal cells, which may accumulate and lead to profound lactic acidosis
- Thiazolidinediones:
  - In the presence of insulin, thiazolidinediones increase glucose uptake and use and decrease gluconeogenesis
- $\alpha$-Glucosidase inhibitors:
  - Lower systemic glucose by decreasing GI absorption of carbohydrates

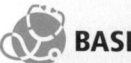 **DIAGNOSIS**

## SIGNS AND SYMPTOMS
- Insulin or sulfonylureas:
  - Overdose causes hypoglycemia.
  - Symptoms most often occur when glucose <40–60 mg/dL (may occur at higher levels in diabetics).
  - Symptoms blunted by $\beta$-antagonists.
  - Facial flushing, diaphoresis, pallor, piloerection
  - Hunger, nausea, abdominal cramping
  - Labored respirations, apnea
  - Headache, blurred vision
  - Paresthesias, weakness, incoordination, tremor
  - Anxiety, irritability, bizarre behavior, confusion, stupor, coma, seizures
  - Palpitations, tachycardia, bradycardia (late)
  - Hypertension
  - Hypothermia
- Biguanides:
  - Toxicity primarily owing to lactic acid accumulation
  - Nausea, vomiting, abdominal pain
  - Agitation, confusion, lethargy, coma
  - Kussmaul respirations
  - Hypotension, tachycardia

### Pediatric Considerations
- Neonatal hypoglycemia may occur after maternal use of sulfonylureas during labor.
- Ingestion of 1 sulfonylurea tablet may cause hypoglycemia in a child:
  - Death has been reported after ingestion of a single tablet.
- Onset of symptomatic hypoglycemia may be delayed up to 8 hr.

### History
- Diagnosis of diabetes in patient
- Access to diabetic medications:
  - If occurring in a medical setting (hospital, nursing home), consider:
    ○ Dosing error
    ○ Malicious intent

### Physical Exam
- Vital signs:
  - Tachycardia (may be blunted if on $\beta$-blockers)
- Neurologic:
  - Confusion, obtundation, coma
  - Ataxia, other cerebellar signs

## ESSENTIAL WORKUP
- Diagnosis based on clinical presentation and an accurate history
- Monitor serum glucose concentration.
- Monitor vital signs and neurologic status.
- Obtain serum electrolytes and lactate for biguanide ingestion.
- Obtain liver function tests for thiazolidinedione ingestion.

## DIAGNOSTIC TESTS & INTERPRETATION
### Lab
- Serum glucose before and after treatment
- Electrolytes:
  - Check for hypokalemia
  - Anion gap acidosis
- BUN, creatinine:
  - May reveal renal insufficiency, causing drug accumulation
- CBC
- Ethanol level
- Lactate level (especially if biguanide medications involved)
- Liver function tests
- Arterial blood gas
- Assays for immunoreactive insulin and C-peptide levels:
  - Confirms administration of exogenous insulin if insulin level is high and C-peptide is low in the setting of hypoglycemia.
  - Do not correlate with severity of clinical symptoms.

### Imaging
- ECG: Sinus tachycardia, premature ventricular contractions (PVCs), atrial dysrhythmias
- EEG: Diffuse slowing without focal abnormalities
- CT scan: Cerebral edema if prolonged hypoglycemia
- Chest radiograph: Aspiration pneumonia or pulmonary edema

## DIFFERENTIAL DIAGNOSIS
- Addison disease
- Panhypopituitarism
- Sepsis
- Insulinoma
- Neuroendocrine tumors
- Cirrhosis
- Chronic ethanol abuse
- Ethanol ingestion
- Salicylate ingestion
- $\beta$-antagonist ingestion
- Ackee fruit poisoning

**TREATMENT**

### PRE-HOSPITAL
Transport all medications, pills, and pill bottles involved in overdose for identification in ED.

### INITIAL STABILIZATION/THERAPY
- ABCs:
  - Airway control essential
  - Administer supplemental oxygen.
  - IV access
  - Cardiac monitor and pulse oximetry
- Naloxone, thiamine, $D_{50}$ (or Accu-Chek) if altered mental status

### ED TREATMENT/PROCEDURES
- Hypoglycemia:
  - $D_{50}$ bolus, then:
    ○ IV infusion $D_5W$ or $D_{10}W$ to maintain euglycemia or mild hyperglycemia
    ○ Food (if mental status improves or normalizes)
- Neuroglycopenia:
  - May persist shortly after serum glucose corrected
  - Persistent symptoms require further dextrose administration.
- Decontamination:
  - Consider administration of activated charcoal for recent or large ingestion of oral agent (sulfonylurea or biguanide).
- Provide supportive care
- Hypotension:
  - 0.9% NS IV fluid bolus
  - Pressor support with dopamine or norepinephrine as needed:
    ○ Pressors may increase lactate production
    ○ Use cautiously with biguanide-induced lactic acidosis
- Administer sodium bicarbonate for biguanide-induced lactic acidosis if pH <7.0.
- Administer benzodiazepines for seizures.
- Inhibit insulin secretion for sulfonylurea overdose with recurrent hypoglycemia with:
  - Octreotide
  - Diazoxide (watch for hypotension)
- Early hemodialysis may be beneficial in cases of biguanide-induced lactic acidosis:
  - Corrects acid–base abnormalities
  - Enhances elimination of the drug

### MEDICATION
- Activated charcoal: 1 mg/kg PO
- Dextrose: 50–100 mL $D_{50}$ (peds: 2 mL/kg of $D_{25}$ over 1 min) IV; repeat if necessary
- Diazepam: 5–10 mg (peds: 0.2–0.5 mg/kg) IV q10–15min
- Diazoxide: 200 mg PO or 1–3 mg/kg IV (infant: 8–15 mg/kg/24 h q8–12h PO/IV; child: 3–8 mg/kg/24 h q8h PO/IV)
- Glucagon: 1–2 mg (peds: 0.03–0.1 mg/kg) IM/SC/IV
- Lorazepam: 2–4 mg (peds: 0.03–0.05 mg/kg) IV q10–15min
- Octreotide: 50–100 $\mu$g q8–12h SC/IV
- Thiamine (vitamin $B_1$): 100 mg (peds: 50 mg) IV or IM

 **FOLLOW-UP**

### DISPOSITION
#### Admission Criteria
- Hypoglycemia owing to sulfonylurea agents (may require several days of monitoring) or long-acting insulin preparations.
- Any patient requiring a constant infusion of dextrose to maintain euglycemia.
- Intentional overdose or self-injection of insulin warrants admission for 24-hr glucose monitoring.
- All children with accidental ingestion of sulfonylureas
- Metabolic alterations owing to biguanide ingestion or accumulation

#### Discharge Criteria
- Accidental hypoglycemia owing to short-acting insulin injection in the setting of dietary insufficiency:
    Must be tolerating oral intake
  - Ensure return to baseline mental status
- Discharge after glucose correction and a 4-h period of observation.

#### Issues for Referral
- Patients with unintentional (accidental) poisoning require poison prevention counseling.
- Patients with intentional (eg, suicide) poisoning require psychiatric evaluation.

### FOLLOW-UP RECOMMENDATIONS
Close primary care follow-up to help monitor blood sugar and adjust medication dosages.

### PEARLS AND PITFALLS
- Sulfonylureas can have markedly prolonged half-lives and long elimination times:
  - Delayed hypoglycemia and refractory hypoglycemia are common
  - Admit for observation, at a minimum
- Metformin must be held for 48 hr after any study requiring IV contrast media:
  - IV contrast can prolong renal clearance of biguanides.
  - Can induce metformin-associated lactic acidosis.

### ADDITIONAL READING
- Green RS, Palatnick W. Effectiveness of octreotide in a case of refractory sulfonylurea-induced hypoglycemia. *J Emerg Med*. 2003;25(3):283–287.
- Kruse JA. Metformin-associated lactic acidosis. *J Emerg Med*. 2001;20(3):267–272.
- Little GL, Boniface KS. Are one or two dangerous? Sulfonylurea exposure in toddlers. *J Emerg Med*. 2005;28(3):305–310.
- McLaughlin SA, Crandall CS, McKinney PE. Octreotide: An antidote for sulfonylurea-induced hypoglycemia. *Ann Emerg Med*. 2000;36(2):133–138.
- Spiller HA. Management of antidiabetic medications in overdose. *Drug Safety*. 1998;19(5):411–424.
- Wolf LR, Smeeks F, Policastro M. Oral hypoglycemic agents. In: Ford MD, Delaney KA, Ling LJ, et al., eds. *Clinical Toxicology*. Philadelphia: WB Saunders; 2001:423–432.

### See Also (Topic, Algorithm, Electronic Media Element)
- Hypoglycemia

**CODES**

ICD9
962.3 Poisoning by insulins and antidiabetic agents

**H**

# HYPOKALEMIA

*David N. Zull*

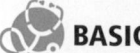 **BASICS**

## DESCRIPTION
- Defined as a serum potassium level <3.5 mEq/L:
  - Mild to moderate 2.5–3.5 mEq/L
  - Moderate to severe <2.5 mEq/L
- Frequency:
  - Up to 20% of inpatients have documented hypokalemia (5% have levels <3.0 mEq/L).
  - Up to 14% of outpatients are mildly hypokalemic (most are related to diuretics or GI loss).
  - 5% of geriatric patients have K <3.0 mEq/L.
- Potassium is the major intracellular cation:
  - Gradient is maintained by Na-K ATPase activity (enhanced by insulin and $\beta$-agonists) and mineralocorticoids.
- Total body potassium is approximately 55 mEq/kg of body weight (98% ICF, 2% ECF).
- Electrophysiologic effects of hypokalemia:
  - Increase in the normal intracellular to extracellular potassium gradient:
    - Alters the depolarization threshold for muscles and nerves
    - Inhibits the termination of action potentials
  - Alterations in intracellular potassium directly affect cellular function.

## ETIOLOGY
### Renal Losses
- Diuretics (thiazides, loop diuretics, carbonic anhydrase inhibitors), usually associated with loss of other cations ($Mg^{2+}$, $Ca^{2+}$, $P^{3+}$, $Na^+$)
- Renal tubular damage:
  - Primary renal tubular disorders (RTA type I and II)
  - Interstitial nephritis, analgesic nephropathy, drug toxicity (amphotericin, gentamicin, toluene, cisplatin), myeloma kidney
  - Overdose toxicity: Acetaminophen, NSAIDs, hydroxychloroquine
- Hyperaldosteronism:
  - Primary (primary hyperaldosteronism, Cushing, pituitary tumor-producing ACTH, congenital adrenal hyperplasia)
  - Secondary (volume depletion, CHF, cirrhosis, nephrotic)
  - Exogenous (steroids; glycyrrhizic acid in licorice and Chinese herbals)
- Hypomagnesemia (increased secretion)
- Polyuria:
  - Osmotic diuresis (mannitol, hyperglycemia)
  - Psychogenic polydipsia
- Congenital disorders:
  - Bartter and Gitelman syndromes—hypokalemic metabolic alkalosis and low BP:
    - Liddle syndrome is the same but with hypertension.
- Delivery of nonreabsorbable anions such that sodium is reabsorbed and potassium is exchanged out and excreted:
  - Bicarbonate in emesis
  - B-hydroxybutyrate in DKA
  - Hippurate in toluene abuse
  - Penicillins—high dose IV therapy
  - Renal artery stenosis with hyperreninism

### GI Losses
- Diarrhea:
  - Proportional to volume and duration
  - Villous adenomas (K losses are more severe)
  - Laxative abuse
- Vomiting and nasogastric suction result in volume depletion and metabolic alkalosis, which increases renal losses of potassium from bicarbonaturia and hyperaldosteronism.
- Ureterosigmoidostomy
- Intestinal fistulae, ileostomy
- Cystic fibrosis

### Intracellular Shift of Potassium
- Alkalosis (metabolic or respiratory)
- Insulin:
  - Insulin administration
  - Stimulation of insulin release by glucose administration
  - Refeeding in prolonged starvation
- Adrenergic excess:
  - Severe stress (trauma, MI, sepsis)
  - Treatment of asthma (frequent $\beta$-agonists and theophylline toxicity)
  - Cocaine, amphetamines
- Hypokalemic periodic paralysis:
  - Familial
  - Thyrotoxic
- $B_{12}$ administration in severely deficient patient
- Barium salt poisoning

### Poor Intake (Rare as a Sole Cause)
- Nutritional (poverty, pica, dementia)
- Eating disorders
- Dental problems/oral lesions
- Esophageal disease

 **DIAGNOSIS**

## SIGNS AND SYMPTOMS
### History
- Neuromuscular:
  - Severe weakness (K <2.5 mEq/L):
    - Begins in the lower extremities and progresses cephalad
  - May progress to paralysis if K <2.0 mEq/L and rapid development
  - Muscle cramps, tetany, and tenderness
  - Rhabdomyolysis
  - Paresthesias
  - Generalized fatigue and malaise
- GI:
  - Constipation
  - Ileus
- Cardiovascular (heart disease increases risk):
  - Ventricular and atrial premature beats
  - AV block, atrial or junctional tachycaridias
  - Ventricular tachycardia or fibrillation
  - Potentiation of digoxin toxicity
- Renal:
  - Impaired urinary concentrating ability resistant to ADH (polyuria, polydipsia)
  - Increased renal bicarbonate reabsorption and ammonia production (worsens alkalosis)

### Physical Exam
- HTN—renal artery stenosis, primary hyperaldosteronism, licorice, congenital adrenal hyperplasia, Liddle syndrome, glucocorticoid use
- Hypotension—GI losses, diuretic use, Bartter and Gitelman syndromes
- Neuromuscular—muscle weakness, decreased reflexes, muscle tenderness if rhabdomyolysis

## DIAGNOSTIC TESTS & INTERPRETATION
### Lab
- Electrolytes, BUN, creatinine, glucose:
  - High $HCO_3$ suggests diuretic abuse, vomiting, mineralocorticoid excess, Bartter, Gitelman.
  - Low $HCO_3$ suggests renal tubular disease or diarrhea
  - Low serum sodium suggests diuretic use or marked volume depletion from GI losses
  - High serum sodium suggests nephrogenic diabetes insipidus or primary hyperaldosteronism
- Urine K (spot sample):
  - <20 mEq/L suggests GI loss, potassium shift into cells, poor intake.
  - >40 mEq/L suggests renal loss.
  - 20–40 mEq/L—calculate transtubular potassium gradient (TTPG) = (urine K × serum osm)/(serum K × urine osm):
    - >7 suggests renal loss; <3 GI loss, poor intake; 3–7, mixed
- Urine Na:
  - <20 mEq/L with elevated urine K suggests secondary hyperaldosteronism.
- Plasma renin if hypertensive:
  - High renin: Secondary hyperaldosteronism, renal artery stenosis
  - Low renin: Primary hyperaldosteronism
- TSH and free T4 if Asian male

### ECG Findings
- Low-voltage T waves
- Sagging of the ST segments
- U waves:
  - In severe hypokalemia, the T disappears and the U wave predominates, giving the illusion of dramatic QT prolongation.
- Diminutive P waves (sometimes misread as a nodal rhythm)
- Dysrhythmias (very prevalent if underlying cardiomyopathy or digoxin toxic):
  - Atrial: Premature atrial contractions [PACs], atrial fibrillation [A fib]
  - Ventricular: Premature ventricular contractions (PVCs), ventricular tachycardia (VT), torsade

## DIFFERENTIAL DIAGNOSIS
- Intrinsic cardiac disease with dysrhythmias
- Causes of muscular weakness:
  - Neuromuscular junction disease (myasthenia gravis, organophosphate poisoning, botulism)
  - Spinal cord disease
  - Polyneuropathies
  - Primary acute myopathies
  - Cataplexy

**TREATMENT**

### INITIAL STABILIZATION/THERAPY
- Establish IV access/volume resuscitation
- ABCs
- Cardiac monitoring

### ED TREATMENT/PROCEDURES
- Total body deficit is 200–300 mEq per 1 mEq/L decrement in serum potassium level.
- Rate of replacement and route dependent on presence of symptoms, severity of hypokalemia, and comorbidities.
- Complete replacement over several days
- Oral potassium preferable to IV therapy whenever possible
- Identify and prevent ongoing K losses:
  - Hold diuretics or laxatives
  - Treat vomiting or diarrhea
  - Minimize nasogastric suction losses by administering H2 blockers or PPI's
  - Avoid glucose containing fluids

### MEDICATION
- Oral potassium chloride:
  - Preferred replacement in almost all cases
  - Liquid (or powder dissolved in water or juice) is more bioavailable, but nausea may occur:
    - 10–40 mEq per dose
    - Rapid rise in K, but will drop after 4 hr from transcellular shift
  - Tablets (wax matrix and microencapsulated):
    - More palatable, more sustained effect
    - Slowly absorbed
    - Potential for small bowel ulceration.
  - Dosage for hypokalemia:
    - Mild to moderate 10–20 mEq q6–12h
    - Moderate to severe 40–60 mEq q8–12h
    - Continue until K remains 3.0–3.5 mEq/L
- Oral potassium gluconate or citrate:
  - Use in acidotic patients (eg, RTA)
  - Ineffective if accompanying metabolic alkalosis
  - Less effective than KCl
  - Can be used as prophylaxis of calcium oxalate renal stones or may dissolve uric acid stones
- IV potassium:
  - Recommended if neuromuscular symptoms, cardiac arrhythmias, ongoing GI losses, or severe hypokalemia
  - Potassium chloride is the preferred replacement:
    - Potassium phosphate is used only if accompanying severe hypophosphatemia.
  - Administration:
    - A potassium rider at 10 mEq/h piggybacked into maintenance 0.9 NS is safest and best tolerated (peds: 0.1–0.2 mEq/kg/h)
    - 15–20 mEq/h are feasible by peripheral vein but not recommended due to risk of phlebitis and pain

- If K is added to maintenance fluids, the concentration should not be >40 mEq/L and dextrose solutions should be avoided
- If sustained life-threatening dysrhythmias, 20–40 mEq/h by central line or 2 peripheral lines can be considered.
- If cardiac arrest occurs in a patient with known severe hypokalemia, 20 mEq could be given IV over 2–3 min
- Frequent monitoring of serum potassium is critical when large amounts of K are used (after every 40 mEq IV)
- Hypokalemic periodic paralysis and other situations in which there is significant transcellular K shifts (adrenergic excess):
  - Small amounts of K are effective (20 mEq IV).
  - More zealous administration may lead to rebound hyperkalemia.
- Electrolyte corrections:
  - Magnesium:
    - Consider if hypokalemia is resistant to K replacement.
    - Magnesium sulfate 2 g slow IV infusion
  - Chloride:
    - Hypokalemia with alkalosis is resistant to replacement unless volume depletion and hypochloremia is corrected by saline administration.

 **FOLLOW-UP**

### DISPOSITION
#### Admission Criteria
- Need of IV potassium repletion
- Cardiac dysrhythmias
- Profound muscle weakness
- Ongoing K losses
- Serum potassium <2.5 mEq/L
- Associated with significant hypotension or severe HTN
- Significant comorbidities or geriatric

#### Discharge Criteria
- Asymptomatic
- Able to replete deficiency with oral potassium
- Early follow-up available and reliable patient
- Repeat electrolyte determination in 2–3 days with the primary care doctor.
- Nephrology referral or consult if suspicion of renal wasting.
- Continue K replacement for 2–3 days if acute, self-limited loss, but ongoing therapy if the cause is not corrected (eg, diuretic therapy, chronic diarrhea).

## PEARLS AND PITFALLS
- If hypokalemia is accompanied by acidosis, correct hypokalemia 1st before treating the acidosis so as to avoid life-threatening hypokalemia from transcellular shifts.
- Minimize glucose administration when treating hypokalemia, since glucose will stimulate insulin release, which will lead to K movement into cells.
- Large doses of oral potassium can by given safely in patients with normal renal function, limited only by GI tolerance.
- Check for hypomagnesemia if hypokalemia is severe or resistant to replacement therapy.
- Relatively small amounts of IV potassium are required to reverse hypokalemia in periodic paralysis and states of adrenergic excess since transcellular shifts are transient.

## ADDITIONAL READING
- Alfonzo AV, Isles C, Geddes C, et al. Potassium disorders—Clinical spectrum and emergency management. *Resuscitation*. 2006;70(1):10–25.
- Grenniee M, Wingo CS, McDonough AA, et al. Narrative review: Evolving concepts in potassium homeostasis and hypokalemia. *Ann Intern Med*. 2009;150:619–625.
- Groeneveld J, Sijpkens Y, Lin S, et al. An approach to the patient with severe hypokalemia: The potassium quiz. *Q J Med*. 2005;98:305–316.
- Diercks DB, Shumaik GM, Harrigan RA, et al. Electrocardiographic manifestations and electrolyte abnormalities. *J Emerg Med*. 2004;27(2):153–160.
- Lin SH, Chiu JS, Hsu CW, et al. A simple and rapid approach to hypokalemic paralysis. *Am J Emerg Med*. 2003;21:487–491.
- Schaefer TJ, Wolford RW. Disorders of potassium. *Emerg Med Clin North Am*. 2005;23(3):723–747.

### See Also (Topic, Algorithm, Electronic Media Element)
- Hyperkalemia

## CODES

**ICD9**
276.8 Hypopotassemia

**H**

# HYPONATREMIA
*Linda Mueller*

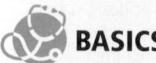 **BASICS**

## DESCRIPTION
- Sodium <136 mEq/L
- Most common electrolyte disturbance (1–4% of hospitalized patients)

## ETIOLOGY
### Pseudohyponatremia
- Low-measured serum sodium but normal measured serum osmolarity
- Occurs secondary to the displacement of sodium to aqueous phase of serum
- Seen with elevated lipids or proteins
- Disease examples include:
  - Multiple myeloma
  - Hyperlipidemia

### Hyponatremia with Normal Osmolarity and Fluid Overload
- Inappropriate retention of water
- Disease examples include:
  - CHF
  - Cirrhosis
  - Renal failure
  - Nephrotic syndrome

### Hyponatremia with Normal Osmolarity and Euvolemia
- Patients tend to have increased total body water without marked edema
- Purest form of dilutional hyponatremia
- Disease examples include:
  - Endocrine abnormalities:
    - Hypothyroid
    - Stress
    - Syndrome of inappropriate ADH (SIADH)
  - Diseases that cause SIADH:
    - Pulmonary disease (tuberculosis, Legionella, Aspergillosis, COPD)
    - CNS disorders (malignancy, sarcoid, infection)
    - Cancer (small cell lung, pancreas, duodenum)
    - HIV infection
  - Water intoxication (3–7% of institutionalized psychotic patients), can also occur in marathon runners
  - Mineralocorticoid abnormalities
  - Postoperative hyponatremia (particularly after transurethral prostatectomy)
  - Consumption of large amounts of beer (beer potomania)

### Hyponatremia with Normal Osmolarity and Hypovolemia
- Deficits in total body water and total body sodium
- Sodium deficits exceed water deficits
- Possible etiologies include:
  - GI losses
  - Sweating
  - Cerebral salt wasting (occurs after head injury or neurosurgical procedures)
  - Burns
  - Cystic fibrosis
  - Salt-wasting nephropathies
  - Diuretics

### Drug-Induced
- Drugs may stimulate antidiuretic hormone (ADH) and cause hyponatremia:
  - Amiodarone
  - Barbiturates
  - Bromocriptine
  - Carbamazepine
  - Clofibrate
  - Cyclophosphamide
  - Opiates
  - Oxytocin
  - Vincristine, vinblastine
- Drugs may increase sensitivity to ADH and cause hyponatremia:
  - Chlorpropamide
  - NSAIDs
- Drugs may stimulate thirst and cause hyponatremia:
  - Amitriptyline
  - Ecstasy
  - Fluoxetine
  - Fluphenazine
  - Haloperidol
  - Sertraline
  - Thiothixene

### Hyponatremia with Hyperosmolarity
- Due to excessive osmotically active substances
- Possible etiologies include:
  - Elevated glucose (most common cause of hyponatremia)
  - Corrected $Na^+ = 0.016 \times$ (measured glucose – to 100) + measured sodium
  - Mannitol infusion
  - Maltose and glycine

### Pediatric Considerations
- More prone to water intoxication
- High incidence of iatrogenic hyponatremia due to dilute formula or rehydration with water only
- If hyponatremia secondary to DKA, follow hydration per pediatric DKA recommendations

### Pregnancy Considerations
Conivaptan and Tolvaptan are class C drugs in pregnancy.

### Geriatric Considerations
- Tend to develop more symptoms
- Hyponatremia more common due to impaired water secretion and low sodium diets

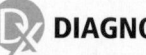 **DIAGNOSIS**

## SIGNS AND SYMPTOMS
- Mild: $Na^+$ >120 mEq/L:
  - Headache
  - Nausea
  - Vomiting
  - Weakness
  - Anorexia
  - Muscle cramps
  - Rhabdomyolysis
- Moderate: $Na^+$ between 110 and 120 mEq/L:
  - Impaired response to verbal stimuli
  - Decreased response to painful stimuli
  - Visual/Auditory hallucinations
  - Bizarre behavior
  - Incontinence
  - Hyperventilation
  - Gait disturbance
- Severe: $Na^+$ <110 mEq/L:
  - Signs of herniation
  - Decorticate/decerebrate posturing
  - Bradycardia
  - HTN
  - Altered temperature regulation
  - Dilated pupils
  - Seizure activity
  - Respiratory arrest
  - Coma/unresponsive

## Chronic
May be asymptomatic

### History
Review patient medication list.

### Physical Exam
- Assess volume status including skin turgor, neck veins, peripheral edema, and signs of ascites
- Perform a complete neurologic exam.

## ESSENTIAL WORKUP
Serum sodium level:
- Recheck sodium to verify.

## DIAGNOSTIC TESTS & INTERPRETATION
### Lab
- Electrolytes, BUN/creatinine
- Glucose:
  - Correct sodium value accordingly if severe hyperglycemia (add 1.6 Na for each 100mg/dl of glucose above normal)
- Calculate osmolality:
  - Plasma osmolality = [2 × NA(mEq L) + Glucose/18 + BUN/2.8]
- Urine sodium
- Serum and urine osmolality
- Thyroid function test
- Adrenal function tests
- CPK for possible rhabdomyolysis

### Imaging
- CXR to rule out CHF, infection, and tumor
- CT of head, particularly if patient has AMS

## DIFFERENTIAL DIAGNOSIS
- Pseudohyponatremia due to:
  - Hyperglycemia
  - Hyperlipidemia
  - Hyperproteinemia
  - Radiocontrast dye particularly in chronic renal insufficient patients

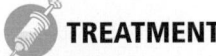 TREATMENT

## PRE-HOSPITAL
- Establish IV
- Supportive care

## INITIAL STABILIZATION/THERAPY
- ABCs
- Initiate IV fluid with 0.9% NS.
- Naloxone, thiamine, $D_{50}W$ (or Accu-Chek) for altered mental status

## ED TREATMENT/PROCEDURES
- Depends on severity and chronicity of hyponatremia and underlying etiology
- Chronic hyponatremia is to be corrected slowly to minimize osmotic demyelination syndrome. Correction should be limited to 10–12 mmol/l in 24 hr

- Acute hyponatremia with severe CNS symptoms/actively seizing:
  - Goal:
    - Raise serum sodium by 8–10mEq/L in 4–6 hr or to level >120–125 mEq/L with administration of hypertonic saline, slow or discontinue when seizure subsides.
    - 200–400 mL of 3% saline solution will be the approximate amount needed in most adults over the 1st 2 hr
    - OR may dose 1–2 mL/kg/h of 3% saline solution
  - Calculate sodium deficit:
    - $Na^+$ deficit = 0.6 (weight in kg)(140 − $Na^+$)
  - Sodium contents:
    - 1 L 0.9% NS = 154 mEq of sodium
    - 1 L 3% saline = 513 mEq of sodium
- Hypovolemic hyponatremia:
  - Correct underlying cause
  - Replete volume with 0.9% NS IV.
  - Primary goals to restore:
    - Extracellular fluid
    - Cardiac output
    - Organ perfusion
- Hypervolemic/euvolemic hyponatremia:
  - Water restriction to <1 L/day with high dietary salt intake
  - For faster correction of sodium:
    - Administer IV 0.9% NS with loop diuretic (furosemide).
  - Maximum rate of correction = 0.5 mEq/L/h

## MEDICATION
- Furosemide: 20–40 mg IV push
- Sodium replacement:
  - Calculate $Na^+$ deficit
  - Replace no more than 1/2 of requirement over 8–12 hr

### First Line
500 mL–1 L of saline for a fluid challenge

### Second Line
- Conivaptan: Arginine vasopressin antagonist
- 20 mg IV loading dose over 30 min followed by 20 mg continuous IV infusion OR
- Tolvaptan: Selective vasopressin V2 receptor antagonist dose 15 mg/d PO and may increase in 24 hr to 30 mg
- Conivaptan and tolvaptan are for the treatment of euvolemic and hypervolemic hyponatremia only

 FOLLOW-UP

## DISPOSITION
### Admission Criteria
- Symptomatic hyponatremia
- Sodium <120 mEq/L
- Asymptomatic, mild hyponatremia ($Na^+$ 120–127 mEq/L), with comorbid factors

### Discharge Criteria
- Sodium >130 mEq/L and asymptomatic
- Known chronic history of hyponatremia with no acute changes
- Asymptomatic, mild hyponatremia ($Na^+$ 120–129 mEq/L) with no comorbid factors; however, must have close outpatient follow-up.

## FOLLOW-UP RECOMMENDATIONS
Have repeat serum sodium with in a week, particularly if related to thiazide diuretics

## PEARLS AND PITFALLS
- Too rapid of correction may cause osmotic demyelination syndrome
- Females, alcoholics, malnuritioned patients, hypokalemia, and history of liver transplant are risk factors for osmotic demyelination syndrome.
- Repeat and document neurologic examinations during correction.
- Beware of false low sodiums drawn near an IV site with hypotonic fluid.
- Thiazide diuretics may cause persistent hyponatremia up to 2 wk after discontinued.

## ADDITIONAL READING
- Fall PJ. Hyponatremia and hypernatremia: A systematic approach to causes and their correction. *Postgrad Med*. 2000;107(5).75–82.
- Fried LF, Palevsky PM. Hyponatremia and hypernatremia. *Med Clin North Am*. 1997;81(3): 585–609.
- Liam YH, Shapiro JI. Hyponatremia: Clinical diagnosis and management. *Am J Med*. 2007;120(8).
- Lin M, Liu S, Lim I. Disorders of water imbalance. *Emerg Med Clin North Am*. 2005;23(3):749–770, ix.
- Palmer B, Gates J, Lader M. Causes and management of hyponatremia. *Ann Phamacother*. 2003;37:1644–1702.
- Verbalis J, Goldsmith SR. Hyponatremia guidelines 2007: Expert panel recommendations. *Am J Med*. 2007;120(11).

## See Also (Topic, Algorithm, Electronic Media Element)
- Hypernatremia

 CODES

ICD9
276.1 Hyposmolality and/or hyponatremia

H

# HYPOPARATHYROIDISM

*Hugh A. Schuckman*
*Stephen L. Chesser*

 **BASICS**

## DESCRIPTION
- Hypoparathyroidism is owing to a deficiency in parathyroid hormone (PTH).
- Pseudohypoparathyroidism is owing to end-organ unresponsiveness to PTH.
- PTH:
  - Decreases urinary $Ca^{2+}$ loss
  - Increases urinary $PO_4$ loss
  - Stimulates vitamin D conversion from 25(OH)-D to 1,25$(OH)_2$-D in kidney
  - Liberates $Ca^{2+}$ and $PO_4$ from bone
- Calcitonin:
  - Promotes deposition of $Ca^{2+}$ and $PO_4$ into bone (produced primarily in C cells in thyroid)
- Magnesium:
  - Cofactor in production of PTH
  - Essential for action of PTH in target tissues
- Hypoparathyroidism:
  - Primary failure of the parathyroid gland (may have associated Addison disease)
- Pseudohypoparathyroidism:
  - Tissue unresponsiveness with elevated PTH levels
  - Associated with hypothyroidism and hypogonadism
- Genetics:
  - Congenital absence
  - DiGeorge syndrome:
    - Hypoparathyroidism
    - Thymic dysplasia
    - Severe immunodeficiency
  - Wilson disease:
    - Destruction of gland owing to copper deposition
  - Autoimmune polyglandular syndrome type I:
    - Hypoparathyroidism
    - Adrenal insufficiency
    - Mucocutaneous candidiasis
  - Albright syndrome (hereditary osteodystrophy):
    - Short stature
    - Obesity
    - Round face
    - Short neck
    - Short 4th and 5th metacarpals and metatarsals (type I pseudohypoparathyroidism)

## ETIOLOGY
- Failure of parathyroid gland:
  - Autoimmune destruction
  - Surgical interruption of blood supply or gland removal
  - Radiation damage
  - Hypomagnesemia as PTH cofactor
- End-organ unresponsiveness to PTH

# DIAGNOSIS

## SIGNS AND SYMPTOMS

### ALERT
The most common symptomatic presentation is postoperatively after parathyroidectomy.

### Pediatric Considerations
Neonates/infants:
- Transient hypoparathyroidism in 1st yr of life
- Subnormal intelligence proportional to duration of hypocalcemia
- Dental hypoplasia

### History
Most common presentation if in the postoperative period after parathyroidectomy or thyroidectomy:
- Prolonged, severe hypomagnesemia, that is, in the alcoholic or high-dose diuretic patient is the next most common and due to slow onset usually less symptomatic.

### Physical Exam
- Related to severity, rapidity of onset, and duration of hypocalcemia
- General:
  - Weakness
  - Malaise
- Neuromuscular:
  - Paresthesias (especially circumoral and extremities)
  - Carpal pedal spasm
  - Latent spasm elicited by:
    - Chvostek sign (twitching of circumoral muscles after tapping facial nerve in front of the tragus)
    - Trousseau sign (spasm after inflating BP cuff 20 mm above patient's systolic BP for 3 min)
  - Laryngospasm/bronchospasm
  - Blepharospasm
  - Muscle cramps
  - Tetany
  - Seizures (presenting symptom of 1/3 with hypoparathyroidism)
  - Increased intracranial pressure (ICP) with papilledema
  - Parkinson syndrome and other extrapyramidal disorders
  - Myelopathy
- Cardiovascular:
  - Prolonged QT interval (owing to ST segment prolongation)
  - Heart block
  - CHF
  - Ventricular fibrillation (VFib)
  - Vasoconstriction
- Psychiatric:
  - Impaired memory
  - Confusion
  - Hallucinations
  - Dementia
- Dermatologic:
  - Brittle hair and nails
  - Psoriasis
- Hyperpigmentation:
  - Lenticular cataracts

## ESSENTIAL WORKUP
- If *no hypocalcemic symptoms* with hypocalcemia, check albumin level:
  - If still low after correcting for hypoalbuminemia, check ionized $Ca^{2+}$.
- If *hypocalcemic symptoms* with normal total $Ca^{2+}$, check pH for alkalosis:
  - If not alkalotic, check ionized $Ca^{2+}$ (active form).
  - Metabolic or respiratory alkalosis increases the binding to albumin reducing the ionized $Ca^{2+}$.
- If *hypocalcemic symptoms* with low ionized $Ca^{2+}$, check a PTH level:
  - Low in primary hypoparathyroidism and in vitamin D deficiency
  - Elevated in pseudohypoparathyroidism and hypocalcemia from renal failure

## DIAGNOSTIC TESTS & INTERPRETATION
### Lab
- Calcium: Correct for albumin using formula:
  - Corrected $Ca^{2+}$ (mg/dL) = measured $Ca^{2+}$ (mg/dL) + 0.8[4.0 − albumin (g/dL)]
- Ionized $Ca^{2+}$ if symptomatic with low total calcium
- Electrolytes, BUN, creatinine, glucose
- Magnesium
- Arterial blood gas (ABG) if symptomatic with normal total $Ca^{2+}$:
  - Elevation of 0.1 pH unit decreases the ionized $Ca^{2+}$ by 3–8%.
- Phosphorus:
  - Elevated except when hypocalcemia caused by vitamin D deficiency
  - Metastatic calcification can cause hypocalcemia by tissue deposition when the calcium/phosphorus product is >60.

### Imaging
On plain films of the mandible, tooth roots may be absent.

### Diagnostic Procedures/Surgery
ECG:
- Prolonged QT interval:
  - Owing to ST-segment prolongation from hypocalcemia

## DIFFERENTIAL DIAGNOSIS

- Must differentiate from variety of causes of hypocalcemia
- Lab artifact:
  - Low total calcium that is normal when corrected for albumin level with no symptoms of hypocalcemia
- Alkalosis:
  - Symptomatic hypocalcemia with a normal total calcium
- Hypomagnesemia (needed for PTH secretion)
- PTH resistance (congenital)
- Vitamin D deficiency (low $Ca^{2+}$ + low $PO_4$):
  - Anticonvulsant use (decreased vitamin D absorption)
  - Liver disease
  - Resistance to vitamin D
  - Malabsorption or dietary deficiency
- Gram-negative sepsis
- Renal failure or nephrotic syndrome
- Chelation:
  - Pancreatitis (fatty acids chelate calcium)
  - Ammonium bifluoride (tire cleaner spray)
  - Hydrofluoric acid
  - Citrated blood
  - Acute hyperphosphatemia:
    - Fleet enemas
    - Rhabdomyolysis
    - Acute renal failure

## TREATMENT

### PRE-HOSPITAL
- Administer calcium in refractory VFib or status epilepticus in addition to usual medications if known hypoparathyroidism or suspected hypocalcemia.
- Stridor may herald laryngospasm.

### INITIAL STABILIZATION/THERAPY
- Airway, breathing, and circulation management (ABCs):
  - Manage airway if laryngospasm.
- Administer IV calcium bolus (chloride or gluconate) if unstable cardiac rhythm or tetany:
  - Slow infusion much safer unless patient markedly symptomatic
- Prepare for ventricular dysrhythmias including ventricular fibrillation.
- Seizure precautions

### ED TREATMENT/PROCEDURES
- Calcium replacement:
  - Calcium chloride 10% (27.2 mg elemental $Ca^{2+}$/mL):
    - For life-threatening conditions: 10 mL (1 gram) IV over 5 min OR
  - Calcium gluconate 10% (9 mg elemental $Ca^{2+}$/mL):
    - For life-threatening conditions: 20–30 mL (2–3 g) over 3–5 min

- For non–life-threatening conditions, administer calcium via slow infusion of 500–1,000 mg elemental $Ca^{2+}$ over 6–24 hr (peds: 100 mg elemental $Ca^{2+}$/kg/24h)
  - Continuous cardiac monitoring
  - Stop infusion if bradycardia develops.
  - Perform frequent checks of serum $Ca^{2+}$ levels.
  - Calcium administration may precipitate digitalis toxicity.
  - Supplement to lowest possible $Ca^{2+}$ level keeping the patient asymptomatic, then switch to oral replacement:
    - Soft tissue calcification may occur with calcium/phosphorus product of 60 (Ca × $PO_4$).
- Replace magnesium if low.
- Bind phosphorus:
  - Aluminum hydroxide–containing antacids (Maalox, Mylanta, or Gelusil) if creatinine <2
  - Calcium acetate (Phos-lo) or calcium carbonate when concurrent renal failure if creatinine >2
  - Sevelamer HCl or carbonate (Renagel, Renvela)
- Vitamin D supplementation
- Avoid carbonated beverages (high in phosphorus).
- Assess for associated endocrinopathies.

## MEDICATION

### First Line
- Calcium gluconate: 10% (9 mg elemental $Ca^{2+}$/mL): 20–30 mL over 3–5 min if life-threatening condition; otherwise, slow infusion (peds: 20 mg/kg of calcium gluconate 10% or 2 mg/kg elemental Ca):
  - Follow with slow infusion: Calcium gluconate 10 g in liter of 5% dextrose infused at 1–3 mg/kg/hr in adults
  - Calcium gluconate has lower risk of venous irritation or extravasational injury compared to calcium chloride
- Magnesium sulfate: 2 g IV (peds: 25–50 mg/kg up to 2 g) over 2 hr—if severe, 6 g over 6 hr
- Calcium chloride 10% (27.2 mg elemental $Ca^{2+}$/mL): 10 mL (1 g) IV over 5 min if life-threatening condition; otherwise, slow infusion

### Second Line
- Calcium acetate: 667 mg (169 mg elemental Ca): 1 or 2 tabs t.i.d. with meals
- Calcium carbonate: 1,250 mg (500 mg elemental Ca): 1 or 2 tabs q.i.d. (2–4 g/d) (peds: 45–65 mg elem Ca mg/kg/d divided q.i.d.)
- Sevelamer (Renagel, Renvela) 800 mg: 1 or 2 tablets t.i.d. with meals
- Magnesium oxide 400 mg: 1 tab daily or b.i.d.
- Vitamin D: 400 I.U. PO daily for supplement (If not responsive to standard supplement, then consider calcitriol (1,25(OH)$_2$-D) 0.25 mcg daily; titrate to 0.5–2 mcg/d:
  - Preferred over other long-acting vitamin D analogues due to patient availability and lower cost, quicker onset and offset of action

## FOLLOW-UP

### DISPOSITION

#### Admission Criteria
- Symptomatic hypocalcemia
- Abnormal ECG
- Inability to take vitamin D or calcium orally
- Corrected calcium <5 mg/dL

#### Discharge Criteria
- Asymptomatic hypocalcemia
- Not meeting any admission criteria

### FOLLOW-UP RECOMMENDATIONS
- Any patient requiring therapy or needing follow-up laboratory studies
- Repeat of calcium, phosphorus, magnesium levels in 1–2 days

## PEARLS AND PITFALLS

- Rapid onset of symptoms following surgical excision of the parathyroid glands is the most common symptomatic presentation.
- Symptoms often confused with hyperventilation or anxiety.
- In the absence of surgery or severe hypomagnesium, be sure that hypocalemia is not due to sepsis or rhabdomyolysis.
- With the exception of life-threatening presentations, avoid rapid IV administration of calcium salts.

## ADDITIONAL READING

- Andreoli T, Carpenter C. *Cecil Essentials of Medicine*, 7th ed. Philadelphia: Saunders-Elsevier; 2007.
- Goldman L, Bennett JC, eds. *Cecil's Textbook of Medicine*, 23rd ed. Philadelphia: Saunders-Elsevier; 2008.
- Guyton A, Hall J. *Textbook of Medical Physiology*, 11th ed. Philadelphia: Saunders-Elsevier; 2006
- Wallach J, ed. *Interpretation of Diagnostic Tests*, 8th ed. Boston: Little, Brown and Company; 2007.

### See Also (Topic, Algorithm, Electronic Media Element)
- Hyperparathyroidism

 ## CODES

**ICD9**
252.1 Hypoparathyroidism

H

# HYPOTHERMIA
*Jordan Moskoff*

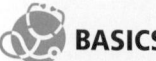 **BASICS**

## DESCRIPTION
- Body temperature <35°C
- Risk factors:
  - Poor temperature regulation:
    - Very young
    - Advanced age
    - Comorbid condition
    - Intoxication
- Pathophysiology:
  - Loss of heat:
    - Radiation: Most rapid, 50% of heat loss
    - Conduction
    - Convection
    - Evaporation
    - Respiration
  - Heat production:
    - Shivering
    - Nonshivering thermogenesis
    - Increased thyroxine
    - Increased epinephrine

## ETIOLOGY
- Dermal disease:
  - Burn
  - Exfoliative dermatitis
  - Severe psoriasis
- Drug-induced:
  - Ethanol
  - Phenothiazines
  - Sedative-hypnotics
- Environmental:
  - Immersion
  - Nonimmersion
- Iatrogenic:
  - Aggressive fluid replacement
  - Heat stroke treatment
- Metabolic:
  - Hypoadrenalism
  - Hypopituitarism
  - Hypothyroidism
- Neurologic:
  - Acute spinal cord transection
  - Head trauma
  - Stroke
  - Tumor
  - Wernicke disease
- Neuromuscular inefficiency:
  - Age extreme
  - Impaired shivering
  - Lack of acclimatization
- Sepsis

### Pediatric Considerations
Infants have a large body surface to mass ratio.

 **DIAGNOSIS**

## SIGNS AND SYMPTOMS
- Mild (35–32.2°C/95–90°F):
  - Initial excitation phase to combat cold:
    - HTN
    - Shivering
    - Tachycardia
    - Early tachycardia followed by bradycardia
    - Tachypnea
    - Vasoconstriction
  - Over time with onset of fatigue:
    - Apathy
    - Ataxia
    - Cold diuresis
    - Defect in distal tubular reabsorption of sodium and water
    - Impaired judgment
- Moderate (32.2–28°C/90–82.4°F):
  - Atrial dysrhythmias
  - Bradycardia:
    - Decreased spontaneous depolarization of pacemaker cells
    - Refractory to atropine
  - Decreased level of consciousness
  - Decreased respiratory rate:
    - Progressive respiratory depression with $CO_2$ retention
  - Dilated pupils
  - Diminished gag reflex
  - Extinction of shivering
  - Hyporeflexia
  - Hypotension
  - J-wave (Osborn wave) on ECG
- Severe (<28°C/<82.4°F):
  - Apnea
  - Coma
  - Decreased or no activity on EEG (electroencephalography)
  - Nonreactive pupils
  - Oliguria:
    - Renal blood flow depressed 50%
  - Pulmonary edema
  - Ventricular dysrhythmias/asystole:
    - Cardiac cycle lengthens, resulting in increased intervals

## History
Time of submersion for near drowning in cold water.

## Physical Exam
- May not be able to palpate pulse
- May not be able to obtain BP
- Pupils dilate <26°C

## ESSENTIAL WORKUP
Accurate core temperature confirms diagnosis.

## DIAGNOSTIC TESTS & INTERPRETATION
### Lab
- Finger stick glucose
- ABG:
  - Temperature correction not needed
- CBC:
  - Hematocrit rises owing to decreased plasma volume.
  - Leukopenia does not imply absence of infection:
    - High-risk groups (eg, neonate, immunocompromised) should receive empiric antibiotics.
- Electrolytes, BUN, creatinine:
  - Vary during rewarming; recheck frequently, especially creatine phosphokinase (CPK) and potassium ($K^+$)
- Serum lactate
- PT, PTT, and platelets:
  - Prolonged clotting times, thrombocytopenia common
- Toxicology screen:
  - Alcohol/drug ingestion common

### Imaging
- CXR:
  - Pneumonia common complication
- EKG:
  - Tachycardia to bradycardia
  - Atrial fibrillation with slow response
  - Ventricular fibrillation
  - Asystole
  - Prolonged PR, QRS, QT intervals
  - J Osborn waves
  - ST elevation mimicking acute coronary syndrome

## DIFFERENTIAL DIAGNOSIS
- Environmental
- Sepsis
- Primary CNS disorder
- Metabolic
- Drug-induced

**TREATMENT**

## PRE-HOSPITAL
- Controversies:
  - CPR not recommended if:
    - Electrical rhythm present without palpable pulse or BP with short transport time
- Cautions:
  - Prolonged palpation/auscultation for cardiac activity: 30–45 sec
  - Apparent cardiovascular collapse may be depressed cardiac output, often sufficient to meet metabolic demands.

## INITIAL STABILIZATION/THERAPY

- ABCs:
  - Supplemental oxygen
  - Oral and nasotracheal intubation are safe.
  - Place nasogastric (NG) tube postintubation.
  - Cardiac monitor
  - Warmed D5.9 NS preferred over lactated Ringer:
    - Shivering depletes glycogen.
- Remove wet clothing and begin passive external rewarming.
- Administer Narcan, $D_{50}W$ (or Accu-Chek), and thiamine to a patient with altered mental status.
- Stress-dose steroids (Solu-Cortef 100 mg IV) for known adrenal insufficiency or treatment failure.
- Obtain accurate core temperatures using rectal thermometer.

## ED TREATMENT/PROCEDURES

- Cardiac arrest resuscitation:
  - Most dysrhythmias correct with rewarming alone.
  - Ventricular fibrillation induction occurs with rough handling, chest compressions, hypoxia, and acid–base changes.
  - CPR is less effective owing to decreased chest wall elasticity.
  - Defibrillation is rarely successful at temperatures <28–30°C:
    - Defibrillate 1–3 times and then again post rewarming.
    - Once >30°C, if ventricular fibrillation persists use amiodarone.
    - Direct current results in myocardial damage.
- Dysrhythmia management:
  - Atrial fibrillation:
    - Common <32°C
    - Usually converts spontaneously
  - Malignant ventricular dysrhythmias:
    - Amiodarone drug of choice
    - Avoid lidocaine and procainamide; may increase ventricular fibrillation.
- Rewarming techniques:
  - Faster rewarming rates (1–2°C/h) generally have better prognosis than slower rewarming rates (<0.5°C/h).
  - Active rewarming is necessary at core temperature of <32°C:
    - Internal thermogenesis insufficient to increase body temperature
    - Shivering extinguished
- Passive external rewarming:
  - Ideal technique for most healthy patients with mild hypothermia
  - Must have intact thermoregulatory mechanisms, normal endocrine function, and adequate energy stores.
  - Cover the patient with dry insulating material.
  - Endogenous thermogenesis must generate an acceptable rate of rewarming:
    - Must increase 0.5–2°C/hr
  - Disadvantage: Core rises very slowly.
- Active external rewarming:
  - Delivers heat directly to the skin
  - Safe in previously healthy, young, acutely hypothermic victims
  - Requires intact circulation to remove peripherally rewarmed blood to core

- Associated with core temperature after-drop
- Rewarming shock: Venous pooling in warmed extremities secondary to vasodilatation
- Cover trunk preferentially.
- Bair Hugger device provides forced warm air: Prevents shock or after-drop.
- Active core rewarming techniques:
  - Airway rewarming (complete humidification at 40–45°C):
    - Administer to all patients.
  - Heated IV (40–42°C) D5.9 NS:
    - Administer to all patients.
    - High flow rates must be maintained.
    - Use blood warmer or calibrated microwave.
  - Heated gastric irrigation via nasogastric or orogastric tubes:
    - Not recommended
    - Low amount of surface area
    - Aspiration risk if airway not secured
  - Pleural irrigation (0.9 NS at 30–42°C):
    - Use in severe hypothermia without cardiac activity.
    - 1–2 chest tubes; midaxillary and midclavicular bilaterally
    - Contraindicated in patients with cardiac rhythm because the chest tube may induce ventricular fibrillation
  - Heated peritoneal lavage (0.9 NS at 40–45°C):
    - Use in unstable hypothermic patients or stable patients with severe hypothermia whose rewarming rates are <1°C/h.
    - 1–2 catheters
    - Advantageous in patients with overdose or rhabdomyolysis
- Extracorporeal rewarming:
  Most effective rewarming method
  - Hemodialysis:
    - Initiate for patients with drug overdoses or severe electrolyte disturbances.
  - Continuous arteriovenous rewarming:
    - BP must be >60 mm Hg.
    - Blood circulated through warmer from percutaneously inserted femoral arterial and contralateral venous catheters
  - Extracorporeal venovenous rewarming:
    - Blood is removed via central venous catheter, heated to 40°C, and returned via 2nd central or large peripheral venous catheter.
  - Cardiopulmonary bypass:
    - Treatment of choice in severe hypothermia with cardiac arrest
- Additional therapy:
  - Methylprednisolone or hydrocortisone for suspicion of adrenocortical insufficiency or steroid dependence
  - Empiric treatment with levothyroxine only for myxedematous patients

## MEDICATION

- Amiodarone: 300 mg IV push (IVP) for ventricular fibrillation followed by 1 mg/kg infusion
- Dextrose: $D_{50}W$ 1 amp—50 mL or 25 g (peds: $D_{25}W$ 2–4 mL/kg) IV
- Hydrocortisone: 250 mg IVP
- Levothyroxine: 50–500 $\mu$g IV over several minutes
- Methylprednisolone: 30 mg/kg IVP
- Naloxone (Narcan): 2 mg (peds: 0.1 mg/kg) IV or IM initial dose
- Thiamine (vitamin $B_1$): 100 mg (peds: 50 mg) IV or IM

 **FOLLOW-UP**

### DISPOSITION

**Admission Criteria**
- Moderate to severe hypothermia (<32°C)
- Young, healthy patients with no comorbid illness who have mild accidental hypothermia (>32°C) that responds well to warming:
  - Admit to an observation area.
  - Discharge if asymptomatic after 8–12 hr and they remain asymptomatic.

**Discharge Criteria**
- Young, healthy patients with no comorbid illness
- Very mild accidental hypothermia (>35°C) that responds well to warming
- Safe, warm environment to go to after discharge

### FOLLOW-UP RECOMMENDATIONS
Social work follow-up for homeless patients with cold exposure and hypothermia

## PEARLS AND PITFALLS

- Defibrillation is rarely successful at temperatures <28–30°C:
  - Defibrillate 1–3 times and then again post rewarming.
- Atrial fibrillation usually converts spontaneously.
- Faster rewarming rates (1–2°C/h) generally have better prognosis than slower rewarming rates (<0.5°C/h).

## ADDITIONAL READING

- Bien J. Out of the cold: Management of hypothermia and frostbite. *CMAJ.* 2003;168(3).
- Cheng D. The EKG of hypothermia. *J Emerg Med.* 2002;22(1):87–91.
- Hanania NA, Zimmerman JL. Accidental hypothermia. *Crit Care Clin.* 1999;15(2):235–249.
- Jurkovich G. Environmental cold-induced injury. *Surg Clin N Am.* 2007;87:247–267.
- Laniewicz M. Rapid endovascular warming for profound hypothermia. *Ann Emerg Med.* 2008;51(2):160–163.
- McCullough L. Diagnosis and treatment of hypothermia. *Am Fam Physician.* 2004;70:2325–2332.

## See Also (Topic, Algorithm, Electronic Media Element)
Frostbite

 **CODES**

ICD9
991.6 Hypothermia

H

# HYPOTHYROIDISM

*Rita K. Cydulka*
*Alix L. Rosenstein*

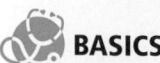 **BASICS**

## DESCRIPTION
- Decreased levels of effective circulating thyroid hormone leads to decreased metabolic rate and decreased sensitivity to catecholamines.
- More common in elderly and women
- Myxedema coma is a rare extreme form of hypothyroidism characterized by altered mental status and defective thermoregulation triggered by a precipitating event in a patient with hypothyroidism.

## ETIOLOGY
- Primary:
  - Idiopathic
  - Congenital
  - Autoimmune:
    ○ Thyroiditis
    ○ Hashimoto disease
  - Iatrogenic:
    ○ Postsurgical
    ○ External radiation
    ○ Radioiodine therapy
    ○ Drugs (iodides, lithium, amiodarone, interferons)
  - Neoplasm: Primary (carcinoma) or secondary (infiltration)
  - Infection: Viral (rarely aerobic or anaerobic bacteria)
  - Iodine deficiency (most common cause worldwide)
- Central:
  - Pituitary or hypothalamic disorder
  - Very rare
  - May have other associated hormone deficiencies
- Myxedema coma:
  - Critical decompensation of a patient with hypothyroidism due to a stress. Stressors include:
    ○ Infection
    ○ Hypothermia
    ○ Intoxication
    ○ Drugs
    ○ Cerebrovascular accident
    ○ CHF
    ○ Trauma

## Pregnancy Considerations
- Postpartum thyroiditis occurs in up to 5% of women:
  - Usually 3–6 mo postpartum
  - Typically resolves without treatment

## Pediatric Considerations
- Thyroid-stimulating hormone (TSH) antibodies and propylthiouracil (PTU) cross placenta
- PTU excreted in small quantities in breast milk

 **DIAGNOSIS**

## SIGNS AND SYMPTOMS
### History
- Exhaustion
- Cold intolerance
- Headaches
- Diminished hearing
- Myalgias
- Menorrhagia
- Infertility
- Carpal tunnel syndrome
- Constipation
- Weight gain
- Depression

### Physical Exam
- Puffy eyelids
- Sparse, coarse hair
- Absent lateral 1/3 of eyebrows (Queen Anne sign)
- Husky or hoarse voice
- Goiter
- Prolonged relaxation phase of deep tendon reflexes (DTRs)
- Yellow, dry, pale skin
- Galactorrhea
- Myxedema (dry, waxy swelling of skin)
- Swelling of hands and feet
- Myxedema coma:
  - Altered mental status
  - Hypotension
  - Hypothermia
  - Respiratory failure
  - Bradycardia

## Geriatric Considerations
Typical symptoms of hypothyroidism may be confused with changes associated with aging.

## ESSENTIAL WORKUP
Laboratory confirmation of the diagnosis of hypothyroidism/myxedema coma may not be available in the ED, and therapy should be initiated based on clinical suspicion.

## DIAGNOSTIC TESTS & INTERPRETATION
Search for the underlying cause of myxedema coma.

### Lab
- Thyroid function studies:
  - Low total and free thyroxine ($T_4$)
  - Low total and free triiodothyronine ($T_3$)
  - TSH:
    ○ Increased in primary hypothyroidism but normal or decreased in central pathology
- Anemia
- Hyponatremia
- Hypoglycemia
- Hypoxemia
- Hypercapnia
- Elevated lactate dehydrogenase (LDH), creatine phosphokinase (CPK), cholesterol

### Imaging
CXR:
- Enlarged cardiac silhouette due to pericardial effusion

### Diagnostic Procedures/Surgery
ECG:
- Profound bradycardia
- Low voltage

## DIFFERENTIAL DIAGNOSIS
- Chronic nephritis
- Chronic renal disease
- CHF
- Depression
- Hypoalbuminemia
- Nephrotic syndrome
- Sepsis

> **ALERT**
> - Euthyroid sick syndrome:
>   - Illness, surgery, fasting may produce abnormal thyroid function test results
>   - Thyroid function tests performed during acute nonthyroid illness may be abnormal and should be interpreted with caution

**TREATMENT**

## INITIAL STABILIZATION/THERAPY
- ABCs:
  - Intubation and ventilation may be necessary
- Cardiac monitor
- BP support
- Supplemental oxygen to meet metabolic needs
- Correct hypothermia:
  - Initiate passive warming measures
  - Aggressive rewarming may precipitate hypotension from vasodilation

## ED TREATMENT/PROCEDURES
- Mild hypothyroidism:
  - Refer for oral thyroid hormone replacement as an outpatient
- Myxedema coma:
  - Life-threatening condition
  - Initiate thyroid hormone replacement therapy if a high index of suspicion:
    - Prompt IV replacement improves survival
    - Controversy over regimen exists
    - Thyroxine ($T_4$) and/or triiodothyronine ($T_3$)
    - Reassess 1 hr after initial dose
    - Use smaller doses of thyroid hormone in the elderly or patients with cardiac disease
  - Hydrocortisone to prevent Addisonian crisis
  - Dextrose for hypoglycemia
  - IV fluid bolus for hypotension:
    - Avoid pressors if possible, may precipitate dysrhythmias
    - Response to pressors is poor until thyroid replacement initiated
    - Thyroid hormone augments pressors
    Consider hypertonic saline for severe hyponatremia
- Correct the underlying precipitant

## MEDICATION
### First Line
Thyroid hormone therapy:
- Administer $T_4$, $T_3$ or a combination:
  - Thyroxine ($T_4$): 200–600 $\mu$g load IV followed by 50–100 $\mu$g IV daily
  - Triiodothyronine ($T^3$): 10–20 $\mu$g load IV followed by 10 $\mu$g IV q4h for 24 hr, then 10 $\mu$g IV q6h for 24–48 hr

### Second Line
- Hydrocortisone: 100 mg (peds: 1 mg/kg/24 h) IV q6–8h
- Dextrose: 50–100 mL $D_{50}$ (peds: 5 mL/kg of $D_{10}$) IV

 **FOLLOW-UP**

## DISPOSITION
### Admission Criteria
All patients with myxedema coma require ICU admission.

### Discharge Criteria
Hypothyroidism is managed in the outpatient setting.

### Issues for Referral
- Primary care providers can generally manage hypothyroidism.
- Pregnant patients, elderly patients, and those with ischemic heart disease require special consideration when initiating thyroid hormone replacement.

## FOLLOW-UP RECOMMENDATIONS
- Patients should be referred to a primary care provider for initiation of oral thyroid hormone replacement therapy.
- Severe untreated maternal hypothyroidism can negatively impact fetal brain development and cause obstetrical complications.

## PEARLS AND PITFALLS
- Signs and symptoms of hypothyroidism are nonspecific and may be confused with other mental or physical disorders.
- Response to treatment for hypothyroidism may take weeks and is best initiated by the primary care physician.
- Consider myxedema coma in patients with altered mental status and underlying hypothyroidism.
- Myxedema coma has a high mortality rate and requires aggressive treatment.

## ADDITIONAL READING
- Hennessey JV, Scherger JE. Evaluating and treating the patient with hypothyroid disease. *J Fam Pract*. 2007;56(8 Suppl Hot Topics):S31–S39.
- Pimentel L, Hansen KN. Thyroid disease in the emergency department: A clinical and laboratory review. *J Emerg Med*, 2005;28(2):201–9.
- Rehman SU, Cope DW, Senseney AD, et al. Thyroid disorders in elderly patients. *South Med J*. 2005;98(5): 543–9.
- Vaidya B, Pearce SH. Management of hypothyroidism in adults. *BMJ* 2008;337:284–9.
- Wartofsky L. Myxedema coma. *Endocrinol Metab Clin North Am*, 2006;35(4):687–98.

### See Also (Topic, Algorithm, Electronic Media Element)
- Hyperthyroidism

**CODES**

ICD9
244.9 Unspecified acquired hypothyroidism

# IDIOPATHIC THROMBOCYTOPENIC PURPURA

*Matthew T. Keadey*

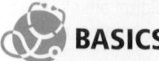 **BASICS**

## DESCRIPTION

- Idiopathic thrombocytopenic purpura (ITP) is thrombocytopenia without apparent cause or abnormalities in other cell lines.
- Incidence is ~2–5/100,000 per year—may be an underestimate owing to undetected, subclinical cases.
- Acute ITP:
  - 1/2 of cases involve children.
  - 80% of children recover within 8 wk with or without therapy.
  - Adult recovery is delayed and requires specific therapy to achieve remission.
- Chronic ITP:
  - Occurs mostly in adults
  - Young women are most susceptible in adult onset ITP
  - Characterized by variable response to corticosteroids and other immune suppressants
  - 60–70% respond to splenectomy
- Chronic refractory ITP:
  - Platelet counts may often wax and wane.
  - Often do not respond to therapy
  - No clear optimal course of treatment
- Genetics:
  - ITP appears to run in families, as do variations in response to corticosteroids for treatment.

## ETIOLOGY

- Autoantibodies produced by B cells and plasma cells cause immune-mediated destruction of circulating platelets
- Macrophages in spleen and liver mediate destruction of platelets via IgG autoantibodies
- IgM and IgA rarely have been seen
- Some patients do not possess autoantibodies, suggesting a role for T-cell-mediated cytotoxicity.
- C3 and C4 complement has also been shown to play a role in patients that lack autoantibodies
- Poor platelet production may also play a role especially in chronic and refractory cases of ITP
- Eradication of *H. pylori* can sometimes be associated with platelet recovery (unclear mechanism).

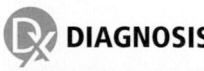 **DIAGNOSIS**

## SIGNS AND SYMPTOMS

### History

- Bleeding is the most common complaint:
  - Common:
    - Mucous membrane: Gingiva, epistaxis, conjunctival, menorrhagia
  - Rare (more common in coagulopathies):
    - GI bleeding, hemarthrosis, hematuria, and hematomas

- 84% of pediatric cases are 2–3 wk following a viral illness
  - Small percentage found following vaccinations
- Most adult cases have an insidious onset
  - Up to 28% of patients are asymptomatic and diagnosed on routine CBC
  - <5% present with life threatening bleeding

### Physical Exam

- Mucosal bleeding often apparent in symptomatic cases:
- Commonly may follow dental procedures, extraction or trauma
- Petechiae (nonblanching)
- Nonpalpable purpura:
- Distinguishes ITP from Henoch-Schönlein purpura (HSP).
- Melena, bright red blood per rectum or Hemoccult positive stools
- Spleen normal size in ITP:
  - Enlarged spleen may be found in leukemia or other platelet sequestration syndromes
- Neurologic deficits from intracranial hemorrhage (ICH):
  - ICH is the most common cause of death in ITP.
  - Risk of ICH in ITP increases with age:
    - Age <40 yr: 2%
    - Age >60 yr: 48%

## ESSENTIAL WORKUP

- Diagnosis of exclusion—other causes of thrombocytopenia must be ruled out.
- Complete blood count with differential
- PT and PTT if actively bleeding to exclude other forms of coagulopathy
- BUN and Creatinine to evaluate renal function
- Liver function to exclude liver disease
- Type and screen if actively bleeding
- Pregnancy test if of child bearing age
- HIV testing should be considered

## DIAGNOSTIC TESTS & INTERPRETATION

### Lab

CBC with differential and peripheral smear:

- Thrombocytopenia
- Increased mean platelet volume
- Normal WBC and RBC morphology and size
- Liver function, coagulation studies, and kidney function should all be within normal limits

### Imaging

CT head without contrast to evaluate for ICH if clinically indicated by focal findings, headache or head trauma.

### Diagnostic Procedures/Surgery

Bone marrow biopsy:

- All adults >60 yr to evaluate for malignancy
- Atypical symptoms and cases refractory to treatment
- Patients considering splenectomy
- Children with persistent thrombocytopenia >6 mo
- Children unresponsive to intravenous immunoglobulin (IVIG)
- Antibody testing is of no clinical value

## DIFFERENTIAL DIAGNOSIS

- Impaired bone marrow production:
  - Bone marrow fibrosis
  - Bone marrow infiltration owing to malignancy
  - Cytotoxic drugs used in chemotherapy
  - Congenital/acquired bone marrow abnormalities
- Splenic sequestration:
  - Portal hypertension
  - Neoplastic infiltration
  - Sickle cell disease
- Accelerated destruction of platelets:
  - Vasculitis
  - TTP/HUS
  - Disseminated intravascular coagulation (DIC)
  - HELLP syndrome
  - Cardiac valvular disease
- Drug induced:
  - Decreased platelet production:
    - Chemotherapy
    - Thiazide diuretics
    - Ethanol
    - Estrogen
  - Increased destruction of platelets:
    - Aspirin
    - Heparin
    - Chlorpropamide
    - Chloroquine
    - Gold salts
    - Sulfonamides
    - Insecticides

**TREATMENT**

## PRE-HOSPITAL

Stabilize ABCs

- Significant oral or laryngeal bleeding my affect airway.
- CNS event may effect ability to control airway
- Establish IV access for cases of significant bleeding
- Control any bleeding with direct pressure

## INITIAL STABILIZATION/THERAPY

- ABCs
- Stabilize life-threatening bleeding:
  - Intracranial hemorrhage:
    - Airway control
    - Neurosurgery consultation: Craniotomy not typically possible until platelet counts >75 K
  - Hemorrhagic shock:
    - 2 large-bore IVs
    - Direct pressure for hemostasis
    - Resuscitation with blood transfusions and isotonic crystalloid
    - Medications and platelets for acute life threatening episodes of bleeding:
    - IV high dose dexamethasone or methylprednisolone
    - IVIG infusion
    - Platelet transfusions: 2–3 times the normal amount
  - Platelets typically infused after steroids and/or IVIG
  - Mucous membrane bleeding:
    - Topical agents
    - Other:
    - IV Aminocaproic acid may be considered
    - In rare cases, plasmapheresis has been proven helpful

## ED TREATMENT/PROCEDURES

- Initial treatment options for ITP are based on:
  - Degree of thrombocytopenia
  - Severity of Illness
  - Duration of symptoms
  - Age
  - Risk factors for bleeding (hypertension, peptic ulcer disease, vigorous lifestyle)
  - Hematologic preference
- Efficacy of treatment is demonstrated in terms of platelet recovery time and not morbidity or mortality.
- Specific treatment options:
  - Observation is recommended for children without bleeding complications or profound thrombocytopenia (<20–30 K)
  - Profound thrombocytopenia (<20 K)
    - High-dose corticosteroids: 75% response
    - IVIG: 80% response, but costly so reserved in time critical emergencies
    - Anti-D IG: 70% response (used only in Rh⁺ patients)
  - Splenectomy:
    - Second-line therapy if inadequate response to a course of glucocorticoid therapy
    - Two thirds of adult patients respond, three fourths of pediatric patients respond.
    - No specific indications for emergent splenectomy

### Pregnancy Considerations

- Differential diagnosis of thrombocytopenia during pregnancy:
  - Gestational thrombocytopenia (75%):
    - Usually of no clinical significance
    - Does not cause neonatal thrombocytopenia
    - Remits 1–2 wk after delivery
    - Platelets typically >50 K

- HELLP syndrome (*h*emolysis, *e*levated *l*iver enzymes, and *l*ow *p*latelets)
- ITP (15%)
  - Platelets typically < 50 K
  - Maternal platelet count does not correlate to neonatal thrombocytopenia.
  - Treatment with steroids or IVIG does not alter incidence of neonatal thrombocytopenia.
  - Degree of thrombocytopenia should not alter decision of vaginal birth versus C-section.
  - Measure neonatal CBC and check brain ultrasound for ICH.
  - Treat neonatal thrombocytopenia with IVIG and steroids

## MEDICATION

### First Line

- Glucocorticoids (high dose over 2–3 wk)
- Dexamethasome: 40 mg PO daily
- Prednisone: 1–2 mg/kg/24 hr PO per day
- Methylprednisolone: 1g IV q8h (30 mg/kg/24 hr pediatric dose)
- IVIG: 1–2 g/kg IV × 1 dose and possible repeated in 24 hr:
- Used only for critical bleeding or when the need to acutely raise platelets is required such as emergency surgery
  - Anti-D immunoglobulin 50 $\mu$g/kg/24 h IV:
- Used only presplenectomy and in Rh+ positive patients

### Second Line

- Chronic long-term suppression and steroid bolus therapy
- Immunosuppressive agents:
    Azathioprine
  - Cyclosporin
  - Mycophenylate
  - Chemotherapeutic agents:
  - Vinca alkaloids
  - Cyclophosphamide
  - Combinational chemotherapy
  - Other:
  - Rituximab: monoclonal antibody directed against B-cell antigens
  - Danazol: antiandrogen
  - Experimental:
    - Other monoclonal antibodies directed at B cells
    - Stem cell transplants
    - Thrombopoietin and Thrombopoietin-like agonists

## FOLLOW-UP

### DISPOSITION

#### Admission Criteria

- Life-threatening bleeding regardless of platelet count
- Any bleeding with platelet count <20 K
- Asymptomatic patient with platelet count <20 K with issues of noncompliance or poor follow-up

#### Discharge Criteria

- Asymptomatic patients
- Patients with minor bleeding and platelets >30 K

### FOLLOW-UP RECOMMENDATIONS

Hematology referral is indicated in all cases (either outpatient or inpatient consultation).

## PEARLS AND PITFALLS

- Before low platelet counts are evaluated, pseudothrombocytopenia should be excluded.
- Spontaneous bleeding usually does not occur until platelet counts are <10 K.

## ADDITIONAL READING

- Godeau B, Provan D, Bussel J. Immune thrombocytopenia pupura in adults. *Curr Opin Heamatol*. 2007; 14:535–556.
- Fogarty PF, Segal JB. The epidemiology oif Immune Thrombocytopenic Purpura. *Curr Opin Heamatol*. 2007;14:515–519.
- George J, Woolf S, Raskob G, et al. Idiopathic thrombocytopenic purpura: A practice guideline developed by explicit methods for the American Society of Hematology. *Blood*. 1996;88:3.
- Provan D, Norfolk D, Bolton-Maggs P. Guidelines for the investigation and management of idiopathic thrombocytopenic purpura in adults, children and in pregnancy. *Br J Haematol*. 2003;120:574.
- Sukenik-Halevy R, Ellis MH, Fejgin MD. The management of immune thrombocytopenic purpura in Pregnancy. *Obstet Gynecol*. 2007;63(3):182–188.

### See Also (Topic, Algorithm, Electronic Media Element)

- HELLP Syndrome;
- Thrombotic Thrombocytopenic Purpura

## CODES

**ICD9**

287.31 Immune thrombocytopenic purpura

# IMMUNIZATIONS
*Ghazala Q. Sharieff*

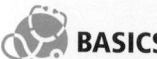 **BASICS**

## DESCRIPTION
- Immunization enhances or initiates resistance to infectious diseases.
- Passive immunization occurs by administration of antibody or through placental antibody transmission from the mother to the fetus.
- Transplacental antibodies can protect the newborn for the 1st few months of life.
- Active immunization results in stimulation of the immune system:
  - Antibody response is seen after 7–10 days.
  - IgM is followed by IgG response.
  - The IgG antibodies (which confer resistance) peak between 2 and 6 wk.
  - The route of vaccine administration is important in immune response: Improper administration may result in decreased immunity.
- Parenteral vaccines, unlike oral vaccines, may not induce mucosal secretory IgA antibodies, which prevent organism absorption in the intestines.

## ETIOLOGY
- Several types of vaccines are available:
  - Attenuated (weakened) live virus is used in measles, mumps, and rubella (MMR) vaccine and varicella (chicken pox) vaccine:
    - May cause serious infections in people with compromised immune systems.
    - Killed (inactivated) viruses or bacteria are used in some vaccines:
    - Polio, pertussis, and influenza vaccines use killed virus and therefore are safe even in people with compromised immune systems. Acellular pertussis vaccine causes fewer local and systemic reactions and has replaced the whole-cell pertussis vaccine.
  - Toxoid vaccines contain a toxin produced by the bacterium or virus (diphtheria and tetanus).
  - Hepatitis B vaccine is made with recombinant DNA technology.
  - Biosynthetic vaccines contain synthetic substances conjugated with an immunogenic carrier protein, which appear to be antigens to the immune system (*Haemophilus influenzae* type B [Hib] vaccine and pneumococcal vaccines).
- Meningococcal group C conjugate vaccine (Menjugate) is available for active immunization of children >2 yr of age, adolescents, and adults for the prevention of *Neisseria meningitis* serogroup C.
- Human papillomavirus vaccine is available.
- Several combination vaccines are also available but have an increased cost:
  - Pediarix (diphtheria and tetanus toxoids and acellular pertussis adsorbed, hepatitis B [recombinant], and inactivated poliovirus vaccine combined) is a combination vaccine providing protection against 5 serious diseases simultaneously, thereby reducing the total number of shots infants receive by up to 6.
  - Comvax combines the hepatitis B and Hib vaccines into 1 shot.
- TriHIBit combines Hib and DTaP. Unfortunately, this vaccine is licensed only for use as the 4th dose of the vaccination series at age 15–18 mo.
- Twinrix combines hepatitis A and hepatitis B vaccines into 1 shot and is given as a 3-dose series.
- Epidemiology:
  - Incidence of several life-threatening illnesses has been markedly reduced with widespread immunization use.
  - Polio caused by wild-type viruses has been eliminated from the Western Hemisphere.
  - Hib, diphtheria, and tetanus vaccines have nearly eliminated these invasive diseases among children.
  - Incidence of measles, rubella, and varicella has also declined; rubella is now very uncommon.
  - 7-valent conjugate vaccine (Prevnar) contains serotypes 4, 6B, 9V, 14, 18C, 19F, and 23F and is 80–100% effective against vaccine-type invasive disease and 50–60% effective against vaccine-type pneumococcal otitis media.
  - 2 vaccines that provide passive immunity to respiratory syncytial virus (RespiGam and palivizumab) are already in use for infants <24 mo with a history of prematurity <35 wk gestation, chronic lung disease (bronchopulmonary dysplasia), severe congenital heart disease, or severe immunodeficiencies.
  - Tdap is now recommended for children >7 yr, adolescents, and adults.
  - A rotavirus vaccine (RotaTeq) is available.
  - H1N1 as well as seasonal influenza vaccination are available in 2 forms: The flu shot, an inactivated vaccine containing fragments of killed influenza virus, and a nasal spray, which is made using a weakened live flu virus.

 **DIAGNOSIS**

## SIGNS AND SYMPTOMS
- Review prior immunization reactions:
  - The most common events associated with vaccination are mild febrile and local reactions.
- Hib:
  - Sterile abscesses may occur at the site of an intramuscular injection. Nerve and vascular injuries are uncommon. Specific side effects to routine vaccinations are listed below.
- Diphtheria-tetanus-pertussis:
  - Historically, many of the significant reactions were associated with DTP rather than DTaP.
  - Mild local reactions (redness, induration, and tenderness at the injection site):
    - Constitutional symptoms (fever <40.5°C, fussiness, drowsiness, crying)
  - Brief, generalized seizures may occur after administration of DTaP:
    - Usually seen in febrile children after the 3rd or 4th dose of the vaccine series
  - Hypotonic-hyporesponsive episodes (collapse or shocklike state) are less common after DTaP vaccination.
- Episodes of persistent, inconsolable crying for ≥3 hr have been observed following DTP injection and rarely after DTaP.
  - Encephalopathy
  - Guillain-Barré syndrome (GBS) within 6 wk of vaccination
- Hepatitis B:
  - Premature infants with birth weights of <2 kg may have a decreased response to vaccination:
    - Current recommendations advise that preterm low-birth-weight infants receive hepatitis B vaccine at 1 mo chronologic age.
    - Full-term infants may begin the series in the nursery.
- Influenza:
  - Febrile reactions occur in children <2 yr of age between 6 and 24 hr following injection.
  - There is a slight increase in cases of GBS in adults.
- Polio:
  - Several cases of oral vaccine–associated paralytic polio had been reported in the United States annually using attenuated vaccine.
  - Inactivated poliovirus vaccine (IPV), which does not carry a risk of paralysis, was introduced into the routine immunization schedule in 2000.
  - IPV contains 3 types of poliovirus inactivated with formaldehyde. Immunity postvaccination is expected to be lifelong.
- Measles-mumps-rubella:
  - Transient rash or fever ≥39°C 6–12 days after vaccination
  - Transient thrombocytopenia within 2 mo of vaccination. Other precautions to future immunization include the recent administration of immune globulin and active tuberculosis.
- Varicella:
  - A few children may develop a mild varicellalike illness with the development of fewer lesions (either vesicular or maculopapular) and lower rates of fever than unimmunized children with varicella disease.
  - Children who develop a postvaccination rash may rarely transmit the virus to others.

## ESSENTIAL WORKUP
- Take an immunization history of status of immunizations:
  - If incomplete, take a good history as to the reason why immunizations have not been administered.
- Reasons to defer vaccine administration:
  - All patients who are acutely ill with or without fever >38.5°C
  - Defer pertussis for 3 wk after a convulsion.
  - Recent administration of immune globulin is a precaution to immunization.

- True contraindications to vaccination:
  - Anaphylactic reaction to a previous dose of the vaccine:
    - Anaphylaxis to baker's yeast contraindicates immunization with hepatitis B vaccine.
    - Anaphylaxis to chicken or egg protein contraindicates influenza and H1N1 vaccination.
    - Anaphylaxis to neomycin or gelatin contraindicates MMR immunization.
    - Anaphylaxis to neomycin, streptomycin, or polymyxin contraindicates inactivated polio vaccine
  - Specific reactions within 48 hr of vaccine of a previous vaccine:
    - Severe, inconsolable screaming for 3 hr
    - Distinctive high-pitched cry
    - Hyporesponsive episode
    - Temperature >40.5°C unexplained by other cause
    - Severe local reaction involving the circumference of the injected limb unless owing to inadvertent subcutaneous injection
  - Encephalopathy within 7 days of vaccine:
    - Severe acute neurologic illness with prolonged seizures and/or unconsciousness and/or focal signs
  - Progressive neurologic disease excluding epilepsy
  - Immunocompromised hosts should not receive the varicella vaccine.
  - Severely immunocompromised patients (non-HIV related) should not receive the MMR vaccine.
  - Pregnant patients should not receive the varicella vaccine, and the hepatitis A vaccine should be used with caution. Live virus vaccines are not routinely recommended during pregnancy.
- Vaccines may be given with the following: Mild acute illness with or without fever
  - Mild to moderate local reaction (ie, swelling, redness, soreness), low-grade or moderate fever after previous dose
  - Lack of previous physical examination in well-appearing person
  - Current antimicrobial therapy
  - Convalescent phase of illness
  - Premature birth (hepatitis B vaccine is an exception)
  - Recent exposure to an infectious disease
  - History of penicillin allergy, other nonvaccine allergies, relative with allergies, receiving allergen extract immunotherapy
  - HIV-infected children who are either asymptomatic or not severely immunocompromised should be vaccinated.
- Review the immunization status and refer if catch-up immunizations are necessary.
- Specific discussion with the parents is required to review the risks and benefits of tetanus vaccination, particularly given the frequent occurrence of trauma and the need to provide both passive and active immunity at that time:
  - Documentation in the chart that the risks and benefits have been thoroughly discussed. A formal informed consent is used in some settings.
  - The National Childhood Vaccine Injury Act requires that a copy of the Vaccine Information Statements be provided before administering each dose of the vaccine.

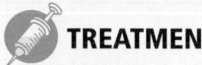 **TREATMENT**

### PRE-HOSPITAL
Attention should be focused on the airway and circulation.

### INITIAL STABILIZATION/THERAPY
Initial medications include IM or IV epinephrine for patients with anaphylaxis, diphenhydramine for urticaria, albuterol for wheezing, and intravenous fluids for hypotension.

### ED TREATMENT/PROCEDURES
- Route and timing of vaccine administration per Advisory Committee on Immunization Practices schedule.
- Prophylaxis with acetaminophen at the time of injection and again at 4–8 hr later may reduce the incidence of fever and local reactions but may reduce immunologic response.
- Children who receive varicella vaccine should avoid salicylates for 6 wk postvaccination because of the association of varicella infection and salicylates to Reye syndrome.

### MEDICATION
**First Line**
- Diphenhydramine
- Steroids
- Albuterol
- IV or IM epinephrine

**Second Line**
- H2 blockers

 **FOLLOW-UP**

### DISPOSITION
**Admission Criteria**
- Patients with serious adverse reactions following immunization should be admitted.
- Patients with anaphylaxis and encephalopathy may require admission to a pediatric ICU.
- Unexpected adverse events should be reported to the Vaccine Adverse Event Reporting System.

**Discharge Criteria**
Patients may be discharged home after routine immunizations unless an immediate adverse reaction occurs.

## PEARLS AND PITFALLS

Failure to continue diphenhydramine for 48 hr following an allergic reaction. Steroids may also be considered.

## ADDITIONAL READING

- Advisory Committee on Immunization Practices, Centers for Disease Control and Prevention. Recommended Guidelines. Available at: http://www.cdc.gov/vaccines/recs/acip/
- American Academy of Pediatrics. Available at: http://www.aap.org
- Black S, Shinefield H, Fireman B, et al. Efficacy, safety, and immunogenicity of heptavalent pneumococcal vaccine in children. *Pediatr Infect Dis J.* 2000;19:187–195.
- Black SB, Shinefield HR, Hansen J, et al. Postlicensure evaluation of the effectiveness of seven valent pneumococcal conjugate vaccine. *Pediatr Infect Dis J.* 2001;20:1105–1107.
- Halsey NA, Hyman SL. Measles-mumps-rubella vaccine and autistic spectrum disorder: Report from the New Challenges in Immunization Conference. *Pediatrics.* 2001;107:e84.
- National Immunization Hotline. Phone 800-232-2522.
- Recommended Childhood and Adolescent Immunization Schedule, by Vaccine and Age—United States, 2009. Available at http://www.cdc.gov/nip/recs/child-schedule.htm

### See Also (Topic, Algorithm, Electronic Media Element)
- Anaphylaxis
- Encephalitis
- Hepatitis
- Influenza
- Measles
- Mumps
- Pertussis
- Polio
- Seizure, Adult
- Seizure, Pediatric
- Tetanus
- Varicella

 **CODES**

### ICD9
- V03.6 Need for prophylactic vaccination and inoculation against pertussis alone
- V03.81 Need for prophylactic vaccination and inoculation against hemophilus influenza, type b {hib}
- V03.82 Need for prophylactic vaccination and inoculation against streptococcus pneumoniae {pneumococcus}

# IMMUNOSUPPRESSION

*Lara K. Kulchycki*

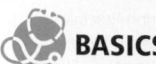 **BASICS**

## DESCRIPTION
Congenital or acquired deficiency in the ability to fight infection:
- Antibody production (B cell)
- Cellular immunity (T cell)
- Phagocytic dysfunction
- Complement deficiency
- Breach of skin/mucosal barriers

## ETIOLOGY
- Congenital disorders
- Immunosuppressive medications
- Aging:
  - Immunosenescence
  - Poor circulation and wound healing
- Chronic (lung, kidney, or heart) disease
- HIV infection:
  - CD4 count determines susceptibility to pathogens.
- Diabetes:
  - Hyperglycemia impairs immune response.
  - Vascular insufficiency
- Malnutrition:
  - Poverty and homelessness
  - Alcoholism
- Asplenia:
  - Functional asplenia (sickle cell disease) or surgical removal of spleen increases risk of infection with encapsulated organisms.
- Organ transplantation:
  - Antirejection medications suppress immune response.
  - Infections may be donor derived, recipient derived, or nosocomial.
  - Increased risk of viral pathogens, such as cytomegalovirus, Epstein-Barr virus, and human herpes viruses
  - The time elapsed since transplantation is crucial, as different patterns of infection arise in early, intermediate, and late posttransplantation periods.
- Malignancy
- Cytotoxic chemotherapy
- Increased risk of infection with pyogenic bacteria and fungi
- Infection risk related to the length and severity of neutropenia

- Neutropenia defined as absolute neutrophil count (ANC) <500/mm$^3$ or <1,000/mm$^3$ with an anticipated nadir of <500/mm$^3$:
  - In the U.S., gram-positive organisms are the leading etiology of infection.
  - Gram-negative organisms are somewhat less common but often virulent.
  - Polymicrobial infections are increasingly frequent.
  - Anaerobic isolates remain relatively rare.
  - The risk of fungal pathogens increases with prolonged neutropenia (>1 wk), prior use of broad-spectrum antibiotics, or intense chemotherapy.

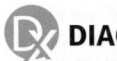 **DIAGNOSIS**

## SIGNS AND SYMPTOMS
### History
- Fever may be the only symptom of a life-threatening infection in an immunocompromised host.
- Perform a careful review of systems to identify any localizing symptoms.
- Identify risk factors for nosocomial infections, such as recent hospitalization or nursing home residence.
- Ask about close contacts with transmissible illnesses, such as influenza.
- Review medications for the presence of immunosuppressive agents, such as steroids.
- Recognize that prophylactic medicines, such as trimethoprim/sulfamethoxazole or fluconazole, will alter both the spectrum of likely pathogens and their resistance patterns.

### Physical Exam
- Examine the patient from head to toe.
- Some clinicians advise avoiding digital rectal exams in patients with febrile neutropenia.
- Inflammation may be subtle or absent:
  - Surgical abdomen without peritoneal signs
  - Meningitis without nuchal rigidity
  - Infected wounds or indwelling lines without induration, erythema, or purulent discharge

## ESSENTIAL WORKUP
- Choice of studies must be tailored to the patient and the presenting complaint.
- Test interpretation may be difficult since inflammatory responses are often blunted in immunosuppressed patients:
  - Pulmonary infections without radiographic infiltrates
  - UTIs without pyuria
  - Meningitis without CSF pleocytosis

## DIAGNOSTIC TESTS & INTERPRETATION
### Lab
- CBC with differential:
- Identify leukocytosis, left shift, bandemia, or neutropenia
- Risk of infection begins to increase once ANC <1,000/mm$^3$.
- Blood cultures:
  - 2 sets of bacterial cultures
  - Draw 1 culture from an indwelling line, if present.
  - Obtain fungal cultures if there is concern for a fungal pathogen.
- Urinalysis/urine culture:
  - Obtain by clean catch, if possible, as catheterization may introduce infection.
- Serum lactate:
  - Useful for identifying occult hypoperfusion in sepsis
- Arterial blood gas:
  - Useful in determining the need for steroids in suspected cases of *Pneumocystis carinii* pneumonia.
- Pregnancy testing in women of childbearing age

### Imaging
- CXR recommended if patient is neutropenic, hypoxic, or has abnormal pulmonary signs.
- Further imaging, such as CT or MRI, can be tailored to the patient's presentation and risk factors.

### Diagnostic Procedures/Surgery
- Lumbar puncture should be performed if there is a clinical suspicion for meningitis:
  - Check platelet counts and coagulation studies prior to procedure if thrombocytopenia or coagulopathy is suspected
  - Consider cryptococcal antigen testing even in the absence of CSF pleocytosis

## DIFFERENTIAL DIAGNOSIS
- Infection:
  - Oropharynx
  - Sinuses
  - Lung
  - Gastrointestinal tract
  - Perineum/anus
  - Urinary tract
  - Skin/soft tissue
  - Bone
  - Indwelling catheters/devices

- Noninfectious etiology of fever:
  – Drug fever
  – Allograft rejection
  – Malignancy
  – Vasculitis
  – Rheumatologic disease
  – Pulmonary embolism
  – Thyroid dysfunction

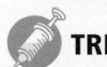 **TREATMENT**

### PRE-HOSPITAL
- Establish IV access.
- IV fluid bolus

### INITIAL STABILIZATION/THERAPY
- Aggressive fluid resuscitation for patients with hypovolemia
- Goal-directed therapy for patients with sepsis
- Consider central access with central venous pressure monitoring to assess volume status
- Cardiac ultrasound can be used to evaluate for suspected malignant pericardial tamponade, as well as IVC filling to quickly assess volume status.
- Administer pressors for hypotension that fails to respond to IV fluids:
  – Dopamine 5–20 mcg/kg/min IV
  – Norepinephrine 2–12 mcg/min IV

### ED TREATMENT/PROCEDURES
- Institute appropriate infection control precautions, such as neutropenic or contact precautions.
- Rapidly collect appropriate cultures and administer broad-spectrum antibiotics.
- Low-risk patients with fever may be candidates for outpatient treatment with oral antibiotics.
- Low-risk:
  – Age >16 and <60 yr
  – Outpatient status at time of fever
  – ANC >100 cells/mm$^3$
  – Duration of neutropenia <7 days
  – Expected resolution of neutropenia <10 days
  – Well appearing
  – No hypotension
  – No change in mental status
  – No dehydration
  – Lack of comorbid conditions:
    ○ Chronic pulmonary disease
    ○ Diabetes
    ○ Renal failure
  – Malignancy in remission
  – No history of fungal infections
  – Normal CXR

### MEDICATION
- Treatment regimens should, if possible, be tailored to the patient.
- Empiric therapy with broad-spectrum agents must be rapidly administered in febrile neutropenia or sepsis.
- Oral antibiotic therapy:
  – Produces comparable results in low-risk adults with febrile neutropenia
  – Ciprofloxacin 750 mg PO b.i.d. plus amoxicillin-clavulanate 875 mg PO b.i.d.
- Parenteral monotherapy options:
  – Ceftazidime: 2 g IV q8h (peds: 150 mg/kg/24 h IV div. q8h)
  – Cefepime: 2 g IV q8h (peds: 150 mg/kg/24 h IV div. q8h)
  – Imipenem-cilastatin: 500 mg IV q6h (peds: dose based on age/weight)
  – Meropenem: 1 g IV q8h (peds: dose based on age/weight)
  – Piperacillin-tazobactam: (less well studied in neutropenia) 4.5 g IV q6h (peds: dose based on age)
- For high-risk patients, consider adding an aminoglycoside (AG) for synergism:
  – Gentamicin: 1 2.5 mg/kg IV q8h–12h (peds: dose based on age)
  – AG use increases risk of adverse events, such as acute renal failure and ototoxicity.
- Empirical vancomycin is usually not indicated in febrile neutropenia:
  – Consider adding if suspected line sepsis or history of methicillin-resistant *Staphylococcus aureus*.
  – Vancomycin: 1 g IV q12h (peds: dose based on age/weight)
- Anaerobic coverage may be added if there is concern for oral or abdominal/perianal infections:
  – Clindamycin: 600–900 mg IV q8h (peds: dose based on age)

 **FOLLOW-UP**

### DISPOSITION
#### Admission Criteria
- ANC <100 cells/mm$^3$
- Immunocompromised patients with infection who do not meet low risk criteria
- Patients with inadequate access to outpatient medical care
- Maintain lower admission criteria for:
  – Elderly
  – Diabetics
  – Children

#### Discharge Criteria
- Low-risk patients that are well appearing and can tolerate oral antibiotics and fluids may be considered for outpatient management.
- Discuss the disposition with the responsible hematology/oncology, infectious disease, or transplant physician prior to discharge.

### FOLLOW-UP RECOMMENDATIONS
24-hr follow-up must be available in order to reassess the patient and monitor culture results.

## PEARLS AND PITFALLS
- Failure to learn institutional/regional infection and antibiotic resistance patterns
- Failure to recognize that a vague symptom or isolated fever may be the sole warning sign of serious infection in an immunocompromised host
- Failure to rapidly administer broad-spectrum antibiotics in febrile neutropenia or sepsis
- Failure to involve the appropriate primary care and specialty physicians who are familiar with the patient and can help tailor therapy and ensure follow-up

## ADDITIONAL READING

- Fishman JA. Infection in solid-organ transplant recipients. *N Engl J Med*. 2007;357(25):2601–2614.
- Hughes WT, Armstrong D, Bodey GP, et al. 2002 guidelines for the use of antimicrobial agents in neutropenic patients with cancer. *Clin Infect Dis*. 2002;34(6):730–751.
- Kamana M, Escalante C, Mullen CA, et al. Bacterial infections in low-risk, febrile neutropenic patients. *Cancer*. 2005;104(2):422–426.
- Sipsas NV, Bodey GP, Kontoyiannis DP. Perspectives for the management of febrile neutropenic patients with cancer in the 21st century. *Cancer*. 2005;103(6):1103–113.
- Wingard JR. Empirical antifungal therapy in treating febrile neutropenic patients. *Clin Infect Dis*. 2004;39(Suppl 1):S38–S43.

### See Also (Topic, Algorithm, Electronic Media Element)
- Sepsis

 **CODES**

**ICD9**
279.3 Unspecified immunity deficiency

# IMPETIGO
*Irving Jacoby*

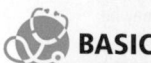 **BASICS**

## DESCRIPTION
- Impetigo is a common infection of the skin.
- Primary infection:
  - Infection of minor breaks in the skin
- Secondary infection:
  - Infection of previously existing skin lesions, known as "impetiginization"
- Most prevalent in children ages 2–5 yr
- More common in summer months and warm and humid climates
- Predisposing factors:
  - Minor trauma
  - Burns
  - Insect bites
  - HIV infection
  - Diabetes
  - Existing skin disease
  - Varicella infection
- Complications:
  - Acute poststreptococcal glomerulonephritis
    - 1–5% in patients with nonbullous impetigo
  - Sepsis
  - Cellulitis
  - Endocarditis
  - Toxic shock syndrome
  - Staph scaled-skin syndrome

## ETIOLOGY
- Classic impetigo:
  - The result of bacteria entering through traumatic skin portal from scratch, abrasion, or insect bite
  - Caused by *Staphylococcus aureus,* group A β-hemolytic streptococci, or both
  - More prevalent in warm climates and warm seasons
  - Often associated with poor hygiene
  - Treatment of both streptococci and *S. aureus*
- Bullous impetigo:
  - Caused by *S. aureus*, phage group II
  - Epidermal cleavage is caused by two staphylococcal exfoliative toxins A and B.

## DIAGNOSIS

### SIGNS AND SYMPTOMS
- Classic (nonbullous) impetigo:
  - Begins as a single 2–4-mm erythematous macule or papule that may evolve into a vesicle or pustule, on a red base
  - Rupture of the vesicle, usually within 24 hr, leaves a honey-colored, dark brown, or reddish-black exudative crust.
  - Highly contagious
  - Often pruritic, may be spread from the original site of infection by scratching
  - Mild lymphadenopathy may be seen, usually not lymphadenitis.
  - Systemic manifestations are rare.
  - Rheumatic fever does not occur following streptococcal skin infection.
  - Skin infections with nephritogenic strains of group A streptococci are major antecedents of poststreptococcal glomerulonephritis.
- Bullous impetigo:
  - Occurs most commonly in the neonate, but can occur at any age
  - Lesions begin as vesicles that turn into flaccid bullae with clear yellow fluid.
  - Nikolsky sign is absent.
  - Large, fragile bullae rupture quickly, leaving only a shiny, erythematous base with peeling edges.

### History
Fever and constitutional symptoms are uncommon.

### Physical Exam
- Common sites of infection:
  - Face
  - Extremities
  - Scalp
- The diagnosis is made based on observation of the classic exam findings, especially appearance, and distribution.

### ESSENTIAL WORKUP
Cultures of fluid from bullae or pustules may be considered in those cases refractory to traditional therapy or if methicillin-resistant *S. aureus* (MRSA) is of particular concern during an outbreak.

## DIAGNOSTIC TESTS & INTERPRETATION
### Lab
- Anti–streptolysin O titer after streptococcal impetigo is scant
- Anti–DNase B response readily occurs; 90% of patients with nephritis complicating streptococcal skin infections have elevated titers.
- Urinalysis to evaluate for hematuria or proteinuria which might suggest onset of poststreptococcal glomerulonephritis

### Imaging
Not usually indicated

### Diagnostic Procedures/Surgery
- Biopsy in this entity is not needed for diagnosis.
- If biopsy is performed, it would show subcorneal epidermal cleavage plane, inflammatory infiltrate of neutrophils and lymphocytes in the upper dermis, and subcorneal blisters with occasional acantholytic cells.
- Gram stain of blister fluid may show PMNs and gram-positive cocci in chains or clusters

## DIFFERENTIAL DIAGNOSIS
- Herpes simplex
- Varicella zoster
- Atopic dermatitis
- Contact dermatitis
- Dermatophytosis
- Erysipelas
- Candidiasis
- Scabies
- Folliculitis
- Pediculosis
- Pemphigus vulgaris
- Bullous pemphigoid
- Seborrheic dermatitis
- Thermal burns
- Stevens-Johnson syndrome
- Bullous erythema multiforme
- Staphylococcal scalded skin syndrome (SSSS; caused by systemic spread of exfoliatin in susceptible individuals)
- Pemphigus neonatorum (Ritter's disease), or SSSS in the newborn
- Toxic epidermal necrolysis
- Cutaneous anthrax

**TREATMENT**

### PRE-HOSPITAL
- Apply dressings to cover for transport.
- Gloves must be worn, as agents can be transmitted person to person.
- Cautions:
  - Maintain universal precautions.
  - Siblings of affected children in same household should be checked for lesions.

### INITIAL STABILIZATION/THERAPY
In healthy children or adults, classic or bullous impetigo is not a life-threatening condition and does not require resuscitative measures.

### ED TREATMENT/PROCEDURES
- Small lesions may be treated with topical therapy alone.
- Larger, widespread lesions, or presence of bullous impetigo, or presence of lymphadenopathy should be treated with systemic therapy.
- Systemic treatment should include a $\beta$-lactamase–resistant penicillin, cephalosporin, or macrolide antimicrobial for 10 days:
  - If no response, check for MRSA and switch antibiotic to cover for MRSA.
- Systemic antibiotic advisable during epidemics of acute poststreptococcal glomerulonephritis or in communities with widespread MRSA
- Local care should include cleansing, removal of crusts, and application of wet dressings to the affected areas.

### MEDICATION
- All treatment regimens are 10 days, except for topical retapamulin, which is used for 5 days and may enhance compliance.
- Avoid use of erythromycin if high incidence of erythromycin resistance of streptococci or staphylococci in the community.
- Oral:
  - Amoxicillin/clavulanic acid: 250 mg PO q8h (peds: 30 mg/kg/d PO in div. doses q8h)
  - Azithromycin: 500 mg PO on day 1; 250 mg PO days 2–5 (peds: 10 mg/kg PO on day 1; 5 mg/kg PO days 2–5)
  - Cephalexin: 500 mg PO q.i.d. (peds: 25–50 mg/kg/d PO in div. doses q8h–q12h)
  - Clarithromycin: 250 mg PO q12h (peds: 15 mg/kg in div. doses q12h)
  - Clindamycin: 150 mg PO t.i.d. (peds: 5 mg/kg. t.i.d.)

- Dicloxacillin: 250 mg PO q6h (peds: 25–50 mg/kg/d PO in div. doses q6h)
  - Erythromycin ethylsuccinate: 250 mg PO q6h (peds: 40 mg/kg/d PO in div. doses q6h)
  - Trimethoprim-sulfamethoxazole DS: 1 tab PO b.i.d. for 10 days. (peds: 5 mL suspension/10 kg (up to 20 mL)/dose PO b.i.d.: Useful when MRSA suspected.
  - Linezolid: 600 mg PO b.i.d.—expensive, used only for multiallergic patients or MRSA (peds: not approved for children)
- Topical:
  - Mupirocin (2% ointment [Bactroban]): adult and peds: Apply topically to affected area t.i.d. (nonbullous impetigo only).
  - Retapamulin (1% ointment) (Altabax): adult and peds >9 mo: Apply topically to affected areas b.i.d. for 5 days.

### First Line
Topical:
- Mupirocin

### Second Line
- Topical:
  - Retapamulin
- Oral antibiotics:
  - Amoxicillin/clavulanic acid
    Cephalosporins
  - Dicloxacillin
  - Erythromycin

 **FOLLOW-UP**

### DISPOSITION
#### Admission Criteria
- Admission for impetigo alone is rarely necessary.
- Patients with disease that is widespread, especially widespread bullae, or refractory to outpatient therapy
- Toxic, ill-appearing, or immunocompromised patients require admission.
- Nephritis may already be present at time patients present for care if presentation is delayed >4–5 days.
- More typically, nephritis, if seen, occurs 2–4 wk after a streptococcal skin infection.

#### Discharge Criteria
- Patients should not be toxic appearing.
- Patients/caregivers should be able to comply with the recommended treatment regimen.
- Follow-up for re-evaluation

### Issues for Referral
Periorbital edema, leg swelling, or hematuria or proteinuria should suggest poststreptococcal glomerulonephritis and referral to nephrologist.

### FOLLOW-UP RECOMMENDATIONS
- Follow-up with primary care physician should be arranged to assure resolution without complications.
- Return for failure of lesions to respond.
- Return for development of hematuria, periorbital edema, or leg swelling.

## PEARLS AND PITFALLS

- Treat with systemic antibiotics in the presence of bullous impetigo or if lymphadenopathy is present.
- Increasing antibiotic resistance continues to limit ability to use historic standard antibiotic protocols.
- Mupirocin resistance is starting to be reported.
- Cultures and sensitivity must be checked for recalcitrant lesions.
- Relapse, representing reinfection, may occur if other affected family members are not treated at the same time

## ADDITIONAL READING

- Yun HJ, Lee SW, Yoon GM, et al. Prevalence and mechanisms of low- and high-level mupirocin resistance in staphylococci isolated from a Korean hospital. *J Antimicrob Chemother*. 2003;51: 619–623.
- Koning S, van der Wouden JC, Chosidow O, et al. Efficacy and safety of retapamulin ointment as treatment of impetigo: Randomized double-blind multi-center placebo-controlled trial. *Br J Dermatol* 2008;158:1077–1082.
- Wolfson AB, Hendey GW, Ling LJ, et al., eds. *Harwood Nuss' Clinical Practice of Emergency Medicine*, 5th ed. Philadelphia: Lippincott, 2010.

### See Also (Topic, Algorithm, Electronic Media Element)
- Cellulitis
- Erysipelas
- Toxic Epidermal Necrolysis

 **CODES**

ICD9
684 Impetigo

# INBORN ERRORS OF METABOLISM

*David A. Perlstein*
*David H. Rubin*

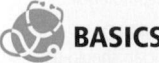 **BASICS**

## DESCRIPTION
- Defect in the type, amount, and toxicity of metabolites that accumulate due to an inherited abnormal pathway in children; result in a variety of clinical findings; >400 human diseases are caused by inborn errors of metabolism
- Epidemiology:
  - Incidence:
    - Variable: 1:10,000–1:200,000 births
- Genetics:
  - Common inherited metabolic diseases:
    - Amino acid disorders
    - Urea cycle defects
    - Organic acidemias
    - Defects in fatty acid oxidation
    - Mitochondrial fatty acid defects and carnitine transport defects
    - Mitochondrial disease
    - Carbohydrate disorders
    - Mucopolysaccharidoses
    - Sphingolipidoses
    - Peroxisomal disorders
    - Protein glycosylation disorders
    - Lysosomal disorders
    - Rhizomelic chondrodysplasia punctata
- Pathophysiology:
  - Related to defect in a metabolic pathway

## ETIOLOGY
Diverse group of disorders involving genetic deficiency of an enzyme of an intermediary metabolite or a membrane transport system.

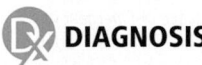 **DIAGNOSIS**

## SIGNS AND SYMPTOMS
- Disorders may present with either a rapid decompensation or a chronic indolent course
- Neonates, initial presentation:
  - Asymptomatic
  - Hypothermia (mitochondrial defects)
  - Hypotonia/hypertonia (peroxisomal disorders)
  - Apnea (urea-cycle defects, organic acidosis)
  - Seizures (peroxisomal disorders, glucose transporter defects)
  - Coma (numerous)
  - Vomiting (numerous)
  - Poor feeding, growth (numerous)
  - Jaundice (galactosemia, Niemann-Pick C)
  - Hypoglycemia (galactosemia, maple syrup urine)
  - Dysmorphic features (lysosomal storage disorders, congenital adrenal hyperplasia, Smith-Lemli-Opitz)

- Older children, untreated:
  - Failure to thrive (urea-cycle defects)
  - Dehydration (organic acidosis)
  - Vomiting (urea-cycle defects and others)
  - Diarrhea (numerous)
  - Food intolerance (lipid defects, amino acid defects)
  - Lethargy (urea-cycle defects)
  - Ataxia (urea-cycle defects)
  - Seizures (numerous)
  - Mental retardation (phenylketonuria and others)

### History
Complete history of current and concomitant illness:
- Newborn screening
- Dietary
- Family
- Consanguinity
- Other

### Physical Exam
- Abnormal odor
- Altered mental status
- Tachypnea
- Abnormal facies
- Cataract
- Cardiomyopathy
- Hepatomegaly
- Splenomegaly
- Dermatitis
- Jaundice

## ESSENTIAL WORKUP
Key is to consider in differential diagnosis:
- Deteriorating neurologic status
- Unexplained failure to thrive, with dehydration, persistent vomiting, or acidosis
- Shock unresponsive to conventional resuscitative measures

## DIAGNOSTIC TESTS & INTERPRETATION
### Lab
- Bedside glucose determination
- Electrolytes, BUN/creatinine, glucose
- CBC with differential
- Calcium level
- LFTs, fractionated bilirubin, prothrombin time
- Arterial or venous blood gas
- Lactate and pyruvate level
- Uric acid
- Urinalysis
- Chemistries, as indicated:
  - Ammonia level
  - Quantitative serum amino acids
  - Urine organic and amino acids
- Cultures:
  - Blood
  - CSF

### Imaging
- CT scan of head for altered mental status
- CXR

### Diagnostic Procedures/Surgery
Lumbar puncture

## DIFFERENTIAL DIAGNOSIS
- Often misdiagnosed as sepsis, dehydration, failure to thrive, toxic ingestion, or nonaccidental trauma
- Infection:
  - Sepsis
  - Meningitis
  - Encephalitis
- Metabolic:
  - Reye syndrome
  - Hepatic encephalopathy
  - Hyperinsulinemia
  - Hormonal abnormality
- Renal:
  - Renal failure
  - Renal tubular acidosis
- Toxic ingestion
- Central nervous system mass lesions
- Nonaccidental trauma

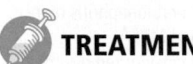 **TREATMENT**

## PRE-HOSPITAL

**ALERT**
- ABCs
- Bedside glucose, if possible
- Intravenous glucose infusion takes precedence over fluid boluses unless patient in shock. Correction can occur concurrently.
- Avoid lactated Ringer solution.
- Keep child NPO.

## INITIAL STABILIZATION/THERAPY
For altered mental status, administer Narcan, glucose (ideally after Accu-Chek and thiamine.)

## ED TREATMENT/PROCEDURES
- Establish airway, breathing, and circulation.
- For fluid boluses, use normal saline and avoid lactated Ringer and avoid hypotonic fluid.
- Initiate IV glucose at rate of 8–10 mg/kg/min to prevent catabolism:
  - Corresponds to $D_{10}$ at 1.5 times maintenance.
  - Do not delay glucose infusion to give a "bolus" of isotonic saline; may be given concurrently in a child in shock.
  - If patient is severely hypoglycemic, give IV glucose bolus of $D_{25}$.

- Rehydrate if patient is hypoglycemic:
  – Restore normal acid-base balance.
- Administer bicarbonate if pH is <7.0:
  – Initiate dialysis if severe acidosis does not improve quickly.
- Increase urine output to help in removal of some toxins.
- Initially, stop all oral intake; amino acid metabolites may be neurotoxic.
- Treat severe hyperammonemia (≥500–600 mmol/L) with immediate dialysis or with ammonia-trapping drugs such as:
  – Arginine hydrochloride
  – Sodium benzoate
  – Sodium phenylacetate
  – Sodium phenylbutyrate
  – Doses vary with disease; consult metabolic physician before use.
- Identify and treat intercurrent or precipitating infection/illness.
- Consult metabolic physician when any child presents with suspected inherited metabolic disease.

## MEDICATION
- D$_{25}$: 2–4 mL/kg IV
- Sodium bicarbonate: 1–2 mEq/kg IV
- Other disease-specific drugs, including pyridoxine and levocarnitine as indicated

### First Line
Glucose:
- NS

### Second Line
Bicarbonate therapy for pH <7.0:
- Hemodialysis as needed

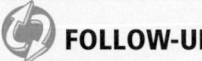

# FOLLOW-UP

## DISPOSITION
### Admission Criteria
- Infants and children presenting with new onset of suspected inherited metabolic disease
- Significant urinary ketones or not tolerating oral intake
- ICU:
  – Significant altered mental status
  – Severe or persistent acidosis
  – Unresponsive hypoglycemia
  – Hyperammonemia
- Transfer to specialized pediatric center may be indicated.

### Discharge Criteria
- Normal mental status
- Normal hydration with unremarkable labs
- No evidence of significant intercurrent illness
- Close follow-up arranged with primary care physician

### Issues for Referral
Neurodevelopment:
- Diet
- Medications

## FOLLOW-UP RECOMMENDATIONS
Primary care physician:
- Metabolic disease specialist

## PEARLS AND PITFALLS
Watch for dehydration:
- Treat dehydration with normal saline fluid bolus:
  – Follow glucose level carefully; avoid hypoglycemia.
  – Use bicarbonate cautiously and only consider if pH <7.0.
  – Hemodialysis may be necessary for hyperammonemia.

## ADDITIONAL READING
- Barness LA. An approach to the diagnosis of metabolic diseases. *Fetal Pediatr Pathol*. 2004;23:3–10.
- Fernhoff PM. Newborn screening for genetic disorders. *Pediatr Clin N Am*. 2009;56:505–513.
- Weiner DL. Metabolic emergencies. In Fleisher GL, ed. *Textbook of Pediatric Emergency Medicine*. 5th ed. Lippincott. Philadelphia; 2006.
- Leonard JV. Inborn errors of metabolism around time of birth. *Lancet*. 2000;356:583–587.
- Levy PA. Inborn errors of metabolism; part 1: overview. *Pediatr Rev*. 2009;30(4):137–138.
- Levy PA. Inborn errors of metabolism; part 2: specific disorders. *Pediatr Rev*. 2009;30(4):E22–E28.
- Wolf AD, Lavine JE. Hepatomegaly in neonates and children. *Pediatr Rev*. 2000;21:303–310.

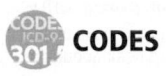

# CODES

## ICD9
277.9 Unspecified disorder of metabolism

# INFLAMMATORY BOWEL DISEASE

*Shayle Miller*

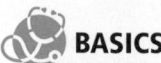 **BASICS**

## DESCRIPTION

- Idiopathic, chronic inflammatory diseases of intestines, which can involve extraintestinal sites as well.
- Differentiation between ulcerative colitis (UC) and Crohn is not always clear; intermediate forms of inflammatory bowel disease (IBD) exist.
- May present as initial onset of disease or exacerbation of existing disease.
- Maintain high index of suspicion owing to frequent, subtle presentation of Crohn disease.
- Pediatric considerations:
  - Can occur in 1st few years of life.
  - Extraintestinal manifestations may predominate.
- Differences between Crohn and UC:
  - Rectum is almost always involved in UC with continuous inflammation proximally in colon.
  - Small intestine is not involved in UC.
  - Crohn can occur anywhere from mouth to anus, often with normal GI tract segments between affected areas.
  - Crohn involves transmural inflammation, whereas UC is confined to submucosa.
- Similarities between Crohn and UC:
  - Higher rate of colon cancer with disease >10 yr
  - Bimodal age distribution, with early peak between teens and early 30s and second peak about age 60 yr
- Crohn disease clinical pattern:
  - Ileocecal: ~40%
  - Small bowel: ~30%
  - Colon: ~25%
  - Other: ~5%
- UC clinical pattern on presentation:
  - Pancolitis: 30%:
    - Most severe clinical course
  - Proctitis or proctosigmoiditis: 30%:
    - Relatively mild clinical course
  - Left-sided colitis (up to splenic flexure): 40%:
    - Between the above 2 in severity

## ETIOLOGY

- Unknown
- Crohn disease and UC are separate entities with common genetic predisposition.
- A positive family history is very common.
- Multifactorial origin involving interplay among the following factors:
  - Genetic
  - Environmental
  - Immune
- Pathogenesis:
  - Gut wall becomes unable to downregulate its immune responses, ultimately resulting in chronic inflammation.
- There is no definitive evidence for the etiologic role of infectious agents.
- Psychogenic factors may play a role in some symptomatic exacerbations.

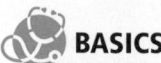 **DIAGNOSIS**

## SIGNS AND SYMPTOMS

- Crohn disease can present with any clinical correlates of chronic inflammatory, fibrostenotic, or fistulizing illness.
- Ulcerative colitis may begin subtly or as catastrophic illness.
- Constitutional, GI, and extraintestinal manifestations are common with both Crohn and UC.

### History

- Constitutional:
  - Crohn:
    - Low-grade fever
    - Night sweats
    - Weight loss
    - Fatigue
    - Pediatric: growth or pubertal delay
  - UC:
    - Fever usually only in fulminant disease
    - Weight loss
    - Fatigue
- Gastrointestinal:
  - Abdominal pain/tenderness—Crohn disease:
    - Episodic
    - Periumbilical; may localize to right lower quadrant (RLQ) with ileal disease
    - Generalized with more diffuse intestinal involvement
    - Can localize to area of intra-abdominal abscesses or fistulous involvement
    - Tenderness and distension suggest obstruction or toxic megacolon
  - Abdominal pain/tenderness—UC:
    - More generalized than Crohn disease
    - Often limited to predefecatory period
    - Tenderness with distension—suspect toxic dilation
- Stool:
  - Crohn disease:
    - Mild, loose stool, rarely >5/d
    - ~50% bloody
  - UC:
    - Diarrhea is variable, can be severe.
    - Vast majority are bloody, sometimes with severe hemorrhage.
    - Mucus
    - Tenesmus and urgency are common.
- Nausea/vomiting:
  - Crohn disease:
    - Obstruction common with ileocolonic disease
  - UC:
    - Obstruction rare
    - Diminished bowel sounds with toxic dilation
- Liver:
  - Sclerosing cholangitis can be seen.
  - Cholelithiasis can be seen in 35–60% of Crohn.
- Renal:
  - Nephrolithiasis
  - Obstructive hydronephrosis

- Musculoskeletal:
  - Peripheral arthritis/arthralgias—follows disease activity.
  - Pediatric—May be confused with juvenile rheumatoid arthritis, idiopathic growth failure, anorexia nervosa.

### Physical Exam

- Perianal:
  - Crohn disease:
    - Perianal abscesses
    - Fissures—characteristically painless
    - Fistulas—seen in up to 50% of patients with colonic disease.
    - May present prior to other manifestations.
  - UC:
    - No perianal involvement
- RLQ pain/mass often mistaken for appendicitis.
- Severe toxicity/abdominal pain—must exclude toxic megacolon.
- Extraintestinal:
  - Eye:
    - Uveitis
    - Episcleritis
    - Keratitis
  - Oral:
    - Aphthous stomatitis
  - Dermatologic:
    - Erythema nodosum
    - Pyoderma gangrenosum

## ESSENTIAL WORKUP

- May present as initial onset of disease or exacerbation of existing disease.
- Maintain high index of suspicion because of subtle presentation of Crohn disease.

## DIAGNOSTIC TESTS & INTERPRETATION

### Lab

- Nothing diagnostic
- CBC:
  - Anemia secondary to chronic or acute blood loss
- Electrolytes, BUN/creatinine, glucose
- Stool exam:
  - Occult blood
  - *Clostridium difficile*
  - Fecal leukocytes may be present.
  - O & P and culture to rule out infectious cause of enteritis
- Erythrocyte sedimentation rate is always elevated.
- Newer, investigational, serologic tests may have use as adjunctive diagnostic aids, screening testing, or predictors in therapy.

### Imaging

- Upright chest and abdominal radiographs for:
  - Toxic megacolon (>6 cm dilation)
  - Obstruction
  - Air in wall of colon (may indicate impending perforation)
  - Perforation—subdiaphragmatic air or free air outlining liver or gall bladder

- CT abdomen:
  - Distinguish abscess from localized inflammatory mass in Crohn.
- Colonoscopy with biopsy can confirm diagnosis of UC or Crohn:
  - Can be withheld with severe symptoms owing to perforation risk.
- Contrast imaging of small bowel, especially terminal ileum, may confirm diagnosis of Crohn.
- MRI can be useful in Crohn perianal disease and avoids ionizing radiation but requires appropriately trained radiologists.

## DIFFERENTIAL DIAGNOSIS

- Infectious enteritis
- Pseudomembranous colitis (*C. difficile*)
- Appendicitis
- Diverticulitis
- Diverticulosis
- Functional bowel disease
- Lymphoma involving bowel
- Ischemic colitis
- Gonococcal or chlamydial proctitis
- HIV
- Colon cancer
- Vasculitis
- Amyloidosis

 **TREATMENT**

### PRE-HOSPITAL
Vital sign stabilization as per BLS

### INITIAL STABILIZATION/THERAPY
- IV 0.9% NS volume replacement if dehydrated
- Transfusion if significant blood loss

### ED TREATMENT/PROCEDURES
- Nasogastric (NG) suction if obstruction or toxic dilation suspected
- Broad-spectrum antibiotics for fulminant UC or suspected perforation
- Consider steroid replacement if stress doses are required for those recently on oral steroids.
- Surgical evaluation indications:
  - Free perforation
  - Intestinal obstruction
  - Massive, unresponsive hemorrhage
  - Toxic dilation:
    - Not an absolute indication for surgical intervention
    - Intensive medical management with small bowel decompression and close radiographic monitoring and surgical consultation
- Walled-off perforation with abscess:
  - Usually not an indication for emergent surgery
  - Careful observation for peritonitis
- Medical therapy:
  - Treatment is usually not initiated unless diagnosis is already established.
  - Refill or restart medications in patient with known disease.

- ED-prescribed medical regimen should be individualized, and consultation with gastroenterologist strongly recommended:
  - Aminosalicylate (sulfasalazine mesalamine) is used for mild to moderate disease.
  - Antidiarrheal agent (diphenoxylate) is used—but withhold if severe disease or suspect toxic megacolon.
  - Steroid (prednisone, budesonide or hydrocortisone enema, ACTH) is used for moderate to severe disease.
  - Antibiotics (metronidazole and/or ciprofloxacin) aid in treatment of Crohn with colon/perineal involvement.
  - Immunosuppressive agents (azathioprine, methotrexate) are used in severe disease.
  - Monoclonal antibodies neutralize cytokine tumor necrosis factor (TNF)-alpha and inhibit binding to TNF-alpha receptors (infliximab [Remicade]). Used as parenteral therapy in disease unresponsive to other modalities. Not ED drug, but be aware of potential severe adverse reactions, infusion reactions, autoimmune diseases, and infections.

### Pediatric Considerations
If nonaccidental trauma is suspected, prompt referral to appropriate child protective agencies is required along with medical treatment.

### MEDICATION
- Ciprofloxacin: 500 mg (peds: 10–20 mg/kg q12) PO q12h
- Hydrocortisone enema: 60 mg
- Mesalamine enemas: 1–4 g retention enema—retain overnight. Adult.
- Mesalamine suppository: 500 mg per rectum b.i.d. Adult.
- Mesalamine tablets (Asacol sustained release 400 mg; Pentasa 250 mg): 800 mg PO t.i.d.; 1000 mg PO q.i.d. Adult.
- Methylprednisolone: 125–250 mg IV load (peds: 2 mg/kg IV load, maintenance as adult), then 0.5–1 mg/kg/dose q6h for 5 d
- Metronidazole: 250–500 mg (peds: 30 mg/kg/24h) PO t.i.d.
- Prednisone: 40–60 mg (peds: 1–2 mg/kg) PO daily
- Sulfasalazine (Azulfidine): 500 mg (peds: 30 mg/kg) PO q.i.d.

 **FOLLOW-UP**

### DISPOSITION

#### Admission Criteria
- Surgical indication:
  - Massive, unresponsive hemorrhage
  - Perforation
  - Toxic dilation
  - Obstruction
- Severe flare-up:
  - Electrolyte imbalance
  - Severe dehydration
  - Severe pain
  - High fever
  - Significant bleeding

### Discharge Criteria
- Initial presentation of diarrhea, mild pain, without toxicity, with close follow-up
- Mild to moderate exacerbation of known disease without obstruction, severe bleeding, severe pain, dehydration, with close follow-up, on renewed therapy or with addition of steroid

### Issues for Referral
Extraintestinal manifestations
- Ocular
- Dermatologic

### FOLLOW-UP RECOMMENDATIONS
Gastroenterologist or primary care as managing physician with surgical consultation as indicated

## PEARLS AND PITFALLS

- With severe flare, rule out toxic meagacolon.
- Consider Crohn in children with growth/puberty delay.
- Consider Crohn with perianal disease.
- Rule out *C. difficile* with flares; the incidence of *C. difficile* complicating IBD is increasing.
- Avoid antidiarrheals/spasmodic with severe UC disease.

## ADDITIONAL READING

- Ananthakrishnan AN. *Clostridium difficile* and inflammatory bowel disease. *Gastroenterol Clin N Am.* 2010;38(4):711–728.
- Sauer CG. Pediatric Inflammatory bowel disease: highlighting pediatric differences in IBD. *Med Clin N Am.* 2010;94(1):35–52.
- Sanborn WJ. New concepts in anti tumor necrosis factor therapy for inflammatory bowel disease. *Rev Gastroenterol Disord.* 2005;5(1):10–18.
- Zisman TL. Prognostic modalities in inflammatory bowel disease. *Med Clin N Am.* 2010;94(1):155–178.

### See Also (Topic, Algorithm, Electronic Media Element)
- Abdominal Pain
- Diarrhea

 **CODES**

ICD9
558.9 Other and unspecified noninfectious gastroenteritis and colitis

# INFLUENZA

*Philip Shayne*
*Stephen Roy Pitts*

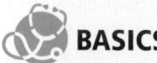 **BASICS**

## DESCRIPTION

- Acute, usually self-limited, viral infection
- Transmission: by dispersion in small-particle aerosols created by sneezing, coughing, and talking
- Virus is deposited on respiratory tract epithelium and absorbed.
- Incubation period: 1–2 days
- Mean duration in adults: 4 days
- Seasonal outbreaks most common in February.
- 2009 novel H1N1 pandemic peaked in fall and early winter of that year. Children and pregnant women had particularly high complication rates.
- Complications:
  - Primary influenza viral pneumonia
  - Secondary bacterial pneumonia
  - Exacerbations of COPD
  - Otitis and sinusitis in children
  - Reactive airway disease
  - Rare complications: Myositis, myocarditis, pericarditis, and aseptic meningitis
  - ARDS and multisystem organ failure
- Key features:
  - Seasonal epidemics are spread by high attack rates in immunologically naive children.
  - Intermittent unpredictable pandemics
  - Mortality results largely from pulmonary complications.

### Pediatric Considerations
- Children exhibit more lower-respiratory involvement (croup, bronchitis, bronchiolitis, pneumonitis) and higher temperatures than adults.
- Children were particularly susceptible to complications of novel H1N1 influenza virus.
- Myalgias in the calf muscle
- Febrile convulsions occur in ~10% of children <5 yr of age with influenza infection.
- Reye syndrome:
  - Influenza may be predisposing factor.
  - Rare and severe complication associated with salicylate use
  - Acute liver and brain injury

## ETIOLOGY
- Caused usually by 1 of 2 influenza types, A or B, the latter usually less severe.
- Influenza A subtypes are classified by hemagglutinin antigens H1, H2, or H3 and less importantly by the neuraminidase subtype.
- Vaccine targets the subtype antigen, which is also the target of natural immunity.

- Annual epidemics are seasonal:
  - Caused by *antigenic drift*—new variants from minor changes in surface protein
  - Duration of epidemic <6 wk
- Pandemics:
  - Unpredictable
  - Caused by *antigenic shift*—major changes in virus structure
- Waterfowl reservoir of influenza virus
- Avian flu has proven difficult to transmit to humans and between humans, but infection is often very severe.

 **DIAGNOSIS**

- Complicated by similar acute infections caused by other respiratory viruses
- CDC defines Influenza-like illness (ILI) as cough or sore throat in a patient with fever >100°F and no alternative diagnosis.

## SIGNS AND SYMPTOMS
- Local status of the epidemic (see CDC weekly status update <URL>http://www.cdc.gov/flu/weekly/</URL>) is by far the most important predictor of influenza in a patient with ILI.
- Despite poor discriminating properties of specific symptoms, a rise in ILI cases accurately predicts onset of the seasonal influenza epidemic.

### History
- No single finding on history has much predictive power. Influenza can be asymptomatic or fatal.
- Fever and cough together is somewhat specific for influenza but insensitive.
- Specificity of findings depends on prevalence of other circulating viruses. For example, RSV epidemics are also accompanied by high frequency of fever.

### Physical Exam
- Fever: Degree of fever is correlated with likelihood of influenza in randomized trials of persons with ILI.
- There is no consistent relationship between physical findings and influenza positivity across multiple studies, but there are very few studies of ED patients.
- Many patients have evidence of reactive airway disease with bronchoconstriction.

### Geriatric Considerations
Elderly may present with high fever, lassitude, and confusion without pulmonary complications.

## ESSENTIAL WORKUP
Clinical diagnosis based on the signs and symptoms of influenza during the winter months in the setting of a known outbreak

## DIAGNOSTIC TESTS & INTERPRETATION
### Lab
- CBC (optional):
  - WBC: Normal to mildly decreased
- Pulse oximetry/arterial blood gas for significant pulmonary symptoms

### Imaging
CXR for prominent lower respiratory signs or symptoms:
- Normal (50–90%)
- Bilateral interstitial infiltration

### Diagnostic Procedures/Surgery
- Culture of nasopharyngeal swab or aspirate is more sensitive than pharynx.
- Yield declines rapidly with duration of symptoms. Infrequently positive after day 2.
- Rapid influenza diagnostic tests and direct fluorescent antibody tests are inexpensive, rapid, and specific but often of very low sensitivity. Some are able to discriminate between A and B but not subtypes of A.
- Polymerase chain reaction (PCR) tests have short turnaround time, are both sensitive and specific, and can discriminate H1 from H2 antigens, and combination of H1 negative and H2 negative is very specific for 2009 H1N1.
- Viral culture: Turnaround time too long for ED use, although OK for local surveillance.

## DIFFERENTIAL DIAGNOSIS
- Other respiratory viruses
- Bronchitis
- Atypical pneumonia
- Epstein-Barr infection (infectious mononucleosis)
- Anthrax is very rare and much more likely to include dyspnea and nausea.

**TREATMENT**

**PRE-HOSPITAL**
Vaccination and respiratory hygiene for EMS personnel during outbreaks

**INITIAL STABILIZATION/THERAPY**
Aggressive fluid resuscitation, supplemental oxygen, and positive-pressure ventilation as clinical circumstances dictate

**ED TREATMENT/PROCEDURES**
- Supportive and symptomatic:
  - Antipyretics (acetaminophen or nonsteroidal anti-inflammatory drugs)—avoid aspirin
  - Cough suppressants (rarely useful)
  - Rehydration
- Antivirals are effective if given within 48 hr of symptom onset:
  - Antiviral resistance patterns vary each season; confirm at CDC update page.
  - The neuraminidase inhibitors (NI) zanamivir and oseltamivir are generally active against types A and B. Peramivir (in development) is the only parenteral NI.
  - The adamantanes amantadine and rimantadine are only effective against influenza A.
  - Antivirals reduce symptom duration by 1 day. Indirect evidence of benefit in severe illness.
  - Costly, except for amantadine
  - Recommended for:
    - Patient with severe illness
    - Immunocompromised patients
    - Patients at high risk for complications
- PREVENTION:
  Inactivated, polyvalent influenza vaccine recommended annually for:
    - Adults >65 yr
    - Residents of nursing homes and long-term care facilities
    - Children age 6–23 mo
    - Children age 6 mo to 18 yr on chronic aspirin therapy
    - High-risk individuals (asthma, COPD, cardiovascular disease, immunocompromised, diabetics)
    - Health care workers
    - Caretakers of children <6 mo old
    - Women who will be pregnant during influenza season
  - Attenuated-live intranasal vaccine (FluMist) is currently approved for healthy people age 2–65 yr.
  - Contraindicated for:
    - Pregnant women
    - Close contacts and health care workers for severely immunocompromised patients

- Chemoprophylaxis in the following settings:
  - Postexposure prophylaxis for exposed family members, especially high risk
  - Short-term prophylaxis during outbreak of influenza A in high-risk patients who did not receive vaccine
  - In conjunction with vaccine in high-risk patients (including those with HIV infections) expected to respond poorly to vaccine
  - In lieu of vaccine when vaccine is contraindicated in high-risk individuals
  - In individuals providing care for high-risk persons
  - Extended-duration, season-long prophylaxis of health care workers is effective but consumes large quantity of stockpiled drug.
  - Exceptions:
    - Could interfere with live-virus vaccine.
    - Should not be started for at least 2 wk after inoculation.
    - Should be stopped 48 hr before administration
- Patients with evidence of bronchoconstriction and reduced breath sounds may benefit from bronchodilators such as albuterol.

**Pregnancy Considerations**
- Inactivated vaccine is recommended for women expected to be pregnant during influenza season.
- Live-attenuated virus is contraindicated in pregnancy.

**MEDICATION**
- Oseltamivir: 75 mg PO b.i.d. for 3–4 days
  - Postexposure prophylaxis: 75 mg PO daily for 7 days.
- Zanamivir: 10 mg nasal insufflation b.i.d. for 3–5 days
- Amantadine: 200 mg PO initially, then 100 mg PO b.i.d. for 3–5 days (halve dose if age >65 yr)
- Rimantadine: 200 mg PO initially, then 100 mg PO b.i.d. for 3–5 days
- Albuterol 2.5 mg in 3 mL by nebulizer or metered-dose inhaler with spacer

 **FOLLOW-UP**

**DISPOSITION**
**Admission Criteria**
- Hypoxia (pneumonia or reactive airway disease)
- Severe dehydration
- Alteration in mental status

**Discharge Criteria**
Most patients will have a short, self-limited course provided they are able to tolerate fluids and antipyretics.

**Issues for Referral**
Consultation with infectious disease specialist when uncertain of local disease status, diagnostic uncertainty, local antiviral resistance patterns

**FOLLOW-UP RECOMMENDATIONS**
Call back for PCR test result.

## PEARLS AND PITFALLS

- Become familiar with online CDC weekly update since flu changes each season.
- In most patients, neither testing nor antiviral treatment is necessary.
- In patients with respiratory distress or hypoxia, consider concurrent reactive airway disease.
- ED policy: Institute respiratory hygiene:
  - Etiquette posters and alcohol hand soap available

## ADDITIONAL READING

- IDSA guideline. Seasonal influenza in adults and children—diagnosis, treatment, chemoprophylaxis, and institutional outbreak management. *Clin Infect Dis.* 2009;48:1003–32.
- CDC 2009 H1N1 flu update: http://www.cdc.gov/h1n1flu/clinicians/
- Prevention and control of influenza. *Morb Mortal Wkly Rep.* 2008;57(RR07):1–60.
- Call SA, Vollenweider MA, Hornung CA, et al. Does this patient have influenza? *JAMA.* 2005;293:987–997.
- CDC. Notice to readers: considerations for distinguishing influenza-like illness from inhalational anthrax. *MMWR Morb Mortal Wkly Rep.* 2001;50(44):984–986.

**See Also (Topic, Algorithm, Electronic Media Element)**
- Anthrax
- Asthma, Pediatric and Adult
- Pneumonia, Pediatric and Adult

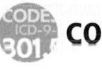 **CODES**

**ICD9**
- 487.0 Influenza with pneumonia
- 487.1 Influenza with other respiratory manifestations
- 488.1 Influenza due to identified novel H1N1 influenza virus

# INTRACEREBRAL HEMORRHAGE

*Atul Gupta*
*Rebecca Smith-Coggins*

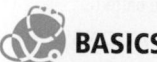 **BASICS**

## DESCRIPTION
Hemorrhage into brain parenchyma:
- Compression of brain tissues
- Secondary injury results from:
  - Cerebral edema
  - Increased intracranial pressure (ICP)
  - Potential of brain herniation

## ETIOLOGY
Intracerebral hemorrhage can occur spontaneously or from trauma:
- Uncontrolled or acute HTN (most common)
- Vascular malformations:
  - Arteriovenous malformation
  - Venous angiomas
  - Ruptured cerebral aneurysms
- Neoplasm (particularly melanoma and glioma)
- Anticoagulant therapy (Coumadin, heparin)
- Thrombolytic agents
- Illicit drugs (cocaine, amphetamines)
- Bleeding disorders (hemophilia)
- Cerebral amyloid angiopathy
- Traumatic hemorrhage secondary to blunt or penetrating injury

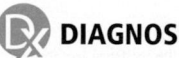 **DIAGNOSIS**

## SIGNS AND SYMPTOMS
### History
- Severe headache, typically sudden in onset
- Seizure
- Evidence of head injury
- Neck stiffness
- Vomiting
- Anticoagulation therapy
- Altered level of consciousness (may be comatose):
  - Altered mental status may occur as late as 24–48 hr after head injury.

### Physical Exam
- HTN
- Nuchal rigidity
- Altered mental status
- Variable neurologic deficits depending on site of intracerebral hemorrhage:
  - Putamen hemorrhage (35%):
    - Contralateral hemiparesis
    - Contralateral hemisensory loss
    - Occasional dysphagia
    - Occasional neglect
  - Lobar hemorrhage (30%):
    - Variable signs depending on involved area
  - Cerebellar hemorrhage (15%):
    - Vomiting
    - Ataxia
    - Nystagmus
  - Thalamic hemorrhage (10%):
    - Similar to putamen, but may also have eye movement abnormalities
  - Caudate hemorrhage (5%):
    - Confusion
    - Memory loss
    - Hemiparesis
    - Gaze paresis
  - Pontine hemorrhage (5%):
    - Quadriplegia
    - Pinpoint pupils
    - Ataxia
    - Sensorimotor loss

## ESSENTIAL WORKUP
- Manage airway if indicated
- Immediate noncontrast head CT:
  - Acute hemorrhage appears as high-density lesion.

## DIAGNOSTIC TESTS & INTERPRETATION
### Lab
- CBC
- Coagulation studies (PT/PTT, INR, platelets)
- Electrolytes; BUN, creatinine
- Pregnancy test in women of childbearing age
- EKG
- Consider toxicology screen

### Imaging
- CT as above
- MRI may be useful but currently not as available or rapid as CT.

### Diagnostic Procedures/Surgery
Cerebral angiography:
- Rarely indicated

## DIFFERENTIAL DIAGNOSIS
- Seizure:
  - Todd's paralysis
- CNS infection
- CNS mass
- Electrolyte or acid-base abnormality
- Intoxication
- Wernicke's encephalopathy
- Migraine headache
- Transient ischemic attack
- Nonhemorrhagic acute cerebrovascular accident
- Air embolism
- Differential diagnosis once bleed is seen on CT:
  - Spontaneous hemorrhage:
    - Hypertensive hemorrhage
    - Arteriovenous malformation
    - Neoplasm
  - Traumatic hemorrhage:
    - Subarachnoid hemorrhage
    - Subdural hematoma
    - Epidural hematoma

### Pediatric Considerations
Additional differential diagnoses include:
- Moyamoya disease
- Acute infantile hemiplegia

**TREATMENT**

### PRE-HOSPITAL
- C-spine precautions if head or neck injury is suspected
- Elevation of head with C-spine control
- Initial pre-hospital responder must ascertain neurologic defect to be able to note progression of symptoms.

### INITIAL STABILIZATION/THERAPY
- Manage airway and resuscitate as needed:
  - Patients with depressed level of consciousness should be intubated immediately for controlled ventilation.
- Early neurosurgical consultation

### ED TREATMENT/PROCEDURES
- Prompt neurosurgery and/or neurology consultation
- BP management:
  - Must use caution in BP control because acute lowering of BP to normal in setting of increased ICP could reduce cerebral perfusion to ischemic levels.
  - Use labetalol, nicardipine, esmolol, enalapril to lower diastolic BP initially by 10%.
  - Normotensive levels should be achieved over 12–24 hr.
  - May use nitroprusside, nitroglycerin, or hydralazine as an alternative
- Treatment of elevated ICP:
  - Controlled ventilation to $PaCO_2$ of 35 torr Fluid restriction; elevate head of bed 30°
  - Mannitol—osmotic diuresis
    Use furosemide as an alternative.
- Correct coagulopathies
- Consider anticonvulsants: phenytoin, fosphenytoin.

### MEDICATION
- Esmolol: 0.5–1 mg/kg initial bolus IV, followed by 50–150 mg/kg/min infusion
- Enalapril: 1.25–5 mg every 6 hr (risk of precipitous BP lowering, test dose 0.625 mg)
- Fosphenytoin: 15–20 mg/kg phenytoin equivalents (PE) at rate of 100–150 mg/min IV/IM
- Furosemide: 20–40 mg (peds: 0.5–1.0 mg/kg per dose) IV; may repeat as necessary
- Hydralazine: 10–40 mg (peds: 0.1–0.2 mg/kg per dose) IV; may repeat as necessary
- Labetalol: 20 mg (peds: 0.3–1.0 mg/kg per dose) IV; may give additional 40–80 mg IV q10min to max 300 mg
- Mannitol: 1 g/kg IV
- Nicardipine: 5–15 mg/hr infusion
- Nitroprusside: Start 0.25–0.3 mg/kg/min IV initially and titrate to effect (max 10 mg/kg/min)
- Phenytoin: 15–20 mg/kg per dose (peds: 0.5–1.0 mg/kg/min) at rate of 40–50 mg/hr

 **FOLLOW-UP**

### DISPOSITION
#### Admission Criteria
- To OR if surgical intervention is indicated
- To ICU if intubated, altered level of consciousness, or on IV infusion for BP control
- Admit to neurologic observation unit if normal neurologic exam without evidence of progression of bleed and hemodynamically stable.

#### Discharge Criteria
All patients with intracerebral hemorrhage should be admitted.

### Issues for Referral
Rehabilitation is a key aspect of recovery.

### FOLLOW-UP RECOMMENDATIONS
- Treating HTN in the nonacute setting is the most important step to reduce the risk of intracerebral hemorrhage.
- Discontinuation of smoking, alcohol use, and cocaine use prevents recurrence of intracerebral hemorrhage.

## PEARLS AND PITFALLS
- Brain imagining is a crucial part of emergent evaluation of patients with headache, HTN, and/or altered level of consciousness.
- Cautious BP control because acute lowering of BP to normal in setting of ICP could reduce cerebral perfusion to ischemic levels
- Consider delayed intracranial bleed in patients on anticoagulation with head trauma.

## ADDITIONAL READING
- Broderick J, Connolly S, Feldmann E, et al. Guidelines for the management of spontaneous intracerebral hemorrhage in adults: 2007 update: A guideline from the American Heart Association/American Stroke Association Stroke Council, High Blood Pressure Research Council, and the Quality of Care and Outcomes in Research Interdisciplinary Working Group. *Stroke.* 2007;38:2001–2023.
- Naval NS, Nyquist PA, Carhuapoma JR. Management of spontaneous intracerebral hemorrhage. *Neurol Clin.* 2008;26:373–384.
- Panagos PD. Intracerebral hemorrhage. *Emerg Med Clin North Am.* 2002;20:631–655.

### See Also (Topic, Algorithm, Electronic Media Element)
- Headache
- Hypertensive Emergencies
- Seizure

 **CODES**

ICD9
431 Intracerebral hemorrhage

# INTUSSUSCEPTION

*Roger M. Barkin*

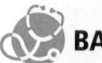 **BASICS**

## DESCRIPTION
- The proximal bowel invaginates into the distal bowel, producing infarction and gangrene of the inner bowel:
  - >80% involve the ileocecal region.
- Often occurs with a pathologic lead point in children >2 yr:
  - Hypertrophied lymphoid patches may be present in infants.
  - Children >2 yr: 1/3 of patients have pathologic lead point.
  - Children >6 yr: lymphoma is the most common lead point.
  - Adults usually have a pathologic lead point.
- The most common cause of intestinal obstruction within the 1st 2 yr of life
- Epidemiology in the United States:
  - Most frequently between 5 and 9 mo of age
  - Incidence is 2.4 cases per 1,000 live births.
  - Male > female predominance of 2:1
  - Mortality <1%
- Morbidity increases with delayed diagnosis.

### ALERT
Patients, particularly those in the pediatric age group, with a picture of potential intestinal obstruction, especially with Hematest-positive stool or altered mental status, need to have intussusception considered.

## ETIOLOGY
- Most cases (85%) have no apparent underlying pathology.
- Predisposing conditions that create a lead point for invagination:
  - Masses/tumors:
    - Lymphoma
    - Lipoma
    - Polyp
    - Hypertrophied lymphoid patches
    - Meckel diverticulum
  - Infection:
    - Adenovirus or rotavirus infection
    - Parasites
  - Foreign body
  - Henoch-Schönlein purpura
  - Celiac disease and cystic fibrosis (small intestine intussusception)

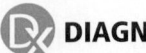 **DIAGNOSIS**

## SIGNS AND SYMPTOMS
### History
- Classic triad (present in <50% of patients):
  - Abdominal pain
  - Vomiting, often bilious
  - Stools have blood and mucus ("currant jelly" stools)
- Recurrent painful episodes accompanied by pallor and drawing up of the legs; intermittent fits of sudden intense pain with screaming and flexion of legs:
  - Occur in 5–20-min intervals
- Mental status changes:
  - Irritability
  - Lethargy or listlessness; child can be limp or have a rag doll appearance.
  - May precede abdominal findings.
- Stool variable:
  - Heme-positive (occult), bloody, or "currant jelly"
- Preceding illness several days or weeks prior to the onset of abdominal pain:
  - Diarrhea
  - Viral syndrome
  - Henoch-Schönlein purpura
- Recurrent intussusception occurs in <10% of patients.

### Physical Exam
- Fever
- Abdomen distended and swollen:
  - A "sausage" mass may be palpated in the right upper quadrant.
  - May have absent cecum in right iliac fossa.
  - Peristaltic wave may be present.
  - Rectal examination may reveal bloody stool and palpable mass.
- Dependent on the time from onset to diagnosis; perforation with peritonitis and sepsis may be present.

## ESSENTIAL WORKUP
- The diagnosis is suggested by the history and is proven radiographically.
- A heme-positive stool may aid in the diagnosis, particularly in the presence of lethargy or listlessness.

## DIAGNOSTIC TESTS & INTERPRETATION
### Lab
- CBC
- Serum electrolytes, BUN
- Type and cross-match

### Imaging
- Abdominal radiograph:
  - Abnormal in 35–40% of patients
  - Decreased bowel gas and fecal material in the right colon
  - Abdominal mass
  - Apex of intussusceptum outlined by gas
  - Small bowel distention and air-fluid levels secondary to mechanical obstruction
  - May aid in excluding intestinal perforation.
- Enema:
  - Often both diagnostic and therapeutic. Reoccurrences do happen.
    - 74% successful if intussusception present ≤24 hr
    - 32% effective when present >24 hr
    - The more distal the intussusception, the lower is the ability to reduce it radiographically.
    - Recurrent disease (up to 10%) has similar success to initial episode.
  - Complications include bowel perforation, reduction of necrotic bowel, incomplete reduction with delay in surgery, and overlooking pathologic lead point.
  - Hypovolemic shock reported following reduction secondary to endotoxins and cytokines.
  - Barium:
    - Traditional standard for diagnosis and treatment
    - Characteristic coiled-spring appearance
  - Air:
    - Fluoroscopic guidance
    - Avoids peritoneal contamination if perforation
    - Increasingly used for diagnosis and treatment
  - Contraindications:
    - Peritonitis
    - Perforation
    - Unstable patients secondary to sepsis or shock
- US is highly accurate and may be useful as a screening technique; operator dependent:
  - Typical appearance is a "donut" structure, with hyperechoic core surrounded by hypoechoic rim of homogeneous thickness.

*Diagnostic Procedures/Surgery*

If enema is unsuccessful in reducing, surgery is required on an emergent basis.

## DIFFERENTIAL DIAGNOSIS

- Infection
- Acute gastroenteritis
- Appendicitis
- Inflammatory bowel disease
- Infectious mononucleosis
- Pneumonia
- Pharyngitis/group A streptococcal
- Pyelonephritis
- Colic
- Intestinal obstruction/peritonitis
- Strangulated hernia
- Malrotation/volvulus
- Hirschsprung disease
- Trauma
- Intestinal vascular/hemorrhagic disorder
- Anal fissure/hemorrhoids
- Ulcer disease
- Vascular malformations
- Henoch-Schönlein purpura
- Polyp
- Protein-sensitive enterocolitis
- Diabetes mellitus
- Coagulopathy

 TREATMENT

## PRE-HOSPITAL

- IV access
- IV bolus of 20 mL/kg of 0.9% NS or lactated Ringer's (IR) if evidence of hypovolemia, abdominal distention, peritonitis, sepsis
- Diagnosis rarely confirmed in prehospital setting

## INITIAL STABILIZATION/THERAPY

- IV access and initiation of 0.9% NS or LR at 20-mL/kg bolus
- Nasogastric tube

## ED TREATMENT/PROCEDURES

- Stabilize patient hemodynamically.
- Surgical consultation
- Abdominal radiograph film series
- Interventional radiography for reduction if no contraindications:
  - Enemas are 75–80% successful at reduction, reflecting duration of condition.
  - Recurrences may also be reduced radiographically.
- Antibiotics:
  - Initiate if evidence of peritonitis, perforation, or sepsis.
  - Ampicillin, clindamycin, and gentamicin
  - Ampicillin/sulbactam
- Laparotomy:
  - Indications:
    - Enema is unsuccessful.
    - Enema is contraindicated.
    - Pathologic lead point
    - Multiple recurrences
  - Procedure:
    - Gentle milking of the intussusceptum
    - Resection of any nonviable bowel as well as any lead points that are identified

## MEDICATION

### First Line

- Ampicillin: 100–200 mg/kg/d q4h IV
- Clindamycin: 30–40 mg/kg/d q6h IV
- Gentamicin: 5.0–7.5 mg/kg/d q8h IV
- Ampicillin/sulbactam 100–200 mg/kg/d q6h IV

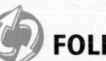 FOLLOW-UP

## DISPOSITION

### Admission Criteria

- Patients undergoing successful enema reduction should be observed for complications or recurrence.
- Patients undergoing surgery

### Discharge Criteria

- May be considered after a *very prolonged* period of observation following successful enema reduction:
  - Stable patient with normal mental status
  - Symptomatic relief of abdominal pain during the postreduction period

### Issues for Referral

Surgeon should be aware of patients with potential diagnosis of intussusception.

## PEARLS AND PITFALLS

- Infants with intermittent abdominal pain, impaired mental status, and blood in stools should generally have intussusception considered.

## ADDITIONAL READING

- Bajaj L, Roback MG. Postreduction management of intussusception in a children's hospital emergency department. *Pediatrics*. 2003;112:1302.
- Daneman A, Alton DJ. Intussusception: issues and controversies in diagnosis and reduction. *Radiol Clin North Am*. 1996;34:743.
- Fecteau A, Flageole H, Nguyen LT, et al. Recurrent intussusception: Safe use of hydrostatic enema. *J Pediatr Surg*. 1996;31(6):859.
- McCabe IB, Singer JI, Love T, et al. Intussusception. A supplement to the mnemonic for coma. *Pediatr Emerg Care*. 1987;3:118.
- Willetts IE, Kite P, Barclay GR, et al. Endotoxins, cytokines and lipid peroxides in children with intussusception. *Br J Surg*. 2001;88:878.

 CODES

ICD9
560.0 Intussusception

# IRITIS

*Jessica Freedman*

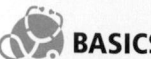 **BASICS**

## DESCRIPTION
- Inflammation of anterior uveal tract
- Iritis and anterior uveitis are synonymous.
- Uveitis secondary to trauma is also called *traumatic iritis*.

## ETIOLOGY
- Most cases are idiopathic, but may be traumatic or associated with numerous infectious and noninfectious systemic diseases.
- May be acute or chronic.
- Noninfectious systemic diseases include the following:
  - Ankylosing spondylitis
  - Reiter syndrome
  - Sarcoidosis
  - Behçet disease
  - Inflammatory bowel disease
  - Juvenile rheumatoid arthritis
  - Kawasaki syndrome
  - Interstitial nephritis
  - IgA nephropathy
  - Drug reactions
  - Sjögren syndrome
  - Psoriatic arthritis
- Infectious conditions include the following:
  - Viral:
    o Rubella
    o Measles
    o Adenovirus
    o Herpes simplex virus
    o Herpes zoster virus
    o HIV
    o Mumps
    o Varicella
    o Cytomegalovirus
    o West Nile virus
  - Bacterial:
    o Tuberculosis
    o Syphilis
    o Pertussis
    o Brucellosis
    o Lyme disease
    o Chlamydia
    o Rickettsia
    o Gonorrhea
    o Leprosy
  - Fungal:

- Malignancies include the following:
  - Leukemia
  - Lymphoma
  - Multiple sclerosis
  - Malignant melanoma
- Other causes include the following:
  - Cocaine use
  - Exposure to pesticides
  - Corneal foreign body
  - Blunt trauma

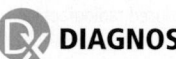 **DIAGNOSIS**

## SIGNS AND SYMPTOMS
- Acute presentation:
  - Ocular pain, red eye
  - Photophobia (consensual)
  - Lacrimation
  - Decreased visual acuity (usually mild)
  - Cells and flare in anterior chamber; hypopyon
  - Posterior synechiae (adhesions of iris to lens)
  - Miosis
  - Low intraocular pressure (occasionally may be high)
  - Injection of perilimbal vessels (ciliary flush)
- Chronic presentation:
  - Recurrent episodes
  - Few or no acute symptoms

## ESSENTIAL WORKUP
- History and review of systems:
  - Up to 50% may be associated with systemic disease.
- Slit-lamp exam:
  - Inflammatory cells (leukocytes) or "flare" in the anterior chamber are diagnostic.
  - Flare is a homogeneous fog secondary to protein leakage into aqueous humor.
  - Use short, wide beam to best appreciate cells and flare.
  - Cellular deposits with more severe inflammation
- Intraocular pressure measurement
- If topical anesthesia relieves pain, probably *not* iritis.

## DIAGNOSTIC TESTS & INTERPRETATION
- None usually indicated
- Tailored outpatient workup if history, signs, and symptoms point strongly to a certain cause (with referral to ophthalmology, rheumatology, or internal medicine)

### Lab
- TB:
  - Purified protein derivative (PPD)
- Sarcoidosis:
  - PPD
- Ankylosing spondylitis:
  - Erythrocyte sedimentation rate
  - HLA-B27
- Inflammatory bowel disease:
  - HLA-B27
- Reiter syndrome:
  - HLA-B27
  - Cultures of conjunctiva and urethra
- Psoriatic arthritis:
  - HLA-B27
- Lyme disease:
  - Immunoassays
- Juvenile rheumatoid arthritis:
  - Antinuclear antibody
  - Rheumatoid factor
- Sarcoidosis:
  - Angiotensin-converting enzyme
  - Serum lysozyme level
- STI:
  - Rapid plasma reagin or VDRL test
  - Fluorescent treponemal antibody absorption test
  - Appropriate cultures

### Imaging
- Ankylosing spondylitis:
  - Sacroiliac spine radiograph
- Sarcoidosis:
  - CXR
- TB:
  - CXR

### Diagnostic Procedures/Surgery
US biomicroscopy can be used to can help to diagnose pathologies.

## DIFFERENTIAL DIAGNOSIS
- Acute angle-closure glaucoma
- Conjunctivitis
- Corneal abrasion
- Corneal foreign body
- Episcleritis
- Intraocular foreign body
- Keratitis
- Posterior segment tumor

 TREATMENT

## INITIAL STABILIZATION/THERAPY
- Goal:
  - Reduce inflammation and prevent complications
- Cycloplegic agent (short-acting):
  - Decreases pain, photophobia
  - Prevents development of posterior synechiae

## ED TREATMENT/PROCEDURES
- Cycloplegia
- Topical steroids if indicated:
  - Use with caution, in consultation with ophthalmologist.
  - May cause significant complications (ie, progression of herpes simplex virus keratitis).
- Treat secondary glaucoma.
- Supportive measures:
  - Warm compresses
  - Dark glasses
  - Analgesia
- Identification of cause:
  - Initiate appropriate management.
- Ankylosing spondylitis:
  - Systemic anti-inflammatory agents
  - Physical therapy
- Inflammatory bowel disease:
  - Systemic steroids
  - Sulfadiazine
  - Vitamin A
- Reiter syndrome:
  - Treat urethritis (and sexual contacts).
- Behçet disease:
  - Systemic steroids or immunosuppressive agents
- Infectious causes:
  - Appropriate management of underlying infection

## MEDICATION
- Cycloplegic:
  - Cyclopentolate 1–2% for mild to moderate inflammation: 1 drop t.i.d. for (lasts up to 24 hr)
  - Homatropine 2% or 5% for moderate inflammation: 1 drop t.i.d. (lasts up to 3 days)
  - Atropine 1% for moderate to severe inflammation (should only be used in consultation with ophthalmologist): 1 drop t.i.d. (lasts 7–14 days)
- Topical steroid (should only be used in consultation with ophthalmologist):
  - Prednisolone acetate 1%: 1 drop q1–6h, depending on severity
- Analgesic:
  - Tylenol or Tylenol with codeine

### Pediatric Considerations
Cycloplegics not recommended in children <6 yr:
- May cause systemic anticholinergic toxicity with blurred vision, flushing, tachycardia, hypotension, and hallucinations.

 FOLLOW-UP

## DISPOSITION
### Admission Criteria
Not indicated unless significant systemic illness

### Issues for Referral
- Iritis:
  - Refer to ophthalmologist within 24 hr for follow up care and possible steroid therapy.
- Inflammatory bowel disease:
  - Gastroenterology consult
- Reiter syndrome:
  - Rheumatology consult
- Psoriatic arthritis:
  - Rheumatology consult
- Juvenile rheumatoid arthritis:
  - Rheumatology consult

## PEARLS AND PITFALLS
- If topical anesthesia relieves pain, probably *not* iritis.
- Must be differentiated from other, vision-endangering forms of eye pain:
  - Keratitis
  - Herpes simplex conjunctivitis
  - Bacterial conjunctivitis
  - Acute-angle closure glaucoma
  - Traumatic globe rupture

## ADDITIONAL READING
- Bertolini J, Pelucio M. The red eye. *Emerg Med Clin North Am.* 1995;13:561–579.
- Dargin JM, Lowenstein RA. The painful eye. *Emerg Med Clin North Am.* 2008; 26:199–216, viii.
- Kunimoto D, Kanitkar K, Makar M. *The Wills Eye Manual: Office and Emergency Room Diagnosis and Treatment of Eye Diseases.* 4th ed. Philadelphia: Lippincott Williams & Wilkins; 2004.
- Leibowitz HM. The red eye. *New Engl J Med.* 2000;343:345–351.
- Ventura A, Hayden B, Taban M, et al. Ocular Inflammatory Diseases. *Ultrasound Clin.* 2008; 3(2):245–255.
- Weinberg RS. Uveitis. *Ophthalmol Clin North Am.* 1999;12:71–79.

### See Also (Topic, Algorithm, Electronic Media Element)
- Conjunctivitis
- Red Eye

 CODES

ICD9
- 364.00 Acute and subacute iridocyclitis, unspecified
- 364.3 Unspecified iridocyclitis
- 364.10 Chronic iridocyclitis, unspecified

I

# IRON POISONING

*Sean M. Bryant*

## BASICS

### DESCRIPTION
- Peak concentrations are 2–4 hr postingestion
- Serum concentrations not reliable if obtained >4–6 hr after ingestion:
  - Enteric coated or sustained release—erratic and may warrant serial levels
- Postabsorption: Iron redistributes into tissues, and fall in serum iron occurs as free iron shifts intracellularly, causing damage at cellular level.
- Injury patterns:
  - Corrosive injury to intestinal mucosa may result in profound fluid loss (shock), hemorrhage, and perforations.
  - Liver receives largest load of iron because of portal venous circulation—has highest injury (hemorrhagic periportal necrosis).
- Free iron:
  - Concentrates in mitochondria, disrupting oxidative phosphorylation; catalyzes lipid peroxidation and free radical formation, resulting in cell death; and increases anaerobic metabolism and acidosis
  - Causes myocardial depression, venodilation, and cerebral edema
- Hydration of ferric form liberates 3 protons, resulting in acidemia.

### ETIOLOGY
Elemental iron ingestion:
- Nontoxic <20 mg/kg
- Moderate to severe >40 mg/kg
- Lethality possible >60 mg/kg
- Elemental iron equivalents:
  - Ferrous sulfate, 20% (325 mg = 65 mg Fe)
  - Ferrous gluconate, 12%
  - Ferrous fumarate, 33%
- Prenatal vitamins vary from 60–90 mg elemental iron per tablet.
- Children's vitamins may contain 5–18 mg elemental iron per tablet.

#### Pediatric Considerations
- Historically notorious for the highest mortality rate among pediatric accidental exposures (adult iron products).
- Children's chewable iron products have been shown to be safe.

## DIAGNOSIS

### SIGNS AND SYMPTOMS
- Classically divided into 5 stages:
  - **Stage 1: GI** (0.5–6 hr):
    - Abdominal pain
    - Vomiting
    - Diarrhea
    - Hematemesis
    - Hematochezia
  - **Stage 2: Latent/quiescent** (6–24 hr):
    - Resolution of GI symptoms
    - Deceptive phase
    - Possible hypotension and acidosis
  - **Stage 3: Shock and organ failure** (6–72 hr):
    - Hypoperfusion
    - Metabolic acidosis
    - Coma
    - Coagulopathy
  - **Stage 4: Hepatic failure** (2–3 days):
    - Coagulopathy
    - Hypoglycemia
    - Jaundice
    - Elevated LFTs (transaminases) and bilirubin
  - **Stage 5: Obstruction** (2–4 wk):
    - Gastric outlet and small bowel obstruction
    - Abdominal pain, vomiting
- Patient may present in or skip any of the 5 stages.
- If onset of stage 1 does not occur within 6 hr, likely not significant ingestion.

### ESSENTIAL WORKUP
Acute iron poisoning is a clinical diagnosis, regardless of laboratory results

### DIAGNOSTIC TESTS & INTERPRETATION
#### Lab
- Serum iron levels (mg/dL):
  - Peak absorption 2–6 hr
  - 4 hr is the most common time for peak level.
  - Delayed peak with enteric coated/sustained release
- Electrolytes, BUN/creatinine, glucose:
  - Anion gap metabolic acidosis
  - Hyperglycemia early
  - Hypoglycemia late
- Arterial blood gas:
  - Metabolic acidosis
- CBC:
  - Anemia with significant hemorrhage
  - Leukocytosis
- Liver function
- Coagulation profile
- Lactate
- Type and screen if hemorrhage
- Total iron-binding capacity is not useful and not recommended.

#### Imaging
Abdominal radiograph check for:
- Tablets (children's chewables rarely visible)
- Absence of pill fragment interpretation:
  - Patient did not ingest iron.
  - Iron was in solution or has already dissolved.
  - Patient ingested pediatric multivitamin product
  - Absence of radiopacities does not rule out significant or lethal ingestion.
- Perforation

### DIFFERENTIAL DIAGNOSIS
- Sepsis
- Acetaminophen toxicity
- Toxic ingestions causing anion gap acidosis:
  - Salicylate
  - Cyanide
  - Methanol
  - Ethylene glycol
- Mushrooms
- Heavy metals
- Theophylline toxicity
- GI bleed from other causes (alcoholic liver disease)

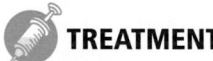

## TREATMENT

### PRE-HOSPITAL
Collect prescription bottles/medications for identification in the ED.

### INITIAL STABILIZATION/THERAPY
- ABCs:
  - Intubate if profoundly unstable.
  - Venous access and fluids for hypotension
  - Cardiac monitor and pulse oximetry
- Naloxone, thiamine, dextrose (or Accu-Chek) as indicated for altered mental status

## ED TREATMENT/PROCEDURES

- Decontamination:
  - Iron is poorly adsorbed to activated charcoal.
  - Gastric lavage has not been shown to change outcome.
  - $NaHCO_3$, phospho soda, and oral deferoxamine are not recommended.
  - If pill fragments are visualized on x-ray, or history of significant ingestion:
    - Consider whole bowel irrigation (with NG Go-Lytely: peds: 10–15 mL/kg/hr; adult: 1–2 L/hr) while monitoring progression with radiograph (KUB).
    - Caution with GI bleed
  - Endoscopy or gastrotomy can remove bezoar formation after massive ingestions (> 240 mg/kg).
- Chelation with deferoxamine (DFO):
  - DFO is a highly specific chelator of parenteral iron.
  - IV infusion results in more constant DFO levels and is route of choice:
    - Must be given as soon as possible (<24 hr).
  - Administration techniques:
    - Increase IV infusion rate to 15 mg/kg/hr over 20 min, monitoring for hypotension.
    - Decrease infusion rate if hypotension occurs.
    - Infusion rates as high as 45 mg/kg/hr have been tolerated.
    - Disregard manufacturer's recommendation of maximum daily doses of 6 g in serious iron exposures.
  - IM DFO challenge test is not advocated.
  - Indication for administration:
    - Sustained GI symptoms
    - Altered mental status
    - Hypotension, lethargy, metabolic acidosis, or shock
    - Serum iron > 500 mg/dL
    - Serum iron >350 mg/dL *and* pills seen on KUB.
    - Rising serum iron levels
    - Interpret serum levels cautiously—time since ingestion must be considered: Treatment may be indicated in patient who presents late, after distribution stage (>8 hr postingestion), with serum iron level <350 mg/dL
    - If serum iron levels are not readily available, base treatment decisions on clinical status.

- Length of infusion (controversial):
  - DFO–iron complex causes urine to turn *vin rose* color; this suggests continuing infusion until urine returns to normal.
  - Resolution of signs and symptoms of significant toxicity is criterion for discontinuing DFO.
  - Prolonged DFO therapy >24–48 hr may precipitate adult respiratory distress syndrome.
  - In severe cases with continued signs and symptoms, infusion may be continued cautiously at lower dose.
- Controversies:
  - Safety of DFO infusions given for >24 hr
  - Maximal infusion rates and total amount of DFO given
  - What serum iron concentration warrants treatment.
  - Endpoint of treatment (best endpoint is resolution of poisoning, ie, acidemia)
  - Role of extracorporeal elimination
- Contact regional poison center for moderate to severe iron exposures.

## MEDICATION

- Dextrose: $D_{50}W$ 1 amp (50 mL or 25 g; peds: $D_{25}W$ 2–4 mL/kg) IV
- Naloxone (Narcan): 2 mg (peds: 0.1 mg/kg) IV or IM initial dose
- Thiamine (vitamin $B_1$): 100 mg (peds: 50 mg) IV or IM

 **FOLLOW-UP**

### DISPOSITION

#### Admission Criteria

- GI symptoms or dehydration
- Patients treated with deferoxamine
- ICU admission for coma, shock, metabolic acidosis, or iron levels >1,000 mg/dL

#### Discharge Criteria

- Asymptomatic with negative radiograph
- Minimal to no symptoms after 6-hr observation
- Mild GI symptoms that have resolved without evidence of metabolic acidosis and serum iron <350 mg/dL

### Issues for Referral

Contact regional poison center for mild to moderate toxicity.

## FOLLOW-UP RECOMMENDATIONS

- Follow-up after discharge may be indicated in patients who are at risk of developing gastric outlet obstruction.
- Psychiatric referral for patients with intentional overdose

## PEARLS AND PITFALLS

- DFO may be indicated in patients who present late, after distribution stage (>8 hr postingestion), or with serum iron level <350 mg/dL and signs of intracellular poisoning (eg, anion gap metabolic acidosis).
- The resolution of GI symptoms does not indicate that there is not significant iron toxicity that will progress over time.

## ADDITIONAL READING

- Anderson BD, Turchen SG, Manoguerra AS, et al. Prospective analysis of ingestions of iron containing products in the United States: Are there differences between chewable vitamins and adult preparations?. *J Emerg Med*. 2000;19:255–258.
- Bryant SM, Leikin J. Iron. In: Brent J, Wallace KL, Burkhart KK, et al., eds. *Critical Care Toxicology*. St. Louis, MO: Mosby; 2005.
- Leikin J, Paloucek F. Iron. In: *Poisoning and Toxicology Handbook*. Hudson, OH: Lexi-Comp; 2002.
- Mills KD, Curry SG. Acute iron poisoning. *Emerg Med Clin North Am*. 1994;12(2):397–413.
- Tenenbein M. Benefits of parenteral deferoxamine for acute iron poisoning. *J Toxicol Clin Toxicol*. 1996;34(5):485–489.

 **CODES**

### ICD9

964.0 Poisoning by iron and its compounds

I

# IRRITABLE BOWEL
*Scott A. Miller*

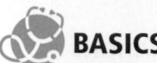 **BASICS**

## DESCRIPTION
- Syndrome of abdominal pain or discomfort associated with altered bowel habits and no other pathology explaining symptoms
- Prevalence estimated to be 10–20%
- Symptom-based diagnosis

## ETIOLOGY
- Uncertain pathophysiology, but many possibilities
- Altered GI motility:
  - Increased motility associated with diarrhea (IBS-D)
  - Decreased motility associated with constipation (IBS-C)
- Increased gut sensitivity (visceral hyperalgesia):
  - Exaggerated response to normal GI physiology
- Mucosal inflammation:
  - Postinfectious:
    ○ After bacterial enteritis, 10% have persistent IBS symptoms
  - Mucosal lymphocyte infiltration
- Altered microflora in small bowel or feces
- Some theorize carbohydrate malabsorption is a cause.
- Psychosocial dysfunction:
  - More anxiety, somatoform disorders, and history of abuse in patients who seek care
  - No evidence of increased psychiatric illness in those who do not seek care

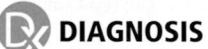 **DIAGNOSIS**

## SIGNS AND SYMPTOMS
- Abdominal pain or discomfort:
  - Relief with defecation
- Altered stool frequency
- Altered stool consistency:
  - May be predominately diarrhea (IBS-D) or constipation (IBS-C) or mixed (IBS-M)
- Bloating or distention

- Passage of mucus
- Feeling of incomplete emptying

### ALERT
- Consider further diagnostic workup if any of the following "alarm" features are present:
  - Onset >50
  - Nocturnal symptoms
  - Unintentional weight loss
  - Iron-deficiency anemia
  - Hematochezia
  - Family history of colorectal cancer, inflammatory bowel disease, or celiac sprue

## History
- Rome III diagnostic criteria: Recurrent abdominal pain or discomfort 3 days per month in the last 3 mo associated with ≥2 of:
  - Improvement with defecation
  - Onset associated with a change in frequency of stool
  - Onset associated with a change in form (appearance) of stool
- Manning (1978), Kruis (1984), Rome I and II (1990, 1999) criteria exist.
- Other symptoms consistent with IBS:
  - Abdominal distention or bloating
  - Passage of mucus in stools
  - Altered stool passage (straining, urgency, or feeling of incomplete evacuation)
  - Postprandial upper abdominal discomfort
  - Symptoms of gastroesophageal reflux
  - Flatulence
- Female < Male, 1.5–2:1 overall, higher in those who seek care

## Physical Exam
- Usually well appearing
- Normal physical exam
- May have tender sigmoid or palpable sigmoid cord

## ESSENTIAL WORKUP
Clinical diagnosis: Careful history crucial

## DIAGNOSTIC TESTS & INTERPRETATION
### Lab
- Typically no abnormalities found
- Labs to be considered (to exclude other pathology), but not required:
  - CBC:
    ○ Should not have leukocytosis or anemia
  - Normal ESR and CRP useful in excluding inflammatory conditions
  - Serum chemistry, thyroid studies unlikely to be useful
  - Stool for ova and parasites:
    ○ Most useful for diarrhea workup
  - Serum testing for celiac disease should be considered in all IBS-D and IBS-M patients (not necessary in ED).
  - Lactose breath testing:
    ○ Try dietary modification empirically 1st

### Imaging
Only necessary if excluding emergent pathology

### Diagnostic Procedures/Surgery
- Colonoscopy/flexible sigmoidoscopy for select patients (outpatient)
- Upper GI endoscopy if other pathology is considered

## DIFFERENTIAL DIAGNOSIS
- Celiac disease
- Inflammatory bowel disease:
  - Ulcerative colitis/proctitis
  - Crohn disease
- Infectious enteritis
- Small-intestinal bacterial overgrowth
- Lactose intolerance
- Colorectal cancer
- Diverticular disease
- Biliary disease
- Diabetic gastroparesis
- Pancreatitis
- Thyroid malfunction
- Obstruction
- Peptic ulcer disease
- Acute intermittent porphyria

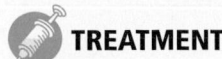

# TREATMENT

## PRE-HOSPITAL
No specific treatment required

## INITIAL STABILIZATION/THERAPY
- Symptomatic treatment
- Pain control
- Administer fluids if dehydrated

## ED TREATMENT/PROCEDURES
- Empathetic approach and therapeutic physician–patient relationship is most important.
- Exercise:
  - Improves gastric emptying
  - Improves constipation
- Diet:
  - Many IBS patients believe symptoms have a food trigger, but studies are mixed.
  - Exclusion diets starting with gluten or lactose can be empirically considered.
  - Avoid beans, cabbage, uncooked broccoli, other flatulent foods if symptomatic.
  - Specific carbohydrate diet can be considered.
- Constipation symptoms:
  - High-fiber diet, fiber supplements
  - Psyllium shows some effectiveness.
  - Polyethylene glycol helps stool frequency but not abdominal pain.
  - Lubiprostone may help women with IBS-C
- Diarrhea symptoms:
  - Loperamide improves stool frequency, but not abdominal pain.
- Abdominal pain:
  - Treat acute pain appropriately.
  - Antispasmodics may be helpful short-term
    - Hyoscine, hyoscyamine, dicyclomine, peppermint oil
- Bloating:
  - Rifaximin (nonabsorbable antibiotic) may be useful (off-label)

- Probiotics:
  - Frequently used empirically
  - Bifidobacteria appear more effective than lactobacilli
- Antidepressants:
  - TCAs and possibly SSRIs appear to be effective at relieving global IBS symptoms and reducing abdominal pain.
- Other effective drugs:
  - Alosetron is effective in IBS-D but may cause ischemic colitis—only available under tight control.
  - Tegaserod was found to be effective, but removed from general market because of the possibility of cardiovascular side-effects.
- Psychological therapies appear effective.

## MEDICATION
### First Line
- Dicyclomine: 10–20 mg PO q6h
- Hyoscyamine: 0.125–0.25 mg PO or sublingual
- Loperamide: 2 mg PO q4h PRN
- Polyethylene glycol: 17 g/d PO
- Psyllium: 1–2 tsp/d PO

### Second Line
- Amitriptyline: 25 mg PO at bedtime (or another TCA)
- Fluoxetine: 20 mg PO daily (or another SSRI)
- Bifidobacteria probiotic

# FOLLOW-UP

## DISPOSITION
### Admission Criteria
- Uncertain diagnosis with suspicion of an emergent abdominal condition
- Severe symptoms with associated psychiatric disorder

### Discharge Criteria
Almost all patients can be managed as outpatients.

### Issues for Referral
Some may benefit from GI or psychiatric referral.

## FOLLOW-UP RECOMMENDATIONS
Most important is follow-up with primary care physician to foster a therapeutic physician–patient relationship.

## PEARLS AND PITFALLS
- Beware of other emergent pathology.
- IBS is common, so it is likely the underlying cause of many abdominal workups done in the ED.

## ADDITIONAL READING
- American College of Gastroenterology IBS Taskforce. An evidence-based position statement on the management of irritable bowel syndrome. *Am J Gastroenterol*. 2009;104(Suppl 1):S1.
- Cash BD, Chey WD. Diagnosis of irritable bowel syndrome. *Gastroenterol Clin North Am*. 2005;34(2):205–220.
- Longstreth GF, et al. Functional bowel disorders. *Gastroenterology*. 2006;130(5):1480–491.
- Schoenfeld P. Efficacy of current drug therapies in irritable bowel syndrome: What works and does not work. *Gastroenterol Clin North Am*. 2005;34(2): 319–335.
- Videlock EJ, Chang, L. Irritable bowel syndrome: Current approach to symptoms, evaluation, and treatment. *Gastroenterol Clin*. 2007;36(3): 665–685, x.

## See Also (Topic, Algorithm, Electronic Media Element)
- Constipation
- Diarrhea
- Gastroenteritis
- Inflammatory Bowel Disease

# CODES

## ICD9
564.1 Irritable bowel syndrome

I

# IRRITABLE INFANT
*David H. Rubin*

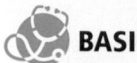 **BASICS**

## DESCRIPTION
- Most children have some period of the day when they are most irritable, usually toward the evening:
  - Normal infant crying ranges from 1–4 hr by 6 wk of age.
  - During the 1st 6 mo of life, 1-mo-olds have the highest prevalence of crying.
- Defining a child as irritable is based on a comparison with the child's normal pattern.
- Colic is the most common cause of inconsolable crying in infants, occurring in as many as 25% of healthy children:
  - Episodes of paroxysmal screaming accompanied by drawing up knees and often passage of flatus
  - Usually begins at 2–3 wk and may continue through 12 wk.
  - Diagnosis of exclusion

## ETIOLOGY
- Infection/inflammation:
  - Minor acute infections (upper respiratory infection, otitis media, thrush, gingivostomatitis)
  - UTI
  - Meningitis
  - Osteomyelitis
  - Pneumonia
  - Gastroenteritis
- Burn
- Teething
- Parental anxiety
- Trauma:
  - Foreign body
  - Fracture
  - Tourniquet (hair around digit or penis)
  - Corneal abrasion/foreign body (eyelash) in eye
  - Child abuse
  - Diaper pin
  - Splinter
- Sickle cell crisis
- Genitourinary (incarcerated hernia, testicular torsion, genital tourniquets, urinary retention)
- GI (colic, gastroesophageal reflux, esophagitis, constipation, cow's milk protein intolerance, anal fissure, volvulus, peritonitis, intussusception, appendicitis, malnutrition)
- Medications: aspirin, antihistamines, atropine, adrenergics, home remedies, new prescription
- Diphtheria, pertussis, and tetanus vaccine
- Iron deficiency/anemia
- Cardiac (supraventricular tachycardia, CHF, aberrant left coronary artery, coarctation of the aorta, endocarditis, myocarditis)
- Pulmonary (pneumothorax, pneumonia, foreign body)
- Neurologic (increased intracranial pressure: mass, hydrocephalus, intracranial hemorrhage, hematoma—subdural, epidural, skull fracture), skull fracture
- Endocrine/metabolic (inborn errors of metabolism, metabolic acidosis, hypernatremia, hypoglycemia, hypocalcemia)
- Vascular

 **DIAGNOSIS**

## SIGNS AND SYMPTOMS
- Vital signs
- Chief complaint
- Chronology of events

### History
Obtain complete history (including neonatal history) and information regarding routine feeding, crying.

### Physical Exam
- Assess vital signs, including rectal temperature and pulse oximetry.
- Measure and plot for percentiles: height, weight, and head circumference.
- Perform a thorough physical exam with infant completely undressed to exclude potential etiologies.

## ESSENTIAL WORKUP
This is usually directed by a comprehensive history and physical examination.

## DIAGNOSTIC TESTS & INTERPRETATION
### Lab
- CBC, urinalysis, chemistries, and cultures as indicated by history and physical examination
- Stat blood glucose at bedside if indicated.

### Imaging
- Fluorescein eye exam
- CXR to exclude cardiopulmonary disease
- ECG
- Electrolytes
- Urinalysis
- CT scan of the head, chest, etc., usually directed by history and physical exam
- Contrast radiograph studies such as barium enema for specific indications

*Diagnostic Procedures/Surgery*
- Skeletal survey
- Stool hemoccult test

## DIFFERENTIAL DIAGNOSIS
See "Etiology."

# TREATMENT

### PRE-HOSPITAL
As determined by history, physical examination, and laboratory studies

### INITIAL STABILIZATION/THERAPY
- Manage underlying conditions; stabilize airway, breathing, and circulation.
- Immediate removal of hair tourniquets and/or splinters

### ED TREATMENT/PROCEDURES
- Initial evaluation of the child focusing on parent–child interaction and then on potential underlying conditions
- Colic responds to soothing, rhythmic activities, avoiding stimulants (coffee, cola), minimizing daytime sleep:
  - Soy or hydrolyzed casein formula may be transiently beneficial.
  - Parents must reduce stress.
  - No proven pharmacologic therapy.
- Support, empathy, close follow-up
- Prolonged observation of the child is usually appropriate.

## MEDICATION
Dependent on the underlying condition

### First Line
Dependent on the underlying condition

### Second Line
Dependent on the underlying condition

# FOLLOW-UP

### DISPOSITION
### Admission Criteria
- Life-threatening underlying condition
- Significant parental stress secondary to crying infant

### Discharge Criteria
- No serious condition
- Functional and supportive family
- Excellent follow-up is essential; parents must feel that their observations and concerns are not being ignored; close follow-up and ongoing observation will occur.

### Issues for Referral
Determined by specific specialty-related issues

### FOLLOW-UP RECOMMENDATIONS
Long term is follow-up strongly recommended.

## PEARLS AND PITFALLS
- Address life-threatening/serious causes of irritability first.
- Detailed history and complete physical examination in the non–critically ill child is crucial prior to obtaining any laboratory or radiologic studies.

## ADDITIONAL READING
- Garrison MM, Christakis DA. A systematic review of treatments for infant colic. *Pediatrics.* 2000;106 (1 pt 2):184–190.
- Herman M, Le A. The crying infant. *Emerg Med Clin North Am.* 2007;25:1137–1159.
- Hiscock H, Jordan B. 1. Problem crying in infancy. *Med J Aust.* 2004;181(9):507–512.
- Pawel BB, Henretig FM. Crying and colic in early infancy. In: Fleisher GR, Ludwig S, Henretig FM, eds. *Textbook of Pediatric Emergency Medicine*, 5th ed. Lippincott, Philadelphia; 2006:229–231.
- Ruiz-Contreras J, Urquia L, Bastero R. Persistent crying as predominant manifestation of sepsis in infants and newborns. *Pediatr Emerg Care.* 1999;15(2):113–115.
- Swischuk LE. Irritable infant and left lower extremity pain. *Pediatr Emerg Care.* 1997;13(2):123–126.

 CODES

### ICD9
- 780.91 Fussy infant (baby)
- 780.92 Excessive crying of infant (baby)

# IRRITANT GAS EXPOSURE

*Patrick M. Whiteley*
*Sean M. Bryant*

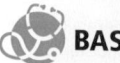 **BASICS**

## DESCRIPTION

- An irritant is any noncorrosive substance that on immediate, prolonged, or repeated contact with respiratory mucosa will induce a local inflammatory reaction.
- Respiratory irritants are inhaled as gases, fumes, particles, or liquid aerosols.
- Inhaled irritants:
  - Pulmonary toxicity is determined primarily by their water solubility.
- Inhalation accidents frequently involve a mixture of irritant gases as well as chemical asphyxiants:
  - Carbon monoxide
  - Hydrogen cyanide
  - Hydrogen sulfide
  - Oxides of nitrogen
- Risk factors include exposure to potential irritants:
  - Occupational
  - Leisure
  - Intentional
  - Accidental
- Pathophysiology:
  - Cellular injury through interaction with respiratory mucosal water with subsequent formation of acids, alkalis, and free radicals

## ETIOLOGY

- Settings:
  - Industrial: Chemical manufacturing, mining, plastics, and petroleum industries
  - Home: improper use or storage of cleaning chemicals
  - Fires: Combustion yields toxic gases.
- ***Immediate onset*** of upper airway inflammation with highly water-soluble irritant gases or with aerodynamic diameter >5 mm:
  - Ammonia (fertilizers, refrigerants, dyes, plastics, synthetic fibers, cleaning agents):
    ○ Immediate symptoms range from mild edema and erythema to full-thickness burns and airway obstruction.
  - Sulfur dioxide (fumigants used on produce, bleaching, tanning, brewing, wine making, combustion of coal, and smelting of sulfide-containing ores):
    ○ Combines with water, forming sulfuric acid.
  - Hydrogen chloride (formed during combustion of chlorinated hydrocarbons such as polyvinyl chloride):
    ○ Combines with water, forming hydrochloric acid.
  - Chloramine (generated when ammonia and bleach are mixed):
    ○ When exposed to moist surfaces, releases hydrochlorous acid.

- Acrolein (production of plastics, pharmaceuticals, synthetic fibers; formed during combustion of petroleum products, cellulose, wood, paper):
  ○ May cause protein damage via free radical production and sulfhydryl binding.
- Formaldehyde (production of plywood, particle board, insulation; combustion product of gas stoves and heaters):
  ○ Combines with water to form sulfuric acid and formic acid.
- Hydrogen fluoride (combustion of fluorinated hydrocarbons):
  ○ Depletes calcium stores, resulting in cell death.
- ***Latent period*** of minutes to hours before onset of symptoms with irritant gases of intermediate water solubility or aerodynamic diameter of 1–5 mm:
  - Chlorine (product of chlorinated chemicals; bleaching agent):
    ○ Upper and lower airway damage after reacting with water to form hydrochloric and hydrochlorous acids
- ***Delayed onset*** of symptoms up to 24 hr after inhalation with irritant gases of poor water solubility or aerodynamic diameter <1 mm (with little or no warning of exposure):
  - Oxides of nitrogen produced:
    ○ In manufacture of dyes and fertilizers
    ○ By electric arc welding and gas blowing
    ○ By fermentation of nitrogen-rich silage (silo-filler's disease)
    ○ In combustion of nitrocellulose and polyamides
  - Phosgene/carbonyl chloride (arc welding and pesticide production: Combustion of chlorinated hydrocarbons and solvents)
  - Ozone (produced during arc welding)
  - Cadmium oxide (oxyacetylene welding and electroplating)

 **DIAGNOSIS**

## SIGNS AND SYMPTOMS

- Dependent on water solubility
- Highly water-soluble gases:
  - Eye, nose, throat burning
  - Shortness of breath
  - Wheezing
  - Cough
  - Hoarseness
  - Stridor
  - Obstruction

- Intermediate water solubility:
  - Upper and lower tract involvement
  - Mucosal irritation
  - Bronchospasm
  - Dyspnea
  - Wheezing
  - Cough
  - Rales
  - Possible delayed pulmonary edema
- Other:
  - Dermal irritation
  - Headache
  - Nausea
  - Vomiting
  - Confusion
  - Seizures
  - Syncope

### History
- Known exposures
- Type of chemical/industry
- Rapidity of symptom
- Material Safety Data Sheet from exposure site
- Water solubility of agent

### Physical Exam
- HEENT:
  - Conjunctival injection
  - Lacrimation
  - Chemosis
- Respiratory
- Stridor
  - Voice changes
  - Dyspnea
  - Wheezing
  - Cough
- GI:
  - Vomiting
- Dermatologic:
  - Skin erythema/irritation
  - Erythematous rash
- Neurologic:
  - Confusion
  - Seizure activity

## ESSENTIAL WORKUP
History of exposure to irritant gases in addition to noted symptoms confirms diagnosis.

## DIAGNOSTIC TESTS & INTERPRETATION
ECG in the following patients:
- Elderly
- Cardiac history
- Evidence of significant pulmonary symptoms

### Lab

- Arterial blood gas to assess:
  - Oxygenation
  - Ventilation status
  - pH
  - Pulse oximetry is unreliable.
- Carbon monoxide level:
  - If smoke inhalation with concomitant irritant gas inhalation (see "Carbon Monoxide Poisoning")
- Methemoglobin level:
  - If oxides of nitrogen are suspected
- Serum calcium level:
  - If hydrogen fluoride is suspected
- Lactate:
  - Elevation may indicate cellular poisoning from carbon monoxide or cyanide.
- Pregnancy test in all females of childbearing age
- Rapid dextrose
- Cardiac enzyme levels if acute coronary syndrome suspected

### Imaging

CXR:

- Frequently normal on initial presentation
- May take up to 24 hr to reveal pulmonary edema or evidence of diffuse injury.

### Diagnostic Procedures/Surgery

- Spirometry:
  - Assess evidence suggesting airway narrowing and bronchoconstriction.
- Direct laryngoscopy:
  - Assess evidence of upper airway edema.
- Corneal fluorescein:
  - Assess evidence of corneal burns/injury.

### DIFFERENTIAL DIAGNOSIS

- Asthma exacerbation
- Allergic stimuli (pollen)
- Physical stimuli (cold air)
- Bronchitis
- Pneumonia
- Occupational asthma
- Hypersensitivity pneumonitis
- Congestive heart failure

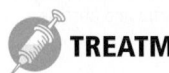 ## TREATMENT

### PRE-HOSPITAL

Rescuer's goal is to prevent self-contamination with use of protective clothing or equipment (self-contained breathing apparatus).

### INITIAL STABILIZATION/THERAPY

- ABCs:
  - 100% oxygen through a tight-fitting, nonrebreathing face mask
  - Early intubation may be necessary to protect airway from edema.
  - Mechanical ventilation
  - Continuous positive airway pressure or positive end expiratory pressure may enhance oxygenation.
- Decontaminate by removing clothes and irrigating skin and ocular tissues.

### ED TREATMENT/PROCEDURES

- Inhaled nebulized $\beta_2$-adrenergic agonists (albuterol) for bronchoconstriction
- Inhaled/IV/PO corticosteroids: beclomethasone, methylprednisolone, prednisone:
  - Controversial
  - No controlled trials that document benefit of acute corticosteroids after irritant gas inhalation.
- Nebulized sodium bicarbonate (3.75% solution) after chlorine gas exposure:
  - Reported to improve oxygenation in several case reports/series.
- Nebulized calcium gluconate after acute hydrogen fluoride inhalation:
  - Reported, but with no proven benefit
- Cyanide antidote kit if hydrogen cyanide is suspected (see "Cyanide Poisoning")
- Oxygen or hyperbaric oxygen therapy if carbon monoxide poisoning documented

### MEDICATION

- Albuterol: 0.5 mL (peds: 0.03 mL or 0.15 mg/kg per dose) of 0.5% solution diluted in NS to 3 mL aerosolized
- Beclomethasone MDI: 1–2 sprays (40–80 mcg/spray) b.i.d.
- Calcium gluconate: Nebulized (2.5–3% solution) prepared by adding 0.15 g of calcium gluconate to 6 mL of NS
- Metaproterenol: 0.3 mL (peds: 0.1–0.3 mL) of 5% solution diluted in NS to 3 mL aerosolized
- Methylprednisolone: 80–125 mg (peds: 1–2 mg/kg) IV
- Prednisone: 40–80 mg (peds: 1–2 mg/kg) PO
- Sodium bicarbonate: Nebulized (3 mL of 8.4% sodium bicarbonate mixed with 2 mL of NS to prepare 5 mL of 5% solution)

 ## FOLLOW-UP

### DISPOSITION

#### Admission Criteria

- ICU admission:
  - Intubated patients
  - Significant respiratory insufficiency or potential upper airway obstruction
- Persistently symptomatic with bronchospasm or oxygen requirement

- Exposure to irritant gases that affect peripheral airways:
  - Delayed pulmonary edema and respiratory failure may occur.
- Conservative treatment for children, pregnant women, elderly patients, or those with pre-existing chronic obstructive pulmonary or coronary disease

#### Discharge Criteria

- Mild exposures that respond well to supportive care and have no oxygen requirement or bronchospasm after 4–6 hr of observation
- Follow-up chest radiograph during observation and prior to discharge, especially if any symptoms are present or clinically worsening

#### Issues for Referral

Intensive care for patients with early evidence of acute lung injury

### FOLLOW-UP RECOMMENDATIONS

- Occupational medicine referral for work-related exposures.
- Pulmonary follow-up for repeated symptomatic exposures.

## PEARLS AND PITFALLS

- Beware of delayed-onset of low-solubility agents. These exposures may require 23-hr observation for delayed respiratory symptoms.
- Avoid exposure of agent to first responders, with appropriate decontamination.

## ADDITIONAL READING

- Bosse GM. Nebulized sodium bicarbonate in the treatment of chlorine gas inhalation. *J Toxicol Clin Toxicol.* 1994;32:233–241.
- Newman-Taylor AJ. Respiratory irritants encountered at work. *Thorax.* 1996;51:541–545.
- Rorison DG, McPherson SJ. Acute toxic inhalations. *Emerg Med Clin North Am.* 1992;10:409–435.
- Vinsel PJ. Treatment of acute chlorine gas inhalation with nebulized sodium bicarbonate. *J Emerg Med.* 1990;8:327–329.
- Weiner AL, Bayer MJ. Inhalation: Gases with immediate toxicity. In: Ford MD, Delaney KA, Ling LJ, et al., eds. *Clinical Toxicology.* Philadelphia: WB Saunders; 2001.
- Weiss SM, Lakshminarayan S. Acute inhalation injury. *Clin Chest Med.* 1994;15:103–116.

### See Also (Topic, Algorithm, Electronic Media Element)

- Carbon Monoxide Poisoning
- Cyanide Poisoning

 ## CODES

### ICD9

987.9 Toxic effect of unspecified gas, fume, or vapor

# ISONIAZID POISONING

Sean M. Bryant

 **BASICS**

## DESCRIPTION

- Complexes with and inactivates pyridoxal-5 phosphate, the active form of pyridoxine (vitamin $B_6$).
- After it complexes with pyridoxine, it is renally eliminated.
- Inhibits pyridoxine phosphokinase, hindering the conversion of pyridoxine to its active form.
- Interfering with pyridoxine levels yields a net decrease in g-aminobutyric acid (GABA) production.
- Depressed GABA causes cerebral excitability and seizures.
- Inhibits lactate dehydrogenase, decreasing the conversion of lactate to pyruvate:
  - Contributes to the profound anion gap metabolic acidosis.
- Chronic toxicity:
  - Interferes with synthesis of nicotinic acid (niacin).
  - Causes syndrome indistinguishable from pellagra after months of therapy (niacin deficiency).
- Some actions similar to the monoamine oxidase inhibitors:
  - Reports of a tyramine-like reaction to isoniazid (INH)
  - Rare cases of mania, diaphoresis, depression, obsessive-compulsive disorder, and psychosis
- Pharmacokinetics:
  - Rapidly absorbed, reaching peak levels within 1–2 hr.
  - Volume of distribution is 0.6 L/kg and protein binding is low (10%).
  - Renally excreted within 24 hr after acetylation in the liver.
  - Half-life is <1 hr in fast acetylators and 2–4 hr in slow-acetylating individuals.

## ETIOLOGY

- High-risk groups include immigrants, homeless, HIV infected, alcoholics, and lower socioeconomic status populations.
- Slow acetylators (60% of African Americans and whites compared to 20% of Asians) are more prone to chronic effects/toxicity.
- LD50 estimated to be 80–150 mg/kg.
- Ingestions less than 1.5 g lead to mild toxicity, and those of 10 g or more often result in fatality.

 **DIAGNOSIS**

## SIGNS AND SYMPTOMS

- Acute toxicity:
  - Neurologic:
    - Altered mental status
    - Seizures refractory to standard therapy
    - Agitation
    - Coma
    - Dizziness
    - Ataxia
    - Hyperreflexia
    - Slurred speech
    - Hallucinations
    - Psychosis
  - GI:
    - Nausea
    - Vomiting
  - Renal:
    - Anuria
    - Oliguria
  - Cardiovascular:
    - Hypotension
    - Tachycardia
    - Shock
    - Cyanosis
  - Metabolic:
    - Profound anion gap metabolic acidosis (elevated lactate)
    - Hyperthermia
- Chronic toxicity:
  - Neurologic:
    - Peripheral neuropathy
    - Optic neuritis, optic atrophy
    - Psychosis
    - Insomnia
    - Vertigo
    - Pellagra
  - GI hepatitis:
    - Liver failure, hepatitis
    - Nausea, vomiting, constipation
    - Anorexia

## ESSENTIAL WORKUP

Without specific history of ingestion, initiate general workup for:

- Altered mental status
- Seizures
- Metabolic acidosis

## DIAGNOSTIC TESTS & INTERPRETATION

### Lab

- Arterial blood gas:
  - Profound metabolic acidosis
- Electrolytes, BUN/creatinine, glucose:
  - Elevated anion gap acidosis
  - Hyperglycemia
- CBC:
  - Acute toxicity:
    - Leukocytosis
    - Eosinophilia
  - Chronic toxicity:
    - Agranulocytosis
    - Eosinophilia
    - Hemolysis
    - Anemia

### Imaging

- CXR:
  - Evidence of tuberculosis increases suspicion for ingestion/toxicity.
  - Evaluate for aspiration pneumonia.
- CT/lumbar puncture if indicated and questionable history

## DIFFERENTIAL DIAGNOSIS

- Toxins:
  - Tricyclic antidepressants
  - Salicylates (aspirin)
  - Theophylline
  - Methanol/ethylene glycol
  - Lithium
  - Carbon monoxide
  - Cocaine/cyanide
  - Agents that cause metabolic acidosis
- CNS:
  - Cerebrovascular accident
  - Intracranial hemorrhage/mass/trauma/abscess
- Hypoglycemia
- Uremia
- Thyrotoxicosis

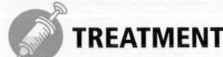 **TREATMENT**

## PRE-HOSPITAL
Collect prescription bottles/medications for identification in the ED.

## INITIAL STABILIZATION/THERAPY
- ABCs:
  - Supplemental oxygen
  - Intubate if necessary for airway protection
  - Secure IV access
  - Cardiac monitor
  - 0.9% NS access
- Naloxone, thiamine, D50W (Accu-Chek) if altered mental status

## ED TREATMENT/PROCEDURES
- Vitamin $B_6$ (pyridoxine):
  - Specific antidotal treatment for INH toxicity
  - Goal: 1 g of pyridoxine for each gram of INH ingested (1 g q2–3min)
  - Administer 5 g for unknown amount ingested.
  - May repeat in 20 min for refractory seizures or persistent coma.
    If insufficient quantity of pyridoxine available, contact other hospital pharmacies and the regional poison control center to obtain more.
  - If no parenteral pyridoxine available, crush tablets and give as a slurry via NG tube.
- Seizure control:
  - Pyridoxine restores deficiency in GABA.
  - Benzodiazepines are synergistic with pyridoxine.
  - Phenytoin has no role.
- Gastric decontamination after stabilization:
  - Consider gastric lavage only in life-threatening ingestions presenting within 1 hr with a protected airway (being aware of potential seizure activity and obtundation).
  - Activated charcoal (AC) dosed at 10:1 ratio (AC:drug)

- Hemodialysis:
  - Persistent symptoms despite adequate therapy
  - Renal insufficiency in symptomatic patients
- Sodium bicarbonate:
  - For severe metabolic acidosis.
  - Acidosis usually resolves spontaneously after elimination of seizures

## MEDICATION
- Dextrose: D50W 1 amp (50 mL or 25 g) (peds: D25W 2–4 mL/kg) IV
- Diazepam (benzodiazepine): 5–10 mg (peds: 0.2–0.5 mg/kg) IV
- Lorazepam (benzodiazepine): 2–6 mg (peds: 0.03–0.05 mg/kg) IV
- Naloxone (Narcan): 2 mg (peds: 0.1 mg/kg) IV/IM initial dose
- Pyridoxine (vitamin $B_6$): 1 g IV for each gram of INH ingested (see above)
- Thiamine (vitamin $B_1$): 100 mg (peds: 50 mg) IV/IM

 **FOLLOW-UP**

## DISPOSITION
### Admission Criteria
- ICU admission for refractory seizures, severe acidosis, coma, altered mental status
- Uncontrolled nausea/vomiting, unclear history of ingestion, or suicidal

### Discharge Criteria
- Symptoms are usually observed within 45 min of an acute overdose but may be delayed for $\geq 2$ hr.
- Discharge if asymptomatic after 6 hr.

## FOLLOW-UP RECOMMENDATIONS
Psychiatric referral for intentional overdoses or suicidal patients.

## PEARLS AND PITFALLS
Inadequate appreciation and management of INH poisoning:
- Refractory seizures to standard treatments should be a clue.
- Severe acidemia with elevated lactate in altered patients with seizures should be a clue.
- Never paralyze a seizing patient without the use of continuous EEG monitoring.
- Goal of pyridoxine therapy is gram for gram of INH.
- If pyridoxine adequately treats seizures, may give more if patient still obtunded or comatose.

## ADDITIONAL READING
- Boyer EW. Antituberculous agents. In: Goldfrank LR, ed. *Goldfrank's Toxicologic Emergencies*. New York: McGraw-Hill; 2002.
- Brent J, Vo N, Kulig K, et al. Reversal of prolonged isoniazid-induced coma by pyridoxine. *Arch Intern Med*. 1990;150:1751–1753.
- Leikin J, Paloucek F. Isoniazid. In: *Poisoning and Toxicology Handbook*. Hudson, OH: Lexi-comp; 2002.
- Mcfee RB, Mofenson HC, Carracio TR. Isoniazid poisoning. *Emerg Med*. 2000;32:57–58.

**See Also (Topic, Algorithm, Electronic Media Element)**
Seizures

 **CODES**

ICD9
961.8 Poisoning by other antimycobacterial drugs

# ISOPROPANOL POISONING

*Paul Kolecki*

 **BASICS**

## DESCRIPTION

- CNS depressant effect of isopropanol is two to three times as potent as that of ethanol.
- Many products that contain isopropanol also contain methanol, ethylene glycol, and ethanol.
- Rapidly absorbed following oral ingestion
- Ketogenic, but does not cause significant acidosis
- Metabolized by alcohol dehydrogenase to acetone (a CNS depressant):
  - Concomitant ethanol ingestion doubles half-life of isopropanol but not that of acetone.
  - Acetone eliminated by lung and kidney
- Half-life:
  - Isopropanol: 3–16 hr
  - Acetone: 7.5–26 hr

## ETIOLOGY

- Isopropanol (isopropyl alcohol): clear, colorless, volatile liquid with faint odor of acetone and bitter taste
- Available as 70% rubbing alcohol solution:
  - May contain blue dye that was added to inhibit its abuse (cblue heavend)
- Found in:
  - Various toiletries
  - Disinfectants
  - Window-cleaning solutions
  - Paint remover
  - Solvents
  - Jewelry cleaners
  - Detergents
  - Antifreeze
- Typical adult patient: Chronic alcoholic who has been on drinking binge and recently depleted his or her ethanol supply
- Dermal and rectal administration can cause systemic toxicity.

# DIAGNOSIS

## SIGNS AND SYMPTOMS

- Usually occur within 30–60 min of ingestion
- Neurologic:
  - Lethargy
  - Weakness
  - Headache
  - Inebriation
  - Vertigo
  - Ataxia
  - Apnea
  - Coma
  - Initial excitation phase seen with ethanol ingestion is absent.
- GI:
  - Nausea/vomiting
  - Abdominal pain
  - Gastritis
  - Hematemesis
- Cardiovascular:
  - Hypotension
  - Tachycardia
  - Myocardial depression
  - Peripheral vascular dilation
- Pulmonary:
  - Respiratory depression
  - Hemorrhagic tracheobronchitis
- Dermatologic:
  - Skin irritation
  - Burns
- Ocular:
  - Irritation
  - Lacrimation

### Pediatric Considerations
- Accidental ingestions common in <6-yr-olds.
- Rubbing alcohol sponge baths may cause inhalational toxicity.

## ESSENTIAL WORKUP
- History of ingestion
- Odor of isopropanol or acetone on patient's breath

## DIAGNOSTIC TESTS & INTERPRETATION
### Lab
- Electrolytes, BUN, creatinine (Cr), glucose:
  - Hypoglycemia occurs.
  - Does *not* produce significant acidosis unless accompanied by end-organ hypoperfusion.
  - Acetone can produce false elevation of serum Cr:
    - When acetone level >40 mg/dL, Cr values rise at ~1 mg Cr/100 mg/dL acetone.
    - Cr returns to baseline following acetone metabolism.
- CBC:
  - Decreased hematocrit with significant hemorrhagic gastritis
- Arterial blood gas:
  - Acidosis rare unless owing to hypoperfusion or coingestant.
- Urinalysis:
  - Ketones present.
- Serum ketones are present.
- Isopropanol level:
  - Coma with level >150 mg/dL
- Serum osmolarity:
  - Osmolar gap: difference between measured and calculated osmolarity
  - Calculated osmolarity = 2 $Na^+$ BUN/2.8 + glucose/18 + ethanol/4.6.
  - Osmolar gap is present if measured minus calculated osmolality is >10.
  - Gap increases by 1 mOsm/kg for each 5.9 mg/dL of isopropanol and 5.5 mg/dL of acetone.

### Imaging
- CXR: For aspiration pneumonia with altered mental status and vomiting
- CT head: Concomitant head injury occurs.

## DIFFERENTIAL DIAGNOSIS

- For CNS depression and elevated osmolar gap includes:
  - Ethanol
  - Ethylene glycol
  - Methanol
  - Glycerol
  - Mannitol

### Pediatric Considerations

- Prone to hypoglycemia following exposure

 **TREATMENT**

### PRE-HOSPITAL

Search for and transport all bottles and medications that may have been ingested by the patient when an overdose is suspected.

### INITIAL STABILIZATION/THERAPY

- ABCs:
  - Maintain airway and assist in ventilation if necessary.
- Hypotension:
  - Treat initially with 0.9% NS IV fluid bolus.
  - Initiate dopamine or norepinephrine infusion if hypotension persists.
    Packed RBCs with significant hemorrhagic gastritis
- Place NG tube and irrigate for patients with hematemesis.
- Naloxone, thiamine, dextrose (or Accu-Chek) if altered mental status

## ED TREATMENT/PROCEDURES

- Primarily supportive therapy—no specific antidote
- Irrigate skin/eyes for dermal or ocular exposure.
- Consider activated charcoal:
  - For coingestants
  - Large doses can absorb significant amounts of isopropanol.
- Do **not** treat with ethanol infusion or 4-methylpyrazole.
- Hemodialysis:
  - Effectively removes isopropanol and acetone.
  - Most managed with supportive care alone.
  - Indications:
    ○ Hemodynamic instability despite fluid replacement and use of pressors
    ○ Levels >400 mg/dL (associated with severe hypotension and prolonged coma)

## MEDICATION

- Activated charcoal slurry: 1–2 g/kg up to 90 g PO
- Dextrose: D50W 1 amp: 50 mL or 25 g (peds: D25W 2–4 mL/kg) IV
- Dopamine: 2–20 mg/kg/min IV
- Naloxone (Narcan): 2 mg (peds: 0.1 mg/kg) IV or IM initial dose
- Sorbitol: 1–2 g/kg to max 150 g (peds >1 yr: 1–1.5 g/kg as 35% solution to max 50 g) PO mixed in activated charcoal slurry
- Thiamine (vitamin B$_1$): 100 mg (peds: 50 mg) IV or IM

 **FOLLOW-UP**

### DISPOSITION

#### Admission Criteria

Moderate to severe isopropanol toxicity (altered mental status, hypotension)

### Discharge Criteria

- Observe asymptomatic patients following ingestion for 2–4 hr before discharge.
- Mild intoxication that resolves over 4–6 hr

### Issues for Referral

GI referral for endoscopy for patients with recurrent hematemesis.

### FOLLOW-UP RECOMMENDATIONS

Alcohol detox or psychiatry referral for patients with intentional ingestion

## PEARLS AND PITFALLS

- Supportive care is the primary treatment.
- Do **not** treat with ethanol infusion or 4-methylpyrazole.

## ADDITIONAL READING

- Burkhart KK, KuligK. The other alcohols. Methanol, ethylene glycol, and isopropanol. *Emerg Med Clin North Am*. 1990;8:913–928.
- Kraut JA, KurtzI. Toxic alcohol ingestions: Clinical features, diagnosis, and management. *Clin J Am Soc Nephrol*. 2008;3:208–225.
- Sharma AN. Toxic alcohols. In: Goldfrank LR, Flomenbaum NE, Lewin NA, et al., eds. *Goldfrank's Toxicologic Emergencies*. 7th ed. New York: McGraw-Hill; 2002:980–990.

### See Also (Topic, Algorithm, Electronic Media Element)

- Alcohol Poisoning
- Ethylene Glycol Poisoning
- Methanol Poisoning

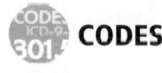 **CODES**

### ICD9

980.2 Toxic effect of isopropyl alcohol

# JAUNDICE

*Andrew K. Chang*
*Antonio Napolitano*

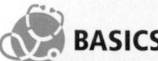 **BASICS**

## DESCRIPTION
Yellow pigmentation of tissues and body fluids due to hyperbilirubinemia, usually present at levels of >3 mg/dL

## ETIOLOGY
- Unconjugated (indirect) hyperbilirubinemia: Unconjugated bilirubin is the direct breakdown product of heme, is water insoluble, and is measured as indirect bilirubin:
  - Hemolytic:
    ○ Excessive production of unconjugated bilirubin
  - Hepatic:
    ○ Decreased hepatobiliary excretion of bilirubin by:
      a. Defective uptake (drugs, Crigler-Najjar syndrome)
      b. Defective conjugation (Gilbert syndrome, drugs)
      c. Defective excretion of bilirubin by the liver cell (drugs, Dubin-Johnson syndrome)
- Conjugated (direct) hyperbilirubinemia:
  - Conjugated bilirubin is water soluble and measured as direct bilirubin.
  - In conjugated hyperbilirubinemia, bilirubin is returned to the bloodstream after conjugation in the liver instead of draining into the bile ducts.
  - Hepatocellular dysfunction:
    ○ Hepatitis
    ○ Cirrhosis
    ○ Tumor invasion
    ○ Toxic injury
  - Intrahepatic (nonobstructive) cholestasis
  - Extrahepatic (obstructive) cholestasis

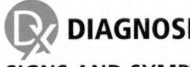 **DIAGNOSIS**

## SIGNS AND SYMPTOMS
### History
- Cholestasis:
  - Pruritus
  - Pale stools
  - Dark urine
- Malignancy:
  - Anorexia
  - Weight loss
  - Malaise
- Abdominal pain

### Physical Exam
- Icterus of sclera and tongue base (levels >2.5 mg/dL)
- Right upper quadrant tenderness:
  - Courvoisier's rule:
    ○ Painless jaundice and a palpable, nontender gallbladder represent malignant common duct obstruction.
- Stigmata of cirrhosis:
  - Abdominal collateral circulation including caput medusae, hepatosplenomegaly, or hepatic atrophy
  - Ascites
  - Spider telangiectasis
  - Palmar erythema
  - Dupuytren contractures
- Palpable gallbladder
- Hepatomegaly
- Splenomegaly
- Abdominal mass
- Evidence of cachexia
- Excoriations (primary biliary cirrhosis, obstruction)
- Kayser-Fleischer rings:
  - Wilson disease

## ESSENTIAL WORKUP
- History and physical examination, together with routine laboratory tests, will suggest the diagnosis in ~80% of patients with jaundice.
- Bilirubin level—severity may suggest cause.
  - Malignancy causes highest levels (10–30 mg/dL).
  - Choledocholithiasis rarely exceeds 15 mg/dL.

## DIAGNOSTIC TESTS & INTERPRETATION
### Lab
- Urine dipstick is 74% sensitive for bilirubin.
- Alkaline phosphatase:
  - If no bone disease and not pregnant, then elevation suggests impaired biliary tract function.
  - 2': hepatitis and cirrhosis
  - 3': extrahepatic biliary obstruction (ie, choledocholithiasis) and intrahepatic cholestasis (ie, drug-induced and biliary cirrhosis)
- Aminotransferases—provide evidence of hepatocellular damage:
  - Alanine aminotransferase (ALT, SGPT): primarily in the liver
  - Aspartate aminotransferase (AST, SGOT): liver, heart, kidney, muscle, and brain
- $\gamma$-Glutamyl transpeptidase—throughout hepatobiliary system, pancreas, heart, kidneys, and lungs:
  - May be the most sensitive indicator of biliary tract disease.
  - Confirms hepatic origin of an elevated alkaline phosphatase.

- 5'-Nucleotidase—widespread tissue distribution:
  - Confirms hepatic origin of an elevated alkaline phosphatase level.
- Albumin: Decreased with severe liver disease
- Prothrombin time: Elevation is an important prognostic indicator in patients with acute hepatitis.

### Imaging
- US: Most effective initial imaging technique:
  - > 90% effective in identifying cholelithiasis
  - Ductal dilation is a reliable indicator of extrahepatic obstruction:
    ○ A dilated common bile duct (CBD) and gallbladder suggest distal obstruction, whereas dilation of the intrahepatic ducts (without CBD dilation) suggests proximal obstruction.
  - Tumors of the liver and head of pancreas are usually well visualized.
  - Distinguishes solid liver tumors from cystic structures.
- Plain radiographs:
  - May show evidence of hepatic and splenic enlargement or biliary calcifications
- Hepatic nuclear scan (hepatobiliary iminodiacetic acid scan):
  - Accurate method of diagnosing acute cholecystitis or cystic duct obstruction
  - Time consuming (usually several hours)
- CT:
  - Superior to US in detecting pancreatic and intra-abdominal tumors.
  - Can help differentiate fluid-containing structures.

### Diagnostic Procedures/Surgery
Endoscopic retrograde cholangiopancreatography (ERCP):
- Diagnostic:
  - Stones are seen as filling defects within bile duct lumen.
  - Malignancies are seen as strictures.
- Therapeutic:
  - Extraction of common bile duct stones and insertion of stents to bypass malignant obstructions
  - Biopsy under direct vision

## DIFFERENTIAL DIAGNOSIS
- Prehepatic:
  - Hemolysis (sickle cell, other hemoglobinopathies)
  - Ineffective erythropoiesis
  - Drugs
  - Gilbert syndrome: Usually benign inherited form of unconjugated hyperbilirubinemia
  - Crigler-Najjar syndrome
  - Prolonged fasting

- Hepatocellular:
  - Hepatitis (infectious, alcoholic, autoimmune, toxin, drug induced)
  - Cirrhosis
  - Postischemic
  - Hemochromatosis
- Intrahepatic cholestasis:
  - Idiopathic cholestasis of pregnancy
  - Drugs
  - Dubin-Johnson syndrome
  - Rotor syndrome
  - Benign recurrent cholestasia
  - Familial syndromes
  - Sepsis
  - Postoperative jaundice
  - Lymphoma
- Extrahepatic obstruction:
  - Common duct stone
  - Biliary stricture
  - Bacterial cholangitis
  - Sclerosing cholangitis
  - Carcinoma (ampulla, gallbladder, pancreas), cholangiosarcoma
  - Pancreatitis, pancreatic pseudocyst
  - Hemobilia
  - Duodenal diverticula
  - Ascariasis
  - Post–laparoscopic cholecystectomy complications
  - Congenital biliary atresia
  - Congenital choledochal cyst

### Pediatric Considerations
Intrahepatic cholestasis:

- Cardiovascular (congenital heart disease, congestive heart failure, shock, asphyxia)
- Metabolic or genetic ($\alpha_1$-antitrypsin deficiency, trisomy 18 and 21, cystic fibrosis, Gaucher disease, Niemann Pick disease, glycogen storage disease type IV)
- Infectious (bacterial sepsis, cytomegalovirus, enterovirus, herpes simplex virus, rubella, syphilis, TB, varicella, viral hepatitis)
- Hematologic (severe isoimmune hemolytic disease)

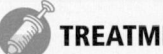 **TREATMENT**

### INITIAL STABILIZATION/THERAPY
- Isotonic IV fluid therapy if dehydrated
- Toxic-appearing patients:
  - Supplemental oxygen, cardiac monitoring
  - Nasogastric suction and bladder catheterization

### ED TREATMENT/PROCEDURES
- For bacterial cholangitis/sepsis, obtain blood cultures and administer parenteral antibiotics:
  - Ampicillin, gentamicin, and metronidazole *or*
  - Ticarcillin, or piperacillin, and metronidazole *or*
  - Cefoxitin and tobramycin
- Obstructive extrahepatic jaundice:
  - Surgical consult
- Choledocholithiasis:
  - ERCP papillotomy, balloon or basket retrieval, or open surgery
- Obstructive intrahepatic or nonobstructive jaundice:
  - Medical management:
    ○ Withdraw causative drug, ethanol.
    ○ Interferon for chronic hepatitis B and C
    ○ Penicillamine and phlebotomy for Wilson disease and hemochromatosis
    ○ Corticosteroids for chronic hepatitis of autoimmune origin

### Pediatric Considerations
- Exchange transfusion:
  - Emergent treatment of markedly elevated bilirubin (>20 mg/dL in full-term infants) and for correction of anemia caused by isoimmune hemolytic disease
- Phototherapy—for neonatal jaundice when bilirubin = 17 mg/dL:
  - Measure bilirubin once to twice daily and stop when bilirubin has been reduced by about 4–5 mg/dL.
- Phenobarbital: In sepsis and drug-induced causes; decreases conjugated bilirubin.
- Metalloporphyrins: Investigational inhibitors of heme oxygenase

### MEDICATION
- Ampicillin: 2 g IV q6h (peds: 25 mg/kg IV q6h–q8h)
- Cefoxitin: 2 g IV q6h (peds: 40–160 mg/kg/d div. q6h–q12h)
- Gentamicin: 2–5 mg/kg IV q8h (peds: same)
- Metronidazole: 1 g IV q12h (peds: 30 mg/kg/d div. q12h)
- Piperacillin/tazobactam: 3 g IV q6h (peds: 300 mg/kg/d div. q6h [>2 months of age])
- Ticarcillin/clavulanate: 3 g IV q6h (peds: 75–100 mg/kg/d div. q6h)
- Tobramycin: 2–5 mg/kg IV q6h (peds: same)

 **FOLLOW-UP**

### DISPOSITION
**Admission Criteria**
- Bacterial cholangitis
- Intractable pain
- Intractable emesis
- Associated pancreatitis
- Elevated prothrombin time

**Discharge Criteria**
- No evidence of infection (evaluate as outpatient)
- Tolerating liquids

## ADDITIONAL READING

- Dennery PA, Seidman DS, Stevenson DK. Neonatal hyperbilirubinemia. *N Engl J Med*. 2001;344: 581–590.
- Faust TW, Reddy KR. Postoperative jaundice. *Clin Liver Dis*. 2004;8:151–166.
- Frank BB. Clinical evaluation of jaundice: a guideline of the Patient Care Committee of the American Gastroenterological Association. *JAMA*. 1989; 262(21):3031–3034.
- Maisels MJ, McDonagh AF. phototherapy for neonatal jaundice. *N Engl J Med*. 2008;358: 920–928.
- Roche SP, Kobos R. Jaundice in the adult patient. *Am Fam Physician*. 2004;69:299–304.
- Wang Q, Gurusamy KS, Lin H, et al. Preoperative biliary drainage for obstructive jaundice. *Cochrane Database Syst Rev*. 2008;16(3):CD005444.

 **CODES**

### ICD9
782.4 Jaundice, unspecified, not of newborn

J

# KAPOSI SARCOMA
*Matthew T. Keadey*

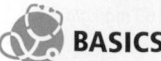 **BASICS**

## DESCRIPTION

- A mesenchymal tumor involving blood and lymphatic vessels
- Lesions are typically found on the skin, mucous membranes, GI and respiratory tracts, lymphatic system, and visceral organs.
- Tumors consist of spindle-shaped cells between collagen bundles, neovascular spaces, extravasated erythrocytes, and an infiltrate of lymphocytes.
- Staging is based on AIDS Clinical Trials Group classification:
  - Characterizes patients as good or poor risk based on:
    - Tumor burden
    - Immune function
    - Presence or absence of systemic illness
    - Recent studies have shown that only tumor burden and systemic illness affect prognosis in the highly active antiretroviral therapy (HAART) medication era. Immune function measured as CD4 count does not affect outcome of disease.
    - Systemic pulmonary involvement has the worse outcome.
- Four epidemiologic manifestations:
  - Classic Kaposi sarcoma (KS):
    - Initially described by Moritz Kaposi in 1872 in males in Mediterranean region.
    - Cutaneous disease, occurring after 6th decade of life, with an indolent course
  - Endemic African KS:
    - Prevalence of 12% in sub-Saharan Africa
    - More likely to affect women and children
    - Varied clinical pattern from benign to fulminate lymphadenopathic disease.
  - Iatrogenic immunosuppressive KS:
    - Chronic immunosuppressive therapy (transplant patients)
  - AIDS-related KS:
    - The most common HIV malignancy
    - Incidence has declined due to HAART.
    - Unpredictable clinical course, even in patients with well-controlled HIV disease

## ETIOLOGY

- Pathogenesis
- Associated with human herpes virus 8 (HHV-8), also known as Kaposi sarcoma herpes virus (KSHV):
  - HHV-8 is found in all KS lesions, yet not all those infected with HHV-8 have KS:
    - HHV-8 is felt to be necessary but not sufficient by itself to cause KS.
  - Host genetic factors likely contribute.
  - HHV-8 genome codes for viral cyclins, cytokines, and antiapoptotic factors:
    - Believed to disrupt mitosis, interrupt apoptosis, and increase angiogenesis

- Risk of developing KS increases with degree of immunosuppression in HIV patients:
  - Measured by lower CD4 counts and higher HHV-8 and HIV viral loads
  - AIDS-KS lesions tend to flare during opportunistic infections.
- Iatrogenic KS has been observed to regress during withdrawal of immunosuppression.
- Survival for patients with HIV-related KS is influenced more heavily by the depth of immunosuppression and the control of the underlying HIV disease than by tumor burden.
- Modes of transmission of HHV-8:
  - Sexual contact, especially among homosexual males, who have much higher risk of KS than other HIV patients
  - Vertical transmission from mother to child
  - Saliva appears to be most frequent form of transmission in endemic African form.
  - Blood products
  - Donated transplanted organs

 **DIAGNOSIS**

## SIGNS AND SYMPTOMS

- Cutaneous:
  - Lesions may arise quickly within a few days.
  - Red, pink, purple, or brown macular lesions with occasional yellow halos
  - Irregularly shaped, ranging from several millimeters to few centimeters in size
  - Frequently lesions are symmetric and arranged along lines of skin tension.
  - Painless and nonpruritic
  - Common sites include face, especially adnexal structures of eyes and nose, trunk, and lower extremities.
  - Lymphatic obstruction can lead to severe edema, pain, and ulceration, especially in lower extremities, groin, and periorbital areas.
- Oral:
  - Most common site of initial involvement
  - Purplish lesions on palate and gingiva
  - Can be easily traumatized from normal chewing, causing bleeding, ulceration, and secondary infection
- Visceral:
  - Gastrointestinal:
    - Common, but usually asymptomatic
    - Does not typically affect prognosis
    - Can occur anywhere in GI tract but most commonly in stomach
    - Lesions begin as macular and submucosal.
    - Lesions may progress to become nodular and bulky with central ulceration.
    - Advanced disease may present with pain, intestinal obstruction, and bleeding.

- Respiratory:
  - Found in ~1/3 of KS patients
  - Lesions in tracheobronchial tree, pulmonary parenchyma, or pleura
  - More at lower range of CD4 counts
  - 85% of patients have evidence of cutaneous disease.
  - Frequently presents concomitantly with opportunistic infections
  - Symptoms: Dyspnea, nonproductive cough
  - Chest pain, fever, and hemoptysis are less common.
  - Symptoms may persist for weeks and then progress rapidly to pulmonary failure.
  - Lung sounds often clear, but may have crackles, wheezes, or signs of pleural effusion
- Systemic:
  - Lymphatic obstruction is the most common cause of morbidity; can occur in the absence of cutaneous involvement.
  - Solid organs such as liver, spleen, heart, bone marrow, and urogenital tract are less commonly affected.

## ESSENTIAL WORKUP

- History should focus on symptoms by system, and examiner should assess degree of immune compromise.
- Physical exam:
  - Careful examination of skin, oral mucosa for lesions
  - Fecal occult blood in patients with suspected GI bleed
  - Lung exam for signs of crackles or dullness to percussion that may suggest a pleural effusion

## DIAGNOSTIC TESTS & INTERPRETATION
### Lab

- Punch biopsy of skin lesions with histologic examination is the gold standard of diagnosis:
  - Not usually performed in ED
  - Demonstrates angioproliferation with spindle cells, cleft-like spaces, and extravasation of RBCs
- CBC may show leukopenia, thrombocytopenia from AIDS, anemia in setting of GI bleed.
- Arterial blood gas in setting of respiratory distress may demonstrate hypoxemia or respiratory alkalosis.
- Electrolytes, liver panel, blood cultures, sputum smear and culture, lactate dehydrogenase in setting of fever and respiratory symptoms to rule out other causes
- Thoracocentesis in setting of pleural effusion typically exudative or frankly bloody

*Imaging*
- CXR:
  - Bilateral opacities in a central or perihilar distribution
  - Nodular densities
  - Pleural effusions
  - Intrathoracic adenopathy
- Thallium/gallium scan:
  - KS lesions are thallium avid and gallium negative.
  - Opposite pattern of opportunistic infections and non-Hodgkin lymphoma
- Chest CT can guide biopsy of extrabronchial lesions.
- Acute abdominal x-ray series or CT of abdomen to look for small bowel obstruction if suspected

*Diagnostic Procedures/Surgery*
- Bronchoscopy with lesional biopsy:
  - Gold standard for diagnosis of pulmonary KS
- GI endoscopy to evaluate source of bleeding or upper GI obstruction

## DIFFERENTIAL DIAGNOSIS
- Cutaneous disease:
  - Bacillary angiomatosis (*Bartonella* spp. infection of the skin)
  - Purpura
  - Hematoma
  - Hemangioma
  - Arteriovenous malformation
  - Angiosarcoma
  - Dermatofibroma
  - Nevi
- GI disease:
  - Peptic ulcer disease
  - Pancreatitis
  - Hepatobiliary tract disease
  - Carcinoid tumor
  - Stomach cancer
  - Variceal disease
- Pulmonary disease:
  - Community-acquired pneumonia
  - Active tuberculosis
  - Opportunistic infections such as *Pneumocystis carinii*, aspergillosis, *Coccidioides*
  - Lung carcinoma
  - Non-Hodgkin or Hodgkin lymphoma

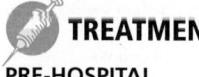 **TREATMENT**

### PRE-HOSPITAL
- ABCs
- Determination of the existence of any advanced directives for patients with advanced AIDS

## INITIAL STABILIZATION/THERAPY
- Universal precautions
- Initial therapy depends on manner of presentation.
- Airway: Assess for stability.
- Breathing: Assess respiratory status and measure pulse oximetry:
- Consider supplemental oxygen.
- Endotracheal intubation and mechanical ventilation if respiratory failure evident
- Circulation: Assess pulse, BP, and perfusion.
- Consider a cardiac monitor.
- Consider IV access with 0.9% NS.
- Resuscitation with IV crystalloid, blood products as needed if hypotensive from GI bleed

## ED TREATMENT/PROCEDURES
- Care of KS must take into account type of KS, extent of tumor, and organs involved.
- ED care is focused on stabilizing acute manifestations of disease and appropriate referral for management of nonemergent lesions.

## MEDICATION
Goal of outpatient treatment for AIDS-KS is palliation of symptoms:
- Cosmetically disfiguring lesions
- Problematic oral lesions
- Pain and edema from lymphadenopathy

*First Line*
- Intensification of HAART medications is first line of treatment in AIDS-KS.
- Local therapy of cutaneous lesions:
  - Cryotherapy
  - Radiation therapy
  - Laser therapy
  - Local excision surgery for troublesome lesions at carefully selected sites
    Topical treatment with alitretinoin gel
  - Intralesional chemotherapy with vinblastine or vincristine.
- Vinblastine: 0.1–0.5 mg/cm$^2$ of lesion intralesional, up to 2 mg; repeat once in 3 wk.
- Systemic therapy:
  - Liposomal anthracyclines (pegylated liposomal doxorubicin):
    ○ First-line therapy for advanced KS
    ○ 20 mg/m$^2$ body area IV every 3 wk

*Second Line*
Systemic therapy:
- Paclitaxel:
  - High response rate in patients who have failed anthracyclines
  - 100 mg/m$^2$ body area IV every 2 wk

- Interferon-$\alpha$:
  - Indicated for HIV-related KS if CD4 count is >400 and KS in early stages.
  - 30 million U/m$^2$ body area SC 3 times weekly
- Experimental:
  - Thalidomide: 100mg PO daily for 8 wk
  - Angiogenesis inhibitors
  - Anti–HHV-8 therapy with ganciclovir, cidofovir, or foscarnet

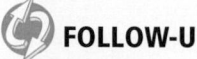 **FOLLOW-UP**

## DISPOSITION
*Admission Criteria*
- Respiratory failure
- Unstable GI bleed
- Bowel obstruction
- Secondary infection of lesion or sepsis

*Discharge Criteria*
Patients with uncomplicated KS lesions may be discharged with referral to a hematologist/oncologist or HIV specialist.

*Issues for Referral*
Uncomplicated mucocutaneous lesions for local therapy as indicated for palliation.

## ADDITIONAL READING

- Belleza WG, Browne B. Pulmonary considerations in the immunocompromised patient. *Emerg Med Clin North Am*. 2003;21(2):499–531, x–xi.
- Bower M, Palmieri C, Dhillon T. AIDS-related malignancies: Changing epidemiology and the impact of highly active retroviral therapy. *Curr Opin Infect Dis*. 2006;19:14–19.
- Levine AM, Hancock BW, MacPhail P, et al. The treatment of AIDS-related cancer. *Lancet Oncol*. 2003;4(9):576 581.
- Mbulaiteye SM, Parkin DM, Rabkin CS. Epidemiology of AIDS-related malignancies: An international perspective. *Hematol Oncol Clin North Am*. 2003;17(3):673–696.
- Noy A. Update in Kaposi sarcoma. *Curr Opin Oncol*. 2003;15:379–381.
- Panthowitz L, Dezube BJ. Advances in the pathobiology and treatment of Kaposi sarcoma. *Curr Opin Oncol*. 2004;16:443–449.
- VonRoenn JH. Clinical presentations and standard therapy of AIDS-associated Kaposi's sarcoma. *Hematol Oncol Clin North Am*. 2003;17(3): 747–762.

## See Also (Topic, Algorithm, Electronic Media Element)
AIDS

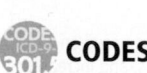 **CODES**

**ICD9**
176.9 Kaposi's sarcoma, unspecified site

K

# KAWASAKI DISEASE

*Adam Z. Barkin*

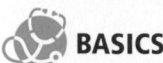

## BASICS

### DESCRIPTION
- Acute inflammatory process involving multiple organs
- Leading cause of childhood-acquired heart disease in developed countries
- Vasculitis is most severe in medium-sized arteries.
- Acute cardiac sequelae:
  - Coronary artery aneurysm:
    - Often lead to stenosis after healing
  - Giant aneurysm:
    - May rupture
  - Myocarditis
  - Pericardiitis
- Stages:
  - Acute (lasts 1–2 wk):
    - Fever
    - Oral mucosal erythema
    - Conjunctival injection
    - Erythema and edema of hands and feet
    - Cervical adenopathy
    - Aseptic meningitis
    - Hepatic dysfunction
    - Diarrhea
    - Myocarditis
    - Pericardial effusion (20–40%)
    - No aneurysms by ECG
  - Subacute (when fever, rash, and lymphadenopathy resolve until about 4 wk):
    - Anorexia
    - Irritability
    - Desquamation of hands and feet
    - Thrombocytosis
    - Coronary artery aneurysms visible on ECG (20% if untreated)
    - Risk for sudden death is highest.
  - Convalescent phase (about 6–8 wk):
    - Clinical signs are absent.
    - ESR normalizes.
- Epidemiology:
  - 80% of cases occur in children <4 yr old; peak at 1–2 yr; rare in infants <3 mo old.
  - Adult cases have been reported.
  - Asians are at highest risk.
  - Males > females 1.5:1.
- Genetics:
  - Possible genetic predisposition
- Risks for nonresponse to standard therapy (10–15%):
  - Elevated band count
  - Low albumin level
  - Abnormal initial ECHO

### ETIOLOGY
Unknown—believed to be infectious based on manifestations of disease, epidemics, and increased numbers of cases in winter and early spring

## DIAGNOSIS

- Classic diagnostic criteria:
  - Fever for 5 days plus 4 of the 5 following criteria:
  - Bilateral conjunctival injection
  - Changes in oral mucosa
  - Polymorphous erythematous rash
  - Changes in hands or feet—edema, erythema, desquamation
  - Cervical lymphadenopathy >1.5 cm
- Atypical cases can be seen without meeting diagnostic criteria.
- Diagnosis can be made before 5 days of fever.

### SIGNS AND SYMPTOMS
#### History
- Temperature >38.5°C (often spiking) for at least 5 days:
  - Begins abruptly and may last >2 wk.
- Cardiac:
  - Shortness of breath
  - Chest pain
- HEENT:
  - Eyes:
    - Conjunctivitis
    - Photophobia
  - Mouth:
    - Erythema
    - Dry and fissured lips
- Skin rash
- Musculoskeletal:
  - Arthralgia, arthritis
- Neurologic:
  - Extreme irritability
- Gastrointestinal:
  - Diarrhea
  - Vomiting
  - Abdominal pain

#### Physical Exam
- Cardiac:
  - Evidence of congestive heart failure
  - Evidence of pericarditis
    - Rub
  - Evidence of valvular disease
    - Murmur
- HEENT:
  - Eyes:
    - Bilateral conjunctival injection without exudates
    - Bulbar conjunctiva is more frequently involved than palpebral conjunctiva.
    - Usually within 2 days of onset of fever and lasting 1–2 wk
    - Photophobia, uveitis, iritis
  - Mouth:
    - Erythema, dry and fissured lips, strawberry tongue, pharyngeal erythema
  - Lymph:
    - Cervical lymphadenopathy (node diameter >1.5 cm)
- Neurologic:
  - Irritability
  - Meningismus
- Skin:
  - Rash, primarily on the trunk
  - May be maculopapular, scarlatiniform, or erythema multiforme–like; erythroderma
  - Changes in the hands or feet—erythema, edema (acute phase); unwilling to bear weight
  - Desquamation (subacute phase) of the tips of fingers and toes 2–3 wk after onset of illness
- Genitourinary:
  - Urethritis
  - Meatitis
- GI:
  - Hydrops of the gallbladder

### ESSENTIAL WORKUP
Must think of the diagnosis in a febrile child with rash

### DIAGNOSTIC TESTS & INTERPRETATION
#### Lab
- CBC:
  - WBC—normally elevated with shift to left in acute phase
  - Normocytic anemia
  - Thrombocytopenia if myocardial infarction or severe coronary disease
  - Thrombocytosis usually in 2nd to 3rd week
- Urinalysis:
  - Sterile pyuria
  - Proteinuria
- ESR elevated from 1st week until 4–6 wk
- Increased C-reactive protein
- CSF pleocytosis
- Cultures: Negative blood, urine, CSF, throat
- Increased transaminases and bilirubin

*Imaging*
- ECG to evaluate for coronary artery aneurysm:
  - Acute phase (baseline)
  - 2–3 wk
  - 6–8 wk
- CXR

*Diagnostic Procedures/Surgery*
- ECG if concern about MI or pericarditis
- Slit-lamp exam—uveitis

## DIFFERENTIAL DIAGNOSIS
- Viral infections:
  - Adenovirus
  - Enterovirus
  - Measles
  - Epstein-Barr virus
  - Rubella
  - Rubeola
- Bacterial infection:
  - Scarlet fever (responds rapidly to penicillin)
  - Staphylococcal scalded-skin syndrome
  - Rickettsial disease, including Rocky Mountain spotted fever and leptospirosis
- Drug reaction:
  - Stevens-Johnson syndrome
  - Erythema multiforme

 TREATMENT

## PRE-HOSPITAL
- ABCs
- Oxygen

## INITIAL STABILIZATION/THERAPY
ABCs with focus on cardiovascular system

## ED TREATMENT/PROCEDURES
- Initiate IV gammaglobulin (IVIG) and aspirin therapy:
  - Do not generally need to monitor salicylate levels because decreased absorption and increased clearance

- Treatment within the 1st 10 days of illness reduces cardiac sequelae from range of 20–25% to range of 2–4%.
- Cardiology consultation
- Treatment of MIs as in adults

## MEDICATION
*First Line*
- IVIG: 2 g/kg IV over 10–12 hr; retreatment may be required for persistent (>48–72 hr) or recrudescent fever:
  - Requires close cardiac monitoring
  - Should be started within the 1st 10 days of illness
- Aspirin: 80–100 mg/kg/d PO q6h until about day 14 when fever has resolved; then 3–5 mg/kg/d PO daily for 6–8 wk:
  - Anti-inflammatory
  - Antiplatelet
  - Potentiates the action of IVIG
  - Reduces the occurrence of aneurysms when given with IVIG
  - Alternative dosing at 30 mg/kg/d during acute and subacute phases

*Second Line*
- Corticosteroids:
  - Controversial
  - May improve outcome in conjunction with IVIG
- Remicade:
  - Studies are underway

 FOLLOW-UP

## DISPOSITION
*Admission Criteria*
- Admit all patients who fulfill diagnostic criteria for Kawasaki disease.
- Admit toxic-appearing patients who do not yet meet the criteria for Kawasaki disease.

*Discharge Criteria*
- Nontoxic children who do not fulfill diagnostic criteria
- Close follow-up is required.

*Issues for Referral*
Cardiology consultation for all patients

## PEARLS AND PITFALLS
- Prompt diagnosis and therapy can prevent coronary aneurysms in 95%
- Aspirin and IVIG are mainstays of therapy
- Must consider the diagnosis in febrile children presenting to the ED for multiple visits.

## ADDITIONAL READING
- Ashouri N, Takahashi M, Dorey F, et al. Risk factors for nonresponse to therapy in Kawasaki disease. *J Pediatr.* 2008;153:365–368.
- Harnden A, Takahashi M, Burgner D. Kawasaki disease. *BMJ.* 2009;338:b1514.
- Inoue Y, Okada Y, Shinohara M, et al. A multicenter prospective randomized trial of corticosteroids in primary therapy for Kawasaki disease: Clinical course and coronary artery outcome. *J Pediatr.* 2006;149:336–341.
- Marx JA, Hockberger RS, Walls RM, et al. *Rosen's Emergency Medicine: Concepts and Clinical Practice.* 7th ed. St. Louis, MO: Mosby; 2009.
- Newburger JW, Sleeper LA, McCrindle BW, et al. Randomized trial of pulsed corticosteroid therapy for primary treatment of Kawasaki disease. *N Engl J Med.* 2007;356:663–675.
- Newburger JN, TakahashiM, Gerber MA, et al. Diagnosis, treatment, and long-term management of Kawasaki disease: A statement for health professionals from the Committee on Rheumatic Fever, Endocarditis, and Kawasaki Disease, Council on Cardiovascular Disease in the Young, American Heart Association. *Pediatrics.* 2004;114:1708–1733.
- Pinna GS, Kafetzis DA, Tselkas OI, et al. Kawasaki disease: An overview. *Curr Opin Infect Dis.* 2008;21:263–270.
- Wood LC, Tulloh RMR. Kawasaki disease in children. *Heart.* 2009;95:787–792.

### See Also (Topic, Algorithm, Electronic Media Element)
Myocardial Infarction

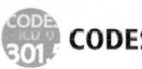 CODES

## ICD9
446.1 Acute febrile mucocutaneous lymph node syndrome (mcls)

K

# KNEE DISLOCATION

*Kelly Anne Foley*

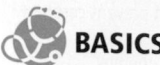

## BASICS

### DESCRIPTION
- Defined by the position of the tibia in relation to the distal femur:
  - Anterior dislocation:
    - Most common dislocation, accounts for 60%
    - Hyperextension of the knee
    - Rupture of the posterior capsule at 30 degrees
    - Rupture of the posterior cruciate ligament (PCL) and popliteal artery (PA) occurs at 50 degrees
  - Posterior dislocation:
    - Direct blow to the anterior tibia with the knee flexed at 90 degrees, "dashboard injury"
    - Anterior cruciate ligament (ACL) is usually spared.
  - Medial dislocation:
    - Varus stress causing tear to the ACL, PCL, and lateral collateral ligament (LCL)
  - Lateral dislocation:
    - Valgus stress causing tear to the ACL, PCL and medial collateral ligament (LCL)
- Associated injuries:
  - Popliteal artery (PA) injury
    - Occurs in 35% of dislocations.
    - Anterior dislocations place traction on PA and cause contusion or intimal injury, which may result in delayed thrombosis.
    - Posterior dislocations cause direct intimal fracture and transection of the artery with immediate thrombosis.
  - Peroneal nerve injury:
    - Less common than PA injury
    - If present, must rule out concomitant arterial insult
    - Medial dislocation causes injury by traction of the nerve.
    - Rotary injuries have a high incidence of traction and transection.

### ETIOLOGY
High-energy injuries such as motor vehicle crashes, auto–pedestrian accidents, and athletic injuries (football most common)

## DIAGNOSIS

### SIGNS AND SYMPTOMS
- Grossly deformed knee
- Grossly unstable knee in AP plane or on varus/valgus stress
- Lack of distal pulse:
  - Popliteal artery injury is primary concern.
- Signs of distal ischemia:
  - Pallor, paresthesias, pain, paralysis

### History
Mechanism of injury with high level of suspicion

### Physical Exam
- Distal pulses
- Distal nerve function:
  - Hypesthesia of first web space, inability to dorsiflex foot
- Ligamentous laxity

### ESSENTIAL WORKUP
- History of mechanism of injury
- Complete and careful physical exam:
  - Pulses—palpation, Doppler, ankle–brachial index (ABI), and cap refill
  - Neurologic—sensation to first web space and great toe, movement of toes, dorsiflexion of foot
- AP and lateral knee radiographs
- Documented repeat exam if any closed reduction is attempted

### DIAGNOSTIC TESTS & INTERPRETATION
#### Imaging
- AP/lateral radiograph of knee:
  - Essential to rule out concominant fractures
- MRI within 1 wk of injury to define ligamentous injury

#### Diagnostic Procedures/Surgery
- ABI—likelihood of significant arterial injury requiring surgery low if $\geq 0.9$
- Peripheral vascular ultrasonography
- Arteriogram should be considered:
  - High suspicion of PA injury
  - Poor pulses or distal perfusion after reduction
  - Peroneal nerve injury
  - Ischemic symptoms despite normal pulses

### DIFFERENTIAL DIAGNOSIS
- Tibial plateau fracture
- Supracondylar femoral fracture
- Ligamentous/tendonous avulsion fracture

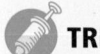

# TREATMENT

## PRE-HOSPITAL
- Management of ABCs
- Documentation of pulses and motor response essential
- Splint knee in slight flexion to prevent PA traction or compression.

## INITIAL STABILIZATION/THERAPY
- ABCs especially when motor vehicle crash or auto–pedestrian accident
- Fluid resuscitation; hypotension may alter distal pulses and perfusion.
- Closed reduction immediately for any limb ischemia
- Early surgical consult in an open injury or high suspicion or arterial injury

## ED TREATMENT/PROCEDURES
- Closed reduction by longitudinal traction and lifting femur into normal alignment without placing pressure on popliteal fossa
- Posterior leg splint/knee immobilizer with knee in 15–20 degrees of flexion
- Repeat neurovascular exam after manipulation and at frequent intervals.
- IV analgesia for patient comfort
- Surgical consult (orthopedic and vascular): open injury, PA injury, or unable to reduce

## MEDICATION
### First Line
- Narcotic analgesia IV
- Avoid PO meds, as surgery may be necessary.

# FOLLOW-UP

## DISPOSITION
### Admission Criteria
All patients require admission for observation of limb perfusion and PA repair if necessary.

### Discharge Criteria
All patients should be admitted.

### Issues for Referral
Eventual repair of ligamentous injuries:
- Usually at 3 wk
- Arthroscopic surgery is contraindicated for 2 wk after injury to prevent compartment syndrome.

## FOLLOW-UP RECOMMENDATIONS
- Orthopedics for ligamentous repair
- Vascular for PA injury

# PEARLS AND PITFALLS

- Failure to revascularize PA within 6–8 hr: amputation rate approaches 90%.
- Peroneal nerve injury:
  – Poor prognosis for recovery
- Delayed compartment syndrome may occur.

# ADDITIONAL READING

- Kelleher HB, Mandavia D. Dislocation, knee. *eMedicine* [serial online]. 2009. Available at www.emedicine.medscape.com/article/823589-overview
- Mills JW. The value of ankle-brachial index for diagnosing arterial injury after knee dislocation: A prospective study. *J Trauma*. 2004;56(6): 1261–1265.
- Nicandri GT, Chamberlain AM, Wahl CJ. Practical management of knee dislocations: a selective angiography protocol to detect limb-threatening vascular injuries. *Clin J Sport Med*. 2009;19(2): 125–129.
- Seroyer ST, Musahl V, Harner CD. Management of the acute knee dislocation: The Pittsburgh experience. *Injury*. 2008;97(7):710–718.

# CODES

## ICD9
- 836.50 Closed dislocation of knee, unspecified part
- 836.51 Anterior dislocation of tibia, proximal end, closed
- 836.52 Posterior dislocation of tibia, proximal end, closed

K

# LABOR

Jonathan B. Walker
James S. Walker

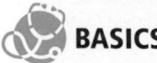

## BASICS

Labor denotes the sequence of physiologic occurrences that result in a fetus being transported from the uterus through the birth canal.

### DESCRIPTION
- Labor brings about changes in the cervix to allow passage of fetus through birth canal.
- Synchronous, coordinated contractions of the uterus
- Contractions progress in magnitude, duration, and frequency to produce dilation of the cervix and ultimate delivery.
- Labor is divided into three stages:
  - Stage 1 (cervical stage): From onset of uterine contractions to full dilation of cervix
  - Stage 1 is further divided into latent and active phases:
    - In the *latent phase*, uterine contraction with little change in cervical dilation or effacement; contractions are mild, short (<45 sec), and irregular.
    - This is followed by the *active phase*, which begins around time of cervical dilation of 3–4 cm; contractions are strong, regular (every 2–3 min), and last longer (>45 sec).
  - Stage 2: From onset of complete cervical dilation to time of delivery of infant
  - Stage 3: From time of delivery of baby to time of placental delivery
- Total duration of labor varies with each woman.
- Generally, lengths of 1st and 2nd stages of labor are significantly longer for nulliparous woman:
  - Nulliparous: Mean length for 1st stage of labor is 14.4 hr and for second stage of labor is 1.0 hr.
  - Parous: Mean length of 1st stage of labor is 7.7 hr and for 2nd stage of labor is 0.2 hr.
- Length of 2nd stage of labor is greatly influenced by "3 Ps":
  - Passenger (infant size and presentation)
  - Passageway (size of bony pelvis and soft tissues)
  - Powers (uterine contractions)
- Problems with any of these 3 Ps can cause abnormal progression of labor:
  - Fetal malposition, uterine dysfunction, cephalopelvic disproportion
- False labor (Braxton-Hicks contractions):
  - Irregular, nonsynchronous contractions of uterus several weeks to days before onset of true labor, and do not cause cervical dilation

## ETIOLOGY
- Premature labor occurs in 8–10% of pregnancies.
- ~30–40% of premature labor is caused by uterine, cervical, or urinary tract infections.
- Premature rupture of membranes is defined as rupture of amniotic/chorionic membranes at least 2 hr before onset of labor in patient before 37 wk gestation:
  - This occurs in only 3% of pregnancies but accounts for 30–40% of all premature births.

## DIAGNOSIS

### SIGNS AND SYMPTOMS
- Symptoms of labor:
  - Intermittent low abdominal pain with or without low back pain
  - Occurring regularly at least every 5 min
  - Lasting 30–60 sec
- Preterm labor is of sufficient frequency and intensity to bring about changes in dilation or effacement of cervix before 37 wk.
- Labor is not associated with vaginal bleeding:
  - Patients with 3rd-trimester abdominal pain or vaginal bleeding should raise suspicion of placenta previa or placental abruption.
- Sudden release of clear fluid from vagina or feeling of constant perineal wetness can represent rupture of membranes:
  - This is not always associated with labor but often leads to onset of labor.

### History
- Gestational age
- Prenatal care
- Previous pregnancies:
  - Complications
  - C-section
- Recent infections

## Physical Exam
- Assess fundal height:
  - Centimeters from pubic bone to top of uterus
  - Correlates with number of weeks after 2nd trimester
  - Can help determine gestational age if unknown
- Sterile pelvic exam to assess cervical dilation and effacement

### ALERT
Do not perform a pelvic exam if vaginal bleeding is present.

### ESSENTIAL WORKUP
- All patients presenting in possible labor should have *immediate sterile pelvic exam* to assess dilation, effacement of cervix, and possibility of imminent delivery.
- Bimanual pelvic exam should not be done in third-trimester patient with vaginal bleeding until US can be done to assess for placenta previa or placental abruption.
- Patients with suspected rupture of membranes should have sterile speculum exam with visual examination of cervix and collection of fluid from vaginal area.
- Suggestive of rupture of membranes:
  - Presence of *ferning* when fluid is allowed to dry on a slide
  - Presence of *pooling* of fluid in vagina
  - *Change of color of litmus paper* from yellow to blue
- Patients with preterm labor and with cervical changes should have urinalysis with culture and cervical cultures.
- Fetal monitoring should be initiated.

### DIAGNOSTIC TESTS & INTERPRETATION
*Lab*
- If patient is in labor, CBC, type, and screen should be sent.
- Urinalysis for proteinuria
- In patients with no prenatal care, obtain Rh factor and antibody screen.
- Cervical cultures and urine culture in patients with preterm labor

### Imaging
- Not generally needed
- 3rd-trimester patients with abdominal pain and vaginal bleeding should have emergent US to evaluate for placenta previa or abruption.

## DIFFERENTIAL DIAGNOSIS
- Braxton-Hicks contractions (false labor) are irregular uterine contractions without associated cervical changes:
  - Contractions can be every 10–20 min.
- Round uterine ligament pain, musculoskeletal back pain
- Other common causes of abdominal pain, such as appendicitis, ovarian cyst, diverticulitis, nephrolithiasis, UTI

 TREATMENT

## PRE-HOSPITAL
- Emergency medical services personnel should place patients in labor on oxygen and in left lateral recumbent position to maximize delivery of oxygen to uterus.
- Maternal transport of high-risk obstetric patients before delivery results in improved outcomes instead of transfer of neonate after delivery.
- Air transport of high-risk obstetric patients has been shown to be beneficial and cost effective.
- Patients in labor who are transported by aircraft should have high-flow oxygen available in the event of cabin decompression at high altitudes.

## INITIAL STABILIZATION/THERAPY
If delivery is imminent (presenting part visible), prepare for immediate vaginal delivery in ED (see "Delivery, Uncomplicated").

## ED TREATMENT/PROCEDURES
- Unless delivery is imminent, patient should be sent directly to the labor and delivery unit.
- If transport to labor and delivery will be delayed, or if transfer to another facility is necessary, these steps should be taken:
  - Consider IV antibiotics for unknown group B *Streptococcus* status.
  - IV hydration with 1 L NS or 5% dextrose in lactated Ringer's over 30–60 min
  - Maternal monitoring
  - Fetal monitoring
  - If labor needs to be arrested (premature fetus), begin tocolytic such as b-agonist terbutaline or magnesium sulfate:
    ○ Magnesium toxicity is suggested by loss of deep tendon reflexes.
    ○ High doses of magnesium can cause cardiac dysrhythmias and respiratory depression.

## MEDICATION
- Magnesium sulfate: 4–6 g IV over 30 min, followed by 2–6 g/hr
- Terbutaline: 0.25 mg SC; may repeat same dose in 30 min.

### ALERT
Consider antibiotic prophylaxis for patients with history of cardiac lesions.

 FOLLOW-UP

## DISPOSITION
### Admission Criteria
- All patients in labor who are not at risk for imminent delivery should be admitted to the labor and delivery department.
- Preterm patients in labor demand immediate obstetric consultation and should be admitted to the labor and delivery department for further treatment.

### Discharge Criteria
Patients with false labor may be discharged only after obstetric consultation, confirmation of fetal well-being, and close follow-up is arranged:
- False labor may progress to true labor.

## PEARLS AND PITFALLS
- If vaginal bleeding is present, must rule out placental abruption or previa.
- Do not perform a digital exam if bleeding is present.
- Pelvic exam must be sterile in a patient in labor.
- False labor may progress to true labor.

## ADDITIONAL READING

- Berghella V, Baxter JK, Chauhan SP. Evidence-based labor and delivery management. *Am J Obstet Gynecol*. 2008;199:445–454.
- DeCherney A, Nathan L, Goodwin TM, et al., eds. *Current Diagnosis and Treatment Obstetrics and Gynecology*, 10th ed. New York: McGraw-Hill; 2007.
- Liao JB, Buhimschi CS, Norwitz ER. Normal labor: Mechanisms and duration. *Obstet Gynecol Clin North Am*. 2005;32:145–164.
- Wilson W, Taubert KA, Gewitz M, et al. Prevention of infective endocarditis: Guidelines from the American Heart Association: A guideline from the American Heart Association Rheumatic Fever, Endocarditis, and Kawasaki Disease Committee, Council on Cardiovascular Disease in the Young, and the Council on Clinical Cardiology, Council on Cardiovascular Surgery and Anesthesia, and the Quality of Care and Outcomes Research Interdisciplinary Working Group. *Circulation*. 2007;116:1736–1754.
- Wolfson AB, Hendey GW, Ling LJ, et al., eds. *Harwood Nuss' Clinical Practice of Emergency Medicine*, 5th ed. Philadelphia: Lippincott, Williams, & Wilkins; 2010.

## See Also (Topic, Algorithm, Electronic Media Element)
- Delivery, Uncomplicated
- Placental Abruption
- Placenta Previa

 CODES

ICD9
650 Normal delivery

# LABYRINTHITIS

*Harish Raj Seetha Rammohan*
*Charles V. Pollack*

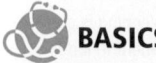 **BASICS**

## DESCRIPTION
- An inflammation that decreases afferent firing from the labyrinth
- The CNS interprets this decreased signal as head rotation away from the diseased labyrinth.
- The imbalance in firing from the labyrinth results in spontaneous nystagmus with the fast phase away from the pathologic side.
- Labyrinthitis:
  - No consensus on definition
  - Peripheral vertigo, sudden onset
  - Single episode of prolonged vertigo lasting days to weeks
  - Peak onset 30–60 yr old
  - Recent upper respiratory tract infection in 50% of patients
  - Symptoms predominantly with head movement but also persist at rest
  - Recovery phase gradual over weeks to months
- The three most common causes of peripheral vertigo are:
  - Benign paroxysmal positional vertigo (BPPV)
  - Ménière disease
  - Labyrinthitis

## ETIOLOGY
- Labyrinthitis:
  - Serous—viral or bacterial
  - Suppurative—bacterial
  - Autoimmune—Wegener or polyarteritis nodosa
  - Vascular ischemia
  - Medications:
    ○ Aminoglycosides
    ○ Loop diuretics
    ○ Antiepileptics
  - Chronic
- BPPV:
  - Dislodgement of otoconia debris:
  - Idiopathic—49%
  - Posttraumatic—18%
  - Sequela of labyrinthitis—15%
  - Sequela of ischemic insult

### Pediatric Considerations
- Suppurative and serous labyrinthitis:
  - Usually secondary to acute otitis media, mastoiditis, or meningitis
- BPPV:
  - Onset 1–5 yr of age
  - Symptoms: Abrupt onset of crying, nystagmus, diaphoresis, emesis, ataxia
  - Recurrences for up to 3 yr
  - Migraine–BPPV complex is the most common etiology of pediatric vertigo.
- Ménière disease:
  - Rare before 10 yr of age

## DIAGNOSIS
### SIGNS AND SYMPTOMS
#### History
- Vertigo:
  - Timing and duration
  - Associated with movement, head position
  - Sensation of room spinning or off balance
- Nausea and vomiting
- Episodes of hearing impairment:
  - Unilateral or bilateral
  - Mild or profound
  - Tinnitus—consider Ménière disease
- Otorrhea—consider otitis media, tympanic membrane (TM) perforation
- Otalgia—consider otitis media, mastoiditis, cholesteatoma
- Recent infections or sick contacts
- Ear surgery
- Diabetes mellitus, stroke, migraine are predisposing factors.
- Head/cervical spine trauma is a direct causal agent, as it dislodges inner ear particles.
- Family history of hearing loss or ear diseases
- Facial weakness or asymmetry: Consider Ramsay Hunt syndrome or stroke.
- Neck pain or stiffness for meningitis
- Visual changes

#### Physical Exam
- Inspect TM and middle ear for perforation, cholesteatoma, middle ear effusion, or otitis media.
- Mastoid tenderness
- Ocular examination, including range of movements, pupillary response, and fundoscopy, to assess for papilledema
- Nystagmus:
  - Augmented by head movement or rapid head shaking
  - Positional
  - Horizontal, frequently with rotational component
  - Direction is constant.
  - Attenuates with fixation
  - Fatigable
- Caloric testing:
  - Irrigate external ear canal with cold water for 20 sec (inspect to confirm absence of TM perforation 1st).
  - Normal response causes horizontal nystagmus with the fast phase away from the irrigated ear.
  - Labyrinthitis produces partial or complete loss of response.
- Dix-Hallpike maneuver:
  - Tests for evidence of BPPV

## ESSENTIAL WORKUP
- Careful neurologic exam to exclude focal findings
- Exclude underlying infections:
  - Acute otitis media
  - Meningitis
  - Mastoiditis
  - Ramsay Hunt syndrome (herpetic lesions on the tympanic membrane)
- Orthostatics
- Auditory evaluation

## DIAGNOSTIC TESTS & INTERPRETATION
- Indicated only if evaluating patients for central vertigo or more unusual etiologies of peripheral vertigo
- Once performed, ensure appropriate follow-up for delayed lab results, such as syphilis screening.

### Lab
- Finger-stick glucose
- Syphilis screening
- Rheumatoid factor

### Pediatric Considerations
Lumbar puncture if clinical suspicion of meningitis

### Imaging
- Indications:
  - Findings suggestive of central nystagmus
- Acute or gradual onset
- Not positional but may be exacerbated by head movements
- Pure direction—vertical, horizontal, or torsional
- Direction may change.
- Nonfatigable
- Minimal effect with fixation:
  - High cardiovascular risk factors
  - Focal neurologic findings
- Head CT:
  - Fine cuts through the cerebellum
- MRI and MRA:
  - Evaluate the posterior fossa, the eighth cranial nerve, and the vestibulobasilar circulation
  - Imaging study of choice in patients suspected of central vertigo

### ALERT
Consider brain imaging in patients >45 yr, children, and patients with cardiovascular risk factors.

### Diagnostic Procedures/Surgery
- Electronystagmography: May help in diagnosing difficult cases.
- Infrared nystagmography: Torsional eye movement can be demonstrated directly.

## DIFFERENTIAL DIAGNOSIS
- Peripheral vertigo:
  - Acoustic neuroma
  - Autoimmune inner-ear disease
  - BPPV
  - Cholesteatoma
  - Ménière disease (associated tinnitus, "fullness," or hearing loss)

- Otosyphilis
- Ototoxic drugs (loop diuretics, aminoglycosides, streptomycin, salicylates, ethanol)
- Perforated tympanic membrane
- Perilymph fistula (symptoms accentuated with Valsalva)
- Posttraumatic vestibular concussion
- Suppurative labyrinthitis (toxic appearance)
- Temporal bone fracture
- Central vertigo—often presents with symptoms indistinguishable from peripheral vertigo because the labyrinth has a monosynaptic connection to the brainstem:
  - Brainstem ischemia
  - Cerebellar hemorrhage
  - Inferior cerebellar ischemia
  - Multiple sclerosis (paresthesias, optic neuritis)
  - Partial seizures of temporal lobe
  - Vestibular-masseter syndrome (associated masseter muscle weakness)
  - Vestibular migraine (30% have vertigo independent of headaches)
  - Wallenberg syndrome (associated Horner syndrome, crossed sensory signs)
- Cardiac arrhythmia (presyncopal symptoms)
- Hypoglycemia (gradual onset, not positional)
- Hypotension (exacerbated with standing)
- Cervicogenic disease (onset with rotational neck movement)
- Hypothyroidism

 **TREATMENT**

**PRE-HOSPITAL**
- Antiemetics for nausea and vomiting
- IV fluids for dehydration
- Fall precautions
- Assessment for acute stroke
- Telemetry for arrhythmia
- Finger-stick glucose to exclude hypoglycemia
- BP check for hypotension

**INITIAL STABILIZATION/THERAPY**
- Bed rest and hydration
- Falls precautions

**ED TREATMENT/PROCEDURES**
- Medications are minimally beneficial for BPPV.
- Avoid chronic use to encourage development of vestibular compensation.
- Medications for symptomatic relief:
  - Vestibular suppressants: Diazepam, meclizine, scopolamine
  - Antiemetics: Ondansetron, prochlorperazine, promethazine
  - Corticosteroids: Poor evidence for efficacy
- Debris repositioning is primary therapy for BPPV. Effective relief in 50–80% of patients:
  - Epley maneuver
- Vestibular enhancement exercises
- Surgery for failed medical and physical therapy:
  - Posterior canal plugging to occlude canal
  - Nerve section

**MEDICATION**
- Diazepam (benzodiazepine): 2–10 mg IV; 5–10 mg (0.1–0.3 mg/kg/24 hr) PO q6h–q12h
- Dimenhydrinate: 5 mg/kg/24 hr PO, IM, IV, or PR
- Meclizine (antihistamine): 25 mg (50 mg/24 hr for patient >12 yr) PO q6h
- Lorazepam: 0.5–2 mg IV, IM, or PO q6h (peds: 0.05 mg/kg IV/PO q4–8h)
- Ondansetron: 4–8 mg IV, IM, or PO q8h (peds: 1 mo–12 yr and <40 kg: 0.1 mg/kg IV; >12 yr and >40 kg: 4 mg IV)
- Prochlorperazine: 5–10 mg (peds: 0.3 mg/kg/24 hr IM or PO for patient >2 yr old) IV, IM, or PO q6h–q8h
- Promethazine: 12.5–25 mg (peds: 1.5–2.0 mg/kg/24 hr) IV or PO q4h–q6h
- Scopolamine (anticholinergic, not approved in pediatrics): 0.6 mg PO q4h–q6h; 1.5-mg transdermal patch q3d

**Pediatric Considerations**
Bacterial labyrinthitis:
- Antibiotics IV
- Surgical debridement

**Pregnancy Considerations**
- Class D medication: Diazepam, lorazepam
- Class C medication: Prochlorperazine
- Class B medication: Famciclovir
- Class B medication: Corticosteroids

**First Line**
- Meclizine
- Ondansetron for nausea/vomiting

**Second Line**
- Diazepam or lorazepam
- Prochlorperazine or promethazine (beware dystonic or dysphoric reactions)

 **FOLLOW-UP**

**DISPOSITION**
**Admission Criteria**
- Intractable nausea and vomiting
- Severe dehydration
- Unsteady gait
- Symptoms concerning for an acute stroke or central etiology of vertigo

**Discharge Criteria**
- Tolerate oral fluids
- Steady gait
- Normal neurologic exam
- Avoid driving, heights, and operating dangerous equipment.
- Fall precautions
- Arrange neurology or otolaryngology follow-up.

**Issues for Referral**
- Recurrent symptoms
- Concern for cholesteatoma
- Possible severe underlying condition such as vertebrobasilar ischemia or brainstem tumor will need referral to neurologist or neurosurgeon.

**FOLLOW-UP RECOMMENDATIONS**
- Vestibular rehabilitation for patients with persistent vestibular symptoms and chronic vertigo due to peripheral vestibular etiology
- Auditory brainstem response test is indicated in younger children.
- Surgical therapy in the form of labyrinthectomy/posterior canal occlusion/vestibular nerve section, etc., can be considered in cases of refractory vertigo and unsuccessful canalith repositioning procedure.

**PEARLS AND PITFALLS**
- Counsel patients regarding occupation and driving.
- Failure to diagnose life-threatening conditions like meningitis, cerebrovascular ischemia, or brain tumors
- Take caution while performing physical maneuvers for BPPV, as violent hyperextension at cervical spine can cause vertebral artery dissection.

**ADDITIONAL READING**
- Baloh RW. Vestibular neuritis. *N Engl J Med.* 2003;348:1027–1032.
- Charles J, Fahridin S, Britt H. Vertigionous syndrome. *Aust Fam Physician.* 2008;37:299–304.
- Kerber KA. Vertigo and dizziness in the emergency department. *Emerg Med Clin North Am.* 2009;27:39–50, viii.
- Korres SG, Balatsouras DG. Diagnostic, pathophysiologic, and therapeutic aspects of benign paroxysmal positional vertigo. *Otolaryngol Head Neck Surg.* 2004;131(4):438–444.
- Newman-Toker DE, Camargo CA Jr, Hsieh YH, et al. Disconnect between charted vestibular diagnosis and emergency department management decisions: A cross-sectional analysis from a nationally representative sample. *Acad Emerg Med.* 2009;16:970–977.

**See Also (Topic, Algorithm, Electronic Media Element)**
- Dizziness
- Vertigo
- Ménière Disease
- Otitis Media
- Mastoiditis

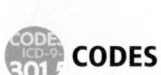 **CODES**

**ICD9**
386.30 Labyrinthitis, unspecified

# LACERATION MANAGEMENT
*Gordon S. Chew*

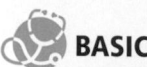 BASICS

## DESCRIPTION
- A laceration is a disruption in skin integrity most often resulting from trauma.
- May be single or multiple layered

## ETIOLOGY
Multiple causes

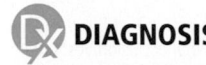 DIAGNOSIS

## SIGNS AND SYMPTOMS
Lacerations may be accompanied by:
- Bleeding
- Tissue foreign bodies
- Hematoma
- Pain or numbness
- Loss of motor function
- Diminished pulses, delayed capillary refill

### History
- Mechanism and circumstances of injury
- Time of injury
- History of foreign body (glass, splinter, teeth)
- Tetanus immunization
- Comorbid condition or medications that may impede wound healing

### Physical Exam
- Evaluate nerve and motor function.
- Document associated neurovascular injury.
- Assess presence of devitalized tissue, debris from foreign materials, bone or joint violation, tendon injury:
  - Avoid digital exploration if the object is believed to be sharp.

## ESSENTIAL WORKUP
- Consider repair in OR if unable to be performed safely within the ED, especially for children requiring deep sedation.
- Consider surgical consultation for complex lacerations, especially involving eyes and face.

### Pediatric Considerations
Assess for possible nonaccidental trauma.

## DIAGNOSTIC TESTS & INTERPRETATION
### Imaging
- Evaluation for possible foreign bodies
- Plain radiography:
  - Soft-tissue views may aid in visualization.
  - Objects with the same density as soft tissue may not be seen (wood, plants).
- US
- CT scan
- MRI with metal precautions

## DIFFERENTIAL DIAGNOSIS
- Skin avulsion
- Contusion
- Abrasion

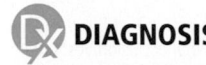 TREATMENT

## PRE-HOSPITAL
- Obtain hemostasis, or control of bleeding with direct pressure.
- Straighten any flaps of skin whose blood supply may be strangulated.
- Apply splint if needed.
- Universal precautions

## INITIAL STABILIZATION/THERAPY
- Airway, breathing, and circulation management (ABCs)
- Control hemostasis.
- Remove rings or jewelry if needed.

## ED TREATMENT/PROCEDURES
- Time of onset:
  - Lacerations may be closed primarily ≤8 hr old in areas of poorer circulation.
  - Lacerations may be closed ≤12 hr old in areas of normal circulation.
  - On face, lacerations may be closed ≤24 hr if clean and well irrigated.
  - If not closed, wound may heal by secondary intention or by delayed primary closure (DPC) in 3–5 days.
- Analgesia and conscious sedation:
  - Adequate analgesia is crucial for good wound management.
  - Conscious sedation may be required (see "Conscious Sedation").
- Local anesthetics:
  - Topical:
    - TAC (tetracaine, adrenaline, cocaine)
    - EMLA (eutectic mixture, lidocaine, prilocaine)
    - LET (lidocaine, epinephrine, tetracaine)
  - Local/regional:
    - Lidocaine, bupivacaine
    - Epinephrine will cause vasoconstriction and improve duration of action of anesthetic.
    - Avoid epinephrine in the penis, digits, toes, ears, eyelids, tip of nose, skin flaps (necrosis), and severely contaminated wounds (impairs defense).
    - For patient comfort, inject slowly with small-gauge needle; buffer every 9 mL of 1% lidocaine with 1 mL 8.4% sodium bicarbonate.
    - Consider a 1% diphenhydramine solution in the lidocaine-allergic patient.

- Exploration and removal of foreign body:
  - Indications for removal of a foreign body include:
    - Potential or actual injury to tendons, nerves, vasculature
    - Toxic substance or reactive agent
    - Continued pain
- Irrigation and debridement:
  - Surrounding intact skin may be cleaned with an antiseptic solution (povidone-iodine, chlorhexidine):
    - Do not use antiseptic solution within the wound itself because it may impair healing.
  - Scrub with a fine-pore sponge only if significant contamination or particulate matter.
  - Irrigation with ≥200 mL of normal saline (NS):
    - Optimal pressure (5–8 psi) generated with 30-mL syringe through 18–20-gauge needle
    - Debride devitalized and contaminated tissue.
- Wound repair:
  - Universal precautions
  - Wounds that cannot be cleaned adequately should heal by secondary intention or DPC.
  - Reapproximate all anatomic borders carefully (eg, skin–vermilion border of lip).
  - Consider tissue adhesive for wounds with clean borders, low tension.
- Single-layered closure:
  - Simple interrupted sutures:
    - Avoid in lacerations under tension.
  - Horizontal mattress sutures (running or interrupted):
    - Edematous finger and hand wounds
    - Ideal in skin flaps where edges at risk for necrosis
  - Vertical mattress:
    - For wounds under greater tension
- Multiple-layered closure:
  - Closes deep tissue dead space
  - Lessens tension at the epidermal level, improves cosmetic result
  - Buried interrupted absorbable suture, simple or running nonabsorbable sutures for epidermis

- Dressing:
  - Dress wound with antibiotic ointment and nonadherent semiporous dressing.
  - Inform patient about scarring and risk for infection, use of sunscreen.
  - Apply splint if needed.
- Antimicrobial agents:
  - Uncomplicated lacerations do not need prophylactic antibiotics.
  - If antibiotics are used, initiate before wound manipulation or as early as possible.
  - Lacerations with high likelihood of infection:
    o Animal, human bites, especially to hand (see "Hand Infection")
    o Contaminated with dirt, bodily fluids, feces
  - Tetanus immunization

## MEDICATION

- See "Conscious Sedation."
- Tetanus (Td adults, DT peds): 0.5 mL IM
- Local anesthetics:
  - Topical, applied directly to wound with cotton, gauze:
    o EMLA (eutectic mixture, 5% lidocaine, and prilocaine): Apply for 60 min.
    o TAC (0.5% tetracaine, 1:2,000 adrenaline, 11.8% cocaine): Apply for 20–30 min.
    o LET (4% lidocaine, 1:1,000 epinephrine, 0.5% tetracaine): Apply for 20–30 min.
- Injected:
  - Bupivacaine (max.: 2 mg/kg; duration 3–10 hr)
  - Lidocaine (max.: 4.5 mg/kg; duration 1.5–3.5 hr)
- Suture materials:
  - Absorbable:
    o For use in mucous membranes and buried muscle/fascial layer closures
    o Natural: Dissolve <1 wk, poor tensile strength, local inflammation: Plain gut, chromic gut, fast-absorbing gut (for certain facial lacerations where cosmesis is important)
    o Synthetic braided: Tensile strength diminishing over 1 mo, mild inflammation: Polyglycolic acid (Dexon), polyglactin 910 (Vicryl)
    o Synthetic monofilament: Tensile strength 70% at 1 mo: Polydioxanone (PDS), polyglyconate (Maxon)

- Nonabsorbable:
  o Greatest tensile strength
  o Monofilament: Nylon (Ethilon, Dermalon), polypropylene (Prolene), polybutester (Novafil) can stretch with wound edema, polyethylene (stainless steel)
  o Multifilament: Cotton, Dacron, silk (local inflammation)
- Needle types:
  - Cutting (cuticular and plastic) types are most often used in outpatient wound repair.
- Staples:
  - For linear lacerations of scalp, torso, extremities
  - Avoid in hands, face, and areas requiring CT or MRI.
- Adhesive tapes (Steri-Strips):
  - For lacerations that are clean, small, and under minimal tension
  - Avoid in wounds that have potential to become very swollen.
  - Pretreat wound edges with tincture of benzoin to improve adhesion.
- Tissue adhesives:
  - Good cosmetic results have been achieved in simple lacerations with low skin tension.
  - An alternative to sutures/staples, especially in children

 **FOLLOW-UP**

## DISPOSITION
### Admission Criteria
- Few lacerations by themselves necessitate admission unless they require significant debridement or ongoing IV antibiotics, or are complicated by extensive wound care issues or comorbid processes (head injury, abdominal trauma)
- It is unsafe for a child to return home when nonaccidental trauma is suspected

### Discharge Criteria
- Wounds at risk for infection or poor healing require a wound check within 48 hr.
- Time of suture removal dependent on location and peripheral perfusion:
  - Scalp: 7–10 days
  - Face: 3–5 days

- Oral: 7 days
- Neck: 4–6 days
- Abdomen, back, chest, hands, feet: 7–10 days
- Upper extremity: 7–10 days
- Lower extremity: 10–14 days
- Overlying joints: 10–14 days

### Issues for Referral
- Complicated lacerations (tendon involvement) may require further repair in the outpatient surgical office.
- Be sure to discuss temporary skin closure and splinting with your surgical consultant.
- Specific follow-up should be arranged prior to patient discharge.

## ADDITIONAL READING

- Beam JW. Tissue adhesives for simple traumatic lacerations. *J Athl Train*. 2008;43(2):222–224.
- Chisolm C, Howell JM. Soft tissue emergencies. *Emerg Med Clin North Am*. 1992;10(4):665–705.
- Hollander JE, Singer AJ. Laceration management. *Ann Emerg Med*. 1999;34(3):356–367.
- Roberts PA, Lamacraft G. Techniques to reduce the discomfort of pediatric laceration repair. *MJA* 1996;164(1):32–35.
- Stone S, Carter WA. Wound preparation. In: Tintinalli JE, Kelen GD, Stapczynski JS, eds. *Emergency medicine: A comprehensive study guide*, 6th ed. New York: McGraw-Hill; 2004:41.

### See Also (Topic, Algorithm, Electronic Media Element)
Hand Infection

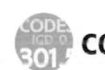 **CODES**

ICD9
879.8 Open wound(s) (multiple) of unspecified site(s), without mention of complication

L

# LARYNGITIS

*Yi-Mei Chng*

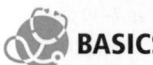

## BASICS

### DESCRIPTION
- Inflammation of the mucosa of the larynx
- In adults, laryngopharyngeal reflux is a common cause, but in children the most common cause is viral or bacterial infection.
- Peaks parallel epidemics of individual viruses
- Most common during late fall, winter, early spring

### ETIOLOGY
- Viral upper respiratory infections most common in acute laryngitis in children:
  - Influenza A and B
  - Parainfluenza types 1 and 2
  - Adenovirus
  - Coronavirus
  - Coxsackie virus
  - Respiratory syncytial virus
  - Measles
  - Rhinovirus
- Bacterial infections in 10% of cases:
  - β-Hemolytic streptococcus
  - *Streptococcus pneumoniae*
  - *Haemophilus influenzae* (HiB)
  - *Moraxella catarrhalis*
  - *Bordetella pertussis*
  - Diphtheria
  - Tuberculosis
  - Syphilis
  - Leprosy
- Fungal infections (often associated with inhaled steroid use or immunocompromise)
- Allergic
- Voice abuse or misuse
- Inhalation or ingestion of caustic substances or other irritants
- Autoimmune (rheumatoid arthritis, relapsing polychondritis, Wegener granulomatosis, or sarcoidosis)
- Gastroesophageal reflux disease (GERD) (especially in adults)
- Trauma
- Idiopathic

### Pediatric Considerations
- Acute spasmodic laryngitis (spasmodic croup)
- More likely to be infectious. Consider HiB, diphtheria, etc., if not immunized.
- Consider foreign body.

## DIAGNOSIS

### SIGNS AND SYMPTOMS
#### History
- Hoarseness
- Abnormal-sounding voice
- Throat swelling
- Throat tickling
- Feeling of throat rawness
- Constant urge to clear the throat
- Cough
- Fever
- Malaise
- Dysphagia

#### Physical Exam
- Regional lymphadenopathy
- Stridor in infants
- Hoarse voice
- Pharyngeal erythema, exudates, and/or edema

### ESSENTIAL WORKUP
- Acute laryngitis:
  - In most cases, the history and inspection of the throat suffice to distinguish between infectious and noninfectious laryngitis.
  - Have increased suspicion for epiglottitis in persons who have not had HiB vaccine.
- Chronic laryngitis (>3 wk):
  - The workup should be directed toward chronic infections, GERD, neurologic disorders, and tumors.
  - Visualization of the larynx should be performed but may not need to be done in the ED.
  - The patient should be referred to an ear-nose-throat specialist for biopsy.
  - Visualization of nodules indicates the need to admit to rule out TB.

### DIAGNOSTIC TESTS & INTERPRETATION
#### Lab
- Blood tests are not generally indicated:
  - An elevated WBC count is not a reliable way to distinguish between bacterial and viral illness.
- Throat culture:
  - Indicated when throat inspection suggests a bacterial infection

#### Imaging
Soft-tissue neck films:
- Rarely indicated because direct laryngoscopy provides a more comprehensive assessment

#### Diagnostic Procedures/Surgery
Direct laryngoscopy:
- Red, inflamed vocal cords, with rounded edges
- Occasionally hemorrhage or exudates
- Demonstration of laryngeal pseudomembrane to distinguish diphtheria from other infectious forms of laryngitis
- This procedure is mainly used to rule out epiglottitis in the ED.

### DIFFERENTIAL DIAGNOSIS
- Asthma
- Epiglottitis
- Esophageal reflux
- Vocal nodules
- Laryngeal or thyroid malignancy
- Croup/laryngotracheobronchitis
- Foreign-body inhalation or other trauma

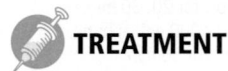

## TREATMENT

### PRE-HOSPITAL
Supportive care and ambulance transport are not generally indicated.

#### ALERT
- Stridor can mean obstruction of the laryngeal or tracheal parts of the airway, particularly in children.
- An otolaryngologist should evaluate laryngitis after trauma to the neck.
- Beware of esophageal injuries in laryngitis associated with caustic ingestions.
- If there are signs of respiratory distress, epiglottitis should be suspected:
  - Transport sitting up.
  - Provide supplemental oxygen.
  - Intubation may be difficult or impossible and should only be attempted in patients in extremis.

## INITIAL STABILIZATION/THERAPY

Stabilization is only required if the patient shows signs of respiratory distress:

- The patient should be managed for epiglottitis.
- Supplemental oxygen via a nonrebreather mask
- Orotracheal intubation when time permits in the OR
- The neck should be prepped and the equipment ready for a surgical airway.

## ED TREATMENT/PROCEDURES

- Antibiotics are not first-line therapy in adults with acute laryngitis. In a systematic review of randomized controlled trials investigating the use of antibiotics vs. placebo, antibiotics offered no objective improvement in symptoms over placebo, although there was some subjective improvement in symptoms with erythromycin.
- Vocal rest (avoid whispering, as it promotes hyperfunctioning of the larynx)
- Humidified air
- Increase fluid intake.
- Analgesics
- Avoid smoking.
- Symptoms usually resolve in 10–14 days, if viral cause.
- Use of inhaled steroids for laryngitis is controversial and not part of current best practices.

## MEDICATION

Depends on cause of laryngitis.

### First Line

- Mucolytics like guaifenesin if related to upper respiratory infection or allergy
- Tylenol or NSAIDs for symptomatic relief if associated with viral syndrome
- Proton pump inhibitors for GERD-related laryngitis:
  – Esomeprazole magnesium: 20–40 mg (peds: 10 mg for patients 1–11 yr) PO daily
  – Omeprazole: 20 mg PO b.i.d.
- Diflucan for candidal laryngitis
- If caused by croup: Dexamethasone (0.6 mg/kg) PO or IM ×1

### Second Line

For bacterial laryngitis:

- Erythromycin: 250 mg (peds: 30–50 mg/kg/d div. q.i.d.) q.i.d. PO
- Penicillin V: 250 mg (peds: 25–50 mg/kg/d div. b.i.d.–q.i.d.) q.i.d. PO for 5 days

 FOLLOW-UP

## DISPOSITION

### Admission Criteria

- Tuberculous laryngitis:
  – Highly contagious requiring isolation
- Signs of epiglottitis, respiratory distress, neck trauma, or anaphylaxis
- Respiratory compromise

### Discharge Criteria

Most patients with uncomplicated laryngitis can be discharged if they have no difficulty breathing and are able to keep adequately hydrated.

### Issues for Referral

Refer patients with chronic laryngitis to otolaryngologist. Patients with >3 wk of laryngitis without obvious benign cause should be evaluated with laryngoscopy to rule out more serious conditions such as carcinoma.

## FOLLOW-UP RECOMMENDATIONS

- With otolaryngology if not improved in 2–3 wk
- With gastroenterology if symptoms of GERD

## PEARLS AND PITFALLS

History is very important in determining the cause of laryngitis:

- Patients with chronic or nonresolving laryngitis should follow up with otolaryngology.

## ADDITIONAL READING

- Behrman RE, Kliegman R, Jenson H, eds. *Nelson Textbook of Pediatrics*, 18th ed. Philadelphia: WB Saunders; 2007.
- Heidelbaugh JJ, Gill AS, Van Harrison R, et al. Atypical presentations of gastroesophageal reflux disease. *Am Fam Physician*. 2008;78:483–488.
- Mehanna HM, Kuo T, Chaplin J, et al. Fungal laryngitis in immunocompetent patients. *J Laryngol Otol*. 2004;118:379–381.
- Reveiz L, Cardona AF, Ospina EG. Antibiotics for acute laryngitis in adults. *Cochrane Database Syst Rev*. 2007;CD004783.

## See Also (Topic, Algorithm, Electronic Media Element)

- Croup
- Epiglottitis

 CODES

### ICD9

- 464.00 Acute laryngitis without mention of obstruction
- 476.0 Chronic laryngitis

L

# LARYNX FRACTURE

Diane DeVita
David Della-Giustina

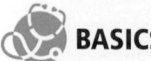 **BASICS**

## DESCRIPTION
- Direct transfer of severe forces to the larynx
- Simple mucosal tears to fractured and comminuted cartilage:
  - Epiglottis, thyroid, arytenoid, cricoid, corniculate, and cuneiform cartilages

## ETIOLOGY
- Rare: 1/14,000–30,000 ED visits
- <1% of all blunt trauma
- Blunt trauma to the anterior neck associated with motor vehicle or motorcycle crash, assault, or recreational activities
- The typical mechanism is hyperextension of neck with a direct blow to the exposed anterior neck.
- "Clothesline" injury is a classic mechanism (victim struck in neck by cord, wire, or branch hung across path of travel).

### Pediatric Considerations
Bicycle handlebars:
- Extended neck hits the bar, compressing structures between the bar and vertebral column.

 **DIAGNOSIS**

## SIGNS AND SYMPTOMS
- May be subtle or delayed for hours
- Neck tenderness
- Bruising or abrasions over the anterior neck
- Hoarseness or voice changes
- Hemoptysis
- Dysphonia
- Stridor
- Subcutaneous emphysema
- Dyspnea
- Loss of normal cartilaginous landmarks of neck

## ESSENTIAL WORKUP
- Cervical spine radiograph:
  - Examine for concomitant spinal injury as well as soft-tissue swelling and subcutaneous emphysema.
- CXR:
  - Identify pneumothorax, pneumomediastinum, and subcutaneous emphysema.
- Fine-cut CT scan of larynx:
  - Recommended unless the patient is going directly to surgery
  - Useful even in cases of apparently less severe symptoms and minor abnormalities on indirect laryngoscopy
- Pulse oximetry

### ALERT
MRI has not gained acceptance:
- Length of time
- Physical demands on injured patient
- Less helpful for skeletal structures

## DIAGNOSTIC TESTS & INTERPRETATION
### Lab
Arterial blood gas if the patient is having respiratory difficulty:
- Identifies hypoxia, hypercarbia

### Diagnostic Procedures/Surgery
- Fiberoptic laryngoscopy:
  - Allows visualization of injuries involving the airway, vocal cords
- Angiography:
  - Penetrating injuries
  - Only when concerned with possible vascular injuries
- CT angiogram offers advantages to conventional angiography:
  - Readily accessible and less invasive
  - Can be rapidly performed
  - Few complications
  - Provides useful information on cervical soft tissues, aerodigestive tract, spinal canal and cord
- Fiberoptic bronchoscopy and esophagoscopy
- Surgical exploration
- Surgery:
  - As indicated by severity of injury
  - Emergent surgical repair if necessary

## DIFFERENTIAL DIAGNOSIS
Associated injuries:
- Intracranial injuries (13%)
- Open neck injuries (9%)
- Cervical spine injuries (8%)
- Esophageal injuries (3%)
- Carotid artery injury
- Phrenic nerve injury
- Hypoxic cerebral injury
- Airway edema
- Aspiration pneumonitis
- Air embolism

### Pediatric Considerations
- Pediatric larynx is located higher in the neck and is more cartilaginous and mobile than in adults; thus, pediatric patients are more resistant to laryngeal fractures.
- Loosely attached submucosal tissue allows for greater soft-tissue trauma, massive edema, and hematoma formation:
  - With smaller airway diameters, rapid airway compromise can occur.
- Neck tenderness is a more common complaint than dysphagia or dyspnea.

 **TREATMENT**

## PRE-HOSPITAL
- Cautions:
  - Aggressive airway management is necessary: oxygen, suction
  - Cervical spine immobilization
  - Injury may be overlooked if patient is intubated prehospital for other injuries owing to loss of subjective complaints.
- Controversies:
  - Elective intubation is not advocated.

## INITIAL STABILIZATION/THERAPY

Airway management is of primary concern:

- Severe injuries may require operative management.
- Early intubation to preclude respiratory embarrassment
- Formal tracheostomy under local anesthesia may be required rather than endotracheal intubation when more severe neck injury is present.
- *Avoid* repeated orotracheal intubation attempts:
  - Proceed to surgical airway.
- Cricothyrotomy for severe maxillofacial injuries and injury is superior to cricothyroid cartilage.
- *Avoid* cricothyrotomy if hematoma present over the cricothyroid membrane or there is evidence of cricotracheal disruption.
- Emergent tracheostomy may be the only option to secure an airway.

### Pediatric Considerations

- Elective intubation is not recommended.
- Mandatory flexible fiberoptic laryngoscopy
- CT scan if management course in doubt

## ED TREATMENT/PROCEDURES

- Supplemental humidified air (or oxygen as needed)
- Elevate head of bed to decrease cerebral and neck soft tissue edema.
- Maintain NPO status.
- Voice rest as much as possible
- Intravenous access
- Consult otolaryngologist for surgical evaluation.
- Positive end expiratory pressure and volume-controlled ventilation for severe pulmonary injury associated with acute respiratory distress syndrome or aspiration pneumonitis

## MEDICATION

- For laryngeal injury with subcutaneous emphysema:
  - Assume that the mucosa of the upper airway has communicated with the deep tissue of the neck:
    - Ampicillin/sulbactam: 1.5 to 3.0 g IV (peds: 50 mg/kg IV) q6h
    - Clindamycin: 600–900 mg IV q8h (peds: 25–40 mg/kg/24 hr IV)
    - Histamine-2 blockers to prevent irritation to mucosal injuries (eg, ranitidine 150–300 mg IV; peds: 2–4 mg/kg/day div. q6h IV) or proton-pump inhibitors (eg, pantoprazole 40 mg IV, no pediatric dosing)
- For laryngeal edema, the following may be used:
  - Steroids:
    - Not routinely used, but may be used for massive edema.
    - Dexamethasone: 4–10 mg IV (peds: 0.15–0.6 mg/kg per dose IV)

### Pediatric Considerations

If stridor present, consider nebulized racemic epinephrine: 2.25% 0.25–0.5 mL in 2.5 mL NS.

 **FOLLOW-UP**

### DISPOSITION

#### Admission Criteria

- Patients with true laryngeal injuries must be admitted to a monitored setting for observation and airway management; prepare for emergent surgical repair of laryngeal defect.
- Patients with suspected laryngeal injury or highly suspicious mechanism must be admitted to a monitored setting for observation and serial flexible fiberoptic laryngoscopic examinations.

#### Pediatric Considerations

Mandatory admission is recommended in all patients for oximetry, oxygen, and serial fiberoptic laryngoscopy examinations.

### Discharge Criteria

Patients without evidence of serious laryngeal injury or airway edema or compromise after an appropriate period of observation in the ED (usually 6 hr):

- Patients can appear deceptively normal for several hours after injury; if there is any doubt, admit to a monitored setting.

## ADDITIONAL READING

- Atkins Z, Abbate S, Fisher S, et al. Current management of laryngotracheal trauma: Case report and literature review. *J Trauma.* 2004;56:185–190.
- Bell B, Verschueren S, Dierks E. Management of laryngeal trauma. *Oral Maxillofacial Surg Clin North Am.* 2008;20(3):415–430.
- Francis S, Gaspard D, Rogers N, et al. Diagnosis and management of laryngotracheal trauma. *J Natl Med Assoc.* 2002;94:21–24.
- Gold SM, Gerber ME, Hott SR, et al. Blunt laryngotracheal trauma in children. *Arch Otolaryngol Head Neck Surg.* 1997;123:83–87.
- Levy D, Gruber B. Neck trauma: Differential diagnoses and workup. *Emed Trauma Orthoped.* Available at: http://emedicine.medscape.com/article/827223-diagnosis. Updated December 12, 2008.
- Pancholi S, Robbin W, Desai A, et al. Laryngeal fracture: Treatment. *Emed Otololaryngol Facial Plastic Surg.* Available at: http://emedicine.medscape.com/article/865277-treatment. Updated January 9, 2009.

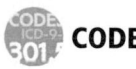 **CODES**

**ICD9**
807.5 Closed fracture of larynx and trachea

**ICD10**
S12.8

# LEAD POISONING

*Harry C. Karydes*

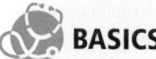 **BASICS**

## DESCRIPTION
- Lead has multiple mechanisms:
  - Binds sulfhydryl groups and affects multiple enzymatic processes
  - Resembles $Ca^{2+}$ and therefore can interfere with $Ca^{2+}$-dependent processes, including cell signaling
  - Mutagenic potential—not known to be a human carcinogen
- Distribution:
  - Up to 99% of lead is bound to erythrocytes after initial absorption.
  - Ultimately redistributed into bone:
    - 95% of total body lead in adults
    - 70% of total body lead in children
  - High lead levels in the serum will compromise the blood–brain barrier and result in lead entry into the CNS and neurotoxicity.
- Often coexists with iron deficiency; this allows for increased lead absorption in the gut.
- Impairs heme synthesis, leading to elevated erythrocyte protoporphyrin; these complex with zinc, causing elevated zinc protoporphyrin (ZPP).

## ETIOLOGY
- Acute toxicity:
  - Most often due to environmental exposure or ingestion of substance containing high lead levels
  - Pottery glaze
  - Certain folk remedies
  - Jewelry
  - Weights
  - Home-distilled alcoholic beverages
- Chronic toxicity:
  - Occupational exposures:
    - Most common via inhalation route
    - Smelting
    - De-leading
    - Bridge painting
  - Home exposures:
    - Lead paint ingestion by children
  - Contamination of drinking water or food
  - Use of folk remedies containing high lead concentrations
- In the U.S., lead intoxication is primarily due to ingestion of leaded paints and most frequently affects children age 1–6 yr.
- May also be seen when a retained bullet enters synovium or other body cavity, where it is systemically absorbed.

 **DIAGNOSIS**

## SIGNS AND SYMPTOMS
- Neurologic:
  - Seizures (may be prolonged and refractory)
  - Encephalopathy
  - Learning disabilities/decreased intelligence
  - Cerebral edema
  - Peripheral neuropathy (wrist drop), classic (but rarely seen) finding with chronic toxicity
- GI:
  - Colicky abdominal pain (lead colic)
  - Ileus
  - Nausea/vomiting
  - Lead lines in gums (Burton lines) appear as bluish tint to gingival line.
  - Hepatitis/pancreatitis
- Cardiovascular:
  - HTN (generally secondary to renal failure)
  - Myocarditis and conduction defects
- Renal:
  - Chronic renal insufficiency with long-term exposure
  - Saturnine gout
- Hematologic:
  - Anemia (due to interference with globin chain synthesis)
  - Elevated ZPP
  - Increases RBC fragility, so decreased RBC life span
- Musculoskeletal:
  - Lead lines from increased $Ca^{2+}$ deposition (not actually lead itself)
  - May lead to decreased bone strength and growth

## ESSENTIAL WORKUP
Blood lead level

## DIAGNOSTIC TESTS & INTERPRETATION
*Lab*
- Whole-blood lead level:
  - Normal <10 mcg/dL
  - 100 mcg/dL—severe encephalopathy; cognitive effects increase with rising levels
  - Expect that lead levels may rise again after treatment is completed as lead redistributes into the serum again.
  - Levels correlate poorly with symptoms:
    - Acute exposures may be symptomatic with levels of 40–50 mcg/dL.
    - Chronic exposures may have minimal findings at levels of 70 mcg/dL.

- CBC:
  - For presence of anemia
  - RBC indices
- Electrolytes, BUN, creatinine, glucose:
  - For renal insufficiency
- Transaminases, liver function tests
- Iron studies
- ZPP

*Imaging*
- Plain abdominal radiographs to look for radiopaque foreign body
- Long-bone series to look for lead lines (specifically in children)
- Cranial CT and other studies as indicated by patient's condition

## DIFFERENTIAL DIAGNOSIS
- Heavy metal intoxications
- Cyclic antidepressants or other seizure-inducing toxins
- Encephalopathy, meningitis, encephalitis
- Causes of increased intracranial pressure
- Reye syndrome
- Status epilepticus
- Bowel obstruction
- Guillain-Barré syndrome
- Addison disease
- Cholera
- Peripheral neuropathies

**TREATMENT**

## PRE-HOSPITAL
- Support airway/breathing and circulation.
- Cardiac monitoring
- Seizure management

### ALERT
- If possible to do so safely, bring containers in suspected overdose or poisoning.
- Decontaminate skin for obvious dermal exposures.

## INITIAL STABILIZATION/THERAPY
- ABCs:
  - Cardiac monitor
  - Isotonic crystalloids as needed for hypotension; vasopressors for refractory hypotension
- Naloxone, thiamine, and dextrose (D50W) as indicated for altered mental status
- Cardiovascular:
  - Isotonic crystalloids to support BP
  - Vasopressors for refractory hypotension (rare)
- Neurologic:
  - Treat seizures with benzodiazepines.
  - Assist ventilation as needed for respiratory insufficiency due to neuromuscular weakness.
- Renal:
  - Hemodialysis for renal failure

## ED TREATMENT/PROCEDURES
- Decontamination:
  - If opacities are seen on upright abdominal film, institute whole-bowel irrigation at 1–2 L/hr of polyethylene glycol until abdominal films are clear.
  - Activated charcoal is not effective.
- Evaluate need for chelation therapy, based on:
  - Levels
  - Acuity of exposure
  - Symptoms
  - Consultation with a medical toxicologist (advised)
- All symptomatic patients need chelation:
  - Begin with British antilewisite (BAL) and continue for 5 days:
    - Stop BAL at 3 days if lead level is <50 mcg/dL and clinically improved.
  - Start calcium disodium ethylenediamine tetra-acetate (CaNa$_2$ EDTA) after 2nd dose of BAL.
- Asymptomatic patients with lead levels >70 mcg/dL should be chelated in a fashion similar to symptomatic patients.
- Asymptomatic patients with levels <70 mcg/dL may be treated with an oral chelating agent (dimercaptosuccinic acid [DMSA]).

- Some experts recommend using CaNa$_2$ EDTA for chelation if levels >50 mcg/dL.
- Some controversy as to when to begin chelation if levels <45 mcg/dL and asymptomatic

### Pediatric Considerations
- Currently, lead levels >10 mcg/dL are considered the action level:
  - Level at which investigation into the cause of the exposure and monitoring must occur
- Much controversy as to long-term cognitive effects of lead and at which level to chelate asymptomatic children with elevated lead levels

### Pregnancy Considerations
- Much controversy about fetal lead toxicity
- Consultation with maternal–fetal medicine and medical toxicology is recommended in pregnant patients with elevated lead levels.

## MEDICATION
- CaNa$_2$ EDTA:
  - Multiple regimens; for acute encephalopathy, 50 mg/kg/d as continuous IV infusion (adults and peds) or 1 g/m$^2$ q12h
  - Treat for 5 days.
- Dextrose 50%: 25 g (50 mL; peds: 0.5 g/kg D25W) IV for hypoglycemia
- Diazepam: 5–10 mg (peds: 0.1 mg/kg) IV for seizure control
- Dimercaprol (BAL):
  - 3 mg/kg IM q4h for 3–5 days if mild to moderate symptoms; 4 mg/kg IM q4h for 5 days for severe symptoms (seizure, encephalopathy)
  - Caution: Cannot use if patient has peanut allergy
- DMSA (succimer): 10 mg/kg PO q8h for 5 days, then q12h for 14 days (adults and peds)
- Lorazepam: 2–4 mg IV or IM
- Naloxone: 0.4–2.0 mg (peds: 0.1 mg/kg) IV
- Thiamine: 100 mg (peds: 1 mg/kg) IM or IV

 FOLLOW-UP

## DISPOSITION

### Admission Criteria
- Symptomatic lead intoxications
- Children at high risk for re-exposure in their current environment
- Pregnant patients with elevated lead levels—consult obstetrics and toxicology.

### Discharge Criteria
- Asymptomatic patients not requiring IV chelation therapy (generally <50 mcg/dL)
- Patients with suspected chronic intoxications who do not require admission should be referred for outpatient evaluation.
- Ensure that home environment is safe for patient prior to discharge.

## FOLLOW-UP RECOMMENDATIONS
Follow up with medical toxicologist or primary care physician.

## PEARLS AND PITFALLS
- Must ensure safe living environment prior to discharge.
- Inquire and test siblings or family members in a patient with lead toxicity.
- Do not give BAL if patient has peanut allergy.

## ADDITIONAL READING
- Henretig F. Lead. In: Flomenbaum NE, Goldfrank LR, Hoffman RS, et al., eds. *Goldfrank's Toxicologic Emergencies*, 8th ed. New York: McGraw-Hill; 2006:1308–1322.
- Morgan BW, Todd K. Elevated lead levels in urban moonshine drinkers. *Ann Emerg Med.* 2001; 37(1):51–54.
- Needleman H. Lead poisoning. *Annu Rev Med.* 2004;55:209–222.
- Shannon M. Severe lead poisoning in pregnancy. *Ambul Pediatr.* 2003;3(1):37–39.

*A special thanks to Dr. Gerald Maloney, who contributed to the previous edition.*

## CODES

### ICD9
- 984.0 Toxic effect of inorganic lead compounds
- 984.1 Toxic effect of organic lead compounds
- 984.8 Toxic effect of other lead compounds

L

# LEGG-CALVÉ-PERTHES DISEASE

*Brandon H. Backlund*

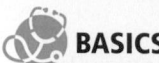 **BASICS**

## DESCRIPTION
- Avascular necrosis of all or part of femoral head in children
- Genetics:
  - Association with factor V Leiden mutation and anticardiolipin antibodies

### Pediatric Considerations
Exclusively a pediatric disease

## ETIOLOGY
- Multiple episodes of infarction causing characteristic findings
- Disruption of vascular supply to femoral head with exact underlying cause unknown
- Growing evidence implicating hypercoagulable states
- May be multifactorial
- Risk factors include growth hormone therapy, exposure to 2nd hand smoke, and low birth weight.
- Progression through 4 stages of disease:
  - Synovitis: Brief duration (weeks), reaction to ischemia
  - Necrosis and collapse of femoral head
  - Fragmentation: Resorption of avascular bone; deformation of femoral head often occurs at this stage.
  - Reconstitution: Formation of new bone
- More common in boys: Male > Female, 4:1
- More common among Caucasians
- Most commonly occurs between ages of 3–9 yr:
  - Range, 2–18 yr
- Bilateral in 10–15% of cases.
- Associated with short stature and delayed skeletal maturation

 **DIAGNOSIS**

## SIGNS AND SYMPTOMS
### History
- Frequently insidious onset
- Limp often presenting complaint
- Pain:
  - Aching in hip, groin, anteromedial thigh, or anteromedial knee
  - May be mild
  - Aggravated by activity, relieved by rest
  - Muscle spasm common complaint early in course of disease

### Physical Exam
- Tenderness over anterior aspect of hip joint
- Joint stiffness:
  - Limitation of internal rotation seen earliest
  - Limited abduction
  - Contractures of adductors
- Muscle atrophy and shortening of leg on affected side are late findings.
- Otherwise well-appearing and afebrile
- May be asymptomatic

## ESSENTIAL WORKUP
- Radiographs of hip most important study for diagnosis in ED
- Consider and exclude septic arthritis (usually an acute febrile illness).

## DIAGNOSTIC TESTS & INTERPRETATION
### Lab
- No specific laboratory studies diagnostic of Legg-Calve-Perthes (LCP)
- CBC, C-reactive protein (CRP), or ESR, if septic arthritis a concern

### Imaging
- Characteristic imaging findings combined with consistent history and physical establish diagnosis.
- Plain radiographs, MRI, and nuclear scintigraphy (bone scan) are the main diagnostic modalities used.
- Hip radiographs:
  - Anteroposterior and frog-leg views of hip
  - Usually abnormal at time of presentation
  - Staging is based on plain radiographs.
  - Early findings:
    - Minimal joint effusion, prominence of soft tissues over capsule
    - Subchondral fracture (Caffey sign): Crescentic subchondral radiolucency
    - Coxa magna: Cartilaginous overgrowth of femoral head; may see joint space widening or lateral shift of femoral head in acetabulum
  - Over subsequent weeks:
    - Sclerosis of affected bone
    - Increased opacity, fragmentation of femoral head
    - May see metaphyseal "cysts" (also known as physeal bridge): Radiolucent areas in metaphysis representing ingrowth of cartilage from growth plate
    - Flattening of femoral head (coxa plana)
- CT:
  - No clear advantage over plain radiographs for establishing diagnosis
  - May have role in operative planning, staging
- MRI:
  - Detects abnormalities earlier than plain radiographs
  - Demonstrates cartilaginous and soft tissue changes
  - Variety of findings depending on imaging protocol used

- Bone scan:
  - As with MRI, abnormal earlier in disease than plain films
  - Initially shows decreased uptake in femoral head on affected side
  - Later increased uptake on affected side due to revascularization
- US:
  - Can identify joint effusion
  - Evaluate articular cartilage for thickening and enlargement.
  - Evaluate deformity and containment of femoral head.

### Diagnostic Procedures/Surgery
Arthrocentesis of hip definitive test to exclude septic arthritis if significant concern for this; may need orthopedic consultation.

### DIFFERENTIAL DIAGNOSIS
- Unilateral involvement:
  - Transient (a.k.a. toxic) synovitis
  - Septic arthritis
  - Osteomyelitis
  - Juvenile rheumatoid arthritis
  - Rheumatic fever
  - Trauma:
    ○ Femoral neck fracture
    ○ Hip dislocation
    ○ Slipped capital femoral epiphysis
  - Tuberculosis
  - Tumor
- Bilateral involvement:
  - Hypothyroidism
  - Epiphyseal dysplasia
  - Gaucher disease

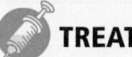 TREATMENT

### PRE-HOSPITAL
Clinical course is subacute; less likely to present via ambulance.

### INITIAL STABILIZATION/THERAPY
Not a life-threatening condition; clinical instability mandates identification of alternative diagnosis

### ED TREATMENT/PROCEDURES
- Main ED intervention is pain control.
- May need crutches if weight-bearing painful

### MEDICATION
#### First Line
Ibuprofen: 10 mg/kg per dose PO q6–8h PRN pain
#### Second Line
Diazepam: 0.1–0.2 mg/kg per dose (max. 5 mg) PO q6–8h PRN muscle spasm

 FOLLOW-UP

### DISPOSITION
#### Admission Criteria
Need for admission rare, indicated for:
- Severe pain or muscle spasm not controlled by PO medications
- Social considerations; bedrest/care at home not possible

#### Discharge Criteria
- Adequate pain control with PO medications
- Orthopedic follow-up arranged

### Issues for Referral
- Very young patients or those with minimal involvement often have good outcome with minimal intervention.
- For more severe disease, a range of treatment options exists, including conservative treatment, orthotics, traction, and surgical osteotomy, determined by consulting orthopedist.
- Osteoarthritis of hip with chronic pain or disability is the main long-term complication.

### FOLLOW-UP RECOMMENDATIONS
Orthopedic consultation to determine further management; may be outpatient

## PEARLS AND PITFALLS

Abrupt onset, presence of fever, unstable patient, or toxic appearance suggest diagnosis other than LCP.

## ADDITIONAL READING

- Balasa V, et al. Legg-Calve-Perthes disease and thrombophilia. *Am J Bone Joint Surg.* 2004;86-A(12):2642–2647.
- Jaramillo D. What is the optimal imaging of osteonecrosis, Perthes, and bone infarcts?. *Pedatr Radiol.* 2009;39(Suppl 2):S216–S219.
- Nelitz M, Lippacher S, Krauspe R, et al. Perthes disease: Current principles of diagnosis and treatment. *Deutsches Arzteblatt International.* 2009;106(31–32):517–523.
- Staheli L. *Practice of Pediatric Orthopedics.* Philadelphia: Lippincott Williams & Wilkins, 2001;146–151.
- Wall E. Legg-Calve-Perthes disease. *Curr Opin Pediatr.* 1999;11(1):76–79.

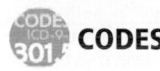 CODES

### ICD9
732.1 Juvenile osteochondrosis of hip and pelvis

L

# LEUKEMIA
*Linda Mueller*

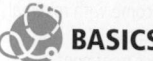 **BASICS**

## DESCRIPTION
- Neoplasms of WBCs that have undergone a malignant transformation
- Hyperleukocytosis:
  - Occurs with WBC >100,000/mm$^3$
  - Leads to occlusions of small vessels primarily in brain or lungs
  - Present with confusion, stupor, or shortness of breath

### Chronic Myelogenous Leukemia (CML)
- Overproduction of granulocytic WBCs (neutrophils)
- Neutrophil function preserved
- Thrombocytosis
- Basophilia
- Philadelphia chromosome present in bone marrow of >95%

### Chronic Lymphocytic Leukemia (CLL)
- Most common leukemia in adults
- Overproduction of monoclonal lymphocytes
- Cells accumulate in lymph nodes, bone marrow, liver, spleen
- Particularly prone to herpes virus infections

### Acute Leukemias
- Proliferation of undifferentiated immature cells:
  - Acute myelogenous leukemia (AML)—immature myeloid cells
  - Acute lymphocytic leukemia (ALL)—immature lymphoid cells (blasts)
- Rapidly fatal

## ETIOLOGY
- Cause unknown
- Familial clustering in CLL
- Increased incidence of AML, ALL, and CML with ionizing radiation

### Pediatric Considerations
- Usually have ALL:
  - Most common pediatric cancer
- 60–80% remission in those who are standard risk
- Better overall prognosis, except if <1 yr of age
- May develop leukostasis at lower levels
- Allopurinol dose is 3 mg/kg.
- Ceftazidime dose is 50 mg/kg.

### Pregnancy Considerations
- 90% of leukemias are AML or ALL.
- Myeloid leukemias are more common.
- CLL is very rare in pregnancy.
- Chemotherapeutics may cause birth defects and/or preterm labor.
- Same prognosis as nonpregnant; do not delay therapy.
- Transfuse earlier than nonpregnant; keep hemoglobin >9.8 mg/dL.

### Geriatric Considerations
More likely to present with CLL and CML

## DIAGNOSIS

### SIGNS AND SYMPTOMS
#### Chronic Myelogenous Leukemia
- Asymptomatic
- Fatigue
- Weight loss
- Left upper quadrant pain, tenderness
- Abdominal fullness
- Splenomegaly (most common)
- Later stage:
  - Headaches
  - Bone pain
  - Arthralgias
  - Fever
  - Leukotactic symptoms:
    ○ Dyspnea
    ○ Drowsiness
    ○ Confusion

#### Chronic Lymphocytic Leukemia
- Asymptomatic
- Fatigue
- Lethargy
- Weight loss
- Lymphadenopathy
- Splenomegaly
- Hepatomegaly

#### Acute Myelogenous Leukemia
- Fever
- Fatigue
- Pallor
- Headache
- Angina
- Congestive heart failure, dyspnea on exertion
- Bone pain
- Granulocytic sarcoma (isolated mass of leukemic blasts)
- Easy bleeding (thrombocytopenia):
  - Petechiae
  - Ecchymosis
  - Epistaxis
  - Hemorrhage
- Infections (granulocytopenic)
- Organ involvement with advanced ALL:
  - Lymphadenopathy
  - Hepatomegaly
  - Splenomegaly
  - Leukemic meningitis:
    ○ Headache
    ○ Nausea
    ○ Seizures

### History
- Radiation exposure
- Exposure to alkylating agents
- Recent viral infection, particularly Epstein-Barr

### Physical Exam
- Signs of bleeding (petechiae, purpura)
- Hepatomegaly and splenomegaly
- Presence of chloromas (AML blast tumors)
- Sausage-like hemorrhagic retinal veins are pathognomic for hyperviscosity.

### ESSENTIAL WORKUP
CBC/platelets:
- CML:
  - WBC range, 10,000–1 million/mm$^3$
  - Neutrophils predominate.
  - Thrombocytosis in 50%
- CLL:
  - Absolute lymphocytosis >5,000
  - WBC range, 40,000–150,000/mm$^3$
- Acute leukemia (AML/ALL):
  - Anemia
  - Thrombocytopenia
  - Elevation/depression of WBCs

### DIAGNOSTIC TESTS & INTERPRETATION
#### Lab
- Electrolytes, BUN, creatinine, glucose, calcium
- Uric acid level:
  - Frequently elevated, especially in ALL
- Lactate dehydrogenase:
  - Increased in acute leukemias
- Coagulation profile:
  - Prothrombin time, partial thromboplastin time, fibrinogen, fibrin-split products
  - If disseminated, suspect intravascular coagulation.
- Blood/urine cultures if fever
- Arterial blood gases/pulse oximetry for shortness of breath

#### Imaging
CXR for infectious workup

#### Diagnostic Procedures/Surgery
- Bone marrow biopsy:
  - Required to make diagnosis
  - CML—hypercellular with myeloid hyperplasia
  - CLL—lymphocytosis (30–100%)
  - Acute leukemia—hypercellular with blast cells, which replace normal marrow
- Leukocyte alkaline phosphatase test:
  - Decreased in neutrophils in CML
- Ph1 chromosome present in CML

## DIFFERENTIAL DIAGNOSIS

- CML:
  - Lymphoma
  - Myeloproliferative syndromes
  - Systemic lupus erythematosus
  - Infection—bacterial, fungal, mycobacterial
- CLL:
  - Pertussis
  - Infectious lymphocytosis
  - Cytomegalovirus
  - Epstein-Barr virus/mononucleosis
  - Hepatitis
  - Rubella
- Acute leukemia:
  - Aplastic anemia
  - Leukemoid reactions to infections

 **TREATMENT**

### INITIAL STABILIZATION/THERAPY

- 100% oxygen for hypoxia/shortness of breath
- IV access with 0.9% NS
- Initiate platelet transfusion for severe bleeding from thrombocytopenia.
- Begin broad-spectrum antibiotics for fever and granulocytopenia.
- Treat disseminated intravascular coagulation (see "Disseminated Intravascular Coagulation").

### ED TREATMENT/PROCEDURES

- Treat leukostasis:
  - Rehydrate with 500-mL bolus (20 mL/kg) IV 0.9% NS
  - Administer acetazolamide to alkalinize urine.
  - Initiate allopurinol.
  - Arrange for leukapheresis.
  - Whole-brain radiation for CNS effects
  - Administer hydroxyurea for CML: 20–30 mg/kg single dose daily
- Transfuse packed RBCs for symptomatic anemia:
  - May require irradiated, filtered, and HLA-type-specific blood

- Post-ED treatment:
  - CLL:
    - Chemotherapy
    - Prednisone for immune-mediated thrombocytopenia
    - Radiation to localized nodular masses/enlarged spleen
  - CML:
    - Interferon therapy
    - Chemotherapy
    - Bone marrow transplantation
  - ALL:
    - Chemotherapy
    - CNS prophylaxis with intrathecal–methotrexate/cranial radiation
    - Bone marrow transplantation
  - AML:
    - Chemotherapy
    - Bone marrow transplantation

### MEDICATION

#### First Line

- IVF, start with normal saline, then alkalinize
- Packed RBC and platelets as needed

#### Second Line

- Ceftazidime if febrile
- Allopurinol if at risk for tumor lysis

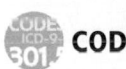 **FOLLOW-UP**

### DISPOSITION

#### Admission Criteria

- Newly diagnosed leukemia with:
  - Symptomatic anemia
  - WBC >30,000
  - Thrombocytopenia
- ICU admission for unstable patients with disseminated intravascular coagulation, blast crisis, or bleeding

#### Discharge Criteria

Asymptomatic patients without significant laboratory abnormalities

### Issues for Referral

Hematology for any patient presenting with new leukemia

## PEARLS AND PITFALLS

- Monitor for tumor lysis and secondary hyperkalemia.
- Hyperleukocytosis may present as respiratory failure or hemorrhage.

## ADDITIONAL READING

- Abramson N. Leukocytosis: Basics of clinical assessment. *Am Fam Physician.* 2000;62: 2053–2060.
- Higdon ML, Higdon JA. Treatment of oncologic emergencies. *Am Fam Physician.* 2006;74(11): 1873–1880.
- Hurley TJ, McKinnell JV, Irani MS. Hematologic malignancies in pregnancy. *Obstet Gynecol Clin North Am.* 2005;32(4):595–614.
- Lowenberg B. Acute myeloid leukemia. *N Engl J Med.* 1999;341:1051–1062.
- Naemi KJ, Malempati S. Emergency department presentation of childhood cancer. *Emerg Med Clin North Am.* 2009;27(3):477–495.
- Pui C. Acute lymphoblastic leukemia. *N Engl J Med.* 1998;339:605–614.
- Sawyers C. Chronic myeloid leukemia. *N Engl J Med.* 1999;340:1330–1340.
- Tsiodras S. Infection and immunity in chronic lymphocytic leukemia. *Mayo Clin Proc.* 2000;75: 1039–1054.

### See Also (Topic, Algorithm, Electronic Media Element)

Hyperviscosity Syndrome

 **CODES**

### ICD9

- 205.00 Myeloid leukemia, acute, without mention of having achieved remission
- 205.10 Myeloid leukemia, chronic, without mention of having achieved remission
- 208.90 Unspecified leukemia, without mention of having achieved remission

L

# LIGHTNING INJURIES

*Tarlan Hedayati*

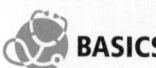

##  BASICS

### DESCRIPTION
- Lightning is a stream of negative energy that occurs cloud to cloud (90%) or cloud to ground (10%).
- Exposure to lightning:
  - Brief duration (1–100 msec)
  - Typically occurs during outdoor activity
  - Highest incidence in summer months, between 3 and 6 PM
  - Fatality rate of 8–10%

### ETIOLOGY
- Mechanism of injury—electrical:
  - Direct strike (3–5%)
  - Contact potential (15–25%):
    - Current passes through an object the victim is touching.
  - Side splash (20–30%):
    - Current jumps from nearby object to the victim.
  - Earth potential rise/ground current (40–50%):
    - Current moves through the ground surface and may injure multiple victims.
    - Current moves through hard-wired telephone lines, metallic pipes, or a structure's electrical equipment, causing lightning injury to victims indoors.
  - Upward streamer (10–15%):
    - Negatively charged lightning strikes from a cloud and induces positive current from the ground to rise and meet it to complete the lightning channel.
- Mechanism of injury—trauma:
  - Barotraumas
  - Blunt trauma:
    - Muscle contractions can throw the victim and/or cause a fall.
  - Thermal burn

## DIAGNOSIS

### SIGNS AND SYMPTOMS
#### History
- Consider lightning strike in unwitnessed falls, cardiac arrests, or unexplained coma in an outdoor setting.
- Conscious patients may report:
  - Muscle aches and pains
  - Chest pain
  - Shortness of breath
  - Extremity pain or discoloration
  - Burns
  - Neurologic deficits including:
    - Parasthesias
    - Dysesthesias
    - Weakness or paralysis
    - Visual disturbance or blindness
    - Headache
    - Confusion or amnesia
    - Hearing loss or deafness
    - Dizziness

#### Physical Exam
- HEENT:
  - Blunt head trauma
  - Ruptured tympanic membrane with ossicular disruption (up to 50%)
  - Ophthalmic injuries:
    - Cataracts
    - Corneal lesions
    - Intraocular hemorrhages
    - Retinal detachment
- Neck:
  - Cervical spine injury
- Cardiopulmonary injuries:
  - Primary cardiac arrest:
    - Cardiac asystole
    - Due to direct current injury
    - May resolve spontaneously as the heart's intrinsic automaticity resumes.
  - Hypertension: Transient
  - Pulmonary contusion or hemorrhage
  - Respiratory arrest:
    - Caused by paralysis of medullary respiratory center
    - May persist longer than primary cardiac arrest and lead to hypoxia-induced secondary cardiac arrest and/or brain injury
- Extremities:
  - Fractures/dislocations
  - Muscle tears, contusions
  - Compartment syndromes
  - Mottled or cold:
    - Caused by autonomic vasomotor instability
    - Usually resolves spontaneously in a few hours
- Skin:
  - Burns:
    - May evolve over several hours after injury
    - Discrete entrance and exit wounds are uncommon.
    - Superficial in nature; deep burns uncommon
    - Direct thermal injury is uncommon due to the brevity of electrical currents.
    - Thermal burns can arise from evaporation of water on skin, ignited clothing, and heated metal objects (buckles, jewelry).
    - Feathering pattern of fernlike "burns" are pathognomonic of lightning injuries and resolve within 24 hrs.
- Neurologic injuries:
  - Confusion, cognitive or memory defects
  - Altered level of consciousness (>70% of cases)
  - Flaccid motor paralysis
  - Seizures
  - Fixed dilated pupils due to either serious head injury or autonomic dysfunction
- Shock:
  - Neurogenic (spinal injury)
  - Hypovolemic (trauma)

### ESSENTIAL WORKUP
Confirmatory history from bystanders or rescuers of the circumstances of the injury

### DIAGNOSTIC TESTS & INTERPRETATION
#### Lab
- CBC
- Urinalysis for myoglobin (rare)
- Electrolytes for acidosis
- BUN, creatinine for renal function
- Troponin, creatine kinase, and cardiac enzymes for muscle/cardiac damage

#### Imaging
- CXR:
  - Pulmonary edema
  - Pulmonary contusion/hemorrhage
  - Rib fractures
- Cervical spine radiograph
- Head CT for altered mental status or significant head trauma
- Relevant imaging for specific injuries

#### Diagnostic Procedures/Surgery
EKG:
- Prolonged QT (most common)
- Nonspecific ST changes
- Premature ventricular contractions
- Atrial fibrillation
- Ventricular tachycardia
- Acute MI (rare)

### DIFFERENTIAL DIAGNOSIS
Other causes of coma, cardiac dysrhythmias, or trauma:
- Hypoglycemia
- Intoxication
- Drug overdose
- Cardiovascular disease
- Cerebrovascular accident
- Seizure
- Syncope

644

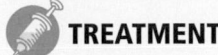 **TREATMENT**

### PRE-HOSPITAL
- Field triage should rapidly focus on providing ventilatory support to unconscious victims or those in cardiopulmonary arrest:
  - Prevents primary cardiac arrest from degenerating into hypoxia-induced secondary cardiac arrest
  - Conscious victims are at lower risk for imminent demise.
- Spine immobilization for:
  - Cardiopulmonary arrest (suspected trauma)
  - Significant mechanical trauma
  - Suspected loss of consciousness at any time
- Cover superficial burns with sterile saline dressings.
- Immobilize injured extremities.
- Rapid extrication to decrease risk for repeat lightning strikes

### INITIAL STABILIZATION/THERAPY
- ABCs
- Standard advanced cardiac life support measures for cardiac arrest
- Diligent primary and secondary survey for traumatic injuries and other causes of collapse/injury:
  - Maintain cervical spine precautions until cleared.
- Treat altered mental status with glucose, naloxone, or thiamine as indicated.
- Hypotension requires volume expansion, blood products, and/or pressor agents.

### ED TREATMENT/PROCEDURES
- IV access
- Cardiac monitor and pulse oximetry
- Clean and dress burns.
- Tetanus prophylaxis
- Treat myoglobinuria if present:
  - Diuretics, such as furosemide or mannitol
  - Alkalinize urine to a pH of 7.45 with intravenous sodium bicarbonate
- Volume expansion:
  - Do not follow burn treatment formulas because lightning burns are rarely the cause of fluid loss.
  - Occult deep burn injury is rare when compared with other types of electrical current injury.
  - Titrate volume administration to urine output.
  - Fluid loading may be dangerous if patient has concomitant head injury.

- Compartment syndrome:
  - Must be distinguished from vasospasm, autonomic dysfunction, and paralysis, which are usually self-limited phenomena.
  - Fasciotomy will rarely be necessary.
- NSAIDs and high-dose steroids have been proposed to reduce long-term neurologic and corneal damage.

### MEDICATION
- Furosemide: 1 mg/kg IV slow bolus q6h
- Mannitol: 0.5 mg/kg IV, repeat PRN
- Sodium bicarbonate: 1 amp IV push (peds: 1 mEq/kg) followed by 2–3 amps/L D5W IV fluid

 **FOLLOW-UP**

### DISPOSITION
#### Admission Criteria
- Post–cardiac arrest patients
- History of change in mental status/altered level of consciousness
- History of chest pain, dysrhythmias, or ECG changes:
  - May not resolve spontaneously
  - 24–48-hr observation period to identify potentially unstable cases
  - Myoglobinuria
  - Acidosis
  - Extremity injury with or at risk for compartment syndrome

#### Discharge Criteria
Asymptomatic patients with no injuries

### FOLLOW-UP RECOMMENDATIONS
- Close follow-up with subspecialists may be required due to the risk for delayed sequelae:
  - Neurology:
    - Memory deficit
    - Attention deficit
    - Aphasia
    - Sleep disturbance
    - Prolonged parasthesias and dysesthesias
  - Ophthalmology
  - ENT
- Psychology/psychiatry:
  - Anxiety
  - Depression
  - Personality changes
  - Posttraumatic stress disorder

## PEARLS AND PITFALLS
- Do not follow burn treatment formulas for lightning burns and injuries.
- Be diligent in the primary and secondary survey so as not to miss occult injuries.
- Have a low threshold to admit and monitor patients with cardiopulmonary complaints, as unstable dysrhythmias may occur 24–48 hr postinjury.

## ADDITIONAL READING
- Cooper MA. A fifth mechanism of lightning injury. *Acad Emerg Med.* 2002;9(2):172–174.
- Cooper MA, Andrews CJ, Holle RL. Lightning injuries. In: Auerbach PS, ed. *Wilderness Medicine*, 5th ed. St. Louis, MO: Mosby; 2007:67–108.
- Cooper MA, Holle RL, Andrews CJ. Distribution of lightning injury mechanisms. Presented at the 20th International Lightning Detection Conference, April, Tucson, AZ.
- O'Keefe Gatewood M, Zane RD. Lightning injuries. *Emerg Med Clin North Am.* 2004;22(2):369–403.
- Price T, Cooper MA. Electrical and lightning injuries. In: Marx JA, Hockenberger RS, Walls RM, et al., eds. *Rosen's Emergency Medicine*, 6th ed. Philadelphia: Mosby, 2006.

### See Also (Topic, Algorithm, Electronic Media Element)
Electrical Injury

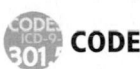 **CODES**

**ICD9**
994.0 Effects of lightning

# LITHIUM POISONING
*Sean M. Bryant*

## 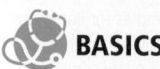 BASICS

### DESCRIPTION
- GI absorption is rapid:
  - Regular release: Peak serum levels 2–4 hr
  - Sustained release: Peak serum levels 4–12 hr
- Half-life 24 hr
- Slow distribution (at least 6 hr)
- Volume of distribution 0.6–0.9 L/kg
- Elimination:
  - *Not* metabolized
  - Renal excretion (unchanged)
  - Reabsorbed in the *proximal* tubules by sodium transport mechanism
  - Elimination half-life (therapeutic) is 20–24 hr and prolonged in chronic users.
- Therapeutic and toxic indices:
  - Therapeutic and toxic effects occur *only* when lithium is intracellular.
  - Narrow toxic-to-therapeutic ratio
  - Therapeutic level 0.6–1.2 mEq/L (after intracellular/extracellular equilibration)
  - Because of its size, renal handling is similar to sodium, potassium, and magnesium.
- Risk factors:
  - Acute conditions increasing risk of toxicity:
    - Dehydration (larger percent reabsorbed)
    - Overdose
  - Chronic conditions increasing risk of toxicity:
    - Hypertension
    - Diabetes mellitus
    - Renal failure
    - Congestive heart failure
    - Advanced age
    - Dose change
    - Drug interactions
    - Lithium therapy
    - Low-salt diet
  - The following may result in increased serum lithium levels due to decreased renal clearance or exacerbated effects:
    - NSAIDs
    - Thiazide diuretics
    - Angiotensin-converting-enzyme inhibitors
    - Phenytoin
    - Tricyclic antidepressants
    - Phenothiazines

### ETIOLOGY
- Acute or chronic conditions affecting lithium clearance
- Overdose

## DIAGNOSIS

### SIGNS AND SYMPTOMS
- Acute toxicity:
  - Less common and less serious than chronic toxicity
  - Neurologic (mild):
    - Weakness
    - Fine tremor
    - Light-headedness
  - Neurologic (moderate):
    - Ataxia
    - Slurred speech
    - Blurred vision
    - Tinnitus
    - Weakness
    - Coarse tremor
    - Fasciculations
    - Hyperreflexia
    - Apathy
  - Neurologic (severe):
    - Confusion
    - Coma
    - Seizure
    - Clonus
    - Extrapyramidal symptoms
  - GI:
    - Very common
    - Nausea/vomiting
    - Diarrhea
    - Abdominal pain
  - Cardiac:
    - Prolonged QT, ST depression
    - T-wave flattening *most common* ECG abnormality
    - U waves
    - Serious dysrhythmias (rare)
- Chronic toxicity:
  - Neurologic:
    - Most common
    - Same symptoms as acute
    - Severe toxicity includes parkinsonian symptoms, psychosis, and memory deficits.
  - Renal:
    - Nephrogenic diabetes insipidus
    - Interstitial nephritis
    - Distal tubular acidosis
    - Direct cellular damage
  - Dermatologic:
    - Dermatitis
    - Ulcers
    - Localized edema
  - Endocrine:
    - Hypothyroidism
  - Hematologic:
    - Leukocytosis
    - Aplastic anemia

### History
- Time of last dose ingested
- Ingestion history:
  - Acute (1-time overdose)
  - Chronic (scheduled dosing)
  - Acute on chronic (overdose in patients who regularly take lithium)

### Physical Exam
Perform complete neurologic exam.

### ESSENTIAL WORKUP
- Lithium level: Goal = postdistribution:
  - Because of prolonged distribution, repeat every 2 hr to detect trend.
- Stratify patient into one of three categories of toxicity to interpret level and predict toxicity: Acute, acute on chronic, chronic:
  - Acute toxicity:
    - Intentional overdose in patient not previously taking lithium
    - Poor correlation between lithium level and symptoms because intracellular distribution has not yet occurred
    - Toxic levels may appear in asymptomatic patients.
    - Lithium level >4 mEq/L is toxic because clearance is slow and complications are possible.
  - Acute on chronic toxicity:
    - Intentional or accidental overdose in patient on lithium therapy
    - Lithium level >3 mEq/L usually associated with symptoms.
  - Chronic toxicity:
    - Patients on lithium therapy who progressively develop toxicity secondary to factors other than acute ingestion
    - Stronger correlation between lithium level and symptoms
    - Lithium level >1.5 mEq/L may be toxic.

### DIAGNOSTIC TESTS & INTERPRETATION
#### Lab
- Electrolytes, BUN, creatinine, and glucose levels to determine electrolyte disturbances/renal function
- Aspirin and/or acetaminophen levels as indicated by history
- Urinalysis:
  - Specific gravity

## DIFFERENTIAL DIAGNOSIS
- Consider lithium toxicity with altered mental status and fasciculations.
- Endocrine:
  - Hypoglycemia
- Toxicologic:
  - Cholinergic substances
  - Heavy-metal poisoning
  - Neuroleptic overdose
  - Black widow/scorpion envenomation
  - Strychnine poisoning

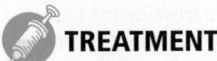 **TREATMENT**

### PRE-HOSPITAL
- Transport all appropriate pill bottles to the hospital.
- IV access, oxygen, and cardiac monitoring

### INITIAL STABILIZATION/THERAPY
- ABCs
- Secure IV access with 0.9% NS.
- Cardiac monitor
- Naloxone, thiamine, dextrose (or Accu-Chek) if altered mental status
- Benzodiazepines for seizures

### ADDITIONAL TREATMENT
#### General Measures
- Correct electrolyte abnormalities.
- Maintain well-hydrated state.
- Continuous cardiac monitoring
- Observe for neurologic changes.
- Prevent absorption:
  - Consider gastric lavage only if patient presents within 1 hr of acute life-threatening ingestion and has protected airway.
  - Activated charcoal:
    - Lithium is not absorbed by charcoal.
    - Administer one dose of activated charcoal if possible coingestants.
  - Whole-bowel irrigation:
    - Polyethylene glycol (PEG) solution (GoLytely)
    - Indicated with sustained-release products
    - Flushes lithium through gut
    - Administer (2 L/hr per nasogastric tube) until rectal effluent is clear.
    - Contraindications include bowel obstruction or perforation, ileus or hypotension, and unprotected airway in obtunded or seizing patient.

- Enhance elimination:
  - IV fluids:
    - Rapidly correct any preexisting fluid deficit with 0.9% NS at 150–300 mL/h (or 2× maintenance).
    - Saline hydration improves glomerular filtration and decreases proximal tubule reabsorption of lithium.
    - Maintain urine output between 1 and 2 mL/kg/hr.
    - Limited value once glomerular filtration rate maximized
    - Sodium bicarbonate offers no additional advantage.
  - Loop, thiazide, and osmotic diuretics not recommended:
    - Dehydration may result in worsening toxicity.
    - No direct effect on renal reabsorption because lithium is reabsorbed in proximal tubules.
  - Kayexalate (sodium polystyrene sulfonate):
    - Animal studies indicate efficacy.
    - Only very large doses have been studied.
    - Complications may include hypokalemia, hyperkalemia, fluid overload, and dysrhythmias.
  - Dialysis:
    - Peritoneal dialysis is not recommended.
    - Hemodialysis may be recommended for augmenting elimination (see below).
- Hemodialysis is recommended for severe cases or acute ingestions with high levels indicating imminent toxicity:
  - Controversial indications (valid criteria not established):
    - Severe and progressive neurologic abnormalities
    - Renal insufficiency
    - Altered mental status
    - Ventricular dysrhythmia/cardiogenic shock
    - History of congestive heart failure or pulmonary edema
    - Acute ingestions with levels >4 mEq/L
    - Chronic ingestions with levels >2.5 mEq/L
  - Standard endpoint is lithium level <1 mEq/L.
  - Repeat lithium level 6 hr after dialysis checking for evidence of redistribution.
  - May need to repeat dialysis due to rebound effect (redistribution of intracellular lithium)
  - May reduce the potential for developing permanent neurologic sequelae with chronic toxicity

### MEDICATION
- Dextrose: D50 1 amp: 25 g (peds: D25W 4 mL/kg) IV
- Diazepam: 5 mg (peds: 0.2–0.4 mg/kg) IV q5min until seizures controlled
- Naloxone: 2 mg (peds: 0.1 mg/kg) IV or via endotracheal tube
- PEG: 2 L/hR (peds: 2 mL/kg/hr) via nasogastric tube
- Thiamine: 100 mg IV

 **FOLLOW-UP**

### DISPOSITION
#### Admission Criteria
- Symptomatic
- Requiring hemodialysis
- Lithium level unchanged, increased, or >2 mEq/L despite ED intervention
- Moderate to severe symptoms with chronic levels >4 mEq/L warrant admission to ICU.
- Intentional ingestion

#### Discharge Criteria
Decreasing lithium levels every 2–4 hr in *asymptomatic* patient *and* serum lithium level <2 mEq/L (nonsuicidal patients)

#### Issues for Referral
Intentional overdose:
- Psychiatry consultation

### FOLLOW-UP RECOMMENDATIONS
Psychiatry follow-up to ensure correct dosing regimen in those with chronic poisoning

## PEARLS AND PITFALLS
- Erroneously interpreting a predistribution lithium concentration as "toxic" in patients without symptoms or history of overdose
- Aggressive hydration in patients with pulmonary edema, renal insufficiency, or mental status changes

## ADDITIONAL READING
- Bailey B, McGuigan M. Comparisons of patients hemodialyzed for lithium poisoning and those for whom dialysis was recommended by PCC but not done: What lesson can we learn? *Clin Neurol.* 2000;54:388–392.
- Belanger DR, Tierney MG, Dickinson G. Effect of sodium polystyrene sulfonate on lithium bioavailability. *Ann Emerg Med.* 1992;21:1312–1315.
- Bosse GM, Arnold TC. Overdose with sustained release lithium preparation. *J Emerg Med.* 1992;10:719–721.
- Leikin J, Paloucek F. *Lithium: Poisoning and Toxicology Handbook.* Hudson, OH: Lexi-Comp; 2002.
- Scharman EJ. Methods used to decrease lithium absorption or enhance elimination. *Clin Toxicol.* 1997;35:601–608.

 **CODES**

**ICD9**
985.8 Toxic effect of other specified metals

L

# LUDWIG ANGINA

*Paul Blackburn*

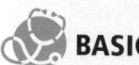 **BASICS**

## DESCRIPTION
- A life-threatening infection of submandibular, sublingual spaces
- Rapidly spreading gangrenous cellulitis, necrotizing fasciitis of the submaxillary, sublingual, submandibular spaces
- First described by von Ludwig in 1836
- Mortality exceeded 50% in pre antibiotic era.
- Most deaths due to airway, respiratory compromise
- Improved dental care, antibiotics reduce incidence
- Four cardinal aspects:
  – Bilateral involvement of >1 deep-tissue space
  – Gangrene with serosanguineous, putrid infiltration; little or no frank pus
  – Involvement of connective tissue, fascia, and muscles; not glandular structures
  – Spread by fascial space continuity, not lymphatics
- Brawny, painful induration of suprahyoid, submandibular areas creates tense edema of sublingual tissues forcing tongue, soft-tissues superiorly, posteriorly.
- Rapid respiratory obstruction (asphyxia) can occur.

## ETIOLOGY
- Odontogenic: 50–90% of reported cases:
  – Most common origin 2nd, 3rd mandibular molars
  – Children less likely to have an odontogenic source
- Less commonly:
  – Mandibular fractures
  – Oral lacerations
  – Peritonsillar abscess
  – IV drug injections into neck veins
  – Sialadenitis
  – Tongue piercing
- Invariably polymicrobial:
  – Most common pathogens:
    ○ *Streptococcus viridans*
    ○ *Staphylococcus aureus*
    ○ *Staphylococcus epidermidis*
    ○ *Gram-negative rods*
    ○ Anaerobes: Most commonly *Bacteroides* species

### Pediatric Considerations
- 27–30% of cases of Ludwig angina occur in children.
- Odontogenic source of infection in only 50%
- Frequently occurs in children without a predisposing cause
- 35% may have positive blood cultures.

 **DIAGNOSIS**

## SIGNS AND SYMPTOMS
### History
- Fever
- Malaise
- Poor oral intake
- Tongue or throat pain
- Jaw pain
- Dyspnea
- Neck stiffness
- Dysphonia; "hot potato" voice
- Dysphagia
- Protruding tongue
- Anxiety

### Physical Exam
- Toxic appearing:
  – Tachypnea
  – Tachycardia
  – Fever
- Cyanosis
- Stridor
- Salivary incontinence
- Patient prefers sitting or "sniffing" position
- HEENT exam:
  – Progressive bilateral submandibular and submental neck swelling
  – Firm induration of floor of mouth
  – Posterior and superior displacement of tongue
  – Examination of mouth, pharynx may be hindered by altered anatomy, trismus.

## ESSENTIAL WORKUP
- Diagnosis is often made clinically, and delay in treatment and/or airway control should not depend on imaging.
- Rapid administration of IV antibiotics is the most important treatment.
- Prepare immediately for airway management:
  – Consider calling for subspecialist backup and/or other arrangements for surgical airway

## DIAGNOSTIC TESTS & INTERPRETATION
### Lab
- Values consistent with systemic infection, but none is specific:
  – Elevated WBC
- Assess renal function and electrolytes for signs of dehydration.

### Imaging
- Soft tissue films of neck: Gas, altered submandibular, retropharyngeal anatomy
- CXR has low yield for intrathoracic extension.
- Panorex detects odontogenic abscesses, mandibular pathology.
- CT scan can help define extent of abscess, cellulitis and bony involvement:
  – Best for mediastinal area
- MRI may provide similar information to CT but requires more time for patient in a supine position.
- US can detect abscess, gas, altered anatomy.

### Diagnostic Procedures/Surgery
Fiberoptic evaluation:
- Inspection of upper airway architecture, compromise
- Low patient tolerance in the ill patient

## DIFFERENTIAL DIAGNOSIS
- Cellulitis
- Epiglottitis
- Bacterial tracheitis
- Peritonsillar abscess
- Salivary gland abscess
- Lymphadenitis
- Angioneurotic edema
- Lingual carcinoma
- Sublingual hematoma secondary to anticoagulation, mandibular fractures

**TREATMENT**

## PRE-HOSPITAL
- Transport in sitting position:
  – Supplemental oxygen, suction secretions as needed
- Early, appropriately aggressive, airway protection

### Pediatric Considerations
Avoid any agitation of patient, which may further compromise airway until patient is in a setting where airway can be expertly managed:
- IV access
- Physical exam

## INITIAL STABILIZATION/THERAPY

- Anticipate and prepare for difficulty maintaining a patent airway:
  - Monitored bed
  - Primary and rescue noninvasive intubation items
  - Surgical airway tools at the bedside
- Skillful airway management is critical, but a safe method of airway control is yet to be established.
- PO route for airway control is not reliable.
- LMA and Combitube will likely be unsuccessful due to lack of access.
- Keep patient sitting up, suctioning own secretions as desired.
- Expect difficulty:
  - Altered anatomy
  - Copious secretions
  - Trismus
  - Respiratory intolerance of positioning other than upright "sniff" posture
- Preoxygenate maximally prior to attempting this difficult airway.
- Rapid-sequence intubation (RSI) may result in loss of soft-tissue supporting structures; loss of visualization and expected anatomical landmarks.
- Preferred technique:
  - Awake, fiberoptic laryngoscopic intubation is recommended as a 1st-line approach:
    - Nasal route may provide more reliable access.
  - Sedation-assisted intubation:
    - Short-acting agents (etomidate, midazolam, ketamine, propofol)
- Other options:
  - Blind nasotracheal intubation
  - Retrograde wire intubation with Seldinger techniques
  - Cricothyrotomy
  - Tracheostomy is the "gold standard" for more definitive, longer-term airway management.

## ED TREATMENT/PROCEDURES

- IV fluids (salivary, insensible losses)
- Initiate broad spectrum antibiotics:
  - Aerobic/anaerobic/polymicrobial infection
- Steroids: Value is unclear.
- Hyperbaric oxygen if mediastinitis, necrotizing fasciitis of the chest wall

## MEDICATION

- Antibiotics:
  - Ampicillin/sulbactam: 1.5–3 g IM/IV q6h (peds: 300 mg/kg/day divided q6h if <1 yr, <40 kg; 1.5–3 g IV q6h if >1 yr, >40 kg); dose not to exceed 12 g/day
  - Cefoxitin: 1–2 g IV q6–8h (peds: 80–160 mg/kg/day divided q4–6h); max 12 g/d
  - Clindamycin: 600–900 mg IM/IV q8h (peds: 15–25 mg/kg/day divided q6–8h)

- Penicillin G: 4 million UIM/IV q4h (peds: 100,000–400,000 U/kg/day IM/IV divided q4–6h) *PLUS*
- Metronidazole: 500 mg IV q6–8h (peds: 30 mg/k/day IV divided q6h)
- Piperacillin/tazobactam: 3.375 g IV q6h (peds: If >9 mo and <40 kg; 300 mg/kg/day IV divided q8h)
- Ticarcillin/clavulanate: 3.1 g IV q4–6h (peds: If >3 mo and <60 kg; 200–300 mg/kg/day divided q4–6h); max 18–24 g/day
- Sedation for airway management:
  - Etomidate: 0.1–0.15 mg/kg IV
  - Ketamine: 1–4.5 mg/kg IV; 6.5–13 mg/kg IM (peds >3 mo: 1.5 mg/kg IV; 4.5 mg/kg IM; consider adding benzodiazepine and antisialagogue (atropine or glycopyrrolate))
  - Midazolam: 2–5 mg IV (peds: 0.05–0.1 mg/kg IV)
  - Propofol: 0.5–1 mg/kg IV
- Analgesia
- Antipyretics

### First Line
- Ampicillin/sulbactam
- Cefoxitin
- Clindamycin
- Penicillin G *PLUS* metronidazole

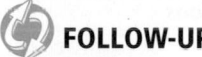 **FOLLOW-UP**

### DISPOSITION

#### Admission Criteria
- All are admitted.
- ICU or monitored setting; airway compromise can be precipitous.

#### Issues for Referral
Immediate communication with the specialist(s) most adept at treating this complex condition:

- Anesthesia
- General surgery
- Otolaryngology

#### Pregnancy Considerations
Primary concerns: Airway patency, oxygenation, constitutional effects of sepsis (hypotension) on mother and fetus. Otherwise, little deviation from approach to nongravid patients.

#### Geriatric Considerations
Therapeutic interventions are less predictable: Comorbid conditions, chronic medications, diminished physiologic reserve

## COMPLICATIONS

- Spread into the thoracic cavity:
  - Empyema
  - Mediastinitis
  - Thoracic abscess
- Pericarditis
- Aspiration
- Lung abscess
- Internal jugular vein thrombosis
- Carotid artery erosion and/or infection
- Sepsis/bacteremia
- Subphrenic abscess

## PEARLS AND PITFALLS

- Prepare to manage airway immediately upon presentation:
  - Arrange for backup airway techniques, including surgical airway.
  - Call consultants early.
  - Best chance for survival is managing the airway while patient is still well-oxygenated.
- Avoid agitation, especially in children, until airway is secure.
- Early broad-spectrum antibiotics are the mainstay of treatment, in addition to monitoring the airway.

## ADDITIONAL READING

- Abramowicz S, Abramowicz JS, Dolwick MF. Severe life-threatening maxillofacial infection in pregnancy presented as Ludwig's angina. *Infect Dis Obstet Gynecol*. 2006:519–531.
- Barton ED, Bair AE. Ludwig's angina. *J Emerg Med*. 2008;34:163–169.
- Lin HW, O'Neill A, Cunningham MJ. Ludwig's angina in the pediatric patient. *Clin Pediatr*. 2009;48:583–587.
- Marx JA, Hockberger RS, Walls RM, et al. *Rosen's Emergency Medicine: Concepts and Clinical Practice*, 7th ed. St. Louis, MO: Mosby; 2009.
- Ovassapian A, Tuncbilek M, Weitzel EK, et al. Airway management in adult patients with deep neck infections: A case series and review of the literature. *Anesth Analg*. 2005;100:585–589.
- Reynolds SC, Chow AW. Life-threatening infections of the peripharyngeal and deep fascial spaces of the head and neck. *Infect Dis Clin North Am*. 2007;21:557–576.
- Singhal P, Kejriwal N, Lin Z, et al. Optimal surgical management of descending necrotising mediastinitis: Our experience and review of literature. *Heart Lung Circ*. 2008;17:124–128.

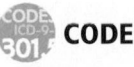 **CODES**

**ICD9**
528.3 Cellulitis and abscess of oral soft tissues

# LUNATE DISLOCATION
*Emi Latham*

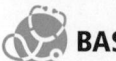

## BASICS

### DESCRIPTION
- Dislocation of the lunate relative to the radius and distal row of metacarpals, either dorsally or volarly
- Usually from high-energy hyperextension with ulnar deviation of the wrist

### ETIOLOGY
- Implies disruption of all four perilunate ligaments and radiocarpal ligament
- In volar dislocations, median nerve injury occurs in the carpal tunnel.
- Associated fractures of the radial styloid, scaphoid, capitate, and triquetrum are common and, if present, should raise suspicion of an occult perilunate ligamentous injury.

## DIAGNOSIS

### SIGNS AND SYMPTOMS
Frequently missed injury

#### History
- Often from fall or motor vehicle accident
- Pain and tenderness in the wrist

#### Physical Exam
- Mass or swelling in the wrist, either dorsally or volarly, depending on direction of dislocation
- Gross deformity can be masked by swelling.
- May display signs of median nerve injury.

### ESSENTIAL WORKUP
- Clinical exam is frequently not diagnostic.
- Assess skin integrity and neurovascular status, including two-point discrimination.
- Radiographs as outlined below

### DIAGNOSTIC TESTS & INTERPRETATION
#### Imaging
- Radiographic imaging to include 3 views of the wrist
- Lateral view most useful:
  - Disruption of the normal imaginary longitudinal line through the centers of the radius, lunate, and capitate indicates dislocation or subluxation.
  - In volar dislocations, the lunate is frequently tilted with the opening of the "cup" toward the palm (spilled-teacup sign)
- Posteroanterior (PA) view:
  - The dislocated lunate has a triangular (as opposed to the usual quadrangular) appearance.
  - Disruption of a smooth and continuous arc formed by the radiocarpal row suggests lunate dislocation.

#### Pediatric Considerations
Radiograph can be difficult to interpret unless full ossification is present.

#### Geriatric Considerations
Other fractures are common.

### DIFFERENTIAL DIAGNOSIS
- Lunate fracture
- Perilunate dislocation
- Scapholunate dissociation
- Scaphoid fracture

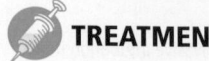

## TREATMENT

### PRE-HOSPITAL
- Dress open wounds.
- Immobilize in neutral position.

### INITIAL STABILIZATION/THERAPY
Immobilize in position of comfort with a volar or "sugar tongs" splint.

### ED TREATMENT/PROCEDURES
- Identify multiple trauma or other injuries.
- Contact a hand surgeon for immediate reduction and possible operative intervention.
- Closed reduction can be difficult or unstable.
- Open reduction and internal fixation are frequently required.

#### Pediatric Considerations
Although serious injury is unusual, children with wrist pain should be splinted and referred for ongoing evaluation of possible occult fractures.

## MEDICATION

### First Line

Analgesics:

- Morphine:
  - Pediatrics: 1 mg/kg IV
  - Adults: 4–8 mg IV
- Acetaminophen with codeine:
  - Pediatrics: 0.5–1 mg/kg/dose PO q4–6 hr
  - Adults: 30–60 mg/dose PO q4–6 hr
- Hydrocodone and acetaminophen:
  - Pediatrics <12 yr old: 10–15 mg/kg apap/dose PO q4–6 hr
  - Pediatrics >12 yr old: 750 mg apap PO q4h, not to exceed 10 mg hydrocodone per dose
  - Adults: 1–2 tabs PO q4–6 h

### Second Line

NSAIDs:

- Ibuprofen:
  - Pediatrics: 20–70 mg/kg/day PO div t.i.d./q.i.d.
  - Adults: 600 mg PO q6h
- Naproxen:
  - Pediatrics >2 yr old: 2.5 mg/kg/day PO b.i.d. (not to exceed 10 mg/kg/day)
  - Adults: 250–500 mg PO b.i.d.

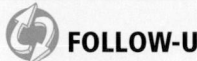 FOLLOW-UP

### DISPOSITION

#### Admission Criteria

- Admission is often necessary for definitive care.
- Open fracture, presence of multiple trauma, or other more serious injuries mandates admission.

#### Discharge Criteria

Patients with closed dislocations or fractures that have been adequately reduced and immobilized in the ED may be discharged with orthopedic follow-up.

### FOLLOW-UP RECOMMENDATIONS

- For those reduced and discharged with splint, follow-up with orthopedics.
- No return to play until fully healed

## PEARLS AND PITFALLS

- Failure to diagnose wrist dislocations
- Missed medial nerve injury
- Avascular necrosis of the lunate (Kienböck disease)
- Degenerative joint disease

## ADDITIONAL READING

- American Society for Surgery of the Hand. *The Hand: Primary Care of Common Problems,* 2nd ed. New York: Churchill Livingstone; 1990:637–649.
- Budoff JE. Treatment of acute lunate and perilunate dislocations. *J Hand Surg Am.* 2008t;33(8): 1424–1432.
- Eisenhauer MA. Forearm and wrist. In: Rosen P, et al., eds. *Emergency Medicine: Concepts and Clinical Practice,* 4th ed. St. Louis: Mosby–Year Book; 2002:535–542.
- Mital RC. The wrist and forearm. In: Schwartz D, et al. *Emergency Radiology.* New York: McGraw-Hill; 2000:48–63.
- Perron AD. Orthopedic pitfalls in the ED: Lunate and perilunate injuries. *Am J Emerg Med.* 2001;19(2): 157–162.
- Uehara DT. The hand in emergency medicine. *Emerg Clin North Am.* 1993;11(3):781–796.

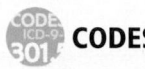 CODES

### ICD9

- 833.00 Closed dislocation of wrist, unspecified part
- 833.09 Closed dislocation of other part of wrist

L

# LYME DISEASE

*Moses S. Lee*

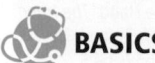 **BASICS**

## DESCRIPTION
- Most common tick-borne illness in North America
- Endemic in Northeast, Upper Midwest, and northwestern California

## ETIOLOGY
- Peak April–November; 80–90% in summer months
- Spirochete *Borrelia burgdorferi* introduced by *Ixodes* tick:
  - *Ixodes dammini* (deer tick) most common
- <50% of patients recall tick bite.
- Pathogenesis—combination of:
  - Organism-induced local inflammation
  - Cytokine release
  - Autoimmunity
- No person-to-person transmission

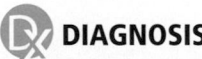 **DIAGNOSIS**

## SIGNS AND SYMPTOMS
Stage I (Early):
- Onset few days to month after tick bite (arthropod transmission)
- 30–50% of patients recall tick bite.
- Erythema chronicum migrans (ECM):
  - Pathognomonic finding:
    - Bull's-eye rash
  - Maculopapular, irregular expanding annular lesion:
    - Single or multiple
    - Central clearing with red outer border
    - Diameter >5 cm
- Regional adenopathy
- Low-grade, intermittent fever
- Headache
- Myalgia
- Arthralgias
- Fatigue
- Malaise

Stage II (Secondary, disseminated):
- Days to weeks after tick bite
- Intermittent and fluctuating symptoms with eventual disappearance
- Triad of aseptic meningitis, cranial neuritis, and radiculoneuritis:
  - Facial (Bell) palsy most common cranial neuritis
  - May present without rash
  - Prognosis generally good

- Cardiac:
  - Tachycardia
  - Bradycardia
  - Atrioventricular block
  - Myopericarditis

Stage III (Tertiary, late):
- Onset >1 yr after disease onset
- Acrodermatitis chronica atrophicans:
  - Extensor surfaces of extremities, especially lower leg
  - Initial edematous infiltration evolving to atrophic lesions
  - Resembles scleroderma
- Arthritis:
  - Brief arthritis attacks
  - Monoarthritis
  - Oligoarthritis
  - Occasionally migratory
  - Most common joints (descending order):
    - Knee
    - Shoulder
    - Elbow

Other:
- GI:
  - Hepatitis
  - Right upper quadrant pain
- Ocular:
  - Keratitis
  - Uveitis
  - Iritis
  - Optic neuritis
- Jarisch-Herxheimer reaction:
  - Worsening of symptoms a few hours after treatment initiated
  - More common in patients with multiple ECM lesions
- Babesiosis occurs simultaneously in endemic areas.

Persistent Lyme Disease:
- Articular and neurologic symptoms despite treatment:
  - Chronic axonal polyneuropathy or encephalopathy

Recurrent Lyme Disease:
- Relapse despite treatment
- Second episodes less severe

### Pediatric Considerations
- More likely than adults to be febrile
- Only 50% of children with arthralgias have history of ECM.
- Facial palsy is accompanied by aseptic meningitis in 1/3.
- Asymptomatic cardiac involvement with abnormal ECGs
- Appropriately treated children have excellent prognosis for unimpaired cognitive functioning.
- Untreated children may have keratitis, joint pain, or chronic encephalopathy.

### History
- History of tick bite in endemic areas
- Flu-like illness in the summer

### Physical Exam
- Rash
- Joint, cardiac, and neurologic findings in later organ involvement

## ESSENTIAL WORKUP
- Clinical diagnosis:
  - Presence of ECM obviates serologic tests.
- Careful search for tick
- Lumbar puncture when meningeal signs
- Arthrocentesis for acute arthritis
- ECG

## DIAGNOSTIC TESTS & INTERPRETATION
### Lab
- CBC:
  - Leukocytosis
  - Anemia
  - Thrombocytopenia
- Erythrocyte sedimentation rate:
  - >30 mm/hr
  - Most common laboratory abnormality
- Electrolytes, BUN, creatinine, glucose
- Liver function tests:
  - Elevated liver enzymes ($\gamma$-glutamyl transferase most common)
- Culture:
  - Low yield
  - Not indicated
- CSF:
  - Pleocytosis
  - Elevated protein
  - Obtain CSF spirochete antibodies.

- Special tests:
  - Serology:
    - Obtain enzyme-linked immunosorbent assay, immunofluorescence assay, and Western blot when disease is suggested without ECM lesion.
    - Antibodies may persist for months to years.
    - Positive serology or previous Lyme disease does not ensure protective immunity.
  - Polymerase chain reaction assay:
    - Highly specific and sensitive
    - Not available for routine use
  - Joint fluid:
    - Cryoglobulin increased fivefold compared with serum
  - Joint films may show soft tissue, cartilaginous, osseous changes.

## DIFFERENTIAL DIAGNOSIS

- Other tick-borne illnesses:
  - Deer tick usually larger (1 cm) than ixodid ticks (1–2 mm)
  - Rocky Mountain spotted fever
  - Tularemia
  - Relapsing fever
  - Colorado tick fever
  - Tick-bite paralysis
- Rheumatic fever:
  - Rash of erythema marginatum
  - Temporomandibular joint arthritis more common than in Lyme disease
  - Valvular involvement rather than heart block
  - Chorea may be isolated finding.
- Viral meningitis
- Syphilis
- Septic arthritis
- Parvovirus B19 infection—polyarticular arthritis
- Infectious endocarditis
- Juvenile rheumatoid arthritis
- Reiter syndrome
- Brown recluse spider bite
- Fibromyalgia
- Chronic fatigue syndrome

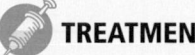 **TREATMENT**

### INITIAL STABILIZATION/THERAPY

- 20 mL/kg of 0.9% NS IV fluid bolus for dehydration
- IV access for neurologic and cardiac involvement
- Cardiac monitoring
- Temporary pacemaker for heart block

### ED TREATMENT/PROCEDURES

- Remove tick:
  - Disinfect site.
  - With blunt instrument, grasp tick close to skin and pull upward with gentle pressure.
- Medications:
  - Aspirin as adjunctive therapy for cardiac involvement
  - NSAIDs for arthritis or arthralgias
- Vaccine (Lymerix) for prevention of disease:
  - A recombinant surface protein
  - For persons in high/moderate risk areas
  - For travelers to endemic areas
  - 3 doses (0 to 1 mo to 12 mo)
- Stage I:
  - Amoxicillin, doxycycline (for those ≥8 yr of age), or cefuroxime (21 days)
  - Azithromycin (14–21 days)
  - Parenteral therapy in pregnant patients
- Stage II:
  - Oral therapy for isolated Bell palsy and mild involvement:
    - Amoxicillin with probenecid (30 days) or doxycycline (avoid if pregnant or ≥8 yr old; 10–21 days)
  - Parenteral therapy for more severe involvement (meningitis, carditis, severe arthritis):
    - Ceftriaxone, cefotaxime (14–21 days), or penicillin G (14–28 days)
- Stage III:
  - Parenteral therapy:
    - Penicillin G, cefotaxime (14–21 days), or ceftriaxone (14–28 days)

### MEDICATION

#### First Line

- Amoxicillin: 500 mg (peds: 50 mg/kg/24 hr) PO t.i.d. for those <8 yr of age or unable to tolerate doxycycline.
- Aspirin: 80–100 mg/kg/d (peds: 50–100 mg/kg/d in 6 div. doses) PO

- Doxycycline: 200 mg PO b.i.d. for 3 days, then 100 mg PO b.i.d. for 21–28 days for children ≥8 yr
- Ceftriaxone: 2 g (peds: 100 mg/kg/24 hr) IV daily (1st line for late-term disease)

#### Second Line

- Azithromycin: 500 mg PO daily
- Cefuroxime axetil, 500 mg b.i.d. (all ages)
- Cefotaxime: 2 g (peds: 100–150 mg/kg/24 hr) IV q8h
- Penicillin G: 20–24 mIU IV q4h–q6h
- Probenecid: 500 mg PO t.i.d.

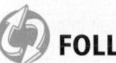 **FOLLOW-UP**

### DISPOSITION

#### Admission Criteria

- Meningoencephalitis
- Telemetry/ICU admission for carditis

#### Discharge Criteria

Patients treated with oral therapy

## PEARLS AND PITFALLS

- Duration of treatment for later organ involvement will be ≥30 days.
- Be aware of coinfections with *Anaplasmosis* and *Babesiosis*.

## ADDITIONAL READING

- Steere AC. Lyme disease. *N Engl J Med*. 2001;345: 115–125.
- Steere AC, Coburn C, Glickstein L. The emergence of Lyme disease. *J Clin Invest*. 2004;113(8): 1093–1101.
- Wormser GP, Dattwyler RJ, Shapiro ED, et al. The clinical assessment, treatment and prevention of Lyme disease, human granulocytic anaplasmosis, and babesiosis: Clinical practice guidelines by the Infectious Diseases Society of America. *Clin Infect Dis*. 2006;43:1089–1134.

 **CODES**

ICD9
088.81 Lyme disease

L

# LYMPHADENITIS

John Mahoney
Dolores Gonthier

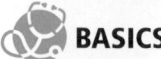 **BASICS**

## DESCRIPTION

- Lymph nodes may be swollen and tender as part of the systemic response to infection:
  - Become engorged with lymphocytes and macrophages
  - May be primarily infected
  - Infection in distal extremity may result in painful tender adenopathy proximally.
- Acute suppurative lymphadenitis may occur after pharyngeal or skin infection.

## ETIOLOGY

- Most frequently caused by bacterial infection.
- Most common organisms in pyogenic lymphadenitis:
  - *Staphylococcus aureus*—including resistant strains such as community-acquired, methicillin-resistant *S. aureus* (CA-MRSA):
    - CA-MRSA risk factors include prior MRSA infection, household contact of CA-MRSA patient, military personnel, incarcerated persons, athletes in contact sports, IV drug users, men who have sex with men.
    - Different antibiotic susceptibility than nosocomial MRSA
    - Variable, rising local prevalence of CA-MRSA should be considered when starting empiric antibiotic therapy.
    - Suspect CA-MRSA in unresponsive infections.
  - Group A $\beta$-hemolytic *Streptococcus*
- Cervical lymphadenitis:
  - Usually pharyngeal or periodontal process
  - *Streptococcus* and anaerobes
- Axillary lymphadenitis:
  - *Streptococcus pyogenes* (group A $\beta$-hemolytic *Streptococcus*)
- Nosocomial MRSA:
  - Risk factors: Recent hospital or long-term care admission, surgery, injection drug use, vascular catheter, dialysis, recent antibiotic use, unresponsive infection.
  - Resistant to most antibiotics (see "Treatment")

### Pediatric Considerations
Acute unilateral cervical suppurative lymphadenitis:

- Most common at age <6 yr
- Group A *Streptococcus*, *S. aureus*, and anaerobes are most common causes.

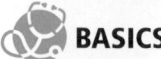 **DIAGNOSIS**

## SIGNS AND SYMPTOMS

- Painful swelling, inflammation/infection of lymph nodes
- Commonly presents simultaneously with acute cellulitis or abscess if pyogenic cause.
- Axillary lymphadenitis:
  - Fever, axillary pain, and acute lymphedema of arms and chest, without features of cellulitis or lymphangitis; ipsilateral pleural effusion may be present.

### History
- Occupation
- Exposure to pets
- Sexual behavior
- Drug use
- Travel history
- Associated symptoms:
  - Sore throat, cough
  - Fever
  - Night sweats
  - Fatigue
  - Weight loss
  - Pain in nodes
- Duration of lymphadenopathy

### Physical Exam
- Extent of lymphadenopathy (localized or generalized)
- Size of nodes:
  - Abnormal size by site:
    - General: >1 cm
    - Epitrochlear: >0.5 cm
    - Inguinal: >1.5 cm
- Presence or absence of nodal tenderness
- Signs of inflammation over node
- Skin lesions
- Splenomegaly
- Enlargement of supraclavicular or scalene nodes is always abnormal.

## ESSENTIAL WORKUP
- Acute regional lymphadenitis is clinical diagnosis, often part of larger syndrome (cellulitis).
- History and physical exam to reveal infectious source

## DIAGNOSTIC TESTS & INTERPRETATION
### Lab
- WBC is not essential:
  - Possible leukocytosis with left shift or normal
- Complete blood count, Epstein-Barr virus (EBV), cytomegalovirus (CMV), HIV, and other serologies based on clinical findings

### Imaging
US or CT in patients who do not improve or progress to suppuration

### Diagnostic Procedures/Surgery
Consider percutaneous needle aspiration or surgical drainage in patients who do not improve or progress to suppuration.

## DIFFERENTIAL DIAGNOSIS
- Common infections:
  - Adenovirus
  - Scarlet fever
  - Cat scratch disease
  - Fungal
  - Herpes zoster
- Unusual infections:
  - Sporotrichosis (rose thorns)
  - Diphtheria
  - West Nile fever
  - Plague
  - Anthrax
  - Typhoid
  - Rubella
- Venereal infections:
  - Syphilis
  - Genital herpes
  - Chancroid
  - Lymphogranuloma venereum
- Other systematic infections causing generalized lymphadenitis:
  - HIV
  - Infectious mononucleosis (EBV or CMV)
  - Toxoplasmosis
  - Tuberculosis
  - Infectious hepatitis
  - Dengue
- Drug reaction:
  - Phenytoin
  - Allopurinol
- Silicone implants
- Malignancy
- Rheumatologic disorders
- Systemic lupus erythematosus
- Sarcoidosis
- Amyloidosis
- Serum sickness

### Pediatric Considerations
- Kawasaki disease
- PFAPA syndrome (periodic fever, aphthous stomatitis, pharyngitis, cervical adenitis)

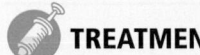 **TREATMENT**

**INITIAL STABILIZATION/THERAPY**
Ensure airway, breathing, and circulation management and hemodynamic stability.

**ED TREATMENT/PROCEDURES**
- General principles:
  - Antibiotics based on involved primary organ/suspected pathogen (see also "Cellulitis")
  - Consider local prevalence of MRSA and other resistant pathogens in addition to usual causes.
  - Usual outpatient treatment: 7–10 days
  - Elevation
  - Application of moist heat
  - Analgesics
- Drainage of abscesses if present:
  - Obtain culture if drainage performed, especially to help identify resistant pathogens.
- Skin origin:
  - Outpatient:
    - Oral cephalexin plus trimethoprim/sulfamethoxazole (TMP/SMX) (to cover CA-MRSA)
    - Alternatives to cephalexin: Oral dicloxacillin, macrolide, or levofloxacin
    - Alternative to TMP/SMX: Clindamycin
  - Inpatient:
    - IV nafcillin or equivalent
- Pharyngeal or periodontal origin:
  - Outpatient:
    - Oral penicillin VK
    - Alternatives: Oral clindamycin or amoxicillin/clavulanate
  - Inpatient:
    - IV penicillin G (aqueous) and IV metronidazole
    - Alternatives: IV ampicillin/sulbactam or IV clindamycin
- Axillary lymphadenitis:
  - Outpatient:
    - Oral penicillin VK
    - Alternatives: Oral macrolide or amoxicillin/clavulanate
  - Inpatient:
    - IV penicillin G (aqueous)
    - Alternatives: IV ampicillin/sulbactam
- Acute unilateral cervical suppurative lymphadenitis:
  - Outpatient:
    - Oral penicillin VK
    - Alternatives: Oral clindamycin or amoxicillin/clavulanate

- MRSA:
  - Nosocomial MRSA:
    - IV vancomycin or linezolid
  - Community-acquired MRSA:
    - Oral doxycycline or combination of oral TMP/SMX and rifampin may be effective for cases not responding to TMP/SMX alone
    - Severe CA-MRSA: IV clindamycin or IV vancomycin

**MEDICATION**
- Amoxicillin/clavulanate: 500–875 mg (peds: 45 mg/kg/24 hr) PO b.i.d. or 250–500 mg (peds: 40 mg/kg/24 hr) PO t.i.d.
- Ampicillin/sulbactam: 1.5–3 g (peds: 100–300 mg/kg/24 hr up to 40 kg; >40 kg, give adult dose) IV q6h
- Cephalexin: 500 mg (peds: 50–100 mg/kg/24 hr) PO q.i.d.
- Clindamycin: 450–900 mg (peds: 20–40 mg/kg/24 hr) PO or IV q8h
- Dicloxacillin: 125–500 mg (peds: 12.5–25 mg/kg/24 hr) PO q6h
- Doxycycline: 100 mg PO b.i.d. for adults
- Erythromycin base: (adult) 250–500 mg PO q.i.d.
- Linezolid: 600 mg PO or IV q12h (peds: 30 mg/kg/d div. q8h)
- Metronidazole: (adult) 15 mg/kg IV once, followed by 7.5 mg/kg IV q6h
- Nafcillin: 1–2 g IV q4h (peds: 50–100 mg/kg/24 hr divided q6h); max. 12 g/24 hr
- Penicillin VK: 250–500 mg (peds: 25–50 mg/kg/24 hr) PO q6h
- Penicillin G (aqueous): 4 mIU (peds: 100,000–400,000 U/kg/24 hr) IV q4h
- Rifampin: 600 mg PO b.i.d. for adults
- TMP/SMX: 2 DS tabs PO q12h (peds: 6–10 mg/kg/24 hr TMP div. q12h)
- Vancomycin: 1 g IV q12h (peds: 10 mg/kg q6h, dosing adjustments required age <5 yr); check serum levels.

 **FOLLOW-UP**

**DISPOSITION**
**Admission Criteria**
- Toxic appearing
- History of immune suppression
- Concurrent chronic medical illnesses
- Unable to take oral medications
- Unreliable patients

**Discharge Criteria**
- Mild infection in a non–toxic-appearing patient
- Able to take oral antibiotics
- No history of immune suppression or concurrent medical problems
- Has adequate follow-up within 24–48 hr

**Issues for Referral**
- If not found in context of acute infection and not quick to resolve with course of antibiotics, evaluate for more serious underlying causes (eg, malignancy).
- Lymph node biopsy may be helpful in the following circumstances:
  - Clinical findings indicate likely malignancy.
  - Lymph node size >1 cm
  - Supraclavicular location

**FOLLOW-UP RECOMMENDATIONS**
- Follow-up within 24–48 hr for response to treatment
- If symptoms worsen—including new or worsening lymphangitis, new or increasing area of redness over the node, worsening fever—patient should be instructed to return sooner.

## PEARLS AND PITFALLS

- Staph species are the most common cause of acute regional lymphadenitis due to pyogenic bacteria.
- Empiric antibiotic coverage must extend to include CA-MRSA, in addition to coverage for other staph species and strep.

## ADDITIONAL READING

- Abrahamian FM, Talan DA, Moran GJ. Management of skin and soft-tissue infections in the emergency department. *Infect Dis Clin North Am*. 2008;22: 89–116.
- Boyce JM. Severe streptococcal axillary lymphadenitis. *N Engl J Med*. 1990;323:655–658.
- Henry PH, Longo DL. Enlargement of lymph nodes and spleen. In: Fauci AS, Braunwald E, Kasper DL, et al., eds. *Harrison's Principles of Internal Medicine*, 17th ed. New York: McGraw-Hill; 2008:370–375.
- Pasternack MS, Swartz MN. Lymphadenitis and lymphangitis. In: Mandell GL, Bennett JE, Dolin R, eds. *Mandell, Douglas and Bennett's Principles and Practice of Infectious Diseases*, 7th ed. New York: Elsevier/Churchill Livingstone; 2010:1323–1334.
- Thomas KT, Feder HM, Lawton AR, et al. Periodic fever syndrome in children. *J Pediatr*. 1999;135: 15–21.

**See Also (Topic, Algorithm, Electronic Media Element)**
- CA-MRSA
- Cellulitis
- Lymphangitis

 **CODES**

**ICD9**
- 289.3 Lymphadenitis, unspecified, except mesenteric
- 683 Acute lymphadenitis

L

# LYMPHANGITIS

*John Mahoney*

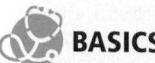 **BASICS**

## DESCRIPTION
- Lymphangitis is the infection of lymphatics that drain a focus of inflammation.
- Histologically, lymphatic vessels are dilated and filled with lymphocytes and histiocytes:
  - Inflammation frequently extends into perilymphatic tissues and may lead to cellulitis or abscess formation.

## ETIOLOGY
- Acute lymphangitis:
  - Likely caused by bacterial infection
  - Most commonly group A β-hemolytic *Streptococcus*
  - Less commonly due to other strep groups, and occasionally *Staphylococcus aureus,* including resistant strains such as community-acquired, methicillin-resistant *S. aureus* (CA-MRSA):
    - CA-MRSA risk factors include prior MRSA infection, household contact of CA-MRSA patient, military personnel, incarcerated persons, athletes in contact sports, IV drug users, men who have sex with men.
    - Different antibiotic susceptibility than nosocomial MRSA
    - Variable, rising local prevalence of CA-MRSA should be considered when starting empiric antibiotic therapy.
    - Suspect CA-MRSA in unresponsive infections or if multiple or recurrent abscesses.
  - Other organisms:
    - *Pasteurella multocida* (cat or dog bite)
    - *Spirillum minus* (rat-bite fever)
    - *Wuchereria bancrofti* (filariasis): Consider in immigrants from Africa, Southeast Asia/Pacific, and tropical South America with lower extremity involvement.
- Chronic lymphangitis:
  - Usually caused by mycotic, mycobacterial, and filarial infections
  - *Sporothrix schenckii* (most common cause of chronic lymphangitis in U.S.):
    - Inoculation occurs while gardening or farming (rose thorn).
    - Organism is present on some plants and in sphagnum moss.
    - Multiple SC nodules appear along course of lymphatic vessels.
    - Typical antibiotics and local treatment fail to cure lesion.

- *Mycobacterium marinum*:
  - Atypical *Mycobacterium*
  - Grows optimally at 25–32°C in fish tanks and swimming pools
  - May produce a chronic nodular, single wartlike or ulcerative lesion at site of abrasion
  - Additional lesions may appear in distribution similar to sporotrichosis.
- *Nocardia brasiliensis*
- *Mycobacterium kansasii*
- *Wuchereria bancrofti*

## DIAGNOSIS

### SIGNS AND SYMPTOMS
- Acute lymphangitis:
  - Warm, tender erythematous streaks develop and extend proximally from the source of infection.
  - Regional lymph nodes often become enlarged and tender (lymphadenitis).
  - Peripheral edema of involved extremity
  - Systemic manifestations:
    - Fever
    - Rigors
    - Tachycardia
    - Headache
- Chronic (nodular) lymphangitis:
  - Erythematous nodule, chancriform ulcer, or wartlike lesion develops in subcutaneous tissue at inoculation site.
  - Often presents without pain or evidence of systemic infection
  - Multiple lesions possible along lymphatic chain

### History
History and physical directed at discovering source of infection.

### Physical Exam
- Fever
- Erythematous streaks from source of infection proceeding toward regional lymph nodes

### ESSENTIAL WORKUP
Lymphangitis is a clinical diagnosis.

## DIAGNOSTIC TESTS & INTERPRETATION
### Lab
- WBC is unnecessary but often elevated.
- Gram stain and culture of initial lesion to focus antimicrobial selection and reveal resistant pathogens (MRSA):
  - Aspirate point of maximal inflammation or punch biopsy.
  - Essential if treatment failure
- If sporotrichosis or *M. marinum* infection is suspected, diagnosis should be confirmed by culture of organism from wound.
- Blood culture may reveal organism.

### Imaging
- Imaging is not commonly performed.
- Plain radiographs may reveal abscess formation, subcutaneous gas, or foreign bodies if these are suspected.
- Extremity vascular imaging (Doppler US) can help rule out deep venous thrombosis.

## DIFFERENTIAL DIAGNOSIS
- Thrombophlebitis; deep venous and superficial:
  - Differentiation from lymphangitis:
    - Absence of initial traumatic or infectious focus
    - No regional lymphadenopathy
- IV line infiltration
- Smallpox vaccination, normal variant of usual reaction to vaccination
- Phytophotodermatitis:
  - Linear inflammatory reaction, mimics lymphangitis
  - Lime rind, lime juice, and certain plants can act as photosensitizing agents.

**TREATMENT**

### INITIAL STABILIZATION/THERAPY
If patient is septic, manage airway and resuscitate as indicated.

### ED TREATMENT/PROCEDURES
- Antimicrobial therapy should be initiated with first dose in ED.
- General principles:
  - Consider local prevalence of MRSA and other resistant pathogens in addition to usual causes.
  - Usual outpatient treatment: 7–10 days
  - Elevation
  - Application of moist heat
- Acute lymphangitis, empiric coverage:
  - Outpatient:
    ○ Oral cephalexin plus trimethoprim/sulfamethoxazole (TMP/SMX) (to cover CA-MRSA)
    ○ Alternatives to cephalexin: oral dicloxacillin, macrolide, or levofloxacin
    ○ Alternative to TMP/SMX: clindamycin
  - Inpatient: IV nafcillin or equivalent
- Lymphangitis after dog or cat bite: IV ampicillin/sulbactam
- MRSA:
  - Nosocomial MRSA: IV vancomycin or linezolid
  - Community-acquired MRSA:
    ○ Oral doxycycline or combination of oral TMP/SMX and rifampin may be effective for cases not responding to TMP/SMX alone.
    ○ Severe CA-MRSA: IV clindamycin or IV vancomycin
- Sporotrichosis:
  Itraconazole or saturated solution of potassium iodide (SSKI)
- *Mycobacterium marinum*:
  - Localized granulomas are usually excised.
  - Antimicrobial therapy is usually reserved for more severe infections:
    ○ Limited data on what combination of agents should be used
    ○ Rifampin and ethambutol may be best choice.

### MEDICATION
- Ampicillin/sulbactam: 1.5–3 g (peds: 100–300 mg/kg/24 hr up to 40 kg; >40 kg, give adult dose) IV q6h
- Cephalexin: 500 mg (peds: 50–100 mg/kg/24 hr) PO q.i.d.
- Clindamycin: 450–900 mg (peds: 20–40 mg/kg/24 hr) PO or IV q8h
- Dicloxacillin: 125–500 mg (peds: 12.5–25 mg/kg/24 hr) PO q6h
- Doxycycline: 100 mg PO b.i.d. for adults
- Erythromycin base: (adult) 250–500 mg PO q.i.d.
- Itraconazole (adult): 200 mg PO daily, continue until 2–4 wk after all lesions resolve (usually 3–6 mo); peds: not approved for use
- Levofloxacin: (adult only) 500–750 mg PO or IV daily
- Linezolid: 600 mg PO or IV q12h (peds: 30 mg/kg/24 hr div. q8h)
- Nafcillin: 1–2 g IV q4h (peds: 50–100 mg/kg/24 hr div. q6h); max. 12 g/24 hr
- Rifampin: 600 mg PO b.i.d. for adults
- SSKI: 5–10 drops, increase to 40–50 drops (peds: 5–10 drops, increase to 25–40) PO t.i.d.; taken in milk, juice, or carbonated beverage to avoid bitter taste
- TMP/SMX: 2 DS tabs PO q12h (peds: 6–10 mg/kg/24 hr TMP div. q12h)
- Vancomycin: 1 g IV q12h (peds: 10 mg/kg IV q6h, dosing adjustments required for age <5 yr); check serum levels.

 **FOLLOW-UP**

### DISPOSITION
#### Admission Criteria
- Toxic appearing
- History of immune suppression
- Concurrent chronic medical illnesses
- Unable to take oral medications
- Unreliable patients

#### Discharge Criteria
- Mild infection in a non–toxic-appearing patient
- Able to take oral antibiotics
- No history of immune suppression or concurrent medical problems
- Adequate follow-up within 24–48 hr

### FOLLOW-UP RECOMMENDATIONS
- Follow-up within 24–48 hr
- Sooner if worsening symptoms, including worsening fever or other systemic symptoms

## PEARLS AND PITFALLS
Empiric antibiotic coverage must extend to include CA-MRSA, in addition to coverage for other staph species and strep.

## ADDITIONAL READING

- Pasternack MS, Swartz MN. Lymphadenitis and lymphangitis. In: Mandell GL, Bennett JE, Dolin R, eds. *Mandell, Douglas and Bennett's Principles and Practice of Infectious Diseases*, 7th ed. New York: Elsevier/Churchill Livingstone; 2010:1323–1334.
- Rex JH, Okhuysen PC. *Sporothrix schenckii*. In: Mandell GL, Bennett JE, Dolin R, eds. *Mandell, Douglas and Bennett's Principles and Practice of Infectious Diseases*, 7th ed. New York: Elsevier/Churchill Livingstone; 2010:3271–3276.
- Smego RA, Castiglia M, Asperilla MO. Lymphocutaneous syndrome: A review of non-*Sporothrix* causes. *Medicine*. 1999;78(1): 38–63.

### See Also (Topic, Algorithm, Electronic Media Element)
- CA-MRSA
- Cellulitis
- Lymphadenitis

 **CODES**

**ICD9**
457.2 Lymphangitis

# LYMPHOGRANULOMA VENEREUM

*Joel Kravitz*

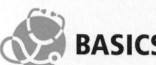 **BASICS**

## DESCRIPTION

- Sexually transmitted disease
- Primary stage:
  - Painless papule, pustule, or ulcer
- Secondary stage:
  - Spread to regional lymph nodes
  - Fluctuant inguinal lymphadenopathy (buboes)
  - Lymphadenopathy may be unilateral or bilateral
- Responsive to antibacterial therapy
- Tertiary stage:
  - If untreated, significant tissue damage and destruction may result.
- Endemic in Southeast Asia, Latin America, parts of Africa, and the Caribbean
- Increasing incidence among men who have sex with men
- Also known as:
  - Struma
  - Tropical bubo
  - Nicolas-Favre-Durand disease

## ETIOLOGY

*Chlamydia trachomatis* serotypes L1, L2, and L3

 **DIAGNOSIS**

## SIGNS AND SYMPTOMS

### History

- Primary genital lesions:
  - Incubation: 3–30 days after sexual exposure to *Chlamydia trachomatis*
  - Painless genital chancre lasts 2–3 days (rarely, a papule or vesicle)
  - Often transient and not noticed
  - May present as proctitis
- Secondary stage:
  - Systemic symptoms:
    ○ Fever and malaise
    ○ Myalgias
  - Lymphadenopathy; usually inguinal:
    ○ May ulcerate and drain pus
  - Proctitis:
    ○ Rectal bleeding
    ○ Tenesmus
    ○ Constipation
- Tertiary stage:
  - Symptoms mimicinflammatory bowel disease or proctocolitis
  - Elephantiasis
  - Strictures

### Physical Exam

- Primary stage:
  - Painless papule, pustule, or ulcer
  - Usually anogenital region
- Secondary stage:
  - Tender inguinal adenopathy:
    ○ Occurs 1–3 wk after initial inoculation
    ○ Adenopathy is unilateral in 2/3 of cases.
    ○ Buboes (large inguinal lymph nodes) form in inguinal and femoral chains.
    ○ Groove sign: Scarred or coalescent buboes above and below inguinal ligament give a linear depression parallel to the inguinal ligament (seen in 30%).
    ○ Anal-receptive patients may develop hemorrhagic proctocolitis.
    ○ Perirectal lymphatic inflammation causes fistulae and strictures.
- Tertiary disease:
  - Chronic proctocolitis:
    ○ Abdominal pain
    ○ Rectal bleeding
  - Genital strictures
  - Perineal and perianal fistulae
  - Elephantiasis of the ipsilateral leg

## DIAGNOSTIC TESTS & INTERPRETATION
### Lab
- Standard *Chlamydia* DNA probes *do not* test for lymphogranuloma venereum (LGV) strain.
- False-positive VDRL in 20%
- Serologic testing and culture are the standard.
- Complement fixation titers >1:64 are consistent with LGV infection.

### Diagnostic Procedures/Surgery
Bubo aspiration—specific but expensive and impractical

## DIFFERENTIAL DIAGNOSIS
- Genital herpes (ulcers usually not seen in LGV)
- Syphilis—nodes nontender, longer incubation
- Chancroid—multiple ulcers, no systemic symptoms
- Granuloma inguinale—lesions painless and bleed easily

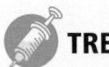 TREATMENT

### PRE-HOSPITAL
No pre-hospital issues

### INITIAL STABILIZATION/THERAPY
No field or ED stabilization required

### ED TREATMENT/PROCEDURES
If large, buboes may need to be aspirated or drained to avoid or minimize scarring.

## MEDICATION
### First Line
Doxycycline: 100 mg PO b.i.d. for 3 wk

### Second Line
- Azithromycin: 1,000 mg PO daily for 3 wk
- Erythromycin: 500 mg PO q.i.d. for 3 wk

### Pregnancy Considerations
Erythromycin is the recommended regimen in pregnancy and during lactation.

 FOLLOW-UP

### DISPOSITION
#### Admission Criteria
Hospitalization is rarely needed (ie, severe systemic symptoms).

#### Discharge Criteria
Immunocompetent patient without systemic involvement

#### Issues for Referral
- Outpatient follow-up is required to confirm diagnosis and cure.
- Rectal infection may require retreatment.

### FOLLOW-UP RECOMMENDATIONS
Ensure that sexual partners are tested and treated.

## PEARLS AND PITFALLS
- Diagnosis is based on clinical suspicion, epidemiologic patterns, and exclusion of other etiologies.
- Consider this diagnosis in men who have sex with men.
- Treat to avoid tertiary disease which is not responsive to antibiotic therapy alone.
- Treatment course is at least 3 wk of antibiotics.

## ADDITIONAL READING
- Centers for Disease Control and Prevention: 2002 guidelines for treatment of sexually transmitted diseases. Available at: http://www.cdc.gov/std/treatment/2006/genital-ulcers.htm#genulc5
- McLean CA, Stoner BP, Workowski KA. Treatment of lymphogranuloma venereum. *Clin Infect Dis*. 2007; 44:S147–S152.
- White JA. Manifestations and management of lymphogranuloma venereum. *Curr Opin Infect Dis*. 2009;22:57–66.
- White J, Ison C. Lymphogranuloma venereum: What does the clinician need to know? *Clin Med*. 2008;8:327–330.

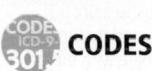 CODES

### ICD9
099.1 Lymphogranuloma venereum

# MALARIA
*Jordan Moskoff*

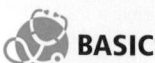 **BASICS**

## DESCRIPTION
- Protozoan infection transmitted through the *Anopheles* mosquito
- Incubation period 8–16 days
- Periodicity of the disease is due to the life cycle of the protozoan:
  - Exoerythrocytic phase: Immature sporozoites migrate to liver, where they rapidly multiply into mature parasites (merozoites).
  - Erythrocytic phase: Mature parasites are released into circulation and invade RBCs.
  - Replication within RBCs followed 48–72 hr later by RBC lysis and release of merozoites into circulation, repeating cycle
  - Fever corresponds to RBC lysis.
- *Plasmodium falciparum*:
  - Cause of most cases and almost all deaths
  - Usually presents as an acute, overwhelming infection
  - Able to infect red cells of all ages:
    ○ Results in greater degree of hemolysis and anemia
  - Causes widespread capillary obstruction:
    ○ Results in end-organ hypoxia and dysfunction
  - More moderate infection in people who are on or who have recently stopped prophylaxis with an agent to which the *P. falciparum* is resistant
  - Posttraumatic immunosuppression may cause relapse of malaria in patients who have lived in endemic areas.
- *Plasmodium vivax* and *Plasmodium ovale*:
  - May present with an acute febrile illness
  - Dormant liver stages (hypnozoites) that may cause relapse 6–11 mo after initial infection
- *Plasmodium malariae*:
  - May persist in the bloodstream at low levels up to 30 yr

## ETIOLOGY
- Transmission usually occurs from the bite of infected female *Anopheles* mosquito.
- North American transmission possible:
  - *Anopheles* mosquitoes on east and west coasts of U.S.
  - Transmission may also occur through infected blood products and shared needles.

### Pediatric Considerations
- Sickle cell trait protective
- Cerebral malaria more common in children
- In highly endemic areas with minimal lab capability, all children presenting with febrile illness may be treated.

### Pregnancy Considerations
Pregnant patients, especially primigravid, at higher risk

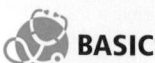 **DIAGNOSIS**

## SIGNS AND SYMPTOMS
- Timing:
  - *P. falciparum*—exhibits within 8 wk of return
  - *P. vivax*—delayed several months
  - Most symptomatic within 1 yr
- General:
  - Malaise
  - Chills
  - Fever—usually >38°C
  - Classic malaria paroxysm:
    ○ 15 min to 1 hr of chills
    ○ Followed by 2–6 hr of nondiaphoretic fever ≤39–42°C
    ○ Profuse diaphoresis followed by defervescence
    ○ Pattern every 48 hr (*P. vivax* and *P. ovale*) or every 72 hr (*P. falciparum*)
    ○ Fever pattern may be varied; rare to have classical fever.
  - Orthostatic hypotension
  - Myalgias/arthralgias
  - Hematology
  - Hemolysis:
    ○ Blackwater fever; named from the dark color of the urine partially due to hemolysis in overwhelming *P. falciparum* infections
  - Jaundice
  - Splenomegaly:
    ○ More common in chronic infections
    ○ May cause splenic rupture
- CNS—cerebral malaria:
  - Headache
  - Focal neurologic findings
  - Mental status changes
  - Coma
  - Seizures
- GI:
  - Emesis
  - Diarrhea
  - Abdominal pain
- Pulmonary:
  - Shortness of breath
  - Rales
  - Pulmonary edema
- Severe malaria:
  - One or more of the following:
    ○ >20% mortality even with optimal management
    ○ Prostration; unable to sit up by oneself
    ○ Impaired consciousness
    ○ Respiratory distress or pulmonary edema
    ○ Seizure
    ○ Circulatory collapse
    ○ Abnormal bleeding
    ○ Jaundice
    ○ Hemoglobinuria
    ○ Severe anemia

## ESSENTIAL WORKUP
Oil emersion light microscopy of a thick-smear Giemsa stain:
- Demonstrates intraerythrocytic malaria parasites
- Cannot exclude diagnosis without three negative smears in 48 hr
- Only high degrees of parasitemia will be evident on a standard CBC smear.

## DIAGNOSTIC TESTS & INTERPRETATION
### Lab
- CBC:
  - Anemia—25%
  - Thrombocytopenia—70% <150
  - Leukocytopenia
- Electrolytes, BUN, creatinine, glucose:
  - Renal failure
  - Hypoglycemia (rare)
  - Lactic acidosis
  - Hyponatremia
- Urinalysis
- Liver function tests:
  - Increased in 25%
  - Increased bilirubin, lactate dehydrogenase signs of hemolysis

### Imaging
Chest radiograph—for pulmonary edema

### Diagnostic Procedures/Surgery
- Immunofluorescence assay, enzyme-linked immunosorbent assay, or DNA probes:
  - Differentiates the type of *Plasmodium* present
  - 5–7% will have mixed infections.
- Lumbar puncture/cerebrospinal fluid (CSF) analysis:
  - Performed to distinguish cerebral malaria from meningitis
  - CSF lactate/protein elevated with malaria
  - CSF pleocytosis/hypoglycemia absent with malaria

## DIFFERENTIAL DIAGNOSIS
- Meningitis
- Encephalitis
- Stroke
- Acute renal failure
- Acute hemolytic anemia
- Sepsis
- Hepatitis
- Viral diarrheal illness
- Hypoglycemic coma
- Heat stroke

**TREATMENT**

### INITIAL STABILIZATION/THERAPY
- ABCs
- 0.9% NS fluid bolus for hypotension
- Immediate cooling if temperature >40°C
- Acetaminophen
- Mist/cool-air fans
- Naloxone, D50W (or Accu-Chek), and thiamine if altered mental status

### ED TREATMENT/PROCEDURES
- Dependent on considering this diagnosis and identifying the type of malaria present and geographic area of acquisition
- Assume drug resistant until proven otherwise.
- *P. vivax, P. ovale, P. malariae*, and non–chloroquine-resistant *P. falciparum*:
  - Treated with oral chloroquine in both adults and children:
    - Chloroquine—safe in pregnant women
  - Chloroquine sensitive for *P. falciparum*, including Central America, Caribbean, and Middle East
  - Eradicate persistent hypnozoites in *P. vivax* and *P. ovale* with primaquine beginning after completion of course of chloroquine.
- Chloroquine-resistant *P. falciparum* infection: PO treatment options:
  - Atovaquone–proguanil
  - Artemether–lumefantrine
  - Mefloquine—safety unproved in pregnancy
  - Quinine, *plus*:
    - Doxycycline (avoid in pregnant women and children <8 yr old)
    - Clindamycin (use in pregnant women and children <8 yr old)
    - Pyrimethamine–sulfadoxine
- Chloroquine-resistant *P. vivax* infection:
  - Atovaquone–proguanil *plus* primaquine
- Severe *falciparum*—IV treatment:
  - Chloroquine if known susceptible
  - If chloroquine resistant:
    - Quinidine (rotary isomer of quinine) or quinine *plus* doxycycline or clindamycin
- Exchange transfusion:
  - Rapidly removes parasitic RBCs, toxins, and red cell debris, replacing them with fresh plasma and RBCs
  - Efficacy not proved in randomized trials
  - Consider in seriously ill with *P. falciparum* parasitemias >10%.
- Steroids are not recommended for cerebral malaria:
  - Dexamethasone worsens both duration of coma and prognosis.
- Supportive therapy for complications
- *P. falciparum* antibiotic resistance:
  - Chloroquine sensitive in the Caribbean, Central America, and the Middle East
  - Pyrimethamine–sulfadoxine resistance in South America, Africa, southern and southeast Asia, and Indonesia
  - Mefloquine resistance in Southeast Asia

- Chemoprophylaxis:
  - Chloroquine:
    - Drug of choice for travel to areas without chloroquine resistance
    - 300 mg PO weekly
    - Begin 2 wk prior to departure and continue for 4 wk after return.
  - Mefloquine:
    - For chloroquine-resistant areas
    - 250 mg PO weekly
    - Begin 2 wk before departure and continue for 4 wk after return.
  - Doxycycline:
    - For chloroquine/mefloquine–resistant areas
    - 100 mg PO daily
    - 1 day prior to entering area
    - Continue for 4 wk after return
  - Primaquine:
    - 30 mg PO every day
    - 1 day prior to entering area
    - Continue 1 wk after return.
- Vaccine is not available, but several are in field trials.

### MEDICATION
- Acetaminophen: 1 g (peds: 15–20 mg/kg) PO
- Artemether (20 mg)– lumefantrine (120 mg): 6 doses of 4 tabs each; 2 tablets time 0 and 8 hr on day 1, then 4 tabs b.i.d. days 2 and 3
- Chloroquine: 600-mg base initially (1,000 mg of chloroquine phosphate) followed by an additional 300 mg (500 mg salt) 6 hr later and again on days 2 and 3 (peds: 10 mg/kg base PO, followed by 5 mg/kg base 6 hr later and on on days 2 and 3)
- Clindamycin: 20 mg/kg/24 hr t.i.d. for 7 days (peds: 20 mg/kg/24 hr t.i.d. for 7 days)
- Dextrose: D50W 1 amp—50 mL or 25 g (peds: D25W 2–4 mL/kg) IV
- Doxycycline: 100 mg PO b.i.d. for 7 days; >8 yr only, 1.5–2 mg/kg (max. 100 mg) b.i.d. for 5–7 days
- Malarone (atovaquone/proguanil):
  - Prophylaxis: 250 mg/100 mg PO per day
  - Treatment: 1,000 mg/400 mg (4 tabs) PO per day for 3 days
- Mefloquine: 750 mg followed 12 hr later by 500 mg (peds: 15 mg/kg followed 12 hr later by 10 mg/kg)
- Naloxone (Narcan): 2 mg (peds: 0.1 mg/kg) IV or IM initial dose
- Primaquine phosphate: 30-mg base (peds: 0.6-mg base/kg/24 hr) PO for 14 days
- Pyrimethamine-sulfadoxine (Fansidar): 3 tabs PO on last day of quinine treatment
- Quinidine gluconate: 10 mg/kg loading dose (max. 600 mg) in normal saline infused slowly over 1–2 hr, followed by continuous infusion of 0.02 mg/kg/min until patient is able to begin oral therapy
- Quinine: 650 mg PO t.i.d. for 3–7 days
- Quinine dihydrochloride: 20 mg salt/kg loading dose in 5% dextrose over 4 hr, followed by 10 mg salt/kg over 2–4 hr q8h (max. 1,800 mg/d) until patient is able to begin oral treatment
- Thiamine (vitamin $B_1$): 100 mg (peds: 50 mg) IV or IM

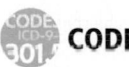 **FOLLOW-UP**

### DISPOSITION
#### Admission Criteria
- ICU admission for severe *P. falciparum* infection
- Suspected acute *P. falciparum* infection
- Severe dehydration
- Inability to tolerate oral solution/medication
- >3% of RBC containing parasites

#### Discharge Criteria
- Non–*P. falciparum* infection
- Able to tolerate oral medications

## PEARLS AND PITFALLS

Consider in patients with appropriate exposure/ epidemiology and in patients with fever and consistent signs and symptoms.

## ADDITIONAL READING

- American Academy of Pediatrics, Committee on Infectious Diseases. *Red Book*, 28th ed. Elk Grove Village, IL: American Academy of Pediatrics; 2009.
- Centers for Disease Control and Prevention. Malaria. Available at: www.cdc.gov/malaria/
- Centers for Disease Control and Prevention. Malaria hotline: 770-488-7788.
- Centers for Disease Control and Prevention. Traveler's Health. Available at: www.cdc.gov/ travel/contentYellow Book.aspx
- Garner P. Systemic reviews in malaria: Global policies need global reviews. *Infect Dis Clin North Am*. 2009;23:387–404.
- Pasvol G. Management of severe malaria: Interventions and controversies. *Infect Dis Clin North Am*. 2005;19:211–240.
- Suh K. Malaria. *Can Med Assoc J*. 2004;170(4): 1693–1702.

**CODES**

ICD9
084.6 Malaria, unspecified

M

# MALGAIGNE FRACTURE

Theodore C. Chan

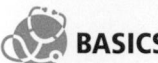 **BASICS**

## DESCRIPTION

- Among the most unstable pelvic fractures:
  - Displacement or potential displacement of entire hemipelvis
  - Involves at least two breaks in continuity of pelvic ring
- Vertical shear forces result in anterior and posterior disruption with real or potential displacement of intervening fragments or hemipelvis:
  - Anterior disruption of symphysis pubis or 2–4 pubic rami
  - Posterior displacement and instability through sacrum, sacroiliac joint, or ileum
- Type C: Unstable pelvic ring injury—rotationally and vertically unstable:
  - C1: Unilateral vertical shear fracture
  - C2: Unilateral vertical shear combined with contralateral type B injury
  - C3: Bilateral vertical shear fracture
- High risk for associated injuries, including: Pelvic hemorrhage and hemorrhagic shock:
  - Intra-abdominal and GI tract
  - Genitourinary and urinary tracts
  - Gynecologic, including uterine and vaginal
  - Neurologic
  - Arterial and venous plexus injuries

## ETIOLOGY

- Malgaigne fracture indicates significant energy force applied to pelvic bones.
- Fractures often occur from vehicular trauma, pedestrian struck by automobile, or falls from heights:
  - As many as 20% of all vehicular trauma fatalities have associated Malgaigne fracture.

### Pediatric Considerations

- Children can have proportionately greater blood loss with pelvic fractures.
- Nonaccidental trauma should always be considered.

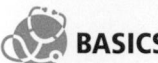 **DIAGNOSIS**

## SIGNS AND SYMPTOMS

- Gross pelvic instability
- History of significant traumatic mechanism of injury

### History

- Often presents in setting of multiple trauma
- Severe pain on pelvic movement, tilt, and compression

### Physical Exam

- Pelvic instability, often with anterior iliac and crest displacement or mobility
- Shortening of legs from migration of hemipelvis
- Ecchymoses, swelling, abrasions, and open wounds involving hips, groin, buttocks, perineum, pelvis
- Evidence of perineal, urethral, rectal, and vaginal injuries
- In hemorrhagic shock:
  - Tachycardia, hypotension, narrowed pulse pressure
  - Altered mental status
  - Cool and pale extremities

## ESSENTIAL WORKUP

- Pelvic radiography is the most valuable initial diagnostic test.
- Single AP view of pelvis should be done early for any major trauma victim in whom pelvic fracture is suspected:
  - Most Malgaigne fractures will be seen on AP view of pelvis.
- Other radiographic signs suggesting Malgaigne fracture:
  - Pubic symphysis disruption with diastasis >15 mm
  - Symphysis disruption associated with overlapping of pubis
  - Symphysis disruption associated with unilateral fracture of both rami
  - Bilateral breaks of both pelvic rami or markedly displaced unilateral fractures of both rami
  - Vertical fracture of sacrum (these fractures rarely occur as isolated pelvic fractures)
  - Asymmetry of iliac wings
  - Avulsion of ischial spine or L-5 transverse process associated with hemipelvis migration
- Inlet projection (30° caudal angulation) allows visualization of posterior pelvis:
  - May aid in assessment of posterior displacement

## DIAGNOSTIC TESTS & INTERPRETATION
### Lab

- Type and cross-match.
- Hemoglobin/hematocrit, platelet count, and coagulation studies (prothrombin time, partial thromboplastin time)

### Imaging

- CT scan may further delineate pelvic fracture(s), retroperitoneal hematoma, visceral injuries:
  - CT contrast angiography may delineate source of bleeding (particularly arterial), but should be considered only in hemodynamically stable patients.
- Abdominal US focused abdominal sonography for trauma (FAST) in patients with significant traumatic injury, but differentiation of intraperitoneal from extraperitoneal hemorrhage from pelvic fracture can be difficult.
- MRI indicated with evidence of neurologic injury

### Diagnostic Procedures/Surgery

- Diagnostic peritoneal lavage (DPL) is a rapid bedside evaluation for intraperitoneal hemorrhage:
  - In the setting of pelvic fracture, the supraumbilical open approach for DPL should be used.
- Angiography and selective vessel embolization in setting of pelvic hemorrhage:
  - Particularly for small-vessel arterial bleeding
- Surgery:
  - As indicated on basis of clinical findings and orthopedic/surgical consult
  - Surgical stabilization with pelvic packing
  - Direct operative control of pelvic bleeding

## DIFFERENTIAL DIAGNOSIS

- Other pelvic fractures:
  - Straddle fracture
  - Open-book fracture
  - Severe multiple pelvic fractures; see "Pelvic Fracture"
- Intra-abdominal injury and hemorrhage

**TREATMENT**

## PRE-HOSPITAL

- ABCs of trauma care
- IV fluid resuscitation as indicated
- Consider stabilization or immobilization measures for pelvis (see below):
  - Pneumatic antishock garment (PASG) may be considered, but controversial:
    - Indication: Prolonged transport time or hemodynamic instability
    - Caution: Aggressive fluid resuscitation must occur before deflation of PASG abdominal compartment if it has been used.

## INITIAL STABILIZATION/THERAPY

- ABCs of trauma care
- IV fluid resuscitation with blood or crystalloid, O-negative or type-specific blood if hemodynamically unstable:
  - Avoid using lower extremity IV sites.
- Stabilize and immobilize the pelvis to prevent further injury and decrease bleeding:
  - Compression device: Folded sheet with clamp or commercial compression device wrapped circumferentially around greater trochanters to stabilize and compress pelvis
    PASG: Use in ED is controversial, but allows rapid pelvic immobilization and pelvic compression to slow bleeding.
  - External fixator: Requires more time to place than PASG but "splints" pelvis in a similar manner; contraindicated in severely comminuted pelvic fracture.
  - Contraindicated in severely comminuted Malgaigne fracture
- Placement of stabilization device should not interfere with further workup and care.

## ED TREATMENT/PROCEDURES

- Immediate trauma surgery and orthopedics consultation
- Nothing by mouth
- Prioritization of studies: CT, angiography, or surgery:
  - In hemodynamically *unstable* patient, rapidly performed US FAST or DPL can determine treatment course:
    - If US or DPL aspirate is positive for bleeding, patient should undergo surgery for celiotomy with external pelvic fixation or pelvic packing, followed by selective angiography.
    - If DPL or US is negative, patient should undergo external fixation as appropriate, followed by selective angiography embolization.
  - In the hemodynamically *stable* patient, the patient can go to CT scan for evaluation of the abdomen, pelvis, and retroperitoneum with external fixation as appropriate:
    - IV contrast may be used to assess for bleeding and source, prior to selective angiography as indicated.

## MEDICATION

- Crystalloid fluids: 2-L IV bolus of normal saline or lactated Ringer (peds: 20 mL/kg)
- Blood products: 4–6 U cross-matched, type-specific, or O-negative blood (peds: 10 mL/kg)

 **FOLLOW-UP**

## DISPOSITION

### Admission Criteria

- All patients with Malgaigne fractures because of the magnitude of the insult, instability of the fracture, and likelihood of hemorrhage and concomitant injury
- Admit to ICU or monitored setting.

### Discharge Criteria

Stable patients without Malgaigne fracture

## PEARLS AND PITFALLS

- Malgaigne fracture results from significant major traumatic injury resulting in an unstable pelvis with potential displacement of hemipelvis.
- Injury to underlying intra-abdominal and pelvic organs and tissue is common, including high risk for pelvic hemorrhage and shock.
- All patients with Malgaigne fracture should be admitted with consultation by trauma surgery and orthopedic services.

## ADDITIONAL READING

- American College of Surgeons, Committee on Trauma. *Advanced Trauma Life Support for Doctors*, 8th ed. Chicago: American College of Surgeons; 2008.
- Dyer GS, Vrahas MS. Review of the pathophysiology and acute management of haemorrhage in pelvic fracture. *Injury.* 2006;37:602–613.
- Geeraerts T, Chhor V, Cheisson G, et al. Clinical review: Initial management of blunt pelvic trauma in patients with haemodynamic instability. *Crit Care.* 2007;11:204–213.
- Rice PL, Rudolph M. Pelvic fractures. *Emerg Med Clin North Am.* 2007;25:795–802.

### See Also (Topic, Algorithm, Electronic Media Element)

- Hemorrhagic Shock
- Pelvic Fracture

**CODES**

ICD9

808.43 Multiple closed pelvic fractures with disruption of pelvic circle

M

# MALLORY-WEISS SYNDROME

Robert C. Montana
Jeffrey J. Schaider

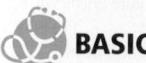 **BASICS**

## DESCRIPTION
- Partial-thickness intraluminal longitudinal mucosal tear of distal esophagus or proximal stomach
- Sudden increase in intra-abdominal and/or transgastric pressure causes:
  - Mild to moderate submucosal arterial and/or venous bleeding:
    o May be related to underlying pathology
    o "Mushrooming" of stomach into esophagus during retching has been observed endoscopically.

## ETIOLOGY
- Associated with:
  - Seizures
  - Forceful coughing/laughing
  - Lifting
  - Straining
  - Blunt abdominal trauma
  - Childbirth
  - Cardiopulmonary resuscitation
- Risk factors:
  - Alcoholics:
    o Especially after recent binge
  - Patients with hiatal hernia
  - Hyperemesis gravidarum
- Greater bleeding associated with:
  - Portal hypertension
  - Esophageal varices
  - Coagulopathy

 **DIAGNOSIS**

## SIGNS AND SYMPTOMS
### History
- Multiple bouts of nonbloody vomiting and/or retching followed by hematemesis:
  - Most bleeding is small and resolves spontaneously.
  - Massive life-threatening hemorrhage can occur.
- Epigastric pain
- Back pain
- Dehydration:
  - Dizzy, light-headed; syncope

### Physical Exam
- Hematemesis
- Melena
- Postural hypotension
- Shock

## ESSENTIAL WORKUP
- CBC
- Rectal exam for occult blood

## DIAGNOSTIC TESTS & INTERPRETATION
### Lab
- Prothrombin time (PT), partial thromboplastin time (PTT), INR
- Electrolytes, BUN, creatinine, glucose
- Amylase/lipase if abdominal pain
- Type and cross-match:
  - At least four units of packed red blood cells (PRBCs) if bleeding is severe
- ECG if elderly or with cardiac history

### Imaging
- Upright chest radiograph for free air from esophageal or gastric perforation
- Upper endoscopy (esophagogastroscopy):
  - Procedure of choice to locate, identify, and treat source of bleeding

## DIFFERENTIAL DIAGNOSIS
- Nasopharyngeal bleeding
- Hemoptysis
- Esophageal rupture (Boerhaave syndrome)
- Esophagitis
- Gastritis
- Gastroenteritis
- Duodenitis
- Ulcer disease
- Varices
- Carcinoma
- Vascular-enteric fistula
- Hemangioma

**TREATMENT**

## PRE-HOSPITAL
- Airway control:
  - 100% oxygen or intubate if unresponsive or airway patency in jeopardy
- If hemodynamically unstable or massive hemorrhage:
  - Initiate 2 large-bore IV catheters.
  - 1-liter bolus (peds: 20 mL/kg) lactated Ringer (LR) solution or 0.9% normal saline (NS)
  - Trendelenburg position

## INITIAL STABILIZATION/THERAPY

- ABCs:
  - IV access with at least 1 large-bore catheter; more if unstable
  - Central catheter placement if unstable for more efficient delivery of fluids and monitoring of central venous pressure
  - IV fluids of either 0.9% NS (or LR) at 250 mL/h if stable; wide open if hemodynamically unstable
  - Dopamine for persistent hypotension unresponsive to aggressive fluid resuscitation
- Large-bore Ewald tube placement with evidence of large amount of bleeding:
  - Safe
  - Will not aggravate Mallory-Weiss tear
  - Lavage blood from stomach with water while patient is on side in Trendelenburg position.
- Nasogastric (NG) tube placement to check for active bleeding
- Transfuse O-negative red blood cells immediately if hypotensive and not responsive to 2 L of crystalloid.
- Most bleeding stops spontaneously with conservative therapy.

## ED TREATMENT/PROCEDURES

- NPO
- Transfuse PRBCs if unstable or lowering hematocrit with continued hemorrhage.
- Place Foley catheter to monitor urine output.
- Monitor fluid status closely.
- With continuing hemorrhage, arrange for immediate endoscopy:
  - Control bleeding endoscopically via:
    - Electrocoagulation
    - Injection therapy (epinephrine)
    - Band ligation
    - Hemoclips
    - Application of blood-clotting agents

- Intravenous vasopressin in massive bleeding and unavailable endoscopy
- In persistent/unresponsive hemorrhage, angiographic infusion of vasopressin
- Surgery—last but definitive treatment modality using techniques to oversew bleeding site or perform gastrectomy
- Failure of above may require gastric arterial embolization in patients of poor surgical risk.
- Avoid Sengstaken-Blakemore tubes (especially in presence of hiatal hernia).
- Antiemetics, antacids, and $H_2$ blockers are helpful.

## MEDICATION

- Dopamine: 2–20 bcg/kg/min IV piggyback (IVPB)
- Vasopressin: 0.1–0.5 IU/min IVPB titrating up to 0.9 IU/min as necessary

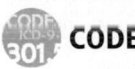

# FOLLOW-UP

## DISPOSITION

### Admission Criteria

- ICU admission for:
  - Continued or massive hemorrhage
  - Hemodynamic instability
  - Extreme age
  - Poor underlying medical condition
  - Complications
- General floor admission if never unstable and minimal bleed that has since cleared

### Discharge Criteria

- History of minimal bleed that has stopped
- Hemodynamically stable
- Normal/stable hematocrit
- Negative or trace heme-positive stool
- Negative or trace gastric aspirate

### Issues for Referral

Consult GI in ED if significant upper GI bleeding suspect that requires urgent endoscopy.

## FOLLOW-UP RECOMMENDATIONS

GI follow up for outpatient endoscopy if clinically stable for discharge.

# PEARLS AND PITFALLS

- Place 2 large bore IVs for patients with upper GI bleed.
- For massive GI bleed, initiate blood transfusion early.
- Contact GI early for emergent endoscopy with significant bleeding.

# ADDITIONAL READING

- Michel L, et al. Mallory-Weiss syndrome: Evolution of diagnostic and therapeutic patterns over two decades. *Ann Surg.* 1980;192:716–721.
- Sugawa C, et al. Mallory-Weiss syndrome: A study of 224 patients. *Am J Surg.* 1983;145(1):30–33.
- Takhar SS. Upper gastrointestinal bleeding. In *Clinical Practice of Emergency Medicine*, Fifth Edition. Wolfson AB, Hendey GW, Ling LJ, et al., Eds. 2010;548–550.
- Wu JC, Chan FK. Esophageal bleeding disorders. *Curr Opin Gastroenterol.* 2004;20:386–390.
- Younes Z, et al. The spectrum of spontaneous and iatrogenic esophageal injury: Perforations, Mallory-Weiss tears, and hematomas. *J Clin Gastroenterol.* 1999;29(4):306–317.

## See Also (Topic, Algorithm, Electronic Media Element)

Gastrointestinal Bleeding

# CODES

## ICD9

530.7 Gastroesophageal laceration-hemorrhage syndrome

M

# MALROTATION

Andrea Bracikowski
Sally Santen

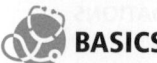 **BASICS**

## DESCRIPTION

- Incomplete rotation and fixation of intestine during embryogenesis during transition from extracolonic position during week 10 of gestation
- Risk factor:
  - Congenital defect
- Associated conditions:
  - Gastrointestinal anomalies:
    ○ Duodenal stenosis, atresia, web
    ○ Meckel diverticulum
    ○ Intussusception
    ○ Gastroesophageal reflux
    ○ Omphalocele or gastroschisis
    ○ Congenital diaphragmatic hernia
    ○ Hirschsprung disease
  - Metabolic acidosis
  - Congenital cardiac anomalies; present in 27% of patients with malrotation; increases morbidity to 61%

## ETIOLOGY

- Duodenojejunal junction remains right of midline.
- Cecum remains in the upper left abdomen with abnormal mesenteric attachments.
- Abnormal anatomy predisposes to obstruction and other conditions.
- Usually found in combination with other congenital anomalies (70%): Cardiac, esophageal, urinary, anal
- Epidemiology:
  - 1 in 500 live births
  - High mortality in infants: Up to 24%
  - Necrotic bowel at surgery increases mortality by 25×.
  - Incidence:
    ○ In neonates, male-to-female ratio 2:1
    ○ 40% of patients present within 1st yr.
    ○ 50% diagnosed by age 1 mo
    ○ 75% diagnosed by age 1 yr of life

## DIAGNOSIS

### SIGNS AND SYMPTOMS

- Neonates:
  - Bilious emesis
  - Abdominal distention
  - Bloody stools
  - Constipation/obstipation
  - Difficulty feeding
  - Poor weight gain
- >1 yr: Abdominal pain followed by bilious emesis
- Older children and adolescents:
  - Chronic vomiting
  - Intermittent colicky abdominal pain
  - Diarrhea
  - Hematemesis
  - Constipation
  - May not exhibit abnormal *physical* findings at time of presentation (50–75%)
- Adults: Symptoms vague and nonspecific
- General:
  - Dehydration, acidosis
  - Peritonitis
  - Ischemic bowel
  - Sepsis, shock

### History

- Bilious vomiting is hallmark.
- Other pertinent history—acute or chronic abdominal pain, poor feeding, lethargy

### Physical Exam

- Abdominal examination
- Evaluate for congenital anomalies.

### ESSENTIAL WORKUP

Diagnosis is suggested by history and physical exam findings and is delineated by contrast radiography.

## DIAGNOSTIC TESTS & INTERPRETATION

### Lab

- CBC
- Venous blood gas
- Electrolytes, BUN, creatinine, glucose; hypoglycemia in infants with poor feeding and emesis
- Urinalysis/urine culture
- Type and screen
- Prothrombin time, partial thromboplastin time, International Normalized Ratio

### Imaging

- Plain abdominal radiographs:
  - Diagnostic in <30%
  - Volvulus likely if accompanied by:
    ○ Duodenal obstruction (requiring no further studies)
    ○ Gastric distention with paucity of intraluminal gas distally
    ○ Generalized distention of small-bowel loops
  - Plain films in neonate to demonstrate obstruction of duodenum:
    ○ Triangular gas shadows in right upper quadrant from liver edge overlying air-filled duodenum
- Upper GI contrast studies:
  - 95% sensitive and 86% accurate
  - Findings:
    ○ Absence of ligament of Treitz
    ○ Dilation of proximal duodenum with termination in conical or beak shape
    ○ Spiral or corkscrew appearance of duodenum
    ○ Proximal jejunum on right side of abdomen (although readily displaced in neonates)
    ○ Thickening of small-bowel folds
- Contrast enema:
  - If obstruction equivocal
  - Evaluates position of cecum in midline of upper abdomen or to left of midline
  - >20% false-negative results
- Adjuncts:
  - US very sensitive in experienced hands
  - CT of little benefit
  - Angiogram (barber pole sign)

## DIFFERENTIAL DIAGNOSIS

- Early life:
  - Midgut volvulus
  - Hirschsprung disease
  - Necrotizing enterocolitis
- Children with acute abdominal pain and peritoneal signs:
  - Appendicitis
  - Intussusception
  - Overwhelming sepsis
- Older children and adults with vague abdominal pain:
  - Irritable bowel syndrome
  - Peptic ulcer disease
  - Biliary and pancreatic disease
  - Psychiatric disorders

#  TREATMENT

### ALERT
Midgut volvulus may result in need for rapid volume and electrolyte replacement/resuscitation to correct severe hypovolemia and metabolic acidosis.

### PRE-HOSPITAL
Rapid transport to ED

### INITIAL STABILIZATION/THERAPY
- ABCs
- NS (0.9%) IV fluid bolus (20 mL/kg) for shock, sepsis, or dehydration
- Consider nasogastric tube
- 2 IVs and/or CV catheter
- Initiate broad-spectrum antibiotics for signs of sepsis or peritonitis.

## ED TREATMENT/PROCEDURES

- Emergent surgical correction. May require transfer to facility with pediatric surgical expertise when associated with midgut volvulus for:
  - Detorsion of volvulus
  - Restoration of intestinal perfusion
  - Resection of obviously necrotic areas
  - Replacement of long segments with questionable vascular integrity back into abdominal cavity for return evaluation and possible celiotomy in 36 hr
- Diet:
  - NPO

### MEDICATION
- Broad-spectrum antibiotics prior to OR
- Correct fluid and electrolyte abnormalities.
- Vasopressors

#  FOLLOW-UP

### DISPOSITION

#### Admission Criteria
- Acute abdomen
- Surgical intervention
- Significant dehydration
- Acidosis
- Sepsis
- Shock

#### Discharge Criteria
Stable, minimally symptomatic, without associated conditions (unusual):
- Pediatric surgical evaluation prior to discharge

### Issues for Referral
Diagnostic evaluation often requires tertiary care pediatric hospital with pediatric surgical and pediatric radiologic expertise.

### FOLLOW-UP RECOMMENDATIONS
As dictated by pediatric surgical service

## PEARLS AND PITFALLS

- Early recognition of child with acute abdomen
- Prompt treatment of acidosis and shock
- Prompt referral to appropriate facility

## ADDITIONAL READING

- Kamal I. Defusing the intra-abdominal ticking bomb: Intestinal malrotation in children. *Can Med Assoc J.* 2000;162:1315–1317.
- Kouwenberg M, Severijnen RS, Kapusta L. Congenital cardiovascular defects in children with intestinal malrotation. *Pediatr Surg Int.* 2008;24(3): 257–263.
- Maxson RT, Franklin PA, Wagner CW. Malrotation in the older child: Surgical management, treatment, and outcome. *Am Surg.* 1995;61:135–138.

# 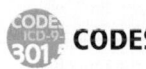 CODES

### ICD9
751.4 Congenital anomalies of intestinal fixation

M

# MANDIBULAR FRACTURES
*David W. Munter*

## 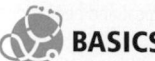 BASICS

### DESCRIPTION
- Typically owing to a direct force
- The most common area fractured is the angle, followed by the condyle, molar, and mental regions.
- Because of its thickness, the mandibular symphysis is rarely fractured.
- Multiple fractures are seen in >50% of cases owing to the ringlike structure of the mandible.
- Bilateral mandibular fractures most commonly result from motor vehicle accidents (MVAs).
- Open fractures are common, including lacerations of the gum overlying a fracture.

### ETIOLOGY
- The mandible is the third most common facial fracture following nasal and zygomatic fractures.
- MVAs, personal violence, contact sports, or industrial accidents
- Patients are often intoxicated and unable to give a clear history of events.
- Facial and head lacerations and facial fractures are the most commonly associated injuries.

#### Pediatric Considerations
- Mandibular fractures are uncommon in children <6 yr of age; when they do occur, they are often greenstick fractures and can be managed with soft diet alone.
- Inform parents that because any fracture of the mandible may damage permanent teeth, follow-up with a specialty consultant is advisable.

## 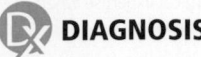 DIAGNOSIS

### SIGNS AND SYMPTOMS
- Mandibular pain
- Facial asymmetry, deformity, and dysphagia
- Malocclusion, decreased ROM of the temporomandibular joint (TMJ), trismus, or a grating sound conducted to the ear

#### History
- Mechanism of injury
- Malocclusion, dental pain, associated injuries

#### Physical Exam
- Inspect maxillofacial area for deformity, including ecchymosis or swelling.
- Malocclusion, trismus, or facial asymmetry
- Loose, fractured, or missing teeth; gross malalignment of teeth; separation of tooth interspaces, bleeding at the base of teeth; gum lacerations between teeth; and ecchymosis or hematoma of the floor of the mouth
- Step-off, bony disruption, or point tenderness with palpation along the entire length of the mandible
- Protrusion or lateral excursion of the jaw
- Interference with normal mandibular function, including decreased ROM or deviation of the mandible with opening:
  - The examiner should be able to insert three fingers between the mandible and maxilla.
  - Inability of patient to hold a tongue depressor laterally between teeth when pulled by the examiner or attempted to be broken by twisting (positive tongue-blade test)
- Paresthesia of the lower lip or gums indicates secondary damage to the inferior alveolar nerve.
- Inability to note motion of the mandibular condyles when palpated through the external ear canals suggests mandibular fracture.
- Tenderness of the condyle at the TMJ

### ESSENTIAL WORKUP
Diagnosis of mandibular fractures requires radiographs: Mandibular series, Panorex, or, if indicated for associated facial fractures, CT

### DIAGNOSTIC TESTS & INTERPRETATION
#### Lab
Indicated only if immediate operative intervention is required or for evaluation of other injuries

#### Imaging
- Plain films or dental panoramic views should be obtained.
- Plain films including an anteroposterior (AP), bilateral obliques, and Towne view should be obtained:
  - Mandibular views are best for evaluating the condyles and neck of mandible (more common site of fracture).
- Dental panoramic view may be obtained:
  - Panorex best evaluates the symphysis and body (less common fracture site).
- If condylar fracture is still suspected and not noted on initial radiographs, obtain CT of the condyles in the coronal plane.
- Missing teeth that cannot be found mandate a chest radiograph to rule out aspiration.
- Obtain cervical spine films if the neck cannot be cleared clinically.

### DIFFERENTIAL DIAGNOSIS
- Contusions
- Dislocation of the mandible:
  - If a single condyle is dislocated, the jaw will deviate away from the side of the dislocation.
  - If fractured, the jaw will deviate toward the fractured side.
- Isolated dental trauma

# TREATMENT

## PRE-HOSPITAL
Cautions:
- Protect the airway.
- Protect the cervical spine.
- Preserve any avulsed teeth.

## INITIAL STABILIZATION/THERAPY
- 20–40% of patients with mandibular fractures have associated injuries:
  - Treatment is directed toward immediate, potentially lethal injuries such as airway obstruction, aspiration, major hemorrhage, cervical spine injury, and intracranial injury.
- Airway must be protected.
- Cervical spine precautions
- If oral intubation cannot be performed, nasotracheal intubation should be performed unless associated facial injuries are present, in which case cricothyrotomy may be indicated.

## ED TREATMENT/PROCEDURES
- With the exception of condylar fractures, many mandibular fractures are associated with mucosal, gingival, or tooth socket disruption and should be considered open fractures:
  - Antibiotics such as penicillin, clindamycin, amoxicillin, amoxicillin/clavulanate, or erythromycin to cover intraoral anaerobic pathogens
- Tetanus prophylaxis for open fractures
- Analgesia such as acetaminophen, ibuprofen, or narcotic medications
- Definitive care usually consists of reduction and fixation by wiring upper and lower teeth in occlusion for 4–6 wk:
  - Linear, nondisplaced, or greenstick fractures may be treated with soft diet without wiring.
- If mandibular dislocation is present, while the jaw is open, apply bilateral downward pressure on the occlusal surface of the posterior lower teeth while grasping the mandible:
  - The goal is to free the condyle from its anterior position to the eminence.
  - Reduction is facilitated by muscle relaxants (diazepam or midazolam) or anesthetic injection of the masticatory muscles.
  - A bite block should be used, or the examiner's fingers should be wrapped in gauze to prevent injury.

## MEDICATION
- Acetaminophen: 650 mg (peds: 10–15 mg/kg) PO q4h
- Amoxicillin/clavulanate: 500/125-875/125 mg PO b.i.d. (peds: 40 mg/kg/day of amoxicillin) PO b.i.d.
- Amoxicillin: 500 mg PO t.i.d. (peds: 40 mg/kg PO div t.i.d.)
- Clindamycin: 150–450 mg PO q.i.d. (peds: 10–20 mg/kg/24 hr)
- Diazepam: 5–10 mg (peds: 0.1–0.2 mg/kg) IV
- Erythromycin: 250–500 mg (peds: 30–50 mg/kg/24 hr) PO q.i.d.
- Ibuprofen: 600–800 mg (peds: 20–40 mg/kg/24 hr) PO t.i.d.–q.i.d.
- Midazolam: 2–5 mg (peds: safety not established, but 0.02–0.05 mg/kg per dose has been used) IV
- Penicillin: 250–500 mg (peds: 25–50 mg/kg/24 hr) PO q.i.d.

# FOLLOW-UP

## DISPOSITION
### Admission Criteria
- Significant displacement or associated dental trauma—open fractures require urgent specialty consultation for possible admission.
- The severity of associated trauma may indicate admission.
- Any patient with the potential for airway compromise should be admitted.
- An unreliable patient with nondisplaced fractures should be admitted for definitive fixation.
- In the pediatric population, if the mechanism of injury is not appropriate to the injuries seen, pediatric or consultation with child protective services should be obtained.

### Discharge Criteria
Patients with nondisplaced closed fractures may be discharged on analgesics and a soft diet.

## FOLLOW-UP RECOMMENDATIONS
Oral or maxillofacial surgeon within 2–3 days for uncomplicated fractures

# PEARLS AND PITFALLS
- Failure to recognize that a gum laceration overlying a mandibular fracture represents an open fracture
- Missing mandibular condylar fractures when only a Panorex film is obtained. If there is condyle tenderness or malocclusion, obtain plain films or CT.

# ADDITIONAL READING
- Alpert B, Tiwana PS, Kushner GM. Management of comminuted fractures of the mandible. *Oral Maxillofac Surg Clin North Am*. 2009;21(2):185–192.
- Cole P, Kaufman Y, et al. Principles of pediatric mandibular fracture management. *Plast Reconstr Surg*. 2009;123(3):1022–1024.
- Ellis E. Management of fractures through the angle of the mandible. *Oral Maxillofac Surg Clin North Am*. 2009;21(2):163–174.
- Laskin DM. Management of condylar process fractures. *Oral Maxillofac Surg Clin North Am*. 2009;21(2):193–196.
- Luyk NH, Ferguson JW. The diagnosis and initial management of the fractured mandible. *Am J Emerg Med*. 1991;9:352–359.
- Myall RW. Management of mandibular fractures in children. *Oral Maxillofac Surg Clin North Am*. 2009;21(2):197–201.

### See Also (Topic, Algorithm, Electronic Media Element)
- Dental Trauma
- Facial Fractures

# CODES

## ICD9
- 802.20 Closed fracture of unspecified site of mandible
- 802.21 Closed fracture of condylar process of mandible
- 802.25 Closed fracture of angle of jaw

M

# MARINE ENVENOMATION

*Adam Black*
*Timothy B. Erickson*

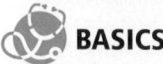

## BASICS

### DESCRIPTION
Marine envenomation refers to poisoning caused by sting or bite from a vertebrate or invertebrate marine species.

### ETIOLOGY
- Sponges:
  - Contain sharp spicules with irritants that cause pruritic dermatitis
- Coelenterates (Cnidaria jellyfish):
  - Contain stinging cells known as nematocysts on their tentacles
  - Fluid-filled cysts eject sharp, hollow thread-tube on contact.
  - Thread-tube penetrates skin and envenomates the victim.
  - Box jellyfish can kill within 60 sec.
- Starfish:
  - Sharp, rigid spines are coated with slimy venom.
- Sea urchins:
  - Hollow, sharp spines filled with various toxins
- Sea cucumbers:
  - Hollow tentacles secrete holothurin, a liquid toxin.
- Cone shells:
  - Venom injected through dartlike, detachable tooth
  - Active peptides interfere with neuromuscular transmission.
  - Presents with puncture wounds similar to wasp stings
- Stingrays:
  - Most common cause of human marine envenomations
  - Tapered spines attached to tail inject venom into victim.
- Scorpion fish:
  - Lionfish usually mild; stonefish can be life threatening.
  - Sharp spines along dorsum and pelvis of fish
  - Often stepped on inadvertently
  - Neurotoxic venom
- Catfish:
  - Dorsal and pectoral spines contain venom glands.
- Sea snakes:
  - Hollow fangs with associated venom glands
  - Highly neurotoxic venom blocks neuromuscular transmission.

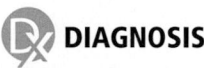

## DIAGNOSIS

### SIGNS AND SYMPTOMS
- Sponges:
  - Itching and burning a few hours after contact
  - Local joint swelling and soft tissue edema
  - Fever
  - Malaise
  - Dizziness
  - Nausea
  - Muscle cramps
  - In severe cases, desquamation in 10 days to 2 mo

- Coelenterates (Cnidaria jellyfish):
  - Mild envenomation:
    - Immediate stinging sensation
    - Pruritus
    - Paresthesia, burning sensation
    - Throbbing
    - Blistering/local edema/wheal formation
  - Moderate/severe:
    - Neurologic: Ataxia, paralysis, delirium, seizures
    - Cardiovascular: Anaphylaxis, hemolysis, hypotension, dysrhythmias
    - Respiratory: Bronchospasm, laryngeal edema, pulmonary edema, respiratory failure
    - Musculoskeletal: Muscle cramps or spasm, arthralgias
    - Gastrointestinal: Nausea, vomiting, diarrhea, dysphagia, hypersalivation/thirst
    - Ophthalmologic: Conjunctivitis, corneal ulcers, elevated intraocular pressure
- Echinodermata:
  - Starfish:
    - Immediate pain
    - Bleeding
    - Mild edema
    - Paresthesias, nausea, vomiting if severe
  - Sea urchins:
    - Intense pain and severe local muscle aches
    - Nausea, vomiting
    - Paresthesias, hypotension, or respiratory distress with multiple stings
  - Sea cucumbers:
    - Mild contact dermatitis
    - Corneal and conjunctival involvement: Severe reactions can lead to blindness.
- Mollusks:
  - Cone shells:
    - Puncture wounds similar to wasp stings
    - Sharp burning and stinging
    - Paresthesias indicate severe envenomation.
    - Can evolve into muscular paralysis and respiratory failure, dysphagia, syncope, disseminated intravascular coagulation
- Stingrays:
  - Puncture wounds or jagged lacerations
  - Local, intense pain, edema, bleeding; necrosis if severe
  - Nausea, vomiting, diarrhea
  - Diaphoresis
  - Headache
  - Tachycardia
  - Seizures
  - Paralysis
  - Hypotension
  - Dysrhythmias
- Scorpion fish:
  - Intense local pain for 6–12 hr
  - Erythema may progress to cellulitis.
  - Headache
  - Nausea, vomiting, diarrhea
  - Pallor
  - Delirium
  - Seizures
  - Fever
  - Hypertension

- Catfish:
  - Local pain, ischemic appearance progressing to erythema
  - Swelling, bleeding, and edema
  - Local muscle spasms
  - Diaphoresis
  - Neuropathy, fasciculations, weakness, syncope
- Sea snakes:
  - Bite initially causes very little pain.
  - Pinlike pairs of fang marks
  - Onset from 5 min to 6 hr
  - Muscle pain, lower extremity paralysis, arthralgias
  - Trismus, blurred vision, dysphagia, drowsiness
  - Severe signs include:
    - Ascending paralysis
    - Aspiration
    - Coma
    - Renal and liver failure
  - If untreated, 25% mortality

### History
- Time of envenomation
- Body part envenomated
- Activity when envenomated (scuba diving, swimming, surfing, fishing, boating, pet care)
- Type of water (salt water, fresh water, aquarium)
- Geographic location (resort, international, remote, local, aquarium, zoo, pet store)
- Onset of symptoms, pain
- Mental status changes
- Near drowning

### Physical Exam
- Vital signs
- Airway
- Mental status
- Cardiopulmonary exam
- Dermatologic exam, foreign bodies, cellulitis, blistering

### ESSENTIAL WORKUP
- Careful history, repeated evaluation of wound sites
- Assessment of ABCs

### DIAGNOSTIC TESTS & INTERPRETATION
#### Lab
- CBC
- Electrolytes, BUN, creatinine, and glucose levels
- LFT
- Urinalysis
- Arterial blood gases if severe symptoms

#### Imaging
Soft tissue radiographs to detect foreign body

### DIFFERENTIAL DIAGNOSIS
- Allergic reaction
- Cellulitis
- Gastroenteritis
- Aspiration pneumonia
- Near drowning

# TREATMENT

## PRE-HOSPITAL
- Remove victim from water source.
- Control airway, breathing.
- Control hemorrhage.
- Detoxify venom with proper wound irrigation as discussed below.

## INITIAL STABILIZATION/THERAPY
- Airway, breathing, and circulation management (ABCs)
- Establish IV access with 0.9% NS.

## ED TREATMENT/PROCEDURES
- General:
  - Prepare for anaphylactic reactions (epinephrine/steroids).
  - Prepare for intubation if needed.
  - Benadryl for itch, burn, hives
  - Tetanus prophylaxis
  - Corticosteroids for severe local reactions
  - Narcotic analgesia for severe pain
  - Antibiotic prophylaxis for the following:
    o Large lacerations or burns
    o Deep puncture wounds
    o Grossly contaminated wounds
    o Elderly or chronically ill
  - Antibiotic choices:
    o Trimethoprim/sulfamethoxazole (TMP-SMX; Bactrim)
    o Tetracycline
    o Ciprofloxacin
    o Third-generation cephalosporin
- Sponges:
  - Gently dry skin and remove spicule:
    o Adhesive tape may aid in removal.
  - 5% acetic acid (vinegar) (or 40–70% isopropyl alcohol) soaks q.i.d. for 10–30 min
- Coelenterates (Cnidaria jellyfish):
  - Rinse wound with salt water or seawater:
    o Hypotonic (fresh or tap water solutions), trigger more nematocysts
  - Do not rub skin to avoid release of nematocysts.
  - Inactivate toxin with 30-min soak of 5% acetic acid (vinegar)
  - Remove remaining nematocysts with razor, clam shell.
  - Apply topical anesthetics once nematocysts are removed.
  - Sea Safe jellyfish sun block products are available.
  - Box-jellyfish sting envenomation (Australia) emergent cases:
    o Administer *Chironex* antivenin: 1 amp (20,000 units) IV diluted 1:5 with crystalloid.
  - Corticosteroids for severe reactions
- Starfish:
  - Immerse in nonscalding hot water for pain relief.
  - Irrigate and explore all puncture wounds.
  - Prophylactic antibiotics for significant wounds

- Sea urchins:
  - Immerse in nonscalding hot water for pain relief.
  - Remove any remaining spines.
  - Prophylactic antibiotics for significant wounds
- Sea cucumbers:
  - Immerse in nonscalding hot water for pain relief.
  - 5% acetic acid soaks
  - Ocular involvement:
    o Proparacaine for pain
    o Copious irrigation with normal saline
    o Careful slit-lamp exam
- Cone shells:
  - Hot water immersion for pain relief
  - Be prepared for cardiac or respiratory support.
- Stingrays:
  - Copious irrigation with removal of any visible spines
  - Local suction is controversial.
  - Hot water soaks for pain relief
  - Narcotics for pain control
  - High incidence of bacterial infection:
    o Administer prophylactic antibiotics for significant wounds.
- Scorpion fish:
  - Hot water soaks for pain relief and venom inactivation
  - Copious irrigation, removal of any visible spines
  - Local lidocaine or regional block for severe pain
  - Surgical exploration for deep penetration/foreign bodies
  - Stonefish antivenin for severe envenomations:
    o One 2-mL amp diluted in 50-mL saline IV slow
    o May cause serum sickness
- Catfish:
  - Hot water soaks for pain relief and venom inactivation
  - Copious irrigation, removal of any visible spines
  - Consider local lidocaine, regional block, or narcotics for severe pain.
  - Surgical exploration for deep penetration, foreign bodies
  - Leave puncture wounds open to heal.
  - Consider prophylactic antibiotics for hand, foot, or deep wounds.
- Sea snakes:
  - Immobilize bitten extremity.
  - Apply pressure bandage for venous occlusion (prehospital).
  - Keep victim warm and still.
  - Polyvalent sea snake antivenin reduces mortality to 3%:
    o May require 3–10 amps (1000 U each)
    o Prepare early for assisted ventilation.

## MEDICATION
- Cefixime: 400 mg (peds: 8 mg/kg/24 hr) PO daily
- Ciprofloxacin: 500 mg PO b.i.d.
- Epinephrine: 0.3–0.5 mL SC 1:1,000 (peds: 0.01 mL/kg)
- Tetracycline: 500 mg PO q.i.d. (caution with photosensitivity)
- TMP-SMX (Bactrim DS): 1 tab [peds: 5 mg liquid (40/200/5 mL)/10 kg per dose] PO b.i.d. (caution with photosensitivity)

# FOLLOW-UP

## DISPOSITION
### Admission Criteria
Significant signs of systemic involvement or need for antivenom administration

### Discharge Criteria
No signs of systemic illness after 8 hr of observation

### Issues for Referral
- Zoos, aquariums for available supplies of antivenom; poison control centers: 800-222-1222
- Wound checks within 48 hr

## PEARLS AND PITFALLS
- Following marine envenomations, proper wound care is essential; antibiotic therapy as indicated.
- Most toxins are detoxified with either temperature change (hot water) or pH alteration (more acidic).
- Specific antivenoms for box jellyfish, stone fish, and sea snake envenomations are available but in limited supply; acquire early in treatment course.

## ADDITIONAL READING
- Atkinson PR, Boyle A, Hartlin D, et al. Is hot water an effective treatment for marine envenomation? *Emerg Med J.* 2006;23(7):503–508.
- Bedry R, de Haro L. Venomous and poisonous animals. V. Envenomations by marine invertebrates. *Med Trop.* 2007;67(3):223–231.
- Brenneke F, Hatz C. Stonefish envenomation: A lucky outcome. *Travel Med Infect Dis.* 2006,4(5): 281–285.
- Clark RF, Girard RH, Roa D, et al. Stingray envenomation: A retrospective review of clinical presentation and treatment in 119 cases. *J Emerg Med.* 2007;33(1):33–37.
- Fernandez I, Valladolid G, Varon J, et al. Encounters with venomous sea-life. *J Emerg Med.* 2009; December 31 (Epub ahead of print).
- Vohra R, Clark R, Shah N. A pilot study of occupational envenomations in North America zoos and aquaria. *Clin Toxicol.* 2008;46(9):790–793.

# CODES

## ICD9
989.5 Toxic effect of venom

M

# MASTITIS

*Marco Coppola*
*Arun V. Raghavan*

 **BASICS**

## DESCRIPTION
- Infection of the breast causing pain, swelling, and erythema
- Most commonly in women who are breast-feeding
- Often with systemic symptoms also:
  - Malaise
  - Fever
- Incidence may be as high as 33% in lactating woman.
- Most common during second and third weeks postpartum
- 75–95% occur before infant is 3 mo old.
- More common in advanced maternal age and patients with diabetes
- Complications:
  - Recurrence
  - Abscess
  - Sepsis
  - Necrotizing fasciitis
  - Fistula
  - Scarring
  - Breast hypoplasia

## ETIOLOGY
- *Staphylococcus aureus* most common
- Other causes:
  - Coagulase-negative *Staphylococcus*
  - *Streptococcus* spp.
  - *Escherichia coli*
  - *Haemophilus influenzae*
  - *Candida albicans*

- Risk factors:
  - Cleft lip or palate
  - Cracked nipples
  - Infant attachment issues
  - Local milk stasis
  - Nipple piercing
  - Poor maternal nutrition
  - Previous mastitis
  - Primiparity
  - Restriction from a tight bra
  - Sore nipples
  - Short frenulum in infant
  - Use of a manual breast pump
  - Yeast infection

 **DIAGNOSIS**

## SIGNS AND SYMPTOMS
- Fever and chills
- General malaise
- Tachycardia
- Breast pain, induration, erythema, warmth; usually unilateral
- Onset typically 2–3 wk to months postpartum while breast-feeding
- Rare during first postpartum week

### History
- Flu-like symptoms
- Fever, malaise, and myalgia
- Breast redness, swelling
- Breast pain
- Decreased milk outflow

### Physical Exam
- Breast warmth and tenderness
- Breast firmness
- Breast tenderness
- Breast erythema

## ESSENTIAL WORKUP
Physical exam with special attention to detecting abscess:
- Abscess is frequently difficult to detect, but is more common in periareolar area.
- Purulent nipple discharge with palpation

## DIAGNOSTIC TESTS & INTERPRETATION
### Lab
Breast milk culture is usually not required.

### Imaging
Consider breast US if abscess is suspected:
- Mammography is not indicated acutely.

## DIFFERENTIAL DIAGNOSIS
- Breast engorgement:
  - Transient fever <39°C of 4–16 hr duration
  - Appearing 48–72 hr postpartum
  - Bilateral nonerythematous engorgement
- Carcinoma (inflammatory)
- Cyst, tumor
- Abscess formation

 **TREATMENT**

## INITIAL STABILIZATION/THERAPY
No specific stabilization

## ED TREATMENT/PROCEDURES
- Continue breast-feeding:
  - Child and mother are colonized with the same organisms.
  - Milk from a breast with mastitis may be protective.
  - If an infant does not like the taste of milk from a breast with mastitis, then encourage the mother to pump and discard.

- Improve breast-feeding technique:
  – May need a lactation consultant
- Maintain good maternal hydration.
- If mild symptoms and early in disease, antibiotics may not be necessary.
- Oral antibiotics for 10 days:
  – β-Lactamase–resistant penicillin, eg, dicloxacillin
  – First-generation cephalosporin, eg, cephalexin
  – Clindamycin, trimethoprim/sulfamethoxazole (TMP/SMX) or erythromycin if penicillin allergic
- Surgical consultation if evidence of abscess
- If considering methicillin-resistant *S. aureus* (MRSA), treat according to local susceptibility patterns:
  – Clindamycin
  – TMP/SMX
  – Vancomycin

### ALERT
Vertical transmission of HIV (mother to infant) may be increased in mothers with mastitis.

### MEDICATION
- Amoxicillin/clavulanate: 875 mg PO q12h
- Cephalexin: 500 mg PO q6h for 10 days
- Clindamycin: 300 mg PO q6h for 10 days
- Dicloxacillin: 500 mg PO q6h for 10 days (first-line treatment)
- Erythromycin: 500 mg PO q6h for 10 days
- Mupirocin 2% ointment t.i.d.
- TMP/SMX: 160 mg/800 mg PO q12h:
  – Avoid in compromised infants and healthy infants <2 mo old
- If MRSA positive: Vancomycin 1 g IV q12h

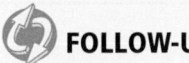

## FOLLOW-UP

### DISPOSITION
#### Admission Criteria
- Incision and drainage under general anesthesia may be necessary and require admission.
- Immunocompromised or evidence of septicemia
- Patients with diabetes may account for 1/3 of mastitis cases.

#### Discharge Criteria
- Most patients may be managed in outpatient setting.
- Most symptoms resolve within 48 hr of therapy.
- In simple mastitis, breast-feeding may be continued, including using affected breast:
  – Gently massage to enhance drainage.
  – Counsel that this will not harm baby.
- Breast support, warm compresses, and analgesia for comfort
- In frank abscess, discontinue breast-feeding until purulent discharge resolves.
- Follow-up should be arranged to exclude diagnosis of inflammatory carcinoma.

### FOLLOW-UP RECOMMENDATIONS
- Patients should follow up with primary care physician.
- International Lactation Consultant Association provides a list of lactation consultants: http://www.ilca.org
- La Leche League offers numerous resources: http://www.llli.org

## PEARLS AND PITFALLS
- Most cases respond to lactation and warm compresses without antibiotics.
- Cessation of breast-feeding will lead to increased milk stasis and increased risk for abscess formation.
- One of the most common complications of mastitis is cessation of breast-feeding.

## ADDITIONAL READING
- Jahanfar S, Ng CJ, Teng CL. Antibiotics for mastitis in breastfeeding women. *Cochrane Database Syst Rev.* 2009;(1):CD005458.
- Spencer JP. Management of mastitis in breastfeeding women. *Am Fam Physician.* 2008;78:727–731.

### See Also (Topic, Algorithm, Electronic Media Element)
- Abscess
- Cellulitis
- Community-Acquired MRSA

 CODES

### ICD9
- 675.20 Nonpurulent mastitis associated with childbirth, unspecified as to episode of care
- 675.21 Nonpurulent mastitis associated with childbirth, delivered, with or without mention of antepartum condition
- 675.22 Nonpurulent mastitis associated with childbirth, delivered, with mention of postpartum complication

M

# MASTOIDITIS

*Jonathan Fisher*

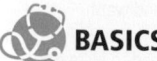

## BASICS

### DESCRIPTION
- Inflammation of the mastoid air cells of the temporal bone, generally caused by direct extension of acute purulent otitis media
- Middle ear and mastoid air cells are contiguous via the aditus and antrum.
- Fluid accumulation from closure of channel due to otitis media creates opportunity for infection.
- Manifestation ranges from clinically insignificant inflammation of mastoid air cells to infection and destruction of the bone.
- Acute mastoiditis:
  - Occurs to some degree in all cases of otitis media
  - Early signs and symptoms are those of acute otitis media.
  - Usually secondary to contamination with infectious material trapped in the mastoid by inflammatory obstruction of the channel between middle ear and mastoid air cells
- Acute mastoiditis with periostitis:
  - As infection progresses, periosteum of the mastoid bone is involved, causing periostitis.
  - Subperiosteal abscess may be present.
- Acute mastoid ostitis (also called coalescent mastoiditis):
  - Progression of the infection within the mastoid air cells leads to destruction of the mastoid trabeculae, causing coalescence of bony trabeculae.
  - Mastoid empyema or a draining fistula may be present.
  - May progress to severe head and neck complications if untreated
- Masked mastoiditis:
  - Mastoid infection, which lingers after an acute otitis media has been treated
  - May progress to acute or coalescent mastoiditis
- Chronic mastoiditis:
  - Infection lasting >3 mo
- Mastoiditis can be a complication of a primary disorder:
  - Leukemia
  - Mononucleosis
  - Sarcoma of the temporal bone
  - HIV
  - Kawasaki disease
- Mastoiditis used to be more common prior to the use of antibiotics for acute otitis media.
- More common in young children and infants

## ETIOLOGY
- Organisms in acute mastoiditis are similar to those in acute otitis media, but differ in frequency:
  - *Streptococcus pneumoniae*
  - Group A streptococcus
  - *Staphylococcus aureus*
  - *Haemophilus influenzae*
- Gram-negative enteric bacteria most common with chronic mastoiditis:
  - *Pseudomonas aeruginosa*
  - *Escherichia coli*
  - *Proteus mirabilis*
  - Bacteroides species
- Other less common causes:
  - *Mycobacterium tuberculosis*
  - Aspergillus species in immunocompromised states

### Pediatric Considerations
- More frequently seen in the pediatric population due to strong association with otitis media
- *S. pneumoniae* most common cause in children

## DIAGNOSIS

### SIGNS AND SYMPTOMS
#### History
- Ear pain
- Otorrhea
- Mild to severe hearing loss
- Fever
- Headache
- History of irritability in a child
- History of recurrent otitis media

#### Physical Exam
- Tenderness, edema, and erythema over the mastoid
- Lateral and inferior displacement of the auricle
- Loss of the postauricular crease
- Swelling of the posterior and superior ear canal wall
- Tympanic membrane abnormalities consistent with severe otitis media
- Purulent fluid drainage from the auditory canal
- Bulging tympanic membrane

### ESSENTIAL WORKUP
Mastoiditis is a clinical diagnosis.

## DIAGNOSTIC TESTS & INTERPRETATION
### Lab
- CBC:
  - Leukocytosis
- Cultures of drainage important owing to diversity of organisms:
  - If spontaneous drainage present or after surgical drainage
- Blood cultures if patient appears toxic

### Imaging
- Mastoid plain radiographs:
  - Early stage of disease may show hazy or cloudy but intact mastoid.
  - May reveal opacification or coalescence of the mastoid air cells or coalescence as disease progresses
  - Unreliable due to low sensitivity
- CT scan:
  - More useful, especially if abscess formation present
  - Can determine presence and extent of destruction of trabeculae as well as evaluate for the complications of mastoiditis
- MRI:
  - If intracranial involvement suspected but not confirmed by CT

### Pediatric Considerations
Conservative use of CT in children may be warranted. The diagnosis can often be made on clinical grounds and avoids radiation exposure.

### Diagnostic Procedures/Surgery
Lumbar puncture:
- Cerebrospinal fluid evaluation for signs of meningitis

### DIFFERENTIAL DIAGNOSIS
- Otitis media
- Cellulitis
- External otitis media
- Scalp infection with inflammation of posterior auricular nodes
- Rubella: Posterior auricular node enlargement
- Trauma to pinna or postauricular area
- Meningitis

**TREATMENT**

### INITIAL STABILIZATION/THERAPY
- ABCs
- Airway management for signs of airway compromise
- 0.9% NS IV fluid bolus for hypotension/volume depletion

### ED TREATMENT/PROCEDURES
- Initiate IV antibiotics
- Otolaryngologist consult for surgical drainage:
  - Drainage is the definitive therapy for acute or coalescent mastoiditis.
  - Emergent drainage if the patient appears toxic
  - Types of surgical procedures:
    ○ Myringotomy drainage and tympanostomy tube placement
    ○ Mastoidectomy and drainage for severe extension (needed in ~50% of cases)

### MEDICATION
- Initiate IV antibiotics:
  - Given increasing proportion of *S. aureus* as causative organism, consider including antistaphylococcal agent before culture results.
  - Parenteral antibiotics can be switched to PO after patient afebrile for 36–48 hr.
  - Consider antipseudomonal coverage when appropriate.
- Administer pain medications:
  - NSAIDs
  - PO or parenteral narcotics

#### First Line
- Ceftriaxone: 1–2 g (peds: 50–75 mg/kg/24 h) IV q12–24h
- Cefotaxime: 1–2 g (peds: 50–180 mg/kg/24 h) IV q4–6h

#### Second Line
- Ampicillin sulbactam: 1.5–3 g IV q6h
- Chloramphenicol: 50–100 mg/kg/24h IV or PO q6h
- Clindamycin: 600–2,700 mg/d IV divided q6–12h or 150–450 mg PO q6–8h; (peds: 20–40 mg/kg/d IM/IV divided q6–8h or 10–25 mg/kg/d PO divided q6–8h)
- Imipenem: 250 mg–1 g IV q6–8h
- Ticarcillin clavulanate: 3.1 g IV q4–6h
- Piperacillin/tazobactam: 3.375 g IV q6h
- Vancomycin: 1 g q8h (peds 40 mg/kg/24h) IV q6–8h

 **FOLLOW-UP**

### DISPOSITION
#### Admission Criteria
- Clinical suspicion of acute or coalescent mastoiditis
- Subperiosteal abscess
- Toxic appearing

#### Discharge Criteria
Patients with acute or coalescent mastoiditis should not be discharged.

#### Issues for Referral
- Otolaryngologist consult for possible surgical drainage
- Audiography should be performed after resolution of mastoiditis to assess hearing loss.

### FOLLOW-UP RECOMMENDATIONS
Patients should follow-up with otolaryngologist after discharge, if not admitted.

### COMPLICATIONS
- Bezold abscess:
  - Extension of infection to soft tissue below pinna or behind the sternocleidomastoid muscle of neck after erosion through the mastoid tip
- Petrositis:
  - Spread of the infection to the petrous air cells
- Osteomyelitis of the calvarium
- Intracranial complications:
  - Subperiosteal abscess
  - Subdural empyema:
    ○ Extension of infection to CNS with empyema around the tentorium
  - Sinus thromboses

## PEARLS AND PITFALLS

- It is important to maintain a high index of suspicion for mastoiditis in setting of persistent or untreated acute otitis media.
- Failure to recognize meningitis or intracranial involvement, which require more aggressive management, is a pitfall.

## ADDITIONAL READING

- Anderson KJ. Mastoiditis. *Pediatr Rev*. 2009;30: 233–234.
- Chase KS, Doty CI. Mastoiditis. Emergency medicine. Emedicine. Available at http://emedicine.medscape.com/article/784176-overview. Accessed January 10, 2010.
- Marx JA, Hockberger RS, Walls RM, et al. *Rosen's Emergency Medicine: Concepts and Clinical Practice*, 7th ed. St. Louis, MO: Mosby, 2009.
- Tamir S, Schwartz Y, Peleg U, et al. Acute mastoiditis in children: Is computed tomography always necessary? *Ann Otol Rhinol Laryngol*. 2009;118:565–569.
- Tamir S, Schwartz Y, Peleg U, et al. Shifting trends: Mastoiditis from a surgical to a medical disease. *Am J Otolaryngol*. 2009; Epub.

**CODES**

### ICD9
- 383.00 Acute mastoiditis without complications
- 383.1 Chronic mastoiditis
- 383.9 Unspecified mastoiditis

M

# MDMA POISONING

*Mark B. Mycyk*

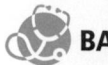

## BASICS

### DESCRIPTION
- MDMA: 3,4-methylenedioxymethamphetamine ("ecstasy")
- Schedule I drug manufactured illegally
- Used recreationally:
  - Rave parties
  - Dance clubs
  - College campuses
- Onset of effects: 15–30 min after ingestion
- Duration of effects: 2–6 hr
- Pills commonly contain contaminants:
  - Caffeine
  - Ephedrine
  - Dextromethorphan
  - Ketamine
  - Related methylated amphetamines: 3,4-methylenedioxyamphetamine (MDA), 3,4-methylenedioxy-*N*-ethylamphetamine (MDEA), 3,4-methylenedioxy-*N*-butylamphetamine (MDBA), *para*-methoxyamphetamine (PMA)
- Pathophysiology:
  - Amphetamine-like structure stimulates catecholamine release.
  - Mescaline-like ring structure enhances serotonergic and dopaminergic activity.

### ETIOLOGY
Deliberate or accidental ingestion of MDMA

## DIAGNOSIS

### SIGNS AND SYMPTOMS
- Overdose:
  - Altered mental status
  - Severe sympathomimetic symptoms
- Central nervous system:
  - Excitation
  - Coma
  - Seizures
  - Cerebral edema
- Cardiovascular:
  - Hypertension (early)
  - Hypotension (late)
  - Palpitations
  - Ventricular tachycardia and ectopy
- Pulmonary:
  - Pulmonary edema
- Metabolic:
  - Hyponatremia
  - Hypoglycemia
  - Syndrome of inappropriate antidiuretic hormone
- Musculoskeletal:
  - Bruxism
  - Restlessness
  - Rigidity
- Renal:
  - Rhabdomyolysis
- Hepatic:
  - Jaundice
  - Hepatitis
- Hematologic:
  - Disseminated intravascular coagulation
- Gastrointestinal:
  - Vomiting
  - Diarrhea
  - Abdominal cramping
- Psychiatric:
  - Euphoria
  - Flight of ideas
  - Delirium/hallucinations
- Other:
  - Hyperthermia
  - Mydriasis
  - Nystagmus

### ESSENTIAL WORKUP
- Diagnosis based on clinical presentation and an accurate history
- Obtain core temperature.
- Exclude toxic coingestants or contaminants.

### DIAGNOSTIC TESTS & INTERPRETATION
*Lab*
- Electrolytes, BUN, creatinine, and glucose levels
- Prothrombin time, partial thromboplastin time, International Normalized Ratio
- Urine dip for blood and myoglobin
- Urine toxicology screen to exclude coingestants:
  - May cause positive amphetamine and methamphetamine screen
- Quantitative MDMA levels rarely helpful
- Creatine phosphokinase level if rhabdomyolysis suspected
- Liver function tests for significant overdose or suspected hepatitis

*Imaging*
- CXR if suspected aspiration pneumonia
- Head CT if suspected intracranial hemorrhage

*Diagnostic Procedures/Surgery*
ECG:
- Sinus tachycardia (most common)
- Dysrhythmias, conduction disturbances

### DIFFERENTIAL DIAGNOSIS
- Cocaine overdose
- Amphetamine overdose
- Anticholinergic overdose
- Serotonin syndrome
- Occult head injury
- Sepsis
- Thyroid storm
- Pheochromocytoma

## TREATMENT

### PRE-HOSPITAL
- Transport all pills/pill bottles involved in overdose for identification in ED.
- Watch for MDMA paraphernalia:
  - Pacifiers
  - Glow sticks
  - Surgical masks

### INITIAL STABILIZATION/THERAPY
ABCs:
- Airway control is essential.
- Administer supplemental oxygen.
- Intubate if indicated.
- IV access
- Naloxone, thiamine, dextrose (or Accu-Chek), if altered mental status

## ED TREATMENT/PROCEDURES

- Supportive care
- Monitor core temperature and cardiac rhythm for at least 6 hr.
- Hydrate with 0.9% normal saline (NS) IV.
- Hypertension:
  – Nitroprusside
  – Phentolamine
  – Esmolol
- Hypotension:
  – 0.9% NS IV bolus
  – Trendelenburg position
  – Pressors titrated to blood pressure
- Anxiety, restlessness, agitation:
  – Diazepam or lorazepam as needed
- Seizures:
  – Treat initially with benzodiazepines.
  – Phenobarbital for persistent seizures
- Rhabdomyolysis:
  – Hydrate aggressively with 0.9% NS IV.
  – Consider sodium bicarbonate administration.
  – Hemodialysis if renal failure
- Hyperthermia:
  – Standard cooling measures
  – Treat agitation with benzodiazepines.
  – Consider dantrolene in refractory cases.

## MEDICATION

- Dantrolene: 1–2 mg/kg to max 10 mg/kg IV
- Diazepam: 5–10 mg (peds: 0.2–0.5 mg/kg) IV q10–15min
- Esmolol: 500 mg/kg IV bolus, then 50 mg/kg/min IV
- Lorazepam: 2–6 mg (peds: 0.05–0.1 mg/kg) IV q10–15min

- Naloxone: 0.4–2 mg (peds: 0.1 mg/kg; neonatal: 10–30 mg/kg) IV or IM
- Nitroprusside: 0.3 mg/kg/min to max 10 μg/kg/min
- Phenobarbital: 10–20 mg/kg IV (loading dose)
- Phentolamine: 1–5 mg (peds: 0.02–0.1 mg/kg) IV bolus q5–10min
- Propofol: 0.5–1.0 mg/kg IV (loading dose), then 5–50 mg/kg/min (maintenance dose)

# FOLLOW-UP

## DISPOSITION

### Admission Criteria

- Altered mental status
- Seizures
- Persistent cardiovascular instability
- Rhabdomyolysis
- Loss of behavioral control
- Disseminated intravascular coagulation

### Discharge Criteria

Asymptomatic 6 hr after oral overdose

## FOLLOW-UP RECOMMENDATIONS

- Substance abuse referral for patients with recreational drug abuse
- Patients with unintentional (accidental) poisoning require poison prevention counseling.
- Patients with intentional (eg, suicide) poisoning require psychiatric evaluation.

## PEARLS AND PITFALLS

- Always obtain a core temperature.
- Concomitant recreational drugs might not be present on a routine hospital drug screen.
- For persistent altered mental status, assess electrolytes for hyponatremia.
- Consider nontoxicologic causes for altered mental status.

## ADDITIONAL READING

- Ben-Abraham R, Szold O, Rudick V, et al. "Ecstasy" intoxication: Life-threatening manifestations and resuscitative measures in the intensive care setting. *Eur J Emerg Med*. 2003;10(4):309–313.
- Gahlinger PM. Club drugs: MDMA, gamma-hydroxybutyrate (GHB), Rohypnol, and ketamine. *Am Fam Physician*. 2004;69:2619–2626.
- Kalant H. The pharmacology and toxicity of "ecstasy" (MDMA) and related drugs. *Can Med Assoc J*. 2001;165:917–928.
- Patel MM, Wright DW, Ratcliff JJ, et al. Shedding new light on the "safe" club drug: Methylenedioxymethamphetamine (ecstasy)-related fatalities. *Acad Emerg Med*. 2004;11(2):208–210.
- Rosenson J, Smollin C, Sporer KA, et al. Patterns of ecstasy-associated hyponatremia in California. *Ann Emerg Med*. 2007;49(2):164–171.
- Shannon MW. Methylenedioxymethamphetamine (MDMA, "ecstasy"). *Pediatr Emerg Care*. 2000;16:377–380.

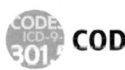 **CODES**

### ICD9

969.72 Poisoning by amphetamines

# MEASLES

*Austen Chai*

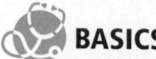 **BASICS**

## DESCRIPTION
- Childhood vaccine—preventable infectious disease characterized by fever, cough, coryza, conjunctivitis, and erythematous maculopapular rash
- Also known as rubeola
- Incidence is low secondary to widespread immunization.

## ETIOLOGY
- *Morbillivirus*, a negative-strand paramyxovirus
- Humans are the only known reservoir.
- Highly contagious; outbreaks seen in nonimmunized or underimmunized

### Pregnancy Considerations
- Increased risk of spontaneous abortion and premature contractions if infected during pregnancy
- Does not appear to cause birth defects.
- Women should not be vaccinated during pregnancy.

### Geriatric Considerations
Those born before 1957 are generally considered immune. However, those in health care should receive vaccination if serologic testing reveals negative titer.

### Pediatric Considerations
Measles, mumps, and rubella (MMR) vaccine should be administered to children on or after 12 mo of age. A 2nd dose is administered at age 4–6 yr, before start of school.
   Catch-up doses should be separated by at least 4 wk between vaccinations.

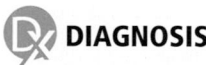 **DIAGNOSIS**

## SIGNS AND SYMPTOMS
- Incubation (7–14 days) before appearance of rash:
  - Transmission via direct contact or inhalation of infectious droplet
  - Children usually have incomplete or no immunization.
- Prodrome (2–8 days):
  - Mild respiratory illness, conjunctivitis, fever
  - Koplik spots:
    - Small white to grayish-blue specks on buccal mucosa
    - Pathognomonic for rubeola
    - Transient and disappear within 48 hr after onset of rash

- Active disease:
  - Cough, coryza, conjunctivitis ("Three C's")
  - Fever of 101°F or greater
  - Rash appears on day 3–7, lasting 4–7 days
    - Begins on head and spreads centrifugally downward
    - Initially pale, then discrete and maculopapular, and, ultimately, confluent
    - Clinical improvement seen in 48 hr of appearance of rash
    - Rash clears in 3–4 days and may desquamate as rash fades.
- Complications:
  - Respiratory:
    - Cough may persist for 1–2 wk after measles infection.
    - Pneumonia seen most commonly in immunocompromised
    - Most common cause of fatality
    - Laryngotracheobronchitis in patients <2 yr old
  - CNS:
    - Encephalomyelitis:
      - 1–14 days after onset of rash
      - Fever, headache, vomiting, and stiff neck
      - Lethargy, stupor, and seizure followed by coma
    - Subacute sclerosing panencephalitis (SSPE):
      - Very rare but serious complication that develops 7–10 yr after infection
      - Insidiously progressive degeneration of CNS functions
      - Personality change, intellectual deterioration, motor and visual deficits, seizures, coma, and death
  - Cardiovascular:
    - Transient myocarditis, pericarditis, and conduction defects
    - Rarely clinically significant
    - Congestive heart failure in elderly patients
  - Thrombocytopenic purpura
  - Otitis media
  - Sinusitis
  - Diarrhea

## ESSENTIAL WORKUP
- Diagnosis is based on clinical findings.
- Cough, coryza, and conjunctivitis with fever and subsequent rash

## DIAGNOSTIC TESTS & INTERPRETATION
### Lab
- CSF analysis for suspected encephalitis
- Viral cultures and antibody testing generally not needed
- Serologic tests for measles IgM and IgG titers, and PCR of measles viruses RNA available

### Imaging
Chest radiograph for suspected pneumonia

## DIFFERENTIAL DIAGNOSIS
- Rubella
  - Milder course, postauricular nodes, pinker rash, no conjunctivitis
- Scarlet fever:
  - Sandpaper-textured rash, strawberry tongue, sore throat
- Infectious mononucleosis:
  - Serologic test available
- Roseola:
  - Rash appears after temperature falls.
- Erythema infectiosum ("fifth disease"):
  - No prodrome and without fever
  - Red, flushed cheeks with lacelike rash when fading
- Enterovirus:
  - No respiratory complaints
- Kawasaki disease:
  - Rash on palm and soles
- Secondary syphilis
- Toxic shock syndrome
- Drug reactions:
  - Usually without high fever and upper respiratory infection symptoms

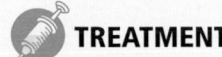 **TREATMENT**

### PRE-HOSPITAL
Nonimmunized prehospital care personnel should be advised of potential risks described above.

### ED TREATMENT/PROCEDURES
- Prevention with vaccination is cornerstone of therapy:
  - 2 doses of measles vaccine given as MMR
  - 1st dose at 12–15 mo and 2nd dose typically before school entry
- Antipyretics
- IV hydration as needed
- Isolate suspected cases.
- Postexposure prophylaxis for the nonimmune:
  - Give MMR if <72 hr after exposure:
    ○ Avoid if pregnant or immunocompromised.
  - Immunoglobulin 0.25 mL/kg IM up to 15 mL (max):
    ○ If given <6 days after exposure, may prevent or modify severity of symptoms
    ○ Indicated for susceptible household or other close contacts, particularly those <1 yr, pregnant women, or immunocompromised
    ○ For patients who receive immune globulin IV (IGIV) regularly, the usual dose of 400 mg/kg should be adequate for measles prophylaxis after exposure occurring within 3 wk of receiving IGIV.
    ○ Patients receiving IG should subsequently receive vaccine if not contraindicated.
- Oxygenation and airway protection for:
  - Pneumonia
  - Encephalitis

### MEDICATION
WHO now recommends vitamin A once a day for 2 days for children with measles. It may reduce the risk of measles mortality:
- 50,000 IU for <6 mo
- 100,000 IU for 6–11 mo
- 200,000 IU for ≥12 mo
- Parenteral and oral formulations are available in the U.S.

 **FOLLOW-UP**

### DISPOSITION
#### Admission Criteria
- Severe pneumonia
- Dehydration
- Encephalitis
- SSPE
- Immunocompromised patients:
  - AIDS
  - Immunosuppressive therapy
- Elderly patients with comorbid conditions

#### Discharge Criteria
Duration of infectivity information:
- 4 days before symptoms and up to 4 days after onset of rash
- Immunocompromised are contagious for duration of illness

## PEARLS AND PITFALLS
- One of the most highly communicable of infectious diseases; death occurs in 1–3/1,000 cases in the U.S.
- Severely immunocompromised patients or those on immunotherapy should not receive MMR vaccine or measles, mumps, rubella, and varicella vaccine.
- Characteristic rash may not develop in immunocompromised patients.

## ADDITIONAL READING
- American Academy of Pediatrics. Measles. In: Pickering LK, ed. *Red Book 2009: The Report of the Committee on Infectious Diseases*, 27th ed. Elk Grove Village, IL: American Academy of Pediatrics; 2009:455–463.
- Centers for Disease Control and Prevention. Update: Recommendations from the Advisory Committee on Immunization Practices (ACIP) regarding administration of combination MMRV vaccine. *MMWR Morb Mort Wkly Rep.* 2008;57:1–4.
- Mason WH. Measles. In: Kliegman RM, ed. *Nelson Textbook of Pediatrics*, 18th ed. Philadelphia: Saunders Elsevier; 2007:1331–1337.

### See Also (Topic, Algorithm, Electronic Media Element)
http://www.cdc.gov/measles

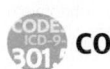 **CODES**

#### ICD9
055.9 Measles without mention of complication

M

# MECKEL DIVERTICULUM

*John Bailitz*
*Brandon C. Tudor*

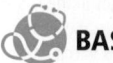 **BASICS**

## DESCRIPTION
- Most common congenital abnormality of the GI tract
- True diverticula (contains all layers):
  - 50% contain normal ileal mucosa.
  - 50% contain either gastric (most common), pancreatic, duodenal, colonic, endometrial, or hepatobiliary mucosa.
- Rule of 2's:
  - 2% prevalence in general population
  - 2% lifetime risk for complications, decreasing with age
  - Symptoms commonly occur around 2 yr of age:
    - 45% of symptomatic patients <2 yr old
  - Average length 2 in.
  - About 2 ft from the ileocecal valve
- Male-to-female ratio approximately equal
- Complications:
  - Obstruction and diverticulitis in adults
  - Hemorrhage and obstruction in children
  - Mean age 10 yr
  - Current mortality rate 0.0001%
  - Occurs more frequently in males
- Obstruction:
  - Diverticulum attached to the umbilicus, abdominal wall, other viscera, or is free and unattached, leading to:
    - Intussusception: Diverticulum is the leading edge.
    - Volvulus: Persistent fibrous band leads to bowel rotation.
- Diverticulitis:
  - Opening obstructed
  - Bacterial infection follows.
  - Presents like appendicitis (most common preoperative diagnosis with Meckel diverticulum)

### Pediatric Considerations
- Most common cause of significant lower GI bleeding in children
- Presents at age <5 yr with episodic painless, brisk, and bright-red rectal bleeding.
- Ectopic gastric tissue with secretions leading to erosions and bleeding

## ETIOLOGY
Remnant of the omphalomesenteric duct that typically regresses by week 7 of gestation

## DIAGNOSIS

### SIGNS AND SYMPTOMS
- 3 different types of presentation:
  - *Rectal bleeding* due to hemorrhage
  - *Vomiting* due to obstruction secondary to volvulus, intussusceptions, or intraperitoneal bands
  - *Abdominal pain* (appendicitis like) due to an inflamed or perforated diverticulum
- General:
  - Fever
  - Malaise
  - Weakness
  - Fatigue
- GI:
  - Classically painless rectal bleeding
  - Abdominal pain:
    - Location depends on cause
    - Appendicitis like
  - Vomiting
  - Distention
  - Changes in bowel movements
  - Hematochezia or melena (depending on briskness or location of diverticulum)
  - Peritonitis and septic shock (late complications)
- Cardiovascular:
  - Tachycardia (due to pain or blood loss)
  - Hypotension and shock (due to bleeding)

### ESSENTIAL WORKUP
- May cause a variety of signs and symptoms:
  - <10% diagnosed preoperatively
  - Consider in patient with recurrent nonspecific abdominal pain, nausea and vomiting, or rectal bleeding.
- History and physical exam narrow diagnosis, but will not give specific findings for Meckel diverticulum.
- Rectal exam mandatory
- Nasogastric (NG) tube placement to rule out upper GI Bleed

## DIAGNOSTIC TESTS & INTERPRETATION
### Lab
- CBC:
  - Decreased hematocrit due to bleeding
  - Rarely a cause of chronic anemia
  - Leukocytosis with diverticulitis, perforation, or gangrene
- Electrolytes, BUN, creatinine, coagulation studies
- Type and screen/cross-match when significant GI bleeding.

### Imaging
- CT abdomen/pelvis:
  - For suspected infection (appendicitis/diverticulitis) or bowel obstruction
- Abdominal radiographs:
  - Screening for bowel obstruction
  - Cannot diagnose Meckel diverticulum
- Tc-99m pertechnetate radioisotope scan:
  - Noninvasive scan that identifies Meckel diverticulum containing heterotopic gastric mucosa
  - 90% accurate in children
  - 45% accurate in adults
- Small bowel enteroclysis:
  - 75% accuracy
  - Barium/methyl cellulose introduced through NG tube into distal duodenum or proximal jejunum
  - Increases the ability to detect Meckel diverticulum in adults
  - Diverticulum may be short and wide-mouthed, making diagnosis difficult.
- Barium enema:
  - Introduces fluid into distal small bowel
  - Look for diverticulum.
- Angiogram for further evaluation of Meckel diverticulum if radioisotope scan and enteroclysis normal:
  - Blood supply is not always abnormal (vitelline artery).
- US may be useful in nonbleeding presentations.
- Laparoscopic evaluation may provide both diagnosis and definitive treatment.
- ECG:
  - Eliminate myocardial ischemia as cause of abdominal pain.
- Colonoscopy:
  - Not useful in diagnosing Meckel diverticulum

## DIFFERENTIAL DIAGNOSIS
- Adults:
  - Adhesions
  - Appendicitis
  - Arteriovenous malformation
  - Bowel obstruction
  - Diverticulitis
  - Hemorrhoids
  - Inflammatory bowel disease
  - Internal hernias
  - Intestinal polyps
  - Intussusception
  - Peptic ulcer disease
  - Pseudomembranous colitis
  - Volvulus
- Pediatric:
  - Adhesions
  - Anal fissures
  - Appendicitis
  - Atresia
  - Gastroenteritis
  - Hemolytic-uremic syndrome
  - Henoch-Schönlein purpura
  - Intestinal polyps
  - Intussusception
  - Malrotation
  - Milk allergy
  - Strictures
  - Volvulus

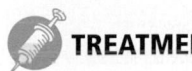 **TREATMENT**

### PRE-HOSPITAL
Establish IV access for patients with rectal bleeding or abdominal pain.

### INITIAL STABILIZATION/THERAPY
- Stabilization followed by early surgical evaluation
- Hypotension:
  - Aggressive fluid resuscitation
  - Packed RBC transfusion with brisk rectal bleeding (more common in children)
  - Pressors for septic shock

## ED TREATMENT/PROCEDURES
- GI bleeding:
  - Fluid resuscitate and transfuse PRBC as indicated
  - Foley to follow urine output
  - NG tube to exclude brisk upper GI bleeding
  - Surgical consult for surgical intervention as indicated
- Obstruction:
  - NG tube
  - Foley
  - Surgical consult
- Diverticulitis/perforation:
  - NPO
  - Preoperative antibiotics
  - Surgical consult

### MEDICATION
- Ampicillin/sulbactam (Unasyn): 3 g (peds: 100–200 mg ampicillin/kg/24 hr) q8h IV
- Cefoxitin (Mefoxin): 1–2 g (peds: 100–160 mg/kg/24 hr) IV q6h
- Dopamine: 2–20 mg/kg/min IV

 **FOLLOW-UP**

### DISPOSITION
**Admission Criteria**
Presumptive diagnosis of Meckel diverticulum with diverticulitis, obstruction, intussusception, hemorrhage, or volvulus requires admission and surgical evaluation.

**Discharge Criteria**
None

### FOLLOW-UP RECOMMENDATIONS
Postoperative surgical follow-up

## PEARLS AND PITFALLS
- Painless, brisk, bright-red blood per rectum in an infant is often caused by Meckel's diverticulum.
- Presents with a wide range of complications, including obstruction, intussusception, and hemorrhage.
- Often diagnosed in the OR for patients undergoing surgery for a presumptive appendicitis.
- Rule of 2's:
  - 2% of the population
  - 2% risk of complications
  - Most <2 yr old
  - 2 in. long
  - 2 ft from the ileocecal valve

## ADDITIONAL READING
- McCollough M, Sharieff GQ. Abdominal pain in children. *Pediatr Clin North Am.* 2006;53(1): 107–137.
- Sagar J, Kumar V, Shah DK. Meckel's diverticulum: A systematic review. *J R Soc Med.* 2006;99(10): 501–505.
- Sharma RK, Jain VK. Emergency surgery for Meckel diverticulum. *World J Emerg Surg.* 2008;3:27.
- Yachouchy EK, Marano AГ, Etienne JC, et al. Meckel's diverticulum. *J Am Coll Surg.* 2001;192(5): 658–662.
- Zani A, Eaton S, Rees CM, et al. Incidentally detected Meckel diverticulum: To resect or not to resect? *Ann Surg.* 2008;247(2):276–281.

**See Also (Topic, Algorithm, Electronic Media Element)**
- Abdominal Pain
- Appendicitis
- Bowel Obstruction
- Diverticulitis
- Intussusceptions

 **CODES**

ICD9
751.0 Meckel's diverticulum

M

# MEDIAL COLLATERAL LIGAMENT STRAIN

*Richard A. Craven*

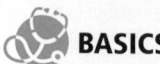 **BASICS**

## DESCRIPTION
Most commonly injured knee ligament

## ETIOLOGY
- Direct trauma to lateral knee
- Most common: Valgus stress with external rotary component on flexed knee:
  – From catching a ski tip
  – Side tackle (football)
- When accompanied by other ligament injury:
  – Hyperextension with external rotation (anterior cruciate ligament [ACL] and posterior cruciate ligament [PCL] injured first)
  – Anterior stress (ACL injured first)

### Pediatric Considerations
- Medial collateral ligament (MCL) attaches distal to tibial epiphysis and proximal to femoral epiphysis.
- Isolated MCL injury infrequent before growth plate closure (<14 yr old)
- MCL injury may accompany underlying fracture.
- Most injuries owing to direct trauma-producing valgus stress (sports, auto–pedestrian)

 **DIAGNOSIS**

## SIGNS AND SYMPTOMS
- Tearing sensation and immediate pain in medial aspect of knee:
  – Medial pain and tenderness may be more pronounced with partial tears than with complete tears.
- Localized swelling:
  – Hemarthrosis signifies tear of capsular portion of MCL or cruciate injury.
- Variable ability to bear weight:
  – May be able to bear weight with complete tear
  – Patients often describe buckling sensation on weight bearing.
  – Additional findings with involvement of other ligaments

### History
- Mechanism of injury
- Weight bearing or rotational forces increase likelihood of meniscal injury.
- Valgus strain stresses MCL.

### Physical Exam
Complete knee examination:
- Palpate medial femoral condyle (most common site for MCL tear).
- Valgus stress testing:
  – In flexion: Grasp lateral aspect of knee and abduct while externally rotating at ankle with knee in 30 degrees of flexion.
  – In extension: Same as above but with knee extended
  – Joint laxity
- Classification of ligament injuries (sprains):
  – Grade 1: Stretched fibers without tear; firm endpoint on stress testing
  – Grade 2: Extracapsular fibers tear without complete rupture; mild instability but firm endpoint on stress testing; inability to extend knee fully
  – Grade 3: Complete rupture; no fixed endpoint on stress testing; hemarthrosis
  – Check function of deep peroneal nerve.
  – 1st dorsal web-space sensation
  – Ankle and toe dorsiflexion

### ALERT
- Underlying fracture should be ruled out before stress test.
- Examine ipsilateral hip and ankle.
- Suspect ACL injury if knee opens medially in extension or if hemarthrosis is present.
- Re-exam in >24 hr may be necessary if severe muscle spasm and pain are present.
- Intra-articular instillation of anesthetic and analgesic may be required to perform adequate exam.

## ESSENTIAL WORKUP
- Complete knee examination
- Check for concomitant neurovascular injuries.

## DIAGNOSTIC TESTS & INTERPRETATION
### Imaging
- Standard radiographs give no clues to MCL tears but can reveal fractures, effusions, tendon calcifications, osteophytes, and foreign bodies:
  – Views: AP, lateral, oblique, notch view
  – Fat–fluid level is pathognomonic of fracture.
- MRI accurately detects collateral ligament injuries and other intra-articular structures and disorders (menisci, ACL, PCL, osteonecrosis, occult fractures).
- Arteriograms to evaluate vascular integrity for severe associated injuries (eg, knee dislocation)
- US useful to diagnose cysts and popliteal artery aneurysms

### Diagnostic Procedures/Surgery
- Aspiration of joint effusion may be therapeutic (relieve pain) and diagnostic (hemarthrosis with cruciate tears, fat globules with fractures).
- Arthroscopy used by consultant for diagnosis and repair of meniscal and cruciate injuries

## DIFFERENTIAL DIAGNOSIS
- Meniscal, other ligament injuries, and fractures may be concomitant.
- Hip injury may present with knee pain.
- Arthritis (rheumatoid, osteoid, septic), cellulitis, bursitis

### Pediatric Considerations
- Examine hip and obtain radiograph if any concern for hip pathology (especially slipped capital femoral epiphysis).
- Epiphyseal plate tenderness may signify nondisplaced Salter I fracture.

 **TREATMENT**

### PRE-HOSPITAL
Immobilize in slight flexion.

> ### ALERT
> - Evaluate for knee dislocation.
> - Document neurovascular status.
> - MCL injury may be overlooked in the multiple trauma victim.

### INITIAL STABILIZATION/THERAPY
Maintenance of joint immobilization in neutral position or position of comfort by prehospital personnel

### ED TREATMENT/PROCEDURES
- Grade 1 or 2: Intermittent ice, elevation, rest, crutches, compression (splint or knee immobilizer)
- Grade 3: As grade 1 or 2 but requires definitive orthopedic referral
- Joint aspiration of large hemarthrosis may help relieve pain.

### MEDICATION
- Oral analgesics: Acetaminophen, NSAIDs, opioids as needed
- Joint instillation of anesthetic (eg, bupivacaine 0.25%, 5 mL) with an analgesic (eg, morphine 1–5 mg diluted to 30 mL) may be required for severe pain.

 **FOLLOW-UP**

### DISPOSITION
**Admission Criteria**
To manage severe associated injuries

**Discharge Criteria**
- Absence of associated injuries requiring admission
- Ensure compliance with splinting and adequate follow-up.

**Issues for Referral**
- Grade 1 or 2 sprain: PCP or orthopedic physician within 2–4 wks
- Grade 3 sprain: Orthopedic physician, urgent referral

## PEARLS AND PITFALLS
- Most frequently injured ligament of the knee
- Conservative, nonoperative management for most isolated injuries
- Rule out associated injuries to the knee:
  – ACL, PCL, meniscus, fracture

## ADDITIONAL READING
- Chen L, Kim PD, Ahmad C, et al. Medial collateral ligament injuries of the knee: Current treatment concepts. *Curr Rev Musculoskelet Med*. 2008;1(2):108–113.
- Noyes FR. *Noyes' Knee Disorders: Surgery, Rehabilitation, Clinical Outcomes*. Philadelphia: Saunders-Elsevier; 2010.
- Phisitkul P, James SL, Wolf BR, et al. MCL injuries of the knee: Current concepts reiview. *Iowa Orthop J*. 2006;26:77–90.
- Simon R, Sherman S, Koenigsknecht SJ. *Emergency Orthopedics: The Extremities*, 5th ed. New York: McGraw-Hill; 2007.

 **CODES**

### ICD9
844.1 Sprain of medial collateral ligament of knee

M

# MEDIAL MENISCUS INJURY

*Nicholle D. Bromley*

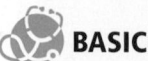 **BASICS**

## DESCRIPTION

- Among most common adult knee injuries
- Medial meniscus injury 10 times more common than lateral
- Sudden rotary motion of knee associated with squatting, pivoting, turning, and bending
- Common in those sports with low stance positions:
  - Wrestling and football
  - Occupations such as carpet installers and plumbers

## ETIOLOGY

- Medial meniscus is more firmly attached to the joint capsule:
  - Less mobile than the lateral meniscus
  - Predisposes it to injury when tensile/compressive forces are applied
- Tears are the result of tensile or compressive forces between the femoral and tibial condyles:
  - With knee flexion, the femur rotates internally on the flexed tibia, displacing the medial meniscus toward the center of the joint.
  - With rapid forceful extension, the meniscus may be trapped centrally, resulting in peripheral segment stretching or tear.
  - Extension of the tear may result in a free segment that may become displaced into the joint, resulting in a true locked joint.
  - More common in men than in women

 **DIAGNOSIS**

## SIGNS AND SYMPTOMS

- Usually present within 24 hr of acute injury
- May report hearing a pop, feeling a tear, catch, lock, or a click
- Usually occurs with rotational force, often when knee is flexed

### History

- Patient may recall the knee "giving way."
- Inability to fully extend knee is common.
- Effusion is found in 50% and usually occurs over 6–12 hr.
- Pain is often intermittent/localized to the joint line.
- Unlike ligamentous injury, patients often report completion of activities at time of injury.

### Physical Exam

- Pay special attention to joint line tenderness:
  - High predictive value of 75–85% and neurovascular system
- Effusion is found in 50% and is typically delayed in onset.
- Inability to extend the joint at 20–45° secondary to true or pseudo locking is a common finding.

## ESSENTIAL WORKUP

- Limitation of extension owing to severe pain from muscle spasm/effusion suggests pseudo locked joint.
- True locked joint from torn fragment within the joint occurs in only 30%.
- Provocative testing should be deferred until severe pain resolves:
  - McMurray, Apley, Steinmann, Childress, and Helfet
- Recent systematic review concludes that physical diagnostic tests have low diagnostic accuracy.

## DIAGNOSTIC TESTS & INTERPRETATION

### Lab

If arthrocentesis is performed, send joint fluid for cell count, protein and glucose, Gram stain, culture, and crystals, as indicated.

### Imaging

- Plain radiograph may demonstrate effusion or associated bony abnormalities.
- MRI has replaced arthrography:
  - Diagnostic accuracy >90–98%, depending on type of injury

### Diagnostic Procedures/Surgery

- Arthroscopy is the standard for diagnostic accuracy.
- Arthrocentesis:
  - May afford significant symptomatic relief when effusion is present
  - Aspiration of bloody fluid suggests cruciate ligament tear or injury to peripheral vascular part of meniscus.

## DIFFERENTIAL DIAGNOSIS

- Osteochondral fractures
- Osteochondritis desiccans
- Patellofemoral joint syndromes
- Anterior and posterior cruciate ligament injury
- Medial/lateral collateral ligament injury
- Iliotibial band syndrome
- Lumbar radiculopathy
- Gout and other inflammatory arthropathies

# TREATMENT

## PRE-HOSPITAL
- Application of ice packs
- Immobilization in a position of comfort
- Careful neurovascular exam
- Assess for dislocations and associated injuries.

## INITIAL STABILIZATION/THERAPY
Assess for significant associated injuries.

## ED TREATMENT/PROCEDURES
- Arthrocentesis may afford relief with large effusions and assist in reducing locked joint.
- Arthrocentesis should be followed by application of compressive dressing.
- Reduction of locked joint should be performed within 1st 24 hr after injury:
  - With patient seated, hang extremity off edge of exam table at 90°:
    - This alone may reduce locked joint.
  - Applying gentle traction and rotation of tibia; usually results in reduction of the locked joint.
- NSAIDs, both parenteral and oral
- Weight-bearing and range of motion are permitted as tolerated.
- Individuals unable to bear weight or those with severe restriction of range of motion may be placed in a knee immobilizer or crutches as needed.
- Definitive treatment by orthopedic consultant:
  - Operative vs. nonoperative treatment depends on multiple factors.

## MEDICATION
- NSAIDs
- Supplement with narcotic analgesia for breakthrough pain

# FOLLOW-UP

## DISPOSITION
### Admission Criteria
- Intractable pain is suggestive of true locked joint and may require emergent orthopedic consult.
- Evidence of potential for neurovascular compromise
- High-risk elderly patients unable to manage splinting devices

### Discharge Criteria
- Patients capable of following a structured discharge plan
- No comorbid conditions likely to negatively impact outcome

### Issues for Referral
Refer all patients for close orthopedic follow-up.

## FOLLOW-UP RECOMMENDATIONS
- With orthopedics or primary care physician
- Definitive treatment is not urgent.

# PEARLS AND PITFALLS
- Unlike ligamentous injury, patients often report completion of activities at time of injury.
- Symptoms such as catching, clicking, or locking should raise suspicion for the possible presence of an unstable bucket handle or flap tear.
- Degenerative meniscal tears tend to have a more insidious, atraumatic presentation, with mild swelling, vague joint line pain, and sometimes with mechanical symptoms.

# ADDITIONAL READING

- Allen JE, Taylor KS. Physical exam of the knee. *Prim Care*. 2004;31:887–907.
- Brockmeier SF, Rodeo SA. *Delee & Drez's Orthopaedic Sports Medicine*, 3rd ed. Philadelphia: Saunders; 2009.
- Karachalios T, Hantes M, Zibis AH, et al. Diagnostic accuracy of a new clinical test (the Thessaly test) for early detection of meniscal tears. *J Bone Joint Surg Am*. 2005;87:955–962.
- Lyn ET, Pallin DJ. *Rosen's Emergency Medicine: Concepts and Clinical Practice*, 7th ed. St. Louis, MO: Mosby; 2009.
- Scholten RJ. The accuracy of physical diagnostic tests for assessing meniscal lesions of the knee: A meta-analysis. *J Fam Pract*. 2001;50:938–944.
- Solomon DH. The rational clinical exam: Does this patient have a torn meniscus or ligament of the knee? *JAMA*. 2001;286:1610–1620.

# CODES

ICD9
836.0 Tear of medial cartilage or meniscus of knee, current

# MÉNIÈRE DISEASE

*Ming Valerie Lin*
*Charles V. Pollack, Jr.*

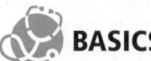 **BASICS**

## DESCRIPTION
- Disease of the inner ear
- Classically unilateral ear involvement (may be bilateral in up to 40% of cases)
- Characterized by recurrent spontaneous and episodic vertigo, sensorineural hearing loss, "roaring" tinnitus, and aural fullness
- Estimated incidence about 15/100,000 in U.S.
- Slight female > male (1.3:1)
- Positive family history up to 20%
- May develop at any age: Peak incidence is age 40–60 yr.
- Affects more whites of northern European decent than Africans or blacks
- A benign disease without cure, and can be associated with significant morbidity

## ETIOLOGY
- Idiopathic
- Endolymphatic hydrops: Blockage of the endolymphatic sac and duct leading to endolymphatic outflow obstruction and increase hydraulic pressure within the endolymphatic system:
  – Increased pressure causes a break in the membrane that separates the perilymph (potassium [K]-poor extracellular fluid) and the endolymph (K-rich intracellular fluid). The resultant chemical mixture bathes the vestibular nerve receptors, leading to a depolarization blockade and transient loss of function.
- May be associated with structural abnormalities such as atrophy of the sac, hypoplasia of the vestibular aqueduct, narrowing of the endolymphatic duct, forwardly located lateral sinus causing compression, and obstruction of the endolymphatic sac
- Autoimmune processes suggested as an etiology, with immune complex deposition in endolymphatic sac and autoantibodies directed against endolymphatic sac
- Other proposed mechanisms are subclinical viral infection causing hydrops, many decades later, and ischemia of the endolymphatic sac and the inner ear.
- Need to differentiate Ménière syndrome from other disease processes that interfere with normal production or resorption of endolymph (eg, thyroid disease, inner ear inflammation due to syphilis, medication)

 **DIAGNOSIS**

Diagnostic criteria (1995 American Academy of Otolaryngology guidelines):
- Recurrent spontaneous and episodic vertigo, $\geq$20 min
- Hearing loss documented by audiograms on at least one occasion
- Tinnitus or aural fullness in the affected ear
- *Certain Ménière disease*: Definite disease with histopathologic confirmation
- *Definite Ménière disease*: 2 or more definitive episodes of vertigo with hearing loss, plus tinnitus, aural fullness, or both
- *Probable Ménière disease*: Only 1 definitive episode of vertigo and the other symptoms and signs
- *Possible Ménière disease*: Definitive vertigo with no associated hearing loss or hearing loss with nondefinitive disequilibrium

## SIGNS AND SYMPTOMS
### History
- Classical tetrad of symptoms: Vertigo, hearing loss, tinnitus, and aural fullness
- Vertiginous attacks lasting minutes to hours, often associated with severe nausea and vomiting (96.2%)
- Sensorineural hearing loss is typically fluctuating and progressive. Low frequencies are affected more severely than high frequencies (87.7%).
- Aural fullness is described as pressure, discomfort, fullness sensation in unilateral ear.
- Attacks reach maximum intensity within minutes, slowly subside over hours.
- After the acute attack, patients generally feel tired, unsteady, and nauseated for hours to days.
- Between episodes, some patients are completely symptom free.
- Sudden, unexplained falls without loss of consciousness or associated vertigo may also occur.
- Symptoms may not be present simultaneously or in the same pattern, particularly in the early phases of disease.
- Close clustering of attacks may occur.

### Physical Exam
- Examination results vary, depending upon the phase of disease.
- During acute attack, patients are often in significant distress, diaphoretic, and pale.
- Vital signs may show elevated blood pressure, pulse, and respiration.
- Horizontal nystagmus

- Impaired hearing
- Pneumo-otoscopy may elicit symptoms or cause nystagmus.
- Weber tuning fork test usually lateralizes away from the affected ear.
- Rinne test usually indicates better air than bone conduction.
- Positive Romberg test, with instability, especially when eyes are closed
- Must exclude central CNS lesion, peripheral pathology in ear (ruptured tympanic membrane, cholesteatoma, cerumen impaction, etc.)

## ESSENTIAL WORKUP
- Complete history and neurologic exam
- Patients with central vertigo or focal neurologic findings require neuroimaging.
- Focal findings include new unilateral hearing loss, usually with tinnitus.

## DIAGNOSTIC TESTS & INTERPRETATION
### Lab
When indicated:
- CBC
- Sedimentation rate
- Thyroid function
- Fasting lipid profiles
- Fasting blood glucose, hemoglobin A1c
- Treponemal antibody-absorption test
- Chemistry panel
- Urinalysis for proteinuria or hematuria

### Imaging
- MRI of the brain with views of internal auditory canal
- CT scan of temporal bone
- Standard lateral mastoid radiographs

### Diagnostic Procedures/Surgery
- Audiometric assessment
- Bithermal caloric testing
- Transtympanic electrocochleography
- Electronystagmography
- None of these tests are necessary during the ED evaluation.

## DIFFERENTIAL DIAGNOSIS
- Otologic:
  – Chronic suppurative otitis media
  – Benign positional vertigo
  – Acoustic neuroma
  – Vestibular neuronitis
  – Otosclerosis
  – Otic capsule dysplasia
  – Perilymphatic fistula
  – Labyrinthitis

- Systemic:
  - Vertebrobasilar insufficiency
  - Stroke
  - Basilar artery thrombosis
  - Intracranial hemorrhage
  - Head trauma
  - CNS lesions (tumors)
  - Epilepsy
  - Multiple sclerosis
  - Paget disease
  - Thyroid dysfunction
  - Drugs/medications
  - Autoimmune disorders (eg, systemic lupus erythematosus)
  - Viral meningitis/encephalitis
  - Lyme disease
  - Neurosyphilis
  - Electrolyte imbalance

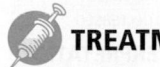 TREATMENT

### PRE-HOSPITAL
- Vertigo and neurologic symptoms can represent a stroke.
- Rapid transport to ED
- Protect patient from falling.
- Maintain patient in comfortable position.
- IV isotonic fluids for patients with vomiting
- Monitor for dysrhythmia.

### INITIAL STABILIZATION/THERAPY
- IV hydration with isotonic fluids
- IV benzodiazepines
- IV antiemetics

### ED TREATMENT/PROCEDURES
Supportive therapy

### MEDICATION
- Symptomatic:
  Meclizine: 12.5–25 mg PO q8h
  - Diazepam: 5–10 mg PO/PR/IV
  - Lorazepam: 0.5–2.0 mg PO/IV/IM
  - Ondansetron: 4 mg IV/IM/PO
  - Metoclopramide: 10 mg IV/IM
  - Promethazine: 10–25 mg PO/PR/IV/IM
  - Prochlorperazine: 10 mg IV
- Therapeutic:
  - Hydrochlorothiazide: 25–50 mg PO daily
  - Triamterene: 100 mg PO daily
  - Acetazolamide: 250 mg PO daily
  - Furosemide: 20 mg PO daily
  - Prednisone: 1 mg/kg PO daily with taper over 7–14 days
  - Dexamethasone: 4 g/L transtympanic injection
  - Gentamicin transtympanic perfusion
  - Pressure pulse treatment
  - Surgery

### First Line
- Diazepam or lorazepam
- Ondansetron for nausea, vomiting
- IV fluid

### Second Line
- Meclizine
- Prochlorperazine

 FOLLOW-UP

### DISPOSITION
#### Admission Criteria
Patient refractory to acute control of vertigo and associated effects (eg, dehydration from protracted vomiting)

#### Discharge Criteria
- Patient with normal neurologic examination
- Symptoms adequately controlled in ED
- Refer to neurology or ear-nose-throat clinic for outpatient audiometry and electronystagmography testing.
- Recurrent attacks are typical.
- Restrict sodium, caffeine, chocolate, tobacco, and alcohol intake.
- Patient needs to avoid driving, operating dangerous equipment, and working at heights until attacks have resolved and sedating medications have been withdrawn.

#### Issues for Referral
- Persistent/intractable symptoms and medical treatment failures
- Presence of ear pathology

### FOLLOW-UP RECOMMENDATIONS
- Proper education in terms of dietary control and avoidance techniques is helpful.
- Vestibular rehabilitation can be helpful in teaching patients to cope with vertigo and imbalance.
- Because of the unpredictable nature of the disease, balance-intensive, dangerous tasks (eg, especially climbing ladders) should be avoided.

## PEARLS AND PITFALLS
- Ménière disease typically presents with the classic tetrad of vertigo, hearing loss, tinnitus, and aural fullness.
- It is a clinical diagnosis; diagnostic studies are not helpful.
- Inpatient care is generally unnecessary and is reserved for patients refractory to acute control of their symptoms or associated effects such as dehydration and vomiting.
- Surgery is reserved for patients who fail medical therapy with intractable symptoms.

## ADDITIONAL READING
- James A. Ménière's disease. *Clin Evid*. 2004;11: 664–672.
- Kerber KA. Vertigo and dizziness in the emergency department. *Emerg Med Clin North Am*. 2009;27: 39–50.
- Kim HH. Trends in the diagnosis and management of Ménière's disease. *Otolaryngol Head Neck Surg*. 2005;132:722–726.
- Li JC. Endolymphatic hydrops. *Emedicine*. Updated Mar 12, 2009. Available at: http://emedicine medscape.com/article/1159069-overview
- Sajjadi H, Paparella M. Ménière's disease. *Lancet*. 2008;372:406–414.
- Semaan MT, Alagramam KN, Megerian CA. The basic science of Meniere's disease and endolymphatic hydrops. *Curr Opin Otolaryngol Head Neck Surg*. 2005;13:301–307.

### See Also (Topic, Algorithm, Electronic Media Element)
- Dizziness
- Labyrinthitis

 CODES

#### ICD9
- 386.00 Meniere's disease, unspecified
- 386.01 Active meniere's disease, cochleovestibular
- 386.02 Active meniere's disease, cochlear

M

# MENINGITIS

Austen Chai
Patricia Shipley

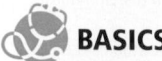 **BASICS**

## DESCRIPTION
CNS infection with inflammation of leptomeninges defined by an increased number of WBC in the CSF often associated with fever, nuchal rigidity, headache, and altered mental status

## ETIOLOGY
- Bacterial:
  - Neonates: Group B *Streptococcus*, *Escherichia coli* and other enteric bacilli, *Listeria monocytogenes*
  - Children/adults: *Streptococcus pneumoniae*, *Neisseria meningitides*, *Haemophilus influenzae* (now rare due to vaccination)
  - Elderly/alcoholic: *S. pneumoniae*, gram-negative bacilli, *Listeria* spp.
  - Neurosurgical patients: *Staphylococcus*- and gram-negative organisms
  - Transplant recipients and dialysis patients: Increased incidence of *Listeria* spp. infection
  - AIDS: Above, plus tuberculosis, syphilis
- Viral
- Fungal
- Chemical, drug, or toxin induced

 **DIAGNOSIS**

## SIGNS AND SYMPTOMS
- General:
  - Fever
  - Nuchal rigidity:
    - Kernig: Flexed knee resists extension (bilateral).
    - Brudzinski: Flexion of neck produces flexion at hips.
    - Kernig and Brudzinski signs are neither sensitive nor specific for meningitis.
  - Altered mental state
  - Headache
  - Photophobia
  - Papilledema
  - Focal CNS abnormalities
  - Seizures
  - Petechial and palpable purpuric rash (meningococcal infection)
  - Associated infections: Sinusitis, otitis media, pneumonia
- Infant/pediatric:
  - Fever or hypothermia
  - Lethargy
  - Weak suck
  - Vomiting
  - Dehydration
  - Respiratory distress
  - Apnea
  - Cyanosis
  - Bulging fontanel
  - Hypotonia
  - Meningismus, commonly absent in <1-yr-old
- Elderly and immune compromised:
  - Confusion with or without fever
  - Less-striking symptoms overall

### History
- Neonates: Prematurity, intrapartum complications as fever, prolonged rupture of membrane, antibiotic use, group B *Streptococcus* infection
- Adults: Recent travels
- Elderly: Pneumococcal vaccination status

- Immunologic competency suggested by frequent infections
- Recent trauma or ENT, facial, or neurologic surgery
- Shunt

## ESSENTIAL WORKUP
- Initiate treatment immediately based on clinical suspicion of meningitis.
- Give antibiotic therapy if at all possible after blood cultures but before other diagnostic procedures if patient is unstable.
- Routine CT before lumbar puncture (LP) not always required. Generally indicated with:
  - Immune deficiency/HIV
  - History of CNS disease (abscess, bleed, mass lesion, stroke, shunt)
  - History of seizure <7 days
  - Focal neurologic deficit
  - Altered level of consciousness
  - Age >60 yr
  - Papilledema
- LP: Every suspected meningitis patient unless contraindicated:
  - Do not delay antibiotics for LP.
  - May delay LP when:
    - Risk for herniation (see above)
    - Unstable patient
    - Thrombocytopenia or bleeding diathesis
    - Spinal epidural abscess
    - Overlying soft tissue infection
- Cerebrospinal fluid (CSF) analysis:
  - Tube 1: Cell count and differential
  - Tube 2: Protein and glucose
  - Tube 3: Gram stain, culture, and sensitivity.
- May add acid-fast bacillus smear, TB culture, India ink and fungal cultures, counter-immunoelectrophoresis (CIE), VDRL, cryptococcal antigen as needed:
  - Tube 4: Repeat cell count or save for additional tests.
  - Check for elevated opening pressure: Normal up to 200 mm $H_2O$
  - Latex agglutination (optional):
    - Useful if patient with prior antibiotic treatment
    - Best if urine and blood also tested
    - Detects: *Meningococcus*, *Pneumococcus*, group B *Streptococcus*, *H. influenzae*, *E. coli*, *Cryptococcus*
  - Polymerase chain reaction (optional):
    - Useful for virus and bacteria: *N. meningitides*, *S. pneumonia*, *H. influenza* a and b
    - Highly sensitive and specific for herpes simplex virus
  - CSF Interpretation:
    - Culture is diagnostic
    - ≥5 WBC/mL in CSF is highly sensitive for meningitis beyond neonatal period.
    - Cell count may be normal in HIV/AIDS.
    - Neonatal considerations: Up to 25 WBC/mL and protein up to 170 mg/dL may be normal.
  - Typical bacterial meningitis:
    - Glucose <40% of serum
    - WBC >500/mL (usually 1,000–20,000)
    - Differential >80% polymorphonuclear neutrophils (PMNs)
    - Protein >200 mg/dL
  - Typical viral meningitis:
    - WBC <500/mL
    - Nearly all mononuclear

- Differential: Initially PMNs, then after 24 hr, predominantly lymphocytes
- Protein mildly increased, <200 mg/dL
- Glucose normal
- Repeat LP within 24 hr may provide suggestive confirmation of viral etiology.
  - Typical fungal meningitis:
    - WBC <500/mL
    - Differential, lymphocytes
    - Protein >200 mg/dL
    - Glucose low
  - Typical tuberculosis meningitis:
    - WBC range, 100–400/mL
    - Differential mixed
    - Protein variable, but usually increased
    - Glucose variable, but usually decreased

## DIAGNOSTIC TESTS & INTERPRETATION
### Lab
- Blood cultures (1 or 2 sets): Before antibiotics initiated
- Urine culture and urinalysis
- CBC with differential and platelets
- Electrolytes/glucose:
  - CSF glucose to serum glucose ratio: <0.4 is indicative of bacterial meningitis
  - Assess for metabolic acidosis
  - Syndrome of inappropriate antidiuretic hormone hypersecretion
  - BUN/Cr for medication dosing
- Prothrombin time, partial thromboplastin time, and platelet: Particularly in patients with petechiae or purpura:
  - Obtain before LP in severe sepsis or disseminated intravascular coagulation
- Serum C-reactive protein:
  - Useful for gram-negative meningitis in pediatric patients
  - Elevated levels very suggestive of bacterial meningitis
- Toxicology studies as needed
- Latex agglutination or CIE of urine, blood, or CSF may be helpful in partially treated meningitis cases.

### Imaging
- CT: See essential workup section above.
- CXR: Pneumonia, TB if suspected

## DIFFERENTIAL DIAGNOSIS
- Encephalitis
- Brain, spinal, epidural abscess
- Febrile seizure
- CNS/systemic lupus erythematosus cerebritis
- Intracranial bleed
- Primary or metastatic CNS malignancy
- Stroke
- Venous sinus thrombophlebitis
- Trauma
- Toxic/metabolic

 **TREATMENT**

## PRE-HOSPITAL
- IV, $O_2$, and transport
- Treat hypotension, seizures. Protect airway.
- Administer prophylactic antibiotics to any close personal contacts of patient diagnosed with meningococcal meningitis:
  - Adults:

- ○ Rifampin: 600 mg PO bid for 2 days, *or*
- ○ Ciprofloxacin: 500 mg PO single dose, *or*
- ○ Ceftriaxone: 250 mg IM (if pregnant)
- – Children:
  - ○ Ceftriaxone: 250 mg IM, *or*
  - ○ Rifampin: 5 mg/kg if <1 mo old and 10 mg/kg if >1 mo old, b.i.d. for 4 doses

## INITIAL STABILIZATION/THERAPY
- Isolate patient as appropriate.
- Airway protection for patients with altered mental status; oxygen
- 0.9% normal saline to treat dehydration, hypotension, shock
- Treat seizures: Benzodiazepines. Consider phenytoin (15 mg/kg) or phenobarbital load.

## ED TREATMENT/PROCEDURES
- Ideally perform LP and give antibiotic +/− steroids promptly.
- If LP is delayed, give antibiotic +/− steroids empirically before LP.
- If CT is indicated prior to LP, empiric antibiotic +/− steroids should be given prior to CT.
- Steroids: If given, should be given prior to or concurrently with administration of antibiotics.
- Antibiotics:
  - Obtain blood cultures (2 sets) before administering antibiotics.
  - Do not delay giving antibiotics to obtain LP or CT unless absolutely necessary.
- IV empiric antibiotic(s) for presumed bacterial infection:
  - Neonates:
  - 0–7 days old: Ampicillin 50–100 mg/kg q8h; plus cefotaxime 50 mg/kg q8h or gentamicin 2.5 mg/kg q12h
  - >7 days old: Ampicillin 50–100 mg/kg q6h; plus cefotaxime 50 mg/kg q6h or gentamicin 2.5 mg/kg q8h
  - Add acyclovir 10–20 mg/kg q8h for suspected herpes simplex encephalitis.
  - Age 1–3 mo:
    - ○ Ampicillin 50–100 mg/kg q6h; plus ceftriaxone 75 mg/kg load, then 50 mg/kg q12h thereafter or cefotaxime 50 mg/kg q6h; plus vancomycin 15 mg/kg q8h (if cephalosporin-resistant *S. pneumoniae* prevalent) +/− dexamethasone (0.15 mg/kg q6h for 4 days)
  - Children >3 mo:
    - ○ Ceftriaxone 75 mg/kg load, then 50 mg/kg q12h thereafter or cefotaxime 50 mg/kg q6h; plus vancomycin 15 mg/kg q8h +/−dexamethasone 0.15 mg/kg q6h for 4 days
    - ○ Immune deficient: Add aminoglycoside like gentamicin 2.5 mg/kg q8h or amikacin 7.5 mg/kg q12h or 5 mg/kg q8h.
    - ○ CNS surgery: Vancomycin 15 mg/kg q8h; plus meropenem 40 mg/kg q8h or ceftazidime 50 mg/kg q8h or cefepime 50 mg/kg q8h
    - ○ Penetrating head trauma: Vancomycin 15 mg/kg q8h; plus cefepime 50 mg/kg q8h or ceftazidime 50 mg/kg q8h or meropenem 40 mg/kg; plus gentamicin 2.5 mg/kg q8h or amikacin 5–10 mg/kg q8h
  - Adults:
    - ○ Ceftriaxone 2 g q12h or cefotaxime 2 g q4–6h; plus vancomycin 15 mg/kg q12h; plus dexamethasone 10 gq6h IV, continue for 4 days if causative agent is *S. pneumoniae*
    - ○ >50 yr: Add ampicillin 2 g q4h to above regimen for adults.
    - ○ Immune impaired: Vancomycin 15 mg/kg q12h plus ampicillin 2g q4h; plus meropenem 2 g q8h or cefepime 2 g q8h

- ○ CNS surgery, shunt, head trauma: Vancomycin 15 mg/kg q12h; plus meropenem 2 g q8h or ceftazidime 2 g q8h or cefepime 2 g q12h
- ○ Vancomycin dosing for patients with normal renal function: 50–89 kg (1 g q12h), 90–130 kg (1.5 g q12h), >130 kg (2 g q12h)
- Other medication considerations
  - Dexamethasone:
    - ○ If given, it should be given prior to or concurrently with the 1st dose of antibiotic.
    - ○ Benefits are not yet conclusive.
    - ○ May be beneficial for children with *H. influenza* meningitis and may be beneficial in children >6 wk with *S. pneumonia meningitis*. May reduce neurologic sequelae, including hearing loss.
    - ○ Reduces risk of death or persistent neurologic deficits in adults with bacterial meningitis, *S. pneumoniae* in particular.
    - ○ Not effective, possibly toxic, in patients without bacterial meningitis.
    - ○ Give before or with antibiotics if patient has altered mental status or with focal neurologic deficit, papilledema, CNS trauma or surgery, space-occupying lesion. Also give if CSF is cloudy, has positive Gram stain, or >1,000 WBC/mm³.
    - ○ Dosage: 10 mg IV q6h for adults and 0.15 mg/kg q6h for peds for 4 days
    - ○ Discontinue when bacterial meningitis has been excluded.
  - Penicillin allergy (severe):
    - ○ Aztreonam or chloramphenicol may be used in place of cephalosporins.
    - ○ Do not delay therapy for lesser allergy history.
    - ○ Consult infectious disease specialist.
  - Vancomycin:
    - ○ Add when concerned about penicillin-resistant pneumococcal infection.

## MEDICATION
- Acyclovir: Peds: 10–20 mg/kg q8h IV
- Amikacin: Peds: 7.5 mg/kg q12h or 5 mg/kg q8h IV. Newborn: Load 10 mg/kg followed by 7.5 mg/kg q12h IV
- Ampicillin: 2 g q4h (peds: 50–100 mg/kg q6h–q8h) IV, max 12 g/d
- Aztreonam: 2 g (peds: 30 mg/kg) q6h–q8h, max 6–8 g/d IV
- Bactrim: 5–10 mg/kg trimethoprim q12h IV
- Cefepime: 2 g q8h, max 6 g/d IV
- Cefotaxime: 2 g (peds: 50 mg/kg) q6h, max 8–12 g/d IV
- Ceftazidime: 2 g q8h, max 6 g/d IV
- Ceftriaxone: 2 g (peds: 50–75 mg/kg) q12h, max 4 g/d IV
- Chloramphenicol: 1–1.5 g (peds: 12.5 mg/kg) q6h, max 4–6 g/d IV
- Dexamethasone: 10 mg (peds: 0.15 mg/kg) q6h IV for 4 days
- Gentamicin: Peds: 2.5 mg/kg q8h IV
- Meropenem: 2 g (peds 40 mg/kg) q8h IV, max 6 g/d
- Tobramycin: Peds: 2.5 mg/kg q8h IV
- Vancomycin: 1–2 g q12h IV (peds: 15 mg/kg q8h)
- Vancomycin and aminoglycosides: Adjust for renal function and serum concentration levels.

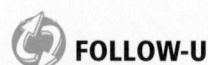

## FOLLOW-UP

### DISPOSITION
### Admission Criteria
- All known or suspected cases of bacterial infections

- Immune-compromised host
- Any toxic-appearing patient

### Discharge Criteria
- Clear viral infection with well-controlled symptoms.
- Thorough and specific discharge instructions
- Careful follow-up plan discussed with primary care physician prior to discharge

## PEARLS AND PITFALLS
- Meningitis generally does not present as uncomplicated febrile seizure in children.
- Failure to diagnose or delay in treatment of meningitis results in catastrophic outcome for patients, and not infrequently, negative medicolegal consequences for the physicians involved.
- Clinical suspicion should generally be associated with a lumbar puncture.

## ADDITIONAL READING

- American Academy of Pediatrics. *Red Book: 2009 Report of the Committee on Infectious Diseases*, 28th ed. Elk Grove Village, IL: American Academy of Pediatrics; 2009.
- Chavez-Bueno S, McCracken GH. Bacterial meningitis in children. *Pediatr Clin North Am*. 2005;52(3):795–810.
- de Gans J, van de Beek D. Dexamethasone in adults with bacterial meningitis. *N Engl J Med*. 2002;347:1549–1556.
- Fitch MT, van de Beek D. Emergency diagnosis and treatment of adult meningitis. *Lancet Infect Dis*. 2007;7(3):191–200.
- Greenwood BM. Corticosteroids for acute bacterial meningitis. *N Engl J Med*. 2007;357:2507–2509.
- Hasbun R, Abrahams J, Jekel J, et al. Computed tomography of the head before lumbar puncture in adults with suspected meningitis. *N Engl J Med*. 2001;345:1727–1733.
- Nelson JD, McCracken GH. Treatment of neonatal meningitis. *Pediatr Infect Dis J*. 2005;24(7).
- Seupaul RA. Evidence-based emergency medicine/rational clinical examination abstract. How do I perform a lumbar puncture and analyze the results to diagnose bacterial meningitis? *Ann Emerg Med*. 2007;50(1):85–87.
- Tunkel AR, Hartman BJ, Kaplan SL, et al. Practice guidelines for management of bacterial meningitis. *Clin Infect Dis*. 2004;39:1267–1284.
- Upadhye S. Corticosteroids for acute bacterial meningitis. *Ann Emerg Med*. 2008:52:291–293.
- van de Beek D, de Gans J, Tunkel AR, et al. Community-acquired bacterial meningitis in adults. *N Engl J Med*. 2006;354(1):44–53.

### See Also (Topic, Algorithm, Electronic Media Element)
Seizures

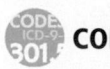

## CODES

### ICD9
- 047.9 Unspecified viral meningitis
- 320.9 Meningitis due to unspecified bacterium
- 322.9 Meningitis, unspecified

M

# MENINGOCOCCEMIA

*Ann M. Buchanan*

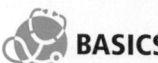 **BASICS**

## DESCRIPTION
- Bacterial illness caused by *Neisseria meningitides*
- Several forms of illness may occur.
- Mild meningococcemia
- Overwhelming meningococcal sepsis
- Meningococcal meningitis
- Chronic/occult meningococcemia
- Septic arthritis
- Acquired from close contact with an infected individual or an asymptomatic carrier
- Intimate kissing and cigarette smoking are independent risk factors.

## ETIOLOGY
- *Neisseria meningitidis*:
  - Serotypes A, B, C, D, H, I, K, L, X, Y, Z, 29E, and W135
  - Serotype B most common in U.S.
  - >95% of infections caused by A, B, C, Y, and W135
- Bacteria attach to and enter nasopharyngeal epithelial cells.
- Bacteria spread from the nasopharynx through the bloodstream via entry of vascular endothelium.
- Most circulating meningococci are eliminated by the spleen.
- Meningococci produce an endotoxin (lipo-oligosaccharide):
  - Involved in pathogenesis of the skin, adrenal manifestations, and vascular collapse
- Human oropharynx/nasopharynx is the only reservoir.
- Carrier usually has developed immunity to serotype-specific antibody (not immune to all serotypes):
  - Age <5 yr: 1% carrier rate
  - Age 20–40 yr: 30–40% carrier rate
  - Lower rate of immunity in children, which is reflected by the higher rates of infection
- Most common in fall and spring
- Increased incidence in military recruits and close living conditions
- Epidemics—ages 5–9 yr most/earliest affected

## DIAGNOSIS

### SIGNS AND SYMPTOMS
- "Mild" meningococcemia:
  - Most common
  - Preceded by upper respiratory infection
  - Fever, chills, myalgias/arthralgias, malaise
  - Often self-limited, resolving in several days
  - Can progress to meningitis (mortality rate 2–10%) or overwhelming sepsis without meningitis
- Overwhelming meningococcal sepsis:
  - 10% of overall meningococcemia cases
  - High mortality rate (20–60%)
  - Most deaths occur in 1st 48 hr.
  - Sudden onset of illness and rapid progression of clinical course

- Initial presentation may be mild:
  - Mild tachycardia
  - Mild tachypnea/respiratory symptoms
  - Mild hypotension
- Fever, chills, vomiting, headache, rash, muscle tenderness
- Toxic appearing
- Infants: Lethargy, poor feeding, bulging fontanel
- Rash:
  - Combination of purpura/ecchymosis
  - May later exhibit coalescence, necrosis/sloughing of the involved skin (purpura fulminans)
  - Petechiae (over skin, mucous membranes, conjunctivae) seen in 50–60%
  - Macules
  - Papules (scrapings of papules demonstrate the organism on Gram stain)
- Deteriorate quickly over several hours:
  - Hypotension/shock
  - Acidosis
  - Acute respiratory distress syndrome (ARDS)
  - Disseminated intravascular coagulation (DIC)
- Meningitis may or may not be present.
- Waterhouse-Friderichsen syndrome:
  - Bilateral hemorrhagic destruction of adrenal glands
  - Vasomotor collapse
- Acute renal failure:
  - From prolonged hypotension (low renal perfusion causing acute tubular necrosis)
- Chronic meningococcemia:
  - Uncommon
  - Well appearing
  - Recurrent fevers, chills, arthralgias over weeks to months
  - Intermittent rash—painful on the extremities
  - Migratory polyarthritis
  - Splenomegaly (20%)
  - Meningococcal meningitis (25%):
    - Headache
    - Fever
    - Neck stiffness
    - Confusion
    - Lethargy
    - Obtundation
- Septic arthritis:
  - Occurs during active meningococcemia
  - Multiple joints involved
  - Joint pain, redness, swelling, effusion, fever, chills
  - Extremely limited or no range of motion
- Other meningococcal Infections:
  - Occur with meningococcal infection elsewhere
  - Conjunctivitis—may occur alone
  - Sinusitis
  - Panophthalmitis
  - Urethritis
  - Salpingitis
  - Prostatitis
  - Pneumonia
  - Myocarditis/pericarditis:
    - Occurs late in onset
    - Usually associated with serogroup C

### History
Progression of illness is variable and classifies illness into mild, overwhelming, and chronic.

### Physical Exam
- Tachycardia
- Hypotension, which may be mild initially
- Progressive, rapid deterioration
- Respiratory failure with ARDS picture
- Petechial rash 50–80%:
  - Involves axillae, flanks, wrists, ankles

### ESSENTIAL WORKUP
- Do not allow workup (including delay in lumbar puncture) to postpone resuscitation and administration of antibiotics in suspected cases of meningococcemia.
- Suspect diagnosis in setting of dramatic clinical presentation.
- Gram stain and culture of:
  - Peripheral blood, CSF, sputum, urine, joint aspirate, or petechial/papular scrapings
  - Gram stain: Intracellular or extracellular gram-negative diplococci

### DIAGNOSTIC TESTS & INTERPRETATION
#### Lab
- CBC:
  - Elevated WBCs initially, later may be suppressed in severe disease
  - Decreased platelet count when large areas of purpura/petechiae or DIC
- Electrolytes, BUN, creatinine, glucose
- CSF:
  - Gram stain, culture, protein and glucose, cell count with differential
  - Consistent with bacterial infection in meningococcal meningitis
- Arterial blood gases for acidosis, hypoxia
- Fibrinogen levels, fibrin degradation products, prothrombin time), partial thromboplastin time if DIC suspected
- Throat/nasopharyngeal swab:
  - Positive swab does not establish the diagnosis of meningococcemia.
- Analysis of buffy-coat layer of peripheral blood for bacteria if sepsis is suspected
- Blood culture:
  - Often negative with chronic meningococcemia
  - Positive in mild and overwhelming meningococcemia
- Immunoassays (beware false negatives)
- Polymerase chain reaction, especially useful when antibiotics given before specimen collection

#### Imaging
CXR: For ARDS/pneumonia

#### Diagnostic Procedures/Surgery
Amputations and debridement of necrotic tissue and/or extremities may be necessary.

## DIFFERENTIAL DIAGNOSIS
- Viral exanthem
- Vasculitis
- Mycoplasma
- Rocky Mountain spotted fever
- Toxic shock syndrome
- Henoch-Schönlein purpura
- Idiopathic thrombocytopenic purpura
- Dengue fever
- Disseminated gonococcal infection
- Influenza
- *Streptococcus* group A and B
- Thrombotic thrombocytopenic purpura

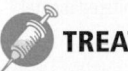 TREATMENT

### PRE-HOSPITAL
Postexposure prophylaxis needed for prehospital personnel in close contact with patient

### INITIAL STABILIZATION/THERAPY
- Wear mask and gloves, observe droplet precautions.
- Notify department of health.
- ABCs
  - Immediate endotracheal intubation for severe acidosis, hypoxia, or decreased mental status:
  - Hyperventilate to treat acidosis (target $PCO_2$ about 25 mm Hg)
- Treat hypotension:
  - 0.9% normal saline bolus of 20 mL/kg; cautious rehydration with ARDS, CHF
  - Begin dopamine or norepinephrine (epinephrine if no response) if hypotensive after 2 L of IV fluids.
- Naloxone, thiamine, dextrose (Accu-Chek) for altered mental status
- Initiate IV antibiotics:
  - 1st line: High dose penicillin (proven meningococcemia) or 3rd-generation cephalosporin (broader coverage pending definitive diagnosis)
  - 2nd line: Ampicillin
  - 3rd line: Chloramphenicol (penicillin-allergic patients)

### ED TREATMENT/PROCEDURES
- Overwhelming meningococcal sepsis
- Severe acidosis (pH <7.0-7.1 or serum $HCO_3$ <8-10):
  - Administer IV $NaHCO_3$ along with hyperventilation.
- Insert Foley catheter to monitor urine output.
- Place in respiratory isolation.
- High-dose steroids:
  - To protect against cranial nerve injury in the setting of ongoing infection (controversial)
  - Administer with adrenal gland injury.
- DIC treatment:
  - Administer fresh-frozen plasma and platelet transfusions.
  - Heparin is not indicated unless significant thrombotic complications are evident clinically (eg, cyanosis or cold digits, low urine output despite adequate volume status, and blood pressure).

- Prophylaxis options for close contacts:
  - Ideally, prophylaxis should be given within 1st 24 hr.
  - 10-day window of observation
  - Serogroup-specific vaccine as adjunct only
- Vaccine:
  - Vaccine recommended in military recruits, travelers to endemic areas, complement-deficient or asplenic patients, 1st-year college dormitory residents
  - Vaccine recommended routinely for ages 11-18 yr

### Pregnancy Considerations
The safety of meningococcal vaccine is unclear in pregnancy.

### MEDICATION
#### First Line
- Cefotaxime: 2 g (peds: 50 mg/kg) IV q6h
- Ceftriaxone: 2 g (peds: 50 mg/kg) IV q12h
- Penicillin G: 4 MU (peds: 250,000 IU/kg/24 hr) IV q4h

#### Second Line
- Ampicillin: 2-3 g (peds: 200-400 mg/kg/24 hr) IV q6h
- Chloramphenicol: 50-100 mg/kg/24 hr IV q6h (max 4 g/d)
- Prophylaxis:
  - Single-dose ceftriaxone:
    - 125 mg IM for age <15 yr
    - 250 mg IM for age >15 yr
  - Ciprofloxacin: 500 mg PO
  - Rifampin: 600 mg (peds: 5-10 mg/kg) PO b.i.d. for 2 days
  - Zithromax 500 mg PO single dose
- Dexamethasone: 0.15 mg/kg IV for pediatric meningitis
- Dopamine: 5-20 mg/kg/min IV titrate to blood pressure (BP)
- Epinephrine: 2-10 mg/min IV titrate to BP
- Heparin: 3,000-5,000 IU (peds: 80 IU/kg) IV bolus followed by 600-1,000 IU/hr (peds: 18 IU/kg/hr) IV drip
- Hydrocortisone (Solu-Cortef): 100 mg (peds: 2 mg/kg) bolus IV for adrenal insufficiency q8h
- Meningococcal polysaccharide 0.5 mL IM × 1
- Meningococcal vaccine 0.5 mL SC × 1
- Norepinephrine: 0.5-30 mg/min IV titrate to BP
- Sodium bicarbonate: 2-5 mEq/kg (peds: 0.5-1.0 mEq/kg) IV over 30 min to 4 hr

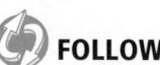 FOLLOW-UP

### DISPOSITION
#### Admission Criteria
- ICU admission for overwhelming sepsis with respiratory isolation
- Respiratory isolation admission for mild meningococcemia

### Discharge Criteria
Prophylaxis for close patient contacts

### Issues for Referral
- Consider transfer to tertiary care center, as multisystem organ failure is common.
- Late neurologic, cardiovascular, and orthopedic complications may necessitate follow-up with specialists.

### FOLLOW-UP RECOMMENDATIONS
- Complete antibiotic course.
- Respiratory precautions may be discontinued after 24 hr.
- All close contacts need prophylaxis.

## PEARLS AND PITFALLS
- Notify department of health in any suspected case.
- Watch for late development of pericardial tamponade.
- Do not wait to give antibiotics.

## ADDITIONAL READING
- American Academy of Pediatrics. *Red Book: 2009 Report of the Committee on Infectious Disease.* Elk Grove Village, IL: American Academy of Pediatrics; 2009.
- Apicella M. *Neisseria meningitidis.* In: Mandell GL, Bennett JE, Dolin R, eds. *Principles and Practice of Infectious Disease,* 6th ed. New York: Churchill Livingstone; 2004:2498-2513.
- Centers for Disease Control and Prevention. Control and prevention of meningococcal disease and control and prevention of serogroup C meningococcal disease: Evaluation and management of suspected outbreaks: Recommendations of the Advisory Committee on Investigation Practices (ACIP). *MMWR Morb Mort Wkly Rep.* 2007;56(31).
- Leclerc F, Leteurtre S, Cremer R, et al. Do new strategies in meningococcemia produce better outcomes? *Crit Care Med.* 2000;28(9 suppl): S60-S63.

### See Also (Topic, Algorithm, Electronic Media Element)
Meningitis

 CODES

### ICD9
036.2 Meningococcemia

M

# MERCURY POISONING

*Keri L. Carstairs*
*David A. Tanen*

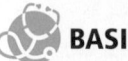

## BASICS

### DESCRIPTION
Mercury:
- 3 forms: Elemental, inorganic salts, and organic
- Reacts with sulfhydryl groups, causing enzyme inhibition and alterations in cellular membranes
- Binds to phosphoryl, carboxyl, amide, and amine groups of enzymes

### ETIOLOGY
- Exposure is usually thorough the GI tract and inhalation and less frequently dermal exposure.
- Exposure through manufacturing of chlorine and caustic soda, diuretics, antibacterial agents, antiseptics, thermometers, batteries, fossil fuels, plastics, paints, jewelry, lamps, explosives, fireworks, vinyl chloride, and pigments
- Exposure through taxidermy, photography, dentistry, mercury mining
- Contaminated seafood

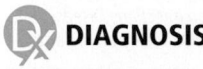

## DIAGNOSIS

### SIGNS AND SYMPTOMS
- Naturally occurring mercury is converted into 3 primary forms, each with its toxicologic effects:
- Elemental mercury:
  - Symptoms from inhalation occur within hours:
    - Cough and dyspnea, which may progress to pulmonary edema
    - Metallic taste, salivation
    - Weakness, nausea, diarrhea, fever, headaches, visual disturbances
  - SC deposits may present as granulomas or abscesses.
  - IV exposure presents with symptoms consistent with pulmonary embolization.
  - Relatively nontoxic from oral ingestion, although appendicitis has been reported
- Inorganic mercurial salt ingestion:
  - Caustic GI injury:
    - Abdominal pain with nausea, vomiting, and diarrhea
    - Metallic taste, sore throat
    - Hemorrhagic gastroenteritis with hematochezia and hematemesis
  - Acute tubular necrosis
  - Acrodynia (pink disease):
    - Idiosyncratic, occurs mainly in children
    - Painful extremities
  - Pink discoloration with desquamation

- Organic mercury ingestion:
  - Historically, infants exposed in womb are most severely affected (eg, Minamata Bay, Japan)
  - May see GI symptoms acutely
  - Delayed CNS toxicity predominates and may take weeks to months to manifest:
    - Paresthesias
    - Ataxia
    - Paralysis
    - Visual field constriction
    - Dysarthria
    - Hearing loss
    - Mental deterioration
    - Death

### History
- Ask about possible workplace, environmental, or accidental exposure to mercurial products.
- Document the patient's ingestion of seafood over the last few weeks.

### Physical Exam
- Elemental mercury:
  - Cough progressing to respiratory distress if inhaled or intravenously injected
  - Ataxia
  - SC nodules or granulomas if injected
- Inorganic mercury:
  - Oral burns
  - Abdominal tenderness
  - Heme-positive stools
- Organic mercury:
  - CNS abnormalities:
    - Progressive cognitive deterioration

### ESSENTIAL WORKUP
- Good history for workplace or environmental exposure
- Physical exam looking for:
  - Respiratory distress
  - Caustic GI injury
  - Neuropsychiatric impairment
- Laboratories tests:
  - Renal failure
  - Urine and blood mercury levels:
    - Not reliable with recent seafood ingestion

### DIAGNOSTIC TESTS & INTERPRETATION
#### Lab
- Inorganic mercury exposure:
  - CBC
  - Electrolytes, BUN, creatinine, glucose
  - 24-hr urine mercury collection:
    - Normal urine levels <20 mg/dL
  - Whole-blood mercury level:
    - Normal blood <10 mg/dL
- Organic mercury exposure:
  - CBC with peripheral smear
  - Electrolytes, BUN, creatinine, glucose
  - Whole-blood mercury level:
    - Normal blood <10 mg/dL

### Imaging
- Chest radiograph:
  - For noncardiac pulmonary edema
  - Evidence of IV mercury in pulmonary vascular tree
- Abdominal radiograph:
  - For presence of mercury with intentional oral ingestion
- Head CT:
  - May detect cerebellar atrophy

### Diagnostic Procedures/Surgery
- Lumbar puncture in the workup of altered mental status

### DIFFERENTIAL DIAGNOSIS
- Multisystem involvement is often confused with other heavy-metal intoxications.
- Cerebrovascular accident
- Senile dementia, Alzheimer disease
- Parkinson disease
- Peptic ulcer disease
- Gastrointestinal bleeding
- Pancreatitis
- Sepsis
- Acute respiratory distress syndrome

## TREATMENT

### PRE-HOSPITAL
- Remove from toxin exposure.
- Decontamination:
  - Wash exposed skin.
- For altered mental status:
  - Dextrose
  - Thiamine
  - Naloxone (Narcan)
  - Oxygen

### INITIAL STABILIZATION/THERAPY
- Secure ABCs and monitoring.
- 0.9% NS
- IV fluid resuscitation for hypotension:
  - Blood transfusion for significant gastrointestinal hemorrhage
- Naloxone, D50W, thiamine for altered mental status

## ED TREATMENT/PROCEDURES

- Elemental mercury:
  - For inhalation exposure, observe closely for several hours for development of noncardiogenic pulmonary edema.
  - Ingested elemental mercury passes through normal intestinal tract with minimal absorption.
  - Consider chelation for symptomatic patients with oral dimercaptosuccinic acid (DMSA).
  - For SC nodules/abscess, perform an incision and drainage.
- Inorganic mercury salt ingestion:
  - Administer activated charcoal.
  - Aggressive 0.9% NS IV fluid resuscitation/blood products for hypovolemic shock:
    ○ Hydrate and maintain urine output (1 mL/kg/hr).
  - Chelate symptomatic patients:
    ○ IM dimercaprol (British antilewisite [BAL])
    ○ Oral DMSA efficacy may be limited secondary to caustic GI injury.
- Organic mercury:
  - Administer activated charcoal.
  - Chelate with oral DMSA.

## MEDICATION

### First Line

- Dextrose: D50W 1 amp: 50 mL or 25 g (peds: D25W 2–4 mL/kg) IV
- Dimercaprol (BAL): 5 mg/kg IM q4h for 48 hr, then 2.5 mg/kg q6h for 48 hr, then 2.5 mg/kg q12h for 7 days
- DMSA: 10 mg/kg PO q8h for 5 days, then q12h for 2 wk
- Naloxone (Narcan): 2 mg (peds: 0.1 mg/kg) IV/IM initial dose
- Thiamine (vitamin B$_1$): 100 mg (peds: 50 mg) IV or IM

### Second Line

- D penicillamine:
  - Adult: 250 mg PO q.i.d. for 7–14 days
  - Peds: 5–7 mg/kg PO q.i.d. for 7–14 days
- 2,3-Dimercapto-1-propanesulfonate:
  - IV or PO formulations. Contact your poison center at 1 800-222-1222 for availability.

 FOLLOW-UP

### DISPOSITION

#### Admission Criteria

Acutely symptomatic patients:

- Any evidence of respiratory compromise
- Ingestion of inorganic mercury salt that may lead to a caustic GI injury
- Renal impairment
- Any patient starting chelation therapy

#### Discharge Criteria

- Asymptomatic patient with history of ingestion of elemental mercury and intact intestinal tract
- Patient with history of inhalation exposure to elemental mercury who remain asymptomatic after 6 hr of observation

#### Issues for Referral

- Medical toxicology referral for symptomatic patients or where chelation is considered
- Gastroenterology for caustic GI injury
- Pulmonary/ICU care for patients with symptomatic inhalational injury
- Neurology in the evaluation of progressive cerebral deterioration
- Poison center for all suspected exposures

### FOLLOW-UP RECOMMENDATIONS

- For discharged patients with possible workplace or environmental exposures, follow up with their primary care provider for results of 24-hr urine or whole-blood mercury levels.
- Outpatient referral to medical toxicology for suspected or confirmed cases
- For the asymptomatic patient, have the patient refrain from eating seafood for 2 wk before repeating the 24-hr urine for mercury.

## PEARLS AND PITFALLS

- Obtain a good history for workplace, environmental or accidental exposure in patients with gastrointestinal and/or neuropsychiatric complaints.
- Monitor patients for at least 6 hr if they were exposed to inhalational elemental mercury.
- Ingestion of inorganic mercurial salts can lead to significant caustic GI injury.
- Lab tests may yield false positives especially in patients who eat seafood.

## ADDITIONAL READING

- Young-Jin S. Mercury. In: Flomenbaum NE, Goldfrank LR, Hoffman RS, et al., eds. *Goldfrank's Toxicologic Emergencies*, 8th ed. New York: McGraw-Hill; 2006;1334–1344.
- Clarkson TW, Magos L, Myers GJ. The toxicology of mercury: current exposures and clinical manifestations. *N Engl J Med*. 2003;349:1731–1737.
- Ruha AM, Curry CS, Gerkin RD, et al. Urine mercury excretion following meso-dimercaptosuccinic acid challenge in fish eaters. *Arch Pathol Lab Med*. 2009;133:87–92.

### See Also (Topic, Algorithm, Electronic Media Element)

- Respiratory Distress
- Caustic Ingestion
- Renal Failure
- Psychosis, Medical vs. Psychiatric

 CODES

ICD9
985.0 Toxic effect of mercury and its compounds

M

# MESENTERIC ISCHEMIA
*Tamara Espinoza*

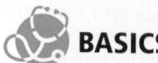

## BASICS

### DESCRIPTION
- Decreased or occluded blood flow through the mesenteric vessels leading to ischemic or infarcted bowel
- Can be from arterial or venous blockage, or low flow state
- 1 in 1,000 of all hospital admissions
- 1–2% of all admissions for abdominal pain:
  - Most cases occur in patients >50.
  - Mortality 60–70%

### ETIOLOGY
- Acute mesenteric arterial embolism:
  - 50% of cases of acute mesenteric ischemia
  - Mean age 70 yr
  - Emboli most commonly arise in left atria or ventricle, from a dysrhythmia, valvular lesions, or ventricular thrombus from a prior MI
  - Typically lodge 3–10 cm distal to the origin of the superior mesenteric artery (SMA):
    - Preserves blood flow to proximal small and large bowel
  - Risk factors include dysrhythmia (especially atrial fibrillation), valvular heart disease, prior MI, aortic aneurysm, or dissection.
- Mesenteric artery thrombus:
  - SMA thrombus in 15% of cases of acute mesenteric ischemia
  - Rare in other vessels
  - Develops from plaque rupture of mesenteric atherosclerotic disease
  - 50–80% may have longstanding intestinal angina (chronic mesenteric ischemia).
  - Risk factors include age, atherosclerotic disease, HTN.
- Mesenteric venous thrombosis:
  - 5–15% of cases of acute mesenteric ischemia
  - Subacute/indolent presentation
  - 20–40% mortality
  - Typically occurs in younger patients with underlying hypercoagulable state
  - Risk factors include:
    - Hypercoagulable state (lupus, protein C and S deficiency)
    - Sickle cell disease
    - Antithrombin III deficiency
    - Malignancy
    - Pregnancy
    - Sepsis
    - Renal failure on dialysis
    - Estrogen therapy
    - Recent trauma or inflammatory conditions

- Nonocclusive mesenteric ischemia:
  - 20–30% of cases of acute mesenteric ischemia
  - Occurs in low cardiac output states with decreased mesenteric blood flow
  - Risk factors include CHF, sepsis, diuretic use, volume depletion, recent surgery (especially cardiac), hypotension or recent vasopressor requirement.
- Chronic mesenteric ischemia:
  - "Intestinal angina":
    - Postprandial, diffuse abdominal pain occurring ~1 hr after eating, lasts 1–2 hr
    - Patients may develop food aversions and eat small meals to avoid pain.
- Uncommon causes:
  - Spontaneous mesenteric arterial dissection
  - Median arcuate ligament syndrome—compression of the celiac axis or SMA by the arcuate ligament of the diaphragm
  - Extrinsic compression from tumors
  - Medications:
    - Digitalis
    - Ergotamine
    - Cocaine
    - Pseudoephedrine
    - Vasopressin

## DIAGNOSIS

### SIGNS AND SYMPTOMS
- Sudden-onset, severe, diffuse abdominal pain in acute ischemia:
  - Pain out of proportion to exam:
    - Patients may have relatively benign abdominal exam despite severe pain.
- Nausea
- Vomiting
- Diarrhea
- Occult GI bleeding
- Elderly patients can have nonspecific symptoms such as altered mental status, tachypnea, or tachycardia.
- Late findings:
  - Peritoneal signs owing to irreversible bowel ischemia
  - Abdominal distention
  - Hypoactive bowel sounds

### History
Rapidity of onset of pain

### Physical Exam
Abdominal pain out of proportion to physical exam during the acute phase of illness

### ESSENTIAL WORKUP
Maintain a high level of suspicion in patients >50 yr with unexplained abdominal pain.

### DIAGNOSTIC TESTS & INTERPRETATION
#### Lab
- Often nonspecific and nondiagnostic
- CBC:
  - Elevated WBC count (90% >15,000)
- Chemistry panel:
  - Approximately 50% have a metabolic acidosis.
- Amylase:
  - Hyperamylasemia found in 50% of cases
- Creatine phosphokinase (CPK) may be elevated.
- Lactate:
  - Elevated in 90% of patients
  - High levels correlate with mortality.

#### Imaging
- Flat and upright abdominal radiographs:
  - Often obtained to rule out acute obstruction or perforation
  - Frequently normal
  - Late findings:
    - Thumbprinting from bowel wall edema and hemorrhage
    - Pneumatosis intestinalis: Air in bowel wall from tissue necrosis
    - Pneumobilia is a late finding associated with poor outcomes.
- Doppler US:
  - Can detect decreased blood flow in SMA but more helpful in chronic mesenteric ischemia
  - For optimal results the patient should be NPO for 8 hr, limiting the utility of this study in the ED
- Abdominal CT scan:
  - Can detect bowel wall edema, pneumatosis
  - Newer helical and multidetector CT (MDCT) scanners can directly visualize mesenteric vascular anatomy and identify sites of occlusion
  - MDCT angiography is more frequently the imaging modality of choice
- MRI:
  - Excellent images of mesenteric vasculature especially with MR angiography
  - Acquisition time and availability limits utility
- Angiography:
  - Historically the gold standard diagnostic modality, now being replaced by MDCT
  - Allows for direct visualization of emboli and administration of vasodilating or fibrinolytic agents
  - Invasive, time-consuming, and potentially nephrotoxic

## DIFFERENTIAL DIAGNOSIS
- Bowel obstruction
- Volvulus
- GI malignancy
- Diverticulitis
- Inflammatory bowel disease
- Peptic ulcer disease
- Perforated viscus
- Cholecystitis
- Ascending cholangitis
- Pancreatitis
- Appendicitis
- Abdominal aortic aneurysm
- MI
- Renal stones

 **TREATMENT**

### PRE-HOSPITAL
Initiate fluid replacement for dehydrated or hypotensive patients.

### INITIAL STABILIZATION/THERAPY
- Airway, breathing, and circulation management (ABCs) with fluid resuscitation as needed
- Caution:
  - Early diagnosis is critical to decrease mortality.

### ED TREATMENT/PROCEDURES
- General measures:
  - Nasogastric suction to decompress the stomach and intestine
  - NPO
  - Electrolyte replacement as needed
  - Cardiac monitor for dysrhythmia
  - Consider invasive cardiac monitoring if patient is unstable.
  - Monitor urine output.
  - Analgesics
  - Broad-spectrum antibiotics to cover bowel flora (may need to adjust dose if concomitant renal failure):
    - Piperacillin/tazobactam
    - Ampicillin/sulbactam
    - Ticarcillin/clavulanate
    - Alternatives include imipenem, meropenem, 3rd-generation cephalosporins plus metronidazole
  - Anticoagulation with heparin
  - Surgical consultation: All patients with peritoneal signs should have exploratory laparotomy.

- Specific therapies:
  - Papaverine 30–60 mg/h intra-arterial:
    - Phosphodiesterase inhibitor causes mesenteric vasodilatation.
    - Administered through angiography catheter
  - Intra-arterial thrombolytics can be used.
  - Surgical revascularization often indicated
- Caution:
  - Avoid vasoconstrictive medications, which may worsen ischemia:
    - If vasopressors are needed, use lowest dose possible.

### MEDICATION
- Ampicillin/sulbactam: 3 g IV q6h (peds: 100–200 mg/kg/d)
- Heparin sulfate: 80 units/kg IV bolus followed by 18 U/kg/h infusion
- Metronidazole: 1.0 g IV bolus followed by 500 mg IV q6h (peds: 12 mg/kg IV bolus, then 7.5 mg/kg IV q6h)
- Piperacillin/tazobactam: 3.375 g IV q6h (peds: 240–400 mg/kg/d)
- Ticarcillin/clavulanate: 3.1 g IV q4–6h

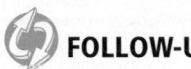 **FOLLOW-UP**

### DISPOSITION
**Admission Criteria**
Admit all patients with mesenteric ischemia.

**Discharge Criteria**
None

### FOLLOW-UP RECOMMENDATIONS
Surgical consultation

## PEARLS AND PITFALLS
- Aggressive pursuit of diagnosis is mandatory.
- Mortality rises to 80% when the diagnosis is made >24 hr after symptom onset.
- Early surgical evaluation for emergent operative intervention is mandatory.

## ADDITIONAL READING
- Cangemi JR, Picco MF. Intestinal ischemia in the elderly. *Gastroenterol Clin North Am.* 2009;38: 527–540.
- Krupski WC, Selzman CH, Whitehall IA. Unusual causes of mesenteric ischemia. *Surg Clin North Am.* 1997;77(2):471–499.
- Martinez JP, Hogan GJ. Mesenteric ischemia. *Emerg Med Clin North Am.* 2004;22:909–928.
- McKinsey JF, Gewertz BL. Acute mesenteric ischemia. *Surg Clin North Am.* 1997;77(2):307–317.
- Tekwani T, Sikka R. High-risk chief complaints III: Abdomen and extremities. *Emerg Med Clin North Am.* 2009;4:747–765.

### See Also (Topic, Algorithm, Electronic Media Element)
Abdominal Pain

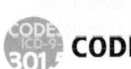 **CODES**

### ICD9
- 557.0 Acute vascular insufficiency of intestine
- 557.1 Chronic vascular insufficiency of intestine
- 557.9 Unspecified vascular insufficiency of intestine

M

# METACARPAL INJURIES

*Davut J. Savaser*
*David Palafox*

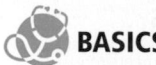 **BASICS**

## DESCRIPTION
- Most metacarpal injuries are caused by crush injuries, a direct blow with hand vs. object, or burns.
- Most common fracture is boxer's fracture of distal 5th metacarpal neck.

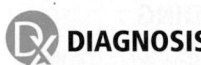 **DIAGNOSIS**

## SIGNS AND SYMPTOMS
- Pain or swelling at the site of injury
- Deformity at the site of injury
- Malalignment of the distal tip of the finger on flexion indicates rotational deformity.
- Lines drawn down the longitudinal axis of each digit in flexion normally should converge on the scaphoid volarly.
- Limitation of movement secondary to pain and anatomic deformity

## ALERT
Have a high suspicion for "fight bite." This injury is the direct blow of a closed fist against a human tooth:
- Concern is violation of the extensor sheath, metacarpophalangeal (MCP) joint, or metacarpal head by a tooth, with subsequent infection by oral flora.

*History*
Not all patients are truthful as to cause of injury.

## ESSENTIAL WORKUP
Examination should pay specific attention to skin integrity and alignment of the distal phalanges in flexion and extension.

## DIAGNOSTIC TESTS & INTERPRETATION
*Imaging*
- Hand radiographs when fracture suspected, and/or to rule out opaque foreign body
- Special radiographic views (CT) of the proximal metacarpals and the carpometacarpal joints may be necessary for patients with a suggestive physical exam and no definite fracture on a standard 3-view series.

## DIFFERENTIAL DIAGNOSIS
Fracture of the metacarpal may be accompanied by dislocation of adjacent phalanges or carpal bones.

 **TREATMENT**

## PRE-HOSPITAL
- Most do not require EMS transport solely for metacarpal injury.
- Cautions:
  - Metacarpal injuries should be splinted in position of comfort.

## INITIAL STABILIZATION/THERAPY
- Other, more serious injuries should be treated 1st.
- Immobilize hand pending evaluation.
- Lacerations should be cleaned as soon as possible, and consideration should be given to the possibility of foreign body.
- Thermal burns are treated with early analgesia.

## ED TREATMENT/PROCEDURES
- Elevation, rest, and intermittent application of ice for the 1st 24 hr are appropriate treatment for all hand injuries (RICE).
- Boxer's fractures usually have some volar flexion of the distal fragment:
  - Reduction should be attempted for volar angulation of 40° or more.
  - Fractures of the 4th and 5th metacarpals that are stable and with no significant rotational component can be treated with a padded ulnar gutter splint.
- Fractures of the index and middle finger metacarpals are more difficult to stabilize:
  - Radial gutter splint and early orthopedic referral
- Thumb metacarpal fractures are uniformly complicated and all should be referred early to a hand surgeon or orthopedist:
  - Place in thumb spica splint.
- Dislocations should be reduced immediately and splinted; metacarpal dislocations are rare and frequently need open reduction and pinning.

- Appropriate splinting position for the MCP joint is the intrinsic plus, or "cobra" position (20–30° wrist extension):
  – MCP joint as close to 90° of flexion as possible
  – Proximal interphalangeal (PIP) and distal interphalangeal (DIP) joints in extension
- Antibiotics for oral flora should be started early for any open injury to the metacarpals suspicious for injury against a tooth, and may require curettage of the impaction site in the operating room.
- Simple torus (buckle) fractures may be splinted and may be followed by a primary care physician.

## MEDICATION

- Check for tetanus status and vaccinate per immunization schedule.
- Silvadene cream or bacitracin ointment is appropriate for thermal burn injury.
- Analgesics may be necessary; NSAIDs or hydrocodone is usually sufficient.
- For human bites or dirty wounds, administer amoxicillin/clavulanate (Augmentin), *or:*
  – A cephalosporin or other penicillinase-resistant antibiotic given parenterally is appropriate.

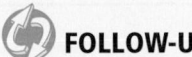 **FOLLOW-UP**

### DISPOSITION

#### Admission Criteria

- Open fractures or dislocations require urgent surgical intervention and should be admitted.
- All thumb metacarpal fractures or dislocations should be seen by an orthopedist or hand surgeon because of the special importance of the thumb in all activities of the hand.
- Infection from a bite wound requires prompt orthopedic consultation, admission for irrigation, debridement, and IV antibiotics.

#### Discharge Criteria

- Patients with a stable transverse or oblique fracture in a good splint may be discharged for early orthopedic follow-up.
- Metacarpal–carpal dislocations are usually unstable enough to require surgery even if reduction is achieved, but this may be semiurgent rather than emergent.
- If a metacarpal fracture produces impaired range of motion or misalignment of the finger, the patient will require surgical repair in the 1st several days after injury.

#### Pediatric Considerations

Epiphyseal injuries mandate orthopedic referral.

## PEARLS AND PITFALLS

With all metacarpal injuries assure proper rotational alignment.

## ADDITIONAL READING

- American College of Radiology, Expert Panel on Musculoskeletal Imaging. Acute hand and wrist trauma. 2001.
- American Society for Surgery of the Hand. *The Hand: Examination and Diagnosis,* 3rd ed. New York: Churchill Livingstone; 1990.
- American Society for Surgery of the Hand. *The Hand: Primary Care of Common Problems,* 2nd ed. New York: Churchill Livingstone; 1990.
- Harrison B, Holland P. Diagnosis and management of hand injuries in the ED. *Emerg Med Pract.* 2005;7(2):28.

 **CODES**

### ICD9

- 815.00 Closed fracture of metacarpal bone(s), site unspecified
- 815.01 Closed fracture of base of thumb (first) metacarpal
- 815.02 Closed fracture of base of other metacarpal bone(s)

M

# METHANOL POISONING

*Kirk L. Cumpston*

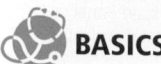 **BASICS**

## DESCRIPTION
- Colorless, volatile liquid
- Absorbed in 30–60 min
- Metabolized by liver
- Half-life 4–8 hr
- Mechanism:
  - Inebriating
  - Nontoxic
  - Metabolites of formaldehyde and formic acid produce toxic effects.
  - Uncouples oxidative phosphorylation
- Formic acid:
  - Determines degree of acidosis, visual symptoms, and mortality
  - Directly toxic to retinal and optic nerve tissue
- Methanol metabolism:
  - Step 1: Methanol is converted to formaldehyde by liver enzyme alcohol dehydrogenase.
  - Step 2: Formaldehyde is then rapidly converted by aldehyde dehydrogenase to formic acid.
  - Step 3: Formic acid is degraded to carbon dioxide and water by folate-dependent mechanism.
  - Steps 1 and 3 are rate-limiting steps.

## ETIOLOGY
Common sources of methanol:
- Wood alcohol
- Windshield washer fluid
- Inhalational abuse of carburetor cleaners
- Fuel antifreeze solutions
- Formalin
- Gasoline
- Paint solvents
- Household cleaners
- Sterno cans
- Moonshine

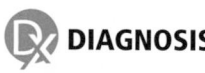 **DIAGNOSIS**

## SIGNS AND SYMPTOMS
- GI:
  - Anorexia
  - Nausea/vomiting
  - Abdominal pain
- CNS:
  - Headache
  - Dizziness
  - Confusion
  - Inebriation
  - Coma
  - Seizures
- Ophthalmologic:
  - Blurry vision
  - Photophobia
  - "Snow fields"
  - Blindness

### History
- Intentional or unintentional methanol ingestion
- No history, but a patient with an unexplained high anion gap metabolic acidosis
- Elevated unexplained osmol gap

### Physical Exam
- Optic disc:
  - Hyperemia or pallor
  - Papilledema
- Tachypnea
- Altered mental status

## ESSENTIAL WORKUP
- History of all substances ingested
- Inquire about visual symptoms.
- Funduscopic examination
- Drawn simultaneously:
  - Arterial blood gas
  - Serum methanol, ethylene glycol, isopropyl alcohol, and ethanol levels
  - Electrolytes, BUN, creatinine, and glucose
  - Measured serum osmolality (by freezing-point depression is preferred)

## DIAGNOSTIC TESTS & INTERPRETATION
### Lab
- Calculate anion gap $= (Na^+) - (Cl^- + HCO_3^-)$:
  - Normal $= 8-12$.
- Determine serum osmol gap:
  - Osmol gap = measured osmolality − calculated osmolarity:
  - Calculated osmolarity $= 2(Na^+) +$ glucose/18 + BUN/2.8 + ethanol (in mg/dL)/4.6.
- Osmol gap:
  - Screens for methanol
  - Most sensitive early in poisoning and normalizes as methanol is metabolized or with concurrent ethanol ingestion
  - Traditionally an osmol gap >10 is considered indication for ruling out occult methanol ingestion. However, potentially toxic serum concentrations of methanol can be present with osmol gap <10.
  - A negative osmol gap **DOES NOT** rule out a methanol exposure.
  - With concurrent ethanol ingestion, osmol gap tends to be larger and acidosis tends to be less severe because relatively less methanol has been converted to acid-producing metabolites.
- Serum methanol concentrations *confirm* methanol poisoning:
  - Late after ingestion, no parent compound may be detected and severe high anion gap metabolic acidosis will be present.
- Ethanol concentration may have clinical implications and is pertinent in interpreting laboratory tests.

### Imaging
CT brain

## DIFFERENTIAL DIAGNOSIS
- Increased osmol gap:
- *ME DIE A*:
  - Methanol
  - Ethanol
  - Diuretics/diluents (mannitol, glycerin, sorbitol, propylene glycol),
  - Isopropyl alcohol
  - Ethylene glycol
  - Acetone, ammonia
- Elevated anion gap metabolic acidosis: *ACAAT MUDPILES*:
  - Alcoholic ketoacidosis
  - Cyanide, CO, $H_2S$, others
  - Acetaminophen:
    - Rare in acute ingestion
    - Rare in chronic ingestion
    - Fulminant hepatic failure
- Antiretrovirals (nucleoside reverse transcriptase inhibitors):
  - Toluene
  - Methanol, metformin
  - Uremia
  - Diabetic ketoacidosis
  - Paraldehyde, phenformin, propylene glycol
  - Iron, isoniazid
  - Lactic acidosis
  - Ethylene glycol
  - Salicylate, acetylsalicylic acid (aspirin), starvation ketosis

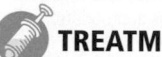 **TREATMENT**

## PRE-HOSPITAL
- Transport all possibly ingested substances.
- Dermal decontamination of a methanol spill by clothing removal, irrigation with soap and water
- Monitor airway and CNS depression.

## INITIAL STABILIZATION/THERAPY
- Airway, breathing, and circulation (ABCs)
- Dextrose, naloxone, and thiamine for altered mental status
- Prevent further methanol absorption:
  - Gastric lavage:
    - Likely not helpful because of rapid absorption of methanol and delay in presentation >1 hr
  - Ipecac-induced emesis not recommended
  - Activated charcoal:
    - For potential coingestants
    - Poorly adsorbs methanol

## ED TREATMENT/PROCEDURES
- Prevent methanol conversion to toxic metabolites with fomepizole (preferable) or ethanol infusion
- Fomepizole (4-MP, Antizol):
  - Competitive inhibitor of alcohol dehydrogenase
  - Indications:
    - Intentional methanol ingestion
    - Accidental methanol ingestion of more than a sip
    - Altered mental status or visual symptoms associated with unexplained osmol gap and/or elevated anion gap metabolic acidosis
  - Initiate before serum methanol level returns if intentional ingestion or more than a sip.
  - Continue until methanol level is <25 mg/dL.
  - Advantages:
    - No need for continuous infusion
    - No inebriation/CNS depression
    - Ease of dosing
    - No hypoglycemia, no hyponatremia, no hyperosmolality
    - No checking serum concentrations
    - Reduced nursing care and monitoring
    - Occult methanol exposure can often be ruled out before second dose is needed.

– Disadvantages:
  ○ Blurry vision
  ○ Transient elevation of liver function tests
• Ethanol therapy:
  – Not FDA approved for treatment of methanol
  – Ethanol has greater affinity than methanol for alcohol dehydrogenase:
    ○ Slows metabolism to formaldehyde and formic acid by competitive inhibition
  – Ethanol is the second-choice antidote if fomepizole is not available.
  – Initiate before methanol level returns if potentially toxic ingestion is highly suspected or confirmed by history:
    ○ Therapeutic range is 100–150 mg/dL.
  – Continue until methanol level is <25 mg/dL.
  – Indications for ethanol therapy:
    ○ Intentional methanol ingestion
    ○ Accidental methanol ingestion of more than a sip
    ○ Altered mental status or visual symptoms associated with unexplained osmol gap and or elevated anion gap metabolic acidosis
  – Advantages:
    ○ Easily accessible
    ○ Oral and IV routes
  – Disadvantages:
    ○ CNS depression especially in children
    ○ Respiratory depression
    ○ Hyponatremia or hypernatremia
    ○ Hypoglycemia
    ○ Hyperosmolarity
    ○ Continuous infusion
    ○ Frequent laboratory testing
    ○ Contraindicated in pregnancy
• Enhance elimination of methanol and toxic metabolites with hemodialysis:
  – Decreases elimination half-life of methanol
  – Removes formaldehyde and formic acid
  – Indications:
    ○ Ingestion of >1 mL/kg of 100% methanol
    ○ Ophthalmologic manifestations
    ○ Severe metabolic acidosis unresponsive to bicarbonate therapy
    ○ Persistent electrolyte or metabolic acidosis
    ○ Renal insufficiency
    ○ Serum methanol level >25 mg/dL
  – Continue hemodialysis until methanol level approaches <25 mg/dL and the metabolic acidosis has resolved.
• Folic acid and folinic acid (leucovorin):
  – Folic acid: Cofactor required for conversion of formic acid to carbon dioxide and water
  – Supplemental folate important in malnourished individuals (alcoholics)
• Correct acid-base abnormalities:
  – Sodium bicarbonate for severe acidosis (pH <7.1)
  – The goal of the sodium bicarbonate drip is to maintain a normal serum pH.

## MEDICATION

• Activated charcoal: 1 g/kg PO
• Dextrose: D50W 1 amp: 50 mL or 25 g (peds: D25W 2–4 mL/kg) IV
• Fomepizole:
  – Loading dose: 15 mg/kg slow infusion over 30 min
  – Maintenance dose: 10 mg/kg q12h for 4 doses, then 15 mg/kg q12h until methanol levels reduced <25 mg/dL
  – Dosing related to hemodialysis:
    ○ Do not administer dose at beginning of dialysis if last dose was <6 hr previously.
    ○ Administer next dose if last dose was >6 hr previously.
    ○ Dose q4h during dialysis.
    ○ If time between last dose and end of dialysis was <1 hr from last dose, do not administer new dose.
    ○ If time between last dose and end of dialysis was 1–3 hr from last dose, administer 1/2 of next scheduled dose.
    ○ If time between last dose and end of dialysis was >3 hr from last dose, administer next scheduled dose.
• Ethanol:
  – Oral: 50% ethanol solution (100-proof liquor) via nasogastric tube:
    ○ Loading dose 2 mL/kg
    ○ Maintenance dose 0.5 mL/kg/hr
    ○ Maintenance dose during hemodialysis 1 mL/kg/hr
  – IV: 10% ethanol in D5W:
    ○ Loading dose 8 mL/kg over 30–60 min
    ○ Maintenance infusion 2 mL/kg/hr
    ○ Maintenance infusion during hemodialysis 4 mL/kg/hr
• Folic acid: 50 mg IV q4h for 24 hr
• Sodium bicarbonate: 1–2 mEq/kg in 1 L of D5W with 40 mEq KCl at 250 mL/hr

##  FOLLOW-UP

### DISPOSITION

#### Admission Criteria

• Significant historical methanol ingestion even if initially asymptomatic
• ICU admission for seriously ill patients
• Transfer to another facility if hemodialysis or antidote is indicated but not readily available.

#### Discharge Criteria

Asymptomatic patient with isolated methanol ingestion if serum methanol level is <25 mg/dL; normal acid/base status and electrolytes

### FOLLOW-UP RECOMMENDATIONS

Psychiatric follow-up for suicidal/depressed patients

## PEARLS AND PITFALLS

• An osmol gap <10 mmol/L does not rule out a methanol exposure.
• If you have a patient with an elevated anion gap and methanol exposure is in the differential diagnosis, administer fomepizole immediately and confirm exposure with a serum concentration.
• If you cannot confirm a methanol exposure, or do not have hemodialysis capabilities 24/7, or have no antidote, transfer the patient to a facility that has all of these capabilities.
• Not all patients will have an elevated osmol and anion gap. Early presenters will have an osmol gap only, and late presenters may have an anion gap only. Patients who present in between will have a combination of an anion gap and an osmol gap.

## ADDITIONAL READING

• Brent J, McMartin K, Phillips S, et al. Fomepizole for the treatment of methanol poisoning. *N Engl J Med.* 2001;344:424–429.
• Hovda KE, Froyshov S, Gudmundsdottir H, et al. Fomepizole may change indication for hemodialysis in methanol poisoning: Prospective study in seven cases. *Clin Nephrol.* 2005;64(3):190–197.
• Leikin J, Paloucek F. Ethyl alcohol. In: *Leikin and Paloucek's Poisoning and Toxicology Handbook,* 4th ed. New York: Lexi-Comp; 2008:294–295.
• Leikin J, Paloucek F. Fomepizole. In: *Leikin and Paloucek's Poisoning and Toxicology Handbook,* 4th ed. New York: Lexi-Comp; 2008:989.
• Leikin J, Paloucek F. Methanol. In: *Leikin and Paloucek's Poisoning and Toxicology Handbook,* 4th ed. New York: Lexi-Comp; 2008:817–819.
• Mycyk MD, Aks SE. A visual schematic for clarifying the temporal relationship between anion and osmol gaps in toxic alcohol poisoning. *Am J Emerg Med.* 2003;21(4):333–335.

##  CODES

ICD9
980.1 Toxic effect of methyl alcohol

M

# METHEMOGLOBINEMIA

*Gerald Maloney*

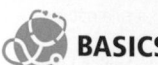 **BASICS**

## DESCRIPTION

- Iron molecule in hemoglobin is oxidized from $Fe^{2+}$ to $Fe^{3+}$, resulting in a form of hemoglobin that cannot transport oxygen.
- Oxygen-carrying capacity of blood is reduced and cyanosis is generally present with significant levels.
- Normal methemoglobin levels are $\leq 1\%$; symptoms usually occur with levels $>20\%$.
- Methemoglobin:
  - Oxidation of hemoglobin iron from ferrous ($Fe^{2+}$) to ferric ($Fe^{3+}$) state
  - Decreases total oxygen-carrying capacity (functional anemia)
  - Shifts hemoglobin oxygen-dissociation curve to the left, impairing $O_2$ release to tissues
  - Maintained at physiologic level (1–2%) by nicotinamide adenine dinucleotide (NADH)-methemoglobin (cytochrome $B_5$) reductase in RBCs
- Congenital methemoglobinemia:
  - NADH-methemoglobin (cytochrome $B_5$) reductase deficiency (homozygous or heterozygous)
  - Heterozygous hemoglobin M and other abnormal hemoglobins
- Acquired methemoglobinemia results from oxidant stress on RBCs:
  - Some methemoglobin-inducing agents are direct oxidants (eg, nitrites)
  - Many substances produce oxidant injury via N-hydroxylamine metabolites.
  - Methemoglobinemia may be delayed relative to initial substance exposure.
- Many methemoglobin-inducing agents also cause Heinz body hemolytic anemia (HA):
  - Caused by oxidant injury of RBC proteins
  - Glucose-6-phosphate dehydrogenase (G6PD)–deficient patients have higher risk.
  - Patients with methemoglobinemia should be worked up for HA.
- Methemoglobinemia may serve as marker for genetic abnormalities:
  - Heterozygous NADH-methemoglobin (cytochrome $B_5$) reductase deficiency

## ETIOLOGY

- More serious with coexisting anemia
- Cyanide (CN) antidote kit:
  - Induces methemoglobinemia via amyl and sodium nitrite
  - CN will preferentially complex with methemoglobin, which can then be chelated by sodium thiosulfate.

- Nitrates/nitrites (most common):
  - Nitrites ($NO_2$)
  - Nitrates ($NO_3$), eg, nitroglycerine, via metabolic conversion to nitrites
  - Nitric oxide (NO)
- Dyes:
  - Aniline dyes
  - Methylene blue (excessive)
- Antiparasitic drugs (high potential for MetHb formation):
  - Dapsone
  - Primaquine
  - Chloroquine
- Local anesthetics (high potential for MetHb formation):
  - Benzocaine
  - Lidocaine
  - Prilocaine
- Analgesics:
  - Phenazopyridine (Pyridium)
  - Phenacetin
- Antibiotics:
  - Nitrofurantoin
  - Sulfones
  - Sulfonamides
- Others:
  - Metoclopramide
  - Naphthalene (mothballs)
  - Paraquat (herbicide)
  - Arsine gas ($AsH_3$)
  - Chlorates ($ClO_4$)
  - Phenols (eg, dinitrophenol, hydroquinone)

 **DIAGNOSIS**

## SIGNS AND SYMPTOMS

- Central cyanosis, refractory to oxygen administration:
  - Cyanosis evident at methemoglobin (MetHb) of 10–15% of total hemoglobin in nonanemic patient (or 1.5 g methemoglobin/dL blood)
- Dyspnea/tachypnea
- Chest pain/dysrhythmias
- Syncope
- Altered mental status with levels $>50\%$

## History

- Exposure to methemoglobin-inducing agent
- All substances ingested and time(s) of ingestion
- G6PD deficiency
- Medical conditions vulnerable to impaired oxygen delivery (eg, coronary artery disease)

### Physical Exam

- Cyanosis
- Emphasis on mental status and cardiovascular findings
- Icterus or dark-colored urine with accompanying hemolytic anemia

## ESSENTIAL WORKUP

- Pulse oximetry is *inaccurate* in methemoglobinemia:
  - MetHb interferes with pulse oximetry measurement of hemoglobin oxygen saturation.
  - Saturation decreases to ~85% with increasingly more severe methemoglobinemia.
  - Pulse oximetry cannot be used to guide management.
- ABG for:
  - Methemoglobin level
  - Carboxyhemoglobin level
  - $PaO_2$ and $PaCO_2$
- ECG

## DIAGNOSTIC TESTS & INTERPRETATION
### Lab

- Blood classically described as chocolate-colored
- CBC with manual differential count and smear analysis for evidence of hemolytic anemia
- Urinalysis for blood versus intact RBCs to detect presence of free hemoglobin in urine

### Imaging
CXR to rule out other pulmonary pathology

## DIFFERENTIAL DIAGNOSIS

- Hypoxia:
  - CHF
  - COPD
  - Pulmonary embolism
- Irritant gas exposure
- Blue discoloration:
  - Hypoxia
  - Sulfhemoglobinemia
  - Cyanide poisoning
  - Hydrogen sulfide poisoning
  - Excess methylene blue administration
  - Tellurium toxicity
  - Skin contact/staining with blue dye

# TREATMENT

## PRE-HOSPITAL
- Bring to hospital all substances patient may have ingested.
- Question witnesses and observe scene for household products and other potential coingestants:
  - Document and relay findings to emergency medical staff.
- Commercial or industrial sites:
  - Obtain relevant Material Safety Data Sheets (MSDSs) if available to identify commercial or chemical products.
  - Avoid dermal exposures.

## INITIAL STABILIZATION/THERAPY
- ABCs:
  - Cardiac monitor
  - Isotonic crystalloids as needed for hypotension
- Naloxone, thiamine, and dextrose ($D_{50}W$) as indicated for altered mental status
- Supplemental oxygen

## ED TREATMENT/PROCEDURES
- Decontamination:
  - If owing to acute ingestion/overdose within previous 1–2 hr, and protective airway reflexes are intact, administer 75 g of activated charcoal PO.
- Remove source of oxidant stress.
- Methylene blue:
  - Indications:
    - Asymptomatic with levels >30%
    - Symptomatic patients with levels >10–20%, especially if comorbid diseases are present
  - Expect transient worsening of saturations on pulse oximetry after methylene blue is administered:
    - No specific intervention required
  - Use with caution in patients with glucose-6 pyruvate decarboxylase deficiency.
    - May cause hemolysis
- If no improvement with methylene blue, consider that source of oxidant stress is not eliminated, or that sulfhemoglobinemia is present:
  - Sulfhemoglobin is sulfur molecule bound to hemoglobin; presents similar to methemoglobin, but is self-limited.

- RBC transfusion:
  - May be necessary to increase blood oxygen-carrying capacity
  - Especially if hemolytic anemia is present
- Exchange transfusion:
  - Especially with neonates/infants
- Hyperbaric oxygen therapy:
  - Increases oxygen delivery to tissues by mass effect, independent of hemoglobin
  - Use in life-threatening methemoglobinemia if immediately available.

## Pediatric Considerations
- Children may develop significant methemoglobinemia from apparently minor ingestions.
- Symptoms delayed several hours after ingestion, so prolonged observation necessary
- Neonates are also at higher risk of methemoglobinemia (owing to decreased stores of NADH methemoglobin reductase).

## MEDICATION
- Dextrose 50%: 25 g (50 mL) (peds: 0.5 g/kg $D_{25}W$) IV for hypoglycemia
- Methylene blue: 1 mg/kg of 1% solution IV over 5 min (adult and peds):
  - May repeat if no improvement in 1 hr
- Naloxone: 0.4–2.0 mg (peds: 0.1 mg/kg) IV, may repeat up to 10 mg for suspected opioid intoxication
- Thiamine: 100 mg (peds: 1 mg/kg) IM or IV

# FOLLOW-UP

## DISPOSITION
### Admission Criteria
- Severely symptomatic patients
- Patients requiring multiple doses of methylene blue
- Dapsone may cause prolonged recurrent methemoglobinemia.

### Discharge Criteria
Methemoglobin levels <20% and falling with no symptoms or comorbid disease

## Issues for Referral
Toxicology consult for significant exposures

## FOLLOW-UP RECOMMENDATIONS
Occupational medicine referral for work-related exposures

# PEARLS AND PITFALLS
- Pulse oximetry is *inaccurate* in methemoglobinemia.
- Obtain an ABG.
- Administer methylene blue for significant levels/symptoms.

# ADDITIONAL READING
- Bradberry SM, Aw TC, Williams NR, et al. Occupational methaemoglobinemia. *Occup Environ Med*. 2001;58:611–615.
- Price D. Methemoglobinemia. In: Goldfrank L, Flomenbaum N, Lewin N, et al., eds. *Goldfrank's Toxicologic Emergencies*, 8th ed. New York: McGraw-Hill; 2006.
- Ward KE, McCarthy MW. Dapsone-induced methemoglobinemia. *Ann Pharmacother*. 1998;32(5):549–553.
- Wright RO, Lewander WJ, Woolf AD. Methemoglobinemia: Etiology, pharmacology, and clinical management. *Ann Emerg Med*. 1999;34:646–656.

# CODES

ICD9
289.7 Methemoglobinemia

M

# MITRAL VALVE PROLAPSE
*Liudvikas Jagminas*

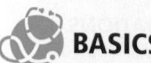

## BASICS

### DESCRIPTION
- Clinical syndrome resulting from diverse pathogenic mechanisms of ≥1 portions of the mitral valve apparatus
- Occurs when the leaflet edges of the mitral valve do not coapt
- Commonly due to abnormal stretching of 1 of the mitral valve leaflets during systole:
  - Myxomatous proliferation of the spongiosa layer within the valve causing focal interruption of the fibrosa layer
  - Excessive stretching of the chordae tendineae, leading to traction on papillary muscles
- Theoretical explanations for associated chest pain:
  - Focal ischemia from coronary microembolism due to platelet aggregates and fibrin deposits in the angles between the leaflets
  - Coronary artery spasm
- Mitral regurgitation (MR) may occur in some patients.
- Age of onset is 10–16 years.
- Female > Male (3:1)
- Typically benign in young women, whereas men >50 years tend to have serious sequelae
- Can be identified by ECG in 2–4% of the general population and in 7% of autopsies
- A variety of neuroendocrine and autonomic disturbances occur in some patients.
- Genetics:
  - Strong hereditary component
  - Sometimes transmitted as an autosomal dominant trait with varying penetrance

### ETIOLOGY
- Marfan syndrome
- Relapsing polychondritis
- Ehlers-Danlos syndrome (ie, types I, II, IV)
- Osteogenesis imperfecta
- Pseudoxanthoma elasticum
- Stickler syndrome
- Systemic lupus erythematosus
- Polyarteritis nodosa
- Polycystic kidney disease
- Von Willebrand syndrome
- Duchenne muscular dystrophy

## DIAGNOSIS

### SIGNS AND SYMPTOMS
Separated into 3 categories:
- Symptoms related to autonomic dysfunction
- Symptoms related to the progression of MR
- Symptoms that occur as a result of an associated complication (ie, stroke, endocarditis, or arrhythmia)

#### History
- Palpitations in up to 40% of cases:
  - Usually ventricular premature beats or paroxysmal supraventricular tachycardia
  - Up to 40% have symptoms of dysautonomia
- Chest pain occurs in 10%:
  - Sharp, localized, of variable duration, and nonexertional
  - Rarely may respond to nitroglycerin
- Panic attacks
- Anxiety
- Fatigue
- Depression in up to 70%
- Nervousness
- Migraine headaches
- Irritable bowel
- Syncope/presyncope:
  - Occurs in 0.9% of patients
- Orthostasis
- Dyspnea and fatigue relatively uncommon

#### Physical Exam
- Mid to late systolic click at the cardiac apex:
  - Standing or Valsalva moves click closer to S1.
  - S1 may be accentuated when prolapse occurs early in systole.
  - Squatting moves click closer to S2.
- Late systolic murmur
- Skeletal abnormalities are observed in 2/3 of patients:
  - Asthenic body habitus: Height-to-weight ratio > normal
  - Arm span > height (dolichostenomelia)
  - Scoliosis or kyphosis
  - Pectus excavatum
  - Arachnodactyly
  - Joint hypermobility
- Hypomastia
- Cathedral palate

### ESSENTIAL WORKUP
- History and auscultation of a midsystolic click are often sufficient to make the diagnosis.
- ECG confirms the diagnosis when clinical information is insufficient.

## DIAGNOSTIC TESTS & INTERPRETATION
### Lab
Not required to establish the diagnosis

### Imaging
- EKG:
  - Usually normal
  - Occasionally ST-T wave depression and inversion in leads III and aVF
  - Premature atrial and ventricular contractions
- CXR:
  - Typically normal
  - If MR is present, may show both left atrial and ventricular enlargement
  - Calcification of the mitral annulus in patients with Marfan syndrome
- ECG:
  - Classic MVP: The parasternal long-axis view shows >2 mm superior displacement of the mitral leaflets into the left atrium during systole, with a leaflet thickness of at least 5 mm.
  - Nonclassic MVP: Displacement is >2 mm, with a maximal leaflet thickness of <5 mm.
  - Other ECG findings that should be considered as criteria are leaflet thickening, redundancy, annular dilatation, and chordal elongation.
  - Minor criteria:
    - Isolated mild to moderate superior systolic displacement of the posterior mitral leaflet
    - Moderate superior systolic displacement of both mitral leaflets

### Diagnostic Procedures/Surgery
Cardiac studies may be indicated in patients with chest pain when the etiology is uncertain.

### DIFFERENTIAL DIAGNOSIS
- MI/ischemia
- Hypertrophic cardiomyopathy with obstruction
- Idiopathic hypertrophic subaortic stenosis
- Tachyarrhythmias
- Atrial fibrillation/flutter
- Ventricular septal defect
- Papillary muscle dysfunction
- Hypokalemia
- Hypomagnesemia
- Valvular heart disease
- Pheochromocytoma
- Anemia
- Thyrotoxicosis
- Pregnancy
- Toxicity from cocaine, amphetamines, or other sympathomimetics
- Ventricular tachycardia
- WPW syndrome
- Rheumatic endocarditis
- Anxiety/panic disorder
- Stress
- Menopause

# TREATMENT

## PRE-HOSPITAL
- ABCs
- IV access
- Supplemental oxygen
- Cardiac monitoring
- Pulse oximetry

## INITIAL STABILIZATION/THERAPY
- Cardiac monitoring
- Supplemental oxygen
- IV catheter placement

## ED TREATMENT/PROCEDURES
- Medications generally are not necessary. $\beta$-blockers may be helpful if palpitations are severe.
- Antiplatelet agents (aspirin, aspirin with extended-release dipyridamole, or clopidogrel) are indicated for patients with transient ischemic attack or stroke symptoms.
- Orthostatic hypotension and presyncope symptoms may be treated with sodium chloride tablets; however, if this treatment is not successful, fludrocortisone may be used.
- Magnesium supplementation may improve symptoms of the classic MVP syndrome.
- Significant MR in the setting of HTN (systolic blood pressure >140 mm Hg) may be improved with the use of ACE inhibitors.
- $\beta$-Blockers:
  - Patients with tachycardia or severely symptomatic chest pain
- Digoxin is an alternative for supraventricular tachycardia and prevention of chest pain and fatigue.
- Antibiotic prophylaxis.
  - When performing surgical procedures (eg, contaminated wound repair, abscess incision and drainage)
  - Indicated in the following settings:
    ○ Presence of a murmur
    ○ Evidence of nontrivial MR on ECG
    ○ Men >45 years with valve thickening
  - Prophylaxis is not suggested for patients who have an isolated click without a murmur or for patients without evidence of MR on an ECG.

## MEDICATION

### First Line
- Amoxicillin: 2 g PO 1 hr before the procedure (peds: 50 mg/kg PO 1 hr before procedure)
- Ampicillin: 2 g IV/IM 30 min before the procedure (peds: 50 mg/kg IV/IM 30 min before the procedure)
- Clindamycin: 600 mg PO 1 hr before procedure (peds: 20 mg/kg PO 1 hr before procedure; not to exceed 600 mg)
- Propranolol: 1–3 mg IV at 1 mg/min, 80–640 mg/d PO (peds: 1–4 mg/kg/d PO div. b.i.d./q.i.d.)
- Isoproterenol: 0.02–0.06 mg IV × 1, 0.01–0.02 mg IV or 2–20 mg/min infusion
- Atenolol: 0.3–2 mg/kg/d PO, max. 2 mg/kg/d

### Second Line
- Digoxin: 0.5–1 mg IV/IM div. 50% initially then 25% × 2 q6–12h or 0.125–0.5 mg/d PO
- Fludrocortisone: 0.05–0.10 mg/d PO

# FOLLOW-UP

## DISPOSITION

### Admission Criteria
- Severe MR
- Severe chest pain with ischemic symptoms
- Syncope or near syncope
- Life-threatening dysrhythmias
- Cerebral ischemic events, including transient ischemic attack

### Discharge Criteria
- Asymptomatic
- No laboratory abnormalities
- No significant MR or dysrhythmias

### Issues for Referral
- Cardiology consultation is warranted in cases of ventricular dysrhythmia or risk of sudden death, as well as when symptoms of severe MR are present.
- Cardiothoracic surgery follow-up is recommended for patients with hemodynamically significant MR.
- Pilots with mitral valve prolapse may develop MR under positive G force and be at risk for dysrhythmia or syncope.

### Pediatric Considerations
Dysrhythmias, sudden death, and bacterial endocarditis have been reported.

### Geriatric Considerations
- Often present in an atypical manner:
  - More likely to have holosystolic murmurs and a greater degree of MR.
- Heart failure may be presenting symptom complex associated with ruptured chordae tendineae.

### Pregnancy Considerations
- Consideration of valve replacement:
  - Symptomatic patients
  - Atrial fibrillation
  - Ejection fraction <50–60%
  - Left ventricular end-diastolic dimension >45–50 mm
  - Pulmonary systolic pressure >50–60 mm Hg
- Valve repair rather than replacement is preferred to avoid the need for anticoagulation.

## FOLLOW-UP RECOMMENDATIONS
- Repeat evaluations are necessary every 3–5 years to identify any progression of disease.
- Infective endocarditis prophylaxis is indicated in patients with MVP and MR while undergoing at-risk procedures.
- Coronary artery anomalies should be excluded in patients with chest pain before they participate in sports.

- Patients with MVP and a murmur should avoid high-intensity competitive sports in the following settings:
  - Syncope associated with dysrhythmia
  - A family history of sudden death associated with MVP
  - Significant supraventricular or ventricular dysrhythmias
  - Moderate-to-severe MR

# PEARLS AND PITFALLS
- The diagnosis of MVP should not be an excuse to terminate further diagnostic evaluation of patients with symptoms of chest pain, palpitations, dyspnea, or syncope.
- MVP does not predispose women to any increased risk during pregnancy.
- MVP is the 3rd most common cause of sudden death in athletes.

# ADDITIONAL READING

- Avierinos JF. Risk, determinants, and outcome implications of progression of mitral regurgitation after diagnosis of mitral valve prolapse in a single community. *Am J Cardiol*. 2008;101(5):662–667.
- Bobkowski W, Siwińska A, Zachwieja J. A prospective study to determine the significance of ventricular late potentials in children with mitral valvular prolapse. *Cardiol Young*. 2002;12(4):333–338.
- Guntheroth W. Link among mitral valve prolapse, anxiety disorders, and inheritance. *Am J Cardiol*. 2007;99(9):1350.
- Salem DN. Valvular and structural heart disease: American College of Chest Physicians Evidence-Based Clinical Practice Guidelines (8th edition) *Chest*. 2008;133(6 Suppl):593S–629S.
- Theal M, Sleik K, Anand S. Prevalence of mitral valve prolapse in ethnic groups. *Can J Cardiol*. 2004;20(5):511–515.
- Weisse AB. Mitral valve prolapse: Now you see it; now you don't: Recalling the discovery, rise and decline of a diagnosis. *Am J Cardiol*. 2007;99(1):129–133.

# CODES

## ICD9
424.0 Mitral valve disorders

M

# MOLLUSCUM CONTAGIOSUM

*Christopher E. Anderson*
*Deepi G. Goyal*

 **BASICS**

## DESCRIPTION
- Molluscum contagiosum (MC) is a generally benign human disease characterized by multiple small, painless, pearly lesions.
- MC appears on epithelial surface and spreads through close contact or autoinoculation.
- 5–18% of patients with HIV have coinfection with MC.

## ETIOLOGY
- MC is caused by a double-stranded DNA poxvirus.
- Transmission in children is by direct skin-to-skin contact, fomites, or pool or bath water.
- Transmission in adults is most often by sexual contact; autoinoculation is common at any age.
- There are rare reports of transmission to infants during childbirth.

 **DIAGNOSIS**

## SIGNS AND SYMPTOMS
### History
- Incubation period: 14–50 days
- Patients are usually asymptomatic, with occasional pruritus or tenderness.
- 10–25% of patients may have eczematous reaction surrounding the lesions.
- Untreated lesions in immunocompetent hosts usually resolve within several months but can last up to 5 yr.

### Physical Exam
- Lesions are smooth-surfaced, firm, spherical papules 3–5 mm in diameter.
- May be flesh colored, white, translucent, or light yellow
- Distinctive central umbilication in 25%
- Atypical presentations include nonumbilicated, persistent, disseminated, or giant lesions, usually in the setting of immunosuppression.
- Distribution in children: Face, trunk, and extremities; healthy adults: Genitals and lower abdomen; occasionally perioral; rarely on palms and soles
- MC is commonly seen with HIV infection, causing atypical involvement of face, neck, and trunk, lesions to 1.5 cm, and a progressive course. Lesions may also appear with initiation of highly active antiretroviral therapy (HAART) as a manifestation of the immune reconstitution inflammatory syndrome.
- Occasional intraocular or periocular involvement presenting as trachoma or chronic follicular conjunctivitis

## ESSENTIAL WORKUP
- History and careful skin examination
- Skin biopsy for confirmation
- Lesions in adult men necessitate evaluation for an immunocompromised state.
- MC in children is rarely associated with immunodeficiency, and usually no further evaluation is needed.

## DIAGNOSTIC TESTS & INTERPRETATION
### Lab
- Test for immunocompromised state if no clear etiology:
  - CBC with differential
  - HIV if indicated
- If anogenital lesions:
  - Consider syphilis, hepatitis C, HIV

### Diagnostic Procedures/Surgery
Skin biopsy for confirmation

## DIFFERENTIAL DIAGNOSIS
- Basal cell carcinoma
- Histiocytoma
- Keratoacanthoma
- Intradermal nevus
- Darier disease
- Nevoxanthoendothelioma
- Syringoma
- Epithelial nevi
- Sebaceous adenoma
- Atopic dermatitis
- Dermatitis herpetiformis
- Mycosis fungoides
- Jessner lymphocytic infiltration

TREATMENT

**PRE-HOSPITAL**
Maintain universal precautions.

**INITIAL STABILIZATION/THERAPY**
Not applicable in routine cases

**ED TREATMENT/PROCEDURES**
- Aimed at destruction or removal of virus-infected epithelial cells and is indicated to prevent autoinoculation and transmission:
  - Intervention is not always indicated: Lesions are self-limited in immunocompetent hosts.
- If treatment is necessary, consider referral to dermatology.
- If dermatology referral is not an option, physical treatment modalities generally most effective:
  - Curettage after local anesthesia with EMLA (eutectic mixture, lidocaine, prilocaine) or ethyl chloride
  - Cryotherapy with liquid nitrogen
  - Podophyllin, trichloroacetic acid, cantharidin, tretinoin, and cidofovir applied topically are variably effective.
- Griseofulvin and methisazone orally for extensive disease have given mixed results.
- HAART has been effective in reducing incidence in HIV-infected patients.
- Topical imiquimod has shown effectiveness in several small studies.

- Examine sexual partners for MC and other sexually transmitted diseases:
  - Patients should avoid contact sports, swimming pools, shared baths and towels, scratching, and shaving until lesions have resolved.
- Reexamine treated patients for recurrence every 2–4 wk; 2–4 treatments are often needed to clear lesions completely.

**MEDICATION**
- Cantharidin 0.9% solution with equal parts acetone and flexible collodion: Apply topically 1–3 treatments every 7 days or until resolution.
- Imiquimod 5%: Apply topically daily for 3–5 consecutive days for 16 wk.
- Podophyllin (podofilox 0.5%): Apply topically q12h for 3 days, withhold for 4 days; repeat 1-wk cycle up to 4 times until resolved.
- Tretinoin 0.1%: Apply topically q12h for 10 days or until resolution of lesions.
- Trichloroacetic acid (50–80%): Apply and cover with bandage 5–6 days.

 FOLLOW-UP

**DISPOSITION**
*Admission Criteria*
Widespread disease with extensive superinfection in an immunocompromised host

*Discharge Criteria*
Patients without extensive superinfection may be safely treated as outpatients.

*Issues for Referral*
Consider referral to dermatology if treatment or confirmatory testing is necessary.

**FOLLOW-UP RECOMMENDATIONS**
Re-examine treated patient for recurrence every 2–4 wk.

## PEARLS AND PITFALLS

- Active nonintervention is an option in immunocompetent hosts.
- Search for an immunocompromised state if no clear etiology.
- Physical destruction of lesions is often most effective treatment versus medication.

## ADDITIONAL READING

- Allen AL, Siegfried EC. Management of warts and molluscum in adolescents. *Adolesc Med*. 2001;12(2):vi, 229–242.
- Brown MR, Paulson CP, Henry SL. Treatment for anogenital molluscum contagiosum. *Am Fam Physician*. 2009;80:864–865.
- Sladden MJ, Johnston GA. Common skin infections in children. *Br Med J*. 2004;329:403.
- van der Wouden JC, van der Sande R, Van Suijlekom-Smit LWA, et al. Interventions for cutaneous molluscum contagiosum (review). *Cochrane Database Syst Rev*. 2009;CD004767.

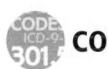 CODES

**ICD9**
078.0 Molluscum contagiosum

M

# MONOAMINE OXIDASE INHIBITOR POISONING

Brenden L. Hansen
James W. Rhee

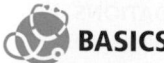 **BASICS**

## DESCRIPTION
- Primarily for depression
- Selegiline, a selective monoamine oxidase B inhibitor, is sometimes used to treat Parkinson disease, and also comes in a transdermal preparation.
- Monoamine oxidase inhibitor (MAOI) pharmacologic actions:
  - Disruption of equilibrium between endogenous monoamine synthesis and degradation, resulting in:
    - Increased neural norepinephrine levels
    - Downregulation of several receptor types
  - Inhibition of irreversible (noncompetitive) enzyme
  - Inhibition of other $B_6$-containing enzymes
- MAO: Principal inactivator of neural bioactive amines:
  - MAO A:
    - Present in the gut and liver
    - Protects against dietary bioactive amines
  - MAO B:
    - Present in neuron terminals and platelets
    - Sympathomimetic amines: Types of bioactive amines

## ETIOLOGY
- MAOI overdose:
  - Toxicopharmacology poorly understood
  - MAO inhibitors: Amphetamine-like in structure:
    - Early: Indirect sympathomimetic effect
    - Late: Sympatholytic response (hypotension)
- MAOI hypertensive crisis syndrome:
  - Results from impaired norepinephrine degradation and large norepinephrine release precipitated by an indirect- or mixed-acting sympathomimetic agent
  - Common precipitants: Tyramine, cocaine, amphetamines
- Serotonin syndrome (SS):
  - Commonly results from exposure to combinations of agents that affect serotonin metabolism or action
  - Increases serotonin synthesis: Tryptophan
  - Increase serotonin release:
    - Indirect- and mixed-acting sympathomimetic agents and dopamine receptor agonists
  - Decrease serotonin reuptake:
    - Selective serotonin reuptake inhibitors
    - Tricyclic antidepressants
    - Newer antidepressants: Trazodone, nefazodone, venlafaxine
    - Phenylpiperidine opioids: Meperidine, dextromethorphan, tramadol, methadone, propoxyphene
  - Direct serotonin receptor agonists:
    - Buspirone, sumatriptan, lysergic acid diethylamide
  - Decrease serotonin breakdown:
    - MAOIs
  - Increases nonspecific serotonin activity:
    - Lithium

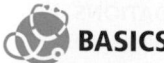 **DIAGNOSIS**

## SIGNS AND SYMPTOMS
- MAOI overdose:
  - Delayed onset (6–12 hr)
  - Initial hypertension with headache
  - Hyperadrenergic activity:
    - Tachycardia
    - Hypertension
    - Mydriasis
    - Agitation
  - Neuromuscular excitation:
    - Nystagmus
    - Hyperreflexia
    - Tremor
    - Myoclonus
    - Rigidity
    - Seizures
  - Hyperthermia
  - Associated complications:
    - Rhabdomyolysis
    - Renal failure
    - Disseminated intravascular coagulation (DIC)
    - Acute respiratory distress syndrome (ARDS)
- MAOI hypertensive crisis syndrome (MAOI interaction with drug or food):
  - Hypertension
  - Tachycardia or bradycardia
  - Hyperthermia
  - Headache, usually occipital
  - Altered mental status
  - Intracranial hemorrhage
  - Seizures
- SS:
  - Increased neuromuscular activity
  - Increased deep tendon reflexes:
    - Lower extremity may be greater than upper
  - Tremor
  - Myoclonus
  - Rigidity (when severe)
  - Autonomic nervous system hyperactivity:
    - Hyperthermia
  - CNS:
    - Agitation
    - Hallucinations
    - Delirium
    - Coma
  - Diarrhea
  - SS versus neuroleptic malignant syndrome (NMS):
    - Both present along a spectrum of severity (mild to severe)
    - Onset: Hours (SS) versus days (NMS)
    - Gastrointestinal symptoms: May be present (SS) versus absent (NMS)
    - Only drug/medication history may differentiate in many cases.

## History
- Time of ingestion
- Bottle available
- Intentional or accidental
- Coingestions

## Physical Exam
- Neuromuscular hyperactivity:
  - Myoclonus
  - Rigidity
  - Tremors
  - Hyperreflexia
- Autonomic hyperactivity:
  - Tachycardia or bradycardia
  - Fever
  - Diaphoresis
- Altered mental status:
  - Agitation, confusion, or excitement

## ESSENTIAL WORKUP
- History of ingested substances
- Rectal temperature monitoring as indicated
- Blood pressure/cardiac monitoring

## DIAGNOSTIC TESTS & INTERPRETATION
### Lab
- Urinalysis:
  - Blood
  - Myoglobin
- Electrolytes, BUN/creatinine, glucose:
  - Hypoglycemia may contribute to altered mental status.
  - Acidosis may accompany severe toxicity.
  - Rhabdomyolysis may cause renal failure.
  - Hyperkalemia—life-threatening consequence of acute renal failure
- Coagulation profile to monitor for potential DIC:
  - INR, prothrombin time, partial thromboplastin time, platelets
- Creatinine kinase:
  - Markedly elevated in rhabdomyolysis
- Urine toxicology screen:
  - May be positive for amphetamines, given the structural similarities between some MAOIs and amphetamines
- Aspirin and acetaminophen levels if suicide attempt a possibility
- Arterial blood gas

### Imaging
- Chest radiograph:
  - ARDS
- Head CT if significant headache or altered mental status or focal neurologic signs:
  - Subarachnoid hemorrhage, intracerebral bleed

### *Diagnostic Procedures/Surgery*

Lumbar puncture for:

- Suspected meningitis (headache, altered mental status, hyperpyrexia)
- Suspected subarachnoid hemorrhage and CT normal

## DIFFERENTIAL DIAGNOSIS

- Hyperthermia:
  - Infection
  - Hyperthyroidism
  - Heat stroke
  - Anatomic thalamic dysfunction
  - Neuroleptic malignant syndrome
  - Malignant hyperthermia
  - Malignant catatonia
  - Ethanol or drug withdrawal
  - Anticholinergic toxicity
  - Sympathomimetic overdose
  - Cocaine-associated delirium/rhabdomyolysis
  - Salicylate toxicity
  - Theophylline toxicity
  - Nicotine toxicity
- Hypertension:
  - Hypoglycemia
  - Carcinoid syndrome
  - Pheochromocytoma
  - Accelerated renovascular hypertension
  - Ethanol or drug withdrawal
  - Sympathomimetic toxicity

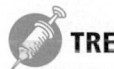 **TREATMENT**

## PRE-HOSPITAL

- Patient may be uncooperative or violent.
- Secure IV access.
- Protect from self induced trauma.

## INITIAL STABILIZATION/THERAPY

- Airway, breathing, and circulation (ABCs)
- IV access and fluid resuscitation if hypotensive
- Oxygen
- Cardiac monitor
- Naloxone, thiamine, D50W (or Accu-Chek) if altered mental status

## ED TREATMENT/PROCEDURES

- Gastrointestinal decontamination:
  - Gastric lavage if within *1 hr* of ingestion or if clinical condition mandates endotracheal intubation
  - Administer activated charcoal.
- Hyperthermia:
  - Benzodiazepines if agitated
  - Active cooling if temperature >40°C:
    - Tepid water mist
    - Evaporate with fan
  - Paralysis:
    - Indicated if muscle rigidity and hyperactivity contributing to persistent hyperthermia
    - Nondepolarizing agent (eg, vecuronium)
    - Avoid succinylcholine
    - Intubation; mechanical ventilation
  - Administer acetaminophen.
  - Apply cooling blankets.

- Severe, malignant hypertension:
  - Nitroprusside (for MAOI overdose)
  - Calcium-channel blocker or phentolamine (for MAOI + food interaction)
  - Use short-acting IV agent that can be rapidly "turned off."
- Hypotension:
  - Initially bolus with isotonic crystalloid solution
  - If no response, administer norepinephrine.
  - Dopamine theoretically contraindicated
- Dysrhythmias (premorbid sign in MAOI overdose):
  - Treat with lidocaine or procainamide.
- Seizures:
  - Benzodiazepines
  - Barbiturates if benzodiazepines unsuccessful
  - Pyridoxine for refractory seizures
- Rigidity:
  - Benzodiazepines
  - Paralysis with vecuronium, endotracheal intubation, and mechanical ventilation
- ARDS:
  - Oxygen
  - Intubation and positive end-expiratory pressure as indicated
- DIC:
  - Fresh-frozen plasma
  - Platelets
  - Whole-blood transfusions
- Rhabdomyolysis:
  - IV isotonic crystalloid solution
  - Maintain hydration.
  - Maintain adequate urine output.
- Specific treatment for SS:
  - Human data limited to case reports and series
  - Mainstay: Supportive care, discontinuation of offending agents
  - Nonselective serotonin antagonist:
    - Cyproheptadine

## ALERT

Phentolamine *contraindicated in MAOI overdose* (results in unopposed beta agonist)

## MEDICATION

- Activated charcoal: 1–2 g/kg PO
- Cyproheptadine: 4–8 mg PO/nasogastric tube q1h–q4h until therapeutic response; max daily dose: 0.5 mg/kg (peds: 0.25 mg/kg/d; max 12 mg/d; safety not established age <2 yr)
- Dextrose: D50W 1–2 amp (50–100 mL or 25–50 g) (peds: D25W 2–4 mL/kg) IV push (IVP)
- Diazepam: 5–10 mg (peds: 0.1 mg/kg slowly) increments IVP
- Lidocaine: 1–1.5 mg/kg IV bolus at 25–50 mg/min followed by infusion at 20–50 mg/kg/min (peds: 1 mg/kg IV bolus at 25–50 mg/min followed by infusion at 20–50 mg/kg/min)
- Lorazepam: 1–2 mg increments IVP
- Nitroprusside: 0.3–10 mg/kg/min IV
- Norepinephrine: 2–4 mg/min (peds: 0.05–0.1 mg/kg/min) IV
- Phentolamine: 5 mg (peds: 0.05–0.2 mg/kg/dose) increments IVP
- Sodium bicarbonate: Bolus 1–2 mEq/kg IVP; adult infusion: 3 amp sodium bicarbonate in 1,000 mL D5W at 2–3 mL/kg/hr IV
- Vecuronium: 0.1 mg/kg IVP

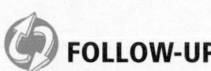 **FOLLOW-UP**

## DISPOSITION

### *Admission Criteria*

- All MAOI overdose patients require admission to a monitored unit for 24 hr.
- ICU admission for seriously ill patients

### *Discharge Criteria*

Resolved mild hypertensive syndrome or resolved mild serotonin syndrome:

- Discharge after several hours of ED observation.

### *Issues for Referral*

Intentional overdoses should receive a psychiatry consult for suicide attempt.

## FOLLOW-UP RECOMMENDATIONS

Following significant MAOI toxicity, medications need to be reassessed to prevent future crises.

## PEARLS AND PITFALLS

- Delayed onset of 6–12 hr prior to symptoms
- Linezolid and methylene blue are MAOIs.
- Phentolamine is contraindicated in MAOI overdose secondary to unopposed beta agonist.

## ADDITIONAL READING

- Boyer EW, Shannon M. The serotonin syndrome. *New Engl J Med*. 2005;352:1112–1120.
- Brush DE, Bird SB, Boyer EW. Monoamine oxidase inhibitor poisoning resulting from Internet misinformation on illicit substances. *J Toxicol Clin Toxicol*. 2004;42:191–195.
- Gillman PK. Monoamine oxidase inhibitors, opioid analgesics and serotonin toxicity. *Br J Anaesth*. 2005;95:434–441.
- Oates JA, Sjoerdsma A. Neurologic effects of tryptophan in patients receiving a monoamine oxidase inhibitor. *Neurology*. 1960;10:1076–1078.
- Ramsay RR, Dunford C, Gillman PK. Methylene blue and serotonin toxicity: Inhibition of monoamine oxidase A (MAO A) confirms a theoretical prediction. *Br J Pharmacol*. 2007;152:946–951.

### See Also (Topic, Algorithm, Electronic Media Element)

Sympathomimetic Poisoning

 **CODES**

### ICD9

969.01 Poisoning by monoamine oxidase inhibitors

**M**

# MONONUCLEOSIS

*Roger M. Barkin*
*Ian Greenwald*

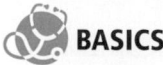

## BASICS

### DESCRIPTION
- Results in most cases from infection with the Epstein-Barr virus (EBV) (a herpesvirus):
  - Non-EBV cases of infectious mononucleosis (IM) caused by:
    - Adenovirus
    - Cytomegalovirus (CMV)
    - Group A β-hemolytic streptococci
    - Hepatitis A
    - Human herpesvirus
    - HIV
    - Rubella
    - *Toxoplasma gondii*
- >90% of adults on serologic testing demonstrate prior infection with EBV:
  - Vast majority of people do not recollect specific IM syndrome.
- Mode of transmission is contact with saliva (usually from an asymptomatic individual):
  - Nickname "kissing disease"
- Incubation period: 4–6 wk
- Viral shedding in saliva can persist intermittently for life.
- Immunologic response:
  - Recruitment and activation of cytotoxic T cells:
    - T cell response is largely responsible for an elevated absolute lymphocyte count.
    - Subtype of the T cell lineage, cytotoxic CD8 cells (Downey cells), contain eccentrically placed and lobulated nuclei with vacuolated cytoplasm: The "atypical lymphocytes" seen on differential.
  - B cell response:
    - B cells are transformed into plasmacytoid cells that secrete immunoglobulins.
  - IgM antibody secreted: The heterophile antibody
  - Clinically manifested by an inflammatory response in the posterior pharynx, regional adenopathy, and splenomegaly.
- Mortality from IM is rare, but secondary to:
  - Splenic rupture
  - Airway edema
  - Secondary bacterial infection
  - Hepatic failure
  - Myocarditis
- EBV infection has also been strongly linked to African Burkitt lymphoma and nasopharyngeal carcinoma.

### Pediatric Considerations
- In children <4 yr, infection with EBV is often asymptomatic.
- In children who do become symptomatic, there is propensity toward atypical presentations:
  - Mesenteric lymphadenopathy and splenomegaly can cause the illness to present with abdominal pain.
  - Infants and toddlers can present with only irritability and failure to thrive.
- Children with splenomegaly should not return to contact sports until exam has normalized.

## DIAGNOSIS

### SIGNS AND SYMPTOMS
#### History
- Insidious onset over several days to weeks
- Prodromal fatigue, malaise, arthralgias, and myalgias
- Prominent sore throat and fever. Progression of airway edema may be associated with respiratory distress.
- Swollen lymph nodes
- Headache
- Significant abdominal pain is uncommon but when present should raise concern about marked splenic enlargement or splenic rupture.
- Development of rash associated with administration of ampicillin or amoxicillin.

#### Physical Exam
- Exudative pharyngitis and tonsillitis (similar appearance to streptococcal pharyngitis)
- Airway compromise associated with edema
- Fever
- Periorbital edema occurs in 15–35% of patients
- Symmetric tender lymphadenopathy
- Hepatomegaly occurs in 15–25% of patients.
- Splenomegaly occurs in 5–60% of patients.
- Nonspecific maculopapular rash can develop.
- Macular erythematous rash can develop if the patient has been given ampicillin:
  - Typically develops 5–9 days after the onset of antibiotic therapy and should not be interpreted as a penicillin-like allergy
- Petechia can occur on the skin or at the junction between the hard and soft palate.

- Complications:
  - Hepatitis:
    - Most common complication, and jaundice occurs in ~5% of patients.
  - Neurologic including:
    - Encephalitis
    - Meningitis
    - Guillain-Barré syndrome
    - Optic neuritis
    - Bell's palsy
- Hemolytic anemia, thrombocytopenia, agranulocytosis, hemophagocytic lymphohistiocytosis (HLH)
- Orchitis
- Secondary infection such as group A strep pharyngitis

### DIAGNOSTIC TESTS & INTERPRETATION
#### Lab
- WBC with differential:
  - Modest elevation in total WBC between 10,000 and 20,000, which peaks during week 2 of the illness
- Lymphocyte count—findings suggestive of IM:
  - >50% lymphocytes on differential
  - Absolute lymphocyte count >4,500
  - Elevated lymphocyte count with >10% atypical lymphocytes
- Liver function tests:
  - Elevated with transaminases up to 3 times normal found in 80–85% of patients
  - Significant elevations in bilirubin to the point of causing clinical jaundice in approximately 5% of cases
- Monospot test detects presence of heterophile antibodies:
  - Most patients develop heterophile antibodies after ~1 wk of illness.
  - Small percentage of patients never develop heterophile antibodies.
  - Heterophile antibodies peak at 2–5 wk and may persist for several months.
  - Positive test relates to a titer >1:40.
  - Rare false positives can be seen with CMV, leukemia, lymphoma, rubella, hepatitis, or lupus.
  - Results often negative in children <4 yr old
- Testing does exist for EBV-specific antibodies but is expensive, time consuming, and rarely needed.

## *Imaging*

Focused abdominal sonography for trauma/CT scan of abdomen for significant abdominal pain looking for evidence of splenic rupture

## DIFFERENTIAL DIAGNOSIS

Divided into infectious and noninfectious causes:

- Infectious:
  - Adenovirus
  - CMV
  - Streptococcal pharyngitis
  - HIV
  - Hepatitis A, B, C
  - Diphtheria in nonimmunized populations
  - Mumps
  - Toxoplasmosis
- Noninfectious:
  - Leukemia
  - Lymphoma
  - Medication-induced syndrome—phenytoin, sulfa drugs

 **TREATMENT**

## PRE-HOSPITAL

### ALERT
- Follow standard universal precautions.
- ABCs. Assess airway patency.
- Initiate IV hydration with normal saline if patient is clinically dehydrated secondary to pharyngitis symptoms.

## INITIAL STABILIZATION/THERAPY
- ABC management. Airway edema may require intervention.
- If possible, avoid placing patient in the same general area as posttransplant and other immunocompromised patients.

## ED TREATMENT/PROCEDURES
- Supportive therapy:
  - Hydration with IV or PO fluids
  - Antipyretics for fever control
  - Analgesics for pain of sore throat
- Steroids (methylprednisolone or prednisone) if there is significant pharyngeal/tonsillar edema with concern about impending obstruction. May also be considered for massive splenomegaly, myocarditis, hemolytic anemia. Treatment is usually continued for up to 7 days with subsequent tapering.
- Antiviral therapy has no effect on clinical course.
- Antibiotics if concerned for bacterial superinfection:
  - Avoid ampicillin because of associated rash.
- Counsel patient on athletic activity limitations.

### *Pediatric Considerations*
Advise parents of athletic activity limitations and the need to be cleared by pediatrician prior to returning to gym and contact sports.

## MEDICATION
- Methylprednisolone: 125 mg IV (peds: 2 mg/kg IV)
- Prednisone: 20-40 mg PO daily for 7 days (peds: 1 mg/kg) with subsequent tapering

 **FOLLOW-UP**

## DISPOSITION

### *Admission Criteria*
- Significant airway edema that represents any level of potential airway compromise
- Neurologic or severe hematologic/hepatic complications
- Inability to take PO

### *Discharge Criteria*
- No airway compromise
- Mild hematologic complications or mild hepatitis
- Ability to take PO fluids
- Patients with splenomegaly need close outpatient follow-up with several weeks of resolved splenomegaly before return to full activity.
- Fever usually resolved within 10 days and lymph nodes and spleen within 4 wk. Fatigue may continue for several weeks, although it may go on for 2–3 mo

## *Issues for Referral*
- Infectious disease consultation may be useful if serology is not conclusive.
- Significant complications

## FOLLOW-UP RECOMMENDATIONS
Contact sports should be avoided until patient is fully recovered and spleen is no longer palpable.

## PEARLS AND PITFALLS

Although usually self-limited, significant complications occur and require consultation.

## ADDITIONAL READING

- American Academy of Pediatrics. *Red Book: 2009 Report of the Committee on Infectious Disease*, 28th ed. Elk Grove Village, IL: American Academy of Pediatrics; 2009.
- Auwaerter PG. Infectious mononucleosis: Return to play. *Clin Sports Med*. 2004;23(3):485–497.
- Ebell MH. Epstein-Barr virus infectious mononucleosis. *Am Fam Physician*. 2004;70(7): 1279–1287.
- Fafi-Karemer S, Morand P, Brion JP, et al. Long-term shedding of infectious Epstein-Barr virus after infectious mononucleosis. *J Infect Dis*. 2005;191(6): 985–989.
- Hanna BC, McMullan R, Hall SJ. Corticosteroids and peritonsillar abscess formation in infectious mononucleosis. *J Laryngol Otol*. 2004;118(6): 459–461.
- Hurt C, Tammaro D: Diagnostic evaluation of mononucleosis-like illness. *Am J Med*. 2007;120: 911.
- Melio F. Pharyngitis. In: Marx JA, Hockberger RS, Walls RM, eds. *Rosen's Emergency Medicine: Concepts and Clinical Practice*, 5th ed. St. Louis, MO: Mosby; 2002.

 **CODES**

### ICD9
075 Infectious mononucleosis

# MRSA, COMMUNITY ACQUIRED

*Benjamin S. Heavrin*

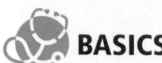 **BASICS**

## DESCRIPTION

- Methicillin-resistant *Staphylococcus aureus* (MRSA) has historically been a pathogen endemic within healthcare settings, usually affecting the elderly and chronically ill. This strain of *S. aureus* has been termed "healthcare-associated MRSA" (HA-MRSA).
- Throughout the past decade, MRSA has become an increasingly common pathogen among younger, healthier populations who do not have a healthcare related exposure history. This type of MRSA pathogen has been termed "community-acquired MRSA" (CA-MRSA).
- CA-MRSA is the most common cause of skin and soft tissue infections seen in the ED.
- While CA-MRSA may cause skin and soft tissue infection, it may also lead to severe multisystem disease, including sepsis and necrotizing pneumonia.

### Geriatric Considerations
Healthcare Associated MRSA (HA-MRSA, see below) is a different genotypic form of MRSA that frequently causes morbidity among the elderly, especially those living within extended-care facilities or those with healthcare-related exposures.

## ETIOLOGY

- *S. aureus* is a gram-positive cocci frequently colonizing the skin.
- MRSA refers to a specific strain of *S. aureus* that has resistance against the antimicrobial properties of numerous antibiotics, including methicillin.
- Prisoners, athletes, soldiers, children in daycare, IV drug users, and those with prior treatment for MRSA or exposure to MRSA are at highest risk for colonization and subsequent infection.

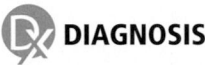 **DIAGNOSIS**

## SIGNS AND SYMPTOMS

- Skin and soft tissue infection:
  - Abscess
  - Cellulitis
- Sepsis
- Pneumonia

### History
- Skin and soft tissue infections:
  - Increasing redness, pain, warmth, and swelling along the skin
  - Recent fever, chills, and malaise
- Sepsis/pneumonia:
  - Weakness, dyspnea, fever, rigors, productive cough, chest pain
- Inquire about prior diagnosis of MRSA infections, MRSA exposures, and family members or close contacts with a history of MRSA, as such a patient is at risk for CA-MRSA infection.

### Physical Exam
- Skin and soft tissue infection:
  - Abscess: Tender, raised boil with underlying induration and fluctuance
  - Cellulitis: Warm erythema possibly with lymphangiitic streaking
- Sepsis:
  - Vital sign abnormalities including tachycardia and hypotension, respiratory failure, mental status changes, petechiae, systemic signs of toxicity
- Pneumonia:
  - Tachypnea, crackles, retractions, hypoxia
  - Alveolar opacities on chest radiographs

### Pediatric Considerations
MRSA is the leading cause of skin and soft tissue infections among children presenting to the emergency department.

## ESSENTIAL WORKUP
- Abscess:
  - I&D with packing and prompt follow-up is warranted for abscess.
  - Microbiology often performed for antibiotic sensitivity given the changing antimicrobial resistance patterns
- Sepsis:
  - Source identification, including blood culture/urine culture, chest x-ray, is indicated as resuscitation begins.
- Pneumonia:
  - Chest radiographs and continuous vital sign monitoring is indicated.

## DIAGNOSTIC TESTS & INTERPRETATION
### Lab
- Skin and soft tissue infection:
  - Bacterial culture is often warranted to monitor for CA-MRSA resistance patterns.
- Sepsis and pneumonia:
  - Blood, urine, and body fluid cultures. CBC, CMP to assess for organ dysfunction.

### Imaging
- Bedside US:
  - Abscess: Anechoic fluid collection
  - Cellulitis: "Cobblestoning" within the soft tissue
- CXR:
  - Indicated for patients with presumed sepsis, systemic illness, or pneumonia

### Diagnostic Procedures/Surgery
Cultures of skin and soft tissue infections are frequently obtained to monitor microbiology and antimicrobial resistance patterns should a patient fail a course of therapy.

## DIFFERENTIAL DIAGNOSIS
Skin and soft tissue infections:
- Pathogens beyond MRSA which cause abscesses and cellulites should be considered.

### ALERT
Empiric antimicrobial treatment of skin and soft tissue infections should cover for common skin pathogens beyond MRSA (ie, streptococcus):
- Necrotizing fasciitis
- Contact dermatitis
- Deep vein thrombosis
- Spider/insect bites
- Drug reactions

## TREATMENT

### PRE-HOSPITAL
- Contact precautions for all providers if MRSA is suspected.
- IV access and fluid resuscitation if sepsis is suspected.

### INITIAL STABILIZATION/THERAPY
Begin resuscitation and administer early empiric antibiotics if pneumonia, fasciitis, or sepsis is suspected:
- Include early coverage with antibiotics effective against MRSA.

### ED TREATMENT/PROCEDURES
- Skin and soft tissue infections:
  - Abscess:
    - I&D with packing
    - Antibiotics may not be necessary if there is no evidence for deep tissue infection or cellulitis.
  - Cellulitis:
    - Cellulitis caused by CA-MRSA in a healthy, well-appearing patient may be treated with oral antibiotics in the outpatient setting.
    - Ill appearing patients, patients with underlying medical conditions, and patients failing outpatient therapy require IV antibiotics with coverage against CA-MRSA.
- Sepsis and pneumonia:
  - Early administration of broad-spectrum antibiotics with anti-MRSA activity should be given if the patient could be at risk for CA-MRSA.

### MEDICATION

#### ALERT
Review Antimicrobial Resistance Patterns of CA-MRSA within your community prior to choosing a specific antibiotic regimen, as many antibiotics listed below may not be 100% effective against CA-MRSA.

### First Line
- Bactrim:
  - Adults: Bactrim DS 160/800 PO b.i.d.
  - Children: 10 mg/kg PO b.i.d.
- Clindamycin:
  - Adults: 150–450 mg PO b.i.d.
  - Children: 5 mg/kg po/IV t.i.d.–q.i.d.
- Doxycycline:
  - Adults: 100 mg PO b.i.d.
  - Children: 2.2 mg/kg PO b.i.d.
- Vancomycin:
  - Adults: 1 g IV q8–12h
  - Children: 15 mg/kg IV q8–12h

### Second Line
- Rifampin:
  - Should not be used as monotherapy due to inducible resistance
  - Adults: 300 mg PO b.i.d.
  - Children: 5–10 mg PO b.i.d.
- Linezolid:
  - Adults: 600 mg PO/IV q12h
  - Children: 10 mg/kg PO/IV q8h

### Pregnancy Considerations
Avoid the use of tetracyclines in pregnancy.

## FOLLOW-UP

### DISPOSITION

#### Admission Criteria
- Patients with signs/symptoms of bacteremia, progressive infection, or systemic illness should be admitted.
  - Fever, chills, lymphangiitic streaking
- Patients with underlying comorbid diseases such as diabetes or immunodeficiency should be admitted.
- Individuals who have failed a course of outpatient therapy should be admitted and given IV antibiotics effective against MRSA.

#### Discharge Criteria
Healthy, well-appearing patients with simple skin and soft tissue infections may be followed in the outpatient setting.

#### Issues for Referral
MRSA infection refractory to multiple medications may require infectious disease consultation.

### FOLLOW-UP RECOMMENDATIONS
- All skin and soft tissue infections should be re-evaluated within 24–48 hr to monitor for clinical improvement.
- Individuals failing outpatient therapy require hospital admission and IV antibiotics.

## PEARLS AND PITFALLS
- CA-MRSA is the most common cause of skin and soft tissue infections seen in the ED.
- CA-MRSA is a rare but serious cause of rapidly progressive pneumonia and sepsis.
- Antibiotic resistance patterns are dynamic and vary widely across geographic boundaries.
- Be cautious with long-term use of tetracyclines in children.

## ADDITIONAL READING

- Moran GJ, Krishnadasan A, Gorwitz RJ, et al. Methicillin-resistant S. aureus infections among patients in the emergency department. *N Engl J Med.* 2006;355:666–674.
- Klevens RM, Morrison MA, Nadle J, et al. Invasive methicillin-resistant Staphylococcus aureus infections in the United States. *JAMA.* 2007;298: 1763–1771.
- Frazee BW, Lynn J, Charlebois ED, et al. High prevalence of methicillin-resistant Staphylococcus aureus in emergency department skin and soft tissue infections. *Ann Emerg Med.* 2005;45:311–320.
- Wallin TR, Hern HG, Frazee BW. Community-associated methicillin-resistant Staphylococcus aureus. *Emerg Med Clin North Am.* 2008;26:431–455.

### See Also (Topic, Algorithm, Electronic Media Element)
- Abscess
- Cellulitis
- Pneumonia
- Sepsis

## CODES

### ICD9
- 041.12 Methicillin resistant Staphylococcus aureus
- V02.54 Carrier or suspected carrier of Methicillin resistant Staphylococcus aureus

M

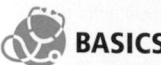

## BASICS

### DESCRIPTION
- Normal cells transform into myeloma cells at the hematopoietic stem cell level.
- Pathologic derangements:
  - Tumor cells within marrow lead to bone destruction and cytopenia.
  - Immunodeficiency develops secondary to suppression of normal immune functions.
  - Myeloma proteins lead to hyperviscosity and amyloidosis.
  - Multifactorial renal failure
- Plasma cell secretions activate osteoclasts, leading to:
  - Bone lysis, pathologic fractures, and neurologic impairment
  - Hypercalcemia (exacerbated by impaired renal function)
- Anemia due to marrow infiltration and renal insufficiency
- Immunocompromised due to:
  - Decrease in the number of normal immunoglobulins
  - Qualitative and quantitative defects in T and B cell subsets
  - Granulocytopenia
  - Decreased cell-mediated immunity
- Hyperviscosity secondary to protein accumulation:
  - Leads to high-output congestive heart failure
- Myeloma light chains accumulate in the renal epithelial cells and destroy the entire nephron.
- Clinical signs such as anemia, renal insufficiency, or lytic bone lesions
- Complications:
  - Pathologic fractures
  - Hypercalcemia
  - Renal failure
  - Recurrent infection
  - Anemia
  - Spinal cord compression (10% of all multiple myeloma (MM) patients

### ETIOLOGY
- Incidence: 4/100,000 population:
  - 1% of all cancers
  - 15% of all hematopoietic malignancies
  - 10,000 deaths/yr
- Mean age at diagnosis is 70 yr
- Slightly higher incidence in men and African Americans (reason unknown)

### *Pediatric Considerations*
- Rarely seen in children.
- <2% in patients <40 yr of age

## DIAGNOSIS

### SIGNS AND SYMPTOMS
- Bone pain predominates (with secondary disuse or neurologic sequelae):
  - Ribs/sternum
  - Spine
  - Clavicle
  - Skull
  - Shoulder
  - Hip
- Constitutional symptoms:
  - Anemia
  - Weakness
  - Fatigue
  - Recurrent infection
  - Weight loss
- Asymptomatic (20%):
  - MM found on follow-up of routine blood screening
- Multiple bouts of sepsis secondary to the encapsulated organisms (*Streptococcus pneumoniae, Haemophilus influenzae,* and *Staphylococcus*).

### ESSENTIAL WORKUP
- CBC, ESR, electrolytes, BUN, creatinine, urinalysis
- Plain radiographs related to bone pain:
  - Skeletal survey: Lateral skull, AP/lateral spine, AP of pelvis, humeri, and femori
- CT or MRI for persistent bone pain with negative plain radiographs
- Confirmation of diagnosis:
  - Serum and urine protein electrophoresis
  - Serum and urine protein immunofixation (diagnostic when electrophoresis is normal or nonspecific)
  - Vitamin D levels
  - Bone marrow biopsy

### DIAGNOSTIC TESTS & INTERPRETATION
#### *Lab*
- CBC:
  - Normochromic, normocytic anemia
  - Thrombocytopenia
  - Leukocytosis
- Rouleaux formation on peripheral blood smear (stacks of red blood cells)
- Electrolytes, BUN, creatinine, glucose:
  - Renal insufficiency
- Serum calcium:
  - Hypercalcemia due to bone resorption

- Urinalysis:
  - Dipstick selects for albumin and not light-chain proteinuria.
  - False-negative screening urinalysis for Bence Jones protein is common.
- Elevated erythrocyte sedimentation rate (ESR)
- Urinary and serum electrophoresis show a monoclonal protein spike:
  - Quantitative screening for light chain is diagnostic.

#### *Imaging*
- Plain radiographs demonstrate:
  - Lytic bone lesions
  - Pathologic fractures
- CT:
  - More sensitive for small lesions
  - Can differentiate malignant from benign vertebral compression fractures in non-MRI candidates
- MRI:
  - Preferred to detect spinal compression or soft-tissue plasmacytomas
- PET with MR or CT: May have future role in surveying response to treatment
- Technetium pyrophosphate bone scan:
  - Lights up bone deposition
  - False-negative scan with MM due to an uncoupling of bone absorption and deposition that results in a negative bone scan even when lytic lesions are present
- Bone marrow biopsy: Increase in plasma cells
- Cytogenetic screening may offer prognostic significance.

### DIFFERENTIAL DIAGNOSIS
- Monoclonal gammopathy of undetermined significance
- Amyloidosis
- Chronic lymphocytic leukemia
- Non-Hodgkin lymphoma
- Waldenström macroglobulinemia
- Bone marrow plasmacytosis includes collagen vascular disease, cirrhosis, immune complex disease, viral illness, and papular mucinosis.

TREATMENT

## PRE-HOSPITAL

Immobilize appropriately patients with MM who present with back pain or neurologic symptoms:

- Presume to have a pathologic spinal fracture

## INITIAL STABILIZATION/THERAPY

Recognition and treatment of:

- Hypercalcemia
- Renal failure
- Sepsis
- Spinal cord compression
- Anemia

## ED TREATMENT/PROCEDURES

- Opiate analgesics are the mainstay of therapy in ED (NSAIDS may worsen renal insufficiency).
- Splint pathologic fracture; immobilize pathologic spine fractures.
- Aggressive normal saline hydration with bisphosphonate therapy for hypercalcemia
- Symptomatic anemia may be managed with transfusions or erythropoietin therapy.
- Hematology/oncology consultation for chemotherapy—administer on inpatient/outpatient basis:
  - Early or asymptomatic stages do not need treatment.
  - Chemotherapy in early stage shows no benefit.
  - Melphalan and prednisone combination chemotherapy is the most common treatment:
    - Symptom relief and decrease in M protein levels in up to 70% of patients
  - Alternative chemotherapy includes cyclophosphamide with or without prednisone or VAD (vincristine, doxorubicin [Adriamycin], and dexamethasone).
- Prolonged melphalan use may lead to a secondary leukemia.
- High-dose chemotherapy with stem cell transplantation has shown promise.
- Thalidomide is useful for salvage therapy.

 FOLLOW-UP

## DISPOSITION

### Admission Criteria

- Refractory pain requiring systemic analgesics
- Life-threatening complications of MM, including acute renal failure, hypercalcemia, sepsis, spinal cord compression, hyperviscosity, neutropenia, and cardiac tamponade

### Discharge Criteria

Pain controlled with oral analgesics

### Issues for Referral

- Oncology referral for all patients regardless of stage of disease discovery
- Neurosurgery and orthopedic referral for persistent vertebral pain that may require percutaneous vertebroplasty or kyphoplasty

## PEARLS AND PITFALLS

- Infectious complications are the major cause of morbidity and mortality such that febrile illness should be treated with empiric therapy for common respiratory and urinary tract infections.
- Consider diagnosis of multiple myeloma for any persistent neurologic complaints or unknown mobility in the elderly.

## ADDITIONAL READING

- Altundag K, Altundag O, Gundeslioglu O, et al. Multiple myeloma. *N Engl J Med.* 2005;352: 840–841.
- Blade J. Complications of multiple myeloma. *Hematol Oncol Clin North Am.* 2007;21(6): 1231–1246, xi
- Bortezomib compared with dexamethasone in treating patients with relapsed or refractory multiple myeloma. Paper presented at the Annual Meeting of the American Society of Clinical Oncology, June 5, 2004, New Orleans, LA.
- Cheong HW. Imaging of diseases of the axial and peripheral skeleton. *Radiol Clin North Am.* 2008;46(4):703–733, vi.
- Grethlein SJ, Thomas, LM. Multiple myeloma. Treatment and medication. Emedicine. Updated Nov 19, 2009. Available at: http://emedicine.medscape. com/article/204369-treatment
- Nau KC. Multiple myeloma: Diagnosis and treatment. *Am Fam Physician.* 2008;78(7):853–859.

### See Also (Topic, Algorithm, Electronic Media Element)

- Anemia
- Hypercalcemia
- Renal Failure
- Sepsis

 CODES

ICD9

203.00 Multiple myeloma, without mention of having achieved remission

M

# MULTIPLE SCLEROSIS
*Richard S. Krause*

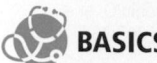

## BASICS

### DESCRIPTION
- Pathophysiology: Recurrent episodes of CNS demyelinization:
  - Signs and symptoms depend on location of lesions and timing of demyelinization.
- Multiple sclerosis (MS) occurs in distinct patterns:
  - *Relapsing recurring multiple sclerosis:* Two or more episodes lasting ≥24 hr separated by ≥1 mo
  - *Primary progressive multiple sclerosis:* Slow or stepwise progression over at least 6 mo
  - *Secondary progressive multiple sclerosis:* Initial exacerbations and remissions followed by slow progression over at least 6 mo
  - *Stable multiple sclerosis:* No progression (without treatment) over at least 18 mo

### ETIOLOGY
- MS is a chronic demyelinating disease of CNS:
  - Etiology is not well understood.
- Presumed to be T cell–mediated autoimmune disease
- There is evidence for a viral trigger.
- Plaques in white matter:
  - Characterized by infiltrate of T cells and macrophages
- Persons of northern European origin most often affected (in U.S.)
- Increased prevalence is seen moving away from equator.

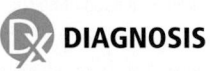

## DIAGNOSIS

### SIGNS AND SYMPTOMS
- Initial attacks usually (~85%) represent single lesions, are abrupt in onset, and are seen in characteristic patterns (in order of decreasing frequency):
  - Optic neuritis:
    - Eye pain exacerbated by movement progressing to visual loss
  - Paresthesias (or changed sensory level) in one limb
  - Limb (usually leg) weakness
  - Diplopia:
    - Intranuclear ophthalmoplegia from lesion of medial longitudinal fasciculus
    - Results in unilateral or bilateral paralysis of adduction of eye on horizontal gaze
  - Trigeminal neuralgia
  - Urinary retention

- Vertigo
- Transverse myelitis:
  - Acute onset of motor and sensory findings at specific spinal cord level
  - Often associated with bladder or bowel incontinence
  - Can be early manifestation of MS
  - Unusual initial manifestations include psychosis, aphasia, etc.
  - Initial symptoms may be minor and only be recognized as due to MS in retrospect
- Symptoms typically develop abruptly (minutes to hours) and last 6–8 wk
- Most common in young women of northern European descent:
  - Increased risk in first-degree relatives
  - Peak age: 30 yr
  - Female-to-male ratio, 2:1
- Pain is uncommon symptom in MS:
  - Exceptions: Trigeminal neuralgia, early optic neuritis

### Physical Exam
Physical exam: Focused on "hard" neurologic signs:
- Focal neurologic deficits
- Afferent pupillary defect
- Internuclear ophthalmoplegia
- Sensory level or sphincter disturbance (transverse myelitis)

### ESSENTIAL WORKUP
- MS is suspected based on history and physical exam.
- Definitive diagnosis is not typically made in ED; requires observation over time and confirmatory testing.

### ALERT
Infection, especially with fever, is a common cause of MS exacerbation.

## DIAGNOSTIC TESTS & INTERPRETATION
### Lab
CSF analysis:
- ~90% of MS patients' CSF gel electrophoresis reveals "oligoclonal bands" not present in serum.
- Not completely specific for MS

### Imaging
MRI most useful imaging test:
- Lesions appear as areas of high signal, in cerebral white matter or spinal cord on T2-weighted images.
- Abnormal in almost all patients who have clinically diagnosed MS
- May also see plaques on CT (less sensitive)

### Diagnostic Procedures/Surgery
Sensory-evoked potential testing:
- Not an ED test

### DIFFERENTIAL DIAGNOSIS
- Signs and symptoms of MS are usually *focal*; diffuse symptoms (seizures, syncope, and dementia) are seldom due to MS.
- Cerebrovascular accident and transient ischemic attack
- Usually older patients with risk factors for atherosclerotic disease or atrial fibrillation
- Systemic lupus erythematosus:
  - CNS involvement usually in setting of known disease and usually nonfocal
- Sarcoid:
  - CNS manifestations usually with known disease and lung involvement and nonfocal
- Lyme disease:
  - May mimic MS
  - Seek history of rash and tick exposure in geographic areas of high risk.
  - Lyme titers may aid in diagnosis.
- Psychiatric illness is diagnosis of exclusion.
- Postinfectious or postimmunization demyelination may mimic MS, usually in children.

- Guillain-Barré is usually ascending and symmetric and progresses over hours to days
- MS unlikely in patients with:
  - Normal neurologic exam
  - Abrupt hemiparesis (stroke)
  - Aphasia (stroke)
  - Pain predominating
  - Very brief symptoms (seconds to minutes)
  - Age <10 or >50 yr

 **TREATMENT**

### INITIAL STABILIZATION/THERAPY
Fever in MS patients should be treated aggressively because it can worsen the neurologic manifestations of MS.

### ED TREATMENT/PROCEDURES
- Acute optic neuritis or transverse myelitis:
  - High-dose parenteral steroids possibly effective
  - Oral steroids *contraindicated* (oral prednisone has been reported to exacerbate symptoms)
- Exacerbations:
  - High-dose IV methylprednisolone (up to 1 g/d) or other parenteral corticosteroid regimen
- Symptomatic treatment:
  - Spasticity: Baclofen, tizanidine
  - Tremor: Clonazepam
  - Urinary symptoms:
    o Treat infection.
    o Self-catheterization for increased postvoid residual
    o Oxybutynin may promote continence between catheterizations.
  - Trigeminal neuralgia: Carbamazepine
  - Fatigue, general weakness: Amantadine and modafinil have been used.
  - Depression: SSRIs are effective.

### MEDICATION
- Amantadine: 100 mg PO b.i.d.
- Baclofen: 10 mg PO t.i.d. initially; may increase to 25 mg PO t.i.d.
- Carbamazepine: 100 mg PO b.i.d. to 200 mg PO q.i.d.
- Clonazepam: 0.5 mg/d PO, increase in 0.5-mg increments and up to three times a day
- Methylprednisolone: 1 g IV daily (first-line treatment)
- Modanifil: 100–200 mg PO daily in AM
- Oxybutynin: 5 mg PO b.i.d. to t.i.d.
- Tizanidine: 2–8 mg PO t.i.d.

 **FOLLOW-UP**

### DISPOSITION
#### Admission Criteria
- Acute exacerbation that requires IV therapy
- Patients unable to care for themselves due to severity of their illness
- Another condition requiring inpatient treatment cannot be effectively ruled out.

#### Discharge Criteria
- *Suspected MS:* Patients may be referred for outpatient evaluation if their general condition permits and other serious conditions requiring admission have been effectively ruled out.
- *Complication of known MS:* Discharge if effective outpatient treatment is available for complication or exacerbating factor.

### FOLLOW-UP RECOMMENDATIONS
Patients with suspected MS should be referred to their primary care provider or a neurologist for further evaluation.

## PEARLS AND PITFALLS
- Signs and symptoms of MS are usually focal.
- Diffuse symptoms are rarely MS.
- Oral steroids are contraindicated.
- Treat fever in MS patients aggressively.

## ADDITIONAL READING
- Balcer LJ. Optic neuritis. *N Eng J Med*. 2006;354:1273–1280.
- Courtney AM, Tredaway K, Remington G, et al. Multiple sclerosis. *Med Clin North Am*. 2009;93:451–76, ix–x.
- Frohman EM, Racke MK, Raine CS. Multiple sclerosis: The plaque and its pathogenesis. *N Engl J Med*. 2006;354:942–955.
- Leary S, Porter B, Thompson A. Multiple sclerosis: Diagnosis and the management of acute relapses. *Postgrad Med J*. 2005;81:302–308.

### See Also (Topic, Algorithm, Electronic Media Element)
- Cerebrovascular Accident
- Guillain-Barré Syndrome
- Lyme Disease

 **CODES**

**ICD9**
340 Multiple sclerosis

M

# MUMPS

*Austen Chai*

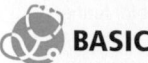 **BASICS**

## DESCRIPTION
Childhood, vaccine-preventable infectious diseases characterized by swelling of ≥1 salivary glands, in particular the parotid glands

## ETIOLOGY
- Rubulavirus, single stranded RNA virus, in the Paramyxovirus family
- Humans only known reservoir

### Pediatric Considerations
- Mumps vaccine with measles and rubella (MMR) should be administered to children on or after 12 mo of age. 2nd dose is usually administered at age of 4–6 yr, before the start of school.
- Catch-up MMR vaccination should include 2 doses separated by at least 4 wk between vaccinations.
- Systemic symptoms and serious complications are less common in children when compared to adults with the infection.

### Pregnancy Considerations
Infection during 1st trimester of pregnancy is associated with increased spontaneous abortion. Although mumps virus may cross the placenta, there is no evidence that mumps virus causes congenital malformation.

### Geriatric Considerations
Adults born before 1957 are considered to have been exposed to mumps and are considered immune. However, during outbreaks, healthcare workers born before 1957 and without laboratory evidence of immunity to mumps should receive 2 doses of the MMR vaccine.

 **DIAGNOSIS**

## SIGNS AND SYMPTOMS
- Incubation period from exposure to onset of symptoms (12–25 days):
  – Viral transmission via respiratory droplets, saliva, contact with contaminated fomites
  – Replication in nasopharynx and regional lymph nodes
  – Viremia to meninges and glands; salivary, pancreas, testes, and ovaries
- Contagious 1–7 days prior to symptoms onset and 6 days afterward
- Often history of no or incomplete immunization
- Active Illness (1–10 days):
  – Nonspecific prodromal symptoms such as low-grade fever, headache, malaise, myalgia, anorexia, otalgia, jaw pain
  – Up to 20% of infections are asymptomatic but still contagious.
  – Up to 50% of cases have nonspecific symptoms of upper respiratory tract infection along with fever, malaise, anorexia, and headache without apparent salivary gland swelling.
  – *Parotitis* (30–40% of patients):
    ○ Most common manifestation of mumps
    ○ Painful and tender unilateral or bilateral enlargement of parotid gland
    ○ May begin as earache or pain at angle of jaw
    ○ Any salivary gland may be affected.
    ○ Stensen's duct is often edematous and erythematous and exudes a clear fluid.
    ○ Skin overlying swollen gland is nonerythematous.
    ○ Symptoms decrease after 1 wk and resolve by 10th day.
    ○ Considered contagious until swelling resolves

- *Orchitis* (20–50% of postpubertal males):
  ○ Most common complication in postpubertal males
  ○ May occur alone, before, during, but most commonly, after parotitis
  ○ Unilateral or bilateral (up to 30%)
  ○ Abrupt, painful, tender swelling with nausea, vomiting, and fever
  ○ Pain and swelling resolve in 1 wk.
  ○ Testicular atrophy in up to 50% of patients
  ○ Sterility rare
- *Oophoritis* (5% of postpubertal females):
  ○ May mimic appendicitis if right-sided
  ○ Fertility not impaired
- Pancreatitis (2–5%):
  ○ May occur without any other manifestations of mumps
  ○ Fever, nausea, vomiting, and epigastric pain
  ○ May see transient hyperglycemia
  ○ May be complicated by pseudocyst formation and shock
- CNS involvement:
  ○ Aseptic meningitis (10–15% of patients)
  ○ Usually resolves without sequelae in 3–10 days
  ○ Encephalitis (very rare)
  ○ Deafness (80% unilateral) with permanent hearing impairment
  ○ Cerebellar ataxia
  ○ Transverse myelitis
- Other:
  ○ Myocarditis (rarely with symptomatic involvement)
  ○ Glomerulonephritis
  ○ Polyarthralgia and arthritis
  ○ Thrombocytopenic purpura
  ○ Ocular complaints
  ○ Thyroiditis
  ○ Mastitis

## ESSENTIAL WORKUP
Diagnosis is based on clinical findings of parotitis and associated signs and symptoms and complications.

## DIAGNOSTIC TESTS & INTERPRETATION
### Lab
- Laboratory tests as needed
- Cerebrospinal fluid (CSF) for symptomatic CNS involvement
- Hyperamylasemia usually due to parotitis
- Mumps nucleic acid detection using PCR assays, mumps viral cultures, or enzyme immunoassays for mumps IgM antibody:
  - Provides definitive diagnosis
  - From blood, throat swab, salivary gland secretions, CSF, or urine
  - Not indicated unless need to confirm diagnosis in absence of parotitis
- Enzyme immunoassay

## DIFFERENTIAL DIAGNOSIS
- Bacterial parotitis:
  - Commonly *Staphylococcus aureus*
  - Erythematous and tender parotid gland
  - Usually in elderly or immunocompromised
- Calculus parotid:
  - Stone may be palpable or may be seen on sialogram (CT)
- Cervical adenitis
- Tumors:
  - Older patients
    History of indolent course
- Testicular torsion
- Bacterial epididymo-orchitis
- Other viral cause of parotitis; influenza A, parainfluenza, cytomegalovirus, coxsackieviruses, HIV

 **TREATMENT**

### PRE-HOSPITAL
Nonimmunized prehospital care personnel exposed to mumps should be advised of potential risks.

### INITIAL STABILIZATION/THERAPY
IV fluids for vomiting/dehydration

### ED TREATMENT/PROCEDURES
- Prevention with mumps vaccination is cornerstone of therapy:
  - MMR at 1 yr of age
  - Second MMR at 4–6 yr of age, no later than 12 yr of age
- Supportive and symptomatic:
  - Antipyretics
  - Analgesia:
    ○ Acetaminophen, NSAIDs, narcotics (for severe pain)
  - IV fluids for vomiting and dehydration
  - Ice pack
  - Scrotal support

 **FOLLOW-UP**

### DISPOSITION
#### Admission Criteria
- Seriously ill who may require supportive care
- Severe vomiting and dehydration
- Encephalitis
- Severe pancreatitis
- Isolate admitted patients.

### Discharge Criteria
- Virtually all patients
- Contagious until about a week after onset of symptoms

## PEARLS AND PITFALLS
- Mumps virus is the only cause of epidemic parotitis.
- Vaccines are highly effective, and confer ~90% immunity.
- Mumps virus is endemic to many parts of the world and may pose a risk to travelers without immunity to mumps.

## ADDITIONAL READING
- American Academy of Pediatrics. Mumps. In: Pickering LK, ed. *2009 Red Book: Report of the Committee on Infectious Diseases*, 27th ed. Elk Grove Village, IL: American Academy of Pediatrics; 2006;468–472.
- Madsen KM, et al. A population-based study of MMR vaccination and autism. *N Engl J Med*. 2002;347(19):1477–1482.
- Mason WH. Mumps. In: RM Kliegman et al., eds., *Nelson Textbook of Pediatrics*, 18th ed. Philadelphia: Saunders Elsevier; 2007;1342–1344.

### See Also (Topic, Algorithm, Electronic Media Element)
www.cdc.gov/mumps

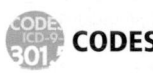 **CODES**

### ICD9
072.9 Mumps without mention of complication

M

# MUNCHAUSEN SYNDROME

*J.C. Huffman*
*T.A. Stern*

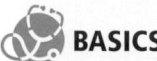

## BASICS

### DESCRIPTION
Intentional production/feigning of physical symptoms motivated by a need to assume the sick role

### ETIOLOGY
- No universal etiology
- Patients often have a history of gaining support/attention via illness during childhood and an abusive or neglectful upbringing.

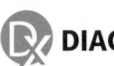

## DIAGNOSIS

Difficult to make a definitive diagnosis, but several common features exist.

### SIGNS AND SYMPTOMS
- Frequent visits to EDs for what appears to be an acute illness
- Numerous hospital admissions (often prolonged)
- A plausible but dramatic case history
- Escalating demands for diagnostic testing and therapeutic interventions
- A hostile/bullying manner and evasiveness regarding specifics
- Arrival with numerous medical reports, hospital cards, or insurance forms
- Masochistic acceptance of painful procedures
- Use of medically sophisticated language
- Employment in a medically related field
- A paucity of verifiable history
- Pseudologia fantastica (the telling of wild, untrue stories)
- A vast array of possible presenting medical complaints and signs
- Gastrointestinal:
  – Vomiting
  – Diarrhea
  – Abdominal pain
- Hematologic:
  – Dizziness
  – Weakness associated with bleeding
  – Anemia (from self-phlebotomy or abuse of anticoagulants)
- Neurologic:
  – Feigned seizures
  – Loss of consciousness
- Musculoskeletal:
  – Self-induced wounds
  – Multiple scars
- Cardiac:
  – Complaints of chest pain
  – Palpitations
  – Dysrhythmias
- Renal:
  – Renal colic
  – Dysuria
  – Hematuria
- Endocrine:
  – Hypoglycemia (from self-administration of insulin)
  – Hyperthyroidism:
    ○ Secondary to exogenous administration of thyroxine
    ○ See "Hyperthyroidism."
  – Hyperdynamic states (from use of epinephrine):
    ○ Tachycardia
    ○ Hypertension
    ○ Diaphoresis
- Infectious:
  – From injection of sputum or feces
  – Factitious fever from manipulation of thermometers
- Pulmonary:
  – Shortness of breath

### Pediatric Considerations
- "Munchausen syndrome by proxy"
- A parent provides a misleading history or induces illness in his or her child to obtain attention
- A form of child abuse

### History
- Frequent homelessness and significant wandering between cities and states
- An absence of close interpersonal relationships
- A history of sadistic and rejecting parents
- A history of chronic childhood illness

### Physical Exam
Findings correspond to the affected organ system.

### ESSENTIAL WORKUP
- The diagnosis is suggested by inconsistencies in the history or the pattern of illness and by the recognition of the above patterns of behavior.
- Diligent detective work, including retrieval of records from other hospitals and calling on family members who can provide evidence of similar prior presentations
- Direct observation of the patient and a search of the patient's room/belongings may reveal the method of deception (eg, insulin vials and syringes)
- Critical to perform tests/workup that focus on objective findings of illness on exam

### DIAGNOSTIC TESTS & INTERPRETATION
Depend on organ system involved and on objective findings

### Lab
- Testing stool for phenolphthalein may detect laxative abuse.
- Testing blood for C3 peptide reveals exogenous insulin administration.

### Imaging
Do not rely on imaging brought by the patient to make diagnoses or treatment plans.

### Diagnostic Procedures/Surgery
Avoid unless there are clear objective findings that indicate the necessity of a procedure

## DIFFERENTIAL DIAGNOSIS

- True primary physical illness:
  - Munchausen patients often with comorbid primary medical illness
- True illness secondary to self-destructive acts or surgical interventions:
  - Small bowel obstruction, infection, dehydration
- Malingering:
  - Also has intentional symptom production
  - In this case, a clear-cut secondary gain (eg, meals/room, disability benefits) is present.
  - The patient is usually much less willing to undergo painful procedures.
- Conversion disorder:
  - Symptoms not consciously/intentionally produced
  - Typically with neurologic symptoms:
    - Blindness
    - Hemiparesis
    - Seizures
- Somatization disorder
  - Symptoms not consciously produced
  - Multiple somatic complaints
  - Multiple organ system involvement

# TREATMENT

### INITIAL STABILIZATION/THERAPY

Treat obvious threats to life or limb:

- Hypoglycemia, bleeding, or wounds

### ED TREATMENT/PROCEDURES

- Identify objective physical illness and treat as appropriate.
- Document history/findings suggestive of factitious illness.
- Flag the chart or create a list to identify such patients.
- Refer for psychiatric care
- Report Munchausen syndrome by proxy to child protective services.

### MEDICATION

Treat comorbid psychiatric conditions with appropriate pharmacologic agents.

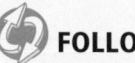

# FOLLOW-UP

## DISPOSITION

### Admission Criteria

- Often requires medical admission to treat or stabilize physical conditions
- Psychiatric admission may be of benefit, but it is rarely accepted by the patient.

### Discharge Criteria

- Medical stability
- Not an active threat to harm self
- Appropriate referral for medical and psychiatric follow-up arranged

### Issues for Referral

- May offer psychiatric referral as a method of dealing with stress caused by illness
- Psychiatric providers located directly in medical settings (eg, primary care physician office) may be more accepted.
- Overall, this is a chronic illness with poor prognosis.

## FOLLOW-UP RECOMMENDATIONS

Maintain contact between the patient and an identified provider for that patient

## PEARLS AND PITFALLS

- Be aware of your emotional reaction to the patient to prevent inappropriate treatment.
- Avoid premature discharge or abandonment when the patient is not yet stabilized/safe.

## ADDITIONAL READING

- Feldman MD, Ford CV. Factitious disorders. In: Sadock BJ, Sadock VA, eds. *Kaplan and Sadock's Comprehensive Textbook of Psychiatry*, 7th ed. Philadelphia: Lippincott Williams & Wilkins; 2000:1533–1543.
- Robertson MM, Cervilla JA. Munchausen's syndrome. *Br J Hosp Med.* 1997;58(7):308–312.
- Souid AK, Keith DV, Cunningham AS. Munchausen syndrome by proxy. *Clin Pediatr.* 1998;37(8): 497–503.
- Stern TA. Munchausen's syndrome revisited. *Psychosomatics.* 1980;21:329–336.
- Walker EA. Dealing with patients who have medically unexplained symptoms. *Semin Clin Neuropsychiatry.* 2002;7:187–195.

**See Also (Topic, Algorithm, Electronic Media Element)**

Abuse, Pediatric

 CODES

**ICD9**
301.51 Chronic factitious illness with physical symptoms

M

# MUSHROOM POISONING

*Adam Black*
*Timothy B. Erickson*

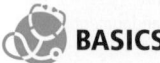 **BASICS**

## DESCRIPTION

- Amanitin/phalloidin:
  - Species:
    - *Amanita phalloides* ("death cap")
    - *Amanita virosa/verna* ("destroying angel")
    - *Galerina marginata, Galerina venenata*
  - Mechanism:
    - Cyclopeptide toxins inhibit RNA polymerase 2, which kills GI epithelium, hepatocytes, nephrocytes
- Gyromitrin:
  - Species:
    - *Gyromitra esculenta* ("false morels")
    - Other *Gyromitra* spp.
  - Mechanism:
    - Inhibits pyridoxal phosphate
    - Damage to RBCs, hepatocytes, neurons
- Muscarine:
  - Species:
    - *Inocybe* (several species)
    - *Clitocybe* (several species)
  - Mechanism:
    - Parasympathomimetic
- Coprine:
  - Species:
    - *Coprinus atramentarius* ("inky caps")
  - Mechanism:
    - Blocks acetaldehyde dehydrogenase
    - Causes disulfiram-like reaction if mixed with alcohol
- Ibotenic acid/muscimol:
  - Species:
    - *Amanita pantherina* ("the panther")
    - *Amanita muscaria* ("fly agaric")
  - Mechanism:
    - GABA agonists
- Psilocin/psilocybin:
  - Species:
    - *Psilocybe* and *Panaeolus* spp. as well as others
  - Mechanism:
    - Similar structure to lysergic acid diethylamide
- Gastric irritants:
  - Many various mushrooms, including those normally considered edible
- Orellanine:
  - Species:
    - *Cortinarius* (several species)
  - Mechanism:
    - Direct renal toxicity
- *Tricholoma equestre* ("man on horse"):
  - Rhabdomyolysis-inducing mushrooms
  - Can lead to acute rhabdomyolysis.

## DIAGNOSIS

### SIGNS AND SYMPTOMS

- Amanitin/phalloidin:
  - Nausea
  - Vomiting
  - Abdominal cramps
  - Bloody diarrhea
  - Clinical course:
    - Onset of symptoms delayed 6–36 hr
    - Transient latent phase may last 2 days (no pain)
    - Can progress to hepatic or renal failure and death in 4–7 days
    - Most-lethal mushroom toxins
- Gyromitrin:
  - First 6 hr:
    - Abdominal cramps
    - Vomiting
    - Watery diarrhea
  - Later symptoms:
    - Weakness
    - Cyanosis
    - Confusion
    - Seizures
    - Coma
- Muscarine:
  - Cholinergic symptoms include:
    - Miosis
    - Salivation
    - Lacrimation
    - Sweating
    - Diarrhea
    - Flushed skin
    - Nausea
    - Bradycardia
    - Bronchoconstriction
  - Onset usually within 1 hr (may be delayed)
- Coprine:
  - Disulfiram-like reaction when combined with alcohol:
    - Flushing
    - Sweating
    - Nausea
    - Vomiting
    - Palpitations
    - Chest pain
  - Begins minutes after combining this toxin with ethanol
- Ibotenic acid/muscimol:
  - Anticholinergic symptoms include:
    - Hallucinations
    - Dysarthria
    - Ataxia
    - Muscle cramps
    - Vomiting
    - Seizures
    - Coma
  - Clinical course:
    - Relatively rapid onset of 30–60 min
- Psilocin/psilocybin:
  - Visual hallucinations
  - Alteration of perception
  - Nausea
  - Mydriasis
  - Tachycardia
  - Fever and seizures in children:
    - Rarely fatal unless mixed drug ingestions
- Gastric irritants:
  - Group of toxins that cause nausea, vomiting, intestinal cramps, and watery diarrhea
  - Onset 30 min to 2 hr, usually resolved in 6–12 hr
- Orellanine/*Amanita smithiania*:
  - Nausea
  - Headache
  - Sweating
  - Chills
  - Low-back pain
  - Thirst
  - Clinical course:
    - May progress to oliguria and acute renal failure
    - Markedly delayed onset of symptoms (2–14 days)
- *Tricholoma equestre*:
  - Acute rhabdomyolysis:
    - Myalgias/arthralgias
    - Hematuria/dark urine
    - Decreased urine output
  - Dehydration
  - Fever

### History

- Time of ingestion
- Time of symptom onset
- Quantity ingested
- Preparation: Raw or cooked
- Picked in the wild or store-bought
- Coingestants, other mushrooms
- Alcohol/drug use history
- Symptoms of family members, friends

### Physical Exam

- Vital signs
- Changes in mental status
- Pupillary response
- Cardiopulmonary exam
- Abdominal exam
- Neurologic exam

### ESSENTIAL WORKUP

- Mushroom description:
  - Pileus (cap); margin shape
  - Stipe (stem)
  - Lammallea (gills)
  - Veil
  - Annulus (ring)
  - Volva
- Store mushroom in brown paper bag for future identification:
  - <3% of cases result in an exact mushroom identification.
  - Digital photography and electronic image transfer to poison control center or regional mycologist

### DIAGNOSTIC TESTS & INTERPRETATION
*Lab*
- CBC
- Prothrombin time (PT), partial thromboplastin time (PTT)
- Electrolytes, BUN, creatinine, glucose
- Urinalysis
- LFTs, creatine phosphokinase (CPK)
- Imaging
- Spore print: Mycologist needed for specific genus/species interpretation

### DIFFERENTIAL DIAGNOSIS
- Symptoms with late onset (>6 hr) indicate more-lethal toxins.
- Always entertain possibility of multiple species ingestion.
- Combination with ethyl alcohol may suggest coprine (disulfiram reaction).
- Consider other illicit drugs with visual hallucinations.
- Fertilizers, insecticides, fungicides, if mushrooms were found in a public place
- Botulism if canned mushrooms

## TREATMENT

### PRE-HOSPITAL
Bring any unconsumed mushrooms or mushroom pieces to hospital to aid in diagnosis:
- Refrigerate specimens if possible, place in brown paper bag.

### INITIAL STABILIZATION/THERAPY
- ABCs
- Establish IV 0.9% NS saline
- Monitor
- Naloxone, D50W (or Accu-Chek), and thiamine for altered mental status

### ED TREATMENT/PROCEDURES
*General Measures*
- Decontamination:
  - Activated charcoal (50–100 g)
  - Gastric decontamination if early after ingestion and patient:
    ○ Has not yet vomited.
    ○ Has normal mental and respiratory status
    ○ Is not undergoing hallucinations
- Fluid rehydration and electrolyte replacement as necessary
- Call local poison control center at 800-222-1222 and request mycologist—digital picture may be electronically sent for identification.
- Obtain specimens (vomitus if needed) for identification.

*Mushroom-Specific Therapy*
- Amanitin/phalloidin:
  - Consider gastric lavage evacuation of mushroom fragments if 1–2 hr postingestion and no previous vomiting.
  - Administer activated charcoal PO q2–4h.
  - Hypoglycemia and elevated PT:
    ○ Signs of liver failure
    ○ Administer fresh-frozen plasma and vitamin K for coagulation disorders with active bleeding.

- Administer calcium in presence of hypocalcemia.
- Liver transplant for severe hepatic necrosis
- Consider *N*-acetylcysteine, high-dose penicillin G, or silibinin if available (thioctic acid controversial)

- Gyromitrin:
  - Administer pyridoxine (vitamin $B_6$) in severely symptomatic patients.
  - Treat seizure with benzodiazepines.
  - Treat liver dysfunctions as outlined for amanitin/phalloidin group.
  - Dialysis for renal failure
- Muscarine:
  - Administer atropine in severe cases.
- Coprine:
  - Self-limited toxicity—supportive care
  - Avoid syrup of ipecac (contains alcohol).
  - Beta-blockers for cardiac dysrhythmias
- Ibotenic acid/muscimol:
  - Usually self-limited toxicity
  - Provide supportive care.
  - Monitor for hypotension.
  - Treat moderate symptoms with benzodiazepines, if severe anticholinergic symptoms; consider physostigmine.
- Psylocin/psilocybin:
  - Self-limited toxicity
  - Monitor if tachycardic.
  - Dark, quiet room and reassurance
  - No aggressive oral decontamination if hallucinating
  - External cooling measures if needed in children
- GI Irritants:
  - When poisoning from above groups not suspected, administer fluids and antiemetics.
  - Provide supportive care
- Orellanine and *Amanita smithiana*:
  - Closely monitor BUN, creatinine, electrolytes, and urine output.
  - Forced diuresis with Lasix contraindicated Diuresis with alkalinization of urine with NaHCO₃ if signs of rhabdomyolysis
  - Hemodialysis/renal transplantation may be needed.
  - Monitor LFTs in cases in which cyclopeptide-containing mushrooms are suspected.
- *Tricholoma equestre* ("man on horse"):
  - Check and follow CPK.
  - Monitor urine output.

### MEDICATION
- Activated charcoal slurry: 1–2 g/kg up to 100 g PO
- Atropine: 0.5 mg (peds: 0.02 mg/kg) IV; repeat 0.5–1.0 mg IV (peds: 0.04 mg/kg) q10min if secretions recur, to max 1 mg/kg in children and 2 mg/kg in adults
- Dextrose: D50W 1 amp: 50 mL or 25 g (peds: D25W 2–4 mL/kg) IV
- Diazepam (benzodiazepine): 5–10 mg (peds: 0.2–0.5 mg/kg) IV
- Lorazepam (benzodiazepine): 2–6 mg (peds: 0.03–0.05 mg/kg) IV
- Naloxone (Narcan): 2 mg (peds: 0.1 mg/kg) IV or IM initial dose
- Physostigmine: 0.5–2 mg IM or IV in adults
- Propranolol: 1 mg (peds: 0.01–0.1 mg/kg) IV
- Pyridoxine: 25 mg/kg over 30 min
- Thiamine (vitamin $B_1$): 100 mg (peds: 50 mg) IV or IM

## FOLLOW-UP

### DISPOSITION
*Admission Criteria*
- All symptomatic patients:
  - Protracted vomiting, dehydration, liver or renal toxicity, or seizures
- Transfer to tertiary medical center for early signs of renal or hepatic failure.
- Symptomatic infants and young children found with mushrooms:
  - Assume ingestion.
- ICU admission for known ingestion of an amanitin-containing mushroom:
  - Early liver service consultation

*Discharge Criteria*
Asymptomatic during 6–8 hr with 24 hr of close home observation (if reliable caregivers)

*Issues for Referral*
Potential liver or renal transplantation

### FOLLOW-UP RECOMMENDATIONS
Drug detoxification programs if chronic recreational use

## PEARLS AND PITFALLS

- Delayed presentations
- Lack of proper mycologic identification
- Timely organ transplant referrals when indicated

## ADDITIONAL READING

- Beuhler MC, Sasser HC, Watson WA. The outcome of North American pediatric unintentional mushroom ingestions with various decontamination treatments. An analysis of 14 years of TESS data. *Toxicon*. 2009;53(4):437–443.
- Matsuura M, Saikawa Y, Inui K, et al: Identification of the toxic trigger in mushroom poisoning. *Nat Chem Biol*. 2009;5(7):465–467.
- West PL, Lindgren J, Horowitz BZ. *Amanita smithiana* mushroom ingestion: A case of delayed renal failure and literature review. *J Med Toxicol*. 2009;5(1):32–38.

### See Also (Topic, Algorithm, Electronic Media Element)
Anticholinergic Poisoning

## CODES

**ICD9**
988.1 Toxic effect of mushrooms eaten as food

**M**

# MYASTHENIA GRAVIS
*Kelley Ralph*

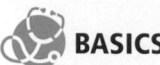

## BASICS

### DESCRIPTION
- Antibody-mediated condition that results in painless, fatigable muscle weakness
- Ocular or generalized:
  - Ocular muscle weakness:
    - Most common initial symptom (60%)
    - ~80% of myasthenia gravis (MG) patients who present with ocular weakness initially will progress to general weakness within 2 yr.
  - Generalized:
    - Usually affects proximal limbs, axial muscle groups such as neck, face, bulbar muscles
- Acute or subacute, with relapses and remissions
- Associated with thymoma in 15%
- Myasthenic crisis:
  - Respiratory failure or inability to protect airway due to weakness
  - Triggers:
    - Infection
    - Surgery
    - Trauma
    - Pregnancy
    - Medication changes (eg, rapid tapering of steroids)
  - Difficult to distinguish from cholinergic crisis resulting from excessive doses of acetylcholinesterase (AChE) inhibitors:
    - Cholinergic crisis may also include muscarinic effects such as sweating, lacrimation, salivation, and GI hyperactivity in addition to weakness.

### EPIDEMIOLOGY
Bimodal distribution:
- 1 peak in 2nd and 3rd decades affecting mostly women
- 2nd peak affecting men in 6th and 7th decades

### ETIOLOGY
- Antibody-mediated attack on nicotinic acetylcholine receptors
- Up to 20% of patients may be acetylcholine receptor antibody (AChR Ab) negative
- Many medications may worsen myasthenic weakness:
  - Aminoglycosides, macrolides, quinilones, antimalarials
  - Local anesthetics
  - Antidysrhythmics (propafenone, quinidine, procainamide)
  - Beta-blockers, calcium-channel blockers
  - Anticonvulsants (phenytoin, carbamazepine)
  - Antipsychotics (phenothiazine, atypicals)
  - Neuromuscular blocking agents
  - Iodine-containing radiocontrast
  - Penicillamine can cause MG as well as other autoimmune conditions.

## DIAGNOSIS

### SIGNS AND SYMPTOMS
Fluctuating focal weakness

#### History
- Symptoms worsen with repeated activity:
  - Improve with rest
- Ocular weakness:
  - Diplopia
  - Ptosis while driving or reading
- Bulbar and facial muscle weakness:
  - Trouble chewing, speaking, swallowing
  - Inability to keep jaw closed after chewing
  - Slurred, nasal speech
- Limb weakness:
  - Difficulty climbing stairs, rising from chair, reaching up with arms

#### Physical Exam
- Ocular findings:
  - Ptosis, diplopia
  - Inability to keep eyelid shut against resistance
  - No pupillary changes
- Bulbar and facial findings:
  - Ask patient to count to 100; look for changes in speech.
  - Decreased facial expression
  - Head droop
- Limb findings:
  - Repetitive testing of proximal muscles or small muscles of hand results in weakness.
  - Reflex and sensory exam are normal.

### ESSENTIAL WORKUP
- Assess for respiratory compromise.
- Search for secondary triggers (eg, infectious source)

### DIAGNOSTIC TESTS & INTERPRETATION
#### Lab
- CBC
- Electrolytes
- LFTs
- Thyroid function tests
- Anti-AChR Ab:
  - Positive in 90% with generalized disease
  - Positive in 50% with ocular disease
- Other tests for initial diagnosis:
  - Antistriated muscle antibody
  - Antinuclear antibody
  - Rheumatoid factor
  - ESR

#### Imaging
- Head CT or MRI to rule out compressive lesions causing cranial nerve findings
- Chest CT with contrast to look for associated thymoma
- CXR as needed to evaluate for infectious source

#### Diagnostic Procedures/Surgery
- Edrophonium (Tensilon) test:
  - Short-acting AChE inhibitor
  - A positive test produces rapid, short-lived (2–5 min) improvement in strength
  - Sensitivity 95% in generalized MG and 86% in ocular MG
  - False positives possible with Lambert-Eaton, Guillain-Barré, MS, botulism, and others
  - Keep patient on cardiac monitor during test.
  - Atropine at bedside for possible bradycardia
  - Suction at bedside for possible increased secretions
- Ice test:
  - Place ice on eyelid for 2 min.
  - Improvement in ptosis suggests myasthenia gravis.

### DIFFERENTIAL DIAGNOSIS
- Amyotrophic lateral sclerosis
- Botulism
- Electrolyte abnormalities
- Graves disease
- Guillain-Barré syndrome
- Hyperthyroidism
- Inflammatory muscle disorders
- Intracranial mass lesions
- Lambert-Eaton syndrome
- Multiple sclerosis
- Periodic paralysis

## TREATMENT

### PRE-HOSPITAL
Attention to airway management

### INITIAL STABILIZATION/THERAPY
Myasthenic crisis:
- Most important is early intubation and mechanical ventilation.
- Signs of impending failure:
  - Vital capacity <20 mL/kg
  - Peak inspiratory pressure <−30 cm $H_2O$
  - Peak expiratory pressure <40 cm $H_2O$

- Considerations regarding paralytics:
  - Decreased sensitivity to depolarizing agents may necessitate higher dose; consider doubling the usual dose of succinylcholine.
  - Nondepolarizing agents can cause extended paralysis; consider halving the usual dose.
  - Others recommend midazolam, etomidate, or thiopental instead.

## ED TREATMENT/PROCEDURES
- Treat infections aggressively.
- Search for and remove triggers.
- Myasthenic crisis may require plasmapheresis or IV gammaglobulin (IVIG).
  - Plasmapheresis: Remove 1–1.5 plasma volume each session × 5 sessions
  - IVIG: 0.4 mg/kg/d × 5 days
- Initiate high-dose corticosteroids.
- Discontinue AChE inhibitors while intubated.
- Atropine for AChE inhibitor effects (bradycardia, GI symptoms, increased bronchial or oral secretions)

## MEDICATION
### First Line
- Edrophonium (Tensilon): 2 mg IV over 15–30 sec; if no effect after 45 sec, can give 2nd dose of 3 mg IV. If still no response, final dose of 5 mg IV can be given (total 10 mg).
- Prednisolone 1 mg/kg/day for crisis
- Atropine for cholinergic crisis 0.5 mg IV or IM

### Second Line
Other medications that may be initiated by neurologist:
- Prednisone, AChE inhibitors, azathioprine, mycophenolate, mofetil, cyclosporine, tacrolimus, rituximab

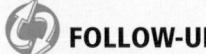 **FOLLOW-UP**

## DISPOSITION
### Admission Criteria
- Myasthenic crisis or questionable respiratory status mandates admission to ICU.
- Myasthenic patients with worsening symptoms
- New-onset myasthenic symptoms
- Diagnosis unclear, but myasthenia a possibility

### Discharge Criteria
Myasthenic patients who are improving can be considered for discharge in consultation with neurology.

### FOLLOW-UP RECOMMENDATIONS
Any discharged patient should have neurology follow-up arranged.

## PEARLS AND PITFALLS
- Always look for signs of myasthenic crisis in any MG patient who presents to ED.
- Always have patient on monitor and atropine and suction at bedside when performing edrophonium test.

## ADDITIONAL READING
- Abel M, Eisenkraft J. Anesthetic implications of myasthenia gravis. *Mt Sinai J Med.* 2002;69(1/2): 31–37.
- Chaudhuri A, Behan PO. Myasthenic crisis. *Q J Med.* 2009;102:97–101.
- Drachman DB. Myasthenia gravis. *N Engl J Med.* 1994;330:1797–1810.
- Gilhus NE. Autoimmune myasthenia gravis. *Expert Rev Neurother.* 2009;9(3):351–358.

- Kothari M. Myasthenia gravis. *J Am Osteopath Assoc.* 2004;104(9):377–384.
- Lang B, Vincent A. Autoimmune disorders of the neuromuscular junction. *Curr Opin Pharmacol.* 2009;9(3):336–340.
- Mahadeva B, Phillips L, Juel V. Autoimmune disorders of neuromuscular transmission. *Semin Neurol.* 2008;28(2):212–227.
- Marx J, Hockberger R, Walls R, eds. *Rosen's Emergency Medicine*, 6th ed. Philadelphia: Mosby Elsevier; 2006.
- Meriggioli MN. Myasthenia gravis with anti-acetylcholine receptor antibodies. *Front Neurol Neurosci.* 2009;26:94–108.
- Vincent A, Palace J, Hilton-Jones D. Myasthenia gravis. *Lancet.* 2001;357:2122–2128.

## See Also (Topic, Algorithm, Electronic Media Element)
- Amyotrophic Lateral Sclerosis
- Botulism
- Guillain-Barré Syndrome
- Hyperthyroidism
- Multiple Sclerosis

*The author gratefully acknowledges Angela Loh's contribution for the previous edition of this chapter.*

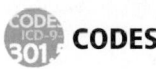 **CODES**

### ICD9
- 358.00 Myasthenia gravis without (acute) exacerbation
- 358.01 Myasthenia gravis with (acute) exacerbation

# MYOCARDIAL CONTUSION

*Sean Patrick Nordt*

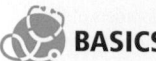

## BASICS

### DESCRIPTION
- Also known as blunt cardiac injury
- Pathologically characterized by discrete and well-demarcated area of hemorrhage
- Usually subendocardial
- May extend in pyramidal transmural fashion
- Most commonly involves anterior wall of right ventricle or atrium due to anatomic location

### ETIOLOGY
- Blunt trauma to chest:
  - High-speed deceleration accidents
  - May occur in accidents with speeds as low as 20–35 mph
- Auto–pedestrian injuries
- Falls
- Prolonged closed-chest cardiac massage
- Heart may be compressed between sternum and vertebrae.
- Heart strikes sternum during deceleration.
- Heart is damaged by abdominal viscera upwardly displaced by force on abdomen.
- Concussive forces (eg, explosion)
- Associated conditions:
  - Life-threatening dysrhythmias
  - Cardiogenic shock/CHF
  - Hemopericardium with tamponade
  - Valvular/myocardial rupture
  - Intraventricular thrombi
  - Thromboembolic phenomena
  - Coronary artery occlusion from intimal tearing or adjacent hemorrhage and edema may rarely occur.

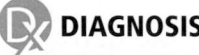

## DIAGNOSIS

### SIGNS AND SYMPTOMS
- Clinical picture is varied and nonspecific:
  - Chest pain
  - Cardiogenic shock
  - Subtle EKG changes without clinical symptoms
- Most common sign is tachycardia out of proportion to degree of trauma or blood loss.
- Friction rub may occur rarely.
- Retrosternal chest pain unrelieved by nitroglycerin:
  - Often delayed up to 24 hr
  - May respond to oxygen
- Evidence of significant thoracic trauma:
  - Contusions, abrasions
  - Palpable crepitus
  - Sternal fracture
  - Visible flail segments
- Other injuries may mask signs and symptoms of myocardial contusion.

### History
- Mechanism of injury (eg, MVA, fall, explosion, missile to chest wall)
- Any syncope or loss of consciousness suggests possible dysrhythmia.
- Crush injury

### Geriatric Considerations
Obtain and consider preexisting cardiac disease and concurrent medications in elderly patients following blunt cardiac injury.

### Pediatric Considerations
Due to increased compliance of pediatric chest wall, significant cardiac compression and contusion may be present with minimal or no external signs of trauma.

### Physical Exam
Complete physical exam as in any trauma patient:
- Evaluate for jugular venous distention (JVD)
- Decreased or muffled heart sounds
- Extra heart sounds
- Crepitus
- Pulsus paradoxus
- Evidence of chest wall trauma

### ESSENTIAL WORKUP
- No single diagnostic study (other than autopsy findings!) confirms presence of myocardial contusion.
- Only abnormal EKG and creatine phosphokinase (CK)-MB have been shown to correlate directly with complications requiring treatment. However, CK-MB fraction may be increased secondary to elevated CK levels from skeletal muscle injury. Troponin is more specific.
- EKG:
  - Best initial screening tool
  - Most common rhythm is sinus tachycardia (70%).
  - Normal EKG does not rule out myocardial damage.
  - EKG changes may be subtle or include nonspecific findings such as ST changes, right bundle branch block, and premature atrial and ventricular contractions.
  - At least 1 repeat EKG is recommended because changes may occur over time.
  - Serious dysrhythmias may result in hemodynamic instability:
    ○ Atrial fibrillation/atrial flutter
    ○ Ventricular tachycardia/ventricular fibrillation (commotio cordis)
- Echocardiography should be performed on all patients with any EKG changes, elevated CPK-MB, or elevated troponin-I or troponin-T.
- Transesophageal ECG (TEE) more sensitive than transthoracic ECG (TTE) but technically more difficult and time-consuming.

## DIAGNOSTIC TESTS & INTERPRETATION
### Lab
- CK-MB, troponins:
  - Levels should be sent on all patients being admitted.
  - Sensitivity varies from 11–97%.
  - Specificity decreased in multiple trauma
- Cardiac troponins are more specific than CK-MB for cardiac injury.

### Imaging
- Radiographs, CT, MRI detect associated injuries:
  - Pulmonary contusion
  - Rib or sternal fractures
  - Acute pulmonary edema
  - No specific findings in cardiac contusion
- Focused assessment with sonography for trauma (FAST) should be performed on all patients to assess pericardium and possible concurrent intraabdominal injuries.
- ECG:
  - Generally regarded as best imaging study for detecting cardiac contusion
  - Detects wall-motion abnormalities and effusions
  - Allows direct visualization of cardiac chambers and valves
  - May not visualize small (possibly clinically insignificant) contusions
  - TEE preferable to TTE if patient stable enough for procedure.
  - TTE may be performed although may also visualize great vessels.
- Radionuclide ventriculography:
  - Has been largely abandoned owing to wide availability of ECG
- Thallium[201] scintigraphy (single photon emission CT [SPECT]):
  - Sensitive and specific to left ventricular injury
  - Unable to evaluate right ventricle, which is most commonly injured

### Diagnostic Procedures/Surgery
- Pericardiocentesis:
  - For treatment of cardiac tamponade, preferably under US guidance
- Thoracotomy:
  - Consider in patient with acute cardiac arrest or decompensation in ED or after unsuccessful pericardiocentesis

## DIFFERENTIAL DIAGNOSIS

- Cardiac rupture
- Tamponade
- Valvular damage
- Other traumatic chest wall injury
- Angina or MI

 TREATMENT

### PRE-HOSPITAL

Prehospital personnel should convey accurate information to emergency department personnel:

- Mechanism of injury
- Motor vehicle status
- Steering wheel and dashboard damage
- Use of restraint devices
- Vehicle speed
- Patient position
- Time to extrication
- Any loss of consciousness

### INITIAL STABILIZATION/THERAPY

Manage airway and resuscitate as indicated:

- Oxygen:
  – IV access
  – Cardiac monitoring

### ED TREATMENT/PROCEDURES

- Dysrhythmias may be treated with same pharmacologic agents used for nontraumatic dysrhythmias:
  – Supraventricular tachycardia:
    ○ Adenosine or calcium channel blocker if patient not hypovolemic
  – Bradycardia:
    ○ Atropine
    ○ Pacing
  – Ventricular dysrhythmias:
    ○ Electrical conversion
    ○ Amiodarone
    ○ Lidocaine
    ○ Procainamide
  – Cardiac arrest:
    ○ Epinephrine
    ○ Atropine
    ○ Other interventions as appropriate
  – Rapid atrial fibrillation or flutter:
    ○ Diltiazem, or digoxin if patient not hypotensive
- Prophylactic treatment of dysrhythmias is not indicated.
- Cardiogenic shock caused by myocardial contusion:
  – Judicious fluid administration
  – Inotropic support (dopamine or dobutamine)
  – Intra-aortic balloon counterpulsation may be necessary.

## MEDICATION

- Medications used in cardiac contusion are supportive for dysrhythmias or hemodynamic compromise secondary to injury.
- There is no primary therapy for cardiac contusion.
- Adenosine: 6 mg rapid IVP (peds: 0.1–0.2 mg/kg rapid IVP), may repeat 12 mg q1–2min twice if no response
- Amiodarone: Load 150 mg IV over 10 min (peds: 5 mg/kg), then 1 mg/min for 6 hr, then 0.5 mg/min (peds: 5 $\mu$g/kg/min)
- Atropine: 0.5–1.0 mg (peds: 0.02 mg/kg per dose, minimum 0.1 mg) IV or endotracheal tube (ET)
- Digoxin: Load 0.5 mg (peds: 0.02 mg/kg) IV, then 0.25 mg (peds: 0.01 mg/kg) IV q6h for 2 more doses
- Diltiazem: 10–20 mg (peds: 0.25 mg/kg) IV over 2 min, may rebolus 0.35 mg/kg (adult and peds) 15 min later
- Dobutamine: 2–15 $\mu$g/kg/min (adult and peds)
- Dopamine: 2–20 $\mu$g/kg/min (adult and peds)
- Epinephrine: 1 mg (peds: 0.01 mg/kg) IV or ET for cardiac arrest (1:10,000 solution)
- Lidocaine: Load 1 mg/kg IV, then 0.5 mg/kg q8–10min to max. 3 mg/kg (adult and peds); infusion 1–4 mg/min (peds: 20–50 $\mu$g/kg) IV
- Procainamide: 100 mg (peds: 15 mg/kg per dose) IV q10min up to 17 mg/kg
- Verapamil: 0.1–0.3 mg/kg up to 5–10 mg IV over 2 min (not approved in children)

 FOLLOW-UP

### DISPOSITION

- Adverse outcomes, particularly dysrhythmias, are uncommon but generally occur within 1st 24 hr.
- No single test or combination of tests will accurately predict which patients can be discharged safely from ED:
  – All patients in whom diagnosis is seriously being entertained should be admitted to a monitored setting.

### Admission Criteria

- EKG abnormalities
- Cardiac enzyme abnormalities
- Hemodynamic instability
- Other studies suggesting cardiac contusion
- Admit to monitored unit for close observation.

### Discharge Criteria

Asymptomatic patients with no EKG abnormalities or dysrhythmia and with normal cardiac enzymes after 6-hr period may be discharged.

### Issues for Referral

Immediate surgical consultation:

- Suspected myocardial wall rupture
- Suspected valve or papillary muscle rupture
- Suspected septal rupture
- Coronary artery thrombosis
- Pericardial effusion
- Cardiac tamponade

## FOLLOW-UP RECOMMENDATIONS

Discharged patients:

- Should have follow-up within 24 hr of injury

## PEARLS AND PITFALLS

- Obtain EKG in patients following chest wall trauma.
- Perform FAST exam on all patients to assess pericardium.
- External signs of chest wall trauma should increase concern of blunt cardiac injury.
- Pediatric patients may have little or no external signs of chest wall trauma.
- Do not administer thrombolytics to patients with ST elevation MI following trauma.
- Negative cardiac markers and normal EKG make significant blunt cardiac injury unlikely.

## ADDITIONAL READING

- Adams J, Davilla Roman V, Bessey P, et al. Improved detection of cardiac contusion with cardiac troponin I. *Am Heart J.* 1996;131:308–312.
- El Chami MF, Nicholson W, Helmy T. Blunt cardiac trauma. *J Emerg Med.* 2008;127–133.
- Elie MC. Blunt cardiac injury. *Mount Sinai J Med.* 2006;73:542–552.
- Rajan GP, Zellweger R. Cardiac troponin I as a predictor of arrhythmia and ventricular dysfunction in trauma patients with myocardial contusion. *J Trauma.* 2004;57:801–808.
- Sybrandy KC, Cramer MJ, Burgersdijk C. Diagnosing cardiac contusion: Old wisdom and new insights. *Heart.* 2003;89(5):485–489.

 CODES

### ICD9

861.01 Contusion of heart without mention of open wound into thorax

**M**

# MYOCARDITIS
*Liudvikas Jagminas*

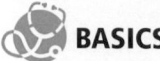 **BASICS**

## DESCRIPTION
- An inflammatory change in the heart muscle characterized by myocyte necrosis and subsequent myocardial destruction
- Direct cytotoxic effect of causative agent followed by a secondary immune response
- True incidence is unknown because many cases are asymptomatic.
- Autopsy studies have demonstrated evidence of myocarditis in 0.5–1% of cases.
- Male > Female (1.5:1)
- Average age of patients with myocarditis is 42 years.

## ETIOLOGY
- Viral:
  - Enteroviruses (coxsackie B)
  - Adenovirus
  - Herpesvirus (including cytomegalovirus [CMV])
  - Hepatitis C
  - Influenza
  - Echovirus
  - Herpes simplex virus
  - Varicella-zoster
  - Epstein-Barr virus
  - Cytomegalovirus
  - Mumps
  - Rubeola
  - Variola/vaccinia
  - Yellow fever
  - Rabies
  - HIV
- Bacteria:
  - Diphtheria
  - Tuberculosis
  - Brucellosis
  - Psittacosis
  - Meningococcus
  - Mycoplasma
  - Group A streptococcus
- Protozoa:
  - Leishmaniasis
  - Malaria
  - Toxoplasmosis in the immunocompromised host
  - *Treponema cruzi* (Chagas disease):
    ○ Most common cause of heart failure and myocarditis worldwide
    ○ 20 million persons infected in Central and South America
  - Trichinosis
  - Trypanosomiasis
- Spirochetes:
  - *Borrelia burgdorferi,* the spirochete agent in Lyme disease
  - Syphilis
- Rickettsial:
  - Scrub typhus
  - Rocky mountain spotted fever
  - Q fever
- Fungal:
  - Candidiasis
  - Aspergillosis
  - Cryptococcosis
  - Histoplasmosis
  - Actinomycosis
  - Helminthic
  - Trichinosis
  - Echinococcosis
  - Schistosomiasis
  - Cysticercosis
- Drugs:
  - Acetaminophen
  - Ampicillin
  - Chemotherapeutic agents (anthracyclines)
  - Cocaine
  - Hydrochlorothiazide
  - Lithium
  - Methyldopa
  - Penicillin
  - Sulfamethoxazole
  - Sulfonamides
  - Zidovudine
  - Radiation
  - Hypersensitivity
  - Heavy metals
  - Hydrocarbons
  - Carbon monoxide
  - Arsenic
- Autoimmune disorders:
  - Systemic lupus erythematosus (SLE)
  - Wegener granulomatosis
  - Kawasaki disease
  - Giant cell arteritis
  - Sarcoidosis
- Peripartum cardiomyopathy
- Bites/stings:
  - Scorpion
  - Snake
  - Black widow venom

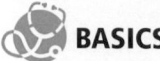 **DIAGNOSIS**

## SIGNS AND SYMPTOMS
Arrhythmias (18%), dyspnea (72%), and chest pain (35%)

### History
- Fatigue
- Myalgias/arthralgias
- Malaise
- Fever
- Chest pain:
  - Reported in 35%
  - Most commonly pleuritic, sharp, stabbing, precordial
- Dyspnea on exertion is common.
- Orthopnea and shortness of breath if congestive heart failure (CHF) is present
- Palpitations are common
- Syncope:
  - May signal high-grade aortic valve block or risk for sudden death

### Physical Exam
- Fever
- Tachypnea
- Tachycardia:
  - Often out of proportion to fever
- Cyanosis
- Hypotension:
  - Due to left ventricular dysfunction
  - Uncommon in the acute setting and indicates a poor prognosis when present
- Bibasilar crackles
- Rales
- Jugular venous distention (JVD)
- Peripheral edema
- Hepatomegaly
- Ascites
- $S_3$ or a summation gallop if significant biventricular involvement
- Intensity of $S_1$ may be diminished
- Murmurs of mitral or tricuspid
- Pericardial friction rub when associated with pericarditis

### Pediatric Considerations
- Most common cause of heart failure in previously healthy children
- Particularly infants, present with nonspecific symptoms:
  - Fever
  - Respiratory distress
  - Poor feeding or, in cases with CHF, sweating while feeding
  - New onset murmur
  - Cyanosis in severe cases

## ESSENTIAL WORKUP
- Physical exam
- EKG
- CXR

## DIAGNOSTIC TESTS & INTERPRETATION
### Lab
- Cardiac enzyme levels:
  - Levels are only elevated in a minority of patients.
- Erythrocyte sedimentation rate (ESR) is elevated in 60% during the acute phase.
- Leukocytosis is present in 25%.
- Viral titers; cultures rarely positive
- Mycoplasma, antistreptolysin titers, cold agglutinin titer
- Hepatitis panels
- Lyme titer
- Monospot testing
- CMV serology
- Blood cultures

## Imaging
- EKG:
  - Sinus tachycardia most frequent finding
  - Transient, nonspecific ST- and T-wave changes
  - Atrial and ventricular dysrhythmias
  - Heart block and conduction defects:
    o 20% have a conduction delay.
    o 20% have a left bundle branch block.
- CXR:
  - Normal cardiac silhouette
  - Pulmonary edema
  - Pleural effusion
- ECG:
  - Impairment of left ventricular systolic and diastolic function
  - Segmental wall motion abnormalities
  - Impaired ejection fraction
  - Pericardial effusion
  - Ventricular thrombus has been identified in 15% of patients
- Gallium[67] and indium[111]-labeled antimyosin antibody scans
- Gadolinium-enhanced MRI:
  - Indicate cardiac inflammation and myocyte necrosis
- Cardiac MRI:
  - Abnormal signal areas correlate with regions of myocarditis
  - Reported 76% sensitivity, 96% specificity, and 85% diagnostic accuracy
  - Considered in patients in whom the diagnosis is unclear and endocardial biopsy is planned

## Diagnostic Procedures/Surgery
- Right ventricular endomyocardial biopsy:
  - Appropriate in heart transplant recipients
  - Polymerase chain reaction (PCR) amplification of viral genome in endomyocardial tissue
- PCR identification of a viral infection from pericardial fluid, or other body fluid sites

## DIFFERENTIAL DIAGNOSIS
- Acute MI
- Acute and chronic pulmonary embolus
- Aortic dissection
- Adrenal insufficiency
- Environmental challenges
- Esophageal perforation/rupture/tear
- Hyperpyrexia
- Hypothermia
- Kawasaki disease
- Pericarditis
- Pneumonia
- Viral
- Bacterial
- Sepsis
- Severe hypothyroidism and hyperthyroidism
- Toxin-mediated disease

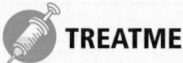 TREATMENT

### ALERT
- Avoid sympathomimetic and β-blocker drugs.
- Patients presenting with Mobitz II or complete heart block require pacemaker placement.

### INITIAL STABILIZATION/THERAPY
- ABCs
- Supplemental oxygen
- Cardiac monitor
- Pulse oximetry
- IV access

### ED TREATMENT/PROCEDURES
- Treat dysrhythmias.
- Transthoracic or transvenous pacing for symptomatic heart block
- Supplemental oxygen
- ACE inhibitors (captopril):
  - Reduce afterload and inflammation.
- Digoxin:
  - CHF or atrial fibrillation
- Diuretics (furosemide, bumetanide)
- Hyperimmunoglobulin therapy in CMV-associated myopericarditis.
- NSAIDs contraindicated in early and acute-phase myocarditis
- Heparin and warfarin for patients with depressed LV function or intracardiac thrombus

### Pediatric Considerations
- IV immunoglobulin is an effective treatment option in pediatric viral myocarditis.
- Improved LV function and trend toward better survival

### MEDICATION
- Captopril:
  - Adult dose: Initial dose 6.25 mg; can titrate to 50 mg/dose
  - Pediatric dose:
    o Infants: 0.15–0.3 mg/kg/dose (max. 6 mg/kg)
    o Children: 0.5–1.0 mg/kg/24h
- Digoxin:
  - Adult dose: Load: 0.4–0.6 mg IV, then 0.1–0.3 mg q6–8 hours. Maintain: 0.125–0.5 mg/d IV/PO
  - Pediatric dose:
    o <2 years: 15–20 μg/kg IV
    o 2–10 years: 10–15 μg/kg IV
    o >10 years: 4–5 μg/kg IV
- Furosemide:
  - Adult dose: 20–80 mg/d PO/IV/IM; titrate up to 600 mg/d for severe edematous states
  - Pediatric dose: 1–2 mg/kg PO; not to exceed 6 mg/kg; do not administer >q6h 1 mg/kg IV/IM slowly under close supervision; not to exceed 6 mg/kg
- Immunoglobulin IV (Gamimune, Gammagard, Gammar-P, Sandoglobulin):
  - Adult dose: 2 g/kg IV over 2–5 d

 FOLLOW-UP

### DISPOSITION

**Admission Criteria**
Symptomatic patients with myocarditis:
- New-onset
- CHF
- Dysrhythmia
- Mobitz II or complete heart block
- Embolic events
- Cardiogenic shock

**Discharge Criteria**
Asymptomatic patient with no evidence of dysrhythmia or cardiac dysfunction

**Issues for Referral**
Cardiac transplant for patients with intractable CHF:
- Approximately 50% of patients die within 5 years of diagnosis.
- Best prognosis for lymphocytic myocarditis

## PEARLS AND PITFALLS
- Myocarditis should be considered in a patient who presents with dyspnea and chest pain, particularly if the history includes a recent viral illness.
- Careful physical examination for signs of CHF and pericarditis is paramount.
- EKG should be obtained when considering the diagnosis and is especially sensitive for pediatric cases.
- Patients with evidence of dysrhythmia, CHF, or thromboembolism must be admitted.

## ADDITIONAL READING
- Brady WJ, Ferguson JD, Ullman EA, et al. Myocarditis: Emergency department recognition and management. *Emerg Med Clin North Am.* 2004; 22(4):865–885.
- Cooper LT. Myocarditis. *N Engl J Med.* 2009;360: 1526–1538.
- Durani Y. Pediatric myocarditis: Presenting clinical characteristics. *Am J Emerg Med.* 2009;27(8): 942–947.
- Magnani JW, Dec GW. Myocarditis: Current trends in diagnosis and treatment. *Circulation.* 2006;113: 876–890.

### See Also (Topic, Algorithm, Electronic Media Element)
Congestive Heart Failure

 CODES

### ICD9
- 422.91 Idiopathic myocarditis
- 422.92 Septic myocarditis
- 429.0 Myocarditis, unspecified

M

# NASAL FRACTURES

*David W. Munter*

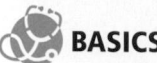 **BASICS**

## DESCRIPTION
- Fractures of the nasal skeleton are the most common body fractures.
- Most nasal fractures result from blunt trauma, frequently from motor vehicle crashes, sports injuries, and altercations.
- Lateral forces are more likely to cause displacement than are straight-on blows.
- Characteristics that suggest associated injuries:
  – History of trauma with significant force
  – Loss of consciousness
  – Findings of facial bone injury
  – Frontal bone crepitus
  – CSF leak

## ETIOLOGY
- The vast majority of nasal fractures are from direct trauma.
- Altercations account for most nasal fractures in adults.
- Direct blows, especially in sports, account for most nasal fractures in children.

 **DIAGNOSIS**

## SIGNS AND SYMPTOMS
- Nasal deformity, asymmetry, swelling, or ecchymosis
- Epistaxis
- Periorbital ecchymosis ("raccoon eyes") from damage to branches of the ethmoid artery:
  – May indicate nasofrontoethmoid complex injury
- Palpable sharp edges, depressions, or other irregularities suggest nasal fracture.
- Crepitus or mobility of skeletal parts on palpation
- Septal hematoma:
  – Bluish fluid-filled sac overlying nasal septum
  – Critical to detect because it must be drained
  – Failure to drain can result in necrosis of the septum

- Flattening of nasal root and widening of intercanthal distance (telecanthus):
  – Indicative of serious injury to the nasofrontoethmoid complex
- Clear rhinorrhea indicates possible CSF leak:
  – Rhinorrhea may be delayed.
- Loss of sense of smell suggests significant injury.
- Tear duct injuries may be present, with abnormal tearing.
- Associated eye injuries:
  – Subconjunctival hemorrhage
  – Hyphema
  – Retinal detachments

### History
- Direct blow
- Associated injuries or symptoms
- Presence of epistaxis
- Changes in vision or smell

### Physical Exam
- Physical examination with visual inspection and palpation is most important.
- It is critical to identify a septal hematoma:
  – Bluish bulging mass on nasal septum
- Septal deviation
- Epistaxis or intranasal laceration
- Examine closely for telecanthus:
  – Intercanthal width >30–35 mm
  – Wider than width of an eye
  – May indicate nasofrontoethmoid fracture
  – Usually associated with depressed nasal bridge
- CSF rhinorrhea:
  – Indicates more serious fracture of underlying facial bone or skull
  – CSF mixed with blood will cause double-ring sign when placed on filter paper.

## ESSENTIAL WORKUP
- If there is concern for anything other than a simple nasal fracture:
- Evaluate nasolacrimal duct for patency:
  – Instill fluorescein into eye and look for it in nasopharynx under the inferior turbinate.
  – Absence implies duct injury.
- Eyelash traction test:
  – Grasp eyelashes on eyelid and pull laterally:
  – If eyelid margin does not become taut or "bowstring," medial portion of tendon has been disrupted.
  – This test is performed on both upper and lower eyelids.
    ○ It is possible for only one portion of the tendon to be selectively injured.

## DIAGNOSTIC TESTS & INTERPRETATION
### Lab
Coagulation studies if patient is on anticoagulants with uncontrolled epistaxis

### Imaging
- Nasal radiographs are rarely indicated:
  – Normally do not alter initial or subsequent management
  – Gross deformities will need referral.
  – Fractures without deformity will be treated conservatively regardless of radiographic findings.
  – Patients with associated facial bone deformity, crepitus, or tenderness may require radiographs.
- CT is test of choice if facial bone, nasofrontoethmoid, or depressed skull fractures are suspected.

## DIFFERENTIAL DIAGNOSIS
- Other facial injuries such as orbital, frontal sinus, maxillary sinus, or cribriform plate fractures
- Nasofrontoethmoid fracture

**TREATMENT**

### PRE-HOSPITAL
- Management of airway takes precedence.
- Nasotracheal intubation is contraindicated.
- Consider orotracheal intubation or cricothyroidotomy if definitive airway control is needed.
- Cervical spine precautions are indicated if there is associated trauma.
- Epistaxis can normally be controlled with direct pressure; pinch nares together.

### INITIAL STABILIZATION/THERAPY
- Airway management with orotracheal intubation or cricothyroidotomy:
  - Nasotracheal intubation is contraindicated.
- Cervical spine precautions
- Other injuries take precedence.

### ED TREATMENT/PROCEDURES
- Abrasions and lacerations:
  - Proper cleansing of facial wounds is essential.
  - Lacerations may be sutured.
- Epistaxis must be controlled if it does not stop spontaneously:
  - Anesthetize/vasoconstrict with topical cocaine, lidocaine, or neosynephrine spray.
  - Identify bleeding source; cauterize anterior source if necessary.
  - Pack nares with petroleum jelly–impregnated gauze or a commercial pack.
  - Posterior packs are rarely needed.
  - Prophylactic antibiotics to prevent sinus infection are indicated if packed: amoxicillin, amoxicillin/clavulanate, or trimethoprim-sulfamethoxazole in penicillin-allergic patients.
  - Displaced fractures do not need reduction in the ED unless the airway is compromised.
  - It is generally recommended to let swelling go down and reduce the fracture in 3–5 days

- Septal hematoma must be drained immediately in the ED:
  - Anesthetize with topical cocaine or lidocaine and vascular constriction with neosynephrine.
  - Attempt to aspirate with 18- to 20-gauge needle on 3-mL syringe.
  - Rolling a cotton swab down the septum may facilitate drainage.
  - Holding mucosa down against cartilage must be done to prevent reaccumulation.
  - This can be done with petroleum jelly gauze packing.
  - Both nares should be packed to ensure adequate pressure:
    - Packing is left in place for 3–5 days or until follow-up with ENT.
  - Prophylactic antibiotics are prescribed.

### MEDICATION
- Amoxicillin: 500 mg PO t.i.d. (peds: 40 mg/kg PO div t.i.d.)
- Amoxicillin/clavulanate: 500/125–875/125 mg PO b.i.d. (peds: 40 mg/kg/day of amoxicillin PO b.i.d.)
- Cocaine: topical 4%
- Lidocaine: 1–2% without epinephrine
- Neosynephrine nasal spray
- Trimethoprim–sulfamethoxazole: double strength (DS) PO b.i.d. (peds: 40 mg/kg/day sulfamethoxazole PO b.i.d.)

 **FOLLOW-UP**

### DISPOSITION
#### Admission Criteria
- Most nasal fractures do not require admission.
- Admit patients with nasoethmoid fractures or more significant craniofacial injuries.

#### Discharge Criteria
- No evidence of significant head, neck, or other injuries
- Epistaxis controlled
- Reliable companion or caregiver

### *Pediatric Considerations*
- Follow up with specialist sooner because fibrous union begins in only 3–4 days.
- Consider contacting child protective services if any suspicion of nonaccidental trauma:
  - History does not fit injury.
  - Always consider nonaccidental trauma as potential mechanism of injury.
- Fractures are rare in children; nasal injuries in children are more likely to be cartilaginous.
- Significant injuries in children are not always fully appreciated.

### FOLLOW-UP RECOMMENDATIONS
- Follow up with ENT, plastic surgery, or oral maxillofacial (OMF) surgeon in 3–5 days for management:
  - Patients with septal hematoma should follow up in 24 hr for re-evaluation after drainage.
- Return for signs of clear rhinorrhea, difficulty breathing, fever, or signs associated with head injury.

## PEARLS AND PITFALLS

The absence of a septal hematoma must be documented in every case.

## ADDITIONAL READING

- Friese G, Wojciehoski RF. The nose: Bleeds, breaks and obstructions. *Emerg Med Serv*. 2005;34(80):129–135.
- Ondik MP, Lipinski L, et al. The treatment of nasal fractures: A changing paradigm. *Arch Facial Plast Surg*. 2009;11(5):296–302.
- Kucik CJ, Clenney T, Phelan J. Management of acute nasal fractures. *Am Fam Physician*. 2004;70:1315–1320.
- Ziccardi VB, Braidy H. Management of nasal fractures. *Oral Maxillofac Surg Clin North Am*. 2009;21(2):203–208.

### See Also (Topic, Algorithm, Electronic Media Element)
- Epistaxis
- Facial Fractures

 **CODES**

### ICD9
- 802.0 Closed fracture of nasal bones
- 802.1 Open fracture of nasal bones

N

# NEAR DROWNING
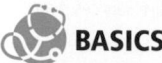

*Colleen N. Hickey*
*Janet M. Poponick*

## 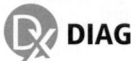 BASICS

### DESCRIPTION
- Definitions:
  - Drowning:
    - Death by asphyxia after submersion in a liquid
    - Death within 24 hr of the accident
  - Near drowning:
    - Survival beyond 24 hr of a submersion accident
- Scenario of drowning:
  - "Wet" drowning (90%):
    - Aspiration of small amount of water
  - "Dry" drowning (10%):
    - Laryngospasm
  - End result: hypoxia
  - No significant difference between fresh water and salt water submersion
- Pathophysiology:
  - Aspiration:
    - Small volume of water
    - Decreased lung compliance causing ventilation/perfusion mismatch and intrapulmonary shunting
    - No significant electrolyte changes
    - Grossly contaminated water: Risk for pulmonary infection
  - Hypoxemia:
    - Metabolic lactic acidosis
    - Multisystem organ dysfunction
    - Noncardiogenic pulmonary edema
    - Myocardial dysfunction (arrhythmias)
    - Coagulation abnormalities (disseminated intravascular coagulation)
    - Renal failure (usually acute tubular necrosis)
    - Cerebral hypoxia: Cerebral edema, increased intracranial pressure

### Pediatric Considerations
- Hypothermia:
  - More common in young children
  - Larger body surface-to-mass ratio
  - Decreases the metabolic rate
  - Survival with full recovery is possible (neuroprotective).
- Diving reflex:
  - Young children are more susceptible.
  - Triggered by submersion of face in cold water
  - Bradycardia ensues: Redistribution of blood flow to the heart and brain
  - Delays onset of hypoxia-related damage

### ALERT
Risk factors:
- Lack of proper supervision
- Alcohol or other drug abuse
- Limited swimming ability or exhaustion
- Trauma
- Risky behavior
- Pre-existing medical problem
- Attempted suicide

##  DIAGNOSIS

### SIGNS AND SYMPTOMS
- Cardiopulmonary arrest
- Cyanosis
- Dyspnea
- Copious pulmonary secretions
- Loss of consciousness
- Cerebral edema/injury
- Evidence of trauma:
  - Cervical spine injury
  - Intracranial hemorrhage
- Hypothermia

### ESSENTIAL WORKUP
- Information from witnesses or emergency medical services personnel at the scene
- Early airway management and CPR
- Rectal temperature for hypothermia

### DIAGNOSTIC TESTS & INTERPRETATION
#### Lab
- Arterial blood gas (pH)
- CBC
- Electrolytes, BUN, creatinine, glucose:
  - Usually normal
  - Hyperkalemia
  - Hypernatremia or hyponatremia
- Alcohol and toxicology screen

#### Imaging
- CXR:
  - Diffuse or focal infiltrates, acute respiratory distress syndrome
  - May be normal initially
- Cervical spine series

- ECG:
  - Long QT interval
  - Sinus bradycardia
  - Atrial fibrillation
- CT scan:
  - Brain: Abnormality at any time during hospitalization is associated with poor neurologic outcome.
  - Cervical spine: traumatic injury

### DIFFERENTIAL DIAGNOSIS
- Consider reason for submersion:
  - Dysrhythmia (long QT syndrome, familial polymorphic ventricular tachycardia)
  - Myocardial infarction
  - Seizure
  - Syncope
  - Trauma
  - Suicide attempt

### Pediatric Considerations
Consider child abuse/neglect:
- Especially infants in bathtub near drowning

## TREATMENT

### PRE-HOSPITAL
- Attention to ABCs:
  - Avoid further aspiration.
  - Apply cricoid pressure during bag-to-mask ventilation.
  - Secure airway—intubate
  - Early CPR
- Strict cervical spine precautions
- Early rewarming attempts
- 90% survival with appropriate intervention
- All near-drowning victims need ED evaluation
- Controversies:
  - Abdominal thrusts to remove water:
    - Increases risk for aspiration
    - Delays effective CPR
    - Useful only if foreign body in airway

## INITIAL STABILIZATION/THERAPY

- ABCs
- Core temperature:
  - Initiate rewarming (see "Hypothermia")
  - Remove wet clothing

## ED TREATMENT/PROCEDURES

- Correct hypoxemia:
  - Titrate to oxygen saturation
  - Intubate and provide mechanical ventilation with positive end-expiratory pressure
- Evaluate and treat traumatic injuries
- Correct acidosis
- Cardiopulmonary arrest:
  - Initiate advanced cardiac life support measures.
  - Continue rewarming efforts:
    - Passive: Blankets, insulators
    - Active external: Warm blankets, radiant heat, warm baths
    - Active internal: Pleural or peritoneal irrigation, cardiopulmonary bypass
  - Continue resuscitation until core temperature >32°C or until spontaneous pulse and respirations return.
- No value to steroids
- Poor prognostic signs:
  - Severe acidosis (pH ≤7.0)
  - Ventricular fibrillation
    Low oxygen saturation
  - Low Glasgow coma score (GCS)

## MEDICATION

- Atropine: 1 mg (peds: 0.02 mg/kg) IV
- Epinephrine: 1 mg (peds: 0.01 mg/kg) IV
- Vasopressin: 40 U (peds: 0.04 U/kg) IV
- Lidocaine: 1 mg/kg IV
- Sodium bicarbonate: 1 mEq/kg IV

### Pediatric Considerations

- Hypothermia may be protective:
  - Aggressive rewarming
  - Aggressive resuscitation
- Evaluate for abuse/neglect
- Family history: Sudden death, similar episode:
  - Long QT syndrome
  - Familial polymorphic ventricular tachycardia
- Prevention is key to treatment:
  Supervision around water
  - Empty pails and buckets

## ALERT

Controversial: Therapeutic hypothermia

- Optimize neurologic outcome.
- Suppress reperfusion injury.

 FOLLOW-UP

## DISPOSITION

Delayed symptomatology occurs:

- Pulmonary edema (up to 12 hr later)
- Neurologic abnormalities

### Admission Criteria

- ICU:
  - Patients who required CPR or artificial ventilation
  - Abnormal chest radiograph
  - Arterial blood gas abnormalities
  - GCS <13
- Admit observation status:
  - All symptomatic patients
  - Submersion for >1 min
  - History of cyanosis or apnea
  - Patients who required brief assisted ventilation

### Discharge Criteria

- Questionable history of submersion:
  - Observe in ED for 8 hr:
    - No respiratory distress
    - No neurologic impairment
- Discharge to reliable home
- Home-going instructions:
  - Return for shortness of breath or mental status changes.

## FOLLOW-UP RECOMMENDATIONS

Primary care follow-up for all patients discharged from ED

## PEARLS AND PITFALLS

- All patients with near drowning require at least 8 hr of observation
- Indicators of poor prognosis:
  - Acidemia (pH <7.1 on presentation)
  - Age <3 yr
  - Submersion >10 min
  - Time to basic life support care >10 min
  - GCS ≤ 5
  - Long transportation time to ED
  - Persistent apnea or need for cardiopulmonary resuscitation in the ED
  - Water temperature >10°C

## ADDITIONAL READING

- Layon, AJ, Modell JH. Drowning. *Anesthesiology.* 2009;110(6):1390–1401.
- Rafaat KT, Spear RM, Kuelbs C, et al. Cranial computed tomographic findings in a large group of children with drowning: Diagnostic, prognostic, and forensic implications. *Pediatr Crit Care Med.* 2008;9(6):567–572.
- Wagner C. Pediatric submersion injuries. *Air Med J.* 2009;28(3):116–119.
- Youn CS, Choi SP, Yim HY, et al. Out-of-hospital cardiac arrest due to drowning: An Utstein Style report of 10 years of experience from St. Mary's Hospital. *Resuscitation.* 2009;80(7):778–783.

### See Also (Topic, Algorithm, Electronic Media Element)

Hypothermia

 CODES

### ICD9

994.1 Drowning and nonfatal submersion

# NECK INJURY BY STRANGULATION/HANGING

David Della-Giustina
Brooks T. Laselle

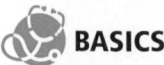 **BASICS**

## DESCRIPTION
- Strangulation:
  - Ligature: Material used to compress structures of neck
  - Manual: Physical force used to compress structures of neck
  - Postural: Airway obstruction from body weight (over an object) or position (typically in infants)
- Hanging is a form of strangulation:
  - Complete (judicial-type): Victim's entire body is suspended off the ground
  - Incomplete (nonjudicial): Some part of victim's body contacts the ground
  - Typical: The point of suspension is placed centrally over the occiput.
  - Atypical: The point of suspension is in any position other than over the central occiput.
  - Intentional: Suicide, homicide, autoerotic, "the choking game"
  - Accidental: Often children or clothing caught in machinery
  - Near-hanging: Survival following nonjudicial hanging

## ETIOLOGY
- Hanging (judicial):
  - Victim is dropped a distance at least equal to his or her height:
  - Forceful distraction of head from torso results in a decapitation type of injury (fracture of cervical spine and transection of spinal cord)
- Hanging (nonjudicial):
  - Typically occurs from a lower height
  - Injuries mimic nonjudicial strangulation
- Strangulation:
  - External neck pressure causes cerebral hypoxia secondary to venous and arterial obstruction.
  - Pressure on neck structures may cause airway, soft tissue, and vascular injuries.
  - Cervical spine injuries are uncommon except with judicial-type hanging.
- Death:
  - Secondary to mechanical closure of blood vessels or airway
  - Secondary to cardiac arrest from extreme bradycardia due to increased vagal tone from carotid sinus pressure
  - Secondary to direct neurologic injury to the spinal cord
  - Secondary to pulmonary complications in near-hanging victims
  - Secondary to cerebral hypoxia

## COMMONLY ASSOCIATED CONDITIONS
- Cervical spine injury
- Hypoxic cerebral injury
- Vascular injury:
  - Arterial or venous dissection/thrombosis
- Hyoid bone fracture:
  - Typically seen in nonjudicial strangulation

- Cricoid cartilage disruption (rare)
- Thyroid cartilage disruption:
  - More common in nonjudicial strangulation deaths
- Phrenic nerve injury
- Airway edema
- Aspiration pneumonitis (may be late)
- Neurogenic pulmonary edema (may be late):
  - Due to massive central sympathetic discharge
- Postobstructive pulmonary edema (may be rapid onset):
  - Due to negative intrapleural pressure resulting from inspiration against an external airway obstruction
- Air embolism:
  - Consider when subcutaneous air and vascular injuries are present

 **DIAGNOSIS**

## SIGNS AND SYMPTOMS
- Airway disruption:
  - Subcutaneous emphysema
  - Dyspnea
  - Dysphonia or stridor
  - Loss of normal cartilaginous landmarks
- Cervical spine injury:
  - Respiratory arrest
  - Paralysis
- Neurologic injury:
  - Hoarseness
  - Dysphagia
  - Altered mental status
  - Neurologic deficit
- Pulmonary sequelae:
  - Respiratory distress
  - Pulmonary edema, ARDS, pneumonia
- Soft tissue injury:
  - Abrasions, contusions, ecchymoses, ligature or hand marks
- Vascular injuries:
  - Expanding hematoma
  - Pulse deficits or bruits
  - Evidence of cerebral infarction
  - *Tardieu's spots:* Petechial hemorrhages of the skin, mucous membranes and conjunctiva cephalad to the ligature marks

### Pediatric Considerations
- Structures of neck are more cartilaginous and mobile than in adults
- More resistant to crush injuries and fractures
- Rapid airway compromise can occur with relatively little edema of soft tissues secondary to smaller airway diameter.

## History
- Strangulation method:
  - Patient position:
    - To determine mechanism of strangulation
    - Predict potential injuries
  - Higher fall implies greater force:
    - Decapitation-type injury more common
  - Knot position:
    - Arterial occlusion more likely in typical hanging
  - Ligature material:
    - Elasticity limits force applied
    - Venous occlusion may still produce unconsciousness and death
- Circumstance:
  - Accidental, suicide/homicide, NAT, sexual, "choking game"

## Physical Exam
- ABCs:
  - Airway or respiratory compromise
  - C-spine precautions
- Disability:
  - Coma, AMS, neurologic deficit, paralysis
- Secondary survey:
  - Assess for traumatic injury to the neck:
    - Soft tissue, aero-digestive, vascular
  - Other traumatic injury due to fall, self-inflicted wounds (suicidal), injury sustained in conflict (homicidal/NAT)

## ESSENTIAL WORKUP
- Plain radiography:
  - Cervical spine/soft-tissue neck to evaluate for bony injuries as well as soft tissue swelling and subcutaneous emphysema
  - Chest to evaluate for subcutaneous emphysema, as well as aspiration pneumonitis, pulmonary edema
- Pulse oximetry
- Cardiac monitor

## DIAGNOSTIC TESTS & INTERPRETATION
### Lab
- ABG (may be considered):
  - Evaluate for evidence of hypoxia or respiratory compromise.
- Hematocrit for significant blood loss
- Type and cross-match in anticipation of transfusion for vascular injuries.
- Coagulation profile for significant blood loss or coagulopathy
- Toxicology studies (ASA/APAP/ETOH):
  - Consider for suicide-related ingestions

### Imaging
- CT scan of the neck:
- Further defines aero-digestive, vascular and bony injuries
- CT angiography for potential vascular injury
- CT scan of the brain for suspected cerebral insult
- Arteriography:
  - Definitive evaluation for potential vascular injuries
- Carotid duplex imaging with flow studies for suspected vascular injury

### Diagnostic Procedures/Surgery
- Fiberoptic endoscopy:
  - Allows direct visualization for evaluation of aero-digestive injury
  - May aid in intubation
- Surgical exploration

## DIFFERENTIAL DIAGNOSIS
Etiology of strangulation:
- Accidental, homicidal, suicidal, NAT, auto-erotic, choking game

 TREATMENT

### PRE-HOSPITAL
- ABCs
- Early and aggressive airway management: Oxygen, suction, intubation, as indicated:
  - Remove ligature.
- Cardiac monitor
- Cervical spine stabilization:
  - Patient position, strangulation method, drop involved, knot location, signs of foul play

### INITIAL STABILIZATION/THERAPY
- ABCs
- Aggressive airway management with cervical spine precautions is paramount:
  - Early intubation for respiratory compromise
  - Supplemental oxygen
  - Cricothyrotomy or tracheostomy may be required if severe maxillofacial injuries are present:
    - Avoid cricothyrotomy if hematoma over cricothyroid membrane or evidence of cricotracheal disruption is seen.
    - Arrange for emergent tracheostomy in above scenario (see Larynx Fracture).
- Control bleeding with application of direct pressure:
  - Do *not* explore in the ED

### ED TREATMENT/PROCEDURES
- IV access
- Consult otolaryngologist or trauma surgeon in management of neck soft-tissue injuries.
- Consult vascular surgery in management of vascular injuries.
- Consult neurology for suspected cerebral ischemic insults (thrombosis, embolism, dissection).
- Supportive care for suspected elevated intracranial pressure/cerebral edema:
  - Elevate head of bed.
  - Ensure adequate oxygenation and cerebral perfusion.
  - Prevent secondary neurologic injury/insult.
  - Consult neurosurgery for intracranial pressure monitoring and surgery as indicated.

- Neck injury with subcutaneous emphysema:
  - Assume that mucosa of upper airway communicates with deep tissues of neck.
  - Administer antibiotics.
- Laryngeal edema:
  - Consider steroids.
- Evaluate for associated injuries or harm:
  - Consider ingestions in suicidal cases.

## MEDICATION
- Hypoxic brain injury:
  - Mannitol: 0.25–1 g/kg/dose IV (consider for elevated intracranial pressure; not routinely used in pediatric cases)
  - Hypertonic saline: Dosing regimens vary (consider for elevated intracranial pressure)
  - Phenytoin: 15–20 mg/kg IV (loading dose) as needed for seizures
- Neck injury with subcutaneous emphysema:
  - Ampicillin/sulbactam: 1.5–3 g (peds: 100–400 mg/kg/d) IV q6h
  - Clindamycin: 600 mg (peds: 20–40 mg/kg/d) IV q8h
- Airway edema:
  - Dexamethasone: 0.5–2 mg/kg/d (peds: 0.25–0.5 mg/kg) IV q6h

 FOLLOW-UP

### DISPOSITION
#### Admission Criteria
- Admit patients with strangulation or hanging-mechanism injuries to a monitored setting to observe for airway compromise (may have delayed onset).
- Surgical correction of laryngeal, esophageal or vascular neck injuries
- Altered level of consciousness, new neurologic deficit, coma
- Respiratory distress:
  - Supportive care for pulmonary edema, ARDS, pneumonia
- All patients with suspected suicidal or homicidal strangulation injury should have psychiatric or social work consultation.

#### Discharge Criteria
Only patients without strangulation or hanging injuries may be discharged after appropriate observation in the ED to ensure absence of airway compromise, vascular injury, neurologic deficit, and suicidal/homicidal ideation.

### FOLLOW-UP RECOMMENDATIONS
- Neuropsychiatric evaluation:
  - Consider in evaluation for hypoxic encephalopathy
- Psychiatry/psychology:
  - Suicidal or homicidal patients
  - Auto-erotic or "choking game" patients for medical/cognitive/behavioral therapy
- Surgical follow-up:
  - As indicated, based on injuries sustained

## PEARLS AND PITFALLS
- Cervical spine injury is uncommon in nonjudicial hanging victims:
  - Cerebral hypoxia is the probable cause of death in the majority of victims.
- Aggressive airway management is paramount.
- Thoroughly evaluate for associated injuries.
- Consider admission for observation of all strangulation/hanging victims.
- Prognosis:
  - GCS on arrival dose not predict prognosis.
  - Poor prognosis is suggested by:
    - Anoxic brain injury on head CT
    - Increased hanging time
    - Cardiac arrest at the scene AND on arrival to the ED

## ADDITIONAL READING
- Iserson KV. Strangulation: A review of ligature, manual and postural neck compression injuries. *Ann Emerg Med.* 1984;13:179–185.
- Kaki A, Crosby ET, Lui AC. Airway and respiratory management following non-lethal hanging. *Can J Anesth.* 1997;44:445–450.
- Matsuyama T, Okuchi K, Seki T, et al. Prognostic factors in hanging injuries. *Am J Emerg Med.* 2004;3:207–210.
- McClane GE, Strack GB, Hawley D. A review of 300 attempted strangulation cases. Part II: Clinical evaluation of the surviving victim. *J Emerg Med.* 2001;21:311–315.
- Sabo RA, Hanigan WC, Flessner K, et al. Strangulation injuries in children. Part I: Clinical analysis. *J Trauma.* 1996;40:68–72.
- Salim A, Martin M, Sangthong B, et al. Near-hanging injuries: A 10-year experience. *Injury.* 2006;37:435–439.
- Wahlen BM, Thierbach AR. Near-hanging. *Eur J Emerg Med.* 2002;9:348–350.
- White H, Cook D, Venkatesh B. The use of hypertonic saline for treating intracranial HTN after traumatic brain injury. *Anesth Analg.* 2006;6:1836–1846.

 CODES

### ICD9
- 959.09 Other and unspecified injury to face and neck
- 994.7 Asphyxiation and strangulation

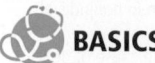 **BASICS**

## DESCRIPTION
- Blunt anterior neck trauma may result in various injuries to structures in the neck:
  - Vascular:
    - Carotid artery injury (internal, external, common carotid)
    - Vertebral artery injury
    - Intramural hematoma, intimal tear, thrombosis, and pseudoaneurysm
    - Hemorrhage or neck hematoma
  - Laryngotracheal:
    - Laryngeal Injuries: Fracture of hyoid bone, thyroid cartilage, cricoid cartilage, cricotracheal separation
    - Vocal cord disruption
    - Dislocation of arytenoid cartilage
    - Tracheal injuries: Hematoma or transection
  - Pharyngoesophageal:
    - Pharynx: Hematoma, perforation
    - Esophagus: Hematoma, perforation
  - Nervous system:
    - Thoracic sympathetic chain wraps around carotid artery: Disruption can result in Horner syndrome
    - Vagus nerve and recurrent laryngeal nerve
    - Cervical nerve roots and spinal cord
  - Cervical spine:
    - Fracture of vertebral body, Transverse process, spinous process, etc.
    - Dislocation

## ETIOLOGY
- Motor vehicle accidents (Most common cause):
  - Unrestrained occupants involved in frontal collisions may strike neck on dashboard or steering wheel: "padded dash syndrome"
  - Shoulder harness (seatbelt) can also cause shearing injury to anterior neck.
- Assault: Blows to anterior neck from fists, kicks, or objects
- "Clothesline injury":
  - Motorcycle, snowmobile, jet ski, or all-terrain vehicle (ATV)
  - Drivers strike neck on cord or wire suspended between two objects.
- Strangulation:

### Pediatric Considerations
- Head is proportionally larger in children, increasing risk of acceleration-deceleration injury to neck
- Intraoral blow to soft palate may cause carotid thrombosis (popsicle in mouth of child who falls, pushing the object into soft palate).

## DIAGNOSIS

### SIGNS AND SYMPTOMS
- Presentation varies depending on mechanism of injury and structures involved:
  - Vascular injury:
    - Hemorrhage, ecchymosis, edema
    - Carotid bruit or thrill (pathognomic for vascular injury)
    - Neurologic deficits (often delayed)
  - Laryngotracheal injury:
    - Voice changes, hoarseness, aphonia
    - Dyspnea, inspiratory stridor, labored breathing, "air hunger"
    - Subcutaneous emphysema, tenderness to palpation
  - Pharyngoesophageal injury (rarely isolated):
    - Dysphagia, odynophagia, hematemesis, blood in saliva
    - Tenderness to palpation
    - Infection, sepsis (delayed presentation)
  - Neurologic injury:
    - Central or peripheral nervous system deficits

### History
- Detailed history (if patient is able to provide) based on signs and symptoms:
  - Cover all structures of the neck, as well as structures outside the neck (neck trauma usually associated with injures to chest, head, etc.)

### Physical Exam
- Ensure airway protection and patency.
- Inspect neck for hemorrhage, hematoma, ecchymosis, edema, or distortion of anatomy.
- Auscultate for carotid bruits, stridor.
- Palpate to detect tenderness or subcutaneous emphysema.
- Neurologic exam to detect evidence of ischemic event, spinal cord injury, or peripheral nerve damage
- Complete physical exam to detect associated injuries to the chest, abdomen, etc.

### ESSENTIAL WORKUP
Depends on history and physical exam findings

### DIAGNOSTIC TESTS & INTERPRETATION
#### Lab
- Type and cross-match
- Baseline CBC
- BUN/creatinine may be needed prior to radiologic testing (contrast with CT or MRI)

### Imaging
- Cervical spine and lateral neck radiographs
- Limited value but may show subglottic narrowing, prevertebral soft tissue swelling, subcutaneous air, fractured calcified larynx
- CXR to rule out associated injury to thorax (pneumothorax, pneumomediastinum, etc.)
- Carotid duplex US is noninvasive, rapid screening test for arterial injury:
  - Sensitivity as high as 92% in retrospective studies for dissection, operator-dependent, poor visualization above carotid bifurcation
- CT may be used in stable patients to evaluate laryngotracheal injury, cartilage disruption, or cervical spine injury.
- CT angiography:
  - Low sensitivity (50%) and high specificity (99%) on initial studies with early-generation CT scanner compared with angiography for carotid and vertebral artery injury, may have improved rates of detection with newer generation CT scanners
- Magnetic resonance arteriography (MRA):
  - Low sensitivity (49%) and high specificity (99%) on initial studies with MRA compared with angiography for carotid and vertebral artery injury
  - 4-vessel angiography is considered gold standard for evaluation of arterial injury.
- Indications for angiography:
  - Presence of carotid bruit
  - Expanding neck hematoma
  - Neurologic deficit without Intracranial pathology on CT
  - Horner syndrome
  - Decreased level of consciousness

### Diagnostic Procedures/Surgery
- Unstable patients must go directly to surgery.
- Laryngotracheal injuries:
  - Fiberoptic laryngoscopy can visualize subglottic airway, facilitate intubation, assess airway patency and injury.
- Esophageal injuries:
  - Initial study of choice: Gastrografin swallow study (less pleural irritation with extravasation) or barium swallow study
- Indications for endoscopy:
  - Odynophagia
  - Hematemesis or blood in saliva
  - Subcutaneous emphysema

### DIFFERENTIAL DIAGNOSIS
- Peripheral or central nervous system injury
- Cervical spine injury
- Associated head or thoracic trauma

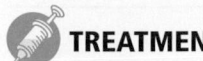 **TREATMENT**

### PRE-HOSPITAL
- Airway must be vigilantly monitored:
  - Edema or expanding hematoma can progress to airway compromise.
- Orotracheal intubation preferred 1st-line technique for airway control
- Clinical signs of respiratory distress:
  - Stridor
  - Air hunger
  - Labored breathing
  - Expanding neck hematoma
- Blind nasotracheal intubation should be avoided:
  - Owing to anatomy distortion and risk of hematoma rupture
- Cervical spine must be stabilized.

### INITIAL STABILIZATION/THERAPY
Airway management with cervical spine control:
- Immediate intubation indicated for patients with signs of airway compromise or impending compromise
- Cricothyroidotomy or emergent tracheostomy may be needed if oral intubation is unsuccessful.
- Contraindicated if bruising or hematoma noted over thyroid/cricoid cartilage
- Bleeding into pharynx can be reduced by packing throat with heavy gauze after airway is secured by intubation.
- Unstable patients must go directly to OR.

### ED TREATMENT/PROCEDURES
- Surgical consultation should be obtained for patients with suspicion of vascular, tracheal, or esophageal injury.
- Immediate surgical repair is required for symptomatic vascular injury, tracheal injury, pharyngeal or esophageal injury.

- Laryngeal injury may not require immediate surgical repair.
- Anticoagulation is recommended for vascular injuries due to consequent luminal narrowing and thrombosis:
  - Results in improved neurological outcomes
  - Requires surgical consultation prior to initiation of therapy

### MEDICATION
- Anticoagulation (see above)
- Prophylactic antibiotics recommended in presence of an esophageal injury to prevent abscess formation (anaerobic coverage):
  - Cefoxitin: 2 g (peds: 80–160 mg/kg/d div. q6h) IV q8h or
  - Clindamycin: 600–900 mg (peds: 25–40 mg/kg/d div. q6–8h) IV q8h or
    Penicillin G: 24 mIU/d (peds: 150,000–250,000 IU/kg/d div. q4–6h) IV div. q4–6h plus
  - Metronidazole: 1 g load, then 500 mg (peds: 30 mg/kg/d div. q12h) IV q6h

 **FOLLOW-UP**

### DISPOSITION
#### Admission Criteria
- Patients who are symptomatic, have abnormal studies, or have significant blunt trauma mechanism must be admitted and observed for at least 24 hours.
- Patients with suspicion of airway or vascular injury must be admitted to ICU.

> **ALERT**
> Patients on anticoagulation medications should be observed in ED for 6 hours from injury to look for signs of delayed neck hematoma.

#### Discharge Criteria
Only patients with most trivial injuries who have negative studies may be discharged from ED after thorough evaluation.

### FOLLOW-UP RECOMMENDATIONS
Patients should be given return precautions to the ED for delayed signs of vascular, tracheal, neurologic injury.

## PEARLS AND PITFALLS
- Vascular injuries frequently have delayed presentation.
- Look for vascular injuries in blunt neck trauma patients with neurologic deficit and normal head CT.
- Always prepare for difficult airway and have specialty intervention (anesthesia, ENT) on standby (if available).

## ADDITIONAL READING
- Miller PR, Fabian TC, Bee TK, et al. Blunt cerebrovascular injuries: Diagnosis and treatment. *J Trauma*. 2001;279–286.
- Miller PR, Fabian TC, Croce MA, et al. Prospective screening for blunt cerebrovascular injuries: Analysis of diagnostic modalities and outcomes. *Ann Surg*. 2002;236(3):386–393.
- Rathlev NK, Medzon R. Evaluation and management of neck trauma. *Emerg Med Clin North Am*. 2007;679–694.
- Ullman E. Blunt neck trauma. In Wolfson AB, et al., eds., *Harwood-Nuss' clinical practice of emergency medicine*. Philadelphia: Lippincott Williams & Wilkins, 2005.

 **CODES**

### ICD9
959.09 Other and unspecified injury to face and neck

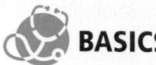

## BASICS

### DESCRIPTION
- Wound severity gauged by violation of platysma muscle
- Neck is divided into 3 zones:
  - Zone I: Between clavicles and cricoid cartilage:
    - Involves vessels, lungs, trachea, esophagus, thyroid
    - Penetrating trauma in this zone carries highest mortality owing to injury to thoracic structures.
  - Zone II: Between cricoid cartilage and angle of mandible:
    - Involves vessels, trachea, esophagus, C-spine, and spinal cord.
    - Injuries are most common in this zone because it is the most exposed region.
  - Zone III lies above the angle of the mandible to base of skull:
    - Injuries are difficult to access surgically.

*Pediatric Considerations*
Larynx is located higher in neck and receives better protection from mandible and hyoid bone.

### ETIOLOGY
- Gunshot wounds
- Stab wounds
- Miscellaneous (eg, glass shards, metal fragments, animal bites)

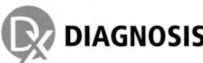

## DIAGNOSIS

### SIGNS AND SYMPTOMS
- Vascular:
  - Active/persistent hemorrhage or hematoma
  - Pulse deficit
  - Horner syndrome (carotid injury)
  - Vascular bruit or thrill
  - Venous air embolism
- Aerodigestive:
  - Respiratory distress
  - Stridor
  - Hemoptysis
  - Tracheal deviation
  - Subcutaneous emphysema
  - Pneumothorax
  - Sucking wound
  - Hoarseness, aphonia, dysphonia
  - Dysphagia/odynophagia
- Neurologic:
  - Deficits of CNS or PNS

### History
- Wounds across midline increase injury significance
- Stab wound:
  - Size of instrument
  - Mostly low-energy penetration
- Gunshot wound:
  - Type of gun used
  - Long range vs close range

### Physical Exam
- Careful examination of wound to determine extent of injury and whether it penetrates the platysma
- Wounds should never be probed blindly:
  - May result in uncontrolled hemorrhage

### ESSENTIAL WORKUP
Platysma violation
- No: Wound care, discharge
- Yes:
  - Unstable: Emergent airway, OR
  - Stable: Workup depends on zone violation

### DIAGNOSTIC TESTS & INTERPRETATION
#### Lab
- Type and cross-match
- Baseline CBC, chem panel, coags

#### Imaging
- Lateral neck radiograph to evaluate soft tissue injury and detect foreign bodies
- Chest radiograph to detect hemopneumothorax, mediastinal air
- Zone I:
  - Angiography: Gold standard to evaluate vessel injury, invasive
  - Helical CT angiography: speed, noninvasive
    - Aware of streak artifact from shoulder, poor view of subclavian vessels
  - Esophagram with water-soluble contrast or dilute barium:
    - Low sensitivity
    - Combine with esophagoscopy to exclude injury.
    - Indications: Wound approaches/crosses midline, SC air
- Zone II:
  - Asymptomatic: observation
  - Symptomatic: OR
- Zone III:
  - Symptomatic: Angiography or CT angiogram

### Diagnostic Procedures/Surgery
- Bronchoscopy can be helpful in evaluating tracheal injury.
- Surgical consult for all wounds that penetrate the platysma muscle:
  - Surgical exploration:
    - Expanding or pulsatile hematoma
    - Active bleeding
    - Absence of peripheral pulses
    - Hemoptysis
    - Horner syndrome
    - Bruit
    - Subcutaneous emphysema
    - Respiratory distress
    - Air bubbling through wound

### DIFFERENTIAL DIAGNOSIS
- Peripheral or CNS injury
- Cervical spine injury
- Associated head or thoracic trauma

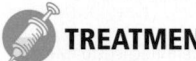

## TREATMENT

### PRE-HOSPITAL
- Frequent suctioning to clear airway of blood, secretions, or vomitus
- 2 large-bore IVs
- High-flow $O_2$ should be provided
- Bag-valve-mask should be avoided for potential distortion of neck anatomy and airway compromise due to forced air through tracheolaryngeal wound into tissues
- Airway must be vigilantly monitored, as edema or expanding hematoma can progress to airway compromise.
- Indications for early oral intubation:
  - Clinical signs of respiratory distress
  - Stridor
  - Air hunger
  - Labored breathing
  - Expanding neck hematoma

- Nasotracheal intubation has not been shown to worsen penetrating wounds.

### ALERT

- Occlusive dressings should be applied to lacerations over major veins to prevent air embolism.
- Cervical spine immobilization in the absence of focal neurologic deficits is not indicated:
  - Blocks direct visualization/palpation of neck; increases likelihood of missing life-threatening signs

### INITIAL STABILIZATION/THERAPY

- Emergent intubation is indicated:
  - Patients who are in respiratory distress or comatose.
  - Be aware of voice change or odynophagia.
  - Patients who are stable without evidence of respiratory distress may be managed aggressively with prophylactic intubation or observed closely with airway equipment at bedside.
  - Orotracheal intubation with rapid-sequence induction is method of choice for securing airway in penetrating neck trauma.
  - Blind nasotracheal intubation is contraindicated with apnea, severe facial injury, or airway distortion.
  - Fiberoptic bronchoscopic intubation is advantageous as patient may stay awake; allows direct visualization of vocal cords and injuries.
  - Percutaneous transtracheal ventilation may be useful when oral or nasotracheal intubation fails:
    ○ This is contraindicated in cases of upper airway obstruction.
    ○ May cause barotrauma
    Cricothyroidotomy contraindicated if significant hematoma overlying cricothyroid membrane
    ○ Tracheostomy is warranted in this setting
    Breathing:
  - Zone I injury can cause pneumothorax or subclavian vein injury and hemothorax:
    ○ May require needle decompression and tube thoracostomy

- Circulation:
  - External hemorrhage:
    ○ Control with direct pressure.
    ○ If failed, insert and inflate Foley catheter balloon within wound to tamponade bleeding
    ○ Blind clamping of vessels is contraindicated owing to risk of further neurovascular injury.
  - Uncontrolled bleeding or hemodynamic instability: Send directly to OR.
  - After intubation, throat can be packed with heavy gauze to tamponade bleeding.
  - Hemothorax: tube thoracostomy

### ED TREATMENT/PROCEDURES

- Nasogastric tube should *not* be placed because of risk of rupturing pharyngeal hematoma.
- Prophylactic antibiotics are recommended (cefoxitin, clindamycin, penicillin G plus metronidazole).
- Tetanus prophylaxis

### MEDICATION

- Cefoxitin: 2 g (peds: 80–160 mg/kg/day div q6h) IV q8h *or*
- Clindamycin: 600–900 mg (peds: 25–40 mg/kg/day div q6–8h) IV q8h *or*
- Penicillin G: 2.4 mIU (peds: 150,000–250,000 IU/kg/d div q4–6h) IV per day div q4–6h *plus*
- Metronidazole: 1 g load, then 500 mg (peds: 30 mg/kg/day div q12h) IV q6h

 FOLLOW-UP

### DISPOSITION

#### Admission Criteria

- All patients with penetrating neck trauma should be admitted and observed for at least 24 hr.
- Observation must take place in facility capable of providing definitive surgical care
- Patients with injuries suggesting airway or vascular injury must be admitted to ICU.

#### Discharge Criteria

- Asymptomatic patients who have negative studies may be discharged after 24 hr of observation.
- Patients with wounds superficial to the platysma may be discharged directly from the ED.

### PEARLS AND PITFALLS

- Failure to anticipate difficulties in airway management
- Failure to recognize impending airway compromise

### ADDITIONAL READING

- Wolfson A, et al. *Harwood-Nuss' Clinical Practice of Emergency Medicine*. Philadelphia: Lippincott Williams & Wilkins, 2005.
- Tisherman SA, Bokhari F, Collier B, et al. Clinical practice guideline: Penetrating zone II neck trauma. *J Trauma*. 2008;64(5):1392–1405.
- Ramasamy A, Midwinter M, Mahoney P, et al. Learning the lessons from conflict: Pre-hospital cervical spine stabilisation following ballistic neck trauma. *Injury*. 40(12):1342–1345.
- Munera F, Cohn S, Rivas LA. Penetrating injuries of the neck: Use of helical computed tomographic angiography. *J Trauma*. 2005;58(2):413–418.
- Woo K, Magner DP, Wilson MT, et al. CT angiography in penetrating neck trauma reduces the need for operative neck exploration. *Am Surg*. 2005;71(9):754–758.

 CODES

#### ICD9

- 874.00 Open wound of larynx with trachea, uncomplicated
- 874.01 Open wound of larynx, uncomplicated
- 874.8 Open wound of other and unspecified parts of neck, without mention of complication

N

# NECROTIZING SOFT TISSUE INFECTIONS

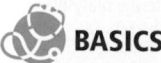

Adam Z. Barkin
Karen B. Van Hoesen

## BASICS

### DESCRIPTION
- Necrotizing soft-tissue infections (NSTI) are infections of any layer of the skin associated with necrotizing changes.
- Characterized by:
  - Widespread fascial and muscle necrosis with relative sparing of the skin
  - High mortality
  - Systemic toxicity
- Crepitant anaerobic cellulitis:
  - Necrotic soft-tissue infection with abundant connective tissue gas
- Progressive bacterial gangrene:
  - Slowly progressive erosion affecting the total thickness of skin but not involving deep fascia
- Nonclostridial myonecrosis (synergistic necrotizing cellulitis):
  - Aggressive soft-tissue infection of skin, muscle, subcutaneous tissue and fascia
- Fournier gangrene:
  - Mixed aerobic-anaerobic soft-tissue necrotizing fasciitis of the skin of the scrotum and penis in men and the vulvar and perianal skin in women
- *Necrotizing fasciitis:*
  - Progressive, rapidly spreading infection with extensive dissection and necrosis of the superficial and deep fascia
- Accounts for 500–1,500 cases per year in the U.S.
- Often difficult to recognize.
- 24–34% mortality
- Also high morbidity:
  - Amputations
  - Renal failure

### ETIOLOGY
- Conditions that lead to the development of necrotizing soft-tissue infections:
  - Local tissue trauma with bacterial invasion
  - Local ischemia and reduced host defenses:
    - More frequently in diabetics, alcoholics, immunosuppressed patients, IV drug users, and patients with peripheral vascular disease
- Type I NSTI:
  - Polymicrobial
  - Anaerobic and aerobic
  - After surgical procedures
  - Existing diabetes or peripheral vascular disease

- Type II NSTI:
  - Monomicrobial
  - Typically anaerobic *Streptococcus*
  - Can occur in any patient
- Bacteria involved include:
  - Group A $\beta$2-hemolytic streptococcus (GABHS)
  - Group B streptococcus
  - Staphylococc*i*
  - Enterococci
  - *Bacillus*
  - *Pseudomonas*
  - *E. coli*
  - *Proteus*
  - *Klebsiella*
  - *Enterobacter*
  - *Bacteroides*
  - *Pasteurella multocida*
  - *Clostridium* sp.
  - *Vibrio* sp.
  - Fungi
- Possible relationship between the use of NSAIDs and severe invasive GABHS infections has been suggested.

### Pediatric Considerations
- Neonates: Omphalitis and circumcision are predisposing factors.
- Children: Surgery, trauma, varicella, and congenital and acquired immunodeficiencies are major factors for the development of necrotizing fasciitis.
- GABHS necrotizing fasciitis as a complication of varicella has been reported

## DIAGNOSIS

### SIGNS AND SYMPTOMS
#### History
- Fever
- Altered mental status
- Chronic medical conditions
- IV drug use
- Skin:
  - Rapid progression of pain and swelling of involved area
  - In 1st 24 hr, rapid development of local swelling, heat, erythema, and tenderness
  - 24–48 hr: Purple and blue discoloration, blisters and bullae develop (often hemorrhagic)
  - Foul-smelling thin fluid (from necrosis of fat and fascia)

#### Physical Exam
- Systemic toxicity:
  - Fever
  - Tachycardia
  - Tachypnea
  - Hypotension
  - Altered mental status
- Pain out of proportion to physical findings
- Skin:
  - Erythema
  - Tense edema
  - Grayish or other discolored wound drainage
  - Vesicles or bullae
  - Necrosis
  - Ulcers
  - Crepitus (pathognomonic but present in only 10–37% of cases)
  - Pain that extends past margin of infection

### ESSENTIAL WORKUP
- Diagnosis can be difficult.
- Careful exam for the aforementioned signs and symptoms in high-risk patients
- Necrotizing soft-tissue infections must be suspected in patients who appear very ill and have pain out of proportion to physical findings.
- Diagnosis may require incision and probing of tissue.

### DIAGNOSTIC TESTS & INTERPRETATION
#### Lab
- CBC with differential
- Electrolytes:
  - WBC >15,400 cells/mm$^3$ and Na <135 mmol/L are associated with NSTI; combination of both increases the likelihood:
    - This data has a high negative predictive value (99%), but a low positive predictive value (26%)
- BUN and creatinine
- Disseminated intravascular coagulation panel
- Calcium level: Hypocalcemia can develop from extensive fat necrosis.
- Parameters to assess risk of mortality:
  - Age >50 (3 points)
  - WBC >40,000 cells/mm$^3$ (3 points)
  - Hematocrit >50% (3 points)
  - Heart rate >110 bpm (1 point)
  - Temperature >36°C (1 point)
  - Creatinine >1.5 mg/dL (1 point)
    - 6% mortality if 0–2 points
    - 24% mortality if 3–5 points
    - 88% mortality if >6 points
- Gram stain and aerobic/anaerobic cultures of wound or tissue biopsy

## Imaging

- X-rays to detect soft-tissue gas: Pathognomonic, but present in only 39–57% of cases
- CT scan:
  - May be more helpful than plain x-rays in detecting subcutaneous air
  - May also identify deep abscess or other cause of infection
- MRI:
  - Can delineate extent of spread of the infection
- US:
  - Fascial thickening
  - Fluid in the fascial plane
  - Subcutaneous soft-tissue edema

### ALERT
Imaging of any kind should never delay surgical debridement.

## Diagnostic Procedures/Surgery

- All patients with suspected NSTI must undergo surgical debridement.
- Deep incisional biopsy and cultures are the gold standard for diagnosis.

## DIFFERENTIAL DIAGNOSIS

- Cellulitis
- Gas gangrene

 **TREATMENT**

### PRE-HOSPITAL
- IV fluid resuscitation
- Manage airway as necessary.

### INITIAL STABILIZATION/THERAPY
Manage airway and resuscitate as indicated:
- Rapid-sequence intubation as needed
- Supplemental oxygen, monitor, evaluate for acid–base disturbances
- IV access, CVP line may be needed
- Aggressive volume expansion including crystalloid, plasma, packed RBCs, and albumin

### ED TREATMENT/PROCEDURES
- Antibiotics: Broad coverage of aerobic gram positive and gram-negative organisms and anaerobes:
- Acceptable combination therapy:
  - Penicillin or cephalosporin *PLUS* an aminoglycoside or fluoroquinolone *PLUS* anaerobic coverage with either clindamycin or metronidazole
- Acceptable monotherapy:
  - Imipenem cilastatin
  - Meropenem
  - Piperacillin/tazobactam
  - Tigecycline
- Penicillin G if strep or clostridium

- Treat methicillin-resistant staphylococcal aureus (MRSA) until excluded:
  - Vancomycin
  - Linezolid
  - Daptomycin
- Surgical consultation:
  - Early debridement of all necrotic tissue with fasciotomy and drainage of fascial planes is paramount.
- Hyperbaric oxygen as an adjunct:
  - Early transfer to hyperbaric facility may result in greater tissue salvage.
- IV immunoglobulin (IVIG):
  - Controversial
  - May be beneficial in NSTI caused by group A streptococcal infection
- Observe for major complications including acute respiratory distress syndrome, renal failure, myocardial irritability, and DIC.

### ALERT
Clindamycin therapy should be initiated as soon as possible when group A strep infection is suspected.

### MEDICATION
- Ceftriaxone: 2 g (peds: 100 mg/kg/24h; max. 4 g) IV q24h
- Clindamycin: 900 mg (peds: 40 mg/kg/d q6h) IV q8h
- Daptomycin: 4 mg/kg IV q24h
- Gentamicin: 2 mg/kg (peds: 2 mg/kg IV q8h) IV q8h
- Imipenem/cilastatin: 250–1,000 mg IV q6–8h
- Levofloxacin: 750 mg IV q24h
- Linezolid: 600 mg PO/IV q12h (peds: 30 mg/kg/d PO/IV divided q8h)
- Meropenem 1 g (peds: 20–40 mg/kg up to 2 g/dose) IV q8h
- Metronidazole: 500 mg (peds: Safety not established) IV q8h
- Penicillin G: 24 mIU/24 h (peds: 250,000 IU/kg/24 h) IV q4–6h
- Piperacillin/tazobactam 3.375–4.5 g (peds: 240 mg/kg/d of piperacillin divided q8h) IV q6h
- Tigecycline: Start 100 mg IV x 1; 50 mg IV q12h
- Vancomycin: 10–15 mg/kg IV q12h (peds: 10–15 mg/kg IV q6–8h)

 **FOLLOW-UP**

### DISPOSITION
#### Admission Criteria
- All patients with a NSTI *must be admitted* for surgical debridement and IV antibiotics.
- Early hyperbaric oxygen therapy may be an important adjunct.

#### Discharge Criteria
No patient with NSTI should be discharged.

#### Issues for Referral
After stabilization with antibiotics and surgical debridement, consider referral for hyperbaric oxygen treatment as an adjunct.

## PEARLS AND PITFALLS

- The clinician must have a high index of suspicion for NSTI, as initial skin findings may be unimpressive.
- Pain out of proportion to exam may be a key finding.
- Mortality will be near 100% if treatment is ONLY with antimicrobials.
- Early and complete debridement is essential.

## ADDITIONAL READING

- Anaya DA, Bulger EM, Kwon YS, et al. Predicting death in necrotizing soft tissue infections: A clinical score. *Surg Infect.* 2009;10;517–522.
- Anaya DA, Dellinger EP. Necrotizing soft-tissue infection: Diagnosis and management. *Clin Infect Dis.* 2007;44:705–710.
- Cainzos M, Gonzalez-Rodriguez FJ. Necrotizing soft tissue infections. *Curr Opin Crit Care.* 2007;13:433–439.
- Ramirez-Schrempp D, Dorfman DH, Baker WE, et al. Ultrasound soft tissue applications in the pediatric emergency department: To drain or not to drain? *Pediatr Emer Care.* 2009;25:44–48.
- Rogers RL, Perkins J. Skin and soft tissue infections. *Prim Care Clin Office Pract.* 2006;33:697–710.
- Wilkinson D, Doolette D. Hyperbaric oxygen treatment and survival from necrotizing soft tissue infection. *Arch Surg.* 2004;139:1339–1345.

### See Also (Topic, Algorithm, Electronic Media Element)
- Cellulitis
- Erysipelas
- MRSA, Community Acquired
- Gangrene

 **CODES**

### ICD9
- 686.9 Unspecified local infection of skin and subcutaneous tissue
- 709.8 Other specified disorders of skin

N

# NECROTIZING ULCERATIVE GINGIVITIS

Stephen K. Epstein
Laura B. Glicksman

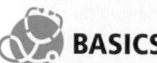 **BASICS**

## DESCRIPTION
- Periodontal disease
- Characterized by the "punched-out" appearance of the gingival papillae
- Synonym(s):
  - Acute necrotizing ulcerative gingivitis
  - Trench mouth
  - Vincent disease
  - Fusospirochetal gingivitis
- Not contagious
- Occurs most often in children and young adults in developing nations.
- Mainly occurs in sub-Saharan Africa
- Rare; seen mostly in severely immunocompromised patients
- Males > females
- Can progress to more advanced disease:
  - Necrotizing stomatitis:
    ○ Similar to necrotizing ulcerative gingivitis with extension to the tongue and buccal mucosa
  - Necrotizing ulcerative periodontitis:
    ○ Similar to necrotizing ulcerative gingivitis with periodontal attachment loss and alveolar bone involvement
  - Orofacial gangrene (noma)

## ETIOLOGY
- Caused by an overgrowth of oral flora
- *Prevotella intermedia*
- Spirochetes
- Predisposing factors (not required for diagnosis):
  - Poor oral hygiene/gingivitis
  - Immunodeficiencies (eg, HIV)
  - Immunosuppression
  - Malnutrition
  - Smoking
  - Emotional and physical stress

## DIAGNOSIS

### SIGNS AND SYMPTOMS
- Essential clinical features:
  - Painful gingival lesions
  - "Punched-out," crater-like ulcers of the papillae
  - Ulcers bleed easily or spontaneously
- Nonessential clinical features:
  - "Pseudomembrane" of necrotic debris covering the ulcerated area
  - Foul breath
  - Fever/malaise

### History
- Acute, generalized oral pain
- Bleeding gums:
  - Spontaneous or with minimal manipulation
- Foul breath
- Malaise
- Low-grade fever

### Physical Exam
- Loss of interdental papillae (key clinical feature)
- "Punched-out," crater-like ulcers of the papillae
- Necrotic debris often present over ulcerated surfaces
- "Pseudomembrane" of inflammatory and necrotic cells
- Covers ulcerative lesions
- Leaves a bleeding surface when removed
- Lymphadenopathy, particularly submandibular
- Foul breath
- Low-grade fever

## ESSENTIAL WORKUP
- Consider systemic disease:
  - Neutropenia
  - HIV
- Other reasons for immunosuppression or immunocompromise
- Rule out complications:
  - Progression to necrotizing stomatitis or ulcerative periodontitis
  - Lesions extending to periodontal ligament and alveolar bone
  - Alveolar bone destruction
  - Progression to orofacial gangrene (noma)

## DIAGNOSTIC TESTS & INTERPRETATION
### Lab
Laboratory tests not clinically helpful

### Imaging
Generally not indicated

## DIFFERENTIAL DIAGNOSIS
- Other diseases rarely have the essential clinical feature of "punched-out" interdental papillae with ulcerations
- Infectious diseases:
  - Acute herpetic gingivostomatitis:
    ○ Affects entire gingival, not just papillae
    ○ Low-grade fever commonly present
    ○ Contagious

- Viral:
  - Viral infections: Epstein-Barr, varicella zoster virus
  - Thrush
  - Actinomycosis
  - Streptococcal/gonococcal gingivitis/stomatitis
  - Secondary syphilis
  - Diphtheria
  - Vesiculobullous disease
  - Pemphigoid
  - Pemphigus
  - Oral lichen planus
  - Systemic lupus erythematosus
- Trauma:
  - Toothpicks
  - Vigorous tooth brushing/flossing
- Immunocompromise:
  - Leukemia
  - Agranulocytosis (malignant neutropenia)
  - HIV

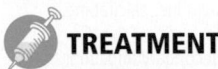 **TREATMENT**

### INITIAL STABILIZATION/THERAPY
IV fluids for dehydration

### ED TREATMENT/PROCEDURES
- Administer systemic and topical pain management:
  - Narcotics rarely necessary
  - Viscous lidocaine
- Debride pseudomembrane:
  Use gauze or cotton-tip applicator soaked in diluted H$_2$O$_2$.
- Antibiotics (penicillin/metronidazole or clindamycin) when indicated:
  - Fever
  - Lymphadenopathy
  - Consider broad-spectrum antibiotics, antifungals, and antivirals in the immunosuppressed patient

- Institute outpatient therapy:
  - Remove predisposing factors.
  - Dilute hydrogen peroxide rinses.
  - Chlorhexidine gluconate (Peridex)
  - Antibiotics if indicated
  - Avoid irritants (spicy foods, hot beverages).
  - Analgesics for pain control
  - Improve oral hygiene with daily brushing and flossing of teeth.

### MEDICATION
#### First Line
- Oral rinses:
  - Chlorhexidine gluconate (Peridex): 15 mL swish/spit b.i.d.
  - Hydrogen peroxide (3% solution diluted in half): rinse up to 12 times daily
- Viscous lidocaine
- NSAIDs:
  - Ibuprofen, acetaminophen

#### Second Line
- Metronidazole: 250–750 mg (peds: 30 mg/kg/ 24 hr) PO q.i.d. × 7 days
- Penicillin VK: 500 mg (peds: <12 yr, 25–50 mg/kg/24 hr) PO q.i.d. × 10 days
- Clindamycin: 300 mg PO (peds: 6–8 mg/kg/24 hr) t.i.d.
- Narcotic pain control

 **FOLLOW-UP**

### DISPOSITION
#### Admission Criteria
- Extensive disease with systemic signs
- Severe dehydration/inability to tolerate PO fluids
- Evidence of orofacial gangrene (noma): infection of mouth/face:
  - 70% mortality with no treatment

#### Discharge Criteria
Able to maintain hydration

### FOLLOW-UP RECOMMENDATIONS
Urgent referral to a dentist or periodontist for deep scaling and debridement

## PEARLS AND PITFALLS
- Consider HIV or immunosuppression.
- If untreated, can progress rapidly.

## ADDITIONAL READING
- American Academy of Periodontology. Parameter on acute periodontal diseases. *J Periodontol.* 2000;71 (5 suppl):863–866.
- American Academy of Periodontology. Periodontal diseases of children and adolescents. *J Periodontol.* 2003;74:1696–1704.
- Bermejo-Fenoll A, Sanchez-Perez A. Necrotising periodontal diseases. *Med Oral Patol Oral Cir Bucal.* 2004;9(suppl):S108–S119.
- Crystal CS, Coon TP, Kaylor DW. Images in emergency medicine. Acute necrotizing ulcerative gingivitis. *Ann Emerg Med.* 2006;47:225, 229.
- Dachs RJ, Tun Y. Painful oral ulcerations in a 51-year-old woman. *Am Fam Physician.* 2009;80: 875.
- Mintz L. Diagnosis and treatment of acute periodontal conditions. *Compend Contin Educ Dent.* 2006;27:8–11.
- Shiboski CH, Patton LL, Webster-Cyriaque JY, et al. The Oral HIV/AIDS Research Alliance: updated case definitions of oral disease endpoints. *J Oral Pathol Med.* 2009;38:481–488.

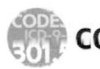 **CODES**

### ICD9
101 Vincent's angina

# NEEDLE STICK

*Gordon S. Chew*

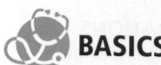 **BASICS**

## DESCRIPTION

- Mechanisms of exposure to blood or body fluid:
  - Percutaneous
  - Mucous membrane
  - Skin
- General prevention:
  - Universal precautions
  - Avoid recapping of needles
  - Wear gloves: Decreases amount of blood exposure by 50%
  - Double gloving
  - Follow body–substance isolation protocols.
  - Hepatitis B virus vaccination
- Risk factors:
  - Risk of seroconversion from a single needle-stick exposure without prior immunization:
    - Hepatitis B virus: 37–62% from HBsAg-positive and HBeAg-positive source, 23–37% from HBsAg-positive and HBeAg-negative source
    - Hepatitis C virus: 1.8%
    - HIV: Blood 0.3%, mucous membrane 0.09%
  - Infectiousness of various body fluids for HIV:
    - Plasma/serum: 10–5,000 ppm
    - Cerebrospinal fluid: 10–1,000 ppm
    - Semen: 10–50 ppm
    - Vaginal secretions, urine, saliva, tears, breast milk: <1 ppm
  - Factors affecting risk:
    - Viral load
    - Actual injection volume
    - Type and size of needle
    - Portal of entry (depth of inoculation)
    - Duration of contact
    - Level of disease in source patient
    - Host susceptibility
    - Barriers (eg, through gloves)

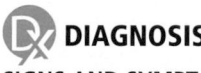 **DIAGNOSIS**

## SIGNS AND SYMPTOMS

### History

Exposure to blood or body fluid:

- Date, time, circumstances, details of exposure, source
- Immunizations

## DIAGNOSTIC TESTS & INTERPRETATION

Women with body-fluid exposure who are considering antiviral therapy must have serum or urine pregnancy testing.

### Lab

To be done with occupational health if possible:

- Baseline serology for HIV (enzyme immunoassay, Western blot), hepatitis B virus, hepatitis C virus (anti-HCV), ALT
- Assess adequacy of hepatitis B virus vaccination.
- Obtain consent from source patient for HIV (consider rapid HIV-antibody test), hepatitis B virus, hepatitis C virus (anti-HCV) testing.

### Imaging

Not applicable unless concerned for retained tissue foreign body

## DIFFERENTIAL DIAGNOSIS

Principally concerned with transmission of hepatitis B virus, hepatitis C virus, and HIV

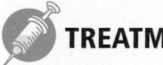 **TREATMENT**

## PRE-HOSPITAL

### ALERT

- Prehospital personnel should always maintain universal precautions to prevent needlestick or other body fluid exposure.
- Patients with exposure should be evaluated within hours for prophylactic therapy.

## INITIAL STABILIZATION/THERAPY

- Copious cleaning, wound care
- Direct and immediate referral to occupational health, when available, to ensure strictest confidentiality in laboratory testing and treatment
- In the ED, after hours, patients with needlestick exposure must be triaged with high priority. It is important to initiate prophylactic therapy quickly after exposure.

## ED TREATMENT/PROCEDURES

- If referral to occupational health is unavailable, initiate prophylactic therapy in ED.
- Tetanus prophylaxis if necessary
- HIV:
  - Begin basic vs. expanded antiretroviral prophylaxis regimen after considering HIV status of source and severity of exposure. Some organizations advocate only the expanded 3-drug regimen. Treat for 28 days.
  - CDC guidelines: For less severe percutaneous exposure, if source patient is:
    - HIV negative: No prophylaxis
    - Unknown source: Consider basic regimen
    - Patient with risk factors: Consider basic regimen
    - HIV positive, low viral load: Recommend basic regimen
    - HIV positive, high viral load: Recommend expanded regimen ≥3 drugs
  - CDC guidelines: For more severe percutaneous exposure, if source patient is:
    - HIV negative: No prophylaxis
    - Unknown source: Consider basic regimen
    - Patient with risk factors: Consider basic regimen
    - HIV positive, low viral load: Recommend expanded regimen 3 drugs
    - HIV positive, high viral load: Recommend expanded regimen ≥3 drugs
  - CDC preferred basic regimen:
    - Zidovudine (AZT) plus lamivudine (3TC); sold as combination drug Combivir; or
    - Zidovudine (AZT) plus emtricitabine (FTC); or
    - Lamivudine (3TC) plus tenofovir DF (TDF); or
    - Tenofovir DF (TDF) plus emtricitabine (FTC);

- CDC alternative basic regimen:
  - Lamivudine (3TC) plus stavudine (d4T); or
  - Emtricitabine (FTC) plus stavudine (d4T) or
  - Lamivudine (3TC) plus didanosine (ddI) or
  - Emtricitabine (FTC) plus didanosine (ddI)
- CDC preferred expanded regimen: Basic regimen and:
  - Lopinavir/ritonavir (Kaletra®)
- CDC alternative expanded regimen: Basic regimen and:
  - Atazanavir (ATV) + ritonavir (RTV) or
  - Fosamprenavir + ritonavir (RTV) or
  - Indinavir (IDV) + ritonavir (RTV) or
  - Saquinavir (SQV) plus ritonavir (RTV) or
  - Nelfinavir or
  - Efavirenz or
  - Consider others after expert consultation: These include abacavir, delavirdine, zalcitabine, nevirapine, enfuvirtide.
- Counseling to prevent secondary infection:
  - Safer sex advice
  - Avoid becoming pregnant
  - Do not donate blood/tissue.
  - Do not breast-feed.
- Hepatitis B virus:
  - Known HBsAg-positive source:
    - Complete vaccination confirmed by titer: No prescription
    - Incomplete vaccination: Hepatitis B virus vaccine booster
    - Unvaccinated: Hepatitis B immune globulin asap, begin hepatitis B virus vaccine series.
    - Nonresponder to vaccine: Hepatitis B immune globulin ASAP, may repeat in 30 days; consider revaccination with 3-dose series.
    - Unknown responder to vaccine with inadequate titer: Hepatitis B immune globulin asap, vaccine booster
  - Known HBsAg-negative source:
    - Vaccinated: No prescription
    - Unvaccinated: Begin hepatitis B virus vaccine series
  - Unknown source:
    - Complete vaccination confirmed by titer: No prescription
    - Incomplete vaccination: Hepatitis B virus vaccine booster
    - Unvaccinated: Begin vaccine series.
    - Nonresponder to vaccine: Hepatitis B immune globulin asap with revaccination 3-dose series, repeat hepatitis B immune globulin in 30 days if high-risk exposure.
    - Unknown responder to vaccine with inadequate titer: Vaccine booster and recheck titer in 1–2 months
  - Hepatitis C virus:
    - Use of immunoglobulins or antivirals (interferon, ribavirin) inconclusive as prophylaxis, but possibly beneficial if initiated early when infection evident

## MEDICATION

- HIV:
  - Zidovudine:
    - 300 mg PO b.i.d. or 200 mg PO t.i.d.
    - Side effects: GI symptoms, headache, fatigue, myalgias, marrow suppression, seizure
  - Lamivudine:
    - 300 mg PO q.d. or 150 mg PO b.i.d.
    - Side effects: GI symptoms, headache, fatigue, neuropathy, congestion, cough (caution with trimethoprim/sulfamethoxazole)
  - Combivir (combination zidovudine plus lamivudine) (300 mg + 150 mg tab):
    - 1 tablet PO b.i.d.
    - Side effects: See side effect profiles of zidovudine and lamivudine
  - Emtricitabine:
    - 200 mg/d PO
    - Side effects: Rash, hyperpigmentation
  - Tenofovir DF:
    - 300 mg/d PO
    - Side effects: GI symptoms, headache, fatigue, neuropathy, dizziness
  - Didanosine:
    - 400 mg/d PO or 200 mg PO b.i.d.; or
    - If wt <60 kg, then 200 mg/d PO or 125 mg PO b.i.d.
    - Side effects: Pancreatitis, GI symptoms, lactic acidosis, neuropathy
  - Stavudine:
    - 40 mg PO b.i.d.; or
    - If wt <60 kg, then 30 mg PO b.i.d.
    - Side effects: Peripheral neuropathy, GI symptoms, headache, pancreatitis, elevated liver function tests, neutropenia, anemia
  - Lopinavir/ritonavir (Kaletra®) (200 mg + 50 mg cap):
    - 2 capsules PO b.i.d
    - Side effects: GI symptoms, hyperlipidemia

- Atazanavir:
  - 400 mg/d PO
  - If used with tenofovir, then decrease to 300 mg/d PO and add ritonavir 100 mg/d PO
  - Side effects: Be wary with medications that prolong PR interval, hyperbilirubinemia
- Fosamprenavir:
  - 1,400 mg PO b.i.d
  - If used with ritonavir, then decrease to 1,400 mg/d PO or 700 mg PO b.i.d.
  - Side effects: GI symptoms, rash, drug interactions, depression
- Ritonavir:
  - 200 mg/d PO or 100 mg PO b.i.d.
  - Side effects: GI symptoms, rash, drug interactions
- Indinavir:
  - 800 mg PO q8h
  - If used with ritonavir, then decrease to 800 mg PO b.i.d.
  - Side effects: Nephrolithiasis, hyperbilirubinemia, GI symptoms
- Saquinavir:
  - 1000 mg PO b.i.d.
  - Side effects: GI symptoms, hepatitis
- Nelfinavir:
  - 1,250 mg PO b.i.d.
  - Side effects: Potential carcinogenic and teratogenic warning, GI symptoms, weakness, rash
- Efavirenz:
  - 600 mg PO at bedtime
  - Side effects: Stevens-Johnson syndrome, rash, sleep disruption, dizziness, psychiatric, teratogen
- For some of the antiretroviral agents, the oncogenic and teratogenic effects are unknown.
- NRTIs and NtRTIs can result in lactic acidosis with hepatic steatosis.
- All can have serious drug interactions that lead to significant harm or death.

- Hepatitis B:
  - Hepatitis B immune globulin: 0.06 mL/kg IM
  - Hepatitis B virus booster: Unit-dose vial

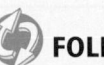

## FOLLOW-UP

**DISPOSITION**

***Admission Criteria***
Admission not necessary

***Discharge Criteria***
Manage as outpatients with appropriate follow-up in occupational medicine clinic

## ADDITIONAL READING

- Beltrami EM, Williams IT, Shapiro CN, et al. Risk and management of blood-borne infections in health care workers. *Clin Microbiol Rev.* 2000;13:385–407.
- Centers for Disease Control and Prevention. Updated U.S. Public Health Service Guidelines for Management of Occupational exposures to HIV and Recommendations for Postexposure Prophylaxis. *MMWR Recomm Rep.* 2005;54(RR-09):1–17.
- Centers for Disease Control and Prevention. Updated U.S. Public Health Service Guidelines for Management of Occupational Exposures to HBV, HCV, and HIV and Recommendations for Postexposure Prophylaxis. *MMWR Recomm Rep.* 2001;50(RR-11):1–42.
- Henderson DK. Risk for exposures to and infection with HIV among health care providers in the emergency department. *Emerg Med Clin North Am.* 1995;13:199–211.
- Lutwick L. Postexposure prophylaxis. *Infect Dis Clin North Am.* 1996;10:899–915.
- National Clinicians' Postexposure Prophylaxis Hotline: Phone (888) 448-4911; Internet: Http://www.ucsf.edu/hivcntr. Accessed 12/17/09; *MMWR Recomm Rep.* 2001;50(RR-11).
- *MMWR Recomm Rep.* 2005;54(RR-09).
- *MMWR Weekly Rep.* 2007;56(49).

## CODES

**ICD9**
883.0 Open wound of fingers, without mention of complication

# NEONATAL JAUNDICE
*Michele Chetham*

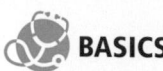 **BASICS**

Produced by a transient imbalance between rates of bilirubin production and bilirubin elimination:

- Newborns have higher rates of bilirubin production than adults because of increased RBC mass and shorter RBC life span.
- Newborns, especially preterm infants, have rate limitations in hepatic conjugation and biliary excretion of bilirubin, increased enterohepatic circulation, and diminished bilirubin binding to albumin- and bilirubin-binding protein.

## DESCRIPTION

- In the vast majority of newborns, this represents *physiologic jaundice* and is not pathologic:
  - Bilirubin normally increases from 1.5 mg/dL in cord blood to a mean of 6.5 mg/dL on day 3, followed by a gradual decline to normal adult levels of 1.5 mg/dL by day 10 or 12 of life.
- However, serum bilirubin may rise to dangerous levels exceeding neuroprotective defenses, causing bilirubin toxicity to the basal ganglia, hippocampus, brainstem nuclei, and cerebellum:
  - *Bilirubin-induced neurologic dysfunction (BIND)* refers to the wide spectrum of disorders caused by increasingly severe hyperbilirubinemia from mild dysfunction to acute bilirubin encephalopathy (ABE) and kernicterus.
    - *ABE* describes the acute manifestations of bilirubin toxicity seen in the 1st weeks after birth.
    - *Kernicterus* is the chronic form of BIND, resulting in significant mortality; survivors have serious neurologic consequences, including a choreoathetoid type of cerebral palsy, gaze abnormalities, hearing loss, and dental dysplasia.
  - Rate of progression of BIND depends on rate of increase of bilirubin levels, duration of hyperbilirubinemia, albumin-binding reserves, unbound bilirubin level, host susceptibility, and comorbidities.
  - Death is due to respiratory failure and progressive coma or intractable seizures.
- Neurotoxic effects of hyperbilirubinemia are seen more commonly with hemolytic disease and less commonly in healthy newborns.
- Severe hyperbilirubinemia may be caused by pathologic conditions.
- Risk factors for hyperbilirubinemia:
  - Hemolytic disease
  - Gestation 35–38 wk
  - Low birth weight
  - Large weight loss after birth
  - Breast-feeding
  - Ethnicity: Asian, Native American, Pacific Islander
  - Siblings with hyperbilirubinemia
  - Family history of glucose-6-phosphate dehydrogenase (G6PD) deficiency or hereditary spherocytosis and elliptocytosis
  - Maternal diabetes
  - Perinatal factors: Polycythemia, birth trauma, infection
- Early discharge of newborns has resulted in more problematic jaundiced newborns due to delayed diagnosis and increased breast-feeding failure.
- Postphototherapy bilirubin rebound to bilirubin levels of concern may occur:
  - At high risk are newborns <37 wk gestation, patients with hemolytic disease, patients treated for <72 hr.

## ETIOLOGY

- Unconjugated hyperbilirubinemia:
  - Physiologic jaundice
  - Jaundice in breast-fed infants:
    - *Breast-feeding failure jaundice*: Exaggeration of physiologic jaundice due to inadequate ingestion of sufficient volume of breast milk in the 1st week of life
    - *Breast-milk jaundice*: Begins days 3–5, peaks within 2 wk but lasts up to 8 wk; caused by increased β-glucuronidase in breast milk
    - May be exacerbated by dehydration
  - Specific hemolytic conditions:
    - Blood group isoimmunization due to ABO, Rh, and minor blood group incompatibility; ABO is most common: Rh disease is unusual (RhoGAM prevents).
    - Red cell membrane defects: Hereditary spherocytosis and elliptocytosis
    - Red cell enzyme deficiencies: G6PD deficiency
  - Sepsis: Bacterial, viral, or protozoal
  - Birth trauma:
    - Increased heme load from resolving cephalohematoma or ecchymosis
  - Polycythemia:
    - Caused by maternal–fetal transfusion
    - Fetal–fetal transfusion
    - Infants of diabetic mothers
  - Congenital hypothyroidism
  - Defective hepatic conjugation:
    - Gilbert syndrome (familial partial defect in glucuronyl transferase activity) is a common benign condition.
    - Crigler-Najjar syndrome (congenital absence of glucuronyl transferase causes lifelong unconjugated hyperbilirubinemia)
  - Intestinal obstruction such as ileus or anatomic obstruction:
    - Increases enterohepatic circulation
- Conjugated hyperbilirubinemia:
  - Failure of hepatic excretion of conjugated bilirubin
  - Causes include neonatal hepatitis, congenital biliary atresia, extrahepatic biliary obstruction, shock liver from neonatal asphyxia, neonatal hemosiderosis

## DIAGNOSIS

### SIGNS AND SYMPTOMS
#### History
- Sleepiness, poor intake, and inadequate urine output may be present.
- Early phase of ABE:
  - Feeding difficulties with poor suck; decreased urine output
  - Fussiness and irritability
  - Lethargy with altered awake–sleep pattern
  - Hypotonia
- Intermediate phase of ABE:
  - High-pitched cry, irritability
  - Increased tone with backward arching of neck (retrocollis) and trunk (opisthotonos) alternating with hypotonia
  - Fever
- Signs of advanced ABE:
  - Pronounced retrocollis-opisthotonos
  - Semicoma, seizures
  - Bicycling movements

### Physical Exam
- Yellowish discoloration of skin, tissues such as sclerae, and body fluids in the newborn infant indicates an elevated serum bilirubin level.
- Evidence of dehydration may exist.
- Increasing levels of bilirubin affect skin color progressing from the face downward:
  - Blanch skin with digital pressure to reveal underlying skin color—only approximates level
  - Face: Bilirubin levels >6–8 mg/dL
  - Feet: Bilirubin levels >12–15 mg/dL
  - Visual diagnosis of jaundice is unreliable, especially in darkly pigmented infants.
- Neurologic dysfunction is identified by abnormal tone—hypotonia, hypertonia, or variability; setting sun sign—sclera visible below upper eyelid.
- Physical exam clues to some causes:
  - Sepsis: Temperature instability, lethargy, poor feeding, vomiting, apnea or tachypnea
  - Hemolytic disease: Pallor, hepatosplenomegaly
  - Extravascular hemolysis: Birth trauma associated with cephalohematoma or bruising
  - Polycythemia: Ruddy complexion
  - Cholestatic jaundice: Persistent jaundice for >3 wk, dark urine, or light-colored stool

### ESSENTIAL WORKUP
- Clinical diagnosis
- Total serum bilirubin (TSB) mandatory in any infant with suspected or obvious jaundice
- Direct (conjugated) and indirect (unconjugated) bilirubin levels
- Interpret TSB according to infant's age in hours, not days, to determine risk and need for treatment.
- Determine if TSB level drawn prior to birth hospitalization discharge.
- Transcutaneous measurement of bilirubin correlates well with TSB if available.
- Further evaluation is recommended for these newborns with jaundice:
  - Occurs in the 1st 24 hr of life
  - Persists beyond the 1st week of life
  - TSB levels reach level to initiate intensive phototherapy.
  - Bilirubin is >10% or >2 mg/dL conjugated.
  - Any signs of ABE

### DIAGNOSTIC TESTS & INTERPRETATION
#### Lab
- Serum albumin, electrolytes, BUN, creatinine, calcium
- CBC with differential and smear for RBC morphology
- Reticulocyte count
- Maternal and infant blood type
- Direct Coombs test on cord blood:
  - Hospital routines vary: Some will test newborns from all type O mothers.
  - If not available, direct Coombs test on infant's blood
- Further workup is directed at suspected cause:
  - Red cell enzyme assay: G6PD
  - Liver function tests
  - Sepsis evaluation
  - Urine-reducing substances

### Imaging

- Evaluation for obstructive liver disease (direct hyperbilirubinemia): Consultation and imaging studies
- MRI scan of brain with abnormal globus pallidus is pathognomonic of kernicterus; not indicated for emergency management.

## DIFFERENTIAL DIAGNOSIS

- See "Etiology."
- Essential to differentiate unconjugated from conjugated hyperbilirubinemia.

 **TREATMENT**

### ALERT

- Significant newborn hyperbilirubinemia with signs of encephalopathy is a neurologic emergency that requires immediate treatment, as outcome is related in part to duration of exposure.
- Hydration should be initiated if any evidence of fluid deficit.

## INITIAL STABILIZATION/THERAPY

0.9% normal saline 20 mL/kg, bolus if signs of dehydration

## ED TREATMENT/PROCEDURES

- Treatment guidelines for infants ≥35 wk gestation based on TSB plotted versus age in hours for infants at lower, medium, or higher risk.
- Higher risk are 35–37 6/7 wk plus risk factors.
- Medium risk are ≥38 wk plus risk factors, or 35–37 6/7 wk and well.
- Lower risk are ≥38 wk and well.
- Risk factors: Isoimmune hemolytic disease, G6PD deficiency, asphyxia, significant lethargy, temperature instability, sepsis, acidosis, albumin <3.0 g/dl
- Depending upon the risk group, hospitalization for intensive phototherapy is indicated when TSB (mg/dL) is above:

|       | High | Medium | Low  |
|-------|------|--------|------|
| 12 hr | 6.0  | 7.5    | 9.0  |
| 24 hr | 7.5  | 9.5    | 11.5 |
| 36 hr | 9.5  | 11.5   | 13.0 |
| 48 hr | 11.0 | 13.0   | 15.0 |
| 60 hr | 12.5 | 14.5   | 16.5 |
| 72 hr | 13.5 | 15.0   | 18.0 |
| 96 hr | 14.5 | 17.0   | 20.0 |
| 5–7 d | 15.0 | 18.0   | 21.0 |

- *Intensive* phototherapy should decrease TSB >0.5 mg/dL/h. Begin as soon as possible.
- Indications for exchange transfusions are also determined by age in hours and risk stratification:
  - For example, at 48 hr, exchange transfusion recommended if higher risk with TSB ≥16 mg/dL, medium risk with TSB ≥19 mg/dL, and low risk with TSB ≥22 mg/dL.
- Immediate exchange transfusion is recommended regardless of TSB level if infant shows signs of acute bilirubin encephalopathy:
  - Type and cross-match for 170 mL/kg of irradiated blood for double-volume exchange transfusion.
  - Albumin infusion 1 g/kg if serum albumin is low (<3.4 g/dL) prior to exchange transfusion.

- If isoimmune hemolytic disease, IV immunoglobulin 0.5–1 g/kg over 2 hr if TSB level is nearing exchange criteria
- Immediate consultation with neonatologist recommended to determine treatment.
- If any delay in admission/transfer, initiate intensive phototherapy in ED.
- Intensive phototherapy implies the use of high level of irradiance in the 430- to 490-nm band delivered to as much of infant's surface area as possible, as close as possible per manufacturer. Eyes must be shielded.
- Encourage feeding with increased frequency, whether breast-fed or bottle-fed; supplemental dextrose-water is not useful.
- If not feeding well, initiate enteral feeds to decrease enterohepatic circulation and increase intestinal bilirubin clearance. If unable to tolerate feeding, consider intravenous fluids
- Treat comorbid illness (sepsis, liver dysfunction, polycythemia, hypothyroidism, etc.)
- Breast-feeding failure and breast milk jaundice:
  - Most infants can continue to breast-feed.
  - Encourage mothers to nurse at least 8–12 times per day for 1st several days.
  - Temporary supplementation with formula until breast milk flow adequate may be needed.
  - May need supplemental IV hydration if dehydrated.
  - 2–3 day cessation of breast-feeding is recommended for those infants with breast milk jaundice and levels not responding to phototherapy.
  - Encourage mother to maintain lactation by use of breast pump or manual expression during period of cessation.
- Physiologic jaundice: Reassurance and arrange appropriate follow-up

## MEDICATION

### First Line

IV immunoglobulin 0.5–1 g/kg over 2 hr in isoimmune hemolytic disease if TSB level is nearing exchange criteria and not responding to intensive phototherapy.

### Second Line

- Phenobarbital increases conjugation and excretion of bilirubin; it may adversely effect cognitive development, and so is not routinely used.
- Ursodeoxycholic acid increases bile flow and is useful in treatment of cholestatic jaundice.
- Tin-mesoporphyrin is a heme-oxygenase inhibitor; not approved for use in U.S.

 **FOLLOW-UP**

## DISPOSITION

### Admission Criteria

- Infants requiring intensive phototherapy
- NICU admission for infants requiring exchange transfusion
- Evidence of significant anemia, sepsis, dehydration, or evidence of obstructive liver disease that may require hospitalization for diagnostic evaluation
- Rapid transport to NICU; transport phototherapy if transport time >30 min

### Discharge Criteria

- Stable infant with hyperbilirubinemia not requiring phototherapy
- Stable term infant with uncomplicated nonhemolytic hyperbilirubinemia not meeting intensive phototherapy guidelines; may have home

phototherapy arranged if appropriate follow-up can be ensured.
- Direct communication with primary care provider and often neonatal consultant is essential.
- Frequently asked questions with answers for parents in English and Spanish available at: http://www.aap.org/family/jaundicefaq.htm. Updated June 2008.

### Issues for Referral

Breast-feeding failure: Lactation consultants are available at many hospitals with outpatient follow-up clinics.

## FOLLOW-UP RECOMMENDATIONS

Follow-up with primary care provider recommended:

- Within 12 hr: Stable infant with hyperbilirubinemia not requiring phototherapy and with no risk factors
- Within 8 hr: Stable infant with uncomplicated nonhemolytic hyperbilirubinemia with home phototherapy arranged

## PEARLS AND PITFALLS

- TSB must be interpreted according to the newborn's age in hours, not days, and with regard for risk factors for severe hyperbilirubinemia.
- Phototherapy needs to be initiated when the TSB exceeds the threshold level based upon an hour of life-specific bilirubin nomogram and the presence or absence of additional risk factors, in order to prevent *bilirubin-induced neurologic dysfunction*.
- Hydration must be assessed and corrected.

## ADDITIONAL READING

- AAP Subcommittee on Hyperbilirubinemia. Clinical practice guideline: Management of hyperbilirubinemia in the newborn infant 35 or more weeks of gestation. *Pediatrics*. 2004;114:297–316
- Kaplan M, Kaplan E, Hammerman C. Post-phototherapy neonatal bilirubin rebound: A potential cause of significant hyperbilirubinemia. *Arch Dis Child*. 2006;91:31–34.
- Shapiro SM, Bhutani VK, Johnson LH. Hyperbilirubinemia and kernicterus. *Clin Perinatol*. 2006;33:387–410.

### See Also (Topic, Algorithm, Electronic Media Element)

Online access to AAP guidelines available at: http://aappolicy.aappublications.org/cgi/content/full/pediatrics;114/1/297

- Online calculators are available to help clinicians assess the risks toward the development of hyperbilirubinemia in newborns:
  - http://bilitool.org/. Required values include the age of the child in hours (between 18 and 168 hr) and the total **bilirubin** in either U.S. (mg/dL) or SI (μmol/L) units.
- Additional information about kernicterus available at: http://www.cdc.gov/ncbddd/dd/kernicterus/ker_healthcare.htm. Updated March 2009.

 **CODES**

### ICD9

- 774.2 Neonatal jaundice associated with preterm delivery
- 774.6 Unspecified fetal and neonatal jaundice

# NEONATAL SEPSIS

*Lazaro Lezcano*

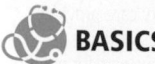 **BASICS**

## DESCRIPTION
### Mechanism
- Life-threatening infection of the newborn, rarely occurring as late as 3 mo of age
- Overwhelmingly bacterial:
  - Rarely viral or fungal infection
  - Organisms usually present in the maternal perineal flora
- Occurs in 3–5 newborns per 1000 live births
- Risk factors:
  - Perinatal:
    ○ History of recent fever (>37.5°C)
    ○ UTI
    ○ Chorioamnionitis
    ○ Prolonged rupture of membranes (>18 hr)
    ○ Foul lochia
    ○ Uterine tenderness
    ○ Intrapartum asphyxia
  - Neonatal:
    ○ Prematurity
    ○ Fetal tachycardia (>180 beats/min)
    ○ Male
    ○ Twinning (especially second twin)
    ○ Developmental or congenital immune defects
    ○ Administration of intramuscular iron
    ○ Galactosemia
    ○ Congenital anomaly (urinary tract, asplenia, myelomeningocele, sinus tract)
    ○ Omphalitis

## ETIOLOGY
### Sepsis
- Bacterial:
  - Group B *Streptococcus*
  - *Escherichia coli*
  - *Listeria monocytogenes*
  - Coagulase-negative *Staphylococcus*
  - *Treponema pallidum*
- Viral:
  - Herpes simplex is a common viral etiology.
  - Enterovirus
  - Adenovirus
- Fungi:
  - *Candida* species
- Protozoa:
  - Malaria
  - *Borrelia*

### Meningitis
- Bacterial:
  - Group B *Streptococcus*
  - *E. coli* type K1
  - *L. monocytogenes*
  - Other streptococci
  - Nontypeable *Haemophilus influenzae*
  - Coagulase-positive and coagulase-negative
  - *Staphylococcus*
  - Less commonly: *Klebsiella, Enterobacter,*
  - *Pseudomonas, T. pallidum,* and *Mycobacterium tuberculosis*
  - *Citrobacter diversus* (important cause of brain abscess)
  - Additional pathogens: *Mycoplasma hominis* and *Ureaplasma urealyticum*
- Viral:
  - Enteroviruses
  - Herpes simplex virus (type 2 more commonly)
  - Cytomegaloviruses
  - *Toxoplasma gondii*
  - Rubella
  - HIV
- Fungi:
  - *Candida albicans* and other fungi

 **DIAGNOSIS**

## SIGNS AND SYMPTOMS
### History
- Nonspecific history:
  - "Not acting normal"
  - Feeding poorly
  - Irritable or lethargic
- General:
  - Toxic appearing
  - Altered mental status: irritable or lethargic
  - Apnea or bradycardia
  - Mottled, ashen, cyanotic, or cool skin

### Physical Exam
- Vital signs:
  - Hyperthermia/hypothermia
  - Tachypnea
  - Tachycardia
  - Prolonged capillary refill time
- Abdominal distention
- Jaundice
- Bruising or prolonged bleeding
- Sepsis syndrome in the neonate:
  - Septic shock
  - Hypoglycemia
  - Seizures
  - Disseminated intravascular coagulation (DIC)
  - If untreated, cardiovascular collapse and death

## ESSENTIAL WORKUP
- Sepsis evaluation followed by empiric antibiotics and support
- Determine a source for the infection.
- Identify metabolic abnormalities.

## DIAGNOSTIC TESTS & INTERPRETATION
### Lab
- Bedside glucose determination
- CBC:
  - WBCs elevated or suppressed
  - Shift to the left
  - Thrombocytopenia
- Urinalysis
- Cultures as soon as the diagnosis is entertained:
  - Blood, CSF, catheterized or suprapubic urine, stool
- Lumbar puncture:
  - May need to delay if hemodynamically unstable
  - Cell count, protein, glucose, culture
- Serum glucose needed to exclude hypoglycemia
- Arterial blood gas and oximetry
  - Metabolic acidosis is common.
- Electrolytes and calcium:
  - Hyponatremia
  - Hypocalcemia
- DIC panel:
  - Coagulopathy is a late complication.
  - Monitor prothrombin time, partial thromboplastin time, and fibrinogen-split products

### Imaging

CXR to rule out pneumonia

### DIFFERENTIAL DIAGNOSIS

- Heart disease:
  - Hypoplastic left heart syndrome
  - Myocarditis
- Metabolic disorders:
  - Hypoglycemia
  - Adrenal insufficiency (congenital adrenal hyperplasia)
  - Organic acidoses
  - Urea cycle disorders
- Intussusception
- Child abuse
- CNS:
  - Intracranial hemorrhage
  - Perinatal asphyxia
- Neonatal jaundice
- Hematologic emergencies:
  - Neonatal purpura fulminans
  - Severe anemia
  - Methemoglobinemia
  - Malignancy (congenital leukemia)

 TREATMENT

### PRE-HOSPITAL

#### Cautions

- Ventilatory support if obtunded, apneic, or respiratory distress
- IV access
- Continuous monitoring

### ED TREATMENT/PROCEDURES

- Implement empiric treatment for neonatal sepsis if presentation at all consistent, particularly if any risk factors are present.
- Administer antibiotics:
  - Ampicillin and gentamicin or cefotaxime
  - Add vancomycin if the patient's condition continues to deteriorate or any suggestion of *Streptococcus pneumoniae*.
  - Cefotaxime may be substituted for gentamicin.
- Support for septic shock if present

### MEDICATION

- Ampicillin: 200 mg/kg/day q6h IV/IM for infant >2 kg birth weight and >2 wk old; 150 mg/kg/day q8h if <7 days old
- Cefotaxime: 150 mg/kg/day q6h IV/IM for infants >2 kg birth weight and >1 wk old; 150 mg/kg/day q8h IV/IM if 8–28 days old; 100 mg/kg/d IV/IM. q12h if 0–7 days old
- Gentamicin: 2.5 mg/kg/dose q8h IV/IM if postconceptual age >37 wk and >7 days old; 2.5 mg/kg/dose q12h if <7 days old
- Vancomycin: 15 mg/kg/dose IV q8h if postconceptual age >37 wk and >7 days old; 15 mg/kg IV q12h if <7 days old

 FOLLOW-UP

### DISPOSITION

#### Admission Criteria

- All patients with suspected sepsis are admitted to the hospital for supportive care, IV antibiotic therapy, and close monitoring.
- All children <1 mo with a fever are generally admitted even in the absence of significant suspicion of sepsis. Older children are admitted based upon the clinical presentation.

### Initial Stabilization

- Airway management indicated if obtundation, apnea, or respiratory distress
- IV access to administer fluids and pressors as needed
- Continuous monitoring

## ADDITIONAL READING

- American Academy of Pediatrics. *Red Book. 2009 Report of the Committee on Infectious Diseases*, 28th ed. Elk Grove Village, IL: American Academy of Pediatrics; 2009.
- Edwards MS. Postnatal bacterial infections. In: Fanaroff AA, Martin RJ, eds. *Neonatal-Perinatal Medicine. Diseases of the Fetus and Infant*, 7th ed. St. Louis, MO: Mosby; 2002:706–722.
- Polin RA, Parravicini E, Regan JA, et al. Bacterial sepsis and meningitis. In: Taesch HW, Ballard RA, Gleason CA. *Avery's Diseases of the Newborn*, 8th ed. Philadelphia: Elsevier Saunders; 2005:551–568.
- Shapiro NI, Zimmer GD, Barkin AZ. Sepsis syndrome. In: Marx JA, Hockberger RS, Walls RM, eds. *Rosen's Emergency Medicine: Concepts and Clinical Practice*, 5th ed. St. Louis, MO: Mosby; 2002:1957–1969.
- Van de Hoogen A, Gerards LJ, Verboon-Maciolek MA, et al. Long-term trends in the epidemiology of neonatal sepsis and antibiotic susceptibility of causative agents. *Neonatology*. 2009;97(1):22–28.
- Young TE, Mangum B (eds.). *Neofax: A Manual of Drugs Used in Neonatal Care*, 22nd ed. Williston, VT: Physicians' Desk Reference; 2009:2–88.

 CODES

### ICD9

771.81 Septicemia {sepsis} of newborn

### ICD10

P36.9

# NEPHRITIC SYNDROME
*Maureen L. Joyner*

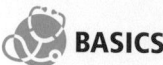 **BASICS**

## DESCRIPTION
- Acute glomerulonephritis (AGN) is acute inflammatory damage to glomerulus, associated with:
  - Abrupt onset of hematuria with or without RBC casts
  - Acute renal failure manifested by edema, hypertension, azotemia, decline in urine output
  - Variable proteinuria
  - Active urine sediment (RBC casts)
- Exact mechanism of AGN unclear:
  - Combination of autoimmune reactivity to specific antigens at renal glomeruli
  - Characterized by crescent formation secondary to nonspecific injury at the glomerular wall

## ETIOLOGY
- Poststreptococcal glomerulonephritis (PSGN):
  - A postinfectious cause of acute nephritic syndrome, resulting from group A $\beta$-hemolytic streptococci
  - Considered a nonsuppurative complication (antibiotic treatment does not prevent this complication)
  - Occurs when immune complexes create hump-shaped subepithelial deposits in renal glomeruli
  - Most commonly affects patients between ages 3 and 15 yr but can occur at any age
  - Incidence of nephritis is 5–10% after pharyngitis and 25% after skin infections.
  - Consider PSGN in the setting of new-onset proteinuria, RBC casts, edema, and any recent infection.
  - Latent period between infection and onset of nephritis helps differentiate between PSGN and IgA nephropathy:
    ○ 1–3 wk in pharyngeal infection
    ○ 2–4 wk in cutaneous infection
  - Renal biopsy is usually not necessary for diagnosis.
  - Low complement (C3) for 6–8 wk
  - Can progress to severe renal failure if underlying infection goes untreated
  - Prognosis:
    ○ Excellent; >95% recover spontaneously with normalization of renal function within 6–8 wk, even with dialysis.
    ○ Hematuria usually resolves in 3–6 mo.
    ○ Transient nephrotic phase in 20% of patients during resolution of illness
    ○ End-stage renal disease occurs <5%
    ○ Rapidly progressive glomerulonephritis (RPGN) is rare, occurring in <1% cases.
    ○ Most cases resolve spontaneously with no long-term sequelae.

- Other infectious sources of glomerulonephritis (GN):
  - Sepsis, pneumonia, endocarditis, viruses, HIV
  - Pulmonary, intra-abdominal or cutaneous infections
  - Syphilis, leprosy, schistosomiasis, and malaria
  - Goal: Treat underlying infection.
- Hepatitis virus–related glomerular disease:
  - Can present with either nephritic or nephrotic symptoms
  - Causes membranoproliferative GN
  - Complements remain low indefinitely (compared to PSGN)
- Noninfectious causes of GN (due to immune complex formation):
  - Systematic lupus erythematosus, Henoch-Schönlein purpura, vasculitis, Wegener granulomatosis
  - Goodpasture syndrome
- IgA nephropathy (IgA-N)
  - Most common cause of AGN (>25%) worldwide
  - Antibody-antigen causes immune complex deposition of IgA and C3
  - Complement levels are usually normal.
  - IgA-N has different presentations:
    ○ Gross hematuria following upper respiratory infection (URI)
    ○ Microscopic hematuria with proteinuria
    ○ Hematuria during viral illness or after exercise
    ○ Prognosis is related to serum creatinine, BP, and proteinuria.
    ○ 50% of patients with proteinuria may develop progressive renal disease.
    ○ ACE inhibitors or angiotensin-receptor blockers (ARBs) may help
- RPGN:
  - Certain patients with AGN may progress rapidly to renal failure.
  - Hallmarks are crescents on renal biopsy.

## DIAGNOSIS

### SIGNS AND SYMPTOMS
- Hematuria:
  - Abrupt onset gross hematuria in 30–40% (coffee- or cola-colored urine)
- Edema:
  - Periorbital edema
  - Generalized edema more common in infants and children
- Infectious source or recent infection: upper respiratory tract or skin common, eg, PSGN
- Symptoms of congestive heart failure:
  - 40% occurrence in patients >60 yr
  - Rare in children

- Arthritis, arthralgias, and various skin rashes: PSGN, systemic disease
- Nonspecific manifestations:
  - Malaise
  - Weakness
  - Anorexia
  - Nausea/vomiting

### History
- Recent URI or skin or other infection
- Change in urine color

### Physical Exam
- Hypertension
- Edema

## ESSENTIAL WORKUP
Urinalysis with sediment evaluation to detect:
- RBCs, proteinuria, and RBC casts
- RBC casts are diagnostic of an active glomerular inflammation.

## DIAGNOSTIC TESTS & INTERPRETATION
### Lab
- CBC:
  - Anemia (seen in more chronic cases of GN or other systemic disease)
  - Acute leukocytosis (may suggest infectious process)
- Basic metabolic panel:
  - Assess baseline renal function
  - Check for electrolyte abnormalities
- Serum albumin
- Cultures (throat, skin, urine, blood):
  - As clinically suspected for infectious source
- Serum complement level (C3): decreased in infectious endocarditis, shunt nephritis, and PSGN
- Streptococcal antibodies:
  - Antistreptolysin (ASO), antistreptokinase (ASK), anti–deoxyribonuclease B (ADNase B), anti–nicotinyl adenine dinucleotidase (ANADase), and antihyaluronidase (AH)
  - ASO more reactive in pharyngeal infections
  - ADNase B, ANADase, and AH more reactive in cutaneous infections
  - ASK elevated in recent hemolytic *Streptococcus* infections
  - Titers do not correlate with prognosis of disease
- Urine osmolality, sodium, creatinine
- 24-hr urine collection:
  - Proteinuria initially present in 5% of children, 20% of adults with PSGN

### Imaging
- Renal ultrasound: kidney size abnormality
- Chest radiograph: cardiomegaly, pulmonary edema, infection

### Diagnostic Procedures/Surgery
Renal biopsy:
- Generally not done for PSGN, as symptoms typically resolve after a brief illness
- Recommended if atypical features of PSGN, persistently abnormal complement levels, persistent hypertension, and proteinuria >3 g/d
- Facilitates diagnosis for other causes of nephritis

## DIFFERENTIAL DIAGNOSIS
- (See Glomerulonephritis for further information on types of GN)
- Renal:
  - Primary glomerular disease
- Systemic:
  - Goodpasture syndrome
  - Vasculitis
  - Henoch-Schönlein purpura
- Other (rare):
  - Hemolytic-uremic syndrome
  - Thrombotic thrombocytopenic purpura
  - Acute hypersensitivity interstitial nephritis
  - Serum sickness

 TREATMENT

### PRE-HOSPITAL
Support ABCs

### INITIAL STABILIZATION/THERAPY
ABCs

### ED TREATMENT/PROCEDURES
- Antibiotics for streptococcal infection:
  - Penicillin (erythromycin, if penicillin allergic)
  - Prophylactic antibiotics to siblings of PSGN patients
- Restrict of salt and fluid intake
- Administer loop diuretics (furosemide)
- Restore urine flow in oliguric patients:
  - Mannitol
- Treat pulmonary edema:
  - Oxygen
  - Morphine
  - Loop diuretics
- Stabilize BP to decrease proteinuria, retard progression of GN:
  - ACEIs, ARBs
  - Hypertensive emergency: nitroprusside or other titratable antihypertensive medication
- Hemodialysis for:
  - Severe hyperkalemia
  - Fluid overload
  - Uremia
  - Severe acidosis
  - Correct electrolyte abnormalities

## MEDICATION
- Erythromycin: 250–500 mg (peds: 30–50 mg/kg/d) PO q 6h for 7–10 days
- Furosemide: 20–80 mg (peds: 1–6 mg/kg) PO daily/b.i.d.
- Lisinopril (ACEI): 10–40 mg (peds: >6 yr: 0.07 mg/kg) PO daily
- Losartan (ARB): 25–100 mg (peds: >6 yr: 0.7 mg/kg) PO daily
- Mannitol: 12.5–100 g (peds: 0.25–0.5 g/kg) IV:
  - May use single or repeat dosing; consider test dosing 1st.
- Morphine sulfate: 0.1 mg/kg/dose IV q4h
- Nitroprusside: 0.3–4 mcg/kg/min IV
  - Titrate to goal mean arterial pressure for hypertensive emergency.
- Penicillin:
  - Benzathine penicillin: 1.2 million units (peds: 0.3–0.9 million units, based on weight) IM as single dose
  - Penicillin VK: 250–500 mg (peds: <12 yr 25–50 mg/kg/d) PO q6–8h for 10 days
- Other agents, including fish oil (omega-3 fatty acids for anti-inflammatory effects) and immunosuppressive agents (glucocorticoids, cyclophosphamide), may be used in consultation with specialists.

 FOLLOW-UP

### DISPOSITION
#### Admission Criteria
- Evidence of infectious cause for GN
- Oliguria, anuria
- Uremia
- Elevated creatinine, BUN levels
- Edema
- Electrolyte abnormalities
- Severe hypertension
- CHF

#### Discharge Criteria
Mild cases of clinical nephritis in healthy patients with:
- No comorbid illness
- Strict supervision/monitoring of symptoms, diet, urine output, and medication
- Close follow-up with PMD and nephrology referral

### Issues for Referral
Nephrology:
- Within 2–3 days

### FOLLOW-UP RECOMMENDATIONS
- Adherence to antibiotic and antihypertensive therapy, as indicated
- Restrict salt and fluid intake.

## PEARLS AND PITFALLS
- Diagnosis is confirmed by biopsy showing characteristic crescent formation within renal glomeruli.
- Must obtain thorough history of ongoing or recent infections as possible etiology of nephritis
- IgA nephropathy is most common cause of nephritis.
- Patients require aggressive management of BP and volume status.

## ADDITIONAL READING
- Couser W. Glomerulonephritis. *Lancet.* 1999;353:1509–1515.
- Ikee R, Kobayashi S, Saigusa T, et al. Impact of hypertension and hypertension-related vascular lesions in IgA nephropathy. *Hypertens Res.* 2006;29(1):15–22.
- Kanjanabuch T, Kittikowit W, Eiam-Ong S. An update on acute postinfectious glomerulonephritis worldwide. *Nat Rev Nephrol.* 2009;5:259–269.
- Kunz R, Friedrich C, Wolbers M, et al. Meta-analysis: Effect of monotherapy and combination therapy with inhibitors of the renin angiotensin system on proteinuria in renal disease. *Ann Intern Med.* 2008;148(1):30–48.

### See Also (Topic, Algorithm, Electronic Media Element)
- Acute Renal Failure
- Glomerulonephritis
- Nephrotic Syndrome

 CODES

### ICD9
- 580.0 Acute glomerulonephritis with lesion of proliferative glomerulonephritis
- 580.9 Acute glomerulonephritis with unspecified pathological lesion in kidney

# NEPHROTIC SYNDROME

*Maureen L. Joyner*

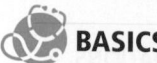

## BASICS

### DESCRIPTION
- Diseases causing defect in glomerular filtration barrier, producing proteinuria:
  - Proteinuria >3.0 g in 24 hr
  - Hypoalbuminemia (serum albumin <3 g/dL)
  - Peripheral edema due to hypoalbuminemia
  - Hypogammaglobulinemia
  - Hyperlipidemia (fasting cholesterol >200 mg/dL)
- Urine fat (oval fat bodies, fatty/waxy casts)
- Glomerular basement membrane altered by:
  - Immune complexes
  - Nephrotoxic antibodies
  - Nonimmune mechanisms
  - Result: More permeable glomerular membranes and excretion of albumin and large protein

### PATHOPHYSIOLOGY
- Proteinuria due to increased filtration within renal glomeruli
- Edema due to sodium retention and hypoalbuminemia
- Postural hypotension, syncope, and shock due to severe hypoalbuminemia
- Hyperlipidemia due to hepatic lipoprotein synthesis stimulated by decreased plasma oncotic pressure
- Cumulative thromboembolism risk increased if:
  - Hypovolemia
  - Low serum albumin
  - High protein excretion
  - High fibrinogen levels
  - Low antithrombin III levels

### ETIOLOGY
- Due to primary renal or systemic diseases
- Membranous nephropathy:
  - Primary cause of nephrotic syndrome in adults
  - Other causes include chronic infection (hepatitis B virus, hepatitis C virus, autoimmune disorders).
  - Renal biopsy shows involvement of all glomeruli.
  - Women have better prognosis.
  - 30% may slowly progress to renal failure.
  - Renal vein thrombosis causes sudden loss of renal function.
  - Treat with steroids and cytotoxic agents in severe cases.
- Minimal change disease:
  - Most common cause (90%) of nephrotic syndrome in children
  - Other causes: Idiopathic, NSAIDs, paraneoplastic syndrome associated with malignancy (often Hodgkin lymphoma)
  - Urine sediment shows Maltese cross in polarized light.
  - Best prognosis among all nephrotic syndromes
  - Good response to steroids
- Focal segmental glomerulosclerosis (FSGS):
  - Young patients (15–30 yr) with nephrotic syndrome
  - Presents with high blood pressure, renal insufficiency, proteinuria, microscopic or gross hematuria.
  - Causes include HIV, heroin abuse, obesity, hematologic malignancies.
  - Primary FSGS responds to steroids.
  - Secondary FSGS treated with angiotensin-converting-enzyme inhibitors (ACEI)
  - Collapsing FSGS usually seen in HIV patients
- Membranoproliferative glomerulonephritis:
  - May present with nephrotic, nonnephrotic, or nephritic sediment
  - Complement levels are persistently low,
  - Supportive care: Steroids may be helpful in children.
  - Aspirin and dipyridamole may slow progression.
- Diabetes mellitus/diabetic nephropathy:
  - Most common secondary cause of nephrotic range proteinuria in adults
  - Microalbuminuria (30–300 mg/24 hr) is primary indicator of renal disease.
  - Worsening of renal function in 5–7 yr
  - Does not cause rapid decline in renal function
  - Strict control of blood sugar and ACEI therapy slow progression.
- Monoclonal gammopathies:
  - Include amyloidosis, multiple myeloma, and light-chain nephropathy
  - Renal manifestations include proteinuria, nephrotic syndrome, nephritic syndrome, and acute renal failure.
  - Lab findings include pseudohyponatremia, low anion gap, hypercalcemia, and Bence-Jones proteinuria.
  - Congo red stain of amyloid shows apple green birefringence in polarized light.
  - Supportive care: Steroids and melphalan have some benefit.
- Systemic lupus erythematosus (SLE):
  - Can present initially as a nephritic process, with progression to nephrotic syndrome
- HIV-associated nephropathy:
  - Focal segmental glomerulosclerosis is most common nephropathy.
  - Collapsing glomerulopathy in seropositive HIV carriers with supernephrotic syndrome results in end-stage renal failure that is rapidly progressive (months).
- Other causes include preeclampsia, hepatitis, and drug reactions (culprits include NSAIDs, gold, penicillamine).

## DIAGNOSIS

### SIGNS AND SYMPTOMS
- Many patients are asymptomatic.
- Proteinuria
- Peripheral edema:
  - Mild pitting edema to generalized anasarca with ascites
- Hyperlipidemia
- Lipiduria (urine fatty casts and oval fat bodies)
- Postural hypotension, syncope, shock
- Hypertension
- Hematuria:
  - Microscopic or gross hematuria (secondary to renal vein thrombosis)
- Renal insufficiency to acute renal failure in some cases
- Tachypnea, tachycardia, with or without hypotension:
  - Acute onset: Suggests pulmonary embolus (PE), secondary to renal or deep venous thrombosis and hypercoagulable state
  - Up to 30% occurrence of PE in membranous glomerulonephritis
  - Chronic or exertional tachypnea due to:
    - Pulmonary edema
    - Pleural effusions
    - Infection risk due to immunosuppressive treatment and frequent exposure to infections such as *Pneumococcus*
    - Ascites
- Protein malnutrition

### History
- Systemic disease such as diabetes, SLE, HIV
- Use of NSAIDS, gold, or penicillamine

### Physical Exam
Varies depending on degree of hypoalbuminemia, hemodynamic status, and etiology of nephrotic syndrome:
- Edema
- Hypotension/hypertension
- Shock

### ESSENTIAL WORKUP
Urinalysis:
- Dipstick protein largely positive:
  - Urine specific gravity >1.025 lowers the diagnostic significance of proteinuria.
- Microscopic analysis for urinary casts and the presence of cellular elements:
  - Oval fat bodies
  - Free lipid droplets

### DIAGNOSTIC TESTS & INTERPRETATION
*Lab*
- CBC plus differential:
  - Anemia common
  - Leukocytosis: Infection
  - Leukopenia: Neoplastic disease or sepsis
  - Thrombocytopenia: Liver disease
- Prothrombin time, partial thromboplastin time, International Normalized Ratio:
  - Coagulation profiles abnormal with concurrent liver disease
- D-dimer, fibrinogen, antithrombin III
  - Suspected thromboembolic event:
    - Often patients are asymptomatic with PE or renal vein thrombosis; therefore need high clinical suspicion.
- 24-hr urine protein, total protein to creatinine ratio
- Serum albumin: <3 g/dL
- Serum total protein
- Basic metabolic panel with Ca, Mg, P
- Lipid profile: Elevated total cholesterol, LDL, and VLDL

- Additional lab tests may be necessary for systemic diseases:
  - Examples include antinuclear antibody, serum and urine protein electrophoresis, hepatitis profile, syphilis, cryoglobulins, complement levels

### Imaging
Renal US:

- Used in suspected secondary causes of nephrotic syndrome

### Diagnostic Procedures/Surgery
- Renal biopsy:
  - Definitive test for patients who do not respond to a short course of corticosteroids
  - Helps discern primary versus secondary pathology
- Renal angiography, CT scan, or MRI for suspected renal vein thrombosis

## DIFFERENTIAL DIAGNOSIS
Proteinuria resulting from other causes:

- Renal parenchymal disease:
  - Chronic renal disease
  - Mechanical nephropathy (outlet obstruction/reflux)
  - Acute pyelonephritis
  - Sickle cell disease
- Other causes:
  - CHF
  - Essential hypertension
  - Acute febrile illness
  - Pregnancy (preeclampsia)
    Severe obesity

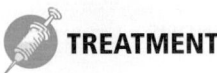

## TREATMENT

### PRE-HOSPITAL
Support ABCs

### INITIAL STABILIZATION/THERAPY
ABCs:

- Supplemental oxygen if respiratory distress
- IV fluids:
  - Slow rehydration for decreased BP or orthostatic hypotension due to decreased intravascular volume
  - Active rehydration in the presence of severe hypotension, shock

### ED TREATMENT/PROCEDURES
- Control edema:
  - Restrict sodium intake: 2 g NaCl/d
  - Loop diuretic (furosemide): Titrate dose until response seen
  - Thiazides and potassium-sparing diuretics
  - Goal: *Slow* diuresis:
    - Aggressive diuresis can precipitate acute renal failure due to hypovolemia and increase the risk of thromboembolic complications.
- Thromboembolic prevention/treatment:
  - Heparin: 80-IU/kg bolus followed by 18-IU/kg/h drip IV for thromboembolic event
  - No prophylactic anticoagulation
  - Consider low-dose aspirin 81 mg.
  - Support stockings

- Plasmapheresis, for severe cases
- Glucocorticosteroid: Mainstay of treatment for primary nephrotic syndrome
- ACEIs/ARBs: Decreases proteinuria, prevents worsening of renal function:
  - Adverse effects of ACEI include renal failure and hyperkalemia.
- Cholesterol-lowering agents/dietary manipulation (eg, bile acid resin, statins)
- Other agents to be considered, under supervision of a specialist:
  - Cytotoxic agents/cyclosporine
  - Recombinant erythropoietin for anemia

## MEDICATION
- Enoxaparin (Lovenox): 30–40 mg (peds: 0.5–0.75 mg/kg) SC q12h
- Furosemide: 20–80 mg (peds: 1–6 mq/kg) PO daily/b.i.d.
- Heparin: 80-IU/kg bolus followed by 18-IU/kg/hr drip IV
- Lisinopril (ACEI): 10–40 mg (peds: >6 yr: 0.07 mg/kg) PO daily
- Losartan (ARB): 25–100 mg (peds: >6 yr: 0.7 mg/kg) PO daily
- Metolazone: 5–20 mg (peds: 0.2–0.4 mg/kg) PO daily
- Prednisone: 5–60 mg (peds: 0.5–2 mg/kg) PO daily

 FOLLOW-UP

### DISPOSITION
### Admission Criteria
- Moderate to severe heart failure, ascites, respiratory compromise
- Signs of comorbid illness, such as undiagnosed malignancy, poorly controlled diabetes, immunocompromised patients
- Acute renal failure
- Evidence of thromboembolic event

### Discharge Criteria
- Patients with no comorbid disease, normal vital signs, and normal blood work
- Close follow-up with a nephrologist for further evaluation and treatment is mandatory.

### Issues for Referral
Nephrology:

- Routine follow-up for BP and disease management
- Renal biopsy for appropriate patients

## FOLLOW-UP RECOMMENDATIONS
- In addition to nephrology, patients should follow-up with rheumatology, infectious disease, hematology/oncology, or endocrine specialist (dependent on underlying disorder contributing to nephritic syndrome).
- Strict BP control and attention to low cholesterol diet allow for best prognosis in long-term disease management.

## PEARLS AND PITFALLS
- Characterized by proteinuria, hypoalbuminemia, and peripheral edema
- Most common causes are minimal change disease in pediatric patients and diabetic nephropathy in adults.
- May present along spectrum from hypertensive to severe hypotension and shock; maintain high index of suspicion in the appropriate setting.
- Consider associated risks of thromboembolic disease.

## ADDITIONAL READING
- Braden GL, Mulhern JG, O'Shea MH, et al. Changing incidence of glomerular diseases in adults. *Am J Kidney Dis*. 2000;35(5):878–883.
- Crew RJ, Radhakrishnan J, Appel G. Complications of the nephrotic syndrome and their treatment. *Clin Nephrol*. 2004;62(4):245–259.
- Huerta C, Castellsague J, Varas-Lorenzo C, et al. Nonsteroidal anti-inflammatory drugs and risk of ARF in the general population. *Am J Kidney Dis*. 2005;45(3):531–539.
- Wheeler DC, Bernard DB. Lipid abnormalities in the nephrotic syndrome: Causes, consequences, and treatment. *Am J Kidney Dis*. 1994;23(3):331–346.

### See Also (Topic, Algorithm, Electronic Media Element)
- Acute Renal Failure
- Glomerulonephritis
- Nephritic Syndrome

*The author gratefully acknowledges the contribution of Anwer Hussain.*

 CODES

### ICD9
581.9 Nephrotic syndrome with unspecified pathological lesion in kidney

# NEUROLEPTIC MALIGNANT SYNDROME

*Gary A. Johnson*

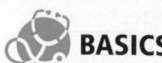 **BASICS**

## DESCRIPTION

- May develop any time during therapy with neuroleptics—from a few days to many years:
  - Typically occurs in the 1st mo of therapy
- Muscular rigidity from dopamine antagonism in the nigrostriatal pathway
- Hyperthermia due to blockage of hypothalamic thermoregulation
- More likely in the setting of benzodiazepine withdrawal
- May be indistinguishable from other causes of drug-induced hyperthermia (malignant hyperthermia, serotonin syndrome, anticholinergic toxins, or sympathomimetic poisoning)
- Most episodes resolve within 2 wk after cessation of offending agent.
- Diagnostic criteria:
  - Development of elevated temperature and severe muscle rigidity in association with use of antipsychotic/neuroleptic medication
  - 2 or more of the following:
    - Diaphoresis
    - Dysphagia
    - Tremor
    - Incontinence
    - Altered mental status (range from confusion to coma)
    - Mutism
    - Tachycardia
    - Elevated of labile blood pressure
    - Leukocytosis
    - Lab evidence of muscle injury
  - Symptoms are not caused by another disease process

## ETIOLOGY

- Rare complication of treatment with neuroleptics:
  - Phenothiazines
    - Chlorpromazine (Thorazine)
    - Prochlorperazine (Compazine)
    - Promethazine (Phenergan)
  - Butyrophenones
    - Haloperidol
    - Droperidol
  - Atypical antipsychotics
    - Risperidone (Risperdal)
    - Olanzapine (Zyprexa)
    - Quetiapine (Seroquel)
    - Clozapine (Clozaril)
    - Aripiprazole (Abilify)
- Occurs in approximately 1% of patients treated with neuroleptics (especially haloperidol)
- Has also been associated with withdrawal from dopamine agonists in Parkinson disease
- Serotonin reuptake inhibitors along with neuroleptic medication may be associated with an increased risk
- Risk factors:
  - Rapid drug loading
  - High-dose antipsychotics
  - High-potency antipsychotics
  - IV administration of drug
  - Dehydration
  - Prior neuroleptic malignant syndrome (NMS)
  - Preceding psychomotor agitation

 **DIAGNOSIS**

## SIGNS AND SYMPTOMS

- Life-threatening condition
- Hallmarks of the disease:
  - Hyperthermia (temperature may be as high as 106–107°F, 41°C)
  - Altered level of consciousness
  - Significant skeletal muscle rigidity—lead-pipe rigidity
  - Autonomic instability (tachycardia, labile BP)

## History

- Neuroleptic use
- Discontinuation of antiparkinsonian drugs
- Change in mental status

### Physical Exam

- Fever
- Tachycardia, labile BP
- Delirium
- Muscle rigidity

## ESSENTIAL WORKUP

- An accurate history (especially current medications) and physical exam confirm the diagnosis.
- Creatine phosphokinase, WBC determination, and liver function tests

## DIAGNOSTIC TESTS & INTERPRETATION

### Lab

- Electrolytes, glucose
- BUN, creatinine
- Prothrombin time, partial thromboplastin time Urinalysis and urine myoglobin
- Creatine kinase

### Imaging

CT scan, EEG if the cause of altered level of consciousness is unclear

### Diagnostic Procedures/Surgery

Lumbar puncture to rule out other causes of fever or altered mental status

## DIFFERENTIAL DIAGNOSIS

- Meningitis or encephalitis
- Sepsis
- Malignant hyperthermia, severe dystonic reaction
- Serotonin syndrome
- Anticholinergic poisoning
- Sympathomimetic poisoning
- Tetanus
- Heat stroke
- Strychnine poisoning
- Vascular CNS event
- Thyrotoxicosis
- Rabies

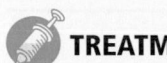 TREATMENT

### PRE-HOSPITAL
- Ventilation may be difficult because of chest wall rigidity.
- Cool the patient, and treat seizures if they occur.
- Check fingerstick glucose.

### INITIAL STABILIZATION/THERAPY
- Airway intervention and circulatory support as needed
- IV, supplemental O$_2$, cardiac monitor
- Immediate IV benzodiazepines (diazepam, lorazepam):
  – May require repeated large doses
- If symptoms are not controlled within a few minutes, rapid-sequence intubation (RSI) and neuromuscular blockade are necessary:
  – Nondepolarizing neuromuscular blockers (vecuronium, rocuronium, pancuronium) are preferable to succinylcholine.
- Measures to control hyperthermia:
  – Ice packs, mist and fan, cooling blankets, etc.
- Aggressive IV fluid therapy with lactated Ringer solution or normal saline

### ED TREATMENT/PROCEDURES
- Relief of muscle rigidity
- Benzodiazepines are the drug of choice:
  – Bromocriptine is a dopamine agonist that may play a role in longer-term management.
  – Dantrolene is a direct skeletal muscle relaxant that may play a role in longer-term management.
  – Neither bromocriptine nor dantrolene has a rapid onset and neither has been demonstrated to alter outcome.

- Discontinue neuroleptics.
- Recognize complications (rhabdomyolysis, respiratory failure, acute renal failure); mortality can be as high as 20%

### MEDICATION
*First Line*
- Diazepam: 5 mg IV q5 min
- Lorazepam: 1 mg IV q5 min
- Rocuronium: 600–1200 mcg/kg IV × 1 for RSI
- Pancuronium: 60–100 mcg/kg IV × 1 for intubation

*Second Line*
- Bromocriptine: 5–10 mg PO t.i.d.–q.i.d. (start 2.5 mg)
- Dantrolene: 1 mg/kg IV q4-6h × 24–48 hr
- Amantadine: 100 mg PO b.i.d.

 FOLLOW-UP

### DISPOSITION
*Admission Criteria*
- Patients with NMS should be admitted.
- Patients will often require intensive care.

### FOLLOW-UP RECOMMENDATIONS
Patients and families must be counseled on the future use of any drug that may trigger NMS.

## PEARLS AND PITFALLS
- Must rule out other causes of fever and altered mental status (ie, meningitis, encephalitis).
- Medication history is essential when considering NMS.
- Stopping offending agent is a key step in treatment.

## ADDITIONAL READING
- Bellamy CJ, Kane-Gill SL, Falcione BA, et al. Neuroleptic malignant syndrome in traumatic brain injury patients treated with haloperidol. *J Trauma*. 2009;66:954–958.
- Marx JA, Hockberger RS, Walls RM, et al. *Rosen's Emergency Medicine: Concepts and Clinical Practice*, 7th ed. St. Louis, MO: Mosby; 2009.
- Seitz DP, Gill SS. Neuroleptic malignant syndrome complicating antipsychotic treatment of delirium or agitation in medical and surgical patients: Case reports and a review of the literature. *Psychosomatics*.2009;50:8–15.
- Stevens DL. Association between selective serotonin-reuptake inhibitors, second-generation antipsychotics, and neuroleptic malignant syndrome. *Ann Pharmacother*. 2008;42:1290–1297.

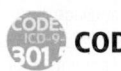 CODES

### ICD9
333.92 Neuroleptic malignant syndrome

# NEUROLEPTIC POISONING

*Timothy D. Heilenbach*

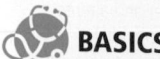 **BASICS**

## DESCRIPTION

- Neuroleptics (antipsychotics) used for management of:
  - Psychotic disorders
  - Agitation
  - Dementia in the elderly
  - Behavioral problems in children
  - Antiemetic
- Acute overdose:
  - Symptoms usually mild to moderate
  - CNS symptoms predominate
- Dystonic reactions (dystonia):
  - Most common adverse effect
  - Occurs during chronic therapy or within 48 hours of starting medication
- Akathisia:
  - Patient has motor restlessness and feels a need to pace or move constantly
  - Occurs within days to weeks of starting medication
- Neuroleptic malignant syndrome (NMS):
  - Idiosyncratic, life-threatening event
  - Occurs in cases of overdose, iatrogenic dose increase, and during the 1st weeks of usage
- Tardive dyskinesia:
  - Movement disorder usually affecting patients after years of taking neuroleptics
  - Treated by decreasing, discontinuing or changing the drug

## ETIOLOGY

- Typical neuroleptics (phenothiazines, butyrophenones) strongly antagonize dopaminergic receptors:
  - Haloperidol (Haldol)
  - Chlorpromazine (Thorazine)
  - Prochlorperazine (Compazine)
  - Thioridazine (Mellaril)
  - Fluphenazine (Prolixin)
  - Promethazine (Phenergan)
  - Droperidol (Inapsine)
  - Hydroxyzine (Atarax)

- Typical neuroleptics also have varying degrees of antagonism for histamine, acetylcholine, and adrenergic receptors.
- Atypical neuroleptics have weaker dopaminergic antagonism and moderate serotonergic antagonism:
  - Clozapine (Clozaril)
  - Risperidone (Risperdal)
  - Olanzapine (Zyprexa)
  - Quetiapine (Seroquel)
  - Ziprasidone (Geodon)

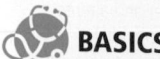 **DIAGNOSIS**

## SIGNS AND SYMPTOMS

- Acute overdose:
  - Peak levels at 4 hours
  - CNS:
    - Ranges from mild sedation to coma
    - Delirium possible (anticholinergic)
    - Extrapyramidal symptoms (dystonia, akathisia)
    - Seizures (clozapine)
  - Cardiovascular:
    - Tachycardia (anticholinergic)
    - Hypotension (antiadrenergic)
    - QT prolongation
    - Torsades de pointes
  - Respiratory:
    - Respiratory depression
  - GI:
    - Constipation
    - Dry mouth
  - Genitourinary:
    - Urinary retention
- Dystonic reactions:
  - Involuntary muscle spasms of face, neck, back, and limbs
  - Dramatic appearance is frightening to patient and family
  - Laryngeal dystonia is a rare form that may cause stridor and dyspnea.

- NMS:
  - Hyperthermia
  - Skeletal muscle rigidity
  - Altered mental status
  - Autonomic dysfunction
  - Rhabdomyolysis
- Agranulocytosis:
  - Seen with clozapine and olanzapine
  - Occurs in the 1st few months of treatment
- Diabetes:
  - Hyperglycemia, new-onset diabetes, and DKA have all been reported with initiation of neuroleptics.

## ESSENTIAL WORKUP

- Monitor vital signs with significant ingestions.
- Cardiac monitor
- Pulse oximetry

## DIAGNOSTIC TESTS & INTERPRETATION
### *Lab*

- Electrolytes, BUN, creatinine, glucose
- CBC for clozapine overdose
- Urinalysis:
  - Dip for myoglobin if rhabdomyolysis suspected
- Creatine phosphokinase (CPK) levels if NMS suspected, agitation, or prolonged immobilization
- Urine toxicologic screen to exclude coingestants
- Quantitative levels are rarely helpful.

### *Imaging*

- EKG:
  - QT prolongation
  - Conduction disturbances
- Head CT:
  - Indicated for significant mental status change

## DIFFERENTIAL DIAGNOSIS

- Antidepressant overdose
- Antihistamine overdose
- Cocaine overdose
- Amphetamine overdose
- MDMA overdose
- Opioid overdose
- Occult head injury
- Endocrine disorder
- Sepsis

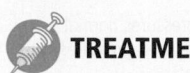 TREATMENT

### PRE-HOSPITAL
Bring medication bottles when transporting patient to hospital.

### INITIAL STABILIZATION/THERAPY
Airway, breathing, and circulation management (ABCs):

- Administer supplemental oxygen.
- Administer naloxone, thiamine, D$_{50}$ (or Accu-Chek) for altered mental status.
- Intubate if respiratory depression.

### ED TREATMENT/PROCEDURES
- Supportive care
- Decontamination:
  - Administer single dose of activated charcoal if recent ingestion.
- Hypotension:
  - 0.9% normal saline (NS) IV fluid bolus
  - Trendelenburg
  - Treat resistant hypotension with norepinephrine or phenylephrine.
  - Dopamine may be ineffective.
- Ventricular dysrhythmias:
  - Avoid class 1a antidysrhythmics: Potential exacerbation of QT prolongation. Magnesium for prolonged QT
  - Cardioversion if hemodynamically unstable

- Dystonic reactions:
  - Administer diphenhydramine or benztropine mesylate.
  - Treatment should be continued for 3 days to prevent recurrence.
- NMS:
  - Recognition and cessation of neuroleptics is critical.
  - Active cooling for hyperthermia
  - Consider dantrolene (a direct acting muscle relaxant ) or bromocriptine (dopamine agonist) for severe cases.
- Seizures:
  - Treat initially with diazepam or lorazepam.
  - Phenobarbital for persistent seizures

### MEDICATION
- Activated charcoal: 1–2 g/kg PO
- Benztropine mesylate: 1–2 mg IV or PO
- Bromocriptine: 2.5–10 mg q8h PO
- Dantrolene: 1–2 mg/kg q10min IV (10 mg/kg max.)
- Diazepam: 5 mg IV
- Diphenhydramine: 25–50 mg IV (1 mg/kg)
- Lorazepam: 2–4 mg (peds: 0.03–0.05 mg/kg) IV q10–15min
- Magnesium sulfate: 1–2 g IV over 5–15 minutes
- Norepinephrine: 1–2 $\mu$q/kg/min IV titrate to blood pressure (BP)
- Phenobarbital: 10–20 mg/kg IV (loading dose)

 FOLLOW-UP

### DISPOSITION

#### Admission Criteria
- Admit overdose with CNS sedation, agitation, dysrhythmias, or vital sign abnormalities to monitored bed.
- Admit if neuroleptic results in new-onset diabetes with severe hyperglycemia and/or ketoacidosis.

#### Discharge Criteria
Asymptomatic after 6 hours of observation

#### Issues for Referral
- Patients with unintentional (accidental) poisoning require poison prevention counseling.

- Patients with intentional (eg, suicide) poisoning require psychiatric evaluation.
- New-onset diabetes requires primary care/endocrine follow-up.

### FOLLOW-UP RECOMMENDATIONS
- Psychiatric referral for intentional overdoses
- Primary care follow-up for accidental ingestions or medication side-effect follow-up.

## PEARLS AND PITFALLS

- Neuroleptics represent a group of drugs with diverse indications and a wide range of toxicity.
- Most overdoses are mild, and CNS depression predominates.
- Dystonic reactions are the most common side effect of neuroleptics. These reactions are dramatic in appearance but easily treatable.
- NMS is a poorly understood, potentially fatal reaction that can be seen in acute or chronic usage of neuroleptics.

## ADDITIONAL READING

- Lipscombe LL. Antipsychotic drugs and hyperglycemia in older patients with diabetes. *Arch Intern Med*. 2009;169:1282–1289.
- Ngo A. Acute quetiapine overdose in adults: A 5 year retrospective case series. *Ann Emerg Med*. 2008;52:541.
- Reulbach U. Managing an effective treatment for neuroleptic malignant syndrome. *Crit Care*. 2007;11:R4.
- Wittler MA. Antipsychotics. In *Marx: Rosen's emergency medicine*, 7th ed. St. Louis: Mosby, 2009.

 CODES

### ICD9
969.3 Poisoning by other antipsychotics, neuroleptics, and major tranquilizers

# NONCARDIOGENIC PULMONARY EDEMA
*David Jerrard*

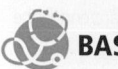 **BASICS**

## DESCRIPTION
- Functional disruption of the capillary–alveolar membrane from a noncardiac source
- Diffuse injury to either the alveolar epithelium or to the vascular endothelium
- Pulmonary parenchymal changes mimic CHF:
  – Cephalad redistribution of blood flow, pulmonary effusions, and cardiomegaly do *not* develop.
- Typically, onset of this edema is within 1–2 hours of noxious insult.
- First described by William Osler in 1889 in a patient "poisoned" by morphine.
- ~250,000 cases occur each year in the U.S.
- Cause of capillary leak or alveolar membrane damage is uncertain.
- Proposed mechanisms include hypoxia, immunologic effects, or direct toxic effects.

## ETIOLOGY
- Smoke inhalation
- Salicylate intoxication
- Toxic gas inhalation
- Transfusion reaction
- Near drowning
- Disseminated intravascular coagulation
- High-altitude pulmonary edema (HAPE)
- Radiation pneumonitis
- Narcotic abuse
- HCTZ
- Uremia
- Cardiopulmonary bypass
- Major trauma
- Aspiration
- Bacterial pneumonia

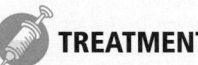 **DIAGNOSIS**

## SIGNS AND SYMPTOMS
- Fatigue
- Weakness
- Anxiety
- Shortness of breath
- Cough
- Malaise

### Physical Exam
- Tachycardia:
  – Characteristically seen secondary to decreasing $PO_2$ levels
- Scattered rhonchi and rales
- Dyspnea
- Tachypnea
- Cyanosis
- Pink, frothy sputum
- The stigmas of left- and right-sided heart failure will *not* be found.

## ESSENTIAL WORKUP
- History and physical to identify severity and determine underlying etiology
- The CXR is essential in confirming the diagnosis and in assessing severity.

## DIAGNOSTIC TESTS & INTERPRETATION
### Lab
- General lab abnormalities are not specific to noncardiogenic pulmonary edema.
- Serum protein levels:
  – Hypoproteinemia may be useful for differentiating permeability-induced pulmonary edema (noncardiogenic) from cardiogenic pulmonary edema.
- Interleukin-8 level in lung lavage washings:
  – Rapid increase in the early stages of acute lung injury before full development of acute respiratory distress syndrome
  – Elevated BNP levels indicate cardiac cause

### Imaging
CXR:
- Initially normal
- Classic butterfly pattern of pulmonary edema
- Unilateral patchy infiltrates resembling pneumonia
- Lack of cardiomegaly

### Diagnostic Procedures/Surgery
Pulmonary artery catheter:
- Pulmonary capillary wedge pressures normal or near-normal in contrast to elevated pressures with cardiogenic pulmonary edema

## DIFFERENTIAL DIAGNOSIS
- Cardiogenic pulmonary edema
- Chronic obstructive pulmonary disease exacerbation
- Pulmonary embolus
- Restrictive lung disease
- Pneumonia

**TREATMENT**

## PRE-HOSPITAL
- Patent airway
- Adequate oxygenation
- Cautions:
  – Patients will not typically respond to usual measures to treat CHF.

## INITIAL STABILIZATION/THERAPY
- Supplemental oxygen (high-flow oxygen)
- IV catheter
- Continuous cardiac monitor
- Continuous pulse oximetry

## ED TREATMENT/PROCEDURES

- The treatment of noncardiogenic pulmonary edema (NCPE) is supportive.
- NCPE associated with drug overdose usually responds to high-flow $O_2$.
- Diuretics are *not* used.
- Removal of trigger that may have caused NCPE:
  - Noxious gas
  - Having patient descend from elevation in cases of HAPE. Sildenafil has shown promise in the prevention and acute treatment of altitude-induced NCPE
- Noninvasive ventilatory support (BiPAP, CPAP) may be used if immediately available:
  - Measure blood gases frequently.
  - If unable to provide adequate oxygenation or ventilation, intubation is required
  - Useful in NCPE caused by drug overdose
- Endotracheal intubation is often necessary:
  - Positive end-expiratory pressure (PEEP) of 5–10 cm $H_2O$
    - NCPE of a neurogenic etiology has a worsened prognosis when PEEP is employed.
  - Improves oxygenation
  - Decreases work of breathing
  - To reduce the likelihood of atelectasis, tidal volumes should be on order of 12–15 mL/kg.
  - Initially place on 100% $O_2$:
    - Measure $PO_2$ and decrease $FIO_2$ accordingly.
- Steroids and cyclooxygenase inhibitors have not been proven effective.

## FOLLOW-UP

### DISPOSITION
#### Admission Criteria
All symptomatic patients should be admitted to ICU:

- Symptoms may worsen at any point for up to 3 days after noxious insult.

#### Discharge Criteria
Asymptomatic patients (especially narcotic overdose, HAPE, or aspiration):

- Observe in ED for 6–12 hours and then discharge with close follow-up scheduled if no evidence of pulmonary edema is present and adequate oxygenation is demonstrated.

### FOLLOW-UP RECOMMENDATIONS
Patients, when discharged from the hospital, should seek medical follow-up within 48 hours.

## PEARLS AND PITFALLS

- Utilizing diuretics in the acute setting may worsen patient condition.
- Failure to distinguish between cardiac and noncardiac etiologies is a pitfall, as treatment is different.

## ADDITIONAL READING

- Fagenholz PJ, Gutman JA, Murray AF, et al. Treatment of high altitude pulmonary edema at 4240 m in Nepal. *High Alt Med Biol*. 2007;8(2): 139–146.
- Macias DJ, Brillman JC. Adult respiratory distress syndrome. In: Harwood-Nuss A, Linden C, Luten R, et al., eds. *The clinical practice of emergency medicine*, 2nd ed. Philadelphia: JB Lippincott, 1996:640–643.
- McIntyre RC Jr. Thirty years of clinical trials in acute respiratory distress syndrome. *Crit Care Med*. 2000;28(9):3314–3331.
- Perina DG. Noncardiogenic pulmonary edema. *Emerg Med Clin North Am*. 2003;21(2):385–393.
- Richalat JP, Gratadour P, Robach P, et al. Sildenafil inhibits altitude-induced hypoxemia and pulmonary HTN. *Am J Respir Crit Care Med*. 2005;171(3): 275–281.

## CODES

### ICD9
- 508.8 Respiratory conditions due to other specified external agents
- 508.9 Respiratory conditions due to unspecified external agent
- 518.4 Acute edema of lung, unspecified

N

# NONSTEROIDAL ANTI-INFLAMMATORY POISONING

*Michele Zell-Kanter*

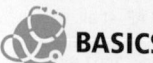 **BASICS**

## DESCRIPTION
- Inhibit cyclo-oxygenase (COX), thereby blocking the conversion of arachidonic acid to prostaglandin.
- Typically, ingestion of an NSAID is benign.
- Fatalities have been reported with large ingestions.
- Greater potential for toxicity with underlying CHF or renal failure:
  - NSAIDs cause sodium and water retention and decrease renal blood flow.
  - Little overdose experience with the COX-2 inhibitors (celecoxib); treatment should be the same as for the traditional NSAIDs.
  - Patients may ingest rofecoxib and valdecoxib from stored supplies even though both are no longer available.

## ETIOLOGY
- Nonsteroidal medications are available by prescription and over the counter.
- NSAID include:
  - Ibuprofen
  - Naproxen
  - Ketoprofen
  - Ketorolac
  - Indomethacin
  - Meclofenamate
  - Phenylbutazone

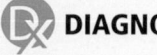 **DIAGNOSIS**

## SIGNS AND SYMPTOMS
- GI:
  - Nausea
  - Vomiting
  - Epigastric pain
- CNS:
  - Drowsiness
  - Dizziness
  - Lethargy
  - Seizures
- Cardiovascular:
  - Hypotension
  - Tachycardia
- Pulmonary:
  - Eosinophilic pneumonia
  - Apnea
  - Hyperventilation
- Renal:
  - Acute renal failure
  - Acute tubular necrosis
  - Acute interstitial nephritis
- Liver:
  - Hepatocellular injury
  - Cholestatic jaundice
- Metabolic:
  - Mild, short-lived metabolic acidosis
- Hypersensitivity:
  - Aseptic meningitis
  - Asthma exacerbation

## ESSENTIAL WORKUP
- Generally, NSAID ingestion results in mild toxicity.
- Exact identification of drug helpful:
  - Subtle toxicologic differences among the NSAIDs

## DIAGNOSTIC TESTS & INTERPRETATION
### Lab
- Electrolytes, BUN/creatinine, glucose:
  - Baseline renal function
  - Check for metabolic acidosis.
- CBC
- Arterial blood gas for large overdoses
- Prothrombin time and partial thromboplastin time:
  - False-positive bilirubin/ketone dipstick with etodolac ingestion
- Acetaminophen and salicylate level
- NSAID difficult to detect on toxicology screens

## DIFFERENTIAL DIAGNOSIS
Agents causing metabolic acidosis, altered mental status, and GI irritation:
- Salicylates
- Isoniazid
- Ethylene glycol
- Methanol
- Isopropanol

**TREATMENT**

**PRE-HOSPITAL**
Collect prescription bottles/medications for identification in the ED.

**INITIAL STABILIZATION/THERAPY**
- ABCs
- Naloxone, thiamine, dextrose (or Accu-Chek) for altered mental status

**ED TREATMENT/PROCEDURES**
- Supportive care and GI decontamination
- Administer activated charcoal.
- Extracorporeal methods to enhance elimination are not beneficial due to high degree of plasma protein binding.

**MEDICATION**
- Activated charcoal slurry: 1–2 g/kg up to 90 g PO
- Dextrose: D50W 1 amp (50 mL or 25 g; peds: D25W 2–4 mL/kg) IV
- Naloxone (Narcan): 2 mg (peds: 0.1 mg/kg) IV or IM initial dose
- Thiamine (vitamin $B_1$): 100 mg (peds: 50 mg) IV or IM

*Pediatric Considerations*
Piroxicam, naproxen, ketoprofen, and mefenamic acid have caused seizures in children.

 **FOLLOW-UP**

**DISPOSITION**
*Admission Criteria*
- Protracted vomiting, hematemesis
- CNS depression, seizure activity
- Metabolic acidosis
- CHF, hypotension, hypertension
- Renal failure

*Discharge Criteria*
Nontoxic ingestion in a patient who is asymptomatic 6–8 hr after ingestion

**FOLLOW-UP RECOMMENDATIONS**
Psychiatry follow-up/referral for intentional ingestion.

## PEARLS AND PITFALLS

- Investigate for coingestions for all NSAID overdoses.
- Obtain acetaminophen level on all patients who present with suspected NSAID ingestion.
- NSAID poisoning is generally benign, except with massive overdoses.

## ADDITIONAL READING

- Dajani EZ, Islam K. Cardiovascular and gastrointestinal toxicity of selective cyclo-oxygenase-2 inhibitors in man. *J Physiol Pharmacol*. 2008;59(suppl 2):117–133.
- Halen PK, Murumkar PR, Giridhar R, et al. Prodrug designing of NSAIDs. *Minirev Med Chem*.2009;9: 124–139.
- Seifert SA, Bronstein AC, McGuire TH. Massive ibuprofen ingestion with survival. *J Toxicol Clin Toxicol*. 2000;38:55–57.
- Zuckerman GB, Uy CC. Shock, metabolic acidosis, and coma following ibuprofen overdose in a child. *Ann Pharmacother*. 1995;29:869–871.

 **CODES**

**ICD9**
965.9 Poisoning by unspecified analgesic and antipyretic

N

# NURSEMAID'S ELBOW

*Neha P. Raukar*
*Daniel L. Savitt*

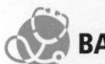 **BASICS**

## DESCRIPTION
The most common elbow injury in children <5 yr old

## ETIOLOGY
- Sudden traction of the distal radius leads to a portion of the annular ligament slipping over the radial head and becoming trapped between the radius and the capitellum.
- By the time the child is 5, the annular ligament is thick and strong and resists tearing and/or displacement.

 **DIAGNOSIS**

## SIGNS AND SYMPTOMS
- Child refuses to use arm.
- Elbow is slightly flexed, with forearm held close to the trunk.
- Pain with flexion of the elbow
- Pain with forearm supination or pronation
- Absence of point tenderness
- Minimal to no swelling

### History
- Child not using affected arm
- 50% report the classic history of pulling the arm.
- Can also be due to a fall, minor trauma to the elbow, or twisting of the forearm
- In children <6 mo, can be due to the child rolling onto the arm.

### Physical Exam
- Affected arm is held close to the body.
- Arm is usually pronated.
- Elbow is either fully extended or slightly flexed.
- Child will not use the elbow.
- Can be mildly tender over anterolateral radial head, but the rest of the elbow is nontender.
- Painless passive range of motion
- Painful with supination

## ESSENTIAL WORKUP
Clinical diagnosis:
- Classic history, passive position of arm, and physical exam are sufficient for diagnosis.

## DIAGNOSTIC TESTS & INTERPRETATION
Imaging:
Radiographs:
- Not routinely indicated
- Obtain to exclude or diagnose other injuries if any of the following are present:
  - Point tenderness
  - Soft tissue swelling
  - Deformity
  - Ecchymosis of the elbow
  - Failed reduction
  - Child continues to favor extremity after reduction maneuver.

## DIFFERENTIAL DIAGNOSIS
- Humerus, radius, or ulna fracture
- Elbow dislocation
- Joint infection
- Osteomyelitis
- Tumor

 **TREATMENT**

## PRE-HOSPITAL
Cautions:
- Place ice on the injured elbow to reduce pain and swelling.
- Immobilize in a sling or splint to facilitate transport and prevent further injury.
- Assess distal neurovascular status.

## INITIAL STABILIZATION/THERAPY
Assess distal motor, sensory, and vascular function.

## ED TREATMENT/PROCEDURES
- 2 common reduction techniques:
  - Supination/flexion:
    ○ More commonly used
  - Hyperpronation/extension:
    ○ Nurses and caretakers perceive this method to be less painful
    ○ More successful
- Supination/flexion technique:
  - Grasp child's hand in handshake position and apply mild axial traction.
  - Stabilize injured elbow with the other hand with the thumb over the radial head exerting moderate pressure.
  - In one smooth, swift motion, fully supinate the forearm and flex the elbow.
- Hyperpronation/extension technique:
  - Grasp child's hand in handshake position and apply mild axial traction.
  - Stabilize injured elbow with the other hand with the thumb over the radial head exerting moderate pressure.
  - Hyperpronate the arm and extend if arm is not already extended.

- Placing the examiner's thumb over the radial head may allow palpation of a click.
- Child may cry during the reduction, but is frequently pain free and using the arm shortly thereafter.
- Attempt reduction a 2nd time if the child does not use arm 15 min after 1st attempt.
- One of the attempts should be the hyperpronation method.
- Consider opposing technique for 2nd reduction attempt.
- Radiographic studies indicated if the 2nd reduction attempt is unsuccessful, to evaluate for fractures.
- Perform postreduction neurovascular assessment.

## MEDICATION
- Usually unnecessary
- Acetaminophen: 15 mg/kg PO q4h
- Ibuprofen 10 mg/kg PO q6h–q8h

 **FOLLOW-UP**

## DISPOSITION
### Admission Criteria
None

### Discharge Criteria
- Discharge to home after child regains full, unrestricted use of the arm.
- Patient instructions:
  – Inform parents not to pull or lift the child by the hand, wrist, or forearm.
  – Recurrence rate of 27–39% until the child reaches 5 yr of age.

### Issues for Referral
Unsuccessful reduction:
- If radiologic evaluation is also negative, child should be referred to an orthopedist.
- Place arm in a sling or a posterior splint for outpatient follow-up.
- No long-term sequelae have been reported with unreduced nursemaid's elbow.

## FOLLOW-UP RECOMMENDATIONS
- None required for successful reduction
- Orthopedics within 24 hr for unsuccessful reduction

## PEARLS AND PITFALLS
- Suspect nursemaid's elbow with a classic history.
- Radiographs are not necessary unless the elbow is focally tender or swollen or history does not suggest nursemaid's elbow.
- Reduction attempt should include the hyperpronation method.
- 2 unsuccessful reductions should prompt radiographic evaluation.

- Unsuccessful reductions should be referred to the orthopedist after the arm is placed in a sling or posterior splint.

## ADDITIONAL READING
- Bachman D, Santora S. Orthopedic trauma. In: Fleisher GR, Ludwig S, Henretig FM, eds. *Textbook of Pediatric Emergency Medicine*, 5th ed. Philadelphia: Lippincott Williams & Wilkins; 2006:1525.
- Green DA, Linares MY, Garcia Pena BM, et al. Randomized comparison of pain perception during radial head subluxation reduction using supination-flexion or forced pronation. *Pediatr Emerg Care*. 2006;22:235.
- Macias CG, Wiebe R, Bothner J. History and radiographic findings associated with clinically suspected radial head subluxations. *Pediatr Emerg Care*. 2000;16(1):22–25.

 **CODES**

### ICD9
832.2 Nursemaid's elbow

# OCULOMOTOR NERVE PALSY

James M. Leaming
Spencer A. Adoff

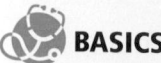 **BASICS**

## DESCRIPTION

- Cranial nerve (CN) III controls 7 ocular muscles:
  - Lesions categorized as:
  - Complete vs. incomplete
  - Pupil involving vs. pupil sparing
- Complete: total loss of CN III function ("down and out"):
  - Compressive lesions:
    ○ Aneurysms
    ○ Tumors
    ○ Brainstem herniation with compression
    ○ Increased intracranial pressure
- Incomplete: partial loss of CN III function:
  - Vascular infarction of vasa vasorum
- Pupil involving:
  - 95–97% of compressive lesions (aneurysm, tumor, etc.) involve the pupil.
- Pupil sparing:
  - Ischemic injury to nerve
  - Diabetics, uncontrolled hypertension

## ETIOLOGY

- Intracranial or orbital tumor
- Aneurysm (particularly posterior communicating artery)
- Trauma
- Intracranial hemorrhage
- Diabetes mellitus
- Migraine headache
- Infection, meningitis
- Arteriovenous malformation or fistula
- Cavernous sinus thrombosis
- Neuropathy (eg, myasthenia gravis, Guillain-Barré)
- Collagen vascular diseases (eg, sarcoidosis)
- Idiopathic

### Pediatric Considerations

Trauma is most common cause of acquired oculomotor nerve palsies.

## DIAGNOSIS

### SIGNS AND SYMPTOMS

A careful history and physical exam are vital to narrow down the differential diagnosis.

### History

History is of utmost importance in determining cause:

- Headache
- Pupillary dilation
- Eye pain
- Diplopia
- Blurry vision
- History of longstanding diabetes mellitus
- Head trauma, either recent or distant
- Unintentional weight loss
- Signs and symptoms of infection
- Sudden onset of severe headache, meningeal signs, photophobia

### Physical Exam

- Ophthalmologic exam:
  - Extraocular movements
  - Fundoscopic exam for papilledema
  - Ipsilateral and contralateral pupillary reaction
  - Ptosis
  - Diplopia
  - Chemosis or conjunctival injection
  - Tenderness
  - Visual acuity
  - Exophthalmos
- CN III functions:
  - Pupillary constrictor:
    ○ Miosis
  - Ciliary muscles:
    ○ Accommodation
  - Levator palpebrae superioris:
    ○ Open eyelid
  - Superior rectus:
    ○ Superolateral gaze
  - Inferior rectus:
    ○ Inferolateral gaze
  - Inferior oblique:
    ○ Superomedial gaze
  - Medial rectus:
    ○ Adduction

- Look for associated symptoms:
  - Extremity weakness
  - Changes in speech
  - Dysfunction of other cranial nerves
  - Gait or coordination

### ESSENTIAL WORKUP

CT/MRI of brain, orbit, sinuses

### DIAGNOSTIC TESTS & INTERPRETATION

#### Lab

When indicated based on history and exam:

- CBC with differential
- ESR
- Antinuclear antibodies, rheumatoid factor to evaluate for vasculitis
- Lumbar puncture

#### Imaging

- MRI brain and cerebral vessels
- CT angiogram
- Cerebral arteriogram: has associated risk of neurologic morbidity and mortality.
- Doppler imaging for arteriovenous malformations, dural sinus thrombosis

#### Diagnostic Procedures/Surgery

- Intraocular pressure to exclude glaucoma
- Slit-lamp exam:
  - Observe structural abnormalities of iris or anterior chamber

### DIFFERENTIAL DIAGNOSIS

- Intracranial infections
- Malignancy
- Vasculitis
- Aneurysms
- Myasthenia gravis
- Botulism
- Orbital infections
- Trauma
- Lens pathology
- Retinal pathology
- Glaucoma
- MS

### Pediatric Considerations

Consider congenital oculomotor nerve palsy.

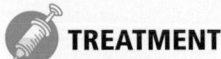 **TREATMENT**

## PRE-HOSPITAL

Without associated trauma, no specific pre-hospital care issues exist.

## INITIAL STABILIZATION/THERAPY

- Initial stabilization of posttraumatic patient should concentrate on underlying traumatic condition.
- Any patient with evidence of herniation should have the following measures to control intracranial pressure:
  – Intubation using rapid-sequence induction and controlled ventilation to a $PCO_2$ level of 35–40 mm Hg
  – Elevate head of bed 30°.
  – Mannitol

## ED TREATMENT/PROCEDURES

- Differentiation between incomplete and complete oculomotor or pupil-involving vs. pupil-sparing nerve palsy guides focus of ED treatment.
- If pupil is involved, neuroimaging is indicated as well as consultation to determine cause.
- If pupil is spared and the patient has diabetes or other risk for an ischemic 3rd nerve, discharge is likely reasonable with outpatient follow-up:
  – If partial sparing or patient does not have these risk factors, consultation and neuroimaging is indicated.
- Medication regimen determined by cause:
  – Aneurysm:
    ○ Control severe HTN.
    ○ Decrease intracranial pressure with intubation.
    ○ Controlled ventilation
    ○ Elevation of head
    ○ Mannitol

– Intracranial tumor: Control increasing intracranial pressure as above.
– Inflammation and edema: Decrease with IV steroids.
– Meningitis:
  ○ Rapid administration of IV antibiotics
  ○ IV steroids may be useful to decrease inflammatory response and edema.
– Vasculitis and collagen vascular diseases: Decrease inflammatory cell infiltration with IV steroids.
– Neuropathy: Myasthenia gravis—edrophonium chloride test
- Neurosurgical consult as appropriate

## MEDICATION

- Ceftriaxone: 1–2 g (peds: 50–100 mg/kg) IV
- Dexamethasone: 10 mg IV (peds: 0.15–0.5 mg/kg IV single dose in ED)
- Edrophonium chloride: 5–8 mg IV (peds: 0.15 mg/kg IV; 1/10 test dose given first)
- Mannitol: 1 g/kg IV (peds: not routinely recommended)
- Methylprednisolone: adults/peds: 1–2 mg/kg IV single dose in ED

 **FOLLOW-UP**

## DISPOSITION

### Admission Criteria

- Complete oculomotor nerve palsy of any cause requires admission and emergency neurosurgical evaluation.
- Incomplete oculomotor nerve palsy with abnormal CT or MRI, abnormal laboratory studies, or other focal neurologic or constitutional symptoms should receive prompt neurologic consult and imaging.

### Discharge Criteria

- Incomplete oculomotor nerve palsy with negative CT or MRI, normal laboratory studies, and no other symptoms can be referred for urgent outpatient neurologic evaluation.
- Complete pupil-sparing oculomotor palsy in patients with risk factors for microvascular disease (ie, diabetic) can receive outpatient neurologic workup.

## FOLLOW-UP RECOMMENDATIONS

If the patient is being discharged, prompt neurologic follow-up is required

## PEARLS AND PITFALLS

- Complete lesions must be assessed rapidly.
- If the pupil is involved, compressive lesions are often the cause.

## ADDITIONAL READING

- Chen CC, Pai YM, Wang RF, et al. Isolated oculomotor nerve palsy from minor head trauma. *Br J Sports Med*. 2005;39(8):e34.
- Woodruff MM, Edlow JA. Evaluation of third nerve palsy in the emergency department. *J Emerg Med*. 2008;35:239–246.

 **CODES**

### ICD9

- 378.51 Third or oculomotor nerve palsy, partial
- 378.52 Third or oculomotor nerve palsy, total

# OPIATE POISONING

*Mark B. Mycyk*
*Amy V. Kontrick*

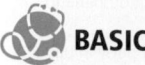 **BASICS**

## DESCRIPTION

- Bind to $\mu$, $\kappa$, and $\delta$ opiate receptors in the central nervous system (CNS) and peripheral nervous system (PNS)
- Physical and psychological dependence occurs.
- Peak plasma levels:
  - PO: 1–2 hr
  - Intramuscular: 0.5–1 hr
  - Intravenous or intranasal: seconds to minutes

## ETIOLOGY

- Overuse or abuse of oral prescription analgesics for moderate to severe pain
- Street preparations of narcotic analogs may contain adulterants:
  - Cocaine
  - Clenbuterol
  - Phencyclidine
  - Strychnine
  - Dextromethorphan
  - Quinine
  - Scopolamine

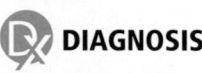 **DIAGNOSIS**

## SIGNS AND SYMPTOMS

- CNS:
  - CNS depression
  - Coma
  - Seizures
- GI:
  - Nausea
  - Vomiting
  - Constipation
- Cardiovascular:
  - Hypotension
  - Bradycardia
  - Palpitations
- Pulmonary:
  - Respiratory depression
  - Bronchospasm
  - Pulmonary edema
  - Apnea
- Other:
  - Miosis
  - Hypothermia
- Withdrawal:
  - HTN
  - Tachycardia
  - Tachypnea
  - Abdominal cramps
  - Diarrhea
  - Piloerection
  - Yawning

### Pediatric Considerations

- Neonatal withdrawal:
  - Infants born to addicted mothers
  - Onset: 12–72 hr after birth
  - Irritability, tremors, poor feeding, and dehydration
- Diphenoxylate (Lomotil): Toxicity more severe in children than adults and may be fatal

## ESSENTIAL WORKUP

Monitor vital signs and pulmonary status with significant exposure:

- Pulse oximetry or arterial blood gases
- CXR if persistent hypoxia or possible aspiration
- Abdominal radiograph if body packing suspected
- Perform a complete exam for occult sticky patches (eg, fentanyl).

## DIAGNOSTIC TESTS & INTERPRETATION
### Lab

- Plasma opiate levels not clinically useful:
  - Treatment based on clinical presentation, not opiate level
- Urine toxicity screen for opioids may not identify some synthetic opioids (eg, methadone).
- Acetaminophen level for overuse or abuse of oral prescription analgesic products

## DIFFERENTIAL DIAGNOSIS

- Clonidine overdose
- Barbiturate overdose
- Benzodiazepine overdose
- $\gamma$-Hydroxybutyrate overdose
- Neuroleptic overdose
- Occult head injury

 **TREATMENT**

## PRE-HOSPITAL

- Transport all pills/pill bottles involved in overdose for identification in ED.
- Provide respiratory support.
- Administer naloxone.

## INITIAL STABILIZATION/THERAPY

- Check ABCs:
  - Airway control is essential.
  - Administer supplemental oxygen.
- Administer naloxone:
  - Reverses respiratory depression and coma in opiate overdoses
  - Intubate if naloxone does not reverse respiratory depression.

## ED TREATMENT/PROCEDURES

- Naloxone administration:
  - Start with low doses for opiate-habituated patients.
  - High doses (10 mg) may be required to reverse the effects of propoxyphene, methadone, and fentanyl.
  - Administer repeated doses that reversed symptoms, as needed every 20–60 min.
  - For long-acting opioids, consider an hourly infusion of 2/3 the dose needed to reverse symptoms.

- Decontamination:
  - Administer activated charcoal for oral ingestion.
  - Administer whole-bowel irrigation with polyethylene glycol for asymptomatic body packers.
- Treat opiate withdrawal with clonidine or methadone.
- Hypotension:
  - 0.9% normal saline IV fluid bolus
  - Trendelenburg test
  - Initiate dopamine for resistant hypotension.
- Seizures:
  - Treat initially with diazepam.
  - Administer phenobarbital for persistent seizures.

## MEDICATION

- Activated charcoal: 1–2 g/kg PO
- Clonidine: 0.1–0.3 mg PO b.i.d. for 10 days; 0.1–0.2 mg/kg/d transdermal patch
- Diazepam: 5–10 mg IV (peds: 0.2–0.5 mg/kg IV) q10–15min
- Dopamine: 2–20 mg/kg/min; titrate to effect.
- Methadone: 15–40 mg/d
- Naloxone: 0.4–2 mg (peds: 0.1 mg/kg; neonates: 10–30 mg/kg) IV or IM
- Phenobarbital: 10–20 mg/kg IV (loading dose)
- Polyethylene glycol: 2 L/hr until clear rectal effluent and/or passage of packets

### ALERT
Opioid patches can be abused in various ways (transdermally, orally, smoked, injected). Even used patches still contain a significant dose of drug.

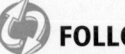 **FOLLOW-UP**

### DISPOSITION
#### *Admission Criteria*
- Symptomatic after oral overdose
- Repeated naloxone dosing or infusion needed to reverse symptoms
- Children <5 yr postdiphenoxylate ingestion should be observed for 24 hr.
- Opiate body packers
- Persistent symptoms from concomitant toxin exposure (eg, clenbuterol)

#### *Discharge Criteria*
- Asymptomatic 6 hr after oral overdose
- Asymptomatic 4 hr after naloxone administration
- Complete elimination of opiate packets

### FOLLOW-UP RECOMMENDATIONS
- Substance abuse referral for patients with oral narcotic abuse.
- Patients with unintentional (accidental) poisoning require poison prevention counseling.
- Patients with intentional (eg, suicide) poisoning require psychiatric evaluation.

## PEARLS AND PITFALLS

- Consider occult acetaminophen poisoning in chronic oral narcotic–abusing patients.
- Buprenorphine may cause prolonged sedation in pediatric patients.
- Semisynthetic and synthetic opioids will not provide a positive opiate hospital drug screen result.

## ADDITIONAL READING

- Bailey JE, Campagna E, Dart RC, et al. The underrecognized toll of prescription opioid abuse in young children. *Ann Emerg Med*. 2009;53(4): 419–424.
- Coon TP, Miller M, Kaylor D, et al. Rectal insertion of fentanyl patches: A new route of toxicity. *Ann Emerg Med*. 2005;46(5):473.
- Hoffman RS, Kirrane BM, Marcus SM, et al. A descriptive study of an outbreak of clenbuterol-containing heroin. *Ann Emerg Med*. 2008;52(5): 548–553.
- Kelly AM, Kerr D, Dietze P, et al. Randomised trial of intranasal versus intramuscular naloxone in prehospital treatment for suspected opioid overdose. *Med J Aust*. 2005;182(1):24–27.
- Kleinschmidt KC, Wainscott M, Ford MD. Opioids. In: Ford MD, Delaney KA, Ling LJ, et al., eds. *Clinical Toxicology*. Philadelphia: WB Saunders; 2001: 637–639.
- Sporer KA. Acute heroin overdose. *Ann Intern Med*. 1999;130:584–590.

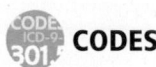 **CODES**

### ICD9
965.00 Poisoning by opium (alkaloids), unspecified

# OPPORTUNISTIC INFECTION

Colleen M. Birmingham
Jennifer V. Pope

 **BASICS**

## DESCRIPTION
Unusual infections that occur when host suffers a decrease in resistance against normally nonpathogenic organisms

## ETIOLOGY
- Occurs in HIV patients when the CD4 T-lymphocyte count falls below 200 cells/mm$^3$ or <14% of the total lymphocyte count:
  – *Pneumocystis jiroveci* pneumonia (PCP)
  – Cryptococcal infection
  – Disseminated tuberculosis
  – Cryptosporidiosis
  – Microsporidiosis
  – Isosporiasis
  – Toxoplasmosis
  – Histoplasmosis
  – Cryptococcosis
  – *Mycobacterium avium* complex
  – Tuberculosis pericarditis or meningitis
  – Cytomegalovirus
  – Human herpesvirus-8 (Kaposi sarcoma)
  – JC virus (progressive multifocal leukoencephalopathy)
  – Bacterial species
- Cell-mediated deficiency:
  – Hematologic malignancies
  – Lymphoma
  – High-dose glucocorticoid therapy
  – Autoimmune disorders
  – Viral infections
  – Cytotoxic drugs/chemotherapy
  – Radiation therapy
  – Associated with:
    ○ *Legionella*
    ○ *Nocardia*
    ○ *Salmonella*
    ○ *Mycobacteria*
- Neutrophil impairment/depletion:
  – Cytotoxic drugs
  – Aplastic anemia
  – Drug reactions:
    ○ Dapsone
  – Neoplastic invasion of bone marrow
  – Arsenic
  – Penicillin
  – Chloramphenicol
  – Procainamide
  – Vitamin deficiencies
  – Associated with:
    ○ *Staphylococcus* and $\alpha$-hemolytic *Streptococcus*
    ○ Enteric organisms and anaerobes
    ○ Invasive aspergillosis

 **DIAGNOSIS**

## SIGNS AND SYMPTOMS
- New or worsening fatigue
- Tachypnea
- Fever
- Chills
- Night sweats
- Pulmonary source of infection:
  – Cough
  – Congestion
  – Rales
- Genitourinary source of infection:
  – Dysuria
  – Increased frequency
  – Urinary retention
- GI source of infection:
  – Abdominal pain
  – Vomiting
  – Diarrhea
  – Bleeding
  – Jaundice
- CNS sources of infection:
  – Confusion
  – Focal neurological deficits
  – Headache
  – Seizure

### History
- History for HIV/AIDS (recent CD4 count)
- History of malignancy with active treatment
- History of organ transplant
- History of autoimmune disorder
- Use of cytotoxic drugs
- Use of high-dose glucocorticoid therapy

### Physical Exam
- Complete, detailed physical exam indicated as signs of infection in the immunocompromised patient may be subtle.
- Signs of systemic inflammatory response syndrome:
  – Temperature >38°C or <36°C
  – Heart rate >90 bpm
  – Respiratory rate >20 breaths per minute or PCO$_2$ <32 mm Hg
- Septic shock
- Focal neurologic deficits
- New murmur
- Ambulatory hypoxia in PCP pneumonia
- Inspect skin and mucosa carefully for a portal of entry.
- Examine oral mucosa and perianal area for erythema and palpate for tenderness or crepitus.
- Oropharyngeal candidiasis as an indicator of immune suppression

## ESSENTIAL WORKUP
Full workup indicated owing to impaired immunity:
- Signs of infection in the immunocompromised patient may not be present.
- Can present with subtle signs with rapid deterioration
- Signs such as fever must lead to a full evaluation of patient.
- Thorough physical exam is critical to search for site of infection.

## DIAGNOSTIC TESTS & INTERPRETATION
### Lab
- CBC with differential for neutropenia or leukocytosis:
  – WBC >12,000 is a criteria for the systemic inflammatory response score
  – Neutropenia:
    ○ ANC (absolute neutrophil count) <1,500/$\mu$L
    ○ ANC = WBC (cells/$\mu$L) × percent (PMNS + bands)/100
- Cultures (aerobic, anaerobic, fungal, viral as indicated):
  – Urine
  – Blood
  – Wound
  – Fecal
  – CD4 count:
    ○ ALC (absolute lymphocyte count) <1,000/$\mu$L predicts CD4 <200 if CD4 unknown
    ○ ALC = WBC (cells/$\mu$L) × percent lymphocytes/100
- Urinalysis for presence of WBC, nitrite, leukocyte esterase
- Electrolytes, BUN/creatinine glucose; anion gap acidosis suggests severe infection.
- ABG for hypoxia/acidosis
- Lactate level; elevated value suggests serious infection.
- PT/PTT for evidence of disseminated intravascular coagulation
- Lactate dehydrogenase (LDH); elevated in patients with PCP

### Imaging

- CXR:
  - Nonspecific for predicting a particular infectious etiology
  - Pneumonia:
    - Segmental or subsegmental infiltrate
    - Air bronchograms
    - Abscess
    - Cavitation
    - Empyema
    - Pleural effusion
  - PCP:
    - Classically reveals bilateral interstitial or central alveolar infiltrates
    - Radiograph normal in up to 25% of patients
- High-resolution chest CT:
  - Early studies show high sensitivity for PCP in HIV-positive patients
  - Reveals patchy ground-glass attenuation
  - Head CT: Contrast-enhancing lesions in *Toxoplasma gondii* encephalitis
- Abdominal CT with contrast:
  - Indicated if a GI source of infection is suggested by the clinical exam

### Diagnostic Procedures/Surgery

Lumbar puncture:

- CSF analysis if signs of CNS infection

## TREATMENT

### INITIAL STABILIZATION/THERAPY

- Check airway, breathing, and circulation.
- Initiate 0.9% normal saline IV 500 mL bolus for hypotension.
- Oxygen
- Cardiac monitor for unstable vital signs
- Early initiation of antibiotic therapy

### ED TREATMENT/PROCEDURES

- Strict isolation
- Antibiotics: Combination of expanded-spectrum penicillin (mezlocillin, ticarcillin, piperacillin) and aminoglycoside (amikacin, tobramycin):
  - Monotherapy with a 3rd-generation cephalosporin (ceftazidime, cefepime), fluoroquinones (levofloxacin, gatifloxacin), or other broad-spectrum antimicrobials (imipenem/cilastatin) may be considered if aminoglycosides contraindicated.

- Vancomycin if there is a high prevalence of methicillin-resistant organisms in the area.
- Antifungals (amphotericin B, fluconazole) if patient is on adequate antibiotics for 1 week.
- Trimethoprim/sulfamethoxazole for suspected PCP (alternatives: Pentamidine, clindamycin plus primaquine)

### MEDICATION

- Amphotericin B: 025 mg/kg/d IV
- Cefepime: 1–2 q12h IV
- Ceftazidime:
  - Adults: 1–2 g IV q8–12h
  - Pediatric: 100–150 mg/kg/24 hrs IV q8–12h
- Fluconazole: 400 mg 1st dose, then 200–400 mg/d IV (peds: 3–6 mg/kg/24 hrs IV q12h)
- Gatifloxacin: 400 mg/d IV
- Imipenem/cilastatin: 500–1,000 mg IV q6–8h, max. 50 mg/kg/d or 4,000 mg/d
- Levofloxacin: 500 mg/d IV
- Piperacillin: 3 g over 30 minutes q4h
- Ticarcillin: 3 g IV q4h over 30 minutes (peds: 200–300 mg/kg/24 hrs IV over 30 minutes q4h)
- Vancomycin: 1–2 g IV q12h (peds: 10–50 mg/kg/24 hrs IV q6h)
- Trimethoprim: 15–20 mg/kg plus sulfamethoxazole: 75 mg/kg PO or IV div. q8h

## FOLLOW-UP

### DISPOSITION

#### Admission Criteria

Suspected or confirmed systemic infection

#### Discharge Criteria

Systemic infection excluded

#### Issues for Referral

Consider infectious disease consultation.

### FOLLOW-UP RECOMMENDATIONS

Patients with systemic opportunistic infections should be admitted to the hospital.

## PEARLS AND PITFALLS

- Signs of infection in the immunocompromised patient may not be present.
- Can present with subtle signs with rapid deterioration

## ADDITIONAL READING

- Daar ES, Meyer RD. Bacterial and fungal infections. *Med Clin North Am*. 1992;17:173–195.
- Emmanouilides C, Glaspy J. Opportunistic infections in oncologic patients. *Hematol Oncol Clin North Am*. 1996;10:841–860.
- Fishman J. Infection in solid-organ transplant recipients. *N Engl J Med*. 2007;357(25):2601–2614.
- Giamarellou H. Empiric therapy for infections in the febrile, neutropenic, compromised host. *Med Clin North Am*. 1992;79:559–578.
- Kaplan JE, Benson C, et al. Guidelines for prevention and treatment of opportunistic infections in HIV-infected adults and adolescents: Recommendations from CDC, the National Institutes of Health, and the HIV Medicine Association of the Infectious Diseases Society of America. *MMWR Recomm Rep*. 2009;58(RR-4):1–207; quiz CE1-4.
- Pizzo PA. The compromised host. In: Bennett JC, et al., eds. *Cecil's textbook of medicine*. Philadelphia: WB Saunders, 1996:908–915.
- Shapiro N, Karras D, et al. Absolute lymphocyte count as a predictor of CD4 count. *Ann Emerg Med*. 1998;32(3):323–328.
- Rothman RE, Marco CA, Yang S. AIDS and HIV infection. In: Marx JA et al., eds. *Rosen's emergency medicine*, 7th ed. Boston: Elsevier, 2009:130.
- Rubin ZA, Somani J. New options in the treatment of invasive fungal infections. *Semin Oncol*. 2004;31 (2 Suppl 4):91–98.

# OPTIC ARTERY OCCLUSION

Yasuharu Okuda
Braden J. Hexom

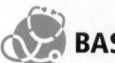 **BASICS**

## DESCRIPTION

- Obstruction of the central retinal artery associated with sudden painless loss of vision
- Usually occurs in persons 50–70 yr old
- Opthalmic artery is 1st branch of carotid
- Risk factors include hypertension, atherosclerotic disease, sickle cell disease, vasculitis, valvular heart disease, lupus, trauma, and coronary artery disease
- Incidence of 1–10/100,000.
- Often described as a "stroke of the eye"

## ETIOLOGY

- Embolic:
  - Occlusion by intravascular material from a proximal source:
    - Atherosclerotic disease (majority)
    - Carotid artery stenosis
    - Valvular heart disease (cardiogenic emboli)
    - Atrial myxoma
    - Dissection of the ophthalmic artery
    - Carotid artery dissection
- Thrombotic:
  - Obstruction of flow from the rupture of a pre-existing intravascular atherosclerotic plaque
  - Hypercoagulable states (sickle cell)
- Inflammatory:
  - Due to temporal arteritis, lupus, vasculitis
- Arterial spasm:
  - Associated with migraine headaches
- Decreased perfusion:
  - Low-flow conditions such as in severe hypotension or high-pressure situations seen in acute angle-closure glaucoma or retrobulbar hemorrhage

 **DIAGNOSIS**

## SIGNS AND SYMPTOMS

- History:
  - Sudden, painless, monocular loss of vision
  - Prior episodes of sudden visual loss:
    - May last a few seconds to minutes (amaurosis fugax)
    - Caused by transient embolic phenomena or decreased ocular blood flow
- Physical exam:
  - Significantly decreased visual acuity
  - Afferent pupillary defect usually present
  - Retinal appearance:
    - Emboli visualized within vascular tree of the retina
    - Appears as glinting white or yellow flecks (Hollenhorst plaques) within the vessels
    - Ischemic edema visible within 15–20 min of occlusion
    - "Cherry-red spot" remains over the fovea (only area where there is very thin retina allowing the vascular choroids to show through).
    - Affected arteries empty or showing dark-red stationary or barely pulsatile segmented rouleaux ("box-carring")
    - Within 1–2 hr opacification of the usually transparent infarcting retinal nerve layer occurs.
  - Partial field deficits:
    - Occur if only if branch of central retinal artery involved

## ESSENTIAL WORKUP

- Visual acuity
- Visual field testing
- Fundoscopic exam
- Intraocular pressure testing
- Emergent ophthalmologic consult

## DIAGNOSTIC TESTS & INTERPRETATION

### Lab

Directed to evaluating underlying etiology of occlusion

- CBC with differential and platelet count
- Prothrombin time, partial thromboplastin time (PTT)
- Electrolytes, BUN/creatinine, glucose
- ESR for giant cell arteritis (in patients >55 yr old)
- ANA, rheumatoid factor, C-reactive protein, ESR
- Rapid plasma regain
- Hemoglobin electrophoresis
- Serum protein electrophoresis

### Imaging

Directed to evaluating underlying etiology of occlusion

- Carotid artery US/Doppler
- Possibly echocardiography
- Fluorescein angiography or electroretinography to confirm the diagnosis

## DIFFERENTIAL DIAGNOSIS

- Acute angle-closure glaucoma
- Central retinal vein occlusion
- Giant cell arteritis (temporal arteritis)
- Optic neuritis
- Retinal detachment

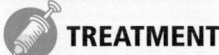 **TREATMENT**

## INITIAL STABILIZATION/THERAPY

### ALERT
Initiate treatment immediately because irreversible visual loss occurs at 90 min:
- Only immediate treatment may help to salvage or restore sight to the affected eye.
- Goals of therapy include dislodging or dissolving the embolus, arterial dilation to improve forward flow, and reduction of intraocular pressure to improve the profusion gradient.

### ED TREATMENT/PROCEDURES
- Immediate global massage in an attempt to dislodge the embolus:
  - Lay patient flat and apply digital global massage.
  - On closed eyelid, apply constant pressure for 15 sec and remove for 15 sec. Repeat for 5 cycles.
- Increase $PCO_2$ to dilate retinal vessels:
  - Have patient breath into paper bag for 10 min each hour or use inhaled carbogen (see below).
  - Administer IV acetazolamide to decrease intraocular pressure.
- Apply topical timolol maleate to reduce intraocular pressure.
- Administer aspirin and IV heparin for prevention of clot propagation.
- Obtain emergent ophthalmology consultation for:
  - Anterior chamber paracentesis to help reduce intraocular pressure
  - Possible intra-arterial fibrinolysis for clot lysis
- Administer high-dose systemic steroids in suspected cases of inflammatory arteritis.

## MEDICATION
### First Line
- Acetazolamide: 500 mg IV or PO
- Carbogen: Inhalation of 95% oxygen and 5% $CO_2$ mixture (Meduna mixture, a mixture of $CO_2$ and oxygen gas. Meduna's original formula was 30% $CO_2$ and 70% oxygen, but the term carbogen can refer to any mixture of these 2 gases, from 1.5% to 50% $CO_2$)
- Heparin: 80-U/kg IV bolus, then 18-U/kg/hr continuous infusions (rate adjusted based on PTT level)
- Timolol maleate 0.5% solution: 1 drop topically to affected eye

### Second Line
- Methylprednisolone: 250 mg IV in suspected cases of inflammatory arteritis
- Aspirin: 325 mg PO
- Mannitol
- Sublingual nitroglycerin

 **FOLLOW-UP**

## DISPOSITION
### Admission Criteria
Required for workup of proximal cause in acute cases (source of embolism, thrombosis, or inflammatory)

### Discharge Criteria
Chronic retinal artery occlusion with no evidence of active disease can be worked up as an outpatient.

### Issues for Referral
- All suspected cases warrant emergent ophthalmology consultation.
- Most cases will require follow-up carotid US to exclude atherosclerotic disease.

## PEARLS AND PITFALLS
- Amaurosis fugax (transient, possibly resolved retinal artery occlusion) is sentinel event and may lead to complete occlusion or stroke requiring further workup.
- Retinal artery occlusion is a medical emergency requiring immediate treatment to prevent loss of the eye.

## ADDITIONAL READING
- Arnold M, Koerner U, Remonda L, et al. Comparison of intra-arterial thrombolysis with conventional treatment in patients with acute central retinal artery occlusion. *J Neurol Neurosurg Psychiatry.* 2005;76(2):196–199.
- Fraser SG, Adams W. Interventions for acute non-arteritic central retinal artery occlusion. *Cochrane Database Syst Rev.* 2009 Jan 21;(1):CD001989.
- Hazin R, Daoud YJ, Khan F. Ocular ischemic syndrome: Recent trends in medical management. *Curr Opin Ophthalmol.* 2009;20:430–433.
- Morgan A, Hemphill R. Acute visual change. *Emerg Med Clin North Am.* 1998;16(4):825–843.

 **CODES**

ICD9
362.30 Retinal vascular occlusion, unspecified

# OPTIC NEURITIS
*Vinh D. Ngo*

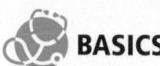 **BASICS**

## DESCRIPTION
- Optic nerve dysfunction due to an inflammatory process, commonly associated with myelin destruction
- Highly associated with multiple sclerosis (MS); presenting feature in 15–20% of patients
- Grouped by site of inflammation:
  - Papillitis: Inflammation of the optic disk
  - Retrobulbar neuritis: Inflammation of the optic nerve proximal to the globe
- 5-yr risk for clinically definite MS following optic neuritis:
  - Normal MRI—16%
  - >3 lesions on MRI—51%
- Recurrence is seen in 35% of patients.

## RISK FACTORS
### Genetics
High prevalence of A23, B7, and DR2 HLA alleles in patients with optic neuritis:
- Especially those that progress to clinically definite MS

## ETIOLOGY
- Idiopathic:
  - Most common
  - Single isolated events
- MS:
  - 20–50% of patients with optic neuritis
- Viral infections:
  - Chicken pox
  - Measles
  - Mononucleosis
  - Herpes zoster
  - Encephalitis
- Postviral optic neuritis:
  - Usually occurs 4–6 wk after a nonspecific viral illness
- Granulomatous inflammation:
  - TB
  - Syphilis
  - Sarcoidosis
  - Cryptococcal infection
- SLE
- HIV:
  - Cytomegalovirus
  - Toxoplasmosis
  - Histoplasmosis
  - Cryptococcus
- Lyme disease
- Contiguous inflammation of meninges, orbit, sinuses, and intraocular inflammation
- Drug induced:
  - Ethambutol
  - Tamoxifen

## DIAGNOSIS

### SIGNS AND SYMPTOMS
- Vision loss and pain most common symptoms
- Visual loss occurring over days (rarely over hours), peaks in 1–2 wk:
  - Adults usually unilateral
  - Bilateral visual loss more common in children
- Retrobulbar pain: Increased with movement of the affected eye
- Light, color vision, and depth perception loss more pronounced than visual acuity loss
- Afferent pupillary defect almost always occurs in unilateral cases if other eye is healthy.
- Visual field defects:
  - Usually characterized by central scotoma
  - Deficits resolve by 1 yr in 56% of patients, and 73% resolve by 10 yr
- Funduscopic exam usually reveals either swollen (papillitis) or normal disk
- Uhthoff sign:
  - Visual deficit occurring with exercise or increased body temperature
  - Unusual sign seen occasionally

### History
- Age (typically women 18–45 yr)
- Pain on eye movement
- Speed of onset of symptoms
- Associated symptoms
- Previous episodes
- Family history of optic neuritis, MS

### Physical Exam
- Check BP.
- Complete ophthalmologic and neurologic examination, especially assessment of:
  - Pupillary function
  - Afferent pupillary defect
  - Visual field defect
  - Color vision (Ishihara color plates)
  - Evaluation of the vitreous body for cells
  - Dilated retinal exam (swollen optic disk)

### DIAGNOSTIC TESTS & INTERPRETATION
#### Lab
- CBC
- ESR
- Rapid plasma reagin, fluorescent treponemal antibody-absorption (FTA–ABS)
- Lyme titer
- Antinuclear antibody
- Purified protein derivative
- HIV

#### Imaging
- CXR for TB, sarcoid
- CT scan or MRI of brain and orbits:
  - Inflammation of the retrobulbar optic nerve during the acute phase may appear as enlargement, thus falsely raising the issue of an optic nerve mass.
  - Optic nerve inflammation is seen in 95% of gadolinium-enhanced MRIs.
  - Visual field testing (preferably automated testing, such as Octopus or Humphrey)

### DIFFERENTIAL DIAGNOSIS
- Acute papilledema
- Ischemic optic neuropathy
- Severe systemic hypertension
- Intracranial tumor compressing the afferent visual pathway
- Orbital mass compressing the optic nerve
- Toxic or metabolic neuropathy:
  - Heavy metal poisoning
  - Anemia
  - Malnutrition
  - Alcohol
  - Chloroquine
  - Ethambutol
- Isoniazid
- Leber hereditary optic atrophy

### Pediatric Considerations
In children, infectious and postinfectious causes should be considered.

### Geriatric Considerations
In patients >50 yr, ischemic optic neuropathies (ex. diabetes and giant cell arteritis) are more common, and appropriate workup should be obtained.

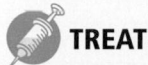 TREATMENT

#### ED TREATMENT/PROCEDURES
- Early ophthalmologic and neurologic consultations
- IV steroid pulse followed by oral steroids:
  - Recommended for those with ≥2 demyelinating lesions on MRI without a prior history of MS or optic neuritis, or severe vision loss
  - Decreases recurrence and progression to MS over 2 yr and shortens duration of visual impairment, but does not affect rate of progression at 5 yr or visual outcome at 1 yr
  - Treatment should be individualized for those with one lesion on MRI.
  - Oral steroids used alone increases recurrence and should be avoided.

#### MEDICATION
Methylprednisolone: 250 mg IV q6h for 3 days, followed by oral prednisone (1 mg/kg/d) for 11 days with subsequent 4-day taper

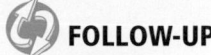 FOLLOW-UP

#### DISPOSITION
##### Admission Criteria
- Bilateral vision loss
- If other sources of acute vision loss cannot be ruled out
- IV steroid pulse treatment needed

##### Discharge Criteria
- Unilateral visual impairment
- Good home support systems
- Neurology and ophthalmology follow-up arranged

##### Issues for Referral
Referral for interferon b-1a treatment as outpatient for high-risk patients (those with ≥2 demyelinating lesions on MRI):
- Reduces progression to MS

#### FOLLOW-UP RECOMMENDATIONS
Needs ophthalmology referral

## PEARLS AND PITFALLS

- Must rule out space-occupying lesions before making the diagnosis of optic neuritis.
- Acute bilateral loss with a severe headache or diplopia should raise concern for pituitary apoplexy.
- IV steroids have been shown to speed the recovery of vision without affecting the final visual outcome and may also decrease the symptom onset of MS over the 1st 2–3 yr after optic neuritis.
- Brain MRI is the most useful predictor of subsequent development of MS.

## ADDITIONAL READING

- Balcer LJ. Clinical practice. Optic neuritis. *N Eng J Med*. 2006;354:1273–1280.
- Beck RW, Cleary PA, Anderson MM, et al. Optic Neuritis Study Group. A randomized controlled trial of corticosteroids in the treatment of acute optic neuritis. *N Eng J Med*. 1992;326:581–588.
- Beck RW, Gal RL, Bhatti MT, et al. Visual function more than 10 years after optic neuritis: Experience of the optic neuritis treatment trial. *Am J Ophthalmol*. 2004;137:77–83.
- CHAMPIONS Study Group. IM interferon β-1a delays definite multiple sclerosis 5 years after a first demyelinating event. *Neurology*. 2006;66:678–684.
- Ehlers JP, Shah CP, Fenton GL, eds. *The Wills Eye Manual*. 5th ed. Philadelphia: Lippincott Williams & Wilkins; 2008.
- Germann CA, Baumann MR, Hamzavi S. Ophthalmic diagnoses in the ED: optic neuritis. *Am J Emerg Med*. 2007;25(7):834–837.

### See Also (Topic, Algorithm, Electronic Media Element)
- *Visual Loss*

*The author gratefully acknowledges Alexander T. Limkakeng Jr's contribution for the previous edition of this chapter.*

 CODES

#### ICD9
377.30 Optic neuritis, unspecified

# ORGANOPHOSPHATE POISONING

Matthew Valento

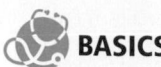 **BASICS**

## DESCRIPTION
- Organophosphates (pesticides and nerve agents) irreversibly bind to cholinesterases, causing deactivation of acetylcholinesterase.
- Initial accumulation of acetylcholine at neural synapse results in cholinergic overdrive (central and peripheral).
- Predominate effects (muscarinic, nicotinic, CNS) may vary and can overlap.
- Death usually secondary to respiratory failure resulting from weakness of respiratory muscles, pulmonary edema, and central depression of respiratory drive.

### Pediatric Considerations
- Symptoms are difficult to differentiate in toddlers.
- Common symptoms: Miosis, salivation, and muscle weakness
- Seizures found in 25% (3% of adults).

## ETIOLOGY
- Exposure to insecticides (organophosphorus compounds)
- Exposure to chemical nerve agents (sarin, soman, VX, tabun)
- Extremely well absorbed from lung, GI tract, skin, mucosa, eyes

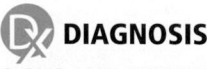 **DIAGNOSIS**

## SIGNS AND SYMPTOMS
- Classic presentation: Cholinergic toxidrome:
  - DUMBELS:
    - **D**iarrhea/diaphoresis
    - **U**rination
    - **M**iosis/muscle fasciculations
    - **B**radycardia, bronchorrhea, bronchospasm
    - **E**mesis
    - **L**acrimation
    - **S**alivation
  - May have garlic odor
- Chronic intermittent exposure, nonspecific symptoms:
  - Weakness
  - Fatigue
  - Malaise
  - Anorexia
- Mild exposure:
  - Visual:
    - Miosis
    - Decreased visual acuity
  - CNS:
    - Headache
    - Dizziness
    - Tremors of tongue and eyelids
    - Weakness

  - GI:
    - Anorexia
- Moderate exposure:
  - CNS:
    - Muscle fasciculation followed by flaccid paralysis
    - Respiratory muscle weakness
    - Incoordination
  - GI:
    - Nausea/vomiting
    - Abdominal cramps
  - Exocrine glands:
    - Salivation
    - Lacrimation
- Severe exposure:
  - Visual:
    - Pinpoint nonreactive pupils
  - Respiratory:
    - Respiratory difficulty
    - Pulmonary edema
  - Cardiovascular:
    - Bradycardia
    - Heart block
  - CNS:
    - Convulsion
    - Coma
    - Centrally mediated respiratory depression
  - GI:
    - Diarrhea
  - Muscarinic manifestations:
  - Respiratory:
    - Bronchoconstriction
    - Wheezing
    - Dyspnea
    - Increased bronchial secretion
    - Cough
    - Pulmonary edema
  - Cardiovascular:
    - Bradycardia (tachycardia may follow pulmonary edema and hypoxia)
    - Cyanosis
  - GI:
    - Nausea, vomiting
    - Abdominal pain
    - Diarrhea
    - Fecal incontinence
  - Exocrine glands:
    - Diaphoresis
    - Salivation
    - Lacrimation
  - Eye:
    - Miosis, occasionally anisocoria
    - Blurred vision
  - Bladder:
    - Frequency
    - Urinary incontinence
  - Nicotinic manifestations:
  - Striated muscle:
    - Fasciculation
    - Weakness, including respiratory muscles

  - Sympathetic ganglia:
    - Mydriasis
    - Tachycardia
    - HTN
    - Bronchodilation
  - CNS:
    - Agitation
    - Restlessness
    - Tremors
    - Confusion
    - Ataxia
    - Weakness
    - Coma
    - Seizures
    - Death

## ESSENTIAL WORKUP
Inquire about possible exposure, occupation, recent insecticide in home, mislabeled, or poorly stored insecticides:
- Obtain original container if suicide attempt.
- Look for parasympathetic and CNS signs with muscle weakness or paralysis.

## DIAGNOSTIC TESTS & INTERPRETATION
### Lab
- RBC and plasma cholinesterase levels to confirm diagnosis:
  - RBC (true) cholinesterase level is best reflection of synaptic inhibition (a send-out lab).
  - Plasma (pseudo) cholinesterase level not as reliable but more timely:
    - These are markers for poisoning, but there is tremendous variation within patients/agents.
  - Cholinesterase levels:
    - Latent exposure: >50% of normal value
    - Mild exposure: 20–50% of normal value
    - Moderate exposure: 10–20% of normal value
    - Severe exposure: <10% of normal value
  - Do not wait for cholinesterase results before administering treatment.
- CBC
- Electrolytes, glucose, BUN, creatinine
- ABG when respiratory symptoms

### Imaging
- CXR if respiratory difficulty is present or suspect pulmonary edema:
  - Pneumonitis from hydrocarbon aspiration
- EKG:
  - Dysrhythmias (atrial fibrillation, ventricular tachycardia, torsades de pointes, QT prolongation)
  - Bradycardia
  - Heart block
  - ST-T–wave abnormalities
- CT scan of head for altered mental status when diagnosis is uncertain

## DIFFERENTIAL DIAGNOSIS

- Mild to moderate exposure:
  - Gastroenteritis
  - Asthma
  - Venomous arthropods bite (black widow, scorpion)
  - Progressive peripheral neuropathy (Guillain-Barré syndrome)
  - Carbon monoxide
- Severe exposure:
  - Narcotic overdose
  - Coma and miosis:
    ○ PCP, meprobamate, phenothiazine, clonidine
    ○ Muscarinic-containing mushrooms—cholinergic crisis without nicotinic symptoms
    ○ Nicotine poisoning
  - Metabolic and infectious:
    ○ Ketoacidosis, sepsis, meningitis, encephalitis
    ○ Hypoglycemia
    ○ Reye syndrome
  - Neurologic:
    ○ Cerebrovascular accident
    ○ Subdural or epidural hematoma
    ○ Postictal state

 **TREATMENT**

### PRE-HOSPITAL

- Decontamination is initial priority:
  - DABC: Decontaminate, airway, breathing, circulation
  - Remove all clothes and store as toxic waste (double bagged)
- Protection of healthcare workers of utmost importance:
  - Impenetrable gloves (neoprene, nitrile), gowns, eye protection
- Decontaminate skin with soap and water:
  - Shower or gentle scrubbing ideal if done before entrance into the ED
- Maintain airway and oxygenate.
- IV access and place on cardiac monitor

### INITIAL STABILIZATION/THERAPY

- Decontaminate ABCs:
  - Decontamination and protection of staff
  - Maintain airway and oxygenate.
  - For unstable airway, intubate, and ventilate.
  - IV access with $D_5W$ 0.9% NS
- Altered mental status: Administer thiamine, glucose, and naloxone (Narcan)

### ED TREATMENT/PROCEDURES

- Atropine:
  - Blocks acetylcholine at muscarinic receptor sites.
  - No effect on nicotinic receptors
  - Onset of action is 1–4 min, peaks at 8 min.
  - Goal of therapy/end point:
    ○ Drying secretions of tracheobronchial tree
  - Administer test dose 1–2 mg IV/IM:
    ○ No clinical response: Double dose q5min until muscarinic findings subside

- Dose: 1–4 mg IV q5min (peds: 0.05–0.2 mg/kg)
- Common pitfalls in therapy:
  ○ Not giving enough atropine
  ○ Using pupillary findings (mydriasis) as end point of atropine therapy
  ○ Dilated pupils or tachycardia are not contraindications to the administration of atropine.
- Pralidoxime (2-PAM):
  - Regenerates cholinesterase by reversing the phosphorylation of the enzyme.
  - Synergistic with atropine, and muscarinic signs and symptoms will start to resolve within 10–40 min.
  - Side effects include neuromuscular blockade with rapid infusion, respiratory arrest, HTN, nausea/vomiting, dizziness, and blurred vision.
  - End point is resolution of muscle weakness and fasciculations.
  - Effective only if given before enzyme aging occurs (point at which cholinesterase is permanently inactivated)
  - Onset of aging varies between products
  - No restriction to its use even if 24–48 hr have passed
- Supportive care:
  - Dermal decontamination: Remove clothes and flush skin with water
  - Gastric lavage (considered in early presentation of life-threatening ingestion):
    ○ Gastric emptying should be done with continuous suction via a nasogastric tube.
    ○ Handle contents with care and avoid coming in direct contact with it to prevent exposure.
  - Respiratory difficulty:
    ○ Frequent respiratory secretion suction required
    ○ Treat bronchospasm with atropine and not bronchodilators.
    ○ Tachycardia may result from hypoxia induced by pulmonary secretions and bronchospasm.
    ○ Atropine will dry secretions and paradoxically lower the heart rate in light of more effective oxygenation.
    ○ Intubate and ventilate if necessary.
    ○ Avoid succinylcholine; this is metabolized by cholinesterase and may have markedly prolonged duration.

### MEDICATION

- Atropine: 1–4 mg (peds: 0.05–0.2 mg/kg) IV q5min (see previous section for details)
- Dextrose: $D_{50}W$, 1 amp (25 g) of 50% dextrose (peds: 2–4 mL/kg $D_{25}W$) IV push
- Naloxone (Narcan): 2 mg (peds: 0.1 mg/kg) IV/IM
- Pralidoxime: 1–2 g (peds: 20–40 mg/kg) dissolved in 0.9% NS over 30-min IV; repeat in 1 hr if necessary, then q3–8h as needed:
  - Some propose a continuous infusion of 500 mg/h to obtain a necessary serum concentration of 4 mg/L.

 **FOLLOW-UP**

### DISPOSITION

#### Admission Criteria

- ICU admission for mild, moderate, or severe exposure confirmed with a response to atropine.
- Any symptomatic patient should be admitted for monitoring.
- Avoid CNS-depressive effects of opioids, phenothiazines, and antihistamines, as these may potentiate toxicity of organophosphates.

#### Discharge Criteria

- Asymptomatic for 6–12 hr after exposure
- Ensure close reliable follow-up and specific instructions when to return for evaluation.

#### Issues for Referral

Contact toxicologist or poison center for patients with significant exposures requiring repeat atropine administration.

### FOLLOW-UP RECOMMENDATIONS

Psychiatry referral for intentional ingestions.

## PEARLS AND PITFALLS

- Treatment failure often secondary to inadequate atropine dosing
- Recognize nicotinic manifestations (tachycardia, seizures).

## ADDITIONAL READING

- Clark RF. Insecticides: Organic phosphorous compounds and carbamates. In Goldfrank LR, ed. *Goldfrank's Toxicologic Emergencies*. New York: McGraw-Hill; 2006, 1497–1512.
- Minton NA, Murray SG. A review of organophosphate poisoning. *Med Toxicol*. 1988;3:350–75.
- Tafuri J, Toberts J. Organophosphate poisoning. *Ann Emerg Med*. 1987;16:193–202.
- Eddleston M, Eyer P, Worek F, et al. Pralidoxime in acute organophosphate insecticide poisoning—A randomised controlled trial. *PLoS Med*. 2009; 6(6):1–2.
- Zwiener RJ, Ginsburg CM. Organophosphate and carbamate poisoning in infants and children. *Pediatrics*. 1988;81:121–26.

 **CODES**

### ICD9

989.3 Toxic effect of organophosphate and carbamate

# OSGOOD-SCHLATTER DISEASE

Beth A. Zelonis

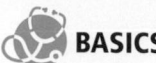
## BASICS

### DESCRIPTION
- Most frequent cause of knee pain in children aged 10–15 yr
- Pain and edema of the tibial tuberosity:
  - Tenderness at insertion site for patellar tendon just below the knee joint
- Extra-articular disease:
  - Pain is worse with activity and improves with rest
  - Caused by repetitive stress and is common in children participating in sports
- Benign, self-limited knee condition

### ETIOLOGY
- Etiology is controversial
- Leading theory: Microfractures caused by traction on the apophysis
- Pain occurs during activities that stress the patellar tendon insertion onto tibial tubercle.

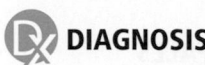
## DIAGNOSIS

### SIGNS AND SYMPTOMS
- Pain and swelling over tibial tuberosity
- Pain exacerbated by running, jumping
- Pain relieved by rest

### History
- Risk factors:
  - Age: 10–15 yr of age, associated with growth spurt in puberty
  - More common in boys
  - Sports: Activities with running, jumping, swift changes in direction (ie, soccer, basketball, figure skating)
- Knee pain is worse with activity and improves with rest.
- Usually unilateral, with 20% occurring bilateral

### Physical Exam
- Prominence and soft tissue swelling over the tibial tuberosity
- Pain reproduced by extending the knee against resistance
- Tenderness over tibial tuberosity at patellar tendon insertion site
- Tight quadriceps and hamstrings compared to unaffected side
- Erythema of tibial tuberosity may be present.
- Knee joint exam is normal.

### ESSENTIAL WORKUP
Diagnosis is clinical:
- Pain, swelling, and tenderness localized to the tibial tubercle

### DIAGNOSTIC TESTS & INTERPRETATION
#### Imaging
Knee x-ray:
- Irregular ossification and fragmentation at the tibial tuberosity may be seen.

### DIFFERENTIAL DIAGNOSIS
- Patellar stress fracture
- Patellar or quadriceps tendonitis
- Prepatellar or infrapatellar bursitis
- Osteochondritis dissecans
- Osteomyelitis
- Patellofemoral pain syndrome
- Septic joint
- Inferior patellar pole traction apophysitis (Sinding-Larsen-Johansson disease)
- Fat pad impingement (Hoffa disease)
- Referred pain, especially from the hip

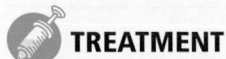 **TREATMENT**

## INITIAL STABILIZATION/THERAPY
- Stabilize lower extremity in position of comfort.
- Apply ice to affected knee.

## ED TREATMENT/PROCEDURES
- Rest from painful activities:
  - Limited activity for 2–4 mo
  - Avoid cutting and jumping sports, such as basketball, soccer, volleyball, etc.
- Ice affected area.
- Analgesic medications
- Stretch the quadriceps and hamstrings.
- Apply protective padding to knee during activities.
- Infrapatellar tendon strap may be worn for 6–8 wk.
- Avoid corticosteroid injections.
- Reassurance; it is a benign, self-limited condition.

## MEDICATION
### First Line
Analgesic medications:
- Ibuprofen: 10 mg/kg PO q6h
- Acetaminophen: 15 mg/kg PO q4h

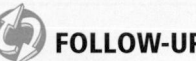 **FOLLOW-UP**

## DISPOSITION
### Admission Criteria
No admission is necessary.

### Discharge Criteria
Discharge home.

### Issues for Referral
If patient fails nonoperative therapy, then refer to pediatric orthopedic surgery:
- Rarely, surgical excision is required but is delayed until after skeletal maturity.

## FOLLOW-UP RECOMMENDATIONS
Rest from painful activities and follow-up with pediatrician in 2–3 wk for repeat exam.

## PEARLS AND PITFALLS
- Diagnosis is clinical:
  - Pain, swelling and tenderness at the tibial tuberosity:
    ○ Tenderness and pain worse during and after exercise
  - Risk factors:
    ○ 10–15 yr of age
    ○ Sports activities with running, jumping

- Treatment is conservative:
  - Treat with rest, ice, and NSAIDs
  - Avoid sports activities until pain resolves.

## ADDITIONAL READING
- Bloom OJ, Mackler L, Barbee J. What is the best treatment for Osgood-Schlatter disease? *J Fam Pract.* 2004;53(2):153–156.
- Cassas KJ, Cassettari-Wayhs A. Childhood and adolescent sports-related overuse injuries. *Am Fam Physician.* 2006;73(6):1014–1022.
- Gholve PA, Scher DM, et al. Osgood-Schlatter syndrome. *Curr Opin Pediatri.* 2007;19(1):44–50.
- Patel DR, Nelson TL. Sports injuries in adolescents. *Med Clin N Am.* 2000;84:983–1007.
- Weiss IM, Jordan SS, et al. Surgical treatment of unresolved Osgood-Schlatter disease: Ossicle excision with tibial tubercleplasty. *J Pediatr Orthoped.* 2007;27(7):844–847.

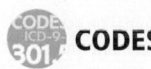 **CODES**

### ICD9
732.4 Juvenile osteochondrosis of lower extremity, excluding foot

# OSTEOGENESIS IMPERFECTA

*Daniel Davis*

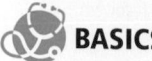 **BASICS**

## DESCRIPTION

- Inherited abnormality of procollagen amino acid sequence
- Bone hypomineralization and incomplete ossification result in brittle bones.
- Abnormal collagen affects all connective tissue to varying degrees.
- Time course is variable:
  - Most cases involve fractures during childhood followed by quiescence during adolescence and early adulthood.

## ETIOLOGY

- Procollagen defects result in abnormalities of bone and connective tissue matrix.
- Defects in different sites on procollagen protein chain result in more severe forms.
- Defects are inherited, either autosomal recessive (generally milder) or autosomal dominant (more severe).
- Lethal cases involve sporadic or new mutations.
- Ehlers–Danlos syndrome involves mutations of same procollagen protein in different location.

### *Pediatric Considerations*

- Most cases involve pathologic fractures during childhood.
- Multiple fractures often initiate evaluation for abuse, but the possibility of pathologic fractures also should be considered.

 **DIAGNOSIS**

## SIGNS AND SYMPTOMS

- Multiple heritable defects that lead to brittle bones:
  - Often associated with other connective tissue abnormalities
- Bones:
  - Multiple recurrent fractures (especially in long bones) are the hallmark of this disease.
  - Fractures may be present at birth or may recur in the elderly.
  - All bones are affected to some extent (see "Imaging/Special Tests").
- Eyes:
  - *Blue sclerae* are another hallmark of this disease.
  - No visual changes are reported.
- Ears:
  - Hearing loss usually begins in adolescence; >90% of patients have some deficit by age 30 yr.
  - Hearing loss is generally sensorineural, although some middle ear abnormalities have been demonstrated.
- Other:
  - Yellow-brown or blue-gray discoloration and abnormal shape of teeth
  - Shares several features with Ehlers–Danlos syndrome:
    - Loose joints
    - Valve problems
    - Vascular abnormalities
- Thyroid abnormalities may be seen.
- Extreme cases may result in perinatal death.

### *History*

- A suspected fracture with a relatively minor mechanism or a history of multiple fractures in a child suggests the diagnosis.
- A careful social history must be obtained to screen for the possibility of nonaccidental trauma.

### *Physical Exam*

Exam findings are related to the acute fracture rather than the disease itself.

## ESSENTIAL WORKUP

- Diagnosis is usually made as combination of clinical and radiographic findings.
- History of repeated fractures or fractures with unimpressive mechanism
- Thorough search for other tender areas and evaluation of eyes, teeth, and joints is important for diagnosis.
- Careful examination of neurovascular status distal to fracture

## DIAGNOSTIC TESTS & INTERPRETATION

### *Lab*

- Evaluate for metabolic derangements such as hyperparathyroidism, vitamin C or D deficiencies, and calcium/phosphate abnormalities.
- DNA studies may be indicated for familial analysis, prenatal testing, and genetic counseling.
- Tissue biopsy is controversial but may help differentiate from tumors.

### Imaging
- Radiographs of fracture sites:
  - May reveal osteopenia (usually mild)
  - Crumpled long bones ("accordion femora")
  - Incomplete ossification at physes
- Skeletal survey is mandatory, especially in children.
- Skull films may show wormian appearance of irregular ossification.
- Popcornlike deposits on long-bone ends is poor prognostic finding.
- Formal audiologic testing as outpatient is required in older patients.

### DIFFERENTIAL DIAGNOSIS
- Nonaccidental trauma in children
- Ehlers–Danlos syndrome
- Hypophosphatasia
- Achondroplasia
- Scurvy
- Congenital syphilis
- Celiac disease

## TREATMENT

### PRE-HOSPITAL
Personnel should obtain information about mechanism or social factors that point toward pathologic fracture vs nonaccidental trauma.

### INITIAL STABILIZATION/THERAPY
- Airway management and resuscitation as indicated
- Fracture immobilization/splinting

### ED TREATMENT/PROCEDURES
- Specific fracture management dictated by type and location of injury
- Orthopedic consultation regarding need for traction or operative fixation
- No specific treatment for osteogenesis imperfecta exists at present.

### MEDICATION
- Pain medications as indicated
- Elderly women may benefit from calcium (1–1.5 g/day) and estrogen replacement (0.625 mg/day)

 FOLLOW-UP

### DISPOSITION
#### Admission Criteria
- Admission is determined by multiple trauma or operative needs for fracture repair.
- Pediatric patients may need admission to investigate possibility of nonaccidental trauma.

#### Discharge Criteria
- Patients may be considered for outpatient management if isolated fracture is present and appropriate home resources are available.
- Most patients should be discharged with orthopedic and primary physician follow-up.

#### Issues for Referral
- Orthopedic referral is driven by the acute injury.
- The presence of fractures in multiple locations or at different times also suggests nonaccidental trauma, which should prompt acute consultation and/or referral per local protocol.

### FOLLOW-UP RECOMMENDATIONS
- Follow-up is generally driven by the acute injuries.
- Follow-up with the primary physician should be instituted to encourage treatment and monitoring of the disease.

## PEARLS AND PITFALLS

The most challenging aspect of caring for these patients is differentiating between pathologic fractures associated with osteogenesis imperfecta and nonaccidental trauma. With any questions, acute consultation and/or referral should be initiated per local protocol.

## ADDITIONAL READING

- Shapiro JR, Sponsellor PD. Osteogenesis imperfecta: Questions and answers. *Curr Opin Pediatr.* 2009;21(6):709–716.
- Chandrasoma P, Taylor CR. *Concise Pathology.* East Norwalk, CT: Appleton & Lange; 1991.
- Cole WG. Advances in osteogenesis imperfecta. *Clin Orthop Rel Res.* 2002;401:6–16.
- McKusick VA. *Heritable Disorders of Connective Tissue,* 4th ed. St. Louis: Mosby; 1972.
- Prockop DJ. Heritable disorders of connective tissue. In: Wilson JD, et al., eds. *Harrison's Principles of Internal Medicine,* 12th ed. New York: McGraw-Hill; 1991:1860.

### See Also (Topic, Algorithm, Electronic Media Element)
Specific orthopedic injuries

 CODES

### ICD9
756.51 Osteogenesis imperfecta

# OSTEOMYELITIS
*Jamila Danishwar*

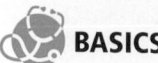 **BASICS**

## DESCRIPTION
- Osteomyelitis (OM): Infection of bone with ongoing inflammatory destruction
- Usually bacterial, but fungal OM does occur
- Could be acute or chronic

## ETIOLOGY
- Hematogenous OM:
  - Primarily in children, elderly, IV drug abuse (IVDA) patients
  - Seeding of bacteria to bone from remote site of infection via bloodstream
  - Children have acute OM and adults subacute or chronic.
  - Hematogenous OM of long bones rarely occurs in adults.
  - Most children with acute hematogenous OM have no preceding illness.
  - 1/3 have history of trauma to affected area.
  - *Staphylococcus aureus* is most common cause of OM in all ages.
  - Neonates: *S. aureus*, Enterobacteriaceae, group A and B streptococci, and *Escherichia coli*
  - Children: *S. aureus*, group A streptococci, *Haemophilus influenzae*, Enterobacteriaceae
  - *Salmonella*: Common in sickle cell disease
  - Adults: *S. aureus*, Enterobacteriaceae, *Pseudomonas*, gram-negative rods, *Staphylococcus epidermidis*, gram-positive anaerobes, especially *Peptostreptococcus*
  - Illicit drug users: *Candida, Pseudomonas, Serratia marcescens*
  - Prolonged neutropenia: *Candida, Aspergillus, Rhizopus, Blastomyces*, coccidioidomycosis
- Hematogenous vertebral OM:
  - Uncommon
  - Most prevalent in adults >45
  - Involves the disk and vertebra above and below
  - Often in setting of long-term urinary catheter placement, IVDA, cancer, hemodialysis, or diabetes
  - IVDA: OM of pubic symphysis, sternoclavicular, and sacroiliac (S-I) joints
  - Lumbar vertebrae most common, followed by thoracic, then cervical
  - Posterior extension leads to epidural/subdural abscess or meningitis.
  - Anterior extension may lead to paravertebral, retropharyngeal, mediastinal, subphrenic, retroperitoneal, or psoas abscess.

- Direct or contiguous OM:
  - Organism(s) directly seeded in bone due to trauma, especially following open fractures:
    - Spread from adjacent site of infection or from surgery
  - More common in adults and adolescents
  - *S. aureus*, Enterobacteriaceae, *Pseudomonas*
  - Normal vascularity:
    - *S. aureus* and *S. epidermidis*, gram-negative bacilli, and anaerobic organisms
  - Vascular insufficiency/diabetes:
    - Small bones of feet are common sites.
    - Infection resulting from minor trauma, infected nail beds, cellulitis, or skin ulceration
    - Polymicrobial, including anaerobes
  - Puncture wound through tennis shoe: *S. aureus, Pseudomonas*
  - Clavicular OM can occur as complication of subclavian vein catheterization.
- Chronic OM:
  - Osteomyelitis that persists or recurs
  - Distinguishing characteristic is necrotic bone (sequestrum) that must be debrided.
  - *S. epidermidis, S. aureus, Pseudomonas aeruginosa, Serratia marcescens*, and *E. coli*

 **DIAGNOSIS**

## SIGNS AND SYMPTOMS
Vary with duration of disease

### History
- Mainly nonspecific symptoms
- Pain: Localized, deep, dull, and throbbing; occurs with and without movement
- Fever and chills; may be absent in chronic OM
- Malaise, nausea, vomiting
- Reluctance to use extremity
- Nonhealing ulcers despite proper therapy
- Consider OM as a cause of fracture nonunion
- Predisposing factors: DM, vasculopathy, IVDA, invasive procedures, trauma

### Physical Exam
- Tenderness to palpation, warmth, erythema, edema, decreased range of motion
- Drainage of sinus tract
- Deep ulcers and palpable bone (+ "probe to bone" test has very high positive predictive value)
- If ulcer size $>2$ cm$^2$ and $>3$ mm in depth, bone involvement is likely.

## ESSENTIAL WORKUP
- CBC
- ESR and C-reactive protein
- Radiographs
- Blood and wound cultures and sensitivities

## DIAGNOSTIC TESTS & INTERPRETATION
### Lab
- CBC; WBC may be elevated but often normal
- ESR; elevated in >90% of cases
- C-reactive protein (usually elevated)
- Blood cultures (positive in ~50% of cases)

### Imaging
- Plays a central role in evaluation
- Start with plain films; other tests often required
- Radiographs:
  - May be normal for the 1st 2–3 wk of symptoms
  - Earliest finding is periosteal elevation, followed by cortical erosions, then new bone formation.
  - 40–50% of focal bone loss needed to detect lucency on radiograph; fewer than 1/3 of cases have diagnostic findings at 10 days
  - Obtain CXR if TB suspected
- MRI:
  - Best modality to obtain detailed anatomy and extension of soft-tissue and bone narrow involvement
  - Sensitivity and specificity of ~90%
  - Reveals bone edema, cortical destruction, periosteal reaction, joint surface damage, and soft-tissue involvement before x-rays
  - Effective in early detection (3–5 days from onset of infection)
  - Test of choice to identify vertebral OM and OM in diabetic foot ulcers
  - Occasional false-positive results in trauma, previous surgical procedures, or neuropathic joint disease
  - Negative study after 1 wk of symptoms rules out acute OM
- CT:
  - Modality of choice when MRI can't be done
  - Reveals bone edema, cortical destruction, periosteal reaction, small foci of gas or foreign bodies, joint surface damage, and soft-tissue involvement when plain films not helpful
  - Useful in OM of vertebrae, sternum, calcaneus, pelvic bones
  - Useful to surgeons in guiding debridement and biopsy

- Bone scan:
  - Technetium$^{99m}$ methylene diphosphonate ($^{99m}$Tc-MDP)
  - Measures increase in bone metabolic activity
  - ~95% sensitive but less specific than MRI
  - Bone scan abnormal after 2–3 days of symptoms
  - False-positive may occur in trauma, surgery, chronic soft-tissue infection, tumor
  - High radiation burden, useful if suspect multifocal disease
- Leukocyte scintigraphy:
  - Indium$^{111}$-labeled WBCs
  - More specific but less sensitive than bone scan
  - Difficult to distinguish bone inflammation from soft-tissue inflammation (ie, cellulitis, tumors, inflammatory arthritis)
- US:
  - An emerging modality for OM especially in children
  - Periosteal elevation or thickening, fluid collections adjacent to bone often seen
  - May show findings of OM days prior to plain films
  - Useful in guiding biopsy

### Diagnostic Procedures/Surgery
- Gold standard for diagnosis is bone biopsy with histology and tissue Gram stains, including culture and sensitivities.
- Needle aspiration has lower sensitivity than open biopsy.
- Culture of sinus or drainage from wound can be misleading; correlates well with *S. aureus*, but not as reliable for other organisms.

### Pediatric Considerations
- 70–85% of children have fever higher than 38.5°C.
- Neonates are commonly afebrile.
- Only ~1 in 3 of children will have leukocytosis.
- Blood cultures positive in ~50%
- US

## DIFFERENTIAL DIAGNOSIS
- Cellulitis
- Paronychia/felon
- Bursitis, toxic synovitis, septic arthritis
- Extremity fracture
- Bone infarction in sickle cell patients
- Acute leukemia, malignant bone tumors
- Mechanical back pain
- Spinal epidural abscess
- Brucellosis, especially in S-I joint
- TB, more common in thoracic spine (Pott disease)

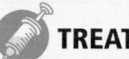 **TREATMENT**

### INITIAL STABILIZATION/THERAPY
Emergent stabilization if septic or if neurologic deficits from spine involvement

### ED TREATMENT/PROCEDURES
- Empiric antibiotic treatment in ED
- Cultures should guide subsequent antibiotic regimen.
- Antibiotics: Depend on patient's age and organism (see Medications section)
- Orthopedic and infectious disease consultation
- Surgical intervention may be needed to optimize treatment (eg, infected fracture or hardware, bone necrosis).
- Parenteral antibiotic treatment for 4–6 wk

### MEDICATION
- Newborn–4 mo: Penicillinase-resistant synthetic penicillin (eg, nafcillin: 37 mg/kg IV q6h) plus a 3rd-generation cephalosporin (eg, ceftriaxone: 50–75 mg/kg/d IV); if suspect methicillin-resistant *S. aureus* (MRSA) then vancomycin (40–60 mg/kg IV q6h) plus a 3rd-generation cephalosporin. (Note: Doses are based on age >28 days)
- Children (>4 mo): Penicillinase-resistant synthetic penicillin (eg, nafcillin: 37 mg/kg IV q6h to max. 8–12 g/d). If suspect MRSA, then vancomycin (40–60 mg/kg IV q6h to max. 2–4 g/d). Add 3rd-generation cephalosporin if suspicion for gram-negative rods, or presence on Gram stain noted (eg, ceftriaxone: 50–75 mg/kg IV per day to max. 2–4 g/d)
- Adult: Penicillinase-resistant synthetic penicillin (eg, nafcillin: 2 g IV q4h); if suspect MRSA, vancomycin (15 mg/kg IV q12h)
- Sickle cell anemia with OM: Ciprofloxacin 400 mg IV q12h, or levofloxacin 750 mg IV q24h (not in children); alternative: 3rd-generation cephalosporin
- Post–nail puncture through tennis shoe: Ciprofloxacin 750 mg PO b.i.d. or levofloxacin 750 mg PO q24h; alternative: Ceftazidime 2 g IV q8h
- Involving orthopedic prosthesis or hardware: Add rifampin (10 mg/kg/d PO/IV to maximum of 600 mg/d) to regimen for *S. aureus*. Hardware removal generally required.
- Post-traumatic OM: Vancomycin and ceftazidime
- If vancomycin-resistant enterococcus present: Linezolid 600 mg IV q12h × 6 wk

### Pediatric Considerations
Children with hematogenous OM may undergo short-course IV antibiotics and then be changed to oral for additional 1–2 mo.

 **FOLLOW-UP**

### DISPOSITION
#### Admission Criteria
- Patients with acute OM should be admitted.
- Patients with chronic osteomyelitis usually require admission for surgical procedures, debridement, and obtaining bone cultures and histology.

#### Discharge Criteria
Subacute or chronic OM patients may be considered for outpatient management if home IV antibiotics arranged, bone specimens obtained, and necrotic bone debrided.
- Cases refractory to debridement and antibiotics benefit from hyperbaric oxygen as an adjunct to standard treatment.
- ~2/3 of these cases will demonstrate benefit.

## PEARLS AND PITFALLS
- WBC may be normal in many cases.
- Radiographs may be normal in the 1st 2–3 wk of symptoms.
- Wound cultures are low yield in guiding antibiotic therapy.

## ADDITIONAL READING
- Butalia S, Palda VA, Sergeant RJ, et. al. Does this patient with diabetes have osteomyelitis of the lower extremity? *JAMA*. 2008;299(7):806–813.
- Lalani T, Sexton D. Overview of osteomyelitis in adults. In: Rose BD, ed. *UpToDate*. Waltham, MA: UpToDate, 2010.
- Weichert S, Charland M, Clark NMP, et al. Acute haematogenous osteomyelitis in children: Is there any evidence for how long we should treat? *Curr Opin Infect Dis*. 2008;21:258 262.
- Winters ME, Kluetz P, Zilberstein J. Back pain emergencies. *Med Clin N Am*. 2006;90:505–523.

 **CODES**

### ICD9
730.20 Unspecified osteomyelitis, site unspecified

# OSTEOPOROSIS

*Daniel Davis*

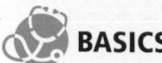 **BASICS**

## DESCRIPTION
- Overall decrease in skeletal mass, generally diffuse
- Trabecular bone (especially vertebrae and femur) affected more commonly and earlier
- Disease begins in adolescence, but fractures do not usually manifest until age ≥50.
- Females affected much more commonly than males, especially after menopause.

## ETIOLOGY
- Overall increase in resorption over formation of new bone
- Advanced age is the most important risk factor.
- Inadequate dietary calcium an important factor, especially early in life
- Sedentary lifestyle is a risk factor (weight bearing on bone favors new bone formation).
- Decrease in estrogen with menopause key factor in women.
- Other causes include long-term steroid use, alcoholism, methotrexate.
- Familial or hereditary factor may coexist.

### Pediatric Considerations
Although disease appears to start in adolescence, pediatric patients are asymptomatic.

 **DIAGNOSIS**

## SIGNS AND SYMPTOMS
- Usually asymptomatic until pathologic fractures occur
- Fractures with insignificant mechanism or recurrent fractures are hallmark.
- Vertebral column most commonly involved
- Multiple compression fractures of vertebral column often lead to kyphosis and scoliosis.
- Hip fractures (femoral neck and intertrochanteric fractures) also common

### History
- A suspected fracture with a relatively minor mechanism or a history of multiple fractures suggests osteoporosis.
- A family history of osteoporosis is an important risk factor.

### Physical Exam
Exam findings are related to the acute fracture rather than the disease itself.

## ESSENTIAL WORKUP
- Fracture without significant mechanism and identification of risk factors is most important.
- Careful neurovascular examination distal to femur or other extremity fracture
- Rectal tone and postvoid residual should be determined in patients with vertebral fractures.
- Radiographs of suspected fracture may show osteopenia (late finding in disease).
- Spine films may show old compression fractures.
- CT scan should be performed to better evaluate vertebral fractures:
  – Retropulsion, spinal canal compromise is not always apparent on plain films.
  – Make sure CT cuts extend full level above and below injuries on spine radiographs.

## DIAGNOSTIC TESTS & INTERPRETATION
### Lab
Serum chemistries—such as calcium, parathyroid hormone, and alkaline phosphatase—may help differentiate this from other illnesses.

### Imaging
- Plain films can identify fractures; however, age of each fracture may be difficult to determine.
- Bone scan or CT can help determine age of fractures, especially in spine.

### Diagnostic Procedures/Surgery
Bone densitometry can provide prognostic information and help guide therapy.

## DIFFERENTIAL DIAGNOSIS
- Multiple myeloma or other metastatic tumor
- Osteogenesis imperfecta (usually apparent in childhood)
- Hyperparathyroidism
- Other demineralizing bone diseases

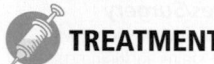 **TREATMENT**

## PRE-HOSPITAL
Cautions:
- Obtain prehospital information on mechanism to help diagnose pathologic fracture.
- Avoid aggressive manipulation or movement of patient, as this may exacerbate bony injury.

## INITIAL STABILIZATION/THERAPY
Immobilize fractures

## ED TREATMENT/PROCEDURES

- Fractures are treated with expectation of delayed or incomplete healing.
- Prevention is far more effective than treatment.
- Long-term therapy is beneficial (see "Medications").
- Use of orthotic back braces and vests should be arranged in conjunction with orthopedic spine consultation.
- Exercise is also helpful.
- Balance must be achieved between osteoporosis risk and steroid or methotrexate therapy.

## MEDICATION

- <Alendronate: 10 mg/day
- Calcitonin: 0.5 mg/day SC of human, 100 IU/day SC of salmon; alternative: nasal spray (100 IU) 1 spray per day in alternate nostrils
- Calcium supplementation (often with vitamin D): 1–1.5 g/day
- Estrogen: 0.625 mg/day (with or without medroxyprogesterone)
- Etidronate: 400 mg/day for 2-wk cycles q15wk
- Raloxifene (selective estrogen receptor modulator): 60 mg PO qd
- Sodium fluoride: 25 mg b.i.d. with calcium

### Pediatric Considerations

Ensure adequate calcium in diet from early age.

 **FOLLOW-UP**

## DISPOSITION

### Admission Criteria

- Per normal orthopedic protocols, with special considerations for age and social situation
- Compression fractures are generally stable, but possibility of burst fracture with cord compression must be ruled out.

- Any cervical fracture or fracture with neurologic symptoms requires admission with emergent consultation with neurosurgery or orthopedics.
- Admission may be necessary for pain control and because of decreased ambulation.

### Discharge Criteria

- Per normal orthopedic protocols with special considerations for age and social situation
- Patients with minimal injuries, able to care for themselves at home or with appropriate assistance, and adequate postoperative pain control may be discharged with orthopedic follow-up.

### Issues for Referral

Orthopedic referral is driven by the acute injury.

## FOLLOW-UP RECOMMENDATIONS

- Follow-up is generally driven by the acute injuries.
- Follow-up with the primary physician should be instituted to encourage treatment and monitoring of the disease.

# PEARLS AND PITFALLS

- A history of recurrent fractures, particularly with a low-energy mechanism, suggests the possibility of osteoporosis.
- Reduced bone density on plain radiographs is highly suggestive and warrants referral back to the PCP for further workup and treatment.

# ADDITIONAL READING

- Unnanuntana A, Gladnick BP, Donnelly E, Lane JM. The assessment of fracture risk. *J Bone Joint Surg Am*. 2010;92(3):743–753.
- Chandrasoma P, Taylor CR. *Concise Pathology*. East Norwalk, CT: Appleton & Lange, 1991.
- Krane SM, Holick MF. Metabolic bone disease. In: Wilson JD, et al, eds. *Harrison's Principles of Internal Medicine*. 12th ed. New York: McGraw-Hill, 1991:19–21.
- North American Menopause Society. Management of postmenopausal osteoporosis: Position statement. *Menopause*. 2002;9(2):84–101.
- Papaioannou A, et al. Diagnosis and management of vertebral fractures in elderly adults. *Am J Med*. 2002;113(3):220–228.

## See Also (Topic, Algorithm, Electronic Media Element)

Specific orthopedic injuries.

 **CODES**

**ICD9**
- 733.00 Osteoporosis, unspecified
- 733.01 Senile osteoporosis

# OTITIS EXTERNA
*Assaad J. Sayah*

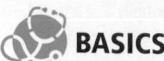 **BASICS**

## DESCRIPTION
- Inflammation or infection of the auricle, auditory canal, or external surface of the tympanic membrane (TM):
  – Spares the middle ear
  – Affects 4/1,000 persons in the U.S.
- Also called "swimmer's ear" due to the usual history of recent swimming:
  – Occasional cases after normal bathing
- Necrotizing (malignant) otitis externa:
  – Infection starts at the ear canal and progresses through periauricular tissue toward the base of the skull.
  – Occurs in elderly, diabetic, or other immunocompromised patients
  – Caused by *Pseudomonas aeruginosa*
  – Can lead to cellulitis, chondritis and osteomyelitis

## ETIOLOGY
- Often precipitated by an abrasion of the ear canal or maceration of the skin from persisting water or excessive dryness
- Predisposing factors include:
  – History of ear surgery or TM perforation
  – Narrow or abnormal canal
  – Humidity
  – Allergy
  – Trauma
  – Abnormal cerumen production
- *P. aeruginosa, Staphylococcus aureus,* streptococcal species, and rarely fungi

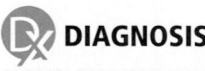 **DIAGNOSIS**

## SIGNS AND SYMPTOMS
### History
- Recent swimming or prolonged water exposure
- History of diabetes
- History of chemotherapy, prolonged steroid use, HIV/AIDS, or other process that compromises immune system
- Itching of the external ear canal is usually the 1st symptom.
- 1–2-day history of progressive pain
- Ear drainage
- Decreased auditory acuity
- Clogged sensation in ear

### Physical Exam
- Pain in ear or with motion of pinna/tragus
- Swollen, erythematous external ear canal
- Ear drainage
- Decreased auditory acuity
- Pain/swelling in preauricular area
- Necrotizing (malignant) otitis externa:
  – Pain, tenderness, swelling in periauricular area
  – Headache
  – Otorrhea
  – Cranial nerve palsy
    o Facial nerve most affected

## ESSENTIAL WORKUP
Clinical diagnosis with typical signs/symptoms:
- Pain in ear or with motion of pinna/tragus
- Otoscopic examination
- Swollen, erythematous external ear canal
- Ear drainage
- Cheesy white or gray green exudate

## DIAGNOSTIC TESTS & INTERPRETATION
### Lab
- None usually indicated, except when possibility of necrotizing otitis externa:
  – Signs of systemic toxicity or local spread of infection should be checked.
- WBC count
- ESR
- Glucose (check for diabetes)
- Cultures

### Imaging
CT/MRI to exclude osteomyelitis if the patient has signs of toxicity or bony involvement

### Diagnostic Procedures/Surgery
- Remove debris with a soft plastic curette or gentle irrigation with peroxide/water mix.
- Wick placement may be needed to facilitate medication delivery.

## DIFFERENTIAL DIAGNOSIS
- Necrotizing otitis externa
- Otitis media
- Folliculitis from obstruction of sebaceous glands
- Otic foreign bodies
- Herpes zoster infection of the geniculate ganglion
- Parotitis
- Periauricular adenitis
- Mastoiditis
- Dental abscess
- Sinusitis
- Tonsillitis
- Pharyngitis
- Temporomandibular joint pain
- Viral exanthems

### Pediatric Considerations
Consider ear canal foreign bodies in children with purulent drainage from edematous, painful ear canals.

 **TREATMENT**

## ED TREATMENT/PROCEDURES
- Clean external ear canal:
  – Remove the inflammatory debris by gentle curettage with a cotton-tipped wire applicator.
  – Occasional suction with a Fraser suction tip may be necessary.
- Insert a cotton or gauze wick 10–12 mm into the canal after cleansing if the ear canal is very edematous.
- Management of otitis externa focuses on pain control, eradication of infection, and prevention of reoccurrence.

## MEDICATION
- Most cases respond well to topical treatment:
  – Antiseptic, anti-inflammatory, and drying otic drops eliminate the pathogenic bacteria and allow for rapid healing of the canal.
  – Acetic acid solutions such as Domeboro otic (2% acetic acid): 4–6 drops q4–6h.
  – Corticosporin otic (hydrocortisone 1%, polymyxin + neomycin) suspension: 4 drops to ear canal q.i.d. (use suspensions and not solutions with suspected TM perforation)
  – Ofloxacin: 5 drops b.i.d. (drug of choice in perforated TM)

- Oral antibiotics:
  - Administer to patients with cellulitis of the face or neck, severe edema of the ear canal, concurrent otitis media, or when the tympanic membrane cannot be visualized.
  - Treat diabetics and other immunocompromised patients with oral ciprofloxacin and follow closely for symptoms of malignant otitis externa.
  - Amoxicillin: 500 mg (peds: 40 mg/kg/d) PO t.i.d.
  - Ciprofloxacin: 500 mg PO b.i.d.
- IV antibiotics for patients with necrotizing otitis externa, severe cellulitis, or septic appearing
- Prophylaxis:
  - Apply rubbing alcohol or acetic acid (2%) to keep the external ear canal dry and prevent recurrence of infection.
- Pain management with acetaminophen or NSAID. Consider opioids if severe pain.
- Surgical debridement of granulation tissue and bony sequestration or drainage of associated abscess may be necessary in necrotizing otitis externa.

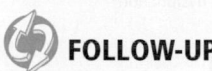 **FOLLOW-UP**

## DISPOSITION
### Admission Criteria
- Necrotizing otitis externa
- Significant involvement of the pinna
- Signs of systemic illness

### Discharge Criteria
- Most patients
- Close follow-up for patients at risk of otitis externa
- Patient instructions:
  - Avoid swimming and keep ears completely dry for 3–4 wk.
  - Apply medications as directed.
  - Return if worse pain, fever, hearing loss develops, or there is any change in mental or neurologic status.
  - Follow-up if symptoms are not improved within 2–3 days

### Issues for Referral
Ear-nose-throat follow-up for:
- Perforated TM
- Worsening of symptoms
- Conductive hearing loss
- Failure of initial management

## FOLLOW-UP RECOMMENDATIONS
Follow up with primary care physician or a return ED visit within 2–3 days for removal of the wick or if symptoms are worse.

## PEARLS AND PITFALLS

- Concomitant and often erroneous diagnoses of acute otitis externa and otitis media are common because the TM in acute otitis externa is erythematous.
- Avoid ear canal lavage until tympanic integrity is documented.
- Regardless of the topical medications, penetration to the epithelium is key to therapy; any obstruction should be cleared.
- Recurrence will be largely prevented by counseling the patient and explaining how it can be avoided by minimizing ear canal moisture, trauma, or exposure to material that incites local irritation or contact dermatitis.

- Necrotizing otitis externa should be suspected in immunocompromised patients and diabetics who have severe otalgia, purulent otorrhea, and granulation tissue or exposed bone in the external auditory canal.

## ADDITIONAL READING

- Birchall JP. Managing otitis externa. *Practitioner.* 2006;250:78–82.
- Carfrae MJ, Kesser BW. Malignant otitis externa. *Otolaryngol Clin North Am.* 2008;41:537–549.
- Osguthorpe JD, Nielsen DR. Otitis externa: Review and clinical update. *Am Fam Physician.* 2006;74: 1510–1516.
- Stone KE. Otitis externa. *Pediatr Rev.* 2007;28: 77–78.

### See Also (Topic, Algorithm, Electronic Media Element)
- Otitis Media
- Mastoiditis
- Tympanic Membrane Perforation

 **CODES**

**ICD9**
380.10 Infective otitis externa, unspecified

# OTITIS MEDIA
*Assaad J. Sayah*

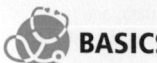

## BASICS

### DESCRIPTION
- Inflammation of the middle ear
- Most commonly occurs in children 6–36 mo
- Rapid onset of local and/or systemic symptoms

### ETIOLOGY
- Usually associated with (or as a result of) upper respiratory tract infections
- Viral:
  - Parainfluenza
  - Respiratory syncytial virus
  - Influenza
  - Adenovirus
  - Rhinovirus
- Bacterial:
  - *Staphylococcus pneumoniae*
  - *Moraxella catarrhalis*
  - *Haemophilus influenzae*
  - *Streptococcus pyogenes*
  - *Mycoplasma pneumoniae*
- Associated with blockage of eustachian tube
- Predisposing factors:
  - Deficient mucus, cilia, or antibodies
  - Intubation, especially nasotracheal
  - American Indians, Eskimos
  - Down syndrome
  - Cleft palate

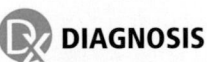

## DIAGNOSIS

### SIGNS AND SYMPTOMS
- **Definition**
- Acute onset (<48 hr)
- Middle ear effusion
- Middle ear inflammation
- **Risk Factors**
- Family history
- Daycare
- Parental smoking
- Pacifier use

### *History*
- Ear pain
- Irritability
- Rhinitis
- Vomiting, diarrhea
- Poor feeding
- Fever
- Sensation of plugged ear
- Pulling at ear
- Vertigo, tinnitus
- Conjunctivitis

### *Physical Exam*
- Tympanic membrane (TM) inflammation, bulging, and limited mobility
- Decreased visibility of the landmarks of the middle ear

### ESSENTIAL WORKUP
- Exclude associated conditions.
- Otoscopic examination for appearance and mobility of TM:
  - Full visualization essential
  - Increased vascularity, erythema, purulence
  - Obscured landmarks—bony, light reflex
  - Pneumatic otoscopy—bulging, retracted, decreased mobility

### DIAGNOSTIC TESTS & INTERPRETATION
#### *Lab*
Cultures unhelpful unless done by tympanocentesis

#### *Imaging*
CT scan if associated mastoiditis is suspected

#### *Diagnostic Procedures/Surgery*
- Tympanocentesis—indications:
  - Severe pain or toxicity
  - Failure of antimicrobial therapy
  - Suspicion of suppurative complication
  - Sick neonate
  - Immunocompromised patient
- Tympanometry and acoustic otoscopy may be useful with difficult examinations

### DIFFERENTIAL DIAGNOSIS
- Infection:
  - Otitis externa
  - Mastoiditis
  - Dental abscess
  - Peritonsillar abscess
  - Sinusitis
  - Lymphadenitis
  - Parotitis
  - Meningitis
- Trauma:
  - Perforation of the TM
  - Foreign body in ear
  - Barotrauma
  - Instrumentation
- Serous otitis media or eustachian tube dysfunction
- Impacted ear cerumen
- Impacted third molar
- Temporomandibular joint dysfunction

## TREATMENT

### ED TREATMENT/PROCEDURES
- Most mild cases could resolve without antibiotics.
- Antibiotics are indicated for all infants <6 mo and for older children with certain diagnosis or severe illness.
- For otherwise normal healthy patients ≥6 mo with mild symptoms and/or uncertain diagnosis, consider no antibiotics and repeat evaluation in 2–3 days:
  - For reliable parents, may provide a prescription for oral antibiotics, which the family can fill if the child's symptoms get worse or persist after 2 days.
- Considerations should include recurrent nature of otitis media, lack of clinical response, and resistance patterns in community.
- Parenteral antibiotics are indicated in febrile toxic children <1 yr or with immunocompromise.
- Antihistamines, decongestants, and steroids have no proven efficacy.
- Antipyretics and analgesics are important (avoid local analgesics in perforated TMs).

## MEDICATION

- Antibiotics:
  - Amoxicillin: 500–875 mg PO q12h (peds: 80–90 mg/kg/d PO div q12h) for 10 days
  - Amoxicillin-clavulanic acid: 500–875 mg PO q12h (peds: 90 mg/kg/d PO q12h) for 10 days
  - Azithromycin: 10 mg/kg PO day 1, then 5 mg/kg/d PO days 2–5
  - Cefuroxime: 500 mg PO q12h (peds: 30 mg/kg/d PO div. q12h)
- Analgesia:
  - Acetaminophen 15 mg/kg per dose orally/rectally every 4 hr as needed
  - Antipyrine/benzocaine (5.4%/1.4% solution): 2–4 drops in ear q.i.d. PRN
  - Ibuprofen 10 mg/kg per dose orally every 6 hr as needed

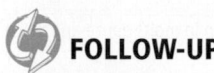 **FOLLOW-UP**

### DISPOSITION

#### Admission Criteria
Febrile toxic children who are:

- <1 yr, immunocompromised
- Moderately or severely dehydrated
- Unable to tolerate oral fluids or medications
- Suspected or proven associated significant infection
- Suspected abuse
- Unreliable caretaker

#### Discharge Criteria
Children without any of the aforementioned criteria

### FOLLOW-UP RECOMMENDATIONS

- Follow-up in 10–14 days to ensure resolution
- Indications for earlier follow-up:
  - Child does not get better in 24–48 hr
  - Any progression of signs or symptoms
  - New problems develop, including a rash
  - Any concerns arise

### COMPLICATIONS

- Recurrent otitis media:
  - 3 episodes within 6 mo or ≥4 episodes within 1 yr
- Perforated TM
- Serous otitis media
- Conductive hearing loss
- Facial nerve injury
- Mastoiditis
- Cholesteatoma
- Meningitis
- Subdural empyema
- Venous sinus thrombosis

## PEARLS AND PITFALLS

For otherwise normal healthy patients ≥6 mo with mild symptoms and/or uncertain diagnosis, consider no antibiotics and repeat evaluation in 2–3 days.

## ADDITIONAL READING

- American Academy of Pediatrics. Diagnosis and management of acute otitis media. *Pediatrics*. 2004;113:1451–1465.
- Gunasekera H, Morris PS, McIntyre P, et al. Management of children with otitis media: A summary of evidence from recent systematic reviews. *J Paediatr Child Health*. 2009;45:554–562.
- Jung TT, Hunter LL, Alper CM, et al. Recent advances in otitis media. 9. Complications and sequelae. *Ann Otol Rhinol Laryngol Suppl*. 2005;194:140–160.
- Powers JH. Diagnosis and treatment of acute otitis media: Evaluating the evidence. *Infect Dis Clin North Am*. 2007;21:409–426.
- Rosenfeld RM, Lous J, Bluestone CD, et al. Recent advances in otitis media. 8. Treatment. *Ann Otol Rhinol Laryngol Suppl*. 2005;194:114–39.
- Spiro DM, Arnold DH. The concept and practice of a wait-and-see approach to acute otitis media. *Curr Opin Pediatr*. 2008;20:72–78.

 **CODES**

**ICD9**
382.9 Unspecified otitis media

# OTOLOGIC TRAUMA
*Michael W. Nielsen*

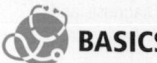

## BASICS

### DESCRIPTION
- Ear cartilage has no blood supply and is nutritionally dependent on perichondrium.
- Hematomas often disrupt perichondrium and cartilage; can lead to ischemia, perichondritis, necrosis, and cauliflower ear
- Penetrating injuries or bite wounds may lead to infection of cartilage.

### ETIOLOGY
- Blunt trauma:
  - Contact sports such as wrestling
  - Motorcycle helmets
- Penetrating trauma such as tympanic membrane (TM) perforation from cotton swabs
- Blast injury
- Lightning injury:
  - TM and ossicular disruptions occur in 50% of lightning strikes.
- Chemical exposure
- Thermal injury
- Diving injuries:
  - Inner ear barotrauma
  - Tympanic membrane rupture

### *Pediatric Considerations*
Consider nonaccidental trauma.

## DIAGNOSIS

### SIGNS AND SYMPTOMS
- Severe ear pain
- Bleeding
- Auricular deformity:
  - Edema
  - Hematoma
    - Bluish, fluctuant, or doughy swelling of auricle
  - Laceration
  - Amputation
  - Loss of contour of the pinna
- Decreased hearing:
  - Partial loss suggests tympanic membrane rupture
  - Complete hearing loss suggests additional injuries to ossicles or inner ear

- Hemotympanum
- Purulent or bloody discharge from ear canal
- Tinnitus
- Vertigo:
  - May be result of inner ear injury or tympanic membrane perforation

### *History*
- Mechanism
- Associated injuries
- Past otologic history
- Medications and allergies

### *Physical Exam*
- Head
- Cranial nerves
- Vascular structures
- Temporal bone
- Pinna
- External ear canal
- Tympanic membrane
- Hearing
- Consider Weber and Rinne test to evaluate for conductive hearing loss due to TM rupture or perforation:
  - Rinne test: Place a struck tuning fork to mastoid tip, hold until patient no longer hears ringing, then place fork near external auditory opening:
    - Normal: Patient still hears ringing; air conduction > bone conduction
    - Abnormal: No sound heard; air conduction < bone conduction; implies a conductive hearing loss
  - Weber test: Place a struck tuning fork to center of forehead:
    - Normal: Equal sound perception in both ears
    - Abnormal due to neurosensory loss: Patient will have decreased sound perception in the impaired ear.
    - Abnormal due to conductive loss: Increased sound perception in the impaired ear
- Be sure to evaluate for concomitant injuries.

## DIAGNOSTIC TESTS & INTERPRETATION
### *Lab*
Wound culture if signs of infection

### *Imaging*
Consider head and/or facial CT to evaluate for intracranial injury or bone fracture.

### DIFFERENTIAL DIAGNOSIS
- Infection
- Hemangioma
- Foreign body in ear

## TREATMENT

### PRE-HOSPITAL
If auricle is amputated, wrap in moist gauze and place in plastic bag.

### INITIAL STABILIZATION/THERAPY
- Check ABCs; full trauma evaluation; resuscitation as appropriate.
- Sterile dressing to injured site

### ED TREATMENT/PROCEDURES
- All injury types:
  - Anesthesia:
    - Local anesthesia via nerve block to auriculotemporal branch of mandibular nerve, lesser occipital nerve, greater auricular nerve, and auricular branch of vagus nerve; use 1% lidocaine or 0.25% marcaine.
    - Alternative: Inject ring of anesthetic around base of pinna.
- Management of TM perforation
- Tetanus prophylaxis if necessary
- For human and animal bites:
  - Treat with amoxicillin-clavulanate

- Specific injury types:
  - Auricular hematoma: Drainage imperative to reapproximate perichondrium to cartilage to prevent cartilage necrosis, ideally within 72 hr; however, no clearly defined best treatment based on meta-analysis
    - Antistaphylococcal antibiotics for 7–10 days
    - Aspiration: Preferred alternative if clot not yet formed; use 18–20 gauge needle for aspiration; milk hematoma until totally evacuated; apply pressure dressing.
    - Incision and drainage: More effective with larger and/or clotted hematomas; Incise along curvature of pinna with #15 scalpel, evacuate, and irrigate; apply pressure dressing.
    - Vaseline gauze: Place to fill crevices of pinna; place over and behind pinna; wrap soft gauze firmly around head.
    - Alternatively, suture dental rolls into place over incised area.
    - If patient has 2nd presentation due to reaccumulation, hematoma should be reaspirated and a wick placed for drainage.
- Laceration:
  - Prophylactic antibiotics are controversial.
  - Clean and debride wound, anesthetize as necessary.
  - Superficial abrasions: Clean, dress with antibiotic ointment.
  - Simple lacerations: 5.0 or 6.0 monofilament nylon or polypropylene suture, then pressure dressing; may use absorbable suture to avoid having to bend ear for suture removal
  - Exposed auricular cartilage: Carefully debride jagged edges; completely cover cartilage to prevent perichondritis; can remove small amount of cartilage to allow skin coverage; approximate cartilage 1st with absorbable sutures at major landmarks; include anterior and posterior perichondrium in stitch.
  - Avulsions:
    - <2 cm total avulsions may be used as graft and survive.
    - >2 cm: Consult or urgently refer to otolaryngologist or plastic surgeon; save in SC pocket.

## MEDICATION

- Amoxicillin-clavulanate: Adults: 875/125 mg PO t.i.d. (peds: 40 mg/kg/day PO t.i.d.)
- Dicloxacillin: 250–500 mg PO q.i.d. (peds: 30–50 mg/kg/d PO div. q6h)

 FOLLOW-UP

### DISPOSITION

#### Admission Criteria

- Concomitant serious traumatic injuries
- Need for IV antibiotics
- Immunosuppressed persons with serious infections, perichondritis, or chondritis

#### Discharge Criteria

- Able to tolerate oral antibiotics
- Able to arrange close follow-up

### FOLLOW-UP RECOMMENDATIONS

- Follow up wound suture repair in 5 days.
- Follow up hematomas in 24 hr to evaluate for reaccumulation

## ADDITIONAL READING

- Ghanem T, Rasamny JK, Park SS. Rethinking auricular trauma. *Laryngoscope*. 2005;115:1251.
- Jones SE, Mahendran S. Interventions for acute auricular haematoma. *Cochrane Database Syst Rev*. 2004;(2):CD004166.
- McKay MP, Mayersak RJ. Facial trauma. In: Marx J, Hockberger R, Walls R. *Rosen's Emergency Medicine*, 7th ed. St. Louis, MO: Mosby; 2009.
- Riviello RJ, Brown NA. Otolaryngologic procedures. In: Rogers JR, Hedges J, eds. *Clinical Procedures in Emergency Medicine*, 5th ed. Philadelphia: WB Saunders; 2009.
- Spring PM, Amedee RG. Ear pain and drainage. In: Calhoun KH, ed. *Expert Guide to Otolaryngology*. Philadelphia: American College of Physicians; 2001.

### See Also (Topic, Algorithm, Electronic Media Element)

- Barotrauma
- Tympanic Membrane Perforation

 CODES

### ICD9

- 920 Contusion of face, scalp, and neck except eye(s)
- 959.09 Other and unspecified injury to face and neck

# OVARIAN CYST/TORSION

Renee A. King
Lynne M. Yancey

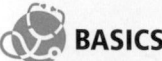 **BASICS**

## DESCRIPTION

- Ovarian cysts:
  - Generally asymptomatic until complicated by hemorrhage, torsion, rupture, or infection
  - Follicular cysts:
    - Most common
    - Occur from fetal life to menopause
    - Unilocular; diameter 3–8 cm
    - Thin wall predisposes to rupture, which usually causes minimal or no bleeding.
    - Rupture during ovulation at midcycle is known as mittelschmerz.
  - Corpus luteal cysts:
    - Most significant
    - Diameter 3 cm, but usually <10 cm
    - Rapid bleeding from intracystic hemorrhage causes rupture.
    - Rupture is most common just before menses begins.
    - Can cause severe intraperitoneal bleeding
    - Gradual bleeding into cyst or ovary distends capsule and may cause pain without rupture.
- Adnexal torsion:
  - 5th-most-prevalent surgical gynecologic emergency
  - Twisting of vascular pedicle of ovary, fallopian tube, or paratubal cyst
  - Causes adnexal ischemia leading to necrosis
  - Occlusion of lymphatics and venous drainage lead to rapid enlargement of adnexa.
  - Greatest risk with cysts 8–12 cm

## RISK FACTORS

Adnexal torsion:

- Reproductive-age women
- Ovarian cysts, especially >5 cm
- Ovarian hyperstimulation
- Tumors: serous cystadenoma most common; teratomas
- Pelvic surgery: tubal ligation; hysterectomy
- Pregnancy
- History of pelvic inflammatory disease

## Pediatric Considerations
15% of adnexal torsions occur in children.

### ALERT
- Anticoagulated patients at increased risk of:
  - Hemorrhagic corpus luteal cyst
  - Significant bleed from ruptured cyst, including with ovulation

## ETIOLOGY

- Ovarian cyst:
  - Follicular cysts result from nonrupture of mature follicle or failure of atresia of immature follicle.
  - Corpus luteal cysts result from unrestrained growth in early pregnancy or from normal intracystic hemorrhage days after ovulation.
  - Other cysts:
    - Theca lutein
    - Cystic teratoma
    - Endometrioma (chocolate cyst)
- Adnexal torsion:
  - Right > left
  - Highest frequency in reproductive women

### ALERT
Cysts found in postmenopausal women suggest carcinoma.

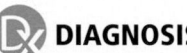 **DIAGNOSIS**

## SIGNS AND SYMPTOMS
### History
- Ovarian cyst:
  - Abdominal pain
    - Sharp, unilateral
    - Intermittent vs. constant
    - Migration
    - Previous episodes
    - May occur with exercise, intercourse, trauma, or pelvic exam
  - Fever is rare.
  - Irregular menses (may suggest polycystic ovary syndrome)
  - Infertility
  - Pregnancy status
  - Previous STDs
  - History of breast or GI cancer (may metastasize)

- Adnexal torsion:
  - Variable history
  - Abdominal pain:
    - Sudden, sharp, colicky
    - Localized vs. diffuse
    - Referred pain to groin or flank
    - May be chronic or recurring with torsion/detorsion
  - Fever
  - Nausea/vomiting
  - Vaginal bleeding
  - UTI symptoms

### Physical Exam
- Ovarian cyst:
  - Abdominal tenderness (mild to severe with peritonitis)
  - Adnexal tenderness
  - Pelvic mass
  - Hemorrhagic shock possible:
    - Usually from corpus luteal cyst rupture
    - Orthostasis, hypotension, tachycardia
- Adnexal torsion:
  - Abdominal tenderness (mild to severe)
  - Adnexal tenderness
  - Adnexal mass

## ESSENTIAL WORKUP
- Pregnancy test essential to rule out ectopic pregnancy
- Rapid hemoglobin or hematocrit

## DIAGNOSTIC TESTS & INTERPRETATION
### Lab
- Urine or serum human chorionic gonadotropin determination
- CBC
- Urinalysis
- If significant hemorrhage, type and cross packed RBCs
- Cervical cultures to rule out PID

### Imaging

- Transvaginal US:
  - Adnexal cysts and masses:
    - Cystic masses <5 cm in premenopausal women generally benign
    - Should be reevaluated at end of menstruation
  - Pelvic free fluid
  - Enlarged, edematous ovary (suggests torsion)
- Doppler:
  - May show decreased flow with torsion
  - Important to document normal blood flow on Doppler in ED, even though does not rule out recent torsion of ovary
- MRI:
  - Consider in pregnant patients with right lower quadrant pain and nondiagnostic US and Doppler
- CT:
  - May demonstrate cysts or evidence of torsion or suggest alternative diagnosis
  - May provide enough information to proceed to laparoscopy if abnormal ovary and no other cause of pain identified
  - Uterus may be shifted to side of torsed adnexa.
  - Ascites may be present.

### ALERT

US sensitivity for diagnosis of ovarian torsion is not well established; continue workup if high clinical suspicion.

### Diagnostic Procedures/Surgery

- Culdocentesis:
  - No longer commonly done
  - May yield serosanguinous fluid with ruptured cyst
  - Hematocrit >15% suggests significant hemoperitoneum.
- Laparoscopy is gold standard for torsed adnexa and definitive diagnosis.

### Pediatric Considerations

Early detorsion of adnexa by laparoscopy is now advocated to preserve ovarian function.

### DIFFERENTIAL DIAGNOSIS

For pelvic pain:

- Ectopic pregnancy
- PID
- Round ligament pain
- Endometriosis
- Neoplasm
- Torsion of uterus
- Appendicitis

### FOLLOW-UP RECOMMENDATIONS

Ovarian cyst

- If pain is resolved and cyst is <4–5 cm, close follow-up is recommend with gynecology for further studies.

## PEARLS AND PITFALLS

Adnexal torsion:

- Torsion is a clinical diagnosis:
  - US may show flow to an ovary that has detorsed.
- Symptoms can be varied and nonspecific.
- Always include adnexal torsion in differential of abdominal pain.

## ADDITIONAL READING

- Becker JH, de Graaf J, Vos CM. Torsion of the ovary: A known but frequently missed diagnosis. *Eur J Emerg Med*. 2009;16:124–126.
- Bottomley C, Bourne T. Diagnosis and management of ovarian cyst accidents. *Best Pract Res Clin Obstet Gynaecol*. 2009;23:711–724.
- Chang, HC, Bhatt S, Dogra VS. Pearls and pitfalls in diagnosis of ovarian torsion. *Radiographics* 2008; 28:1355–1368.
- Houry D, Abbott JT. Ovarian torsion: A fifteen-year review. *Ann Emerg Med*. 2001;38:156–159.
- McWilliams GDE, Hill MJ, Dietrich CS. Gynecologic emergencies. *Surg Clin North Am*. 2008;88: 265–283.
- Moore C, Meyers AB, Capostato J, et al. Prevalence of abnormal CT findings in patients with proven ovarian torsion and a proposed triage schema. *Emerg Radiol*. 2009;16:115–120.

### See Also (Topic, Algorithm, Electronic Media Element)

- Abdominal Pain
- Ectopic Pregnancy
- Endometriosis
- Pelvic Inflammatory Disease

 CODES

ICD9

- 620.2 Other and unspecified ovarian cyst
- 620.5 Torsion of ovary, ovarian pedicle, or fallopian tube

# PAGET DISEASE
*Daniel Davis*

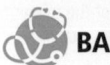

## BASICS

### DESCRIPTION
- Paget disease involves resorption of normal bone and its replacement with fibrous and sclerotic tissue.
- Also known as osteitis deformans
- Usually focal, bones most frequently involved include:
  - Pelvis (70%)
  - Femur (55%)
  - Skull (42%)
  - Tibia 32%)
  - Spine (53%, lumbar spine)
  - Flat bones
- Usually found incidentally and generally asymptomatic
- Occurs in ~1–2% of patients >40
- Starts with resorptive or osteolytic phase, during which osteoclasts remove healthy bone.
- Hypervascularity begins in resorptive phase:
  - Predisposes to hematoma and fracture
- Resorbed bone is eventually replaced by irregular, dense, disorganized trabecular bone in sclerotic or osteoplastic phase.
- Malignant transformation is rare:
  - Osteosarcoma is malignancy of concern.
  - Usually malignant transformation occurs in 1%.
- More common in men
- Typically involves 1 bone (monostotic)
- May involve a few bones (polyostotic)

### ETIOLOGY
- Unknown
- May represent vascular hyperplasia with subsequent inflammation
- Presence of nucleocapsids from measles, canine distemper, or respiratory syncytial virus may implicate viral cause.
- Genetic component
- Environmental influences may also play a role.

### *Pediatric Considerations*
Generally not seen in children

## DIAGNOSIS

### SIGNS AND SYMPTOMS
- Many patients are asymptomatic, with disease discovered by incidental radiographs or elevated alkaline phosphatase levels.
- Deep, aching bone pain occurs late in the clinical course.
- Pain with weight-bearing if femur or tibia involvement
- Acute (resorptive/osteolytic) phase:
  - Pathologic fractures
  - Pain from acute lysis, pathologic fracture, or resultant arthritis
  - Hypercalcemia or renal stones
  - Hypervascularity may result in significant bleeding if affected bone is fractured.
  - Widespread disease:
    ○ Increased vascularity and blood flow may result in high-output cardiac failure.
- Secondary (sclerotic/osteoplastic) phase:
  - Long-bone involvement may present with swelling or deformity and gait abnormality.
  - Skull involvement may lead to headaches or abnormal skull contours (change in hat size).
  - Severe skull or spine involvement may result in CNS compression.
  - Hearing loss may result from nerve compression or ossicle involvement.

### ESSENTIAL WORKUP
- Diagnosis usually suggested by radiographs
- Thorough neurologic exam must be documented, especially with vertebral or pelvis involvement.

## DIAGNOSTIC TESTS & INTERPRETATION
### *Lab*
- Alkaline phosphatase is most dramatic marker of disease activity (especially resorptive phase).
- Calcium and phosphate levels should be checked as well, but are usually normal.
- EKG if suspect hypercalcemia and CXR with evidence of high-output cardiac failure
- Increased bone formation may lead to elevations in urine hydroxyproline or serum osteocalcin or procollagen fragments.
- Alterations in parathyroid hormone (PTH) levels occur as secondary changes during resorptive/osteolytic phase (low PTH) and sclerotic/osteoplastic phase (high PTH).

### *Imaging*
- Plain x-rays:
  - During resorptive phase, lytic lesions are often not seen, except in skull, where lesions are well demarcated (osteoporosis circumscripta).
  - Bowing of long bones may occur with resorption and strength loss.
  - New bone initially appears irregular and spotty, and later becomes homogeneous and dense ("ivory pattern").
  - Excess bone may be deposited along stress lines, leading to cortical irregularities.
- CT or MRI defines margins and helps evaluate for neoplasm or hematoma:
  - Spiral CT to detect renal calculi
- Bone scan is most sensitive for diagnosis of Paget disease.
- Radionuclide scans (technetium$^{99m}$, gallium$^{67}$) may help guide therapy by assessing response to therapy.

## DIFFERENTIAL DIAGNOSIS
- Primary hyperparathyroidism
- Multiple myeloma
- Hodgkin variants
- Acromegaly
- Osteosarcoma

 ## TREATMENT

### PRE-HOSPITAL
- Prehospital personnel should obtain information about mechanism of injury or social factors that suggest pathologic fracture.
- Adequate immobilization can limit excessive bleeding around fracture site.

### INITIAL STABILIZATION/THERAPY
- Airway management and resuscitation, as indicated
- High-output cardiac failure should be treated as outlined in CHF chapter.
- Prompt immobilization of fractures will limit excessive bleeding around fracture site.

### ED TREATMENT/PROCEDURES
- Analgesia for pain of lytic lesions, fractures, or arthritis includes NSAIDs and narcotics.
- High-dose prednisone can suppress disease.
- Fracture treatment is often more conservative, owing to difficulties with bleeding during operative repair.
- Orthopedic consultation for severe arthritis and definitive fracture management
- Hypercalcemia may be treated with IV fluids, furosemide (Lasix), calcitonin, inorganic phosphate, etidronate, mitramycin.

- Long-term chemotherapy may provide temporary or prolonged remission.
- CNS compression requires emergent neurosurgical consultation and possible decompression.

### MEDICATION
- Alendronate: 40 mg/d for 6 mo
- Calcitonin: 0.5 mg/d SC of human, 100 IU/d SC of salmon
- Chemotherapy with plicamycin/mitramycin, dactinomycin, diphosphonate
- Etidronate: 400 mg/d for 6-mo cycles
- Furosemide (Lasix): 20–80 mg IV for hypercalcemia
- Inorganic phosphate
- Pamidronate: 30 mg/d IV for 3 days
- Risedronate: 30 mg PO for 2 mos

 ## FOLLOW-UP

### DISPOSITION
#### Admission Criteria
- Admission as indicated for major trauma or injury, or excessive bleeding
- Orthopedic procedures
- Hypercalcemia
- CNS compressive symptoms

#### Discharge Criteria
- No evidence of significant bleeding, neurologic compromise, or hypercalcemia, and adequate pain control
- Appropriate fracture immobilization and orthopedic follow up

#### Issues for Referral
Referral is driven by any acute injuries.

## FOLLOW-UP RECOMMENDATIONS
- Follow-up is generally driven by the acute injury that led to the radiographs on which the diagnosis of Paget disease was made.
- Follow-up with the primary physician should be adequate.

## PEARLS AND PITFALLS
- The diagnosis of Paget disease is usually made as an incidental finding on radiographic imaging.
- Prompt immobilization of fractures will limit excessive bleeding around fracture site.
- Consider Paget disease if elevation of alkaline phosphatase is present without any other explanation.

## ADDITIONAL READING
- Ralston SH, Langston AL, Reid IR. Pathogenesis and management of Paget's disease of bone. *Lancet*. 2008;372:155–163.
- Schneider D, et al. Diagnosis and treatment of Paget's disease of bone. *Am Fam Physician*. 2002;65:2069–2072.
- Whyte MP. Paget's disease of bone. *N Engl J Med*. 2006;355:593–600.

### See Also (Topic, Algorithm, Electronic Media Element)
Specific Orthopedic Injuries

 ## CODES

### ICD9
731.0 Osteitis deformans without mention of bone tumor

# PANCREATIC PSEUDOCYST

*Trevor Lewis*

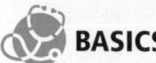 **BASICS**

## DESCRIPTION

- Cystic collection of fluid with high content of pancreatic enzymes surrounded by a wall of fibrous tissue lacking a true epithelial lining
- Localized in parenchyma of pancreas or adjacent abdominal spaces (lesser peritoneal sac)
- Requires 4–6 wk to form from onset of acute pancreatitis

## ETIOLOGY

- Ethanol abuse accounts for 70–80% cases.
- Other causes include trauma, biliary tract disease, hypertriglyceridemia, and recent surgery.
- Average age at diagnosis 45 yr
- Men > women
- Complication in 5–16% of acute pancreatitis; 20–40% of chronic pancreatitis

### Pediatric Considerations

- >60% result from blunt trauma.
- Usually can palpate a mass

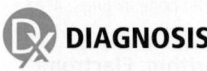 **DIAGNOSIS**

## SIGNS AND SYMPTOMS

- Frequency:
  - Abdominal pain: 86%
  - Nausea/vomiting: 72%
  - Palpable mass: 49%
  - Weight loss: 35%
  - Pleural effusion: 15%
  - Jaundice: 13%
  - Ascites: 11%
  - Internal hemorrhage: 7%

- GI:
  - In chronic pancreatitis, pseudocyst is heralded by change in typical pain pattern.
  - Symptoms reflecting structural compression by pseudocyst:
    - Nausea, vomiting, weight loss: Duodenal or gastric outlet obstruction
    - Jaundice: Common bile duct compression
    - Patients can be asymptomatic with pseudocyst.
- Respiratory:
  - Left lung pleural effusion common
- Cardiac:
  - Commonly occurs with pseudocyst rupture or hemorrhage
  - Tachycardia
  - Hypotension
  - Shock (depending on fluid losses)
- Infected pseudocyst:
  - Fever
  - Chills
  - Leukocytosis
- Pseudocyst hemorrhage:
  - Hypotension
  - Expanding abdominal mass
  - Usually erodes into splenic or gastroduodenal arteries
- Ruptured pseudocyst:
  - Abdominal rigidity, severe pain
  - Occurs when cyst ruptures into peritoneal cavity
  - Can rupture into GI tract

## ESSENTIAL WORKUP

- Laboratory tests not helpful in diagnosis
- Useful to anticipate complications

## DIAGNOSTIC TESTS & INTERPRETATION

### Lab

- Amylase/lipase:
  - Normal value in up to 50% of pseudocysts
- CBC:
  - Leukocytosis suggests infected pseudocyst
  - Low hematocrit with pseudocyst hemorrhage
- Electrolytes, BUN, creatinine, glucose:
  - Hypocalcemia
  - Hypokalemia with extensive fluid losses
  - Hypomagnesemia with underlying ethanol abuse
  - Hyperglycemia

### Imaging

- CT scan:
  - Imaging test of choice
  - Indicated for all cases of newly suspected pseudocyst
  - Can evaluate wall surrounding cyst and adjacent structures
- US:
  - Useful for follow-up of previously diagnosed pseudocyst to assess pseudocyst dimensions
  - May miss smaller cysts
- Angiography:
  - Helpful in cases of pseudocyst hemorrhage
  - Usually impractical due to instability of patient

## DIFFERENTIAL DIAGNOSIS

- Pancreatic abscess
- Neoplastic pancreatic cysts
- Perforated ulcer
- Ruptured abdominal aortic aneurysm (pseudocyst hemorrhage)
- Myocardial infarction
- Biliary colic
- Intestinal obstruction

**TREATMENT**

### PRE-HOSPITAL
- Initiate IV access in cooperative patients.
- Apply cardiac monitor.

### INITIAL STABILIZATION/THERAPY
- ABCs
- Supplemental oxygen
- Cardiac monitor
- IV fluids

### ED TREATMENT/PROCEDURES
- Fluid resuscitation:
  - Fluid losses may necessitate large fluid volumes.
  - Continuously assess vitals, urine output, and electrolytes to ensure rapid and adequate replacement of intravascular volume.
- Correct electrolytes abnormalities (hypocalcemia, hypokalemia, hypomagnesemia).
- Blood products:
  - Transfuse immediately in cases of pseudocyst hemorrhage pending definitive surgical treatment.
- Analgesia (opiate analgesia drug of choice)
- Nasogastric suction if intractable nausea/vomiting
- Antiemetics (promethazine)

### Geriatric Considerations
Consider central venous pressure monitoring in elderly.

### MEDICATION
#### First Line
Analgesics, antiemetics:
- Morphine 2–4 mg IV
- Meperidine (Demerol) 25–50 mg IV, 50–75 IM q3h–q4h
- Compazine 5–10 mg PO/IV/IM
- Zofran 4 mg IV/IM

#### Second Line
Electrolyte replacement:
- Potassium chloride: 10 mEq/h IV over 1 hr
- Calcium gluconate: 10%: 10 mL IV over 15–20 min
- Magnesium 2 g IV

 **FOLLOW-UP**

### DISPOSITION
#### Admission Criteria
- All newly diagnosed pseudocysts >6 cm
- Pseudocysts <6 cm if symptoms of acute pancreatitis
- Previously known pseudocysts if cyst is increasing in size compared with old studies
- Hemodynamic instability
- Severe abdominal pain
- Fever/infected pseudocyst

#### Discharge Criteria
Refer stable, asymptomatic patient with pseudocyst <6 cm for urgent surgical clinic follow-up.

#### Issues for Referral
- Surgical consultation:
  - Emergent surgical consultation mandatory in cases of suspected ruptured pseudocyst or pseudocyst hemorrhage, as definitive treatment is emergent laparotomy
- Surgical treatment options (pseudocyst >6 cm or persists for >6 wk):
  - Observation (no acute intervention):
    ○ Usually reserved for asymptomatic patients
  - Surgical excision:
    ○ Used infrequently
  - External drainage:
    ○ CT- or US-guided percutaneous drainage
  - Internal drainage:
    ○ Open vs. endoscopic technique

### FOLLOW-UP RECOMMENDATIONS
Patients discharged with small pseudocyst need coordinated follow-up with surgery and gastroenterology.

## PEARLS AND PITFALLS
- Majority of pseudocysts occur in chronic pancreatitis with a history of alcohol use.
- Intractable vomiting or jaundice in a patient with a history of pancreatitis may indicate bile duct or gastric outlet obstruction from a pseudocyst.
- Abdominal rigidity or hypotension in a patient with a history of pseudocysts mandates urgent surgical evaluation for pseudocyst rupture or hemorrhage.
- CT scan is the best imaging modality for newly suspected pseudocysts.

## ADDITIONAL READING

- Aghdassi A, Mayerle J, Kraft M, et al. Diagnosis and treatment of pancreatic pseudocysts in chronic pancreatitis. *Pancreas.* 2008;36(2):105–112.
- Baillie J. Pancreatic pseudocysts. *Gastrointest Endosc.* 2004;59:873–879.
- Cooperman AM. An overview of pancreatic pseudocysts: The emperor's new clothes revisited. *Surg Clin North Am.* 2001;81:391–397.
- Habashi S, Draganov P. Pancreatic pseudocyst. *World J Gastroenterol.* 2009;15(1):38–47.

### See Also (Topic, Algorithm, Electronic Media Element)
Pancreatitis

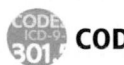 **CODES**

### ICD9
577.2 Cyst and pseudocyst of pancreas

# PANCREATIC TRAUMA

*Vaishal M. Tolia*
*Chirag A. Dholakia*

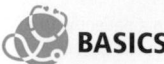

## BASICS

### DESCRIPTION
- Direct epigastric blow compressing pancreas against vertebral column resulting in blunt trauma
- Injury to pancreas from penetrating object

#### Pediatric Considerations
- Trauma affects proportionately larger areas, leading to multisystem injuries.
- Children have less protective muscle and subcutaneous tissue.
- Malpositioned seat belts and child abuse need to be considered in small children.
- Children will less often present with hypotension.

### ETIOLOGY
- Penetrating trauma: Most common mechanism
- Blunt trauma: Deep location of pancreas requires significant force to cause injury:
  – Steering wheel, seat belts, or bicycle handlebars to abdomen
  – In children, evaluate for nonaccidental trauma

### COMMONLY ASSOCIATED CONDITIONS
90% of pancreatic injuries associated with injuries to adjacent structures:
- Liver, stomach
- Major arteries and veins
- Spleen, kidney
- Duodenum, colon, small bowel
- Common bile duct, gallbladder
- Spine: Chance fracture

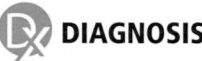

## DIAGNOSIS

### ALERT
Extent of pancreatic injury may not be apparent on initial evaluation.

### SIGNS AND SYMPTOMS
- Abdominal pain:
  – Diffuse or epigastric
  – Often out of proportion to physical exam and vital signs
- Soft-tissue contusion in upper abdomen
- Injury to lower ribs or costal cartilage
- Acute abdomen, often associated with other intra-abdominal injuries
- Concomitant splenic injury can present initially as dull back pain
- Hypotension
- Grey-Turner sign:
  – Flank ecchymosis
- Cullen sign:
  – Periumbilical ecchymosis

#### History
Concise; details of incident especially important for blunt trauma

#### Physical Exam
- Inspect for abrasions, contusions, penetrating wounds:
  – Must log roll patient for full inspection.
  – Look for seat belt–related injuries.
- Auscultate for presence or absence of bowel sounds.
- Palpate to determine location and severity of pain, presence of guarding, and rebound tenderness.
- Rectal exam for occult blood, vaginal exam, or penile exam
- Serial physical exams and vital signs for unidentified injuries

### ALERT
Vascular injury is the most common cause of mortality related to pancreatic injury. Suspicion necessitates immediate evaluation and possible surgical exploration.

### ESSENTIAL WORKUP
- Pace of workup is dictated by patient condition and other injuries.
- Abdominal CT with IV contrast is essential to evaluate for pancreatic trauma.
- MRCP is being used more frequently in trauma centers to better evaluate ductal injury.

### DIAGNOSTIC TESTS & INTERPRETATION
#### Lab
- Blood type, screen, or cross-match
- Hematocrit, WBC with differential, complete metabolic profile
- Amylase:
  – Not a reliable indicator of pancreatic trauma
  – Serial levels may increase sensitivity, but specificity still poor.
  – Elevated amylase may be early indicator of potential pancreatic injury.
  – Normal amylase does not rule out pancreatic injury.
  – More sensitive and specific if detected in diagnostic peritoneal lavage (DPL) fluid
- Lipase:
  – No more specific for pancreatic injury
- Urinalysis
- Pregnancy test
- Alcohol and drug screening if indicated
- Prothrombin time/partial thromboplastin time, BUN, and creatinine

#### Imaging
- Note that all imaging tests may miss pancreatic injury.
- Cervical spine, CXRs, and pelvis films as for all blunt trauma patients
- Bedside US/FAST scan
- CT scan with IV contrast, helical CT if available:
  – Shows better contrast enhancement of pancreatic parenchyma than standard scanning
- Magnetic retrograde cholangiopancreatography:
  – Noninvasive evaluation of injury to ductal components
- Endoscopic retrograde cholangiopancreatography:
  – Useful for patients with persistent hyperamylasemia
  – Unexplained abdominal symptoms
  – Some advocating early use to minimize complications
- Operative exploration and intraoperative cholangiogram remains the ideal diagnostic modality, particularly if patient is unstable.

#### Diagnostic Procedures/Surgery
Diagnostic peritoneal lavage to identify intraperitoneal injuries:
- Check fluid for amylase level.
- May still miss significant pancreatic injury

### DIFFERENTIAL DIAGNOSIS
Other or associated abdominal traumatic injuries

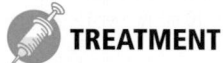

## TREATMENT

### PRE-HOSPITAL
Transport to closest trauma center.

### INITIAL STABILIZATION/THERAPY
- Airway management, resuscitation as indicated with crystalloids, colloids, or blood products
- Nasogastric-tube suction may be especially helpful in setting of pancreatic trauma.

## GENERAL MEASURES

Follow standard trauma treatment for blunt abdominal trauma:

- Penetrating trauma:
  - Tetanus prophylaxis and broad-spectrum antibiotic therapy
- Intra-abdominal injury requiring operative intervention:
  - Broad-spectrum antibiotic therapy
- Must cover for colonic bacteria:
  - Aerobic: *Escherichia coli, Enterobacter, Klebsiella, Enterococcus*
  - Anaerobic: *Bacteroides fragilis, Clostridium, Peptostreptococcus*

## ED TREATMENT/PROCEDURES

Follow ABCDE of trauma and resuscitate unstable patient with emergent surgical consultation or transfer to trauma center as indicated:

- Evaluate for associated abdominal injury.
- Choose imaging modality for rapid evaluation (CT and/or MRCP).
- Early identification of ductal injuries has been shown to reduce morbidity and mortality.
- Surgical: Pancreaticoduodenectomy, distal pancreatectomy, endoscopic stent (controversial), sump/closed suction drainage
- East Trauma Guidelines 2009
- Level III evidence: Grade I and II injuries: Drainage Grade III–V injuries: Resection and drainage

## MEDICATION

- Adults:
  - Piperacillin/tazobactam 3.375 g IV
  - *OR*
  - Cefotetan: 2 g IV *PLUS* gentamicin 2 mg/kg IV *OR*
  - Cefoxitin: 2 g IV plus gentamicin 2 mg/kg IV *OR*
  - Ceftriaxone: 1–2 g IV *PLUS* Flagyl 15 mg/kg IV *OR* Clindamycin: 600 mg IV *PLUS* gentamicin 2 mg/kg IV
- Children:
  - Cefotetan: 20 mg/kg IV *PLUS* gentamicin 2 mg/kg IV *OR*
  - Cefoxitin: 40 mg/kg IV *PLUS* gentamicin 2 mg/kg IV *OR*
  - Ceftriaxone: 50 mg/kg per dose IV *PLUS* Flagyl 15 mg/kg IV

### First Line

Ceftriaxone and Flagyl or piperacillin/tazobactam or carbapenem:

- Goal is to choose broad-spectrum coverage with both aerobic and anaerobic coverage, particularly of enteric gram-negative organisms.

### Second Line

Addition of an aminoglycoside, as it has good activity in an alkaline environment:

- Particularly useful if patient is unstable for broader gram-negative coverage

 **FOLLOW-UP**

## DISPOSITION

### Admission Criteria

- All patients with suspected pancreatic injuries must be admitted.
- Abdominal pain after blunt trauma requires serial exam and observation for 24–72 hr.
- Intoxicated trauma patient requires admission and serial exams for unidentified injury.

### Discharge Criteria

Only for very minor trauma and with no evidence of pancreatic or any other intra-abdominal injury with appropriate follow-up and return precautions

### Issues for Referral

- Patient with surgical drains or complications such as fistula formation, may need further surgical, GI, and wound care evaluations
- Most patients need close monitoring and follow-up within 1 wk.

## FOLLOW-UP RECOMMENDATIONS

Delayed presentation of pancreatic injury is rare, but complications may arise and should be considered:

- Pancreatitis, pseudocysts, vascular aneurysms (such as splenic artery)
- Rare for exocrine or endocrine dysfunction to occur unless a majority of the pancreas is resected/destroyed:
  - Evaluate for glucose intolerance and digestive abnormalities

## PEARLS AND PITFALLS

- Always consider pancreatic injury when evaluating abdominal or back trauma, both blunt and penetrating
- Beware of nearby vascular injuries.
- Assess for related injuries.
- Choose the best imaging modality and obtain as rapidly as possible.
- Penetrating trauma or unstable patients should be rapidly prepared for surgical exploration.

## ADDITIONAL READING

- Ahmed N, Vernick JJ. Pancreatic injury. *South Med J.* 2009;102(12):1253–1256.
- Beckingham IJ. ABC of diseases of liver, pancreas and biliary system: Liver and pancreatic trauma. *BMJ.* 2001;322:783–785.
- Bradley EL, Young PR, Chang MC, et al. Diagnosis and initial management of blunt pancreatic trauma. *Ann Surg.* 1998;6:861–869.
- Emmick RH Jr., Peterson SR. Evaluation of pancreatic injury after blunt abdominal trauma. *Ann Emerg Med.* 1996;27:658–661.
- Gupta A, Stuhlfaut JW, Fleming KW, et al. Blunt trauma of the pancreas and biliary tract: A multimodality imaging approach to diagnosis. *Radiographics.* 2004;24(5):1381–1395.
- Jurkovich J. Injury to the duodenum and pancreas. In: Feliciano DV, Mattox KL, Moore EE, eds. *Trauma*, 3rd ed. Norwalk, CT: Appleton & Lange; 1996:473–494.
- Novelline RA, Rhea JT, Bell T. Helical CT of abdominal trauma. *Radiol Clin North Am.* 1999;37:591–612.
- Rekhi S, Anderson SW, Rhea JT, et al. Imaging of blunt pancreatic trauma. *Emerg Radiol.* 2010;17(1):13–19.
- Shanmuganathan K. Multi-detector row CT imaging of blunt abdominal trauma. *Semin Ultrasound CT MR.* 2004;25(2):180–204.
- Vasquez JC, Coimbra R, Hoyt DB, et al. Management of penetrating pancreatic trauma: An 11-year experience of a level 1 trauma center. *Injury.* 2001;32(10):753–759.
- Wolf A, Bernhardt J, Patrzyk M, et al. The value of endoscopic diagnosis and the treatment of pancreas injuries following blunt abdominal trauma. *Surg Endosc.* 2005;19(5):665–669.

 **CODES**

### ICD9

- 863.81 Injury to pancreas head without mention of open wound into cavity
- 863.82 Injury to pancreas body without mention of open wound into cavity
- 863.83 Injury to pancreas tail without mention of open wound into cavity

# PANCREATITIS
*Trevor Lewis*

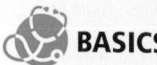 **BASICS**

## DESCRIPTION
- Inflammation of pancreas due to activation, interstitial liberation, and digestion of gland by its own enzymes
- Acute pancreatitis:
  - Exocrine and endocrine function of gland impaired for weeks to months
  - Glandular function will return to normal.
- Chronic pancreatitis:
  - Exocrine and endocrine function progressively deteriorate with resultant steatorrhea and malabsorption.
  - Dysfunction progressive and irreversible

## ETIOLOGY
- Gallstones and alcohol abuse most common causes of *acute pancreatitis* (75–80%)
- Alcohol abuse accounts for 70–80% of *chronic pancreatitis.*
- Acute:
  - Biliary tract disease
  - Chronic alcoholism
  - Obstruction of pancreatic duct
  - Ischemia
  - Medications
  - Infectious
  - Postoperative
  - Metabolic diseases
  - After renal transplant
  - Scorpion venom
  - Penetrating peptic ulcer
  - Hereditary
- Chronic:
  - Chronic alcoholism
  - Obstruction pancreatic duct
  - Tropical
  - Hereditary
  - Shwachman disease
  - Enzyme deficiency
  - Idiopathic
  - Hyperlipedemia
  - Hypercalcemia

### Pediatric Considerations
Cause mainly viral, trauma, and medications

## DIAGNOSIS

### SIGNS AND SYMPTOMS
- Frequency:
  - Abdominal pain: 95–100%
  - Epigastric tenderness: 95–100%
  - Nausea and vomiting: 70–90%
  - Low-grade fever: 70–85%
  - Hypotension: 20–40%
  - Jaundice: 30%
  - Grey Turner/Cullen sign: <5%
  - Subcutaneous fat necrosis: <1%
- GI:
  - Severe, persistent epigastric pain radiating to back:
    - Colicky or rebound tenderness suggests nonpancreatic source.
    - Worse when supine
  - Bowel sounds usually decreased or absent
  - Significant GI bleed in patients with acute severe pancreatitis is uncommon.
  - Cullen sign:
    - Bluish discoloration at umbilicus secondary to hemorrhagic pancreatitis
  - Grey Turner sign:
    - Bluish discoloration at flank secondary to hemorrhagic pancreatitis
- Respiratory:
  - Pleuritic chest pain
  - Dyspnea
  - Lung exam:
    - Left pleural effusion (most common)
    - Atelectasis
    - Pulmonary edema
  - Hypoxemia (30%)
- Cardiac:
  - Tachycardia
  - Hypotension
  - Shock
- Neurologic:
  - Irritability
  - Confusion
  - Coma
  - Chvostek and Trousseau signs are rare despite laboratory evidence of hypocalcemia.

### Ranson Criteria
- Indicators of morbidity and mortality:
  - 0–2 criteria: 2% mortality
  - 3 or 4 criteria: 15% mortality
  - 5 or 6 criteria: 40% mortality
  - 7 or 8 criteria: 100% mortality
- Criteria on admission:
  - Age >55 yr
  - WBC count >16,000 mm$^3$
  - Blood glucose >200 mg/dL
  - Serum lactate dehydrogenase >350 IU/L
  - AST >250 IU/L
- Criteria during 1st 48 hr:
  - Hematocrit fall >10%
  - BUN increase >5 mg/dL
  - Serum calcium <8 mg/dL
  - Arterial PO$_2$ <60 mm Hg
  - Base deficit >4 mEq/L
  - Estimated fluid sequestration >6 L

### ESSENTIAL WORKUP
Laboratory tests to confirm physical diagnosis

### DIAGNOSTIC TESTS & INTERPRETATION
*Lab*
- Lipase:
  - Rises within 4–8 hr of pain onset
  - More reliable indicator of pancreatitis than amylase
- Amylase:
  - Rises within 6 hr of pain onset
  - Levels >3 times limit of normal suggest pancreatitis.
  - Levels >1,000 IU suggest biliary pancreatitis.
  - May be normal during acute inflammation due to significant pancreatic destruction
  - Secreted from various sources
- Electrolyte, BUN, creatinine, glucose:
  - Hypokalemia occurs with extensive fluid losses.
  - Hyperglycemia
- CBC:
  - Increased hematocrit with fluid losses
  - Hematocrit >47% at risk for pancreatic necrosis
  - Decreased hematocrit with retroperitoneal hemorrhage
  - WBC count >12,000 unusual

- Calcium/magnesium:
  - Hypocalcemia indicates significant pancreatic injury.
  - Hypomagnesemia occurs with underlying alcohol abuse.
- Liver function tests:
  - Useful for prognostic indicators if suspected biliary cause
- Pregnancy test
- Arterial blood gases:
  - Indicated if hypoxic (assess $PO_2$) or toxic appearing (assess base deficit)
- ECG:
  - Assess electrolyte imbalances, ischemia

### Imaging
- Abdominal series radiograph:
  - Excludes free air
  - May visualize pancreatic calcifications
  - Most common finding is isolated dilated bowel loop (sentinel loop) near pancreas.
- Chest radiograph:
  - Pleural effusion
  - Atelectasis
  - Infiltrate
- US:
  - Useful if gallstone pancreatitis suspected
- Abdominal CT indications:
  - High-risk pancreatitis (>3 Ranson criteria)
  - Hemorrhagic pancreatitis
  - Suspicion for pseudocyst
  - Diagnosis in doubt

### Diagnostic Procedures/Surgery
Endoscopic retrograde cholangiopancreatography (ERCP):
- Indicated for severe pancreatitis with cholangitis or biliary obstruction

## DIFFERENTIAL DIAGNOSIS
- Mesenteric ischemia/infarction
- Myocardial Infarction
- Biliary colic
- Intestinal obstruction
- Perforated ulcer
- Pneumonia
- Ruptured aortic aneurysm
- Ectopic pregnancy

 **TREATMENT**

### PRE-HOSPITAL
- Initiate IV access in cooperative patients.
- Apply cardiac monitor.

### INITIAL STABILIZATION/THERAPY
- ABCs
- Supplemental oxygen
- Cardiac monitor
- IV fluids

## ED TREATMENT/PROCEDURES
- Airway management:
  - Pulmonary complaints necessitate supplemental oxygen.
  - Endotracheal intubation for adult respiratory distress syndrome or severe encephalopathy
- Fluid resuscitation:
  - Large fluid volumes (up to 5–6 L in 1st 24 hr) to compensate for fluid losses
  - Continuously assess vitals, urine output, and electrolytes to ensure rapid and adequate replacement of intravascular volume.
- Correct electrolyte abnormalities if present:
  - Hypocalcemia (calcium gluconate)
  - Hypokalemia occurs with extensive fluid losses.
  - Hypomagnesemia occurs with underlying alcohol abuse.
- Blood products:
  - In hemorrhagic pancreatitis, transfuse to hematocrit level of 30%.
  - Fresh-frozen plasma and platelets if coagulopathic and bleeding
- Analgesia:
  - Opiate analgesia is drug of choice.
- Nasogastric suction:
  - Not useful in cases of mild pancreatitis
  - Beneficial in severe pancreatitis or intractable vomiting
- Antiemetics
- Antibiotics:
  - Indicated if pancreatic necrosis >30% on abdominal CT

### Geriatric Considerations
Consider central venous pressure monitoring when fluid overload is concern.

### MEDICATION
#### First Line
Analgesics, antiemetics:
- Morphine 2–4 mg IV
- Meperidine (Demerol): 25–50 mg IV, 50–75 IM q3h–q4h
- Compazine 5–10 mg PO/IV/IM
- Zofran 4 mg IV/IM

#### Second Line
Electrolyte replacement, antibiotics:
- Potassium chloride: 10 mEq/hr IV over 1 hr
- Calcium gluconate 10%: 10 mL IV over 15–20 min
- Magnesium sulfate: 2 g IV piggyback
- Imipenem: 500 mg IV q6h

 **FOLLOW-UP**

### DISPOSITION
#### Admission Criteria
- Acute pancreatitis with significant pain, nausea, vomiting
- ICU admission for hemorrhagic/necrotizing pancreatitis

#### Discharge Criteria
- Mild acute pancreatitis without evidence of biliary tract disease and able to tolerate oral fluids
- Chronic pancreatitis with minimal abdominal pain and able to tolerate oral fluids

#### Issues for Referral
Surgical consultation for ERCP in severe pancreatitis with cholangitis or biliary obstruction

#### FOLLOW-UP RECOMMENDATIONS
All discharged mild pancreatitis should have scheduled follow-up within 24–28 hr.

## PEARLS AND PITFALLS
- Gallstones and alcohol account for etiologies of 75–80% of acute pancreatitis.
- Early aggressive fluid therapy is essential to replace large volume losses.
- Nasogastric suction is not beneficial in routine pancreatitis.
- Consider early CT of abdomen when diagnosis in doubt or patient appears ill by clinical scoring scale (Ranson criteria ≥3).

## ADDITIONAL READING
- Frossard D, Steer ML, Pastor CM. Acute pancreatitis. Lancet. 2008;371:143–152.
- Go VLW. The Pancreas. New York: Raven Press; 1993:575–635.
- Heinrich S, Schäfer M, Rousson V, et al. Evidence-based treatment of acute pancreatitis: A look at established paradigm. Ann Surg. 2006;243(2): 154–168.
- Mayerle J, Simon P, Lerch MM. Medical treatment of acute pancreatitis. Gastroenterol Clin North Am. 2004;855–869.
- Tenner S. Initial management of acute pancreatitis: Critical issues during the first 72 hours. Am J Gastroenterol. 2004;99:2489–2494.

### See Also (Topic, Algorithm, Electronic Media Element)
Pancreatic Pseudocyst

 **CODES**

### ICD9
- 577.0 Acute pancreatitis
- 577.1 Chronic pancreatitis

# PANIC ATTACK

*B.J. Beck*

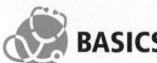

## BASICS

### DESCRIPTION
- Characteristic, acute episodes of physical symptoms and intense fear that rapidly peak within 10 min and resolve in ~20 min
- There may be a nonfearful variant in medical patients.

### Panic Disorder
- Recurrent, unexpected panic attacks with ≥1 mo of persistence:
  - Concerns about having another attack
  - Worry about the implications or consequences of the attacks
  - Behavioral change, such as phobic avoidance, related to the attacks
- Episodic, recurrent, or chronic attacks
- Frequently comorbid with depression, substance abuse, disability, suicidal tendency

### Genetics
- Probably genetic
- Family history of panic or anxiety is common.
- Altered serotonin- and benzodiazepine-receptor function

### ETIOLOGY
#### Mechanism
Limbic system, norepinephrine release, other neurotransmitters (eg, serotonin) implicated

### RISK FACTORS
- Major life events in year preceding onset
- Family history of panic or anxiety
- Childhood shyness or separation anxiety
- May develop in the course of predisposing physical illness or cocaine abuse:
  - May persist after the illness or substance use has resolved
- Twice as common in women

## DIAGNOSIS

### SIGNS AND SYMPTOMS
- Multiple systems suggest autonomic arousal
- Cardiac:
  - Palpitations
  - Tachycardia
  - Chest pain
- Respiratory:
  - Shortness of breath
  - Smothering
  - Choking

- Neurologic:
  - Tremor
  - Dizziness
  - Light-headedness
  - Feeling faint
  - Numbness
  - Tingling
  - Sweating
  - Chills
  - Flushing
  - Feelings of unreality or detachment
- GI:
  - Nausea
  - Cramps
  - Abdominal pain
- Intense fears:
  - Automatic, stereotypic
  - Imminent death
  - Having a heart attack
  - Humiliation
  - Loss of control—"going crazy"

### History
- Known medical conditions
- All medications, including over the counter
- Herbal supplements
- Recreational drugs/alcohol use
- Caffeine consumption
- Age at onset
- Family history of panic, anxiety
- Initiating life events
- Childhood antecedents
- Resultant avoidance
- Response to previous medication trials

### Physical Exam
- Thorough physical and neurologic exam
- Guided by particular symptoms

### ESSENTIAL WORKUP
Detailed history, appropriate physical exam:
- Guided by presentation and initial findings, may be minimal, depending on presentation

### DIAGNOSTIC TESTS & INTERPRETATION
#### Lab
- Toxicology screen
- CBC
- Electrolytes, BUN/creatinine, glucose
- Thyroid-stimulating hormone
- Pulse oximetry or arterial blood gases

#### Diagnostic Procedures/Surgery
- ECG for suspected mitral valve prolapse (MVP) or to exclude underlying cardiac disease:
  - Age >40 yr
  - Cardiac symptoms
- Holter monitor:
  - If associated with palpitations, near-syncope
- Sleep-deprived EEG if seizure suspected

### DIFFERENTIAL DIAGNOSIS
- Consider organic causes if:
  - Panic presents late in life (>50 yr)
  - No childhood antecedents or family history
  - No initiating or major life events
  - Without avoidance or significant fear
  - With a history of poor response to previous trials of antipanic or antidepressant medication
- Medications:
  - Neuroleptics (akathisia)
  - Bronchodilators
  - Digitalis
  - Anticholinergic agents
  - Psychostimulants
  - Diet pills
  - Herbal supplements
- Respiratory:
  - Hyperventilation
  - Chronic obstructive pulmonary disease
  - Pulmonary embolus
  - Bacterial pneumonia
  - Costochondritis
- Cardiovascular:
  - Angina
  - Arrhythmia
  - Anemia
  - MVP may be comorbid with panic.
- Substances:
  - Stimulant abuse
  - Withdrawal (alcohol, sedative-hypnotics)
  - Excessive caffeine intake
- Endocrine:
  - Hyperthyroidism
  - Hypoglycemia
  - Hypoparathyroidism
  - Pheochromocytoma
- Other metabolic derangements:
  - Hypokalemia
  - Hypomagnesemia
  - Hypophosphatemia

- Neurologic:
  - Complex partial or limbic seizures (fear, physical symptoms, perceptual distortions)
  - Transient ischemic attack
  - Labyrinthitis
  - Benign positional vertigo
- Psychiatric:
  - Other anxiety, stress, or phobic disorders, eg, obsessive-compulsive disorder, posttraumatic stress disorder, or social phobia
- Domestic violence

### Pediatric Considerations
Tachycardia

 TREATMENT

### PRE-HOSPITAL
- If diagnosis is supported by previous events, history and workup:
  - Reassurance and diversion
  - Does not require emergent care
- If 1st episode, treat and transport as appropriate to presentation.

### INITIAL STABILIZATION/THERAPY
- Be calm and reassuring.
- Most panic attacks resolve within 20–30 min without any treatment.
- Fear may trigger another panic attack.

### ED TREATMENT/PROCEDURES
- Patient education, new cognitions:
  - Normal response to abnormal alarm
  - Physiologic explanations for symptoms
- High-potency benzodiazepines (drugs of choice):
  - Clonazepam:
    - Slow for emergency use
    - Long-acting without rapid onset/offset phenomena
    - Best choice in this class for maintenance therapy of recurrent panic attacks
  - Alprazolam:
    - Rapid onset
    - Rebound anxiety occurs due to short duration and rapid offset.
    - May lead to escalating doses with continued use
  - Lorazepam:
    - Quick onset
    - Advantage of sublingual (SL) use
    - Longer effect and less abrupt offset than alprazolam
- Avoid low-potency benzodiazepines:
  - Diazepam
  - Chlordiazepoxide
- Treat recurrent panic attacks and panic disorder with selective serotonin reuptake inhibitors (SSRIs) (or tricyclic antidepressants [TCAs]), with or without clonazepam:
  - Will not work immediately
  - Do not need to be started emergently, especially if there is no clear, established access to follow-up management
- There are preliminary case reports on the efficacy of olanzapine for treatment-resistant panic disorder.

- Discharge therapy:
  - Several clonazepam tablets in case of repeated attacks

### ALERT
Rapid offset (withdrawal) of alprazolam may trigger further attacks.

### MEDICATION
#### First Line
- Clonazepam: 0.5 mg PO in the ED; 0.25–0.5 mg PO b.i.d. for initial outpatient therapy
- SSRI:
  - To be started as an outpatient
  - May require higher doses and longer time to therapeutic response for panic than for depression

#### Second Line
- Lorazepam: 1 mg PO or SL
- TCA:
  - To be started as an outpatient

### Pregnancy Considerations
- Limit use of benzodiazepines.
- Risk/benefit discussion about the relative safety of SSRIs and less anticholinergic TCAs, eg, nortriptyline or desipramine
- Physiologic and autonomic effects of pregnancy and postpartum period may trigger attacks in predisposed women.

 FOLLOW-UP

### DISPOSITION
#### Admission Criteria
- As medically indicated to rule out organic cause
- Meets criteria for psychiatric admission (suicidal, homicidal)

#### Discharge Criteria
Most panic attacks do not require inpatient level of care.

### Issues for Referral
- Managed care mental health carve-outs
- Psychopharmacologic and cognitive behavioral therapy evaluation for repeated attacks, or interepisode fear or avoidance
- Stigma
- Primary care follow-up may be an acceptable alternative to specialty, mental health/psychiatry referral.

### FOLLOW-UP RECOMMENDATIONS
- Appointment with primary care physician or referral to mental health specialty treatment
- Avoid precipitants, eg, caffeine, stimulants, alcohol.

## PEARLS AND PITFALLS
- Panic is "contagious"; try not to be infected by the patient's sense of urgency to stop the symptoms: They will resolve spontaneously.
- Be calm, to not add to the patient's alarm, but diligent, so patient feels attended to and reassured.
- Cognitive–behavioral therapy (CBT) can start in the ED with brief explanation of the physiologic cause of symptoms.
- Be cautious not to start adolescents and young adults on a lifetime course of benzodiazepines; CBT (± SSRI therapy) is associated with good outcomes and fewer deleterious side effects.
- Avoid the use of alprazolam, especially for ongoing treatment.

## ADDITIONAL READING
- Fleet RP, Martel J-P, Lavoie KL, et al. Non-fearful panic disorder: A variant of panic in medical patients? Psychosomatics. 2000;41:311–320.
- Furukawa TA, Watanabe N, Churchill R. Psychotherapy plus antidepressant for panic disorder with or without agoraphobia: Systematic review. Br J Psychiatry. 2006;188:305–312.
- Huffman JC, Pollack MH. Predicting panic disorder among patients with chest pain: An analysis of the literature. Psychosomatics. 2003;44:222–236.
- Khaldi S, Korreich C, Dan B, et al. Usefulness of olanzapine in refractory panic attacks. J Clin Psychopharm. 2003;23:100–101.
- Neumeister A, Bain E, Nugent AC. Reduced serotonin type 1A receptor binding in panic disorder. J Neurosci. 2004;24:589–591.
- Rayburn NR, Otto MW. Cognitive-behavioral therapy for panic disorder: A review of treatment elements, strategies, and outcomes. CNS Spectrum. 2003;8: 356–362.
- Roy-Byrne PP, Clary CM, Miceli RJ, et al. The effect of selective serotonin reuptake inhibitor treatment of panic disorder on emergency room and laboratory resource utilization. J Clin Psychiatry. 2001;62: 678–682.
- Wulsin L, Liu T, Storrow A, et al. A randomized, controlled trial of panic disorder treatment initiation in an emergency department chest pain center. Ann Emerg Med. 2002;39:139–143.

### See Also (Topic, Algorithm, Electronic Media Element)
- Psychosis, Medical vs. Psychiatric
- Withdrawal, Drug

 CODES

### ICD9
300.01 Panic disorder

# PARAPHIMOSIS

*Nicole M. Franks*

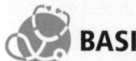

## BASICS

### DESCRIPTION
- The entrapment of the retracted foreskin proximal to the glans of the penis
- Leads to lymphatic congestion and venous obstruction, which may result in arterial compromise to the glans
- Paraphimosis is a urologic emergency.

### ETIOLOGY
- A number of conditions of the foreskin may predispose to paraphimosis, including:
  - Phimosis
  - Inflammation
  - Trauma
  - Sexually naive may be unaware of the need to reduce foreskin after intercourse
- Commonly iatrogenic, from failure to replace the foreskin after exam, catheterization, or cleaning

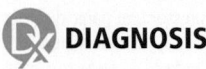

## DIAGNOSIS

### SIGNS AND SYMPTOMS
- Retracted prepuce (foreskin)
- Pain
- Swollen, edematous glans
- Local cellulitis
- Necrosis of glans in untreated cases

### Physical Exam
Examination of the genitalia should include a search for constricting foreign bodies or constricting bands.

### ESSENTIAL WORKUP
- Paraphimosis is a clinical diagnosis with the clinical findings described earlier.
- Treatment must not be delayed pending diagnostic laboratory or radiographic studies.

### DIAGNOSTIC TESTS & INTERPRETATION
*Imaging*
If history suggests penile foreign body, radiographs may be obtained once the vascular compromise has been relieved.

### DIFFERENTIAL DIAGNOSIS
- Foreign bodies constricting the penile shaft may mimic paraphimosis; these include:
  - Hair tourniquets
  - Wire, string, or other material used for sexual enhancement or punishment
- Balanoposthitis
- Trauma (zipper injuries)
- Acute idiopathic penile edema

## TREATMENT

### PRE-HOSPITAL
- Patients should be transported promptly; do not attempt reduction in the field.
- Prehospital personnel can be advised to apply an ice pack to the glans with adequate protection of the skin.
- Pain control

### INITIAL STABILIZATION/THERAPY
- Ice can be applied to the glans while preparing to reduce the prepuce:
  - Use the thumb of a glove as an ice-filled condom to aid in direct application.
- The incarcerated foreskin must be released as soon as possible to prevent ischemia and necrosis of the glans.
- The pain associated with reduction techniques must be managed with some combination of conscious sedation, adequate analgesia, and local anesthesia.

### ED TREATMENT/PROCEDURES
- Medical therapy for paraphimosis involves reassuring the patient, reducing the preputial edema, and restoring the prepuce to its original position and condition.
- The following sequence of procedures should be followed:
  - Paraphimosis can most frequently be reduced using a penile block and compressing the glans manually while applying traction on the foreskin.
  - Penile block is performed by infiltrating 5 mL of 1% lidocaine *without* epinephrine in the angle between the inferior rami of the symphysis pubis:
    - Then use another 5 mL to infiltrate a wheel along the sides of the penis.
    - This produces a block after 5 min.
  - Successful reduction requires steady circumferential pressure on the distal edema with simultaneous manual reduction of the foreskin.
  - In children, conscious sedation is usually required.

– If manual reduction is unsuccessful, then the technique of multiple punctures may facilitate reduction:
  o Make ~20 holes in the swollen foreskin with a small sterile needle (26 g), allowing expression of edema fluid, then resume manual reduction.
– If this fails to return the foreskin to its original position, it will be necessary to incise the constricting ring of tissue with a dorsal longitudinal slit in the foreskin after sterile preparation:
  o If the incision made is too long, after reduction it may be necessary to suture the incision transversely with 3.0 absorbable sutures.
• If a delay is likely before the paraphimosis can be treated (eg, NPO status), then applying a gauze swab soaked in 50% dextrose will reduce edema by osmosis and facilitate reduction.
• For patients who want to retain uncircumcised phallus steroid therapy can be attempted to reduce fibrose ring. Consult urology for close follow-up:
  – Triamcinolone cream 0.1% to affected area ×6 wk
  – If unsuccessful, circumcision may still be required.

## MEDICATION
• Appropriate analgesics or anesthetics as required
• Antibiotics generally not required unless treating associated cellulitis or balanoposthitis.

 **FOLLOW-UP**

### DISPOSITION
**Admission Criteria**
Necrosis or cellulitis of the penis

**Discharge Criteria**
• Successful reduction with relief of symptoms
• Close urologic follow-up

**Issues for Referral**
• Urologic consultation is required.
• Subsequent circumcision to prevent recurrence is an area of clinical debate; historically, it has been common practice.

### FOLLOW-UP RECOMMENDATIONS
• Education regarding importance of replacement of the foreskin after retraction for instrumentation or cleaning
• Emphasis on prepuce hygiene

## PEARLS AND PITFALLS
• Goal is to reduce penile edema enough to allow the foreskin to return to original position over the glans.
• Generally, noninvasive reduction methods (at least 2 or 3 attempts) are successful. and dorsal slit incision is required only mostly in severe cases.

## ADDITIONAL READING
• Donohoe JM, Burnette JO, Brown JA. Paraphimosis treatment. *eMedicine*. Available at: http://www.emedicine.medscape.com/article/442883. Updated October 7, 2009.
• Ghory HZ, Sharma R. Phimosis and paraphimosis. *eMedicine*. Available at: http://www.emedicine.medscape.com/article/777539. Updated April 28, 2010.
• Huang CJ: Problems of the foreskin and glans penis. *Clin Pediatr Emerg Med*. 2009;10:56–59.
• Marx JA, Hockberger RS, Walls RM. *Rosen's Emergency Medicine: Concepts and Clinical Practice*, 7th ed. St. Louis, MO: Mosby; 2009:2201–2202.
• Roberts JR, Hedges J. *Clinical Procedures in Emergency Medicine*, 5th ed. Philadelphia: Saunders; 2009:1003–1005.

### See Also (Topic, Algorithm, Electronic Media Element)
• Phimosis
• Priapism

 **CODES**

**ICD9**
605 Redundant prepuce and phimosis

# PARKINSON DISEASE

James M. Leaming
Spencer A. Adoff

 **BASICS**

## DESCRIPTION
- Gradually progressive neurologic disorder of middle or late life
- Aggregates of melanin-containing nerve cells in the brainstem:
  - Substantia nigra locus ceruleus
- Reactive gliosis with nerve cell loss
- Lewy bodies:
  - Eosinophilic intracytoplasmic inclusions
- Decreased dopamine in the caudate nucleus and putamen
- Accelerated cortical atrophy
- Can begin unilaterally, but generalizes to symmetric

## ETIOLOGY
- Sporadic or idiopathic
- Disorders presenting with parkinsonism:
  - Drug induced:
    - Parkinsonism-hyperpyrexia syndrome (dopaminergic drug withdrawal)
    - Amphotericin B
    - Chemotherapeutic drugs
    - Neuroleptic treatment induced
  - Toxins:
    - Carbon monoxide
    - Methanol
    - Cyanide
    - Organophosphate poisoning
    - 1-Methyl-4-phenyl-1,2,3,6-tetrahydropyridine
  - Brain lesions:
    - Basal ganglia stroke
    - Midbrain lesions
    - Hydrocephalus
  - Infections:
    - *Mycoplasma*
    - Viral encephalitis
  - Other:
    - Central pontine myelinosis
    - Encephalitis lethargica (autoantibodies against basal ganglia antigens)

## DIAGNOSIS

### SIGNS AND SYMPTOMS
- Nonmotor vs. motor symptoms:
  - Nonmotor:
    - Orthostatic hypotension
    - Constipation
    - Delayed gastric emptying
    - Dysphagia
    - Pain sensory dysfunction
    - Depression
    - Hallucinations
    - Dementia
    - Sleep disorders
- Motor symptoms:
  - "Pill-rolling" resting tremor
  - "Cog-wheel" rigidity due to increased muscular tone
  - Stooped posture and instability of posture
  - Stiffness and slowness of movement, hypokinesia
  - "Masked face" appearance

### History
- Sudden change in baseline motor function or mental status:
  - May be the only indication of systemic disease such as infection
- Noncompliance (sudden withdrawal) of dopaminergic medications can lead to parkinsonism-hyperpyrexia syndrome:
  - Rigidity, pyrexia, reduced consciousness
  - Complications: Acute renal failure, deep vein thrombosis, pulmonary embolism, disseminated intravascular coagulation, rhabdomyolysis, autonomic instability

### Physical Exam
- Cog-wheel rigidity:
  - Jerking movements when a muscle is passively stretched
- Stooped posture
- Pill-rolling tremor

## ESSENTIAL WORKUP
- History is of primary importance:
  - Diagnosis is made based on clinical findings.
- Important historical information includes:
  - Onset of symptom, whether gradual or sudden
  - History of potential causes of a Parkinson-like syndrome. Patients with established Parkinson disease:
    - Sudden change in baseline motor function
    - Change in mental status
    - Should prompt workup for infectious process

## DIAGNOSTIC TESTS & INTERPRETATION
### Lab
- No specific or recommended laboratory studies necessary to confirm the diagnosis
- Disorders presenting as Parkinson disease may require directed laboratory studies as appropriate for suspected cause.
- Directed labs if suspect parkinsonism-hyperpyrexia syndrome

### Imaging
- CT and MRI are not required to diagnose Parkinson disease but are often elements of evaluation for dementia.
- CXR may be indicated for any signs of respiratory tract infection.

## DIFFERENTIAL DIAGNOSIS
- Benign familial tremor
- Major depression
- Wilson disease
- Huntington disease
- Alzheimer disease
- Creutzfeldt-Jacob disease
- Carbon monoxide poisoning
- $B_{12}$ deficiency
- Hydrocephalus
- Multi-infarct dementia
- Essential tremor disorders
- Hypothyroidism

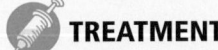 **TREATMENT**

### ED TREATMENT/PROCEDURES

- Treatment with antiparkinsonian medications can be initiated in the ED to alleviate symptoms.
- Consultation with neurology for recommended medication regimens and ongoing support and monitoring is prudent.
- For patients with mild disease, no medication may be required.
- For moderate disease, anticholinergic medications and dopaminergic medications should be used.
- Treat underlying infection, if present.
- Treat parkinsonism-hyperpyrexia syndrome:
  – Replace levodopa or bromocriptine.
  – Supportive
  – Treat complications.

### MEDICATION

- Parkinson:
  – Amantadine: 100 mg b.i.d.
  – Benztropine: 0.5–1 mg t.i.d.
  – Bromocriptine: 15 mg every day
  – Levodopa/dopa carboxylase inhibitor (carbidopa) combination: 25/100 mg every day
  – Trihexyphenidyl: 1–2 mg q.i.d.
- Parkinsonism-hyperpyrexia syndrome:
  – Levodopa: 50–100 mg IV over 3 hr
  – Bromocriptine: 7.5–15.0 mg PO t.i.d.

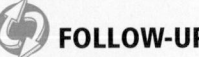 **FOLLOW-UP**

### DISPOSITION

#### Admission Criteria

- Patients with previously diagnosed Parkinson with infections, trauma, cardiovascular emergencies, cerebrovascular emergencies, GI emergencies, electrolyte disturbances, altered mental status, or other medical problems
- Depression with intent to do self-harm
- Confirm diagnosis and levodopa responsiveness
- Medication complications (parkinsonism-hyperpyrexia syndrome)
- Management of motor fluctuations and dyskinesias
- Inability to go home secondary to elder abuse
- Complications from deep brain stimulation devices (eg, headache, infection, mental status change)
- Failure to thrive

#### Discharge Criteria

- Mild to moderate disease without medications
- Moderate to severe disease with medications and urgent neurologic outpatient follow-up

### FOLLOW-UP RECOMMENDATIONS

Discuss prevention strategies in disease management.

## PEARLS AND PITFALLS

Sudden withdrawal of dopaminergic medications can result in parkinsonism-hyperpyrexia syndrome, a medical emergency.

## ADDITIONAL READING

- Grinberg LT, Rueb U, Alho A, et al. Brainstem pathology and non-motor symptoms in PD. *J Neurol Sci*. 2010;289:81–88.
- Kipps CM, Fung VSC, Grattan-Smith P, et al. Movement disorder emergencies. *Mov Disord*. 2005;20:322–334.
- Newman EJ, Grosset DG, Kennedy PGE. The parkinsonism-hyperpyrexia syndrome. *Neurocrit Care*. 2009;10:136–140.
- Understanding Parkinson's disease: An update on current diagnostic and treatment strategies. *J Am Med Dir Assoc*. 2006;7(suppl 2):4–10.
- Temlett JA, Thompson PD. *Intern Med J*. 2006;36:524–526.

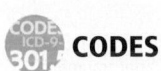 **CODES**

**ICD9**
332.0 Paralysis agitans

# PARONYCHIA
*Gene Ma*

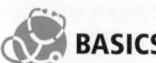

## BASICS

### DESCRIPTION
- Disruption of the seal between the nail plate and the nail fold may allow entry of bacteria into the eponychial space.
- Inflammation of the nail folds surrounding the nail plate

### ETIOLOGY
- Acute paronychia: Predominantly *Staphylococcus aureus* but also streptococci, *Pseudomonas*, and anaerobes
- Chronic paronychia: Multifactorial due to allergens and irritants in addition to fungal etiologies, predominantly *Candida albicans*, which commonly coexist with *Staphylococcus* species

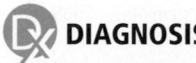

## DIAGNOSIS

### SIGNS AND SYMPTOMS
- Pain, warmth, and swelling to the proximal and lateral nail folds, often 2–5 days after trauma
- Symptoms must be present for 6 wk to meet criteria for a chronic paronychia.

### History
- Acute paronychia: Nail biting, finger sucking, aggressive manicuring or manipulation, and trauma predispose to development.
- Chronic paronychia: Occupations with persistent moist hands; dish washers, bartenders; also increased in patients with peripheral vascular disease or diabetes

### *Pediatric Considerations*
Frequently anaerobic mouth flora in children from nail biting

### *Physical Exam*
- Begins as swelling, pain, and erythema in the dorsolateral corner of the nail fold bulging out over the nail plate
- Progresses to subcuticular/subungual abscess

### ESSENTIAL WORKUP
- History and physical exam with special attention to evaluating for concomitant infections such as felon or cellulitis
- Assess tetanus status.

### DIAGNOSTIC TESTS & INTERPRETATION
### *Lab*
- No specific tests are useful.
- Cultures are not routinely indicated.

### *Imaging*
Soft tissue radiographs if foreign body is suspected; routine films if osteomyelitis suspected

### *Diagnostic Procedures/Surgery*
Digital pressure test (opposing the thumb and the affected finger) may help identify the margins of an early subungual abscess

### DIFFERENTIAL DIAGNOSIS
- Felon
- Herpetic whitlow
- Trauma or foreign body
- Primary squamous cell carcinoma
- Metastatic carcinoma
- Osteomyelitis
- Psoriasis
- Reiter syndrome
- Pyoderma gangrenosum

## TREATMENT

### ED TREATMENT/PROCEDURES
### *Acute Paronychia*
- Early paronychia without purulence may be managed with warm-water soaks 4 times a day with or without oral antibiotics; may also consider topical antibiotics and corticosteroids.
- Early superficial subcuticular abscess:
  - Elevation of the eponychial fold by sliding the flat edge of a no. 11 blade (18-gauge needle or small clamps may be used) gently between the proximal nail fold and the nail plate near the point of maximal tenderness
  - A digital nerve block or local anesthesia may be necessary.
- Partial nail involvement:
  - If the lesion extends beneath the nail, remove a longitudinal section of the nail.
  - Petroleum jelly or iodoform gauze packing for 24 hr
- Runaround abscess:
  - If the lesion extends beneath the base of the nail to the other side, remove one quarter to one third of the proximal nail with two small incisions at the dorsolateral edges of the nail fold and pack eponychial fold with petroleum jelly or iodoform gauze to prevent adherence.

- Extensive subungual abscess:
  – Remove entire nail.
- Early paronychia without purulence present may be managed with warm soaks alone; beyond that, antibiotics are recommended if there is any apparent cellulitis, abscess, or systemic sign of infection.
- Trimethoprim–sulfamethoxazole, dicloxacillin, and amoxicillin–clavulanate are appropriate first-line agents, with treatment regimens ranging from 5–10 days, depending on severity.
- Clindamycin or amoxicillin–clavulanate if associated with nail biting or oral contact

### Chronic Paronychia

- Avoidance of predisposing exposures and irritants/chemicals
- Topical steroids should be considered first line therapy, with or without broad spectrum topical antifungal agent
- Consideration for antistaphylococcal regimen
- For recalcitrant cases:
  – Eponychial marsupialization involving removal of a crescentic piece of skin just proximal to the nail fold, including all thickened tissue down to but not including germinal matrix
  – Oral antifungal therapy

### MEDICATION

- Amoxicillin–clavulanate: 875 mg PO b.i.d. for 7 days (peds: 25 mg/kg/d PO q12h)
- Trimethoprim–sulfamethoxazole (Bactrim DS) b.i.d. for 7 days
- Clindamycin: 300 mg PO q.i.d. for 7 days (peds: 20–40 mg/kg/d div q6h PO, IV, IM)
- Dicloxacillin: 500 mg PO q.i.d. for 7 days (peds: 12.5–50 mg/kg/d PO q6h)

- Topical antibiotics: Bacitracin–neomycin–polymyxin B (Neosporin), mucipurin topical (Bactroban), or gentamicin t.i.d. for 5–10 days
- Topical antifungal/steroid combination: nystatin–triamcinolone b.i.d.–t.i.d. until resolution, no longer than 1 mo

## FOLLOW-UP

### DISPOSITION

#### Admission Criteria
Admission is not needed for paronychia alone.

#### Discharge Criteria
- Patients with uncomplicated paronychias may be discharged with appropriate follow-up instructions.
- Patients with packings should be re-evaluated in 24 hr.

#### Issues for Referral
Chronic paronychias refractory to treatment

## PEARLS AND PITFALLS

- Acute paronychias respond well to decompression with or without antibiotics.
- Chronic paronychias are largely a result of chronic exposure to allergens/irritants.
- Reiter syndrome and psoriasis can mimic paronychia.
- Recurrent paronychia should raise suspicion for herpetic whitlow.
- Assess for felons.

## ADDITIONAL READING

- Canales FL, Newmeyer WL, Kilgore ES. The treatment of felons and paronychias. *Hand Clin.* 1989;5(4):515–523.
- Hochman LG. Paronychia: More than just an abscess. *Int J Dermatol.* 1995;34(6):385–386.
- Jebson PJ. Infections of the fingertip. Paronychias and felons. *Hand Clin.* 1998;14:547–55, viii.
- Moran GJ, Talan DA. Hand infections. *Emerg Med Clin.* 1993;11(3):601–619.
- Rigopoulos D, Larios G, Gregoriou S, et al. Acute and chronic paronychia. *Am Fam Physician.* 2008;77(3):339–348.
- Rockwell PG. Acute and chronic paronychia. *Am Fam Physician.* 2001;63(6):1113–1116.
- Tosti A, Piraccini BM, Ghetti E, et al. Topical steroids versus systemic antifungals in the treatment of chronic paronychia: An open randomized, double-blind and double dummy study. *J Am Acad Dermatol.* 2002;47(1):73–76.

 ## CODES

### ICD9
- 112.3 Candidiasis of skin and nails
- 681.02 Onychia and paronychia of finger
- 681.11 Onychia and paronychia of toe

# PATELLAR INJURIES
*Stephen R. Hayden*

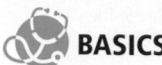 **BASICS**

## DESCRIPTION
### Dislocation
- Usually caused by sudden flexion and external rotation of tibia on femur, with simultaneous contraction of quadriceps muscles
- Lateral dislocation of patella most common, with patella displaced over the lateral femoral condyle
- Uncommon dislocations include superior, medial, and rare intra-articular dislocation.
- Direct trauma to patella

### Fracture
- Direct trauma:
  - Most common mechanism of injury
  - Secondary to direct blow or fall on patella
  - Usually results in comminuted or minimally displaced fracture
- Indirect forces
  - Avulsion injury secondary to sudden contraction of the quadriceps tendon
  - Usually results in transverse or displaced fracture (often both)
- Types of patellar fractures:
  - Transverse: 50–80% (usually middle or lower third of patella)
  - Comminuted (or stellate): 30–35%
  - Longitudinal: 25%
  - Osteochondral

### Patellar Tendon Rupture
- Usually caused by forceful eccentric contraction on a flexed knee (eg, jump landing and weight lifting)
- Often occurs in middle-aged athlete

### Patellar Tendinitis
Overuse syndrome from repeated acceleration, deceleration, jumping, landing

## ETIOLOGY
### Dislocation
- Risk factors for patellar dislocation:
  - Genu valgum (knock-knee)
  - Genu recurvatum (hyperextension of knee)
  - Shallow lateral femoral condyle
  - Deficient vastus medialis
  - Lateral insertion of patellar tendon
  - Shallow patellar groove
  - Patella alta (high-riding patella)
  - Deformed patella
  - Pes planus (flatfoot)
- Common injury in adolescents, especially girls
- The younger the patient at the time of initial dislocation, the greater the risk of recurrent dislocation.

### Fracture
- Direct trauma
- Indirect forces caused by forcible quadriceps tendon contraction
- Male:female ratio 2:1
- Highest incidence in those 20–50 yr old

### Patellar Tendon Rupture
- Peak incidence in third and fourth decades:
  - Often athletically active individual
- Risk factors:
  - History of patellar tendinitis
  - History of diabetes mellitus, previous steroid injections, rheumatoid arthritis, gout, systemic lupus erythematosus
  - Previous major knee surgery

### Patellar Tendinitis
- Microtears of tendon matrix from overuse
- Seen in high jumpers, volleyball and basketball players, runners

 **DIAGNOSIS**

## SIGNS AND SYMPTOMS
### Dislocation
- History of feeling knee "go out"; popping, ripping, or tearing sensation
- Pain
- Inability to bear weight
- Obvious lateral deformity of patella
- Mild to moderate swelling
- Often reduces spontaneously before ED evaluation
- Tenderness along patella
- Positive apprehension or Fairbanks sign:
  - Attempts to push the patella laterally elicit patient apprehension.

### Fracture
- Pain over anterior knee
- Difficulty ambulating
- Increased pain with movement of patella
- Tenderness and swelling over patella
- Difficulty or inability to extend knee
- Palpable defect, crepitus, or joint effusion/hemarthrosis

### Patellar Tendon Rupture
- Abrupt onset of severe pain
- Decreased ability to bear weight
- Occasionally hemarthrosis
- Proximally displaced patella
- Incomplete extensor function
- Inability to maintain knee extension against force

### Patellar Tendinitis
- "Jumper's knee"
- Pain in area of patellar tendon
- Pain worse from sitting to standing or going up stairs
- Point tenderness at distal aspect of patella or proximal patellar tendon

## ESSENTIAL WORKUP
- Radiographs essential
- For patellar tendon rupture, a high-riding patella (ie, patella located superior to level of intercondylar notch) observed
- For patellar tendinitis, radiographic findings unlikely with symptom duration of <6 mo

## DIAGNOSTIC TESTS & INTERPRETATION
### Imaging
- Anteroposterior (AP) and lateral views of knee should be obtained.
- Postreduction radiographs should include AP, lateral, and sunrise (or skyline, axial) views to exclude osteochondral fracture (in patellar dislocations).
- Bipartite patella (patella with accessory bony fragment connected to main body by cartilage) may be mistaken for fracture; comparison view may help differentiate.

## DIFFERENTIAL DIAGNOSIS
- Patellar subluxation
- Femoral or tibial fracture
- Traumatic bursitis
- Quadriceps tendon rupture

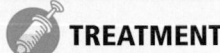 **TREATMENT**

**PRE-HOSPITAL**
Patient should be transported in supine position with knee flexed and supported.

**INITIAL STABILIZATION/THERAPY**
Appropriate history and physical exam to identify any associated injuries (eg, femoral fracture, hip fracture, posterior hip dislocation) and assess extensor mechanism

**ED TREATMENT/PROCEDURES**
*Dislocation*
- For simple lateral patellar dislocation, reduce dislocation by extending the knee gently to 180 degrees:
  – Occasionally simultaneous pressure may have to be applied over the lateral aspect of patella in a medial direction.
- For other types of patellar dislocation (superior, medial, intra-articular), do not attempt reduction; obtain orthopedic consultation.
- Aspiration of joint with sterile technique is necessary if reduction is difficult secondary to hemarthrosis.
- If osteochondral fracture is present (28–50% of cases), obtain orthopedic consultation.
- Although reduction is typically easy to accomplish, procedural sedation or parenteral analgesia may facilitate it.

*Fracture*
- Orthopedic consultation when patellar fracture is confirmed
- Initial treatment often consists of long-leg bulky splint and subsequent operative repair.

*Patellar Tendon Rupture*
Orthopedic consultation, with surgical repair within 2–6 wk

**MEDICATION**
- Fentanyl citrate: 1–2 $\mu$g/kg (peds: 0.5–1.0 $\mu$g/kg) IV
- Midazolam Hcl: 1–3 mg (peds: 0.05–0.1 mg/kg, max dose 2.5 mg) IV
- Morphine sulfate: 2–5 mg per dose (peds: 0.1–0.2 mg/kg per dose) IV
- Meperidine: 50–150 mg (peds: 0.5–0.8 mg/lb) IM
- Ketorolac: 60 mg IM; 30 mg IV (peds: 0.5–1 mg/kg IV, max 15 mg dose if <50 kg; max. 30 mg dose if >50 kg, IV)
- Methohexital: 1–2 mg/kg IV (or adult; 20 mg bolus q45sec)
- Propofol: 1–2 mg/kg IV (or adult; 20 mg bolus q45sec) push slow IV to avoid dec BP

 **FOLLOW-UP**

**DISPOSITION**
*Admission Criteria*
- Patients with superior, medial, or intra-articular dislocation or in whom a lateral dislocation cannot be reduced require orthopedic consultation in the ED and possible admission.
- Patellar dislocation associated with a fracture (osteochondral or lateral femoral condyle) requires orthopedic consultation in the ED.
- Operative intervention indicated if fragments are displaced >4 mm, if patient is unable to raise extended leg off bed, or if articular step-off >3 mm
- All open fractures require debridement and irrigation; such patients should be admitted.
- For patellar tendon rupture, discuss case with orthopedics.

*Discharge Criteria*
- Patients with successful reduction of lateral patellar dislocation and normal postreduction radiographs may be discharged with knee immobilization, crutches, and orthopedic follow-up.
- Fracture is displaced <3 mm and patient has full active knee extension:
  – Knee immobilizer, or bulky long-leg splint, partial to full weight bearing as tolerated with crutches, and orthopedic follow-up within a few days
- For patellar tendonitis. Rest, avoidance of inciting activity, heat, and NSAIDs

**PEARLS AND PITFALLS**
- Lateral patella dislocations often reduce spontaneously prior to arrival in ED; do not dismiss patient's history of dislocation.
- In patella tendon ruptures, tendon defect may not be palpable if sufficient time has elapsed and swelling has occurred.

**ADDITIONAL READING**
- Ahmad CS, McCarthy M, Gomez JA, et al. The moving patellar apprehension test for lateral patellar instability. *Am J Sports Med.* 2009;37(4):791–796. Epub Feb 3, 2009.
- Atkin DM, Fithian DC, Marangi KS, et al. Characteristics of patients with primary acute lateral patellar dislocation and their recovery within the first 6 months of injury. *Am J Sports Med.* 2000;28:472–479.
- Cash JD, Hughston JC. Treatment of acute patellar dislocation. *Am J Sports Med.* 1988;16:244–249.
- Enad JG. Patellar tendon ruptures. *South Med J.* 1999;92:563–566.
- Jackson JL, O'Malley PG, Kroenke K. Evaluation of acute knee pain in primary care. *Ann Intern Med.* 20037;139(7):575–588.
- Palmu S, Kallio PE, Donell ST, et al. Acute patellar dislocation in children and adolescents: A randomized clinical trial. *J Bone Joint Surg Am.* 2008r;90(3):463–470.

 **CODES**

**ICD9**
- 726.64 Patellar tendinitis
- 822.0 Closed fracture of patella
- 836.3 Dislocation of patella, closed

# PATENT DUCTUS ARTERIOSUS
*Steven Lelyveld*

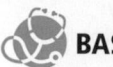 **BASICS**

## DESCRIPTION
- Patent vessel in the fetal heart connects the pulmonary trunk to the descending aorta.
- Shortly after birth, changes normally provoke contraction, closure, and fibrosis:
  - Sudden increase in the partial pressure of oxygen
  - Changes in the synthesis and metabolism of vasoactive eicosanoids
- In the preterm infant, persistent patency of the ductus may be a normal life-saving response.
- The patent ductus usually has a normal structural anatomy.
- Patency results from hypoxia and immaturity.
- In the full-term newborn, patency of the ductus is a congenital malformation.
- Deficiency of both the mucoid endothelial layer and the muscular media of the ductus
- As pulmonary vascular resistance falls, aortic blood is shunted into the pulmonary artery.
- Extent of the shunt reflects the size of the ductus and the ratio of the pulmonary to systemic vascular resistances.
- Up to 70% of the left ventricular output may be shunted through the ductus to the pulmonary circulation.
- Risk factors:
  - Premature birth
  - Coexisting cardiac anomalies
  - Conditions resulting in hypoxia
  - High altitude
  - Maternal rubella infection
  - Female-to-male ratio, 3:1

## ETIOLOGY
- Prematurity
- Congenital anomaly
- Hypoxia
- Prostaglandins

## DIAGNOSIS

### SIGNS AND SYMPTOMS
*History*
- Isolated patent ductus arteriosus (PDA), an unanticipated event
- PDA, as part of a larger congenital cardiac anomaly, may be diagnosed by US during pregnancy.

*Physical Exam*
- Asymptomatic when the patent ductus arteriosus is small, but otherwise may present with a range of findings.
- Congestive heart failure (CHF)
- Wide pulse pressure
- Prominent apical impulse
- Thrill
- Maximal in the 2nd left intercostal space
- Radiates toward the left clavicle, down the left sternal border, or toward the apex
- Systolic and continuous
- Continuous murmur
- Sounds like a humming top or rolling thunder
- Begins soon after onset of the 1st sound, reaches maximal intensity at the end of systole, and wanes in late diastole
- Localized to the 2nd left intercostal space or radiates down the left sternal border or to the left clavicle
- Recurrent pulmonary infections
- Retardation of physical growth

### ESSENTIAL WORKUP
- Establish the diagnosis with imaging studies.
- Rule out complications such as heart failure and endocarditis.

## DIAGNOSTIC TESTS & INTERPRETATION
*Lab*
Unhelpful in making the diagnosis

*Imaging*
- CXR:
  - Usually normal in infants
  - In children and adults:
    - Increased intrapulmonary markings
    - Calcifications
    - Left ventricle and left atrial enlargement
    - Dilated ascending aorta
    - Dilated pulmonary arteries
- EKG:
  - Abnormal if the ductus is large:
    - Left ventricular hypertrophy
    - Right ventricular hypertrophy is a sign of severity.
- Echocardiography:
  - Normal if the ductus is small
  - Left atrial enlargement
  - Size of the ductus can be determined by scanning from the suprasternal notch.
  - Doppler studies will determine aortic to pulmonary artery flow during diastole.
- Cardiac catheterization:
  - Normal or increased right-sided pressure
  - Oxygenated blood in the pulmonary artery confirms left-to-right shunting.
  - Injection of contrast into the ascending aorta shows opacification of the pulmonary arteries.

### DIFFERENTIAL DIAGNOSIS
- Venous hum:
  - Common insignificant bruit
  - Heard in the neck or anterior portion of the chest
  - Soft humming sound in systole and diastole
  - Decreased by light compression of the jugular venous system

- Total anomalous pulmonary venous connection to the innominate vein:
  - Continuous murmur like venous hum
- Aorticopulmonary septal defect:
  - Murmur is often only systolic.
  - Heard at the right sternal border
- Ruptured sinus of Valsalva
- Coronary arteriovenous fistulas
- Anomalous origin of left coronary artery from the pulmonary artery
- Absence or atresia of pulmonary valve
- Aortic insufficiency with ventricular septal defect
- Peripheral pulmonary stenosis
- Truncus arteriosus

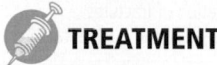 TREATMENT

### ALERT
Supplemental oxygen if CHF

### PRE-HOSPITAL
Monitoring and oxygen

### INITIAL STABILIZATION/THERAPY
- Small, asymptomatic shunts may not need closure.
- Pulmonary support
- Supplemental oxygen

### ED TREATMENT/PROCEDURES
- Sodium and fluid restriction
- Correction of anemia to hematocrit >45%
- Antibiotic prophylaxis for endocarditis
- Preterm infants:
  - Usually closes spontaneously
  - Varies with the magnitude of shunting and severity of respiratory distress syndrome Pharmacologic inhibition of prostaglandin synthesis with indomethacin during the 1st 2–7 days of life.

- Full-term infants and children:
  - Surgical closure is required, even in asymptomatic patients, as spontaneous closure is rare with several options.
  - Ligation and division
  - Transfemoral catheter technique to occlude PDA with foam plastic plug or double umbrella

### MEDICATION
Indomethacin: 0.2–0.25 mg/kg per dose; repeat q12–24h for 3 doses

 **FOLLOW-UP**

### DISPOSITION
*Admission Criteria*
- Heart failure
- Endocarditis
- Pulmonary hypertension

*Discharge Criteria*
- Asymptomatic
- Prophylactic antibiotics
- Close follow-up with plans for early surgical closure

*Issues for Referral*
A pediatric cardiologist/neonatologist should be involved in all patients who have any evidence of heart failure, particularly if pharmacologic management is being considered.

## PEARLS AND PITFALLS
- CHF may cause decrease in glomerular filtration rate and urinary output.
- Indomethacin may cause GI bleeding.

## ADDITIONAL READING
- Dorfman AT, Marino BS, Wernovsky G, et al. Critical heart disease in the neonate: Presentation and outcome at a tertiary care center. *Pediatr Crit Care Med.* 2008;9:193–202.
- Horeczko T, Young KD. Congenital heart disease. In: Strange GR, Ahrens WF, Schafermeyer RW, et al., eds. *Pediatric Emergency Medicine: A Comprehensive Study Guide*, 3rd ed. New York: McGraw-Hill; 2009:420.
- John SD, Swischuk LE. Pediatric chest. In: Brant WE, Helms CA, eds. *Fundamentals of Diagnostic Radiology*, 3rd ed. Philadelphia: Lippincott Williams & Wilkins; 2007:1261–1262.
- Moore P, Brook MM, Heymann MA. Patent ductus arteriosus and aortopulmonary window. In: Allen HD, Gutgesell HP, Clark EB, et al., eds. *Moss and Adams' Heart Disease in Infants, Children, and Adolescents: Including the Fetus and Young Adult*, 7th ed. Philadelphia: Lippincott Williams & Wilkins; 2008:683–701.
- Webb GD, Smallhorn JF, Therrien J, et al. Congenital heart disease. In: Libby P, Bonow RO, Mann DL, et al., eds. *Braunwald's Heart Disease: A Textbook of Cardiovascular Medicine*, 7th ed. Philadelphia: WB Saunders; 2008:1585–1586.

### See Also (Topic, Algorithm, Electronic Media Element)
- http://www.nhlbi.nih.gov/health/dci/Diseases/pda/pda_what.html
- http://www.nlm.nih.gov/medlineplus/ency/article/001560.htm
- http://www.americanheart.org/presenter.jhtml?identifier=1672

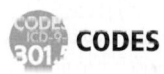 **CODES**

**ICD9**
747.0 Patent ductus arteriosus

# PEDIATRIC TRAUMA

Kevin M. Ban
Grace Kim
Lance Brown

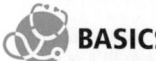 **BASICS**

## DESCRIPTION

- Pathophysiology and anatomy of adolescents and young adults are similar.
- 80% of pediatric trauma is blunt; 80% of multisystem trauma includes head injury.
- Trauma is the leading cause of death and disability in children >1 yr in U.S. and Europe.
- Most victims of child abuse are <3 yr. 1/3 of these patients are <6 mo.

## ETIOLOGY

- Most cases of pediatric trauma are single-system, minor, blunt injuries.
- Common mechanisms of injury include motor vehicle collisions and bicycle accidents, struck by a vehicle as a pedestrian, and fall from height.
- Penetrating injuries are rare in younger children.
- Risk factors include inadequate supervision, developmental inadequacy of child to perform task, inadequate attention to task, risk taking, drugs, and alcohol.

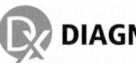 **DIAGNOSIS**

## SIGNS AND SYMPTOMS

### History

- History is often straightforward and provided by the child, parents, witnesses, or paramedics. If inconsistent with injury, consider child abuse.
- Mechanism(s) of injury relatively poor predictor of injury severity, but may suggest type of injury.
- Variables that increase the likelihood of serious injuries include handlebar injuries, significant passenger space intrusion, and failure to use proper restraint during a motor vehicle collision or helmet when riding a bike or skateboard.
- AMPLE history includes *a*llergies, *m*edications, *p*ast medical history, time of *l*ast meal, and *e*vents leading up to injury.

### Physical Exam

- Primary survey:
  - For all children who have sustained a major trauma, a traditional stepwise ABCDE evaluation based on assessing the *a*irway, *b*reathing, *c*irculation, *d*isability, and *e*xposure is appropriate.

- Secondary survey:
  - General:
    - Mass-to-surface ratio may impact insensible water loss and increase the risk of hypothermia.
    - Compensatory mechanisms may delay signs of hypovolemia. Few findings may be present until loss of 25–30% of blood volume, at which time decompensation abruptly occurs.
    - Smaller total blood volume (80 mL/kg)
  - Head:
    - Note bulging fontanel, scalp hematomas, midface instability, auricular and septal hematomas, lacerations, functional or cosmetic deformities to the face, and pupillary abnormalities.
    - Open sutures/fontanelles or multiple skull fractures may delay the onset of other signs and symptoms of increased intracranial pressure.
    - Large head/occiput causes cervical spine flexion when patient is supine on adult backboard.
  - Eye/ears, nose, and throat exam:
    - Look for evidence of blood, trauma, hemotympanum, hyphema, and CSF fluid.
    - Large tongue and tonsillar hypertrophy may obstruct the airway.
  - Neck:
    - Tracheal deviation and posterior neck step-offs are exceedingly unusual in children.
    - Shorter trachea increases risk of right mainstem intubation.
    - Cricoid cartilage is narrowest portion of airway in children <8 yr.
    - Children with altered mental status cannot have their cervical spine precautions cleared in the ED. These children should remain in a cervical collar (and be taken off the spinal board) while in the ED.
    - Pseudo-subluxation (anterior displacement of C-2 on C-3) occurs in 20% of patients.
    - The term spinal cord injury without radiologic abnormality (SCIWORA) is controversial in the MRI era.
  - Chest:
    - Note the overall work of breathing, grunting, asymmetric breath sounds, posterior abrasions, chest wall deformities, and crepitus.
    - Flexible and compliant chest walls make pulmonary contusions more likely than rib fractures in young children. Rib fractures may be a sign of abuse.
    - Diaphragmatic breathing

  - Abdomen:
    - Bruising, abrasions, and tenderness
    - Distention is usually caused by gastric air.
    - Liver and spleen relatively large
    - Rib cage covers less of abdomen.
    - Bladder is intra-abdominal in children <2 yr.
  - Extremities:
    - Palpation and evaluation of joint stability and tenderness
    - Assess pulses and compartments.
    - Salter-Harris classification of fractures
    - Unique injuries: Greenstick and buckle fractures
  - Neurologic exam:
    - Age-appropriate mental status assessment
    - Assess movement of the extremities.
  - Skin:
    - Assess for prolonged capillary refill and pallor.
    - Bruising of the ears, dorsa of the feet, or genitalia may suggest nonaccidental trauma.
  - Patterns of Injury:
    - Car vs. pedestrian: Waddell triad (femur, torso, and head injuries)—uncommon
    - Bicycle handlebar injuries may impale child: Pancreatic or small bowel injury.
    - Lap belt syndrome: Abdominal ecchymoses and intestinal injury with or without lumbar spine fracture (chance fracture)
    - Minor history with major injury: Child abuse

## ESSENTIAL WORKUP

- History and age-appropriate physical exam are the only essential components to a workup for all children who present for an evaluation following trauma.
- Obtaining standard radiographic and laboratory "trauma panels" is not evidence based in children.

## DIAGNOSTIC TESTS & INTERPRETATION

### Lab

- Laboratory tests should generally be individualized, reflecting the patient's clinical presentation.
- A normal initial hemoglobin and hematocrit do not rule out a significant hemorrhage but will provide a baseline value for later comparison; tachycardia may be only sign of fluid/blood loss early in presentation, although it is nonspecific for blood loss.
- Initial electrolyte measurement is unnecessary.
- Amylase and lipase have reasonable test characteristics, but because of the low incidence of pancreatic injuries, the false-positive tests far outnumber the true positives.
- Aspartate aminotransferase and alanine aminotransferase cannot be used as the sole determinant in deciding which children should undergo CT of the abdomen and pelvis.

- Gross hematuria is predictive of urinary tract injuries, but microscopic hematuria is not.
- Blood bank specimen for typing in appropriate patients
- A pregnancy testis indicated for teenage girls.
- Diagnostic peritoneal lavage is not indicated with availability of imaging modalities.

### Imaging

- The traditional "c-spine, chest, pelvis" set of radiographs is no longer universally obtained; selective approach is more appropriate.
- Forgo cervical spine radiographs in children who are awake, alert, cooperative, neurologically intact without neck pain or midline tenderness on palpation of the neck, are without pain on range of motion testing, and are without distracting injury:
  – An unconscious child will not be able to have the cervical spine cleared in the ED and may later need MRI (less often CT) as an inpatient.
- Chest radiographs indicated for grunting respirations, hypoxia, asymmetric breath sounds, dyspnea, crepitus, endotracheal intubation, and thoracostomy tube or central venous catheter placement in the internal jugular or subclavian veins
- Pelvic radiographs are seldom indicated. Children with clinically significant pelvic pain or instability typically undergo CT of the abdomen and pelvis.
- CT of the head is indicated for abnormal mental status, focal neurologic deficit, prolonged loss of consciousness, bulging fontanel, temporal or parietal scalp hematoma, depressed skull fracture, and uncontrollable persistent vomiting.
- CT of the abdomen and pelvis is typically indicated for children with altered mental status, gross hematuria, abdominal bruising above the iliac crests, handlebar injuries, and abdominal tenderness with hemodynamic effect.
- US has limited utility since the presence of free fluid (ie, blood) does not always indicate the need for laparotomy. The usefulness of focused abdominal sonography for trauma exam in young children needs further study.

### DIFFERENTIAL DIAGNOSIS

Nonaccidental trauma should be considered when the history is inconsistent with the injury.

 **TREATMENT**

### PRE-HOSPITAL

- Rapid transport to a facility capable of managing the child's suspected injuries
- Priorities include stabilization of airway (intubation by paramedics in the prehospital setting is controversial), breathing, circulation.
- Immobilization of cervical spine and extremity fractures

### INITIAL STABILIZATION/THERAPY

- Most traumatized children are stable throughout their ED course.
- Stabilization may require:
  – Cardiorespiratory and pulse oximetry monitoring
  – Early oxygen administration
  – Placement of 2 large-bore IVs and aggressive fluid resuscitation with normal saline
  – Laboratories and radiographs as indicated
  – Administration of packed red blood cells if not responding to two crystalloid boluses
  – Endotracheal intubation:
    ○ Tube size based on age in years or length-based tape
    ○ (16+ age in years) divided by 4
    ○ Initial estimate of the depth of insertion is 3 times the size of endotracheal tube.
    ○ Must check placement by auscultation, chest rise, pulse oximetry, and end tidal $CO_2$, then chest radiograph
  – Cervical spine immobilization
  – Thoracostomy tube as indicated
  – Urinary catheter (look for blood at the meatus)
  – Gastric decompression with a nasogastric or orogastric tube

### ED TREATMENT/PROCEDURES

- Risk-stratify based on history and physical exam.
- Acknowledge the limitations of using the mechanism of injury to predict its severity.
- Assess priorities; reassess frequently.
- Provide analgesia; sedate as appropriate.
- Clean wounds and splint fractures.
- Tetanus immunization if indicated
- Allow parents at the bedside during resuscitation and treatment.

### MEDICATION

- Normal saline/lactated Ringer: 20-mL/kg boluses IV
- Packed red blood cells: 10 ml/kg units IV
- Etomidate: 0.3 mg/kg IV
- Morphine sulfate: 0.1 mg/kg IV
- Succinylcholine: 1.5 mg/kg IV
- Lorazepam: 0.1 mg/kg IV
- Propofol: 2 mg/kg IV
- Ketamine: 2 mg/kg IV (generally thought to raise intraocular and intracranial pressure—usually avoided when head injury is suspected)

 **FOLLOW-UP**

### DISPOSITION

#### Admission Criteria

- Persistent altered mental status, endotracheal intubation, thoracostomy tube placement, intra-abdominal or intracranial injury identified on CT, pulmonary contusion, fractures requiring operative management, nonaccidental trauma
- Hemodynamic instability
- Airway concerns

- CT negative for intra-abdominal injury, but persistent abdominal pain as pancreatic or bowel injury is possible
- Failure to identify an appropriate adult to be responsible for the child (eg, both parents are admitted to the hospital for their injuries)

#### Discharge Criteria

- Most traumatized children with normal mental status and normal radiographic tests (if obtained) can be discharged home to a reliable caregiver.
- Posttraumatic stress syndrome may develop, and parents should be advised to seek appropriate counseling should concerns develop.

### FOLLOW-UP RECOMMENDATIONS

- Specialists as indicated by injury
- Psychiatric evaluation may be indicated for evidence of posttraumatic stress.
- Neurologic assessment for evidence of residual from postconcussion syndrome.

### ADDITIONAL READING

- Davis DH, Localio AR, Stafford PW, et al. Trends in operative management of pediatric splenic injury in a regional trauma system. *Pediatrics*. 2005;115: 89–94.
- Dudley NC, Hansen KW, et al. The effect of family presence on the efficiency of pediatric trauma resuscitations. *Ann Emerg Med*. 2009;53:777–784.
- Hutchings L, Willett K. Cervical spine clearance in pediatric trauma: A review of current literature. *J Trauma*. 2009;67:687–691.
- Hutchison JS, Ward RE, Lacroix J, et al. Hypothermia after traumatic brain injury in children. *N Engl J Med*. 2008;358:2447–2456.
- Kupperman N, Holmes JF, Dayan PS, et al. Identification of children at very low risk of clinically-important brain injuries after head trauma: A prospective cohort study. *Lancet*. 2009;374: 1160–1170.
- Tepas JJ 3rd, Mollitt DL, Talbert JL, et al. The pediatric trauma score as a predictor of injury severity in the injured child. *J Pediatr Surg*. 1987;22: 14–18.

### See Also (Topic, Algorithm, Electronic Media Element)

- Abuse, Pediatric
- Fractures, Pediatric
- Trauma, Multiple

 **CODES**

### ICD9

- 959.01 Other and unspecified injury to head
- 959.09 Other and unspecified injury to face and neck
- 959.11 Other injury of chest wall

# PEDICULOSIS

*Andrew B. Ziller*

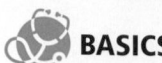

## BASICS

### DESCRIPTION
- Infestation by organisms that live in close association with host
- Bites are painless.
- Signs and symptoms result from host response to saliva and anticoagulant injected during feeding.
- Transmitted by direct contact and fomites (inanimate objects):
- Head lice are transmitted by head-to-head contact:
  - Combs
  - Pillows
  - Hats
- Head lice are more common in children and females.
- Pubic lice are transmitted by sexual contact.
- Obligate human parasites cannot survive away from hosts >7–10 days.

### ETIOLOGY
Infestation by:
- Pediculus capitis (head louse):
  - Most common
  - All socioeconomic groups
- Pediculus corporis (body louse):
  - Associated with poverty, poor hygiene, overcrowding
  - Live in clothing and transfer to human host for feeding
  - Can live up to 30 days off of human
  - Related to bed bugs
- *Phthirus pubis* (pubic or crab louse)

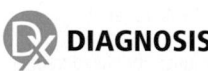

## DIAGNOSIS

### SIGNS AND SYMPTOMS
*History*
- Head lice:
  - Dandruff
  - Pruritus
  - Often asymptomatic
- Body lice:
  - Pruritus
  - Excoriation particularly at belt lines or seams of clothing
- Pubic lice:
  - Intense pruritus, worse at night

*Physical Exam*
- Examine hair for adult lice and nits:
  - Nits are cemented on hair shafts and are not easily removed.
  - Head lice and pubic lice infestation is confirmed by differentiating nits from scales, hair casts, and other easily brushed-off artifacts.
  - Empty nits are not diagnostic of active infection.
- Scalp and posterior neck erythema, scaling, and excoriated papules:
  - May lead to pyoderma, posterior cervical lyphadenopathy, and bacterial superinfection
- Body lice are observed only in very heavy infestation; infestation is confirmed by finding nits in clothing seams:
  - Linear excoriations of neck and trunk
  - Pus or serum stains on clothing
- Pubic lice:
  - Occasional urticaria with typical flare/wheal formation
  - May infest eyelashes and scalp in children
  - Characteristic bluish macules (maculae caeruleae) appear infrequently on trunk and thighs.
  - Prefer the perineum and pubic areas
  - Inguinal adenopathy

### ESSENTIAL WORKUP
- Careful history and physical exam
- Universal precautions

### DIAGNOSTIC TESTS & INTERPRETATION
*Lab*
- Nits may be visualized under low-power microscopy along hair shafts. They are <1 mm long:
  - Fluorescent under Wood lamp
- Mature lice are 3–4 mm long.
- Pubic louse ~1 mm long but wider body than head or body louse

*Imaging*
No imaging indicated

### DIFFERENTIAL DIAGNOSIS
- Scabies
- Contact or allergic dermatitis
- Seborrheic dermatitis
- Bedbugs (Cimicidae)

## TREATMENT

### PRE-HOSPITAL

> **ALERT**
> Maintain universal precautions.

### INITIAL STABILIZATION/THERAPY
Not applicable for routine cases

### ED TREATMENT/PROCEDURES
- Oral antihistamines and topical steroids may help pruritic symptoms of all lice infestations.
- Head lice:
  - Topical pediculicidal agents:
    ○ Permethrin 1% cream rinse (Nix) is the best first-line agent; it has low toxicity and is ovicidal.
    ○ Pyrethrin (Rid) also has low toxicity but is less effective.
    ○ Lindane shampoo is effective but may cause CNS toxicity and seizures if applied incorrectly or overused.
  - All agents require reapplication in 7–10 days if further adult lice or nits noted.
  - Remove nits with fine-toothed comb.
  - Examine all members of household; treat infested individuals.
  - Change clothing and machine wash and dry (using hot cycles) all clothing, towels, linens, and headgear:
    ○ Vacuum floors and furniture.
    ○ Wash combs and brushes in hot water for 10–20 min or coat with pediculicide for 15 min and wash.
  - Temperature >131°F (55°C) for >5 min kills eggs, nymphs, and mature lice.
- Body lice:
  - Wash and dry bedding and clothing using hot cycles.
  - Apply topical pediculicide cream or lotions from chin to toes.
- Pubic lice:
  - Topical pediculicide applied to hairy areas of chest, axilla, and groin
  - Remove nits with fine-toothed comb.
  - Treat sexual contacts simultaneously.
  - Wash and dry bedding and clothing using hot cycles.
  - Treat eyelash involvement with topical petrolatum twice daily for 9 days.

## MEDICATION

### First Line

- Antipruritics:
  - Diphenhydramine: 25–50 mg PO (peds: 5 mg/kg/d) q6h
  - Hydroxyzine: 25 mg PO q8h (peds: 12.5 mg per dose q6h)
- Pediculicides:
  - Permethrin 1% cream rinse (Nix): Apply to scalp and hair, rinse after 10 min; reapply in 7–10 days if needed.
  - Pyrethrin/piperonyl butoxide (Rid): Apply to scalp and hair, wash after 10 min; repeat in 7–10 days; avoid in patients with ragweed allergies.
  - Benzyl alcohol lotion 5% (Ulesfia lotion): Apply to scalp and hair, wash off after 10 min; repeat in 7 days.
  - Mercuric oxide ophthalmic ointment 1%: Use for louse infestation of eyelids: Apply q.i.d. for 14 days.

### Second Line

- Pediculicides:
  - Lindane ($\gamma$-benzene hexachloride) 1% shampoo: Lather for 4 min, then rinse; cream: Apply from chin to toes, wash off after 8 hr.
    - Use if first-line agents (Nix, Rid, Ulesfia) are not tolerated or effective.
    - Avoid use in children, lactation, pregnancy, or seizure disorder
  - Trimethoprim (TMP)-sulfamethoxazole: 8 mg/kg/d of TMP in divided doses is effective for head lice in patients who have previously failed treatment.
- Antihistamine:
  - Cetirizine (Zyrtec): Age >12 yr, 5–10 mg PO (peds: 6–11 yr, 5–10 mg PO; 2–5 yr, 2.5 mg PO) daily

### Pregnancy Considerations

Do not use lindane in pregnancy.

### Pediatric Considerations

Lindane is contraindicated in premature infants.

 FOLLOW-UP

## DISPOSITION

### Admission Criteria

Extensive bacterial superinfection; systemic hypersensitivity reaction with cardiorespiratory compromise

### Discharge Criteria

- Mild to moderate infestation with absence of significant superinfection or hypersensitivity reaction
- Children may return to school after initial treatment if repeat therapy is administered in 7–10 days.
- Pubic lice are often associated with sexually transmitted diseases; prudent screening is recommended. Pubic lice may also indicate sexual abuse in children.

## FOLLOW-UP RECOMMENDATIONS

- Re-evaluation is necessary to observe if treatment has been successful.
- Case management and/or social services may be required if concern for child well-being.

# PEARLS AND PITFALLS

- Diagnosed by direct visualization
- Most of the topical agents need to be reapplied in 7–10 days since unhatched eggs are not killed.
- Clothing and bedding must be washed and dried at a high heat to eradicate the infestation.
- Lindane is a second-line medication and is contraindicated in premature infants and uncontrolled seizure disorders.

## ADDITIONAL READING

- Benzyl alcohol lotion for head lice. *Med Lett.* 2009;51:57.
- Burkhart CG. Relationship of treatment-resistant head lice to the safety and efficacy of pediculicides. *Mayo Clin Proc.* 2004;79:661.
- Drugs for head lice. *Med Lett.* 2005;47:68.
- Lebwohl M, Clark L, Levitt J. Therapy for head lice based on life cycle, resistance, and safety considerations. *Pediatrics.* 2007;119:965.
- Morrell DS, Burkhart CN, Diamantis SA. Pediatric infestations. *Pediatr Ann.* 2009;38:326–332.
- Roberts RJ. Head lice. *N Engl J Med.* 2002;346: 1645.

## CODES

### ICD9

- 132.0 Pediculus capitis (head louse)
- 132.1 Pediculus corporis (body louse)
- 132.2 Phthirus pubis (pubic louse)

# PELVIC FRACTURE

*Theodore C. Chan*

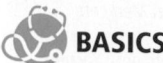 **BASICS**

## DESCRIPTION
- 3% of all bony fractures
- Pelvis is made up of sacrum and two innominate bones:
  - The innominate bones consist of the ilium, ischium, and pubis.
- Bony structures are stabilized by a network of ligaments, musculature, and other soft tissues in the pelvic area.
- Anterior stability and support are provided by the symphysis pubis and pubic rami.
- Posterior stability and support are provided by the sacroiliac complex and pelvic floor.
- Pelvis provides protection for lower urinary tract; GI tract; gynecologic, and vascular, and nervous structures contained in the region:
  - Pelvic fractures have a high associated morbidity and mortality rate and require urgent diagnosis and therapy.

## ETIOLOGY
- 65% of pelvic fractures are caused by vehicular trauma, including pedestrians struck by automobiles.
- 10% caused by falls
- 10% caused by crush injuries
- The remainder caused by athletic, penetrating, or nontraumatic injuries
- Mortality rate from pelvic fractures is 6–19%:
  - Increases with open fractures or evidence of hemorrhagic shock
- Significant pelvic hemorrhage can occur in unstable, high-energy pelvic fractures (Tile type B and C fractures):
  - Bleeding most commonly from posterior injuries involving the vascular plexuses
  - Retroperitoneal hematoma that may tamponade in the enclosed pelvic space

### Tile Classification System
- Includes stable single bone and avulsion fractures as well as pelvic ring fractures
- Predicts need for operative repair
- Type A: Stable pelvic ring injuries:
  - A1: Avulsion fractures of the innominate bone (ischial tuberosity, iliac crest)
  - A2-1: Iliac wing fractures
  - A2-2: Isolated rami fractures; most common pelvic fracture
  - A2-3: Four-pillar anterior ring injuries
  - A3: Transverse fractures of sacrum or coccyx
- Type B: Partially stable pelvic ring injury (rotationally unstable, but vertically stable):
  - B1: Unilateral open-book fracture
  - B2: Lateral compression injury:
    - B2-1: Ipsilateral double rami fractures and posterior injury
    - B2-2: Contralateral double rami fractures and posterior injury (bucket-handle fracture)
    - B2-3: Bilateral type B injuries

- Type C: Unstable pelvic ring injury—rotationally and vertically unstable, *Malgaigne fracture:*
  - Anterior disruption of symphysis pubis or 2–4 pubic rami with posterior displacement and instability thru sacrum, sacroiliac (SI) joint, or ileum:
    - C1: Unilateral vertical shear fracture
    - C2: Unilateral vertical shear combined with contralateral type B injury
    - C3: Bilateral vertical shear fracture
- Acetabular fractures (posterior lip, central/transverse, anterior column, or posterior column fractures)

### Young Classification System
- Based on mechanism of injury
- Only fractures that result in disruption of pelvic ring included; no single bone, avulsion, or acetabular fractures
- Predicts chance of associated injuries and mortality risk:
  - LC: Lateral compression
  - APC: Anteroposterior compression
  - VS: Vertical shear
  - CM: Combination of injury patterns

### Pediatric Considerations
- Children can have proportionately greater hemorrhage.
- Nonaccidental trauma is a concern.

### Pregnancy Considerations
Gravid uterus may be at risk for injury, including uterine rupture.

 **DIAGNOSIS**

## SIGNS AND SYMPTOMS
- Pain, swelling, ecchymoses, tenderness over hips, groin, perineum, and lower back
- Often presents with other traumatic injuries including neurologic, intra-abdominal, genitourinary, perineal, rectal, vaginal, and vascular injury
- Evidence of hemorrhagic shock

### History
- History of trauma mechanism of injury (fall, vehicular trauma, crush injuries, athletic injuries)
- Pain on hip movement, ambulation, sitting, standing, defecation

### Physical Exam
- Ecchymoses, swelling, tenderness over bony prominences, pubis, perineum, pelvic region, lower back
- Lower extremities may be shortened or rotated.
- Inability to actively or passively perform range of motion of involved hip
- Tenderness on lateral compression of pelvis, palpation of symphysis pubis or SI joints

- Gross pelvic instability, deformity, asymmetry in lower extremity
- Wounds over pelvic or bleeding from rectum, vagina, or urethra may indicate open fracture.
- In hemorrhagic shock:
  - Tachycardia, hypotension, narrowed pulse pressure
  - Altered mental status
  - Cool and pale extremities

## ESSENTIAL WORKUP
Pelvic radiograph is most common initial test:
- A single AP view of the pelvis can confirm diagnosis and should be obtained as early as possible when fracture suspected:
  - Most significant unstable pelvic fractures will be seen on the single AP view.
- Other views include:
  - Inlet projection: 30° caudal view; allows visualization of posterior arch
  - Outlet projection: 30° cephalic angulation; allows visualization of sacrum
  - Judet oblique views: Allow evaluation of acetabulum

## DIAGNOSTIC TESTS & INTERPRETATION
### Lab
- Type and cross-match.
- Hemoglobin/hematocrit, platelet count, and coagulation studies (prothrombin time, partial thromboplastin time)

### Imaging
- CT may further delineate pelvic fracture(s), retroperitoneal hematoma, visceral injuries:
  - CT contrast angiography may delineate source of bleeding (particularly arterial), but should be considered only in hemodynamically stable patients.
- Abdominal US focused abdominal sonography for trauma in patients with significant traumatic injury, but differentiation of intraperitoneal from extraperitoneal hemorrhage from pelvic fracture can be difficult
- MRI indicated with evidence of neurologic injury

### Diagnostic Procedures/Surgery
- Diagnostic peritoneal lavage (DPL) is a rapid bedside evaluation for intraperitoneal hemorrhage:
  - In the setting of pelvic fracture, the supraumbilical open approach for DPL should be used.
- Angiography and selective vessel embolization in setting of pelvic hemorrhage:
  - Particularly for small-vessel arterial bleeding
- Surgery:
  - As indicated on basis of clinical findings and orthopedic/surgical consult
  - Surgical stabilization with pelvic packing
  - Direct operative control of pelvic bleeding

## DIFFERENTIAL DIAGNOSIS

- Normal variants (ie, os acetabuli epiphyseal line can mimic type I fracture on radiograph)
- Ligamentous injury
- Spinal injury
- Intra-abdominal injury and hemorrhage

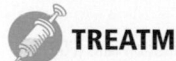 **TREATMENT**

### PRE-HOSPITAL

- ABCs of trauma care
- IV fluid resuscitation as indicated
- Consider stabilization or immobilization measures for pelvis (see below).

### INITIAL STABILIZATION/THERAPY

- ABCs of trauma care
- IV fluid resuscitation with blood or crystalloid, O-negative or type-specific blood if hemodynamically unstable:
  - Avoid using lower extremity IV sites.
- Stabilize and immobilize the pelvis to prevent further injury and decrease bleeding:
  - Compression device: Folded sheet with clamp or commercial compression device wrapped circumferentially around greater trochanters to stabilize and compress pelvis
  - Pneumatic antishock garment (PASG): Use in ED is controversial, but allows rapid pelvic immobilization and pelvic compression to slow bleeding.
  - External fixator: Requires more time to place than PASG but "splints" pelvis in a similar manner; contraindicated in severely comminuted pelvic fracture.
  - Placement of a stabilization device should not interfere with further workup and care (eg, US, DPL).

### ED TREATMENT/PROCEDURES

- Determine which pelvic fractures are stable and which are unstable.
- Type A fractures are generally stable.
- Type B and C fractures are unstable.
- Type A fractures:
  - Treated conservatively with bed rest, analgesics, and comfort measures; management decisions may be made in conjunction with orthopedics.
  - For four-pillar anterior ring injuries, CT should be obtained to evaluate the posterior pelvis.
  - Ensure that there are no other breaks in the pelvic ring.
- Type B and C fractures:
  - Immediate orthopedics consultation; patient should remain NPO.
  - May require ED pelvic stabilization measures
  - Assess for pelvic hemorrhage (see "Pelvic Hemorrhage").

- Acetabular fractures:
  - Immediate orthopedics consultation; patient should remain NPO.
- Pelvic hemorrhage:
  - Mechanical stabilization of unstable pelvic fractures (usually by application of external pelvic fixation)
  - Angiography and selective vessel embolization
  - Direct operative control of pelvic bleeding
- Prioritization of studies: CT, angiography, or surgery:
  - In the hemodynamically *unstable* patient:
    - Open B and C fractures: Surgical exploration
    - Closed fractures: DPL or US can help determine management in terms of need for immediate surgical exploration or selective angiography/embolization.
  - In the hemodynamically *stable* patient, the patient can go to CT for evaluation of the abdomen, pelvis, and retroperitoneum with external fixation as appropriate. IV contrast may be used to assess for bleeding and source, prior to selective angiography as indicated.

### MEDICATION

- Crystalloid fluids: 2-L IV bolus of normal saline or lactated Ringer (peds: 20 mL/kg)
- Blood products: 4–6 U cross-matched, type specific, or O negative (peds: 10 mL/kg)

 **FOLLOW-UP**

### DISPOSITION

#### Admission Criteria

- Hemodynamic instability, and pelvic hemorrhage to the ICU
- Type B or C pelvic fracture
- Acetabular fracture
- Other related injuries (eg, genitourinary, intra-abdominal, neurologic)
- Intractable pain

#### Discharge Criteria

Type A pelvic fracture; hemodynamically stable with no evidence of other injuries

#### Issues for Referral

Close follow-up should be ensured for discharged patients.

### FOLLOW-UP RECOMMENDATIONS

Discharged patients should be referred to an orthopedist for follow-up.

## PEARLS AND PITFALLS

- Pelvic fractures can be a marker for high-energy traumatic mechanism and injury:
  - Assess for underlying abdominal/pelvic injuries including GI, genitourinary, vascular, and neurologic injuries.
- In addition to initial resuscitation measures, immobilization and stabilization of the pelvis should be considered particularly for unstable or open fractures or where underlying hemorrhage is suspected.
- Determination of diagnostic/therapeutic pathways including CT with or without angiography, selective IR angiography, and surgery are dictated by the patient's hemodynamic status, suspected underlying injuries, and type of pelvic fractures.

## ADDITIONAL READING

- American College of Surgeons, Committee on Trauma. *Advanced Trauma Life Support for Doctors*, 8th ed. Chicago: American College of Surgeons; 2008.
- Dyer GSM, Vrahas MS. Review of the pathophysiology and acute management of haemorrhage in pelvic fracture. *Injury.* 2006;37:602–613.
- Geeraerts T, Chhor V, Cheisson G, et al. Clinical review: Initial management of blunt pelvic trauma in patients with haemodynamic instability. *Critical Care.* 2007;11:204–213.
- Rice PL, Rudolph M. Pelvic fractures. *Emerg Med Clinics North Am.* 2007;25:795–802.

### See Also (Topic, Algorithm, Electronic Media Element)

- Malgaigne Fracture
- Hemorrhagic Shock

 **CODES**

### ICD9

- 808.0 Closed fracture of acetabulum
- 808.1 Open fracture of acetabulum
- 808.2 Closed fracture of pubis

# PELVIC INFLAMMATORY DISEASE

*Erich Salvacion*

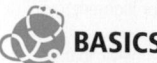 **BASICS**

## DESCRIPTION
- Pelvic inflammatory disease (PID) is an acute, community-acquired, sexually transmitted infection of the upper genital tract, including the uterus, fallopian tubes, ovaries, or adjacent structures.
- Most frequent gynecologic cause for ED visits (350,000 per year)
- Represents a spectrum of infection:
  - No single diagnostic gold standard
  - Requires low clinical threshold for considering the diagnosis and starting empiric antibiotic therapy
- Progressive disease can lead to tubo-ovarian abscess (TOA)
- Fitz-Hugh-Curtis syndrome is a capsular inflammation of the liver associated with PID:
  - Sharp right upper quadrant abdominal pain
  - Worse with inspiration, movement, or coughing

## ETIOLOGY
- Risk factors:
  - Age <25 yr
  - Multiple or symptomatic sexual partners
  - Previous episode of PID
  - Nonbarrier contraception
  - Oral contraception
  - African American ethnicity
- Most common causes of PID are *Chlamydia trachomatis* and *Neisseria gonorrhea*.
- Other organisms include groups A and B streptococci, staphylococci, gram-negative rods (commonly *Klebsiella* spp., *Escherichia coli*, and *Proteus* spp.), and anaerobes.

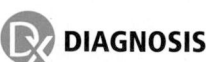 **DIAGNOSIS**

## SIGNS AND SYMPTOMS
- Lower abdominal pain, usually bilateral
- Vaginal discharge
- Abnormal uterine bleeding
- Dysmenorrhea
- Dysuria
- Dyspareunia
- Nausea and vomiting
- Fever and chills
- Proctitis
- Lower abdominal tenderness
- Decreased bowel sounds

- Bilateral adnexal tenderness
- Cervical motion tenderness
- Purulent endocervical discharge
- Adnexal mass or fullness
- Right upper quadrant tenderness

### History
- Lower abdominal pain is the most common symptom in PID, ranging from subtle to severe pain.
- Abdominal pain that worsens during intercourse or onset of pain shortly after or during menses is very suggestive of PID.
- Abdominal pain is usually bilateral and usually present for ≤2 wk.
- New vaginal discharge, urethritis, fever, and chills are common symptoms but are neither sensitive nor specific for the diagnosis.

### Pregnancy Considerations
PID is rare during pregnancy, but if present usually occurs during the 1st trimester before hormonal changes such as mucus plug formation can protect the uterus from ascending bacteria.

### Physical Exam
- Only 50% of patients with PID have fever.
- Abdominal exam reveals diffuse tenderness worse in the lower quadrants, usually but not always symmetric.
- Rebound tenderness and decreased bowel sounds are commonly found.
- Right upper quadrant tenderness is suggestive of perihepatitis (Fitz-Hugh-Curtis syndrome) in the setting of PID.
- Pelvic exam can reveal a purulent endocervical discharge, cervical motion tenderness, or adnexal tenderness.
- If uterine or adnexal tenderness is not prominent, one must consider other diagnoses.

## ESSENTIAL WORKUP
- History and physical exam including pelvic exam
- Pregnancy test to rule out ectopic pregnancy or complications of an intrauterine pregnancy
- Cervical culture for *N. gonorrhea* and *C. trachomatis*
- Minimum criteria for clinical diagnosis:
  - Lower abdominal tenderness *or*
  - Uterine/adnexal tenderness *or*
  - Cervical motion tenderness

- Supportive criteria for diagnosis:
  - Fever >38.3°C (101°F)
  - Abnormal cervical/vaginal discharge
  - Intracellular gram-negative diplococci on endocervical Gram stain
  - Leukocytosis >10,000/mm$^3$
  - Elevated erythrocyte sedimentation rate (ESR) or C-reactive protein
  - WBCs or bacteria in peritoneal fluid obtained by culdocentesis or laparoscopy

## DIAGNOSTIC TESTS & INTERPRETATION
### Lab
- CBC
- Gram stain of endocervix
- Urine polymerase chain reaction tests for *Chlamydia* and *Gonococcus*
- Microscopic exam of vaginal discharge in saline
- Liver enzymes may be elevated in Fitz-Hugh-Curtis syndrome.
- Positive urinalysis or occult blood in stool decreases the probability of PID.
- ESR or C-reactive protein may be elevated, but not routinely recommended

### Imaging
- Patients with adnexal fullness or an adnexal mass on exam should have a transvaginal US to exclude TOA.
- Consider obtaining a pelvic US in patients who use an intrauterine device, fail outpatient antibiotic therapy for PID, or who have inadequate pelvic exams due to pain or obesity.

### Diagnostic Procedures/Surgery
Laparoscopy may be useful in confirming PID in a patient with a high suspicion of competing diagnosis or who failed outpatient treatment for PID.

## DIFFERENTIAL DIAGNOSIS
- Ectopic pregnancy (must be excluded with a pregnancy test in any woman suspected of having PID)
- Acute appendicitis
- Adnexal torsion
- Endometriosis
- Cystitis
- Urolithiasis
- Ovarian tumor

- Adenomyosis uteri
- Chronic pelvic pain
- Benign ovarian cyst
- Diverticulitis
- Inflammatory bowel disease
- Mesenteric vascular disease
- Irritable bowel syndrome

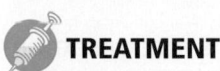

# TREATMENT

## PRE-HOSPITAL
- No specific prehospital considerations
- Appropriate pain management

## INITIAL STABILIZATION/THERAPY
- Resuscitation rarely indicated
- Pain control

## ED TREATMENT/PROCEDURES
### Outpatient
- Ceftriaxone or cefoxitin/probenecid plus doxycycline; with metronidazole when anaerobes are a particular concern
- Alternatives include ceftriaxone plus azithromycin.
- Must evaluate and treat sex partner as appropriate.

### Inpatient
- Doxycycline plus cefoxitin or cefotetan
- Alternatives include gentamicin plus clindamycin; or ampicillin/sulbactam plus doxycycline.
- Continue parenteral antibiotic administration for 24 hr after clinical improvement, then switch to oral antibiotics to finish 14-day course.
- Laparoscopy can be used to lyse adhesions in the acute and chronic stages of Fitz-Hugh-Curtis syndrome.
- Add metronidazole when anaerobes are a particular concern.

## MEDICATION
- Ampicillin/sulbactam: 3 g IV q6h
- Azithromycin: 1 g PO once per week for 2 wk
- Cefotetan: 2 g IV q12h
- Cefoxitin: 2 g IM single dose (outpatient); 2 g IV q6h (inpatient)
- Ceftriaxone: 250 mg IM single dose
- Clindamycin: 450 mg PO q.i.d. for 14 days (outpatient); 900 mg IV q8h (inpatient)

- Doxycycline: 100 mg PO b.i.d. for 14 days (outpatient); 100 mg IV or PO q12h (inpatient)
- Gentamicin: 2-mg/kg loading dose followed by 1.5 mg/kg IV q8h. Single daily IV dosing of gentamicin may also be used.
- Metronidazole: 500 mg PO b.i.d. for 14 days (outpatient); 500 mg IV q8h (inpatient)
- Probenecid: 1 g PO single dose

### First Line
- For outpatient: Ceftriaxone or cefoxitin/probenecid plus doxycycline; with metronidazole when anaerobes are a particular concern
- For inpatient: Doxycycline plus cefoxitin or cefotetan

### Second Line
- For outpatient: Ceftriaxone plus azithromycin with or without metronidazole
- For inpatient: Gentamicin plus clindamycin; or ampicillin/sulbactam plus doxycycline

# FOLLOW-UP

## DISPOSITION
### Admission Criteria
- Uncertain diagnosis and toxic appearance
- Suspected pelvic abscess, including TOA
- Pregnancy
- Immunodeficiency
- Severe illness (eg, vomiting or severe pain)
- Failure of outpatient therapy
- Probable noncompliance with outpatient therapy (eg, adolescents)
- Consider admission if appropriate clinical follow-up cannot be arranged.

### Discharge Criteria
- Patients who do not meet admission criteria may be treated as outpatients.
- Recent studies have shown that in women with mild to moderate PID, there was no difference in reproductive outcomes between women randomized to inpatient vs. outpatient treatment.

### Issues for Referral
TOAs may require drainage or surgical intervention in addition to antibiotics.

## FOLLOW-UP RECOMMENDATIONS
- If outpatient therapy is selected, it is important to have follow-up in 48–72 hr to assess for clinical improvement.
- If the patient has not defervesced by 72 hr, inpatient treatment and further evaluation should be considered.

## PEARLS AND PITFALLS
- PID represents a spectrum of disease from simple endometritis to fatal intra-abdominal sepsis.
- There is no single gold standard in use to establish the diagnosis of PID because no one test is adequate alone; older studies defining PID by a single standard, such as laparoscopic visualization of salpingitis, are now believed to lack sensitivity.
- Quinolones are no longer recommended in the U.S. for the treatment of gonorrhea or associated conditions such as PID, due to increasing rates of resistance.
- Patients with PID should have extensive counseling and testing for other STDs, including HIV.
- Male sex partners of women with PID should be treated if they had sexual contact with the patient during the previous 60 days prior to the patient's onset of symptoms.

## ADDITIONAL READING
- Centers for Disease Control and Prevention. Sexually transmitted disease surveillance, 2006. Available at: http://www.cdc.gov/std/stats/default.htm
- Centers for Disease Control and Prevention. Sexually transmitted diseases treatment guidelines, 2006. *MMWR Recomm Rep.* 2006;55(RR-11):1.
- Drugs for sexually transmitted infections. *Treat Guidel Med Lett.* 2004;2:67.
- Ness RB, Trautmann G, Richter HE, et al. Effectiveness of treatment strategies of some women with pelvic inflammatory disease: A randomized trial. *Obstet Gynecol.* 2005;106:573–580.
- Savaris RF. Comparing ceftriaxone plus azithromycin or doxycycline for pelvic inflammatory disease: A randomized controlled trial. *Obstet Gynecol.* 2007; 110:53.
- Update to CDC's sexually transmitted diseases treatment guidelines, 2006: Fluoroquinolones no longer recommended for treatment of gonococcal infections. *MMWR Morb Mortal Wkly Rep.* 2007;56: 332.

# CODES

## ICD9
614.9 Unspecified inflammatory disease of female pelvic organs and tissues

# PEMPHIGUS

Zachary P. Soucy
Deepi G. Goyal

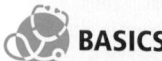

## BASICS

### DESCRIPTION
- Autoantibody (IgG)-mediated blistering disease of the skin and mucous membrane:
  - Characterized by loss of cell-to-cell adhesion called acantholysis
- Mortality is highest in those with mucocutaneous involvement; if untreated, mortality rates average 60–90%.
- Pemphigus is most common in individuals 40–60 yr old but has been reported in people ranging from neonates to 89 yr of age.
- Pemphigus is a rare disease, with a worldwide incidence of 0.076–1.61/100,000.
- Acquired blistering diseases include those caused by drugs (eg, toxic epidermal necrolysis) and idiopathic (eg, bullous diabeticorum).
- Pemphigoid: A term describing the group of syndromes that cause a separation of the epidermis from the dermis
- *Pemphix* is Greek for bubble or blister.
- Incidence: Males = Females
- 2 major subtypes exist:
  - Vulgaris; more serious with deeper involvement:
    - Accounts for 70–80% of all pemphigus
    - Up to 70% with vulgaris present with oral lesions, which is often the presenting complaint
    - Affects most races in middle age and elderly Ashkenazi Jews
  - Foliaceus; milder and more superficial:
    - Very rarely changes to pemphigus vulgaris
    - Often lacks oral lesions and has better prognosis

### Pediatric Considerations
- Pemphigus is rare in neonates and children but may occur in adolescents.
- Early diagnosis and treatment significantly impact growth, psychological, social, and cultural development.
- Histopathology is identical to adult disease.
- Neonates may develop the disease secondary to transplacental transfer of IgG.
- Neonatal pemphigus spontaneously resolves in several weeks as the maternal antibodies are catabolized.

### Pregnancy Considerations
Effective treatment of maternal disease prior to conception lowers the risk of neonatal transmission and gestational complications.

## ETIOLOGY
- IgG autoantibodies are directed against desmosomal cadherins desmoglein 1 and desmoglein 3 found in all keratinocytes.
- Autoantibodies cause histopathologic acantholysis, cytoskeletal derangements, and apoptosis.
- Bullea formation is caused by the loss of cell–cell adhesion and separation of the keratinocytes.
- UV-B from sunlight may increase rapidity of acantholysis and cause flaring of disease.
- Immunogenetic predisposition secondary to higher frequencies of specific human leukocyte antigen HLA haplotypes including DR4 and DRw6
- Drugs such as penicillamine, captopril, rifampin, piroxicam, and phenobarbital can trigger pemphigoid reactions.
- Endemic pemphigus foliaceus (fogo selvagem), most common in South America, may be triggered or transmitted by bites from flying insects.
- Pemphigoid reactions may occur in association with a neoplasm, usually lymphoma (paraneoplastic pemphigus).

## DIAGNOSIS

### SIGNS AND SYMPTOMS
- Generalized or focal flaccid bullae (blisters) of the skin and mucosa
- Painful skin erosions with shreds of detached epithelium
- Painful nonhealing oral, vaginal, or mucosal erosions
- Crusting, partially healing skin erosions from ruptured bullae
- Hypertrophic, hyperplastic erosive plaques with pustules in intertriginous areas (pemphigus vegetans)
- Moist, edematous, exfoliative erosions in seborrheic areas (pemphigus foliaceus)
- Erythematous, scaly, crusting skin lesions in a malar distribution (pemphigus erythematosus)

### History
- Typically features mucocutaneous blisters followed by erosions
- Often appear 1st in mucous membranes and several months later appear cutaneously
- Skin lesions are painful flaccid blisters that may appear anywhere.

### Physical Exam
Nikolsky sign (separation of the epidermis with lateral pressure) is characteristic but not diagnostic.

## ESSENTIAL WORKUP
- Suspected based on clinical presentation
- Biopsy with histologic and immunofluorescence testing is essential for definitive diagnosis (arrange with a dermatologist).

## DIAGNOSTIC TESTS & INTERPRETATION
### Lab
Serum antibody titers, detected by indirect immunofluorescence, are often used as a marker of disease activity; however, the ED physician usually does not order these titers.

### Imaging
No diagnostic imaging test exists.

### Diagnostic Procedures/Surgery
Biopsy

## DIFFERENTIAL DIAGNOSIS
- Bullous pemphigoid
- Contact dermatitis
- Dermatitis herpetiformis
- Erythema multiforme
- Erysipelas
- Erythroderma
- Erythema multiforme
- Toxic epidermal necrolysis
- Epidermolysis bullosa
- Hand, foot, and mouth disease
- Systemic lupus erythematosus
- Systemic vasculitis
- Oral candidiasis
- Herpes simplex gingivostomatitis
- Erosive lichen planus
- Seborrheic dermatitis

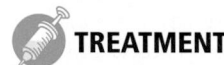

## TREATMENT

### PRE-HOSPITAL
If severe disease, IV access, pulse oximetry monitor, and cardiac monitor

### INITIAL STABILIZATION/THERAPY
- If symptoms of hypotension or sepsis are present, IV fluid resuscitation should be guided by the Parkland burn formula:
  - 4 mL of crystalloid/kg body weight per percentage of body surface area involved per 24 hr
  - Give half of the total calculated fluid over the course of the 1st 8 hr, the remainder over the next 16 hr.
  - Adjust fluids to keep urine output >0.5 mL/kg/hr.

- If signs or symptoms of sepsis are present, initiate broad-spectrum antibiotic coverage:
  - Keep mean arterial pressure >65 mm Hg, keep central venous oxygen saturation >70%, keep central venous pressure 8–12 mm Hg.
  - Vasopressors may be needed to achieve these goals.
- In steroid-dependent patients, administer stress-dose steroids.

### ED TREATMENT/PROCEDURES
- Systemic corticosteroids are the mainstay of therapy.
- *Severe disease:* Conventional high-dose corticosteroids:
  - If severe symptoms are unresponsive to high-dose PO corticosteroids, consider pulse IV corticosteroids and admission for plasmapheresis.
- *Mild to moderate disease* should receive PO prednisone, and intralesional triamcinolone acetonide may be used.
- Adjuvant immunosuppressive therapy may also be added to decrease the symptoms associated with high-dose systemic corticosteroids or in patients with contraindications to steroid therapy:
  - Dapsone, gold, azathioprine, cyclophosphamide, cyclosporine, methotrexate, mycophenolate, and IV immunoglobulins

### MEDICATION
- Hydrocortisone: 100–300 mg IV stress dose steroids
- Methylprednisolone (pulse IV therapy; adults): 1 g IV over 3 hr daily
- Prednisone: 20–400 mg PO daily (adults); severe disease, 200–400 mg PO daily for 5–10 wk, then taper; mild to moderate disease, 20–80 mg PO daily
- Triamcinolone acetonide: 20 mg/mL 0.1-mL injection into each superficial lesion

#### First Line
- Immune suppression:
  - Hydrocortisone: 100–300 mg/day IV stress dose steroids adjusted based on patients known dosage and use habits
  - Methylprednisolone (pulse IV therapy; adults): 1 g IV over 3 hr daily
  - Prednisone: 20–400 mg PO daily (adults); severe disease, 200–400 mg PO daily for 5–10 wk, then taper; mild to moderate disease, 20–80 mg PO daily
- Pain:
  - Opiates, anti-inflammatory agents, acetaminophen
  - Biobrane synthetic dressing
  - Diphenhydramine and Maalox or Xylocaine oral wash

#### Second Line
- Usually performed as an inpatient.
- Immune suppression:
  - Triamcinolone acetonide: 20 mg/mL 0.1-mL injection into each superficial lesion
- Pain:
  - Gabapentin 300 mg daily titrated up to 300 mg t.i.d. over a month
- Other considerations: Patients on high-dose steroids should have diets high in vitamin D and calcium and may benefit from a proton-pump inhibitor or bisphosphonates.

 FOLLOW-UP

### DISPOSITION
#### Admission Criteria
- Admit to the ICU or burn unit if any signs and symptoms of shock or sepsis are present because aggressive fluid resuscitation, wound care, and multiple medications will be required.
- Admit to a floor bed if pulse parenteral steroid therapy or plasmapheresis is indicated.
- Admit 1st-time presentations of disease to facilitate treatment and definitive diagnosis.

#### Discharge Criteria
- Discharge if mild to moderate disease will not require aggressive steroid management, plasmapheresis, or aggressive pain control.
- A follow-up evaluation is essential to monitor the course of the disease and to adjust treatment.

### FOLLOW-UP RECOMMENDATIONS
- A follow-up evaluation with dermatology is essential to monitor the course of the disease and to adjust treatment.
- Rheumatology follow-up may be advantageous to assess risk of osteoporosis via bone scan if on high-dose steroids.

### PEARLS AND PITFALLS
- Patients on immunosuppressive treatment including steroids and immunomodulating agents are at very high risk of complications and may present in adrenal crisis, severe sepsis, or hyperosmolar nonketotoic acidosis secondary to new-onset type 2 diabetes.
- Patients with hypotension require aggressive fluid resuscitation.

### ADDITIONAL READING
- Ahmed AR, Spigelman Z, Cavacini LA, et al. Treatment of pemphigus vulgaris with rituximab and intravenous immune globulin. *N Engl J Med.* 2006; 355:1772–1779.
- Amagai M, Ikeda S. Shimizu, et al. A randomized double-blind trial of intravenous immunoglobulin for pemphigus. *J Am Acad Dermatol.* 2008;60: 595–603.
- Asarch A, Razzaque Ahmed A. Treatment of juvenile pemphigus vulgaris with intravenous immunoglobulin therapy. *Pediatr Dermatol.* 2009;26:197–202.
- Kavusi S, Daneshpazhooh M, Farahani F, et al. Outcome of pemphigus vulgaris. *J Eur Acad Dermatol Venereol.* 2008;22:580–584.
- Lehman JS, Mueller KK, Schraith DF. Do safe and effective treatment options exist for patients with active pemphigus vulgaris who plan conception and pregnancy? *Arch Dermatol.* 2008;144:783–785.
- Rashid RM, Candido KD. Pemphigus pain: A review on management. *Clin J Pain.* 2008;24:734–735.
- Schmidt E, Waschke J. Apoptosis in pemphigus. *Autoimmun Rev.* 2009;8:533–537.

### See Also (Topic, Algorithm, Electronic Media Element)
- Erythema Multiforme
- Rash
- Toxic Epidermal Necrolysis

 CODES

ICD9
694.4 Pemphigus

# PENILE SHAFT FRACTURE

*Ian R. Grover*

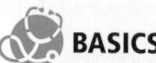 **BASICS**

## DESCRIPTION

- Traumatic rupture of the corpus cavernosum and the encompassing tunica albuginea
- May involve the corpus spongiosum and urethra
- Hematoma formation occurs at rupture site.
- Injury is usually unilateral and transverse.
- Most common fracture site is the proximal shaft of the penis.
- During erection, pressure within the corpus cavernosum is maximal, close to arterial pressure, increasing the volume in each corpus to maximum, which thins the tunica albuginea, making it susceptible to rupture.
- Penile erection stretches the spongiosum to the limit, which limits movement vertically while allowing lateral movements; this forms a bend at the base of the penis, making it vulnerable to lateral swing and rupture of corpus cavernosum.
- 25–30% have associated urethral injury, which may be partial or complete.
- Caused by blunt trauma to erect penis during:
  - Sexual intercourse
  - Manipulation
  - Fall on erect penis
  - Entanglement in clothing
  - *"Taghaandan"*—Middle Eastern practice of forcefully bending the erect penis to cause detumescence

## ETIOLOGY

- Peyronie disease
- Urethritis in past
- Surgical procedure on corpus cavernosum or trauma to corpus cavernosum resulting in weak scar tissue

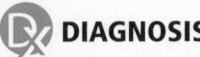 **DIAGNOSIS**

## SIGNS AND SYMPTOMS

- Loud popping or crunching sound heard at the time of injury
- Immediate detumescence
- Severe penile pain
- Deviation of the penis away from the side of injury
- Penile swelling and ecchymosis
- There may be blood at the urethral meatus if there is a urethral injury.
- May have dysuria, inability to void, or an increase in the size of the swelling with voiding due to extravasation of urine

### History

- Cause of the injury
- Sudden painful sensation in erect penis during sexual intercourse or soon after with loss of erection
- Blood at the urethral meatus after intercourse
- Problems with poor erections after the injury if presentation is delayed
- Penile deviation with erection
- Urinary retention or weak urinary stream

### Physical Exam

- Swelling and blue-black discoloration at base of penis, usually on one side
- Ecchymosis may also involve scrotum.
- Penis flaccid and edematous with angulation away from the side of tear
- Defect in the penile shaft may be palpable at the site of the tear.
- Blood at tip of penis or frank hematuria suggests an associated urethral injury.
- Urethrocavernous or urethrocutaneous fistulas may be present as late complications of a penile fracture.

## ESSENTIAL WORKUP

- Urinalysis
- PT/PTT
- Retrograde urethrography if urethral trauma is suspected

## DIAGNOSTIC TESTS & INTERPRETATION

### Lab

Urinalysis to evaluate urethral trauma:

- May have frank blood or microscopic hematuria
- PT/PTT if patient is on Coumadin or has a history of bleeding disorder

### Imaging

- Retrograde urethrography—recommended in all cases of suspected urethral trauma:
  - Should be done with low pressure during injection, before urethral catheterization
- Cavernosography and MRI of penis may be needed to confirm diagnosis and site of tear.
- Ultrasonography may also be done to confirm a suspected tear.

### Diagnostic Procedures/Surgery

Diagnostic exploration of the penis is recommended when cavernosography is negative but clinical suspicion of a fracture is high.

## DIFFERENTIAL DIAGNOSIS

- Cellulitis of penis
- Contusion of penis
- Lymphangitis of penis
- Neoplasm of penis
- Paraphimosis
- Trauma because of constrictive ring or other structure
- Urethral injury
- Vasculature rupture, especially superficial or deep dorsal vein or dorsal artery

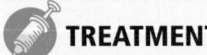 TREATMENT

### PRE-HOSPITAL
- Other injuries take precedence in the setting of multiple trauma.
- Local treatment: Ice packs to the penis; splinting of the penis with tongue blade
- Elevate the area to reduce swelling.

### INITIAL STABILIZATION/THERAPY
- Pain control
- Needle suprapubic cystotomy in patients with urethral trauma and a full bladder to relieve patient discomfort

### ED TREATMENT/PROCEDURES
- Combined efforts of ED physician and urologist are aimed toward restoration of normal shape of penis and sexual and urinary functions.
- ED treatment is directed to reducing hemorrhage, preventing further complications.
- Prophylactic antibiotic use is unnecessary.
- Urethral catheterization in all cases after excluding urethral trauma
- Urologic evaluation and early surgical treatment are essential to prevent complications such as erectile dysfunction, impotence, penile deformity, urethral stricture.
- All patients with suspected or definite diagnosis *must* have early urologic evaluation.

### MEDICATION
- Diazepam: 2–5 mg IV q1–6h PRN anxiety
- Fentanyl: 0.05–0.2 mg IV q1h PRN pain
- Hydromorphone: 0.5–1.0 mg IV q1–2h PRN pain
- Lorazepam: 0.5–1.0 mg IV q1–6h PRN anxiety
- Morphine sulfate: 0.1 mg/kg IV q1h PRN pain

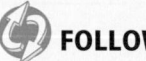 FOLLOW-UP

### DISPOSITION
*Admission Criteria*

> **ALERT**
> *All* patients with penile fracture must be hospitalized for prompt surgery.

### Issues for Referral
If immediate urologic consultation and treatment are unavailable, patient may be transferred to a suitable hospital after initial stabilization and transfer criteria have been met.

### FOLLOW-UP RECOMMENDATIONS
Follow up with urologist to ensure adequate repair and return to normal sexual and urinary function.

## PEARLS AND PITFALLS

- Penile fracture is not a rare occurrence.
- Coitus and penile manipulation are the most common causes.
- Delay in seeking treatment is the major cause of morbidity.
- Mainly a clinical diagnosis:
  – Cavernosography, MRI, and US may be used to confirm the diagnosis.
  – Early surgical repair is important.

## ADDITIONAL READING

- Eke N. Fracture of the penis. *Br J Surg*. 2002;89(5): 555–565.
- Ekwere PD, Al Rashid M. Trends in the incidence, clinical presentation, and management of traumatic rupture of the corpus cavernosum. *J Natl Med Assoc*. 2004;96(2):229–233.
- Kamdar C, Mooppan UM, Kim H, et al. Penile fracture: Preoperative evaluation and surgical technique for optimal patient outcome. *BJU Int*. 2008;102(11):1640–1644.
- Kervancioglu S, Ozkur A, Bayram MM. Color Doppler sonographic findings in penile fracture. *J Clin Ultrasound*. 2005;33(1):38–42.
- Muentener M, Suter S, Hauri D, et al. Long-term experience with surgical and conservative treatment of penile fracture. *J Urol*. 2004;172(2):576–579.

### See Also (Topic, Algorithm, Electronic Media Element)
- Urethral Trauma
- Paraphimosis

 CODES

**ICD9**
959.13 Fracture of corpus cavernosum penis

# PEPTIC ULCER
*Yanina A. Purim-Shem-Tov*

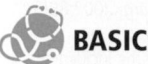 **BASICS**

## DESCRIPTION
- Produced by breakdown in gastric or duodenal mucosal defenses
- Imbalance exists between production of acid and ability of mucosa to prevent damage.

## ETIOLOGY
- *Helicobacter pylori*:
  - Gram-negative spiral bacteria that live in mucous layer
  - Responsible for 90–95% of duodenal ulcers and 80% of gastric ulcers
  - Increases antral gastrin production and decreases mucosal integrity
- NSAIDs:
  - Interfere with prostaglandin synthesis
  - Lead to break in mucosa
- Aspirin
- Cigarette smoking
- Alcohol

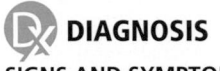 **DIAGNOSIS**

## SIGNS AND SYMPTOMS
- Epigastric pain or tenderness (80–90%):
  - Burning, gnawing, aching pain
  - Location: Midline, xiphoid, or umbilicus
- Duodenal ulcers:
  - Pain occurs 90 min to 3 hr after meals.
  - Usually awakens patient at night
  - Food and antacids relieve pain.
- Gastric ulcers:
  - Pain worsens after meals.
  - Nausea and anorexia
- Difficult to differentiate clinically between gastric and duodenal ulcers
- Relief of pain with antacids
- Heme-positive stools
- Complications of peptic ulcer disease (PUD):
  - Acute perforation:
    ○ Rigid, boardlike abdomen
    ○ Generalized rebound tenderness
    ○ Pain radiation to back or shoulder
  - Obstruction:
    ○ Pain with vomiting
    ○ Succussion splash from retained gastric contents and abdominal distention
  - Hemorrhage:
    ○ Hematemesis
    ○ Melena
    ○ Hypotension
    ○ Tachycardia
    ○ Skin pallor
    ○ Orthostatic changes

## History
- NSAID, Aspirin
- Smoking
- Previous history of PUD
- Family history of stomach cancer
- Abdominal pain
- Diarrhea
- Weakness

## Physical Exam
- Abdominal pain
- Signs of anemia
- Guaiac-positive stool

## ESSENTIAL WORKUP
- Careful physical exam including Hemoccult testing and vital signs with orthostatics
- For stable patients, oral GI cocktail typically relieves pain:
  - Antacid: 30 mL
  - Viscous lidocaine: 10 mL

## DIAGNOSTIC TESTS & INTERPRETATION
### Lab
- Normal lab values in uncomplicated ulcer disease
- CBC:
  - Low hematocrit with bleeding
  - Leukocytosis with perforation/penetration
- Amylase/lipase:
  - Elevated with perforation/penetration
  - Pancreatitis in differential diagnosis
- Electrolytes, BUN/creatinine, glucose for critically ill
- Type and cross-match for significant blood loss.

### Imaging
Chest radiograph/abdominal series:
- Evaluate for perforations/obstructions.

### Diagnostic Procedures/Surgery
- ECG:
  - For elderly patients
  - Myocardial ischemia in differential diagnosis
- Endoscopy:
  - Procedure of choice
  - Outpatient unless significant hemorrhage
  - Allows for biopsies of gastric/duodenal ulcers for presence of *H. pylori*
  - Detects malignant gastric ulcers
- Upper GI series:
  - Single contrast barium diagnoses 70–80%
  - Double contrast diagnoses 90%
- Gastrin level is elevated in Zollinger-Ellison syndrome.

## DIFFERENTIAL DIAGNOSIS
- Gastroesophageal reflux
- Biliary colic
- Cholecystitis
- Pancreatitis
- Gastritis
- Abdominal aortic aneurysm
- Aortic dissection
- Myocardial infarction
- Subset with symptoms and no ulcer on endoscopy called *nonulcer dyspepsia*

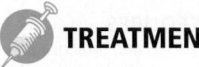 **TREATMENT**

## PRE-HOSPITAL
- ABCs
- IV fluid resuscitation for hypotensive/shock patients

## INITIAL STABILIZATION/THERAPY
- ABCs
- Identify ulcer complications (hemorrhage, perforation, obstruction)
- Treat hypotension with lactated Ringer/normal saline fluid bolus via two large-bore IVs.
- Type and cross early.
- Nasogastric tube (NGT) for gastric decompression/check for hemorrhage

## ED TREATMENT/PROCEDURES
- Pain control with antacids (GI cocktail) or IV $H_2$ antagonists
- Avoid narcotics—may mask serious illness.
- Promotion of ulcer healing:
  - Antacids
  - $H_2$ antagonists (cimetidine, famotidine, ranitidine, nizatidine):
    ○ May continue for 2–5 yr for ulcer suppression therapy
  - Sucralfate
  - Prostaglandin congeners (misoprostol)
  - Proton-pump inhibitors (PPIs; omeprazole, lansoprazole, or pantoprazole):
    ○ If $H_2$ antagonists have failed
  - Sucralfate, $H_2$-receptor antagonists, and PPIs should not be combined because of lack of documented benefit.
- Gastric outlet obstruction:
  - Decompress stomach with NGT.
  - IV hydration
- Gastric hemorrhage:
  - IV fluid resuscitation
  - Blood transfusion depending on loss/hematocrit
  - Foley catheter to monitor volume status
  - GI consultation

- Perforation:
  - IV hydration
  - Foley catheter to monitor hydration status
  - Preoperative antibiotics
  - Emergency surgical consultation
- Treatment of *H. pylori* infection:
  - Invasive or noninvasive testing to confirm infection
  - Oral eradication antibiotic therapy options:
    - PPI (omeprazole 20 mg b.i.d. or lansoprazole 30 mg PO b.i.d.) and two antibiotics (clarithromycin 500 mg b.i.d. plus metronidazole 500 mg b.i.d.) for 14 days
    - H₂ blocker, bismuth subsalicylate (Pepto-Bismol) plus either amoxicillin 1,000 mg b.i.d. or tetracycline 500 mg q.i.d. in combination with either metronidazole 250 mg q.i.d. or clarithromycin 500 mg b.i.d. for 14 days
    - Most common regimen: Omeprazole 20 mg or lansoprazole 30 mg plus clarithromycin 500 mg and amoxicillin 1 g, all taken twice a day for 2 wk
- Stop NSAIDs
- Surgical therapy:
  - Refractory ulcer
  - Complications:
    - Bleeding
    - Perforation
    - Pyloric stenosis

## MEDICATION

- Bismuth subsalicylate: Two 525-mg tabs PO
- Maalox Plus: 2–4 tabs PO q.i.d.
- Misoprostol: 100–200 mg PO q.i.d.
- Mylanta II: 2–4 tabs PO q.i.d.
- Sucralfate: 1 g PO q.i.d. for 6–8 wk
- Famotidine (H₂ blocker): 40 mg PO nightly at bedtime (peds: 0.5–0.6 mg/kg q12h) for 6–8 wk
- Nizatidine (H₂ blocker): 300 mg PO nightly at bedtime for 6–8 wk; 20 mg PO b.i.d. (peds: 0.6–0.7 mg/kg q12–24h) for 2 wk
- Ranitidine (H₂ blocker): 300 mg PO nightly at bedtime (peds: 5–10 mg/kg/24 hr given q12h) for 6–8 wk
- Cimetidine (H₂ blocker): 400 mg PO b.i.d. for 6–8 wk
- Lansoprazole (PPI): 30 mg PO b.i.d. for 2 wk
- Pantoprazol (PPI): 40 mg PO daily for 2 wk
- Omeprazole (PPI): 20 mg PO b.i.d. for 2 wk
- Rabeprazole (PPI): 20 mg PO daily for 6 wk
- Esomeprazole (PPI): 40 mg daily for 4 wk

- *H. pylori* therapy:
  - PPI (omeprazole 20 mg or lansoprazole 30 mg), clarithromycin 500 mg b.i.d. for 2 wk, amoxicillin 1 g, b.i.d. for 2 wk
  - For penicillin-allergic patients: PPI plus clarithromycin 500 mg b.i.d. plus metronidazole 500 mg b.i.d. for 14 days
  - 4-drug therapy: H₂ blocker, bismuth subsalicylate (Pepto-Bismol) plus either amoxicillin 1,000 mg b.i.d. or tetracycline 500 mg q.i.d. in combination with either metronidazole 250 mg q.i.d. or clarithromycin 500 mg b.i.d. for 14 days

### First Line
*H. pylori* eradication regimes:

- PPI (omeprazole 20 mg or lansoprazole 30 mg), clarithromycin 500 mg b.i.d. for 2 wk, amoxicillin 1 g, b.i.d. for 2 wk
- For penicillin-allergic patients: PPI plus clarithromycin 500 mg b.i.d. plus metronidazole 500 mg b.i.d. for 14 days
- 4-drug therapy: H₂ blocker, bismuth subsalicylate (Pepto-Bismol) plus either amoxicillin 1,000 mg b.i.d. or tetracycline 500 mg q.i.d. in combination with either metronidazole 250 mg q.i.d. or clarithromycin 500 mg b.i.d. for 14 days

### Second Line
1 wk quadruple therapy:

- Bismuth subsalicylate 120 mg PO q.i.d., tetracycline PO 500 mg q.i.d., metronidazole 400 mg PO q.i.d., esomeprazole 20 mg PO b.i.d.
- 80% eradication rate

 **FOLLOW-UP**

## DISPOSITION
### Admission Criteria
- Gastric obstruction
- Perforation
- Active upper GI bleed
- Melena
- Uncontrolled pain
- Anemia requiring transfusion

### Discharge Criteria
- Unremarkable physical examination with normal CBC and heme-negative stools
- If heme-positive stools, discharge if stable vital signs, normal hematocrit, and negative NGT aspiration for upper GI hemorrhage

### Issues for Referral
Outpatient GI evaluation and endoscopy

## FOLLOW-UP RECOMMENDATIONS
- Patients with hemorrhage require admission
- High-risk patients include those with the following characteristics:
  - Bleeding with hemodynamic instability
  - Repeated hematemesis or any hematochezia
  - Failure to clear with gastric lavage
  - Coagulopathy
  - Comorbid disease
  - Advanced age
  - Patients with ulcer perforation or penetration require operative repair.
- Hospitalization for gastric outlet obstruction
- All patients require primary care follow-up in 2–6 wk to evaluate efficacy of treatment.
- Patients >55 years and patients with severe symptoms should receive GI referral for endoscopy and testing for *H. pylori*.

## PEARLS AND PITFALLS

- *H. pylori* is the most common cause of PUD.
- NSAID-induced PUD is frequently silent.
- Dyspeptic symptoms are nonspecific.
- Endoscopy is diagnostic, should include *H. pylori* screening.
- Treatment should include *H. pylori* eradication, H₂ blockers, or PPIs.
- Complications include perforations, hemorrhage, anemia
- Failure to follow up may result in failure to diagnose gastric cancer.

## ADDITIONAL READING

- Louw JA, Marks IN. Peptic ulcer disease. *Curr Opinion Gastroenterol.* 2004;20(6):533–537.
- Malfertheiner P, Chan FK, McColl KE. Peptic ulcer disease. *Lancet.* 2009;374:1449–1461.
- Smoot DT, Go MF, Cryer B. Peptic ulcer disease. *Prim Care.* 2001;28(3):487–503.
- Yuan Y, Padol IT, Hunt RH. Peptic ulcer disease today. *Nat Clin Pract Gastroenterol Hepatol.* 2006; 3(2):80–89.

### See Also (Topic, Algorithm, Electronic Media Element)
- Gastroesophageal Reflux Disease
- Gastritis
- Gastrointestinal Bleeding

 **CODES**

### ICD9
- 531.00 Acute gastric ulcer with hemorrhage, without mention of obstruction
- 531.01 Acute gastric ulcer with hemorrhage, with obstruction
- 531.10 Acute gastric ulcer with perforation, without mention of obstruction

# PERFORATED VISCOUS

Ingrid D. Carter
Jeffrey J. Schaider

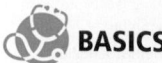 **BASICS**

## DESCRIPTION
- Perforation of viscous structure into peritoneal cavity
- Inflammation
- Ulceration
- Shearing/crushing or bursting forces in trauma
- Obstruction
- Chemical peritonitis occurs as result of disruption of gastric or intestinal lining into peritoneal cavity.

## ETIOLOGY
- Peptic ulcer disease
- Appendicitis
- Inflammatory bowel disease
- Diverticular disease
- Colon carcinoma
- Foreign body ingestion
- Trauma
- Radiation enteritis

### Pediatric Considerations
- Blunt trauma more common cause of bowel rupture than penetrating trauma
- Jejunum is most common site of rupture.

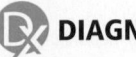 **DIAGNOSIS**

## SIGNS AND SYMPTOMS
- Sudden severe abdominal pain:
  - Initially local
  - Rapidly becoming diffuse
- Rigidity
- Guarding
- Rebound tenderness
- Absent bowel sounds
- Hypovolemic shock:
  - Tachycardia
  - Hypotension

## ESSENTIAL WORKUP
Upright chest radiograph:
- Best demonstrates pneumoperitoneum
- When in upright position for 5–10 min, may detect as little as 1–2 mL of free air under diaphragm

## DIAGNOSTIC TESTS & INTERPRETATION
### Lab
- CBC
- Electrolytes, BUN/creatinine, glucose
- Lipase
- Urinalysis
- Liver function test

### Imaging
- Upright CXR
  - To detect air under diaphragm
- Abdominal radiographs:
  - Left lateral decubitus film more helpful than supine abdomen.
  - Double wall sign of perforated viscous:
    - Air in intestinal lumen and peritoneal cavity allows for visualization of both serosal (not normally seen) and mucosal surfaces of intestine.
- Abdominal CT:
  - Detects small amounts of free air from perforated viscous
- ECG

## DIFFERENTIAL DIAGNOSIS
- Intra-abdominal abscess
- Pneumomediastinum with peritoneal extension
- Pancreatitis
- Peptic ulcer disease
- Inferior wall myocardial infarction
- Cholecystitis

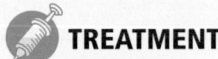 **TREATMENT**

### PRE-HOSPITAL
Initiate IV fluids for patients with history of vomiting or abnormal vital signs.

### INITIAL STABILIZATION/THERAPY
Treat hypotension/tachycardia with 0.9% normal saline:
- Adults: 500 mL to 1 L bolus
- Pediatric: 20 mL/kg bolus

### ED TREATMENT/PROCEDURES
- Nasogastric tube
- Foley catheter
- Administer broad-spectrum antibiotics:
  – Cephalosporin
  – Aminoglycoside plus clindamycin
- Immediate surgical consultation for operative intervention

### MEDICATION
- Amikacin: 15 mg/kg/24 h IV q8h
- Cefoxitin: 2 g (peds: <7 days: 20 mg/kg IV q12h; >1 wk, 80–160 mg/kg IV q6h) IV q6h
- Clindamycin: 600–900 mg (peds: 20 to 40 mg/kg/24 h) IV q8h
- Morphine sulfate: 2–4 mg (peds: 0.1 mg/kg) IV q2h–q3h

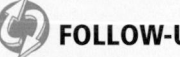 **FOLLOW-UP**

### DISPOSITION
#### Admission Criteria
Suspected or confirmed perforation requires admission and immediate surgical consultation.

#### Discharge Criteria
None

#### Issues for Referral
General surgery consult for operative intervention

### FOLLOW-UP RECOMMENDATIONS
Postoperative surgery follow-up

## PEARLS AND PITFALLS

- Obtain upright CXR and abdominal radiographs for patients with suspected perforated viscous.
- If high clinical suspicion for perforation and plain films normal, obtain CT of abdomen to detect small perforation.
- Obtain immediate surgical consult for operative intervention.

## ADDITIONAL READING

- Ghekier O, Lesnik A, Hoa D, et al. Value of computed tomography in the diagnosis of the cause of nontraumatic gastrointestinal tract perforation. *J Comput Assist Tomogr*. 2007;31:169–176.
- Graff LG, Robinson D. Abdominal pain and emergency department evaluation. *Emerg Med Clin North Am*. 2001;19:123–136.
- Shaffer H. Perforation and obstruction of the gastrointestinal tract. *Radiol Clin North Am*. 1992;30:405–426.
- Sivit C. Gastrointestinal emergencies in older infants and children. *Radiol Clin North Am*. 1997;35:865–877.

### See Also (Topic, Algorithm, Electronic Media Element)
Abdominal Pain

 **CODES**

### ICD9
- 799.89 Other ill-defined conditions
- 868.00 Injury to unspecified intra-abdominal organ without mention of open wound into cavity

# PERICARDIAL EFFUSION/TAMPONADE

Jessica H. Klausmeier
Carlo L. Rosen

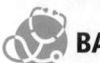 **BASICS**

## DESCRIPTION
- Pericardial effusion:
  - Pericardial sac usually contains 15–40 cc of fluid
  - Collection of additional fluid = effusion
- Pericardial tamponade:
  - Accumulation of pericardial fluid causes an elevation of pressure in the pericardial space, resulting in impairment of ventricular filling and decreased cardiac output.
  - Increase of as little as 80–120 cc of fluid may lead to a rise in pericardial pressure.
  - Potentially lethal
  - Up to 70% present in "early tamponade" and appear clinically stable
  - Occurs in 2% of patients with penetrating chest trauma

## ETIOLOGY
- Medical causes:
  - Pericarditis (20%):
    ○ 90% idiopathic or viral
    ○ Bacterial, fungal, parasitic, tuberculosis, HIV
  - Malignancy (13%):
    ○ Lymphoma, leukemia, melanoma, breast, lung
    ○ Metastatic disease, primary malignancy, postradiation
  - Post–myocardial infarction (8%):
    ○ Acute: 1–3 days after acute myocardial infarction (AMI)
    ○ Subacute (Dressler syndrome): Weeks to months after AMI
  - End-stage renal disease, uremia (6%)
  - Autoimmune/collagen vascular disease (5%): Rheumatoid arthritis, systemic lupus erythematosus, scleroderma
  - Rheumatic fever
  - Radiation therapy
  - Myxedema
  - Congestive heart failure (CHF), valvular heart disease
  - Drug toxicity (isoniazid, doxorubicin, procainamide, hydralazine, phenytoin)
  - Idiopathic
- Surgical causes:
  - Penetrating chest trauma
  - Thoracic aortic dissection
  - Iatrogenic (cardiac catheterization, post–cardiac surgery, central line placement)
  - Blunt trauma rarely causes pericardial effusion.

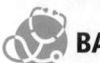 **DIAGNOSIS**

## SIGNS AND SYMPTOMS
- Beck's triad = classic presentation of cardiac tamponade:
  - Hypotension
  - Muffled heart sounds
  - Jugular venous distention
- Dressler syndrome: Pericarditis seen several weeks after a myocardial infarction:
  - Fever
  - Chest pain
  - Pericardial friction rub

### History
- Past medial history is key:
  - History of malignancy?
  - Recent viral illness?
  - Connective tissue disorder?
  - Recent MI?
- History of the present illness:
  - Most are asymptomatic.
  - Pulmonary symptoms: Dyspnea, cough:
    ○ Dyspnea is most common symptom seen in tamponade (87–88% sensitivity).
  - Chest pain is most common symptom:
    ○ Usually sharp, pleuritic, relieved by sitting forward
    ○ Can be referred to scapula
    ○ Can also be dull, aching, constrictive
  - GI symptoms: Nausea or abdominal pain from hepatic and visceral congestion or dysphagia from esophageal compression
  - Generalized symptoms: Fatigue, malaise

### Physical Exam
- Signs of shock or right heart failure:
  - Tachycardia, hypotension
  - Jugular venous distention (may be absent if the patient is also hypovolemic)
- Pericardial friction rub (100% specific):
  - High-pitched "scratchy" sound
  - Best heard at left sternal border
  - Increased by leaning forward
  - Can be transient/intermittent
- Pulsus paradoxus:
  - Fall in systolic blood pressure >10 mm Hg with inspiration
  - When severe, this can manifest as lack of brachial or radial pulse during inspiration.
  - Sensitive but not specific
  - Only present in approximately 1/3 of patients
- Fever >38°C is uncommon; if present, consider purulent pericarditis (can also result from autoimmune/connective tissue disease).
- Lungs should be clear; if not, consider CHF or pneumonia.

## ESSENTIAL WORKUP
- ECG
- CXR
- US:
  - Echocardiography, including evaluation of aortic root
  - Shock US: Include focused assessment with sonography in trauma, aorta, pleural effusion, and pneumothorax views to rule out other causes of hypotension

## DIAGNOSTIC TESTS & INTERPRETATION
### Lab
- CBC
- ESR, C-reactive protein:
  - Usually elevated in pericarditis
- Cardiac enzymes:
  - May be elevated in pericarditis
- Electrolytes:
  - BUN/creatinine in suspected uremic pericarditis
- Coagulation profile:
  - Especially in liver failure, anticoagulation, trauma
- Blood cultures if an infectious source is suspected

### Imaging
- Chest radiograph:
  - Cardiomegaly is 89% sensitive for tamponade.
  - Can be normal even with effusion if developed quickly
- Echocardiography:
  - 97–100% sensitive, 90–97% specific
  - Effusion: Can detect as little as 20–50 cc of pericardial blood/fluid:
    ○ Small effusions will only be seen posteriorly.
    ○ Anterior fat pad may mimic effusion; must also visualize posterior pericardial space for diagnosis of effusion.
  - Tamponade:
    ○ Effusions large enough to cause tamponade should be circumferential.
    ○ Right atrial or ventricular bowing and eventual collapse
    ○ "Sniff" test: During inspiration, the inferior vena cava will not collapse in patients with tamponade.
- Chest CT for detecting hemopericardium
- Transesophageal echocardiography
- MRI with gadolinium (for stable patients only)

### Diagnostic Procedures/Surgery
- ECG:
  - Low voltage
  - Electrical alternans: Alternating beat-to-beat variation of QRS amplitude (usually only seen with large effusions)
  - Evidence of pericarditis:
    ○ Diffuse ST-segment elevation without reciprocal depression
    ○ Can be difficult to distinguish from early repolarization: ST elevation/T wave ratio >0.25 in V6 suggests pericarditis, not early repolarization
    ○ PR depression
    ○ In late presentation ST and PR changes may disappear; ECG may show diffuse T wave inversion.

- Pericardiocentesis and fluid analysis:
  - Therapeutic for tamponade
  - Diagnostic for bacterial effusion (to guide antibiotics) or malignant effusion (for cytology)
- Central venous pressure (CVP) determination:
  - May be used in penetrating chest trauma patients
  - CVP >15 cm $H_2O$ suggests tamponade, but may be normal in the hypovolemic patient.

### DIFFERENTIAL DIAGNOSIS

- Noncardiogenic shock:
  - Hypovolemic, septic, anaphylactic, spinal
- Other cardiac conditions:
  - Myocardial infarction—common misdiagnosis!
  - Pericardial constriction (due to pericardial fibrosis)
  - CHF
- Pulmonary conditions:
  - Pulmonary embolus
  - Tension pneumothorax
  - Hemothorax
- Other causes:
  - Air embolism
  - Aortic dissection
  - Ruptured abdominal aortic aneurysm

 **TREATMENT**

### PRE-HOSPITAL

- 2 large-bore IV lines
- Start IV fluids.
- Supplemental $O_2$

### INITIAL STABILIZATION/THERAPY

- Continue prehospital measures
- Continuous cardiac monitoring
- Pain control:
  - Ketorolac 30 mg IV for pericarditis (if not pregnant, no renal failure, hemopericardium not suspected)
  - Morphine 0.1 mg/kg IV
- In tamponade:
  - IV fluid resuscitation with normal saline or blood (to consider in cases of traumatic tamponade)
  - Pericardiocentesis for unstable patients to decompress the tamponade:
    - US guided if available
    - Consider placing catheter to facilitate further drainage (perform using Seldinger technique).

### ED TREATMENT/PROCEDURES

- Medical causes of tamponade in patients who are unstable:
  - Perform pericardiocentesis with placement of an indwelling catheter for continued drainage:
    - Subxiphoid: 2 cm below and 1 cm to the left of the xiphoid process, needle aimed at 30–45° angle toward the patient's left shoulder
    - Left parasternal approach: Fifth intercostal space just lateral to sternum, needle inserted perpendicular to the skin
    - Needle is advanced with constant syringe aspiration.
    - Remove fluid as needed to improve clinical condition.
    - When assembling supplies, be sure needle is secure on syringe but can be removed easily if needed (for additional syringe or placement of guidewire).

- Traumatic pericardial tamponade:
  - Consult trauma surgeon immediately.
  - Definitive therapy is thoracotomy in the OR.
  - If patient is deteriorating despite resuscitation, ED thoracotomy with pericardotomy is an option.
- Bacterial pericardial effusion:
  - Initiate antibiotic therapy to cover gram-negative and anaerobic organisms and *Staphylococcus aureus*.
  - May ultimately require partial surgical resection of the pericardium
- Uremic pericardial effusion:
  - Arrange urgent dialysis.
- Dressler syndrome and postirradiation pericardial effusion:
  - Initiate NSAIDs
- Aortic dissection:
  - Immediate cardiothoracic surgical consultation for operative repair

### MEDICATION

#### First Line

- Medical treatment is appropriate for *pericarditis* (not tamponade):
  - Aspirin 650 mg PO q4h
  - Also start patients on a proton-pump inhibitor or $H_2$ blocker to prevent gastritis.
- Treat underlying illness (ex: dialysis for uremic pericarditis).
- Purulent pericarditis requires antibiotics:
  - [Nafcillin 2 g IV q4h or vancomycin 15 mg/kg q12h] + aminoglycoside × 4 wk
  - Ampicillin/sulbactam 3 g IV q6h × 4 weeks

#### Second Line

- Ibuprofen: 800 mg PO q8h
- Indomethacin: 25–75 mg PO b.i.d.
- Colchicine is controversial.
- Steroids:
  - Only for refractory cases (more commonly associated with rebound when tapered)
  - Prednisone: 1.0–1.5 mg/kg, continued for at least 1 mo, slowly tapered

 **FOLLOW-UP**

### DISPOSITION

#### Admission Criteria

- ICU admission for acute, symptomatic pericardial effusion/tamponade
- New pericardial effusion

#### Discharge Criteria

- Most patients with pericarditis or hypotension/chest pain in the setting of a pericardial effusion will be admitted.
- Exceptions:
  - Known or incidentally found small pericardial effusion in asymptomatic stable patient
  - Pericarditis without evidence of tamponade in a young, healthy person whose pain is controlled with NSAIDs

#### Issues for Referral

- Trauma surgery:
  - Tamponade in setting of trauma: Will need to go to OR for thoracotomy (or from ED status post ED thoracotomy)

- Cardiothoracic surgery:
  - Tamponade/effusion in setting of aortic dissection/other primary cardiac problem
  - Patients requiring pericardial window
  - Any patients who have had recent cardiac surgery
- Cardiology/interventional cardiology:
  - Dressler syndrome
  - Recent percutaneous intervention
  - Any patients who need pericardiocentesis

### FOLLOW-UP RECOMMENDATIONS

Discharged patients need urgent primary care physician follow-up and repeat echo to evaluate for resolution of effusion.

### PEARLS AND PITFALLS

- ECG changes associated with pericarditis include diffuse ST elevation with PR depression and eventual T wave inversion. Should be contrasted with ECG findings of localized ST elevation with reciprocal ST depression in AMI.
- Relatively small effusions can cause tamponade if rapidly developing (conversely, large effusions can be relatively benign when they develop slowly).
- Cardiac output can be fluid dependent in tamponade—start fluids early.
- Use bedside US to look for pericardial effusion and other signs of tamponade in the setting of hypotension (including in trauma).
- ED thoracotomy should not be employed if there is no OR readily available.

### ADDITIONAL READING

- Bessen HA, Byyne R. Acute pericarditis and cardiac tamponade. In: Wolfson AB, ed. *Harwood Nuss' Clinical Practice of Emergency Medicine*, 4th ed. Philadelphia: Lippincott Williams & Wilkins; 2005:294–297.
- Hoit BD. Pericardial disease and pericardial tamponade. *Crit Care Med*. 2007;35(8):S355–S364.
- Little WC, Freeman GL. Pericardial disease. *Circulation*. 2006;113:1622–1632.
- Roy CL, Minor MA, Brookhart MA, et al. The rational clinical examination: Does this patient with a pericardial effusion have cardiac tamponade? *JAMA*. 2007;297(16):1810–1818.
- Shockley LW. Penetrating chest trauma. In: Wolfson AB, ed. *Harwood Nuss' Clinical Practice of Emergency Medicine*, 4th ed. Philadelphia: Lippincott Williams & Wilkins; 2005:990–999.

### See Also (Topic, Algorithm, Electronic Media Element)

Cardiogenic Shock

 **CODES**

#### ICD9

- 420.90 Acute pericarditis, unspecified
- 423.3 Cardiac tamponade
- 423.9 Unspecified disease of pericardium

# PERICARDITIS

Shamai A. Grossman
Samuel C. Gross

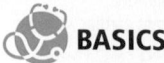

## BASICS

### DESCRIPTION
- Inflammation, infection, or infiltration of the pericardial sac surrounding the heart:
  - Pericardial effusion may or may not be present.
- Acute pericarditis:
  - Rapid in onset
  - Potentially complicated by cardiac tamponade from effusion
- Constrictive pericarditis:
  - Results from chronic inflammation causing thickening and adherence of the pericardium to the heart

### ETIOLOGY
- Idiopathic (most common)
- Viral:
  - Echovirus
  - Coxsackie
  - Adenovirus
  - Varicella
  - Epstein-Barr virus
  - Cytomegalovirus
  - Hepatitis B
  - Mumps
  - HIV
- Bacterial:
  - *Staphylococcus*
  - *Streptococcus*
  - *Haemophilus*
  - *Salmonella*
  - *Legionella*
  - *Tuberculosis*
- Fungal:
  - *Candida*
  - *Aspergillus*
  - Histoplasmosis
  - Coccidioidomycosis
  - Blastomycosis
  - *Nocardia*
- Parasitic:
  - Amebiasis
  - Toxoplasmosis
  - Echinococcosis
- Neoplastic:
  - Lung
  - Breast
  - Renal cell
  - Lymphoma
  - Leukemia
  - Melanoma
- Uremia
- Myocardial infarction:
  - Dressler syndrome
- Connective tissue disease:
  - Systemic lupus erythematosus
  - Rheumatoid arthritis
  - Scleroderma
- Radiation
- Chest trauma
- Postpericardiotomy
- Aortic dissection
- Myxedema
- Pancreatitis
- Inflammatory bowel disease
- Amyloidosis
- Drugs:
  - Procainamide
  - Cromolyn sodium
  - Hydralazine
  - Dantrolene
  - Methysergide
  - Mesalamine
  - Doxorubicin

## DIAGNOSIS

### SIGNS AND SYMPTOMS
- Chest pain
- Fever
- Mild dyspnea
- Cough
- Hoarseness
- Nausea
- Anorexia

### History
- Chest pain:
  - Pain radiating to the ridge of the trapezius from phrenic irritation
  - Central or substernal pain
  - Sudden onset
  - Sharp
  - Pleuritic
  - Worse when supine
  - Worse with cough
  - Improved with leaning or sitting forward
- Previous episodes of pericarditis
- History of fever or infection
- History of malignancy or autoimmune disease

### Physical Exam
- Tachypnea
- Tachycardia
- Odynophagia
- Friction rub:
  - Heard best at lower left sternal border
  - Very specific
  - Triphasic rub is classic
  - Can have any of these 3 components:
    - Presystolic
    - Systolic
    - Early diastolic
  - Intermittent and exacerbated by leaning forward
- Beck's triad with the accumulation of pericardial fluid:
  - Muffled heart sounds
  - Increased venous pressure (distended neck veins)
  - Decreased systemic arterial pressure (hypotension)
- Ewart sign:
  - Dullness and bronchial breathing between the tip of the left scapula and the vertebral column
- Pulsus paradoxus:
  - Exaggerated decrease (>10 mm Hg) in systolic pressure with inspiration
- Constrictive pericarditis:
  - Signs of both right- and left-sided heart failure
  - Pulmonary and peripheral edema
  - Ascites
  - Hepatic congestion

### ESSENTIAL WORKUP
- ECG has 4 classic stages
- Stage 1:
  - Concave ST elevations diffusely except aVR and V1
  - PR segment depressions with elevation in aVR
- Stage 2:
  - Normalization of ST and PR segments
  - T wave flattening
- Stage 3:
  - Diffuse T wave inversions
- Stage 4:
  - T waves normalize, may have some persistent T wave inversions
- Atypical changes may include localized ST elevations or T wave inversions
- Myocardial involvement suggested by intraventricular conduction delay, new bundle branch block, or Q waves

### DIAGNOSTIC TESTS & INTERPRETATION
#### Lab
- CBC:
  - May show leukocytosis
- Erythrocyte sedimentation rate and C-reactive protein:
  - May be elevated, can follow for resolution
- Cardiac enzymes:
  - Helpful in distinguishing pericarditis from myocardial infarction
  - May also be elevated in myopericarditis

#### Imaging
- CXR:
  - Most often normal
  - May show enlargement of the cardiac silhouette
  - No change in heart size until >250 mL of fluid has accumulated in the pericardial sac

- Echocardiography:
  - Diagnostic method of choice for the detection of pericardial fluid
  - Can detect as little as 15 mL of fluid in the pericardial sac
  - Bedside US good screening tool
- Chest CT:
  - Useful for the detection of calcifications or thickening of the pericardium
  - Can help rule out other etiologies

### Diagnostic Procedures/Surgery
Pericardiocentesis:

- Pericardial fluid can help determine underlying etiology.
- Fluid sent for protein, glucose, culture, cytology, Gram and acid-fast stains, and fungal smears

## DIFFERENTIAL DIAGNOSIS
- Acute myocardial infarction
- Pulmonary embolism
- Pneumothorax
- Aortic dissection
- Pneumonia
- Empyema
- Cholecystitis
- Pancreatitis

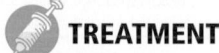 **TREATMENT**

### PRE-HOSPITAL
- ABCs, IV access, O$_2$, monitor
- Consider fluid bolus if no crackles.

### INITIAL STABILIZATION/THERAPY
- ABCs
- Emergent pericardiocentesis:
  - For hemodynamic compromise secondary to cardiac tamponade
  - Removal of a small amount of fluid can lead to a dramatic improvement.
  - US guidance if available

### ED TREATMENT/PROCEDURES
- Treatment dependent on the underlying etiology
- Idiopathic, viral, rheumatologic, and posttraumatic:
  - NSAID regimens effective
  - Corticosteroids reserved for refractory cases
- Bacterial:
  - Aggressive treatment with IV antibiotics along with drainage of the pericardial space
  - Search for primary focus of infection.
  - Therapy guided by determination of pathogen from pericardial fluid tests
- Neoplastic:
  - Treat underlying malignancy.
- Uremic:
  - Intensive 2–6 wk course of dialysis
  - Caution should be used if using nonsteroidal medications.
- Expected course/prognosis:
  - Most patients will respond to treatment within 2 wk.
  - Most have complete resolution of symptoms.
- Few progress to recurrent episodes with eventual development of constrictive pericarditis or cardiac tamponade.

## MEDICATION
### First Line
- Ibuprofen 300–800 mg q6–8h for days to weeks depending on severity:
  - Can also be tapered to prevent recurrence
  - Improves coronary blood flow
  - GI prophylaxis with 20 mg omeprazole
- Aspirin 800 mg PO q6–8h × 7–10 days:
  - Taper to off over 3–4 wk
  - Omeprazole as with ibuprofen
  - Colchicine 1–2 mg × 1 day, then 0.5–1 mg daily × 3 mo
- Colchicine alone: 1–2 mg × 1 day, then 0.5–1 mg daily × 3 mo:
  - Combination with aspirin decreased recurrence rate
  - Lower doses may also be effective.

### Second Line
- Indomethacin 25–50 mg q6h:
  - May restrict coronary blood flow
- Prednisone 1–1.5 mg/kg daily × 2–4 wk with taper:
  - Used for refractory cases
  - For use if contraindication to aspirin/NSAIDs
  - Associated with increased rate of recurrence
  - Also beneficial in uremic and autoimmune pericarditis

### Pregnancy Considerations
- NSAIDs and aspirin are not teratogenic in first 20 wk of pregnancy
- Glucocorticoids may be used during pregnancy.
- Avoid aspirin and high-dose steroids when breast-feeding.
- Colchicine may be a reasonable alternative.

 **FOLLOW-UP**

### DISPOSITION
### Admission Criteria
- ICU:
  - Hemodynamic instability
  - Cardiac tamponade
  - Malignant dysrhythmia
  - Status post pericardiocentesis
- Telemetry unit:
  - Suspicion of myocardial infarction
  - Severe pain
  - Suspicion of bacterial etiology
  - Any high-risk criteria
- High-risk criteria:
  - Large effusion (>2 cm total)
  - Anticoagulant use
  - Malignancy
  - Temperature >38°C
  - Traumatic pericarditis
  - Immunosuppression
  - Pulsus paradoxus
  - Slow onset

### Discharge Criteria
- Mild symptoms in patients without any hemodynamic compromise
- Close follow-up
- Able to tolerate a regimen of oral medication
- Debate on need for ECG to evaluate for effusion prior to discharge

### Issues for Referral
Follow-up with cardiology:

- Recurrent cases
- Admitted patients

### FOLLOW-UP RECOMMENDATIONS
Follow up with primary care physician for reevaluation and verification of resolution of symptoms and absence of complications in 1–2 wk.

## PEARLS AND PITFALLS
- Classic history: Viral illness preceding development of sharp, positional chest pain
- Rub is very specific but not always audible.
- ECG changes help identify etiology.
- The challenge is distinguishing pericarditis from acute MI and other etiologies of chest pain.

## ADDITIONAL READING
- Bessen HA, Byyny R. Acute pericarditis and cardiac tamponade. In: Wolfson AB, ed. Harwood-Nuss' Clinical Practice of Emergency Medicine, 4th ed. Philadelphia. Lippincott Williams & Wilkins; 2005: 294–297.
- Imazio M, Bobbio M, Cecchi E, et al. Colchicine in addition to conventional therapy for acute pericarditis: Results of the colchicine for acute pericarditis (COPE) trial. Circulation. 2005;112: 2012–2016.
- Imazio M, Cecchi E, Demichelis B, et al. Myopericarditis versus viral or idiopathic acute pericarditis. Heart. 2008;94:498–501.
- Maisch B, Seferovic OM, Ristic AD, et al. Guidelines on the diagnosis and management of pericardial diseases. EurHeart J. 2004;25:587–610.
- Spodick DH. Acute pericarditis: Current concepts and practice. JAMA. 2003;289:1150–1153.
- Spodick DH. Risk prediction in pericarditis: Who to keep in hospital? Heart. 2008;94:398–399.

### See Also (Topic, Algorithm, Electronic Media Element)
Pericardial Effusion/Tamponade

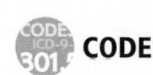 **CODES**

### ICD9
- 074.21 Coxsackie pericarditis
- 115.03 Histoplasma capsulatum pericarditis
- 115.13 Histoplasma duboisii pericarditis

# PERILUNATE DISLOCATION

Ian R. Grover

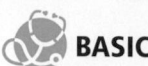

## BASICS

### DESCRIPTION
- Lunate remains located and in line with the radius but the distal carpal bones are displaced dorsally (~95% of the time) or volarly (~5% of the time)
- Early surgical treatment is recommended.
- This injury has a high incidence of posttraumatic arthritis.

### ETIOLOGY
- Mechanism of injury is usually wrist hyperextension with ulnar deviation.
- These are high-energy injuries:
  - Falls from a height
  - Motor vehicle accidents
  - Industrial accidents
  - Sporting accidents

### ALERT
Scaphoid is frequently fractured with perilunate dislocations.

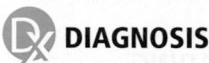

## DIAGNOSIS

### SIGNS AND SYMPTOMS
- Severe wrist pain
- Wrist swelling
- Diffuse wrist tenderness
- Paresthesias in the median nerve distribution

### History
- History of a high-energy injury
- Any concomitant injuries
- Pain in the wrist
- May complain of paresthesias in the median nerve distribution

### Physical Exam
- Wrist swelling
- Possible deformity of the wrist
- Decreased range of motion of the wrist
- Possible decreased sensation in the median nerve distribution
- Special attention should be paid to skin integrity because open fractures are common.
- Neurovascular status should be monitored closely, including 2-point discrimination.
- Check closely for concomitant injuries, specifically of the upper extremity.

### ALERT
Diagnosis is frequently missed on clinical exam.

### ESSENTIAL WORKUP
Radiographs of the wrist

### DIAGNOSTIC TESTS & INTERPRETATION
#### Imaging
- Radiographic imaging that includes 3 views of the wrist
- Perilunate dislocation visualized best on the true lateral view:
  - Distal carpal row, specifically the capitate, seen dorsally (95% of the time) or volarly (5% of the time) in relation to the lunate
  - Lunate is located and in line with the radius
- CT and MRI are not generally needed for diagnosis, but some orthopedists may request them for preoperative planning.

#### Pediatric Considerations
- Wrists are rarely sprained in children.
- Wrist radiographs are difficult to interpret in pediatric patients.
- Comparison view of other wrist may be helpful.

### DIFFERENTIAL DIAGNOSIS
- Lunate fracture
- Lunate dislocation:
  - Dislocation occurs between lunate and distal radius.
- Scapholunate dissociation and other similar ligamentous disruptions
- Distal radius fracture

#### Pediatric Considerations
Consider nonaccidental trauma.

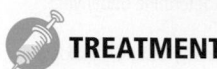

## TREATMENT

### ALERT
Concern is for concomitant, more serious, injuries.

### PRE-HOSPITAL
- Assess for other injuries
- Immobilize
- Pain control
- Elevate

### INITIAL STABILIZATION/THERAPY
- Identify other, more serious, associated injuries.
- Immobilize
- Elevate
- Ice

### ED TREATMENT/PROCEDURES
- Pain control
- Procedural sedation for closed reduction:
  - Etomidate: 0.1–0.15 mg/kg IV
  - Methohexital: 1–1.5 mg/kg IV
  - Propofol: 40 mg IV every 10 sec until induction (2–2.5 mg/kg IV)

- Closed reduction of the dislocation should be done emergently:
  - Arm is hung in traction for 10 min with 10–15 pounds of counterweights and the fingers in traps.
  - The fingers are then removed from the traps and manual traction is continued.
  - One of the physician's thumbs is placed volarly over the lunate and then the injury is recreated with wrist extension.
  - Continued traction is applied to the wrist and then slow flexion of the wrist is performed, which usually locates the distal carpal bones.
- Operative fixation to reduce and maintain wrist stability is required.
- Immobilize wrist using a sugar-tong splint in neutral position.

### Pediatric Considerations
Although perilunate dislocation is unusual in pediatric patients, children with wrist pain should be splinted and referred to a pediatric hand surgeon.

### MEDICATION
- Diazepam: 2–5 mg IV q1–6h (peds: Maximum dose is 0.25 mg/kg q4h) PRN anxiety
- Fentanyl: 0.05–0.2 mg IV q1h PRN pain
- Hydromorphone: 0.5–1.0 mg IV q1–2h (peds: 0.015 mg/kg/dose q4–6h) PRN pain
- Lorazepam: 0.5–1.0 mg IV q1–6h (peds: 0.044 mg/kg q4–6h) PRN anxiety
- Morphine sulfate: 0.1 mg/kg IV q1h PRN pain

## FOLLOW-UP

### DISPOSITION
### Admission Criteria
- Open dislocation, presence of multiple trauma, or other, more serious, injuries
- Inability to reduce dislocation or maintain reduction
- Neurovascular compromise

### Discharge Criteria
- Closed injuries
- Adequate reduction
- No neurovascular involvement
- Orthopedic follow-up within 2–3 days

### Issues for Referral
All patients with perilunate dislocations should be referred to a hand surgeon for surgical stabilization and ligament repair.

### FOLLOW-UP RECOMMENDATIONS
- All patients with a perilunate dislocation must follow-up with a hand surgeon for surgical stabilization and ligament repair.
- Follow-up should be within 2–3 days.

## PEARLS AND PITFALLS

- Up to 25% of these injuries are missed on initial presentation.
- In a patient with wrist pain, swelling, and limited range of motion, it is important to obtain adequate x-rays of the wrist and make sure that the lunate and capitate are located in their fossa on the lateral wrist x-ray.
- Late presentation of these injuries leads to a very poor outcome and often requires a salvage operation.
- Even with appropriate treatment, there is a high incidence of post-traumatic arthritis

## ADDITIONAL READING

- Budoff JE. Treatment of acute lunate and perilunate dislocations. *J Hand Surg*, 2008;33A:1424–1432.
- Escarza R, Chin HW. Wrist injuries. In: Hart RG, Uehara DT, Wagner MJ, eds. *Emergency and primary care of the hand*. Dallas, TX: American College of Emergency Physicians; 2001:139–160.
- Forli A, Courvoisier A, Wimsey S, et al. Perilunate dislocations and transscaphoid perilunate fracture-dislocations: A retrospective study with minimum ten-year follow-up. *J Hand Surg*. 2010;35A:62–68.
- Grabow RJ, Catalano L 3rd. Carpal dislocations. *Hand Clin*. 2006;22:485–500; abstract vi–vii.
- Melsom DS, Leslie IJ. Carpal dislocations. *Curr Orthoped*. 2007;21:288–297.

### See Also (Topic, Algorithm, Electronic Media Element)
- Carpal Fractures
- Lunate Dislocation
- Scaphoid Fracture

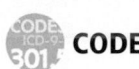 CODES

### ICD9
833.09 Closed dislocation of other part of wrist

# PERIODONTAL ABSCESS

*John Sullivan*

## BASICS

### DESCRIPTION
- Collection of pus in supporting structures of teeth:
  - Periodontal ligament
  - Alveolar bone
- Periodontal pockets result from progression of periodontal disease and resultant bone loss:
  - Food and debris accumulate in periodontal pockets.
  - Coronal epithelial tissues can reattach to tooth while bacteria and food debris remain trapped in pocket, impairing drainage.
  - Food and debris become secondarily infected in setting of impaired drainage.
- Complications:
  - Osteomyelitis
  - Dentocutaneous fistula
  - Cavernous sinus thrombosis
  - Ludwig angina
  - Maxillary sinusitis
  - Mediastinitis
  - Tooth loss
  - Sepsis

### Pediatric Considerations
- Periodontal abscess is rare in children.
- Periapical abscess is more common:
  - Originates in pulp
  - Associated with caries

### ETIOLOGY
- Anaerobic gram-negative rods
- Peptostreptococci
- Usually polymicrobial

## DIAGNOSIS

### SIGNS AND SYMPTOMS
Periodontal abscess is a clinical diagnosis.

### History
- Dental pain
- Malaise
- Fever

### Physical Exam
- Focal swelling or fluctuance of gums and or face
- Tenderness to palpation
- Increased tooth mobility
- Parulis:
  - Pimple-like lesion on gingiva, representing terminal aspect of a sinus tract
  - May be seen in chronic abscess
- Expression of pus from sinus tract
- Heat sensitivity
- Lymphadenopathy
- Trismus is generally absent, unless infection has spread to muscles of mastication.

### ESSENTIAL WORKUP
This is a clinical diagnosis:
- Imaging and lab data are not essential for diagnosis.

### DIAGNOSTIC TESTS & INTERPRETATION
#### Lab
Anaerobic culture of pus:
- Complicated abscess
- Immunocompromised patients

#### Imaging
- Panoramic, periapical, or occlusal radiographs
- Bedside US may also aid in confirming diagnosis.
- CT may help visualize extension of abscess into adjacent structures.
- Imaging can confirm and help define extent of abscess but is not essential to make diagnosis.

#### Diagnostic Procedures/Surgery
Electric pulp testing:
- Performed by dental consultant to verify viability of tooth
- Performed during follow-up visit with dentist

### DIFFERENTIAL DIAGNOSIS
- Periapical abscess
- Aphthous ulcers
- Oral herpes
- Salivary gland tumors
- Mumps
- Blocked salivary gland due to siladenitis or dehydration
- Localized adenopathy due to oral infections
- Facial cellulitis
- Maxillary sinusitis
- Acute otitis media
- Peritonsillar abscess
- Pediatric consideration: Periapical abscess
- For asymptomatic parulis:
  - Fibroma
  - Pyogenic or peripheral ossifying granuloma
  - Kaposi sarcoma

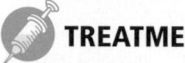

## TREATMENT

### PRE-HOSPITAL
Rarely associated with airway emergencies, but if any signs of airway compromise are present:
- Intubation equipment at bedside
- Transport in sitting position
- Supplemental oxygen
- Suction secretions as needed

### INITIAL STABILIZATION/THERAPY
- Assess for airway patency.
- Establish definitive airway via endotracheal intubation or cricothyrotomy/tracheostomy in presence of:
  - Respiratory distress
  - Inability to handle secretions
  - Oropharyngeal tissue swelling that impairs or threatens airway

### ED TREATMENT/PROCEDURES
- Analgesia with NSAIDs or opiates may be required.
- Incision and drainage:
  - Anesthetize gingiva superficially with 2% lidocaine with 1:100,000 epinephrine until blanching occurs.
  - Make a 1-cm stab incision using a scalpel blade toward alveolar bone.
  - Blunt dissection using mosquito hemostat
  - Irrigate cavity with saline.
  - If abscess cavity sufficiently large, place 1/4–in. iodoform gauze drain or fenestrated Penrose drain for 24–48 hr:
    - To prevent its aspiration, secure gauze or drain with silk suture.

- Antibiotics:
  - Indicated if abscess extensive or if systemic signs present
  - Penicillin considered first-line empiric therapy
  - Erythromycin, azithromycin, clindamycin for penicillin-allergic patients
  - Clindamycin for penicillin-allergic patients or patients not responding to penicillin
  - Ampicillin/sulbactam for severe infections
- Warm salt water rinses hourly while awake for 24–48 hr

## MEDICATION

### First Line

- Penicillin VK: 250–500 mg PO q6h (peds: 25–50 mg/kg/d PO div. q6h)
- Azithromycin: 500 mg (peds: 10 mg/kg) PO 1st day, then 250 mg (peds: 5 mg/kg) PO per day × 4 days (for penicillin-allergic patients)
- Clindamycin: 150–450 mg PO q6h (peds: 10–25 mg/kg/d div. PO q6h)
- Clindamycin: 300–900 mg IV q8h (peds: 15–25 mg/kg/d div. q6–8h IV q8h)
- Erythromycin: 250–500 mg PO q6–8h (peds: 30–50 mg/d div. q6–8h PO q6–8h)

### Second Line

- Ampicillin/sulbactam IV: 1.5–3.0 g IV q6h (peds >1 yr, <40 kg: 300 mg/kg/d IV div. q6h)
- Amoxicillin/clavulanate: 875 mg PO q12h (peds: 25–45 mg/kg/d div. q12h) (oral conversion)
- Penicillin G potassium aqueous: 4 million units IM/IV q4h (peds: 100,000–400,000 units/kg/d div q4–6h IM/IV q4h)

 FOLLOW-UP

## DISPOSITION

### Admission Criteria

- Severe infection or complication requiring parenteral antibiotics
- Necrosis or cellulitis involving areas with potential airway compromise
- Cavernous sinus thrombosis
- Osteomyelitis
- Outpatient therapy failure

- Immunocompromised patients:
  - Neutropenia
  - Uncontrolled diabetes
  - Advanced HIV
  - Cancer patients undergoing chemotherapy
- Ludwig angina
- Systemic involvement with significant dehydration
- Patients unable to handle secretions
- Patients unable to manage infection at home because of physical or mental disability or psychosocial factors

### Discharge Criteria

- Uncomplicated cases
- Dental follow-up available in 24–48 hr

### Issues for Referral

Dental follow-up useful for:

- Viability of affected tooth
- Dental extraction
- Root canal therapy
- Removal of Penrose drain or wic

## FOLLOW-UP RECOMMENDATIONS

Dental follow-up in 24–48 hr:

- Lacking dental follow-up, patients should have alternative follow-up in 24–48 hr with provider familiar with disease process (oral surgeon, ED, urgent care, primary care).

## PEARLS AND PITFALLS

Maxillary sinusitis may be incorrectly diagnosed without adequate oral examination:

- Dental follow-up is essential for short-term resolution of symptoms and long-term tooth viability and oral hygiene issues.

## ADDITIONAL READING

- Caruso PA, Watkins LM, Suwansaard P, et al. Odontogenic orbital inflammation: Clinical and CT findings: Initial observations. *Radiology*. 2006;239: 187–194.
- Marx JA, Hockberger RS, Walls RM, et al. *Rosen's Emergency Medicine: Concepts and Clinical Practice*, 7th ed. St. Louis, MO: Mosby; 2009.
- Roberts J, Hedges J, eds. *Clinical Procedures in Emergency Medicine*, 5th ed. Philadelphia: WB Saunders; 2009.
- Resnick CM, Novelline RA. Cemento-osseous dysplasia, a radiological mimic of periapical dental abscess. *Emerg Radiol*. 2008;15:367–374.
- Robertson D, Smith AJ. The microbiology of the acute dental abscess. *J Med Microbiol*. 2009; 58(pt 2):155–162.
- Schneider K. Dental abscess. *eMedicine*. Updated July 28, 2009.

**See Also (Topic, Algorithm, Electronic Media Element)**

Toothache

 CODES

ICD9

- 522.5 Periapical abscess without sinus
- 523.31 Aggressive periodontitis, localized

# PERIORBITAL AND ORBITAL CELLULITIS

*Shari Schabowski*

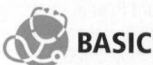 **BASICS**

## DESCRIPTION

### Periorbital Cellulitis
- An inflammatory, typically infectious condition affecting the eyelid(s)
- It is anatomically distinguished by its location, isolated to the tissues anterior to the orbital septum:
  - Orbital septum is the connective tissue extension of the orbital periosteum that is reflected into the upper and lower eyelids.
  - Extension to the deep tissues is rare because the septum represents a nearly impenetrable barrier.
- Most commonly presents as a complication of upper respiratory tract infection (URTI) and sinusitis:
  - Swelling is caused by inflammatory edema from vascular and lymphatic congestion.
- Commonly occurs as a complication of a localized inflammation/infection in the eyelid or adjacent structures:
  - Blepharitis
  - Hordeolum
  - Dacryocystitis
  - Surrounding skin disruptions:
    - Insect bites
    - Minor trauma
    - Impetigo or other dermatologic disorders

### Orbital Cellulitis
- Inflammatory process in the structures deep to the orbital septum
- Occurs secondary to extension from an adjacent structure:
  - Sinusitis:
    - Most commonly ethmoid
  - Dental abscess
  - Retained foreign body in the orbit
  - Puncture wounds
  - Orbital fracture
  - Postoperative infection
  - Hematogenous spread from a remote source
  - Rare cause—extension of periorbital cellulitis

## ETIOLOGY

### Periorbital Cellulitis
- *Streptococcus pneumoniae*
- *Staphylococcus aureus*
- *Streptococcus pyogenes*
- *Moraxella catarrhalis*
- *Haemophilus influenzae*:
  - Previously acommon cause of the most severe form of this disease but rarely seen in the post–Hib vaccine era
- May extend from conjunctivitis or dacryoadenitis:
  - *Gonococcus*
- Consider nonbacterial cause.

### Orbital Cellulitis
- Currently streptococcal and staphylococcal infections are the most common causes:
  - *S. pneumoniae, Streptococcus viridans, S. pyogenes*
  - *S. aureus*:
  - Anaerobes, *Bacteroides*, and gram-negatives may also be seen.
- All forms of orbital cellulitis carry a risk of severe morbidity and possible mortality and are therefore a true emergency:
  - Permanent visual loss may occur, and extension to subperiosteal abscess formation, cavernous sinus thrombosis, and CNS infections may be life threatening.
- Fungal infection are an uncommon but even more lethal form particularly in the immunocompromised:
  - Named cerebrorhino-orbital phycomycosis (CROP)
  - Rapidly fatal in 75% of cases:
    - 80% of cases occur in diabetic patients with a recent episode of diabetic ketoacidosis (DKA).
    - Predisposing factor: Severe metabolic acidosis
    - Toxic appearance in any age group
    - More common in immunocompromised patients
    - Begins in the paranasal sinuses and proliferates in the blood vessels causing thrombosis and necrosis
    - Bloody nasal discharge is common.
    - Frequently presents with evidence of necrosis of the palate and/or nasal mucosa

### Pediatric Considerations
Historically *H. influenzae* is an important and severe form of bacteremic periorbital cellulitis in young children:
- Toxic appearance
- Temperature >39°C
- Erythematous and violaceous swollen eyelids
- Preceded by upper respiratory infection
- Known to progress to orbital cellulitis and meningitis
- Dramatic decrease in incidence by 80% since Hib vaccine:
  - Incidence decreases significantly after two immunizations.

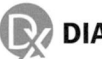 **DIAGNOSIS**

## SIGNS AND SYMPTOMS

### Periorbital Cellulitis/Orbital Cellulitis
- Both present with a unilateral, red, swollen eye:
  - Lid swelling may be profound in both.
- Differences include:
  - Source of inciting infection
  - Toxicity, intraocular manifestations, systemic and neurologic symptoms

### Orbital Cellutis
#### History
- Preceded by sinusitis (most often ethmoid), dental infection, trauma, puncture wound, or recent operation
- Complaint of swelling and redness surrounding eye in addition to eye pain, visual impairment, restricted eye movements
- Headache, meningismus, and symptoms of systemic illness may occur.
- Identify complicating medical problems:
  - Immunocompromise
  - Diabetes

#### Physical Exam
- Toxic appearance:
  - Fever >39°C
- Restricted, painful extraocular movements
- Afferent pupillary defect
- Conjunctival injection
- Chemosis
- Decreased visual acuity
- Diplopia:
  - Proptosis
  - Meningismus and neurologic findings may be seen.

### Periorbital Cellulitis
#### History
- Preceded by local skin injury, insect bite, URTI, or superficial ocular infection
- Ask about Hib vaccination status in young children
- Low-grade fever
- Subacute presentation

#### Physical Exam
- Red, swollen eyelid
- Often single lid involvement but can involve both
- Conjunctival injection common
- Low-grade fever common:
  - Rare systemic symptoms
- Normal visual acuity:
  - No symptoms of deep ocular involvement

## ESSENTIAL WORKUP
- Complete eye exam:
  - External exam
  - Visual acuity
  - Extraocular movements
  - Pupillary exam
  - Fundoscopic exam
- Complete neurologic exam

## DIAGNOSTIC TESTS & INTERPRETATION
### Lab
Supportive but not diagnostic:
- CBC:
  - WBC <15,000 for periorbital cellulitis
  - WBC >15,000 may suggest bacteremic periorbital cellulitis.
- Blood culture
- Gram stain and culture of tissue aspirate or swab of draining purulent material:
  - Chocolate agar plate should be used when gonorrhea suspected.

### Imaging
CT scan orbits:
- Indicated if:
  - Suspect orbital cellulitis or traumatic penetration of the orbital septum
  - Failure to respond to parenteral antimicrobial therapy
- Demonstrates extent of:
  - Orbital cellulitis
  - Sinusitis
  - Orbital emphysema
  - Subperiosteal abscess
  - Presence of foreign body

### Diagnostic Procedures/Surgery
Lumbar puncture:
- Rule out CNS involvement.
- Consider in patients with:
  - Signs or symptoms of meningismus
  - Toxic appearance
  - Patients at risk of *H. influenzae* type B: <4 yr and non-Hib vaccinated

## DIFFERENTIAL DIAGNOSIS
- Allergic reaction
- Dacryoadenitis
- Dacryocystitis
- Graves disease
- Hordeolum
- Inflammatory orbital pseudotumor
- Insect bite
- Orbital rhabdosarcoma
- Periorbital ecchymosis
- Periorbital edema
- Retrobulbar hemorrhage

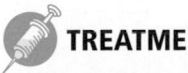

# TREATMENT

## INITIAL STABILIZATION/THERAPY
IV fluids for vomiting, dehydration, toxic appearance, clinical need for parenteral antibiotics

## ED TREATMENT/PROCEDURES
- Antipyretics
- Pain medication as needed
- Antibiotics

### Periorbital Cellulitis
- Typically responds to oral antibiotics unless appears bacteremic or toxic:
  - Augmentin: 500 mg (peds: 45 mg/kg/24 hr) PO t.i.d.
  - Cephalexin: 500 mg (peds: 100 mg/kg/24 hr) PO q.i.d.
  - Clindamycin: 300 mg (peds: 20 mg/kg/24 hr) PO q.i.d.
  - Dicloxacillin: 500 mg (peds: 100 mg/kg/24 hr) PO q.i.d.
- Parenteral antibiotics:
  - Cefotaxime: 1–2 g (peds: 150 mg/kg/24 hr) IV q6–8h
  - Clindamycin: 600 mg (peds: 40 mg/kg/24 hr) IV q6h

### Orbital Cellulitis
- Early administration of parenteral antibiotics
- Ophthalmologic consultation
- If sinusitis is the source, consider ear, nose, and throat consultation.
- Emergent surgical intervention may be necessary:
  - If *Bacteroides* is suspected organism:
    - Surgical debridement
    - Vancomycin
    - Tetanus toxoid when appropriate
- If proptosis leaves the cornea exposed:
  - Lubricating drops (Lacri-Lube: 2 drops q2–4h PRN)
- If you suspect CROP:
  - Amphotericin B IV at highest tolerated dose
  - Topical amphotericin B (1 mg/mL) irrigation or nasal packing
  - Local debridement

### First Line
- Ceftriaxone: 1–2 g (peds: 100 mg/kg/24 hr) IV q12–24h
- Erythromycin ophthalmologic ointment: Applied q4h to lower cul-de-sac

### Second Line
Depending on suspected organism:
- Gentamicin: 5 mg/kg/24 hr IV
- Metronidazole: 15 mg/kg IV load, then 7.5 mg/kg q6h
- Nafcillin: 1–2 g (peds: 100 mg/kg/24 hr) IV q4h
- Vancomycin: 1 g (peds: 40 mg/kg/24 hr) q12h

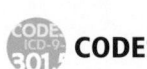

# FOLLOW-UP

## DISPOSITION
### Periorbital Cellulitis
Discharge with oral antibiotics and prompt follow-up unless:
- Evidence of systemic toxicity
- Progression of infection on oral antibiotics
- Unable to arrange follow up within 24–48 hr
- High-risk *H. influenzae* type B
- Unable to tolerate PO antibiotics

### Orbital Cellulitis
Admit for:
- IV antibiotics
- Observation for progression
- Specialist consultation
- Surgical incision and drainage

## PEARLS AND PITFALLS
- Any time a patient presents with a red swollen eye consider the possibility of orbital cellulitis.
- Take a careful history for:
  - Recent sinusitis, particularly ethmoid sinusitis
  - Recent puncture or history of trauma or surgical procedure
  - Recent dental infection, particularly a canine space abscess
  - History of immunocompromise or recent or current episode of DKA
  - Determine Hib vaccination status in children
- Pay careful attention to exclude:
  - Systemic toxicity
  - Eye pain or visual impairment
  - Restriction of eye movements
  - Signs and symptoms of neurologic involvement

## ADDITIONAL READING
- Chang CH, Lai YH, Wang HZ, et al. Antibiotic treatment of orbital cellulitis: An analysis of pathogenic bacteria and bacterial susceptibility. *J Ocul Pharmacol Ther.* 2000;16(1):75–79.
- Danter EM, Jolly BT. Pediatric ophthalmology. *Emerg Med Clin North Am.* 1995;13(3):669–680.
- Ghosh C. Periorbital and orbital cellulitis after *H. influenzae* B vaccination. *Ophthalmology.* 2001; 108:1514–1515.
- Givner L. Periorbital versus orbital cellulitis. *Pediatr Infect Dis J.* 2002;21(12):1157–1158.
- Jain A, Rubin PA. Orbital cellulitis in children. *Int Ophthalmol Clin.* 2001;41(4):71–86.
- Wald E. Periorbital and orbital infections. *Infect Dis Clin North Am.* 2007;21(2):392–408.

### See Also (Topic, Algorithm, Electronic Media Element)
- Dacryoadenitis
- Dacryocystitis
- Hyperthyroidism
- Hordeolum and Chalazion
- Pseudotumor Cerebri

# CODES

### ICD9
- 373.13 Abscess of eyelid
- 376.01 Orbital cellulitis

# PERIPHERAL NEUROPATHY

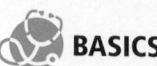

*Minh V. Le*

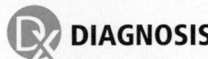

## BASICS

### DESCRIPTION
Peripheral neuropathy is a general term for peripheral nerve disorders of any cause.

### ETIOLOGY
Variable, depending on presentation of symptoms; refer to differential diagnosis

## DIAGNOSIS

### SIGNS AND SYMPTOMS
- Sensory nerve dysfunction:
  - Numbness
  - Localized tingling
  - Paresthesias
  - Dysesthesias
  - Vibration and position sensations are decreased with large-fiber neuropathy.
  - Pain and temperature sensation are decreased with small-fiber neuropathy.
  - Deep tendon reflexes are decreased secondary to decrease sensation of afferent limb.
- Motor nerve dysfunction:
  - Weakness:
    - Distal > proximal
    - Occasionally fasciculations
  - Muscle atrophy, diminished tone with long-standing motor nerve involvement
  - Loss of reflexes secondary to slowing of conduction along motor nerve efferent limb

- Autonomic nerve dysfunction:
  - Orthostasis
  - Constipation
  - Urinary retention
  - Impotence

### History
- Duration of symptoms
- Symmetric or asymmetric symptoms
- Distal or proximal symptoms
- Motor, sensory, or mixed

### Physical Exam
- Thorough head-to-toe physical exam
- Focus on neurologic exam:
  - Motor weakness
  - Sensory loss typically in stocking-glove distribution

### ALERT
Absence of reflexes early in course could represent demyelinating neuropathy such as Guillain-Barré syndrome (acute inflammatory demyelinating syndrome [AIDP]).

### ESSENTIAL WORKUP
- Studies based on acuteness, severity of neuropathy, and most likely diagnosis
- Neurologic consult early if acute and severe symptoms

## DIAGNOSTIC TESTS & INTERPRETATION

### Lab
- Basic metabolic panel
- CBC
- Liver function tests
- Urinalysis
- Thyrotropin-stimulating hormone
- HIV or vitamin $B_{12}$ based on individual presentations
- Electrocardiogram

### Imaging
- CXR if indicated
- Head CT if indicated

### Diagnostic Procedures/Surgery
- Electromyographic studies, nerve conduction studies, and nerve biopsy per neurologic consult on admission or outpatient follow-up
- Lumbar puncture as appropriate for AIDP

### DIFFERENTIAL DIAGNOSIS
- Focal:
  - Entrapment
  - Common sites of compression:
    - Carpal, ulnar tunnel
    - Tarsal tunnel
    - Peroneal
    - Myxedema
    - Rheumatoid arthritis
    - Amyloidosis
    - Acromegaly
  - Compressive neuropathies
  - Trauma
  - Ischemic lesions
  - Diabetes mellitus (DM), vasculitis
  - Leprosy
  - Sarcoidosis
  - Neoplastic infiltration or compression

- Multifocal (mononeuropathy multiplex):
  - DM
  - Vasculitis:
    - Polyarteritis nodosa
    - Systemic lupus erythematosus
    - Sjögren syndrome
  - Sarcoidosis
  - Leprosy
  - Malignancy related
  - HIV/AIDS
  - Hereditary predisposition to pressure palsies
- Symmetric:
  - Endocrine:
    - Most common is DM
    - Hypothyroidism
  - Medications:
    - Isoniazid
    - Lithium
    - Metronidazole
    - Phenytoin
    - Cimetidine
    - Hydralazine
    - Amitriptyline
    - Amiodarone
  - Nutritional diseases:
    - Alcoholism
    - $B_{12}$/folate deficiency
    - Thiamine
  - Critical illness neuropathy
  - Hypophosphatemia
  - Guillain-Barré syndrome (AIDP)
  - Toxic neuropathy:
    - Carbon monoxide
    - Acrylamide
    - Carbon disulfide
    - Ethylene oxide
    - Organophosphate esters
    - Lead
- Myelopathy mimicking peripheral neuropathy
- Back pain
- Saddle anesthesia
- Lower extremity weakness

# TREATMENT

## PRE-HOSPITAL
- Pain control as needed
- Airway protection as indicated

## INITIAL STABILIZATION/THERAPY
Establish airway protection with severe acute peripheral neuropathy, such as Guillain-Barré syndrome.

## ED TREATMENT/PROCEDURES
Variable depending on acuity of symptoms

## MEDICATION
- Variable depending on underlying diagnosis
- Opioid analgesics
- Gabapentin 300 mg PO daily then b.i.d. day 2, then t.i.d. on day 3 up to 1,800 mg/d div. t.i.d.
- Carbamazepine 100 mg PO b.i.d. for trigeminal neuralgia
- IV immunoglobulin for Guillain-Barré syndrome (AIDP)

# FOLLOW-UP

## DISPOSITION
### Admission Criteria
- Respiratory distress or acute gait disturbance
- Intractable pain

### Discharge Criteria
Stable respiratory and gait status with outpatient follow-up

### Issues for Referral
Neurology—based on duration, severity of presentation

## FOLLOW-UP RECOMMENDATIONS
Primary care or neurology depending on etiology and severity of symptoms

# PEARLS AND PITFALLS
Failure to diagnose Guillain-Barré syndrome (AIDP)

# ADDITIONAL READING
- Marx JA, Hockberger RS, Walls RM, et al. *Rosen's Emergency Medicine: Concepts and Clinical Practice*, 7th ed. St. Louis, MO: Mosby; 2009.
- Pascuzzi RM. Peripheral neuropathy. *Med Clin North Am.* 2009;93:317–342.
- Gilron I, Watson CP, Cahill CM, et al. Neuropathic pain: A practical guide for the clinician. *CMAJ.* 2006;175:265–275.

# CODES

## ICD9
356.9 Unspecified idiopathic peripheral neuropathy

# PERIPHERAL VASCULAR DISEASE

*Sally Santen*

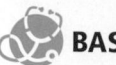 **BASICS**

## DESCRIPTION

- Obstruction of ≥1 of the peripheral arteries secondary to embolism or thrombus
- Caused by atherosclerosis
- Patients with PAD may also have coronary artery and cerebrovascular disease.
- Chronic arterial insufficiency (CAI):
  - Progressive obstructing atherosclerotic disease causing subacute ischemia and pain (claudication)
  - 10% develop critical leg ischemia.
  - Risks factors (selected):
    ○ Age
    ○ Smoking
    ○ Diabetes
    ○ Hyperlipidemia
    ○ HTN
  - Associated with morbidity and mortality from other forms of atherosclerosis (coronary artery disease, stroke)
  - Complications:
    ○ Aneurysm
    ○ Thrombosis
    ○ Ulceration
    ○ Limb loss
- Acute arterial insufficiency (AAI):
  - Caused by arterial thrombosis (50%) or embolism
  - Causes acute limb ischemia with signs and symptoms of the 6 Ps (below)
- Atheroembolism:
  - Caused by rupture or partial disruption of an atherosclerotic plaque (aorta, femoral, iliac)
  - Gives rise to cholesterol emboli that shower and obstruct arteriolar networks
  - May be precipitated by invasive arterial procedures such as cardiac catheterization

## ETIOLOGY

- Obstruction by atherosclerotic plaques (CAI)
- Arterial thrombosis
- Arterial emboli:
  - Cardiac emboli from dysrhythmias, valvular heart disease, or cardiomyopathy (80%)
  - Aneurysms
  - Infection
  - Tumor
  - Vasculitis or foreign body
  - Thrombosis of plaques from preexisting CAI
- Atheroembolism

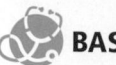 **DIAGNOSIS**

## SIGNS AND SYMPTOMS
### History
- CAI:
  - Claudication:
    ○ Aching pain in the calves (femoropopliteal occlusion) or buttocks and thighs (aortoiliac region)
    ○ Occurs with activity and slowly relieved by rest
    ○ Classic claudication presents in about 1/2 of patients with PVD
  - Severe disease presents with limb pain at rest:
    ○ Usually starting in the foot
    ○ Rapidly progressive claudication or ulceration
- AAI:
  - Extremity pain:
    ○ Sudden onset
    ○ Gradual increase in severity
    ○ Starts distally and moves proximally over time
    ○ Decrease in intensity once ischemic sensory loss occurs
- Atheroembolism:
  - Complaint of cold and painful fingers or toes
  - Small atherosclerotic emboli may affect both extremities.
  - Usually related to recent arteriography, vascular or cardiac surgery
  - Multiorgan involvement is common (renal, mesentery, skin, other)

### Physical Exam

**ALERT**

Sudden onset of pain and pallor in extremity is limb- and life-threatening.

- CAI:
  - Absent or decreased peripheral pulses
  - Delayed capillary refill with cool skin
  - Increased venous filling time
  - Bruits
  - Pallor and dependent rubor of the leg
  - Muscle and skin atrophy
  - Thickened nails and loss of dorsal hair
  - Ulcerations (especially toes or heels) or gangrene with severe disease
- AAI:
  - 6 Ps:
    ○ Pain (1st symptom)
    ○ Pallor
    ○ Pulselessness
    ○ Poikilothermic
    ○ Paresthesias (late finding)
    ○ Paralysis (late finding)
  - Identification of a source of a possible embolic process is crucial (atrial fibrillation, cardiomegaly).
- Atheroembolism:
  - Ischemic and painful digits
  - "Blue toe syndrome"
  - Livedo reticularis

## ESSENTIAL WORKUP
- CAI:
  - Ankle-brachial index (ankle systolic blood pressure [BP] divided by arm systolic BP)
  - Bedside test to determine whether CAI is present (see NEJM video reference)
  - Ratio of <0.9 is abnormal and <0.4 indicates severe disease.
  - Calcific arteries (diabetes) can have false negative ABI or elevated ABI (>1.3).
- AAI:
  - Physical diagnosis using the 6 Ps
  - Those with acute-on-chronic arterial insufficiency tolerate limb ischemia better than those without CAI, due to well-developed collateral circulation.
- Atheroembolism:
  - Clinical diagnosis: Affected areas painful, tender, and may be either dusky or necrotic
  - Workup may investigate source of emboli with duplex US, CT angiogram, cardiac EKG.

## DIAGNOSTIC TESTS & INTERPRETATION
### Lab
- CBC and platelets
- Electrolytes, BUN, creatinine, glucose
- Coagulation studies
- Creatine phosphokinase to evaluate for ischemia.
- Special tests for suspected etiologies:
  - Hold blood for hypercoagulable studies
  - Sedimentation rate, CRP for vasculitis
  - Blood cultures for endocarditis

### Imaging
- Doppler US:
  - Visualizes both venous and arterial systems
  - Identifies level of arterial occlusion, as well as thrombosis and aneurysm
  - Sensitivity and specificity >80–90% for occlusion of vessels proximal to the popliteal vessels
- Plethysmography/segmental pressure measurements:
  - Uses measurements of the volume and character of blood flow to detect areas of CAI
  - Less widely available than US, therefore requires an experienced technician
  - Approximates US in sensitivity and specificity
- Angiography:
  - Determines details about the anatomy, including the level of occlusion, stenosis, and collateral flow
  - Useful where the diagnosis of AAI is uncertain or before emergent bypass grafting
  - Advantage is intervention (atherectomy, angioplasty, or intraluminal thrombolytics) can be done at the time of diagnosis.

- CT angiogram:
  - CT is useful for diagnosis of occlusive aortic disease or dissection.
  - Rapidly available and reliable
  - Many centers have moved to CT angiogram as the 1st-line diagnostic tool. The decision for operative or angiographic intervention is based on the CT angiogram.
  - Requires contrast, therefore may not be 1st line for patients with renal insufficiency
- MRI:
  - Sensitive for evaluation of CAI and dissection
  - Disadvantages are that MRI is time-consuming and expensive.

## DIFFERENTIAL DIAGNOSIS

- Acute thrombosis or emboli
- Arterial dissection
- Deep venous thrombosis
- Venous insufficiency
- Compartment syndrome
- Buerger disease
- Spinal stenosis
- Neuropathy
- Bursitis
- Arthritis
- Reflex sympathetic dystrophy

 TREATMENT

### PRE-HOSPITAL

- Maintain hemodynamic stability with fluids.
- Apply cardiac monitor.
- Place the ischemic limb at rest and in a dependent position.
- Provide oxygen if low oxygen saturation or pulmonary symptoms.

### INITIAL STABILIZATION/THERAPY

- IV fluid bolus for hypotension
- EKG, monitor, pulse oximetry
- Supplemental oxygen

### ED TREATMENT/PROCEDURES

- CAI:
  - Antiplatelet therapy with 75 or 325 mg of aspirin or clopidogrel (75 mg/d) may be used as 1st-line treatment. Dual therapy has not been shown to improve outcomes, although may be indicated in other forms of atherosclerosis.
  - Other approved drugs include: Cilostazol 100 mg b.i.d., dipyridamole 200 mg b.i.d., pentoxifylline 400 mg t.i.d.
  - Revascularization depending on the severity and location of obstruction:
    ○ Balloon angioplasty
    ○ Atherectomy
    ○ Bypass grafting
  - Risk-factor modification:
    ○ Tobacco cessation
    ○ Aggressive management of hyperlipidemia, HTN, diabetes
    ○ Exercise therapy

- AAI:
  - Limit further clot propagation with IV heparin.
  - Do not anticoagulate patients suspected of having an aortic dissection or symptomatic aneurysm.
  - Emergent consultation with a vascular surgeon:
    ○ To determine which diagnostic study is best to make the diagnosis
    ○ To begin arrangements for possible operative therapy or other intervention
    ○ Options for operative therapy include thrombectomy, embolectomy, angioplasty, regional arterial thrombolysis, bypass grafting.
    ○ Blood flow to the affected limb must be reestablished within 4–6 hr after onset of ischemic symptoms.
    ○ Interventional radiology may also play a role.
  - Complications of AAI include:
    ○ Compartment syndrome
    ○ Irreversible ischemia requiring amputation
    ○ Rhabdomyolysis, renal failure
    ○ Electrolyte disturbances
- Atheroembolism:
  - Treat conservatively if a limited amount of tissue is involved and renal function is not significantly compromised.
  - No clear therapy for the ischemic digits besides supportive wound care and analgesia
  - Some studies have tried corticosteroids to decrease inflammation, statins to stabilize plaque, aspirin, or dipyridamole
  - Amputation for irreversibly necrotic toes
  - Vascular surgeon referral within 12–24 hr of ED visit
  - Prevent further embolic events by a thorough investigation and correction of the source of atheroemboli.

### MEDICATION

- Aspirin: 81–325 mg/d
- Cilostazol: 100 mg b.i.d.
- Clopidogrel: 75 mg/d
- Heparin: 80 U/kg bolus IV followed by 18 U/h IV
- Pentoxifylline: 400 mg t.i.d.

 FOLLOW-UP

### DISPOSITION

#### Admission Criteria

- All patients with AAI are admitted for evaluation and revascularization.
- CAI: Consider admission for rapidly progressive claudication or ischemic pain at rest:
  - To undergo heparinization and angiography to rule out an acute thrombosis
- Atheroembolism admission indicated with large areas involved, significant pain, infection, or renal compromise

#### Discharge Criteria

- Atheroembolism:
  - If they have small lesions, adequate pain control, no evidence of renal compromise or superinfection, and follow-up within 24 hr
- CAI:
  - No evidence of rapid progression, critical leg ischemia, gangrene, or infection

#### Issues for Referral

- CAI will need urgent referral to vascular surgery.
- Atheroembolism, depending on the origin of the emboli, may need referral to vascular surgery or to cardiology.

### FOLLOW-UP RECOMMENDATIONS

CAI without acute ischemia and atheroembolism with minimal involvement should have close follow-up to evaluate the extent of their disease.

### ADDITIONAL READING

- Grenon SM, Gagnon J, Hsiang Y. Ankle–brachial index for assessment peripheral arterial disease. *N Engl J Med.* 2009;361:e40, summary and video.
- Hirsch AT, Haskal ZJ, Bakal CW, et al. ACC/AHA guidelines for the management of patients with peripheral arterial disease. *J Vasc Interv Radiol.* 2006;17:1383–398.
- Liewaand YP, Bartholome JR. Atheromatous embolization. *Vasc Med.* 2005;10:309–326.
- Momsen AH, Jensen MB, Norager CB, et al. Drug therapy for improving walking distance in intermittent claudication: A systematic review and meta-analysis of robust randomised controlled studies. *Eur J Vasc Endovasc Surg.* 2009;38:463–474.
- Norgren L, Hiat WR, Dormandy JA, et al. Inter-society consensus for the management of peripheral arterial disease (TASC II). *J Vasc Surg.* 2007;45:SA5–S67.
- White C. Intermittent claudication. *N Engl J Med.* 2007;356:1241–1250.

### See Also (Topic, Algorithm, Electronic Media Element)

- Arterial Occlusion
- Venous Insufficiency

 CODES

#### ICD9

443.9 Peripheral vascular disease, unspecified

# PERIRECTAL ABSCESS

*Scott A. Miller*

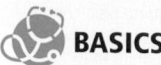 **BASICS**

## DESCRIPTION
Localized infection and accumulation of purulent material adjacent to anus or rectum

## ETIOLOGY
- Predominant theory is anal crypt gland infection, with subsequent spread of infection to adjacent areas separated by muscle and fascia:
  - Perianal:
    - Most common
    - Usually with red bulge near anus
  - Ischiorectal:
    - Large potential space
    - May become very large before diagnosed
    - Can communicate posteriorly with other side forming "horseshoe" abscess
  - Intersphincteric:
    - Contained at primary site of origin between internal and external sphincters
    - May be difficult to diagnose
  - Supralevator:
    - Very deep above levator ani
    - Needs operative debridement under general anesthesia
    - Often systemic symptoms before diagnosis is made
    - Rarely caused by surgery, episiotomies, trauma, or hemorrhoids
- 25–50% develop fistula
- Bacterial cause is typically a mix of stool pathogens:
  - *Escherichia coli*
  - *Bacteroides* sp.
  - *Peptostreptococcus* sp.
  - *Streptococcal* sp.
  - *Staphylococcus* sp., commonly MRSA
- Associated diseases:
  - Diabetes
  - Inflammatory bowel disease
  - Malignancy
  - Immunocompromised host

## DIAGNOSIS

### SIGNS AND SYMPTOMS
- Perianal, pelvic, or rectal pain
- Typical abscess symptoms:
  - Fluctuance, drainage, fever

### History
- Perianal pain:
  - Constant
  - Aggravated by defecation, sitting, coughing, or sneezing
  - Perianal abscesses or ischiorectal abscesses that extend to perineum
- Dull deep pelvic or rectal pain:
  - More likely to have systemic toxicity owing to delayed diagnosis and spread of infection
  - Ischiorectal and supralevator abscesses
- Rectal or perirectal drainage
- Fever/chills
- Constipation
- Urinary retention
- Penile discharge has been described

### Physical Exam
- Perianal swelling, erythema, induration, fluctuance, tenderness:
  - Perianal and large ischiorectal abscesses
- Cellulitis may be present.
- Intra-anal and intrarectal swelling:
  - Intersphincteric and supralevator abscesses
  - May be only clue to abscess
- Pelvic exam:
  - Thickened rectovaginal septum or tenderness
- Hypotension or signs of dehydration if systemic infection present
- Local anesthesia insufficient for thorough rectal exam and determination of extent of abscess on all but small, superficial abscesses (mostly perianal)

### ESSENTIAL WORKUP
- Careful history and physical are paramount in making diagnosis.
- Have high index of suspicion for any constant perirectal pain.

### ALERT
Factors associated with significant morbidity and mortality:
- Delay in diagnosis or treatment:
  - Hemorrhoid most common misdiagnosis
- Inadequate initial exam or treatment
- Associated systemic disease

### DIAGNOSTIC TESTS & INTERPRETATION
No labs or imaging routinely indicated

### Lab
- CBC:
  - Leukocytosis with left shift
- Wound culture:
  - Consider if giving antibiotics, although doesn't often affect management.
- Blood cultures:
  - If concern for bacteremia exists

### Imaging
- CT (with IV contrast, +/– PO contrast)
- MRI (helpful with detecting fistulas)
- US:
  - May be helpful in diagnosis and delineating extent of abscess
- Imaging is important if supralevator or large ischiorectal abscess is considered.

### Diagnostic Procedures/Surgery
- Incision and drainage (I&D) is the definitive management.
- Barium enema or anoscopy/proctoscopy may be helpful to diagnose supralevator or intersphincteric abscess bulging into rectum.

## DIFFERENTIAL DIAGNOSIS
- Anal fissure
- Sentinel pile in the posterior midline or anterior midline
- Thrombosed or inflamed hemorrhoids
- Anal ulcer (ie, HIV)
- Proctitis (ie, gonococcal)
- Anorectal carcinoma

### Pediatric Considerations
Rectal duplication in children should be considered in differential.

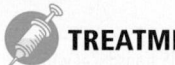

# TREATMENT

## INITIAL STABILIZATION/THERAPY
- IV fluids if septic or dehydrated
- Pain medication

## ED TREATMENT/PROCEDURES
- Antibiotics alone without drainage are contraindicated:
  - Infection may worsen, leading to extensive soft tissue destruction, sepsis, or death.
  - Administer prior to surgery with valvular heart disease.
- Incision and drainage (I&D) for all abscesses
- Bedside drainage under local anesthetic:
  - Differentiation of superficial perianal abscess and deeper abscess is imperative:
    ○ Be sure superficial abscess is not actually the "tip" of a much deeper abscess.
  - Small visible abscess, nontoxic patient (mostly perianal and small superficial ischiorectal abscesses)
  - May attempt needle aspiration initially to localize, but I&D must be done.
  - Radial incision close to anal verge:
    ○ Facilitates surgical excision of potential subsequent fistula
  - Elliptical or cruciate incision:
    ○ Ensure ongoing adequate drainage.
  - Explore cavity, breaking any loculations.
  - Irrigate liberally.
  - Pack with loosely iodoform gauze to ensure continued drainage:
    ○ Remove/replace at 48-hr intervals.
- Follow-up with surgeon in 24–48 hr (evaluate for fistula).

- Operative exam and debridement under general anesthesia:
  - If local anesthesia is inadequate, or there is any question about the extent of the abscess
  - All supralevator and intersphincteric abscesses
  - Ischiorectal abscesses that are large or have extensive necrosis
  - Unable to drain under local anesthetic
  - Immunosuppressed (ie, HIV, diabetics, transplant recipients, patients on chemotherapy)
- Antibiotic administration:
  - Rarely necessary:
    ○ Extensive cellulitis
    ○ Immunosuppression
    ○ Valvular heart disease
    ○ Systemic infection
    ○ Prosthetic device
  - If antibiotics required, often need IV antibiotics and admission
  - PO:
    ○ Amoxicillin clavulanate or fluoroquinolone
    ○ Consider MRSA coverage
  - IV:
    ○ Cefoxitin
    ○ Ampicillin sulbactam
    ○ Combination therapy with ampicillin, gentamicin, and clindamycin or metronidazole
- Postoperative care:
  - Sitz baths t.i.d. 24 hr after I&D
  - High-fiber diet or bulking agent
  - Analgesic

### ALERT
- Large ischiorectal abscesses:
  - Do not I&D if drainage already occurring inside the rectum.
  - I&D of draining abscess may result in high extrasphincteric fistula.
- Beware of inadequately drained abscess:
  - This frequently leads to unnecessary morbidity and mortality.

## MEDICATION
### First Line
- Ampicillin sulbactam: 1.5–3 g IV q6h
- Clindamycin: 600–900 mg IV divided q8h

### Second Line
- Ampicillin: 500 mg IV q6h
- Amoxicillin clavulanate: 875 mg PO q12h or 500 mg PO q8h
- Cefoxitin: 1–2 g IV q6–8h
- Gentamicin: 3–6 mg/kg/d IV divided q8h
- Metronidazole: 7.5 mg/kg IV q6h

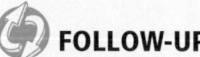

# FOLLOW-UP

## DISPOSITION
### Admission Criteria
- Need for operative drainage
- Systemic toxicity/signs of sepsis

### Discharge Criteria
- Adequate I&D with return of discernible pus
- Ability to ambulate and care for wound

### Issues for Referral
All should be referred to surgeon to evaluate for fistula:
- Fistulas develop in 25–50% of anorectal abscesses.

## FOLLOW-UP RECOMMENDATIONS
Surgeon should be seen within 24–48 hr if discharged.

# PEARLS AND PITFALLS
- Be certain of extent of abscess:
  - Adequate rectal exam is mandatory.
  - Image if any questions.
- Have high index of suspicion for more advanced abscess in immunosuppressed patients and those with comorbidities.

# ADDITIONAL READING
- Janicke DM, Pundt MR. Anorectal disorders. *Emerg Med Clin North Am.* 1996;14:757–788.
- Marcus RH, Stine RJ, Cohen, MA. Perirectal abscess. *Ann Emerg Med.* 1995;25(5):597–603.
- Rizzo JA, et al. Anorectal abscess and fistula-in-ano: Evidence based management. *Surg Clin North Am.* 2010;90(1):45–68.
- The Standards Practice Task Force. Practice parameters for the treatment of perianal abscess and fistula-in-ano (revised). *Dis Colon Rectum.* 2005;48:1337–1342.

## See Also (Topic, Algorithm, Electronic Media Element)
- Abscess
- Anal Fissure
- Hemorrhoid

# CODES

### ICD9
566 Abscess of anal and rectal regions

# PERITONSILLAR ABSCESS

Brad Talley
Maria E. Moreira

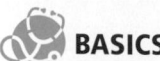

## BASICS

### DESCRIPTION
- Suppurative complication of tonsillitis where infection spreads outside the tonsillar capsule between the palatine tonsil and pharyngeal muscles
- Most common deep infection of the head and neck (incidence of 37/100,000 per year)
- Occurs in all ages, more commonly in young adults (mean age 20–40 yr)
- Occurs most commonly Nov–Dec, April–May
- Complications:
  - Airway compromise (uncommon)
  - Sepsis (uncommon)
  - Recurrence (12–15%)
  - Extension to lateral neck or mediastinum
  - Spontaneous perforation and aspiration pneumonitis
  - Jugular vein thrombosis ("Lemierre disease")
  - Poststreptococcal sequelae (glomerulonephritis, rheumatic fever)
  - Hemorrhage from extension and erosion into carotid sheath
  - Severe dehydration
  - Intracranial extension (meningitis, cavernous sinus thrombosis, cerebral abscess)

### ETIOLOGY
- 2 theories explain the development of peritonsillar abscess (PTA):
  - Direct bacterial invasion into deeper tissues in the patient with acute pharyngitis
  - Acute obstruction and bacterial infection of small salivary glands (Weber glands) in the superior tonsil
- Smoking may be a risk factor.
- Most common pathogens:
  - $\alpha$-Hemolytic *Streptococcus*
  - $\beta$-Hemolytic *Streptococcus*
  - Staphylococcal species
  - Anaerobes (*Prevotella*, *Peptostreptococcus*, *Fusobacterium*)
  - Polymicrobial

## DIAGNOSIS

### SIGNS AND SYMPTOMS
#### History
- Sore throat (100%)
- Fever (26–97%)
- Voice change
- Odynophagia (difficulty swallowing)
- Drooling
- Headache
- Pain radiating to the ear
- Decreased PO intake
- Malaise

#### Physical Exam
- Fever
- Trismus (55–100%)
- "Hot potato" voice
- Tonsils/soft palate erythematous
- Inferior and medial displacement of superior pole of tonsil on affected side
- Uvular deviation away from affected side
- Halitosis
- Cervical lymphadenitis
- Tenderness on ipsilateral side of neck at the angle of the jaw

### ESSENTIAL WORKUP
- Evaluation for deep space infections beyond the peritonsillar abscess, either with additional imaging or physical exam that may require admission and surgery
- Evaluate and ensure airway patency: Look for stridor, tripoding, or inability to handle secretions.
- Definitive management with either needle aspiration or incision and drainage (I&D), followed by a course of antibiotics

### DIAGNOSTIC TESTS & INTERPRETATION
- Usually a clinical diagnosis made by visually examining oropharynx
- May be difficult with severe trismus

### Lab
- Throat culture and monospot (20% incidence of mononucleosis with peritonsillar abscess)
- CBC and culture of the abscess contents may be useful in some cases.
- Basic metabolic panel may be useful in patients with decreased oral intake and clinical signs of dehydration.

### Imaging
- Bedside intraoral US:
  - High-frequency endocavity US transducer with a lubricated latex cover is used.
  - Can aid identification and localization of abscess
  - A cooperative patient can be instructed to place the transducer at the point of maximal tenderness.
- Soft tissue lateral neck:
  - If suspicion for epiglottitis or retropharyngeal abscess exists
- Chest radiograph:
  - With severe respiratory symptoms or draining abscess
- CT scan of neck:
  - If suspicion exists for other deep space infection of the neck, CT may be indicated.
  - CT also may be indicated if unable to obtain a good exam secondary to trismus.
- MRI may be useful to evaluate for complications of deep space infections (internal jugular vein thrombosis or erosion into the carotid sheath).

### Diagnostic Procedures/Surgery
- Needle aspiration is diagnostic and often curative.
- Bedside incision and drainage

### DIFFERENTIAL DIAGNOSIS
- Peritonsillar cellulitis
- Epiglottitis
- Retropharyngeal abscess
- Peripharyngeal abscess
- Tracheitis
- Meningitis
- Retropharyngeal hemorrhage
- Cervical osteomyelitis
- Cervical adenitis
- Epidural abscess
- Infectious mononucleosis
- Internal carotid artery aneurysm
- Lymphoma
- Foreign body
- Other deep space infections of the neck

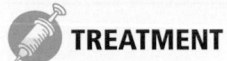 **TREATMENT**

### PRE-HOSPITAL
Rarely associated with airway emergencies, but diagnosis is likely to be uncertain in transport, so suction and intubation equipment should be at the bedside:

- Pulse oximetry, supplemental oxygen
- Cardiac monitor
- IV access

### Pediatric Considerations
- PTA occurs in children (<18 yr) in 24–39% of reported cases.
- Young children may need sedation or general anesthesia if I&D or aspiration of the abscess is attempted.
- Obtain soft-tissue lateral neck radiograph before oral examination in young children with symptoms of upper airway obstruction.

### INITIAL STABILIZATION/THERAPY
- Same as for prehospital
- Airway management may be necessary.
- Equipment for intubation and cricothyroidotomy should be available.

### ED TREATMENT/PROCEDURES
- Antibiotics should be administered.
- IV fluid should be given for dehydration
- Pain control is important.
- A single dose of steroids may improve symptoms.
- Adequate anesthesia prior to aspiration or I&D procedures is important.
- No clear benefit for one drainage technique over another:
  - Needle drainage:
    ○ Successful 87–94%
    ○ Should be performed by person experienced in drainage procedure and adept at advanced airway techniques
    ○ Less painful, less invasive than I&D
    ○ The internal carotid artery lies ~2.5 cm posterolaterally to the tonsil; sheathing the aspiration needle to prevent introduction of the needle to <0.5 cm is prudent.
    ○ The superior pole of the tonsil is the most common place for maximal fluctuance (followed by the middle pole and then the inferior pole)
    ○ Repeat aspiration is necessary in 10%.
  - I&D:
    ○ Successful 90–92%
    ○ An 11- or 15-blade scalpel is used to incise the mucosa for 1 cm from posterior to anterior in the area of maximal fluctuance.
    ○ Avoid >0.5 cm depth.
    ○ Suction should be ready to remove purulent drainage and blood.
    ○ Packing is *not* used.

- Tonsillectomy (indications in children):
  ○ Upper airway obstruction
  ○ Previous episodes of severe recurrent pharyngitis or peritonsillar abscess
  ○ Failure of abscess resolution with other drainage techniques
  ○ Can be performed immediately or after resolution of acute infection

### MEDICATION
- Length of antibiotic treatment should be 14 days (<10-day treatment course may be associated with recurrence).
- Adjunct with steroids can improve symptoms.

### First Line
- Penicillin is the antibiotic of first choice; however incidence of penicillin-resistant organisms is increasing:
  - Penicillin G benzathine: 1 million U IV q6h (peds: 12,500–25,000 U/kg q6h)
  - Penicillin VK 500 mg PO q6h (peds: 25–50 mg/kg/d div. q6–8h)
- For broader coverage, concern for penicillin-resistant organisms or more severe infections requiring admission:
  - Amoxicillin and sulbactam: 1.5–3 g IV q6h
  - Amoxicillin and clavulanate: 500 mg PO q12h (45 mg/kg/d div. q12h)
  - Ceftriaxone: 1–2 g IV (peds: 50 mg/kg)

### Second Line
- To be used for penicillin allergic patients:
  - Clindamycin: 300–450 mg PO q6h (8–16 mg/kg/24 hr)
  - Erythromycin: 250–500 mg/kg/d IV div. q6h (30–50 mg/kg/d PO div. q6–8h)
- Dexamethasone: 10 mg IV/IM/PO single dose (0.6 mg/kg; not to exceed 10 mg) or methylprednisolone 2–3 mg/kg up to 250 mg

 **FOLLOW-UP**

### DISPOSITION

### Admission Criteria
- Airway compromise
- Sepsis
- Altered mental status
- Dehydration and inadequate PO intake
- Extension of infection beyond the peritonsillar abscess (ie, deep space neck infections)

### Discharge Criteria
- Most patients with PTA can be discharged home on oral antibiotics after abscess drainage.
- Must be able to tolerate sufficient oral intake and antibiotics

### Issues for Referral
- Referral to an otolaryngologist or surgeon should be provided.
- Tonsillectomy is recommended 6–8 wk following treatment of the abscess.

### FOLLOW-UP RECOMMENDATIONS
Close follow-up recommended in 24–48 hr:

- Treatment failures and recurrences are relatively common.

## PEARLS AND PITFALLS
- Failure to secure the airway early in a severe infection
- Failure to recognize a more advanced, deep space infection of the neck
- Knowing the anatomy before performing needle aspiration or bedside I&D
- Bedside US is a useful adjunct in differentiating and identifying a peritonsillar abscess vs. peritonsillar cellulitis.

## ADDITIONAL READING

- Khayr W, Taepke J. Management of peritonsillar abscess: Needle aspiration versus incision and drainage versus tonsillectomy. *Am J Ther.* 2005;12(4):344–350.
- Lyon M, Blaivas M. Intraoral ultrasound in the diagnosis and treatment of suspected peritonsillar abscess in the emergency department. *Acad Emerg Med.* 2005;12(1):85–88.
- Marx JA, Hockberger RS, Walls RM, et al. *Rosen's Emergency Medicine: Concepts and Clinical Practice,* 7th ed. St. Louis, MO: Mosby; 2009.
- Millar KR, Johnson DW, Drummond D, et al. Suspected peritonsillar abscess in children. *Pediatric Emerg Care.* 2007;23:431–438.
- Wald ER. Peritonsillar cellulitis and abscess in children and adolescents. *UpToDate for Patients.* September 21, 2009. Available at: http://www.uptodate.com/patients/content/topic.do?topicKey=~9gOQQHXBABXPLQ

### See Also (Topic, Algorithm, Electronic Media Element)
- Epiglottitis
- Retropharyngeal Abscess

 **CODES**

### ICD9
475 Peritonsillar abscess

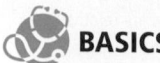

# PERTUSSIS
*Adam Z. Barkin*

## BASICS

### DESCRIPTION
- Acute respiratory tract infection spread by small respiratory droplets
- Bacteria (fimbriae) attach to respiratory epithelial cells and proliferate, producing toxins:
  - Ciliary dysfunction, accumulation of cellular debris, increased mucus production, lymphocytic and granulocytic infiltration
- Bronchiolar congestion, obstruction, and necrosis
- Obstruction of the airway due to mucus plug, leading to hypoxia and hypoventilation
- Increased intrathoracic or intracranial pressure
- Secondary bacterial infection may exacerbate respiratory distress/failure.
- CNS injury caused by encephalitis, increased intracranial pressure, and/or hypoxia
- Uncomplicated cases last 6–10 wk; half of cases last <6 wk.
- Mortality:
  - Mortality greatest in those <1 yr
  - 1.3% for patients <1 mo
  - 0.3% in children 2–11 mo
  - 90% of deaths are secondary to bacterial pneumonia.
- Epidemiology:
  - Incubation period is 6–20 days, usually 7–10 days.
  - Mostly young children; 24% in children <6 mo
  - Increasing incidence in adolescents
  - Adults are the primary reservoir
  - Peak incidence is late summer/fall.
  - Preventable with diphtheria-tetanus-pertussis (Tdap) vaccine

### ETIOLOGY
Bordetella pertussis:
- A fastidious, gram-negative, pleomorphic bacillus

## DIAGNOSIS

### SIGNS AND SYMPTOMS
- Generally 3 recognized phases with progression:
  - Infants may have indistinct stages.
- Catarrhal stage:
  - 1–2 wk duration
  - Rhinorrhea
  - Mild cough
  - Minimal fever
- Paroxysmal stage:
  - 1–6 wk duration
  - Classic "whooping" cough, increasing in severity:
    - Coughing spasm that ends with a sudden inflow of air—the whoop; unremitting paroxysms
  - Cyanosis with respiratory distress/failure
  - Apnea (infants <6 mo)
  - Altered mental status secondary to hypoxia or encephalitis

- Convalescent stage:
  - 2–12 wk duration
  - Waning cough
  - Improving respiratory status
- Atypical presentations:
  - Often atypical in children <6 mo
  - Partially immunized children have less severe disease.
  - Adult manifestations are often only rhinorrhea, sore throat, persistent cough; often in family members.

### History
- Catarrhal phase:
  - Malaise
  - Low-grade fever
  - Rhinorrhea
  - Sore throat
- Paroxysmal phase:
  - "Whooping" cough
  - Posttussive cyanosis
  - Posttussive emesis
- "Whooping" sound during paroxysmal phase
- Catarrhal phase:
  - Persistent cough

### Physical Exam
- Catarrahal phase:
  - Low-grade fever
  - Rhinorrhea
  - Lacrimation
  - Dry cough (late phase)
  - Conjunctival inflammation
- Paroxysmal phase:
  - Paroxysmal whooping cough
- Convalescent phase:
  - Occasional paroxysmal cough

### ESSENTIAL WORKUP
- The ED diagnosis should be made on clinical grounds.
- Attempt to establish a history of a contact.
- Observe the paroxysmal cough with the characteristic whoop.
- Use ancillary studies to further support the clinical diagnosis and exclude complications.

### DIAGNOSTIC TESTS & INTERPRETATION
#### Lab
- Polymerase chain reaction:
  - Varying sensitivity and specificity
  - Expensive
  - Should be used in conjunction with a culture
- Direct immunofluorescence assay of nasopharyngeal mucus:
  - High false-positive rate
- Culture of nasopharynx or cough plate on a Bordet-Gengou medium:
  - Takes 7–12 days
  - High specificity
  - Low sensitivity
- Serology:
  - Useful in later diagnosis

- WBC count:
  - Leukocytosis (20,000–50,000 cells/mm$^3$) with marked lymphocytosis
  - Normalizes during convalescent phase
  - Elevation of WBC and lymphocytosis parallels severity of cough
- Immunofluorescent and enzyme immunoassays to exclude respiratory syncytial virus
- Done on either nasal wash or nasopharyngeal swab (Dacron)

#### Imaging
CXR:
- Most often normal
- Perihilar infiltrates
- Atelectasis
- Occasionally characteristic "shaggy" right heart border
- Secondary bacterial pneumonia

### DIFFERENTIAL DIAGNOSIS
- Infection:
  - Parallel whooping cough syndrome caused by *Bordetella parapertussis, Chlamydia trachomatis, Chlamydia pneumoniae, Bordetella bronchiseptica,* or adenovirus
  - Pneumonia:
    - Bacteria
    - *Mycoplasma*
    - *Mycobacterium*
  - Bronchiolitis:
    - Respiratory syncytial virus
    - Influenza
    - Other virus
- Reactive airway disease
- Foreign body
- Cystic fibrosis

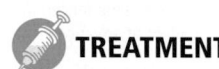

## TREATMENT

### PRE-HOSPITAL
- Oxygen
- Monitor airway.
- Suction

### INITIAL STABILIZATION/THERAPY
- Oxygen and respiratory support
- Suction mucous plugs.

### ED TREATMENT/PROCEDURES
- Universal precautions:
  - Specifically requires droplet precautions for 5 days after initiation of antimicrobial therapy
- Maintenance of adequate hydration
- Monitor oxygenation during paroxysms; supplement oxygen.
- Airway management may be life saving in younger children.

- Antibiotics:
  - Effective in the catarrhal stage
  - Prevent further transmission in the paroxysmal stage
  - Azithromycin is the first-line agent.
  - Alternatively, clarithromycin, erythromycin, or trimethoprim-sulfamethoxazole may be used, although the efficacy is unproven; useful if erythromycin is not tolerated.
- Corticosteroids and albuterol may reduce paroxysms of coughing, but further studies are required.
- With increasing incidence of pertussis among adolescents and adults, emergency physicians can decrease incidence of pertussis by making vaccination routine when also vaccinating against tetanus:
  - Tetanus toxoid, reduced diphtheria toxoid, acellular pertussis (Tdap)

## MEDICATION
Bronchodilators and steroids are generally not recommended for pertussis.

### First Line
- Azithromycin: 500 mg PO day 1, then 250 mg PO QD for 4 days
- Azithromycin <5 mo: 10 mg/kg PO daily for 5 days (max 500 mg daily)
- Azithromycin 5 mo to adult: 10 mg/kg PO day 1 (max 500 mg), then 5 mg/kg PO daily for 4 days (max 250 mg daily)
- Tetanus toxoid, reduced diphtheria toxoid, Tdap vaccine: 0.5 mL IM:
  - Adacel: Approved for age 11–64 yr
  - Boostrix: Approved for age 10–64 yr

### Pregnancy Considerations
Tdap may provide passive immunity to infants:
- Currently Class C

### Second Line
- Clarithromycin: 15 mg/kg/d divided b.i.d. for 7 days (max 1 g/d)
- Erythromycin: 40–50 mg/kg/d divided q.i.d. for 14 days (max 2 g/d)
- Trimethoprim-sulfamethoxazole: 8/40 mg/kg/d divided b.i.d. for 14 days (max 320/1,600 mg/d):
  - Not for infants <2 mo

 **FOLLOW-UP**

## DISPOSITION
### Admission Criteria
- Patients <1 yr
- Apnea
- Cyanosis during paroxysms of cough
- Significant associated pneumonia
- Encephalitis

### Discharge Criteria
- Children without apnea, respiratory compromise, altered mental status, or complications and respiratory distress
- Warm liquids to reduce coughing spasm
- Remove thick secretions with bulb suction in infants.
- Good hydration
- Avoid cough triggers: Cigarette smoke, pollutants, perfumes.
- Postexposure prophylaxis is recommended to all persons with close contact (within 3 ft of a symptomatic person):
  - Antibiotic recommendations are the same as those with disease.
  - Symptomatic children should be excluded from school or work; individuals with pertussis may return after 5 days of full treatment.

## FOLLOW-UP RECOMMENDATIONS
Children who are discharged need close follow-up to monitor hydration status and for respiratory compromise.

### ALERT
Physicians are legally required to report cases of pertussis to state health department.

## COMPLICATIONS
- Head, eyes, ears, neck, throat:
  - Epistaxis
  - Subconjunctival hemorrhage
- Respiratory:
  - Acute respiratory arrest
  - Pneumonia caused by secondary infection
  - Pneumothorax
  - Subcutaneous or mediastinal emphysema with crepitus
  - Bronchiectasis
- GI:
  - Hernia: Inguinal or abdominal
  - Rectal prolapse

- Neurologic:
  - Seizures
  - Encephalitis
  - Coma
  - Intracranial hemorrhage
  - Spinal epidural hemorrhage

### ALERT
The child with pertussis may have significant respiratory distress or apnea

## PEARLS AND PITFALLS
- Infants ≤1 yr need admission for pertussis.
- Tdap should be given to eligible patients requiring tetanus prophylaxis.
- Droplet precautions should be implemented for known or potential patients with pertussis.

## ADDITIONAL READING
- Crowcroft NS, Peabody RG. Recent developments in pertussis. *Lancet.* 2006;367:1926–1936.
- Gregory DS. Pertussis: A disease affecting all ages. *Am Family Physician.* 2006;74:420–426.
- Hitchcok WP. Rationale for use of Tdap booster vaccines for adolescent immunization: Overview of efficacy, safety and clinical use. *Clin Pediatr.* 2006;45:785–794.
- McIntyre P, Wood W. Pertussis in early infancy: Disease burden and preventive strategies. *Curr Opin Infect Dis.* 2009;22:215–223.
- Shah S, Sharieff GS. Pediatric respiratory infections. *Emerg Med Clin North Am.* 2007;25:961–979.
- Wood N, McIntyre P. Pertussis: Review of epidemiology, diagnosis, management and prevention. *Paediatr Respir Rev.* 2008;9:201–211.

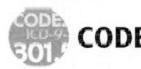 **CODES**

### ICD9
033.0 Whooping cough due to bordetella pertussis (b. pertussis)

Taylor Y. Cardall

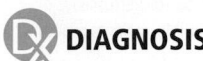 **BASICS**

## DESCRIPTION
- The phalanges of the foot are prone to injury.
- 5th (or small) toe most commonly affected

## ETIOLOGY
- Usually the result of direct trauma
- Stubbing the toe, kicking a hard surface, or dropping a heavy object onto toes most common mechanisms of injury

 **DIAGNOSIS**

## SIGNS AND SYMPTOMS
### History
History may predict the type of injury found and should include:
- Time of injury
- Mechanism
- History of previous trauma
- Status of tetanus immunization if laceration is present

### Physical Exam
- Tenderness, swelling, crepitus, and ecchymosis of affected digit
- Subungual hematomas are often present.
- Lacerations or crush-type wounds
- Document neurovascular status of the affected digit.

## ESSENTIAL WORKUP
Radiographs of involved digit

## DIAGNOSTIC TESTS & INTERPRETATION
### Imaging
- Radiographs of involved digit
- Lateral view may be most sensitive.

## DIFFERENTIAL DIAGNOSIS
- Fracture
- Contusion
- Abrasion/laceration
- Dislocation

**TREATMENT**

## PRE-HOSPITAL
- Ice to affected digit
- Direct pressure and dressing to any wounds

## INITIAL STABILIZATION/THERAPY
- Ice to affected digit
- Direct pressure and dressing to any wounds

## ED TREATMENT/PROCEDURES
- Fractures involving the proximal phalanx and interphalangeal (IP) joint of the hallux:
  - Nondisplaced, non–intra-articular fractures may be placed in a short-leg walking cast with toe extension for comfort.
  - Displaced, non–intra-articular fractures:
- Closed reduction with digital block anesthesia
  - Longitudinal traction
  - Placement in short-leg walking cast with toe extension:
    - Intra-articular fractures of the hallux merit orthopedic consult:
      - Frequently treated with open reduction and internal fixation
- Fractures involving the proximal phalanx and IP joint of the lesser toes:
  - Rarely cause long-term disability
- Nondisplaced fractures:
  - Treat with splinting or buddy taping
  - Gauze padding between the taped toes to prevent skin breakdown
- Displaced fractures:
  - Closed reduction by digital block anesthesia
  - Longitudinal traction
  - Buddy taping or splinting
  - Hard-sole shoe, weight bearing as tolerated
  - Oral analgesics for pain
  - Pain usually resolved by 2–3 wk
- IP joint dislocations:
  - Closed reduction by digital block anesthesia
  - Longitudinal traction with gentle downward pressure on distal phalanx
  - Buddy tape to adjacent toe
  - Unstable or unsuccessful reductions require orthopedic consultation.
  - Oral analgesics for pain

- Distal tuft fractures:
  - Subungual hematomas should be drained.
  - Nail-bed laceration repair may be necessary.
  - Buddy tape digit to adjacent toe.
  - Weight bearing as tolerated
  - Oral analgesics for pain
  - Pain usually resolved in 2–3 wk
- Open fractures:
  - Orthopedic consultation
  - Prophylactic antibiotics

## MEDICATION

- NSAIDs are useful treating acute pain:
  - Ibuprofen 800 mg (peds: 5–10 mg/kg) PO t.i.d.
- Narcotic analgesics may be required for severe pain:
  - Cephalexin: 1 g IM/IV in ED (peds: 50–100 mg/kg IM/IV in ED) for open fractures

 **FOLLOW-UP**

## DISPOSITION

### Admission Criteria

- Unstable or blocked dislocations
- Open fractures require orthopedic consultation in the ED.

### Discharge Criteria

All other fractures may be discharged with orthopedic follow-up in 2–3 wk to evaluate healing.

### Issues for Referral

Patient copies of any radiographs obtained may facilitate early follow-up.

## FOLLOW-UP RECOMMENDATIONS

- Intra-articular fractures involving the proximal phalanx of the great toe require urgent orthopedic or foot and ankle surgery follow-up.
- Simple nondisplaced fractures of the small toes may often be followed by primary care physicians.

## PEARLS AND PITFALLS

Open, displaced, or intra-articular fractures, particularly involving the hallux, merit orthopedic consultation.

## ADDITIONAL READING

- Ho K, Abu-Laban RB. Ankle and foot. In: Marx JA, ed. *Rosen's Emergency Medicine: Concepts and Clinical Practice*, 7th ed. Philadelphia: Mosby/Elsevier; 2010:670–697.
- Mittlmeier T, Haar P. Sesamoid and toe fractures. *Injury*. 2004;35(Suppl 2):87–97.
- Schnaue-Constantouris EM, Birrer RB, Grisafi PJ, et al. Digital foot trauma: Emergency diagnosis and treatment. *J Emerg Med*. 2002;22:163–170.
- Wedmore IS, Charette J. Emergency department evaluation and treatment of ankle and foot injuries. *Emerg Med Clin North Am*. 2001;18:85–113.

 **CODES**

### ICD9

- 826.0 Closed fracture of one or more phalanges of foot
- 924.3 Contusion of toe
- 924.20 Contusion of foot

# PHALANGEAL INJURIES, HAND

*Hetal Bharat Patel*
*David Palafox*

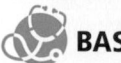 **BASICS**

## DESCRIPTION

- The fingers are the body part most frequently injured in athletic or occupational accidents.
- Children usually present with crush injuries.
- Hyperextension injuries most commonly cause ligamentous injury or chip fractures.
- Hyperflexion injury to the tip of digits may cause mallet finger injury with avulsion fracture at the insertion of the extensor tendon on the distal phalanx.
- Crush injuries most commonly cause fractures and diffuse soft-tissue injury.

### ALERT
Indications for reimplantation in amputation:
- Thumb
- Single digit between proximal interphalangeal (PIP) and distal interphalangeal (DIP) joint
- Multiple digits
- Amputation in child

### *Pediatric Considerations*
- Injuries may be more difficult to diagnose in children who are unable to cooperate for a full exam.
- Open epiphyses make radiographic interpretation less sensitive.
- Careful repeated exam and protective splinting are necessary.

## ETIOLOGY
Accident, trauma

 **DIAGNOSIS**

## SIGNS AND SYMPTOMS
- Pain in the area of injury
- Swelling and ecchymosis
- Deformity, laceration, burn, or amputation of the digit
- Loss of motion in the digit involved

### ALERT
High-pressure injection injury requires immediate consult to orthopedic hand surgeon.

## ESSENTIAL WORKUP
- Careful history and complete physical:
  - Explore all wounds fully to identify tendon injury or foreign body and perform 2-point discrimination testing.
  - Radiographic series of the affected hand for suggestion of greater than minor injury
- Special attention directed at assessing individual tendon status, neurovascular integrity, and identifying rotational deformity
- Examination conducted 1st to assess function, then under anesthesia, and finally with tourniquet if needed to allow a bloodless field for better exam of lacerated areas:
  - For distal digits, an elastic band can be used at the base of the digit.

## DIAGNOSTIC TESTS & INTERPRETATION
### *Imaging*
Plain radiography of involved digits including true lateral and oblique views

## DIFFERENTIAL DIAGNOSIS
- Tendon laceration/rupture; partial/complete
- Complicated open injuries may include several injuries, and the entire hand should be examined carefully.
- Beware of lacerations over dorsal metacarpal-phalangeal areas, which may be "fight bites" (human bites).

### *Pediatric Considerations*
Many fractures in children are torus (buckle) fractures of the phalanges.

 **TREATMENT**

- Most phalangeal dislocations are dorsal or dorsolateral:
  - These may be reduced under digital block.
  - Gentle distraction, hyperextension, and guiding the base of the dislocated phalanx into proper position with mild pressure
  - Always check for stability postreduction by having patient perform active range of motion (ROM).
- Simple impacted transverse or small corner fractures not exceeding 25% of a joint surface and dislocations:
  - Treated with "buddy" splinting in functional position or padded splint in neutral position
  - Splint for several days, with arrangements for appropriate follow-up within a week.
- Unstable fractures (rotational deformity, oblique fractures, fractures involving larger portion of a joint, angulated fractures, or significant epiphyseal injuries):
  - Splinted and referred for urgent orthopedic care

- Subungual hematoma:
  – Blood released by using a heated paper clip, electric cautery, or a hole drilled in the nail with an 18-gauge needle
  – This injury does not have to be treated as an open injury just because of subungual hematoma.
- Nail avulsions:
  – Repair of nail bed lacerations
  – Splinting of the eponychium and germinal matrix to avoid adhesions
  – The avulsed nail can be used or a small piece of gauze or foil can be inserted in the area.
- Many other lacerations can be left open with protective cover and allowed to heal secondarily.

### PRE-HOSPITAL
- Most patients do not require EMS transport solely for phalangeal injury.
- Cautions:
  – Prehospital personnel should not attempt to reduce a phalangeal dislocation at the scene unless there will be an unusually long transport time or there is vascular or neurologic compromise:
    ○ Reduction may be successful but prompt the physician to miss significant ligamentous injuries.

### ALERT
- Amputated digits or tissue should be placed in clean moist saline gauze, placed in plastic bag, and then placed in a separate bag with ice. *Do not place digit in direct contact with ice!*
- Bleeding should be treated with appropriate direct pressure dressings.

### INITIAL STABILIZATION/THERAPY
- Assess for other, more serious injuries.
- Remove all rings from injured hand.
- Immobilize the involved areas by proximal-to-distal splinting.
- Intermittent ice pack application with constant elevation for the 1st 24 hr
- Dislocations or severely deformed fractures producing vascular compromise should be reduced immediately to a neutral position and immobilized.

### MEDICATION
- Evaluate tetanus status and vaccinate per immunization schedule.
- Mild analgesics should be offered, with NSAIDs or hydrocodone usually sufficient.
- Antibiotics are not indicated for simple noncontaminated wounds:
  – Indicated for high-risk wounds such as bite wounds or grossly contaminated injury

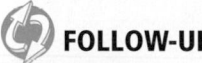 FOLLOW-UP

### DISPOSITION
Patients with a stable fracture in an appropriate splint may be discharged for orthopedic follow-up.

#### Pediatric Considerations
- Simple fractures can be treated with splinting if no significant rotational deformity is present.
- Epiphyseal fractures (Salter-Harris injuries) mandate orthopedic referral.

#### Admission Criteria
- Open joint injuries or fractures are usually admitted for irrigation, debridement, and early repair.
- Closed injuries requiring surgical management may be admitted for early operative intervention:
  – Acceptable to wait 1–2 days for semielective repair of clean injuries

### PEARLS AND PITFALLS
Rotational deformity may not be apparent if finger is straight; finger should be assessed in a flexed position.

### ADDITIONAL READING
- American College of Radiology, Expert Panel on Musculoskeletal Imaging. Acute hand and wrist trauma. 2001.
- American Society for Surgery of the Hand. *The Hand: Examination and Diagnosis*, 3rd ed. New York: Churchill Livingstone.
- American Society for Surgery of the Hand. *The hand: Primary care of common problems*, 2nd ed. New York: Churchill Livingstone.
- Bernstein ML, Chung KC. Hand fractures and their management: An international view. *Injury*. 2006;37(11):1043–1048.
- Cornwall R, Ricchetti ET. Pediatric phalanx fractures: Unique challenges and pitfalls. *Clin Orthop Relat Res*. 2006;445:146–156.

 CODES

#### ICD9
- 816.00 Closed fracture of phalanx or phalanges of hand, unspecified
- 816.01 Closed fracture of middle or proximal phalanx or phalanges of hand
- 816.02 Closed fracture of distal phalanx or phalanges of hand

# PHARYNGITIS

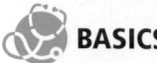

George C. Willis
Brian J. Browne

## BASICS

### DESCRIPTION
- Inflammation/infection of the pharynx
- 3rd-most-common complaint for physician visits
- 200 visits per 1,000 population annually in U.S.
- $300 million annually to diagnose and treat
- Strep throat:
  - 15–30% of childhood pharyngitis
  - 5–10% of adult pharyngitis
  - Unusual in children <3 yr
  - Peak age 4–11 yr
  - Peak months Jan–May; also start of school year
- Centor criteria for strep throat:
  - Criteria:
    ○ Fever by history
    ○ Tonsillar exudates
    ○ Tender anterior cervical lymphadenopathy
    ○ Absence of cough
  - The most widely used decision rule
  - If 3 or 4 criteria are present, the positive predictive value for group A $\beta$-hemolytic streptococci (GABHS) infection is 40–60%.
  - The absence of 3 or 4 of the criteria has an 80% negative predictive value.
  - Patients with none or only 1 of these criteria should not be tested or treated.
  - Patients with ≥2 criteria should be tested:
    ○ Presumptive treatment without testing has led to inappropriate use of antibiotics in about 50% of cases.

### ETIOLOGY
- Viral:
  - Most common cause of infectious pharyngitis
  - Rhinovirus (20%)
  - Coronavirus (>5%)
  - Adenovirus (5%)
  - Herpes simplex virus (4%)
  - Parainfluenza virus (2%)
  - Influenza virus (2%)
  - Coxsackievirus (<1%)
  - Epstein-Barr virus (<1%)
  - Cytomegalovirus (<1%)
  - Acute retroviral syndrome
- Bacterial:
  - *Streptococcus pyogenes* (GABHS) (15–30%)
  - Group C and G $\beta$-hemolytic streptococci (5%)
  - *Neisseria gonorrhoeae* (<1%)
  - *Corynebacterium diphtheriae* (<1%)
  - *Arcanobacterium haemolyticum* (<1%)
  - *Chlamydia pneumoniae*
  - *Mycoplasma pneumoniae* (<1%)
  - Syphilis
  - Tuberculosis
- Fungal:
  - *Candida* (thrush)
- Chemical burns
- Foreign bodies
- Inhalants
- Postnasal drip
- Malignancy
- GERD

## DIAGNOSIS

### SIGNS AND SYMPTOMS
#### History
- Viral:
  - Cough
  - Rhinorrhea
  - Sore throat usually follows.
- GABHS (also group C/G):
  - Sudden-onset sore throat that usually precedes other symptoms
  - Odynophagia
  - Fever
  - Headache
  - Abdominal pain
  - Nausea and vomiting
  - Uncharacteristic symptoms:
    ○ Coryza
    ○ Hoarseness
    ○ Diarrhea

#### Physical Exam
- Viral:
  - Rhinorrhea
  - Pharyngeal erythema
  - Lack of cervical adenopathy
- GABHS:
  - Tonsillopharyngeal erythema/exudates
  - Soft palatal petechiae
  - Beefy red, swollen uvula
  - Anterior cervical lymphadenopathy
  - Scarlatiniform rash
  - Uncharacteristic signs:
    ○ Conjunctivitis
    ○ Anterior stomatitis
    ○ Discrete ulcerative lesions
- Mononucleosis:
  - Often mistaken for GABHS infection due to similar presentation:
    ○ Exudative pharyngitis
    ○ Tender palpable cervical lymphadenopathy
    ○ Fever
    ○ Rash
  - Hepatosplenomegaly
  - Jaundice
- Diphtheria:
  - Consider in nonimmunized patients
  - Airway-threatening gray pharyngeal membrane
  - Myocarditis (2/3 of patients); clinically evident cardiac dysfunction (10–25%)
  - Cranial and peripheral neuritis (5%)
- Gonococcal pharyngitis:
  - Can be asymptomatic
  - Always evaluate children for sexual abuse.
  - Recurrent episodes of pharyngitis

### ESSENTIAL WORKUP
Physical exam:
- Nearly impossible alone to differentiate between viral and bacterial pharyngitis

### DIAGNOSTIC TESTS & INTERPRETATION
#### Lab
- Throat culture:
  - Gold standard
  - 24–48 hr for results, which delays treatment
  - Necessitates contacting patient/family
  - False-negative rate for GABHS is 10%.
  - False-positive rate for GABHS is 20%:
    ○ Often related to GABHS carrier state with superimposed viral pharyngitis
    ○ May have concurrent viral pharyngitis
  - Not cost effective and not routinely recommended for evaluation of adults
  - Throat culture should be collected when *Gonococcus* is being considered.
- Rapid strep test (RST):
  - Results are available within 30 min.
  - Sensitivity 85–95%
  - Specificity 96–99%
  - All patients with positive RST results should be treated.
  - Negative RST results in children and adolescents (not adults) should be confirmed with a conventional throat culture.
  - Use of RST without (or in lieu of) a culture does not increase the risk of suppurative or nonsuppurative complications of GABHS infection.
  - Use of RST without culture confirmation of all negative results is the most cost-effective strategy in the treatment of pharyngitis.
  - The new optical immunoassay is extremely accurate; negative results do not require confirmatory culture.
- Monospot:
  - Detects heterophil antibody for suspected mononucleosis
  - 90% sensitive in patients >5 yr of age
  - 75% sensitive in patients 2–4 yr of age
  - <30% sensitive in patients <2 yr of age
- CBC with peripheral smear for suspected mononucleosis:
  - 50% lymphocytes, 10% atypical lymphocytes
- Loeffler media culture for diphtheria
- Viral loads should be obtained in patients suspicious for acute retroviral syndrome.

#### Imaging
- Lateral neck radiograph for suspected epiglottitis, retropharyngeal abscess, or foreign body
- Contrast-enhanced CT to identify and define the extent of complications such as retropharyngeal abscess

### DIFFERENTIAL DIAGNOSIS
- Epiglottitis
- Peritonsillar/retropharyngeal abscess
- Diphtheria
- Mononucleosis

- Ludwig angina
- *Candida* infection
- Gonorrhea
- HIV acute retroviral syndrome
- Acute leukemia/lymphoma
- Oropharyngeal cancer
- Foreign body
- Inhalants and chemical burns
- Postnasal drip
- GERD

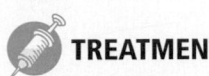 **TREATMENT**

**PRE-HOSPITAL**
- Observe/manage airway for respiratory distress
- Normal saline (NS) hydration for hypotension/dehydration

**INITIAL STABILIZATION/THERAPY**
- ABCs
- 1-L (peds: 20-mL/kg) NS bolus for signs of volume depletion or if patient is unable to tolerate oral solutions

**ED TREATMENT/PROCEDURES**
- Antipyretics/analgesics:
  - Acetaminophen
  - Ibuprofen
  - Topical analgesics (Chloraseptic spray or lozenges)
- GABHS infection:
  - Without treatment, GABHS pharyngitis is often a mild and self-limited infection:
    ○ Antibiotic therapy accelerates symptom relief (fever and pain) by 1–2 days.
  - Although symptom duration may be slightly shortened with antibiotics, the real goal of treatment is prevention of acute rheumatic fever (a complication rarely seen in U.S.).
- Antibiotics:
  - Penicillin V is the drug of choice for GABHS pharyngitis.
  - Amoxicillin in a once-daily regimen may be as effective as the penicillin regimen.
  - For patients who are allergic to penicillin and those who fail therapy with a $\beta$-lactam, macrolides are an acceptable alternative.
  - Oral cephalosporins are reasonable to use in patients with penicillin allergy and inability to tolerate macrolides.
  - A "treat-all" strategy is not recommended because of the extremely low incidence of poststreptococcal sequelae and emergence of antibiotic resistance.
- Corticosteroids:
  - Steroids are efficacious at relieving odynophagia in patients with pharyngitis.
  - Avoid in diabetics or if immunosuppression.
- Possible complications of streptococcal infection:
  - Acute rheumatic fever:
    ○ Rare in industrialized countries, but still the leading cause of cardiac death in 1st 5 decades of life
    ○ A sequela of GABHS; not proven in association with group C or G

- Peritonsillar/retropharyngeal abscess
- Poststreptococcal glomerulonephritis
- Pediatric autoimmune neuropsychiatric disorder associated with streptococcal infection:
  ○ A rare, and controversial, consequence of *Streptococcus* infection
  ○ Sudden onset of symptoms like those of obsessive-compulsive disorder, caused by an autoimmune reaction that affects the basal ganglia
- Treatment failure:
  - A full 10-day course of penicillin is necessary to eradicate infection from the pharynx.
  - Probability of relapse is 50% if penicillin is discontinued after 3 days of therapy.
- Diphtheria:
  - Goals of therapy:
    ○ Prevent airway obstruction
    ○ Treat infection
  - Penicillin or macrolide antibiotic
  - Complications:
    ○ Exotoxin-mediated myocarditis and neuritis (cranial neuropathies)
- Gonococcal pharyngitis:
  - Treat according to the usual sexually transmitted disease protocol.
  - Third-generation cephalosporin (gonorrhea)
  - Always include cotreatment for *Chlamydia* (azithromycin).

**MEDICATION**
**First Line**
- Penicillin:
  - <27 kg: Penicillin G benzathine (Bicillin LA): 0.6 million U IM × 1
  - >27 kg: Penicillin G benzathine (Bicillin LA): 1.2 million U IM × 1
  - <12 yr: 25–50 mg/kg/d PO div. q6–8h × 10 days
  - >12 yr: 250–500 mg PO q6–8hr × 10 days

**Second Line**
- Macrolides:
  - Azithromycin: 500 mg PO, then 250 mg PO daily × 4 days (peds: 12 mg/kg daily × 5 d; max 500 mg/d)
  - Clarithromycin: 250–500 mg (peds: 7.5 mg/kg) PO b.i.d. × 10 days
- Oral cephalosporins:
  - Cephalexin: 500 mg (peds: 12.5 mg/kg) PO q.i.d. × 10 days
  - Cefdinir: 600 mg (peds: 14 mg/kg) PO daily × 10 days
- Steroids:
  - Dexamethasone: 0.6 mg/kg to a max 10 mg IM/PO × 1
  - Prednisone: 40–60 mg PO × 1
- Gonococcal:
  - Ceftriaxone: 125–250 mg IM × 1
  - Azithromycin: 1,000 mg PO × 1

 **FOLLOW-UP**

**DISPOSITION**
**Admission Criteria**
- Airway compromise
- Severe dehydration
- Suspected child abuse

**Discharge Criteria**
Able to tolerate oral intake

**FOLLOW-UP RECOMMENDATIONS**
- Should follow up if symptoms do not improve within 72 hr.
- Patients remain contagious until they have taken antibiotics for at least 24 hr.
- Mononucleosis patients should avoid contact sports.

## PEARLS AND PITFALLS

- Use the Centor criteria to make the decision to test for GABHS pharyngitis.
- Children, but not adults, with negative RST need follow-up throat culture.
- Use of once-daily or one-time dosing regimens increases compliance.
- Evaluate for deep space infections if concerning history or presentation.

## ADDITIONAL READING

- Alcaide AL, Bisno AL. Pharyngitis and epiglotittis. *Infect Dis Clin North Am.* 2007;21:449–469.
- Centor RM, Witherspoon JM, Dalton HP, et al. The diagnosis of strep throat in adult in the emergency room. *Med Decision Making.* 1981;1:239–246.
- Gerber MA, Baltimore RS, Eaton CD, et al. Prevention of rheumatic fever and diagnosis and treatment of acute *Streptococcal pharyngitis.* *Circulation.* 2009;119:1541–1551.
- Mell LK, Davis RL, Owens D. Association between streptococcal infection and obsessive-compulsive disorder, Tourette's syndrome, and tic disorder. *Pediatrics.* 2005;116:56–60.
- Tasar A, Yanturali S, Topacoglu H, et al. Clinical efficacy of dexamethasone for acute exudative pharyngitis. *J Emerg Med.* 2008;35:363–367.

**See Also (Topic, Algorithm, Electronic Media Element)**
- Epiglottitis
- Mononucleosis
- Peritonsillar Abscess
- Retropharyngeal Abscess
- Rheumatic Fever

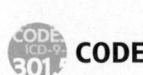 **CODES**

**ICD9**
- 034.0 Streptococcal sore throat
- 462 Acute pharyngitis

# PHENCYCLIDINE POISONING

*Steven Aks*

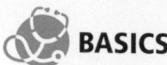 **BASICS**

## DESCRIPTION
- Phencyclidine (PCP) is a dissociative anesthetic structurally related to ketamine:
  - Causes decreased perception of pain and agitation
- Half-life of 21–24 hr, but may be longer in overdose
- Enterohepatic recirculation—recirculated into the stomach

## ETIOLOGY
- Drug of abuse:
  - Frequently encountered as an adulterant of marijuana
- Street names for PCP include:
  - Angel dust
  - Wicky stick
  - Wicky weed
  - Wacky weed
  - Wet
  - Illy
  - Embalming fluid
  - Sherman

### Pediatric Considerations
Exposure in toddlers reported via passive exposure

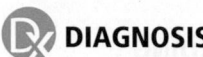 **DIAGNOSIS**

## SIGNS AND SYMPTOMS
- CNS:
  - Altered mental status
  - Agitation
  - Bizarre/violent behavior
  - Belligerence
  - Coma
  - Seizures
  - Nystagmus (vertical, horizontal, or rotatory)
- Cardiovascular:
  - HTN
  - Tachycardia
- Musculoskeletal:
  - Traumatic injury (decreased pain perception)
  - Rhabdomyolysis (due to vigorous muscular contraction)
- Vital signs:
  - Hyperthermia

### History
How was the PCP consumed?:
- Smoked with marijuana
- Ingested

### Physical Exam
- Agitation
- Coma
- Hypertension
- Tachycardia
- Diaphoresis
- Nystagmus (vertical, horizontal, or rotatory)
- Hyperthermia
- Vigorous muscular contraction

## ESSENTIAL WORKUP
- Clinical diagnosis based on presentation supported by urine toxicology screen:
  - Dextromethorphan and ketamine may give false positive.
- Careful physical exam for occult trauma
- Exclude other causes of altered mental status.

## DIAGNOSTIC TESTS & INTERPRETATION
### Lab
- CBC
- Electrolytes, BUN/creatinine, glucose
- Urinalysis:
  - Dip for myoglobin (rhabdomyolysis)
- Creatine phosphokinase:
  - If urine dip for blood is positive
- Ethanol level

### Imaging
- Chest radiograph for aspiration pneumonia
- Extremity/spine radiographs when there is associated trauma
- CT of the head when there is head trauma/altered mental status

## DIFFERENTIAL DIAGNOSIS
- Drugs of abuse:
  - Cocaine
  - Amphetamines
  - Designer drugs:
    - Methcathinone ("Cat")
    - "Ecstasy"
    - "Ice" (methamphetamine)
  - Alcohols
  - Ketamine
  - Sympathomimetics
- Drugs that cause nystagmus:
  - Lithium
  - Carbamazepine
  - Sedative-hypnotics
  - Alcohols
  - Phenothiazines
  - Dextromethorphan

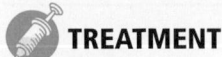 **TREATMENT**

### PRE-HOSPITAL

**ALERT**
Use restraints/additional personnel to control combative patient.

### INITIAL STABILIZATION/THERAPY
- ABCs
- IV
- Cardiac monitor
- Naloxone, thiamine, glucose (or Accu-Chek) if altered mental status
- Protect patient and staff from injury.

### ED TREATMENT/PROCEDURES
- Maintain patient in a quiet place; avoid stimulation.
- Physical restraints for violent patient
- Sedation:
  - Benzodiazepines
  - Butyrophenones (haloperidol) theoretically can lower the seizure threshold.
- Activated charcoal/sorbitol if oral coingestants
- IV 0.9% normal saline for hydration, sodium bicarbonate/mannitol for rhabdomyolysis

### MEDICATION
*First Line*
- Ativan (lorazepam): 2-mg IV increments
- Diazepam: 5-mg IV increments

*Second Line*
- Activated charcoal slurry: 1–2 g/kg up to 90 g PO
- Dextrose: D50W 1 amp: 50 mL or 25 g (peds: D25W 2–4 mL/kg) IV
- Haloperidol: 5-mg IV increments
- Mannitol: 25–50 g IV
- Naloxone (Narcan): 2 mg (peds: 0.1 mg/kg) IV or IM initial dose
- Sodium bicarbonate: 2 amps diluted in 1 L of D5W, given at 125–250 mL/hr (for rhabdomyolysis) to urine pH of 7.0
- Sorbitol: 1–2 g/kg to a max 100 g (peds: >1 yr, 1–1.5 g/kg as 35% solution to max 50 g) PO mixed in activated charcoal slurry—use only for first dose.
- Thiamine (vitamin B$_1$): 100 mg (peds: 50 mg) IV or IM

 **FOLLOW-UP**

### DISPOSITION
*Admission Criteria*
- Prolonged altered mental status
- Significant traumatic injuries
- Rhabdomyolysis
- Hyperthermia

*Discharge Criteria*
Becomes lucid after a period of observation (6 hr)

### FOLLOW-UP RECOMMENDATIONS
Psychiatry or social work referral for suicidal ideation or chronic drug use

## PEARLS AND PITFALLS
- PCP poisoning can lead to traumatic injuries that can become life threatening.
- Adequate chemical restraints with benzodiazepines are needed to prevent excessive muscular activity leading to rhabdomyolysis.
- Dextromethorphan is a common cause for a false-positive PCP urine toxicology screen.
- Ketamine abuse presents with similar signs and symptoms of PCP abuse.

## ADDITIONAL READING
- Hahn I-H. Phencyclidine and ketamine. In: Erickson TB, Ahrens W, Aks SE, et al., eds. *Pediatric Toxicology*. New York: McGraw-Hill; 2004:297–302.
- Pugach S, Pugach IZ. Overdose in infant caused by over-the-counter cough medicine. *South J Med*. 2009;102:440–442.
- Shannon M. Recent ketamine administration can produce a urine toxic screen which is falsely positive for phencyclidine. *Pediatr Emerg Care*. 1998;14:180.
- Wills B, Erickson T. Drug- and toxin-associated seizures. *Med Clin North Am*. 2005;89:1297–1321.

 **CODES**

ICD9
968.3 Poisoning by intravenous anesthetics

# PHENYTOIN POISONING
*Michele Zell-Kanter*

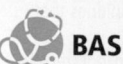 **BASICS**

## DESCRIPTION
- Follows zero-order pharmacokinetics:
  - Small incremental increase in dose can result in a large increase in plasma concentration.
- Half-life in overdose up to 70 hr
- Cardiovascular toxicity from IV administration likely due to the diluent propylene glycol
- Fosphenytoin, a prodrug for parenteral administration, is metabolized to its active moiety.

## ETIOLOGY
- Phenytoin intoxication results from acute, chronic, or acute on chronic ingestion.
- If the cause of the intoxication is unclear in a patient on phenytoin, consider:
  - Change in the brand of phenytoin
  - Change in dosage form
  - Drug interaction
  - Change in serum albumin

# DIAGNOSIS

## SIGNS AND SYMPTOMS
- Level 20–40 mg/mL:
  - Nystagmus
  - Dizziness
  - Ataxia
  - Drowsiness
  - Nausea/vomiting
  - Diplopia
  - Slurred speech
- Level 40–90 mg/mL:
  - Confusion
  - Disorientation
- Level >90 mg/mL:
  - Coma
  - Respiratory depression
  - Paradoxical seizures
- Hypotension/bradycardia with rapid IV administration:
  - Fosphenytoin injection does not contain propylene glycol.
  - Hypotension/dysrhythmia unlikely with fosphenytoin
- Hypersensitivity reaction following chronic use:
  - Rash
  - Fever
  - Neutropenia
  - Agranulocytosis
  - Hepatitis
  - Cholangitis

## ESSENTIAL WORKUP
- Determine the time and amount of ingestion.
- Phenytoin level:
  - After oral overdose, the peak plasma concentration may not be reached until 24 hr or more post–acute ingestion.
  - Absorption differs with various oral preparations
  - Repeat levels every 4 hr until levels have peaked and are declining.
  - Once levels begin declining, check every 24 hr until <30 mg/mL.
  - Free phenytoin level may be required in patients who are hypoalbuminemic or patients who are poor metabolizers.

## DIAGNOSTIC TESTS & INTERPRETATION
### Lab
- Fosphenytoin level:
  - Measured as phenytoin
  - Measure fosphenytoin after conversion to phenytoin is complete (2 hr post–IV infusion/4 hr post–IM injection).
  - Prior to complete conversion to phenytoin, immunoanalytic techniques may overestimate plasma phenytoin concentrations due to cross-reactivity with fosphenytoin.
- Electrolytes, BUN, creatinine, glucose:
  - Check for anion gap metabolic acidosis due to coingestant, seizure activity.
  - Determine glucose with altered mental status.

## DIFFERENTIAL DIAGNOSIS
- Intoxication with other CNS depressants
- Guillain-Barré syndrome
- Botulism
- Posterior fossa tumor
- Acute cerebellitis

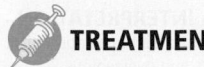 **TREATMENT**

### PRE-HOSPITAL
- Differentiate phenytoin-induced altered mental status from other potentially serious causes:
  - Head trauma common in seizure population
- Collect/transport prescription bottles and medications to aid in identification and quantification of ingestion

### INITIAL STABILIZATION/THERAPY
- ABCs:
  - IV access
  - Cardiac monitor (with IV overdose)
- For altered mental status:
  - Accu-Chek.
  - Administer naloxone, dextrose, and thiamine as indicated.
- Treat hypotension with IV fluids and Trendelenburg position:
  - Dopamine for refractory hypotension
- Treat paradoxical seizures with diazepam.

## ED TREATMENT/PROCEDURES
Activated charcoal:
- Administer single dose.
- Multiple-dose activated charcoal may increase the clearance of phenytoin; does not correlate with clinical improvement in patients with phenytoin toxicity.

### MEDICATION
- Activated charcoal slurry: 1–2 g/kg up to 90 g PO
- Dextrose: D50W 1 amp: 50 mL or 25 g (peds: D25W 2–4 mL/kg) IV
- Dopamine: 2–20 mg/kg/min IV titrated to desired blood pressure
- Naloxone (Narcan): 2 mg (peds: 0.1 mg/kg) IV or IM initial dose
- Thiamine (vitamin $B_1$): 100 mg (peds: 50 mg) IV or IM

 **FOLLOW-UP**

### DISPOSITION
#### Admission Criteria
- Altered mental status, severe ataxia, increasing phenytoin level
- Level >25 mg/mL
- ICU admission with intoxication from IV phenytoin
- Fall precautions

#### Discharge Criteria
- Level ≤25 mg/mL
- Ambulatory without ataxia

## FOLLOW-UP RECOMMENDATIONS
- Psychiatric referral for intentional ingestions/suicide attempts.
- Close primary care follow-up to check phenytoin levels.

## PEARLS AND PITFALLS
- Small incremental increases in dose of phenytoin can result in toxicity since phenytoin follows zero-order kinetics.
- Repeat phenytoin levels every 4 hr until declining.

## ADDITIONAL READING
- Glick TH, Workman TP, Gaufberg SV. Preventing phenytoin intoxication: Safer use of a familiar anticonvulsant. *J Family Pract*. 2004;53:197–202.
- Kawasaju C, Busgu R, Uekihara S, et al. Charcoal hemoperfusion in the treatment of phenytoin overdose. *Am J Kidney Dis*. 2000;35:323–326.
- McCluggage LK, Loils SA, Bullock MR. Phenytoin toxicity due to genetic polymorphism. *Neurocrit Care*. 2009;10:222–224.
- Von Winckelmann SL, Spriet I, Willems L. Therapeutic drug monitoring of phenytoin in critically ill patients. *Pharmacotherapy*. 2008;28:1391–1400.

 **CODES**

**ICD9**
966.1 Poisoning by hydantoin derivatives

# PHEOCHROMOCYTOMA
*David N. Zull*

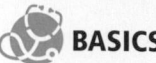 **BASICS**

## DESCRIPTION

- Pheochromocytoma (pheo) is a catecholamine-producing tumor arising from the chromaffin tissues of the sympathetic nervous system.
- Origin from the adrenal medulla or sympathetic ganglia:
  - 80% solitary adrenal (usually the right side)
  - 10% bilateral (usually inherited form)
  - 10% extra-adrenal in location:
    ○ Abdominal, within mesenteric ganglia (86%)
    ○ Thorax (10%), neck (3%), bladder (1%)
  - 10% malignant (usually inherited form)
- Incidence:
  - 0.2–0.4% of hypertensive patients, but higher proportion of patients with severe hypertension
  - 2–8/million population per year
  - Peaks in decades 3–5, 10% in children
  - Male = Female
  - In about half of cases, the diagnosis is made postmortem.
  - 10% asymptomatic, found incidentally by CT
- Genetics:
  - Inherited form 25%, autosomal dominant
  - Usually associated with multiple endocrine neoplasia (MEN) 2A, less so with MEN 2B or von Hippel-Lindau (VHL) disease:
    ○ MEN 2A (medullary thyroid carcinoma [CA], pheo, and hyperparathyroidism)
    ○ MEN 2B (medullary thyroid CA, pheo, oral mucosal neuromas, skeletal and bony abnormalities)
    ○ VHL (hemangiomas of the retina, cerebellum, and brainstem, with renal tumors)
  - Other associated diseases: Neurofibromatosis, tuberous sclerosis, Sturge-Weber syndrome, paragangliomas of the neck

## ETIOLOGY

- The tumor synthesizes and stores catecholamines in the same manner as the normal adrenal medulla.
- Tumors predominantly secrete norepinephrine, and to a lesser extent epinephrine (some tumors are epinephrine predominant, in which hypotensive episodes are characteristic)
- Paroxysmal release of catecholamines:
  - Spontaneously due to changes in blood flow or tumor necrosis
  - Direct pressure on the gland from external forces (trauma, exercise)
  - Precipitation of release (opiates, glucagon, metoclopramide, steroids, foods with tyramine, iodinated contrast media)
  - Augmentation of catecholamine effect (tricyclic antidepressants [TCAs], β-blockers, sympathomimetics)

 **DIAGNOSIS**

## SIGNS AND SYMPTOMS

- Hypertension, moderate to severe, refractory to treatment:
  - 40%: Paroxysms with normal blood pressure (BP) between episodes
  - 30%: Sustained hypertension with paroxysms
  - 30%: Sustained hypertension without paroxysms
  - Sometimes normotensive in familial forms and small tumors: <5%
- Features of paroxysms:
  - Sudden onset, gradual resolution
  - Duration: Minutes to hours (average 20 min)
  - Intervals: Hours to months (average weekly)
  - Increasing frequency, duration, and severity with time

## History

- Clinical characteristics:
  - Hypertensive crisis or urgency
  - Headache
  - Tachycardia/palpitations
  - Profuse diaphoresis
  - Apprehension/anxiety
  - Shock associated with trauma, surgery, parturition, anesthesia
- Associated symptoms:
  - Chest pain (myocardial ischemia, dissection)
  - Syncope (arrhythmia, hypotension)
  - Orthostasis (decreased plasma volume and blunted sympathetic reflexes)
  - Abdominal pain, vomiting (tumor necrosis, mesenteric ischemia):
    ○ Acute hemorrhagic tumor necrosis may lead to an acute abdomen with marked hypertension followed by shock.
  - Constipation can be severe, leading to ileus or pseudo-obstruction (catecholamines inhibit peristalsis)
  - Weight loss/fevers (increased metabolic rate)
  - Lethargy, confusion (hypertensive encephalopathy or catecholamine withdrawal))
  - Focal neurologic symptoms (cerebral vascular accident [CVA])
  - Polydipsia, polyuria (glucose intolerance)
  - Pheochromocytoma multisystem crisis:
    ○ Severe hypertension or shock
    ○ Hyperpyrexia
    ○ Encephalopathy
    ○ Lactic acidosis
    ○ Multiorgan failure

## Physical Exam

- Moderate to severe hypertension, often with orthostatic changes
- Tachycardic, diaphoretic, evidence of weight loss, low-grade fever
- Pallor, cold hands and feet (flushing not seen, except rarely after a paroxysm)
- Tremor, anxiety
- Mydriasis, hypertensive retinopathy
- Café au lait spots, neurofibromas, thyroid nodule
- No palpable masses (tumors tend to be small)

## ESSENTIAL WORKUP

- Accurate blood pressure (BP) determination with orthostatics
- ECG to exclude ischemia or dysrhythmias

## DIAGNOSTIC TESTS & INTERPRETATION

- Overdiagnosis in >20% from misinterpretation of borderline biochemical tests and overzealous imaging
- Underdiagnosis is common from failure to consider the diagnosis or ignoring adrenal masses on CT.

### Lab

- CBC:
  - Elevated hemoglobin due to diminished plasma volume
  - Elevated WBC from demargination
- Electrolytes, BUN, creatinine, glucose:
  - Lactic acidosis
  - Renal failure secondary to hypertensive nephropathy
  - Hyperglycemia due to impaired response to insulin and effect of catecholamines
  - Hypercalcemia due to excess parathyroid hormone
- Urinalysis: Proteinuria and hematuria
- Plasma free metanephrine (fractionated):
  - 96% sensitive, 85% specific—excellent screening, but false positives
  - Least likely to be interfered by medications or stress and no special prep for venipuncture

### Imaging

- CT sensitive for adrenal masses >1 cm (IV contrast may pose a slight risk):
  - 5% of incidental adrenal tumors seen on CT are pheochromocytomas.
- MRI or positron emission tomography more sensitive in identifying adrenal pheos as well as identifying extra-adrenal tumors
- Metaiodobenzylguanidine (radionuclear scintiscan: High specificity for localization, but not sensitive enough to exclude pheo)
- Chest radiograph for pulmonary edema
- CT head for CVA/intracranial bleed

### Diagnostic Procedures/Surgery

- Clonidine suppression test if diagnosis uncertain (levels not suppressed if pheo)
- Provocative testing with glucagon is not recommended.
- 24-hr urine collection for free catecholamines and metanephrine (total and fractionated):
  - 99.7% combined specificity and 87.5% sensitivity
  - Must include creatinine to verify adequate collection
  - Medications that interfere: Levodopa, methyldopa, monoamine oxidase inhibitors (MAOIs), labetalol, propranolol, radiographic contrast media, sympathomimetics, benzodiazepines, TCAs, caffeine, nicotine
  - Should be done at the time of a paroxysm
- Fine-needle aspiration is contraindicated.
- Laparoscopic resection is feasible in many cases.

## DIFFERENTIAL DIAGNOSIS

- Alcohol withdrawal syndromes
- Autonomic hyperreflexia
- Carcinoid syndrome
- Cerebral vascular accident
- Cocaine or amphetamine intoxication
- Hypertensive crisis
- Migraines
- MAOI reaction
- Panic attack
- Postural tachycardia syndrome
- Paroxysmal supraventricular tachycardia
- Subarachnoid hemorrhage
- Thyrotoxicosis
- Toxemia

 TREATMENT

### PRE-HOSPITAL

- IV access, oxygen
- Continuous cardiac/blood pressure monitoring
- Nitroglycerin 0.4 mg SL for chest pain or hypertension

### ED TREATMENT/PROCEDURES

- Hypertensive crisis:
  - $\alpha$-Blockade with phentolamine—first-line agent
  - Vigorous fluid resuscitation required as vasoconstriction is relieved
- $\beta$-Blockade (labetalol or esmolol):
  - For further BP control
    If tachycardia develops during induction of $\alpha$-blockade
  - Never use alone: Institution of $\beta$-blockade without prior $\alpha$-adrenergic blockade may exacerbate hypertension by antagonizing $\beta$-mediated vasodilation in smooth muscle.
- Nitroprusside for uncontrolled hypertension
- Ventricular tachydysrhythmias:
  Lidocaine, $\beta$ blockade, amiodarone

### Management of Hypertensive Paroxysm

- Phentolamine: First-line therapy—$\alpha$-blockade:
  - 2.5–5.0 mg IV bolus at 1 mg/min
  - Repeat bolus q5min to response
  - IV Infusion: 0.5–10 mcg/kg/min (100 mg in 500 mL D5W)
- $\beta$-Blockade (should not be started unless $\alpha$-blockade initiated):
  - Esmolol: Load 500 $\mu$g/kg over 1 min, followed by 50 $\mu$g/kg/min for 4 min; if adequate therapeutic effect not achieved within 5 min, repeat loading dose and increase infusion to 100 $\mu$g/kg/min; repeat loading dose and titrate infusion rate upward at 50 $\mu$g/kg/min q4–q5min as needed; omit further loading doses once nearing therapeutic target.
  - Labetalol: Begin with 10–20 mg IV; BP falls within 5 min, maximum effect at 10 min; can double IV dose q15–q30min until target reached ($\alpha$-blockade inadequate to be relied on as a single agent).
  - Metoprolol: 5 mg IV q15min until response
- Resistance to $\alpha$- and $\beta$-blockade:
  - Nitroprusside 0.5–10 $\mu$g/kg/min IV infusion
  - Nicardipine: Start infusion at 5 mg/hr, titrate up by 2.5 mg/hr every 15 min up to 15 mg/hr.

## MEDICATION

### First Line

- Phenoxybenzamine: Start at 10 mg b.i.d. orally, titrate up 10 mg every other day until desired effect (start at least 7 days pre-op).
- Other $\alpha$-blockers (first dose effect):
  - Doxazosin: 1–8 mg/d (start at 1 mg)
  - Terazosin: 1–10 mg/d (start at 1 mg)
- $\beta$-Blocker to control reflex tachycardia:
  - Metoprolol or atenolol: 25–100 mg/d

### Second Line

- Calcium-channel blockers:
  - Amlodipine, nicardipine or nifedipine
- Inhibition of catecholamine synthesis:
  - Metyrosine: 250–500 mg q6h

### ALERT

The following medications commonly administered in the ED can precipitate hypertensive crisis in pheochromocytoma:

- $\beta$-Blockers
- Glucagon
- Glucocorticoids
- Iodinated contrast media
- Ketamine
- Metoclopramide
- Opiates
- Sympathomimetics, including over-the-counters

### Pregnancy Considerations

- May be confused with toxemia, but proteinuria is usually absent
- MRI is preferred imaging modality.
- Nitroprusside should not be used for hypertensive crisis, but all other BP medications are acceptable.
- Spontaneous vaginal delivery will likely precipitate hypertensive crisis, such that C section should be planned.

 FOLLOW-UP

### DISPOSITION

#### Admission Criteria

- Suspicion of pheo in an ill patient mandates $\alpha$-blockade and aggressive volume expansion in a closely monitored setting.
- Hypertensive urgency or crisis
- Cardiac arrhythmias
- End organ compromise: Congestive heart failure, myocardial infarction, renal insufficiency, CVA, abdominal pain

#### Discharge Criteria

Stable patient with mild hypertension may be referred for prompt outpatient evaluation.

### FOLLOW-UP RECOMMENDATIONS

- Obtain plasma free metanephrine during a hypertensive episode.
- Consider initiating doxazosin or terazosin or a calcium-channel blocker for BP control.
- Arrange close follow-up and contact the physician referral to alert them of your suspicion.

## PEARLS AND PITFALLS

- Paroxysms of severe hypertension, headache, intense diaphoresis, and palpitations comprise a tetrad very suggestive of pheo.
- Pallor, not flushing, is typical of pheo crisis.
- Orthostasis is common in pheo and it is further aggravated by $\alpha$-blockade, unless volume repletion is not done concomitantly.
- Consider pheo in unexplained shock, multisystem organ failure, cardiomyopathy, or glucose intolerance associated with weight loss.
- Never administer $\beta$-blockers (even labetalol) before $\alpha$-blockade.
- If pheo is suspected, send off plasma free metanephrine during an attack.

## ADDITIONAL READING

- Brouwers FM, Lenders JWM, Eisenhofer G, et al. Pheochromocytomas as an endocrine emergency. *Rev Endocr Metab Disord*. 2003;4:121–128.
- Eisenhofer G. Pheochromocytoma: Diagnosis and management update. *Curr Hypertens Rep*. 2004;6: 477–484.
- Kercher KW, Novitsky YW, Park A, et al. Laparoscopic curative resection of pheochromocytomas. *Ann Surg*. 2005;741(6):919–928.
- Lenders JW, Pacak K, Walther MM, et al. Biochemical diagnosis of pheochromocytoma: Which test is best? *JAMA*. 2002;287:1427–1434.
- Manger WM. The protean manifestations of pheochromocytoma. *Horm Metab Res*. 2009;41: 658–663.
- Young WF Jr. Clinical practice: The incidentally discovered adrenal mass. *N Engl J Med*. 2007;356: 601–610.
- Yu R, Nissen NN, Chopra P, et al. Diagnosis and treatment of pheochromocytoma in an academic hospital from 1997 to 2007. *Am J Med*. 2009;122: 85–95.

 CODES

### ICD9

- 194.0 Malignant neoplasm of adrenal gland
- 227.0 Benign neoplasm of adrenal gland

# PHIMOSIS
*Nicole M. Franks*

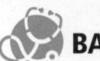 **BASICS**

## DESCRIPTION
- True phimosis is the pathologic inability to retract the foreskin over the glans of the penis as a result of scarring.
- The inability to retract a normal, supple foreskin is not true phimosis.
- The foreskin is rarely retractable at birth due to normal adhesions between the glans and the inner prepuce.
- ~90% are retractable by 3 yr of age, and 99% are retractable by 17 yr, as the epithelial cells that comprise smegma are shed.
- Parents should be instructed not to forcibly retract the foreskin.

## ETIOLOGY
Possible causes of true phimosis include:
- Trauma from forcible retraction of the foreskin
- Repetitive bouts of diaper dermatitis
- Recurrent balanoposthitis
- Poor hygiene
- Poorly performed circumcision
- Congenital anomalies

 **DIAGNOSIS**

## SIGNS AND SYMPTOMS
- Dysuria, hematuria
- Poor urinary stream
- Whitish, narrowed preputial opening of the foreskin
- Edema, erythema, and tenderness of prepuce
- *Balanoposthitis* (inflammation of the glans and foreskin)
- Ballooning of foreskin on urination in severe cases

### Physical Exam
Exam should include an evaluation for potential complications:
- Obstruction and vascular compromise of glans
- Occur only in the most extreme cases

## ESSENTIAL WORKUP
- In the majority of cases, no workup is necessary.
- In patients with severe stenosis, the complication of an *obstructive uropathy* may occur. This should be investigated by:
  - Evaluation of kidney function:
    - BUN and creatinine
  - Renal sonogram

- Phimosis secondary to recurrent balanoposthitis should prompt a workup for *diabetes mellitus*:
  - Urinalysis, serum glucose, or glycosylated hemoglobin (Hgb A1C)

## DIFFERENTIAL DIAGNOSIS
- Preputial adhesions are normal in young children.
- Balanoposthitis without phimosis

 **TREATMENT**

## PRE-HOSPITAL
- Prehospital personnel and family members should be instructed not to attempt retraction of the foreskin prior to medical evaluation.
- Unwarranted attempts may traumatize a normal, nonretractable prepuce or convert the situation to a more emergent *paraphimosis*.

## INITIAL STABILIZATION/THERAPY
None required in most cases

## ED TREATMENT/PROCEDURES

- Relieve obstructive uropathy, if present, with urethral catheterization or suprapubic aspiration.
- If vascular flow to the glans is compromised, a dorsal slit must be made in the foreskin:
  - Performed after achieving adequate penile block (see "Paraphimosis" for more detailed description of procedure)
  - This is rarely necessary in phimosis.
- Potent topical steroids for a multiweek course have been reported to successfully reduce phimosis:
  - Betamethasone dipropionate 0.05–0.1%: Apply to preputial orifice twice daily for 4–6 wk.

### Pediatric Considerations

For foreskin incision, procedural sedation will likely be needed in place of penile block.

## MEDICATION

Pain control as required

# FOLLOW-UP

## DISPOSITION

### Admission Criteria

- Obstructive uropathy
- Severe balanoposthitis with ischemia or necrosis

### Discharge Criteria

- Ability to urinate
- Adequate urologic follow-up

### Issues for Referral

Urologic follow-up for response to steroid therapy, dilation of the preputial opening, operative repair, or elective circumcision as necessary

## FOLLOW-UP RECOMMENDATIONS

Physiologic phimosis requires waiting for age-appropriate development and continued preputial hygiene.

# PEARLS AND PITFALLS

- Foreskin is normally nonretractable from the neonatal period to age 3 yr.
- Do not forcibly retract foreskin especially in children 3–17 yr, as phimosis may still be physiologically normal.
- Vascular compromise of the glans penis requires a dorsal slit to the foreskin to prevent necrosis.

# ADDITIONAL READING

- Donohoe JM, Burnette JO, Brown JA. Paraphimosis treatment. *eMedicine*. Available at: http://www.emedicine.medscape.com/article/442883. Updated October 7, 2009.
- Ghory HZ, Sharma R. Phimosis and paraphimosis. *eMedicine*. Available at: http://www.emedicine.medscape.com/article/777539. Updated April 28, 2010.
- Huang CJ. Problems of the foreskin and glans penis. *Clin Pediatr Emerg Med*. 2009;10:56–59.
- Marx JA, Hockberger RS, Walls RM. *Rosen's Emergency Medicine: Concepts and Clinical Practice*, 7th ed. St. Louis, MO: Mosby; 2009:2201–2202.
- Roberts JR, Hedges J. *Clinical Procedures in Emergency Medicine*, 5th ed. Philadelphia: Saunders; 2009:1003–1005.

## See Also (Topic, Algorithm, Electronic Media Element)

- Paraphimosis
- Priapism

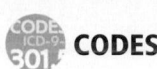 CODES

**ICD9**
605 Redundant prepuce and phimosis

# PITYRIASIS ROSEA

*Benjamin S. Heavrin*

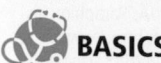 **BASICS**

## DESCRIPTION
- A self-limited skin exanthem of unknown origin primarily affecting children and young adults
- Skin findings often begin with an isolated "herald patch," an ovoid erythematous raised lesion seen along the trunk and extremities.
- A secondary eruption usually follows, where multiple smaller exanthems appear along the Langer lines of the trunk and proximal extremities in a symmetric "Christmas tree pattern."
- Nearly 80% have resolution of symptoms within 2 mo.

## ETIOLOGY
- Unknown, although there is weak evidence for a viral etiology such as herpes 6 and 7.
- Many medications have been associated with a pityriasis-like reaction:
  - Barbiturates
  - Captopril
  - Clonidine
  - Gold
  - Isotretinoin
  - Metronidazole
  - Bismuth
  - Hepatitis B vaccine
  - Gleevec
  - Interferon
- Eczema, asthma, and underlying malignancies may be weakly associated.

 **DIAGNOSIS**

## SIGNS AND SYMPTOMS
Prodromal symptoms and characteristic skin findings are discussed below.

### History
Prodromal symptoms occur in 60–70% of patients:
- Malaise, GI symptoms, respiratory symptoms

### Physical Exam
- Dermatologic findings
- Herald patch:
  - Solitary, erythematous, slightly raised papule 2–10 cm in diameter
  - Seen in 50–90% of cases
- Secondary eruption:
  - Widespread salmon-colored, elliptic, finely scaling papules
  - Usually appear symmetrically along Langer lines in a "Christmas tree" pattern
  - Generally follows herald patch by 7–14 days
  - Lesions are concentrated on the trunk and proximal extremities.
  - Pruritis is common.
- Lesions concentrated on the face and distal extremities with minimal trunk involvement characterize *inverse pityriasis*.

## Pediatric Considerations
- Inverse pityriasis, lesions on the face and distal extremities, characterize *inverse pityriasis* and may be seen more often in pediatric populations.
- Rarely, pediatric presentations may have oral lesions, usually punctate hemorrhage and ulceration.

## ESSENTIAL WORKUP
Exclude other diagnoses, especially when a herald patch is not seen:
- Secondary syphilis can have similar skin findings. Consider rapid plasma reagin (RDR) or venereal disease research laboratory (VDRL).
- KOH prep may diagnose tinea

## DIAGNOSTIC TESTS & INTERPRETATION
### Lab
None required:
- KOH and RPR/VDRL if other diagnoses are considered.

## DIFFERENTIAL DIAGNOSIS

- Herald patch:
  - Nummular eczema
  - Tinea corporis
- Secondary eruption:
  - Secondary syphilis
  - Drug eruption
  - Guttate psoriasis
  - Kaposi sarcoma
  - Lichen planus
  - Occult malignancy
  - Scabies
  - Seborrheic dermatitis
  - Tinea versicolor
  - Dermatomyositis
  - Cutaneous lymphoma
  - Lupus

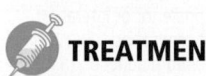 TREATMENT

### INITIAL STABILIZATION/THERAPY
None required

### ED TREATMENT/PROCEDURES
- Pityriasis is self-limiting.
- Pruritis may improve after treatment with steroids, antihistamines, and erythromycin.

## MEDICATION

- Diphenhydramine: Adult: 25–50 mg PO q.i.d. (peds: 5 mg/kg/d div. q.i.d.)
- Erythromycin: 400 mg (peds: 10 mg/kg) PO q.i.d.
- Hydrocortisone: 1% cream t.i.d.
- Prednisone: 15–40 mg (peds 0.25–0.5 mg/kg) daily

### First Line
- Diphenhydramine: Adult: 25–50 mg PO q.i.d. (peds: 5 mg/kg/d div. q.i.d.)
- Hydrocortisone: 1% cream t.i.d.

### Second Line
- Prednisone: 15–40 mg (peds 0.25–0.5 mg/kg) daily
- Erythromycin: 400 mg (peds: 10 mg/kg) PO q.i.d.

 FOLLOW-UP

### DISPOSITION

#### Admission Criteria
Pityriasis rosea is a self-limited disease; admission is not required.

#### Discharge Criteria
Patients with a clear diagnosis of pityriasis rosea may be discharged.

#### Issues for Referral
Severe refractory pruritis may require dermatology follow-up.

### FOLLOW-UP RECOMMENDATIONS
- With primary care provider as needed
- Symptoms usually resolve over 1–2 mo.

## PEARLS AND PITFALLS

- Pityriasis is usually limited to the proximal extremities and trunk. Consider alternative diagnoses beyond *inverse pityriasis* in a patient with mucous membrane or distal extremity involvement.
- Consider alternative diagnoses in those patients who appear toxic or have atypical presentations.

## ADDITIONAL READING

- Browning JC. An update on pityriasis rosea and other similar childhood exanthems. *Curr Opin Pediatr*. 2009;21:481–485.
- Chuh AA, Dofitas BL, Comisel GG, et al. Interventions for pityriasis rosea. *Cochrane Database Syst Rev*. 2007 Apr 18;(2):CD005068.
- Drago F, Broccolo F, Rebora A. Pityriasis rosea: An update with a critical appraisal of its possible herpesviral etiology. *J Am Acad Dermatol*. 2009;61: 303–318.
- Stulberg DL, Wolfrey J. Pityriasis rosea. *Am Fam Physician*. 2004;69:87–91.

 CODES

### ICD9
696.3 Pityriasis rosea

# PLACENTA PREVIA
*Roneet Lev*

 **BASICS**

## DESCRIPTION
- Placental tissue overlying or proximate to the internal cervical os
- Uterine enlargement and cervical dilation cause placental vessels near the cervix to tear, resulting in vaginal bleeding.
- >90% of placenta previa seen on ultrasound (US) before 20 wk "migrate" and does not end up as placenta previa at term.
- Increased amount of placental overlap (>15–23 mm) predicts placenta previa present at birth.
- Cause for 20% of all antepartum hemorrhage
- Classifications:
  - Complete placenta previa: Cervical os is completely covered by placenta.
  - Partial placenta previa: Cervical os is partially covered by placenta.
  - Marginal placenta previa: Edge of placenta is within 2 cm of cervical os.
  - Low-lying placenta: Placenta edge is close to cervical os, 2–3.5 cm.

## ETIOLOGY
- Unknown etiology
- Incidence: 4/1,000 births = 0.4% of pregnancies at term
- Maternal mortality: 0.03%
- Perinatal morbidity and mortality: Triple, due to preterm delivery
- Factors affecting location of implantation:
  - Increased number of curettages from spontaneous or induced abortions
  - Abnormal endometrial vascularization
  - Delayed ovulation
- Risk factors:
  - Multiparity (5% grand multiparous patients vs. 0.2% nulliparous)
  - Multiple gestation
  - Prior C-section (10% after >3 C-sections)
  - Increased maternal age (0.03% age <30 yr, 0.25% age ≥40 yr)
  - Previous placenta previa (4–8% recurrence)
  - Smoking (2–4 times increase)
  - Male fetus (14% increase)
  - Assisted fertilization
  - Residence at higher altitude
  - Asian maternal race

- Associated conditions:
  - Intrauterine growth restrictions (16%)
  - Congenital anomalies
  - Abnormal fetal presentation
  - Preterm premature rupture of the membranes
  - Amniotic fluid embolism; associated with pathologies of the placenta
  - Vasa previa: Fetal vessels course through membranes and cover os.
  - Placenta accreta, increta, percreta (growth of placenta into uterine wall) occur in 5–10% of patients with placenta previa; sustained bleeding may require C-section hysterectomy.

 **DIAGNOSIS**

## SIGNS AND SYMPTOMS
*Painless* vaginal bleeding in pregnancy after 20 wk is placenta previa until proven otherwise.

### History
- Painless bright red vaginal bleeding in 70%
- Uterine contraction in 20%
- Common incidental finding on US in 2nd trimester (6% at 16–18 wk)
- 1st episode of bleeding typically occurs at 27–32 wk.
- Bleeding may range from minor to massive; number of bleeding episodes does not correlate with degree of placenta previa.
- Inciting factors—usually no cause; recent intercourse or heavy exercise may contribute.
- Initial bleeding is often self-limited and not lethal.

### Physical Exam
- Never do a digital exam or instrument probe of the cervix in 2nd-trimester vaginal bleeding until placenta previa is ruled out.
- Sterile speculum exam can be safely performed prior to US.
- Blood seen at patient's feet is a sign of heavy bleeding.
- Hypotension and tachycardia may indicate hemorrhagic shock.
- Fetal heart tones should be monitored along with other vital signs.

## ESSENTIAL WORKUP
Vaginal ultrasonography is diagnostic procedure of choice.

## DIAGNOSTIC TESTS & INTERPRETATION
### Lab
- CBC, platelets
- Type and screen; upgrade to cross match if transfusion is indicated.
- Kleihauer-Betke (KB)—detects >5 mL of fetal cells in maternal circulation (it takes only 0.1 mL to sensitize mother if Rh negative)
- If coagulopathy suspected (rare): Prothrombin time/partial thromboplastin time, fibrin-split products, fibrinogen (<300 mg/dL is abnormal)
- Rh status

### Imaging
- Transabdominal US: 93–97% accurate:
  - False-negative: Obesity, posterior or lateral placenta, fetal head over cervical os
  - False-positive: Overdistended bladder
  - Not sufficient accuracy for placenta previa position, need to obtain transvaginal US if placenta previa is detected or uncertain findings
- Transvaginal US: 100% accurate:
  - Vaginal probe does not exacerbate bleeding.
- Color flow Doppler US: Used to determine placenta accreta
- MRI: May be useful in evaluating placental abnormalities such as accreta and percreta

## DIFFERENTIAL DIAGNOSIS
- Placenta abruption (may occur concurrently)
- Uterine rupture
- Fetal vessel rupture
- Cervical/vaginal trauma
- Cervical/vaginal lesions
- Bleeding disorder
- Spontaneous abortion
- "Bloody show" of labor

 **TREATMENT**

## PRE-HOSPITAL
- Patient with vaginal bleeding at >24 wk should be transported to a facility that can handle high risk and premature delivery.
- Place patient in left lateral recumbent position if hypotensive in 2nd half of pregnancy.
- $O_2$ and IV as with other patients

## INITIAL STABILIZATION/THERAPY

- ABCs
- 2 large-bore IVs with normal saline (NS) or lactated Ringer (LR) for resuscitation
- Left lateral recumbent position if hypotensive in 2nd half of pregnancy
- Fluid resuscitation
- Blood transfusion for hematocrit (Hct) <30 or hypotension not responding to fluids
- Fresh-frozen plasma if coagulopathy
- Fetal monitoring (heart rate <120 or >160 bpm is abnormal)
- Immediate OB consultation for symptomatic patients

## ED TREATMENT/PROCEDURES

- Emergent OB consultation for patients with active bleeding
- Volume resuscitation with 2 large-bore IVs with NS or LR
- Blood transfusion to keep Hct 30–35%
- RhoGAM if mother is Rh negative
- Fetal monitoring
- Keep NPO and on bed rest until considered stable by OB.
- Tocolytics (magnesium sulfate or terbutaline) only for contractions of preterm labor and delivery are not recommended.
- Antenatal steroids at 24–34 wk to stimulate prenatal lung maturity
- Emergency C-section or delivery for continued bleeding or fetal compromise

## MEDICATION

- RhoGAM: 1 vial (300 mg) IM; may need more >1 vial if KB indicates >15 mL of fetal RBS
- Magnesium sulfate: 6 g IV over 20 min, then 2–4 g/hr; adjust to contractions
- Betamethasone: 12 mg IM q24h × 2 doses

 FOLLOW-UP

### DISPOSITION

#### Admission Criteria
- Active bleeding placental previa is a potential obstetric emergency, and all patients should be admitted.
- Select patients may be managed on outpatient basis if bleeding is resolved. Consult OB.

#### Discharge Criteria
- Incidental finding of placenta previa by US at <28 wk with no vaginal bleeding or uterine contractions
- Patients at ≥28 wk with no active bleeding and no uterine contractions may be discharged after OB consultation to ensure follow-up.
- Pelvic rest (no intercourse or tampons in vagina) if placenta previa found after 28 wk or at any time if associated with bleeding. Asymptomatic patients with placenta previa in 2nd trimester can continue normal activities.
- 70% of patients will have a 2nd episode of bleeding.

### FOLLOW-UP RECOMMENDATIONS
Patients with incidental finding of placenta previa found at <28 wk will need regular outpatient US to determine migration of placenta.

## PEARLS AND PITFALLS

- Do not perform digital vaginal exam if suspect vaginal bleeding after 2nd trimester. Do US 1st.
- Sterile speculum exam and transvaginal US are safe and do not increase bleeding.
- Painless vaginal bleeding after 20 wk is placenta previa until proven otherwise.
- Painful vaginal bleeding after 20 wk is placental abruption until proven otherwise.
- The 2 above conditions can occur simultaneously.

## ADDITIONAL READING

- Cunningham FG, Leveno KJ, Bloom SL, et al. *Williams' Obstetrics*, 23rd ed. New York: McGraw-Hill; 2009.
- DynaMed. Placenta previa; 2009. Available at: http://www.DynamicMedical.com
- Lockwood CJ, Russo-Stieglitz K. Clinical manifestations and diagnosis of Placenta Previa. *UpToDate*; 2009. Available at: http://www.uptodate.com/patients/content/topic.do?topicKey=~18112/pmocgerp3
- Marx JA, Hockberger RS, Walls RM, et al. *Rosen's Emergency Medicine: Concepts and Clinical Practice*, 7th ed. St. Louis, MO: Mosby; 2009.

### See Also (Topic, Algorithm, Electronic Media Element)
Placental Abruption

 CODES

### ICD9
- 641.00 Placenta previa without hemorrhage, unspecified as to episode of care
- 641.10 Hemorrhage from placenta previa, unspecified as to episode of care

# PLANT POISONING

*Harry C. Karydes*

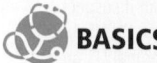 **BASICS**

## DESCRIPTION
- Exposure to plants is among the most common causes of calls to poison centers.
- Vast majority (85%) of cases are in children <6 yr old and are unintentional.

## ETIOLOGY
Positive identification of plants species should be attempted whenever possible.

### Plants with Anticholinergic Properties
- *Atropa, Brugmansia, Datura, Hyoscyamus, Solandra, Solanum*
- Competitive antagonists of acetylcholine at the muscarinic acetylcholine receptor

### Plants with Cardioactive Steroids
- *Acokanthera, Adenium, Adonis*
- *Calotropis, Convallaria, Cryptostegia*
- *Digitalis, Helleborus, Nerium*
- *Ornithogalum, Pentalinon*
- *Scilla, Strophanthus, Thevetia, Urginea*
- Inhibit $Na^+/K^+$-ATPase:
  - Therapeutically, enhance inotropy and slow heart rate
  - In excess, increase myocardial excitability, which can predispose individual to development of ventricular dysrhythmias

### Plants with Nicotine-Like Alkaloids
- *Baptisia, Caulophyllum, Conium*
- *Gymnocladus, Hippobroma, Laburnum*
- *Lobelia, Nicotiana, Sophora*
- Direct-acting agonists at the nicotinic acetylcholine receptor

### Plants with Cyanogenic Compounds
- *Eriobotrya, Hydrangea, Malus, Prunus, Sambucus*
- Metabolized to cyanide, which results in cellular energy failure

### Plants with Calcium Oxalate Crystals
- *Alocasia, Arisaema, Brassaia, Caladium, Caryota, Colocasia, Dieffenbachia*
- *Epipremnum, Monstera, Philadendron, Spathiphyllum*
- Clinical manifestations occur after stimulation/disruption of intracellular packaging (idioblasts):
  - These needles penetrate the mucous membrane and result in histamine release along with other inflammatory mediators.

### Plants with Pyrrolizidine Alkaloids
- *Crotalaria, Echium, Heliotropium*
- Metabolized to pyrroles, which injure the endothelium of the hepatic sinusoids or pulmonary vasculature

### Plants with Sodium Channel Activators
- *Aconitum, Kalmia, Leucothoe, Lyonia*
- *Pernettya, Pieris, Rhodedendron*
- *Schoenocaulon, Veratrum, Zigadenus*
- Cause persistent depolarization due to persistent sodium influx and prevent repolarization

### Plants with Toxalbumins
- *Abrus, Hura, Jatropha, Momordica*
- *Phoradendron, Ricinus, Robinia*
- Inhibit the function of ribosomes, which are responsible for protein synthesis

 **DIAGNOSIS**

## SIGNS AND SYMPTOMS
### Anticholinergic
- Dry, warm, and flushed skin
- Absent bowel sounds
- Urinary retention
- Delirium and hallucination
- Possibly elevated body temperature

### Cardioactive Steroids
- Abdominal pain
- Vomiting
- Multiple cardiac effects, which can span the continuum from junctional bradycardia to ventricular tachycardia/fibrillation
- Hyperkalemia (usually associated with poor patient prognosis)
- Digoxin-like toxicity

### Nicotine-Like Alkaloids
- Hypertension
- Tachycardia
- Diaphoresis
- Salivation
- Vomiting
- Fasciculations
- Muscle weakness
- Neuromuscular blockade (rare)

### Cyanogenic Compounds
- Typically delayed presentation
- Initial symptoms:
  - Abdominal pain
  - Vomiting
  - Lethargy
  - Sweating
- Followed by:
  - Altered mental status
  - Seizures
  - Cardiovascular collapse
  - Multiorgan system failure

### Calcium Oxalate Crystals
- Oropharygeal pain and garbled speech (after biting or chewing)
- Ocular exposure results in keratoconjunctivitis, chemosis, and vision loss (rare).
- Dermal irritation after dermal contact

### Pyrrolizidine Alkaloids
- Right upper quadrant abdominal pain
- Hepatosplenomegaly
- Jaundice
- Acute hepatoxicity
- More indolent course may lead to hepatic venous occlusion.

### Sodium Channel Activators
- Vomiting
- Perioral and distal extremity parasthesias
- Fasciculations, motor weakness leading to paralysis
- Bradycardia, atrioventricular blocks, and ventricular dysrhythmias
- Seizures

### Toxalbumins
- Gastroenteritis, diarrhea, or abdominal pain if ingested
- Localized pulmonary effects if inhaled
- Diffuse organ dysfunction if injected

### Pediatric Considerations
- Often present with lip, tongue, and oropharyngeal irritation and swelling from oxalate crystal–containing plants:
  - Potential for airway compromise
- Usually consume leaves and seeds
- Nicotine group: 1 or 2 cigarettes potentially lethal
- Jimson weed:
  - Seeds highly concentrated
  - 100 seeds equals 6 mg of atropine
  - Lethal at 4–5 g of leaf
- Yellow oleander:
  - 2 leaves lethal in 12.5-kg child

## ESSENTIAL WORKUP
- Identification of ingested material
- Workup depends on plant ingested

## DIAGNOSTIC TESTS & INTERPRETATION
### Lab
- Electrolytes, BUN, creatinine, glucose, liver function tests
- Arterial blood gas:
  - Check pH
  - Oxygen saturation
- Digoxin level for cardioglycoside plants
- Cyanide level for cyanogenic plants

### Imaging
- ECG: Dysrhythmias/bradycardia
- CXR

## DIFFERENTIAL DIAGNOSIS
- Altered mental status:
  – Drug use/alcohol
  – Seizures
  – Trauma
  – Cerebrovascular accident
  – Hypoglycemia
- Digoxin toxicity
- Gastroenteritis
- Agents causing metabolic acidosis (use mnemonic ACAAT MUD PILES, as defined in Acidosis section)
- Cardiotoxic drugs

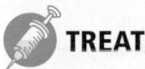

## TREATMENT
### PRE-HOSPITAL
- Nontoxic houseplants:
  – African violet
  – Aluminum plant
  – Baby's tears
  – Bird's nest fern
  – Corn plant
  – Creeping Charlie
  – Creeping Jenny
  – Gardenia
    Grape ivy
  – Jade plant
  – Parlor palm
  – Peacock plant
  – Piggyback begonia
  – Prayer plant
  – Rubber tree
  – Snake plant
  – Spider plant
  – Swedish ivy
  – Velvet plant
  – Wandering Jew
  – Wax plant
  – Zebra plant
- Collect seeds, leaves, spores in paper bag.
- Contact local botanist.
- Syrup of ipecac is not recommended in setting of severe GI distress, altered mental status.

### INITIAL STABILIZATION/THERAPY
- Airway, breathing, and circulation management (ABCs)
- 0.9% normal saline IV:
  – Aggressive volume replacement for dehydration/hypotension
  – Initiate pressors for hypotension unresponsive to fluids
- Cardiac monitoring
- Supportive care for most ingestants

### ED TREATMENT/PROCEDURES
- Supportive care
- Depending on plant exposed, dictates further care or medication/antidotal therapy

### Anticholinergic
- Benzodiazepines for agitation
- Consider physostigmine.

### Cardioactive Steroids
Digoxin-specific Fab indicated in:
- Significant bradycardia
- Tachydysrhythmia
- Hyperkalemia with or without elevated serum digoxin level

### Nicotine-Like Alkaloids
- Parenteral antihypertensives such as nitroprusside or diltiazem for hypertensive crisis
- Treat seizures with benzodiazepines.

### Cyanogenic Compounds
- Correction of electrolyte abnormalities
- Hydroxocobalamin or prepackaged cyanide antidote kit

### Calcium Oxalate Crystals
- Supportive care especially in airway management
- Viscous lidocaine and analgesics for oral ingestions
- Copious irrigation for ocular, oropharyngeal, and dermal exposure

### Pyrrolizidine Alkaloids
Liver transplantation for patients with severe disease

### Sodium Channel Activators
- Atropine for bradycardia and atrioventricular blocks
- Normal saline bolus for hypotension, or vasopressor therapy with normal saline fails

### Toxalbumins
Initiate supportive care based on clinical symptoms such as replacing GI losses with intravenous fluids and restoring electrolytes.

### MEDICATION
- Atropine: 0.5 mg (peds: 0.02 mg/kg) IV, repeat 0.5–1.0 mg IV
- 4-Dimethylaminophenol: 3.25 mg/kg IV
- Hydroxocobalamin: 50 times cyanide dose or 50 mg/kg IV
- Magnesium: 2–4 g IV
- Physostigmine: 0.5–2 mg IV
- Cyanide antidote kit:
  – Inhale amyl nitrite ampule for 30 sec every minute until sodium nitrite given.
  – Sodium nitrite: 10 mL of 3% solution or 300 mg IV over 3–5 min (peds: 0.15–0.33 mL/kg):
    ○ Monitor methemoglobin levels to keep <30%.
  – Sodium thiosulfate: 50 mL IV of 25% solution or 12.5 g (peds: 1.65 mL/kg)
- Digoxin Fab fragments: Empiric dose 5–10 vials
- Sodium bicarbonate 8.4%: 1 amp IV push until narrowing of QRS complex

## FOLLOW-UP
### DISPOSITION
**Admission Criteria**
- Dysrhythmias for cardiac monitoring
- Intractable vomiting
- Refractory hypotension
- Evidence of end-organ damage
- Altered mental status

**Discharge Criteria**
- Baseline mental status
- Tolerating fluids
- Normal cardiac activity
- No delayed sequelae

**Pediatric Considerations**
Lower threshold to admit children:
- Tend to eat more-concentrated parts
- Lower doses are lethal.
- Symptoms more nonspecific

### FOLLOW-UP RECOMMENDATIONS
Follow-up with medical toxicologist or primary care physician

## PEARLS AND PITFALLS
- Death from unintentional exposures is rare.
- Intentional exposures from herbal remedies, attempted abuse or therapeutic misadventures can be deadly.

*A special thanks to Dr. Kirk Cumpston, who contributed to the previous edition.*

## ADDITIONAL READING
- Bryant SM, Aks SE. "Are you taking any medications?" Herbal toxicities and their manifestations in the ED. *Emerg Med Pract.* 2005;7(1):1–24.
- Nelson LS, Shih RD, Balick MJ. *Handbook of Poisonous and Injurious Plants.* 2nd ed. New York: Springer; 2007;21–34.
- Palmer M, Betz JM. Plants. In: Goldfrank LR, Flomenbaum NE, Lewin NA, et al., eds. *Goldfrank's Toxicological Emergencies*, 8th ed. New York: McGraw-Hill; 2006:1577–1602.

### See Also (Topic, Algorithm, Electronic Media Element)
- Acidosis
- Cyanide Poisoning
- Digoxin Poisoning

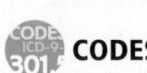

## CODES
**ICD9**
988.2 Toxic effect of berries and other plants eaten as food

# PLEURAL EFFUSION

*Jeremy T. Chou*

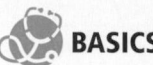 **BASICS**

## DESCRIPTION

- Normal conditions:
  - Pleural space usually contains 0.1–0.2 mL/kg (30 mL in an adult) of clear, low-protein fluid that helps facilitate movement of the pulmonary parenchyma within the thoracic space.
  - Fluid formation and reabsorption are governed by hydrostatic and oncotic forces acting at the parietal and visceral surfaces.
  - Normally, the sum of these forces results in movement of fluid into the pleural space from the parietal surface and reabsorption at the visceral surface.
  - Lymphatics help remove any excess fluid.
- Alteration of any of the above factors results in abnormal fluid accumulation.
- Pleural effusions are classified as transudative or exudative:
  - Transudative effusion:
    ○ An ultrafiltrate of serum, containing low protein and cells
    ○ Results from increase in hydrostatic pressure and/or decrease in oncotic pressure
    ○ Pleural surface is not involved in the primary pathologic process.
  - Exudative effusion:
    ○ Contains high amount of protein and cells
    ○ Results from pathologic disease of the pleural surface leading to membrane permeability and/or disruption of lymphatic reabsorption

## ETIOLOGY

- Transudative effusions:
  - Congestive heart failure (CHF)
  - Peritoneal dialysis
  - Cirrhosis with ascites
  - Pulmonary embolism
  - Acute atelectasis
  - Nephrotic syndrome
  - Myxedema
  - Hypoproteinemia
  - Superior vena cava syndrome
  - Meigs syndrome:
    ○ Triad of ascites, benign ovarian tumor, and pleural effusion
- Exudative effusions:
  - Pulmonary or pleural infection:
    ○ Bacterial, viral, fungal, tuberculosis (TB), parasitic
  - Primary lung cancer
  - Mesothelioma
  - Metastasis (often from breast cancer, ovarian cancer, or lymphoma)
  - Pericarditis
  - Pulmonary embolism
- Intraabdominal disorders:
  - Pancreatitis, hepatitis, cholecystitis
  - Subdiaphragmatic abscess
  - Esophageal rupture
  - Peritonitis
  - Meigs syndrome

- Rheumatologic disease:
  - Systemic lupus erythematosus
  - Rheumatoid arthritis
  - Sarcoidosis
- Trauma:
  - Hemothorax
  - Chylothorax
- Drugs:
  - Drug-induced lupus
  - Nitrofurantoin, methysergide, dantrolene, amiodarone, bromocriptine
  - Crack cocaine

 **DIAGNOSIS**

## SIGNS AND SYMPTOMS

- Small effusions are often asymptomatic.
- Dyspnea, pleuritic chest pain, and/or cough
- Tachypnea, hypoxia, decreased breath sounds, and/or dullness to percussion

### History

- Underlying primary pathologic process (CHF, pneumonia, pulmonary embolus, pancreatitis) is often the source of complaints.
- Dyspnea on exertion or at rest
- Cough with large effusion
- Pleuritic chest pain with inflammation of pleura
- Empyema: Fever, fatigue, weight loss

### Physical Exam

- Decreased breath sounds
- Decreased tactile fremitus
- Increased egophony for large effusions
- Dullness to chest percussion
- Pleural friction rub
- Examine for the primary cause of pleural effusion.

## ESSENTIAL WORKUP

- Cardiac monitor and pulse oximetry
- CBC, comprehensive metabolic panel, coagulation panel
- Chest radiography
- Search for underlying cause

## DIAGNOSTIC TESTS & INTERPRETATION

### Lab

- CBC
- Electrolytes, BUN/creatinine, glucose, serum lactate dehydrogenase (LDH), serum protein
- Pulse oximetry or arterial blood gas
- Coagulation panel
- Pleural fluid analysis to determine if transudative or exudative effusion:
  - Check pleural protein and LDH levels.
  - Light's criteria: Fluid is likely exudative if 1 or more of the following criteria are met:
    ○ Pleural fluid protein/serum protein >0.5
    ○ Pleural fluid LDH/serum LDH >0.6
    ○ Pleural fluid LDH >2/3 upper limit of normal serum LDH

- If effusion is transudative, no further fluid analysis is usually necessary.
- Pleural fluid analysis to determine etiology of exudative effusion:
  - Initial testing: Cell count with differential, Gram stain and culture, acid fast bacilli stain, pH, glucose, and cytology
  - Selective tests based on clinical scenario include triglycerides, amylase, albumin, creatinine, adenosine deaminase, and tumor markers.
  - RBC and Hct:
    ○ 5,000–100,000/mm³ nonspecific
    ○ >100,000/mm³ suggestive of malignancy, trauma, or pulmonary embolus
    ○ Pleural fluid Hct >0.5 serum Hct is by definition a hemothorax.
    ○ Other causes: Malignancy, TB, aortic rupture
    ○ Heparinize and chill hemorrhagic samples to be sent for cytology.
  - WBC:
    ○ 1,000–10,000/mm³ nonspecific
    ○ >10,000/mm³ suggestive of parapneumonic effusion, empyema, pancreatitis, rheumatologic, malignancy, or TB
  - Glucose:
    ○ Glucose <60 mg/dL suggestive of complicated parapneumonic effusion/empyema, malignancy, esophageal rupture, or rheumatologic disease
  - Triglyceride:
    ○ Triglycerides >100 mg/dL suggestive of chylous effusion from disruption of thoracic duct
  - Amylase:
    ○ Amylase >200 IU/L suggestive of pancreatitis, esophageal rupture, malignancy, TB, or empyema
  - pH:
    ○ Send in a chilled heparinized arterial blood gas syringe.
    ○ pH <7.0 suggests complicated parapneumonic effusion or empyema
  - Cytology identifies malignant cells.

### Imaging

- Chest radiograph:
  - Upright chest film:
    ○ Blunting of the costophrenic angle
    ○ Requires at least 200–250 mL of fluid
    ○ Presence of subpulmonic effusions may be indicated by loss of supradiaphragmatic vascular markings or an increased space between the gastric bubble and pulmonary parenchyma.
  - Lateral decubitus film:
    ○ Can identify as little as 5–10 mL of fluid.
    ○ Suspect a loculated effusion or alternative diagnosis if effusion fails to layer.
- US:
  - Has similar sensitivity to lateral decubitus film and can detect as little as 5–10 mL of fluid.
  - Indicated as a guide for thoracentesis, particularly if a difficult tap is anticipated.

- CT chest with IV contrast:
  – Most sensitive study for detecting pleural fluid collections and identifying loculated effusions.
  – Useful for determination of underlying lung process such as masses and pleural thickening

### ALERT
- Consider pulmonary embolism as a cause of unexplained pleural effusion and obtain the correct diagnostic test.
- Obtain lateral decubitus films prior to performing thoracentesis to avoid misdiagnosis and procedural complications.

### Diagnostic Procedures/Surgery
Diagnostic/therapeutic ED thoracentesis:

- Indication:
  – Diagnose new effusion in toxic-appearing patient.
  – Suspected parapneumonic effusions (including patients with previously diagnosed effusions)
  – Symptomatic dyspnea caused by large effusions.
  – Diagnostic thoracentesis of a nonparapneumonic effusion in a stable patient can be deferred until after the patient has been admitted.
- No absolute contraindications.
- Relative contraindications:
  – Platelets <50,000/mm$^3$
  – Prothrombin and partial thromboplastin time >2 × normal level
  – Serum creatinine >6
- Correct coagulopathy if present.
- Position patient upright with arms crossed in front to elevate scapula.
- Identify superior border of effusion via percussion, US, or egophony.
- Mark area 1 interspace below this in the posterior axillary line or the mid-scapular line.
- Prepare area with Betadine, dry, and drape for sterile field.
- Anesthetize with 2% lidocaine.
- Attach 3-way stopcock between needle and syringe. Enter superior border of rib with needle bevel down, gently aspirating while advancing.
- Use a 20-gauge needle for simple diagnostic aspiration.
- Use a 16–18-gauge needle/catheter (commercial kit) for therapeutic aspiration.
- Caution: Entering inferior aspect of rib risks lacerating neurovascular bundle.
- Advance catheter over or through needle once pleural space entered.
- Minimum of 100 cc required for basic studies (protein, LDH, cell count, Gram stain and culture)—more required for cytology and additional studies.
- Avoid withdrawing >1,500 cc to prevent postexpansion pulmonary edema.
- Intraprocedural chest pain may indicate trapped lung or pneumothorax; stop procedure and obtain chest radiograph.
- After obtaining fluid, withdraw needle, apply pressure, dress, and obtain postprocedural chest radiograph for pneumothorax.
- Indications for tube thoracostomy:
  – Loculated effusion
  – Aspiration of pus
  – Complicated parapneumonic effusion with pH <7.0, or pleural glucose <60 mg/dL, or positive pleural Gram stain or culture
  – Hemothorax

## DIFFERENTIAL DIAGNOSIS
- Intraparenchymal densities:
  – Lobar collapse
  – Mass, tumor, infiltrative disease
  – Pneumonia
- Pleural densities:
  – Pleural scaring
  – Mesothelioma, metastatic disease
- Other:
  – Herniated abdominal contents
  – Paralyzed diaphragm

 **TREATMENT**

### PRE-HOSPITAL
- Give high-flow oxygen.
- Apply cardiac monitor and pulse oximeter.
- Initiate IV line access.

### INITIAL STABILIZATION/THERAPY
- ABCs
- High-flow oxygen for shortness of breath
- Emergency thoracentesis for significant respiratory compromise.

### ED TREATMENT/PROCEDURES
- Identify and treat underlying primary pathologic process:
  CHF, pneumonia, intra-abdominal infection
- Surgical consult for tube thoracostomy if empyema found.
- Interventional radiology or pulmonology for loculated effusions.

### MEDICATION
#### First Line
- CHF: Diuresis
- Parapneumonic effusion: Antibiotics
- Pulmonary embolism: Anticoagulation:
  – Bloody effusion is not a contraindication to anticoagulation.

#### Second Line
- Rheumatologic disease: NSAIDs and steroids
- Loculated effusion: Injection of streptokinase or urokinase into pleural space by thoracic surgeon or pulmonologist

 **FOLLOW-UP**

### DISPOSITION
#### Admission Criteria
- Respiratory compromise
- Unknown cause of the effusion
- Primary process requires hospitalization
- Presence or suspected parapneumonic effusion or empyema
- Observation for 6 hr or admission for potential complications of thoracentesis:
  – Pneumothorax
  – Postexpansion pulmonary edema
- ICU admission for severe hemodynamic and respiratory compromise

#### Discharge Criteria
- Source of the pleural effusion is known.
- No evidence of respiratory compromise exists.
- Majority of effusions will resolve if the primary process is treated appropriately.
- Patient must be reliable and have access to a telephone, a supportive social environment, and adequate follow-up.

#### Issues for Referral
Arrange appropriate follow-up with oncologist or pulmonologist prior to discharge.

### FOLLOW-UP RECOMMENDATIONS
Patients should be instructed to return to the ED for worsening dyspnea, fever/chills, or other symptoms of respiratory distress.

## PEARLS AND PITFALLS
- The most common causes of pleural effusion are CHF, pneumonia, and malignancy.
- Identify and treat the underlying cause of the pleural effusion.
- Failure to identify fatal causes of pleural effusion such as pulmonary embolism, esophageal rupture, or hemothorax
- Failure to drain large effusions that are causing respiratory or circulatory compromise

## ADDITIONAL READING
- Blok B. Thoracentesis. In: Roberts JR, Hedges JR. *Clinical Procedures in Emergency Medicine*, 5th ed. Philadelphia, PA: Saunders Elsevier; 2009.
- Kosowsky JM. Pleural disease. In: Marx JA, ed. *Rosen's emergency medicine: Concepts and clinical practice*, 7th ed. Philadelphia, PA: Mosby Elsevier; 2009.
- Light R. Pleural effusion. *N Engl J Med.* 346(25): 1971–1977.

### See Also (Topic, Algorithm, Electronic Media Element)
- Congestive Heart Failure
- Hemothorax
- Pancreatitis
- Pneumonia, Adult
- Pneumonia, Pediatric
- Pulmonary Embolism
- Systemic Lupus Erythematous
- Tube Thoracostomy
- The author gratefully acknowledges the contributions of Scott Murray and Edward Ullman for their previous editions of this chapter.

 **CODES**

#### ICD9
- 511.1 Pleurisy with effusion, with mention of a bacterial cause other than tuberculosis
- 511.9 Unspecified pleural effusion

# Pneumocystis carinii PNEUMONIA
*Alan M. Kumar*

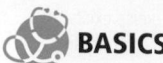

## BASICS

### DESCRIPTION
- Renamed *Pneumocystis jirovecii* pneumonia but still referred to as PCP
- Most common opportunistic infection in patients with HIV, even with PCP prophylaxis and antiretroviral therapy
- Believed to be transmitted by respiratory-aerosol route:
  - Cysts colonize respiratory tract.
  - Cysts rupture and multiple trophozoites release and form foamy exudate in alveoli.
- Most cases are believed to represent reactivation of latent disease, although person-to-person transmission suggested.
- Actual mode of transmission is unclear.

### ETIOLOGY
- Controversy surrounds the classification of *Pneumocystis* as a parasite or fungus.
- *Pneumocystis* occurs in hosts with altered cellular immunity:
  - HIV infection (most common, especially when CD4 count <200 cells/mm$^3$)
  - Cancer
  - Corticosteroid treatment
  - Organ transplantation
  - Malnutrition

### Pediatric Considerations
PCP in children is typically more severe.

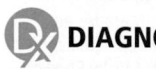

## DIAGNOSIS

### SIGNS AND SYMPTOMS
- Subacute presentation
- Up to 7% of patients can be asymptomatic.
- Patients on inhaled pentamidine prophylaxis may have milder symptoms:
  - Increased incidence of pneumothorax
  - Increased incidence of extrapulmonary disease

### History
- Fever
- Cough with none or minimal amount of white sputum
- Dyspnea on exertion or at rest:
  - Progressive over days (most common in non–HIV-immunocompromised hosts)
  - Indolent, developing over weeks to months (more common in HIV-positive hosts)
  - Oxygen desaturation with exercise
- Chills
- Fatigue
- Weight loss
- Chest pain

### Physical Exam
- Tachypnea
- Tachycardia
- Crackles and rhonchi on lung examination

### ESSENTIAL WORKUP
- CBC
- Electrolytes
- Arterial blood gas (ABG)
- Lactate dehydrogenase (LDH)
- Blood cultures
- Chest x-ray

### DIAGNOSTIC TESTS & INTERPRETATION
#### Lab
- ABG:
  - Obtain in all cases of PCP.
  - Calculate the alveolar-arterial (A-a) gradient (usually increased).
  - Adjunctive corticosteroid therapy for A-a gradient >35 mm Hg or PaO$_2$ <70 mm Hg
- LDH:
  - Elevated in HIV-positive patients with PCP compared to non-PCP pneumonia
  - Higher levels correlate with poorer prognosis.

#### Imaging
- Chest radiograph:
  - Classically reveals bilateral interstitial or central alveolar infiltrates
  - Radiograph normal in up to 25% of patients with PCP
  - Early or mild infection associated with decreased sensitivity
  - Atypical presentations include:
    - Lobar infiltrates
    - Cysts
    - Pneumothoraces
    - Pleural effusions
    - Nodular infiltrates
  - Prophylaxis with aerosolized pentamidine is a risk factor for developing predominantly upper lobe.
  - Chest radiograph abnormalities can persist for months after treatment.
- High-resolution chest CT:
  - High sensitivity for PCP in HIV-positive patients.
  - Reveals patchy ground-glass attenuation

#### Diagnostic Procedures/Surgery
- Induced sputum:
  - Definitive diagnosis requires presence of *Pneumocystis* organisms in an appropriately stained respiratory specimen.
  - Specificity approaches 100%, but sensitivity depends on quality of induced sputum and lab expertise.
  - Less sensitive in patients on inhaled pentamidine prophylaxis and non–HIV-positive patients
- Bronchoalveolar lavage:
  - Perform if the induced sputum is nondiagnostic and the suspicion for PCP is still high.
  - Sensitivity 80–100%

### DIFFERENTIAL DIAGNOSIS
Constellation of dyspnea, fever, diffuse radiographic infiltrates, minimal or nonproductive cough, and slow progressive course suggests atypical cause of the pneumonia:
- *Chlamydia pneumoniae*
- *Legionella*
- *Mycoplasma*
- Tuberculosis
- Viral pneumonia (especially cytomegalovirus)

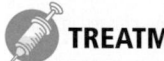

## TREATMENT

### PRE-HOSPITAL
Provide supplemental oxygen for symptomatic patients.

### INITIAL STABILIZATION/THERAPY
- ABCs
- Provide adequate oxygenation with nasal cannula up to 100% nonrebreather.
- Perform endotracheal intubation in those with refractory hypoxemia despite maximal oxygenation or hypercarbic respiratory failure.
- At least 500–1,000 cc 0.9% normal saline IV bolus for hypotension, sepsis, dehydration

## ED TREATMENT/PROCEDURES

- Initiate antibiotics:
  - IV Bactrim is the first-line agent.
  - IV pentamidine for those who cannot tolerate Bactrim
  - Oral therapy is an option for well-appearing patients.
  - Alternative regimens include trimethoprim, dapsone, clindamycin-primaquine, and atovaquone.
  - Continue antibiotics for 21 days.
- Adjunctive corticosteroids in patients with A-a gradient >35 mm Hg or $PaO_2$ <70 mm Hg:
  - Must start within 1st 72 hr of treatment
- Isolate suspected PCP patients from others who are immunocompromised.

## MEDICATION

- Atovaquone: 750 mg (peds: dosing not established) PO q12h
- Clindamycin/primaquine: Clindamycin 900 mg (peds: dosing not established) IV q8h or 300–450 mg PO q6h and primaquine 15–30 mg (peds: dosing not established) PO per day
- Pentamidine: 4 mg/kg/24 hr IV over 1 hr (peds: 150 mg/m$^2$ IV per day for 5 days, then 100 mg/m$^2$ IV per day for 16 days)
- Prednisone: 40 mg (peds: Dosing not established) PO q12h for 5 days, 40 mg PO per day for 5 days, then 20 mg PO per day for 11 days (IV methylprednisolone at 75% of the prednisone dose may be substituted)
- Trimethoprim/dapsone: Trimethoprim 15–20 mg/kg/d IV div. q8h plus dapsone 100 mg PO per day (peds: Dosing not established)
- Trimethoprim/sulfamethoxazole (Bactrim): Trimethoprim 15–20 mg/kg/d IV div. q6h and sulfamethoxazole 100 mg/kg/d IV div. q6h (peds: Dosing same)

### Pediatric Considerations

- Treatment of choice is IV trimethoprim/sulfamethoxazole, followed by IV pentamidine.
- Dosing for alternative medications not yet established (consult pediatric infectious disease specialist).

 FOLLOW-UP

### DISPOSITION

#### Admission Criteria

- Moderate to severe disease ($PaO_2$ <70 mm Hg or A-a gradient >35 mm Hg)
- Inability to digest medications
- Inability to return for careful follow-up

#### Discharge Criteria

- Nontoxic clinical appearance
- Mild disease state (no hypoxemia or A-a gradient)
- Ability to tolerate medications
- Close follow-up arranged
- If results of induced sputum are not available, add macrolide to empirical regimen.

### FOLLOW-UP RECOMMENDATIONS

Close follow-up must be arranged with infectious disease specialist to allow for outpatient management.

## PEARLS AND PITFALLS

- Include PCP in differential diagnosis in any patient presenting with shortness of breath who is immunocompromised or is suspected of having undiagnosed HIV.
- Patients considered for PCP are also more likely to have TB or atypical bacterial pneumonia.
- Well-appearing patients with low oxygen saturations are at higher risk for complications.

## ADDITIONAL READING

- Kovacs JA, Gill VJ, Meshnick S, et al. New insights into transmission, diagnosis and drug treatment of PCP. *JAMA*. 2001;286:2450.
- Santamauro JT, Stover DE. *Pneumocystis carinii pneumonia. Med Clin North Am*. 1997;81(2): 299–318.
- Wolff AJ, O'Donnell AE. HIV-related pulmonary infections: A review of the recent literature. *Curr Opin Pulm Med*. 2003;9:210.

### See Also (Topic, Algorithm, Electronic Media Element)

- HIV/AIDS
- Pneumonia, Adult
- Pneumonia, Pediatric
- Tuberculosis

 CODES

ICD9
136.3 Pneumocystosis

# PNEUMOMEDIASTINUM

*Matthew D. Bitner*

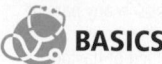

## BASICS

### DESCRIPTION
- Presence of free air or gas within the mediastinum (mediastinal emphysema)
- May originate from esophagus, lungs, or bronchial tree (*aerodigestive* process)
- May occur spontaneously or as result of trauma, surgery, or other pathologic processes
- Spontaneous pneumomediastinum:
  - Caused by extrapleural tracheobronchial tears:
    o Increased alveolar pressure, low perivascular pressures, or both
    o Terminal alveolar rupture into the lung interstitium
    o Dissection of air into the hilum and subsequently the mediastinum along a pressure gradient
    o Mediastinal air then dissects into the fascial planes, most commonly into the tissues of the neck.
  - Often in setting of a Valsalva maneuver, forceful vomiting, in association with bronchospasm or inhalational drug use
  - Men > women (2:1 in some series)
  - Young > old
  - Pediatric patients have a bimodal age distribution of peak incidence (<7 and 13–17 yr)
- Relatively rare, 1/30,000–40,000 hospital admissions

### ETIOLOGY
- Primary or spontaneous pneumomediastinum:
  - Associated with forced Valsalva maneuvers:
    o Illicit inhalation drug use (marijuana, cocaine, methamphetamine)
    o Preexisting lung disorders (interstitial lung disease, pulmonary fibrosis, pneumonitis)
    o Labor and delivery
    o Forceful straining during exercise
    o Straining during defecation
    o Coughing
    o Sneezing
    o Vomiting
    o Inflation of party balloons
    o Pulmonary function testing
    o Anorexia nervosa
    o Obesity
  - Has been rarely described after dental extraction/procedures.

- Secondary pneumomediastinum:
  - Secondary to thoracic barotrauma
  - Common traumatic mechanisms:
    o Motor vehicle collision
    o Fall
    o Blows to chest or neck
  - Positive-pressure ventilation
  - Esophageal rupture (Boerhaave syndrome)
  - In association with mediastinal infection caused by gas-forming organisms
- Tension pneumomediastinum:
  - Rare but life-threatening event
  - Usually in patients on positive-pressure ventilation
- May be associated with pneumopericardium and pneumothorax/tension pneumothorax

## DIAGNOSIS

### SIGNS AND SYMPTOMS
- Chest pain:
  - Sharp
  - Pleuritic
  - Retrosternal
  - Radiating to back and arms
  - Often positional
- Dyspnea
- Neck pain:
  - Occurs in association with dissection of air into soft tissues of neck
  - Often described as "neck swelling," "neck pain," "throat pain," or "difficulty swallowing"
- Subcutaneous emphysema:
  - Most commonly located to the supraclavicular area and anterior neck
- Dysphagia
- Dysphonia/hoarseness
- Hamman crunch: Presence of a precordial crinkling or crepitance during systole:
  - Uncommon but pathognomonic
  - Best heard with patient in left lateral decubitus position
- Meckler triad (esophageal rupture): Vomiting, lower chest pain, and cervical subcutaneous emphysema following overindulgence of food or alcohol

### History
- Inhalational drug use
- Asthma exacerbation
- Preexisting lung disorders
- Forceful vomiting (such as in diabetic ketoacidosis [DKA])
- Preceding athletic activity

### Physical Exam
- Subcutaneous emphysema
- Hamman crunch

### ESSENTIAL WORKUP
- Exclude secondary causes, notably esophageal rupture.
- Chest radiography

### DIAGNOSTIC TESTS & INTERPRETATION
#### Lab
CBC if there is suspicion of mediastinitis (the most concerning consequence of esophageal rupture, with high morbidity and mortality)

#### Imaging
- CXR:
  - Most valuable initial test
  - Important to include lateral view because mediastinal air is often missed on posterior-anterior view
  - Aids in excluding pneumothorax, pneumopericardium
  - Identification of a pleural effusion or parenchymal infiltrate suggests an esophageal rupture.
  - Negative in up to 30% of cases
  - Spinnaker sail sign or "angel wing" sign (produced by air lifting the thymus off the heart and major vessels)
  - Continuous diaphragm sign (air collecting between the diaphragm and the pericardium)
  - Subcutaneous or superior mediastinal emphysema
- Chest CT:
  - Imaging test of choice if suspicion is high but CXR is negative (CXR has high false-negative rate)
- Esophagram with water-soluble contrast material:
  - Study of choice to exclude diagnosis of esophageal rupture

#### Diagnostic Procedures/Surgery
- Esophagoscopy:
  - Limited usefulness (overutilized)
  - May be used to further delineate injuries identified with CT and/or esophagram
- Laryngoscopy/bronchoscopy:
  - Limited usefulness (overutilized)
  - May be used to exclude diagnosis of laryngeal/tracheobronchial injury
- Pericardiocentesis:
  - Only in the setting of tension pneumopericardium in the crashing patient
- Tube thoracostomy:
  - Only in the setting of concomitant pneumothorax of sufficient size or progression to require such

## DIFFERENTIAL DIAGNOSIS

- Aortic dissection
- Coronary ischemia
- Esophageal diverticula
- Esophageal webs
- Mediastinitis
- Myocarditis
- Pericarditis
- Pneumonia
- Pneumopericardium
- Pneumothorax/tension pneumothorax
- Pulmonary embolus
- Schatzki rings

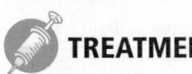 TREATMENT

### PRE-HOSPITAL

- Resuscitation of the acutely ill patient (as in the septic mediastinitis patient)
- In the appropriate setting, standard care of the trauma patient
- Rapid patient evolution and transport to an appropriate facility

### INITIAL STABILIZATION/THERAPY

- IV access
- Oxygen
- Cardiac monitoring
- Pulse oximetry

### ED TREATMENT/PROCEDURES

- Spontaneous pneumomediastinum:
  - Usually a benign, self-limiting condition
  - Does not require specific treatment
  - Efforts should focus on pain relief and reassurance once diagnosis is confirmed.
  - High-flow oxygen may facilitate the reabsorption of nitrogen and provide comfort.
  - Condition is self-limiting and may be expected to resolve over 2–5 days.
- Secondary pneumomediastinum:
  - Once diagnosis is made, direct invasive diagnostic modalities toward the most likely underlying cause (esophagoscopy, laryngoscopy, bronchoscopy).
  - Direct therapy toward underlying cause.

## MEDICATION

- Treat underlying cause aggressively (eg, asthma exacerbation or DKA).
- Oxygen 15 L via nonrebreather mask
- Analgesia (nonnarcotic and narcotic as necessary)
- Antibiotics have limited use, but in the setting of concern for mediastinitis, use broad-spectrum coverage to include GI flora, resistant organisms, and *Pseudomonas*:
  - Vancomycin 1 g IV q12h *and*
  - Piperacillin/tazobactam 3.375 g IV q6h *and*
  - Clindamycin 600 mg IV q8h *or* metronidazole 500 mg IV q8h

 FOLLOW-UP

### DISPOSITION

#### Admission Criteria

- Secondary pneumomediastinum
- Associated pneumothorax
- Possibility of esophageal rupture has not been excluded
- Abnormal vital signs
- Ill/toxic-appearing patient
- Intractable pain
- Underlying disorder requires admission (asthma exacerbation, exacerbation of lung disorder, DKA).
- Social situation prevents compliance or follow up
- Extremes of age (pediatric and elderly)
- Immunosuppression
- Failure of outpatient management

#### Discharge Criteria

- Spontaneous pneumomediastinum
- Normal vital signs
- No pneumothorax
- No significant comorbidities
- Period of observation in the ED with resolution of symptoms
- Close outpatient follow up

## FOLLOW-UP RECOMMENDATIONS

- Patients should be followed up for reevaluation of clinical symptoms and imaging for resolution of the process.
- Recurrent spontaneous pneumomediastinum may warrant cardiothoracic consultation for further diagnostic evaluation (invasive studies).

## PEARLS AND PITFALLS

- Ensure that underlying causes are excluded.
- Be aware of typical presenting features, preexisting conditions, and precipitating factors associated with pneumomediastinum.
- Hamman crunch is pathognomonic but not commonly seen.
- Remember Meckler triad:
  - Vomiting
  - Lower chest pain
  - Cervical subcutaneous emphysema

## ADDITIONAL READING

- Al-Mufarrej F, Badar J, Gharagozloo F, et al. Spontaneous pneumomediastinum: Diagnostic and therapeutic interventions. *J Cardiothoracic Surg.* 2008;59(3):1–4.
- Bullaro F, Bartoletti S. Spontaneous pneumomediastinum in children. *Pediatr Emerg Care.* 2007;23(1): 28–30.
- Dissanaike S, Shalhub S, Jurkovich G. The evaluation of pneumomediastinum in blunt trauma patients. *J Trauma.* 2008;65(6):1340–1345.
- Iyer V, Joshi A, Ryu J. Spontaneous pneumomediastinum. *Mayo Clinic Proc.* 2009;84(5).417–421.

### See Also (Topic, Algorithm, Electronic Media Element)

- Pneumothorax
- Vomiting, Adult
- The author gratefully acknowledges the contributions of Jennifer De la Pena and Leon D. Sanchez for the previous edition of this chapter.

 CODES

### ICD9

518.1 Interstitial emphysema

# PNEUMONIA, ADULT

Jonathan Roberts
Jason Imperato

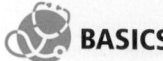

## BASICS

### DESCRIPTION
- Epidemiology:
  - 7th-leading cause of death in U.S., accounting for 1.7 million yearly admissions, with 5.4–22% mortality rate
- Highest mortality in elderly and patients with the following coexisting conditions:
  - Chronic heart, lung, liver, and kidney disease
  - Diabetes mellitus
  - Alcoholism
  - Malignancy
  - Asplenia
  - Immunosuppression
  - Use of antimicrobials within last 3 mo
- Classifications:
  - Source based:
    - Community acquired (CAP)
    - Health care associated (HCAP)
    - Hospital acquired (HAP)
    - Ventilator associated (VAP)
  - Symptom based:
    - Typical
    - Atypical
- Complications:
  - Bacteremia
  - Sepsis
  - Abscess
  - Empyema
  - Respiratory failure

### ETIOLOGY
- CAP (typicals):
  - *Streptococcus pneumoniae*
  - *Haemophilus influenzae*
  - *Klebsiella pneumoniae*
  - *Moraxella catarrhalis*
  - *Streptococcus pyogenes*
  - *Staphylococcus aureus*
- CAP (atypicals):
  - *Mycoplasma pneumoniae*
  - *Chlamydia pneumoniae*
  - *Legionella pneumophila*
  - Viral
- HCAP/HAP/VAP:
  - Gram-negatives (*Pseudomonas, Stenotrophomonas*)
  - Methicillin-resistant *Staphylococcus aureus* (MRSA)
- Immunosuppressed:
  - Fungus
  - *Pneumocystis carinii*
- Aspiration:
  - Chemical pneumonitis ± oral and gastric anaerobes

## DIAGNOSIS

### SIGNS AND SYMPTOMS
#### History
- Typical:
  - Acute onset
  - Fever
  - Chills
  - Rigors
  - Cough
  - Purulent sputum
  - Shortness of breath
  - Pleuritic chest pain
- Atypical:
  - Subacute onset
  - Viral prodrome
  - Nonproductive cough
  - Low-grade fever
  - Headache
  - Myalgias
  - Malaise
  - Absence of pleurisy and rigors

#### Physical Exam
- Vital signs:
  - Tachypnea
  - Tachycardia
  - Hypoxia
  - Fever
- Pulmonary examination:
  - Dullness to percussion
  - Tactile fremitus
  - Egophony
  - Rales
  - Rhonchi
  - Decreased breath sounds
- Note that pneumonia may be present in the absence of the above signs of consolidation.

#### Geriatric Considerations
- Elderly patients have higher morbidity and mortality from pneumonia.
- Atypical presentations are more common.

### ESSENTIAL WORKUP
Combination of clinical and radiographic diagnosis

### DIAGNOSTIC TESTS & INTERPRETATION
#### Lab
- General:
  - CBC with differential:
    - Very high and very low WBC counts predict increased morbidity.
  - Serum chemistry
- Others:
  - Arterial blood gas
  - Blood cultures
  - Sputum cultures and gram stain
  - Urine *Legionella* antigen
  - C-reactive protein possibly helpful

#### Imaging
Chest radiograph:
- General:
  - Findings are nonspecific for particular infectious etiologies.
  - May be deferred in young, healthy patients receiving empiric outpatient management.
  - Negative imaging should not preclude antimicrobial therapy in patients with clinical diagnosis.
- Suggestive findings:
  - Silhouette sign (R. heart border = RML, L. heart border = lingula, R. hemidiaphragm = RLL, L. hemidiaphragm = LLL)
  - Air bronchograms
  - Segmental or subsegmental consolidation
  - Diffuse interstitial opacities
  - Pleural effusion
  - Empyema
  - Abscess
  - Cavitation

#### Diagnostic Procedures/Surgery
Thoracentesis:
- For large effusions, enigmatic pneumonia, and patients who fail to respond to standard therapy

### DIFFERENTIAL DIAGNOSIS
- Asthma
- Bronchitis
- CHF
- COPD
- Foreign-body aspiration
- Occupational or environmental exposure
- Pneumothorax
- Pulmonary embolism
- Tumor

## TREATMENT

### PRE-HOSPITAL
- IV access
- Supplemental oxygen
- Cardiac monitor
- Consider inhaled bronchodilators.
- Consider endotracheal intubation in cases of severe respiratory distress.

### INITIAL STABILIZATION/THERAPY
- IV access and fluid resuscitation as needed
- Supplemental oxygen
- Cardiac monitor
- Inhaled bronchodilators
- Endotracheal intubation in cases of severe respiratory distress as indicated

### ED TREATMENT/PROCEDURES

- American Thoracic Society guidelines for empiric therapy:
- Outpatient:
  - Previously healthy, no coexisting conditions:
    - Macrolide (azithromycin) OR doxycycline
  - Significant coexisting conditions (see prior):
    - Combination $\beta$-lactam (ceftriaxone, cefuroxime, cefpodoxime, high-dose amoxicillin, Augmentin) PLUS macrolide (azithromycin) OR
    - Respiratory floroquinolone (levofloxacin, moxifloxacin) alone
- Inpatient:
  - Noncritical care:
    - Combination $\beta$-lactam (ceftriaxone, cefuroxime, cefpodoxime, ampicillin/sulbactam) PLUS macrolide (azithromycin) OR
    - Respiratory floroquinolone (levofloxacin, moxifloxacin) alone
    - For aspiration, consider adding clindamycin OR metronidazole.
  - Critical care:
    - Combination $\beta$-lactam (ceftriaxone, cefotaxime, ceftazidime, ampicillin-sulbactam) PLUS macrolide (azithromycin) OR respiratory floroquinolone (levofloxacin, moxifloxacin)
    - For Pseudomonas, consider adding antipseudomonal agent (piperacillin/tazobactam, imipenem, meropenem, cefepime) PLUS antipseudomonal fluoroquinolone (high-dose levofloxacin) OR antipseudomonal agent (see above) PLUS aminoglycoside (gentamicin) PLUS macrolide (azithromycin).
    - For MRSA, consider adding vancomycin OR linezolid.
    - For aspiration, consider adding clindamycin OR metronidazole.
    - For drug-resistant Streptococcuspneumoniae, consider adding vancomycin.

### MEDICATION

- Amoxicillin-clavulanate (Augmentin): 500 mg PO q12h
- Ampicillin-sulbactam (Unasyn): 1.5–3.0 g IV q6h
- Azithromycin: 500 mg PO on day 1 and 250 mg PO on days 2–5
- Azithromycin: 500 mg IV daily
- Aztreonam: 1–2 g IV q12h
- Cefepime: 2 g IV q12h
- Ceftazidime: 2 g IV q12h
- Ceftriaxone: 1–2 g IV daily
- Cefuroxime: 0.75 and 1.5 g IV q8h
- Doxycycline: 100 mg PO/IV q12h
- Imipenem: 500 mg IV q6h
- Meropenem: 1 g IV q8h
- Moxifloxacin: 400 mg IV daily
- Piperacillin-tazobactam (Zosyn): 3.375–4.5 g IV q6h
- Levofloxacin: 500–750 mg PO/IV daily
- Vancomycin: 1 g IV q12h

### First Line

- Outpatient:
  - Healthy:
    - Azithromycin: 500 mg PO day 1, 250 mg PO days 2–5
  - Co-morbidities:
    - Levofloxacin: 750 mg PO daily
- Inpatient:
  - Non-ICU:
    - Levofloxacin: 750 mg IV daily
  - ICU:
    - Ceftriaxone 1 g IV daily AND levofloxacin 750 mg IV daily ± piperacillin-tazobactam 4.5 g IV q6h ± vancomycin 1g IV q12h

### Second Line

Aztreonam may be substituted for $\beta$-lactams in confirmed penicillin-allergic patients for the above ICU regimens.

## FOLLOW-UP

### DISPOSITION

### Admission Criteria

- Based on severity of illness, coexisting conditions, ability of home care, and follow-up
- Clinical decision-making rules may aid in stratifying patients but should not supersede clinical judgment.
- CURB-65 rule:
  - Criteria:
    - Confusion (Abbreviated Mental Test <8)
    - Urea >7 mmol/L OR BUN >19
    - Respiratory rate >30/min
    - BP with SBP <90 mm Hg, DBP <60 mm Hg
    - Age ≥65 yr
  - Interpretation:
    - 0–1: Outpatient treatment
    - 2: Close outpatient vs. brief inpatient
    - 3–5: Inpatient
- Pneumonia Severity Index:
  - Demographics:
    - If Male: + age (yr)
    - If Female: + age (yr) – 10
    - If nursing home resident: +10
  - Comorbidity:
    - Neoplastic disease: +30
    - Liver disease: +20
    - Congestive heart failure: +10
    - Cerebrovascular disease: +10
    - Renal disease: +10
  - Physical examination:
    - Arterial pH <7.35: +30
    - BUN ≥30 mg/dL: +20
    - Sodium <130 mmol/L: +20
    - Glucose ≥250 mg/dL: +10
    - Hematocrit <30%: +10
    - $PaO_2$ <60 mm Hg: +10
    - Pleural effusion: +10
  - Interpretation:
    - 0: Class I (outpatient)
    - <70: Class II (home with IV antibiotics vs. short observation)
    - 71–90: Class III (home with IV antibiotics vs. short observation)
    - 91–130: Class IV (inpatient)
    - >130: Class V (inpatient)

- Additional considerations:
  - Previous hospitalization within last year for pneumonia
  - Failed outpatient therapy
  - Social conditions preventing safe outpatient disposition

### Discharge Criteria

- Age <65 yr
- No comorbid illnesses
- Nontoxic appearance
- Normal vital signs
- Normal laboratory studies
- Primary care follow-up within 72 hr

### Issues for Referral

Follow-up with primary care within 72 hr

### FOLLOW-UP RECOMMENDATIONS

Primary care follow up within 72 hr

## PEARLS AND PITFALLS

- Delayed initiation of antibiotics in ill-appearing patients
- Failure to recognize pneumonia in patients assumed to have exacerbations of underlying lung conditions
- Failure to question patients regarding TB and HIV risk factors
- Elderly and immunocompromised patients may not exhibit any classic symptoms of pneumonia when ill.

## ADDITIONAL READING

- Mandell LA, Wunderink RG, Anzueto A, et al. Infectious Disease Society of America/American Thoracic Society consensus guidelines on the management of community acquired pneumonia in adults. Clin Infect Dis. 2007;44(suppl 2):27–72.
- Nazarian DJ, Eddy OL, Lukens TW, et al. Clinical policy: Critical issues in the management of adult patients presenting to the emergency department with community-acquired pneumonia. Ann Emerg Med. 2009;54:704–731.
- Segreti J, House HR, Siegel RE. Principles of antibiotic treatment of community-acquired pneumonia in the outpatient setting. Am J Med. 2005;118:215–285.
- Wolfson AB, ed. Harwood-Nuss' Clinical Practice of Emergency Medicine, 4th ed. Philadelphia: Lippincott Williams & Wilkins; 2001:206–213.

### See Also (Topic, Algorithm, Electronic Media Element)

- Pneumonia, Pediatric
- Pneumocystis carinii Pneumonia

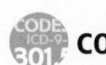 **CODES**

ICD9

- 481 Pneumococcal pneumonia {streptococcus pneumoniae pneumonia}
- 482.9 Bacterial pneumonia, unspecified
- 486 Pneumonia, organism unspecified

# PNEUMONIA, PEDIATRIC

Gary D. Zimmer
Karen P. Zimmer

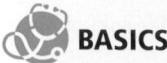 **BASICS**

## DESCRIPTION
- Mechanism is often unknown.
- Source is oropharyngeal aspiration (most common) or hematogenous.
- Distribution depends on the organism: Interstitial (*Mycoplasma pneumonia*, virus), lobar (*Streptococcus pneumoniae*), abscesses (*Staphylococcus aureus*), or diffuse (*Pneumocystis carinii*)

## ETIOLOGY
- <2 wk:
  - Group B *Streptococcus* species
  - Enteric gram-negative organisms
  - Respiratory syncytial virus (RSV)
  - Herpes simplex virus
  - *S. aureus*
- 2 wk to 3 mo:
  - *Chlamydia trachomatis*
  - Parainfluenza virus
  - RSV
  - *S. pneumoniae*
  - *S. aureus*
  - *H. influenza*
  - *Bordetella pertussis*
- 3 mo to 8 yr:
  - Viral (predominate):
    ○ RSV
    ○ Parainfluenza virus
    ○ Influenza virus
    ○ Adenovirus
  - *S. pneumoniae*
  - *H. influenza* in unimmunized children
  - Group A streptococci
  - *S. aureus*
  - *B. pertussis*
- >8 yr:
  - *M. pneumoniae* most common
  - Viral
  - *S. pneumoniae*
- Recent immigrants from developing countries:
  - *Mycoplasma tuberculosis*
  - *H. influenza*
  - *B. pertussis*
- Immunocompromised (eg, HIV, cancer):
  - *P. carinii*
  - *Mycoplasma avium* complex
  - *M. tuberculosis*
  - *Klebsiella pneumoniae*
  - *Pseudomonas aeruginosa*
- Less common:
  - Fungal (coccidioidomycosis, histoplasmosis)
  - *Rickettsia* (Q fever)

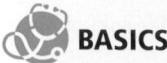 **DIAGNOSIS**

## SIGNS AND SYMPTOMS
- General (in all ages):
  - Cough
  - Rales
  - Fever
  - Hypoxia
  - Tachycardia
  - Tachypnea, retractions, grunting
  - Rash (up to 10% of cases); usually maculopapular
  - Nonspecific symptoms of toxicity
  - Pulmonary exam:
  - Decreased breath sounds, ventilation
  - Dullness to percussion
  - Wheezing, ronchi, rales
- Infants <6 mo:
  - Altered behavior: Listless, irritable
  - Apnea (esp. RSV in premature infants)
  - Conjunctivitis (*Chlamydia* <1 mo old)
  - Cyanosis
  - Grunting
  - Poor feeding
  - Temperature instability (hypothermia/hyperthermia)
  - Vomiting, often with coughing
  - Cough
  - Nasal congestion
  - Nasal flaring
  - Wheezing
  - Staccato cough (*Chlamydia*)
- Children >5 yr:
  - Pleuritic chest pain
  - Productive cough
  - Rigors, chills

## History
- Immunization history
- Past medical history include immune status
- Exposures
- Progression of signs and symptoms

## Physical Exam
- Pulmonary exam may be helpful, particularly in children >5 yr.
- Peripheral and central cyanosis should be assessed.
- Evidence of respiratory compromise, distress, failure

## ESSENTIAL WORKUP
- Pulse oximetry
- Chest radiograph:
  - Gold standard for diagnosis
  - Should be ordered for patients with signs of lower respiratory tract infection and patients <36 mo old with marked leukocytosis or neutrophilia (WBC >15,000 or absolute neutrophil count [ANC] >9,000).
  - Much overlap between viral and bacterial findings
  - Viral and *M. pneumoniae* tend to show interstitial infiltrates, often perihilar and peribronchial.
  - Bacterial pneumonias may show focal lobar consolidation, focal alveolar infiltrates, and possibly effusion or pneumatocele.
  - Round pneumonia pathognomonic of *S. pneumonia*
  - Lateral decubitus films may aid in demonstrating effusion.

## DIAGNOSTIC TESTS & INTERPRETATION
### Lab
- CBC with differential:
  - Patients with bacteremia tend to have leukocytosis with left shift.
  - Sensitivity and specificity are poor.
  - Patients with WBC ≥20,000 or ANC >9000 are at increased risk of pneumococcal bacteremia.
  - *B. pertussis* usually has elevated WBC with lymphocytosis.
- Blood culture:
  - Low yield (<10–20%)
  - Recommended in children <36 mo
  - Probably worthwhile in toxic patients requiring hospitalization
- Arterial blood gas may be useful in determining degree of respiratory insufficiency in critically ill patients.
- Electrolytes to exclude syndrome of inappropriate antidiuretic hormone secretion and in hypotensive children
- Sputum for Gram stain and culture may be obtained in older children with suspected bacterial infection.
- *Mycoplasma* IgM or cold agglutinin titers:
  - Useful if suspecting this organism
  - More likely positive with severe illness
- Nasopharyngeal washes for direct fluorescent antibody and culture:
  - Identify RSV, *Chlamydia trachomatis*, and *B. pertussis* infections

### Imaging
Chest radiographs are still the imaging modality of choice:
- Posteroanterior and lateral films should be obtained whenever possible.
- CT provides additional detail and better identification of underlying lung pathology but adds little as an initial testing modality.

### Diagnostic Procedures/Surgery
Pleural fluid (if present) for culture, Gram stain, protein, glucose, and cell counts

## DIFFERENTIAL DIAGNOSIS

- Reactive airway disease (asthma, bronchiolitis [age <2 yr])
- Aspiration:
  - Gastroesophageal reflux
  - Vascular ring
  - H-type tracheoesophageal fistula
  - Foreign body
  - Hydrocarbon
- Congestive heart failure
- Congenital:
  - Cystic fibrosis
  - Sequestered lobe
  - Congenital lobe absence
  - Hemangioma
- Neoplasm

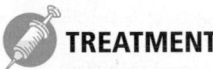 TREATMENT

### PRE-HOSPITAL

- Pulse oximetry
- Administer high-flow oxygen for respiratory distress.
- IV fluids (0.9% normal saline [NS] 20 mL/kg initial bolus) for volume depletion, hypotension
- Support and intubation for respiratory failure

### INITIAL STABILIZATION/THERAPY

- If moderately or severely ill:
  - Secure airway, as appropriate; intubate for clinical respiratory failure. Children with severe sepsis or septic shock benefit from aggressive airway management.
  - High-flow oxygen
  - IV hydration (0.9% NS 20 mL/kg initial bolus) and resuscitation if in shock or hypovolemia
- Monitor
- Ongoing pulse oximetry
- Arterial blood gas if inadequate ventilation
- Check bedside glucose in severely ill appearing infants and toddlers:
  - If hypoglycemic, administer glucose D25 at 2 mL/kg IV for toddlers or D10 at 5 mL/kg IV for neonates.

### ED TREATMENT/PROCEDURES

- Continue prehospital and initial stabilization therapy.
- Early antibiotic therapy should be broad enough to address local resistance patterns in your area.
- Often have concurrent reactive airway disease that needs specific treatment with bronchodilator (albuterol or levalbuterol)
- Perform thoracentesis if pleural effusion is compromising respiratory function or for diagnostic tests.

### MEDICATION

- Empiric therapy with oral antibiotics for most well-appearing children ≥6 mo:
  - Infants <2 mo:
    - Outpatient treatment generally not recommended unless child has no respiratory distress or associated conditions or issues.
  - Children 3 mo to 5 yr:
    - Amoxicillin
    - Amoxicillin-clavulanate
    - Trimethoprim-sulfamethoxazole
    - Erythromycin-sulfisoxazole
    - Macrolide (azithromycin or clarithromycin)
  - Children 5–18 yr:
    - Macrolide (azithromycin or clarithromycin)

- Initiate IV antibiotic therapy for moderate to severely ill children who require admission:
  - Neonate:
    - Ampicillin, and cefotaxime or gentamicin
    - Azithromycin or erythromycin for suspected *C. trachomatis* or *B. pertussis* pneumonia
  - Infants 1–2 mo:
    - Ampicillin and cefotaxime
    - Azithromycin or erythromycin for suspected *C. trachomatis* or *B. pertussis*
  - Children ≥3 mo:
    - Cefotaxime, cefuroxime, or ceftriaxone
    - Vancomycin for suspected or confirmed penicillin-resistant *S. pneumoniae*
    - Macrolide (ie, azithromycin) for suspected *M. pneumoniae*
- Unusual organisms require specific therapy in coordination with infectious disease consultation.
- Albuterol (0.5% solution or 5 mg/mL): Nebulizer 0.015 mg (0.03 mL)/kg per dose up to 5 mg per dose q10–20 min as needed; metered dose inhaler (with spacer; 90 mg per puff) 2 puffs q10–20 min up to total of 10 puffs
- Amoxicillin: 80 mg/kg/24 hr q12h PO
- Amoxicillin-clavulanate: 30 mg/kg/24 hr q12h PO
- Ampicillin: 100–150 mg/kg/24 hr q6h IV
- Azithromycin: 10 mg/kg/24 hr daily for 1 day, then 5 mg/kg/24 hr daily for 4 days
- Cefotaxime: 50–75 mg/kg/24 hr q8h IV, max. 2 g q8h
- Ceftriaxone: 100 mg/kg/24 hr q12–24h IV, max. 2 g q12h
- Cefuroxime: 100 mg/kg/24 hr q8h IV, max. 2 g q8h
- Clarithromycin: 15 mg/kg/24 hr q12h PO, max. 500 g q12h
- Erythromycin: 40 mg/kg/24 hr q6h PO or IV, max. 2 g/d
- Erythromycin-sulfisoxazole: 40 mg/kg/24 hr as erythromycin q8h PO, max. 2 g/d
- Gentamicin: 5–7.5 mg/kg/24 hr q8–12h IV
- Trimethoprim-sulfamethoxazole: 8–10 mg/kg/24 hr as TMP q12h PO
- Vancomycin: 10–15 mg/kg/24 hr q8–12h IV; max. 1,000 mg

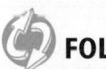 FOLLOW-UP

### DISPOSITION

*Admission Criteria*
- Toxic appearance
- Respiratory distress or failure
- Dehydration/vomiting
- Apnea
- Infants <2 mo
- Infants <6 mo with lobar pneumonia
- Hypoxia ($O_2$ saturation <92% on room air [sea level])
- Pleural effusion
- Poor response to outpatient oral therapy
- Immunocompromised children
- Concern about noncompliant parents

*Discharge Criteria*
- Most cases are mild and can be discharged home if no evidence of hypoxia, significant work-of-breathing, dehydration, vomiting, or noncompliance.
- Ensured follow-up within 1–2 days

*Issues for Referral*
Respiratory failure, effusion, toxicity

### FOLLOW-UP RECOMMENDATIONS
Clinical resolution should be ensured through follow-up.

## PEARLS AND PITFALLS

- Early, aggressive airway management for patients with severe sepsis and septic shock
- Delays to antibiotic therapy should be avoided.
- Discharged patients should have clear evidence of good support, follow-up, and lack of toxicity.
- Local patterns of drug resistance should be known and empiric therapy should take these resistance patterns into consideration.

## ADDITIONAL READING

- Bachur R, Perry H, Harper MB. Occult pneumonias: Empiric chest radiographs in febrile children with leukocytosis. *Ann Emerg Med*. 1999;33:166–173.
- Baraff LJ. Management of fever without source in infants and children. *Ann Emerg Med*. 2000;36:602–614.
- Cevey-Macherel M, Galetto-Lacour A, Gervaix A, et al. Etiology of community-acquired pneumonia in hospitalized children based on WHO clinical guidelines. *Eur J Pediatr*. 2009;168(12):1429–1436.
- Michelow IC, Olsen K, Lozano J, et al. Epidemiology and clinical characteristics of community-acquired pneumonia in hospitalized children. *Pediatrics*. 2004;113(4):701–707.
- Murphy CG, van de Pol AC, Harper MB, et al. Clinical predictors of occult pneumonia in the febrile child. *Acad Emerg Med*. 2007;14(3):243–249.

**See Also (Topic, Algorithm, Electronic Media Element)**
Asthma

 CODES

### ICD9
- 486 Pneumonia, organism unspecified
- 507.0 Pneumonitis due to inhalation of food or vomitus
- 516.8 Other specified alveolar and parietoalveolar pneumonopathies

# PNEUMOTHORAX
*William Porcaro*
*David Feldman*

 **BASICS**

## DESCRIPTION
- Presence of free air in the intrapleural space
- Spontaneous pneumothorax is due to atraumatic rupture of alveolus, bronchiole, or bleb.
- Primary spontaneous pneumothorax (2/3 of incidences):
  - No underlying pulmonary pathology present
  - Rupture of small subpleural cyst or bleb
  - Primarily young, healthy patients (20–40 yr old) with tall, thin body habitus
- Secondary spontaneous pneumothorax from underlying pulmonary pathology (see Etiology)
- Tension pneumothorax:
  - Air continues to enter pleural space through bronchoalveolar disruption and becomes trapped via "ball-valve" mechanism.
  - Intrapleural pressure increases.
  - Venous return to right heart decreases, resulting in decrease in cardiac output.
  - Mediastinum shifts toward uninvolved side, mechanically interfering with right atrial filling.
  - Ventilation compromise and ventilation/perfusion mismatch result in hypoxemia

## ETIOLOGY
- Idiopathic
- Airway disease:
  - Chronic obstructive pulmonary disease (COPD)
  - Asthma
  - Cystic fibrosis
- Infections:
  - Necrotizing bacterial pneumonia
  - TB
  - Fungal pneumonia
  - *Pneumocystis carinii*
- Neoplasm
- Interstitial lung disease:
  - Sarcoidosis
  - Idiopathic pulmonary fibrosis
  - Lymphangiomyomatosis
  - Tuberous sclerosis
  - Pneumoconioses
- Connective tissue diseases
- Pulmonary infarction
- Endometriosis
- Blunt chest trauma
- Penetrating trauma to neck or trunk
- Iatrogenic:
  - Central line placement
  - Other vascular access procedures

## DIAGNOSIS

### SIGNS AND SYMPTOMS
#### History
- Severity of symptoms is generally proportional to size of the pneumothorax.
- Chest pain on the ipsilateral side:
  - Sharp, pleuritic pain
  - Sudden onset
  - Dull ache in delayed presentations
- Shortness of breath
- Rarely cough, asymptomatic, or generalized malaise

#### Physical Exam
- Tachypnea
- Heart rate <120 bpm generally seen in simple spontaneous pneumothoraces
- Jugular venous distention and tracheal deviation to the contralateral side may be evident in tension pneumothorax.
- Cardiac and pulmonary exam:
  - Asymmetric decreased breath sounds
  - Hyperresonance to percussion of ipsilateral side
- Tension pneumothorax:
  - Hypotension
  - Tachycardia, heart rate >120 bpm
  - Diaphoresis
  - Cyanosis
  - Cardiovascular collapse
  - Tracheal deviation

### ESSENTIAL WORKUP
- Imaging is mainstay of the workup
- DO NOT delay chest decompression if the patient is hemodynamically unstable and there is sufficient clinical evidence of pneumothorax.

### DIAGNOSTIC TESTS & INTERPRETATION
#### Lab
Arterial blood gas offers little over oxygen saturation.

#### Imaging
- Chest radiograph:
  - Upright chest radiograph
- Patients unable to tolerate upright chest radiograph can be taken in decubitus position with the suspected side up:
  - Absence of lung markings distal or peripheral to the visceral pleural white line
  - Displacement of mediastinum or anterior junction line
  - Deep sulcus sign

- On frontal view, larger lateral costodiaphragmatic recess than on opposite side
- Diaphragm may be inverted on side with deep sulcus:
  - A rough estimate of pneumothorax size is sufficient to make clinical decisions.
- Expiratory film:
  - May demonstrate small pneumothorax but has not been shown to increase yield of detection
- Chest CT:
  - Very sensitive for small pneumothorax but has little practical advantage over chest radiograph
- US:
  - User experience required
  - Rapid at bedside
  - Lack of lung sliding and comet-tail artifact signifies pneumothorax.
  - M-mode confirms pneumothorax with smooth lines above and below pleural line.

#### Diagnostic Procedures/Surgery
ECG:
- Often necessary to rule out cardiac etiologies of chest pain
- Nonspecific changes include T wave inversion, left axis deviation, and decreased R wave amplitude.

### DIFFERENTIAL DIAGNOSIS
- Acute abdominal processes
- Aortic aneurysm or dissection
- Asthma exacerbation
- Chest wall pain
- COPD exacerbation
- Myocardial infarction
- Pericarditis
- Pleuritis
- Pneumomediastinum
- Pulmonary embolus

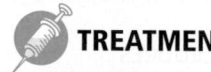 **TREATMENT**

### PRE-HOSPITAL

> **ALERT**
> Unstable patients with a suspected tension pneumothorax require immediate needle thoracostomy.

### INITIAL STABILIZATION/THERAPY
- Cardiac monitor
- Pulse oximetry
- Oxygen 100% via nonrebreather face mask
- IV access

- Suspected tension pneumothorax requires either immediate needle thoracostomy or tube thoracostomy.
- Needle thoracostomy:
  – Immediate placement indicated in unstable patients with a tension pneumothorax
  – 14–18-gauge angiocatheter in the second intercostal space at midclavicular line or 4th or 5th intercostal space at anterior axillary line

### ED TREATMENT/PROCEDURES

- Nontraumatic pneumothorax estimated at <15% collapse and no cardiovascular or respiratory compromise:
  – Observe with 100% oxygen support for 4–6 hr.
  – Repeat chest radiograph and discharge if unchanged.
- Simple aspiration:
  – Indications:
    ○ Simple pneumothorax with only 15–30% collapse
    ○ Increase in size of a small pneumothorax during observation
  – Placement of aspiration catheter (typically 8 Fr) with 3-way stopcock
- Aspirate air until resistance or 3 L of air aspirated.
- If the pneumothorax is no longer visible on 2 subsequent chest radiographs at 4-hr intervals, remove catheter.
- If a final chest radiograph is normal 2 hr after the catheter is removed, the patient may be discharged.
- A second aspiration may be attempted if the pneumothorax does not resolve.
- Heimlich valve:
  – Indicated when <30% collapse after failure of aspiration
    Attach Heimlich valve to aspiration catheter or chest tube.
- Suction:
    Indicated when the Heimlich valve fails
  – Attach aspiration catheter to suction at 20 cm $H_2O$.
  – Observe in ED for 1 hr.
- Tube thoracostomy:
  – Indications:
    ○ Suspicion of a tension pneumothorax
    ○ Gunshot wound to the chest
    ○ Clinical evidence of a pneumothorax following blunt chest trauma or penetrating chest trauma
    ○ Presence of a pneumothorax of any size in patient receiving positive-pressure ventilation
    ○ Pneumothorax with >30% collapse
    ○ Most cases of secondary pneumothorax
    ○ Definitive therapy after needle thoracostomy
  – Tube size:
    ○ Small-caliber (7–14 Fr) tube for primary spontaneous pneumothoraces
    ○ 20–28 Fr for secondary spontaneous pneumothorax
    ○ 28 Fr when there is detectable pleural fluid or an anticipated need for mechanical ventilation
  – Check for tube kinks by fully rotating the inserted tube.

– All side holes in the tube must be within the chest wall to avoid leak.
– Following insertion, the tube should be connected to a water-seal device.
– A Heimlich valve may be used instead of a water-seal device in stable patients without a pleural effusion.
– Reexpansion edema is a rare complication requiring supportive care.
- Possible complications:
  – Intercostal vessel bleeding
  – Inadequate drainage:
    ○ Kinked tube
    ○ Clogged tube
    ○ Communication outside of pleural cavity with leak
  – Reexpansion pulmonary edema:
    ○ Treatment with fluid resuscitation

### MEDICATION

- Local anesthetic:
  – 1% lidocaine with epinephrine 1:100,000
  – Max dose: 7 mg/kg–500 mg
- Consider procedural sedation in stable awake patients
- No indication for antibiotics in a clean procedure

 **FOLLOW-UP**

### DISPOSITION

#### Admission Criteria

- Tension pneumothorax
- Chest tube required

#### Discharge Criteria

- <15% collapse, no expansion while in the ED or successful aspiration with catheter removed:
  – Discharge with follow up in 24 hr and 1 wk for chest radiograph to assure reexpansion.
- Reliable patients with the thoracic vent and successful aspiration or secured catheter and Heimlich valve:
  – Discharge with 24- and 48-hr follow-up.
  – At 48-hr follow-up:
    ○ Clamp catheter, observe for 2 hr, and repeat chest radiograph.
    ○ Remove thoracic vent or catheter if no reexpansion.
    ○ Observe for 2 hr and repeat chest radiograph.
    ○ If no reexpansion, discharge with 24-hr and 1-wk follow-up.
- Discharge instruction should include prompt return for new onset of chest pain or dyspnea.
- Patients without reexpansion at 1 wk require a cardiothoracic surgery consult.

### FOLLOW-UP RECOMMENDATIONS
Pulmonary medicine and/or chest surgery

### PEARLS AND PITFALLS

- Delay in chest decompression in the unstable patient leading to rapid hemodynamic compromise
- Avoid poor tube placement involving kinks or improper depth, which may necessitate repeating the procedure.
- Avoid placement of catheter or tube too low on the lateral chest wall, which may lead to iatrogenic abdominal injuries.
- Failure to detect associated mediastinal or lower neck injuries

### ADDITIONAL READING

- Baumann MH, Strange C, Heffner JE, et al. Management of spontaneous pneumothorax: An American College of Chest Physicians Delphi consensus statement. *Chest.* 2001;119:590–602.
- Gaudio M, Hafner JW. Simple aspiration compared to chest tube insertion in the management of primary spontaneous pneumothorax. *Ann Emerg Med.* 2009;54:458–460.
- Hassani B, Foote J, Borgundvaag B. Outpatient management of primary spontaneous pneumothorax in the emergency department of a community hospital using a small-bore catheter and a Heimlich valve. *Acad Emerg Med.* 2009;16:513–518.
- Kelly AM. Treatment of primary spontaneous pneumothorax. *Curr Opin Pulm Med.* 2009;15: 376–379.
- Sethuraman KN, Duong D, Mehta S, et al. Complications of tube thoracostomy placement in the emergency department. *J Emerg Med.* 2010; in press
- Shen KR, Cerfolio RJ. Decision making in the management of secondary spontaneous pneumothorax in patients with severe emphysema. *Thorac Surg Clin.* 2009;19:233–238.
- Soldati G, Testa A, Sher S, et al. Occult traumatic pneumothorax: diagnostic accuracy of lung ultrasonography in the emergency department. *Chest.* 2008;133:204–211.
- Zehtabchi S, Rios CL. Management of emergency department patients with primary spontaneous pneumothorax. Needle aspiration or tube thoracostomy? *Ann Emerg Med.* 2008;51:91–100.

### See Also (Topic, Algorithm, Electronic Media Element)
- Chest Pain
- Dyspnea

 **CODES**

#### ICD9
- 512.0 Spontaneous tension pneumothorax
- 512.8 Other spontaneous pneumothorax

# POISONING

*Mark B. Mycyk*

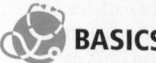 **BASICS**

## DESCRIPTION
- Poisoning may be intentional or unintentional.
- Patients with change in mental status without clear cause should have poisoning (intoxication, overdose) considered in differential diagnosis.

## ETIOLOGY
- Intentional:
  - Depression
  - Suicide
  - Homicide
  - Recreational drug abuse
- Unintentional (accidental):
  - Common cause in children
  - Therapeutic error (eg, double dose)
  - Recreational drug experimentation

### Pediatric Considerations
- Accidental ingestions—typically young children (1–5 yr)
- Consider child abuse if inconsistent or suspicious history.

 **DIAGNOSIS**

## SIGNS AND SYMPTOMS
- Neurologic:
  - Lethargy
  - Agitation
  - Coma
  - Hallucinations
  - Seizures
- Respiratory:
  - Tachypnea, bradypnea, apnea
  - Inability to protect airway
- Cardiovascular:
  - Dysrhythmias
  - Conduction blocks
- Vital signs:
  - Varies depending on toxic substance
  - Hyperthermia, hypothermia
  - Tachycardia, bradycardia
  - Hypertension, hypotension

### Selected Toxidromes (see "Poisoning, Toxidromes")
- Anticholinergic:
  - Altered mental status (confusion, delirium, lethargy)
  - Dry skin and mucous membranes
  - Fixed dilated pupils
  - Tachycardia
  - Hyperthermia
  - Flushing
- Urinary retention
- Cholinergic:
  - Secretory overdrive (salivation, lacrimation, urination, diaphoresis)
  - Miosis
  - Bronchospasm, wheezing
- Opiate:
  - CNS and respiratory depression
  - Pinpoint pupils
- Sympathomimetic:
  - CNS excitation
  - Seizures
  - Tachycardia
  - Hypertension
  - Diaphoresis

## ESSENTIAL WORKUP
- A complete set of vital signs, including core temperature
- A complete physical exam, including eyes, skin, odors

## DIAGNOSTIC TESTS & INTERPRETATION
*Lab*
- Electrolytes, BUN/creatinine, glucose
- Calculate anion gap: $Na + (Cl + HCO_3)$:
  - Normal anion gap: 8–12
  - Use mnemonic *A CAT MUD PILES* for elevated anion gap acidosis:
    - Alcoholic ketoacidosis
    - Cyanide, carbon monoxide
    - Aspirin, other salicylates
    - Toluene
    - Methanol, metformin
    - Uremia
    - Diabetic ketoacidosis
    - Paraldehyde, phenformin
    - Iron, isoniazid
    - Lactic acidosis from other causes
    - Ethylene glycol
    - Starvation ketosis
- Serum osmol gap:
  - Calculate osmol gap if elevated anion gap acidosis from potential toxic alcohol.
  - Most sensitive *early* in poisoning
  - Normal osmol gap does not completely rule out toxic alcohol ingestion.
  - Calculated osmolality = $2(Na^+) + glucose/18 + BUN/2.8 + ethanol$ (in mg/dL)/4.6.
  - Osmol gap = measured osmolality – calculated osmolality.
  - Use mnemonic *ME DIE A* when osmol gap >10:
    - Methanol
    - Ethanol
    - Diuretics (mannitol, glycerin, sorbitol)
    - Isopropyl alcohol
    - Ethylene glycol
    - Acetone

- Pregnancy test
- Acetaminophen level for suicidal ingestions
- Toxicology screen

### Imaging
- ECG for dysrhythmias or QRS/QT changes
- CT of head for altered mental status not clearly due to toxin
- Chest radiograph if suspected aspiration or pneumonia

## DIFFERENTIAL DIAGNOSIS
- Causes of altered mental status
- Intracranial mass, bleeding
- Infection, sepsis
- Endocrine abnormalities
- Hypothermia
- Hypoxia
- Metabolic abnormalities
- Psychogenic

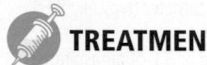 **TREATMENT**

## PRE-HOSPITAL
- Search for clues at scene:
  - Pills/pill bottles
  - Drug paraphernalia
  - Witnesses
  - Transport all drugs and pill bottles for identification.
- Restrain uncooperative patients for patient and health care giver protection.
- Consider comorbid conditions:
  - Trauma
  - Medical illness
  - Environmental exposure
- Prehospital administration of activated charcoal may optimize decontamination if prolonged transport time.

## INITIAL STABILIZATION/THERAPY
- ABCs:
  - Endotracheal intubation as needed for airway protection, oxygenation, ventilation, and orogastric lavage
  - Supplemental oxygen for hypoxia
  - Pulse oximetry
  - Cardiac monitor
  - IV access
- Hypotension:
  - Administer 0.9% normal saline IV fluid bolus.
  - Trendelenburg
  - Vasopressors for persistent hypotension

- Bradycardia:
  - Atropine
  - Cardiac pacing
- If altered mental status, administer coma cocktail: Thiamine, D50W (or Accu-Chek), naloxone

## ED TREATMENT/PROCEDURES

- Decontamination:
  - See "Poisoning, Gastric Decontamination."
  - Prevents systemic absorption of ingested toxin
- Orogastric lavage:
  - Consider in potentially lethal ingestions without known antidote within 1 hr of ingestion.
  - Protected airway *essential* prior to lavage
- Activated charcoal:
  - Most effective within a few hours of most toxic ingestions
  - Contraindicated if caustic ingestion, unprotected airway, or bowel obstruction
  - Drugs not effectively bound to charcoal: Metals (borates, bromide, iron, lithium), alcohols, potassium
- Whole-bowel irrigation:
  - Polyethylene glycol (Colyte, Go-Lytely) evacuates bowel without causing electrolyte disturbances.
  - Consider in toxins not well adsorbed by charcoal (eg, iron and lithium), body packers/stuffers, sustained-release ingestions.
  - Contraindicated if bowel obstruction, perforation, or hypotension
- Enhanced elimination:
  - Enhances removal of systemically absorbed toxin
- Multiple-dose activated charcoal:
  - Theophylline
  - Carbamazepine
  - Phenobarbital
- Urinary alkalinization:
  - Salicylates
  - Phenobarbital
- Hemodialysis/hemoperfusion:
  - Lithium
  - Salicylates
  - Theophylline
  - Toxic alcohols
  - Valproate
- Seizures
  - Treat initially with diazepam or lorazepam.
  - For persistent seizures, consider phenobarbital.
  - Phenytoin *not* indicated in toxicologic seizures:
    - Indicated only if seizures secondary to idiopathic epilepsy, posttraumatic, or status epilepticus

- Antidotes:
  - Acetaminophen: *N*-acetylcysteine
  - Anticholinergic: Physostigmine
  - Benzodiazepines: Flumazenil
  - β-Blockers: Glucagon
  - Calcium-channel blockers: Calcium chloride/gluconate, insulin
  - Carbon monoxide: Oxygen, hyperbaric oxygen
  - Coumadin: Vitamin $K_1$
  - Cyanide: Cyanide antidote kit, hydroxocobalamin
  - Digoxin: Digibind
  - Ethylene glycol: Ethanol, 4-methylpyrazole
  - Iron: Deferoxamine
  - Isoniazid: Pyridoxine (vitamin $B_6$)
  - Methanol: Ethanol, 4-methylpyrazole
  - Methemoglobinemia: Methylene blue
  - Opiates: Naloxone
  - Organophosphates: Atropine, pralidoxime
  - Tricyclic antidepressants: $NaHCO_3$

## MEDICATION

- Activated charcoal slurry: 1–2 g/kg PO
- Dextrose: D50W 1 amp: 50 mL or 25 g (peds: D25W 2–4 mL/kg) IV
- Diazepam: 5–10 mg (peds: 0.2–0.5 mg/kg) IV every 10–15 min
- Lorazepam: 2–6 mg (peds: 0.05–0.1 mg/kg) IV every 10–15 min
- Naloxone (Narcan): 0.4–2 mg (peds: 0.1 mg/kg) IV or IM initial dose
- Thiamine (vitamin $B_1$): 100 mg (peds: 50 mg) IV or IM

 **FOLLOW-UP**

### DISPOSITION

#### Admission Criteria

- Altered mental status
- Cardiopulmonary instability
- Suicidal
- Laboratory abnormalities
- Potential for decompensation from delayed acting substance

#### Discharge Criteria

- Psychiatrically clear
- Detoxified
- Hemodynamically stable

### Issues for Referral

- Patients with unintentional (accidental) poisoning require poison prevention counseling.
- Patients with intentional (eg, suicide) poisoning require psychiatric evaluation.
- Consider substance abuse referral for patients.

### Pregnancy Considerations

In general, treating the mother is also the best treatment strategy for the fetus.

### FOLLOW-UP RECOMMENDATIONS

- Consider substance abuse referral for patients with recreational drug abuse.
- Patients with unintentional (accidental) poisoning require poison prevention counseling.
- Patients with intentional (eg, suicide) poisoning require psychiatric evaluation.

## PEARLS AND PITFALLS

- Do not forget to consider nontoxicologic etiologies for altered mental status.
- Do not rely on the urine drug screen to make a diagnosis: It only provides screening tests for a limited number of drugs.
- Call a toxicologist or a poison center for help: 800-222-1222.

## ADDITIONAL READING

- Hahn I H. Phencyclidine and ketamine. In: Erickson TB, Ahrens W, Aks SE, et al., eds. *Pediatric Toxicology*. New York: McGraw-Hill; 2004:297–302.
- Pugach S, Pugach IZ. Overdose in infant caused by over-the-counter cough medicine. *South J Med*. 2009;102:440 442.
- Shannon M. Recent ketamine administration can produce a urine toxic screen which is falsely positive for phencyclidine. *Pediatr Emerg Care*. 1998;14:180.
- Wills B, Erickson T. Drug- and toxin-associated seizures. *Med Clin North Am*. 2005;89:1297–1321.

### See Also (Topic, Algorithm, Electronic Media Element)

- Poisoning, Antidotes
- Poisoning, Gastric Decontamination
- Poisoning, Toxidromes

 **CODES**

### ICD9

989.9 Toxic effect of unspecified substance, chiefly nonmedicinal as to source

**TREATMENT**

## N-ACETYLCYSTEINE (NAC)
- Indications: Acetaminophen overdose
- Warnings:
  – Unpleasant odor, nausea, vomiting
  – Most effective if given in 1st 8 hr postingestion
- Dose:
  – PO: 140 mg/kg, then 70 mg/kg q4h for 17 doses
  – IV: (consult poison center) 150 mg/kg in 200 mL $D_5W$ over 15 min, then 50 mg/kg in 500 mL $D_5W$ over 4 hr, then 100 mg/kg in 1,000 mL $D_5W$ over 16 hr

### *Pediatric Considerations*
This volume of $D_5W$ may need to be reduced in dosing pediatric patients to avoid fluid overload/hyponatremia.

## ATROPINE
- Indications:
  – Bradycardia owing to drugs
  – Organophosphate insecticides
- Warnings:
  – Myasthenia gravis, narrow-angle glaucoma, HTN, coronary ischemia, and urinary obstruction
- Dose:
  – Adult: 0.5–1.0 mg IV
  – Pediatric: 0.02 mg/kg (min. 0.1 mg) IV
  – Large repeated doses needed in organophosphate poisoning

## BENZTROPINE (COGENTIN)
- Indications: Acute dystonic reactions
- Warnings: Carbamates, myasthenia gravis, narrow-angle glaucoma, HTN, coronary ischemia, and urinary obstruction
- Dose:
  – Adult: 1–2 mg IV (for acute reaction) or PO (to prevent reaction)
  – Pediatric: 0.02 mg/kg IV (for acute reaction) or PO (to prevent reaction)

## BENZODIAZEPINE
- Indications: Agitation, stimulant drugs, seizures
- Warnings: Respiratory/CNS depression
- Dose:
  – Midazolam:
    ○ Adult: 1 mg IV/IM every 2–3 min PRN
    ○ Pediatric: 0.1 mg/kg IV/IM
  – Diazepam:
    ○ Adult: 2–5 mg IV/IM, repeat in 10–15 min
    ○ Pediatrics: 0.1 mg/kg IV/IM

## BICARBONATE, SODIUM
- Indications: Cyclic antidepressant poisoning, metabolic acidosis, urinary alkalinization
- Warnings: May cause CHF, excessive alkalosis, hypokalemia
- Dose:
  – Serum alkalinization:
    ○ 1 mEq/kg IVP
  – Urine alkalinization:
    ○ 100–150 mEq in 1 L DW at 2–3 mL/kg/h IV, goal urine pH 7–8

## BLACK WIDOW SPIDER ANTIVENIN (LACTRODECTUS MACTANS)
- Indications: Severe HTN, muscle spasms not alleviated by analgesics and muscle relaxants; consider in extremes of age (<5 or >65 years), pregnant women with threatened abortion

- Warnings:
  – Equine serum-derived: Immediate hypersensitivity, serum sickness 10–14 days
  – Premedicate for anaphylaxis if know equine serum hypersensitivity.
- Dose: 1–2 vials IV slowly over 15–30 min

## BOTULIN ANTITOXIN TRIVALENT A,B,E
- Indications: Clinical botulism, prior to onset of paralysis
- Warnings:
  – Binds only free toxins
  – Not for infant botulism
  – Equine serum-derived: Immediate hypersensitivity, serum sickness 10–14 days
  – Premedicate for anaphylaxis if know equine serum hypersensitivity.
  – Administer slow IV push.
- Dose: 1–2 vials IV q4h for 4 or 5 doses

## CALCIUM
- Indications:
  – Hyperkalemia with cardiac toxicity
  – Hydrofluoric acid burn
  – Calcium channel blocker overdose
  – Citrate, oxalate, phosphate poisoning
- Warnings:
  – Avoid in digoxin toxicity, hypercalcemia
  – Calcium chloride (CaCl) corrosive to skin, SC tissue
  – Incompatible with certain IV solutions
  – Administer slow IV push.
- Dose:
  – Adult: 5–10 mL of 10% Ca chloride, or 10–20 mL of 10% Ca gluconate
  – Pediatric: 0.1–0.2 mL/kg of 10% Ca chloride, or 0.2–0.3 mL/kg of 10% Ca gluconate

## CALCIUM EDTA (EDETATE DISODIUM)
- Indications: Lead, chromium, nickel, manganese, zinc toxicity
- Warnings: Nausea, vomiting, chill, nephrotoxicity, hypercalcemia
- Dose: 20–30 mg/kg over 24 hr as 6 divided doses or continuous IV infusion, follow lead (Pb) level

## CORAL SNAKE ANTIVENIN (MICRURUS FULVIUS)
- Indications: Eastern or Texas coral snake
- Warnings:
  – Equine serum-derived: Immediate hypersensitivity, serum sickness 10–14 days
  – Premedicate for anaphylaxis if know equine serum hypersensitivity.
- Dose: 4–10 vials IV over 15–30 min

## CYANIDE ANTIDOTE KIT
- Indications: Cyanide poisoning
- Warnings: Hypotension, methemoglobinemia
- Dose:
  – Amyl nitrite: 1–2 amp crushed, inhaled
  – Sodium nitrite:
    ○ Adult: 300 mg in 10 mL IV over 5 min
    ○ Pediatric: 0.3 mL/kg of 3% solution IV
  – Sodium thiosulfate:
    ○ Adult: 12.5 g IV, may repeat in 1 hr
    ○ Pediatric: 50 mg/kg IV

## CYANOKIT® (HYDROXOCOBALAMIN)
- Indications: Cyanide poisoning
- Warnings: Erythema, HTN

- Dose:
  – Adult: 5 g IV over 15 min; may repeat a 2nd 5 g dose depending on severity of poisoning and clinical response. Max: 10 g.
  – Pediatric: Safety and efficacy have not been established in children. Suggested initial dose: 70 mg/kg IV.

## DANTROLENE
- Indications:
  – Malignant hyperthermia
  – Neuroleptic malignant syndrome
  – Serotonin syndrome
  – Muscle rigidity
- Warnings: Muscle weakness, respiratory depression, hepatitis
- Dose: 1–2 mg/kg IV bolus, repeat q10–15 min PRN, max. 10 mg/kg

## DEFEROXAMINE (DESFERAL)
- Indications: Iron toxicity
- Warnings:
  – Do not treat for >24 hours, risk for delayed adult respiratory distress syndrome (ARDS).
  – Hypotension if >15 mg/kg/h, flushing, urticaria
- Dose: 10–15 mg/kg/h IV, may increase in severe iron (Fe) poisoning

## DIGOXIN ANTIBODY (DIGIBIND)
- Indications: Digoxin, digitoxin toxicity
- Warnings:
  – Falsely elevated digoxin levels after use
  – Development of CHF/atrial fibrillation in patients requiring digoxin
- Dose:
  – 1 vial (40 mg) binds 0.6 mg digoxin.
  – Number of vials = digoxin level (ng/mL) × weight (kg)/100
  – Dose estimate: Acute overdose 10–20 vials, chronic overdose 4–6 vials

## DIMERCAPROL (BAL)
- Indications: Arsenic, gold, mercury, lead-induced encephalopathy
- Warnings: Renal toxicity, fever, nausea, vomiting, urticaria, cholinergic symptoms
- Dose:
  – 3 mg/kg deep IM q4h for 2 days, then q12h for 7 days; follow metal levels
  – For Pb level >100 $\mu$g/dL: 4–5 mg/kg IM q4h until Pb <50 $\mu$g/dL, in conjunction with EDTA

## DIPHENHYDRAMINE (BENADRYL)
- Indications: Antihistamine, acute dystonic reaction
- Warnings: Sedation, excitation in children, anticholinergic symptoms
- Dose:
  – Adult: 25–50 mg IV/IM/PO q4–6h
  – Pediatric: 0.5–1 mg/kg IV/IM/PO q4–6h

## DMSA (SUCCIMER, CHEMET)
- Indications: Pediatric lead poisoning
- Warnings:
  – Caution in renal impairment—urinary elimination
  – Nausea, vomiting diarrhea
- Dose: 10 mg/kg PO q8h for 5 days, then q12h for 14 days, then reassess blood lead levels

## EPINEPHRINE
- Indications: Angioedema, anaphylaxis, acute asthma, spinal shock, $\beta$-blocker overdose
- Warnings: Dysrhythmias, HTN, tremor, anxiety

- Dose:
  - Hypotension/shock:
  - Adult: 1–4 $\mu$g/min IV infusion
  - Pediatric: Start IV infusion at 0.1 $\mu$g/kg/min.
  - Mild-moderate reactions:
    ○ Adult: 0.3–0.5 mg SC
    ○ Pediatric: 0.01 mg/kg SC

## ETHANOL
- Indications: Methanol or ethylene glycol toxicity
- Warnings:
  - Disulfiram reaction, CNS sedation
  - Hypoglycemia in pediatric population
  - Increase dose during dialysis, for chronic alcoholics.
- Dose:
  - IV: 10 mL/kg load as 10% solution over 1 hr, then 1 mL/kg/h maintenance
  - PO: 1.5 mL/kg as 100-proof solution, then 0.3 mL/kg/h maintenance
  - Goal: Ethanol level of 100–150 mg/dL

## FLUMAZENIL (ROMAZICON)
- Indications: Benzodiazepine overdose
- Warnings:
  - Contraindicated in tricyclic antidepressant (TCA) overdose
  - Lowers seizure threshold
  - Induces benzodiazepine withdrawal
- Dose:
  - Adult: 0.2 mg IV slow, repeat q2–3min to 1 mg max.
  - Pediatric: 0.01–0.05 mg/kg IV over 30 min to 1 hr

## FOMEPIZOLE (4-MP, ANTIZOL)
- Indications: Methanol or ethylene glycol toxicity
- Warnings: Nausea, dizziness, headache
- Dose: 15 mg/kg load, then 10 mg/kg q12h for 4 doses, then 15 mg/kg q12h

## GLUCAGON
- Indications:
  - $\beta$-Blocker or calcium channel blocker overdose with bradycardia/hypotension
  - Hypoglycemia
- Warnings:
  - Nausea, vomiting, hyperglycemia
  - Hypotension from diluent (phenol-containing)
- Dose:
  - $\beta$-Blocker or calcium channel blocker overdose:
    ○ Adult: 5–10 mg IV over 1 min
    ○ Pediatric: 0.15 mg/kg IV over 1 min
  - Hypoglycemia:
    ○ Adult: 0.5–1 mg IM/IV/SC
    ○ Pediatric: 0.025–0.1 mg/kg IM/IV/SC (max. 1 mg per dose)

## INSULIN/GLUCOSE
- Indications:
  - Calcium channel blocker overdose with severe hypotension/symptomatic bradycardia refractory to other therapies
  - Hyperkalemia
- Warnings:
  - Experimental therapy: Consult a poison control center/medical toxicologist.
  - Follow serum glucose q15min for 1 hr after the 1st bolus or after any increase in dose, then q1h
- Dose:
  - Bolus:
    ○ 0.5–1.0 IU/kg regular insulin, followed by 25 g glucose (1 amp $D_{50}$)
  - Maintenance:
    ○ Insulin 0.5 IU regular insulin per kg/h, titrate to 1.0 IU regular insulin per kg/h

- Glucose $D_{10}$ start at 100 mL/h (10 g/h) and titrate to keep glucose $\geq$ 100 mg/dL

## METHYLENE BLUE
- Indications: Methemoglobinemia with dyspnea or >25%
- Warnings: G6-PD deficiency
- Dose: 1–2 mg/kg slow IV as 1% solution, repeat in 1 hr

## NARCAN
- Indications:
  - Opiate poisoning, empiric treatment of coma
- Warnings:
  - Acute opiate withdrawal, severe agitation
- Dose:
  - Adult: 0.4–2.0 mg IV or IM, repeat to 10 mg
  - Pediatric: 0.1 mg/kg IV or IM

## OCTREOTIDE
- Indications: Sulfonylurea overdose with hypoglycemia
- Warnings: Use with caution in diabetic patients.
- Dose:
  - Adult: 50 $\mu$g SC q6h
  - Pediatric: 4–5 $\mu$g/kg/d SC div. q6h

## OXYGEN, HYPERBARIC
- Indications: Carbon monoxide (CO) poisoning
- Warnings:
  - Tympanic membrane (TM) perforation, seizures owing to oxygen toxicity
  - Difficulty monitoring patient
- Dose: 100% oxygen at 2–3 atm

## PENICILLAMINE
- Indications: Arsenic, copper, lead, mercury with/following BAL or EDTA
- Warnings: Contraindicated in penicillin allergy, renal insufficiency
- Dose:
  - Lead:
    ○ Adult: 250–500 mg per dose PO q8–12h
    ○ Pediatric: 25–40 mg/kg/d PO in 3 div. doses
    Arsenic: 100 mg/kg/d PO divided in 4 doses for 5 days (max. 1 g/d)
  - Mercury:
    ○ Adult: 250 mg PO q.i.d.
    ○ Pediatric: 20–30 mg/kg/d PO in 4 div. doses

## PHENTOLAMINE
- Indications:
  - Hypertensive crisis: Stimulants, sympathomimetics, MAO-tyramine reaction, and extravasated pressors
  - Reversal of cocaine-mediated vasospasm
- Warnings: HTN, tachycardia, dysrhythmias
- Dose:
  - HTN (HTN):
    ○ Adult: 1–5 mg IV bolus
    ○ Pediatric: 0.02–0.1 mg/kg bolus
  - Extravasation:
    ○ Adult: 5 mg diluted in 10–15 mL saline SC
    ○ Pediatric: 0.1 mg/kg diluted in 10–15 mL saline SC

## PHYSOSTIGMINE
- Indications: Severe anticholinergic syndrome
- Warnings: Contraindicated in TCA overdose
- Dose:
  - Adult: 0.5–1.0 mg IV, repeat in 10 min PRN
  - Pediatric: 0.02 mg/kg IV, repeat in 10 min PRN

## PRALIDOXIME (2-PAM, PROTOPAM)
- Indications:
  - Organophosphate toxicity
  - Reversal of nicotinic effects

- Reactivates enzyme
- Use in conjunction with atropine
- Warnings:
  - Myasthenic crisis if myasthenia gravis
  - Nausea, headache, dizziness, laryngospasm, muscle rigidity
- Dose:
  - Adult: 1–2 g in 100 mL NaCl over 15 min, repeat in 1 hr PRN, repeat in 6 hr if nicotinic symptoms return
  - Pediatrics: 25–50 mg/kg over 15 min, repeat in 1 hr PRN, repeat in 6 hr if nicotinic symptoms return

## PROTAMINE
- Indications: Reversal of heparin anticoagulation
- Warnings:
  - Hypersensitivity in patients with fish allergy
  - Avoid benzyl alcohol diluent in neonates.
- Dose: 1 mg for each 100 IU heparin, half dose if 30–60 min, and quarter dose if 2 hr after heparin bolus

## PYRIDOXINE (VITAMIN B₆)
- Indications:
  - Isoniazid-induced seizures
  - *Gyromitra* mushroom
- Warnings: None, nontoxic
- Dose:
  - Isonicotinic acid hydrazide (INH)–induced seizures:
    ○ Unknown ingested amount: 5 g for adult or 1 g for pediatrics
    ○ Dose (mg) = amount INH ingested (mg)
    ○ *Gyromitra*: 25 mg/kg IV over 30 min to 1 hr

## RATTLESNAKE ANTIVENIN (CROTALINE)
- Indications: Significant envenomation by *Crotaline* species. Rattlesnake, cottonmouth, water moccasin, pit viper
- Warnings:
  - Equine or ovine-derived products: Immediate hypersensitivity, serum sickness 10–14 days
  - Premedicate for anaphylaxis if know equine/ovine serum hypersensitivity.
- Dose:
  - Equine derived (Wyeth-Ayerst polyvalent).
    ○ Mild: 5 vials—infuse slowly
    ○ Moderate: 10 vials—infuse slowly
    ○ Severe: 15 vials—infuse slowly
  - Ovine-derived (CroFab):
    ○ 4–6 vials slowly; may repeat dose of 4–6 vials if control of envenomation not achieved, then 2 vials q6h for 3 doses

## VITAMIN K (PHYTONADIONE, AQUA MEPHYTON)
- Indications: Reversal of Coumadin anticoagulation
- Warnings: Hypersensitivity from IV administration
- Dose:
  - 2–10 mg IM/SC/slow IV, may repeat in 8 hr
  - 2–10 mg PO, may repeat in 12–48 hr

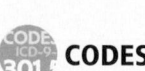 **CODES**

# POISONING, GASTRIC DECONTAMINATION

Frank LoVecchio

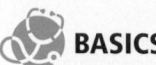 **BASICS**

## DESCRIPTION
Modalities to decontaminate the GI tract of poisons

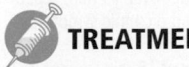 **TREATMENT**

### ALERT
- Ipecac is contraindicated in ambulance setting.
- Controversies:
  - Home use of ipecac in general is not recommended.
  - In extremely rare cases (eg, very prolonged transit times, protecting airway), consider ipecac administration only after consultation with regional poison control center.
  - Decreased time to activated charcoal administration when given in prehospital setting
  - Decreased drug absorption in a simulated ingestion while volunteers were lying in left lateral vs. right lateral decubitus position

### INITIAL STABILIZATION/THERAPY
- Airway, breathing, and circulation management (ABCs):
  - Secure airway for decreased mental status/inability to protect airway.
  - IV access
  - Cardiac monitor
- With altered mental status from overdose:
  - Naloxone
  - Thiamine
  - Dextrose (or Accu-Chek)

### ED TREATMENT/PROCEDURES
- **Ipecac**:
  - General:
    - Derived from the roots of the plant *Cephaelis acuminata*
    - Exerts emetic action by direct gastric irritation and centrally mediated chemoreceptive trigger-zone stimulation
    - Delays administration of activated charcoal
    - Offers no advantage over activated charcoal alone when both treatments are potentially effective

  - Dosage:
    - >12 yr: 30 mL
    - 1–12 yr: 15 mL
    - 6 mo to 1 yr: 5–10 mL plus 15 mL clear fluid
  - Indications:
    - No utility in ED
    - The use should be abandoned.
  - Adverse effects:
    - Vomiting may complicate and worsen clinical presentation.
    - Delay to administration of activated charcoal or oral antidotes
  - Contraindications:
    - Caustics (acids and alkali) ingestion
    - Hydrocarbon ingestion
    - Ingestion of agents that rapidly depress mental status
    - Patient actively vomiting
- **Orogastric lavage**:
  - General:
    - Placement of large-bore tube (32–36 Fr) in stomach for removal of ingested toxins
    - Effectiveness of orogastric lavage depends on time since ingestion, timing of last meal, and toxin ingested.
    - Protected airway is essential prior to any attempts at orogastric lavage.
  - Indications:
    - Presentation within 1 hr of taking a potentially lethal ingestion with no known antidote
    - Poisoned intubated patient
  - Adverse effects:
    - Intubation of respiratory tree
    - Esophageal or gastric perforation
    - Charcoal aspiration
    - Patient discomfort
  - Contraindications:
    - Large pills (limited by lavage-tube port size) ingestion
    - Caustics (acids and alkali) ingestion
    - Hydrocarbon ingestion
    - Ingestion of agents that rapidly depress mental status
    - Unprotected airway

- Pediatric considerations:
  - Avoid in children
  - Unlikely to result in any clinically significant pill extraction secondary to smaller-bore orogastric tube (ie, 18 Fr)
  - Risk of aspiration increased in children
  - Controversies: Several randomized, controlled trials have documented no benefit when lavage plus activated charcoal is compared with activated charcoal alone.
- **Activated charcoal:**
  - General:
    - Prepared by treating heated wood pulp, which creates a large surface area to bind toxins
    - Mainstay of gastric decontamination
    - Effective when contents have reached small intestine
  - Dose:
    - 1–2 g/kg of body weight or an activated charcoal-to-drug ratio of 10:1; often mixed with sorbitol (see below)
    - Oral or nasogastric tube administration
  - Indications:
    - Administer in every toxic ingestion (see below for exceptions).
    - Optimal for toxic ingestions presenting within 1 hr of ingesting a drug that is absorbed by charcoal in a patient with a patent airway
  - Adverse effects:
    - Vomiting and constipation
    - Charcoal aspiration and subsequent charcoal pneumonitis
  - Contraindications:
    - Caustic ingestions
    - Unprotected airway
    - Bowel obstruction or ileus
  - Drugs not effectively bound to charcoal:
    - Metals (borates, bromide, iron, lithium)
    - Alcohols
    - Potassium
    - Potassium cyanide (poorly absorbed)
    - Hydrocarbons
    - Caustics

– Pediatric considerations:
  ○ Mix with palatable substance (cola or juice) to facilitate intake or administer via gastric tube.
– Controversies:
  ○ Randomized, controlled trials have shown a slightly worse outcome and higher complication rate when *asymptomatic* patients received charcoal versus nothing.
  ○ An extremely small minority of patients are likely to benefit from gastric lavage.

• **Multiple-dose activated charcoal:**
  – General:
    ○ Used in toxic ingestions that are well absorbed by charcoal and undergo enterohepatic circulation
  – Dose:
    ○ 1 g/kg followed by 0.5 g/kg q2–6h
    ○ Never use cathartics in conjunction with multiple-dose activated charcoal.
  – Indications:
    ○ Theophylline
    ○ Salicylates
    ○ Multiple-dose activated charcoal may decrease area under the curve for such drugs as phenobarbital, phenytoin, and carbamazepine but has not been proven to improve outcome.

• **Cathartics:**
  – General:
    ○ Used in combination with activated charcoal to prevent constipation and to enhance GI transit time
    ○ Limited data available to demonstrate any decreased absorption when a cathartic (sorbitol) is added to activated charcoal
    ○ Cathartics alone are of no proven benefit and should be avoided.
    ○ *Never* use cathartics in conjunction with multiple-dose activated charcoal.

  – Dose:
    ○ Magnesium citrate: 10% solution: 250 mL (peds: 4 mL/kg)
    ○ Magnesium sulfate: 15–20 g (peds: 250 mg/kg)
    ○ Sorbitol: 0.5–1 g/kg to a max. 100 g of 70% solution (peds: >1 yr old: 0.5–1 g/kg as a 35% solution to a max. 50 g) PO mixed in the activated charcoal slurry—use only in 1st dose.
  – Adverse effects:
    ○ Dehydration
    ○ Hypermagnesemia
    ○ Diarrhea
    ○ Abdominal discomfort
  – Contraindications:
    ○ Preexisting dehydration
    ○ Renal disease (cathartics containing magnesium)
    ○ Avoid in children
  – Controversies:
    ○ No proven benefit and some cases of harm reported

• **Whole-bowel irrigation:**
  – General: Cleansing of bowel
  – Indications:
    ○ Toxins not well absorbed by charcoal, such as toxic iron and lithium ingestions
    ○ Toxins in sealed containers (body packers) without signs of gastrointestinal perforation
    ○ Toxic, sustained-release product ingestions
  – Dose:
    ○ Polyethylene glycol (Colyte, Go-Lytely)
    ○ Solution at 2 L/h in adults (0.5 L/h in children) until rectal excretions clear
    ○ Administer via nasogastric tube with activated charcoal via continuous or bolus method as indicated.
  – Adverse effects:
    ○ Bloating
    ○ Rectal irritation
    ○ Frequent bowel movements
  – Contraindications:
    ○ Mechanical or pharmacologic ileus
    ○ Bowel obstruction
    ○ Intestinal perforation
    ○ Unprotected airway

## PEARLS AND PITFALLS

• Ipecac has no utility in the ED.
• Administer activated charcoal in almost every toxic ingestion.
• Never use multiple doses of cathartic in conjunction with multiple-dose activated charcoal.

## ADDITIONAL READING

• American College of Emergency Physicians. Clinical policy for the initial approach to patients with acute toxic ingestions or dermal or inhalation exposure. *Ann Emerg Med*. 1995;25:570–585.
• Ellenhorn MJ, Schoonwald S, Ordog G, et al. Gut decontamination. In: Ellenhorn MJ, ed. *Ellenhorn's Medical Toxicology*, 2nd ed. Baltimore: Williams & Wilkins; 1997:66–78.
• Perrone J, Hoffman RS, Goldfrank LR. Special considerations in gastric decontamination. *Emerg Med Clin*. 1994;12:285–299.
• Pond SM, Lewis Driver DJ, Williams GM, et al. Gastric emptying in acute overdose: A prospective randomized controlled trial. *Med J Aust*. 1995;163: 345–349.

### See Also (Topic, Algorithm, Electronic Media Element)

• Poisoning
• Poisoning, Antidotes
• Poisoning, Toxidromes

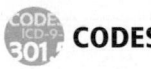 **CODES**

**ICD9**

973.8 Poisoning by other specified agents primarily affecting the gastrointestinal system

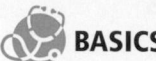 **BASICS**

## DESCRIPTION

- A toxidrome is the constellation of signs and symptoms that result from the effects of a particular toxin.
- The mechanism of action varies with each class of toxin to which the patient may be exposed:
  - Anticholinergic: Results from inhibition of acetylcholine at receptors
  - Cholinergic: Excess parasympathetic stimulation and *cholinergic crisis* result from inhibition of acetylcholinesterase or increased activity at acetylcholine receptor.
  - Opiates: Differ in their agonist and antagonist properties at various opioid receptor sites:
    ○ $\mu$-Receptor stimulation—full agonist
    ○ $\kappa$ and $\delta$ receptors share partial agonist and antagonist properties.
  - Sympathomimetic: Stimulation of sympathetic effector organs (particularly CNS)
  - Withdrawal: Hyperactivity of sympathetic nervous system predominates.

 **DIAGNOSIS**

## SIGNS AND SYMPTOMS

### Toxidromes

- There are 6 classic toxidromes:
  - Anticholinergic
  - Cholinergic
  - Sympathomimetic
  - Opiate
  - Sedative–hypnotic
  - Sedative withdrawal.
- Serotonin syndrome and malignant neuroleptic syndrome are 2 other important toxic syndromes.
- **Anticholinergic**: Mnemonic: *"Blind as a bat, mad as a hatter, red as a beet, hot as a hare, dry as a bone, the bowel and bladder lose their tone, and the heart runs alone"*:
  - Hyperthermia ("hot as a hare")
  - Dry, flushed skin ("dry as a bone" and "red as a beet")
  - Dilated pupils ("blind as a bat")
  - Delirium ("mad as a hatter")
  - Tachycardia ("the heart runs alone")
  - Hypertension
  - Hyperthermia
  - Urgency retention ("bowel and bladder lose their tone")
  - Decreased bowel sounds ("bowel and bladder lose their tone")
  - Seizures
  - Mental status changes
  - Somnolence

- **Cholinergic**: Mnemonic: *DUMBELS for the muscarinic component:*
  - Muscarinic signs:
    ○ Diarrhea, diaphoresis
    ○ Urination
    ○ Miosis
    ○ Bradycardia, bronchorrhea, bronchospasm (the killer B's)
    ○ Emesis
    ○ Lacrimation
    ○ Salivation
  - Nicotinic signs:
    ○ Mydriasis
    ○ Tachycardia
    ○ Weakness
    ○ Hypertension
    ○ Fasciculations
- **Sympathomimetic**: Similar to anticholinergic presentation except for skin and bowel differences (diaphoresis and increased bowel sounds may be present in sympathomimetic presentations):
  - Diaphoresis
  - Mydriasis
  - Tachycardia
  - Hypertension
  - Hyperthermia
  - Seizures
  - Increased peristalsis
- **Opiate**:
  - Classic triad:
    ○ Miosis
    ○ Hypoventilation
    ○ Coma
  - May also present with:
    ○ Bradycardia
    ○ Hypotension
    ○ Hypothermia
    ○ Decreased bowel sounds
- **Sedative–hypnotics and alcohol**:
  - Sedation
  - Mental status changes (confusion, delirium, hallucinations)
  - Vision changes (blurred vision, diplopia)
  - Slurred speech
  - Ataxia
  - Nystagmus
- **Withdrawal** (alcohol, benzodiazepine, barbiturates):
  - Mydriasis
  - Tachycardia
  - Hypertension
  - Hyperthermia
  - Increased respiratory rate
  - Diaphoresis
  - Increased bowel sounds
  - Tremor
  - Agitation
  - Anxiety
  - Hallucinations
  - Confusion
  - Seizures

- **Withdrawal** (opioid):
  - Nausea
  - Vomiting
  - Diarrhea
  - Abdominal cramps
  - Increased bowel sounds
  - Mydriasis
  - Piloerection
  - Tachycardia
  - Lacrimation
  - Salivation
  - Hypertension
  - Yawning
- **Neuroleptic malignant syndrome**:
  - Recent treatment with typical and atypical antipsychotic medications:
    ○ Generally occurs from hours to several weeks of starting or increasing the dose of a medication, but can occur at any time.
  - Hyperthermia
  - Muscular rigidity
  - Diaphoresis
  - Mental status changes
  - Hypertension or hypotension may be seen
  - Sialorrhea
  - Tremor
  - Incontinence
  - Increased creatinine phosphokinase
  - Leukocytosis
  - Metabolic acidosis
- **Serotonin syndrome**:
  - Occurs soon after the increase in dose or addition of serotonergic medications.
  - Syndrome with variable presentation
  - Following are most common, seen 25–57% of the time:
    ○ Mental status changes (confusion, agitation, hypomania, lethargy)
    ○ Seizures
    ○ Myoclonus
    ○ Hyperreflexia
    ○ Muscle rigidity
    ○ Tremor
    ○ Nystagmus
    ○ Hyperthermia
    ○ Diaphoresis
    ○ Tachycardia
    ○ Hypertension
    ○ Mydriasis

### Physical Exam

- **Bradycardia**:
  - $\alpha_2$-Adrenergic agonists (eg, clonidine)
  - $\beta$-Blockers
  - Calcium-channel blockers
  - Digoxin and related substances
  - Cholinergics
  - Opioids
- **Tachycardia**
  - Sympathomimetics
  - Anticholinergics
  - Methylxanthines
  - Tricyclic antidepressant
  - Withdrawal
  - Phenothiazines
  - Atypical antipsychotics
  - $\alpha_1$-Blockade with reflex tachycardia
  - Phosphodiesterase type 5 inhibitor (eg, Sildenafil)

P

- **Hyperthermia:**
  - Anticholinergics
  - Sympathomimetics
  - Serotonin syndrome
  - Neuroleptic malignant syndrome
  - Malignant hyperthermia
  - Dinitrophenol
  - Salicylates
  - Withdrawal
- **Hypothermia:**
  - Carbon monoxide
  - Oral Hypoglycemics
  - Opiates
  - Ethanol
  - Sedative–hypnotics
  - $\alpha_2$-Adrenergic agonists
- **Hypertension:**
  - Sympathomimetics
  - Anticholinergics
  - Nicotine
  - Phencyclidine (PCP)
  - Ergot alkaloids
- **Hypotension:**
  - $\alpha_2$-Agonists
  - $\alpha_1$-Antagonists
  - $\beta$-Blockers
  - Calcium-channel blockers
  - Angiotensin-converting-enzyme inhibitors
  - Methylxanthines
  - Nitrates
  - Opioids
  - Phenothiazines
  - Phosphodiesterase type 5 inhibitors
  - Sedative–hypnotics
  - Ethanol
  - Tricyclic antidepressants
  - Atypical antipsychotic medications
- **Miosis:**
  - Cholinergics
  - Clonidine
  - Reserpine
  - Phenothiozines
  - Atypical antipsychotics
- **Mydriasis:**
  - Anticholinergics
  - Sympathomimetics
  - Withdrawal (esp. opioids)
  - Botulism
- **Seizures:** *Mnemonic with a limited list of causes for toxic seizures* OTIS CAMPBELL:
  - Organophosphates
  - Tricyclic antidepressants
  - Isoniazid, insulin
  - Sympathomimetics, salicylates
  - Camphor, cocaine, citalopram
  - Amphetamines, anticholinergic agents
  - Methylxanthines (theophylline, caffeine), mushrooms (*Gyromitra*: monomethyl hydrazine group)
  - PCP, pethidine (Demerol), propoxyphene, plants (nicotine, water hemlock)
  - Benzodiazepine withdrawal, bupropion
  - Ethanol withdrawal
  - Lithium, lidocaine
  - Lead, lindane
- **Diaphoresis:**
  - Sympathomimetics
  - Cholinergics
  - Salicylates
  - Withdrawal
  - Serotonin syndrome

- **Bradypnea:**
  - Opiates
  - Sedative–hypnotics
  - Ethanol
  - $\gamma$-Hydroxybutyric acid and congeners
  - Botulism
  - Muscular receptor blockade
- **Tachypnea:**
  - Paraquat (and other drugs that cause pneumonitis)
  - Salicylates
  - Sympathomimetics
  - Dinotrophenol
  - Methylxanthines

### *Dermatologic*

- Mee's lines:
  - Arsenic
  - Thallium
  - Chemotherapy agents
  - Radiation
- Bullae:
  - Barbiturates
  - Carbon monoxide
  - Captopril
- Flushed or red appearance:
  - Anticholinergics
  - Disulfiram reactions
  - Niacin
  - Boric acid
  - Scombroid poisoning
  - Monosodium glutamate
  - Carbon monoxide (frequently postmortem)
  - Cyanide (rare)
  - Vancomycin
- Blue skin:
  - Ergotamines
  - Methemoglobinemia from:
    - ○ Nitrite
    - ○ Nitrate
    - ○ Dapsone
    - ○ Aniline dye
    - ○ Phenazopyridine
    - ○ Benzocaine
    - ○ Chloroquine
  - Pseudocyanosis from:
    - ○ Chlorpromazine
    - ○ Amiodarone
    - ○ Minocycline
    - ○ Silver (argyria)
    - ○ Gold (chrysiasis)

### ESSENTIAL WORKUP

Depends on ingested substance:

- CBC
- Electrolytes, BUN, creatinine, glucose
- Urinalysis
- Arterial blood gas, venous blood gas
- Carboxyhemoglobin, methemoglobin levels
- Toxicology screen
- Serum osmols
- Liver function tests

### DIAGNOSTIC TESTS & INTERPRETATION

- **Anion gap acidosis:** Mnemonic: *A CAT MUD PILES (encompasses a limited number of common causes)*:
  - Alcohol ketoacidosis
  - CO/cyanide
  - Acetaminophen in fulminant hepatic failure

- Toluene
- Methanol
- Uremia
- Diabetic ketoacidosis
- Paraldehyde, phenformin/metformin
- Iron, isoniazid
- Lactic acidosis
- Ethylene glycol
- Salicylates, sodium azide, hydrogen sulfide
- **Increased osmolar gap:**
  - Methanol
  - Ethylene glycol
  - Isopropyl alcohol
  - Ethanol
  - Acetone
  - Mannitol

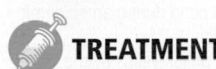 **TREATMENT**

### INITIAL STABILIZATION/THERAPY
ABCs

### ED TREATMENT/PROCEDURES
Depends on ingested substance (see "Poisoning"; "Poisoning, Gastric Decontamination")

## PEARLS AND PITFALLS

- Obtain appropriate laboratory tests.
- Recognize signs and symptoms and laboratory clues to the toxidromes.

## ADDITIONAL READING

- Boyer EW, Shannon M. The serotonin syndrome. *N Engl J Med.* 2005;352:1112–1120.
- Weatherald J, Marrie T. Pseudocyanosis. Drug-induced skin hyperpigmentation can mimic cyanosis. *Am J Med.* 121(5):385–386.
- Benzer TI. Neuroleptic malignant syndrome. *eMedicine.* Available at: http://emedicine.medscape.com/article/816018. Updated Aug 18, 2009.
- Nelson L, Lewin N, Howland MA, et al. *Goldfrank's Toxicologic Emergencies,* 9th ed. New York: McGraw-Hill; 2010.

### See Also (Topic, Algorithm, Electronic Media Element)

- Poisoning
- Poisoning, Gastric Decontamination

 **CODES**

### ICD9

- 965.00 Poisoning by opium (alkaloids), unspecified
- 971.0 Poisoning by parasympathomimetics (cholinergics)
- 971.1 Poisoning by parasympatholytics (anticholinergics and antimuscarinics) and spasmolytics

# POLIO

Philip Shayne
Ann Azcuy

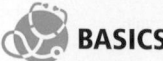 **BASICS**

## DESCRIPTION

- Caused by poliovirus infection
- Incubation period 7–14 days
- Duration <1 wk
- Clinical manifestations are defined as follows:
  - Subclinical (ie, not apparent) 90–95%
  - Abortive poliomyelitis 4–8%:
    ○ Clinically indistinct from many other viral infections (fever, myalgias, malaise)
    ○ Only suspected to be polio during an epidemic
  - Nonparalytic poliomyelitis 1–2%:
    ○ Differs from abortive poliomyelitis by the presence of meningeal irritation
    ○ Course similar to any aseptic meningitis
  - Paralytic poliomyelitis 0.1%, which is further subdivided:
    ○ Spinal paralytic poliomyelitis (frank polio)
    ○ Bulbar paralytic poliomyelitis (10% of paralytic polio): Paralysis of muscle groups innervated by cranial nerves; involves the circulatory and respiratory centers of the medulla with high mortality
    ○ Mixed bulbospinal poliomyelitis
  - Postpoliomyelitis syndrome:
    ○ New onset of increased muscle weakness, pain, and focal or generalized atrophy
    ○ Occurs 8–70 yr after the active illness, usually in the previously affected limb
    ○ Risk factors include age at time of infection and extent of recovery (increased risk with better recovery)
    ○ Gradual progression

## ETIOLOGY

- Polioviruses:
  - Picornaviruses
  - Small, nonenveloped RNA viruses of the enterovirus genera
- Fecal-oral route transmission
- Humans are the only natural host and reservoir.
- Poliovirus selectively destroys motor and autonomic neurons.

- Natural (wild) virus is completely eliminated in the Americas.
- Oral poliovirus vaccine (OPV):
  - Accounts for only poliomyelitis seen in the U.S.
  - 8–10 cases/yr of vaccine-associated paralytic poliomyelitis (VAP): Neurovirulent conversion of vaccine virus; decreased since widespread use of inactivated poliovirus vaccine (IPV)
  - VAP occurs in poorly immunized regions by acquiring properties of wild-type virus.

 **DIAGNOSIS**

## SIGNS AND SYMPTOMS

- Primarily asymptomatic
- Viral symptoms: Fever, headache, sore throat, malaise, fatigue, nausea, vomiting
- Muscle pain and weakness
- Progressive weakness for <1 wk:
  - Dysphagia and dysarthria with bulbar involvement

### History

- Vaccination history
- History of prior polio infection
- Recent exposure to individual vaccinated with OPV
- Recent travel to endemic countries (Nigeria, Pakistan, India, Afghanistan)
- Comorbid conditions affecting immunocompetence

### Physical Exam

- Fever (37–39°C)
- Headache, photophobia
- Nuchal rigidity
- Neurologic changes:
  - Muscle soreness that becomes severe muscle spasm, progressing rapidly to spotty flaccid weakness and paralysis
  - Asymmetric paralysis more prominent in the lower than the upper extremities
  - Urinary retention (50% of paralytic cases)
  - Reflexes initially hyperactive, then absent
  - Apprehensive and irritable, occasionally drowsy
  - No sensory loss associated with the motor deficit

### Pediatric Considerations

More likely to have a biphasic acute course:

- Viral-type syndrome for 1–2 days
- Symptom-free period of 2–5 days
- Then an abrupt onset of the major illness

## ESSENTIAL WORKUP

- Clinical diagnosis
- Differentiate from other causes of acute paralysis.
- Notify public health officials when diagnosis suspected.

## DIAGNOSTIC TESTS & INTERPRETATION
### Lab

- CBC:
  - WBC normal or mildly elevated
- Diagnosis confirmed by:
  - Comparing acute with convalescent sera for antigen titers
  - Isolation of virus from blood, CSF, stool, throat secretions (within week 1 of infection)

### Diagnostic Procedures/Surgery

- Lumbar puncture/CSF analysis:
  - Abnormalities typical of aseptic meningitis (increased lymphocytes and elevated protein)
  - Poliovirus rarely isolated from the CSF
- Electrodiagnostics:
  - Normal to slow motor function
  - Sensory function intact

## DIFFERENTIAL DIAGNOSIS

- Abortive poliomyelitis is similar to many viral illnesses.
- Nonparalytic poliomyelitis is indistinguishable from any viral, aseptic meningitis.
- Paralytic poliomyelitis:
  - Guillain-Barré (not febrile, symmetric, not ill appearing)
  - Acute transverse myelitis
  - Spinal cord compression/infarction
  - Multiple sclerosis
  - Rhabdomyolysis
  - Acute intermittent porphyria
  - West Nile virus
  - Diphtheria
  - Botulism
  - Tick paralysis
  - Encephalitis

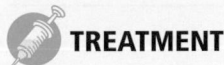 **TREATMENT**

**ALERT**
Rare fatal case comes from respiratory insufficiency, which requires prompt ventilatory support.

**INITIAL STABILIZATION/THERAPY**
Aggressive pulmonary toilet and early intubation mandated for respiratory insufficiency

**ED TREATMENT/PROCEDURES**
- Supportive and symptomatic management
- Analgesics for severe muscle pain and spasm
- Bed rest to prevent augmentation or extension of paralysis
- Paralytic poliomyelitis tends to localize to a limb that has been the site of intramuscular injection or injury within 2–4 wk prior to the onset of infection:
  - Avoid any unnecessary tissue damage in suspected cases.
  - No antiviral agents available
  - Prevention
- IPV:
  - Costly
  - Painful
  - No conferred immunity
  - No VAP, which previously accounted for all poliomyelitis cases in the U.S.
- OPV:
  - Accounted for only poliomyelitis seen in the U.S. (8–10 cases/yr)
  - Incidence of VAP: 1/900,000 (immunocompromised: 1/1,000):
    - Most at risk are the underimmunized young and their caretakers.
  - Confers immunity to unvaccinated contacts by fecal-oral spread.
  - Inexpensive
  - No longer available in the U.S.
  - Still remains vaccine recommended by WHO Expanded Program on Immunization

 **FOLLOW-UP**

**DISPOSITION**
*Admission Criteria*
All acute-phase paralytic poliomyelitis for strict bed rest and observation for respiratory symptoms:
- Isolate from nonvaccinated personnel.

*Discharge Criteria*
No evidence of nervous system involvement and no danger of contact with nonvaccinated population:
- Deterioration of muscle strength usually ends after 3–5 days.

**FOLLOW-UP RECOMMENDATIONS**
Physical therapy:
- Only 1/3 of people with acute flaccid paralysis regain full strength.

## PEARLS AND PITFALLS

- Most cases are asymptomatic, with symptoms ranging from viral illness to acute flaccid paralysis.
- IPV is the only vaccine available in the U.S., but OPV is still the vaccine of choice for global eradication.
- Diagnosis is primarily clinical and is confirmed by virus isolation from blood, CSF, stool, or throat secretions.
- Treatment is supportive; all acute-phase paralytic poliomyelitis patients should be admitted for observation.
- Paralytic poliomyelitis may occur decades after initial infection and manifests with neurologic and nonneurologic symptoms.

## ADDITIONAL READING

- Alexander L, Birkhead G, Guerra F, et al. Ensuring preparedness for potential poliomyelitis outbreaks: Recommendations for the US poliovirus vaccine stockpile from the National Vaccine Advisory Committee (NVAC) and the Advisory Committee on Immunization Practices (ACIP). *Arch Pediatr Adolesc Med.* 2004;158:1106–1112.
- Bouza C, Muñoz A, Amate JM. Postpolio syndrome: A challenge to the health-care system. *Health Policy.* 2005;71(1):97–106.
- Centers for Disease Control and Prevention. Imported vaccine-associated paralytic poliomyelitis—United States, 2005. *MMWR Morb Mortal Wkly Rep.* 2006;55(4):97–99.
- Centers for Disease Control and Prevention. Updated recommendations of the Advisory Committee on Immunization Practices (ACIP) regarding routine poliovirus vaccination. *MMWR Morb Mortal Wkly Rep.* 2009;58(30):829–830.
- Shahzad A, Köhler G. Inactivated polio vaccine (IPV): A strong candidate vaccine for achieving global polio eradication program. *Vaccine.* 2009;27(39):5293–5294.
- White C, Halperin SA, Scheifele DW. Pediatric combined formulation DTaP-IPV/Hib vaccine. *Expert Rev Vaccines.* 2009;8(7):831–840.

**See Also (Topic, Algorithm, Electronic Media Element)**
- Botulism
- Encephalitis
- Guillain-Barré Syndrome
- Multiple Sclerosis
- Rhabdomyolysis
- Spinal Cord Syndromes
- Tick Bite
- West Nile Virus

 **CODES**

**ICD9**
- 045.00 Acute paralytic poliomyelitis specified as bulbar, unspecified type of poliovirus
- 045.10 Acute poliomyelitis with other paralysis, unspecified type of poliovirus
- 045.90 Unspecified acute poliomyelitis, unspecified type poliovirus

# POLYCYTHEMIA

*David N. Zull*

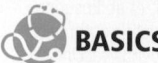 **BASICS**

## DESCRIPTION
- Increase in circulating RBCs above the normal range:
  - Men: Hemoglobin (Hgb) >17 g/dL, hematocrit (Hct) >50%
  - Women: Hgb >15 g/dL, Hct >45%
- Symptoms are related to blood viscosity, which increases exponentially at Hct >60%.

## ETIOLOGY
- Relative (apparent) polycythemia:
  - Resulting from decrease in plasma volume/dehydration
  - Gaisbock syndrome (stress polycythemia): Obese, hypertensive, middle-aged smokers with chronic elevations in Hct
- Primary erythrocytosis:
  - Polycythemia vera (PV): A stem cell disorder characterized by panhyperplasia of all bone marrow elements leading to increased production of RBCs, WBCs, and platelets. Erythrocytosis is the most prominent feature:
    - Proliferative stage: Increase in RBCs, megakaryocytes, platelets
    - Stable phase: Return of blood counts to normal values due to replacement of marrow by fibrosis
    - Spent phase: Extensive marrow fibrosis: Peripheral cytopenias
- Secondary polycythemia:
  - Central hypoxia increasing erythropoietin:
    - Chronic pulmonary disease
    - Sleep apnea
    - Obesity hypoventilation syndrome (Pickwickian syndrome)
    - Congenital heart disease (right-to-left shunt)
    - High altitude (chronic)
    - Smoker's erythrocytosis
    - Carbon monoxide poisoning (chronic)
    - Chronic methemoglobinemia
  - Renal-mediated causes of increased erythropoietin production:
    - Renal artery atherosclerotic narrowing
    - Focal glomerulonephritis
    - Postrenal transplant with or without rejection
    - Renal cell carcinoma
    - Chronic hydronephrosis
    - Polycystic kidney disease and renal cysts
  - Inappropriate autonomous erythropoietin production:
    - Hepatomas
    - Cerebellar hemangioblastoma
    - Wilm tumor
    - Parathyroid carcinoma and adenoma
    - Ovarian tumors
    - Adrenal adenomas and carcinomas (including pheochromocytoma)
    - Uterine leiomyomata
  - Blood doping:
    - Recombinant erythropoietin abuse
    - Autologous transfusions
  - Drug abuse:
    - Chronic cocaine abuse
    - Androgenic steroids
- Genetic disorders with polycythemia:
  - High-affinity hemoglobin variants
  - Bisphosphoglycerate deficiency
  - von Hippel-Lindau syndrome
  - Chuvash polycythemia
  - Erythropoietin-receptor mutations
  - Congenital methemoglobinemia
- Miscellaneous:
  - Viral hepatitis, Cushing syndrome, primary aldosteronism, AIDS, and azidothymidine treatment

## *Diagnostic Criteria for Polycythemia Vera*
- Major criteria:
  - A1: Hemoglobin >18.5 g/dL in men, >16.5 g/dL women, or increased RBC mass (male: >35 mL/kg, female: >32 mL/kg)
  - A2: Presence of JAK2 mutation by polymerase chain reaction (PCR)
  - A3: Oxygen saturation >92% and no other cause for secondary erythrocytosis
  - A4: Splenomegaly
- Minor criteria:
  - B1: Platelets >400,000/mm$^3$
  - B2: ANC >10,000 (WBC >12,000/mm$^3$)
  - B3: CT evidence of splenomegaly
  - B4: Low serum erythropoietin level
- Diagnosis established by any of these combinations:
  - A1 + A2 (consider 1.5 g/dL lower Hgb cutoff if A2 positive)
  - A1, A3, A4
  - A1 + A3 + any 2 category B criteria
- Adjuncts to diagnosis:
  - Bone marrow aspirate and biopsy revealing panhyperplasia
  - Leukocyte alkaline phosphatase elevation
  - B$_{12}$ >900 pg/mL; unbound vitamin B$_{12}$-binding capacity >2,200 pg/mL

 **DIAGNOSIS**

## SIGNS AND SYMPTOMS
### *History*
- General:
  - Dyspnea
  - Weakness/fatigue
  - Excessive sweating
  - Epistaxis/gingival bleeding
  - Pruritus:
    - Generalized
    - Exacerbated by warm bath or shower
    - 40% of PV, uncommon in other causes
    - Excoriations from scratching common in PV
  - Gouty arthritis and tophi
- Neurologic (hyperviscosity):
  - Headache
  - Vertigo/dizziness/tinnitus
  - Lethargy/confusion
  - Paresthesias
  - Cerebrovascular accident/transient ischemic attack
- Visual (hyperviscosity):
  - Amaurosis fugax
  - Scomata/blurred vision
  - Ophthalmic migraine

- Cardiovascular:
  - CHF
  - Angina/myocardial infarction
  - Deep vein thrombosis (DVT)
  - Hypertension
- Extremities:
  - Erythromelalgia:
    - Secondary to capillary sludging
    - Burning pain in the feet or hands
    - Warmth, erythema/cyanosis of the affected areas
    - Acral paresthesias
    - Worse at night
    - Relief with cooling
    - Pulses intact
  - Painful ulcers of fingers and toes (digital ischemia)
- GI (unique to PV):
  - Hepatomegaly/splenomegaly
  - Epigastric discomfort/early satiety
  - Peptic ulcer disease/GI bleed
  - Budd-Chiari syndrome (hepatic vein thrombosis): Ascites and peripheral edema

### *Physical Exam*
- Hypertension
- Conjunctival suffusion
- Fundus: Venous engorgement
- Ruddy complexion/plethora
- Erythema/rubor of hands, feet, nailbeds
- Skin excoriations from severe pruritus
- Splenomegaly (75% in PV)
- Hepatomegaly (30% in PV)
- Thrombotic complications:
  - Evidence of stroke
  - DVT
  - Digital infarcts
  - Ascites from Budd-Chiari syndrome
- Complications of hyperviscosity:
  - Lethargy/confusion
  - Crackles/findings of CHF
- Hemorrhagic complications:
  - Ecchymosis
  - Epistaxis
  - Gingival bleeding

## ESSENTIAL WORKUP
CBC with platelets

## DIAGNOSTIC TESTS & INTERPRETATION
### *Lab*
- 1st priority: Distinguish relative from true erythrocytosis:
  - Volume repletion IV or PO, then repeat CBC
- 2nd priority: Evaluate for secondary causes:
  - Pulse oximetry with pO$_2$ <92%
  - Carboxyhemoglobin level
  - Erythropoietin level (normal or elevated if secondary)
  - CXR, chest CT, pulmonary function tests
  - Sleep study
  - Hemoglobin electrophoresis

- RBC mass:
  – Cr-51–labeled RBCs by nuclear medicine
  – Concomitant plasma volume with I-131–labeled albumin always done
  – Usually elevated and may not be needed if Hgb >18.5 and Hct >56 in men, or Hgb >16.5 and Hct >50 in women
  – Red blood cell mass <35 mg/kg (males) or <31 mg/kg (females) is normal
  – Decreased plasma volume with normal RBC mass verifies relative erythrocytosis.
  – Elevated RBC mass suggests PV or secondary polycythemia.
  – Falsely low:
    ○ GI blood loss
    ○ Obesity
    ○ Very early or end-stage PV
- PV suspected if:
  – Elevated RBC mass
  – WBC >12,000 (more specifically total neutrophils >10,000)
  – Platelet count >400,000
  – Pulse oximetry >92%
  – Low erythropoietin level
  – Vitamin $B_{12}$ level elevated in 30% (unbound vitamin $B_{12}$-binding capacity elevated in 75%)
  – Uric acid elevated in 40%
  – Leukocyte alkaline phosphatase elevated in 70%
  – PCR for JAK2 gene mutation diagnostic of PV (seen in >90%)

### Imaging
Abdominal US or CT can detect a nonpalpable spleen.

### DIFFERENTIAL DIAGNOSIS
See Etiology.

 TREATMENT

#### INITIAL STABILIZATION/THERAPY
ABCs with emphasis on fluid resuscitation if no evidence of CHF

#### ED TREATMENT/PROCEDURES
##### Emergency Management of Hyperviscosity Syndrome or Hct >60%
- Fluid resuscitation to achieve hemodilution:
  – Withhold if evidence of CHF
- Emergency phlebotomy of 250–500 mL of blood over 1–2 hr replacing with an equal amount of 0.9% normal saline (NS)
- Removal of 1,000–1,500 mL of blood over 24 hr with a goal of Hct <60 or relief of symptoms:
  – Keep Hct >45.
  – Replace with an equal amount of 0.9% NS.
- Phlebotomize the elderly and those with cardiovascular disease more slowly:
  – Every-other-day phlebotomy
- Emergent surgery with polycythemia:
  – Phlebotomize to Hct of 45 to avoid thrombotic complications postoperatively.
- Thrombocytosis therapy:
  – Administer aspirin if platelet count is 500,000–1,500,000/mm$^3$ and there are no hemorrhagic complications.
- Treat pruritus with diphenhydramine.

### Long Term Management
- Phlebotomy: Maintain Hct at 45% for men and 42% for women.
- Iron supplementation is contraindicated.
- Interferon-$\alpha$:
  – Especially helpful for refractory pruritus and painful splenomegaly
  – Suggested in symptomatic patients <60 yr
- Anagrelide:
  – Specific for thrombocytosis
  – No risk of leukemia, ideal for younger patients with postphlebotomy thrombocytosis
  – Effective alone and can decrease need for or frequency of chemotherapy
- Hydroxyurea:
  – Mainstay of therapy, especially for patients >60 yr, with frequent phlebotomy requirements, thrombotic episodes, or refractory thrombocytosis
- Imatinib (Gleevec)—possible alternative to hydroxyurea
- Aldylating agents:
  – Severe refractory disease
  – High risk of leukemic transformation

### Pregnancy Considerations
Temporary remission during pregnancy, no treatment usually needed

### Pediatric Considerations
- In the neonate, PV is defined as a peripheral venous Hct >65%, Hgb >22 g/dL:
  – Sample must be obtained >6 hr post delivery
  – Capillary Hgb and Hct are 10% higher than venous (always rely on venous)
  – 1–5% of neonates
  – Up to 50% of neonates with intrauterine growth retardation
- Etiology:
  – Maternal-fetal hypoxemia secondary to maternal heart or lung disease, diabetes, preeclampsia, hypertension, or smoking
  – Delayed clamping of the umbilical cord with increase cord transfusion
- Symptoms and signs (most asymptomatic):
  – Acrocyanosis/plethoric
  – Tachypnea/respiratory distress
  – Irritable, lethargic, poor feeding
- Hypoglycemia and hyperbilirubinemia common
- Treatment:
  – Observation and serial CBCs
  – 0.9 NS 100 mg/kg per day (symptomatic)
  – Partial exchange transfusion: Remove 20 mL/kg blood and infuse equal amount of saline (persistent or severe symptoms)

### Geriatric Considerations
Caution with speed of phlebotomy and fluid resuscitation as noted

 FOLLOW-UP

#### DISPOSITION
##### Admission Criteria
- New diagnosis of polycythemia
- Hct >60% without symptoms
- Symptoms of hyperviscosity
- Unstable vital signs/significant comorbidities
- Inability to comply with outpatient treatment or follow-up

##### Discharge Criteria
- Previous diagnosis of polycythemia, Hct <60, and asymptomatic
- Stable vital signs

##### Issues for Referral
All patients should be referred to a hematologist or primary care physician.

## PEARLS AND PITFALLS
- Criteria for phlebotomy is not clear in polycythemia secondary to hypoxemia. While phlebotomy will decrease viscosity, it may decrease oxygen-carrying capacity.
- It is critical to distinguish PV from secondary causes of erythrocytosis since PV carries a high risk of thrombotic complications if the Hct remains >45; therefore aggressive phlebotomy or myelosuppressive therapy may be needed.

## ADDITIONAL READING
- Adams BD, Baker R, Lopez JA, et al. Myeloproliferative disorders and hyperviscosity syndrome. Emerg Med Clin North Am. 2009; 27:459–476.
- Di Nisio M, Barbui T, DiGennaro L, et al. The hematocrit and platelet target in polycythemia vera. Br J Haematol. 2007;136:249–259.
- Elliott MA, Tefferi A. Thrombosis and haemorrhage in polycythaemia vera and essential thrombocythaemia. Br J Haematol. 2005;128: 275–290.
- Finazzi G, Barbui T. Risk adapted therapy in essential thrombocythemia and polycythemia vera. Blood Rev. 2005;19(5):243–252.
- McMullin MF. The classification and diagnosis of erythrocytosis. Int J Lab Hematol. 2008;30: 447–459.
- Patnaik MM, Tefferi A. The complete evaluation of erythrocytosis: congenital and acquired. Leukemia. 2009;23:834–844.
- Sarkar S, Rosenkrantz TS. Neonatal polycythemia and hyperviscosity. Semin Fetal Neonat Med. 2008;13:248–255.

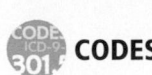 CODES

### ICD9
- 238.4 Polycythemia vera
- 289.0 Polycythemia, secondary

# POSTPARTUM HEMORRHAGE

*Marco Coppola*
*Arun V. Raghavan*

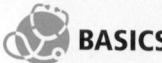 **BASICS**

## DESCRIPTION
- Immediate: Hemorrhage occurring ≤24 hr after delivery
- Delayed: Hemorrhage occurring >24 hr after delivery:
  - Between 24 hr and 6 mo
- Definitions:
  - >500 mL after vaginal delivery
  - >1,000 mL after C-section
  - Blood loss sufficient to cause hypovolemia
  - 10% drop in hematocrit
  - Blood loss requiring transfusion
- Occurs in 4% of vaginal deliveries
- Occurs in 6% of C-sections
- Leading cause of death in pregnancy worldwide
- 95% of postpartum hemorrhage is caused by:
  - Uterine atony (50–60%)
  - Retained placenta (20–30%)
  - Cervical/vaginal lacerations (10%)
- Complications:
  - Hypovolemic shock
  - Blood transfusion
  - Acute respiratory distress syndrome
  - Renal and/or hepatic failure
  - Sheehan syndrome
  - Loss of fertility
  - Disseminated intravascular coagulopathy (DIC)
- Risk factors:
  - Prior postpartum hemorrhage
  - Advanced maternal age
  - Multiple gestations
  - Prolonged labor
  - Polyhydramnios
  - Instrumental delivery
  - Fetal demise
  - Anticoagulation therapy
  - Placental abruption
  - Fibroids
  - Prolonged use of oxytocin
  - C-section
  - Placenta previa and accreta
  - Chorioamnionitis
  - General anesthesia

## ETIOLOGY
- 4 T's:
  - Tone
  - Tissue
  - Trauma
  - Thrombosis
- Immediate:
  - Uterine atony
  - Lower genital lacerations
  - Retained placental tissue
  - Placenta accreta
  - Uterine rupture
  - Uterine inversion
  - Puerperal hematoma
  - Coagulopathies
- Delayed:
  - Retained products of conception
  - Postpartum endometritis
  - Withdrawal of exogenous estrogen
  - Puerperal hematoma
- Coagulopathies:
  - Preexisting idiopathic thrombocytopenic purpura
  - Thrombotic thrombocytopenic purpura
  - Von Willebrand disease
  - DIC
- Associated conditions:
  - If bleeding is present at other sites, consider coagulopathy.

 **DIAGNOSIS**

## SIGNS AND SYMPTOMS
- Ongoing blood loss, usually painless
- Significant hypovolemia, resulting in:
  - Tachycardia
  - Tachypnea
  - Narrow pulse pressure
  - Decreased urine output
  - Cool, clammy skin
  - Poor capillary refill
  - Altered mental status
- Maternal tachycardia and hypotension may not occur until blood loss >1,500 mL.

### History
- Condition is typically recognized by obstetrician soon after delivery.
- Delayed postpartum hemorrhage presents as copious vaginal/perineal bleeding.

- Key historical elements:
  - Complications of delivery
  - Episiotomy
  - Prior clotting disorders
- Symptoms of hypovolemia:
  - Decreased urine output
  - Lightheaded
  - Syncope
  - Pale skin

### Physical Exam
Thorough exam of perineum, cervix, vagina, and uterus:
- External inspection
- Speculum exam
- Bimanual exam

## ESSENTIAL WORKUP
- Abdomen and pelvic examination to assess for uterine atony, retained products, or other anatomic abnormality
- Type and cross-match for packed red blood cells.
- Rapid hemoglobin determination

## DIAGNOSTIC TESTS & INTERPRETATION
Diagnosis is chiefly based on clinical suspicion and exam.

### Lab
- CBC, platelets
- Prothrombin time, partial thromboplastin time
- Fibrinogen level
- Type and cross-match

### Imaging
US may be helpful to evaluate for retained products in delayed postpartum hemorrhage.

### Diagnostic Procedures/Surgery
Manual exam preferred over ultrasonography:
- Greater sensitivity
- Both diagnostic and therapeutic

## DIFFERENTIAL DIAGNOSIS
- Consider puerperal hematomas if perineal, rectal, or lower abdominal pain in conjunction with tachycardia and hypotension.
- Retained products of conception

## TREATMENT

### ALERT
- Patients with postpartum hemorrhage may be hemodynamically unstable.
- IV access and fluid resuscitation is important.

### PRE-HOSPITAL
- Monitor hemodynamics
- Aggressive IV fluids to maintain blood pressure

### INITIAL STABILIZATION/THERAPY
- Attempt to simultaneously control bleeding and stabilize hemodynamic status.
- Manage airway and resuscitate as indicated:
  - Supplemental oxygen
  - Cardiac monitor
- IV fluid resuscitation with normal saline or lactated Ringer solution
- Foley catheter

### ED TREATMENT/PROCEDURES
- Management of uterine atony:
  - Bimanual massage
  - Oxytocin (Pitocin) administered IV/IM
  - Methylergonovine (Methergine) or ergonovine (Ergotrate) IM if oxytocin fails:
    o Avoid if known hypertensive
    o Onset in minutes
  - 15-Methyl prostaglandin $F^{2\alpha}$ ($PGF^{2\alpha}$; Hemabate) IM if above fails:
    o Relatively contraindicated in asthma
  - Surgery if medical intervention fails
- Inspect closely for genital tract laceration: Repair required if $\geq 2$ cm
  - Use 00 or 000 absorbable suture; continuous, locked recommended.
- Management of uterine inversion (acute):
  - Reposition uterus using Johnson maneuver or Harris method:
    o Use left hand on abdominal wall to stabilize fundus of uterus.
    o Place right hand with fingers spread into vagina and push steadily on inverted part to reduce.
  - If unsuccessful, give terbutaline IV or magnesium sulfate to produce cervical relaxation, and reposition.
  - Surgery if unsuccessful or if subacute or chronic inversion
- Uterine balloon tamponade:
  - Various devices have been used, including Sengstaken-Blakemore esophageal catheter

- Management of coagulopathies in childbirth:
  - Fresh-frozen plasma, platelets, cryoprecipitate as indicated
  - Careful attention to volume status
  - Continuous reassessment
  - Active over expectant management
  - Immediate administration of uterotonics after delivery
  - Cord clamping and cutting without delay
  - Cord traction/uterine countertraction (Brandt-Andrews maneuver)

### MEDICATION
- Uterotonics—stimulate uterine contraction to control bleeding:
  - Ergonovine (Ergotrate): 0.2 mg IM; avoid if known hypertensive.
  - Methylergonovine (Methergine): 0.2 mg IM; 0.2 mg PO q6h; avoid if known hypertensive.
  - 15-Methyl $PGF^{2\alpha}$ (Hemabate): 0.25 mg IM; may repeat in 15–60 min.
  - Oxytocin (Pitocin): 10 units IM or 20–40 IU in 1 L normal saline; titrate to achieve uterine contractions.
- Cervical relaxation agents facilitate uterine inversion reduction:
  - Magnesium sulfate 20%: 2 g IM bolus over 10 min
  - Terbutaline: 0.25 mg IV; avoid if hypotensive.

### First Line
- Uterotonics
- Oxytocin
- Methylergonovine

### Second Line
- Surgical intervention:
  - Hysterectomy is required in management of postpartum hemorrhage in 1/1,000 deliveries.
- Radiologic embolization
- Uterine balloon tamponade

## FOLLOW-UP

### DISPOSITION
### Admission Criteria
- All patients with immediate postpartum hemorrhage require admission to a closely monitored setting.
- Early obstetrics consultation is recommended.
- Early surgical intervention is dependent on cause.
- ICU setting if DIC or evidence of hemodynamic compromise
- Patients with endometritis should be admitted for parenteral antibiotics.

### Discharge Criteria
- Delayed postpartum hemorrhage that is easily controlled without excessive bleeding
- Outpatient management with methylergonovine 0.2 mg PO every 6 hr may be considered in consultation and close follow-up with obstetrician.

### FOLLOW-UP RECOMMENDATIONS
- Close follow-up with obstetrician
- Seek immediate care if bleeding recurs.

## PEARLS AND PITFALLS
- Management of postpartum hemorrhage should be active and not expectant.
- Uterotonics are the first line of treatment.
- Aggressive use of fluid and blood products for resuscitation
- Immediate obstetric consult is indicated if significant postpartum hemorrhage.

## ADDITIONAL READING

- Gulmezoglu AM, Forna F, Villar J, et al. Prostaglandins for preventing postpartum haemorrhage. *Cochrane Database Syst Rev.* 2007;(3):CD000494.
- Mercier FJ, Van de Velde M. Major obstetric hemorrhage. *Anesthesiology Clin.* 2008;26:53–66.
- Mousa HA, Alfirevic Z. Treatment for primary postpartum haemorrhage. *Cochrane Database Syst Rev.* 2007;(1):CD003249.
- Oyelese Y, Scorza WF, Mastrolia R, et al. Postpartum hemorrhage. *Obstet Gynecol Clin North Am.* 2007;34:421–441.

### See Also (Topic, Algorithm, Electronic Media Element)
- Vaginal Bleeding
- Placenta Previa
- Placental Abruption
- Pregnancy, Trauma in
- Pregnancy, Uncomplicated
- Labor
- Delivery, Uncomplicated

## CODES

### ICD9
- 666.10 Other immediate postpartum hemorrhage, unspecified as to episode of care
- 666.20 Delayed and secondary postpartum hemorrhage, unspecified as to episode of care

# POSTPARTUM INFECTION

Arun V. Raghavan
Marco Coppola

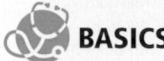 **BASICS**

## DESCRIPTION
- Early postpartum endometritis (PPE):
  - Classic triad:
    - Fever
    - Lower abdominal pain and uterine tenderness
    - Foul-smelling lochia
  - Develops within 48 hr
  - Most often complicating C-section
  - Risk of PPE as high as 85–95% in high-risk nonelective C-section patient
  - Occurs in 1–3% of uncomplicated vaginal deliveries
- Late PPE:
  - Develops after 3 days to 6 wk
  - Usually following vaginal delivery
- Complications of PPE:
  - Pelvic thrombophlebitis
  - Pelvic abscess
  - Bacteremia:
    - All are more common after C-section vs. vaginal delivery.
- Risk factors for PPE:
  - C-section
  - Prolonged labor
  - Prolonged rupture of membranes
  - Increased number of vaginal exams
  - Use of internal fetal monitoring
- Septic pelvic thrombophlebitis is a diagnosis of exclusion with two distinct clinical presentations, either of which may present with postpartum pulmonary embolus:
  - Acute thrombosis: Most common right ovarian vein, usually occurring in 1st 48 hr as acute, progressive lower abdominal pain
  - Enigmatic fever: "Picket fence" spiking fevers and tachycardia
- Septic abortion:
  - Still common in developing countries
  - Usually an ascending infection through an open cervical os
  - Associated with:
    - Nonsterile techniques, instruments
    - Retained products of conception
- Mastitis:
  - Ranges from mild breast redness to fever, systemic illness, and abscess
  - Common (1–30% of postpartum patients)
  - Occurs within the 1st 3 mo postpartum
  - Peaks at 2–3 wk
  - Recurs in 4–8%

- Risk factors:
  - Cracked, sore nipples
  - Ineffective technique with incomplete emptying
  - Use of breast pump
  - Immunocompromise
  - Diabetes
  - Steroid use
  - Prior lumpectomy or radiotherapy
  - Tight-fitting bras/clothing
  - Stress/fatigue
- UTI/pyelonephritis:
  - Along with mastitis accounts for 80% of postpartum infections

## ETIOLOGY
- Postpartum endometritis:
  - Polymicrobial infection result of ascending spread from lower genital tract
  - Anaerobic (up to 80%) and aerobic (~70%):
  - Gram-positive aerobes:
    - Group A, B streptococci
    - Enterococci
    - *Gardnerella vaginalis*
  - Gram-negative aerobes:
    - *Escherichia coli*
    - *Enterobacter*
  - Anaerobes:
    - *Bacteroides*
    - *Peptostreptococcus*
  - Other genital mycoplasmas common in late PPE:
    - *Ureaplasma urealyticum*
    - *Mycoplasma hominids*
    - *Chlamydia trachomatis*
- Septic abortion:
  - Usually polymicrobial
  - *Escherichia coli*
  - *Bacteroides*
  - Anaerobic gram-negative rods
  - Group B streptococci
  - Staphylococcus
  - STD:
    - Gonorrhea
    - *Chlamydia trachomatis*
    - *Trichomonas*
- Mastitis:
  - *Staphylococcus aureus*
  - Group A and B-hemolytic streptococci
  - *Escherichia coli*
  - *Bacteroides*

## DIAGNOSIS

### SIGNS AND SYMPTOMS
*History*
- Careful birth history:
  - C-section
  - Length of labor
  - Complications
  - Exposure to STDs
- Preexisting immunocompromise or disease
- Endometritis:
  - Fever and chills
  - Abdominal pain
  - Foul-smelling lochia
- Septic abortion:
  - Similar to endometritis
  - Fever
  - Abdominal pain
  - May present with symptoms of shock including:
    - Dyspnea (acute respiratory distress syndrome [ARDS], pulmonary edema)
    - Bruising, bleeding (disseminated intravascular coagulation [DIC])
- Mastitis:
  - Fever
  - Breast pain, engorgement, redness
- Other sources of infection:
  - Wound infection:
    - Redness, pain, swelling
  - UTI/pyelonephritis:
    - Fever, dysuria, frequency, flank pain

*Physical Exam*
- Abdominal and/or uterine tenderness
- Foul-smelling lochia
- Unilateral tender, engorged, erythematous breast in cases of mastitis
- Episiotomy infections
- Suprapubic or costovertebral angle tenderness in cases of UTI/pyelonephritis

### ESSENTIAL WORKUP
- Abdominal and pelvic examination
- Cervical cultures for *Chlamydia*
- Transcervical endometrial cultures

## DIAGNOSTIC TESTS & INTERPRETATION

### Lab
- CBC
- Urinalysis and culture
- Blood cultures

### Imaging
- CT or MRI for ovarian vein thrombosis
- US is sensitive for abscess or retained products of conception.
- Plain x-rays may show retained foreign bodies or free air in septic abortion.

### DIFFERENTIAL DIAGNOSIS
- Fever from other sources
- <6 hr:
  - Early streptococcal infection
  - Transfusion reaction
  - Thyroid crisis
- <48 hr:
  - Atelectasis
- <72 hr:
  - UTI
  - Pneumonia
- 3–5 days:
  - Mastitis
  - Breast engorgement
  - Necrotizing fasciitis
- 3–7 days:
  - Mastitis
  - Septic thrombophlebitis
- 7–14 days:
  - Abscess
- >2 wk:
  - Mastitis
  - Pulmonary embolism

 TREATMENT

### PRE-HOSPITAL
- ABCs
- IV and IV fluids if signs of shock or impending shock

### INITIAL STABILIZATION/THERAPY
Manage airway and resuscitate as indicated:
- Prompt evaluation of respiratory and hemodynamic status
- Supplemental oxygen, cardiac monitor, and pulse oximetry, as needed
- Venous access; support circulatory status with crystalloid and pressors, if needed

## ED TREATMENT/PROCEDURES
- IV antibiotics and close observation
- Septic abortion is usually treated with dilatation and curettage and removal of any inciting agents.
- Monitor for signs of impending shock, circulatory failure, ARDS, and/or sepsis.
- Heparin if suspicion or evidence of thrombophlebitis
- Infected wound or abscess should be opened to establish drainage.
- Necrotizing fasciitis requires wide surgical debridement, parenteral antibiotics, and adjunctive hyperbaric oxygen therapy.
- Peritonitis requires imaging to evaluate cause.

## MEDICATION
Per underlying infection. See corresponding chapters for complete list (consider safety in breast-feeding)

### Endometritis
- Cefoxitin: 2 g IV q6h *or*
- Cefotetan: 2 g IV q12h *or*
- Piperacillin/tazobactam: 3.375 g IV q6–8h *or*
- Ampicillin/sulbactam: 1.5–3 g IV q6h *or*
- Clindamycin: 600–900 mg IV q8h *plus*
- Gentamicin: 2-mg/kg load, then 1–1.5 mg/kg IV q8h

### Septic Abortion
- Triple antibiotics
- Gram-positive coverage:
  - Ampicillin/sulbactam: 1.5–3 g IV q6h *or*
  - Cefoxitin: 2 g IV q6h *or*
  - Cefotetan: 2 g IV q12h *or*
  - Piperacillin: 4 g IV q6h *or*
- Gram-negative coverage:
  - Gentamicin: 2-mg/kg load, then 1–1.5 mg/kg IV q8h
- Anaerobic coverage:
  - Clindamycin: 600–900 mg IV q8h *or* Metronidazole: 500 mg IV q8h

### Mastitis
- Dicloxacillin: 250 mg q6h PO for 10 days
- Mupirocin 2% ointment t.i.d.
- Cephalexin: 500 mg q6h PO for 10 days
- Clindamycin: 300 mg q6h PO for 10 days
- Erythromycin: 500 mg q6h PO for 10 days
- If MRSA positive: vancomycin 1 g IV q12h

### UTI/Pyelonephritis (Inpatient)
- Ciprofloxacin: 400 mg IV q12h OR
- Ceftriaxone: 1–2 g IV q24h *or*
- Piperacillin/tazobactam: 3.375 g IV q6–8h

 FOLLOW-UP

### DISPOSITION

#### Admission Criteria
- Patients with endometritis or suspicion for septic pelvic thrombophlebitis should be admitted.
- Septic abortion

#### Discharge Criteria
Nontoxic, mildly symptomatic patient may be considered for outpatient management in consultation and close follow-up with obstetrics.

### FOLLOW-UP RECOMMENDATIONS
Close follow-up with obstetrician and/or primary care physician to evaluate treatment

## PEARLS AND PITFALLS

- Mastitis and urinary tract infections account for 80% of postpartum infections.
- C-section increases risk for postpartum endometritis.
- Entertain broad differential with regard to source of infection.
- Early broad-spectrum antibiotics are often indicated.

## ADDITIONAL READING

- Faro S. Postpartum endometritis. *Clin Prenatal.* 2005;32:803–814.
- French LM. Antibiotic regimens for endometritis after delivery. *Cochrane Database Syst Rev.* 2004;(4): CD000106/.
- Gorgas DL. Infections related to pregnancy. *Emerg Med Clin North Am.* 2008;26:345–366.
- Wong AW, Rosh AJ. Pregnancy, postpartum infections. *eMedicine.* Available at: http://emedicine medscape.com/article/796892-overview. Updated April 14, 2010.

### See Also (Topic, Algorithm, Electronic Media Element)
- Mastitis
- Urinary Tract Infection
- Pyelonephritis

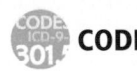 CODES

### ICD9
- 647.94 Unspecified infection or infestation of mother, postpartum
- 670.14 Puerperal endometritis, postpartum

# PRE-ECLAMPSIA/ECLAMPSIA

*Elaine Sapiro*

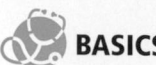 **BASICS**

## DESCRIPTION
- Pregnancy-induced hypertension (PIH)
- Pregnancy-aggravated hypertension (PAH)
- Preeclampsia: PIH or PAH with proteinuria
- Eclampsia: Preeclampsia with seizures
- HELLP syndrome (hemolysis, elevated liver enzymes, low platelet count):
  - Variant of severe preeclampsia
  - Hemolysis, elevated liver function tests (LFTs), thrombocytopenia
  - Affects 20% of women with preeclampsia
  - BP may be normal.
- Timing:
  - Usually occurs late 3rd trimester
  - Can also present up to 30 days postpartum

## ETIOLOGY
- Diffuse arteriolar vasospasm:
  - Secondary endothelial activation
  - Microthrombi formation
  - Tissue ischemia
- Vascular endothelial damage:
  - Increased vascular permeability
  - Edema
  - Proteinuria
- Risk factors:
  - Extremes of reproductive age
  - Primagravida
  - Multiple gestations
  - Molar pregnancy, hydatidiform mole
  - Smoking
  - Increased body mass index
  - Diabetes, collagen vascular diseases
  - Preexisting hypertension or renal disease
  - History of preeclampsia with prior pregnancies

# DIAGNOSIS

- PIH:
  - BP >140/90 mm Hg; *or*
  - SBP >130 mm Hg or DBP >80 mm Hg on two occasions
  - Rapid weight gain (>2 lb/wk)
- Preeclampsia—PIH plus:
  - Proteinuria:
    - May see wide fluctuation
    - Single urine sample may be negative even in severe cases
  - Dependent edema progressing to constant edema
- Severe preeclampsia:
  - Epigastric or right upper quadrant (RUQ) pain mimicking cholelithiasis due to hepatocellular necrosis with edema and stretch of capsule
  - Abdominal pain with nausea and vomiting
  - Thrombocytopenia
  - Hyperreflexia
  - Severe and worsening headache
  - Visual disturbances including blindness
  - Oliguria, proteinuria >3+ dipstick
  - BP >160/110 mm Hg
- Eclampsia—PIH or preeclampsia plus:
  - Seizures, tonic-clonic:
    - Unrelenting, severe headache ± visual changes often precedes seizures.
    - Up to 2% of women with preeclampsia progress to eclampsia.

## SIGNS AND SYMPTOMS
### History
- History of preeclampsia
- Parity
- Weight gain
- Leg swelling
- Abdominal pain
- Shortness of breath
- Headache
- Visual changes

## Physical Exam
- Check serial BP
- Palpate abdomen carefully, especially RUQ
- Assess extremities for edema
- Perform neurologic exam:
  - Deep tendon reflexes
  - Mental status changes
  - Visual acuity

## ESSENTIAL WORKUP
- Serial BP measurements
- Urinalysis
- CBC, LFTs, BUN/creatinine, uric acid
- US, fetal monitoring, head CT depending on severity of presentation

## DIAGNOSTIC TESTS & INTERPRETATION
### Lab
- Urinalysis:
  - Protein >1+ correlates to 30 mg/dL
  - >1+ requires 24-hr urine collection
  - Urine sediment for RBC, WBC, casts
- CBC, LFTs (HELLP syndrome)
- BUN/creatinine, uric acid

### Imaging
- US:
  - Gestational age
  - Fetal viability
- Fetal monitoring, stress test

### Diagnostic Procedures/Surgery
- Head CT: Rule out mass or hemorrhage.
- Lumbar puncture: Rule out infection or subarachnoid hemorrhage.
- Urine toxicology: Rule out substance abuse:
  - Cocaine
  - Methamphetamine

## DIFFERENTIAL DIAGNOSIS
- Essential hypertension
- Pregnancy-aggravated hypertension
- Renal or collagen vascular disease
- Hydatidiform mole, hydrops fetalis
- Drug abuse
- Epilepsy
- Encephalitis
- Meningitis
- Encephalopathy
- Brain tumor
- Intracranial hemorrhage

# TREATMENT

## PRE-HOSPITAL
- ABCs
- Oxygen
- Place patient in left lateral decubitus position

## INITIAL STABILIZATION/THERAPY
- ABCs
- 100% oxygen
- Left lateral decubitus position (reduces pressure on inferior vena cava, enhancing cardiac return/output)
- Maternal cardiopulmonary monitoring
- Magnesium sulfate ($MgSO_4$) for seizures

## ED TREATMENT/PROCEDURES
- $MgSO_4$ for seizure treatment and prophylaxis
- Hydralazine or labetalol for BP control
- Mg toxicity:
  - Hypotension
  - Loss of patellar reflex
  - Respiratory depression
  - Calcium gluconate to reverse
- Intubate for airway protection/hypoxia or if seizures refractory to interventions
- Tocographic and fetal monitoring
- OB consult:
  - All cases along PIH-preeclampsia-eclampsia spectrum
  - Expectant management if <30 wk gestation
  - Delivery >30 wk
  - Emergent delivery for severe symptoms: Induction vs. C-section

## MEDICATION
### First Line
- $MgSO_4$: 10 mg IM or 4 g IV; followed by 2 g/hr IV infusion:
  - $MgSO_4$ bolus should not exceed 1 g/min.
  - Serum Mg goal: 4–7 mEq/L
- Hydralazine: 5–20 mg IV
- Labetalol: 10 mg IV initially, then 5–10 mg increments for desired effect

### Second Line
- Valium: 5–10 mg IV if no response to $MgSO_4$
- Fosphenytoin: 15–20 mg phenytoin equivalents (PE) IV ×1 (max 150 mg PE/min IV)
- Phenytoin: 15–18 mg/kg IV, not to exceed 25–50 mg/min, for persistent seizure activity
- Calcium gluconate: 1 g IV

# FOLLOW-UP

## DISPOSITION
### Admission Criteria
- Preeclampsia
- Eclampsia
- HELLP syndrome
- ICU, labor and delivery, OR

### Discharge Criteria
- Isolated hypertension with workup negative for preeclampsia
- Asymptomatic
- Close obstetric follow-up assured

## FOLLOW-UP RECOMMENDATIONS
- Follow-up with OB as above
- Return to ED:
  - Headache
  - Abdominal pain
  - Leg swelling
  - Decreased urination
  - Shortness of breath

# PEARLS AND PITFALLS
- BP of 130/80 mm Hg in a pregnant woman requires investigation.
- Must rule out other causes of hypertension or seizures.
- Postpartum presentation: Consider preeclampsia/eclampsia in patient up to 30 days postpartum presenting with:
  - Edema
  - Shortness of breath
  - Headache
  - Seizure

- Diuretic use:
  - Avoid in pre- and peripartum patients as can induce placental hypoperfusion and fetal hypoxia
  - Acceptable in postpartum patients
- Airway considerations in severely preeclamptic or eclamptic patients:
  - Reduced internal diameter of airways due to engorgement
  - Airway edema may be present.
  - Use smaller-diameter endotracheal tube.
  - Use fiberoptic guidance if available.
  - Higher risk for aspiration

# ADDITIONAL READING

- Airoldi J, Weinstein L. Clinical significance of proteinuria in pregnancy. *Obstet Gynecol Surv.* 2007;62:117–124.
- Henry CS, Beidermann SA, Campbell MF, et al. Spectrum of hypertensive emergencies in pregnancy. *Crit Care Clin.* 2004;20:1–12.
- Leeman L, Fontaine P. Hypertensive disorders of pregnancy. *Am Fam Physician.* 2008;78:93–101.
- Marx JA, Hockberger RS, Walls RM, et al. *Rosen's Emergency Medicine: Concepts and Clinical Practice,* 7th ed. St. Louis, MO: Mosby; 2009.
- Yoder SR, Thornburg LL, Bisognano JD. Hypertension in pregnancy and women of childbearing age. *Am J Med.* 2009;122:890–895.

## See Also (Topic, Algorithm, Electronic Media Element)
- HELLP Syndrome
- Hydatidiform Mole
- Seizure, Adult

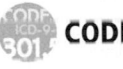

# CODES

## ICD9
- 642.40 Mild or unspecified pre-eclampsia, unspecified as to episode of care
- 642.50 Severe pre-eclampsia, unspecified as to episode of care
- 642.60 Eclampsia complicating pregnancy, childbirth or the puerperium, unspecified as to episode of care

# PRE-EXCITATION SYNDROMES
*Richard E. Wolfe*

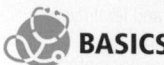 **BASICS**

## DESCRIPTION
- A group of conditions characterized by premature activation of the ventricular myocardium by an impulse that bypasses the physiologic delay in the atrioventricular (AV) junction by means of an accessory pathway
- Preexcitation occurs when an atrial impulse is conducted in an anterograde (atria to ventricle) fashion down an AV accessory pathway before the AV node-His-Purkinje axis begins depolarization.
- Accessory pathways:
  - Small bands of tissue that failed to separate during development
  - Preexcitation syndromes are determined by their accessory pathway's anatomy.
  - These may be atrioventricular, nodofascicular nodoventricular, fasciculoventricular, or atriofascicular
- Wolff-Parkinson-White syndrome (WPW) syndrome:
  - AV bypass tract or bundle of Kent:
    ○ Left lateral accessory pathway is most common.
    ○ 2nd-most-common location, the posteroseptal region of the AV groove, is often mistaken for prior inferior myocardial infarction and can give the appearance of left axis deviation.
  - Commonly presents with orthodromic reciprocating tachycardias:
    ○ The electrical impulse is conducted down the AV node-His-Purkinje axis and reenters the atria through the AV accessory pathway.
    ○ Narrow QRS complex
  - Atrial flutter
  - Atrial fibrillation
  - Antidromic reciprocating tachycardias:
    ○ Uncommon
    ○ The electrical impulse is conducted down the AV accessory pathway and reenters the atria through the AV node-His-Purkinje axis.
    ○ Wide QRS complex
- Lown-Ganong-Levine syndrome:
  - Accessory pathway in the AV node
  - Usually James fibers connect atrium to distal or compact AV node.
  - Rare preexcitation syndrome
- Brechenmacher fibers connect the atrium to the His bundle

- Mahaim fibers connect the atrium (atriofascicular pathways), AV node, or His bundle to distal Purkinje fibers or ventricular myocardium
- The majority of patients with accessory pathways never become symptomatic.
- Risk of death is very low (0.1–4%).
- Preexcitation with wide complex tachycardia is most at risk for ventricular dysrhythmias.
- Prevalence is estimated at 0.1–0.3% of the population.
- Males are affected twice as often as females.
- Most are young and healthy.

### Pediatric Considerations
- Most supraventricular tachycardias in children are the result of AV nodal reentry.
- 10% are the result of an identified preexcitation syndrome.

## RISK FACTORS
### Genetics
- Recent molecular genetic investigations indicate that preexcitation disorders may have a substantial genetic component.
- Preexcitation disorders are sometimes inherited as single-gene disorders.

## ETIOLOGY
- Idiopathic
- In association with structural heart disease:
  - Cardiomyopathy
  - Transposition of the great vessels
  - Mitral valve prolapse
  - Ebstein anomaly

**DIAGNOSIS**

## SIGNS AND SYMPTOMS
### History
- Asymptomatic
- Palpitations:
  - Fast or irregular
- Chest pain
- Dyspnea
- Dizziness
- Nausea
- Diaphoresis
- Syncope

### Physical Exam
- Tachycardia up to 250 bpm:
  - Rapid and regular
  - Supraventricular tachycardia
  - Irregular (atrial fibrillation)
- Signs of instability:
  - Chest pain
  - Hypotension
  - Change in mental status
  - Rales
  - Cyanosis

## ESSENTIAL WORKUP
- The diagnosis is made on the 12-lead ECG
- Pre-existing history
- Stable patients must be carefully monitored and reassessed for signs of instability.

## DIAGNOSTIC TESTS & INTERPRETATION
### Lab
- Cardiac enzymes only if signs of ischemia
- Consider electrolytes

### Imaging
ECG:
- Complications of the preexcitation syndrome:
  - Atrial fibrillation
  - Atrial flutter
  - Supraventricular tachycardia (SVT)
- WPW syndrome:
  - Short pulse rate (PR) <0.12 sec
  - Prolonged QRS >0.10 sec
  - Delta wave: Small slurred upstroke at the beginning of the QRS
- Lown-Ganong-Levine syndrome:
  - PR interval <0.12 sec
  - Normal QRS upstroke and duration
  - Absence of a delta wave
- Mahaim tachydysrhythmia:
  - QRS axis between 0° and −75°
  - QRS duration of ≤0.15 sec
  - R wave in lead 1
  - rS complex in lead V1
  - Precordial transition in lead V4 or later

### Diagnostic Procedures/Surgery

Radiofrequency catheter ablation:

- Definitive diagnosis and therapeutic procedure for accessory pathways that is not performed on an emergent basis

## DIFFERENTIAL DIAGNOSIS

- AV nodal reentry SVT
- Ventricular tachycardia

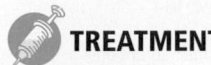 **TREATMENT**

## PRE-HOSPITAL

- Supplemental oxygen
- Monitor
- Synchronized cardioversion:
  - Signs of instability
  - Atrial fibrillation with WPW: Wide complex tachycardia
- Prehospital use of adenosine:
  - Stable patients do not require emergent conversion.
  - Unstable patients should undergo cardioversion, not adenosine.

## INITIAL STABILIZATION/THERAPY

- Unstable patients:
  Synchronized cardioversion starting with 50 J-min
  - Increase incrementally until sinus rhythm is restored.
- Stable patients with wide complex tachycardia:
  - Procainamide
  - Amiodarone
  - Avoid lidocaine, calcium-channel blockers, and β-blockers

## ED TREATMENT/PROCEDURES

- Vagal maneuvers such as a Valsalva:
  - Right carotid artery massage for no more than 10 sec
  - Auscultate the artery 1st for a bruit that would contraindicate this procedure.
- Fluid replacement and Trendelenburg if the patient has mild hypotension
- Pharmacologic conversion if carotid massage fails:
  - Adenosine
  - Verapamil on if narrow complex QRS
- Irregular wide complex tachycardia.
  - Procainamide, amiodarone, or magnesium

### Pediatric Considerations

- Children may develop ventricular rates up to 320 bpm that are poorly tolerated.
- Cardiovert unstable children with 0.5–2 J/kg.
- Vagal maneuvers and adenosine are safe in stable children.

## MEDICATION

- Adenosine: 6 mg rapid IV bolus over 1–2 sec; if ineffective, repeat with 12 mg (peds: 0.1 mg/kg rapid IV push, repeat with 0.2 mg/kg)
- Amiodarone: 150 mg IV over 10 min, 360 mg over the next 6 hr
- Magnesium: 2-g IV bolus
- Procainamide: 6–13 mg/kg IV at 0.2–0.5 mg/kg/min until either arrhythmia controlled, QRS widens 50%, or hypotension, then 2–6 mg/min, max dose of 1,000 mg
- Only to be used in stable narrow complex tachycardia:
  - Diltiazem: 0.25 mg/kg IV over 2 min followed in 15 min by 0.35 mg/kg IV over 2 min
  - Esmolol: 0.5 mg/kg over 1 min; maintenance infusion at 0.05 mg/kg/min over 4 min, then 0.1–0.2 mg/kg/min continuously
  - Verapamil: 2.5–5 mg IV bolus over 2 min; may repeat with 5–10 mg q5–30min to max 20 mg

 **FOLLOW-UP**

## DISPOSITION

### Admission Criteria

- Patients with signs of instability require admission to a monitored bed.
- Failure of outpatient therapy for continuous pharmacologic control or ablation

### Discharge Criteria

- The majority of patients will be stable and can be discharged once converted to sinus rhythm.
- Consider low-dose verapamil prophylaxis.

### Issues for Referral

- Follow-up should be arranged with a cardiologist.
- Electrophysiologic studies with possible ablative therapy during the outpatient workup

## FOLLOW-UP RECOMMENDATIONS

Cardiology for possible radioablation

## PEARLS AND PITFALLS

Never use calcium-channel blockers, β-blockers, or digoxin for wide complex tachycardias.

- These medications block the AV node.
- Conduction occurs exclusively down the faster accessory pathway.
- Precipitation of ventricular dysrhythmias

## ADDITIONAL READING

- Mark DG, Brady WJ, Pines JM. Preexcitation syndrome: Diagnostic considerations in the ED. *Am J Emerg Med*. 2009;27:878–888.
- Rosner MH, Brady WJ Jr, Kefer MP, et al. Electrocardiography in the patient with the Wolff-Parkinson-White syndrome: Diagnostic and initial therapeutic issues. *Am J Emerg Med*. 1999;17: 705–714.
- Redfearn DP, Krahn AD, Skanes AC, et al. Use of medications in Wolff-Parkinson-White syndrome. *Expert Opin Pharmacother*. 2005;6(6):955–963.
- Rubart M, Zipes DP. Genesis of cardiac arrhythmias: Electrophysiological considerations. In: Libby P, ed. *Braunwald's Heart Disease. A Textbook of Cardiovascular Medicine*, 8th ed. Philadelphia: WB Saunders; 2007:727–761.
- Stahmer SA, Cowan R. Tachydysrhythmias. *Emerg Med Clin North Am*. 2006;24(1):11–40.

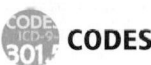 **CODES**

ICD9
426.7 Anomalous atrioventricular excitation

# PREGNANCY, TRAUMA IN

A. Antoine Kazzi
Ziad N. Kazzi

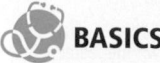

## BASICS

### DESCRIPTION

- Fetal and maternal injury after the 1st trimester:
  - Increased rate of fetal loss, but not maternal mortality
- Likelihood of fetal injury increases with the severity of maternal insult.
- Physiologic hypervolemia of pregnancy may lead to an underestimation of blood loss:
  - Clinical shock may be apparent only after a 30% maternal blood loss.
- Abdominal findings are less evident in the gravid patient.
- Minor trauma can also lead to fetal injuries (at least 50% of fetal losses).
- An Injury Severity Score >9 is associated with a worse outcome.
- Less frequent bowel injury
- More frequent retroperitoneal hemorrhage due to the engorgement of pelvic organs and veins
- Increased morbidity and mortality with pelvic fractures due to pelvic and uterine engorgement
- Fetal or uterine trauma includes:
  - Placental abruption
  - Fetal maternal hemorrhage
  - Premature labor
  - Uterine contusion or rupture
  - Fetal demise
  - Premature membrane rupture
  - Hypoxemic or anatomic fetal injury (skull fracture)
- Abruption occurs in up to 60% of severe trauma and 1–5% of minor injuries:
  - Accounts for up to 50% of fetal loss
  - May occur with no external bleeding (20%)
  - Occurs after 16 wk of gestation
  - Can present with abdominal pain, cramping and/or vaginal bleeding
  - Hallmark is uterine contractions.
- Uterine rupture:
  - Usually inpatients with prior C-section
  - Nearly universal mortality
  - 10% maternal mortality
- Pelvic fracture:
  - May be an independent predictor of fetal death
  - Fatal insults to fetus can occur in all trimesters.
  - 10% fetal mortality in patients with minor injuries
- Fetal/maternal hemorrhage (FMH) occurs in >30% of severe trauma:
  - Isoimmunization of Rh-negative mothers (with as little as 0.03 cc of FMH)
- Penetrating trauma results in direct injury to fetus, maternal shock, and premature delivery.

## ETIOLOGY

- Trauma occurs in ~7% of all pregnancies.
- Most common cause of nonobstetric morbidity and mortality in pregnancy
- Rate of fetal loss 3.4–38%
- Motor vehicle accidents (48–84%)
- Falls
- Domestic violence
- Direct abdominal trauma
- Penetrating (stab or gunshot)
- Electrical or burn
- Higher rate in younger woman

## DIAGNOSIS

### SIGNS AND SYMPTOMS
*History*
- Mechanism of injury
- Last menstrual period
- Abdominal pain
- Uterine contraction
- Vaginal bleeding or leakage of fluid
- Previous pregnancies, C-sections
- Substance use/abuse

*Physical Exam*
- Perform with patient in left lateral recumbent position if possible
- Primary survey
- Secondary survey
- Tertiary survey
- Placental abruption:
  - Uterine tenderness
- Uterine rupture:
  - Uterine tenderness and variable shape
  - Palpation of fetal body parts
- Determine the gestational age (EGA) to assess viability:
  - Estimate last menstrual period
  - EGA = fundal height (FH; distance from pubic bone to top of uterus in cm) × 8/7 after wk 16
- Vaginal exam to assess for:
  - Blood
  - Amniotic fluid
  - Cervical dilation and effacement

## ESSENTIAL WORKUP

- Maintain spinal immobilization
- Identify maternal condition 1st:
  - Airway management and resuscitate as indicated
- Determine the EGA to assess viability:
  - EGA = FH × 8/7 after wk 16
  - Doppler fetal heart tones
  - Sonography (may miss small abruptions)
- Fetal/maternal monitoring for >4–6 hr:
  - Only monitor viable fetuses (typically with an EGA >24 wk)
  - Abruption unlikely if no contractions during 1st 4 hr of monitoring
  - >8 contractions/hr over 4 hr is associated with adverse outcome.
  - If >1 contraction every 10 min, there is a 20% incidence of abruption.
  - The occurrence of bradycardia, poor beat-to-beat variability, or type II "late" deceleration indicates fetal distress.
  - An abnormal tracing has a sensitivity and specificity of 62% and 49%, resp., of predicting adverse fetal outcomes.
  - A normal tracing combined with a normal physical exam has a negative predictive value of nearly 100%.

## DIAGNOSTIC TESTS & INTERPRETATION
*Lab*
- CBC, urinalysis
- Blood gas and electrolyte panel
- Type, Rh, and screening of blood
- The Kleihauer-Betke (KB) stain:
  - Identifies FMH in vaginal fluid or blood
  - Indicated when quantification of FMH is important

*Imaging*
- Shield the uterus if possible, but obtain necessary maternal radiographs.
- *Inform the mother of the potential risks of radiation exposure.*
- No definite evidence of increased risk for congenital malformation or intrauterine death
- Cancer risk is debated.
- Radiation <1 rad (10 mGy) believed to carry little risk
- Increased risk of fetal malformation at 5–10 rad

- The radiation exposure is estimated at the following:
  – CXR (2 views): Minimal
  – Pelvis (anteroposterior): 1 rad
  – Cervical spine x-ray: Minimal
  – Thoracic spine x-ray: Minimal
  – Lumbar spine x-ray: 0.031–4.9 rads
  – CT head: <0.05 rad
  – CT thorax: 0.01–0.59 rads
  – CT abdomen: 2.8–4.6 rads
  – CT pelvis: 1.94–5.0 rads
- Ultrasonography:
  – Focused assessment with sonography for trauma (FAST) exam
  – Evaluate for solid-organ injury or hemoperitoneum
  – Fetal heart activity
  – Gestational age
  – Amount of amniotic fluid (amniotic fluid index)
  – It misses 50–80% of placental abruptions.
- Test vaginal fluid with Nitrazine paper (turns blue) and for ferning.
- With stable penetrating trauma, triple-contrast CT is advocated, particularly with stab wounds.

### Diagnostic Procedures/Surgery
As indicated by traumatic injury

## DIFFERENTIAL DIAGNOSIS
Differential diagnosis is broad and should include careful examination for occult traumatic injuries.

 TREATMENT

### PRE-HOSPITAL
- Maintain spinal immobilization
- Patients in late 2nd and 3rd trimester should be transported to a trauma center.
- Advise trauma center early of pregnancy and EGA to facilitate mobilization of appropriate resources.
- Place patient (while on backboard) in the left lateral recumbent position to avoid supine hypotension (after 20 wk EGA or earlier in multiple gestations).
- Mast suit inflation over the abdomen is contraindicated.

### INITIAL STABILIZATION/THERAPY
- Direct therapy at the mother with no delays due to pregnancy:
  – Manage airway and resuscitate as indicated.
- Cardiac, pulse oximetry, and cardiotocographic monitoring
- Tilt patient or board 15–30° to the left (or manually displace uterus to the left).

### ED TREATMENT/PROCEDURES
- Lactated Ringer preferred for IV fluids:
  – Large volumes of normal saline may induce a hyperchloremic acidosis.

- Replace estimated blood loss in a 3:1 ratio:
  – O-negative packed red blood cells if type-specific blood is not available
- Resort to transfusions after 1 L of estimated blood loss or if hypovolemia persists after 2 L of crystalloid.
- Nasogastric tube decompression (higher risk of aspiration in pregnancy)
- Foley catheterization to assess urinary output
- Tube thoracostomy:
  – Use a higher intercostal space to avoid diaphragm
- Rapid sequence intubation:
  – Safe and preferred method
  – Avoid aspiration and deoxygenation
- If diagnostic peritoneal lavage is necessary, use supraumbilical open technique.
- Use tocolytic therapy only for hemodynamically stable patients:
  – Contraindicated if cervix dilated >4 cm or if FMH and abruption have not been reasonably ruled out.
  – Use tocolytics only when >8 contractions/hr have lasted >4 hr.
- A perimortem cesarean delivery may be attempted within 4–5 min of cardiopulmonary arrest. See "Cesarean Section, Emergency."
- In minor trauma after week 20, fetal and maternal monitoring is best done in the labor and delivery area.

## MEDICATION
- RhoGAM in all Rh-negative women (within 72 hr):
  – 50 mcg IM in women <12 wk pregnant
  – 300 mcg IM in women >12 wk pregnant
- 24-hr recheck for ongoing FMH:
  – Repeat Rh immune globulin if needed (if FMH >30 mL)
- Tocolytics: Magnesium sulfate 4 g IV
- Avoid aspirin, hypnotics, nonsteroidals, vasopressors.

 FOLLOW-UP

### DISPOSITION
### Admission Criteria
- Vaginal bleeding or amniotic fluid leakage
- Fetomaternal hemorrhage
- Abdominal pain
- Uterine contractions
- Evidence of fetal distress
- Abruption placenta
- Hemoperitoneum or visceral or solid organ injury
- Fetal survival begins at week 24 (9.9%):
  – Survival becomes significant after week 26 (54.7%).

### Discharge Criteria
- All the following criteria must be met:
  – No uterine contractions for >4 hr of tocodynamometry
  – No evidence of fetal distress
  – No vaginal bleeding or amniotic fluid leakage
  – No abdominal pain or tenderness
  – Timely obstetric follow-up
- Specific instructions to return if any of the above symptoms occur
- Discharge only in consultation with obstetrics.

## FOLLOW-UP RECOMMENDATIONS
A pregnant trauma patient being discharged after appropriate evaluation and observation needs prompt follow-up with obstetrician.

## PEARLS AND PITFALLS

- Minor trauma can lead to maternal and/or fetal death.
- Stabilization of the mother is 1st priority.
- Maternal stress may not occur until 1,500–2,000 mL of blood loss.

## ADDITIONAL READING

- Chames MC, Pearlman MD. Trauma during pregnancy: Outcomes and clinical management. *Clin Obstet Gynecol.* 2008;51:398–408.
- Cusick SS, Tibbles CD. Trauma in pregnancy. *Emerg Med Clin North Am.* 2007;25:861–872.
- Hill CC, Pickinpaugh J. Trauma and surgical emergencies in the obstetric patient. *Surg Clin North Am.* 2008;88:421–440.
- Muench MV, Canterino JC. Trauma in pregnancy. *Obstet Gynecol Clin North Am.* 2007;34:555–583.

### See Also (Topic, Algorithm, Electronic Media Element)
- Cesarean Section, Emergency
- Placental Abruption

 CODES

### ICD9
- 641.80 Other antepartum hemorrhage, unspecified as to episode of care
- 648.90 Other current conditions classifiable elsewhere of mother, complicating pregnancy, childbirth, or the puerperium, unspecified as to episode of care

# PREGNANCY, UNCOMPLICATED

*James S. Walker*
*Jonathan B. Walker*

## 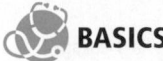 BASICS

### DESCRIPTION
- Pregnancy is not a disease process but rather a physiologic state. It involves severe metabolic stresses on the mother to facilitate the growth and development of the fetus.
- All women of reproductive age with abdominal pain are considered pregnant until proven otherwise even with history of sterilization.
- The changes in pregnancy occur from the production of large amounts of placental hormones:
  - Placental progesterone and estrogen

### Pediatric Considerations
- Range for menarche in U.S. is 11–15 yr old
- Pregnant adolescents who present to the ED may be either unaware of the pregnancy or reluctant to admit it:
  - Assume pregnancy in adolescents, regardless of the chief complaint.
  - Pediatric pregnancies have an increased risk of obstructive labor.

### ETIOLOGY
- Preceding signs and symptoms can be explained by elevations in various hormone levels or changes in anatomy that are a function of the progression of the pregnancy.
- Placental human chorionic gonadotropin (hCG):
  - Prevents the normal involution of the corpus luteum at the end of the menstrual cycle
  - Causes the corpus luteum to secrete even larger quantities of estrogen and progesterone
  - Elevated hCG levels are responsible for nausea and vomiting.
- Placental progesterone:
  - Causes decidual cells in the endometrium to develop and provide nutrition for the early embryo
  - Decreases contractility of the gravid uterus and risk of spontaneous abortion
  - Helps estrogen prepare the breasts for lactation

- Placental estrogen:
  - Responsible for enlargement of uterus, breasts, and mammary ducts
  - Enlargement of female external genitalia, relaxation of pelvic ligaments, symphysis pubis, and sacroiliac joints

##  DIAGNOSIS

The diagnosis of pregnancy and some of its potential complications focus on 3 diagnostic tools:
- History and physical
- Hormonal assays
- Ultrasonography

### SIGNS AND SYMPTOMS
- Amenorrhea accompanied by nausea and vomiting in a sexually active woman
- Amenorrhea:
  - The most common cause of secondary amenorrhea in a woman of reproductive age is pregnancy.
- Nausea and vomiting (morning sickness)
- Breast tenderness (mastodynia)
- Urinary frequency
- Headache
- Low back pain
- Pica
- Edema of feet and ankles
- Weight gain
- Easy fatigability, generalized malaise
- Increase in abdominal girth
- Constipation
- Heartburn
- Excessive eructation
- Skin darkening

### History
- Determine 1st day of last menstrual period (FDLMP).
- 40% of women cannot accurately remember their FDLMP.

### Physical Exam
Pelvic examination:
- Estimate expected date of delivery by determining uterine fundal height.
- Centimeters from pubic bone to top of uterus approximates gestational age after 16 wk.
- Detect abnormal pelvic pain or masses

### DIAGNOSTIC TESTS & INTERPRETATION
#### Lab
- Pregnancy tests:
  - $\beta$ subunit of hCG
  - Quantitative hCG normally doubles every 2 days until 6–7 wk gestation
  - Progesterone
- Measurement of $\beta$-hCG:
  - Most urine pregnancy tests have a sensitivity to 25 mIU/mL:
    - False-negative tests with dilute urine
  - Home pregnancy tests are not that accurate:
    - Detect pregnancy 9–12 days postconception
  - Positive home pregnancy tests should be confirmed by serum hCG levels.
  - Serum level of hCG:
    - Detectable 8–11 days postconception
  - hCG levels may remain detectable up to 60 days after an abortion.
- Serum progesterone level is an indicator of the viability of the pregnancy and may be used to predict the outcome of the pregnancy:
  - A serum progesterone level of <5 ng/mL is indicative of a nonviable pregnancy (spontaneous abortion or ectopic pregnancy).
  - Progesterone level 25 ng/mL denotes a viable pregnancy.

#### Imaging
- Ultrasonography is used to confirm pregnancy in the setting of abdominal pain, vaginal bleeding, or some other potential obstetric complication:
  - Can estimate gestational age
  - Confirm intrauterine or ectopic pregnancy
  - Evaluate fetal viability
  - Identify fetal abnormalities

- Transabdominal US vs. transvaginal US:
  – Transvaginal US is more sensitive but more difficult to perform.
  – Intrauterine pregnancy seen at 4–5 wk in transvaginal US
  – Gestational sac seen at 5.5–6 wk in transabdominal US
  – Transvaginal US is contraindicated in the setting of premature rupture of membranes and 3rd-trimester bleeding.
- When used in combination with hCG levels, US is a very helpful tool in detecting abnormal/problem pregnancy.
- Other imaging modalities
- MRI: No significant side effects have been documented
  – Often study of choice to evaluate for appendicitis in pregnancy
- Plain radiography and CT:
  – Dose-dependent teratogen
  – Slight increase in risk of childhood cancer
  – Goal is to not exceed 5,000 mrad fetal dose of radiation:
    ○ CXR with abdominal shield: <1 mrad
    ○ Abdominal plain film: 240 mrad
    ○ Chest CT: <10 mrad
    ○ Head CT: < 10 mrad
    ○ Abdominal CT with and without contrast: 2,000 and 1,000 mrad
    ○ Cardiac catheterization: 1,300 mrad
    ○ VQ scan: <50 mrad

## DIFFERENTIAL DIAGNOSIS
Any woman who is of the age to be sexually active who presents to the ED should be assumed to be pregnant until proven otherwise.

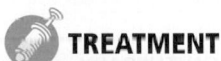

# TREATMENT

## PRE-HOSPITAL
- Assume the patient is pregnant.
- Administer medications only when necessary to avoid teratogenetic side effects or placental fetal compromise (eg, epinephrine).
- If >24 wk gestation, transport in left lateral recumbent position.

## INITIAL STABILIZATION/THERAPY
- Advanced cardiac life support, advanced trauma life support measures as needed: Oxygen, cardiac monitor, IV access, and fluids:
  – 1st objective is to resuscitate mother.
- If >24 wk gestation, place in the left lateral recumbent position.

## ED TREATMENT/PROCEDURES
The goal is to optimize maternal condition to improve fetal condition.

## MEDICATION
- 1st trimester is when organogenesis is occurring.
- Fetal malformation continues beyond the 1st trimester.
- Before using any drug, refer to its Food and Drug Administration safety classification in pregnancy:
  – This classification system categorizes drugs as A, B, C, D, and X, with category A being the safest and category X being the most toxic.
- Analgesics: Acetaminophen is the preferred OTC analgesic.
- Aspirin and NSAIDs are not teratogenic but are best used in consultation with an obstetrician.
- Oxycodone, codeine, hydrocodone, meperidine, and morphine have no known teratogenic affect and can be used for the control of severe pain in pregnancy for short periods of time (3–4 days).
- Antibiotics: Selecting the right antibiotic in a gravid female depends on 3 factors:
  Maternal drug allergies
  – Gestational age
  – Type of infections and associated pathogens
- Consider placing patient on prenatal vitamins.
- Pain control:
  – Acetaminophen: 325–1,000 mg PO q6h
- Antiemetic:
  – Ondansetron: 4 mg IM/IV q8h

# FOLLOW-UP

## DISPOSITION
### Admission Criteria
- Pregnant women with the following obstetric complications should be admitted to the hospital:
  – Hyperemesis gravidarum with inability to tolerate oral fluids
  – Complicated urinary tract infection
  – Ectopic or molar pregnancy
  – Septic abortion
  – Preterm labor
  – Premature rupture of membranes
  – Preeclampsia/eclampsia
  – Severe pregnancy-induced HTN
- Pregnant women with medical conditions that would warrant admission in a nongravid female

### Discharge Criteria
Women without the above conditions may be discharged from the ED.

## FOLLOW-UP RECOMMENDATIONS
Need OB follow up for prenatal care by 6–8 wk gestation

# PEARLS AND PITFALLS
- All women are considered to be pregnant until proven that they are not.
- Minimize radiation exposure to fetus to <5,000 mrad.

# ADDITIONAL READING
- Dighe M, Cuevas C, Moshiri M, et al. Sonography in first trimester bleeding. *J Clin Ultrasound.* 2008;36: 352–366.
- Moschos E, Twickler DM. Endometrial thickness predicts intrauterine pregnancy in patients with pregnancy of unknown location. *Ultrasound Obstet Gynecol.* 2008;32:929–934.
- Marx JA, Hockberger RS, Walls RM, et al. *Rosen's Emergency Medicine: Concepts and Clinical Practice,* 7th ed. St. Louis, MO: Mosby; 2009.

# CODES

## ICD9
- V22.0 Supervision of normal first pregnancy
- V22.1 Supervision of other normal pregnancy

# PRIAPISM

*David Barlas*

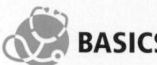 **BASICS**

## DESCRIPTION

- Penile erection (engorgement of corpora cavernosa) in the absence of sexual arousal that is prolonged and frequently painful
- Low-flow priapism:
  - Most common mechanism
  - Poor venous outflow
  - Usually painful
  - Ischemia and thrombosis from stagnant, hypoxic blood can occur after a few hours.
  - Fibrosis and erectile dysfunction are late sequelae.
- High-flow priapism:
  - Rare
  - Penile arterial laceration with uncontrolled inflow of arterial blood
  - Usually painless
  - Presentation may be later than in low-flow priapism.
  - Ischemia and erectile dysfunction are uncommon.

## ETIOLOGY

- Idiopathic
- Pharmacologic agents:
  - Intracavernosal injectables for the treatment of erectile dysfunction:
    - Prostaglandin E1
    - Papaverine
    - Phentolamine
  - Psychotropics:
    - Phenothiazines
    - Butyrophenones
    - Trazodone
    - Sedative–hypnotics
    - Selective serotonin uptake inhibitors
  - Antihypertensives:
    - Prazosin
    - Hydralazine
    - Phenoxybenzamine
    - Guanethidine
- Rarely implicated agents:
  - Phosphodiesterase inhibitors: Sildenafil (Viagra), tadalafil (Cialis), vardenafil (Levitra)
  - Anticoagulants
  - Cocaine
  - Marijuana
  - Ethanol
  - Androstenedione
- Hematologic disorders predisposing to sludging of blood:
  - Sickle cell anemia (most common cause)
  - Leukemia
  - Multiple myeloma
  - Polycythemia
- Penile and perineal trauma (arterial laceration and high-flow priapism)
- Spinal trauma (loss of inhibitory adrenergic tone)
- Rare causes:
  - Pelvic neoplasms and infections
  - Infiltrative diseases (eg, amyloidosis)
  - Dialysis
  - Parenteral nutrition solutions containing a fat emulsion

### *Pediatric Considerations*
Sickle cell anemia is the cause of most priapism in children.

 **DIAGNOSIS**

## SIGNS AND SYMPTOMS
### *History*
- Type of priapism may be determined by history:
- Low-flow priapism:
  - Painful
  - Predisposing condition or medication
- High-flow priapism:
  - Painless
  - Penile trauma

### *Physical Exam*
- Diagnosis is clinically apparent.
- Check for penile implants.
- Evaluate trauma (ie urethral, rectal injuries).
- Urinary retention

## ESSENTIAL WORKUP
Lab tests and imaging should not delay urologic consultation and definitive management.

## DIAGNOSTIC TESTS & INTERPRETATION
### *Lab*
- CBC
- Coagulation studies
- Sickle cell evaluation may be indicated.

### *Imaging*
- Duplex Doppler US can verify and localize the arterial laceration in high-flow priapism.
- Angiography enables localization and embolization of the arterial laceration in high-flow priapism.

### *Diagnostic Procedures/Surgery*
Intracavernosal blood gas analysis can help differentiate type of priapism if unsure:
- Because of the possibility of penile arterial injury, a urologist should perform this procedure.
- High-flow priapism: Near-normal values
- Low-flow priapism: Acidosis and hypoxia (pH $<7.25$; $O_2$ $<30$ torr)

## DIFFERENTIAL DIAGNOSIS
- Penile erection from sexual arousal is usually painless and transient.
- Penile implants are a benign cause of "priapism."

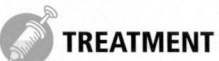 **TREATMENT**

## PRE-HOSPITAL
- IV
- $O_2$
- Analgesia

## INITIAL STABILIZATION/THERAPY
- $O_2$
- Analgesia and sedation
- Intravenous hydration

## ED TREATMENT/PROCEDURES

- Urgent urologic consultation
- Management of specific causes should begin concurrently with specific therapy outlined below:
  - Sickle cell anemia:
    - Packed RBC or exchange transfusion
    - Hyperbaric oxygen if other measures fail
  - Leukemia:
    - Chemotherapy
  - Arterial injury:
    - Expectant management is an option
    - Angiographic localization and embolization
- Terbutaline (β-agonist):
  - May be administered to initiate treatment of low-flow priapism, but may not be effective alone.
- Intracavernosal injection/aspiration is often required for low-flow priapism despite the above measures:
  - Ideally performed by urologist, but the ED physician may perform the procedure as follows if specialty care is not immediately available:
    - Sterile prep area
    - Consider IV sedation and analgesia
    - Administer local anesthesia, or perform a pudendal nerve block or penile nerve block (inject plain lidocaine around the base of the penis)
    - Position yourself to the right of the patient and grasp the penile shaft with your left hand
    - Enter the corpus cavernosum with a 19-gauge butterfly needle and 10-mL syringe inserted laterally at 2- or 10-o'clock position and 45° angle to avoid the ventral urethra and the dorsal neurovascular bundle
    - Aspirate blood <u>slowly</u> while "milking" the penile shaft until arterial blood is obtained, often after 30–50 mL. Irrigation with saline may be necessary.
    - Aspirating both corpora cavernosa is unnecessary as they are connected by shunts.
  - Phenylephrine (preferred to limit systemic effects), epinephrine, or pseudoephedrine may be injected through the butterfly needle if retumescence occurs. Monitor cardiac rhythm and BP if these agents are used and avoid in patients with cardiovascular or cerebrovascular disease, hypertension, or those taking monoamine oxidase inhibitors because of the risk of hypertensive crisis.
  - Repeated injections may be needed 5–15 min apart for 1 hr.
  - Surgical shunt (ie, corpus cavernosum to spongiosum) may be necessary if the above measures fail.

## MEDICATION

### First Line

- Terbutaline: 0.25–0.5 mg SC (may repeat in 15 min) or 5 mg PO
- Phenylephrine: Dilute 1 mg in 100 mL saline; inject 10-mL boluses in the corpus cavernosum.

### Second Line

- Epinephrine: Dilute 1 mg in 100 mL saline; inject 1–3-mL boluses in the corpus cavernosum, up to 10 mL.
- Pseudoephedrine: 60–100 mg in the corpus cavernosum

 **FOLLOW-UP**

## DISPOSITION

### Admission Criteria

- Persistent priapism despite noninvasive treatments
- Serious underlying disease (sickle cell anemia, leukemia)

### Discharge Criteria

- Detumescence is complete and has not recurred after several hours of observation
- Urologic consultation has been obtained

### Issues for Referral

Arrange short-term follow-up with a urologist for all patients.

## FOLLOW-UP RECOMMENDATIONS

- Ensure underlying conditions are addressed.
- Discontinue offending medication(s).
- Advise patient to return to the ED if tumescence recurs.

## PEARLS AND PITFALLS

- Intracavernosal injection of vasoactive medications during partial tumescence increases the risk of a systemic bolus and adverse effects.
- Management of underlying conditions should not delay timely direct therapy to reduce the risk of subsequent erectile dysfunction.
- Always document and warn of the possibility of subsequent complete erectile dysfunction even when timely and successful treatment has occurred.

## ADDITIONAL READING

- Burnett AL, Bivalacqua TL. Priapism: Current principles and practice. *Urol Clin North Am*. 2007;34:631–642.
- Hakim LS, Kulaksizoglu H, Mulligan R, et al. Evolving concepts in the diagnosis and treatment of arterial high flow priapism. *J Urol*. 1996;155:541–548.
- Montagne DK, Jarow J, Broderick GA, et al. American Urological Association guideline on the management of priapism. *J Urol*. 2003;170(4 pt 1): 1318–1324. (Also available at: http://www.auanet. org/content/guidelines-and-quality care/clinical-guidelines/main-reports/priapism/online.pdf.)
- Mulhall JP, Honig SC. Priapism: Diagnosis and management. *Acad Emerg Med*. 1996;3:810–816.

### See Also (Topic, Algorithm, Electronic Media Element)

- Conscious Sedation
- Paraphimosis
- Penile Shaft Fracture
- Sickle Cell Disease

 **CODES**

**ICD9**
607.3 Priapism

# PROCEDURAL SEDATION

*Christopher Ross*
*Theresa Schwab*

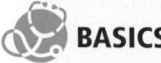 **BASICS**

Procedural sedation is a technique of administration of sedatives or dissociative agents with or without analgesia to induce a state that allows diagnostic and therapeutic procedures to be performed successfully without significant pain and/or anxiety while maintaining cardiorespiratory function.

## Preparation
- Position patient in area accessible to appropriately sized resuscitation equipment and be able to monitor patient's condition to manage airways, allergic reactions, and potential drug overdoses. The following equipment should be readily available:
  - Airway and breathing: Breathing masks, bag-valve ventilation device, oropharyngeal and nasal airways, laryngoscopes, endotracheal tubes, and stylets appropriate for size of patient
  - Circulation: Defibrillator/automated external defibrillator
  - Emergency cart with all available medications necessary to resuscitate the patient by Advanced Cardiac Life Support protocols as well as including reversal medications flumazenil and naloxone
- Apply cardiorespiratory monitor, pulse oximeter, and BP monitor.
- Gather medicines that will be used in procedure, label (preferably color-coded) syringes, and place at bedside.
- Assemble reversal agents if applicable.
- Apply appropriate oxygen delivery device (cannula or mask) and keep oxygen saturation >95%.
- Assemble wall suction unit and catheters and verify operation.
- Acquire informed consent.

## Sedation Agents and Techniques
- Can be administered by various means (eg, IV, IM, PO, sublingual, transmucosal, and intranasal)
- Administer medications and titrate to effect.
- Administer local or regional anesthesia if applicable.
- Perform the procedure.
- Closely observe and monitor patient during entire course of procedure as well as the recovery period afterward.
- Monitor patient until awake, alert, and back to baseline function.

 **DIAGNOSIS**

## SIGNS AND SYMPTOMS
### History
Perform a complete history:
- Focus on past medical history, anesthesia history, medications, allergies, review of systems and last meal.

### Physical Exam
- Focus on BP, heart rate, respiratory rate, pulse oximetry, cardiopulmonary and neurologic exams.
- Airway assessment is mandatory as many medications used for procedural sedation can lead to respiratory depression mandating aggressive airway management:
  - Look for markers of difficult bag-valve mask ventilation (beards, abnormal facial contour, morbid obesity, no teeth, and patients with chronic obstructive pulmonary disease [COPD]/asthma/congestive heart failure).
  - Look for external markers of difficult airways (short neck, large tongue, small mandible), Mallampati scoring, and evidence of airway obstruction (stridor, drooling, and dysphagia).

 **TREATMENT**

## MEDICATION
It is difficult for a single agent to meet both sedation and analgesia requirements, so usually a combination of medications may be used if pain is expected.

### ALERT
Many sedative and analgesic medications cause respiratory depression. Combination of two or more of these agents may have a synergistic effect on respiratory depression that can lead to hypoxia and apnea.

### Suggested Procedural Sedation Agents by Type
- Painless procedures (single agents):
  - Methohexital
  - Choral hydrate (children)
  - Pentobarbital
  - Midazolam
  - Ketamine
- Painful procedures:
  - Fentanyl/remifentanil and midazolam
  - Ketamine ± midazolam (reduce emergence reactions)
  - Nitrous oxide
  - Propofol and fentanyl
  - Etomidate and fentanyl
  - Dexmedetomidine

### Specific Sedation Medications
- **Chloral hydrate**: To be used in procedural sedation in children (<2 yr old) undergoing *painless* diagnostic studies:
  - Dosage (PO): 50–100 mg/kg with usual dose of 50–75 mg/kg (max 2 g)
  - Dosage for rectal administration: Not recommended due to erratic absorption
  - Onset: 30–45 min
  - Duration of action: 2–4 hr (effects can recur up to 24 hr)
  - Side effects:
    - Nausea and vomiting
    - Respiratory depression
    - Prolonged sedation
    - Rarely paradoxical excitation
- **Dexmedetomidine**: A short-acting, rapidly cleared $\alpha_2$-adrenergic agonist with sedative, anxiolytic, and analgesic properties:
  - Dosage IV: 1-$\mu$g/kg loading dose over 5–10 min followed by infusion at 0.2–1.0 $\mu$g/kg/hr (use half dose for elderly or less invasive procedures)
  - Onset: Progressive during loading dose cycle
  - Duration: 6 min after cessation of infusion
  - Side effects:
    - Moderate BP and heart rate reductions should be expected, but alternative agent should be used if bradycardia and/or severe heart block.
- **Etomidate**: Sedative-hypnotic agent to facilitate both painful and nonpainful procedures:
  - Minimal cardiovascular and respiratory effects
  - Dosage IV: 0.2 mg/kg
  - Onset: <1 min
  - Duration: 5 min
  - Side effects:
    - Myoclonus that seems to be related to dose and speed of administration
    - Nausea and vomiting
    - Hypotension and respiratory depression when combined with opioid or benzodiazepine
    - Adrenocortical
- **Fentanyl**: Synthetic opioid with analgesic properties but minimal sedative properties:
  - Dosage (IV): 1–4 $\mu$g/kg (titrate)
  - Onset (IV): 30–60 sec with peak at 1–3 min
  - Transmucosal 10–15 $\mu$g/kg with onset in 15–20 min:
    - Oral lozenge (Oralet) allows patient to suck on drug, which then can be removed by physician or patient when adequate sedation achieved.
  - Duration of action: 30 min
  - Side effects:
    - Respiratory depression with potential apnea
    - Hypotension
    - Chest wall rigidity is a rare complication when large doses given quickly.
    - Use <1/3 dose in children <6 mo.
    - Emesis with transmucosal preparation

- **Methohexital**: A short-acting barbiturate with rapid recovery that produces a state of unconsciousness and profound amnesia but has no analgesic properties:
  - Dosage (IV): 0.75–1.0 mg/kg with subsequent titration at 0.5 mg/kg every 3–5 min to required effect
  - Onset: 30–60 sec
  - Duration of action: 5 min
  - Side effects:
    - Respiratory depression with potential apnea
    - Hypotension due to myocardial depressant effect (caution with underlying myocardial disease)
- **Midazolam**: Provides anxiolysis and amnesia but *not* analgesia, so should not be the sole agent for painful procedures:
  - Dosage (IV): 0.05–0.2 mg/kg (single max dose, 2 mg) with subsequent incremental doses at 3-min intervals to desired effect
  - Dosage (IM): 0.05–0.2 mg/kg
  - Dosage (PO): 0.5–0.75 mg/kg (max of 15 mg)
  - Dosage (nasal): 0.2–0.5 mg/kg (max of 5 mg)
  - Onset/duration:
    - IV: Fast onset (30–60 sec) and short duration of action (20–40 min)
    - IM, PO, and nasally: Slower onset and longer duration of action
  - Cautions for benzodiazepines:
    - Respiratory depression
    - Hypotension
    - Excessive sedation
    - Effects augmented by opioids, so reduce dose by 30–50% if opioid therapy utilized simultaneously
  - Effects may be reversed with flumazenil: 200 $\mu$g every 1–2 min, to effect
- **Ketamine**: Excellent agent for all procedures usually as a sole agent as it produces analgesia, amnesia, and sedation due to its dissociative effect while maintaining spontaneous respirations and airway reflexes:
  - Dosage (IV): 0.5–1.0 mg/kg (use midazolam 0.05 mg/kg and atropine 0.01 mg/kg concurrently) with onset of action 5–10 min
  - Dosage (IM): 2.0–4.0 mg/kg (combine atropine and midazolam in same syringe) with onset of action 15–25 min
  - Dosage (PO): 5–10 mg/kg (use midazolam 0.5 mg/kg and atropine 0.02 mg/kg PO as well) with onset of 30–45 min
  - Duration of action: IV 15–45 min; IM 30–90 min; PO 60–120 min
  - Side effects:
    - Causes hypertension and tachycardia, so do not use if hypertension or cardiovascular disease
    - Increases intracranial and intraocular pressure, so do not use with head injury or penetrating globe injury
    - Stimulates salivary and tracheobronchial secretions, so must be administered with an anticholinergic agent such as atropine
    - Emergence reactions with hallucinations reported, but are less frequent in children <10 yr; the incidence can be reduced by premedication with midazolam

- **Nitrous oxide**: Inhalational agent administered in 50% nitrous oxide/oxygen concentration:
  - Excellent agent for quick procedures, as provides analgesia, anxiolysis, and sedation without the need for IV placement
  - Onset of action: 30–60 sec
  - Duration of action: 3–5 min after ceasing inhalation
  - Side effects are rare but can cause deep sedation with respiratory depression (especially if concurrent narcotic) as well as nausea and vomiting
  - Contraindications: Pregnancy, pneumothorax, and bowel obstruction
- **Pentobarbital**: Barbiturate used only for *painless* procedures as a sole agent for diagnostic modalities:
  - Dosage (IV): 2–5 mg/kg for children, and adults have a loading dose of 100-mg slow bolus repeated/titrated q3–5min to max of 200–500 mg.
  - Dosage (IM): 4 mg/kg
  - Duration of action: 30–60 min
  - Onset: IV mode acts within 30 sec, and patient is appropriately sedated within 5 min.
  - Side effects: Central nervous system, respiratory depression, and bronchospasm (contraindicated in asthma/COPD)
- **Propofol**: Rapid onset and short duration make for excellent ED agent for procedural sedation:
  - Produces amnesia and sedation but *not* analgesia
  - Onset of action: 15–45 sec
  - Dosage (IV): 0.5–1.0 mg/kg bolus (usually given as 20-mg boluses every 10 sec in adults until desired effect is obtained) followed by infusion of 50–75 $\mu$g/kg/min; effective total dose for adults 20–150 mg
  - Duration of action: <2 min
  - Side effects:
    - Dose-related respiratory depression with occasional apnea (care with COPD)
    - Hypotension (care with cardiomyopathy or hypovolemia)
    - Pain at injection site
  - Care with patients in renal failure due to accumulation of active metabolite leading to prolonged sedation
- **Remifentanil**: Potent short acting synthetic opioid with potent sedative and analgesic properties:
  - Dosage (IV): 0.05–2 $\mu$g/kg/min
  - Onset: 30–60 sec
  - Duration of action: 5–10 min
  - Side effects:
    - Bradycardia
    - Hypotension
    - Respiratory depression with potential apnea
    - Chest wall rigidity is rare side effect believed due to large dose and quick bolus administration.

### Reversal agents
- **Naloxone**: Opioid antagonist:
  - For reversal of respiratory depression, apnea, and severe hypotension
  - Dosage: 0.1–0.2 mg/kg IV/IM in incremental doses (to total of 2 mg) q1–2min to the desired reversal effect; usual adult dose of 1–2 mg effective
  - Duration of action: 20–45 min

- **Flumazenil**: Benzodiazepine antagonist:
  - Reverses CNS depression and some degree of respiratory depression
  - Dosage (IV): 0.01 mg/kg per dose (max initial dose 0.2 mg) repeated at 1-min intervals to desired effect or max 0.05 mg/kg or 1.0 mg
  - Duration of action: 20–45 min

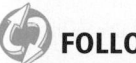 **FOLLOW-UP**

### DISPOSITION
#### Admission Criteria
- Postprocedural sedation
- Inability to walk
- No responsible adult to accompany patient home
- Reason for undergoing conscious sedation still present
- Postprocedure complication

#### Discharge Criteria
- Patient is awake, alert, and at baseline.
- Stable hemodynamically
- Ambulatory 30 min before discharge
- Able to urinate
- Able to retain oral fluids
- Pain controlled
- Discharged with follow-up instructions both for the necessitating procedure and for conscious sedation
- Under observation of a responsible person and have transportation from the hospital

## PEARLS AND PITFALLS
- All airway adjuncts should be readily available in case of respiratory compromise.
- All reversal agents should be readily available in case of inadvertent overdose of medications.
- Patients must have continuous cardiorespiratory monitoring during and after procedural sedation.

## ADDITIONAL READING
- Godwin A, Caro DA, Wolf SI, et al. Clinical policy: Procedural sedation and analgesia in the emergency department. *Ann Emerg Med.* 2005;45(2):177–196.
- Mace S, Brown LA, Francis L, et al. Clinical policy: Critical issues in the sedation of pediatric patients in the emergency department. *Ann Emerg Med.* 2008; 51(4):378–399.
- Marx JA, Hockberger R, Walls R. *Rosen's Emergency Medicine: Clinical Concepts and Practice*, 7th ed. St. Louis, MO: Mosby; 2009.

# PROSTATITIS
*Nicole M. Franks*

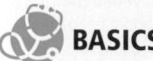

## BASICS

### DESCRIPTION
- Acute (bacterial) prostatitis:
  - Acute febrile illness
  - Systemic symptoms may appear days before localizing urinary symptoms appear.
  - Patients may appear toxic and usually have a concurrent cystitis.
- Prostatic abscess:
  - Once common after acute prostatitis, now rare except in immunocompromised patients
  - Fever, rectal pain, and leukocytosis despite treatment
  - Fluctuant mass on rectal exam
- Chronic bacterial prostatitis:
  - ~10% of cases of prostatitis
  - Most common cause of recurrent urinary tract infection in men
  - WBC and bacteria may be present in expressed prostatic secretions (EPS).
- Chronic nonbacterial prostatitis (also called prostatosis):
  - Same symptoms as chronic bacterial prostatitis but unable to culture organisms from urine or EPS
- Chronic pelvic pain syndrome (CPPS):
  - Symptoms referable to the prostate
  - No inflammatory cells are found
  - No bacteria cultured from the urine or EPS

### ETIOLOGY
- Usually a single-organism bacterial infection of the prostate
- Acute prostatitis:
  - Age <35 yr:
    - *Neisseria gonorrhoeae* and *Chlamydia trachomatis* are usual etiologies.
  - Age ≥35 yr:
    - Enterobacteriaceae or *Escherichia coli* (usual), *Klebsiella, Pseudomonas, Enterococcus,* and *Proteus* also seen
  - Rarely may be caused by *Salmonella, Clostridia,* tuberculosis, or fungi.
  - *Cryptococcus neoformans* in AIDS patients

- Chronic bacterial prostatitis:
  - Enterobacteriaceae (80%), *Enterococcus* (15%), and Pseudomonas aeruginosa
- Chronic nonbacterial prostatitis:
  - Possible role for *Chlamydia, Ureaplasma urealyticum, Trichomonas vaginalis,* and *Mycoplasma hominis*

## DIAGNOSIS

### SIGNS AND SYMPTOMS
#### History
- Irritative voiding symptoms:
  - Frequency, urgency, dysuria
- Low back pain
- Perineal, suprapubic, or testicular pain
- Bladder outlet obstruction and urinary retention
- Ejaculatory symptoms such as hematospermia
- Acute prostatitis:
  - Fever, chills
  - Malaise
  - Arthralgias or myalgias
- Primary symptom in chronic prostatitis is relapsing dysuria.

#### Physical Exam
- Acute prostatitis:
  - Exquisitely prostate tenderness
  - Warm, swollen
  - Firm or boggy prostate
  - Acutely inflamed prostate should not be massaged because may precipitate hematogenous spread of organisms.
- In chronic prostatitis, the examination is usually normal.

### DIAGNOSTIC TESTS & INTERPRETATION
#### Lab
- Urinalysis (with microscopy) and culture
- Acute prostatitis:
  - CBC, electrolytes, and blood cultures may be helpful in the acutely ill patient.
  - If <35 yr old or suspected sexual transmission, test for syphilis:
    - Venereal Disease Research Laboratory or rapid plasma reagin

- Chronic prostatitis/CPPS:
  - Prostatic massage between voiding may be used to capture EPS for Gram stain and culture if organism or white cells not present in the urine.

#### Imaging
- Not indicated in acute prostatitis
- If prostatic abscess suspected, transrectal US or pelvic CT with IV and rectal contrast will confirm diagnosis.

#### Diagnostic Procedures/Surgery
Not applicable in ED

### DIFFERENTIAL DIAGNOSIS
- Benign prostatic hyperplasia
- Cystitis
- Epididymitis
- Orchitis
- Perirectal/perianal abscess
- Proctitis
- Prostatic carcinoma
- Prostatic infarction
- Pyelonephritis
- Seminal vesiculitis
- Urethritis
- Urolithiasis
- Vesicular calculi
- Other causes of lower back pain (strain, disc disease, sacroiliac joint disease, etc.)

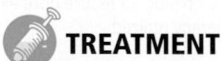

## TREATMENT

### INITIAL STABILIZATION/THERAPY
Initial resuscitative measures as indicated

### ED TREATMENT/PROCEDURES
- Prostatic abscess requires urgent urologic consultation and transrectal US-guided aspiration.
- Antibiotic therapy should be initiated in ED (see Medications).
- Urinary tract instrumentation should be avoided:
  - If patient has painful urinary retention in acute prostatitis, suprapubic needle aspiration or suprapubic catheter placement should be performed.

- Many patients will benefit from IV fluid.
- Pain control with NSAIDs and narcotic analgesics as needed
- Stool softeners
- Bed rest
- Irritative voiding symptoms may persist for months after antibiotic therapy and may be treated with NSAIDs.

## MEDICATION

- Analgesia:
  - Narcotic, analgesic combinations such as hydroxycodone/acetaminophen: 1–2 tabs PO q4h
  - NSAIDs such as ibuprofen: 800 mg PO t.i.d.
- Parenteral antibiotic therapy for acute prostatitis:
  - Levofloxacin: 750 mg IV daily
  - Ampicillin/sulbactam: 3 g IV q6h
  - Cefotaxime: 2 g IV q8h
  - Ceftriaxone: 2 g IV daily
  - Ciprofloxacin: 400 mg IV b.i.d.
  - Ofloxacin: 200 mg IV b.i.d.
  - Piperacillin/tazobactam: 3.375 g IV q6h or 4.5 g IV q8h
  - Ticarcillin/clavulanate: 3.1 g IV q6h
- Antibiotics for outpatient treatment of acute (≤35 yr old) prostatitis, suspected etiology *N. gonorrhoeae* or *C. trachomatis*:
  - Ceftriaxone: 250 mg IM, then doxycycline: 100 mg PO b.i.d. ×10–14 days
  - Levofloxacin: 500 mg PO every day for 10–14 days
  - Ofloxacin: 400 mg PO ×1, then 300 mg PO b.i.d. ×10–14 days
- Antibiotics for outpatient treatment of acute (>35 yr old) prostatitis, suspected etiology Enterobacteriaceae (coliforms); some authorities recommend 3–4 wk of therapy:
  - Ciprofloxacin: 500 mg PO b.i.d. ×14 days
  - Levofloxacin: 500 mg PO every day for 14 days
  - Ofloxacin: 200 mg PO b.i.d. ×14 days
  - Trimethoprim/sulfamethoxazole: 1 double strength (DS) tab or 2 regular-strength tabs PO b.i.d. ×28 days

- Outpatient therapy for chronic bacterial prostatitis (Enterobacteriaceae, *Enterococcus*, or *P. aeruginosa*):
  - Ciprofloxacin: 500 mg PO b.i.d. for 4 wk
  - Levofloxacin: 500 mg PO every day for 4 wk
  - Ofloxacin: 300 mg PO b.i.d. for 6 wk
  - Trimethoprim/sulfamethoxazole DS: 1 tab PO b.i.d. for 1–3 mo
- Chronic pelvic pain syndrome:
  - Tamsulosin: 0.4 mg PO every day
  - Doxazosin: 1 mg PO every day
  - Peripheral β-adrenergic blocking agents have been used with some success; consult a urologist.
  - Prazosin: 1 mg PO b.i.d./t.i.d.
  - Terazosin: 1 mg PO qhs

 **FOLLOW-UP**

## DISPOSITION

### Admission Criteria

- Acute prostatitis:
  - Patients who appear ill or toxic
  - Hypotension
  - Urinary retention
- Chronic prostatitis:
  - Admission generally not warranted unless patient has signs or symptoms of acute prostatitis.

### Discharge Criteria

- Acute prostatitis:
  - Patient must be nontoxic.
  - Able to take fluids and oral medications (analgesia and antibiotics)
  - Urinate without difficulty
  - Immunocompetent
  - Relatively free of concurrent underlying disease
  - Have appropriate follow-up care
- Chronic prostatitis: Appropriate follow-up care should be available.

### Issues for Referral

Patient with either acute or chronic prostatitis should be referred to an urologist.

## PEARLS AND PITFALLS

- Obtain a good history to distinguish acute from chronic prostatitis, as longer antibiotic therapy may be warranted.
- Consider this diagnosis even in sexually active adolescent males.
- Acutely ill males with antibiotic treatment failure for prostatitis should be evaluated for abscess regardless of immunocompetence.

## ADDITIONAL READING

- Benway BM. Bacterial prostatitis. *Urol Clin North Am.* 2008;35(1):23–32, v.
- Hedayati T, Keegan M. Prostatitis. *eMedicine.* Available at: www.emedicine.medscape.com/ article/785418. Updated July 29, 2009.
- Pontari MA. Chronic prostatitis/chronic pelvic pain syndrome. *Urol Clin North Am.* 2008;35(1): 81–89, vi.
- Schaeffer AJ. Chronic prostatitis and the chronic pelvic pain syndrome. *N Engl J Med.* 2006;355: 1690–1698.
- Wagenlehner FM. Current challenges in the treatment of complicated urinary tract infections and prostatitis. *Clin Microbiol Infect.* 2006;12(suppl 3): 67–80.

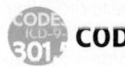 **CODES**

### ICD9

- 601.0 Acute prostatitis
- 601.1 Chronic prostatitis
- 601.2 Abscess of prostate

# PRURITUS
*Christine Tsien Silvers*

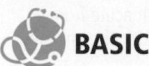

## BASICS

### DESCRIPTION
- Unpleasant sensation that provokes a desire to scratch
- Mediated by unmyelinated C fibers in upper portion of dermis:
  - Transmitted to dorsal horn of spinal cord
  - Via spinothalamic tract to cerebral cortex
- Peripheral mediators (eg, histamine and peptides such as substance P that release histamine) stimulate C fibers and induce itching.
- Prostaglandins ($PGE_2$, $PGH_2$) lower threshold to pruritus.
- Opiates cause pruritus by acting on central receptors.
- No single pharmacologic agent effectively treats all causes of pruritus.
- "Itch–scratch–itch" cycle:
  - Itching triggers scratching.
  - Scratching damages skin and stimulates nerve endings, thereby producing even greater itching.

### ETIOLOGY
4 categories in proposed itch classification:
- Pruritoceptive: Generated in the skin from localized irritation or inflammation
- Neurogenic: Generated in the CNS due to circulating pruritogens
- Neuropathic: Due to CNS or PNS lesions
- Psychogenic

## DIAGNOSIS

### SIGNS AND SYMPTOMS
#### History
- Onset:
  - Shortly after freshwater bathing in swimmer's itch
  - More intense at night with scabies
  - Paroxysmal with multiple sclerosis
  - With sudden changes in temperature in polycythemia vera
- Character: Paroxysmal, burning, pricking
- Time of occurrence, circadian nature
- Duration
- Severity
- Anatomic area (eg, exposed skin only)
- Exacerbating or alleviating factors:
  - Water, heat, dryness, dampness, coolness
- Medications
- New topical products (soap, cosmetics, etc.)
- Laundry detergents, fabric softeners
- Family history of atopic dermatitis or skin disease
- Personal history of allergies or asthma
- Pruritus in other family members
- Systemic or associated symptoms:
  - Night sweats, fever, tremors, weight loss, fatigue
- Sexual history, history of HIV or AIDS
- Social: Occupation, hobbies, pets, travel

### Physical Exam
- Dermatologic:
  - Absence of rash
  - Diffuse or localized rash
  - Location: Genitals, interdigital webs, axilla, wrists, etc.
  - Generalized morbilliform eruptions
  - Discrete weeping patches with vesicles
  - Dry skin
  - Jaundice
  - Follicular (around the hair)
  - Nonfollicular (eg, insect bites, scabies)
  - Primary lesions:
    - Papular, pustular, urticarial, or polymorphic
  - Secondary lesions:
    - Excoriations
    - Lichenification
    - Hyperpigmentation
    - Prurigo papules: Thickened papular areas of skin from constant rubbing
- Psychogenic: Constant rubbing in areas patient can readily reach

### ESSENTIAL WORKUP
- Detailed history is key in the ED workup.
- Physical exam to characterize skin lesions
- Look for evidence of systemic disease.

### DIAGNOSTIC TESTS & INTERPRETATION
#### Lab
Indications for specific studies (eg, CBC and differential, BUN/creatinine, LFTs, TSH, HIV, cancer screening, CXR, CT/MRI) vary based on the clinical presentation and should be guided by clinical judgment.

#### Diagnostic Procedures/Surgery
- Skin scrapings for scabies and dermatophytoses
- Skin biopsy performed by dermatologist at follow-up visit
- Skin culture for bacterial, viral, or fungal infection

### DIFFERENTIAL DIAGNOSIS
#### Dermatologic
- Xerosis (dry skin)
- Insect infestations:
  - Scabies: Vesicles and burrows on intertriginous areas
  - Pediculosis (lice)
- Insect bites: Localized clusters of papules
- Dermatitis:
  - Atopic dermatitis
  - Contact dermatitis (eg, poison ivy contact)
  - Nummular dermatitis: Round eczematous or vesicular eruption
- Drug-induced (suspect when no rash):
  - Opiates and derivatives
  - Aspirin/NSAIDs
  - Quinidine; amiodarone
  - Certain antibiotics, antifungals, antimalarials
  - Phenothiazines
  - Estrogens, progestins, testosterone
  - Statins
  - Others

- Lichen planus: Lichenification, hyperpigmentation, skin thickening
- Urticaria
- Bullous pemphigoid
- Eosinophilic folliculitis
- Psoriasis
- Dermatitis herpetiformis: Burning itch
- Sunburn
- Aquagenic pruritus
- Fiberglass dermatitis
- Seborrheic dermatitis: Scaly plaques on sebaceous gland–bearing areas
- Swimmer's itch, schistosome cercarial dermatitis, or schistosomiasis:
  - Repeated freshwater exposure
  - Itching starts as water evaporates
  - Highly pruritic papules develop hours later
- Miliaria rubra (prickly heat)

#### Pregnancy Considerations
- Polymorphic eruption of pregnancy
- Pemphigoid gestationis
- Intrahepatic cholestasis of pregnancy
- Atopic eruption of pregnancy

#### Infectious
- HIV
- Parasites:
  - Ankylostomiasis/helminthiasis (hookworm)
  - Onchocerciasis/river blindness (nematode)
  - Ascariasis (roundworm)
  - Trichinosis (roundworm)

#### Cholestatic
- Obstructive biliary disease
- Primary biliary cirrhosis
- Hepatic cholestasis secondary to drugs
- Intrahepatic cholestasis of pregnancy
- Extrahepatic biliary obstruction
- Chronic hepatitis, especially hepatitis C

#### Hematologic
- Polycythemia vera
- Iron-deficiency anemia
- Paraproteinemia
- Waldenström macroglobulinemia
- Mastocytosis

#### Neoplastic
- Lymphoma, including Hodgkin disease
- Mycosis fungoides
- Leukemia
- CNS tumors
- Multiple myeloma
- Carcinoid
- Visceral malignancies (breast, stomach, lung)

#### Metabolic-Endocrine
- Uremia
- Hyperthyroidism
- Hypothyroidism
- Hyperparathyroidism
- Diabetes mellitus
- Carcinoid

### Neurologic
- Multiple sclerosis: Paroxysmal itching
- Notalgia paraesthetica: Local itch of back, medial shaft scapula
- Brain abscess
- CNS infarct
- Cerebral tumor
- Creutzfeldt-Jakob disease

### Renal
- Chronic renal failure
- Chronic hemodialysis

### Rheumatologic
- Sjögren syndrome
- Dermatomyositis

### Psychiatric
- Stress, anxiety, neurotic excoriation
- Delusions of parasitosis
- Psychogenic pruritus

## TREATMENT

### ED TREATMENT/PROCEDURES
- Start with antihistamines for pruritus of undetermined etiology.
- Emollients indicated for pruritus secondary to dry skin
- Coolants to alleviate itching: Menthol, camphor, eucalyptus oil, calamine lotion
- Substance P evacuators (capsaicin) block C fibers:
  – Burning sensation during 1st weeks of use
  – Anesthetic can be applied prior
- Topical glucocorticoids for contact dermatitis
- Permethrin cream for scabies and lice when rash is suggestive
- Topical antihistamines (doxepin) for eczema, urticaria, bites
- Swimmer's itch:
  – Control with antihistamines, cool compresses, calamine lotion
  – Topical steroids to suppress intense inflammation
  – Towel dry immediately after leaving water as preventive measure
- Discontinue medications that may cause allergic reaction
- UV light for uremic pruritus
- Treat the underlying cause for pruritus associated with a systemic disease.

### MEDICATION
- Oral antihistamines:
  – Chlorpheniramine 4 mg (peds: 0.35 mg/kg/24 hr div. q 4–6h PRN; 2–6 yr max 4 mg/24 hr; 6–12 yr max 12 mg/24 hr) PO q4–6h PRN; max 24 mg/24 hr
  – Diphenhydramine 25–50 mg (peds: 5 mg/kg/24 hr div. q6h PRN; 2–5 yr max 37.5 mg/24 hr; 6–11 yr max 150 mg/24 hr; >12 yr max 400 mg/24 hr) PO q4–6h PRN; max 400 mg/24 hr
  – Hydroxyzine 25–100 mg (peds: 2 mg/kg/24 hr div. q6h PRN) PO q6–8h PRN; max 600 mg/24 hr

- Topical treatments:
  – Capsaicin 0.025%, 0.075% cream: Apply t.i.d. to q.i.d. PRN
  – Doxepin 5% cream: Apply q.i.d. for up to 8 days (to max of 10% of the body)
  – EMLA (2.5% lidocaine + 2.5% prilocaine): Apply prior to capsaicin Hydrocortisone 0.5%, 1%, 2.5%: Up to q.i.d.
  – Permethrin 5% cream (for scabies):
    ○ Apply from neck down after bath.
    ○ Wash off thoroughly with water in 8–12 hr.
    ○ May repeat in 7 days.
  – Permethrin 1% cream rinse (for lice):
    ○ Shampoo, rinse, towel dry, saturate hair and scalp (or other affected area), leave on 10 min, then rinse.
    ○ May repeat in 7 days.
  – White petroleum emollients: Apply after short bath/shower in warm (not hot) water.
- Other treatments for specific diseases

## FOLLOW-UP

### DISPOSITION
#### Admission Criteria
- Anaphylaxis
- Generalized exfoliating lesions
- Manifestations of systemic diseases requiring admission

#### Discharge Criteria
Vary by etiology

#### Issues for Referral
- Refer patients with skin lesions to primary care physician or dermatologist.
- Stable patients with pruritus without skin lesions should be discharged on antipruritic medication and referred to a physician for an underlying systemic illness.

### FOLLOW-UP RECOMMENDATIONS
- Practical recommendations for dry skin:
  – Take baths with baking soda, bath oils, or colloidal oatmeal.
  – Use moisturizers frequently during day and immediately after bathing.
- Avoid:
  – Dry air (humidity <40%)
  – Contact irritants (wool, cleansers, etc.)
  – Alkaline soaps and overwashing
  – Alcohol, caffeine, peppery foods
  – Overexposure to heat, hot water

## PEARLS AND PITFALLS
- Detailed history is key in the ED workup.
- Pruritus can be indicative of systemic illness.
- No single treatment for all causes of pruritus

## ADDITIONAL READING
- Greaves MW. Recent advances in pathophysiology and current management of itch. *Ann Acad Med Singapore.* 2007;36:788–792.
- Reich A, Stander S, Szepietowski JC. Drug-induced pruritus: A review. *Acta Dermatol Venereol.* 2009; 89.236–244.
- Stander S, Weisshaar F, Luger TA. Neurophysiological and neurochemical basis of modern pruritus treatment. *Exp Dermatol.* 2008;17:161–169.
- Weisshaar E, Dalgard F. Epidemiology of itch: Adding to the burden of skin morbidity. *Acta Dermatol Venereol.* 2009;89:339–350.
- Yosipovitch G, Samuel LS. Neuropathic and psychogenic itch. *Dermatol Ther.* 2008;21:32–41.

### See Also (Topic, Algorithm, Electronic Media Element)
- Anaphylaxis
- Anemia
- Contact Dermatitis
- Eczema/Atopic Dermatitis
- Hepatitis
- HIV/AIDS
- Hyperparathyroidism
- Hyperthyroidism
- Hypothyroidism
- Leukemia
- Multiple Myeloma
- Multiple Sclerosis
- Pediculosis
- Polycythemia
- Psoriasis
- Rash
- Renal Failure
- Scabies
- Seborrheic Dermatitis
- Tinea Infections, Cutaneous
- Urticaria

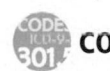

## CODES

### ICD9
- 698.8 Other specified pruritic conditions
- 698.9 Unspecified pruritic disorder

# PSEUDOTUMOR CEREBRI

*Ian Reilly*

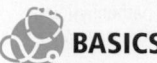 **BASICS**

## DESCRIPTION
- Buildup of cerebrospinal fluid (CSF) pressure without mass lesion and no clear cause
- Also known as idiopathic intracranial hypertension
- Two proposed mechanisms:
  - Increased abdominal pressure may elevate right heart pressures and decrease venous drainage from the head.
  - Vitamin A levels above the saturation of the liver can damage cell membranes in the arachnoid granulations.
- Associated with obesity
- Average age of onset 30 yr
- Female predominance (7:1)

## ETIOLOGY
Proposed causative agents:
- Obesity
- Hypervitaminosis A
- Steroids/steroid withdrawal
- Tetracycline antibiotics
- Oral contraceptive pills
- Hypertension
- Recent weight gain
- Chronic carbon dioxide retention with elevated intracranial pressure

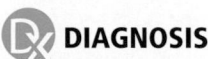 **DIAGNOSIS**

## SIGNS AND SYMPTOMS
### History
- Headache:
  - Typically described as constant, bilateral
  - Pressure-like
  - Worse in the morning
  - Worse with Valsalva maneuver
- Nausea and vomiting
- Pulsatile intracranial noise
- Diplopia
- Dizziness
- Scotoma
- Transient visual obscurations lasting seconds
- Blind spots
- Constriction of vision

### Physical Exam
- Visual field defects (in up to 90%):
  - Typically inferior nasal visual field loss
- Papilledema
- Lumbar puncture improves symptoms
- Sixth cranial nerve palsy
- Loss of visual acuity
- Otherwise normal neurologic exam except:
  - Visual changes
  - Abducens palsy
  - Rarely seventh cranial nerve palsy

### Pediatric Considerations
- Usually presents with strabismus as opposed to headache and visual field loss
- Also associated with obesity and medications (tetracycline antibiotics, steroids)

## ESSENTIAL WORKUP
- Thorough history and physical exam
- Detailed neurologic assessment and fundoscopic exam

## DIAGNOSTIC TESTS & INTERPRETATION
### Lab
- Lumbar puncture: CSF normal or low protein with a normal cell count
- Opening pressure >25 cm $H_2O$ or >20 cm $H_2O$ in nonobese, relaxed patient
- Consider CBC, coagulation studies prior to lumbar puncture.
- Improvement of symptoms with lumbar puncture

### Imaging
- Head CT/MRI to rule out mass lesions (prior to lumbar puncture)
- Classically the head CT will demonstrate slitlike frontal horns of the lateral ventricles.
- MRI recommended in the full workup:
  - Can be done as an outpatient
  - Cerebral venous thrombosis can mimic pseudotumor cerebri in all regards including normal head CT.

### Diagnostic Procedures/Surgery
Modified Dandy criteria for diagnosis:
- Symptoms of raised intracranial pressure
- No localizing symptoms with exception of sixth nerve palsy
- Patient is awake and alert.
- Normal CT/MRI findings without evidence of thrombosis
- Lumbar puncture opening pressure >25 cm $H_2O$ (some suggest >20 cm $H_2O$ in nonobese, relaxed patients)
- Lumbar puncture
- Be sure patient is lying down with legs extended when measuring opening pressure.
- Observing respiratory variation ensures good transmission of pressure.
- Improvement of symptoms may occur with lumbar puncture.

## DIFFERENTIAL DIAGNOSIS
- Migraine headache
- Hypertensive headache
- Anoxic headache
- Tension headache
- Cluster headache
- Subarachnoid hemorrhage
- Aneurysm/arteriovenous malformation
- Meningitis/encephalitis

- Subdural hematoma
- Epidural hematoma
- Tumor
- Abscess
- Trigeminal neuralgia
- Giant cell/temporal arteritis
- Sinusitis
- Glaucoma
- Central retinal vein/artery occlusion
- Congenital optic nerve head elevation
- Optic nerve drusen
- Labyrinthitis
- Optic neuritis
- Cerebral venous thrombosis
- Chronic carbon dioxide retention

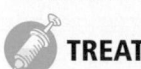 ## TREATMENT

### PRE-HOSPITAL
Pain control as appropriate

### INITIAL STABILIZATION/THERAPY
- Airway and circulation management as indicated
- IV fluid hydration

### ED TREATMENT/PROCEDURES
- Large-volume lumbar puncture of 20–30 mL of CSF:
  - Only if confident of correct diagnosis and head CT demonstrates open basilar cisterns and fourth ventricle
- Acetazolamide
- Pain control
- Neurology consult
- Ophthalmology consult
- Neurosurgery consult for acute or impending visual loss unresponsive to diuretics (for lumboperitoneal shunt)
- Optic nerve fenestration is another surgical option.
- Weight loss
- Discontinue any drugs that could be causative.
- Typically resolves spontaneously

### MEDICATION
- Acetaminophen: 650 mg to 1 g (peds: 15 mg/kg) PO q6h
- Acetazolamide: 500 mg slow-release PO b.i.d. (peds: 25 mg/kg/d div. q.i.d./t.i.d.) PO/IV
- Ibuprofen: 600–800 mg (peds: 10 mg/kg) PO q8h
- Lasix: 0.5–1 mg/kg IV/PO
- Morphine: 0.1 mg/kg IV/IM
- Prednisone: Helpful when severe visual symptoms present, 5-day course recommended

### First Line
- Acetazolamide
- NSAIDs

### Second Line
Topiramate has been suggested as a second-line agent but is not FDA approved for this use.

 ## FOLLOW-UP

### DISPOSITION
#### Admission Criteria
Acute or impending visual loss

#### Discharge Criteria
- Consultation obtained from neurology and ophthalmology
- Appropriate follow-up arranged
- Tolerating oral diuretics
- Pain under control

#### Issues for Referral
Timely referral and return precautions:
- Visual loss
- Focal neurologic deficit
- Worsening headache

### FOLLOW-UP RECOMMENDATIONS
Follow-up is recommended with neurology and ophthalmology.

## PEARLS AND PITFALLS
- Consider this diagnosis in younger patients with chronic headache.
- Consider measuring opening pressure when performing lumbar puncture for headache.
- Visual changes can portend visual loss.

## ADDITIONAL READING
- Bradley WG, Daroff R, Fenichel G, et al., eds. *Neurology in Clinical Practice*, 5th ed. Philadelphia: Butterworth-Heinemann, 2008.
- Irani DN, ed. *Cerebrospinal Fluid in Diseases of the Nervous System*, 1st ed. Philadelphia: WB Saunders; 2009.
- Randhawa S, Van Stavern GP. Idiopathic intracranial hypertension (pseudotumor cerebri). *Curr Opin Ophthalmol*. 2008;19:445–453.

### See Also (Topic, Algorithm, Electronic Media Element)
- Giant Cell Arteritis
- Headache
- Headache, Migraine
- Labyrinthitis
- Trigeminal Neuralgia

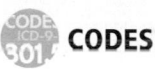 ## CODES

### ICD9
348.2 Benign intracranial hypertension

# PSORIASIS

Adam Z. Barkin
Stephen R. Hayden

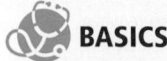 **BASICS**

## DESCRIPTION
- Chronic skin condition presents with erythematous plaques with silver scaling
- Caucasians and atopics most affected
- Majority of cases are diagnosed between 10 and 30 yr.
- Second peak incidence between 50–60 yr
- Equal number of adult male and female cases
- Occurs as the result of defective inhibition of epidermal proliferation
- Several clinical presentations:
  – Plaque-type psoriasis (psoriasis vulgaris):
    ○ Most common form (90%) with classic lesions on the extensor surfaces (elbows, knees, occipital scalp, back)
  – Guttate psoriasis:
    ○ Red drop-like lesions usually on the trunk
    ○ Occurs more commonly in children and often after streptococcal infections
  – Pustular psoriasis:
    ○ Collections of pustules on 1 area of the body, usually palms or soles
    ○ Potentially severe and life-threatening
    ○ Usually treated as inpatients
  – Erythrodermic psoriasis:
    ○ Simple confluent erythroderma, or the patient may exhibit pustules
    ○ Increased risk for infection, dehydration
    ○ Often treated as inpatients
  – Light-sensitive psoriasis:
    ○ Response to sunburning (Koebner phenomenon)
  – Inverse flexural psoriasis:
    ○ A variant that causes lesions in flexural areas that do not exhibit scaling due to moisture in these areas
  – HIV-induced psoriasis:
    ○ May be the 1st manifestation of AIDS with an explosive presentation
  – Keratoderma blennorrhagicum:
    ○ Psoriasis of the penis seen with Reiter syndrome with a distinctive winding pattern to the lesion (balanitis circinata)
- Genetics:
  – 41% chance of a child having psoriasis if both parents have the disease
  – 14% chance if 1 parent has psoriasis
  – 6% chance if a sibling has psoriasis

## ETIOLOGY
- Affects ~1–2% of people in the U.S.
- Triggers include:
  – Drugs:
    ○ Lithium
    ○ β-Blockers
    ○ Antimalarials
    ○ Steroids
    ○ NSAIDs
    ○ Alcohol
    ○ Tetracycline
    ○ Penicillin
    ○ Amiodarone
    ○ Morphine
    ○ Procaine
    ○ Potassium iodide
    ○ Sulfapyridine and sulfonamides
  – Infections:
    ○ Streptococcal pharyngitis
    ○ HIV
    ○ Viral URI
  – Local trauma:
    ○ Frostbite
    ○ Sunburn
    ○ Routine skin breaks (Koebner phenomenon)
  – Stress: Emotional and physical
  – Winter:
    ○ Low light exposure
    ○ Dry weather
  – Cigarette smoking
  – Hormonal changes, such as puberty or menopause

 **DIAGNOSIS**

## SIGNS AND SYMPTOMS
### History
- Patients usually complain of skin lesions that are not intensely pruritic but may itch or burn.
- May give a history of previously diagnosed psoriasis
- May relate 1 of the above triggers
- Age at 1st appearance of lesions
- Specific location of lesions
- Family history of the disease
- History of improvement with sun exposure, or if recurrent, success of prior regimens
- Systemic symptoms like fevers or joint pains

### Physical Exam
- The classic skin lesion is a round red patch with central plaque of silvery white scale that appears on extensor surfaces:
  – The lesions are not intensely pruritic, but do itch.
- Positive Auspitz sign:
  – Erythema and punctuate bleeding when scales are removed
- Scalp lesions may be confused with seborrhea:
  – Lesions that extend beyond the hair borders indicate psoriasis.
- Stippling and pitting of nail and oncolysis:
  – Yellow or brown band across the nail will help differentiate psoriasis (+ band) from onychomycosis (– band)
- ~10% of patients with plaque psoriasis have concomitant psoriatic arthritis:
  – Often affects the DIP joints of the hands and feet
- Asymmetric oligoarticular arthritis:
  – Present in 70% of these patients
  – Swelling of the juxtaarticular tissue
  – "Sausage-shape" to the affected digits

## ESSENTIAL WORKUP
- The diagnosis is clinical.
- Rarely, a biopsy is necessary to confirm the diagnosis or rule out other conditions in unusual cases.

## DIAGNOSTIC TESTS & INTERPRETATION
### Lab
- Elevated sedimentation rate and uric acid
- Decreased serum albumin
- Anemia with vitamin $B_{12}$, folate, and iron deficiency
- Positive streptococcal cultures and titers
- Hypocalcemia and leukocytosis in pustular disease
- Negative rheumatoid factor
- Key biopsy traits:
  – Dilated tortuous capillaries (Auspitz sign)
  – Hyperkeratosis
  – Epidermal hyperplasia
  – Munro micro-abscesses

### Imaging
Plain radiographs of the hands or feet may show osteoporosis and bone loss at the distal phalanx:
- Pencil-in-cup deformation at the MTP or MCP joints
- Sacroiliitis and ankylosing spondylitis may also be seen on radiographs.

## DIFFERENTIAL DIAGNOSIS
- Best thought of by region
- Scalp: Seborrhea
- Flexure creases:
  – Candidiasis
  – Intertrigo
  – Eczema
- Nails: Onychomycosis
- Trunk and extremities:
  – Nummular eczema
  – Pityriasis rosea or rubra pilaris
  – Tinea
  – Systematic lupus erythematosus
  – Syphilis
  – Drug eruption
  – Atopy
  – Mycosis fungoides
  – Squamous cell carcinoma

**TREATMENT**

## PRE-HOSPITAL
- Maintain universal precautions.
- IV access as necessary

## INITIAL STABILIZATION/THERAPY
- General resuscitation efforts aimed at correcting fluid and electrolyte abnormalities
- Treating sepsis if present:
  - Cultures of lesions, blood, and urine
- Soothing moist compresses are appropriate.
- Systemic steroids should not be used as they may predispose to severe complications.

## ED TREATMENT/PROCEDURES
- 3 basic types of treatment for psoriasis:
  - Topical therapy
  - Systemic therapy
  - Phototherapy
- Topical therapy is the most commonly prescribed treatment modality from the ED.
- Systemic therapy is usually employed only after patients have failed topical and phototherapy.
- Exceptions where systemic therapy may be used:
  - Generalized pustular psoriasis
  - Very active psoriatic arthritis
  - Psoriasis that is considered severely disabling
- Phototherapy is not an ED treatment modality.
- Dermatology consult should be obtained in severe cases.

## MEDICATION
- Mild to moderate disease:
  - Usually topical treatment only
  - No single topical agent works best for all people.
  - Emollients:
    - Hydrates and softens plaques
    - Greasier choices work best, but are poorly tolerated by patients.
  - Keratolytics:
    - Help to remove plaques
    - Salicylic acid (2–10%) is the mainstay of treatment (caution must be used in applying near the eyes).
  - Coal-tar preparations:
    - Usually used with topical steroids
    - Ointments and shampoos are available.
  - Anthralin:
    - May be used in complex treatment regimens with other topical agents and ultraviolet light
  - Topical corticosteroids:
    - Mainstay of treatment in the U.S.
    - Best results are obtained by rotating drugs and using occlusive dressings.
    - Small lesions may be treated with intralesional Kenalog, as may psoriatic nails.
    - Steroids have been implicated in serious relapses and pustular psoriasis.

- Vitamin D analogs:
  - Calcipotriene and tacalcitol
- Vitamin A analogs:
  - Tazarotene
  - Particularly useful for scalp lesions
- Moderate to severe disease:
  - The above-named agents may be employed along with phototherapy and systemic medications.
  - Phototherapy:
    - Indicated in patients with very large areas of skin involvement or refractory to topical treatments.
    - Proper facilities are required for this form of treatment.
    - Ultraviolet B light is usually combined with ≥1 topical agents and has reports of 80% remission.
    - Ultraviolet B may be used alone in guttate psoriasis.
    - Ultraviolet A light (PUVA) is combined with a systemic agent (psoralen) that sensitizes the skin to UVA light.
    - Therapy is usually given 2–3 times per week.
  - Systemic agents: May be used in various combinations with the above modalities:
    - Methotrexate (immunosuppressant); assess renal, liver, and hematologic function prior to therapy; not to be used during pregnancy
    - Etretinate: A retinoid, it causes dryness, scaling, redness, and tenderness of the skin.
    - Systemic corticosteroids: Not in favor due to iatrogenic Cushing syndrome; it may have a role in acute erythrodermic psoriasis if patient is extremely ill.
    - Cyclosporine: Use in conjunction with dermatology consult.
  - Psoralens (see above): No effect unless combined with UVA light therapy
  - Etanercept (Enbrel): Injectable agent that works with the immune system to reduce inflammation
  - Alefacept (Amevive): Immunosuppressant given as injection once per week

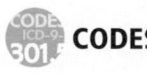 **FOLLOW-UP**

## DISPOSITION

### Admission Criteria
Acute erythroderma and acute pustular psoriasis warrant admission for supportive therapy and systemic treatment, as noted above.

### Discharge Criteria
- Patients without the above-mentioned forms may be discharged.
- Advise patients that the disease is not contagious.
- Warn against excessive scrubbing to loosen scale, as it may worsen the disease.
- Educate the patient on avoiding medications that trigger relapses.
- Refer patients to the National Psoriasis Foundation, www.psoriasis.org

### Pediatric Considerations
- 37% of all psoriasis cases occur before age 20.
- The younger the patient at onset of disease, the worse the course.
- The emotional side of this chronic disease may be paramount in children whose body image is being formed.
- In general, topical agents are well tolerated, but PUVA and systemic agents are generally avoided in children.

### Pregnancy Considerations
Many of the drugs used to treat psoriasis are contraindicated in pregnancy.

### Issues for Referral
- Referral to dermatology is indicated for most patients with psoriasis.
- Patients with psoriasis may also need referral to primary care doctor and/or psychiatry to cope with impaired quality of life.

## FOLLOW-UP RECOMMENDATIONS
Follow-up with dermatology and/or primary care doctor to evaluate efficacy of treatment.

## PEARLS AND PITFALLS
- Patients with pustular psoriasis are at risk for severe systemic infections.
- Patients with erythrodermic psoriasis are at risk for dehydration and may need to be treated similarly to a major burn patient.
- Patients with psoriasis report similar impairments to quality as life to those with diabetes or cancer.

## ADDITIONAL READING
- Camisa C. Psoriasis: A clinical update on diagnosis and new therapies. *Cleve Clin J Med.* 2000;67(2):105–106, 109–113, 117–119, S193.
- Levine D, Gottlieb A. Evaluation and management of psoriasis: An internist's guide. *Med Clin N Am.* 2009;93:1291–1303.
- Nestle FO, Kaplan DH, Barker J. Psoriasis. *N Eng J Med.* 2009;361:496–509.
- Rogers M. Childhood psoriasis. *Curr Opin Pediatr.* 2002;14:404–409.

## CODES

**ICD9**
696.1 Other psoriasis and similar disorders

# PSYCHIATRIC COMMITMENT

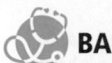

*Jennifer M. Park*
*Lawrence T. Park*

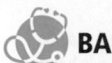

## BASICS

### DESCRIPTION
- Commitment criteria (check specific laws in your state):
  - Individual is mentally ill.
  - Failure to hospitalize or discharge from hospital creates likelihood of serious harm.
  - Likelihood of serious harm defined as:
    - Substantial risk of physical harm to self: Threats or attempts at suicide
    - Substantial risk of physical harm to other persons: Homicidal or violent behaviors, or others are placed in reasonable fear of violent behaviors
    - Very substantial risk of physical impairment due to inability to protect self resulting from impaired judgment; reasonable protection not available in community
- No less-restrictive alternative to hospitalization would attenuate risk.
- Physician usually must sign form attesting that patient meets 1 of above criteria:
  - Often leads to a period of mandatory hospitalization, which may be followed by petition for psychiatric commitment
  - Once the patient is admitted involuntarily, psychiatrist petitions the court for psychiatric commitment.
- If court does not grant petition for commitment, patient must be released from psychiatric facility.
- Civil commitment: Confinement of an individual
- Involuntary commitment: Confinement against patient's will
- Basis of civil commitment: Danger to self or others
- Psychiatric (civil) commitment:
  - Refers to order by judge for continued hospitalization of inpatient in a mental health facility for treatment of psychiatric disease against patient's wishes
  - Based on danger to self or others by reason of mental illness

- Psychiatric commitment not indicated for other causes of dangerous behavior:
  - Anger
  - Antisocial behavior
  - Substance abuse
  - Medical illness
- Psychiatric commitment usually involves 2 steps:
  - Initial involuntary hospitalization in psychiatric facility, most commonly initiated by a psychiatrist
  - Petition to court for psychiatric commitment

### ETIOLOGY
Psychiatric illness results in dangerous behavior or inability to care for self.

## DIAGNOSIS

### SIGNS AND SYMPTOMS
*History*
- Psychiatric evaluation through history/mental status exam:
  - History of psychiatric illness
  - History of previous admissions, psychiatric or medical
  - Recent change in behavior or thinking
  - Medication doses
  - Drugs of abuse: Amount and time of last use
  - Disabling thought patterns: Hallucinations, delusions, disorganization
- Assessment of commitment criteria:
  - Threat of violence toward self
  - Threat of violence toward others
  - Inability to care for self or severe deficits in judgment
- Rule out criminal behavior.

*Physical Exam*
- Complete physical and neurologic exam:
  - Folstein mini–mental state exam may elucidate gross cognitive changes.
- Rule out medical causes for mental status change, commonly delirium or substance intoxication/withdrawal.

### ESSENTIAL WORKUP
- Thorough psychiatric evaluation
- Rule out medical causes of change in thinking or behavior.

### DIAGNOSTIC TESTS & INTERPRETATION
*Lab*
Labs as indicated by history and physical:
- Electrolytes, BUN, creatinine, glucose
- Liver function tests
- CBC and differential
- Toxicology screens and medication levels
- Urinalysis if infection suspected

*Imaging*
CT of head if injury or structural CNS pathology suspected

### DIFFERENTIAL DIAGNOSIS
- Intoxication or withdrawal
- Delirium
- Dementia
- Traumatic brain injury
- Antisocial behavior

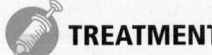 **TREATMENT**

### PRE-HOSPITAL
- Controversies/ethical considerations:
  - Involuntary admission leads to loss of basic rights.
  - *Parens patriae power*: State's authority to care for citizen who cannot care for self
  - *Police power*: State's authority to detain citizen who is danger to self or someone else
- Risk to emergency staff if patient threatens harm to self or others:
  - Enlist police assistance as necessary.

### INITIAL STABILIZATION/THERAPY
- Initial containment by police
- Transport patient to facility for psychiatric evaluation.
- Ensure patient and staff safety.

### ED TREATMENT/PROCEDURES
- Restrain dangerous patients using least restrictive means required to maintain safety:
  - Nurse or security guard standing outside room
  - Medications given PO, IM, or IV
  - Physical restraints
  - Closely observe patients when using physical restraints or involuntary medications.
- Determine if patient requires psychiatric hospitalization.

### MEDICATION
- May be necessary for extremely agitated patient
- Treat alcohol or drug withdrawal as needed.

 **FOLLOW-UP**

### DISPOSITION
#### Admission Criteria
- Patient meets criteria for psychiatric commitment and declines voluntary hospitalization.
- Follow commitment process for your state:
  - Usually involves consultation by a psychiatrist

#### Discharge Criteria
Patients may be discharged after initial psychiatric evaluation if they:
- Can care for themselves adequately *and*
- Have no intention of harm to self or others

### FOLLOW-UP RECOMMENDATIONS
Close psychiatric follow-up for patient with acute psychiatric illness but does not meet criteria for hospitalization

## PEARLS AND PITFALLS
- Civil (psychiatric) commitment involves involuntary hospitalization due to mental illness with:
  - Substantial risk of harm to self
  - Substantial risk of harm to others
  - Or substantial risk of physical impairment due to inability to care for/protect self
- Thorough psychiatric and medical evaluation to substantiate cause of change in patient's behavior
- Physician must weigh the ethical considerations inherent in hospitalization against the patient's will vs. the safety of patient or others.

## ADDITIONAL READING
- Behnke SH, Hilliard JT. *The Essentials of Massachusetts Mental Health Law*. New York: WW Norton; 1998.
- Folstein MF, Folstein FE, McHugh PR. The "mini-mental state": A practical method for grading the cognitive state of patients for the clinician. *J Psychiatr Res*. 1975;12:189.
- Gutheil TG, Appelbaum PS. *Clinical Handbook of Psychiatry and the Law*, 3rd ed. Philadelphia: Lippincott Williams & Wilkins; 2000.
- Linford S. Mental health law: Compulsory treatment in a general medical setting. *Br J Hosp Med*. 2005; 66(10):569–571.
- Schouten R. Psychiatry and the law I: Informed consent, competency, treatment refusal, and civil commitment. In: Stern TA, Herman IB, eds. *Psychiatry Update and Board Preparation*. New York: McGraw-Hill; 2000:415–419.
- Wand T. Duty of care in the emergency department. *Int J Mental health Nurs*. 2004;13(2):135–139.

### See Also (Topic, Algorithm, Electronic Media Element)
- Alcohol Poisoning
- Altered Mental Status
- Delirium
- Dementia
- Traumatic Brain Injury
- Withdrawal, Alcohol
- Withdrawal, Drug

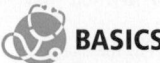

## BASICS

### DESCRIPTION
- A severe mental disorder characterized by derangement of personality and loss of contact with reality causing gross disorganization of a person's mental capacity
- The psychosis may be secondary to functional (psychiatric) or organic (medical) causes.
- Medical psychoses are generally secondary to systemic or neurologic diseases or neuroactive medications.
- Neurodevelopmental abnormalities in the dopaminergic and serotonergic systems are implicated in functional psychosis.

### ETIOLOGY
#### Organic
- Autoimmune disease
- CNS:
  - Alzheimer disease
  - Cerebritis
- Autoimmune disorders:
  - Cerebrovascular accident
  - Encephalitis
  - Encephalopathy
  - Head injury
  - Huntington chorea
  - Migraine
  - Multiple sclerosis
  - Neoplasms
  - Normal pressure hydrocephalus
  - Parkinson disease
  - Seizure
- Endocrine:
  - Addison disease
  - Cushing disease
  - Thyroid dysfunction
  - Parathyroid dysfunction
  - Postpartum psychosis
  - Recurrent menstrual psychosis
  - Sydenham chorea
- Metabolic:
  - Intoxication or withdrawal
  - Hypercarbia
  - Hypoglycemia
  - Hypoxia
  - Porphyria
  - Electrolyte imbalance
- Nutritional deficiencies:
  - Niacin
  - Thiamine
  - Vitamin $B_{12}$ and folate
- Organ failure:
  - Hepatic encephalopathy
  - Renal failure

#### Pharmacologic
- Psychoactive agents
- Benzodiazepines
- Chlordiazepoxide
- Antidepressants
- Antiepileptics
- Antibiotics:
  - Isoniazid
  - Rifampin
- Cardiovascular agents:
  - Captopril
  - Digoxin
  - Methyldopa
  - Procainamide
  - Propranolol
  - Reserpine
- Drugs of abuse:
  - Alcohol
  - Amphetamines
  - Cocaine
  - Opioids
  - Hallucinogens
- Other:
  - Steroids
  - Heavy metals
  - Antihistamines
  - Cimetidine
  - Disulfiram

#### Functional
- Brief psychotic disorder:
  - Usually secondary to acute emotional stress
- Schizophreniform disorder:
  - Symptoms present 1–6 mo
- Schizophrenia
- Mood disorder with psychotic features or schizo-affective disorder

## DIAGNOSIS

### SIGNS AND SYMPTOMS
- Delusions are erroneous beliefs that:
  - Involve a misinterpretation of perceptions
  - Are clearly implausible
  - Are often persecutory, religious, or somatic in nature
- Hallucinations:
  - Sensory experiences that exist only in the mind of the patient
  - Can involve any sense; auditory and visual are most common.

- Disorganized speech:
  - Loose associations
  - Neologisms
  - Perseverations
  - Poverty of content
  - Word salad
- Disorganized or catatonic behavior:
  - Unable to perform goal-directed behavior
  - Unaware of the environment
- Negative symptoms:
  - Flattened affect
  - Poverty of speech
  - Avolition:
    - Unable to maintain goal-directed activities
- Features suggesting an organic etiology:
  - Sudden onset
  - >40 years old
  - Fluctuating course
  - Confusion
  - Headaches
  - Loss of consciousness
  - Focal neurologic symptoms
  - Speech difficulties
  - Abnormal vital signs
  - Disorientation
  - Psychomotor retardation
  - Visual hallucinations
  - Global impairment of attention and cognitive function
  - Delusions are disorganized
  - Labile affect
  - Incoherent speech
  - Social immodesty

### History
- Speed of onset
- Hallucinations
- Suicidal behavior or homicidal threats
- Social situation and ability to care for self
- Past medical and psychiatric history
- Recent increase or cessation of recreational drugs or alcohol
- Medications

### Physical Exam
Look for signs of organic disease:
- Vital signs
- Eye exam:
  - Pupils, EOM, fundi
- General exam with particular attention to the signs and symptoms of endocrine, liver, and renal disease
- Neurologic exam
- Careful assessment for signs of delirium

## ESSENTIAL WORKUP

- The workup is case-specific and primarily based on the suspected etiology.
- Functional and organic etiologies are generally distinguished by features of the history and physical exam described below.
- Collateral history is important, as the patient history is often unreliable.
- Complete physical exam with particular attention to the neurologic exam, vital signs, and mental status exam
- Mental status exam:
  – Orientation
  – Memory (short- and long-term)
  – Attention (or calculation)
  – Recall
  – Language
  – Thoughts
  – Perception
  – Mood/affect
  – Judgment

## DIAGNOSTIC TESTS & INTERPRETATION

### Lab
Laboratory evaluation is needed in patients at risk for an organic etiology:

- Routine "screening labs" not helpful
- Specific studies should be guided by the suspected underlying etiologies.
- Serum glucose
- Toxicologic screen
- Serum electrolytes
- Urinalysis

### Imaging
Head CT scan is indicated in patients at risk for a neurologic etiology.

### Diagnostic Procedures/Surgery
Lumbar puncture is indicated if signs and symptoms suggest delirium.

## DIFFERENTIAL DIAGNOSIS
See "Etiology."

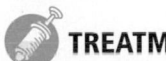 TREATMENT

## PRE-HOSPITAL

- Prevention of violent behavior must be established before transport.
- Consider police backup to reduce risk of violence and to place restraints.
- Controversies:
  – Chemical restraints are rare in field protocols.
  – May be a beneficial adjunct to physical restraints

## INITIAL STABILIZATION/THERAPY
Prevention of violence

## ED TREATMENT/PROCEDURES

- Antipsychotic agents are symptom-specific and therefore useful in both organic or functional psychoses.
- High-potency, IV antipsychotics, such as haloperidol, are most commonly utilized in the ED setting.
- Rapid tranquilization may be achieved with the addition of a benzodiazepine.
- If a specific organic etiology is identified, therapy should be directed toward the treatment of the medical condition.
- Treatment of adverse effects from antipsychotic medications:
  – Extrapyramidal symptoms, dystonia, akathisia, pseudoparkinsonism, and tardive dyskinesia:
    ○ Treat with diphenhydramine or benztropine.
  – Neuroleptic malignant syndrome is a life-threatening complication:
    ○ Characterized by hyperthermia, muscle rigidity, autonomic instability, and altered consciousness
    ○ Treat with supportive measures and dantrolene.
    ○ Droperidol has been reported to cause QT prolongation and dysrhythmias.

## MEDICATION

- Antipsychotics:
  – Droperidol: 2.5–5.0 mg IV or IM
  – Haloperidol: 2–5 mg IV or IM or PO; 0.5–2.0 mg for elderly
  – Risperidone: 1–2 mg PO
- Benzodiazepines:
  – Lorazepam 1.0–2.0 mg IV or IM or PO
- Treatment of medication side effects:
  – Benztropine: 2 mg IM or IV
  – Dantrolene: 1 mg/kg IV repeated to symptom resolution or total of 10 mg/kg
  – Diphenhydramine: 50 mg IV, IM, or PO

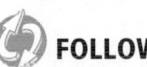 FOLLOW-UP

## DISPOSITION

### Admission Criteria

- If the cause is determined to be medical in origin, admission to the appropriate medical service is indicated.
- Acute psychosis of psychiatric etiology requires admission to a psychiatric service.
- Safety of staff and patient must be maintained in the hospital after disposition from the ED, including possible chemical and physical restraint or a 1-on-1 sitter.

- If the patient is felt to be a danger to either self or others, the patient cannot be discharged.
- Involuntary commitment is required if patient is uncooperative and a threat to self or others.

### Discharge Criteria
If the psychotic behavior was caused by a temporary, reversible organic cause (eg, drug intoxication) and the patient is now deemed to be in control, competent, and not a danger to self or others, the patient may be discharged.

### Issues for Referral
Psychiatric consultation prior to discharge is recommended.

## FOLLOW-UP RECOMMENDATIONS

- When patients with psychiatric disorders do not need to be admitted, plan outpatient management in conjunction with psychiatry.
- Consider referral for detoxification in patients with underlying addiction and problems related to substance abuse.

## PEARLS AND PITFALLS

Assuming that psychosis is psychiatric and not recognizing treatable organic causes is a pitfall.

## ADDITIONAL READING

- Lukens TW, Wolf SJ, Edlow JA, et al. Clinical policy: Critical issues in the diagnosis and management of the adult psychiatric patient in the emergency department. *Ann Emerg Med.* 2006;47(1):79–99.
- Mathias M, Lubman DI, Hides L. Substance-induced psychosis: A diagnostic conundrum. *J Clin Psychiatry.* 2008;69:358–367.
- Richards CF, Gun DE. Psychosis. *Emerg Med Clin North Am.* 2000;18:253–262.

### See Also (Topic, Algorithm, Electronic Media Element)
Violence, Management of

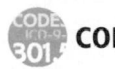 CODES

### ICD9
298.9 Unspecified psychosis

# PSYCHOSIS, MEDICAL VS. PSYCHIATRIC

Kelly E. Irwin
Felicia A. Smith
Kathy M. Sanders

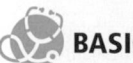 **BASICS**

## DESCRIPTION
- The symptoms of psychosis are listed under Signs and Symptoms.
- A patient with psychotic symptoms does not always have a primary psychiatric disorder.
- A wide variety of medical and neurologic illnesses can present with psychosis at diagnosis or later in the course of the illness.
- It can be difficult to determine whether medical or psychiatric illness is the cause of psychotic behavior.
- Evaluation for underlying medical or neurologic condition is essential, particularly for patients without previous history of psychosis.

## ETIOLOGY
- CNS impairment leading to a psychotic presentation may be due to:
  - Neurological disorders
  - Metabolic conditions
  - Toxins or drug effects
  - Infections
  - Primary psychiatric disorders
- Age factors:
  - Late adolescence/early adulthood presentation more likely to be primary psychiatric etiology
  - Middle- to late-life presentation raises suspicion for a medical cause such as dementia or delirium.

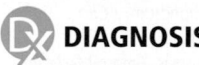 **DIAGNOSIS**

## SIGNS AND SYMPTOMS
- Psychosis characterized by:
  - Impaired reality testing
  - Inappropriate affect
  - Poor impulse control
- Focal and diffuse CNS impairment may result in derangements of:
  - Perception
  - Thought content
  - Thought process
- Hallucinations:
  - Sensory perceptions without external source
  - Auditory, visual, olfactory, tactile
- Delusions:
  - False beliefs held strongly by patient even in face of reasonable evidence to the contrary
- Thought disorder:
  - Disorganized thinking
  - Inability to communicate one's internal experience
- Affective symptoms may include mania, depression, or catatonia.

## History
- Time course: Acute, episodic, chronic
- Collateral from family or outpatient providers
- Substance use
- Medications and medication adherence
- Family history

## Physical Exam
- Vital signs
- Neurologic exam:
  - Cognitive exam: Attention and orientation
  - Motor exam: Tone, abnormal movements

## ESSENTIAL WORKUP
- Detailed history and physical, including neurologic exam
- Use history and physical to guide further workup, including labs and imaging.

## DIAGNOSTIC TESTS & INTERPRETATION
### Lab
- First line:
  - CBC
  - Electrolytes including calcium, BUN/creatinine, glucose
  - Urine and serum toxicology screen
  - Urinalysis
  - Liver function tests
  - Thyroid function tests
  - Vitamin $B_{12}$ and folate
- Second line guided by history and physical findings:
  - Ammonia level
  - HIV testing
  - Fluorescent treponemal antibody-absorption (to rule out neurosyphilis; rapid plasmin reagin not sufficient as screen)
  - Ceruloplasmin
  - Urine heavy metals
  - ESR, C-reactive protein, antinuclear antibody

### Imaging
- Overall yield low without focal neurologic deficits but recommended for 1st episode or atypical presentation
- MRI brain preferred over CT as screen for 1st episode psychosis; higher yield for potentially clinically meaningful lesions:
  - White matter changes
  - Mesial temporal sclerosis
  - Tumors or developmental anomalies

### Diagnostic Procedures/Surgery
- EKG with attention to corrected QT interval, given link between antipsychotics and increased risk for sudden cardiac death
- Not recommended as routine screens:
  - Lumbar puncture/CSF analysis
  - EEG: Past seizure, stereotyped episodes, episodic loss of consciousness, history of serious brain injury, suspicion of narcolepsy, delirium

## DIFFERENTIAL DIAGNOSIS
- Neurologic:
  - Head trauma
  - Space-occupying lesion/structural brain abnormality
  - Cerebrovascular disease
  - Postanoxic encephalopathy
  - Seizure disorders
- Degenerative diseases:
  - Alzheimer disease
  - Pick disease
  - Huntington disease
  - Parkinson disease
  - Wilson disease
- Infectious:
  - HIV
  - Neurosyphilis
  - Viral encephalitis:
    - Herpetiform: Herpes simplex virus, varicella zoster virus; cytomegalovirus, Epstein-Barr virus, rubella
    - Measles (subacute sclerosing panencephalitis), mumps, rabies, influenza
  - Lyme disease: Neuroborreliosis
  - Parasites:
    - Cerebral malaria
    - Neurocysticercosis
    - Schistosomiasis
    - Toxoplasmosis
    - Trypanosomiasis
  - Systemic infection:
    - Delirium due to other infection (eg, urinary tract infection, pneumonia, peritonitis)
    - Sepsis
    - Hepatitis
    - Mononucleosis
- Endocrine:
  - Thyroid disorders
  - Parathyroid disorders
  - Diabetes mellitus
  - Pituitary abnormalities
  - Adrenal abnormalities
- Metabolic:
  - Electrolyte imbalance
  - Hypoglycemia
  - Inborn errors of metabolism
  - Porphyria
- End-organ failure:
  - Cardiac/respiratory
  - Renal
  - Hepatic
  - Pancreatic
- Deficiency diseases:
  - Pernicious anemia
  - Beriberi, Wernicke-Korsakoff syndrome
  - Pellagra
  - Pyridoxine deficiency
- Demyelinating disease:
  - Multiple sclerosis
  - Leukodystrophies
- Autoimmune disorders:
  - Systemic lupus erythematosus
  - Sarcoidosis
  - Myasthenia gravis
  - Paraneoplastic syndromes
- Postoperative states:
  - Delirium
- Chromosomal abnormalities

- Intoxicants:
  – Alcohol
  – Benzodiazepines
  – Barbiturates
  – Stimulants (cocaine, amphetamines)
  – Hallucinogens
  – Opiates
  – Anticholinergic compounds
  – Inhalants
  – Cannabis
- Withdrawal states:
  – Alcohol withdrawal (delirium tremens)
  – Benzodiazepine withdrawal
  – Barbiturate withdrawal
  – Baclofen withdrawal
- Toxins:
  – Bromide
  – Carbon monoxide
  – Heavy metals
  – Organic phosphates
- Medication side effects:
  – Corticosteroids
  – Anticholinergics
  – Sedative–hypnotics
- Psychiatric:
  – Antidepressants
  – Antipsychotics
  – Lithium carbonate
- Antiparkinsonian drugs
- Anticonvulsants
- Antibiotics (quinolones, isoniazid)
- Antihypertensive agents
- Cardiac (digitalis, lidocaine, propranolol, procainamide)
- Interferon
- Muscle relaxants
- Over the counter medications:
  – Pseudoephedrine
  – Antihistamines
- Idiosyncratic drug reaction of any medication
- Psychiatric:
  – Schizophrenia
  – Schizoaffective disorder
  – Delusional disorder
  – Bipolar disorder with psychotic features
  – Major depression with psychotic features
  – Stress reactions including posttraumatic stress disorder
  – Narcolepsy (hallucinations at edge of sleep/wake cycle)
  – Postpartum psychosis

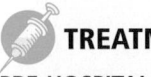

# TREATMENT

## PRE-HOSPITAL
- Ensure safety of patient, bystanders, and medical personnel.
- Know local laws regarding involuntary hospitalization.
- Monitor vital signs, check finger stick.

## INITIAL STABILIZATION/THERAPY
ABCs of psychiatric assessment:
- Safety
- Evaluation
- Management:
  – If uncooperative and dangerous, control behavior with neuroleptics and/or benzodiazepines.
  – Consider need for physical restraint, prioritizing safety and using least restrictive means necessary.

## ED TREATMENT/PROCEDURES
- Determine if medical cause for psychosis.
- Treat underlying medical illness or substance abuse disorder.
- Psychiatric consultation for psychiatric etiology or assistance with management
- Control psychotic behavior with psychotropic medications:
  – Treatment approach based on severity of psychotic features
  – Severe behavioral disturbance of medical psychosis requires sedation to complete medical workup and treatment.
- Haloperidol in combination with lorazepam:
  – Safe, fast; least disruptive of ongoing medical exam of patient
  – Effectively calms and sedates behaviorally agitated, psychotic medical patient
- If medically unstable and sedation not necessary, consider IV Haldol alone.
- Atypical neuroleptics:
  – Few extrapyramidal side effects
  – Olanzapine and ziprasidone can be given IM
  – Olanzapine (Zydis) and Risperdal M-tab are available in dissolving wafer preparations.
  – Avoid IM lorazepam with IM olanzapine due to risk of respiratory depression.

## MEDICATION
### First Line
- Haloperidol 2–10 mg IM or IV with lorazepam 0.5–2 mg IM or IV
- If using IM preparation, consider addition of anticholinergic agent (eg, diphenhydramine 25–50 mg) to prevent dystonic reaction (avoid anticholinergic agent in elderly and delirious patients).

### Second Line
- Neuroleptics:
  – Olanzapine: 5–10 mg PO, SL, or IM
  – Risperidone: 1–2 mg PO or SL
  – Quetiapine: 25–100 mg PO
- Benzodiazepines:
  – Diazepam: 5–10 mg IV

### Geriatric Considerations
- Increased mortality risk in patients >65 yr on typical and atypical antipsychotics; therefore assess risk and benefit, particularly before discharging a patient on an antipsychotic
- Start with lower doses (Haldol 2 mg IV), Zyprexa 2.5–5 mg PO, SL, or IM).
- Use benzodiazepines cautiously, given risk of disinhibition; avoid in delirious patients.

### Pregnancy Considerations
Best evidence of safety of antipsychotic use in pregnancy is for 1st-generation (typical) antipsychotics such as haloperidol.

 # FOLLOW-UP

## DISPOSITION
### Admission Criteria
- If primarily medical etiology, admission to medical service, criteria dictated by specific medical condition
- If primarily psychiatric etiology (eg, schizophrenia), admit to psychiatric service if:
  – Danger to self or others

- – Inability to care for self
- – Deranged thought pattern that can be threat to self or others
- – 1st episode: Evaluation and stabilization
- – Laws for involuntary hospitalization vary by state.

### Discharge Criteria
- Stable medical condition
- Not suicidal/homicidal
- Able to care for self
- Capable of making medical decisions

### Issues for Referral
- Insurance coverage determines inpatient and outpatient psychiatric disposition options.
- Case management or social services necessary for psychiatric disposition.

## FOLLOW-UP RECOMMENDATIONS
- If psychosis is primarily psychiatric, confirm follow-up appointment with mental health provider within 1–2 wk.
- Reassess risk/benefit of continuing on antipsychotic medication at follow-up.

# PEARLS AND PITFALLS

- Patients with psychosis may not be able to explain their symptoms in a typical way. Get collateral and maintain a high degree of suspicion.
- Important to rule out medical and neurologic factors prior to ascribing psychosis to a primary psychotic disorder.
- Age matters: Elderly patients without previous history are more likely to have psychosis due to medical or neurologic illness.

# ADDITIONAL READING

- Freudenreich O, Schulz SC, Goff DC. Initial work-up of a first-episode psychosis: A conceptual review. *Early Interv Psychiatry*. 2009;3:10–18.
- Psychotic patients. In: Stern TA, Fricchione GL, Cassem NH, et al., eds. *MGH Handbook of General Hospital Psychiatry*. St. Louis: Mosby, 2004: 155–174.
- Ray WA, Chung CP, Murray KT, et al. Atypical antipsychotics and the risk of sudden cardiac death. *N Engl J Med*. 2009;360(3):225–235.
- Wang PS, Schneeweiss S, Avorn J, et al. Risk of death in elderly users of conventional vs. atypical antipsychotic medications. *N Engl J Med*. 2005; 353(22):2335–2341.

## See Also (Topic, Algorithm, Electronic Media Element)
- Agitation, Management of
- Psychosis, Acute
- Schizophrenia

 # CODES

### ICD9
- 294.9 Unspecified persistent mental disorders due to conditions classified elsewhere
- 298.9 Unspecified psychosis

# PULMONARY CONTUSION
*Nicholas C. Mosely*

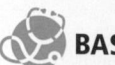 **BASICS**

## DESCRIPTION
- Transfer of kinetic energy to the lung, causing direct damage to the lung parenchyma, resulting in both hemorrhage and edema in the absence of a pulmonary laceration
- Mortality rate is 10–25%.
- Independent risk factor for:
  - Acute respiratory distress syndrome
  - Pneumonia
  - Long-term respiratory dysfunction

## PATHOPHYSIOLOGY
- Development of pulmonary contusion:
  - Takes place in two stages:
    ○ First stage, which is related to the direct injury, results in disruption of the alveolocapillary membrane, which leads to extravasation of blood into the interstitial and alveolar space.
    ○ Second stage is related to the indirect worsening of the injury as a result of measures that occur during the resuscitation of the patient, in particular administration of IV fluids.
- Leads to:
  - Increased intrapulmonary shunting
  - Increased resistance to airflow
  - Decreased lung compliance
  - Increased respiratory work
  - Hypoxemia and acidosis
  - Respiratory failure

## ETIOLOGY
- Blunt or penetrating thoracic trauma
- Sudden deceleration-compression
- Fall from height
- Motor vehicle accident
- Assault
- Missile

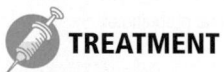 **DIAGNOSIS**

## SIGNS AND SYMPTOMS
### History
- Blunt or penetrating thoracic trauma by any mechanism
- Mechanism as described by patient, family or emergency medical services personnel:
  - Seat belt use
  - Steering wheel damage
  - Air bag deployment
- Chest pain
- Dyspnea
- Hemoptysis

### Physical Exam
- Auscultation:
  - Initially normal or diminished breath sounds
  - Progresses to crackles, rales, absent breath sounds
- Localized ecchymosis, edema, erythema, and tenderness of chest wall
- Bony deformities, crepitus, point tenderness associated with rib fractures
- Ecchymosis from seat belt, aka "seat belt sign"
- Ecchymosis from steering wheel impact
- Splinting respirations
- Cyanosis, tachycardia, hypotension
- Dyspnea, tachypnea

### ALERT
Insidious onset increasing 6–12 hr post injury

## ESSENTIAL WORKUP
CXR:
- Radiographic findings may not appear until 6–12 hr post injury.
- Patchy alveolar infiltrates to frank consolidation.
- Associated intrathoracic injury:
  - Rib fractures
  - Pneumothorax, hemothorax
  - Widened mediastinal silhouette

## DIAGNOSTIC TESTS & INTERPRETATION
### Lab
Arterial blood gas may reveal hypoxemia and elevated alveolar-arterial gradient.

### Imaging
- Chest radiograph:
  - Percentage of contusion can help predict the need for intubation:
    ○ <18%: Usually will not need intubation
    ○ >28%: Usually leads to intubation
- Thoracic CT is useful in detecting pulmonary injury and associated intrathoracic injuries not identified on CXR:
  - Studies have shown injury size on CT can also assist with prognosis.
  - >20% of the total lung volume is predictive of the need of assisted ventilation.
- US has been studied and could prove to be a fast, sensitive method for diagnosing pulmonary contusion.

## DIFFERENTIAL DIAGNOSIS
- Adult respiratory distress syndrome
- CHF
- Hemothorax
- Noncardiogenic causes of pulmonary edema
- Pneumonia, abscess, or other infectious process
- Pneumothorax
- Pulmonary laceration, infarction, or embolism

**TREATMENT**

## PRE-HOSPITAL
Thoracic trauma with significant mechanism or pre-existing pulmonary disease should be routed to the nearest available trauma center.

## INITIAL STABILIZATION/THERAPY
- Manage airway and resuscitate as indicated.
- IV line, O₂, continuous cardiac monitoring, and pulse oximetry

- Control airway:
  - Endotracheal intubation indications:
    - Severe hypoxemia (PaO$_2$ <60 mm Hg on room air, <80 mm Hg on O$_2$)
    - Significant underlying lung disease
    - Impending respiratory failure
  - Early intubation and institution of positive end expiratory pressure:
    - Correct hypoxemia and acidosis.
    - Decrease the work of breathing.

## ED TREATMENT/PROCEDURES

- Maintain adequate oxygenation and ventilation.
- Monitor O$_2$ saturation and respiratory rate.
- In conscious and alert patient, O$_2$ administration via face mask is first-line therapy.
- If patient cannot maintain a PaO$_2$ >80 mm Hg on high-flow oxygen:
  - Continuous positive airway pressure via mask
  - Nasal bilevel positive airway pressure (BiPAP)
- If adequate oxygenation cannot be maintained with face mask:
  - Continuous positive airway pressure (CPAP)
  - BiPAP
  - Early endotracheal intubation and mechanical ventilation

### ALERT

- Avoid excessive fluid administration:
  - IV crystalloid administration needed for resuscitation must be balanced with the risk of increasing interstitial pulmonary edema.
- Frequent reexamination and serial chest radiographs are required to monitor alveolar fluid accumulation.
- Mental status must be appropriate and patient must be alert and cooperative for BiPAP/CPAP:
  - Often this is only a temporizing intervention and should not delay intubation in worsening patients.

### MEDICATION

- Adequate pain control is key for optimal outcome.
- Steroids have no proven benefit.
- Prophylactic antibiotics are not indicated.

### Pediatric Considerations
Increased pliability of the chest wall increases the frequency of pulmonary contusions.

### Geriatric Considerations

- Suboptimal cardiopulmonary reserve in combination with large-volume fluid resuscitation increases the likelihood of worsening of pulmonary contusions in the elderly.
- Pulmonary contusion has been identified as a marker for bad outcomes in elderly patients with isolated blunt chest trauma.

 **FOLLOW-UP**

## DISPOSITION

### Admission Criteria
Patients with pulmonary contusion must be admitted to the hospital for observation in anticipation of delayed-onset respiratory compromise.

### Discharge Criteria

- Patients with minimal chest trauma
- No evidence of respiratory distress or hypoxemia:
  - Normal respiratory rate
  - Reassuring pulse oximetry
  - Negative chest radiograph
- Strict return criteria should be discussed with the patient prior to discharge:
  - Shortness of breath
  - Hemoptysis
  - Inadequate pain control or increased pain
  - Cough

## PEARLS AND PITFALLS

- Avoid underestimating the severity of pulmonary injury based on initial chest x-ray.
- Failure to recognize this injury in the ED can lead to unexpected deterioration.
- Comorbid conditions such as chronic lung disease and renal failure increase the likelihood of requiring mechanical ventilation.
- Careful monitoring and reassessment is key.

## ADDITIONAL READING

- Buchman TG, Bruce HL, Bowling WM, et al. Thoracic trauma. In: Tintinalli JE, Kelen GD, Stapczynski JS, eds. *Emergency Medicine: A Comprehensive Study Guide*, 6th ed. New York: McGraw-Hill; 2004.
- Eckstein M, Henderson S. Thoracic trauma. In: Marx J, Hockberger R, Walls R, eds. *Rosen's Emergency Medicine: Concepts and Clinical Practice*, 6th ed. St. Louis, MO: Mosby; 2006:453.
- Hamrick MC, Duhn RD, Ochsner MG. Critical evaluation of pulmonary contusion in the early post-traumatic period: Risk of assisted ventilation. *Am Surg*. 2009;75(11):1054–1058.
- Lotfipour S, Kaku SK, Vaca FE, et al. Factors associated with complications in older adults with isolated blunt chest trauma. *West J Emerg Med*. 2009;10:79–84.
- Schmittenbecher P. Lung contusion-lacerations after blunt thoracic trauma in children. *J Pediatr Surg*. 2005;40(5):892.
- Wanek S, Mayberry JC. Blunt thoracic trauma: Flail chest, pulmonary contusion, and blast injury. *Crit Care Clin*. 2004;20(1):71–81.

### See Also (Topic, Algorithm, Electronic Media Element)

- Dyspnea
- Chest Trauma, Blunt
- Flail Chest
- Trauma, Multiple

*The author gratefully acknowledges Gregory W. Lampe for his work on the previous edition of this chapter.*

 **CODES**

ICD9
861.21 Contusion of lung without open wound into thorax

# PULMONARY EDEMA

Shamai A. Grossman
Leon Adelman

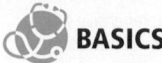 **BASICS**

## DESCRIPTION
- Pathophysiology: Imbalance in Starling forces causes an accumulation of alveolar fluid secondary to leakage from pulmonary capillaries into the interstitium and alveoli of the lung, leading to oxygen desaturation and respiratory distress.
- Cardiogenic (also called acute heart failure syndromes [AHF]): Abnormality in cardiac function leading to inadequate tissue perfusion:
  - Acute decompensated cardiac failure: Acute fluid overload in the setting of chronic HF
  - Acute vascular failure: Decreased contractility and increased vascular resistance
- Noncardiogenic: Diffuse alveolar damage, increased alveolar-capillary membrane permeability, and accumulation of fluid in the alveoli without cardiac etiology:
  - Acute lung injury: Lower severity
  - Acute respiratory distress syndrome (ARDS): $PaO_2/FiO_2$ ratio of $\leq$200 mm Hg
- New York Heart Association classification of congestive heart failure (CHF):
  - Class I: Not limited in normal physical activity by symptoms
  - Class II: Ordinary physical activity results in fatigue, dyspnea, or other symptoms
  - Class III: Marked limitation in normal activity
  - Class IV: Symptoms at rest or with any activity
- Epidemiology:
  - CHF prevalence: 5.2 million patients in the U.S.
  - Incidence of HF increases with increasing age and affects 10% of population >75 yr.
  - 30–40% of patients with HF are hospitalized every year.
  - 11% 1-mo mortality after AHF admission

## ETIOLOGY
- Cardiogenic etiologies:
  - Contractile dysfunction:
    - Ischemic heart disease
    - Idiopathic cardiomyopathy
    - Myocarditis
  - Systolic pressure overload:
    - Aortic stenosis
    - Systemic hypertension
  - Systolic volume overload:
    - Aortic regurgitation
    - Mitral regurgitation
  - Restricted diastolic filling:
    - Mitral stenosis
    - Left atrial myxoma
    - Hypertrophic cardiomyopathy
  - High-output states:
    - Hyperthyroidism
    - Anemia
    - Arteriovenous fistula
    - Wet beriberi
  - Congenital heart disease
  - Endocarditis
  - Rheumatic heart disease

- Noncardiogenic etiologies:
  - Sepsis
  - Acute pulmonary infection, aspiration
  - Inhalation injuries
  - Aspiration
  - Near drowning
  - Disseminated intravascular coagulation
  - Pancreatitis
  - Pulmonary contusion
  - Severe (nonthoracic) trauma
  - Cardiopulmonary bypass
  - Uremia
  - High-altitude pulmonary edema
  - Neurogenic pulmonary edema
  - Narcotic overdose
  - Salicylate overdose
  - Pulmonary embolism
  - Fat embolism
  - Transfusion-related acute lung injury

 **DIAGNOSIS**

## SIGNS AND SYMPTOMS
### History
- Risk factors:
  - CHF diagnosis
  - History of coronary artery disease or myocardial infarction
  - Diabetes
  - Severe systemic illness
- Symptoms:
  - Dyspnea on exertion progressing to dyspnea at rest
  - Orthopnea
  - Peripheral edema
  - Paroxysmal nocturnal dyspnea
  - Acute weight gain
  - Weakness/fatigue
  - Cough

### Physical Exam
- Vitals:
  - May be hypertensive or hypotensive, depending on the balance of cardiac function, vascular constriction and fluid status
  - Tachypnea
  - Low oxygen saturation
- General:
  - Diaphoresis
  - Cold, ashen, or cyanotic skin
- Respiratory:
  - Rales
  - Wheezes
- Cardiovascular:
  - Tachycardia
  - Jugular venous distention
  - Abnormal heart sounds: Increased P2, S3, S4
  - Hepatojugular reflex
- Extremities: Peripheral edema
- Noncardiogenic pulmonary edema presents with similar pulmonary signs as AHF, but rarely exhibits the peripheral signs of AHF.

## ESSENTIAL WORKUP
- An ECG is required to evaluate for cardiac ischemia and arrhythmias.
- The chest radiograph is essential in confirming the diagnosis and assessing illness severity.
- Labs such as B-type natriuretic peptide (BNP), cardiac enzymes, and creatinine should be used to establish the diagnosis, identify underlying triggers, and assess for complications.

## DIAGNOSTIC TESTS & INTERPRETATION
### Lab
- BNP:
  - A proteohormone secreted by the left ventricle in response to wall tension
  - Laboratory parameter for the detection and follow-up of heart failure:
    - <100 pg/mL: CHF unlikely
    - 100–500 pg/mL: Indeterminate
    - >500 pg/mL: Most consistent with CHF
  - Helpful in determining whether dyspnea is secondary to chronic obstructive pulmonary disease or AHF
- N-terminal pro-BNP:
  - BNP precursor
  - Similar test characteristics to BNP
- Cardiac troponins:
  - May be elevated due to myocardial ischemia causing AHF or as result of AHF's effects on cardiac myocytes
  - Elevated in 20% of AHF episodes
  - Strong negative prognostic factor
  - Cardiology consult indicated when troponin is elevated in AHF episodes.
- Serum chemistry panel:
  - Creatinine elevation:
    - Predicts all-cause mortality in chronic heart failure
    - Indication of acute end-organ hypoperfusion
    - Indication for admission or observation
  - Hyponatremia: Marker of severe HF
  - Electrolyte abnormalities are common due to various HF treatments.
- Elevated alanine aminotransferase, aspartate aminotransferase, or bilirubin suggests congestive hepatopathy.
- Serum lipase if pancreatitis is suspected as the underlying cause
- Arterial blood gas: Evaluates hypoxemia, ventilation/perfusion mismatch, hypercapnia, and acidosis.

### Imaging
- CXR:
  - Pulmonary redistribution: Cephalization of vessels
  - Cardiomegaly: Cardiac silhouette >50% of thoracic width
  - Interstitial edema:
    - Pleural effusions
    - Kerley B lines
  - Alveolar infiltrates: Bilateral perihilar alveolar edema producing a characteristic butterfly pattern

– Noncardiogenic: Bilateral interstitial or alveolar infiltrates in a homogeneous pattern, typically without enlarged heart shadow
– Radiographs are often normal in the 1st 12 hr of the disease process.
- ECG:
  – Assess for underlying cardiac disorders:
    ○ Acute dysrhythmias
    ○ Signs of acute coronary syndromes
    ○ Signs of electrolyte abnormalities
    ○ Atrial fibrillation occurs in 30–42% of patients admitted for acute heart failure.
    ○ Both tachy- and bradyarrhythmias can lead to decreased cardiac output.
- Echocardiography:
  – Evaluates left ventricle function
  – Assesses acute valvular or pericardial pathology
  – Measures cardiac output

## DIFFERENTIAL DIAGNOSIS
- COPD exacerbation
- Pneumonia
- Asthma
- Pulmonary embolism
- Pericardial tamponade
- Pneumothorax
- Pleural effusion
- Anaphylaxis
- Acidosis
- Hyperventilation syndrome

 **TREATMENT**

### PRE-HOSPITAL
- IV access
- Supplemental oxygen
- 100% nonrebreather mask
- Cardiac monitor
- Pulse oximetry
- Sublingual nitrates
- Endotracheal intubation may be required in severe cases.

### INITIAL STABILIZATION/THERAPY
- Assess and gain control of airway, breathing, and circulation.
- Control airway as needed: Noninvasive ventilation or endotracheal intubation for impending respiratory failure.
- IV access
- Supplemental oxygen
- Cardiac monitor
- Pulse oximetry
- Place patient in an upright position.
- Inotropic therapy for hypotensive patient with signs of end-organ dysfunction

### ED TREATMENT/PROCEDURES
- Treatment decisions should be based on the underlying cause of pulmonary edema.
- Supplemental O$_2$
- Volume restriction
- Bilevel positive airway pressure (BiPAP)/continuous positive airway pressure (CPAP):

– Improve oxygenation, reduce respiratory work, decrease left ventricular afterload
– Reduce need for intubation, length of stay, and mortality
– Efficacy of BiPAP = CPAP
- Endotracheal intubation for impending respiratory failure
- Noncardiogenic causes: Frequently require positive-pressure ventilation:
  – Low-volume ventilation recommended (6 mL/kg)
- Positive end-expiratory pressure: Most useful strategy for oxygenation
- Hypotensive patients:
  – Avoid nitrates, angiotensin-converting-enzyme inhibitors (ACEIs), and morphine.
  – Initiate inotropes:
    ○ Dobutamine
    ○ Dopamine
    ○ Norepinephrine
    ○ Milrinone
- Normotensive or hypertensive patients:
  – Nitrates (nitroglycerin vs. nitroprusside)
  – Diuretics (furosemide vs. bumetanide)
  – ACEIs (captopril vs. enalapril)
- Noncardiogenic: Treat underlying cause.

## MEDICATION
- Goal of treatments: Improve hemodynamics by reducing preload and afterload; increase contractility. First-line and preferred therapy is with nitrates and then diuretics and other agents.
- Aspirin: 325 mg PO/PR if myocardial infarction suspected
- Bumetanide: 1–3 mg IV
- Captopril: 6.25 mg SL   *ACEI*
- Dobutamine: 2–10 mcg/kg/min IV, titrate. May lower blood pressure due to vasodilatory effects.
- Dopamine: 2 × 20 mcg/kg/min IV; titrate
- Enalapril: 0.625–1.25 mg IV
- Furosemide: 20 × 80 mg IV
- Milrinone: 50 mcg/kg IV; titrate; inotropic effects comparable to dobutamine
- Nitroglycerin: 0.4 mg SL; 1–2 inches; 5–20 mcg/min IV and titrate; Nitropaste is not preferred as it is more difficult to titrate and to use in diaphoretic patients.
- Nitroprusside: 0.3–10 mcg/kg/min IV; titrate
- Norepinephrine: 2–12 mcg/min IV; titrate

 **FOLLOW-UP**

### DISPOSITION
#### Admission Criteria
- ICU:
  – Positive-pressure ventilation
  – Inotropic support
  – Acute cardiac ischemia or infarction
  – ARDS
- Monitored unit:
  – New-onset pulmonary edema
  – Electrocardiographic changes
  – Patients presenting with risk factors for mortality, including advanced age, renal dysfunction, hypotension, digoxin use, and anemia

#### Discharge Criteria
- Most patients with pulmonary edema should be admitted.
- Patients with mild underlying disease and a mild exacerbation that responds fully to ED management and have no risk factors for in-house mortality (see above) may be discharged.
- Ensure close outpatient follow-up.

### FOLLOW-UP RECOMMENDATIONS
- Contact patient's primary physician and/or cardiologist to establish close follow-up.
- Continue diuresis.
- Low-salt diet
- Daily weights

## PEARLS AND PITFALLS
- Nitrates, SL and IV, are first-line therapy to reduce preload.
- BNP can reliably differentiate between AHF syndromes and other causes of dyspnea.
- AHF chest radiography findings can be absent early in disease course.
- Aggressive, early treatment of normotensive and hypertensive patients with nitrates, diuretics, and ACEIs can rapidly reverse the clinical course.
- Positive-pressure ventilation is an essential intervention in noncardiogenic pulmonary edema and can reduce rates of intubation and mortality in AHF.

## ADDITIONAL READING
- Mattu A, Martinez JP, Kelly BS. Modern management of cardiogenic pulmonary edema. *Emerg Med Clin North Am.* 2005;23:1105–1125.
- Nieminen MS, Bohm M, Cowie MR, et al. Executive summary of the guidelines on the diagnosis and treatment of acute heart failure: The Task Force on Acute Heart Failure of the European Society of Cardiology. *Eur Heart J.* 2005;26:384–416.
- Perina DG. Noncardiogenic pulmonary edema. *Emerg Med Clin North Am.* 2003;21:385–393.
- Wang CS, FitzGerald M, Schulzer M. Does this dyspneic patient in the emergency department have congestive heart failure? *JAMA.* 2005;294:1944–1956.
- Ware, LB, Matthay, MA. Clinical practice. Acute pulmonary edema. *N Engl J Med.* 2005;353:2788–2796.

### See Also (Topic, Algorithm, Electronic Media Element)
Congestive Heart Failure

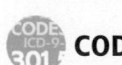 **CODES**

### ICD9
- 428.1 Left heart failure
- 518.4 Acute edema of lung, unspecified

# PULMONARY EMBOLISM
*Alan M. Kumar*

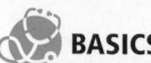 **BASICS**

## DESCRIPTION
- The majority of pulmonary embolisms (PEs) arise from thrombi in the deep veins of the lower extremities and pelvis.
- Thrombi also originate in renal and upper extremity veins.
- After traveling to lungs, the size of the thrombus determines signs and symptoms.

## ETIOLOGY
- Most patients with pulmonary embolism have identifiable risk factor:
  - Recent surgery
  - Pregnancy
  - Previous deep vein thrombosis (DVT)/PE
  - Stroke or recent paraplegia
  - Malignancy
  - Age >50 yr
  - Obesity
  - Smoking
  - Oral contraceptives
  - Major trauma
- Hematologic risk factors:
  - Factor 5 Leiden
  - Protein C or S deficiency
  - Antithrombin III deficiency
  - Antiphospholipid antibody syndrome
  - Lupus anticoagulant

### Pediatric Considerations
- Thromboembolic disease is quite rare.
- Risk factors in children:
  - Presence of central venous catheter
  - Immobility
  - Heart disease
  - Trauma
  - Malignancy
  - Surgery
  - Infection

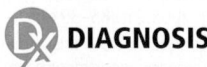 **DIAGNOSIS**

## SIGNS AND SYMPTOMS
- Variability in signs and symptoms make diagnosis difficult
- Most common:
  - Dyspnea
  - Pleuritic chest pain
  - Tachypnea
- General:
  - Fevers (rarely >102.0°F)
  - Diaphoresis
- Pulmonary:
  - Cough
  - Hemoptysis (rarely massive)
  - Rales

- Cardiovascular:
  - Tachycardia
  - Syncope
  - Murmur
- Extremities:
  - Cyanosis
  - Evidence of thrombophlebitis
  - Lower extremity edema
- Abdominal pain
- Symptoms similar in elderly but typically more subtle if age <40 yr

## ESSENTIAL WORKUP
- Routine labs are nonspecific.
- CXR:
  - Used to rule out other causes
  - Most common findings with PE:
    - Normal
    - Nonspecific parenchymal abnormality
    - Atelectasis
  - Other findings with PE:
    - Pleural effusions
    - Pleural-based opacities (Hampton hump)
    - Elevated hemidiaphragm
    - Local oligemia (Westermark sign)
- ECG:
  - To rule out cardiac etiology
  - Usually normal in PE
  - Other findings include:
    - Nonspecific ST-T wave changes (most common abnormality)
    - Sinus tachycardia
    - Left axis deviation
    - Right-bundle-branch-block pattern
    - S1Q3T3 pattern is uncommon and not specific enough to rule in/out diagnosis.
- Modified Wells criteria:
  - Popular decision rule that can assist with risk stratification in combination with D-dimer
  - Each criterion is given numeric value and if total value <4, likelihood of PE in combination with negative D-dimer is ~2%:
    - Clinical signs/symptoms of DVT: 3 pts
    - PE is no. 1 diagnosis: 3 pts
    - Heart rate >100 bpm: 1.5 pts
    - Surgery or Immobilization for 3 days within last 4 wk: 1.5 pts
    - Previous PE or DVT: 1.5 pts
    - Hemoptysis: 1 pt
    - Malignancy with treatment within last 6 mo: 1 pt

## DIAGNOSTIC TESTS & INTERPRETATION
### Lab
- Arterial blood gas:
  - Can show hypoxemia, hypocapnia, respiratory alkalosis, or increased alveolar-arterial (A-a) gradient
  - PE still possible with normal A-a gradient
  - Does not aid in diagnosis of PE
- CBC:
  - Anemia may be contributing factor to dyspnea.
- D-dimer enzyme-linked immunosorbent assay:
  - D-dimers are detectable at levels >500 ng/mL in nearly all patients with PE.
  - High sensitivity (close to 100%) with low specificity for PE
  - Almost always elevated in patients with malignancy or surgery within the last 3 mo
  - Multiple studies confirm that negative enzyme-linked immunosorbent assay D-dimer in combination with low clinical suspicion effectively rules out PE.

### Imaging
- Spiral chest CT with IV contrast:
  - Has ability to also detect alternative pulmonary abnormalities
  - Accurate for identifying PE in proximal pulmonary tree:
    - In patients with high pretest probability, positive predictive value of 96%
    - In patients with low pretest probability, negative predictive value of 96%
- Ventilation-perfusion scan (V/Q):
  - Results reported in probabilities and correlated to clinical suspicion
  - Probability of PE with V/Q results:
    - Normal or near normal V/Q scan: 4% probability for PE
    - Low-probability V/Q scan with low clinical suspicion: 4% probability for PE
    - Low-probability V/Q scan with high clinical suspicion: 16–40% probability for PE
    - Intermediate V/Q scan: 16–66% probability for PE
    - High-probability V/Q scan with low clinical suspicion: 56% probability for PE
    - High-probability V/Q scan with high clinical suspicion: 96% probability for PE

- Lower-extremity duplex US:
  – Used in patients who would otherwise require pulmonary angiogram
  – Presence of DVT requires same anticoagulation as PE.
  – Negative lower extremity duplex does not rule out PE.
- Echocardiogram:
  – Used to assess for right heart strain or patent foramen ovale when thrombolysis is a possibility

### Diagnostic Procedures/Surgery
Pulmonary angiogram:
- Gold standard for diagnosis
- Used when diagnosis not confirmed or excluded
- Higher complication rate than other modalities

### DIFFERENTIAL DIAGNOSIS
- Anxiety disorder
- Aortic dissection
- Asthma
- Cardiac dysrhythmias
- Costochondritis
- Myocardial infarction
- Pericarditis
- Pneumonia
- Pneumothorax
- Rib fracture

 TREATMENT

#### PRE-HOSPITAL
- Initial supplemental oxygen
- Establish IV access
- Cardiac monitor

#### INITIAL STABILIZATION/THERAPY
- Airway, breathing, and circulation
- Provide supplemental oxygen to maintain adequate oxygen saturation.
- Intubate if unable to provide adequate oxygenation.
- Administer IV fluids carefully for hypotensive patients:
  – Excessive fluid expansion may worsen right heart failure.
- IV vasopressor therapy is indicated if hypotension does not resolve with IV fluids.

### ED TREATMENT/PROCEDURES
- Anticoagulation:
  – Prevents additional thrombus from forming
  – Stabilizes existent clot to prevent migration
- Unfractionated heparin:
  – Dose titration fraught with difficulty leading to inadequate therapy
  – Goal to maintain partial thromboplastin time test between 1.5 and 2.5 times the control value (60–80 sec)   *PTT 1.5–2.5*
- Low-molecular-weight heparin:
  – At least as effective as unfractionated heparin in multiple prospective randomized trials
  – Therapeutic goal automatic with weight-based dosing
  – Easier administration and monitoring than heparin with some cost benefit
- Warfarin: *(Coumadin)*
  – Oral therapy for long-term anticoagulation
  – Goal is international normalized ratio (INR) of 2–3   *INR 2–3*
- Thrombolysis:
  – Initiate in hemodynamically unstable patients with confirmed PE.
  – Consider in stable patients with PE and severe hypoxemia, massive PE, or right ventricular dysfunction.
- Inferior vena cava filter:
  – Indicated in patients who have contraindications to anticoagulation or have been therapeutic on anticoagulation but failed prevention of PE
- Surgical or catheter embolectomy:
  – Consider in those with thrombolysis contraindications or failure, or deemed unstable for medical management.
  – Case-by-case basis

### MEDICATION
- Alteplase: 100 mg (peds: N/A) IV over 2 hr
- Enoxaparin: 1 mg/kg (peds: 0.75 mg/kg) SC q12h
- Reteplase: 10 U (peds: N/A) IV bolus q30min ×2
- Streptokinase: 250,000 U (peds: 3,500–4,000 U/kg) IV bolus over 30 min, then 100,000 U (peds: 1,000–1,500 U/kg) IV maintenance over 24 hr
- Unfractionated heparin:
  – Bolus: 80 U/kg (peds: 75 U/kg) IV over 10 min
  – Maintenance: 18 U/kg (peds: 20 U/kg) IV drip
- Warfarin: 5 mg (peds: 0.05–0.34 mg/kg/d) PO per day, adjust for INR goal 2–3

 FOLLOW-UP

#### DISPOSITION
**Admission Criteria**
- Admit all patients with PE for continued anticoagulation and observation.
- Clinically stable patients with a high suspicion for PE, no contraindication to anticoagulation, and a lack of V/Q scanning or angiographic availability may be anticoagulated and studied when resources are available in the morning.

## PEARLS AND PITFALLS
- Clinical presentation is variable and nonspecific, making diagnosis difficult in many cases.
- Patients with malignancy are higher risk for Coumadin failure and recurrent PE even with therapeutic INR.

## ADDITIONAL READING
- Edlow JA, Brown J, eds. Emergency department management of pulmonary embolism. *Emerg Med Clin North Am*. 2001;19:995–1011.
- Goldhaber SZ. Pulmonary embolism. *N Engl J Med*. 1999;339:93–104.
- PIOPED Investigators. Value of the ventilation/perfusion scan in acute pulmonary embolism. *JAMA*. 1990;263:2753–2759.
- Stein P, Fowler S, Goodman LR, et al. Multidetector computed tomography for acute pulmonary embolism. *N Eng J Med*. 2006;354:2317–2327.
- Stein PD, Woodward PK, Weg JG, et al. Diagnostic pathways in acute PE: Recommendations of the PIOPED II investigators. *Am J Med*. 2006;119:1040.
- Wells PS, Anderson DR, Rodger M, et al. Derivation of a simple clinical model to categorize patients' probability of pulmonary embolism: Increasing the model's utility with the SimpliRED D-dimer. *Thromb Haemost*. 2000;83(3):416–420.

### See Also (Topic, Algorithm, Electronic Media Element)
- Chest Pain
- Dyspnea

 CODES

**ICD9**
415.19 Other pulmonary embolism and infarction

# PURPURA

*Richard E. Wolfe*

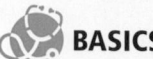 **BASICS**

## DESCRIPTION

- Skin lesions caused by extravasation of blood into the skin or subcutaneous tissue
- Increased fragility of capillaries or dermal support
- The resultant lesions do not blanch completely with pressure (as seen when pressing down through a glass slide).
- Nomenclature varies by the size of the lesions:
  - Petechiae (<2 mm)
  - Purpuric lesions (2–10 mm)
  - Ecchymoses (>10 mm)
- Color determined by depth and time of onset:
  - Red if superficial and of recent onset
  - Purple if deep
  - Deep purple, brown, orange, or blue-green with later presentations
- Nonpalpable purpura:
  - Simple hemorrhage or microvascular occlusion with ischemic hemorrhage
  - Generally due to a platelet disorder:
    ○ Diminished production
    ○ Altered distribution
    ○ Increased destruction
    ○ Abnormal function
- Palpable purpura:
  - Generally due to vasculitis:
    ○ Autoimmune, small-vessel leukocytoclastic vasculitis
    ○ Hypersensitivity to various antigens
    ○ Formation of circulating immune complexes deposited in walls of postcapillary venules; activate complement that is chemotactic for polymorphonuclear leukocytes
    ○ Released enzymes damage vessel walls and cause leakage of blood.
    ○ Vasculitic lesions may not be palpable in immunocompromised patients.

## ETIOLOGY

- Nonpalpable purpura:
  - Viral:
    ○ Echovirus
    ○ Coxsackie
    ○ Measles
    ○ Parvovirus B19
  - Drugs:
    ○ Acetaminophen
    ○ Allopurinol
    ○ Anticoagulants
    ○ Aspirin
    ○ Digoxin
    ○ Furosemide
    ○ Gold salts
    ○ Lidocaine
    ○ Methyldopa
    ○ Penicillin
    ○ Phenylbutazone
    ○ Quinidine
    ○ Quinine

---

    ○ Rifampin
    ○ Steroids
    ○ Sulfonamides
    ○ Thiazides
  - Nutritional deficiencies:
    ○ Vitamin K deficiency
    ○ Scurvy
  - Bone marrow disease
  - Hypersplenism
  - Idiopathic thrombocytopenic purpura (ITP)
  - Disseminated intravascular coagulation (DIC)
  - Thrombotic thrombocytopenic purpura
  - Liver or renal insufficiency
  - Thrombocytosis (>1,000,000 plt/cc spiking elevations of intravascular pressure (childbirth, vomiting, paroxysmal coughing)
  - Hemophilia
  - Solar purpura (limited to sun-exposed areas)
- Palpable purpura:
  - Viral:
    ○ Echovirus type 9
    ○ Coxsackie
    ○ Hepatitis B
  - Streptococcal pharyngitis
  - Drugs:
    ○ Allopurinol
    ○ Aspirin
    ○ Anti-influenza vaccines
    ○ Cephalosporins
    ○ Gold
    ○ Hydralazine
    ○ Iodides
    ○ Metoclopramide
    ○ Nonsteroidal anti-inflammatory drugs
    ○ Penicillin
    ○ Phenylbutazone
    ○ Phenytoin
    ○ Quinidine
    ○ Quinine
    ○ Streptomycin
    ○ Sulfonamides
    ○ Thiazides
    ○ Ticlopidine
  - Malignancies
  - Autoimmune and connective tissue diseases
  - *Gonococcus*
  - *Meningococcus*
  - *Pseudomonas* (ecthyma gangrenosum)
  - Rocky Mountain spotted fever
  - In immunocompromised hosts: *Candida*, *Aspergillus*
  - Occlusion due to organisms living in vessels, generally in immunocompromised patients (mucormycosis, aspergillosis, disseminated strongyloidiasis)
  - Occlusion due to microvascular platelet plugs (heparin necrosis)

---

  - Cold-related gelling or agglutinations (cryoglobulinemia)
  - Local or systemic coagulation abnormalities: Scarlet fever (rarely "strep throat"), *Vibrio vulnificus* bacteremia; "malignant chickenpox" and "black measles" (both rare in U.S.); Coumadin necrosis
  - Embolization: Cholesterol, crystal, thrombus (atrial myxoma, septic endocarditis, multiple myeloma)

### Pediatric Considerations

- Henoch-Schönlein purpura
- Kawasaki disease
- Neonatal:
  - Extramedullary erythropoiesis (blueberry muffin baby)
  - Purpura fulminans (protein C and S deficiency)
  - Maternal ITP
  - Wiskott-Aldrich syndrome

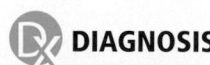 **DIAGNOSIS**

## SIGNS AND SYMPTOMS

- Palpable or nonpalpable nonblanching lesions 0.2–1 cm in diameter:
  - Irregular when caused by infectious emboli
  - Regular lesions with leukocytoclastic emboli
  - Massive bleeding from a platelet disorder may cause palpable hematomas.
- Shape and size:
  - Petechiae (<2 mm)
  - Macular (2–10 mm)
  - Ecchymoses (>10 mm)
  - Annular or erythema multiforme (target lesions)
  - Irregular (retiform)
- Distribution:
  - Generally more frequent in lower extremities (increased hydrostatic force):
    ○ Widespread petechiae and ecchymoses seen with DIC and meningococcemia
    ○ When oral mucous membranes involved, consider idiopathic thrombocytopenic purpura.
- Hypotension
- Altered mental status
- Gingival hemorrhage
- Epistaxis
- Hematuria
- Fever
- Malaise
- Arthralgias
- Myalgias
- Purpura fulminans:
  - Large, irregular ecchymoses
  - Fever
  - Shock
  - DIC

- *Pseudomonas* (ecthyma gangrenosum):
  - Begins as edematous, erythematous papules
  - Bullae formation in girdle region
- Disseminated gonococcal infection:
  - Usually <10 lesions, purpuric papules, or vesicopustules on the extensor surface of hands, dorsal aspect of ankles and toes
  - Fever
  - Arthralgias
- Meningococcemia:
  - Small areas of skin infarction cause purpura in irregular pattern.
  - May involve head, palms, soles, mucous membranes, including conjunctivae
  - Fever
  - Headache
- Rocky Mountain spotted fever:
  - After 4–7 days of generalized symptoms, erythematous macules on distal extremities including palms and soles, then petechial
  - Fever
  - Chills
  - Headache
- Henoch-Schönlein purpura:
  - Appears on extensor aspects of lower extremities and buttocks
  - Fades in ~5 days
  - Fever
  - Arthralgias
  - Abdominal pain
  - Hematuria
- Kawasaki disease:
  - Purpura is rare.
  - Fever, plus 4 of the following: Polymorphous exanthema, peripheral extremity changes, bilateral conjunctivitis, changes of lips and mouth, cervical lymphadenopathy

## ESSENTIAL WORKUP
- Obtain a complete medical history.
- Previous bleeding problems
- Deep venous thrombosis/pulmonary embolism suggesting factor V Leiden mutation
- Splenectomy
- Alcohol abuse
- Family history of bleeding disorders
- High-risk medications

## DIAGNOSTIC TESTS & INTERPRETATION
### Lab
- Platelet count: Abnormal counts must be verified by manual examination of a peripheral smear.
- DIC screen: Indicated when patient appears toxic
- Prothrombin time/partial thromboplastin time
- Rapid strep test
- Urinalysis
- Studies for outpatient management:
  - Bleeding time
  - Hepatitis B and C serologies
  - Strep throat culture or anti–streptolysin O titer
  - Antinuclear antibodies
  - Cryoglobulins
  - Platelet function studies
  - Serum complements
  - Serum protein electrophoresis
  - von Willebrand disease screen

## DIFFERENTIAL DIAGNOSIS
- Disorders with telangiectasias:
  - Cherry angiomas
  - Hereditary hemorrhagic telangiectasia
  - Chronic actinic telangiectasia
  - Scleroderma
  - CREST syndrome
  - Ataxia-telangiectasia
  - Chronic liver disease
  - Pregnancy-related telangiectasia
- Kaposi sarcoma and other vascular sarcomas
- Fabry disease
- Neonatal extramedullary hematopoiesis
- Angioma serpiginosum

 **TREATMENT**

### PRE-HOSPITAL
- IV access
- Monitor for:
  - Fever
  - Hypotension
  - Altered mental status

### ALERT
Take respiratory precautions

### INITIAL STABILIZATION/THERAPY
- For fever, hypotension, altered mental status, or generalized ecchymoses
- Airway support
- IV access
- Fluid resuscitation
- IV antibiotics as soon as possible (ceftriaxone)

### ED TREATMENT/PROCEDURES
- Presumptive treatment of bacterial infection:
  - *Meningococcus*: Ceftriaxone
  - *Pneumococcus*: Ceftriaxone, consider penicillin
- Prophylaxis for meningococcal infection:
  - Rifampin
  - Ciprofloxacin

### MEDICATION
- Adults:
  - Ceftriaxone: 2 g IV q12h
  - Ciprofloxacin (prophylaxis): 500 mg PO single dose
  - Penicillin: 4 million units IV q4h
  - Rifampin (prophylaxis): 600 mg PO q12h for 2 days
- Children:
  - Ceftriaxone: 100 mg/kg/24 hr IV q12h
  - Penicillin: 240,000 U/kg/24 hr IV q4h
  - Neonatal sepsis: Ampicillin 100 mg/kg/24 hr IV q6h *and* gentamicin 7.5 mg/kg/24 hr IV q8h (or cefotaxime 200 mg/kg/24 hr IV q6h)

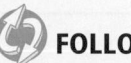 **FOLLOW-UP**

### DISPOSITION
#### Admission Criteria
- Unstable vital signs
- Altered mental status
- Fever

#### Discharge Criteria
Exclusion of life-threatening etiologies:
- Serious bacterial infections
- Critical thrombocytopenia

#### Issues for Referral
Serious hematologic, rheumatologic features and malignancies require an in-depth outpatient assessment if the patient is not admitted.

### FOLLOW-UP RECOMMENDATIONS
- Appropriate close follow-up scheduled
- Consider follow-up with dermatology (skin biopsy) and hematology.

## PEARLS AND PITFALLS

Empiric antibiotics to cover for meningococcemia and Rocky Mountain Spotted fever if any doubt of underlying infection

## ADDITIONAL READING

- Coller BS, Schneiderman PI. Clinical evaluation of hemorrhagic disorders: The bleeding history and differential diagnosis of purpura. In: Hoffman R, Benz EJ Jr, Shattil SJ, et al., eds. *Hematology: Basic Principles and Practice*, 5th ed. New York: Churchill Livingstone; 2008:1975–2000.
- Baselga E. Purpura in infants and children. *J Am Acad Dermatol*. 1997;37:673–705.
- Leung AK, Chan KW. Evaluating the child with purpura. *Am Fam Physician*. 2001;64:419–428.
- Piette WW. Hematologic disorders. In: Freedberg IM, Eisen AZ, Wolff K, et al., eds. *Fitzpatrick's Dermatology in General Medicine*, 5th ed. New York: McGraw Hill; 1999:1867–1881.

### See Also (Topic, Algorithm, Electronic Media Element)
Rash, Pediatric

 **CODES**

#### ICD9
- 287.2 Other nonthrombocytopenic purpuras
- 459.89 Other specified circulatory system disorders
- 782.7 Spontaneous ecchymoses

# PYELONEPHRITIS
*Matthew D. Bitner*

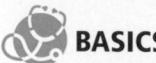 **BASICS**

## DESCRIPTION
- Ascension of bacteria from lower urinary tract infection (UTI) into the upper urinary tract
- Primarily a clinical diagnosis
- Incidence lower in males in every age group
- Male/female ratio:
  - 1:10 in 1st years of life
  - 1:5 in children
  - 1:50 in reproductive years
  - 1:1 in fifth decade and later

## ETIOLOGY
- Bacteriology:
  - *Escherichia coli* 80–95% predominates
  - Uropathogens:
    ○ *Klebsiella* species
    ○ *Citrobacter* species
    ○ *Enterobacter* species
  - Others:
    ○ *Staphylococcus saprophyticus* 5–15%
    ○ *Proteus mirabilis*
    ○ *Serratia* species
    ○ *Pseudomonas* species
    ○ *Staphylococcus aureus* (increasing)
- Predisposing factors:
  - Recent instrumentation:
    ○ Catheterization
    ○ Cystoscopy
  - Urinary retention:
    ○ Mechanical (see Obstruction below)
    ○ Medications (eg, anticholinergics)
    ○ Other infections (eg, herpes simplex)
  - Urinary obstruction:
    ○ Stricture
    ○ Renal calculi
    ○ Prostatic hypertrophy
  - Anatomic abnormalities:
    ○ Hypospadias
    ○ Ureteral ectopia
    ○ Bifid ureter
    ○ Renal scarring
    ○ Ureterovesicular reflux (UVR)
    ○ Posterior urethral valves
  - Neurologic conditions:
    ○ Neurogenic bladder
    ○ Spinal cord injury
  - Abnormal urodynamics
  - Previous UTIs (in childhood, >3 in last year)
  - Recent pyelonephritis (within 1 yr)
  - Diabetes mellitus
  - Immunosuppression
  - Pregnancy

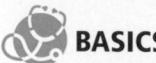 **DIAGNOSIS**

## SIGNS AND SYMPTOMS
- Dysuria, urgency, frequency
- Back, flank, or abdominal pain
- Fever, chills
- Arthralgias, myalgias, malaise
- Nausea and/or vomiting
- Costovertebral angle tenderness or suprapubic tenderness
- Ill/toxic appearing
- Dehydration
- Occult pyelonephritis:
  - Invasion of upper urinary tract without clinical symptoms:
    ○ Suspect in lower UTI that does not resolve with standard treatment.

### Pediatric Considerations
- Fever, irritability, lethargy, poor feeding, or jaundice may be only symptom in infants.
- Enuresis in previously toilet-trained child
- Common cause of a serious bacterial infection (SBI) in neonates, young children, and the immunocompromised (hematogenous spread)
- Renal scarring:
  - More common sequelae in young children than in adults
- Group B streptococci
- Etiologic agents in neonates

### Geriatric Considerations
May present atypically:
- Absence of classic dysuria/frequency
- Instead of nausea/vomiting, diarrhea, fever, or altered mental status may predominate.

## ESSENTIAL WORKUP
- Urinalysis:
  - Clean-catch or catheterized urine specimen; catheterized specimen if:
    ○ Vaginal discharge or bleeding
    ○ Contaminated specimen
  - Pyuria: 5–10 WBCs, plus leukocyte esterase, plus nitrites:
    ○ If not present, consider alternate diagnosis.
    ○ Nitrite represents a gram-negative bacteria is present that is converting dietary nitrates to nitrites.
  - Hematuria:
    ○ White cell cast: Renal origin of pyuria
- Urine culture and sensitivity:
  - Obtain in:
    ○ Suspected pyelonephritis
    ○ Unclear diagnosis
    ○ Treatment failures, recurrent infections
  - >100,000 colony-forming units (CFU)/mL is positive.
  - $10^2$–$10^4$ CFU considered positive in:
    ○ Early infection
    ○ Clinical scenario consistent with UTI
    ○ Catheter or suprapubic specimen
    ○ Males

## DIAGNOSTIC TESTS & INTERPRETATION
*Lab*
- CBC:
  - Leukocytosis
  - Does not rule in or out upper tract infection
- Blood cultures:
  - Not needed unless patient is septic; positive cultures do not correlate with more severe disease.
  - Bacteria identified more readily on urine culture
- Chemistries:
  - For patients with significant risk for electrolytes abnormalities (severe nausea/vomiting, or medication use)

*Imaging*
- Imaging is required to differentiate pyelitis (no parenchymal involvement) and pyelonephritis (parenchymal involvement); however, this typically does not alter ED treatment.
- Bedside renal US:
  - Limited value for characterization except for detecting hydronephrosis/obstruction
- Helical CT:
  - Superior to renal ultrasound in detecting abnormalities and characterizing extent of the disease
  - Consistent or concerning findings:
    ○ Stranding or inflammation and edema of parenchyma
    ○ Perinephric fluid
    ○ Calculi, obstruction
    ○ Renal/perinephric abscess
    ○ Intraparenchymal gas formation (consistent with emphysematous pyelonephritis)
- MRI:
  - Useful in:
    ○ Pregnant patients (lack of radiation)
    ○ Renal failure (lack of iodinated contrast)
  - Cost/availability limit usefulness in the ED
  - Obtain imaging if:
    ○ Concomitant stone or obstruction suspected
    ○ Diagnosis unclear
    ○ Patient very ill, worsening, or failing to improve with standard therapy
    ○ At risk for emphysematous pyelonephritis or abscess (immunocompromised, diabetes mellitus, instrumented, or elderly)
    ○ Elective evaluation of genitourinary tract in males with pyelonephritis

### Pediatric Considerations
- Obtain catheter urine specimen:
  - Vast majority of bag urine specimens will result in positive cultures (contaminants).
  - Helpful only for excluding disease if culture is negative
  - Catheterized or suprapubic specimen with >1,000 CFU is positive.
- Blood cultures usually performed for children <1 yr of age (due to risk for SBI)
- All children with 1st episode of pyelonephritis should have urinary tract imaging performed later.
- Renal US:
  - Within 48 hr if no clinical improvement
  - Within 3–6 wk if clinical improvement

- Girls 4–10 yr old:
  – Radionuclide isocystogram for UVR
- Boys 4–10 yr old:
  – Voiding cystourethrogram after urine is sterile and bladder spasm has subsided

### Diagnostic Procedures/Surgery
Suprapubic bladder aspiration:

- When urethral catheterization is not successful, or not possible (phimosis, urethral stricture, etc.)
- Contraindicated when there is a overlying infection, a known anatomic abnormality (tumor), recent complete voiding/micturition

### DIFFERENTIAL DIAGNOSIS

- Abdominal aortic aneurysm or dissection
- Appendicitis
- Cholecystitis
- Cystitis
- Diverticulitis
- Gynecologic infections:
  – Cervicitis
  – Pelvic inflammatory disease
  – Endometritis
  – Salpingitis
- Inferior pneumonia
- Male genitourinary infections:
  – Prostatitis
  – Epididymitis
- Nephrolithiasis
- Renal/perinephric abscess
- Urethritis

 TREATMENT

### PRE-HOSPITAL
IV access for the ill/toxic-appearing patient with appropriate fluid resuscitation

### INITIAL STABILIZATION/THERAPY
Treat shock with 0.9% normal saline 500-mL to 1-L (peds: 20 mL/kg) IV fluid bolus

- While shock needs to be treated aggressively, be cognizant of fluid overload in patients with comorbidities (renal failure, congestive heart failure).

### ED TREATMENT/PROCEDURES

- Parental antibiotics for:
  – Inability to tolerate oral therapy
  – Extremes of age, immunosuppression, and pregnancy
  – Failure of oral/outpatient therapy
  – Urinary obstruction
  – Suspected antibiotic-resistant organisms
- Empiric IV antibiotics:
  – Aminoglycoside (gentamicin) plus ampicillin
  – 3rd-generation cephalosporin (ceftriaxone)
  – Fluoroquinolones—not approved for children
  – In pregnancy:
    ○ 3rd-generation cephalosporin
    ○ Gentamicin/ampicillin
    ○ Cefazolin
    ○ Aztreonam
- Outpatient oral antibiotics:
  – For nontoxic and otherwise healthy patient:
    ○ Fluoroquinolone: 14-day course
  – May administer 1 dose of parenteral antibiotics prior to oral antibiotics:
    ○ Ensures prompt cessation of bacterial proliferation

- ○ Avoids delays in oral antibiotic administration
- ○ No literature addressing efficacy
- ○ Antiemetics for vomiting
- ○ Analgesia for pain

### MEDICATION

- Oral antibiotics:
  – Ciprofloxacin: 500 mg PO b.i.d.
  – Levofloxacin: 750 mg PO daily (5 days)
  – Ofloxacin: 200 mq PO b.i.d.
  – Amoxicillin/clavulanic acid: 875 mg/125 mg PO b.i.d.
- IV antibiotics:
  – Ceftriaxone: 1 g IV q24h
  – Ciprofloxacin: 400 mg IV q12h
  – Ampicillin/sulbactam: 3 g IV q6h
  – Cefazolin: 1–1.5 g IV q8h
  – Gentamicin: 3–5 mg/kg IV load
  – Levofloxacin: 500 mg IV daily
  – Piperacillin-tazobactam: 3.375 g IV q8h

### Pediatric Considerations

- Oral antibiotic liquid preparations for children:
  – Amoxicillin: 30–50 mg/kg/24 hr PO t.i.d.
  – Amoxicillin/clavulanic acid: 45 mg/kg/24 hr PO t.i.d.
  – Cefixime: 8 mg/kg PO daily
  – Cefpodoxime: 10 mg/kg/24 hr PO b.i.d.
  – Cephalexin: 50–75 mg/kg/24 hr PO QID
  – Erythromycin/sulfisoxazole: 50 mg erythromycin/kg/24 hr PO q.i.d.
- Parenteral antibiotics for admitted children:
  – Age 0–3 mo:
    ○ Cefotaxime (50–180 mg/kg/d t.i.d.) plus ampicillin (50–100 mg/kg/d q.i.d.)
    ○ Gentamicin (1–2.5 mg/kg/d t.i.d.) plus ampicillin
  – Age >3 mo:
    ○ May substitute ceftriaxone (50–100 mq/kq/d b.i.d. to daily) for cefotaxime

 FOLLOW-UP

### DISPOSITION
#### Admission Criteria

- Sepsis, ill/toxic appearance
- Inability to tolerate oral therapy
- Intractable nausea/vomiting
- Social situation prevents compliance.
- Pregnancy
- Indwelling urinary catheter
- Urinary obstruction/anatomic abnormalities
- Proximal obstruction, such as kidney stone (high risk for renal abscess or sepsis and so requires emergent urologic consultation)
- Immunosuppression/diabetes mellitus
- Extremes of age (children <2–6 mo)
- Failure of outpatient therapy/recent antibiotics
- If uncertain of diagnosis
- Immunocompromised

#### Discharge Criteria

- Clinical course improving in ED
- Ability to maintain oral hydration
- Pain controlled with oral analgesic
- Follow-up in 48–72 hr

### FOLLOW-UP RECOMMENDATIONS

- Uncomplicated pyelonephritis in patients without significant comorbidities can safely follow up with their primary care physicians.
- If cultures were obtained, patient will need to follow up on results for possible therapy change once antibiotic sensitivities are known.
- Pediatric patients all need to follow up with their pediatrician for required imaging for anatomic abnormalities (eg, voiding cystourethrogram).
- Pregnant patients need repeat urinalysis to assess for resolution/recurrence and possible suppressive therapy.
- Patients with recurrent infections and those with identified unusual or resistant organisms require close follow-up with urologic and/or infectious disease consultation.

### PEARLS AND PITFALLS

- Primarily a clinical diagnosis with minimal lab work required
- Treat young, old, immunosuppressed, and pregnant patients aggressively.
- Consider other diagnoses (eg, gynecologic etiologies, abdominal aortic aneurysm)

### ADDITIONAL READING

- Czaja C, Scholes D, Hooton T, et al. Population-based epidemiologic analysis of acute pyelonephritis. *Clin Infect Dis*. 2007;45:273–280.
- Piccoli BG, Cresto E, Ragni F, et al. The clinical spectrum of acute uncomplicated pyelonephritis from an emergency medicine perspective. *Int J Antimicrob Agents*. 2008;31(suppl S):S46–S53.
- Stunnell H, Buckley O, Feeney J, et al. Imaging of acute pyelonephritis in the adult. *Eur Radiol*. 2007;17:1820–1828.
- Talan D, Krishnadasan A, Abrahamian F, et al. Prevalence and risk factor analysis of trimethoprim-sulfamethoxazole and fluoroquinolone resistant *E. coli* infection among emergency department patients with pyelonephritis. *Clin Infect Dis*. 2008;47:1150–1158.
- Warren JW, Abrutyn E, Hebel JR, et al. Guidelines for antimicrobial treatment of uncomplicated acute bacterial cystitis and acute pyelonephritis in women. *Clin Infect Dis*. 1999;29:745–758.

#### See Also (Topic, Algorithm, Electronic Media Element)

- Pelvic Inflammatory Disease
- Urinary Tract Infection, Adult
- Urinary Tract Infection, Pediatric

*The author gratefully acknowledges the contribution of Ingrid Carter for the previous edition of this chapter.*

 CODES

#### ICD9
590.80 Pyelonephritis, unspecified

# PYLORIC STENOSIS
*Roger M. Barkin*

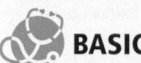 **BASICS**

## DESCRIPTION
- Postnatal hypertrophy and hyperplasia of the circular smooth muscle cell layer causing a thickened pylorus and antrum leading to progressive gastric outlet obstruction
- Neuronal nitric oxide synthase (NOS-1) may be a genetic susceptibility locus.
- Administration of erythromycin in infants may increase risk of hypertrophic pyloric stenosis.
- Jaundice due to transient glucuronyl transferase deficiency
- Adult: Caused by peptic ulcer disease

## ETIOLOGY
- Most common cause of GI obstruction in infants; incidence 1/150 males, 1/750 females (average: 3/100 live births)
- Males affected 5× more commonly than females; firstborn most common
- Familial, 15%:
  - Child of affected parent has 7% incidence.
  - Recurrence risk in subsequent male children is 10%; 2% in females.

 **DIAGNOSIS**

## SIGNS AND SYMPTOMS
### History
- Vomiting:
  - Gradual onset, usually beginning at around 3 wk of age
  - Progressive, usually becoming projectile
  - Nonbilious
  - May be blood tinged (secondary to esophagitis, gastritis, gastric ulceration)
  - Progressively worsening
  - Postprandial
- Represents the hypertrophied pylorus:
  - Confirms diagnosis
- Constipation or small amount of stools
- "Lean and hungry" infant early in course; dehydrated and uninterested in feeding late in course; failure to thrive
- Variable dehydration and wasting depending on duration of symptoms
- Jaundice in 8% of children
- Adult presents with vomiting, anorexia, early satiety, and epigastric pain.

### Physical Exam
- Often normal unless a relaxed abdomen
- May feel olive-shaped mass at lateral margin of the right rectus abdominis muscle in the right upper quadrant (80% of patients), often after vomiting:
  - Best felt immediately after vomiting or after the stomach is emptied via gastric suction as the dilated body of the stomach overlies the pylorus
  - Represents the hypertrophied pylorus:
    - Helps confirm diagnosis
    - Peristaltic waves moving from the left to right in the left upper quadrant, seen best after feeding or just prior to vomiting

## ESSENTIAL WORKUP
If "olive" palpable, further diagnostic evaluation may be unnecessary and surgical consultation should be sought; otherwise, imaging studies are indicated.

## DIAGNOSTIC TESTS & INTERPRETATION
### Lab
- Electrolytes, BUN/creatinine, glucose:
  - Hypokalemic, hypochloremic metabolic alkalosis
  - Normal electrolytes do not exclude the diagnosis.
- Bilirubin elevated
- CBC if blood in emesis
- Urinalysis for hydration

P

## Imaging

- Abdominal US:
  - Study of choice
  - US diagnosis hinges on identification and measurement of pyloric muscle mass (3-mm ring thickness with 1.5-cm pylorus channel) and observation of fluid movement through the pylorus.
  - Positive predictive value approaches 100%; 19% false negatives.
  - Serial US for equivocal or negative study
- Upper GI series:
  - String sign representing contrast passing through a narrowed gastric outlet
  - 95% accurate
  - Remove contrast from the stomach after the study to prevent aspiration.
- Supine abdominal film:
  - Not diagnostic; rarely helpful
  - Dilated stomach and no air distal to the pylorus
  - Most useful with other views to begin evaluation for other abdominal pathology

## DIFFERENTIAL DIAGNOSIS

- GI anatomic/functional disorder:
  - Gastroesophageal reflux
  - Hiatal hernia
  - Obstruction/atresia
  - Gastric or duodenal web
- Infection:
  - Gastroenteritis
  - UTI
  - Sepsis
- Metabolic:
  - Adrenal insufficiency
  - Inborn error of metabolism
- Feeding problems:
  - Psychosocial: Poor maternal interaction or stress
  - Chalasia
  - Formula intolerance
  - Overfeeding
- Drug withdrawal
- Increased intracranial pressure

##  TREATMENT

### PRE-HOSPITAL
Fluid resuscitation if significant volume deficit

### INITIAL STABILIZATION/THERAPY
- IV access
- Rapid bedside glucose test to exclude hypoglycemia
- Correct volume deficit with 20-mL/kg bolus of 0.9% normal saline IV; may repeat.

### ED TREATMENT/PROCEDURES
- Correct electrolyte abnormalities.
- Hydrate with dextrose-containing solution after fluid resuscitation at 1–1.5× maintenance rate:
  - Add potassium after ensuring adequate urine output.
- Insert nasogastric tube to decompress the stomach.
- Restrict oral intake.
- Consult pediatric surgeon for pyloromyotomy.
- Adult: Proton pump antagonist (lansoprazole or omeprazole)

### MEDICATION
#### Adults
- Lansoprazole: 30 mg daily PO
- Omeprazole: 20 mg daily PO

##  FOLLOW-UP

### DISPOSITION
#### Admission Criteria
- All pediatric patients should be admitted to the hospital for rehydration and surgical correction with either an umbilical pyloromyotomy or laparoscopic pyloromyotomy.
- Adult patients: Admit as necessary for rehydration; may be scheduled for elective pyloromyotomy if proton pump inhibitors fail to improve this condition.

#### Discharge Criteria
None

#### Issues for Referral
Surgical consultation concurrent with correction of electrolytes and fluid deficits

### FOLLOW-UP RECOMMENDATIONS
Follow growth pattern after surgery.

## PEARLS AND PITFALLS

Suggestive clinical presentation combined with laboratory evaluation should lead to imaging and correction of electrolyte abnormalities.

## ADDITIONAL READING

- Heller RM, Hernanz-Schulman M. Application of new imaging modalities to the evaluation of common pediatric conditions. *J Pediatr.* 1999;135:632–639.
- Mahon BE, Rosenman MG, Kleiman MB. Maternal and infant use of erythromycin and other macrolide antibiotics as risk factors for infantile hypertrophic pyloric stenosis. *J Pediatr.* 2001;13:380–384.
- Najmaldin A, Tan HL. Early experience with laparoscopic pyloromyotomy for infantile hypertrophic pyloric stenosis. *J Pediatr.* 1995;30–37.
- Touloukian RJ, Higgins E. The spectrum of serum electrolytes in hypertrophic pyloric stenosis. *J Pediatr Surg.* 1983;18(4):394–397.

##  CODES

### ICD9
- 537.0 Acquired hypertrophic pyloric stenosis
- 750.5 Congenital hypertrophic pyloric stenosis

# QT SYNDROME, PROLONGED

*Jason A. Tracy*

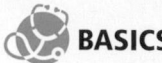

## BASICS

### DESCRIPTION

- Alteration in cardiac sodium, potassium, or calcium channel mechanics
- Prolonged ventricular repolarization results in lengthening of QT interval on surface ECG:
  - "Pause-dependent" lengthening due to short–long–short sequence in which a sinus beat is followed by an extrasystole (short), then a postextrasystolic pause (long), concluding with a ventricular extrasystole (short)
  - "Adrenergic-dependent" pauses found in congenital cases
- Symptoms often preceded by vigorous exercise, emotional stress, or loud noise.
- Nocturnal bradycardia can lengthen QT interval, causing sleep-related symptoms.
- Re-entrant rhythm can lead to torsades de pointes, ventricular tachycardia, and ventricular fibrillation.
- Hemodynamic compromise following dysrhythmia leads to syncope or death.
- Independent risk factor for sudden cardiac death.

### RISK FACTORS
#### Genetics
- 6 genetic loci identified with sporadic cases owing to spontaneous mutations:
  - Autosomal recessive form associated with deafness (Jervell and Lange–Nielsen syndromes)
  - Autosomal dominant form not associated with deafness (Romano–Ward syndrome)
  - Adrenergic stimulation (fright, exertion, delirium tremens, and loud auditory stimulus) becomes prodysrhythmic in certain genotypes, while sleep-related symptoms are found in others.
- 10%–15% of carriers have baseline normal QTc.
- Death occurs in 1%–2% of untreated patients per year.
  - Drug-induced QT prolongation may also have a genetic background.
  - Congenital form occurs in 1 in 3,000–5,000, with mortality of 6% by age 40 yr.

#### Pediatric Considerations
- Diagnosis suspected in the young with syncope, cardiac arrest, or sudden death
- Syncope following emotional stress or exercise suggestive
- Death occurs without preceding symptoms in 10% of pediatric patients.

## ETIOLOGY

- Drugs:
  - Complete list at www.QTDrugs.org
  - Class Ia antidysrhythmics—quinidine, procainamide, disopyramide
  - Class III antidysrhythmics—sotalol, ibutilide, amiodarone
  - Antibiotics—erythromycin, pentamidine, chloroquine, trimethoprim–sulfamethoxazole
  - Antifungal agents—ketoconazole, itraconazole
  - Psychotropic drugs—phenothiazines, haloperidol, risperidone, STCAs
  - Cisapride
  - Antihistamines
  - Organophosphates
  - Narcotics—methadone
- Electrolyte abnormalities
  - Hypokalemia
  - Hypomagnesemia
  - Hypocalcemia
- Cardiac
  - Bradyarrhythmias
  - Arteriovenous block
  - Mitral valve prolapse
  - Myocarditis
  - Myocardial ischemia
- CNS
  - Subarachnoid hemorrhage
  - Stroke
- Congenital (idiopathic)
- Other
  - Protein-sparing fasting
  - Anorexia nervosa
  - Hypothyroidism
  - Hypothermia

## DIAGNOSIS

### SIGNS AND SYMPTOMS
- Palpitations
- Light-headedness
- Dizziness

#### History
- Syncope
- Near syncope
- Seizure
- Family history of syncope or sudden death
- Congenital deafness
- Medication use

## ESSENTIAL WORKUP
Cardiac monitor:
- ECG
- QTc (QT corrected for heart rate) >0.44 sec in men and >0.46 sec in women
- QT measured from beginning of quasi-random signal to end of T wave:
  - Measured best in the limb leads and should be averaged over 3–5 beats
  - There is no expert consensus on best heart rate correction (QTc) formula.
  - Bazett formula (QT divided by square root of RR interval) is most commonly used
  - Increase in QT variability
- T-wave abnormalities (T-wave alternans, biphasic)
- Appearance of U waves
- Ventricular tachycardia
- Ventricular fibrillation
- Torsades de pointes

## DIAGNOSTIC TESTS & INTERPRETATION
### Lab
- Full electrolytes including calcium and magnesium
- Toxicology screen

### Imaging
Echocardiography to exclude other cardiac causes

### Diagnostic Procedures/Surgery
- ECG stress testing to induce a prolonged QT interval in suspected cases
- Holter monitoring of QTc
- Genetic counseling/testing in suspected congenital forms
- Familial ECG testing

## DIFFERENTIAL DIAGNOSIS
- Myocardial infarction
- Hypertrophic cardiomyopathy
- Valvular defect

# TREATMENT

## PRE-HOSPITAL
- Supplemental oxygen
- IV access
- Monitor

### ALERT
- Stable patients with prolonged QT transported without intervention
- Cardioversion for unstable patients with confirmed torsades de pointes
- Magnesium sulfate for stable patients with evidence of torsades de pointes

## INITIAL STABILIZATION/THERAPY
- IV access
- Monitor
- Determine hemodynamic stability
- Unstable patients require immediate cardioversion

## ED TREATMENT/PROCEDURES
- IV magnesium sulfate for torsades de pointes
- IV potassium to serum levels of 4.5–5 mEq/L
- Temporary transvenous cardiac pacing (rates from 100–120 beats per min) for recurrences of torsades de pointes refractory to magnesium sulfate therapy (shortens QTc)
- IV isoproterenol for refractory cases or hemodynamically unstable patients with acquired long QT (ineffective in congenital cases) who do not respond to transvenous pacing
- Remove any offending medications and correct metabolic derangements.
- Consult with cardiology in those with symptomatic long QT regarding use of beta blockers at maximum doses
- No ED treatment needed (In consultation with cardiology) for those with suspected idiopathic long QT and no history of syncope, family history of sudden cardiac death, or ventricular arrhythmias.
- Pacemaker or defibrillator placement with or without cervicothoracic stellectomy (to reduce adrenergic stimulation) may be required in high-risk patients.
- Beta blockers prevent 70% of cardiac events in congenital cases.

## MEDICATION

### First Line
- Magnesium sulfate: 2 g (peds: 25–50 mg/kg) IV bolus over 2–3 min followed by IV infusion at 2–4 mg/min
- Isoproterenol: 1 $\mu$g/min (peds: 0.05–0.1 $\mu$g/kg/min) IV continuous infusion, titrate for effect, up to 10 $\mu$g/min

### Second Line
Propanolol: 2–3 mg/kg/day (peds: 2–3 mg/kg/day) PO (in consultation with cardiology)

# FOLLOW-UP

## DISPOSITION

### Admission Criteria
- Symptomatic prolonged QT
- Syncope
- Cardiac dysrhythmia
- Possible cardiac or ischemic event
- Metabolic abnormality

### Discharge Criteria
Asymptomatic prolonged QT in consultation with cardiology

## FOLLOW-UP RECOMMENDATIONS
Follow-up recommended in all patients with a new diagnosis of prolonged QT

# PEARLS AND PITFALLS

- Suspect prolonged QT in patients with syncope
- Prolonged QT is an independent risk factor for sudden cardiac death.
- Correct electrolyte abnormalities and discontinue offending drugs in those with prolonged QT.
- Magnesium sulfate followed by pacing for torsades de pointes.

# ADDITIONAL READING

- Al-Khatib SM, LaPointe NM, Kramer JM, et al. What clinicians should know about the QT interval. *JAMA*. 2003;289:2120–127.
- Chugh SS, Reinier K, Singh T, et al. Determinants of prolonged QT interval and their contribution to sudden death risk in coronary artery disease: The Oregon sudden unexpected death study. *Circulation*. 2009;119:663–670.
- Meyer JS, Mehdirad A, Salem BI, et al. Sudden arrhythmia death syndrome: Importance of the long QT syndrome. *Am Fam Physician*. 2003;68: 483–488.
- Libby P, Bonow RO, Mann DL, Zipes DP, eds. *Braunwald's Heart Disease: A Textbook of Cardiovascular Medicine*, 8th ed. Philadelphia: Saunders, 2007.
- Zipes DP, Camm AJ, Borggrefe M, et al. ACC/AHA/ESC 2006 Guidelines for Management of Patients With Ventricular Arrhythmias and the Prevention of Sudden Cardiac Death-Executive Summary A Report of the American College of Cardiology/American Heart Association Task Force and the European Society of Cardiology Committee for Practice Guidelines (Writing Committee to Develop Guidelines for Management of Patients with Ventricular Arrhythmias and the Prevention of Sudden Cardiac Death). *J Am Coll Cardiol*. 2006;48:1064.

## See Also (Topic, Algorithm, Electronic Media Element)
- www.QTDrugs.org

# CODES

### ICD9
426.82 Long qt syndrome

# RABIES

*Matthew A. Kippenhan*

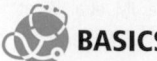 **BASICS**

## DESCRIPTION

CNS infectious disease of mammals caused by the rabies virus:

- Negative-stranded RNA genome, family Rhabdoviridae, genus *Lyssavirus*

## ETIOLOGY

- Epidemiology:
  - Human cases 30,000–70,000/yr worldwide
  - Especially common in Southeast Asia, Philippines, Africa, South America, and Indian subcontinent
  - Dogs and foxes are main reservoirs.
  - U.S. has 2–3 human cases per year.
  - Most clinical cases in U.S. from foreign travel and bat exposures
  - Wild animals 93% of cases, domestic animals 6.8%
  - Raccoons, skunks, bats, foxes, woodchucks, groundhogs are reservoirs.
  - *Lasionycteris* (silver haired) and *Pipistrellus* (eastern pipistrelle) bats are associated with most cases.
  - Though not enough to constitute exposure, squirrel, rat, mouse, hamster, guinea pig, gerbil, chipmunk, rabbit are also reservoirs.
- Pathophysiology:
  - Mode of transmission:
    - Infected saliva of host passed to uninfected animal
    - Bite: Most common
    - Nonbite: Scratch, abrasion, mucous membrane contact with saliva, bat aerosol exposure
    - Corneal and solid-organ transplant procedures
    - Not considered transmission risk: Petting rabid animal; contact with blood, urine, or feces of rabid animal
  - Progression after infection:
    - Virus multiplies in local tissue (ie, muscle)
    - Virus taken up into peripheral nerves through acetylcholine receptors
    - Virus transported to CNS via retrograde axoplasmic flow
    - Once in CNS, rapid replication and dissemination cause encephalitis.
    - Centrifugal spread of virus to peripheral nerves, including salivary glands

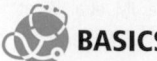 **DIAGNOSIS**

## SIGNS AND SYMPTOMS

- 5 stages: Latent period, prodrome, encephalitis, coma, death (or recovery):
  - Latent period: 1–3 mo (range 10 days to >6 yr):
    - Virus incubation in peripheral tissues
    - Shorter period for head or neck bite
  - Prodrome: Duration 1–7 days:
    - Fever, headache, malaise, myalgias, anorexia, sore throat, nausea, and vomiting
    - Paresthesias or fasciculations around bite site give clue to diagnosis.
  - Encephalitis: Duration 2–7 days:
    - Anxiety, agitation, hallucinations, confusion or delirium, muscle spasms, seizure, persistent high fever
    - Aerophobia: Pharyngeal spasm from draft of air
    - Hydrophobia: Violent involuntary muscle contraction of diaphragm, pharyngeal, laryngeal, and accessory respiratory muscles when attempting to swallow (seen in 2/3 of cases)
    - Autonomic instability, dysrhythmias, myocarditis
    - Brainstem involvement: Diplopia, facial paralysis
  - Coma:
    - Apnea from respiratory center involvement, vascular collapse, flaccid paralysis, adult respiratory distress syndrome, syndrome of inappropriate diuretic hormone
    - Most die within 2 wk
  - Death (or recovery):
    - Fatal if no pre- or postexposure prophylaxis given
    - Single case report in 2004 of survival without prophylaxis
    - Residual neurologic deficits likely persist.
- 3 manifestations of disease:
  - Classic (encephalitic) accounts for ~80% of cases.
  - Dumb rabies (paralytic) accounts for ~20%: Ascending paralysis mimicking Guillain-Barré Syndrome (GBS)
  - Nonclassic (atypical) rabies (<1%): Neuropathic pain, sensory or motor deficits, choreiform movements, myoclonus, and seizures

## History

- Bite wound or other known exposure
- Bat found in room with person unable to give history (eg, child, intoxicated): Assume exposure
- Travel to endemic areas
- Unprovoked attack carries higher risk of infection.

## Physical Exam

- Fever
- Bat bite often not visible on exam
- Altered mental status, seizures, encephalopathy
- Percussion myoedema: Muscle mounds at percussion site
- Autonomic manifestations: Dilated pupils, perspiration, hypersalivation, orthostatic hypotension

## ESSENTIAL WORKUP

- Saliva:
  - Rabies RNA by reverse transcription- polymerase chain reaction (RT-PCR)
  - Virus isolation in cell culture
- Serum: Rabies antibodies:
  - Positive titers are diagnostic if not vaccinated.
  - Earliest positive, day 6
- Cerebrospinal fluid—mildly elevated WBC and protein, normal glucose:
  - Virus isolation
  - Rabies antibodies are diagnostic, even if immunized.

## DIAGNOSTIC TESTS & INTERPRETATION

### Lab

- CBC
- Electrolytes, BUN, creatinine, glucose
- Blood cultures/urinalysis:
  - Search for other infection/illness
- Neck biopsy: RT-PCR, immunofluorescent staining for viral antigen

### Imaging

- CT head: Other causes of altered mental status, seizure, encephalopathy
- Chest radiograph: Other infectious etiologies

*Diagnostic Procedures/Surgery*
Lumbar puncture

## DIFFERENTIAL DIAGNOSIS
- Other causes of encephalitis:
  - Herpesviruses: HSV1, VZV
  - Enterovirus (Coxsackie, echovirus, poliovirus)
  - Arboviruses (West Nile virus, eastern/western equine encephalitis, LaCrosse, St. Louis)
- Tetanus
- Delirium tremens
- Psychosis
- Paralytic form:
  - GBS
  - Polio
  - Tick-bite paralysis
  - Immune-mediated polyneuritis
  - Botulism

 ## TREATMENT

### PRE-HOSPITAL
- Thoroughly wash wound with soap and water.
- If safely able, capture wild animal for sacrifice and testing.

### INITIAL STABILIZATION/THERAPY
- Airway, breathing, and circulation
- Intubation as needed
- Treatment of seizures

### ED TREATMENT/PROCEDURES
- Wound cleansing with soap and virucidal agent
- Tetanus immunization
- Determine if exposure requires treatment:
  - Domestic animal bite:
    - Home monitoring of animal for 10 days
    - If animal displays no signs of illness, patient does not need postexposure prophylaxis (PEP).
  - Wild animal bite:
    - Rabies testing of sacrificed animal head
    - May delay PEP pending results
    - Treat if animal not captured.
  - All unprovoked attacks should be assumed at high risk for exposure.
- PEP:
  - Passive immunization with human rabies immune globulin (HRIG)
  - HRIG: 20 IU/kg:
    - 1/2 infiltrated in and around wound
    - Remainder given IM (gluteus okay)
    - Active immunization with rabies vaccine
  - Rabies vaccine: 1 mL (2.5 IU) IM days 0, 3, 7, 14, 28

- Three vaccines available; equally safe and efficacious:
  - Human diploid cell vaccine (Imovax, Imovax ID: IM, intradermal forms)
  - Rabies vaccine adsorbed
  - Purified chick embryo cell vaccine (RabAvert)
- Administration location:
  - Deltoid in adults or anterior thigh in children
  - Not given in gluteus: reported failures with inadvertent administration into subcutaneous fat
- For those with preexposure prophylaxis and rabies exposure:
  - Do not require HRIG
  - Need vaccine booster on days 0 and 3
- If care delayed after rabies exposure:
  - HRIG not indicated >7 days after exposure
  - Vaccine should be administered as usual.
- Preexposure prophylaxis:
  - Rabies vaccine on days 0, 7, 21, 28
  - Target groups: Veterinarians, animal handlers, virus laboratory workers, foreign travelers in endemic regions

*Pediatric Considerations*
Treat as in adults.

*Pregnancy Considerations*
Treatment considered safe during pregnancy.

 ## FOLLOW-UP

### DISPOSITION
Ensure adequate access for subsequent vaccine administration post rabies exposure.

*Admission Criteria*
Patient with encephalitis or high suspicion of rabies

*Discharge Criteria*
- Stable patient
- No evidence of reaction to vaccine

*Issues for Referral*
Public health and CDC for suspicious cases

### FOLLOW-UP RECOMMENDATIONS
- Ensure access to subsequent vaccine doses
- Patient should follow-up with animal control if source animal has been sacrificed or is being observed.

## PEARLS AND PITFALLS
- PEP is only proven treatment.
- PEP should be given in all high-risk exposures regardless of timing
- Vaccine should only be given in deltoid in adults: Treatment failures reported with inadvertent subcutaneous administration in gluteus injections.

## ADDITIONAL READING
- Centers for Disease Control and Prevention. Human Rabies Prevention—United States 2008. Recommendations of the Advisory Committee on Immunization Practices. *Morb Mortal Wkly Rep.* 2008;57:1–26, 28.
- Centers for Disease Control and Prevention. Recovery of a Patient from Clinical Rabies—Wisconsin. *Morb Mortal Wkly Rep.* 2004;53(50):1171–1173.
- Centers for Disease Control and Prevention. Rabies. Available at: http://www.cdc.gov/rabies/. Updated April 21, 2010.
- World Health Organization. *WHO Expert Consultation on Rabies, First Report.* Geneva: WHO; 2004.

### See Also (Topic, Algorithm, Electronic Media Element)
- Encephalitis
- Meningitis

 ## CODES

### ICD9
- 071 Rabies
- V01.5 Contact with or exposure to rabies
- V04.5 Need for prophylactic vaccination and inoculation against rabies

R

# RADIATION INJURY
*Robert Feldman*

## BASICS

### DESCRIPTION
- *Radiation* in this chapter refers to ionizing radiation.
- Alpha ($\alpha$)—helium nucleus; does not penetrate skin
- Beta ($\beta$)—electron; penetrates tissue a few cm
- Gamma ($\gamma$)—photon; penetrates body
- Neutron—very penetrating; not detected by Geiger counter, but neutron emitters also emit $\gamma$ radiation
- Radioisotope/radionuclide—chemical element that emits radiation from its nucleus:
  - Radioactivity cannot be destroyed, only relocated or shielded.
  - Being radioactive does not change element's other chemical and physical properties, such as heavy metal toxicity.
- Exposure/irradiation—patient has been in presence of ionizing radiation:
  - Whole body or only certain areas may be exposed.
- Contamination—radioactive material where it is not desired:
  - Internal—within body (eg, lung)
  - External—outside body (skin, hair, clothing)
- Dose—amount of radiation energy absorbed by tissue:
  - Units and conversions:
    - 1 gray (Gy) = 100 rad
    - 1 sievert (Sv) = 100 rem
  - For $\beta$ and $\gamma$ radiation:
    - 1 Gy = 1 Sv = 100 rad = 100 rem

### ALERT
Contact regional or federal authorities for guidance if radiation incident is suspected.

### Pediatric Considerations
- Children are more sensitive to radiation injury.
- Potassium iodide is most protective for children and should be given promptly if contamination with radioactive iodine (I-131) is suspected.

### Pregnancy Considerations
- Developing fetus is very sensitive to radiation.
- Pregnant staff should not care for radioactively contaminated patients.

### ETIOLOGY
- Ionizing radiation leads to cellular injury.
- Damage to blood vessels leads to endarteritis and loss of tissue blood supply.
- Higher rates of cell division within an organ make it more sensitive to radiation:
  - Bone marrow and GI tract are very sensitive.
  - Skin and nerve are less sensitive.
- *Acute radiation syndrome* (ARS) occurs in stages following whole-body exposure:
  - Prodromal: Acute radiation injury leads to acute inflammation (0–48 hr).
  - Latent: If the acute phase of injury is survived, inflammation and symptoms subside (0–2 wk).
  - Manifest illness: At higher radiation doses, organ failure then develops.
  - Recovery or death (usually from infection) follows.
- Sources of radiation include medical devices, therapeutics, nuclear weapons, and industry.

## DIAGNOSIS

- Diagnosing contamination is fairly easy.
- Diagnosing and quantifying exposure is more difficult and probably require expert consultation.

### SIGNS AND SYMPTOMS
- Vary based on dose; see: http://www.afrri.usuhs.mil/outreach/pdf/AFRRI-Pocket-Guide.pdf for quick reference.
- Overall:
  - Whole-body exposure: Syndrome similar to high-dose chemotherapy toxicity
  - ARS progresses more rapidly the higher the absorbed dose.
- Local exposure:
  - Early resembles thermal or UV burn
  - Later resembles ischemic ulcer

### History
- Recognized exposure:
  - Occupational, medical, transportation accident
- Unrecognized or clandestine exposure:
  - Radiologic dispersal device (RDD), concealed or unrecognized source
  - Industrial and medical radiography sources may be pellets only a few mm in diameter and are highly radioactive.
  - Suspect if multiple patients present with symptoms of ARS at any stage, burns without history of thermal exposure, or ischemic ulcers in unusual locations (eg, hand from handling unrecognized source, hip from placing source in pocket).

### Physical Exam
- Whole-body exposure:
  - Nausea, vomiting:
    - Within 3–6 hr for >100 rad exposure; sooner with higher exposures
    - Vomiting within 1 hr of exposure indicates potentially lethal injury (>600 rad).
  - Confusion and weakness (>200 rad)
  - Fever:
    - Acutely, from inflammation
    - During manifest illness, from infection
  - Hair loss, hemorrhage, diarrhea may develop with doses >300 rad.
- Dermal exposure:
  - Initial erythema
  - Blistering and ischemic necrosis may follow.

### ESSENTIAL WORKUP
- *Survey for radiation* using a *Geiger counter*, which can be found in any nuclear medicine or radiation therapy department:
  - Any probe style is acceptable for survey.
  - Cover probe with exam glove:
    - Prevents contamination of probe
    - Blocks $\alpha$ radiation but detects b/g
  - Measure background radiation away from patient.
  - Move probe slowly over patient's skin:
    - 1–2 cm from skin
    - Move probe only 2–3 cm/sec.
    - Contamination is >2 × background radiation level.
    - Note any contaminated areas.
    - Follow systematic pattern to avoid missing areas.
    - Remember to survey palms, soles, hair.

- *Absolute lymphocyte count* is best indicator of severity of ARS:
  - <1,000/mm$^3$: Moderate exposure, 200–600 rad
  - <500/mm$^3$: Severe exposure, >600 rad

### DIAGNOSTIC TESTS & INTERPRETATION
#### Lab
- CBC with differential every 4–6 hr (for 24 hr or until stable)
- Swab both nares and survey swab for inhaled contaminants.
- Type and cross-match blood.
- 24-hr stool for radioassay if GI contamination suspected
- 24-hr urine for radioassay if any internal contamination is suspected

#### Imaging
- Diagnostic imaging as clinically indicated
- Whole-body gamma camera (without collimator) is best for ruling out internal contamination with low levels of radioisotopes, if suspicion is high and survey with Geiger counter is negative.

#### Diagnostic Procedures/Surgery
Cytogenetics allows more accurate dose assessment:
- 10 mL blood in lithium-heparin tube (ethylenediaminetetraacetic acid also acceptable)
- Draw 24 hr postexposure.
- Refrigerate (4°C) and ship cold to Radiation Emergency Assistance Center/Training Site (REAC/TS).
- Only limited number of samples can be processed due to resources required.

### DIFFERENTIAL DIAGNOSIS
- Systemic illness: Lymphopenia, weakness, nausea:
  - Psychological effects are common in both exposed and unexposed patients and may mimic ARS:
    - Radiation casualty with vomiting from ARS should have falling absolute lymphocyte count (ALC); if ALC normal and stable, consider psychological stress reaction or other type of illness.
  - Hematologic malignancy
  - Chemical warfare agents (blister/mustard)
  - HIV disease, immunosuppression
- Skin injuries:
  - Ischemic ulcer
  - Brown recluse spider bite
- Pyoderma gangrenosum

## TREATMENT

Personal protective equipment (PPE):
- Must provide protection from dust (particulate respirator, eg, N-95, gown, gloves, hair, and shoe covers)
- Radiography aprons are of no value—they do not protect against most $\gamma$ radiation.

## PRE-HOSPITAL

- Treat life threats (airway, breathing, and circulation management [ABCs]).
- Assess any bombing scene for radioactive contamination (RDD).
- Removing clothing will eliminate about 80% of external contamination.
- Survey for residual contamination:
  - No contamination: Patient may be cared for as usual.
  - If contamination is present, assess medical condition:
    - Stable: Proceed with decontamination.
    - Unstable: Provide necessary care and transport; use sheets to control contamination.

## INITIAL STABILIZATION/THERAPY

- ABCs
- Assess for contamination.
- If patient condition permits, perform decontamination before patient enters (and contaminates) facility.
- Minimize staff exposure:
  - *Time*: Limit time in contaminated area, remove contaminated material often.
  - *Distance*: Use long-handled instruments to handle contaminated material.
  - *Shielding*: Place contaminated material in a lead container (available in nuclear medicine department); radiography lead aprons are not effective.

## ED TREATMENT/PROCEDURES

- Hospital issues:
  - Activate hospital disaster plan, if indicated, to mobilize resources.
  - Designate contaminated and "clean" treatment areas.
  - Appoint a temporary radiation safety officer (RSO) for incident to survey all patients and staff and all materials leaving treatment area:
    - Hospital RSO if available
    - Any staff member who is trained to use Geiger counter and dosimeters may fill RSO role initially if necessary.
  - Patients and materials that are not contaminated do not need decontamination or containment.
  - Call for expert assistance: Hospital radiation safety officer, local department of nuclear safety, health department, or REAC/TS.
- Staff issues:
  - Provide PPE and psychological support as described above.
  - Assign pregnant personnel to "clean" areas only.
- Decontamination:
  - Priorities: Wounds > mucous membranes > intact skin
  - Use fenestrated drapes to shield adjacent skin.
  - Use soap and water; no harsh chemicals.
  - Diaper wipes work well for intact skin; wipe from edges of area to center, then lift away.

- Irrigate wounds—collect and survey runoff, avoid splashing.
- Resurvey frequently to assess effectiveness of decontamination.
- Do not abrade skin.
- If contamination cannot be removed, cover area to prevent spread and move on—residual contamination can be controlled.
- RDD:
  - Necessary surgery must be done immediately (36–48 hr), or else delayed 1–2 mo, with exposure >200 rad.
  - Any bombing victim must be assessed for radioactive contamination until RDD is ruled out by assessment of scene.
  - Preserve evidence for criminal investigation.
- Treat vomiting and dehydration:
  - Antiemetics (ondansetron)
  - IV fluids
- Decorporation agents for internal decontamination are specific to each radionuclide:
  - Contact REAC/TS for guidance (see below).
- Cytokines and transfusions may be needed with doses >200 rad.
- Potassium iodide:
  - Useful only to prevent thyroid uptake of radioactive iodine (found in nuclear reactors), and only if given within a few hours after contamination (see Additional Reading).

## MEDICATION

- Ondansetron 4 mg IV
- Potassium iodide:
  - Adults: 130 mg PO
  - Children:
    - 3–18 yr: 65 mg PO
    - 1 mo to 3 yr: 32 mg PO
    - <1 mo: 16 mg PO

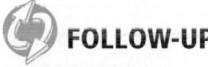 **FOLLOW-UP**

## DISPOSITION
### Admission Criteria

- Lymphocyte count <1,000 at 24–48 hr postexposure
- Lymphocyte count decreased 50% at 24–48 hr
- Suspect acute exposure >200 rad
- Significant trauma or other illness
- Uncontrolled vomiting
- When in doubt, admit for serial CBC and obtain consultation.

### Discharge Criteria

- No residual contamination
- No evidence of acute exposure >100 rad
- Tolerating oral fluids

### Issues for Referral

- Internal contamination: Contact REAC/TS for guidance.
- 24-hr emergency number: 865-576-1005
- External contamination that cannot be removed
- Any patient with radiation exposure requires dose assessment and risk counseling.

## PEARLS AND PITFALLS

- Emergency medical care takes precedence over decontamination:
  - No known case where a live, contaminated patient was so radioactive as to be an immediate hazard to emergency personnel
- Do not underestimate psychological impact of any incident involving "radiation" on staff (and public):
  - Get early support from hospital or outside experts to counsel staff.
- ALC can help differentiate ARS from psychosomatic illness: If vomiting is due to ARS, ALC should be low.

## ADDITIONAL READING

- Armed Forces Radiobiology Research Institute. *Medical Management of Radiological Casualties*. 2nd ed. 2003. Available at http://www.afrri.usuhs.mil/outreach/guidance.htm.
- Centers for Disease Control and Prevention. Emergency Preparedness and Response: Radiation Emergencies. Available at: http://www.bt.cdc.gov/radiation/.
- National Council on Radiation Protection. *Management of terrorist events involving radioactive material. NCRP Report no. 138*. Bethesda, MD: National Council on Radiation Protection; 2001.
- Oak Ridge Institute for Science and Education. Radiation Emergency Assistance Center/Training Site (REAC/TS). Available at http://orise.orau.gov/reacts/.
- 24-hr emergency line: (865) 576-1005 (ask for REAC/TS).
- U.S. Department of Health and Human Services, Food and Drug Administration, Center for Drug Evaluation and Research Guidance. Potassium Iodide as a thyroid blocking agent in radiation emergencies. Available at: http://www.fda.gov/downloads/Drugs/GuidanceCompliance RegulatoryInformation/Guidances/ucm080542.pdf.

## See Also (Topic, Algorithm, Electronic Media Element)

Chemical Weapons Poisoning

 **CODES**

### ICD9

990 Effects of radiation, unspecified

# RAPID SEQUENCE INTUBATION

Christopher Ross
Theresa Schwab

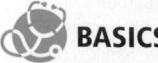

## BASICS

### DESCRIPTION
Combines induction agents with paralytic agents to create optimal conditions during emergency intubation, ideally without interposed mechanical ventilation

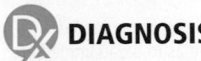

## DIAGNOSIS

### SIGNS AND SYMPTOMS
#### History
- Medication allergies
- Family history of malignant hyperthermia
- History of neuromuscular disease (contraindication for succinylcholine) and/or renal failure (caution regarding potential hyperkalemia)

#### Physical Exam
- Assess the airway for potential anatomic difficulty for intubation:
  - Look for hoarseness, stridor, drooling consistent with upper airway obstruction.
  - Use "3-3-2" rule to assess airway:
    ○ 3 fingers should fit side by side vertically in patient's mouth.
    ○ 3 fingers should fit side by side between the mentum (chin) and the angle of the neck.
    ○ 2 fingers should fit between the angle of the neck and the superior notch of the thyroid cartilage.
- Assess mobility of cervical spine:
  - Patients who cannot move their neck will be difficult in laryngeal visualization. Flexion <35° degrees and extension <80° degrees may predict difficulty.
- Assess faucial pillars, soft palate, and uvula (Mallampati classification) by having patient open mouth:
  - Loss of visualization of posterior anatomic structures is more predictive of difficulty.

### DIAGNOSTIC TESTS & INTERPRETATION
#### Lab
Serum potassium, BUN/creatinine:
- May dictate pharmacologic choices or predicted pharmacokinetics

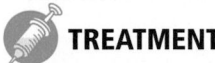

## TREATMENT

### INITIAL STABILIZATION/THERAPY
- Preparation:
  - Place in monitored area where resuscitation procedures may be initiated and monitored.
  - Apply cardiorespiratory monitor, pulse oximeter, and BP monitor.
  - Test laryngoscope blade:
    ○ Adult: no. 3 or no. 4 Macintosh (curved) blade
    ○ Child <8 yr: no. 2 Miller or Macintosh blade depending on preference
    ○ Term infant: no. 1 Miller (straight) blade
    ○ Premature infant: no. 0 Miller blade

- Obtain endotracheal tube (ETT):
  - Adult man: 7.5–8.5 Fr
  - Adult woman: 7.0–8.0 Fr
  - Infants and children: Recommended to use cuffed ETT over the uncuffed tubes of traditional training:
    ○ Size of ETT is most accurate using length-based resuscitation body tapes (Broselow)
  - Infants/children for *cuffed* ETT: (age in years/4) + 3, or length-based (use Broselow tape)
  - Infants/children for *uncuffed* (if only one available) ETT (age in years/4) + 4, or length-based (use Broselow tape).
- Check the balloon of the ETT by inflating, looking for leaks, and then deflating.
- Use stylet for ETT; do not extend beyond distal ETT to avoid soft tissue injury.
- End-tidal $CO_2$ monitor or colorimetric device for ETT verification
- At bedside:
  - Bag-valve mask with functioning high-flow oxygen
  - Functioning suction with Yankhauer tip
- Establish 2 IV lines:
  - 10-mL syringe
  - Water-soluble lubricant
  - Tape or commercial ETT securing device
  - Crash cart

### ALERT
- There must always be an anticipated backup airway management plan to manage unanticipated problems. Backup plans vary with the clinical situation and the availability of devices. A surgical backup tray should always be accessible.
- Assemble appropriate medicines and draw up and label ideally in color-coded manner.

### ED TREATMENT/PROCEDURES
- Preoxygenation:
  - Oxygen in a nonrebreathing mask at 15 L/min for 5 min:
    ○ Allows 3–5 min before desaturation <90% occurs.
    ○ 8 maximal inspirations with 100% oxygen are almost as effective in a cooperative patient.

### ALERT
Physiologically stressed patients may have much less reserve, so that oxygen desaturation may occur much more quickly than expected.

- Do **not** bag, as inflation of stomach increases aspiration risk.
- Pretreatment (3 min before paralytic):
  - Vecuronium (defasciculating dose) or rocuronium
  - Atropine:
    ○ For children <5 yr
    ○ Before succinylcholine administration
  - Lidocaine:
    ○ Increased intracranial pressure (ICP)
    ○ Ocular trauma
    ○ History of reactive airway disease
  - Fentanyl: Reduces reflex sympathetic response, which may be useful for increased ICP

### Pediatric Considerations
Opioids are generally not recommended for children, as sedatives used for induction rapidly cause loss of consciousness and children are more sensitive to hypotension and respiratory depression.

- Induction and paralysis:
  - Induction agent immediately before paralytic agent:
    ○ Etomidate: Minimal hemodynamic effects and is neuroprotective; therefore, best for hypotensive and head-injured patients
    ○ Thiopental: Neuroprotective, so good for increased ICP; may cause hypotension, so use in hemodynamically stable patients
    ○ Ketamine: Preserves airway reflexes, causes catecholamine release, analgesia, and bronchodilation: Good for hypotension and reactive airways disease; caution if hypertension or ischemic heart disease
    ○ Propofol: Limited usefulness in rapid sequence intubation due to vasodilation and myocardial depression and may lead to hypotension and reduced cerebral perfusion
  - Paralytic agent:
    ○ Succinylcholine: Depolarizing agent with rapid onset and short duration makes for ideal paralytic; avoid in ocular trauma, hyperkalemia, 2 days after severe crush injury/burn, or in congenital neuromuscular disorders; if contraindication present, use nondepolarizing agent.
    ○ Succinylcholine can lead to profound bradycardia and sometimes asystole in children, especially if repeated doses are administered; pretreatment with atropine is recommended before succinylcholine in children <5 yr old
    ○ Alternative (nondepolarizing) agents to be used if contraindication to succinylcholine (see below): Rocuronium (most recommended) and vecuronium.
  - Immediately apply cricoid pressure and release only after successful intubation.
  - Position the patient:
    ○ If no suspicion of a cervical spine injury, position the patient in the optimum "sniffing" position (neck flexed forward on shoulders, extended head at atlanto-occipital joint).
    ○ If suspicion of cervical spine injury, an assistant should provide manual in-line stabilization while removing the anterior portion of the cervical spine collar.
- Placement of ETT:
  - Intubate the trachea 1 min after succinylcholine administration.
  - For Macintosh blade:
    ○ Holding the laryngoscope in the left hand, sweep the patient's tongue up and to the left and into the space between the base of the tongue and the epiglottis, which should allow visualization of the glottis and vocal cords.
  - For Miller blade:
    ○ Insert the blade completely, and slowly withdraw blade to allow the airway to fall into view as the epiglottis is held out of the way.
    ○ Lift handle anteriorly and inferiorly to elevate the mandible, tongue, and epiglottis.

- Do not rotate or "crank" on the laryngoscope, or the blade may break the teeth.
- Place tube through vocal cords with direct visualization of glottis.
- Limit attempts to <30 sec and ventilate briefly with bag-valve mask between attempts.
- After placement, cuff should be inflated and placement confirmed with symmetric chest expansion, equal breath sounds bilaterally, end-tidal $CO_2$ monitor (either colorimetric or quantitative), and chest radiograph.
- Secure the ETT with tape or a proprietary tube-holder device.
- Administer adequate sedation and neuromuscular relaxation as necessary.
- Place nasogastric tube to decompress the stomach.
- Special clinical situations:
  - Head injury or penetrating globe injury:
    o Prevent ICP rise: Lidocaine, vecuronium (defasciculating dose) fentanyl to prevent sympathetic discharge.
    o Prevent vagally stimulated bradycardia with atropine.
    o Sedation with etomidate *or* thiopental (if hemodynamically stable)
    o Muscle relaxants/paralytic agents: succinylcholine *or* vecuronium
  - Status asthmaticus: Use ketamine to sedate.
  - Status epilepticus: Use thiopental to sedate (raises seizure threshold) if hemodynamically stable.
  - Multiple trauma/hemorrhagic shock: Use etomidate to sedate.

## MEDICATION
- Atropine: 0.02 mg/kg IV (min dose 0.1 mg to max dose 4 mg):
  - Onset: <1 min
  - Indications:
    o For pediatric intubations in children <5 yr to prevent bradycardia/asystole in patients who receive succinylcholine as a paralytic agent.
- Etomidate: 0.3 mg/kg IV:
  - Onset: 15–45 sec
  - Duration of action: 5 min
  - Indications:
    o For hemodynamically unstable patients of cardiac and hypovolemic etiologies
    o Asthmatics, as it does not release histamine
  - Cautions:
    o Partial seizures (*not* generalized)
    o Nausea and vomiting, myoclonus
    o Patients who have *preexisting* adrenal suppression
- Fentanyl: 3 $\mu$g/kg over 30–60 sec IV:
  - Onset: <90 sec
  - Duration: 20–30 min
  - Indication: Increased ICP or cardiovascular disease that may be exacerbated by elevations of blood pressure
  - Cautions:
    o Respiratory depression (reversed with naloxone 2 mg [adults] or 0.1 mg/kg [ped])
    o Hypotension in hypovolemia
    o "Rigid chest" syndrome, in which patient becomes apneic and cannot be ventilated usually as result of high doses and rapid administration in children. Administration of paralytic is required to intubate.

- Ketamine: 1–2 mg/kg IV:
  - Onset: 30–45 sec
  - Duration: 10–20 min
  - Indication: Preserves respiratory drive, causes sympathetic stimulation and brochodilates, so good for "awake" intubations if concern of difficult airway, hypotension, and asthma.
  - Cautions:
    o Head trauma (increases ICP)
    o Ischemic heart disease (increases BP, heart rate, and myocardial oxygen demand)
    o Emergence reactions
- Lidocaine: 1.5 mg/kg IV:
  - Onset: 1–3 min
  - Duration: 20 min
  - Indication: Attenuate rise in airway pressure (asthma) and ICP (increased ICP)
  - Cautions:
    o Absolute contraindication: High-grade heart block (Mobitz II or third degree) without a functioning pacemaker
- Propofol: 1.5–3.0 mg/kg IV:
  - Onset: 15–45 sec
  - Duration: 5–10 min
  - Indications: Reduces airway resistance and neuroinhibitory effects, so good for asthma and intracranial pathology
  - Cautions: Myocardial depressant and peripheral vasodilation, which can cause precipitous drop in BP (potential worse neurologic outcome), so limited usefulness as induction agent
- Rocuronium: 1.0 mg/kg IV:
  - Onset: 45–60 sec
  - Duration: 30–45 min
  - Indications: When succinylcholine is contraindicated as paralytic agent in ocular trauma, in hyperkalemia, 2 days after crush or burn injury, or in malignant hyperthermia
  - Cautions: Tachycardia and, if hepatic pathology, may have prolonged action
- Succinylcholine: 1.5 mg/kg IV (2.0 mg/kg in infants and young children):
  - Onset: <1 min
  - Duration: 3–8 min
  - Indication: Paralytic of choice due to rapid onset and short duration of onset
  - Contraindications:
    o Malignant hyperthermia
    o Hyperkalemia (renal failure, burns or crush injury >72 hrs old, or rhabdomyolysis)
    o Neuromuscular disease involving denervation
  - Cautions:
    o Bradycardia/potential asystole in children, especially if repeat dosing required, necessitating pretreatment with atropine
- Thiopental: 3.0–5.0 mg/kg IV:
  - Onset: 30–60 sec
  - Duration: 5–10 min
  - Indications: Increased ICP in hemodynamically stable patients
  - Cautions:
    o Hypotension
    o Laryngospasm
    o Bronchospasm via histamine release

- Vecuronium:
  - Defasciculating dose: 1 mg (adults), 0.01 mg/kg (pediatric) to max 1 mg
  - Intubating dose: 0.15 mg/kg
  - Onset: 75–90 sec
  - Duration: 25–40 min
  - Indications: When succinylcholine is contraindicated (see succinylcholine)
  - Cautions: Predicted difficult airway due to prolonged duration of action; prolonged recovery time

## PEARLS AND PITFALLS
- Not being aggressive in airway management early can lead to loss of airway and significant morbidity and mortality.
- Always have a backup airway management plan if unsuccessful with first method.
- Proper patient positioning facilitates intubation.
- Using only sedatives for intubation leads to inadequate visualization and conditions as well as increases risk of aspiration.
- Verification of successful ETT placement requires an end-tidal $CO_2$ detector in either a colorimetric or quantitative manner.
- Physical examination for ETT placement verification is notoriously inaccurate.

## ADDITIONAL READING
- American Heart Association. Part 12. Pediatric advanced life support. *Circulation* 2005;112: 167–187.
- Braude D. *Rapid sequence intubation and rapid sequence airway.* 2nd ed. Albuquerque, NM: University of New Mexico School of Medicine; 2009.
- Walls RM, Murphy MF. *Manual of emergency airway management.* 3rd ed. Philadelphia: Lippincott Williams & Wilkins; 2008.

## See Also (Topic, Algorithm, Electronic Media Element)
Airway Management

# RASH

*Richard E. Wolfe*
*J. Scott Goudie*

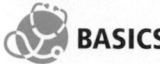 **BASICS**

## DESCRIPTION

- Abnormal skin lesions due to an inflammatory reaction that can be classified into patterns with distinctive clinical features
- Papulosquamous:
  - Papules and scaly desquamation of the skin
  - Lesions may also be red and macular.
  - Classified into psoriasiform, pityriasiform, lichenoid, annular, and erythroderma
- Eczematous:
  - Allergic response secondary to histamine release
  - Acute eczema is an oozing vesicular rash.
  - In subacute eczema, the vesicles have crusted over.
  - In chronic eczema, there is lichenification, hyperpigmentation, and scaling.
- Erythema:
  - Vascular dilatation of the superficial vessels leading to red macular lesions
  - Toxic erythema:
    ○ Diffuse red blanchable rash
  - Figurate erythema:
    ○ Erythema classified by its particular shape
    ○ Erythema chronicum migrans is a large red ring that arises around a tick bite and spreads outward.
    ○ Erythema annulare centrifugum are usually multiple red-ringed lesions; often plaques with central clearing.
    ○ Erythema marginatum are multiple red, slightly indurated evanescent plaques that migrate up to 1 cm/h.
    ○ Erythema gyratum repens is a rare rash with scaly red plaques in zebra-like bands.
    ○ Erythema multiforme is an acute reaction in which red papules with dusky centers appear on the body and mucous membranes.
  - Urticaria
- Vesicobullous lesions:
  - Fluid-filled swelling of the skin
  - Formed by disruption of epidermal/dermal integrity and filling with exudative fluid
- Purpura and petechiae:
  - Failure of normal vascular integrity/hemostatic mechanisms
  - Raised purpura often indicates vasculitis rather than thrombocytopenia.
- Nodules:
  - Secondary to prolonged inflammatory response
  - Histocytic granulomatous:
    ○ "Apple jelly" appearance when pressed with glass slide

## ETIOLOGY

- Papulosquamous:
  - Psoriasiform:
    ○ Psoriasis
    ○ Seborrheic dermatitis
    ○ Mycosis fungoides
  - Pityriasiform:
    ○ Pityriasis rosea
    ○ Secondary syphilis
    ○ Tinea versicolor
  - Lichenoid:
    ○ Lichen planus
    ○ Drug-induced
  - Annular:
    ○ Tinea
  - Erythroderma:
    ○ Psoriasis
    ○ Seborrheic dermatitis
    ○ Mycosis fungoides
    ○ Lymphoma of the skin
- Diffusely erythematous rashes:
  - Viral exanthema
  - Drug reaction
  - Scarlatiniform rash:
    ○ Scarlet fever
    ○ Staphylococcal scalded skin syndrome
    ○ Toxic shock syndrome
    ○ Kawasaki syndrome
    ○ Toxic shock syndrome (TSS)
- Figurate erythema:
  - Erythema chronicum migrans:
    ○ Lyme disease
  - Erythema annulare centrifugum:
    ○ Infections
    ○ Ingestants
    ○ Underlying malignancy
  - Erythema marginatum:
    ○ Rheumatic fever
  - Erythema gyratum repens:
    ○ Underlying malignancy
  - Erythema multiforme:
    ○ *Mycoplasma pneumoniae*
    ○ Herpes simplex
    ○ Drug reaction leading to Steven-Johnson syndrome
  - Urticaria:
    ○ Allergic reaction from drugs, food, infection, pressure, heat, or cold
- Vesicobullous lesions:
  - Stevens-Johnson syndrome
  - Toxic epidermal necrolysis
  - Pemphigus vulgaris fulminant
  - Bullous pemphigoid
  - Smallpox
  - Disseminated herpes simplex
  - Herpes zoster
  - Varicella
  - Vaccinia
- Purpura and petechiae:
  - Meningococcemia
  - Gonococcemia
  - Pneumococcemia
  - DIC
  - Rocky Mountain spotted fever (RMSF):
    ○ Pronounced prodrome of fever, headache, myalgia, rash, peripheral moves to palms/soles, systemic

- Ecthyma gangrenosum:
  ○ *Pseudomonas* infections in critically ill and immunocompromised patients
- Babesiosis: Similar to RMSF, rash less often, frequent coinfection with Lyme
- Henoch-Schönlein purpura
- Multiple systemic illnesses (see chapter on Purpura)
- Nodules:
  - Histocytic granulomatous:
    ○ Sarcoid
    ○ Necrobiosis lipoidica diabeticorum
    ○ Leprosy
    ○ Tuberculosis
  - Generalized exfoliative erythroderma
  - Lupus
  - Cutaneous T-cell lymphoma

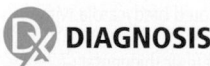 **DIAGNOSIS**

## SIGNS AND SYMPTOMS

### History

- Age of patient
- Immune status (HIV, chemotherapy, diabetes, steroids)
- Previous episodes/prior history of lesions/reactions
- Sick contacts
- Chronologic and physical evolution
- Associated symptoms:
  - Pruritus
  - Fever
  - Abdominal pain
  - Myalgias/arthralgias
- Prodromal symptoms:
  - Fever
  - Headache
  - Cough
  - Odynophagia
  - Rhinorrhea
- Environmental exposure:
  - Tick bite
  - Unusual flora
  - Diet
  - Travel
- Recent change in medication
- Family history

### Physical Exam

- Distribution of the rash:
  - Characterized as central/peripheral, confluent/scattered, mucosal/nonmucosal, presence of palm/sole involvement
- Primary lesion appearance:
  - Macule:
    ○ Nonraised areas of distinct coloration
    ○ Blanching lesions are inflammatory; nonblanching lesions are either altered pigmentation or petechiae/purpura.

- Papule:
  - Raised, palpable lesions <5 mm in diameter, not fluid-filled
  - Hemorrhagic, nonblanching lesions palpable purpura
- Vesicles:
  - Small, raised, clear fluid-filled lesions (<5 mm)
- Bullae:
  - Large, raised, clear fluid-filled lesions (>5 mm)
- Pustules:
  - As vesicles and bullae, but containing purulent fluid
- Nodule:
  - Solid, raised lesion >5 mm seated in deeper layer of skin and tissue
- Secondary changes:
  - Scaling, lichenification, excoriation, fissuring all result from manipulation/scratching or proliferation/shedding of epidermal cells.
  - Erosions/ulcers from varying degrees of tissue loss (superficial to deep) from loss of vascular supply/tissue integrity
- Associated signs/symptoms:
  - Pruritus associated with allergic reactions, systemic and contact
  - Fever with infection/drug reaction/systemic inflammatory response, viral exanthema common in children
- Assess severity of systemic signs:
  - Abnormal vital signs, airway compromise, respiratory distress, hemodynamic instability

## ESSENTIAL WORKUP
- Identify systemic illness
- Signs/symptoms of local infectious source
- Categorize the lesions and type of rash

## DIAGNOSTIC TESTS & INTERPRETATION
### Lab
- Presence of fever, systemic symptoms, or possible infection warrants blood work:
  - CBC with differential, electrolytes, BUN/creatinine Blood cultures, viral cultures
  - Gram stain and culture of purulent lesions
- Tzanck smear for suspected herpetic lesions
- Venereal disease research laboratory (VDRL) or/rapid plasma reagin (RPR) for suspected syphilis
- Suspected autoimmune disorders:
  - CBC
  - ESR
  - Particular assays in consultation with a rheumatologist (ANA, antineutrophil cytoplasmic antibody)
- Petechiae/purpura:
  - CBC with platelets
  - Partial thromboplastin time, prothrombin time, INR
  - Disseminated intravascular coagulation (DIC) screen: Fibrinogen, fibrin split products, haptoglobin, LDH

### Diagnostic Procedures/Surgery
- In febrile and seriously ill patients, suspected sepsis lesions may be opened and sent for cultures.
- Nikolsky test: Expansion of bullous lesion with lateral stress at margin indicates epidermal/dermal disruptive process
- Scrapings: Indicated to rule out topical fungal infections and parasites:
  - Potassium hydroxide preparation from edge of lesion reveal hyphae
  - Plain mineral oil to rule out scabies in pruritic linear lesions of hands
- Biopsy under dermatologic consultation to differentiate allergic/autoimmune/infectious processes

## DIFFERENTIAL DIAGNOSIS
See "Etiology."

 **TREATMENT**

### PRE-HOSPITAL
Universal precautions, masks if infectious etiology suspected

### INITIAL STABILIZATION/THERAPY
Aggressive, presumptive management of potentially lethal presentations:
- Petechial lesions
- Disseminated erythematous or vesicobullous lesions

### ED TREATMENT/PROCEDURES
- Treatment directed by underlying cause
- Immediate empiric antibiotics targeted towards meningococcemia and Rocky Mountain spotted fever in unstable patients with fever and purpura
- Treat disseminated bullous or exfoliative disease as a severe thermal burn.
- Symptomatic treatment of pruritus (diphenhydramine or hydroxyzine)
- Steroid therapy reserved for clear allergic reactions, relapse of known steroid responsive disease, or in consultation with dermatologist
- Allergic reactions:
  - Diphenhydramine
  - H2-blocker
  - Steroids
  - Epinephrine if respiratory compromise

### MEDICATION
- Acetaminophen: 625 mg PO/PR q4–6h (peds: 60 mg/kg/24h)
- Diphenhydramine: 50 mg PO/IM/IV q6h (peds: 5 mg/kg/24h)
- Hydroxyzine: 25–100 mg PO q6h (peds: 50 mg/24h)
- Methylprednisolone: 125 mg IV q24h (peds: 0.5–2 mg/kg/24h)

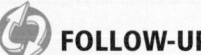 **FOLLOW-UP**

## DISPOSITION
### Admission Criteria
- Patients with significant bullous/exfoliative disorders
- Associated systemic symptoms

### Discharge Criteria
- Limited lesions
- Viral exanthems
- Absence of systemic signs or symptoms

### Issues for Referral
Discharge to follow-up with primary care physician or dermatologist

## FOLLOW-UP RECOMMENDATIONS
- Reassure patients that rashes that cannot be diagnosed in the ED are often due to a mild viral illnesses or allergic reactions
- Stress the importance, however, of a follow-up visit with their physician or a dermatologist to obtain the best possible outcome.
- The patient should see his doctor quickly or return to the ED if the condition worsens:
  - Spreading redness from the rash
  - Increasing pain from the rash
  - Joint pain
  - Spreading of the rash with crusting
  - Fever
  - Severe headache
  - Confusion
  - Signs of a life-threatening allergic reaction:
    - Feeling dizzy or faint
    - Trouble breathing or swallowing
    - Swelling of the tongue

## PEARLS AND PITFALLS
- Treat rapidly with empiric antibiotics in patients with purpura and fever to cover for meningococcemia and Rocky Mountain spotted fever.
- Hyperpigmented scaly papules on the palms and soles require that secondary syphilis be ruled out.

## ADDITIONAL READING
- Brady WJ, DeBehnke D, Crosby DL. Dermatological emergencies. *Am J Emerg Med.* 1994;12(2): 217–237.
- Browne BJ, Edwards B, Rogers RL. Dermatologic emergencies. *Prim Care.* 2006;33(3):685–695, vi.
- Gropper CA. An approach to clinical dermatologic diagnosis based on morphologic reaction patterns. *Clin Cornerstone.* 2001;4(1):1–14.

**See Also (Topic, Algorithm, Electronic Media Element)**
Purpura

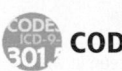 **CODES**

### ICD9
782.1 Rash and other nonspecific skin eruption

# RASH, PEDIATRIC

*Bruce Webster*

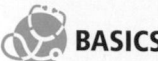 **BASICS**

## DESCRIPTION

- Lesion morphology:
  - Macule:
    - Localized nonpalpable changes in skin color
    - Purpura or petechiae (nonblanching with pressure)
  - Maculopapule:
    - Slightly elevated lesions with localized changes in skin
  - Papule:
    - Solid, elevated lesions <5 mm in diameter
    - Keratotic (rough-surfaced lesion)
    - Nonkeratotic (smooth lesion)
    - Palpable purpura (nonblanching with pressure)
  - Plaque:
    - Solid, elevated lesions >5 mm in diameter
    - Often results from a confluence of papules
  - Nodule:
    - Solid, elevated lesions extending deep into the dermis or subcutaneous tissue >5 mm in diameter
  - Wheal:
    - Circular, irregular lesions varying from red to pale
  - Vesicle:
    - Clear, fluid-filled lesions <5 mm in diameter
  - Bullae:
    - Clear, fluid-filled lesions >5 mm in diameter
  - Pustules:
    - Pus-filled lesions
- Secondary lesions:
  - Scales:
    - Thin plates of dried cornified epithelium partially separated from the epidermis
  - Lichenification:
    - Dried plaques resulting in skin furrowing
  - Erosion:
    - Moist surface uncovered by rupture of vesicles or bullae
  - Excoriation:
    - Linear loss of the skin secondary to trauma
  - Ulcer:
    - Deep loss of the skin involving the epidermis and a variable amount of the dermis and subcutaneous tissue
- Configuration:
  - Circles or arcs
  - Serpiginous (creeping or wormlike)
  - Iris grouping (bull's eye appearance)
  - Irregular grouping
  - Zosteriform grouping
  - Linear grouping
  - Retiform grouping
- The color of a lesion or the entire skin may be due to a number of substances:
  - Red or red-brown lesions result from oxyhemoglobin found in RBCs.
  - The macular erythematous lesions seen in viral exanthema usually represent dilated superficial cutaneous vessels.
  - Purpura and petechiae result from leakage of RBCs out of the vascular space.

- Hypopigmentation or hyperpigmentation represent postinflammatory change from either increases or decreases in melanin production.
- Depigmentation refers to the total loss of pigment secondary to autoimmune effect (vitiligo) or in congenital disorders from a genetic inability to produce melanin (albinism).
- Scales represent a proliferative disorder of epidermal cell turnover.

## ETIOLOGY

- Papulosquamous:
  - Infections:
    - Viral or bacterial
    - Rickettsial or fungal
  - Allergic reactions
  - Autoimmune disorders
- Purpura and petechiae:
  - Clotting or platelet disorder
  - Vascular fragility disease
  - Vasculitis
  - Overwhelming infection
- Vesicobullous:
  - Infection
  - Drug reaction
  - Autoimmune disorder
- Ulcer:
  - Infection
  - Vascular insufficiency

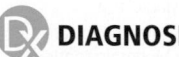 **DIAGNOSIS**

## SIGNS AND SYMPTOMS

- Fever (consider infectious exanthemas)
- Pruritus
- Joint pain
- Abdominal pain
- Heart murmur

### History

Obtain a detailed history:

- Age group: Conditions, distribution, and appearance may vary with age
- Development, progression, pattern and duration of the rash
- Lesions synchronous or asynchronous
- Associated symptoms
- Prodromes—cough, rhinorrhea, pharyngitis, fever, meningismal symptoms, pruritus
- Family history, exposures, immunizations
- Generic dermatoses
- Atopic dermatitis
- Psoriasis

### Physical Exam

- Cardiac:
  - Murmurs/rubs
- Pulmonary:
  - Crackles/wheezing
- Abdominal:
  - Tenderness
  - Hepatosplenomegaly
- Skin:
  - See "Essential Workup."

## ESSENTIAL WORKUP

Classify the rash based on the primary lesions:

- Papulosquamous
- Vesicobullous
- Purpuric

## DIAGNOSTIC TESTS & INTERPRETATION

### Lab

- Indicated if the rash is purpuric:
  - CBC with platelet count
  - Bleeding screen (prothrombin test, partial thromboplastin time, bleeding time, disseminated intravascular coagulation [DIC] screen)
- Indicated if fever present:
  - CBC
  - Electrolytes, BUN, creatinine to evaluate dehydration and scarlatiniform rash (exclude glomerulonephritis)
  - Viral culture and titers for suspected exanthems
  - Bacterial blood cultures for suspected systemic bacterial infection
- Lumbar puncture if meningococcus or other meningitides or encephalitis suspected

### Imaging

- Chest radiograph for suspected pulmonary involvement
- Potassium hydroxide (KOH) preparations:
  - Indicated with scaling lesions to differentiate dermatophytosis from nummular eczema and pityriasis rosea
  - Superficial scale sample from active border of lesion removed from the skin with a scalpel or the edge of a glass slide
  - Place on a slide and add 1 drop of 10% KOH.
  - Place a coverslip and heat slowly without boiling. Allow to set for a few minutes and scan for hyphae.
- Wood lamp:
  - Useful in dermatophytosis and erythrasma
- Scabies preparations:
  - Most of the mite population resides on the hands and feet.
  - Place a drop of mineral oil on the lesion. Scrape with a no. 15 blade to produce speck of blood.
  - Examine under low power for the mite, ova, larva, or fecal matter.

## DIFFERENTIAL DIAGNOSIS

**Maculopapular rash:**

- Solid, skin colored, or yellow:
  - Keratotic
  - Wart
  - Corn or callus
  - Nonkeratotic
  - Molluscum contagiosum
  - Sebaceous cyst
  - Basal and squamous cell carcinoma
  - Nevi
- Solid, brown:
  - Café au lait patch
  - Nevi
  - Freckle
  - Melanoma
  - Photoallergic/phototoxic drug eruption
  - Tinea nigra palmaris hypopigmentation

- Solid, red, nonscaling:
  – Nonpurpuric
  – Exanthems
  – Rubeola, rubella, or roseola
  – Scarlet fever
  – Toxin-producing staphylococcal or streptococcal disease
  – Erythema infectiosum ("fifth disease")
  – Rubella-like rash (echoviruses, Coxsackie A viruses)
  – Varicella (early manifestations)
  – Variola (smallpox: Early manifestations)
  – Epstein-Barr virus
  – Enterovirus or adenovirus
  – *Mycoplasma*
  – Kawasaki disease
  – Erythema multiforme
  – Localized, pruriginous
  – Insect bites
  – Scabies
  – Allergic or irritant contact dermatitis
  – Purpuric
  – Bacteremia sepsis
  – Meningococcemia, pneumococcemia, gonococcemia, *Haemophilus influenzae*
  – Endocarditis
  – Plague
  – DIC
  – Rocky Mountain spotted fever (RMSF)
  – Henoch-Schönlein purpura
  – Idiopathic thrombocytopenic purpura
  – Leukemia
  – Underlying bleeding disorder
  – Ecthyma gangrenosum
  – Rarely, pityriasis rosea
- Solid, red, scaling:
  – Without epithelial disruption:
    ○ Tinea corporis, capitis, pedis, or cruris
    ○ Pityriasis rosea
    ○ Secondary syphilis
    ○ Lupus erythematosus
  – With epithelial disruption:
    ○ Papular urticaria
    ○ Eczema
    ○ Seborrheic, diaper, contact, or stasis dermatitis
    ○ Impetigo
    ○ Candidiasis
    ○ Tinea corporis, capitis, pedis, or cruris
    ○ Vesiculobullous rash
    ○ Herpes virus: Varicella, variola (smallpox)
    ○ Herpes simplex/zoster
    ○ Hand-foot-and-mouth syndrome
    ○ Scabies
    ○ Drug hypersensitivity, toxic epidermal necrolysis
    ○ Staphylococcal scalded skin syndrome (SSS)
    ○ Impetigo, bullous impetigo
    ○ Cat-scratch disease
    ○ Dermatitis herpetiformis
    ○ Eczema
    ○ Erythema multiforme
    ○ Lichen planus
- Pustular:
  - Acne
  - Folliculitis
  - Candidiasis
  - Gonococcemia
  - Meningococcemia
  - With Fever, consider:
    – Infection
    – Drug reaction
    – Systemic inflammatory disease (juvenile rheumatoid arthritis, systematic lupus erythematosus, etc.)

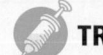 **TREATMENT**

**PRE-HOSPITAL**

Field management is indicated when there are signs of systemic instability:

- Airway management using precautions to avoid exposure to respiratory secretions; IV access
- Identify rashes with a potentially life-threatening illness or need for special isolation.

**INITIAL STABILIZATION/THERAPY**

- Aggressive, empiric management of children with a purpuric rash associated with fever or unstable vital signs:
  – Airway support, IV access, pressors if cardiovascular collapse
  – IV antibiotics should be administered as soon as possible:
    ○ Cefotaxime or ceftriaxone
    ○ Plus doxycycline if RMSF is considered
- Fluid resuscitation as if burn with SSS or toxic epidermal necrolysis

**ED TREATMENT/PROCEDURES**

- Specific ED treatment should be directed to the underlying etiology.
- Diphenhydramine should be used when an allergic reaction is suspected.

**MEDICATION**

- Acetaminophen: 10–15 mg/kg PO/PR q4–6h
- Cefotaxime: 50 mg/kg IV q6h; max dose, 12 g/24 hr
- Ceftriaxone: 50 mg/kg IV q12h; max dose, 4 g/24 hr
- Diphenhydramine: 1.25 mg/kg PO/IM/IV q6h
- RSMF:
  – Doxycycline: 100 mg PO/IV q12h (>8 yr) or chloramphenicol: 12.5 mg/kg/dose q6h (max 500 mg/dose)
- Kawasaki disease:
  – Immune globulin: 2 g/kg IV over 10–12 hr and aspirin: 25 mg/kg/dose PO q6h
- Varicella:
  – Acyclovir: 800 mg PO q.i.d. (peds: 20 mg/kg/dose) with pulmonary or CNS involvement; give 10–12 mg/kg/dose IV q8h in the immunocompromised patient; no aspirin should be used.
- Toxic shock syndrome or SSS:
  – Clindamycin: 8–13 mg/kg IV q8h
  – Vancomycin: 10mg/kg IV q6h *if methicillin-resistant Staphylococcus aureus a possibility*
  – Nafcillin or oxacillin: 2 g IV q4h (peds: 200 mg/kg/d IV q4h) *if methicillin-sensitive S. aureus is cause*; alternative: Cefazolin 2 g IV q8h (peds: 100 mg/kg/d IV q8h)
- Scarlet fever:
  – Penicillin V: 500 mg PO q.i.d. (peds: 250 mg PO q.i.d.) for 10 days; alternative: Erythromycin: 250–500 mg PO q.i.d. (peds: 12.5 mg/kg/dose PO q.i.d.) ×10 days, or azithromycin 500 mg PO per day (peds: 12 mg/kg PO per day) for 5 days

 **FOLLOW-UP**

**DISPOSITION**

***Admission Criteria***

- Hospital admission is determined by the underlying disorder.
- Admit life-threatening conditions: Meningococcemia, RMSF, toxic shock syndrome, Kawasaki disease.
- Other illnesses associated with systemic illness or potential deterioration, SSS, rubeola, and varicella, as well as others, may require inpatient care.

***Discharge Criteria***

Discharge instructions should be based on the underlying disorder.

***Issues for Referral***

- Exanthems associated with self-limited entities in stable children.
- Follow-up with primary care physician or dermatologist should be arranged.

**FOLLOW-UP RECOMMENDATIONS**

Patient should return for reevaluation for any rapidly spreading rash, changes in rash morphology, petechiae or hemorrhage, new onset fever or neck stiffness.

## PEARLS AND PITFALLS

- Note where rash first appeared and how it is spreading.
- Note associated signs and symptoms. They are often key for critical illness.
- Keep meningococcemia in mind in any rash with fever.

## ADDITIONAL READING

- Mancini AJ. Childhood exanthems: A primer and update for the dermatologist. *Adv Dermatol.* 2000;16:337.
- Pomeranz AJ. The systematic evaluation of the skin in children. *Pediatr Clin North Am.* 1998;45:49–63.
- Sanfilippo AM, Barrio V, Kulp-Shorten C, et al. Common pediatric and adolescent skin conditions. *J Pediatr Adolesc Gynecol.* 2003;16:269–283
- Stocker JT. Clinical and pathologic differential diagnosis of selected potential bioterrorism agents of interest to pediatric health care providers. *Clin Lab Med.* 2006;26:329–344.

**See Also (Topic, Algorithm, Electronic Media Element)**

- Henoch-Schönlein Purpura
- Kawasaki disease
- Staphylococcal Scalded Skin Syndrome

 **CODES**

**ICD9**
782.1 Rash and other nonspecific skin eruption

# RECTAL PROLAPSE

*Marilyn M. Hallock*

 **BASICS**

## DESCRIPTION

- Full thickness evagination of the rectal wall outside the anal opening
- 3 types of rectal prolapse:
  - Full-thickness prolapse:
    - Protrusion of the rectal wall through the anal canal; the most common
  - Partial thickness or mucosal prolapse:
    - Only mucosal layer protrudes through anus
  - Occult (internal) prolapse or rectal intussusception:
    - Rectal wall prolapse without protrusion through the anus
    - May be difficult to diagnose

## ETIOLOGY

- Cause unclear and multifactorial:
  - Chronic constipation/excessive straining
  - Laxity of sphincter:
    - Pelvic floor trauma/weakness; childbearing
    - Neurologic disease
- More common in women, peak in 7th decade

### Pediatric Considerations

- Very rare after age 4 years
- True rectal prolapse unusual in children; more likely partial or intussusception
- Consider chronic diarrhea, parasites, cystic fibrosis (CF), malnutrition as contributing causes

 **DIAGNOSIS**

## SIGNS AND SYMPTOMS

- Dark red mass protrudes from the rectum
- Possible mucous or bloody discharge
- Sensation of rectal mass
- Tenesmus
- Constipation or incontinence

### History

- History with emphasis on bowel obstruction and duration of prolapse
- Often progressive symptoms over time with self-reducing prolapse initially

### Physical Exam

- Rectal exam must differentiate prolapse from polyps, hemorrhoids, and intussusception.
- True prolapse shows dark red mass at the anal verge with or without mucus; circumferential circular folds in beefy mucosa of protruding rectum.
- Mucosal prolapse rarely > a few centimeters of protrusion; will not contain circular folds of muscular layer
- Internal hemorrhoids identified by folds of mucosa radiating out like spokes in wheel
- Prolapsed polyps and hemorrhoids don't involve the entire rectal mucosa and don't have a hole in the center.
- Intussusception identified by complaints of intermittent, severe abdominal pain; may appear more ill:
  - Examiner's finger can be passed between the apex of the prolapsed bowel and the anal sphincter; whereas, in rectal prolapse the protruding mucosa is continuous with the perianal skin

## ESSENTIAL WORKUP

Careful physical exam

## DIAGNOSTIC TESTS & INTERPRETATION

### Lab

- No lab test necessary for uncomplicated prolapse
- Preoperative testing for incarcerated rectal prolapse, going to OR

### Imaging

No imaging is necessary for uncomplicated prolapse

## DIFFERENTIAL DIAGNOSIS

- Prolapsed internal hemorrhoids
- Prolapsed rectal polyp
- Intussusception
- Other rectal mass

 **TREATMENT**

## PRE-HOSPITAL

- Position of comfort
- Prevent mucosal desiccation with moist gauze.
- Avoid trauma to mucosa.

## INITIAL STABILIZATION/THERAPY

- Stabilization generally not needed in simple prolapse
- Incarcerated or ischemic prolapse:
  - NPO
  - IV fluids
  - Prepare for surgery

## ED TREATMENT/PROCEDURES

Manual reduction of rectal prolapse:

- Place in knee-chest position.
- Apply gentle steady pressure for 5–15 minutes.
- Invert mucosa through lumen from distal.
- Sedation as needed to relax sphincter
- Finger may be placed in rectum to guide reversal of prolapse.

- Prolapse very large or difficult to reduce:
  – Apply 1/2–1 cup sugar to reduce swelling and assist manual reduction
- Prolapse recurs immediately after reduction:
  – Apply pressure dressing with lubricant, gauze, tape; buttock may be taped together for several hours
- If prolapse incarcerated or ischemic, or if manual reduction fails or prolapse frequently recurs:
  – Admission for emergent surgical correction

### ALERT
- Constriction of blood flow to rectum by anal sphincter can lead to ischemia, venous obstruction and thrombosis, full thickness necrosis, possible loss of gut
- Timely reduction decreases risk
- Surgical intervention required for ischemic mucosa
- Most common complication of spontaneous or manual reduction:
  – Localized pain
  – Self-limited mucosal bleeding

### MEDICATION
Sedation and pain medication only as needed

 ## FOLLOW-UP

### DISPOSITION
#### Admission Criteria
- Necrotic or ischemic mucosa
- Inability to reduce acute prolapse or frequently recurs

#### Discharge Criteria
- Reduced rectal prolapse
- Stable and tolerating PO
- Instructions to treat the presumed underlying cause:
  – Correct constipation:
    ○ Stool softeners
    ○ Increase fluid intake
    ○ Increase dietary fiber
  – Avoid prolonged sitting or straining

#### Issues for Referral
Refer for workup including:
- Search for leading lesion
- Refer for definitive surgical repair of recurrent prolapse
- Testing for CF in children

### FOLLOW-UP RECOMMENDATIONS
Colorectal follow-up.

## PEARLS AND PITFALLS

- Perform careful physical exam to differential rectal prolapsed from polyps, hemorrhoids, and intussuscepted bowel.
- For large or difficult to reduce rectal prolapsed, apply sugar to reduce swelling and assist in manual reduction.

### ADDITIONAL READING
- Bartolo DC. Rectal prolapse. *Br J Surg*. 1996;83(1):3–5.
- Coburn WM 3rd, Russell MA, Hofstetter WL. Sucrose as an aid to manual reduction of incarcerated rectal prolapse. *Ann Emerg Med*. 1997;30(3):347–349.
- Gourgiotis S, Baratsis S. Rectal prolapse. *Int J Colorectal Dis*. 2007;22(3):231–243.
- Kairaluoma MV, Kellokumpu IH. Epidemiologic aspects of complete rectal prolapse. *Scand J Surg*. 2005;94(3):207–210.
- Madiba TE, Baig MK, Wexner SD. Surgical management of rectal prolapse. *Arch Surg*. 2005;140(1):63–73.

### See Also (Topic, Algorithm, Electronic Media Element)
Hemorrhoid

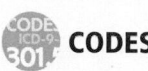 ## CODES

**ICD9**
569.1 Rectal prolapse

R

# RECTAL TRAUMA

*Elaine Sapiro*

## 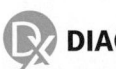 BASICS

### DESCRIPTION
- Injury to rectal mucosa
- Simple contusion to full-thickness laceration with extension into peritoneum or perineum
- 2/3 of rectum is extraperitoneal.

### ETIOLOGY
- Penetrating trauma:
  - Gunshot wounds: 80% penetrating rectal trauma
  - Knife wounds
  - Impalement injuries
- Blunt trauma:
  - Motor vehicle accidents
  - Waterskiing and watercraft accidents:
    - Hydrostatic pressure injury
  - Pelvic fractures:
    - Bony fragments penetrate rectum
- Foreign body:
  - Autoeroticism
  - Anal intercourse
  - Assault
  - Ingestion of sharp objects
- Iatrogenic trauma: Most common cause of rectal injury:
  - Barium enema:
    - Perforation occurs in 0.04% patients
    - 50% mortality
  - Colonoscopy:
    - 0.2% perforation rate
    - Increased risk with polopectomy
  - Hemorrhoidectomy
  - Urologic and ob-gyn procedures:
    - Episiotomy

### Pediatric Considerations
- Rectal injury may result from thermometer insertion.
- Any rectal trauma in young children should raise the suspicion of nonaccidental trauma.

## 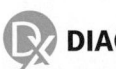 DIAGNOSIS

### SIGNS AND SYMPTOMS
- Perineal, anal, or lower abdominal pain
- Signs of perforation or peritonitis:
  - Guarding
  - Rebound tenderness
  - Fever
- Rectal bleeding
- Obstipation
- Presence of pelvic fracture
- History of anal manipulation, foreign-body insertion, sexual abuse

### History
- Time and mechanism of injury
- Suspect rectal injury in all patients with gunshot wound, stab wound, or impalement injury to trunk, buttocks, perineum, or upper thigh.
- Consider in any patient with history of anal manipulation complaining of lower abdominal or pelvic pain.

### Physical Exam
- Inspect and palpate thoroughly buttocks, anus, and perineum.
- Identify entrance and exit wounds if penetrating trauma.
- Perform digital rectal exam:
  - Assess for gross blood or guaiac-positive stool
  - Note position of prostate
- Assess perineal integrity:
  - Speculum and bimanual exam in all female patients
  - Thorough genitourinary exam in all male patients, including prostate exam

### ESSENTIAL WORKUP
- Labs: CBC, urinalysis
- Acute abdominal series
- CT abdomen and pelvis if blunt trauma
- Sigmoidoscopy: Following extraction of foreign body
- Evidentiary exam: Required in cases of sexual assault

### DIAGNOSTIC TESTS & INTERPRETATION
#### Lab
- CBC:
  - Blood loss
  - Leukocytosis/bandemia suggesting peritonitis
- Type and screen:
  - If evidence of hemorrhage
- Urinalysis:
  - Evaluate for fecal matter

#### Imaging
- Supine/upright abdominal films, pelvic radiographs:
  - Evaluate for pneumoperitoneum or extraperitoneal and extrarectal densities suggesting perforation.
  - Identify location, size, and shape of foreign body.
  - Identify pelvic fracture or diastasis of symphysis pubis, which may accompany rectal injury.
- CT abdomen and pelvis

#### Diagnostic Procedures/Surgery
- Retrograde urethrogram if high-riding prostate noted on rectal exam
- Contrast enema helpful only in situations where perforation is unclear:
  - Water-soluble contrast (eg, gastrografin)

### DIFFERENTIAL DIAGNOSIS
- Colon injuries
- Genitourinary injuries

## 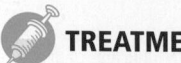 TREATMENT

### PRE-HOSPITAL
- Airway, breathing, and circulation
- Spinal precautions if blunt trauma
- Fluid resuscitation if blood loss, hypotension
- Do not attempt removal of rectal foreign body.
- Control bleeding.

### INITIAL STABILIZATION/THERAPY
Penetrating or blunt abdominal trauma, follow trauma protocols:
- Primary survey
- Resuscitation
- Secondary survey
- Treatment

### ED TREATMENT/PROCEDURES
- Tetanus prophylaxis if needed
- Broad-spectrum antibiotics if significant mucosal disruption or signs of peritonitis are present
- Foley catheter (after excluding urethral injury)
- Rectal foreign body removal in ED:
  - Determine location and type of foreign object
  - Sedation:
    - Avoid conscious sedation if possible
    - Ideally, patient can aid extraction by bearing down during procedure
  - With patient in lithotomy position:
    - Local anesthesia to maximize anal sphincter dilation
    - Gentle digital sphincter dilation
    - Obstetric, ring, or biopsy forceps, tenaculum, or suctioning device to aid extraction
    - Suprapubic pressure
    - Patient Valsalva
  - Foley catheter:
    - Pass above foreign body, inflate balloon, and apply gentle traction to release suction and permit extraction
    - Using 3 catheters, pass each alongside of foreign body, inflate, and gently pull (helpful for smooth objects or if unable to pass Foley above object)
  - Sigmoidoscopy to evaluate mucosal injury following extraction
- Surgical consultation:
  - Peritonitis
  - All traumatic rectal mucosal lacerations
  - Objects >10 cm from anal verge
  - Sharp objects whose removal may provoke mucosal injury
  - Inability to extract foreign body in ED

## MEDICATION

- Antibiotics with coverage against gram-negative and anaerobic organisms:
  - Ampicillin/sulbactam:
    - Adults: 3 g q6h IV (peds: 50 mg/kg IV)
  - Cefotetan:
    - Adults: 2 g q12h IV (peds: 40 mg/kg IV)
  - Cefoxitin:
    - Adults: 2 g q6h IV (peds: 80 mg/kg q6h IV)
  - Piperacillin/tazobactam:
    - Adults: 3.375 g IV (peds: 75 mg/kg IV)
  - Ticarcillin/clavulanate:
    - Adults: 3.1 g IV (peds: 75 mg/kg IV)
- Additional anaerobic coverage:
  - Clindamycin:
    - Adults: 600–900 mg IV (peds: 10 mg/kg IV)
  - Metronidazole:
    - Adults: 1 g IV (peds: 15 mg/kg IV)
- Combination therapy:
  - Adults: Ampicillin 500 mg IV q6h, gentamicin 1–1.7 mg/kg IV, and metronidazole 1 g IV
  - Peds: Ampicillin 50 mg/kg IV q6h, gentamicin 1–1.7 mg/kg IV, and metronidazole 15 mg/kg IV
- Sedation and analgesia:
  - Fentanyl: 2–3 $\mu$g/kg IV (peds and adults)
  - Midazolam: 0.01–0.2 mg/kg IV (peds and adults)
  - Lidocaine: Topical and/or injectable

## SURGERY/OTHER PROCEDURES

- Perforation
- Torn sphincter
- Foreign body:
  - General anesthesia required to remove high-riding or sharp object
  - Laparotomy is last resort

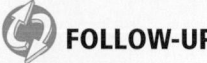 FOLLOW-UP

### DISPOSITION

#### Admission Criteria

- Perforation
- Significant bleeding
- Unstable vital signs
- Abdominal pain
- Torn anal sphincter
- Foreign body that requires extraction in operating room

#### Discharge Criteria

- Stable vital signs
- No abdominal pain
- Normal sigmoidoscopy/anoscopy exam

### FOLLOW-UP RECOMMENDATIONS

- Repeat abdominal exam 12–24 hr
- Return to ER:
  - Abdominal pain
  - Vomiting
  - Fever

## PEARLS AND PITFALLS

- Consider rectal injury in all patients presenting with abdominal pain following lower GI or genitourinary procedure.
- 60% of foreign bodies can be removed in ED.
- Failure to recognize perforation following extraction of foreign body
- Creativity and imagination can aid successful extraction of foreign body in ED.

## ADDITIONAL READING

- Carrillo EH, Somberg LB, Ceballos CE, et al. Blunt traumatic injuries to the colon and rectum. *J Am Coll Surg*. 1996;183:548–552.
- Cleary RK, Pomerantz RA, Lampman RM. Colon and rectal Injuries. *Dis Colon Rectum*. 2006;49(8):1203–1232.
- Coates WC. Anorectum. In: Marx J, ed. *Emergency Medicine: Concepts and Clinical Practice*. 5th ed. St. Louis, MO: Mosby; 2002: 1343–1359.
- Cohen JS, Sackier JM. Management of colorectal foreign bodies. *J R Coll Surg Edinburgh*.1996; 41:312–315.
- Manimaran N, Shorafa M, Eccersley J. Blow as well as pull: An innovative technique for dealing with a rectal foreign body. *Colorectal Dis*. 2009;11: 325–326.

### See Also (Topic, Algorithm, Electronic Media Element)

- Abdominal Trauma, Blunt
- Abdominal Trauma, Imaging
- Abdominal Trauma, Penetrating
- Colon Trauma

 CODES

### ICD9

- 863.45 Injury to rectum without open wound into cavity
- 863.55 Injury to rectum with open wound into cavity

# RED EYE
*Franklin D. Friedman*

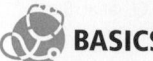 **BASICS**

## DESCRIPTION
- May be caused by almost any eye disorder
- Often benign; may represent systemic disease
- Red eye is due to vascular engorgement of conjunctiva.
- Main causes include inflammatory, allergic, infection, or trauma.
- Conjunctivitis (diffuse injection)

## ETIOLOGY
- Inflammatory:
  - Uveitis:
    ○ Anterior and posterior
  - Iritis (perilimbic injection)
  - Episcleritis (70% are idiopathic)
  - Scleritis (50% associated with systemic disease)
  - Systemic inflammatory reactions
- Allergic:
  - Due to histamine release and increased vascular permeability, resulting in swelling of conjunctiva (chemosis), watery discharge, and pruritus; usually bilateral
- Infectious:
  - Bacterial (purulent mucous discharge), viral (watery or no discharge), or fungal
  - Orbital cellulitis
  - Dacryocystitis
  - Canaliculitis
  - Endophthalmitis
- Traumatic:
  - Corneal abrasion
  - Subconjunctival hemorrhage
  - Foreign body
  - Occult perforation
- Other:
  - Pingueculitis and pterygium
  - Hemorrhage
  - Blepharitis
  - Dry eye syndrome
  - Acute angle-closure glaucoma
  - Ophthalmia neonatorum
  - Conjunctival tumor

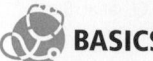 **DIAGNOSIS**

## SIGNS AND SYMPTOMS
### History
- Age (especially neonatal and age >50 yr)
- Time of onset, duration of symptoms
- Exposures (ie, chemicals, allergens)
- Patient's occupation (ie, metal worker)
- Associated signs and symptoms (headache, systemic symptoms, other infections)
- Ocular symptoms:
  - Pain
  - Foreign-body sensation
  - Change in vision
  - Discharge
  - Pruritus
- Contact lens use
- Other comorbidities

### Physical Exam
- Thorough physical exam:
  - Preauricular or submandibular adenopathy
  - Rosacea (may cause blepharitis)
  - Facial or skin lesions (herpes)
- Ophthalmologic:
  - Visual acuity
  - General appearance:
    ○ Universal eye redness or locally
    ○ Conjunctival injection
    ○ Lid involvement
    ○ Purulent or clear discharge
    ○ Obvious foreign body
    ○ Proptosis
    ○ Photophobia
    ○ Eyelash against globe (trichiasis)
  - Pupil exam
  - Confrontational visual field exam
  - Extraocular muscle function
  - Slit-lamp examination with fluorescein:
    ○ Anterior chamber cell or flare
    ○ Corneal abrasion
    ○ Foreign body
  - Lid eversion
  - Fundoscopy and tonometry

## ESSENTIAL WORKUP
- Consider systemic causes of red eye.
- Physical exam as described above.

## DIAGNOSTIC TESTS & INTERPRETATION
Tests should be directed toward the suspected etiology of red eye:
- Dacryocystitis: Culture discharge
- Corneal ulcers: Scrape cornea for culture (often is performed by ophthalmologist)
- Bacterial conjunctivitis:
  - Moderate discharge: Obtain conjunctival swab for routine culture and sensitivity (usually *Staphylococcus aureus*, *Streptococcus*, and *Haemophilus influenzae* in children); however, not always needed, as conjunctivitis is often treated presumptively.
  - Severe discharge: *Neisseria gonorrhoeae*

### Pediatric Considerations
- *Chlamydia trachomatis* is the most common neonatal infectious cause of conjunctivitis (monocular or bilateral, purulent or mucopurulent discharge)
- *N. gonorrhoeae* is the other neonatal infectious etiology; typically presents within 2–4 days after birth; marked purulent discharge, chemosis, and lid edema; complications may be severe.

### Lab
- Often not indicated
- Useful if etiology is thought to be systemic disease
- If bilateral, recurrent, granulomatous uveitis is suspected, send CBC, ESR, antinuclear antibody, Venereal Disease Research Laboratory, fluorescent treponemal antibody–absorption, purified protein derivative, angiotensin-converting-enzyme level, chest x-ray (sarcoidosis and tuberculosis), Lyme titer, and HLA-B27, *Toxoplasma*, and cytomegalovirus (CMV) titers

### Imaging
Obtain plain films and/or CT scan of the orbits if suspect foreign body, orbital disease, or trauma.

### Diagnostic Procedures/Surgery
- Tonometry if glaucoma considered
- Slit lamp examination with fluorescein

## DIFFERENTIAL DIAGNOSIS
- Local: Infection, allergy, trauma (also see Etiology)
- Acute angle-closure glaucoma
- Systemic (generally an inflammatory reaction):
  - Arthritic disease
  - Ankylosing spondylosis
  - Ulcerative colitis
  - Reiter syndrome
  - TB
  - Herpes
  - Syphilis
  - Sarcoidosis
  - Toxoplasma
  - CMV

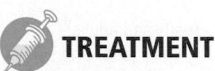 **TREATMENT**

## PRE-HOSPITAL
- Analgesic and comfort measures
- Initiate irrigation for a chemical exposure.

## INITIAL STABILIZATION/THERAPY
- Removal of contact lenses if applicable
- Irrigation for chemical insult
- Treat systemic illness if applicable.

## ED TREATMENT/PROCEDURES
- Direct therapy toward specific etiology.
- Medication as indicated
- Special reminders:
  - Differentiate between a corneal abrasion and a corneal ulcer.
  - Eye patching is no longer routinely recommended for abrasions and is contraindicated for high infection risk (contact lens wearers, abrasions from tree branches or fingernails).
  - Update tetanus immunization for injury.
  - Refrain from contact lens use.
  - Do not spread infection from the affected eye to the unaffected eye or to unaffected individuals.
  - Diagnosis of conjunctivitis caused by *N. gonorrhoeae* or *C. trachomatis* requires treatment of systemic infection for the individual as well as treatment of source individual(s).
  - Always include workup and treatment of systemic disease if this is suspected.

### Special Topics
#### Corneal Abrasion
- Non–contact lens wearer:
  - Ointment or drops:
    ○ Erythromycin ointment every 4 hr
    ○ Polytrim drops 4 times/d
- Contact lens wearers need pseudomonal coverage:
  - Tobramycin ointment every 4 hr
  - Tobramycin, ofloxacin, or ciprofloxacin drops 4 times/d

- Dilate eyes with cyclopentolate 1–2%, 2–4 gtt daily to prevent pain from iritis.
- Abrasions will heal without patching.
- Systemic analgesics, opiate or nonopiate
- Reevaluation if symptomatic at 48 hr

### Corneal Ulcer
- Non–contact lens wearer:
  – Polytrim ointment 4 times/d
  – Ofloxacin, ciprofloxacin drops q2–4h
- Contact lens wearers need pseudomonal coverage (see above)

### Severe or vision-threatening corneal ulcers
- Central, >1.5 mm or with significant anterior chamber reaction
- Treat as aforementioned and add increased frequency of antibiotic drops such as 1–2 gtt every 15 min for 6 hr, then every 30 min around the clock
- Ophthalmology consult for further recommendations, which may include ciprofloxacin 500 mg PO b.i.d. or fortified antibiotic drops made by pharmacist
- Hospitalization is often recommended in consultation with ophthalmologist.

### Acute Angle-Closure Glaucoma
- Symptoms typically include rapid onset of symptoms, severe eye pain, nausea and vomiting, headache, blurred vision and/or seeing haloes around light, lacrimation.
- Diagnosis is further suspected when tonometry detects elevated eye pressure.

### Herpes Simplex or Zoster (HSV)
- Add trifluridine (Viroptic) 1%, 2 gtt 9 times/d or vidarabine 3% ointment 5 times/d (ointment preferred for children)
- Ophthalmology consultation

### Pediatric Considerations
- Usually associated with HSV2 infections
- May be associated with encephalitis or as an isolated lesion
- Neonate onset occurs 1–2 wk after birth
- Presentation: Generally monocular, serous discharge, moderate conjunctival injection

### ALERT
Ocular HSV infection carries significant risk of vision loss

### Trauma or Uveitis
Rule out foreign body.

### MEDICATION
- Antibiotic drops:
  – Ciprofloxacin 0.3%: 1–2 gtt q1–6h
  – Gentamicin 0.3%: 1–2 gtt q4h
  – Ofloxacin 0.3%: 1–2 gtt q1–6h
  – Polytrim: 1 gtt q3–6h
  – Sulfacetamide 10%: 0.3% 1–2 gtt q2–6h
  – Tobramycin 0.3%: 1–2 gtt q1–4h
  – Trifluridine 1%: 1 gtt q2–4h
- Antibiotic ointments (ophthalmic versions):
  – Bacitracin: 500 U/g 1/2-in. ribbon of ointment q3–6h
  – Ciprofloxacin 0.3%: 1/2-in. ribbon of ointment q6–8h

  – Erythromycin 0.5%: 1/2-in. ribbon of ointment q3–6h
  – Gentamicin 0.3%: 1/2-in. ribbon of ointment q3–4h
  – Neosporin: 1/2-inch ribbon of ointment q3–4h
  – Polysporin: 1/2-in. ribbon of ointment q3–4h
  – Sulfacetamide 10%: 1/2-in. ribbon of ointment q3–8h
  – Tobramycin 0.3%: 1/2-in. ribbon of ointment q3–4h
  – Vidarabine: 1/2-in. ribbon of ointment 5 times/d
- Mydriatics and cycloplegics:
  – Atropine 1%, 2%: 1–2 gtt per day to q.i.d.
  – Cyclopentolate 0.5%, 1%, 2%: 1–2 gtt PRN dilation
  – Homatropine 2%: 1–2 gtt b.i.d. to t.i.d.
  – Phenylephrine 0.12%, 2.5%, 10%: 1–2 gtt t.i.d. to q.i.d.
  – Tropicamide 0.5%, 1%: 1–2 gtt PRN dilation
- Corticosteroid antibiotic combination drops (use only with ophthalmology consultation):
  – Blephamide: 1–2 gtt q1–8h
  – Cortisporin: 1–2 gtt q3–4h
  – Maxitrol: 1–2 gtt q1–8h
  – Pred G: 1–2 gtt q1–8h
  – Tobradex: 1–2 gtt q2–6h
- Glaucoma agents (always use with ophthalmology consultation):
  – Acetazolamide: 250–500 mg PO per day to q.i.d.
  – Betaxolol 0.25%, 0.5%: 1–2 gtt b.i.d.
  – Carteolol 1%: 1 gtt b.i.d.
  – Levobunolol 0.25%, 0.5%: 1 gtt daily to b.i.d.
  – Dipivefrin 1%: 1 gtt b.i.d.
  – Mannitol: 1–2 g/kg IV over 45 min
  – Pilocarpine 0.25, 0.5, 1, 2, 3, 4, 6, 8, 10%: 1–2 gtt t.i.d. to q.i.d. (use only if mechanical closure is ruled out)
  – Timolol 0.25, 0.5%: 1 gtt b.i.d.

 FOLLOW-UP

### DISPOSITION
### Admission Criteria
- Endophthalmitis
- Perforated corneal ulcers
- Orbital cellulitis
- Concurrent injuries (eg, trauma)
- If indicated for systemic disease

### Pediatric Considerations
Neonates with conjunctivitis suspected to be due to *N. gonorrhoeae* should be hospitalized for IV antibiotics (cefotaxime), and consideration should be given to septic workup.

### Discharge Criteria
Ability to follow outpatient instructions
### Issues for Referral
- Dacryocystitis
- Corneal ulcer
- Scleritis
- Angle-closure glaucoma
- Uveitis

- Proptosis
- Orbital cellulitis
- Vision loss
- Uncertain diagnosis
- Gonorrheal or chlamydial conjunctivitis

### FOLLOW-UP RECOMMENDATIONS
- Prompt reevaluation if symptoms not resolving over expected time course
- Avoid use of contact lenses until approved by ocular specialist.

## PEARLS AND PITFALLS
- Failure to recognize and treat ulcers, herpetic infections, neonatal bacterial infections, angle-closure glaucoma, and penetrating trauma
- Steroids should only be used with ophthalmology consultation.

## ADDITIONAL READING
- Ehlers JP, Shah CP. *The Wills Eye Manual: Office and Emergency Room Diagnosis and Treatment of Eye Disease*. 5th ed. Philadelphia: Lippincott Williams & Wilkins; 2008.
- Leibowitz HM. The red eye. *N Engl J Med*. 2000; 343:345–351.
- Sethuraman U, Kamat D. The red eye: Evaluation and management. *Clin Pediatr*. 2009;48:588–600.
- Wirbelaur C. Management of the red eye for the primary care physician. *Am J Med*. 2006;119: 302–306.

### See Also (Topic, Algorithm, Electronic Media Element)
- Conjunctivitis
- Corneal Abrasion
- Corneal Burn
- Corneal Foreign Body
- Dacryocystitis
- Glaucoma
- Globe Rupture
- Hordeolum and Chalazion
- Hyphema
- Iritis
- Optic Artery Occlusion
- Optic Neuritis
- Periorbital and Orbital Cellulitis
- Ultraviolet Keratitis
- Visual Loss
- Vitreous Hemorrhage

 CODES

ICD9
379.93 Redness or discharge of eye

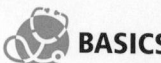

# REITER DISEASE

*Christopher Fischer*

 **BASICS**

## DESCRIPTION

- Syndrome classically includes triad of conjunctivitis, urethritis, arthritis
- More appropriately known as "reactive arthritis":
  – Typically taught as the syndrome where 1 "can't see, can't pee, can't climb a tree"

## ETIOLOGY

- Exact incidence difficult to determine because of lack of standardized diagnostic criteria
- 2 main types:
  – Post-dysentery:
    ○ *Salmonella, Shigella, Campylobacter, Yersinia, Clostridium difficile*
  – Venereal:
    ○ *Chlamydia trachomatis, Neisseria gonorrhoea*
- Has also been described after upper respiratory infections
- M > F (~5:1)
- Peak onset during 3rd decade

## DIAGNOSIS

## SIGNS AND SYMPTOMS

- Urogenital: Occur in >90% of cases, seen in both forms of disease
- Arthritis, tendonitis:
  – Typically polyarticular, asymmetric
  – Knees and ankles most commonly affected
  – May also affect fingers, back, sacroiliac joints
  – Achilles' tendonitis present in 40% of cases
- Ophthalmologic: Occur in 30–60% of cases:
  – Conjunctivitis is most common:
    ○ Usually bilateral
  – Uveitis, keratitis is less common:
    ○ Usually unilateral
    ○ Usually preceded by 1–2 days of eye discomfort
- Mucocutaneous:
  – More common in patients with HLA-B27 positivity

## History

- Symptoms generally within 4 wk of infection, although may be delayed up to 1 yr
- Diagnosis made by history and physical exam findings
- Only 1/3 have the complete triad of conjunctivitis, urethritis, arthritis
- Post-dysentery: Usually preceded by symptomatic GI infection, especially in children
- Venereal: Often follows asymptomatic infection

## Physical Exam

- General:
  – May include fever, fatigue, weight loss, malaise
- Urogenital:
  – Urethritis
  – Cervicitis
  – Prostatitis
- Extremities:
  – Swelling, painful range of motion, erythema may all be present.
  – Sausage digit (diffuse swelling of an entire digit) present in ~15% of cases
- Ophthalmologic:
  – Conjunctivitis:
    ○ Often with mucopurulent discharge
    ○ Symptoms range from mild irritation to severe inflammation.
  – Uveitis:
    ○ Eye pain, redness, photophobia, miosis, blepharospasm
- Skin/mucosa:
  – Keratoderma blennorrhagicum:
    ○ Begins as erythematous macules and vesicles on palms and soles, progresses to pustules and dark plaques
    ○ Similar in appearance to pustular psoriasis
  – Circinate balanitis: Present in >50% of males:
    ○ Plaques, vesicles or papules on glans penis
  – Ulcerative vulvitis may be associated with vaginal discharge
  – Nail changes
  – Oral lesions, usually painless

## ESSENTIAL WORKUP

- Clinical diagnosis is based on characteristic physical exam findings and a history of GI illness, sexually transmitted infection or upper respiratory infection.
- Must exclude other serious time-sensitive diagnoses that require prompt treatment

## DIAGNOSTIC TESTS & INTERPRETATION
### Lab
No laboratory tests can confirm the diagnosis:
- CBC may show leukocytosis and mild anemia
- ESR and CRP are usually elevated
- Urinalysis may show sterile pyuria

### Imaging
- No radiology exams can confirm the diagnosis
- Plain x-ray can be considered of affected extremities to exclude other diagnoses:
  – May show swelling around affected joint, indicating joint effusion

### Diagnostic Procedures/Surgery
Arthrocentesis:
- Should be performed if septic arthritis is considered
- Synovial fluid analysis may show leukocytosis, PMN predominance:
  – Crystals not present, and indicate other pathologies (gout, pseudogout)

## DIFFERENTIAL DIAGNOSIS

- Gonococcal urethritis
- Chlamydial urethritis
- Syphilis
- Gout
- Gonococcal arthritis
- Septic arthritis
- Rheumatoid arthritis
- Pustular psoriasis
- Behçet disease
- Contact dermatitis
- Psoriasis
- Kawasaki disease (in children)

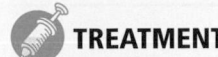 **TREATMENT**

**PRE-HOSPITAL**
No specific prehospital considerations

**ED TREATMENT/PROCEDURES**
- Once other serious infections have been excluded, treatment is symptomatic
- No consensus about the role of antibiotics
- Rationale for antibiotic treatment is that RS is caused by bacterial infection, which may have long-term viability in synovium (especially *Chlamydia*):
  – Studies have demonstrated no long-term benefit with doxycycline, ciprofloxacin, azithromycin
- Arthritis:
  – Rest, ice, elevation
  – NSAIDs
- Conjunctivitis:
  – Topical antibiotics may provide symptomatic relief
- Urethritis:
  – Should be treated if initial infection not recognized or treated

**MEDICATION**
No definite role for medication

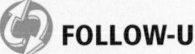 **FOLLOW-UP**

**DISPOSITION**
*Admission Criteria*
Treatment is generally outpatient, once syndrome is recognized and other diagnoses have been excluded.

*Discharge Criteria*
Most patients with Reiter syndrome can be discharged with follow-up with their primary care provider.

*Issues for Referral*
Severe uveitis should be referred to ophthalmology for close follow-up.

**FOLLOW-UP RECOMMENDATIONS**
With primary care provider

## PEARLS AND PITFALLS

Failing to diagnose serious life- or limb-threatening diseases is a pitfall:
- Septic arthritis
- Gonococcal arthritis
- Kawasaki disease

## ADDITIONAL READING

- Carter JD, Hudson AP. Reactive arthritis: Clinical aspects and medical management. *Rheum Dis Clin North Am.* 2009;35(1):21–44.
- Wu IB, Schwartz RA. Reiter's syndrome: The classic triad and more. *J Am Acad Dermatol.* 2008;59(1):113–121.

**See Also (Topic, Algorithm, Electronic Media Element)**
- Conjunctivitis
- Iritis/Uveitis
- Kawasaki Disease
- Septic Arthritis
- Urethritis

 **CODES**

**ICD9**
- 099.3 Reiter's disease
- 372.33 Conjunctivitis in mucocutaneous disease
- 711.10 Arthropathy, site unspecified, associated with reiter's disease and nonspecific urethritis

# RENAL CALCULUS
*Matthew A. Wheatley*

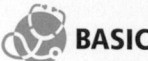

## BASICS

### DESCRIPTION
- Urinary tract obstruction
- Intermittent distention of the renal pelvis of proximal ureter produces pain.
- Kidney stones:
  - Most common cause of renal colic
  - Stone composition:
    - 80%: Calcium stones (calcium oxalate > calcium phosphate)
    - 5% uric acid
    - Others: Magnesium ammonium phosphate (struvite), cystine
  - Associated with infections caused by urea-splitting organisms (eg, *Pseudomonas, Proteus, Klebsiella*) along with an alkalotic urine
  - 90% of urinary calculi are radiopaque.

### ETIOLOGY
- 1% of the population
- Twice as common in men as women
- Theories on stone formation:
  - Urinary supersaturation of solute followed by crystal precipitation
  - Decrease in the normal urinary proteins inhibiting crystal growth
  - Urinary stasis from a physical anomaly, catheter placement, neurogenic bladder, or the presence of a foreign body

#### Pediatric Considerations
- Rare in children
- When present, indication of an overt metabolic or genetic disorder
- Painless hematuria common presentation (up to 30%)
- Pediatric patients <16 yr comprise approximately 7% of all cases of renal stones.
- 1:1 sex distribution
- Causes of stone formation:
  - Metabolic abnormalities (50%)
  - Urologic abnormalities (20%)
  - Infection (15%)
  - Immobilization syndrome (5%)

## DIAGNOSIS

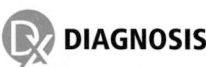

### SIGNS AND SYMPTOMS
#### History
- Sudden onset of severe pain in the costovertebral angle, flank, and/or lateral abdomen
- Colicky or constant pain:
  - Patient cannot find a comfortable position.
- Hematuria:
  - Gross hematuria in 1/3 of patients
- Nausea/vomiting
- Diaphoresis
- History of prior stone formation

#### Physical Exam
- Obtain vital signs:
  - Fever suggests an occult infection.
  - Hypotension with an altered mental status suggests urosepsis.
- Abdominal exam:
  - Pain on palpation, rebound tenderness, and or guarding suggests a more serious intra-abdominal process.
  - Palpate the abdominal aorta for tenderness or pulsatile enlargement suggestive of an aneurysm.
- Genitourinary exam:
  - Examine the genitalia for evidence of hernia, epididymitis, torsion, or testicular masses.

### ESSENTIAL WORKUP
- Urinalysis
- Microscopic hematuria present in >80%
- Gross hematuria
- Absent urinary blood in 10–30%
- No correlation between the amount of hematuria and the degree of urinary obstruction
- WBC/bacteria suggests infection

### DIAGNOSTIC TESTS & INTERPRETATION
#### Lab
- CBC:
  - WBC >15,000 suggests concomitant infection
- Urine culture
- Electrolytes, glucose, BUN, creatinine
- Pregnancy test when suggestive

#### Imaging
- CT:
  - Helical CT has replaced IV pyelogram (IVP) as test of choice.
  - Detects calculi as small as 1 mm in diameter
  - Directly visualizes complications, such as hydroureter, hydronephrosis, and ureteral edema
  - Advantages over IVP:
    - Performed rapidly
    - Does not require IV contrast media
    - Detects other nonurologic causes of symptoms, such as abdominal aortic aneurysms (AAAs)
  - Disadvantages:
    - Does not evaluate flow or renal function
  - Nonenhanced helical CT in the evaluation of renal colic:
    - Sensitivity 95%
    - Specificity 98%
    - Accuracy 97%
  - Indications:
    - 1st-time diagnosis
    - Persistent pain
    - Clinical confusion with pyelonephritis

- IVP:
  - Establishes diagnosis in 95%
  - Demonstrates the severity of obstruction
  - Scout film prior may localize stones that would otherwise be obscured by the dye.
  - Postvoiding film
  - Useful to identify stones at the ureteral vesicular junction or distal ureter that are obscured by a full bladder.
- Kidney, ureter, and bladder (KUB) radiograph:
  - Indicated when allergy to IVP dye and when renal scanning and US not available
  - Distinguishes calcium-bearing stones (radiopaque) from noncalcium stones
  - Assists in locating radiopaque stones and the exclusion of other pathologies in nonpregnant patients
  - Difficult to distinguish radiopaque body:
    - Phlebolith
    - Bowel contents
    - Obstruction within the urinary tract on the KUB
    - Oblique films assist in localizing suspicious calcifications.
- US:
  - For patients who are not candidates for IV contrast
  - Useful in the detection of larger stones and hydronephrosis
  - Provides anatomic information only
  - Helpful in diagnosing obstruction and localizing stones in the proximal and distal portions of the ureter
  - Ability to detect hydronephrosis:
    - Sensitivity 85–94%
    - Specificity 100%
  - Limitations:
    - May miss stones <5 mm in size
    - May miss an obstruction in the early phase of renal colic
    - Time delay until the onset of pyelocaliectasis even after total obstruction

#### Pregnancy Considerations
- Every effort should be made to minimize ionizing radiation exposure to the fetus.
- US is the imaging modality of choice.

#### Diagnostic Procedures/Surgery
Ureteroscopy

### DIFFERENTIAL DIAGNOSIS
- Dissecting or rupturing AAA
- Pyelonephritis
- Papillary necrosis (sickle cell disease, NSAID analgesic abuse, diabetes, or infection)
- Renal infarction (vascular dissection or arterial embolus)

- Ectopic pregnancy
- Ovarian cyst/torsion
- Appendicitis
- Intestinal obstruction
- Biliary tract disease
- Musculoskeletal strain
- Lower lobe pneumonia
- Malingering or narcotic dependence (diagnosis of exclusion)

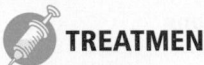

# TREATMENT

## PRE-HOSPITAL
Parenteral opiates may be required for pain control with long transport times.

## INITIAL STABILIZATION/THERAPY
- Rapid dipstick urine test for blood:
  - Positive test in conjunction with clinical findings sufficient to begin analgesic therapy
- Provide adequate analgesia when diagnosis suspected on clinical and laboratory findings.

## ED TREATMENT/PROCEDURES
- Hydration:
  - Initiate IV crystalloid infusion with 1 L of normal saline infused over 30–60 min followed by 200–500 mL/hr.
  - Bolus volume compromised patients with 500-mL increments until urine output adequate
- Analgesics (morphine, ketorolac):
  - Combination of IV NSAIDS and opioids decrease ED stay.
- Antiemetics (prochlorperazine, ondansetron, droperidol, hydroxyzine)
- α-Blockers (tamsulosin) or calcium-channel blockers (nifedipine) have been shown to decrease time to spontaneous stone passage:
  - Most efficacious for stones <5 mm in diameter
  - Tamsulosin and nifedipine equally effective
  - Prescribe on discharge.

### Pregnancy Considerations
Avoid NSAIDs in pregnancy, particularly in 3rd trimester.

## MEDICATION
- Hydromorphone (Dilaudid): 1–4 mg (peds: 0.015 mg/kg/dose) IM/IV/SC q4–6h PRN. Reduce dose in opiate-naive patients.
- Hydroxyzine hydrochloride (Vistaril): 25–50 mg (peds: 0.5–1 mg/kg/dose) IM (not IV) q4–6h
- Ketorolac (Toradol): 30–60 mg IM or 30 mg (peds: 0.5 mg/kg/dose up to 1 mg/kg/24–48 hr) IV (alone or with opiates); reduce dose to 30 mg IM or 15 mg IV if >65 yr or <50 kg.

- Meperidine (Demerol): 50–100 mg (peds: 1–1.75 mg/kg/dose) q3–4h IV/IM
- Morphine sulfate: 2–10 mg (peds: 0.1–0.2 mg/kg/dose q2–4h) IM/IV/SC q2–6h PRN; may redose more frequently if needed.
- Nifedipine 30 mg PO daily.
- Ondansetron (Zofran): 4 mg (peds: 0.1 mg/kg ×1) IM/IV
- Prochlorperazine (Compazine): 5–10 mg IM/IV q4–6h; 25-mg suppository PR
- Promethazine (Phenergan): 12.5–25 mg (peds: 0.25–1 mg/kg) IM/IV q4–6h
- Tamsulosin (Flomax) 0.4 mg PO daily for 4 wk

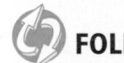

# FOLLOW-UP

## DISPOSITION

### Admission Criteria
- Obstruction in the presence of infection mandates immediate urologic intervention.
- Intractable pain with refractory nausea and vomiting
- Severe volume depletion
- Urinary extravasation
- Hypercalcemic crisis
- Solitary kidney and complete obstruction
- Relative admission indications (discuss with urologist):
  - High-grade obstruction
  - Renal insufficiency
  - Intrinsic renal disease
  - Stones of size <5 mm usually pass spontaneously; those >8 mm rarely do.

### Discharge Criteria
- Normal vital signs
- No evidence of concomitant urinary tract infection
- Adequate analgesia
- Able to tolerate PO fluids to maintain hydration status
- Reliable patient with an adequate home situation
- Appropriate outpatient follow-up arranged
- Normal renal function
- Provide a urine strainer to collect the stone for possible future stone analysis.
- Arrange urologic follow-up.

### Issues for Referral
Imaging if pain persists and diagnosis not established in ED

## FOLLOW-UP RECOMMENDATIONS
All patients should have urology follow-up, especially:
- 1st episode of renal stone
- Large stone >5 mm
- Patients who fail to pass a stone after 4 wk of conservative therapy

# PEARLS AND PITFALLS

- Do not miss a vascular catastrophe mimicking as renal colic.
- Aggressive pain management and hydration promote passage of stones
- The absence of hematuria does not exclude the diagnosis of acute renal colic.

# ADDITIONAL READING

- Bartosh SM. Medical management of pediatric stone disease. *Urol Clin North Am.* 2004;31:575–587.
- Hollingsworth JM, Rogers MA, Kaufman SR, et al. Medical therapy to facilitate stone passage: A meta-analysis. *Lancet.* 2006;368:1171–1179.
- Loughlin KR, Kerr LA. The current management of urolithiasis during pregnancy. *Urol Clin North Am.* 2002;29:701–704
- Marx JA, Hockberger RS, Walls RM, eds. *Rosen's Emergency Medicine: Concepts and Clinical Practice.* 7th ed. St. Louis, MO: Mosby; 2009.
- Teichman J. Acute renal colic from ureteral calculus *N Engl J Med.* 2004;350:684–693.

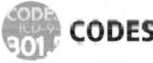

# CODES

ICD9
592.0 Calculus of kidney

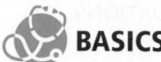 **BASICS**

## DESCRIPTION
- The term renal failure is outdated; the disorder is now known as acute kidney injury (AKI).
- Changes in glomerular filtration rate (GFR) and urine output encompassing a spectrum ranging from normal physiologic response to end-stage renal disease (ESRD) and measured by accumulation of nitrogenous byproducts in the blood
- Defined by the RIFLE criteria:
  - 3 stages of renal injury:
    - Risk: Increased creatinine $\times 1.5$ or GFR decrease $>25\%$, urine output (UO) $<0.5$ mL/kg/hr $\times 6$ hr
    - Injury: Increased creatinine $\times 2$ or GFR decrease $>50\%$, UO $<0.5$ mL/kg/hr $\times 12$ hr
    - Failure: Increased creatinine $\times 3$ or GFR decrease $>75\%$ or creatinine $\geq 4$ mg/dL (acute rise of $\geq 0.5$ mg/dL), UO $<0.3$ mL/kg/hr $\times 24$ hr or anuria $\times 12$ hr
  - 2 stages of outcome:
    - Loss: Complete loss of renal function $>4$ wk
    - ESRD
- The most severe marker defines stage.
- Higher RIFLE stages correlate with higher 1- and 6-mo mortality rates for hospitalized patients.

## ETIOLOGY
- Prerenal AKI:
  - Caused by renal hypoperfusion
  - Renal tissue remains normal unless severe/prolonged hypoperfusion.
- Intrarenal AKI:
  - Caused by diseases of the renal parenchyma
- Iatrogenic causes include:
  - Aminoglycoside antibiotics
  - Radiocontrast material administration
  - NSAIDs
  - Angiotensin-converting-enzyme inhibitors
- Postrenal AKI:
  - Due to acute obstruction of the urinary tract (eg, benign prostatic hyperplasia, prostatitis)

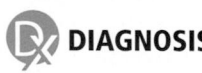 **DIAGNOSIS**

## SIGNS AND SYMPTOMS
### Acute Kidney Injury
- Often asymptomatic and commonly diagnosed with incidental laboratory findings
- Oliguria ($<400$ mL/d urine production)
- Fluid overload:
  - Dyspnea
  - Hypertension
  - Jugular venous distention
  - Pulmonary and peripheral edema
  - Ascites
  - Pericardial and pulmonary effusion
- Nausea/vomiting

### Prerenal AKI
- Absolute or relative volume deficit
- Dry mucous membranes
- Hypotension
- Tachycardia
- Low cardiac output
- Congestive heart failure
- Systemic vasodilation (eg, sepsis, anaphylaxis)

### Intrarenal (Intrinsic) AKI
- Renal artery thrombosis:
  - Flank or abdominal pain
  - Atrial fibrillation
  - Recent myocardial infarction
- Renal vein thrombosis:
  - Nephrotic syndrome
  - Pulmonary embolus
  - Flank or abdominal pain
- Glomerulonephritis, vasculitis
- Hemolytic uremic syndrome (HUS):
- Thrombotic thrombocytopenic purpura (TPP):
  - Mild elevation of BUN/creatinine
  - Fever
  - Altered mental status
  - Headache
  - Seizures
  - Anemia
  - Coma
- Allergic interstitial nephritis fever:
  - Rash
  - Arthralgias

### Postrenal AKI
- Abdominal or flank pain
- Distended bladder
- Oliguria or anuria

### Complications of AKI
- Uremic syndrome:
  - Altered mental status
  - Asterixis
  - Reflex abnormalities
  - Focal neurologic abnormality
  - Seizures
  - Restless leg syndrome
  - Pericarditis
  - Pericardial effusion
  - Cardiac tamponade
  - Ileus
  - Platelet dysfunction
- Hematologic disorders:
  - Anemia
  - Increased bleeding time
  - Leukocytosis

### History
- Prior history of AKI
- Medication history including nephrotoxins
- Weight change

### Physical Exam
- Eyes: Fundoscopy
- CV exam: Jugular venous distention, S3
- Lungs: Rales, crackles
- Abdomen: Flank pain, palpable kidneys
- Edema

### Geriatric Considerations
- Prone to prerenal
- Creatinine will vary by body mass index, so a "normal" range in elderly may represent an elevation.
- Increased risk of contrast- and medication-induced AKI

### Pediatric Considerations
- Prerenal AKI common in neonates
- Anatomic abnormalities

### Pregnancy Considerations
- Intrinsic renal azotemia
- Preeclampsia/eclampsia
- Ischemia: Postpartum hemorrhage, abruptio placentae, amniotic fluid embolus
- Direct toxicity of illegal abortifacients
- Postpartum TTP, HUS

## ESSENTIAL WORKUP
- Electrolytes
- BUN/creatinine:
  - Elevated in ratio determined by cause of AKI
- Urinalysis (UA):
  - Centrifuged specimen helps to distinguish different etiologies of AKI.
  - Exam for casts, blood, WBCs, and crystals
- CBC: Anemia common with chronic disease

## DIAGNOSTIC TESTS & INTERPRETATION
### Lab
**Prerenal**
UA:
- Specific gravity $>1.018$
- Osmolality $>500$ mmol/kg
- Sodium $<10$ mmol/L
- Hyaline casts
- BUN/creatinine ratio $>20$
- Rapid recovery of renal function when renal perfusion normalized

**Intrarenal**
- BUN/creatinine ratio $<10$–$15$
- Glomerulonephritis, vasculitis:
  - UA with red cell or granular casts
  - Complement and autoimmune antibodies
- HUS or TTP:
  - UA normal
  - Anemia
  - Thrombocytopenia
  - Schistocytes on blood smear
- Nephrotoxic acute tubular necrosis (ATN):
  - UA:
    - Brown granular or epithelial cell casts
    - Specific gravity 1.010
    - Urine osmolality $<350$ mmol/kg
    - Urine Na $>20$ mmol/L

- Ethylene glycol ingestion:
  - UA: Calcium oxalate crystals
  - Anion gap metabolic acidosis
  - Osmolar gap
- Rhabdomyolysis:
- UA: Heme positive without red cells:
  - Elevated serum $K^+$, $PO_4$, myoglobin, creatine phosphokinase-MM, uric acid
  - Decreased serum $Ca^{2+}$
- Tubulointerstitial disease
- Allergic interstitial nephritis:
  - UA with WBC casts, WBCs, RBCs, and proteinuria
  - Systemic eosinophilia

**Postrenal**
UA:

- Usually normal
- May have some hematuria but no casts or protein

### *Imaging*

- US:
  - 98% sensitive for excluding obstruction
- Helical CT scan:
  - Without contrast sensitive for obstruction
  - May detect intrarenal changes
- Duplex scan for:
  - Renal artery or vein thrombosis
- Renal arteriogram:
  - Definitive diagnosis of renal artery thrombosis
- Inferior vena cava and renal vessel venogram for renal vein thrombosis
- IV pyelogram:
  - Avoid contrast with renal insufficiency, as it may worsen renal function.

### *Diagnostic Procedures/Surgery*
ECG:

- Hypertension secondary to volume overload may cause ischemia.
- Sensitive for significant, acute electrolyte changes

## TREATMENT

### PRE-HOSPITAL
- Airway, breathing, and circulation (ABCs).
  - Supplemental oxygen for hypoxia
- IV NS for volume depletion

### INITIAL STABILIZATION/THERAPY
- ABCs:
- Supplemental oxygen for hypoxia
- IV NS for volume depletion
- Correct electrolyte disturbances.
- Indications for emergent dialysis:
  - Life-threatening hyperkalemia
  - Intractable hypertension or pulmonary edema
  - Fluid overload unresponsive to other treatments
  - BUN >100 mg/dL
  - Creatinine >10 mg/dL:
    - ESRD patients on regular dialysis may have a baseline elevated creatinine that by itself is not an indication for emergent dialysis.
  - Metabolic acidosis (pH <7.2)
  - Uremia pericarditis
- Avoid nephrotoxic drugs.
- Monitor urine output.

## ED TREATMENT/PROCEDURES
### *Prerenal AKI*
- Treat hypoperfusion:
  - Packed RBC for blood loss, anemia, or lack of response after 2 boluses
- Invasive cardiac monitoring if unable to assess cardiac failure versus hypovolemia
- Response to NS good indicator of the degree to which hypovolemia is a factor

### ALERT
Administer NS fluid challenge cautiously to avoid fluid overload in liver failure with ascites.

### *Intrarenal AKI*
- Glomerulonephritis:
  - Glucocorticoids or plasma exchange
- ATN:
  - Volume replacement
  - Furosemide
- Hyponatremia: Fluid restriction with IV NS
- Hyperkalemia:
  - Sodium polystyrene sulfonate or calcium polystyrene sulfonate for asymptomatic patient with $K^+$ >5.5 mEq/L
  - For $K^+$ >6.5 mEq/L or ECG abnormalities consistent with hyperkalemia:
    - Albuterol via nebulizer
    - Glucose and insulin
    - Furosemide if patient not anuric
    - Calcium stabilizes myocardium in severe hyperkalemia
    - Calcium gluconate for awake patient
    - Calcium chloride for patient without pulse
  - Dialysis for intractable hyperkalemia
- Metabolic acidosis:
  - Consider sodium bicarbonate for pH <7.2 or $HCO_3$ <15 mEq/L in *chronic disease*
  - Hyperphosphatemia:
  - Calcium carbonate
  - Aluminum hydroxide
  - Myoglobinuria:
  - Aggressive fluid resuscitation with NS

### ALERT
- Calcium gluconate is only indicated by ECG for widened PR, QT, or QRS intervals. Peaked T waves alone are *not* an indication.
- Sodium bicarbonate is a considerable sodium load; use caution in anuric/oliguric patients.

### MEDICATION
- Albuterol: 10–20 mg via nebulizer
- Aluminum hydroxide (Amphojel): 0.5–1.5 g PO
- Calcium carbonate (Os-Cal): 0.250–3 g PO
- Calcium gluconate: 10 mL of 10% solution over 5 min IV
- Calcium chloride: 10 mL of 10% solution
- Dextrose: D50W 1 amp (50 mL or 25 g) (peds: D25W 2–4 mL/kg) IV

- Furosemide: 20–400 mg IV push
- Insulin: 10 IU regular IV with dextrose (decrease 50% for severe renal and/or liver disease)
- Mannitol: 12.5–25 g IV push
- Sodium bicarbonate: 1–2 mEq/kg IV
- Sodium polystyrene sulfonate (Kayexalate) or calcium polystyrene sulfonate: 1 g/kg up to 15–60 g PO or 30–50 g retention enema in sorbitol q6h

 **FOLLOW-UP**

### DISPOSITION
### *Admission Criteria*
- New-onset AKI
- Hyperkalemia/significant electrolyte abnormalities
- Fluid overload with hypoxia/congestive heart failure

### *Discharge Criteria*
- Stable
- Normal electrolytes

### *Issues for Referral*
Refer to primary physician for progressive AKI in an otherwise stable patient.

## PEARLS AND PITFALLS

- Insulin dose for hyperkalemia should be reduced for significant liver or renal disease so as to avoid hypoglycemia.
- NSAIDS should be avoided with any degree of AKI if possible.
- Sodium polystyrene sulfonate is a considerable sodium load; therefore, calcium polystyrene sulfonate is preferred when volume overload is a concern.

## ADDITIONAL READING

- Andreoli S. Acute kidney injury In children. *Pediatr Nephrol.* 2009;24:253–263.
- Brady HR, Brenner BM, Clarkson MR, et al. Acute kidney injury. In: Brenner BM, ed. *Brenner and Rector's The Kidney.* 8th ed. Philadelphia: WB Saunders; 2007: 943–975.
- Kellum J. Acute kidney injury. *Crit Care Med.* 2008;36(suppl):S141–S145.

### See Also (Topic, Algorithm, Electronic Media Element)
- Hyperkalemia
- Renal Injury

 **CODES**

### ICD9
- 584.9 Acute kidney failure, unspecified
- 585.9 Chronic kidney disease, unspecified
- 586 Renal failure, unspecified

# RENAL INJURY

*Albert Jin*

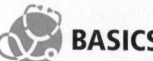

## BASICS

### DESCRIPTION
- Kidneys are located in the retroperitoneal space and are surrounded by adipose tissue and loose areolar connective tissue.
- Kidneys lie along the lower two thoracic vertebrae and 1st 4 lumbar vertebrae.
- Left kidney is positioned slightly higher than the right.
- Kidneys are not fixed:
  - Shift with the diaphragm and are supported by the renal arteries, veins, and adipose tissue to the renal (Gerota) fascia

### ETIOLOGY
- Most common of all urologic injuries
- Occurs in ~8–10% of all abdominal trauma
- Blunt renal trauma accounts for 80–85% of all renal injuries and is 5 times more common than penetrating injury:
  - Mechanisms include motor-vehicle accidents, falls, domestic violence, and contact sports.
  - Pathophysiology includes rapid deceleration and displacement mechanisms.
  - ~20% of cases are associated with intraperitoneal injury.
- Mechanisms responsible for significant renal injury almost never affect the kidney alone:
  - Most often disrupt and injure other vital organs that can be responsible for patient mortality
- Renal injuries are classified according to type and severity of the injury:
  - Grade I
    - Contusion: Microscopic or gross hematuria, urologic studies normal
    - Hematoma: Subcapsular, nonexpanding without parenchymal laceration
  - Grade II:
    - Hematoma: Nonexpanding, perirenal hematoma confined to retroperitoneum
    - Laceration: <1 cm parenchymal depth of renal cortex without urinary extravasation
  - Grade III:
    - Laceration: >1 cm parenchymal depth of renal cortex without collecting system rupture or urinary extravasation
  - Grade IV:
    - Laceration: Parenchymal laceration extending through renal cortex, medulla, and collecting system
    - Vascular: Main renal artery or vein injury with contained hemorrhage
  - Grade V:
    - Laceration: Completely shattered kidney
    - Vascular: Avulsion of renal hilum, devascularizing the kidney

### Pediatric Considerations
- The kidney is the organ most commonly damaged by blunt abdominal trauma.
- Contributing factors:
  - Relatively larger size of kidneys compared with adults
  - 10th and 11th ribs are not completely ossified until the 3rd decade of life.
- Significant abdominal injury occurs in about 5% of nonaccidental trauma cases but is the 2nd most common cause of death after head injury.

## DIAGNOSIS

### SIGNS AND SYMPTOMS
#### History
- Mechanism of injury and kinematics are important factors.
- In blunt trauma, note the type and direction (horizontal or vertical) of any deceleration or compressive forces.
- In penetrating trauma, note the characteristic of the weapon (type and caliber), distance from the weapon, or the type and length of knife or impaling object:
  - Injuries result from a combination of kinetic energy and shear forces of penetrating object.

#### Physical Exam
- Hematuria is the best indicator of traumatic urinary system injury:
  - Severity of renal trauma does not correlate with the degree of hematuria.
- Flank mass or ecchymosis
- Tenderness in the flank, abdomen, or back
- Fracture of the inferior ribs or spinal transverse processes
- Nausea and vomiting

### ESSENTIAL WORKUP
- In 1989, Mee et al. published the hallmark article (10-year prospective study) that established guidelines for the evaluation and treatment of blunt renal trauma:
  - Major renal lacerations represent significant reparable renal injuries.
  - Adult patients at risk for having sustained major lacerations:
    - Gross hematuria, *or*
    - Microhematuria (≥ 3–5 RBCs/HPF) with shock (systolic blood pressure ≤90) in the field or on arrival in the ED, *or*
    - History of sudden deceleration without hematuria or shock
  - IV contrast-enhanced CT scan is the procedure of choice in identifying urologic injury.
  - Guidelines are not applicable in cases of penetrating renal trauma or in children.

- Adults with blunt renal trauma and gross hematuria, or microhematuria in the presence of shock, require renal imaging for further evaluation of renal injury.
- In adults with penetrating renal trauma, significant injuries to the kidney and ureter can occur without hematuria:
  - Location of penetrating wound in relation to urinary tract is most important factor in deciding need for radiographic imaging.
  - Penetrating injuries with any degree of hematuria should be imaged.
- Important to rule out coexisting injuries

### DIAGNOSTIC TESTS & INTERPRETATION
#### Lab
- Urinalysis: Gross hematuria or >50 RBCs/HPF in adults and >20 RBC/HPF in children is suggestive of renal injury.
- Baseline laboratory values including hematocrit and BUN/creatinine should be obtained.

#### Imaging
- Plain abdominal films:
  - May show fractured inferior ribs or transverse processes, a unilateral enlarged kidney shadow, or obscuring of the psoas margin
- IV pyelogram (IVP):
  - Bolus infusion IVP with nephrotomography study of choice in institutions without 24-hr availability of CT
- Rapid injection of 1.5–2 mL of contrast material per kilogram of body weight to a maximum or 150 mL after obtaining a preliminary kidney, ureter, and bladder image
- Postinfusion supine film is obtained followed by 1-, 2-, and 3-min supine films.
  - Allows evaluation for renal viability and function
  - Extravasation reflects injury to the collecting system.
  - Nonvisualization of a kidney may indicate renal pedicle injury or parenchymal shattering.
  - Abnormal findings are often nonspecific and require more definitive studies.
- US:
  - Role in evaluation of renal injury is controversial
  - May show size of perirenal hematoma and whether it is expanding or resolving
  - Otherwise, exam is nonspecific and does not provide enough information
- CT scan:
  - An IV contrast-enhanced helical CT scan is the diagnostic procedure of choice.
  - Superior anatomic detail and diagnostic accuracy of 98% for renal injury
  - Sensitive indicator of minor extravasation, parenchymal laceration, vascular injury, and nonrenal injuries

### Pediatric Considerations
- Major blunt renal trauma can occur in the absence of gross hematuria or shock (as children have a high catecholamine output after trauma, which maintains BP until ~50% of blood volume has been lost).
- Meta-analysis has defined 50 RBC/HPF as the microscopic quantity below which imaging can be omitted and no significant injuries missed.
- CT scan is the imaging modality of choice.

### Diagnostic Procedures/Surgery
- Renal parenchymal injury
- Renal vascular injury
- Ureteral injury
- Bladder or urethral injury

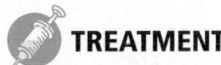 **TREATMENT**

#### PRE-HOSPITAL
- Obtain details of injury from prehospital providers.
- IV access
- Penetrating wounds or evisceration should be covered with sterile dressings.

#### INITIAL STABILIZATION/THERAPY
- Airway management and resuscitation:
  - Adequate IV access
  - Fluid resuscitation, initially with 2 L of crystalloid (NS or lactated Ringer solution), followed by blood products as needed
- Rule out potential life-threatening injuries 1st.

#### ED TREATMENT/PROCEDURES
- Immediate laparotomy in the acutely injured patient who is hemodynamically unstable with presumed hemoperitoneum and renal injury
- All penetrating renal trauma requires renal exploration, unless complete radiographic staging reveals an injury which can be managed nonoperatively.
- Significant injuries (grades II–V) are found in only 5.4% of renal trauma cases.

- 98% of blunt renal injuries can be managed nonoperatively.
- ~80–90% of renal injuries have major associated organ injury that can affect the choice of renal injury management.
- Isolated renal injury without significant associated injuries occurs more commonly from blunt trauma, and in most circumstances, can be managed nonoperatively.
- Management of renal injuries:
  - Classes I and II: Contusions and minor lacerations with stable vital signs and urographically normal renal function can be managed nonoperatively.
  - Class III: Renal lacerations with urinary extravasation:
    - Controversy between operative vs. nonoperative management
    - Management should be based on degree of injury using CT scanning.
  - Classes IV and V: Shattered kidney or renal pedicle injuries and hemodynamically unstable patients require emergent laparotomy.
  - All ureteral injuries require operative repair.

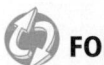 **FOLLOW-UP**

#### DISPOSITION
##### Admission Criteria
Patients with significant renal injury require hospitalization for definitive laparotomy or observation.

##### Discharge Criteria
- Adult trauma patients without hematuria, shock, or no renal injury confirmed radiographically
- Adult blunt trauma patient with microhematuria (≥ 3–5 RBCs/hpf) but no shock (systolic blood pressure ≤90)
- Pediatric blunt trauma patient with <50 RBC/HPF and no other coexisting major organ injuries

### Issues for Referral
Outpatient referral to urologist should be made for microhematuria to ensure that it does not represent a more serious underlying condition.

## ADDITIONAL READING
- Broghammer JA, et al. Conservative management of renal trauma: A review. *Urology.* 2007;70(4): 623–629.
- McAninch JW, Santucci RA. Renal and ureteral trauma. *Campbell-Walsh urology,* 9th ed. Philadelphia: Saunders Elsevier; 2007.
- Mee SL, et al. Radiographic assessment of renal trauma: A ten-year prospective study of patient selection. *J Urol.* 1989;(141):1095.
- Santucci RA, et al. Evaluation and management of renal injuries: Consensus statement of the renal trauma subcommittee. *BJU Int.* 2004;93(7): 937–954.
- Schneider R. Genitourinary system. In: Rosen P, et al., eds. *Emergency medicine: Concepts and clinical practice,* 5th ed. St. Louis: CV Mosby; 2002: 437–456.

 **CODES**

### ICD9
- 866.00 Unspecified injury to kidney without mention of open wound into cavity
- 866.01 Hematoma of kidney, without rupture of capsule, without mention of open wound into cavity
- 866.02 Laceration of kidney without mention of open wound into cavity

R

# REPERFUSION THERAPY, CARDIAC

*Shamai A. Grossman*
*Ethan M. Ross*

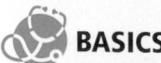 **BASICS**

## DESCRIPTION
- Thrombolytic therapy:
  - Reduces morbidity and mortality in ST-segment elevation myocardial infarction (STEMI)
  - The earlier thrombolytics are started, the more myocardium is salvaged.
  - Goal of thrombolytic therapy is a door-to-needle time of 30 min if percutaneous coronary intervention (PCI) is not planned.
- PCI:
  - Balloon inflation results in overstretching of vessel wall and partial disruption of intima, media, and adventitia, resulting in enlargement of lumen and outer diameter of diseased vessel.
  - Goal of primary PCI is a door-to-balloon time of 90 min from 1st medical contact for STEMI.
  - Stent placement decreases early and late loss in luminal diameter seen with percutaneous transluminal coronary angioplasty (PTCA).
  - PCI provides greater coronary patency and thrombolysis in MI flow than do thrombolytics.
  - Lower risk of bleeding than with thrombolytics
  - Immediate knowledge of extent of disease
  - Meta-analysis suggests improved survival with PCI for STEMI when compared with thrombolytic therapy (6.5% vs. 4.4%); however, improved outcomes may be contingent on operator and institutional expertise.
  - PTCA has a 30% restenosis rate in first 6 mo.
  - Medication-coated stents may reduce revascularization rate to ≤5%.
  - PCI should be strongly considered within 1st 48 hours after a non–ST-segment elevation MI (NSTEMI) with concomitant use of glycoprotein IIb/IIIa inhibitors.
- Glycoprotein IIb/IIIa inhibitors:
  - Antiplatelet agents that bind to platelet receptor glycoprotein IIb/IIIa and inhibit platelet aggregation
  - Reduce mortality and reinfarction rate in patients in whom PCI is planned; reasonable to administer at time of primary PCI
  - Recent data suggest reduced mortality in all patients with unstable angina and non–Q-wave infarction.
  - Not indicated for patients with STEMI, unless also undergoing PCI

- Unfractionated heparin (UH) and low-molecular-weight heparin (LMWH):
  - Adjuncts in treatment with aspirin, clopidogrel, thrombolytics, glycoprotein IIb/IIIa inhibitors, and PCI
  - Anticoagulant therapy with either UFH or LMWH is indicated in patients with either STEMI (with PCI or thrombolytics) or unstable angina/NSTEMI
- Clopidogrel should be added to standard therapy regardless of whether PCI or reperfusion therapy is planned.
- Statin therapy reduces clinical events in patients with stable coronary artery disease. This may also extend to patients experiencing an acute ischemic coronary event.

## ETIOLOGY
Ischemic MI is caused by occlusion of a coronary artery, usually as a result of a thrombotic event.

 **DIAGNOSIS**

## SIGNS AND SYMPTOMS
- Chest pain, heaviness, or pressure feeling
- Shortness of breath
- Arm, neck, or back pain
- Weakness or fatigue
- Nausea, vomiting
- Diaphoresis
- Palpitations
- Dizziness or syncope

## ESSENTIAL WORKUP
- History is critical in assessing window for use of both thrombolytics and PCI.
- ECG:
  - Will be normal ~50% of time
  - Must be compared with prior tracings if available
  - New ST-segment changes or T-wave inversions are suspicious for unstable angina or non–Q-wave infarct.
  - 1-mm depression of the ST segment below the baseline, 80 ms from the J point, is characteristic of unstable angina or non–Q-wave infarct.
  - New left-bundle-branch block or new ST-segment elevation 1 mm in 2 contiguous limb leads or 2 mm in 2 contiguous precordial leads suggests Q-wave infarct.
- Chest radiograph: May be helpful if aortic dissection is being considered
- Heme stool test: Helpful in establishing baseline, especially in setting of anticipated anticoagulation

## DIAGNOSTIC TESTS & INTERPRETATION
*Lab*
- Cardiac enzymes
- Baseline creatinine, hematocrit, and coagulation profile are all appropriate in initial workup.

## DIFFERENTIAL DIAGNOSIS
- Aortic dissection
- Anxiety
- Biliary colic
- Costochondritis
- Esophageal spasm
- Esophageal reflux
- Herpes zoster
- Hiatal hernia
- Mitral valve prolapse
- Peptic ulcer disease
- Psychogenic symptoms
- Panic disorder
- Pericarditis
- Pneumonia
- Pulmonary embolus

 **TREATMENT**

## PRE-HOSPITAL
- IV access
- Oxygen
- Cardiac monitoring
- Sublingual nitroglycerin for symptom relief
- Aspirin
- Controversies:
  - Whether to bypass closer EDs in favor of hospitals capable of primary PCI; follow local emergency medical service protocols.
  - Whether to allow EMS activation of cardiac catheterization labs and administration of thrombolytics.

## ALERT
- All chest pain should be treated and transported as a possible life-threatening emergency.
- Therapy with thrombolytics and glycoprotein IIb/IIIa inhibitors in the field is not currently standard of care.

## INITIAL STABILIZATION/THERAPY

- IV access
- Oxygen
- Cardiac monitoring
- Oxygen saturation
- Continuous blood pressure monitoring and pulse oximetry
- Nitrates

## ED TREATMENT/PROCEDURES

- Aspirin
- Clopidogrel
- Thrombolytics:
  - Unless contraindicated
  - If PCI is not readily available within 90 min
- PCI is preferred for both diagnostic and therapeutic options.
- PCI and thrombolytic therapy must be used with either UFH or a LMWH, such as enoxaparin.
- LMWH:
  - Kinetics more predictable
  - Requires no monitoring
  - Less potential for platelet activation
  - Lower bleeding rate
  - Is at least as effective as UFH in treatment of acute coronary syndromes
- Glycoprotein IIb/IIIa inhibitors

## MEDICATION

- Aspirin: 161–325 mg PO
- Enoxaparin (Lovenox): 1 mg/kg SC q12h
- Clopidogrel (Plavix): 300–600 mg PO load, 75 mg PO per day
- Glycoprotein IIb/IIIa inhibitor:
  - Abciximab (ReoPro): For use before PCI only; 0.25-mg/kg IV bolus
  - Eptifibatide (Integrilin): 100 μg/kg IV over 1–2 min, followed by continuous IV infusion of 2 μg/kg per minute up to 72 hr
  - Tirofiban (Aggrastat): 0.4 μg/kg per minute for 30 min, then 0.1 μg/kg per minute for 48–108 hr
- Heparin 60-units/kg IV bolus (maximum 4,000 U), then 12 units/kg/hr (maximum 1,000 U/hr)
- Metoprolol: 5 mg IV q5–15min followed by 25–50 mg PO starting dose as tolerated (note: β-blockers contraindicated in cocaine chest pain)

- Thrombolytics:
  - Anisoylated plasminogen streptokinase activator complex: 30 mg IV over 2–5 min; patients should also receive methylprednisolone 250 mg IV.
  - Recombinant tissue plasminogen activator (Reteplase): 10 million unit IV bolus, repeat dose after 30 min; patients should also receive heparin 5,000 IU IV bolus, then infuse 1,000 IU per hour for 48 hr, keeping activated partial thromboplastin time (aPTT) 1.5–2.5.
  - Streptokinase: 1.5 million units over 60 min; patients should also receive methylprednisolone 250 mg IV.
  - Tissue plasminogen activator: 15-mg IV bolus, then 0.75 mg/kg (max 50 mg) over 30 min, then 0.5 mg/kg (max 35 mg) over 60 min; patients should also receive heparin 5,000 IU IV bolus, then infuse 1,000 IU per hour for 48 hr keeping aPTT 1.5–2.5
  - Urokinase: 1.5 IU IV over 2 min, then 1.5 IU IV over next 90 min
  - Contraindications:
    ○ Active internal bleeding
    ○ History of cerebrovascular accident in last 6 mo
    ○ History of a hemorrhagic cerebrovascular accident
    ○ Recent (within 2 mo) intracranial or intraspinal surgery or trauma
    ○ Intracranial neoplasm, arteriovenous malformation, or aneurysm
    ○ Known bleeding diathesis
    ○ Severe, uncontrolled hypertension
    ○ Pregnancy
    ○ Head trauma within last month
    ○ Trauma or surgery within last 2 wk that may result in closed-space bleed

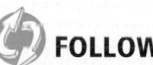 **FOLLOW-UP**

## DISPOSITION

### Admission Criteria

All patients being considered for reperfusion therapy should be admitted to a telemetry or ICU setting.

### Discharge Criteria

No patient being considered for reperfusion therapy should be discharged home from ED

## PEARLS AND PITFALLS

- Goal of reperfusion therapy is primary PCI within 90 min of 1st medical contact. Transfer to a PCI capable facility when this window can be accomplished.
- Goal of thrombolytic therapy is a 30-min door-to-needle time if PCI not possible.

## ADDITIONAL READING

- Anderson JL, Adams, CD, Antman EM, et al. ACC/AHA 2007 guidelines for the management of patients with unstable angina/non-ST-elevation myocardial infarction. *J Am Coll Cardiol.* 2007;50:e1–e157.
- Kushner FG, Hand M, Smith SC, et al. ACC/AHA guidelines for the management of patients with ST-elevation myocardial infarction (updating the 2004 guideline and 2007 focused update) and ACC/AHA/SCAI guidelines on percutaneous coronary intervention (updating the 2005 guideline and 2007 focused update). *Circulation.* 2009;120;2271–2306.
- Sabatine MS, Cannon CP, Gibson CM, et al. CLARITY-TIMI 28 Investigators. Addition of clopidogrel to aspirin and fibrinolytic therapy for myocardial infarction with ST-segment elevation. *N Engl J Med.* 2005;352(12):1179–1189.
- White HD, Braunwald E, Murphy SA, et al. Enoxaparin vs. unfractionated heparin with fibrinolysis for ST-elevation myocardial infarction in elderly and younger patients: Results from ExTRACT-TIMI 25. *Eur Heart J.* 2007;28:1066–1071.

### See Also (Topic, Algorithm, Electronic Media Element)

Acute Coronary Syndrome: Myocardial Infarction

 **CODES**

### ICD9

410.90 Acute myocardial infarction of unspecified site, episode of care unspecified

# REPERFUSION THERAPY, CEREBRAL
*Kama Guluma*

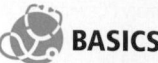

## BASICS

### DESCRIPTION
- An ischemic cerebrovascular accident (CVA), or stroke, is an acute interruption of regional cerebral blood supply:
  - Onset may be sudden or gradual.
  - Course may be progressive or stuttering.
- Cerebral reperfusion therapy involves:
  - Administration of an IV thrombolytic agent to rapidly dissolve a thromboembolic occlusion
  - Site-specific endovascular intra-arterial thrombolysis or mechanical clot removal

### ETIOLOGY
- Caused by occlusion of a cerebral artery:
  - Primarily from a thrombotic or embolic event
- Thrombotic CVA is from an in-situ thrombosis:
  - At an ulcerated atherosclerotic plaque or other prothrombotic endothelial abnormality
  - From hypercoagulable states:
    - ○ Antithrombin III, protein C or S deficiency
  - From sludging:
    - ○ Sickle cell disease
    - ○ Polycythemia vera
- Embolic CVA is caused by acute obstruction by an embolus from:
  - Cardiac mural thrombus formed in:
    - ○ Atrial fibrillation
    - ○ Hypokinetic ventricle (MI, cardiomyopathy, failure)
    - ○ Ventricular aneurysm
  - An abnormal or prosthetic cardiac valve
  - Aortic, carotid, or cerebrovascular atherosclerotic plaques
- Other occlusive events include:
  - Vascular dissection in aorta, cerebral, vertebral, carotid, or innominate arteries
  - Cerebral vasospasm induced by:
    - ○ Subarachnoid hemorrhage (SAH)
    - ○ Vasoconstrictive agents (eg, cocaine)

## DIAGNOSIS

### SIGNS AND SYMPTOMS
#### History
- Acute focal neurological symptoms presenting within 4–5 hr of onset
- Time of symptom onset is critical:
  - If time of onset cannot be firmly established, the time the patient was last known normal should be used as a surrogate.
- Historical elements that may suggest an etiology other than routine thromboembolic stroke:
  - Neck injury in carotid or vertebral dissection
  - Tearing back pain in aortic dissection
  - Drug abuse in vasospastic occlusions

#### Physical Exam
- Consider cerebral reperfusion therapy for symptoms and neurological exam findings consistent with a distinct vascular supply territory.

- Middle cerebral artery:
  - Contralateral hemiplegia and hemisensory deficits (upper > lower)
  - Contralateral homonymous hemianopsia
  - Expressive or receptive aphasia (dominant hemisphere)
  - Contralateral neglect
- Posterior cerebral artery:
  - Cortical blindness in half the visual field
  - Visual agnosia
  - Thalamic syndromes:
    - ○ Abnormal movements (chorea or hemiballismus)
    - ○ Hemisensory deficit
- Vertebrobasilar system:
  - Impaired vision, visual field defects
  - Nystagmus, vertigo, dizziness
  - Facial paresthesia, dysarthria
  - Cranial nerve palsies
  - Contralateral sensory deficits (pain and temperature)
  - Limb ataxia, abnormal gait
- Anterior cerebral artery:
  - Contralateral hemiplegia and hemisensory deficits (lower >upper)
  - Apraxia
  - Confusion, impaired judgment
- Lacunar (deep subcortical):
  - Pure motor hemiplegia (most common), or pure sensory hemiplegia
  - Dysarthria with hand ataxia (clumsy hand), or dysarthria with facial weakness
  - Ataxic hemiparesis
- The National Institutes of Health Stroke Scale (NIH-SS) can be used to delineate severity of a CVA as follows (total of subcategory scores):
  - 1a. Level of consciousness (LOC): Alert = 0; drowsy = 1; stuporous = 2; coma = 3
  - 1b. LOC questions: Answers both correctly = 0; 1 correctly = 1; none correct = 2
  - 1c. LOC commands: Obeys both correctly = 0; 1 correctly = 1; none correctly = 2
  - 2. Best gaze: Normal = 0; partial gaze palsy = 1; forced deviation = 2
  - 3. Visual: No visual loss = 0; partial hemianopia = 1; complete hemianopia = 2; bilateral hemianopia = 3
  - 4. Facial palsy: Normal, symmetric = 0; minor paralysis = 1; partial paralysis = 2; complete paralysis = 3
  - 5 to 8. Best motor (computed for each arm and leg): No drift = 0; drift = 1; some effort against gravity = 2; no effort against gravity = 3; no movement = 4
  - 9. Limb ataxia: Absent = 0; present in 1 limb = 1; present in two or more limbs = 2
  - 10. Sensory (pinprick): Normal = 0; partial loss = 1; dense loss = 2
  - 11. Best language: No aphasia = 0; mild to moderate aphasia = 1; severe aphasia = 2; mute = 3
  - 12. Dysarthria: Normal articulation = 0; mild to moderate dysarthria = 1; unintelligible = 2
  - 13. Neglect/inattention: No neglect = 0; partial neglect = 1; complete neglect = 2

### ESSENTIAL WORKUP
- Stat bedside blood glucose testing
- Immediate noncontrast head CT scan:
  - Can differentiate between ischemic and hemorrhagic CVA
  - Can reveal other etiologies
  - Very likely normal in the hours after symptom onset:
    - ○ Early signs of ischemia (eg, edema) should prompt a reevaluation of time of onset.
- EKG to assess for dysrhythmia, pericarditis, MI

### DIAGNOSTIC TESTS & INTERPRETATION
#### Lab
- CBC, serum electrolytes and glucose, BUN, creatinine, prothrombin time (PT)/partial thromboplastin time (PTT)
- Urine pregnancy test
- Urine toxicology screen
- Liver function tests in patients prone to liver dysfunction

#### Imaging
- Multimodal MRI (with perfusion- and diffusion-weighted protocols):
  - Can detect ischemic CVA almost immediately after onset
- Perfusion brain CT can reveal a perfusion deficit immediately after onset.
- MR angiography or CT angiography can provide anatomical information.
- Carotid US
- CXR

#### Diagnostic Procedures/Surgery
Cerebral angiography may be a useful diagnostic and therapeutic adjunct:

- Consider in consultation with a neurologist and interventional radiologist.

### DIFFERENTIAL DIAGNOSIS
- Intracranial hemorrhage (ICH) or SAH
- Seizure
- Complex migraine
- Bell palsy or other focal neuropathies
- Hypoglycemia and other metabolic abnormalities
- Dural sinus thrombosis
- Intracranial neoplasm
- Intracranial trauma
- Meningitis, encephalitis, or brain abscess
- Vasculitis
- Air embolism or decompression illness
- Spinal cord lesion
- Psychogenic

## 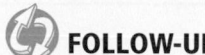 TREATMENT

### PRE-HOSPITAL
- Assess for deficits:
  - Dysarthria, facial weakness
  - Arm or leg weakness
- Notify and mobilize ED and hospital resources.
- Test blood glucose:
  - Hypoglycemia can mimic a CVA.
  - Treat hypoglycemia with dextrose.

### INITIAL STABILIZATION/THERAPY
- Supplemental oxygen to correct hypoxia
- IV access and NS bolus to correct hypotension
- Cardiac monitoring and pulse oximetry
- Rapid-sequence intubation if airway protection is warranted or ventilatory insufficiency is evident

### ED TREATMENT/PROCEDURES
- Exclude other diagnoses in the differential.
- Thrombolytic therapy should be reserved for thromboembolic ischemic strokes.
- Inclusion criteria for IV thrombolytic therapy:
  - Age ≥18 yr of age
  - Defined onset of symptoms within 4.5 hr
  - No hemorrhage on noncontrast head CT
- Absolute contraindications to IV thrombolytic therapy:
  - ICH on pretreatment head CT scan
  - Prior ICH
  - Clinical presentation consistent with SAH
  - Known arteriovenous malformation or aneurysm
  - CVA, serious brain injury, or intracranial surgery within previous 3 mo
    Active internal bleeding
  - Major surgery within previous 14 days
  - Pregnancy
  - Pericarditis
  - Known bleeding diathesis:
    - Platelet count <100,000/mm$^3$
    - INR >1.7, PT >15 sec, or prolonged PTT
    - Current anticoagulant use
    - Use of heparin within 48 hr
  - Uncontrollable HTN >185/110 mm Hg
- Relative contraindications to IV thrombolytics:
  Rapid improvement of neurological symptoms
  - Mild CVA
  - GI or GU bleeding within 21 days
  - Recent lumbar puncture
  - Recent arterial puncture at a noncompressible site
  - Seizure at the time stroke was observed
  - Blood glucose level <50 or >400 mg/dL
- Treat BP >185/110 mm Hg with 1–2 doses of labetalol, nicardipine, or other appropriate agent:
  - Do not aggressively normalize BP
  - Stroke patient may be dependent on an elevated mean arterial pressure for cerebral perfusion.
  - Avoid thrombolytic therapy if BP cannot be reduced to ≤180/110 mm Hg with minimal intervention.
- Administer IV tissue plasminogen activator (TPA); alteplase.
- Avoid antiplatelet agents and anticoagulants for 24 hr.

- Monitor arterial BP during the 1st 24 hr after treatment with TPA and aggressively treat a SBP >180 or a DBP >105:
  - Check BP every 15 min for 2 hr, then every 30 min for 6 hr, then every hour for 24 hr.
  - Keep BP <180/105 mm Hg using medication such as labetalol or nicardipine.
  - Consider nitroprusside for HTN unresponsive to labetalol or nicardipine, or for a DBP >140 mm Hg.
- Monitor for signs of ICH:
  - Decreased LOC
  - Increased weakness
  - Headache
  - Acute HTN or tachycardia
  - Nausea or vomiting
- If ICH suspected, obtain an emergent head CT to confirm diagnosis:
  - If present, treat as follows:
    - Discontinue TPA.
    - Obtain blood samples for PT, PTT, platelet count, fibrinogen level.
    - Prepare cryoprecipitate, fibrinogen, and platelets, and infuse as needed.
    - Obtain neurosurgical consultation.
- For patients who have presented after 3 hr but within 6 hr of symptom onset:
  - Consider intra-arterial thrombolysis or mechanical recanalization if available.

### ALERT
- For patients presenting between 3 and 4.5 hr of onset; there are additional exclusion criteria:
  - Age >80 yr
  - Oral anticoagulant use (regardless of INR)
  - NIH-SS >25 or >1/3 MCA territory involved
  - History of previous stroke and diabetes
- Up to a 6% risk of ICH with TPA that goes up significantly in patients with NIH-SS >20.

### MEDICATION
#### First Line
- Alteplase (TPA): 0.9 mg/kg IV, max. 90 mg, over 1 hr:
  - Give 10% of dose as a bolus over 1 min.
  - Immediately follow with the remainder, infused over the subsequent 59 min
- Labetalol: 10 mg IV over 1–2 min; then, if needed:
  - Repeat or double dose q10–20min up to a max. of 300 mg, or
  - Start a drip at 2–8 mg/min
- Nitropaste: 1–2 inches to anterior chest wall
- Nicardipine: 5 mg/hr as a drip; titrate upward in 2.5 mg/hr increments every 5 min, up to a max. of 15 mg/hr

#### Second Line
- Nitroprusside: 0.5–1.0 mg/kg/min, continuous IV drip, titrated to BP parameters
- Cryoprecipitate and fibrinogen: 6–8 U IV
- Platelets: 6–8 U IV

## 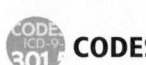 FOLLOW-UP

### DISPOSITION
#### Admission Criteria
All patients given reperfusion therapy for a CVA should be admitted to an intensive care setting for frequent neurological checks and vital sign assessments.

#### Issues for Referral
Not applicable

## PEARLS AND PITFALLS
- Be specific in eliciting time of onset; patient or family may note "time of onset" as the time the stroke was 1st recognized (eg, upon awakening from sleep)
- TPA has a plasma half-life of <5 min; a delay between bolus and infusion, or pause in the infusion, may result in a decrease in plasma levels and effectiveness.
- "Time is brain" (and hemorrhage); initiate treatment as quickly as possible, even if the patient presents early.
- There are additional exclusion criteria for administration of TPA for patients presenting between 3 and 4.5 hr.

## ADDITIONAL READING
- Adams HP Jr., del Zoppo G, Alberts MJ, et al. Guidelines for the early management of adults with ischemic stroke: A guideline from the American Heart Association/American Stroke Association Stroke Council, Clinical Cardiology Council, Cardiovascular Radiology and Intervention Council, and the Atherosclerotic Peripheral Vascular Disease and Quality of Care Outcomes in Research Interdisciplinary Working Groups. Stroke. 2007;38: 1655–1711.
- del Zoppo GJ, Saver JL, Jauch EC, et al. Expansion of the time window for treatment of acute ischemic stroke with IV/IV tissue plasminogen activator: A science advisory from the American Heart Association/American Stroke Association. Stroke. 2009;40:2945–2948.
- Hacke W, Kaste M, Bluhmki E, et al. Thrombolysis with alteplase 3 to 4.5 hours after acute ischemic stroke. N Engl J Med. 2008;359:1317–1329.
- Leary M, Saver JL, Gobin PY, et al. Beyond tissue plasminogen activator: Mechanical intervention in acute stroke. Ann Emerg Med. 2003;41:838–846.
- The NINDS rt-PA Stroke Study Group. Tissue plasminogen activator for acute ischemic stroke. N Engl J Med. 1995;333:1581–1587.

### See Also (Topic, Algorithm, Electronic Media Element)
- Cerebral Vascular Accident
- Transient Ischemic Attack

## CODES

### ICD9
434.91 Cerebral artery occlusion, unspecified with cerebral infarction

R

# RESPIRATORY DISTRESS

*Erik D. Barton*

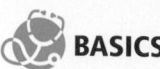 **BASICS**

## DESCRIPTION
Respiratory distress, shortness of breath, or dyspnea is a common complaint for patients presenting to the ED.

## ETIOLOGY
- Upper airway obstruction:
  - Epiglottitis
  - Croup syndromes
  - Laryngotracheobronchitis
  - Foreign body
  - Angioedema
  - Retropharyngeal abscess
- Cardiovascular:
  - Pulmonary edema/CHF
  - Dysrhythmias
  - Cardiac ischemia
  - Pulmonary embolus
  - Pericarditis
  - Tamponade
  - Air embolism
- Pulmonary:
  - Asthma
  - Chronic obstructive pulmonary disease (COPD)/emphysema
  - Pneumonia
  - Influenza
  - Bronchiolitis
  - Aspiration
  - Adult respiratory distress syndrome (ARDS)
  - Pulmonary edema
  - Pleural effusion
  - Toxic inhalation injury
- Trauma:
  - Pneumothorax
  - Tension pneumothorax
  - Rib fractures
  - Pulmonary contusion
  - Fat embolism with long bone fractures
- Neuromuscular:
  - Guillain-Barré syndrome
  - Myasthenia gravis
- Metabolic/systemic/toxic:
  - Anaphylaxis
  - Anemia
  - Acidosis
  - Hyperthyroidism
  - Sepsis
  - Septic emboli from IV drug use or infected indwelling lines
  - Salicylate intoxication
  - Drug overdose
  - Amphetamines
  - Cocaine
  - Sympathomimetic
  - Obesity
- Psychogenic:
  - Anxiety disorder
  - Hyperventilation syndrome
- Bioterrorist threats:
  - Anthrax
  - Pneumonic plague
  - Tularemia
  - Viral hemorrhagic fevers

### Pediatric Considerations
- Respiratory failure is most common cause of cardiac arrest in infants.
- Croup syndromes include:
  - Viral
  - Spasmodic
  - Bacterial
  - Congenital defects
  - Noninflammatory causes (foreign body, gastroesophageal reflux, trauma, tumors)
- Most common cause of upper airway obstruction:
  - <6 months: Congenital laryngomalacia
  - >6 months: Viral croup
- Epiglottitis:
  - Highest incidence at ages 2–4 years
  - Abrupt onset
  - Fever
  - Respiratory distress and stridor
  - Difficulty swallowing oral secretions
  - Restlessness and anxiety

### Pregnancy Considerations
- Amniotic fluid embolism during or after delivery
- Septic embolism from septic abortion or postpartum uterine infection

 **DIAGNOSIS**

## SIGNS AND SYMPTOMS
- Tachypnea
- Dyspnea
- Tachycardia
- Anxiety
- Diaphoresis
- Cough ("barking," productive)
- Stridor
- Hoarse voice
- Difficulty swallowing or handling oral secretions
- Upper airway rhonchi (wheezes)
- Lower airway crackles (rales)
- Increased work of breathing
- Accessory and intercostal muscle use
- Hypoxemia
- Hypocapnia or hypercapnia if severe
- Respiratory acidosis
- Cyanosis
- Lethargy, then obtundation

## History
- Previous history of asthma, COPD, cardiac disease, or dysrhythmia, CHF, foreign-body aspiration, or toxic exposure
- Recent fever or upper respiratory tract infection, cough, sputum production, sore throat, systemic disease, anxiety disorder
- Recent chest or long-bone trauma
- IV drug use or indwelling catheters
- Recurrent fevers, night sweats, weight loss

## Physical Exam
- Observe: Mental status, level of distress, work of breathing, jugular venous pressure, skin color
- Feel/palpate: Distal pulses, heart perioperative MI, chest wall, peripheral edema
- Percuss: Lungs for dullness or resonance, abdominal distention or hepatomegaly
- Auscultate: Heart sounds, murmurs, lung wheezes or crackles, neck for upper airway stridor, abdomen bowel sounds

### Pediatric Considerations
- Evaluate retractions, behavior, respiratory rate, breath sounds, and skin color.
- Weak cry, expiratory grunting, nasal flaring, tachypnea and tachycardia, retractions, and cyanosis in neonates

## ESSENTIAL WORKUP
- Pulse oximetry
- Cardiac and BP monitoring
- EKG if suspected cardiac etiology

## DIAGNOSTIC TESTS & INTERPRETATION
### Lab
- ABG for severity and acid–base determination
- CBC
- Electrolytes, BUN/creatinine, glucose
- Sputum cultures, smears, and Gram stain
- Blood cultures for fever or sepsis
- B-type natriuretic peptide (BNP) for undifferentiated shortness of breath or CHF severity
- Venous thromboembolus test (VTE) for low-risk PE
- HIV
- Seasonal and "novel" flu testing
- Urinary output monitoring for CHF
- Toxicology screen or salicylate level if suspected

### Imaging
- CXR for:
  - Pneumonia
  - Pneumothorax
  - Hyperinflation
  - Atelectasis
  - CHF/pulmonary edema
  - Abscess/cavitary lesions/other infiltrates
  - Tuberculosis
- Spirometry (peak expiratory flow rates) for asthma, COPD
- Neck CT or radiographs to assess epiglottis and soft-tissue spaces, foreign body
- Fiberoptic laryngoscopy to assess epiglottis, vocal cords, and pharyngeal space
- CT angiography or ventilation/perfusion scan for pulmonary embolus

### Pediatric Considerations
- Chest/neck radiograph may show foreign body or "steeple sign" in croup syndromes.
- Chest fluoroscopy may be used to assess inspiratory and expiratory excursions if foreign body is suspected.

### Diagnostic Procedures/Surgery
- Bronchoscopy for foreign body in trachea or bronchus
- Pulmonary artery (Swan-Ganz) catheter for severe CHF, ARDS, pulmonary edema

## DIFFERENTIAL DIAGNOSIS
See "Etiology."

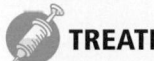

## TREATMENT

### PRE-HOSPITAL
- Assume a position of comfort for patient.
- 100% oxygen:
  - Assisted bag-valve mask (BMV) ventilation if obtunded
- Airway adjunct devices (oral or nasal) to maintain patency if tolerated
- Intubation for severe respiratory distress
- Needle aspiration of suspected tension pneumothorax

### INITIAL STABILIZATION/THERAPY
- ABCs
- Ensure patent airway; BVM assist or intubate for severe distress or arrest
- IV fluids if hypotensive
- 100% oxygen by face mask:
  - Use cautiously in patients with severe COPD or chronic $CO_2$ retention.
- Monitor BP, heart rate, respirations, pulse oximetry
- Advanced cardiac life support for dysrhythmias or arrest

### ED TREATMENT/PROCEDURES
- Treat underlying etiology as appropriate.
- CHF or pulmonary edema:
  - Diuretics
  - Nitroglycerin
  - Nitroprusside if hypertensive
  - Pulmonary artery catheter if severe
  - Noninvasive positive-pressure ventilation (NPPV/BiPAP) or intubation if severe
- Asthma, bronchiolitis, COPD:
  - Bronchodilators
  - Steroids
  - Antibiotics for infection
  - Antivirals for influenza
  - NPPV or intubation if severe
- ARDS, aspiration, toxic lung injury:
  - Mechanical ventilation as needed
  - Steroids controversial
- Pneumonia:
  - Antibiotics
  - Respiratory isolation for TB
- Pneumothorax:
  - Immediate decompression if suspected tension pneumothorax
  - Aspiration or tube thoracostomy (see Pneumothorax)

- Pleural effusion:
  - Determine etiology
  - Diagnostic and symptomatic thoracentesis
- Croup:
  - Cool, misted air or oxygen
  - Steroids
  - Racemic epinephrine
  - Antibiotics for bacterial infection
- Epiglottitis:
  - Immediate airway stabilization with intubation or tracheostomy in OR if possible
  - Antibiotics for *Haemophilus influenzae*
- Anaphylaxis, angioedema:
  - IV steroids
  - $H_1/H_2$-blockers
  - SQ or IV epinephrine
  - Early intubation
- Retropharyngeal abscess:
  - Drainage
  - IV antibiotics
  - ENT consult
- Cardiac:
  - Treat dysrhythmias or ischemia
  - Anticoagulation or thrombolysis for PE
  - Pericardiocentesis for tamponade
  - NSAIDs or aspirin for pericarditis
- Neuromuscular:
  - Support ventilation
  - Pyridostigmine bromide or neostigmine for myasthenia gravis
- Metabolic/toxic:
  - Treat underlying cause
- Psychogenic:
  - Anxiolytics

### Pediatric Considerations
- Transtracheal jet ventilation if unable to intubate (cricothyrotomy not recommended in children <10 yr)
- Bronchiolitis:
  - Bronchodilators
  - Antivirals for respiratory syncytial virus
  - Antibiotics for infection
- Spasmodic croup:
  - Very sensitive to misted air
- Bacterial croup (membranous laryngotracheobronchitis):
  - Treat *Staphylococcus aureus*.

### Pregnancy Considerations
- Supportive oxygen therapy and heparin for PE or amniotic fluid embolism
- IV antibiotics for septic embolism

## MEDICATION
Refer to specific etiologies

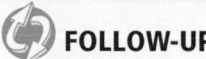

## FOLLOW-UP

### DISPOSITION
#### Admission Criteria
- Continued supplemental oxygen requirement
- Cardiac or hemodynamic instability:
  - Requiring IV therapy or hydration
  - Requiring close airway observation or repeated treatments
  - Respiratory isolation
- As required by underlying cause or significant comorbid disease

#### Discharge Criteria
- Correction of underlying disease
- Stable airway
- Acute supplemental oxygen not required

#### Issues for Referral
Refer to specific etiologies

## PEARLS AND PITFALLS
- Consider immune-compromised state.
- Consider "novel" flu strains (H1N1).
- Start antibiotic treatment within 6 hours of ED arrival (JCAHO Quality Measure).

## ADDITIONAL READING
- Ausiello D, Goldman L. Eds. *Cecil textbook of medicine*, 22nd ed., Philadelphia: WB Saunders; 2004:492–583, 1523–1524.
- Barton ED, Collings J, DeBlieux PMC, et al., eds. *Adams emergency medicine*, 1st ed. Philadelphia: Saunders Elsevier; 2009:455–512, 1935–42.
- Sigillito RJ, DeBlieux PM. Evaluation and initial management of the patient in respiratory distress. *Emerg Med Clin North Am.* 2003;21(2):239–258.
- Williams SA, Hutson HR, Speals HL. Dyspnea. In: *Emergency medicine: Concepts and clinical practice*, 4th ed. St. Louis: Mosby; 1998:1460–1469.

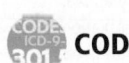

## CODES

### ICD9
- 770.89 Other respiratory problems after birth
- 786.09 Other dyspnea and respiratory abnormalities

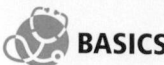

## BASICS

### DESCRIPTION
- Annually, almost 1 million deaths worldwide are related to birth asphyxia.
- 10% of newborns require some assistance at birth.
- 1% of newborns require extensive resuscitation.
- Consider NOT initiating resuscitation if:
  - Newborns confirmed to be <23 wk gestation or 400 g
  - Anencephaly
  - Babies with confirmed trisomy 13 or 18
  - Ideally, discuss with family and health care team prior to delivery.
- APGAR (activity, pulse, grimace, appearance, respiration) scores do not guide resuscitation:
  - Do not wait to assign APGAR scores prior to starting resuscitation.
  - APGAR scores should NOT guide resuscitative efforts.
  - APGAR score: 5 categories with score of 0, 1, or 2 in each at 1 and 5 min
- Heart rate: 0 = absent; 1 = <100 bpm; 2 = >100 bpm
- Respirations: 0 = absent; 1 = slow, irregular; 2 = good, crying
- Muscle tone: 0 = limp; 1 = some flexion; 2 = active motion
- Reflex irritability: 0 = no response; 1 = grimace; 2 = cough, sneeze, cry
- Color: 0 = blue or pale; 1 = pink body and blue extremities; 2 = all pink

### ETIOLOGY
- Newborns transition from dependence on the placenta to dependence on the lungs for oxygen.
- Hypoxia initially causes tachypnea followed by primary apnea.
- Stimulation may cause resumption of breathing during primary apnea.
- Continued hypoxia leads to secondary apnea.
- Secondary apnea requires assisted ventilation.
- Antepartum risk factors associated with need for resuscitation include:
  - Maternal diabetes
  - Pregnancy-induced hypertension
  - Chronic hypertension
  - Anemia
  - Previous fetal or neonatal death
  - Bleeding in 2nd or 3rd trimester
  - Maternal infection
  - Maternal cardiac, renal pulmonary, thyroid or neurologic disease
  - Polyhydramnios
  - Oligohydramnios
  - Premature rupture of membranes
  - Postterm gestation
  - Multiple gestation
  - Size–dates discrepancy
  - Drug therapy
  - Maternal substance abuse
  - Fetal malformation
  - Diminished fetal activity
  - No prenatal care
  - Maternal age <16 or >35 yr
- Intrapartum risk factors associated with need for resuscitation include:
  - Emergency C-section
  - Forceps or vacuum assist
  - Breech or other abnormal presentation
  - Premature labor
  - Precipitous labor
  - Chorioamnionitis
  - Prolonged rupture of membranes
  - Prolonged 2nd stage of labor
  - Fetal bradycardia
  - Non-reassuring fetal heart tracing
  - General anesthesia
  - Uterine tetany
- Narcotics administered to mother within 4 hr:
  - Meconium-stained amniotic fluid
  - Prolapsed cord
  - Abruptio placenta
  - Placenta previa

## DIAGNOSIS

### SIGNS AND SYMPTOMS
Compromised infants requiring resuscitation may exhibit 1 or more of:
- Decreased muscle tone.
- Depressed respiratory drive.
- Bradycardia
- Hypotension
- Tachypnea
- Cyanosis

### History
Risk factors as above predict the need for resuscitation

### Physical Exam
- Respirations—rate and effectiveness
- Heart rate (HR)—by auscultation or palpation of umbilical cord
- Color

### ESSENTIAL WORKUP
ABCs:
- Airway
- Breathing
- Circulation
- Drying and warming child

### DIAGNOSTIC TESTS & INTERPRETATION
#### Lab
- Bedside blood glucose measurement
- Blood gas

#### Imaging
Chest radiograph

#### Diagnostic Procedures/Surgery
- Endotracheal intubation:
  - Straight blades Miller 1 for full term, Miller 0 for preterm
  - Endotracheal tubes (ETTs):
    - 2.5 for <1,000 g or <28 wk
    - 3.0 for 1,000–2,000 g or 28–34 wk
    - 3.5 for 2,000–3,000 g or 34–38 wk
    - 4.0 for >3,000 g or >38 wk
  - Have stylet, end-tidal $CO_2$ detector, suction, tape, meconium aspirator available.
- Umbilical vein catheterization:
  - Tie umbilical tape around base of cord.
  - Prefill syringe attached to umbilical catheter (3.5 or 5 Fr).
  - Cut cord on clean edge below clamp.
  - Identify umbilical vein (large, thin-walled and single).
  - Insert catheter into umbilical vein directed cephalad.
  - Advance 2–4 cm until blood flows freely into syringe.
  - Inject drugs/fluids as appropriate.
  - Secure catheter with suture.

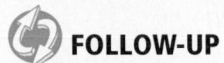

# TREATMENT

## PRE-HOSPITAL
- Resuscitation should be started by prehospital personnel.
- Neonatal resuscitation equipment should be available.
- Pay particular attention to heat retention and warming.

## INITIAL STABILIZATION/THERAPY
- ABCs
- If meconium, poor respiratory effort, poor muscle tone, cyanosis, or prematurity are present, proceed with resuscitation.
- Initial steps include:
  - Warm the baby.
  - Position (neck slightly extended, sniffing position) and clear the airway (meconium may necessitate intubation—see below).
  - Dry thoroughly; stimulate (flick feet, rub trunk or extremities).
  - Provide oxygen.
- Meconium:
  - Meconium present and baby is not vigorous:
    - Insert endotracheal tube (ETT).
    - Suction with endotracheal tube meconium aspiration device.
    - Slowly withdraw tube.
    - Repeat as necessary until little meconium is recovered or HR is not maintained.
  - Meconium present and baby is vigorous.
  - Suction mouth then nose with bulb or suction catheter.
- If reevaluation within 30 sec reveals apnea or HR <100 bpm, proceed with:
  - Positive-pressure ventilation with 100% oxygen
  - Self inflating or flow-inflating (anesthesia type) bag
  - Proper-fitting mask
  - 1st breath may require high pressure, necessitating occlusion of "pop-off" valve.
  - Rate of 40–60 breaths/min
  - Pressure of 20–40 cm H₂O
  - If prolonged, place nasogastric (NG) tube.
- If reevaluation after 30 sec of positive-pressure ventilation with 100% oxygen reveals HR <60 bpm, proceed with:
  - Continued positive-pressure ventilation and chest compressions
  - 2-thumb technique: Hands encircle torso
  - 2-finger technique:
    - Compress ~1/3 the anterior posterior diameter of chest and release.
    - 1 recent study suggests compressing to ~1/2 the diameter of the chest.
  - 3 compressions followed by 1 ventilation
  - 120 events/min (90 compressions and 30 breaths)

- If after 30 sec HR is >60 bpm, stop compressions.
- If after 30 sec HR is >100 bpm, stop positive-pressure ventilator.
- If after 30 sec HR still <60 bpm, administer epinephrine (IV or via ET tube).

## ED TREATMENT/PROCEDURES
- If evidence of blood loss or poor response to resuscitation, administer volume expander.
- NS, lactated Ringer, O-negative blood (cross-matched if time permitting)
- If severe metabolic acidosis is suspected or proven:
  - Ensure adequate ventilation.
  - Administer sodium bicarbonate.
- If hypoglycemia is proven or suspected, treat with IV dextrose.
- If heart rate and color improve but respiratory effort and tone are poor and mother received narcotics within 4 hr, treat with naloxone hydrochloride:
  - Contraindicated in mothers addicted to narcotics or receiving methadone: Can precipitate seizures.
- Persistent distress may indicate pneumothorax.
- Known or suspected diaphragmatic hernias should be treated with immediate endotracheal intubation and placement of NG tube.
- Consider discontinuation of resuscitation if 10 min of asystole.

## MEDICATION
- Dextrose: 2–4 mL/kg of D10W given IV (umbilical vein)
- Epinephrine: 0.1–0.3 mL/kg of 1:10,000 solution, may be given IV or via ETT (0.3–1 mL/kg if giving via ETT)
- Naloxone hydrochloride: 0.1 mg/kg. Administer IV or via ETT; can administer IM or SC, but onset of action is delayed.
- Sodium bicarbonate: 2 mEq/kg (4 mL/kg of 4.2% solution) (0.5 mEq/mL). Administer slowly via IV route (umbilical vein).
- Volume expanders: NS, lactated Ringer, blood. Initial dose 10 mL/kg, may be repeated, all given IV (umbilical vein).
- Other agents as specifically indicated by newborn's underlying condition

# FOLLOW-UP

## DISPOSITION
### Admission Criteria
- All newborns require admission.
- If significant resuscitation is necessary, admit to NCIU.

## PEARLS AND PITFALLS
- Resuscitation and care of low-birth-weight infants may lead to the following complications:
  - Difficulty with thermoregulation
  - Intraventricular hemorrhage
  - Chronic lung disease
  - Retinopathy of prematurity
- Oxygen and the very low birth weight (VLBW) infant:
  - VLBW infant defined as birth weight <1,500 g
  - VLBW infants are at increased risk of oxidative stress and damage including retinopathy of prematurity.
  - Some studies suggest resuscitating with <100% oxygen in this group, possibly even 21% (room air), to avoid oxidative stress and damage.

## ADDITIONAL READING
- Fowlie PW, McGuire W. Immediate care of the preterm infant. *BMJ*. 2004;329(9):845–848.
- Kattwinkel J, ed. *Textbook of neonatal resuscitation*. 5th ed. Elk Grove Village, IL: American Academy of Pediatrics; 2006.

### See Also (Topic, Algorithm, Electronic Media Element)
- Skills may be enhanced with education and practice at a simulation center.
- Resuscitation, Pediatric

# CODES

## ICD9
768.9 Unspecified severity of birth asphyxia in liveborn infant

# RESUSCITATION, PEDIATRIC

Brian Clyne
Brandon Maughan

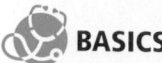

## BASICS

### DESCRIPTION
Emergent treatment of pediatric patients with imminent or ongoing respiratory or circulatory failure

### ETIOLOGY
- Respiratory failure
- Early shock (compensated)
- Late shock (uncompensated)
- Cardiopulmonary arrest
- Respiratory and/or circulatory failure leads to tissue hypoxia, acidosis, and cell death.
- Multisystem organ failure subsequently develops.

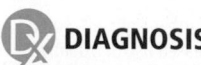

## DIAGNOSIS

### SIGNS AND SYMPTOMS
#### History
- History from caregivers/parents of onset, progression, inciting, contributing, or predisposing trauma/exposure/conditions, associated findings, past medical history, family history, medications, ingestions
- History of immediate preceding events from transporting prehospital personnel
- Respiratory failure:
  - Tachypnea
  - Slow, irregular breathing pattern prearrest
  - Decreased or absent breath sounds; inadequate ventilation
  - Retractions, accessory muscle use, expiratory grunting, nasal flaring
  - Mottled skin, cyanosis
  - Altered level of consciousness (LOC): Irritability, agitation, lethargy, weak or absent cry, decreased response to pain
  - Poor muscle tone
  - Weak or absent cough or gag reflex
- Early shock (compensated):
  - Vital signs initially compensated
  - Orthostatic changes or isolated tachycardia
  - Slightly delayed cap refill (>2 sec)
  - Warm, dry skin in early septic shock
- Late shock (uncompensated):
  - Tachycardia, tachypnea, prearrest bradycardia
  - Hypotension, weak peripheral pulses
  - Mottled, pale, cool extremities with markedly decreased capillary refill
  - Decreased urine output progressing to anuria
  - Decreased LOC, seizures, coma
  - Fever or hypothermia in septic shock
- Cardiopulmonary arrest:
  - Final common pathway of progressive deterioration of respiratory and circulatory function

#### Physical Exam
- Airway assessment:
  - Look, listen, feel for air movement, breath sounds, and chest movement. Observe for stridor or signs of obstruction.

- Breathing assessment:
  - Respiratory rate: Tachypnea or slow/irregular pattern (more ominous)
  - Respiratory effort: Note grunting, nasal flaring, head bobbing, retractions, stridor.
  - Pulse oximetry reflects hemoglobin oxygen saturation, not necessarily oxygen delivery.
  - Auscultation: Assess for wheezing, rales, diminished breath sounds.
- Circulatory assessment:
  - Pulse: Tachycardia or bradycardia (more ominous); orthostatic changes noted easily.
  - Blood pressure: Typical SBP in children is 90 mm Hg plus twice the age (yrs). Hypotension is a late finding; widened pulse pressure in early septic shock.
  - Peripheral pulse presence and strength (brachial/femoral [<1 yr] or carotid [>1 yr])
  - Capillary refill: Delayed >2 sec with poor perfusion
  - Skin: Mottled, pale, or cyanotic with poor perfusion
- Mental status assessment:
  - Observe for signs of decreased CNS perfusion: Decreased responsiveness, irritability, confusion, agitation, poor muscle tone, sluggish pupillary response, posturing.
- Complete set of vital signs including rectal temperature, oximetry, and orthostatics when appropriate

### ESSENTIAL WORKUP
- ABCDE evaluation:
  - Airway: Assess patient ability to speak/cry; look, listen, and feel for air movement. Observe for stridor or signs of trauma.
  - Breathing: Observe for nasal flaring, grunting, head bobbing, retractions, tracheal deviation, signs of chest injury or pneumothorax; auscultate, apply oxygen.
  - Circulation: Evaluate pulses, heart rate, blood pressure, capillary refill, mottling/cyanosis.
  - Disability: Determine mental status with alert/verbal/painful/unresponsive (AVPU) responsiveness scale or Glasgow Coma Scale and assess for neurologic deficits; check stat glucose.
  - Exposure/environment: Fully expose for rapid skeletal survey while preventing hypothermia.
- Obtain pertinent history from emergency medical services or family.

### DIAGNOSTIC TESTS & INTERPRETATION
#### Lab
- Workup directed by history, assessment of airway, breathing, and circulation (ABCs) and differential diagnosis
- Arterial blood gas with oximetry to assess oxygenation, ventilation, acid–base status
- Glucose, electrolytes; use bedside glucometer, rapid electrolyte assay if available.
- Other metabolic/toxicology tests as indicated
- Sepsis evaluation including lumbar puncture, urine and blood cultures as indicated

#### Imaging
- Chest radiograph to evaluate pulmonary or cardiac etiologies
- Lateral decubitus film, inspiratory/expiratory film, or laryngoscopy/bronchoscopy for suspicion of foreign body
- ECG
- Echocardiogram
- Cervical spine, other trauma films as indicated
- CT brain for trauma or abnormal neuro exam
- US as indicated

### DIFFERENTIAL DIAGNOSIS
- Cardiopulmonary failure in children is usually the result of primary respiratory failure but is the potential endpoint of all untreated or unresponsive critical illness.
- Respiratory:
  - Upper airway obstruction: Croup, epiglottitis, peritonsillar or retropharyngeal abscess, foreign body, tracheitis, congenital abnormalities
  - Lower airway obstruction: Asthma, pneumonia, bronchiolitis, foreign body, cystic fibrosis
  - Thoracic trauma, near drowning
- Hypovolemia: Trauma/hemorrhage, diarrhea/vomiting, burns
- Cardiovascular: Congenital/acquired heart disease, myocarditis, pericarditis, CHF, dysrhythmias
- Infectious: Sepsis, meningitis, gastroenteritis, peritonitis
- CNS: Status epilepticus, epidural/subdural hematoma
- Metabolic: Diabetic ketoacidosis, hypoglycemia, hypernatremia, hypo/hyperkalemia, acidosis
- Toxicologic: CO poisoning, cardiotoxic agents
- Near sudden infant death syndrome/apparent life-threatening event
- Consider child abuse when history is inconsistent with the illness or pattern of injury.

## TREATMENT

### PRE-HOSPITAL
- Priority is to stabilize ABCs; monitor.
- Avoid prolonged on-scene times; rapid transport of critically ill child is crucial.
- Gather history from family/bystanders about preceding events, past medical history, medications, and allergies.
- Recognize respiratory or circulatory failure; intervene early.
- Recognize impending arrest and provide life-sustaining procedures during transport.
- Automated external defibrillator for ventricular fibrillation (VF) and pulseless ventricular tachycardia (VT) in children ≥1 yr.
- Timely notification of ED to allow proper preparation

### INITIAL STABILIZATION/THERAPY
- Early recognition and stabilization of respiratory failure or shock
- Glucose, IV, oxygen, cardiac monitoring

- Diagnose and treat immediately life-threatening conditions simultaneously.
- Empirical intervention is required.
- Broselow Pediatric Emergency Tape relates patient's length to weight and thus to appropriate drug doses and equipment sizes.

## ED TREATMENT/PROCEDURES
- Airway:
  - Secure 1st in every resuscitation.
  - Open airway with head tilt/chin lift or modified jaw thrust (if trauma suspected).
  - Clear secretions and blood with suction.
  - Temporary stabilization with oral or nasal airway, bag-valve mask assistance
  - Intubation as necessary using appropriate tube size ([16 + age in years]/4) or size similar to patient's little finger or nares
- Rapid-sequence intubation:
  - Preoxygenate
  - Pretreatment: Atropine to prevent bradycardia, lidocaine if head injury
  - Induction agents: Midazolam, thiopental, etomidate, ketamine
  - Paralytics: Succinylcholine, pancuronium, vecuronium, rocuronium
  - Position of endotracheal tube (ETT) at lips (cm) = 3 times diameter of tube (mm)
  - Postintubation: Confirm tube placement with colorimetric $CO_2$ device, continuous end-tidal $CO_2$ monitoring, auscultation.
- Breathing:
  - Oxygenate with supplemental $O_2$, nonrebreather mask; assist ventilation with bag-valve mask or control ventilation if intubation performed.
  - Treat conditions that limit ability to oxygenate/ventilate: Pneumothorax, hemothorax, cardiac tamponade, circumferential burns.
- Circulation:
  - Obtain access: IV, intraosseous (IO), or central
  - Fluid resuscitate with crystalloid (NS or lactated Ringer) bolus at 10–20 mL/kg; repeat if necessary; correct hypovolemia.
  - Control obvious sources of bleeding: Apply direct pressure; elevate.
  - Consider transfusion of packed RBCs after crystalloid replacement in trauma.
  - Vasopressors in decompensated shock: Epinephrine, dopamine, norepinephrine.
  - Inotropes in compensated shock: Dobutamine, milrinone.
- Cardiopulmonary resuscitation:
  - Provide blood flow to vital organs while restoring spontaneous circulation:
  - Infant <1 yr: Check brachial or femoral pulse.
  - Child 1–8 yr: Check carotid pulse.
- Cardiac dysrhythmias:
  - Usually secondary to respiratory insufficiency or metabolic disturbance
  - Treat dysrhythmias per published algorithms.
  - Unstable tachydysrhythmia may require adenosine, lidocaine, amiodarone, cardioversion, or defibrillation.
  - Unstable bradydysrhythmia may require atropine, epinephrine, or pacing.
  - Pulseless rhythms: VF, pulseless VT, pulseless electrical activity, asystole. May require epinephrine, defibrillation, lidocaine, amiodarone
- Continuously monitor patient.

## MEDICATION
- 1st or loading dose unless otherwise noted
- All IV doses may be given IO if necessary
- LEAN (lidocaine, epinephrine, atropine, Narcan) may be given by endotracheal route
- Epinephrine: Multiple uses:
  - Pulseless arrest/symptomatic bradycardia: 0.01 mg/kg 1:10,000 IV q3–5min (max 1 mg) or 0.1 mg/kg 1:1,000 ETT q3–5 min
  - Asthma: 0.01 mg/kg 1:1,000 SC q15min
  - Anaphylaxis: 0.01 mg/kg 1:1,000 IM in thigh q15min (max 0.5 mg); if hypotensive, 0.01 mg/kg 1:10,000 IV q3–5min
  - Shock with hypotension: 0.1–1 mcg/kg/min IV
  - Toxins/overdose: 0.01 mg/kg 1:10,000 IV; if no response, consider higher doses up to 0.1 mg/kg 1:1,000 IV.
- Rapid-sequence intubation
  - Pretreatment:
    - Atropine: 0.02 mg/kg IV, minimum 0.1 mg
    - Lidocaine: 1–2 mg/kg IV
  - Induction:
    - Etomidate: 0.3 mg/kg IV
    - Ketamine: 1–1.5 mg/kg IV or 4–5 mg/kg IM
    - Midazolam: 0.1–0.2 mg/kg IV
    - Thiopental: 3–5 mg/kg IV
  - Paralytics:
    - Succinylcholine: 1–2 mg/kg IV
    - Rocuronium: 0.6–1.2 mg/kg IV
    - Vecuronium: 0.1–0.2 mg/kg IV
    - Pancuronium: 0.1 mg/kg IV
- Antiarrhythmic agents:
  - Adenosine: 0.1 mg/kg (max 6 mg) IV rapid push; 2nd dose 0.2 mg/kg (max 12 mg).
  - Amiodarone: 5 mg/kg IV, max dose 300 mg. Give as bolus for pulseless VF/VT, load over 20–60 min for supraventricular tachycardia/VT.
  - Lidocaine: For VF or pulseless VT: 1 mg/kg IV bolus, 20–50 mcg/kg/min IV maintenance.
  - Magnesium sulfate: 25–50 mg/kg (max 2 g) for pulseless VT with torsades de pointes
  - Procainamide: 15 mg/kg IV over 30–60 min.
- Inotropes and pressors:
  - Dobutamine: 2–20 mcg/kg/min IV
  - Dopamine: 2–20 mcg/kg/min IV
  - Inamrinone: Load 0.75–1 mg/kg IV over 5 min; maintenance 5–10 mcg/kg/min
  - Milrinone: Load 50–75 mcg/kg IV over 10–60 min; maintenance 0.5 × 0.75 mcg/kg/min
  - Norepinephrine: 0.1–2 mcg/kg/min IV
- Other agents:
  - Albuterol: For asthma or anaphylaxis, multidose inhaler 4–8 puffs q20min or nebulizer 2.5 mg/dose (5 mg/dose if >20 kg) q20min; for severe symptoms: 0.5 mg/kg/hr by continuous nebulizer
  - Alprostadil: 0.05–0.1 mcg/kg/min IV for ductal-dependent congenital heart disease
  - Calcium chloride: 20 mg/kg IV; give as slow push in arrest with suspected hypocalcemia.
  - Dexamethasone: 0.6 mg/kg IV (max 16 mg) for severe croup with impending respiratory failure or for mild-moderate asthma
  - Dextrose: 0.5–1 g/kg IV. D25W 2–4 mL/kg or D10W 5–10 mL/kg.
  - Diphenhydramine: 1–2 mg/kg IV q4–6 hr
  - Ipratropium: 250–500 mcg q20min ×3 doses
  - Naloxone: 0.1 mg/kg IV q2min (max 2 mg)
  - Sodium bicarbonate: 1 mEq/kg IV slow bolus
  - Terbutaline: 10 mcg/kg SC q10–15min or 0.1–10 mg/kg/min IV for status asthmaticus
- Cardioversion: 0.5–1 J/kg, increase to 2 J/kg
- Defibrillation: 2 J/kg, increase to 4 J/kg

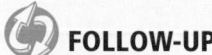 FOLLOW-UP

## DISPOSITION
### Admission Criteria
- All patients with impending or ongoing respiratory or cardiovascular compromise
- Survivors of cardiopulmonary arrest require continuous monitoring for decompensation postresuscitation in an ICU setting.
- Consider transfer to pediatric critical care center.

### Discharge Criteria
Patients with mild dehydration who respond to fluid resuscitation without signs of hemodynamic instability may be considered for discharge. Such children did not require resuscitation beyond fluids.

### Issues for Referral
- Consultation with pediatric intensivist for any patient requiring pressors or intubation
- Consultation as appropriate depending on specific etiology
- Involve authorities if abuse is suspected.

## FOLLOW-UP RECOMMENDATIONS
- Educate patients, parents, and caregivers regarding household products and toxic ingestions.
- Educate patients about self-administration of epinephrine in anaphylaxis (if age appropriate).

## PEARLS AND PITFALLS
- Empiric treatment is often necessary.
- In very young children, examine for signs of early sepsis.
- Consider abuse if exam is inconsistent with history.

## ADDITIONAL READING
- 2005 American Heart Association (AHA) guidelines for cardiopulmonary resuscitation (CPR) and emergency cardiovascular care (ECC) of pediatric and neonatal patients: Pediatric basic life support. *Circulation.* 2005;112(24S):IV1–IV203.
- Cardiopulmonary resuscitation and pediatric advanced life support: Update for the emergency physician. *Pediatr Emerg Care.* 2008;24(8): 561–565.
- Pediatric Advanced Life Support Task Force, ILCOR. Use of automated external defibrillators for children: An update. *Circulation.* 2003;107(25):3250–3255.
- Ralston M, Hazinski MF, Zaritsky AL, et al. *Pediatric Advanced Life Support.* Dallas, TX: American Heart Association; 2006.
- The International Liaison Committee on Resuscitation (ILCOR) consensus on science with treatment recommendations for pediatric and neonatal patients: Pediatric basic and advanced life support. *Pediatrics.* 2006;117(5):e955–e977.

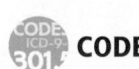 CODES

ICD9
- 518.81 Acute respiratory failure
- 785.50 Shock, unspecified

# RETINAL DETACHMENT

Scott R. Sanderson
Carl G. Skinner

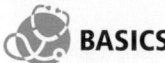 **BASICS**

## DESCRIPTION
- 3 types of retinal detachments with common final pathway:
  - Rhegmatogenous retinal detachments (RRD)
  - Tractional retinal detachments (TRD)
  - Exudative retinal detachments (ERD)
- RRD:
  - Most common
  - Violation of sensory retina allows vitreous to separate the sensory and pigmented parts of retina from each other.
  - Acute event, flashes secondary to tearing of nerve fibers, floaters secondary to bleeding; from ruptured retinal vessels
- TRD:
  - Contraction of fibrous vitreous bands, as a result of previous insult, pulls the sensory retina off the pigmented retina.
  - Chronic and progressive
  - Asymptomatic unless hemorrhage or retinal tear occurs
- ERD:
  - Subretinal collections of serous fluid separate retinal layers without violating either layer.
  - Affected part of retina changes with head position.
  - Usually secondary systemic disease such as severe acute hypertension, sarcoid, cancer

## ETIOLOGY
- RRD:
  - Myopia
  - Cataract surgery
  - Marfan syndrome
  - Structural degeneration of underlying anatomy of vitreous body, sensory or pigmented retina
  - Trauma

- TRD:
  - Proliferative diabetic retinopathy
  - Vasculopathy
  - Perforating injury
  - Chorioretinitis:
    - Retinopathy of prematurity, sickle cell disease, or toxocariasis
  - Trauma
- ERD:
  - Malignant hypertension, preeclampsia
  - Tumors of the choroid or retina (melanoma, retinoblastoma)
  - Inflammatory disorders (Coats or Harada disease, posterior scleritis)

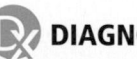 **DIAGNOSIS**

## SIGNS AND SYMPTOMS
- Flashes of light
- Floaters
- "Night shade" obscuring visual field
- Peripheral/central vision loss or other visual field defects
- Asymptomatic

## History
- Symptoms onset, course, description:
  - May progress over hours or weeks
  - Dark curtain or veil
  - Usually begins peripherally
- Associated symptoms: Flashing lights, floaters, painless
- Ophthalmologic history:
  - Baseline eyesight, myopia, surgery, eye disease, trauma
- Systemic disease

## Physical Exam
- Visual acuity, visual fields by confrontation—prior to dilation:
  - May have normal visual acuity if macula spared
  - Detachment is on opposite side of field defect
- May have afferent pupillary defect
- May have loss of red reflex
- Fundoscopy:
  - Pale, opaque, wrinkled retina
  - Cannot rule out detachment on fundoscopy alone
- Slit-lamp exam: Anterior vitreous pigment granules ("tobacco dust") suggest retinal tear.

## ESSENTIAL WORKUP
- Complete ophthalmologic examination
- Thorough neurologic examination to exclude cerebrovascular accident/transient ischemic attack

## DIAGNOSTIC TESTS & INTERPRETATION
### Lab
As needed to work up underlying diseases

### Imaging
Ocular US: 97% sensitive by trained EM physicians

### Diagnostic Procedures/Surgery
- Intraocular pressure (IOP) measurement: IOP usually lower in the affected eye
- Dilating pupil with short-acting mydriateic carries very low risk of acute angle-closure glaucoma.

## DIFFERENTIAL DIAGNOSIS
- Central retinal artery or vein occlusion
- Vitreous hemorrhage
- Senile retinoschisis
- Juvenile retinoschisis
- Choroidal detachment
- Methanol poisoning
- Other retinal or CNS disease

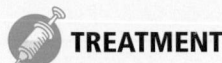 **TREATMENT**

**PRE-HOSPITAL**
- Bed rest
- Consider transport to hospital with neurology and ophthalmology availability.

**INITIAL STABILIZATION/THERAPY**
If suspected ERD, treat systemic disease.

**ED TREATMENT/PROCEDURES**
- Bed rest:
  - Rest head on pillow with side of detachment down, side opposite of field defect
- Emergent ophthalmologic consultation

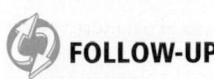 **FOLLOW-UP**

**DISPOSITION**
*Admission Criteria*
Need for surgical repair

*Discharge Criteria*
- Any patient with retinal detachment seen by an ophthalmologist and deemed safe to go home
- Chronic retinal detachments are repaired over the same time course as it took to create them.
- ERD resolves with treatment of the underlying problem.

*Issues for Referral*
Detachments with macula involvement require repair within 1 day.

**FOLLOW-UP RECOMMENDATIONS**
Per ophthalmologist

## PEARLS AND PITFALLS

- Fundoscopy alone does not provide sufficient visualization to rule out detachment.
- Early recognition of retinal tears allows possible prophylactic:
  - 90% risk of retinal tear with "tobacco dust"
- Do not fail to recognize central retinal artery occlusion (CRAO):
  - Increased risk of stroke for patient with CRAO in setting of carotid disease or cardioembolic disease

## ADDITIONAL READING

- Abouzeid H, Wolfensberger TJ. Macular recovery after retinal detachment. *Acta Ophthalmol Scand.* 2006;84:597–605.
- Ehlers JP, Shah CP, et al., eds. *The Wills eye manual: Office and emergency room diagnosis and treatment of disease.* 4th ed. Philadelphia: Lippincott Williams & Wilkins; 2004.
- Kang HK, Luff AJ. Management of retinal detachment: A guide for non-ophthalmologists. *BMJ.* 2008;336:1235–1240.

- Regillo C, Benson W. *Retinal detachment. Opthalmic surgery.* 3rd ed. Philadelphia: Elsevier Science; 2003.
- Shinar Z, Chan L, Orlinsky M. Use of ocular ultrasound for the evaluation of retinal detachment. *J Emerg Med.* 2009; Jul 20; Epub ahead of print.
- Shingleton B, O'Donoghue M. Blurred vision. *N Engl J Med.* 2000;343(8):556–562.
- Vortman M, Schneider JI. Acute monocular visual loss. *Emerg Med Clin North Am.* 2008;26(1):73–96.
- Yanoff M, Duker JS, eds. *Ophthalmology.* 3rd ed. Philadelphia: Elsevier; 2008.

**See Also (Topic, Algorithm, Electronic Media Element)**
- Visual Loss
- Vitreous Hemorrhage

 **CODES**

**ICD9**
- 361.00 Retinal detachment with retinal defect, unspecified
- 361.01 Recent retinal detachment, partial, with single defect
- 361.02 Recent retinal detachment, partial, with multiple defects

R

# RETROPHARYNGEAL ABSCESS

Deborah Vinton
Maria E. Moreira

 **BASICS**

## DESCRIPTION

- Deep tissue infection of the retropharyngeal space:
  - Potential space bound anteriorly by pharyngeal mucosa, posteriorly by prevertebral fascia, superiorly by skull base, and inferiorly by the carina.
- Primarily a disease of children, but increasing frequency in adults:
  - Peak incidence at 3–5 yr when posterior pharyngeal nodes most prominent
  - Most often arises from infection of nasopharynx, paranasal sinuses, or middle ear
  - Infection then spreads to lymph nodes between posterior pharyngeal wall and prevertebral fascia.
- Prognosis is good when promptly diagnosed and aggressively managed with IV antibiotics and/or surgical drainage.
- Complications due to mass effect, rupture, or spread are major source of morbidity and include:
  - Airway compromise (most common)
  - Sepsis
  - Spontaneous perforation
  - Aspiration pneumonia due to rupture
  - Necrotizing fasciitis
  - Mediastinitis
  - Thrombosis of the internal jugular vein
  - Jugular vein suppurative thrombophlebitis (Lemierre syndrome)
  - Erosion into carotid artery (primarily adults)
  - Atlantoaxial dislocation from erosion of ligaments
  - Cranial nerve palsies (typically IX–XII)
  - Recurrent abscess formation (1–5%)

## ETIOLOGY

- Causes:
  - Often preceded by upper respiratory infection in children (45%) and oropharyngeal trauma in adults (27%)
  - 28% idiopathic
- Bacteriology: Predominately polymicrobial
- Most common organisms are:
  - *Streptococcus pyogenes* (33%)
  - *Staphylococcus aureus* (including MRSA)
  - Respiratory anaerobes (including *Fusobacterium*, *Prevotella*, and *Veillonella*)
- Less common organisms are:
  - *Haemophilus* species
  - Acid-fast bacilli
  - *Klebsiella pneumoniae*
  - *Escherichia coli*

## DIAGNOSIS

### SIGNS AND SYMPTOMS
May differ between adults and children

### History
- Most Common:
  - Sore throat (84% of children >1 yr)
  - Fever
  - Neck pain/stiffness
  - Muffled voice
- Additional presenting symptoms:
  - Dysphagia
  - Odynophagia
  - Stridor, dyspnea

### Pediatric Considerations
Young children may present with only:
- Poor oral intake
- Lethargy or Irritability
- Cough

### Physical Exam
- Adults:
  - Posterior pharyngeal edema (37%)
  - Nuchal rigidity
  - Cervical adenopathy
  - Fever
  - Drooling
  - Stridor
  - Dysphonia (cri du canard)
  - Tracheal "rock" sign: Tenderness on moving the larynx and trachea side to side
- Children and infants:
  - Cervical adenopathy (80%)
  - Retropharyngeal bulge (43%)
  - Neck stiffness with extension most frequently limited
  - Torticollis
  - Drooling
  - Agitation
  - Respiratory distress (4%)

### ESSENTIAL WORKUP
Rapid assessment of airway and respiratory status:
- Normal exam does not rule out diagnosis.
- No lab tests make the diagnosis.
- When suspicious, obtain lateral neck x-ray or CT of neck with IV contrast.

## DIAGNOSTIC TESTS & INTERPRETATION
### Lab
- CBC (WBC >12,000 in 91% of children):
  - Nonspecific
- Blood cultures
- Throat cultures

### Imaging
- Portable films appropriate if concern for airway compromise
- Lateral neck radiographs:
  - Film taken in inspiration with neck slightly extended
  - May not get good exposure of soft tissue if cannot adequately extend neck due to pain or difficulty cooperating at young age
  - Increased suspicion if:
    ○ Retropharyngeal space anterior to C2 > 7 mm or 2× the diameter of the vertebral body (sensitivity 90%)
    ○ Space anterior to C6 to >14 mm in preschool children or 22 mm in adults
- Chest radiograph:
  - Indicated if abscess identified to rule out inferior spread of infection
  - Mediastinal widening is suggestive of mediastinitis and possible rupture.
- US of neck:
  - Low sensitivity
  - Not recommended
- CT of neck with IV contrast:
  - Obtain when x-rays nondiagnostic or to determine exact size and location of abscess noted on x-ray
  - Abscess appears as hypodense lesion with peripheral ring enhancement in retropharyngeal space.
  - Sensitivity: 64–100%
  - Specificity: 45–88%
  - Can aid in operative planning, revealing extent of invasion into retro/parapharyngeal spaces
  - Unclear if it reliably can distinguish abscess from cellulitis and lymphadenitis
  - Due to radiation exposure and need for sedation, CT should only be obtained in young children if x-rays are nondiagnostic.
  - Now preferred imagining modality
- MRI:
  - More sensitive than CT
  - Also useful for imaging vascular lesions such as jugular thrombophlebitis

### Diagnostic Procedures/Surgery

- Surgical drainage/needle aspiration should be performed in OR:
  - Presence of pus is gold standard for making diagnosis.
  - Abscess should be completely evacuated.
  - Pus should be sent for Gram stain and culture.
- No role for nasopharyngolaryngoscopy

## DIFFERENTIAL DIAGNOSIS

- Tonsillopharyngitis
- Epiglottitis
- Peritonsillar abscess
- Croup
- Foreign body
- Tracheitis
- Meningitis
- Retropharyngeal hemorrhage
- Dystonic reactions
- Cervical osteomyelitis
- Dental infections
- Mononucleosis
- Epidural abscess
- Other deep space infection of the neck

 TREATMENT

### PRE-HOSPITAL

- Keep child in position of comfort:
  - Forcing child to sit up or flex neck may occlude airway.
- Pulse oximetry, cardiac monitor
- Supplemental oxygen
- Adequate hydration
- Suction, endotracheal tube, tracheostomy equipment ready for potential emergent intubation
- Airway control will be required for:
  - Airway compromise
  - Prior to long transport

### INITIAL STABILIZATION/THERAPY

- Assess and control airway.
- Provide supplemental oxygen.
- IV access:
  - Avoid if signs of airway compromise.

### ED TREATMENT/PROCEDURES

- Early endotracheal intubation or tracheostomy for patients with respiratory distress or impending obstruction:
  - Caution must be used with induction, as sedation medications may lead to relaxation of airway muscles causing complete obstruction.
  - Rescue airway equipment such as a Laryngeal Mask Airway available, as pharyngeal swelling may make intubation difficult
  - Cricothyrotomy may be required if upper airway is obstructed.
- Surgical consultation (ear/nose/throat if available)
- Early administration of IV antibiotics

## MEDICATION

Empiric IV antibiotic therapy to cover group A streptococci, *S. aureus* (including MRSA), and respiratory anaerobes):

- Antibiotic tailored to local preferences and susceptibilities.
- Coverage is narrowed when culture results and sensitivities return.
- Use of corticosteroids is controversial and recommended only after consultation with ear/nose/throat.

### First Line

Clindamycin: 600–900 mg IV (peds: 25–40 mg/kg/d, div. q6h; max 4.8 g/d) alone or in combination with:

- Ampicillin/sulbactam: 1.5–3 g IM/IV q6h (peds: 1–23 mo: 300–450 mg/kg/d IV div. q6h; 2–12 yr: 300–600 mg/kg/d IV q6h)
- Piperacillin/tazobactam: 3.375 g IV q6h (peds:240–300 mg/kg/d IV q8h)
- Cefoxitin: 1–2 g IV q6–8h (peds: 80–160 mg/kg/d IV div. q4–6h)

### Second Line

If patients do not respond or there is concern for MRSA:

- Vancomycin: 1–1.5 g IV q12h (peds: 40–60 mg/kg/d div. q6 8h)
- Linezolid: 600 mg IV/PO q12h (peds: 0–11 yr: 30 mg/kg/d PO/IV div. q8h; >12 yr: 600 mg PO/IV q12h)

 FOLLOW-UP

## DISPOSITION

### Admission Criteria

- All patients with retropharyngeal abscess should be admitted to the hospital for IV antibiotics and possible surgical drainage.
- Criteria for surgical drainage:
  - Airway compromise or other life-threatening complications
  - Large (>2 cm hypodense area on CT)
  - Failure to respond to parenteral antibiotic therapy
- ICU admission for patients with:
  - Airway compromise
  - Sepsis
  - Altered mental status
  - Hemodynamic instability
  - Infants and toxic-appearing children
  - Major comorbidities

### Discharge Criteria

Patients with retropharyngeal abscesses should not be discharged.

### Issues for Referral

Transfer should be considered if facility does not have the ability to drain infection:

- Airway should be stabilized prior to transfer.

## PEARLS AND PITFALLS

- Diagnosis should be considered in all children who present with fever, stiff neck, or dysphagia:
  - High clinical suspicion is required in children, as they present with nonspecific signs and symptoms.
- Adult cases most often present in the setting of underlying illness, recent intraoral procedures, neck trauma, or head and neck infections.
- When imaging isnondiagnostic and clinical suspicion remains high, surgery should be consulted.
- Early surgical consultation and administration of IV antibiotics is essential to prevent complications such as airway compromise and extension into mediastinal structures.

## ADDITIONAL READING

- Chow AW. Deep neck space infections. UpToDate August 18, 2008. Available at: http://www.uptodate.com/patients/content/topic.do?.topicKey=~oaa629_uwVFiXC.
- Cummings CW, Haughey BH, Thomas JR, et al. *Cummings otolaryngology: Head and neck surgery.* 4th ed. St. Louis, MO: Mosby; 2005.
- Marx JA, Hockberger RS, Walls RM, et al. *Rosen's emergency medicine: Concepts and clinical practice.* 7th ed. St. Louis, MO: Mosby; 2009.
- Page NC, Bauer FM, Lien IF. Clinical features and treatment of retropharyngeal abscess in children. *Otolaryngol Head Neck Surg.* 2008;138:300–306.

### See Also (Topic, Algorithm, Electronic Media Element)

- Epiglottitis
- Peritonsillar Abscess

 CODES

ICD9
478.24 Retropharyngeal abscess

# REYE SYNDROME
*Brian D. Euerle*

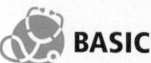 **BASICS**

## DESCRIPTION
- Reversible clinicopathologic syndrome of unknown etiology
- Primary mitochondrial injury
- Decreased enzyme activity:
  - Krebs cycle
  - Gluconeogenesis
  - Urea biosynthesis
- Fatty infiltration:
  - Liver:
    - Hyperammonemia due to decreased conversion from ammonia to urea
    - Hepatorenal syndrome may be the end result.
    - Rapid recovery of liver function in survivors
  - Brain:
    - Encephalopathy of unclear etiology
    - Cytotoxic edema
    - Deteriorating level of consciousness reflects increasing intracranial pressure (ICP).
    - Herniation is the most common cause of death.
    - Normal recovery of neurologic function in survivors
  - Skeletal and myocardial muscle
  - Fatty infiltration and distorted mitochondria
- <10% of cases occur before the age of 1 yr:
  - Average age is 7 yr.
  - Peak age is 4–11 yr.
- Regional differences:
  - Highest incidence in the midwestern states
  - Lower incidence in the states of the southeast and far west
- More common in whites than in blacks
- Peak incidence in winter and early spring
- Reye-like syndrome:
  - Describes conditions resulting in defects in urea and fatty acid metabolism, toxicologic injury, and impaired gluconeogenesis

## ETIOLOGY
- Not known with certainty
- Multifactorial causes have been epidemiologically implicated:
  - Antecedent viral syndrome
  - Influenza A or B
  - Varicella
  - Diarrhea illness
  - Genetic predisposition
  - Exposure to salicylates
  - Other undefined factors

---

# DIAGNOSIS

## SIGNS AND SYMPTOMS
- Usually the patient is afebrile.
- Tachycardia
- Hyperventilation

### History
- Biphasic history marked by an infectious phase (viral illness or prodrome) followed by an encephalopathic stage
- Profuse and repeated vomiting:
  - Typically 4–5 days after the start of the viral illness
- Marked behavioral changes, including delirium and combativeness, disorientation, and hallucination

### Physical Exam
- No focal neurologic signs
- Hepatomegaly in 40% of cases
- Pancreatitis
- Clinical staging of Reye syndrome with Lovejoy classification:
  - Stage 0:
    - Wakeful
  - Stage I:
    - Vomiting
    - Lethargy
    - Sleepiness
  - Stage II:
    - Disorientation
    - Delirium
    - Combative/stuporous
    - Hyperventilation
    - Hyperreflexia
    - Appropriate response to noxious stimuli
  - Stage III:
    - Obtunded
    - Coma
    - Hyperventilation
    - Inappropriate response to noxious stimuli
    - Decorticate posturing
    - Preservation of pupillary light reflexes
    - Preservation of oculovestibular light reflexes

---

  - Stage IV:
    - Deeper coma
    - Decerebrate rigidity
    - Loss of oculovestibular reflexes
    - Dilated, fixed pupils
    - Dysconjugate eye movements in response to caloric stimulation
  - Stage V:
    - Seizures
    - Absent deep tendon reflexes
    - Respiratory arrest
    - Flaccid paralysis
    - No papillary response
- Infants: Atypical presentation:
  - Tachypnea
  - Apnea
  - Irritability
  - Seizures
  - Hypoglycemia

## ESSENTIAL WORKUP
- Establish the presence of encephalopathy and liver abnormalities.
- Laboratory testing to assess for characteristic biochemical abnormalities
- Liver biopsy confirms the diagnosis.

## DIAGNOSTIC TESTS & INTERPRETATION
### Lab
- Liver function tests:
  - $\geq 3\times$ rise in aspartate aminotransferase, alanine aminotransferase
  - Serum ammonia level $>1.5–3\times$ normal:
    - Transient 24–48 hr after mental status changes
    - Level $>300\ \mu g/dL$ is associated with poor prognosis.
  - Serum bilirubin should be normal or slightly elevated.
- Hypoglycemia may be present, especially in infants.
- Elevated BUN
- Ketonuria
- The prothrombin time may be prolonged due to decreased liver-dependent clotting factors (II, VII, IX, X).
- Normal platelet count and blood smear
- Negative toxicology screen

### Imaging
Head CT scan:
- May show diffuse cerebral edema
- Edema is diffuse, and lumbar puncture is not contraindicated.

### Diagnostic Procedures/Surgery
- Lumbar puncture:
  - Perform after head CT
  - Measure opening pressure
  - <8 leukocytes/mm$^3$
- Percutaneous liver biopsy:
  - Useful in patients with atypical presentation (1 yr old, recurrent, familial)

## DIFFERENTIAL DIAGNOSIS
- Inborn errors of metabolism:
  - Disorders of the urea cycle
  - Disorders of fatty acid oxidation
  - Systemic carnitine deficiency
  - Organic acidemias
  - Disorders of the electron transport chain
- Hypoglycemia
- Toxin exposure:
  - Toxic encephalopathy without liver dysfunction (Gall syndrome)
  - Lead
  - Hydrocarbons
- Drug intoxication:
  - Acetaminophen
  - Salicylates
  - Ethanol
- Infection:
  - Sepsis
  - Meningitis
  - Encephalitis
  - Varicella hepatitis
- Trauma, head

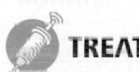 TREATMENT

### PRE-HOSPITAL
- Decreased mental status:
  - Glucose
  - Narcan
- Coma:
  - Assist respirations with bag-valve mask.

### INITIAL STABILIZATION/THERAPY
- Place on a cardiorespiratory monitor.
- Supplemental oxygen
- Rapid-sequence intubation if airway management required

- Glucose if mental status is altered:
  - 10% glucose solution IV
  - Rate of 2/3 maintenance requirement after dehydration is corrected
  - Follow serum glucose hourly; maintain glucose 125–175 mg/dL.
- Avoid early overhydration.

### ED TREATMENT/PROCEDURES
- Institute treatment before the liver biopsy.
- Vitamin K:
  - Indicated if prothrombin time is elevated.
- Fresh-frozen plasma:
  - To control bleeding
  - To correct a severe coagulopathy
- Interventions aimed at lowering ICP:
  - Stage III or greater
  - Stage II with serum ammonia >300 μg/L:
    ○ Intubation using rapid-sequence protocol
    ○ Hyperventilation
    ○ Fluid restriction
    ○ Barbiturate coma
- Osmotically active agents:
  - Mannitol
  - Furosemide
- Monitor ICP:
  - Subarachnoid bolt
  - Intraventricular cannula

### MEDICATION
- D50W: 1–2 mL/kg/dose (0.5–1.0 g/kg) IV for age >3 yr
- D25W: 2–4 mL/kg/dose (0.5–1.0 mg/kg) IV for age of <3 yr; maintenance infusion 10% dextrose solution at a rate of 2/3 maintenance
- Fresh-frozen plasma: 10 mL/kg/dose q12–24h IV or PRN
- Lasix: 1 mg/kg IV
- Mannitol: 0.25–1.0 g/kg IV q4–6h
- Pentobarbital: 3–20 mg/kg IV slowly while monitoring BP; maintenance infusion 1–2 mg/kg/hr; maintain level at 25–40 μg/dL
- Vitamin K: 1–2 mg/dose (infants and children); 2–10 mg/dose (adolescents)

 FOLLOW-UP

### DISPOSITION
#### Admission Criteria
- All children with suspected Reye syndrome should be admitted to the ICU.
- Hospital capable of ICP monitoring

#### Discharge Criteria
Hospital discharge criteria are individualized for each case:
- Mental status and laboratory values have improved and stabilized.

### Issues for Referral
Close follow-up with specialists in gastroenterology (hepatology) and neurology

## FOLLOW-UP RECOMMENDATIONS
Long-term psychological and neuropsychological testing

## PEARLS AND PITFALLS
- Aspirin and salicylates are found in many medications and combination products.
- All efforts must be directed at identifying other possible causes of illness in the patient with suspected Reye syndrome.
- Monitoring and control of intracranial pressure is a key component of treatment.

## ADDITIONAL READING
- Glasgow JF. Reye's syndrome: The case for a casual link with aspirin. *Drug Safety*, 2006;29:1111–1121.
- Gosalakkal JA, Kamoji V. Reye syndrome and Reye-like syndrome. *Pediatr Neurol.* 2008;39: 198–200.
- Hurwitz ES. Reye syndrome. In Feigin RD, Cherry JD, Demmier-Harrison GJ, Kaplan SL, eds. *Feigin & Cherry's textbook of pediatric infectious diseases.* 6th ed. Philadelphia: WB Saunders; 2009: 693–694.
- National Reye's Syndrome Foundation. Available at: www.reyessyndrome.org. Accessed November 11, 2009.
- Pugliese A, Deltramo T, Torre D. Reye's and Reye's-like syndromes. *Cell Biochem Function.* 2008;26:741–746.
- Schror K. Aspirin and Reye syndrome: A review of the evidence. *Paediatr Drugs.* 2007;9:195–204.

### See Also (Topic, Algorithm, Electronic Media Element)
- Altered Mental Status
- Coma
- Influenza
- Varicella

 CODES

ICD9
331.81 Reye's syndrome

# RHABDOMYOLYSIS
*Marcelo Sandoval*

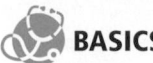 **BASICS**

## DESCRIPTION
Abnormal systemic release of muscle contents—creatine phosphokinase (CPK), myoglobin, potassium, phosphate, urate— caused by trauma, poisoning, infection, primary muscle disorders, and many other disease states. Complications include:
- Myoglobin-induced renal failure in 15%–50% adults, (1) only 5% in children (6)
- Hyperkalemia may lead to sudden death
- Hypocalcemia and acidosis
- Volume loss—fluid sequestration in injured muscle or result of underlying illness
- Compartment syndrome of muscles in crush, worsened by IV fluid sequestration in damaged tissue (3,4)
- Hepatic dysfunction in 25% (9)
- DIC (4,9)

## EPIDEMIOLOGY
### Incidence
- 26,000 per year in the U.S. (7,9)
- Disaster situations lead to hundreds of cases of renal failure. (8)

## RISK FACTORS
- Inherited myopathy (9)
- Alcohol or drug use (9)
- Medications as listed below (7)
- Overexertion with or without risk factors.

## GENERAL PREVENTION
- High-quality buildings in quake zones.
- Furniture affixed to walls (8)

## PATHOPHYSIOLOGY
- Sarcolemma keeps intracellular calcium low.
- Etiologies disrupt cell membrane and lead to following cascade. (1,4,5)
- Breakdown of sarcolemma Na-Ca pumps allows calcium to enter cell.
- Calcium-dependent proteases cause destruction.
- Ischemia and neutrophils cause damage.
- Escape of cell contents: Myoglobin, potassium, phosphate, CPK, lactate, etc.
- Myoglobin causes renal damage by direct toxicity in acidic urine.
- Myoglobin precipitates with other proteins to obstruct renal tubular flow.
- Volume depletion also leads to renal vasoconstriction and failure.
- Hyperkalemia can lead to arrhythmias.
- Calcium precipitates with phosphate, leading to systemic hypocalcemia.

## ETIOLOGY
Cause usually obvious, but not always.
   Adults: Trauma, toxicity, infection (1,4,7,9,11).
   Children: Viral myositis, trauma (6,9)
- Muscle injury—Due to trauma/crush, burn, electrical shock—most common cause overall.
- Muscle exertion: Strenuous exercise; marathon running; exercise in hot, humid conditions; exercise in individuals with an inherited myopathy or with poor physical training; status epilepticus; delirium tremens; tetanus; psychotic agitation
- Muscle ischemia: Extensive thrombosis, multiple embolism, generalized shock, sickle cell crisis
- Surgery: Immobilization, hypotension, ischemia due to vessel clamping
- Massive blood transfusion
- Hypothermia, hyperthermia
- Prolonged immobile state without trauma
- Drugs/toxins: Alcohols, cocaine, amphetamines and analogs (methamphetamine and ecstasy), toluene, opiates, LSD, phencyclidine (PCP), caffeine, carbon monoxide, snake venom, bee/hornet venom, hemlock, buffalo fish, tetanus toxin, mushroom poisoning (*Tricholoma equestre*)
- Medications: Most common—haloperidol, phenothiazines, HMG–CoA reductase inhibitors (statins) and other cholesterol-lowering agents, antihistamines, selective serotonin receptor inhibitors (SSRIs). Others include propofol, succinylcholine, halogenated anesthetic gases, isoniazid (INH), zidovudine, antimalarials, methylxanthines, colchicine, corticosteroids, itraconazole, erythromycin, diuretics, cyclosporine, barbiturates.
- Sports supplements including ephedra, caffeine, androgenic steroids, creatine, diuretics (5).
- Neuroleptic malignant syndrome (idiosyncratic and not dose-related)
- Metabolic disorders: Hypokalemia, hypophosphatemia, hypocalcemia, hyper- and hyponatremia, diabetic ketoacidosis, hyperosmolar state, hypoxia, hyperthyroid state (rare), pheochromocytoma (rare)
- Infections:
  – Viral: Coxsackievirus, herpesviruses, HIV, influenza B, cytomegalovirus, Epstein–Barr virus, adeno/echovirus
  – Bacterial: Legionnaires' disease, pyomyositis, salmonellosis, shigellosis, *Staphylococcus*, *Streptococcus*, *Listeria*, tetanus, toxic shock syndrome, tularemia, gas gangrene, *Bacillus cereus*
  – Parasitic (*Malaria falciparum*), protozoan (leptospirosis), rickettsial
  – Inherited myopathic disorders: McArdle disease, Tarui disease, CPT deficiency. These inherited myopathies can exacerbate any other cause.
- Immunologic disorders: Dermatomyositis, polymyositis
- Idiopathic

## COMMONLY ASSOCIATED CONDITIONS
- Crush syndrome
- Compartment syndrome
- Alcohol and drug abuse
- Elderly and acutely immobile (found on floor)

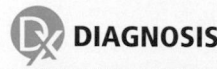 **DIAGNOSIS**

## SIGNS AND SYMPTOMS
### History
- Can vary dramatically, reflecting underlying disease process.
- Trauma or crush usually obvious.
- Consider child abuse in trauma with unclear details.
- If no trauma, consider in drug toxicity, heat illness, immobilization, or overexertion states.
- Ask about reddish brown urine and decreased urine output
- Most nontraumatic cases in children <9 yr old are due to viral illness with myositis (6).

### Physical Exam
- Hypothermia/hyperthermia
- Alert/obtunded
- Muscle pain (only 40%–50%) (4,6).
- Neurovascular status of involved muscle groups if compartment syndrome is suspected.
- Hypovolemic state, dry mucous membranes, poor skin turgor, tachycardia, hypotension
- Decreased urine output
- Urine color (tea-colored) is early sign (1,4,9).
- Children more often have absent physical findings (5,6)

## DIAGNOSTIC TESTS & INTERPRETATION
### Lab
**Initial lab tests**
- History and physical are insensitive in making the diagnosis (6).
- Serum and urine myoglobin levels often normal due to rapid metabolism and excretion.
- Serum CPK level >1,000 (standard) considered positive (6).
- CPK level not always predictive of renal failure but most often associated with level >15,000
- Urine dipstick test positive for heme but absent for RBCs suggests rhabdomyolysis (1).
- Microscopic urinalysis to look for pigmented tubular casts
- Because of rapid urinary excretion of myoglobin, up to 26% of patients with rhabdomyolysis have negative urine dipstick test.
- In children, heme <2+ on urine dip correlates with reduced risk of ARF (6).
- Serum electrolytes (potassium, calcium, magnesium, phosphorus, BUN, creatinine, uric acid, bicarbonate)
- In addition to above consider:
  – Arterial and venous blood gases (ABG/VBG) (baseline pH if considering bicarbonate therapy).

- Urine/serum myoglobin, but may be too transient to be useful
- Serum glucose
- LFTs including GGTP, LDH, albumin
- Toxicology screen in absence of physical injury
- PT/PTT, platelet count, fibrinogen, fibrin split products if DIC is suspected

### Imaging
- Renal US to rule out long-standing renal failure (small, shrunken kidneys) or renal obstruction (hydronephrosis)
- MRI is 90%–95% sensitive in visualizing muscle injury but does not change initial ED treatment.
- Other imaging as indicated

### Diagnostic Procedures/Surgery
- Early ECG: Hyperkalemia or hypocalcemia before serum levels available
- Measure compartment pressure if compartment syndrome is suspected.

## DIFFERENTIAL DIAGNOSIS
Conditions that may present with elevated serum CPK but are not rhabdomyolysis:
- Nontraumatic myopathies including muscular dystrophies and inherited myopathies
- Chronic renal failure
- IM injections
- Myocardial injury
- Stroke

 TREATMENT

## PRE-HOSPITAL
- Rapid extrication in case of crush injury
- Early IV saline before extrication to prevent complications of restored blood flow to injured limb (hypovolemia, hyperkalemia, etc.) (3,8)
- "Crush injury cocktail" during extrication is 1.5 l 0.9% NS per hr; consider adding 1 amp (50 mEq) bicarbonate and 10 g of mannitol to each liter (controversial) (1,3).
- Pediatric recommendation: 10–15 mL/kgm/hr saline initially, then switch to hypotonic (0.45%) saline upon arrival to hospital. Add 50 mEq bicarbonate to each 2nd or 3rd liter to alkalinize urine (8).

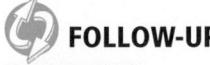 FOLLOW-UP

## DISPOSITION
### Initial Stabilization
- Manage ABCs
- Immobilization of trauma/crush injuries
- Adult crush injury treatment literature extrapolated to children
- IV saline for hypovolemia at rate of 1–1.5 L/hr (10–20 mL/kg/hr). Volume restored within 6 hr helps prevent renal failure (1,8,9).
- May need 12 L/day, 4–6 of which should include bicarbonate. Use CVP, urine output (8).
- Diuretics only after patient's volume restored to keep urine output 200–300 mL/hr (3–5 ml/kg/hr) (1,8).
- Mannitol: Diuretic, free radical scavenger. May help compartment syndrome (1).
- Furosemide and other loop diuretics if indicated in management of oliguric (<500 mL/day) renal failure. Some believe it can be harmful.

- Bicarbonate: Alkalinize urine (pH> 6.5) most studied in crush/trauma. Most authorities recommend its use as long as urine pH and calcium are monitored. A retrospective study suggests benefit only when CPK level >30,000 (2).
- Monitor for hyperkalemia frequently with serum levels and ECG. Higher potassium correlates with more severe injury (8).
- Treat hyperkalemia as usual but do not use calcium unless it is severe (1,8).
- Hypocalcemia: Treat only if symptomatic (tetany or seizures) or arrhythmias present. Calcium infusion can lead to hypercalcemia later as precipitated calcium mobilizes (8).
- bicarbonate can trigger symptoms by increasing free calcium binding to albumin (1,9).

### Admission Criteria
All but the most trivial elevations in CPK (<1,000) should be admitted, since complications can occur at any level and are difficult to predict. Children seem to be less susceptible to renal complications (6).
- Critical Care Admission Criteria
  - Hyperkalemia or CPK levels >15,000–30,000 due to worse prognosis (1)
  - Underlying severe illness

### Discharge Criteria
- Levels decreased to <1,000 after therapy. Generally not applicable to ED.

## MEDICATION
### First Line
- bicarbonate as above to keep urine ph >6.5. Discontinue if urine pH fails to rise after 6 hr or if symptomatic hypocalcemia develops (1).
- Albuterol, insulin/dextrose, polystyrene resin (kayexalate), for hyperkalemia treatment. Avoid calcium if possible.

### Second Line
- Mannitol 20%: 50 ml (10 g added to each liter up to 120–200 g/day (1–2 g/kgm/day) (1,8).
- Discontinue if fail to achieve diuresis and osmolal gap >55 (1).

## SURGERY/OTHER PROCEDURES
- Hemodialysis for refractory hyperkalemia, fluid overload, anuria, acidosis (1).
- Central venous monitoring of volume (1,8).
- Fasciotomy for compartment syndrome (11).

## PROGNOSIS
- No renal failure—almost no mortality
- Renal failure—3.4%–30% mortality (1)
- ICU—59% if renal failure, 22% without (1).

## COMPLICATIONS
- Acute renal failure
- Hyperkalemia
- Compartment syndrome
- Hypocalcemia
- Acidosis

## PEARLS AND PITFALLS
Suspect in unexplained renal failure.

## REFERENCES
1. Bosch X, Poch F, Grau JM. Rhabdomyolysis and acute kidney injury. N Engl J Med. 2009; 361(1):62–72.
2. Brown C, Rhee P, Chan L, et al. Preventing renal failure in patients with rhabdomyolysis: Do bicarbonate and mannitol make a difference? J Trauma. 2004;56:1191–1196.
3. Gonzalez D. Crush syndrome. Crit Care Med. 2005;33(1 Suppl):S34–S41.
4. Huerta-Alardín AL, Varon J, Marik PE. Bench-to-bedside review: Rhabdomyolysis—An overview for clinicians. Crit Care. 2005;9(2): 158–169.
5. Luck RP, Verbin S. Rhabdomyolysis: Review of clinical presentation, etiology, diagnosis and management. Pediatr Emerg Care. 2008; 24:262–268.
6. Mannix R, Tan ML, Wright R, Baskin M. Acute pediatric rhabdomyolysis: Causes and rates of renal failure. Pediatrics. 2006;118(5):2119–2125.
7. Melli G, Chaudhry V, Cornblath DR. Rhabdomyolysis: An evaluation of 475 hospitalized patients. Medicine. 2005; 84(6):377–385.
8. Sever MS, Vanholder R, Lameire N. Management of crush-related injuries after disasters. N Engl J Med. 2006;354:1052–1063.
9. Sauret JM, Marinides G, Wang GK. Rhabdomyolysis. Am Fam Physician. 2002;65: 907–912.
10. Watemberg N, Leshner RL, Armstrong BA, Lerman-Sagie T. Acute pediatric rhabdomyolysis. J Child Neurol. 2000;15(4):222–227.
11. Vanholder R, Sever MS, Erek E, Lameire N. Rhabdomyolysis. J Am Soc Nephrol. 2000; 11(8):1553–1561.

## ADDITIONAL READING
**See Also (Topic, Algorithm, Electronic Media Element)**
- Compartment Syndrome
- Hyperkalemia

 CODES

ICD9
728.88 Rhabdomyolysis

# RHEUMATIC FEVER
*Jon D. Mason*

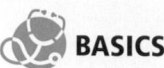 **BASICS**

## DESCRIPTION
- Constellation of symptoms and signs (Jones criteria)
- Follows group A streptococcal infection (GAS); usually pharyngitis.
- Uncommon in U.S.; most cases are in developing nations.
- Remains a major cause of cardiac morbidity and mortality worldwide.
- Most common in 5- to 15-yr-olds

## ETIOLOGY
- GAS infection
- Inflammatory, autoimmune response following GAS infection

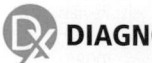 **DIAGNOSIS**

- 2 major or 1 major and 2 minor elements of the Jones criteria plus evidence of a recent GAS infection

## SIGNS AND SYMPTOMS
### Jones Criteria
- Major manifestations:
  - *Migratory polyarthritis* in 60–75% of initial attacks:
    - Can involve knees, ankles, elbows, and wrists
    - Lower extremity joints more commonly involved
    - Rheumatic arthritis generally responds to salicylates.
  - *Carditis* occurs in 1/3 of new cases; prednisone used in severe cases:
    - Pericardium, myocardium, and endocardium may be affected (pancarditis).
    - Myocarditis may lead to heart failure but is frequently asymptomatic.
    - Valvular disease and endocarditis are most serious sequelae of acute rheumatic fever (ARF).
    - Carditis heralded by a new murmur, tachycardia, gallop rhythm, pericardial friction rub, or CHF
    - Echocardiogram may aid in diagnosis.
  - *Chorea* occurs in 10% of cases:
    - Sydenham chorea predominantly affects teenage girls.
    - Purposeless, uncoordinated movements of the extremities
    - Movements are more apparent during periods of anxiety and disappear with sleep.
    - Chorea may be the sole manifestation of ARF.

  - *Erythema marginatum* occurs in <5% of cases:
    - Nonpruritic pink eruptions with central clearing and well-demarcated irregular borders
    - Usually seen on the trunk and the extremities
  - Subcutaneous nodules in 10% of patients:
    - Crops of small subcutaneous, painless nodules located most commonly on extensor surfaces
- Minor manifestations:
  - Clinical:
    - Fever (>38°C)
    - Arthralgia
  - Laboratory:
    - Elevated acute-phase reactants
    - Prolonged P-R interval
- Supporting evidence of recent GAS throat infection:
  - Positive throat culture or rapid antigen test
  - Elevated or increasing antibody test: Anti–streptolysin O (ASO) titer

## History
- Fever
- Sore throat
- Rash
- Joint pains
- Unusual movements of extremities
- Dyspnea
- Lower extremity edema

## Physical Exam
- Pharyngeal erythema
- Rash consistent with erythema marginatum
- Subcutaneous nodules
- New heart murmur consistent with mitral or aortic disease
- Evidence of fluid overload/CHF

## ESSENTIAL WORKUP
- Careful exam to look for skin lesions/joint swelling
- Careful heart and lung exam
- Throat swab for rapid strep test or culture
- ECG
- Chest x-ray
- See other labs below.

## DIAGNOSTIC TESTS & INTERPRETATION
### Lab
- Rapid antigen strep test
- Throat culture
- ASO titer
- CBC
- ESR or C-reactive protein
- Other rheumatic serology tests to rule out other diseases

### Imaging
- Chest radiograph
- Echocardiogram

### Diagnostic Procedures/Surgery
- ECG
- Diagnosis is based on clinical picture and meeting Jones criteria

## DIFFERENTIAL DIAGNOSIS
- Juvenile rheumatoid arthritis
- Infective endocarditis
- Reiter syndrome
- Systemic lupus erythematosus
- Postgonococcal arthritis
- Other infectious causes of arthritis and carditis:
  - Coxsackie B virus and parvovirus

### Pediatric Considerations
Rheumatic fever is primarily a pediatric disease but can occur in young adults. The pediatric drug doses are noted below.

### Pregnancy Considerations
Prenatal counseling recommended if woman has history of rheumatic fever due to increased cardiac risks.

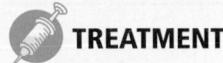 **TREATMENT**

**PRE-HOSPITAL**
- Oxygen as needed
- Monitors if in distress
- IV access may be prudent.

**INITIAL STABILIZATION/THERAPY**
Some patients in CHF will need airway management.

**ED TREATMENT/PROCEDURES**
- Pericardial effusions may need drainage.
- In severe carditis, start steroids.
- In case of severe chorea, start haloperidol.
- Penicillin IM, IV, or PO
- NSAIDS or aspirin

**MEDICATION**
- Aspirin: 4–8 g/d (peds: 100 mg/kg/d) PO q4–6h
- Digoxin: 0.25–0.5 mg (peds: 0.04 mg/kg) IV
- Erythromycin: 250 mg (peds: 30–50 mg/kg/d) q6h PO for 10 days
- Furosemide: 20–80 mg (peds: 1 mg/kg/dose) IV
- Haloperidol: 2–10 mg (peds: 0.01–0.03 mg/kg/d) q6h IM or PO
- Penicillin (benzathine benzylpenicillin): 1.2 million U (peds: 600,000 U for <27 kg) IM acutely and monthly thereafter (prophylaxis)
- Penicillin VK: 500 mg (peds: 250 mg) PO q8h for 10 days (acute treatment)
- Prednisone: 1–2 mg/kg/d for 14 days with taper for the next 2 wk

**First Line**
- Aspirin
- Penicillin
- Haloperidol (for chorea)

**Second Line**
Corticosteroids

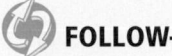 **FOLLOW-UP**

**DISPOSITION**
Most patients with a new diagnosis should be admitted for stabilization and further evaluation of the severity of the heart disease.

**Admission Criteria**
- CHF
- New diagnosis
- Uncontrolled chorea
- Uncontrolled pain
- Pericardial effusion

**Discharge Criteria**
- Pain is controlled
- Stable cardiovascular status
- Education regarding prolonged treatment and endocarditis prophylaxis

**Issues for Referral**
All patients need close follow-up with their primary physician and cardiologist. Consider referral to infectious disease specialist and rheumatologist

**FOLLOW-UP RECOMMENDATIONS**
- Cardiology for echocardiogram and advice on subacute bacterial endocarditis prophylaxis
- Infectious disease specialist to advise on prolonged use of penicillin to prevent recurrence
- Rheumatology if needed for chronic joint problems (uncommon)

## PEARLS AND PITFALLS

- Rheumatic fever is uncommon in U.S., but must be vigilant to treat strep infections to prevent resurgence of disease.
- More common in patients living in poor and crowded conditions

## ADDITIONAL READING

- Carpapetis JR. Acute rheumatic fever. *Lancet* 2005;366:155–168.
- Cilliers AM. Rheumatic fever and its management. *BMJ.* 2006;1153–1156.
- Gerber MA, Baltimore RS, Eaton CB, et al. Prevention of rheumatic fever and diagnosis and treatment of acute streptococcal pharyngitis. A Scientific Statement from the American Heart Association. *Circulation.* 2009;119:1541–1551.
- Miyake CY, Gauvreau K, Tani LY, et al. Characteristics of children discharged from hospitals in the United States in 2000 with the diagnosis of acute rheumatic fever. *Pediatrics.* 2007;120: 503–508.
- Weiner SG, Normandin PA. Sydenham chorea: A case report and review of the literature. *Pediatr Emerg Care.* 2007;23:20–24.

**See Also (Topic, Algorithm, Electronic Media Element)**
Pharyngitis

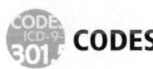 **CODES**

**ICD9**
- 390 Rheumatic fever without mention of heart involvement
- 398.90 Rheumatic heart disease, unspecified

R

# RIB FRACTURE
*Charles W. O'Connell*

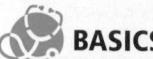 **BASICS**

## DESCRIPTION
- Result of major or minor thoracic trauma
- Can be classified as traumatic or pathologic

## ETIOLOGY
- Blunt thoracic trauma:
  - Simple fall, fall from height
  - Motor vehicle crash
  - Assault
  - Missile
  - CPR-related
- Penetrating trauma is a less likely cause.
- Ribs usually break at the point of impact or the posterior angle:
  - Structurally weakest region
- Stress fractures in upper and middle ribs can occur with recurrent, high force movements:
  - Athletic activities: Golf, rowing, throwing
  - Severe cough
- Pathologic fractures associated with minor trauma or significant underlying disease:
  - Coughing or sneezing
  - Advanced age
  - Osteoporosis
  - Neoplasm

### Pediatric Considerations
- Relatively elastic chest wall makes rib fractures less common in children.
- Consider nonaccidental trauma for infants and toddlers without appropriate mechanism.
- Obtain a skeletal survey to assess for other fractures in infants suspected of being abused

### Geriatric Considerations
- Elderly are more prone to rib fractures as well as atelectasis, pneumonia, respiratory failure, and other associated complications.
- Morbidity and mortality are twice that found in younger populations.

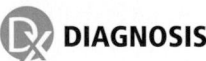 **DIAGNOSIS**

## SIGNS AND SYMPTOMS
### History
- Blunt thoracic trauma by any mechanism
- Mechanism as described by patient, parent or prehospital personnel:
  - Seat belt usage
  - Steering wheel damage
  - Air bag deployment
- Localized chest wall pain that increases with deep inspiration, coughing, movement
- Pleuritic chest pain
- Dyspnea, shortness of breath

### Physical Exam
- Point tenderness
- Pain referred to fracture site with palpation of the involved rib elsewhere
- Bony step-off
- Crepitus
- Localized edema
- Erythema
- Ecchymosis:
  - Ecchymosis from seat belt, aka "seat belt sign"
  - Ecchymosis from steering wheel impact
- Intercostal muscle spasm
- Splinting respirations
- Hypoxia, tachypnea, respiratory distress
- Auscultation shows normal or diminished breath sounds, occasionally an audible click over fracture site.
- Segmental paradoxical movement of chest suggests flail chest indicating multiple, unattached fractured ribs.

## ESSENTIAL WORKUP
- Diagnosis is initially made on clinical grounds.
- Evaluate for injury to underlying structures

### ALERT
- The 1st 3 ribs are relatively protected and require significant impact to fracture, indicating possible intrathoracic injury.
- Ribs 9–12 are relatively mobile; their fracture suggests possible intra-abdominal injury.
- Multiple rib fractures may be associated with flail chest and pulmonary contusion.
- Morbidity correlates with degree of injury to underlying structures and number of ribs fractured.

## DIAGNOSTIC TESTS & INTERPRETATION
### Lab
ABGs may reveal hypoxemia or elevated alveolar–arterial gradient:
- Not indicated for simple, uncomplicated rib fractures
- May consider in patients with multiple rib fractures or pre-existing pulmonary disease

### Imaging
- Chest radiography is indicated to rule out associated intrathoracic injury but misses up to 50% of rib fractures:
  - May reveal associated intrathoracic pathology:
    - Pneumothorax
    - Hemothorax
    - Pneumomediastinum
    - Pulmonary contusion
    - Atelectasis
    - Widened mediastinal silhouette
  - Pulmonary contusion appears within 6–12 hr after injury:
    - Ranges from patchy alveolar infiltrates to frank consolidation

- Indications for rib radiograph series:
  - Suspected fractures of ribs 1–3 or 9–12
  - Multiple rib fractures
  - Elderly patients with pre-existing pulmonary disease or suspected pathologic fractures
- CT is more sensitive for detecting rib fractures and internal injuries.
- CT of the chest may be required to rule out intrathoracic injuries.
- CT or US of the abdomen may be required to rule out associated intra-abdominal injuries.
- Angiography can be used for the detection of vascular injury if signs and symptoms of neurovascular compromise are present
  - Injury to the 1st and 2nd ribs can be associated with vascular injury, particularly with posterior displacement.

## DIFFERENTIAL DIAGNOSIS
- Rib contusion or intercostal muscle strain
- Costochondral separation
- Sternal fracture and dislocation
- Nontraumatic causes of chest pain:
  - Cardiovascular:
    - Myocardial ischemia or infarction
    - Pericarditis
    - Aortic dissection
    - Pulmonary embolism
  - Pulmonary:
    - Infections
    - Inflammation
    - Barotrauma
  - Musculoskeletal:
    - Costochondritis
    - Cervical or thoracic spine disease
  - Gastrointestinal:
    - Esophageal reflux or spasm
    - Mallory–Weiss tear
    - Biliary or renal colic
    - Peptic ulcer disease
    - Gastritis, pancreatitis, hepatitis
  - Dermatologic:
    - Herpes zoster
    - Chest wall tumor

## TREATMENT

### PRE-HOSPITAL
Focus on airway maintenance and supplemental oxygen

### INITIAL STABILIZATION/THERAPY
- For simple fractures, generally no significant stabilization is required.
- Multiple fractures, elderly patients, or significant underlying lung disease:
  - Manage airway and resuscitate as indicated.
  - Endotracheal intubation indicated for patients with severe hypoxemia ($PaO_2$ <60 mm Hg on room air, <80 mm Hg on 100% $O_2$) or impending respiratory failure

### ED TREATMENT/PROCEDURES
- Simple fractures:
  - Pain control:
    - Key to maintaining adequate pulmonary function, avoiding atelectasis and subsequent pneumonia
  - Intercostal nerve blocks with 0.5% bupivacaine are safe and effective:
    - Provides 6–12 hr of pain relief
    - Intercostal nerve block should be performed posteriorly, 2–3 fingerbreadths from the vertebral midline.
    - Inject 0.5–1 mL just under the inferior surface of the rib where the neurovascular bundle is located.
    - Aspirate 1st to be certain the intercostal vessels have not been punctured.
  - Deep breathing or incentive spirometry should be encouraged with adequate pain control.
  - Avoid binders or banding of the chest wall because these restrict ventilation and promote atelectasis.
- Multiple fractures, elderly patients, or significant underlying lung disease:
  - Pain control and pulmonary toilet
  - Search for associated injuries; treat exacerbation of underlying lung disease.
  - Intercostal nerve blocks for multiple fractures are safe and effective providing 6–12 hr of pain relief.
  - For the admitted patient, thoracic epidural analgesia or patient-controlled analgesia (PCA) is effective, with minimal inhibition of respiratory drive.

### MEDICATION
- NSAIDs are first-line with or without opioids
  - Ibuprofen: 600 mg PO q6h (peds: 5–10 mg/kg PO q6–8h)
  - Ketoprofen: 25–50 mg PO q6–8h
  - Naproxen: 250–500 mg PO q12h (peds: 10–20 mg/kg/day PO div q12h)
- Opioid analgesics
- Multiple acetaminophen/narcotic analgesic combinations are available; see "Alert" below.
  - Acetaminophen: 300 mg/codeine 30 mg (peds: 0.5–1 mg/kg codeine) PO q4–6h
  - Acetaminophen: 500 mg/hydrocodone 5 mg PO q4–6h
  - Acetaminophen: 500 mg/hydrocodone 7.5 mg PO q4–6h
  - Acetaminophen: 325 mg/hydrocodone 10 mg PO q4–6h
  - Acetaminophen: 325 mg/oxycodone 5 mg PO q6h
- Hydromorphone: 2–8 mg PO q3–4h (peds: 0.03–0.08 mg/kg PO q4–6h)
- Hydromorphone: 1–4 mg (peds: 0.03–0.08 mg/kg) IV/IM/SC q4–6h
- Morphine sulfate: 2.5–10 mg (peds: 0.1–0.2 mg/kg) IV/IM/SC q2–6h
- Patient-controlled analgesia (PCA) using hydromorphone or morphine sulfate is effective.
- Bupivacaine 0.5%: 0.5–1 mL per injection for intercostal nerve blocks

### ALERT
- Consider thoracic epidural analgesia:
  - Patients with intractable pain
  - Oversedation
  - Hypoventilation from narcotic analgesics
- Avoid NSAIDs when contraindicated due to renal insufficiency or GI bleed
- Use lowest effective dose of NSAID and shortest treatment duration
- The dose of acetaminophen/narcotic analgesic combinations is limited by the hepatic toxicity of acetaminophen.
- The maximum acetaminophen dose is 1 g per dose and 4 g/day (peds: 15 mg/kg per dose).

 FOLLOW-UP

### DISPOSITION
#### Admission Criteria
- Intractable pain
- Inability to cough and clear secretions
- Compromised pulmonary function
- Multiple fractures, fractures of the 1st 3 ribs
- Displaced rib fractures
- Associated pneumothorax, pneumomediastinum, pulmonary contusion, intrabdominal or intrathoracic pathology
- Elderly patients and patients with significant underlying lung disease:
  - Chronic COPD, CHF, pulmonary fibrosis, asthma
- Inadequate pain control on oral analgesics
- ICU care for elderly patients with 6 or more rib fractures

#### Discharge Criteria
- Patients with normal pulmonary function, no underlying pulmonary injury, and adequate pain control on oral analgesics
- Strict return criteria should be discussed with the patient prior to discharge:
  - Shortness of breath
  - Increased pain
  - Inadequate pain control
  - Fever
  - Cough

### FOLLOW-UP RECOMMENDATIONS
- Most rib fractures heal within 6 weeks, but patients should be able to return to regular daily activities much sooner.
- Follow-up chest x-rays are not recommended.

## ADDITIONAL READING

- Ashrafan H, Kumar P, Sarkar PK, et al. Delayed penetrating intrathoracic injury from multiple rib fractures. *J Trauma.* 2005;58:858.
- Eckstein M, Henderson S. Thoracic trauma. In: JA Marx, RS Hockberger, RM Walls, eds. *Rosen's emergency medicine: Concepts and clinical practice*, 6th ed, Philadelphia: Mosby-Elsevier; 2006.
- Sears BW, Luchette FA, Esposito TJ, et al. Old fashion clinical judgement in the era of protocols: Is mandatory chest x-ray necessary in injured patients? *J Trauma.* 2005;59:324.
- Sirmali M, et al. A comprehensive analysis of traumatic rib fractures: Morbidity, mortality and management. *Eur J Cardiothorac Surg.* 2003;24:133.
- Stawicki SP, Grossman MD, Hoey BA, et al. Rib fractures in the elderly: A marker of injury severity. *J Am Geriatr Soc.* 2004;52:805.

## CODES

### ICD9
- 807.00 Closed fracture of rib(s), unspecified
- 807.09 Closed fracture of multiple ribs, unspecified
- 807.10 Open fracture of rib(s), unspecified

# RING/CONSTRICTING BAND REMOVAL

*Gary M. Vilke*

## BASICS

### DESCRIPTION
- *Primary constricting band*: A band tightened around an appendage causes swelling and pain (eg, a hair knotted around a toddler's toe).
- *Secondary constricting band*: Injury or disease process that causes swelling and edema as a result of tightness against the band (eg, impacted ring with an underlying fracture of the finger)
- Untreated, the constricting band may become *embedded* and interrupt skin integrity.

#### Pediatric Considerations
In the preverbal child, a constricting band may be a manifestation of child abuse or neglect.

#### Geriatric Considerations
The cognitively impaired nursing home resident or Alzheimer patient may be unable to give an indication of injury or pain.

### ETIOLOGY
Tourniquet syndrome may result from allergic, dermatologic, iatrogenic, endocrinologic, infectious, malignant, metabolic, physiologic, or traumatic conditions, or it may be related to pregnancy.

## DIAGNOSIS

### SIGNS AND SYMPTOMS
- A constricting band with swollen tissue and skin, most commonly involving a finger
- Other locations include wrist, ankle, toe, umbilicus, earlobe, nipple, septum or nares of nose, penis, scrotum, vagina, labia, uvula, or tongue.
- Pain on manipulation of the appendage or constricting band

#### History
An inconsolable infant may be having pain due to a hair tourniquet.

#### Physical Exam
- Evaluate area of concern.
- If evaluating an inconsolable infant or agitated nonverbal adult, assess fingers, toes, and genitalia.

### ESSENTIAL WORKUP
- Primary constricting band: Diagnosis made by history and physical exam with special attention to neurovascular status.
- Secondary constricting band: Diagnosis of underlying pathology may depend on results of imaging and laboratory test results.

### DIAGNOSTIC TESTS & INTERPRETATION
#### Lab
- Usually not indicated for acute treatment
- Measurement of electrolytes, BUN, and creatinine; thyroid function tests; and Tzanck smear of vesicular lesions may be useful in identifying the underlying diagnosis.

#### Imaging
Plain films for evaluation of underlying fracture or foreign body *after* band removal

### DIFFERENTIAL DIAGNOSIS
*Any* condition causing marked swelling and edema predisposing to the tourniquet syndrome

## TREATMENT

### PRE-HOSPITAL
Remove rings and other potential constricting bands before development of tourniquet syndrome:
- Particularly in regions of extremity trauma

### INITIAL STABILIZATION/THERAPY
Pain management or procedural sedation as needed

### ED TREATMENT/PROCEDURES
- Removal of the constricting band either by advancing the band distally or by division
- The most benign methods should be attempted 1st.
- These adjuvant methods may be used alone or in combination:
  - Elevation of the affected extremity may decrease vascular congestion.
  - *Cooling* the extremity with ice or cold water may reduce edema and erythema.
  - *Lubrication* with soap or mineral oil may allow slippage over an inflamed or edematous area.
  - *Digital block* with 1%–2% lidocaine *without epinephrine* decreases the discomfort of removal and manipulation of an underlying injury.
  - A digital block may, however, increase local swelling.
  - *Gauze* or a *needle holder* may be used to manipulate the band.

- The distal swollen finger, especially the proximal interphalangeal joint, is an important obstacle in constricting band removal.
- Distal to proximal edema reduction by sequential compression:
  - *Self-adherent tape* is wrapped from distal to proximal to form a smooth and decompressed area over which the band is advanced.
  - A *Penrose surgical drain* or a finger cut from a small glove is stretched to fit over the distal swelling before attempted removal.
  - With lubrication, the proximal end of the drain is pulled under the ring to form a cuff around the ring; the cuff with distal traction applied advances the band over the decompressed area.
  - *Suture material* (no. 0 silk, dental floss, or umbilical tape) is wrapped under tension in a tight layer advancing over the edema in a distal-to-proximal direction; the proximal tail of the suture material or floss is tucked under the ring; with lubrication, the tail under tension is pulled distally and unwound, forcing the ring over the layered suture material and decompressed area.
- Constricting band removal by division:
  - *Scissors* may be used to 1st lift and then cut the offending fibrous band constricting a toddler's toe or penis.
  - A *no. 11 scalpel* blade with cutting edge up may be sufficient to cut constricting bands formed by hair, fibers, or plastic ties.
  - A topical commercially available depilatory agent may be used to divide a tourniquet formed by a suspected hair obscured by local edema.
  - A *handheld wire cutter/stripper* may divide small-girth metallic rings with minimal discomfort to the underlying injury; this type of removal may, however, impart a crush defect to the ring, making repair difficult.
  - A *long-handled bolt cutter,* available in most operating rooms or hospital engineering departments, may be used to divide large-girth or broad-sized rings:
    - Long handles provide the significant mechanical advantage needed to cut large rings.
    - The reinforced cutting blades may not easily fit through a constricting band with adjacent swollen tissue and skin.

- A *standard hand-powered, medically approved ring cutter* (Steinmann pin cutter with a MacDonald elevator) may be used to divide small-girth metallic constricting bands made of soft metals (gold/silver):
  - This method has the advantage of a cleaner cut for subsequent repair of the ring.
  - The disadvantage is that the handheld ring cutter is labor-intensive and may aggravate the pain of an underlying injury.
  - A *motorized high-rpm cutting device* may be used to rapidly divide constricting bands irrespective of girth and size of the ring; it may be AC-powered or pneumatically driven in the operating suite.
- Cutting procedure:
  - The initial cut is made on the band on the volar aspect of the extremity.
  - A tenaculum may be used to spread the band in softer metals.
  - For a 2nd cut, the band should be rotated 180° on the extremity, allowing the 2nd cut on the band over the volar aspect of the extremity.
- Motorized cutting:
  - Remove *flammable solvents* from the work area.
  - *Protective eyewear* should be worn by everyone present, including the patient.
  - Place a thin *aluminum splint* (shaped to the curvature of the ring) between the patient's skin and the ring as a shield to protect underlying tissue.
  - Cool splint and cutting surface with ice water irrigations before and during the cutting procedure.
  - Limit cutting with motorized device to 5 sec during intervals of 60–90 sec between ice water irrigations to avoid producing local excessive heat.
- Postdivision care:
  - Underlying injuries should be irrigated thoroughly to remove metallic dust and avoid foreign body reaction and granuloma formation.
  - Tetanus prophylaxis should be provided if indicated.

## MEDICATION

- Tetanus prophylaxis: Tetanus toxoid 0.5 mL IM
- No medications are typically required unless evidence of or at risk for infection

### First Line

- Cefazolin: 1 g IV/IM (peds: 20–40 mg/kg IV/IM single dose in ED)
- Cephalexin: 500 mg PO (peds: 25–50 mg/kg/d) q.i.d. for 7 days *or*
  - Amoxicillin/clavulanate: 875/125 mg PO (peds: 25 mg/kg/day) b.i.d. for 7 days
- Erythromycin: 333 mg PO t.i.d. (peds: 40 mg/kg/day q6h for 7 days)

### Second Line

- If patient is penicillin-allergic:
- EES: 800 mg PO, then 400 mg PO q6h for 7 days *or*
  - Clindamycin: 300 mg PO q6h for 7 days

 **FOLLOW-UP**

### DISPOSITION
#### Admission Criteria

- Neurovascular compromise or injury requiring surgical repair
- Concomitant infection or necrosis

#### Discharge Criteria

Successful band removal with restoration of circulation

#### Issues for Referral

Wounds at high risk for infection should have close follow up in 1–2 days.

### FOLLOW-UP RECOMMENDATIONS

Return to the ED for increasing pain, numbness, tingling, redness, swelling drainage, fevers or other changes in clinical presentation.

## PEARLS AND PITFALLS

- Failure to completely examine the fingers, toes, and genitalia of the irritable infant
- Rings must be removed early after trauma to the distal extremity.

## ADDITIONAL READING

- Chiu TF, Chu SJ, et al. Use of a Penrose drain to remove an entrapped ring from a finger under emergent conditions. *Am J Emerg Med*. 2007;25(6):722–723.
- Krishna S, Paul RI. Hair tourniquet of the uvula. *J Emerg Med*. 2003;24(3):325–326
- Peckler B, Hsu CK. Tourniquet syndrome: A review of constricting band removal. *J Emerg Med*. 2001;20(3):253–262.
- Rosen P, Chan TC, Vilke GM, et al. *Atlas of Emergency Procedures*. St. Louis: Mosby; 2001.
- Venters WB. Ring removal from a swollen finger: A refined technique. *J Surg Orthop Adv*. 2006;15(3):181–183.

 **CODES**

### ICD9

- 915.8 Other and unspecified superficial injury of fingers without mention of infection
- 917.8 Other and unspecified superficial injury of foot and toes, without mention of infection

# ROCKY MOUNTAIN SPOTTED FEVER

*Roger M. Barkin*
*Moses S. Lee*

## 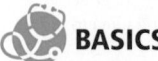 BASICS

### DESCRIPTION
Rickettsial invasion of small blood vessels:
- Causes direct vascular damage
- Superimposed additional vascular damage/vasculitis due to immunologic phenomena

### ETIOLOGY
- Acute infection by *Rickettsia rickettsii* via tick vector:
  - *Dermacentor andersoni* (wood tick) in the western states
  - *Dermacentor variabilis* (dog tick) in the eastern states
- Reported in all states; 1/2 of cases occur in 5 states (NC, SC, TN, OK, AR), as well as parts of Central America and South America
- More common April–September, but can occur any month

##  DIAGNOSIS

### SIGNS AND SYMPTOMS
#### History
- Tick bite reported within 14 days of rash in 60% of patients
- Incubation varies 2–14 days with median 7 days
- Exposure to ticks, often in rural environment

#### Physical Exam
- Rash:
  - Initial rash (3–5 days)
    - Macular, red, and flat
    - Blanches under pressure
    - 1–4 mm diameter
  - In hours to days:
    - Becomes darker, papular, dusky, and palpable
  - In 2–3 days:
    - Petechial or purpuric
    - Positive Rumpel-Leede test
    - May coalesce or ulcerate
  - In severe disease, necrosis of dependent peripheral parts may occur.
  - Location:
    - Begins in flexor surfaces of wrist and ankles, rapidly spreading to palms and soles
    - Spreads centripetally involving extremities; may involve trunk and face
    - 15% with centrifugal spread to palms and soles
  - Often not identified when patient initially presents for care

- Pulmonary:
  - Nonproductive cough
  - Chest pain
  - Dyspnea
  - Rales
- GI:
  - Often associated with fatal Rocky Mountain spotted fever
  - Secondary to vasculitis
  - Nausea/vomiting
  - Abdominal pain/distention
  - Ileus
  - Hepatosplenomegaly
- Neurologic:
  - Focal or generalized neurologic manifestation in 2/3
  - Meningismus
  - Severe, unremitting headache
  - Encephalitis
- Other:
  - Generalized edema
  - Dehydration
  - Malaise
  - Myalgia
  - Retinal hemorrhage and conjunctivitis
- Complications:
  - Disseminated intravascular coagulation (DIC)
  - Noncardiogenic pulmonary edema
  - Acute renal failure
  - Severe or fatal in advanced age, male sex, African American, chronic alcohol abuse, glucose-6-phosphate dehydrogenase deficiency

### ESSENTIAL WORKUP
Clinical diagnosis supplemented by confirmatory laboratory findings such as hyponatremia, anemia, and thrombocytopenia

### DIAGNOSTIC TESTS & INTERPRETATION
#### Lab
- Serology:
  - Diagnose by single titer >1:64 or 4-fold increase
  - Methods:
    - Immunofluorescent antibody
    - Complement fixation
    - Indirect hemagglutination test
    - Indirect immunofluorescence assay is reference standard.

- CBC:
  - Normal WBC count
  - Thrombocytopenia
  - Anemia
- Electrolytes, BUN/creatinine, glucose:
  - Hyponatremia <130 mEq/L
- Liver profile:
  - Elevated aspartate aminotransferase
  - Lactate dehydrogenase
- Arterial blood gas for:
  - Hypoxia
  - Respiratory alkalosis
- Coagulation profile if DIC suspected
- Microbiology:
  - Immunohistologic antibody stain of skin biopsy
  - Isolation of *R. rickettsii* (time-consuming/expensive)
  - Polymerase chain reaction assay
- Cerebrospinal fluid:
  - Pleocytosis and increased protein

#### Imaging
- Chest radiograph for pulmonary edema, pneumonia
- Echocardiography:
  - Decreased left ventricular contractility

#### Diagnostic Procedures/Surgery
Skin biopsy may be confirmatory if immunohistologic antibody studies available.

### DIFFERENTIAL DIAGNOSIS
- Other tickborne diseases:
  - Ehrlichiosis: Older adults
  - Relapsing fever
  - Lyme disease: Erythema chronicum migrans
  - Tularemia
  - Babesiosis
  - Colorado tick fever

- Infectious diseases:
  - Meningococcemia—late winter, early spring; maculopapular or petechial rash
  - Measles—late winter, early spring; severe prodrome
  - Rubella—palms and soles spared
  - Varicella—does not have rash in extremities
  - Viral exanthem
  - Infectious mononucleosis—palms and soles spared
  - Disseminated gonococcal infection—pustular lesions
  - Typhus—rash starts at trunk with centrifugal spread
  - Secondary syphilis
  - Scarlet fever
  - Kawasaki disease—red, cracked lips
  - Toxic shock syndrome
  - Gastroenteritis
  - Staphylococcal sepsis
- Inflammatory causes:
  - Allergic vasculitis
  - Thrombotic thrombocytic purpura
  - Collagen vascular disease
  - Juvenile rheumatoid arthritis
- Heat illness

 ## TREATMENT

### PRE-HOSPITAL
Stabilize as appropriate

### INITIAL STABILIZATION/THERAPY
- ABC management
- 0.9% NS IV fluid bolus for dehydration
- Oxygen for hypoxia

### ED TREATMENT/PROCEDURES
- Correct fluid and electrolyte deficits.
- Initiate antibiotic therapy immediately based on clinical and epidemiologic findings. Should not be delayed until laboratory confirmation is obtained:
  - Doxycycline—drug of choice
  - Chloramphenicol in pregnant and allergic patients
  - Sulfonamides make infection worse.

- Administer acetaminophen for fever.
- Consider high-dose steroids for severe cases complicated by extensive vasculitis, encephalitis, or cerebral edema (controversial).
- Better outcome in children if treatment begins before day 5 of illness
- Treat complications:
  - DIC
  - Adult respiratory distress syndrome
  - CHF
- Medication

### Pediatric Considerations
- Highest incidence in 5–9-yr-olds
- 2/3 of cases occur in children <15 yr.
- Doxycycline is used in children due to potential for fatal cases, the relatively low risk of significant dental discoloration with a short course, and adverse effects of chloramphenicol

### Pregnancy Considerations
Use chloramphenicol in pregnant patients.

### MEDICATION
#### First Line
Doxycycline: 100 mg (peds: 2 mg/kg for <45 kg) PO or IV b.i.d. for 5–7 days. Patient should generally be treated 2–3 days beyond becoming afebrile.

#### Second Line
- Acetaminophen: 1 g (peds: 15 mg/kg) PO q4h
- Chloramphenicol: 75 mg/kg/24 hr PO or IV q6h for 5–7 days and 48 hr after defervescence
- Solu-Medrol: 125 mg (peds: 1–2 mg/kg) IV

 ## FOLLOW-UP

### DISPOSITION
#### Admission Criteria
Moderate to severe symptoms

#### Discharge Criteria
- Mild, early disease with early treatment
- Notify family because of clustering and potential exposures.

### Issues for Referral
Reflective of defined complications

### FOLLOW-UP RECOMMENDATIONS
Reflective of ongoing complications

## PEARLS AND PITFALLS

Early treatment based on the clinical presentation and epidemiology is indicated.

## ADDITIONAL READING

- Buckingham SC, Marshall GS, Schutze GE, et al. Clinical and laboratory features, hospital course and outcome of Rocky Mountain spotted fever in children. *J Pediatr*. 2007;150:180–184.
- Centers for Disease Control and Prevention. Tickborne rickettsial diseases. Rocky Mountain spotted fever. Available at: http://www.cdc.gov/ticks/diseases/rocky_mountain_spotted_fever/. Updated May 14, 2010.
- Chapman AS, Bakken JS, Folk SM, et al. Diagnosis and management of tickborne rickettsial diseases: Rocky Mountain spotted fever, ehrlichioses and anaplasmosis—United States. *MMWR Recomm Rep*. 2006;55(RR-4):1–27.
- Chen LF, Sexton DJ. What's new in Rocky Mountain spotted fever? *Infect Dis Clin North Am*. 2008;22:415–432.
- Masters FJ, Olson GS, Weiner SJ, et al. Rocky Mountain spotted fever: A clinician's dilemma. *Arch Intern Med*. 2003;163:769–774.

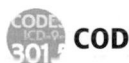 ## CODES

### ICD9
082.0 Spotted fevers

R

# ROSEOLA

*Moses S. Lee*

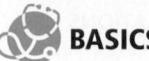 **BASICS**

## DESCRIPTION
- Incubation period of 5–15 days
- Mode of acquisition unknown:
  – Horizontal spread by oral shedding suggested
  – It is spread person to person but is not very contagious.
- Pathophysiology:
  – Complex immune response (cytokines, antibody responses, T cell reactivity)

## ETIOLOGY
- Exanthem subitum
- Human herpesvirus 6 (HHV-6):
  – Large, double-stranded DNA
  – Closely related to human cytomegalovirus
- Peak incidence at 6–12 mo; 90% occurrence within first year
- Highest incidence in late spring and early summer

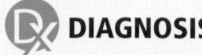 **DIAGNOSIS**

## SIGNS AND SYMPTOMS
- Febrile seizures in 5–35%
- Diarrhea
- Irritability
- Rarely causes severe or fatal disseminating diseases:
  – Infectious mononucleosis syndrome of hepatitis
- Reactivation in immunocompromised individuals

### Pediatric Considerations
- Most newborns are seropositive for HHV-6 due to transplacental antibodies.
- By age 1–2 yr, >90% of infants are seropositive.

### History
- Sudden, high fever 39.4–41.2°C (103–106°F) commonly followed by defervescence and appearance of rash
- Absence of physical findings:
  – Child looks well
  – Temperature normalizes in 3–4 days.

### Physical Exam
- Enlarged lymph nodes
- Maculopapular eruption from trunk to arms and neck after temperature normalizes
- Rash fades within 3 days.
- Erythematous papules in pharynx (Nakayama spots)

## ESSENTIAL WORKUP
Clinical diagnosis:
- High fever in well-appearing child

## DIAGNOSTIC TESTS & INTERPRETATION
### Lab
- CBC:
  – Initial increase in WBC, then normalization with lymphocytosis
- HHV-6 DNA:
  – Detected by polymerase chain reaction
  – Available at research level
  – Immunoglobulin M appears early and declines as immunoglobulin G is produced

## DIFFERENTIAL DIAGNOSIS
- Fever of unknown origin
- Scarlet fever:
  - "Sandpaper" rash, Pastia lines, and strawberry tongue
- Measles (rubeola):
  - Koplik spots, cough, coryza, conjunctivitis, and fever
- Rocky Mountain spotted fever:
  - Rash begins at ankles and wrists.
- Rubella:
  - Fever after rash
- "Fifth disease" (erythema infectiosum)
- Dengue fever
- Pneumococcal bacteremia
- Meningitis

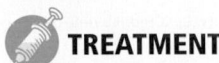 TREATMENT

### PRE-HOSPITAL
- None

### INITIAL STABILIZATION/THERAPY
ABC management

### ED TREATMENT/PROCEDURES
- Supportive
- Antipyretics:
  - Acetaminophen
  - Ibuprofen

### MEDICATION
- Acetaminophen: 650 mg (peds: 15 mg/kg) PO q4h
- Ibuprofen: 200–600 mg (peds: 5–10 mg/kg; suspension 100 mg/5 mL; oral drops 40 mg/mL) PO q6h

 FOLLOW-UP

### DISPOSITION
**Admission Criteria**
Fever in child who is toxic and does not respond to initial supportive care

**Discharge Criteria**
Usually, all patients may be discharged.

### FOLLOW-UP RECOMMENDATIONS
Re-evaluate if persistent fever after 3–4 days

## PEARLS AND PITFALLS
- Child looks well
- Antivirals are not recommended in the immunocompetent child.

## ADDITIONAL READING
- Leach CT. Human herpesviruses 6 and 7. In: Hutto C, ed. *Congenital and Perinatal Infections: A Concise Guide to Diagnosis*. Totowa, NJ: Humana Press; 2006: 101–109.
- Leach CT. Roseola (human herpesviruses 6 and 7). In: Kliegman R, Behrman R, Jenson H, et al., eds. *Nelson Textbook of Pediatrics*. 18th ed. Philadelphia: WB Saunders; 2007: 1380–1383.
- Stoeckle MY. The spectrum of human herpesvirus 6 infection: from roseola infantum to adult disease. *Annu Rev Med*. 2000;51:423–430.

 CODES

### ICD9
057.8 Other specified viral exanthemata

R

# RUBELLA

*Moses S. Lee*

## BASICS

### DESCRIPTION
- Transmission via droplets from respiratory secretions
- Moderately contagious:
  - Especially during rash eruption and infants with congenital rubella syndrome (CRS)
- Up to 50% may be subclinical.
- Infants with congenital rubella shed large quantities of virus for several months.
- Infectious period 7 days before to 5 days after appearance of rash
- Incubation period: 14–21 days

### ETIOLOGY
- Also known as German measles or 3-day measles
- Rubella virus (family: Togaviridae, genus: *Rubivirus*)
- Live, attenuated virus vaccine indications:
  - All children >12 mo and entering school
  - All women of childbearing age

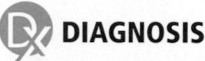

## DIAGNOSIS

### SIGNS AND SYMPTOMS
- Acute viral disease
- Complications:
  - Uncommon, tend to occur more in adults
  - CRS: Infected women in 1st trimester
  - Arthritis:
    - More common in women (up to 79%)
    - Chronic arthritis is rare.
    - Begins after 2–3 days of illness
    - Knees, wrists, fingers affected
  - Hemorrhagic manifestations:
    - Secondary to thrombocytopenia
    - More common in children
  - Neurologic sequelae:
    - Encephalitis most common in adults

### *History*
- Low-grade fever
- Malaise
- Headache
- Upper respiratory tract symptoms

### *Physical Exam*
- Rash:
  - Rash is fainter than measles rash and does not coalesce.
  - Red macular rash evolving to pink-red maculopapules with occasional pruritus
  - Begins in face with rapid caudal spread
  - Completed in 1st day and disappears in 3 days
  - May have hemorrhagic manifestations
- Lymphadenopathy:
  - Postauricular
  - Occipital
  - Posterior cervical

### ESSENTIAL WORKUP
Generally clinical diagnosis

### DIAGNOSTIC TESTS & INTERPRETATION
#### *Lab*
- CBC:
  - Decreased WBC, platelets (more common in children)
- Urinalysis:
  - Hematuria
- Reverse transcriptase–polymerase chain reaction
- Enzyme-linked immunosorbent assay to detect rubella immunoglobulin M
- Rubella antibody titer:
  - Acute and convalescent serum specimens
  - Hemagglutination-inhibition test most common
  - Definitive diagnosis in acute infection
  - Compare infant with maternal sera for CRS.
  - False positives in parvovirus, infectious mononucleosis, rheumatoid factor
  - May be useful to check for immunity of pregnant patients with potential exposure.

- Pharynx:
  - Virus may be isolated from pharynx 1 wk before and until 2 wk after rash onset (valuable epidemiologic tool).
- Cerebrospinal fluid:
  - Few WBCs (monocytes) in encephalitis

#### *Diagnostic Procedures/Surgery*
- Lumbar puncture if suspected encephalitis
- Arthrocentesis in unexplained arthritis.

### DIFFERENTIAL DIAGNOSIS
- Scarlet fever:
  - "Sandpaper" rash, Pastia lines, and strawberry tongue
- Measles (rubeola):
  - Koplik spots, cough, coryza, conjunctivitis, and fever
- Roseola infantum:
  - Spring and fall
- Rocky Mountain spotted fever:
  - Rash begins at ankles and wrists.
- Rheumatoid arthritis

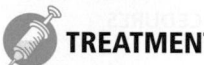

## TREATMENT

### PRE-HOSPITAL
Use N95 filter mask for potential respiratory transmission.

### INITIAL STABILIZATION/THERAPY
ABC management

## ED TREATMENT/PROCEDURES

- Symptomatic therapy
- Antipyretics and antiinflammatory agents:
  - Acetaminophen
  - Ibuprofen
- Isolate rubella patients from susceptible persons (eg, pregnancy).
- Vaccine:
  - Measles-mumps-rubella vaccine
  - Rubella vaccine is live attenuated virus.
  - Indications:
    ○ >12 mo and entry to school
    ○ Susceptible postpubertal females
    ○ High-risk groups (colleges, military, places of employment)
    ○ Unimmunized contacts
    ○ Health care workers and women of childbearing age born before 1957
  - Contraindicated in pregnant women
  - Avoid pregnancy for 3 mo after vaccination.
  - 1 dose confers probable lifelong protection.
  - Common complaints are fever, lymphadenopathy, and arthralgia.
- Immunoglobin:
  - Will not prevent viremia but may modify symptoms

## MEDICATION

- Acetaminophen: 650 mg (peds: 15 mg/kg) PO q4h
- Ibuprofen: 200–600 mg (peds: 5–10 mg/kg; suspension 100 mg/5 mL; oral drops 40 mg/mL) PO q6h
- Immunoglobin: 0.5 mL reconstituted vial SC (0.25–0.50 mL/kg)

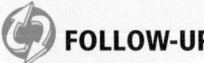 **FOLLOW-UP**

### DISPOSITION

#### Admission Criteria
- Congenital rubella syndrome
- Encephalitis

#### Discharge Criteria
- Most patients may go home.
- Inquire regarding vaccination status of family members.

#### Issues for Referral
- Potential exposure or disease in pregnant women
- Complications
- CRS-suspected child will need comprehensive evaluation.

### FOLLOW-UP RECOMMENDATIONS
Pregnant women with suspected rubella or exposure must be followed with titers and counseling should have obstetric consult.

## PEARLS AND PITFALLS

- Current literature does not support a causal relationship between childhood vaccination with thimerosal-containing vaccines and development of autistic-spectrum disorders.
- Infected individual should be isolated from susceptible (pregnancy, immunocompromised) individual for 7 days.

## ADDITIONAL READING

- American Academy of Pediatrics. *Red Book 2009 Report of the Committee on Infectious Diseases*. Elk Grove IL: American Academy of Pediatrics; 2009.
- Banatvala JE, Brown DW. Rubella. *Lancet*. 2004;363:1127–1137.
- Hviid A, Stellfield M, Melbye M, et al. Association between thimerosal-containing vaccine and autism. *JAMA*. 2003;290:1763–1766.
- Mason WH. Rubella. In: Kliegman RM, Behrman R, Jenson H, et al., eds. *Nelson Textbook of Pediatrics*. 18th ed. Philadelphia: WB Saunders; 2007: 1337–1340.

 **CODES**

### ICD9
- 056.00 Rubella with unspecified neurological complication
- 056.01 Encephalomyelitis due to rubella
- 056.09 Rubella with other neurological complications
- 056.71 Arthritis due to rubella

# SACRAL FRACTURE

Allan V. Hansen
Jaime B. Rivas

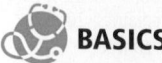 **BASICS**

## DESCRIPTION
- Sacral fractures are rarely isolated injuries (<5%)
- They occur in 45% of all pelvic fractures
- They are defined by the orientation of the fracture line.
- Mechanism:
  - Axial compression
  - Direct posterior trauma
  - Massive crush injury
  - Low-energy fractures in elderly and osteoporotic patients

### *Fracture Classification*
**Transverse**
- High sacral: above S4:
  - Neurologic injury common
  - Can see cauda equina syndrome (CES)
- Low sacral: below S4:
  - Associated rectal tears
  - Rare neurologic injury

**Vertical**
- *Lateral to sacral foramina*:
  - Sciatica
  - L5 root injury
  - Neurologic deficit infrequent
- *Foraminal* (zone 2):
  - Bowel/bladder dysfunction
  - L5, S1, S2 root injury
  - Neurologic deficit frequent
- *Canal* (zone 3):
  - Bowel/bladder dysfunction
  - Sciatica
  - Sexual dysfunction
  - L5, S1 root injury
  - Neurologic deficit often present (>50%)

## ETIOLOGY
- Transverse: Fall from height, flexion injuries, direct blow
- Vertical: Usually high-energy mechanism

 **DIAGNOSIS**

## SIGNS AND SYMPTOMS
- Pain in buttocks, perirectal area, and posterior thigh
- Swelling and ecchymosis over the sacral prominence
- Possible sacral nerve dysfunction:
  - Absent or diminished anal sphincter tone is an important finding.
  - Bowel or bladder incontinence

## ESSENTIAL WORKUP
- History and exam with attention to loss of anal sphincter tone, sensation in the perineum, and bowel and bladder sphincter control.
- Sacral fractures rarely occur in isolation; look for associated injuries.
- Rectal exam will elicit pain in the sacrum; blood in the rectum suggests an open fracture.
- Displacement can be assessed with bimanual rectal exam.

## DIAGNOSTIC TESTS & INTERPRETATION
### Imaging
- Only 30% of sacral fractures are detected on plain radiograph.
- Inlet and outlet views of lumbosacral junction may help.
- CT provides optimal imaging to identify sacral fractures.
- MRI is indicated when neurologic dysfunction is present.

## DIFFERENTIAL DIAGNOSIS
- Contusion
- Lumbar spine fracture
- Pelvic fractures

 TREATMENT

### PRE-HOSPITAL
- Sacral fractures are frequently associated with other spinal and intra-abdominal injuries.
- Immobilize with backboard and C-spine collar.

### INITIAL STABILIZATION/THERAPY
- Manage ABCs as needed.
- Early immobilization in unstable pelvis or spine fractures
- Pain control with NSAIDs or narcotic analgesics

## ED TREATMENT/PROCEDURES
- Vertical unstable fractures require a rapid and thorough assessment for life-threatening injuries as well as orthopedic consultation (see "Pelvic Fracture").
- Nondisplaced isolated transverse sacral fractures are treated symptomatically with touch-down weight bearing on affected side and early orthopedic referral.
- Surgery is often required for fractures associated with neurologic injury.
- Early application of cold compresses

## MEDICATION
### First Line
Analgesia as indicated

 FOLLOW-UP

## DISPOSITION
### Admission Criteria
- Critically injured trauma patient with unstable pelvic fracture
- Neurologic impairment requires orthopedic consultation.

### Discharge Criteria
- Isolated nondisplaced sacral fractures
- Consider intermediate or assisted-care setting for elderly patients.

### FOLLOW-UP RECOMMENDATIONS
- Only nondisplaced, transverse fractures are appropriate for outpatient follow-up
- Prompt surgical evaluation is indicated for displaced fractures.

## PEARLS AND PITFALLS
- Sacral fractures are rarely isolated; consider associated pelvic fractures.
- Detailed neurologic exam, including rectal sphincter tone and perianal sensation, is indicated to assess for associated sacral nerve root injury.
- Foley catheter in a trauma patient may mask voiding problems from sacral nerve root injury.

## ADDITIONAL READING
- Choi SB, Cwinn AA. Pelvic trauma. In: Rosen P, et al., eds. *Emergency Medicine: Concepts and Clinical Practice*, 7th ed. Philadelphia: Mosby-Elsevier, 2009.
- Hak DJ, Baran S, Stahel P. Sacral fractures: Current strategies in diagnosis and management. *Orthopedics*. 2009;32:752–757.
- Simon R, et al. *Emergency Orthopedics: The Extremities*, 5th ed. New York: McGraw-Hill, 2007.

### See Also (Topic, Algorithm, Electronic Media Element)
Pelvic Fracture

 CODES

### ICD9
- 805.6 Closed fracture of sacrum and coccyx without mention of spinal cord injury
- 805.7 Open fracture of sacrum and coccyx without mention of spinal cord injury

S

# SALICYLATE POISONING

*Michele Zell-Kanter*

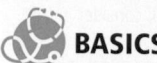 **BASICS**

## DESCRIPTION

- Respiratory alkalosis and metabolic acidosis:
  - Secondary to inhibition of Krebs cycle and uncoupling of oxidative phosphorylation
- Dehydration, hyponatremia or hypernatremia, hypokalemia, hypocalcemia:
  - Owing to increased sweating, vomiting, tachypnea
- Noncardiogenic pulmonary edema:
  - Because of toxic effect of salicylate on pulmonary endothelium resulting in extravasation of fluids
- Pharmacokinetics of salicylate change from first order to zero order in overdose setting; ie, a small dosage increment results in a large increase in salicylate concentration.

### Geriatric Considerations

- Greater morbidity
- Respiratory distress/altered mental status indicative of severe toxicity
- Diagnosis of salicylate intoxication delayed because underlying disease states mask signs and symptoms

### Pediatric Considerations

- Children exhibit faster onset and more severe signs and symptoms than adults:
  - Results from salicylate being distributed more quickly into target organs such as brain, kidney, and liver
- Respiratory alkalosis (hallmark of salicylate poisoning in adults) may not occur in children.
- Metabolic acidosis occurs more quickly in children than in adults.
- Hypoglycemia more common than hyperglycemia
- Ingestion of more than "a taste" of oil of wintergreen (98% methyl salicylate) by children <6 years or greater than 4 mLof oil of wintergreen by patients >6 years warrants ED assessment.

## ETIOLOGY

Sources of salicylate:

- Aspirin
  - Ingestion of >150 mg/kg can cause serous toxicity
- Oil of wintergreen
  - Any exposure should be considered dangerous.
- Bismuth subsalicylate

 **DIAGNOSIS**

## SIGNS AND SYMPTOMS

- Gastrointestinal:
  - Nausea
  - Vomiting
  - Epigastric pain
  - Hematemesis
- Pulmonary:
  - Tachypnea
  - Noncardiogenic pulmonary edema
- CNS:
  - Tinnitus
  - Deafness
  - Delirium
  - Seizures
  - Coma

### History

Ask if taking aspirin or aspirin products:

- Many patients do not list aspirin among their regular medications

## ESSENTIAL WORKUP

Check salicylate level at presentation and then q2hr until level begins to decline.

- Verify that units are correct, generally mg/dL.

## Guidelines for assessing severity of salicylate poisoning

- Acute ingestion with levels of:
  - <150 mg/kg or <6.5 g of aspirin equivalent—considered nontoxic
  - 150–300 mg/kg—mild to moderately toxic
  - >300 mg/kg—potentially lethal
- In the chronic overdose setting:
  - Manage patient on clinical findings and not level alone
  - Clinical findings better indication of severity than plasma salicylate levels
  - Done nomogram not valid
  - Salicylate levels needed to achieve anti-inflammatory effect (20–25 mg/dL) approach toxic levels
  - Enteric-coated aspirin absorbed in intestine; peak level delayed

## DIAGNOSTIC TESTS & INTERPRETATION
### Lab

- Arterial blood gas (ABG):
  - Respiratory alkalosis
  - Metabolic acidosis
- CBC
- Electrolytes, BUN/creatinine, glucose:
  - Anion-gap metabolic acidosis
  - Hypokalemia
  - Baseline renal function
- Urinalysis:
  - Urine pH
- PT/PTT with significant ingestions
- Ferric chloride test:
  - Purple if salicylate present
  - Positive 30 min postingestion
- In the presence of salicylate, Phenistix turn brown-purple; may detect concentrations as low as 20 mg/dL

## Imaging
- Abdominal flat-plate radiograph for concretions
- Chest radiograph for pulmonary edema

## DIFFERENTIAL DIAGNOSIS
- Acute salicylate poisoning:
  - Considered with change in mental status, unexplained noncardiogenic pulmonary edema, mixed acid–base disorder:
  - Methanol
  - Ethylene glycol
  - Conditions causing noncardiogenic pulmonary edema
- Chronic Salicylate Poisoning:
  - Impending myocardial infarction
  - Alcohol withdrawal
  - Organic psychoses
  - Sepsis
  - Dementia

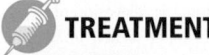

# TREATMENT

## PRE-HOSPITAL
In suspected overdose settings, patient must bring in medications bottles for review

## INITIAL STABILIZATION/THERAPY
- Management of airway, breathing, and circulation (ABCs)
- Naloxone, thiamine, glucose (or Accu-Chek) for altered mental status
- IV rehydration with 0.9% normal saline (NS) for hypotension

## ED TREATMENT/PROCEDURES
- Morbidity and mortality from chronic salicylate poisoning are greater than from acute poisoning
- Manage chronic intoxication more aggressively

### Gastric Decontamination
- Administer activated charcoal
- Whole-bowel irrigation of theoretical benefit:
  - For concretions visible on plain abdominal radiograph
  - For ingestion of sustained-release preparation
  - If salicylate levels continue to increase despite appropriate management
  - Do not use in patients who may develop altered mental status

### Enhanced Elimination
- Alkalinization:
  - Enhances elimination of ionized salicylate
  - Indications:
    - Acidosis
    - Presence of symptoms
    - Elevated salicylate levels
  - One or two ampules of sodium bicarbonate followed by IV $D_5W$ with three ampules sodium bicarbonate
    - Goal: urine pH of 7.5–8 at rate of 3–6 mL/kg/h
    - Add 20–40 mEq KCl per liter to avoid hypokalemia
    - Avoid fluid overload with CHF or CAD
    - Closely monitor serum potassium
- Indications for hemodialysis include:
  - CHF
  - Noncardiogenic pulmonary edema
  - CNS depression
  - Seizures
  - Unstable vital signs
  - Severe acid–base disorder
  - Hepatic compromise
  - Coagulopathy
  - Underlying disease state compromising elimination of salicylate
  - Absolute salicylate level should not be used as sole criterion for deciding to dialyze without considering patient's clinical status unless level is >80–100 mg/dL in acute ingestion.
- Threshold to dialyze is lower in patients with chronic overdose.

## MEDICATION
- Activated charcoal slurry: 1–2 g/kg up to 90 g PO
- Dextrose: $D_{50}W$ 1 amp (50 mL or 25 g) (peds: $D_{25}W$ 2–4 mL/kg) IV
- Naloxone (Narcan): 2 mg (peds: 0.1 mg/kg) IV or IM initial dose
- Thiamine (vitamin $B_1$): 100 mg (peds: 50 mg) IV or IM

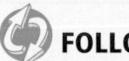 FOLLOW-UP

## DISPOSITION
### Admission Criteria
- Monitor patients with salicylate levels >25 mg/dL until level drops <25 mg/dL and symptoms abate.
- ICU admission for altered mental status, metabolic acidosis, pulmonary edema

### Discharge Criteria
Salicylate level <25 mg/dL and resolution of symptoms

## FOLLOW-UP RECOMMENDATIONS
- Psychiatric referral for intentional ingestions
- Close primary care follow-up for chronic ingestions

## PEARLS AND PITFALLS
- Patients need to maintain their respiratory drive to reverse acidemia, respiratory acidosis:
  - Do not intubate prematurely.
  - It is extremely difficult to achieve and maintain hyperventilation mechanically.
- Salicylate poisoning may result from topical exposure to salicylate-containing lotions or creams.

## ADDITIONAL READING
- Kent K, Ganetsky M, Cohen J, et al. Non-fatal ventricular dysrhythmias associated with severe salicylate toxicity. *Clin Toxicol*. 2008;46:297–299.
- Rivera W, Kleinschmidt KC, Velez LI, et al. Delayed salicylate toxicity at 35 hours without early manifestations following a single salicylate ingestion. *Ann Pharmacother*. 2004;38:1186–1188.
- Stolbach AI, Hoffman RS, Nelson LS. Mechanical ventilation was associated with acidemia in a case series of salicylate-poisoned patients. *Acad Emerg Med*. 2008;15:866–869.

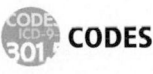 CODES

ICD9
965.1 Poisoning by salicylates

S

# SARCOIDOSIS
*Maureen L. Joyner*

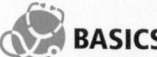
## BASICS

### DESCRIPTION
- Chronic, multisystem disorder characterized in affected organs by an accumulation of T lymphocytes and mononuclear phagocytes, noncaseating epithelioid granulomas, and derangements of the normal tissue architecture
- Prevalence 10–20/100,000 in the U.S. and Europe
- Commonly affects females>males and almost all ages, races, and geographic locations
- Ratio of blacks to whites ranges from 10:1–17:1

### ETIOLOGY
Unknown

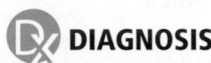
## DIAGNOSIS

### SIGNS AND SYMPTOMS
*History*
- Constitutional:
  - Fatigue
  - Fever
  - Anorexia
  - Weight loss
- Cardiac/Respiratory:
  - Dyspnea
  - Chest pain
  - Palpitations
  - Cough
  - Hemoptysis
- Neurologic:
  - Cranial nerve palsy (usually CN VII)
- Renal:
  - Flank pain
- Musculoskeletal:
  - Joint pain/arthralgia

*Physical Exam*
- Constitutional:
  - Fever
- Skin:
  - Erythema nodosum
  - Subcutaneous nodules
  - Maculopapules
  - Plaques
  - Infiltrative scars
  - Lupus pernio
- EENT:
  - Acute anterior uveitis
  - Keratoconjunctivitis
  - Parotid gland enlargement
- Neurologic:
  - Cranial nerve palsy (usually CN VII)
  - Ataxia
- Respiratory:
  - Adventitious breath sounds
- Cardiac:
  - Dysrhythmias (conduction abnormalities)
  - Signs of CHF (due to restrictive cardiomyopathy)
- Renal:
  - Nephrolithiasis
  - Nephrocalcinosis
- Musculoskeletal:
  - Polyarthralgias
- Löfgren syndrome:
  - Bilateral hilar adenopathy
  - Erythema nodosum
  - Often accompanied by joint symptoms
- Heerfordt–Waldenström syndrome:
  - Fever
  - Uveitis
  - Parotid gland enlargement
  - ±CN VII palsy

*Pediatric Considerations*
- Children <4 yr old classically present with triad of rash, uveitis, and arthritis.
- Children ≥4 yr old present similarly to adults.

### ESSENTIAL WORKUP
- Physical examination with emphasis on lung, skin, eye, heart, and musculoskeletal
- Pulse oximetry/ABG
- ECG (dysrhythmias, conduction delays)
- Slit-lamp eye examination

### DIAGNOSTIC TESTS & INTERPRETATION
*Lab*
- Serum level of angiotensin converting enzyme (ACE) inhibitor
- Basic chemistry panel
- LFTs: mild, usually asymptomatic, elevation of transaminases
- Serum calcium: hypercalcemia due to excessive synthesis of vitamin D
- UA: hypercalciuria
- ESR
- CRP
- CSF analysis: lymphocyte predominance, elevated ACE level

*Imaging*
Chest radiograph:
- Stage 0: normal chest radiograph
- Stage 1: bilateral hilar lymphadenopathy
- Stage 2: lymphadenopathy and parenchymal lung changes
- Stage 3: parenchymal lung changes
- Stage 4: pulmonary fibrosis

*Diagnostic Procedures/Surgery*
- Biopsy:
  - Demonstrates noncaseating granulomas and exclusion of other diseases producing similar histologic picture
- Kveim–Siltzbach test:
  - Rarely used in the U.S. except when affected nodes are inaccessible; requires intradermal injection of lymph node or splenic tissue and subsequent biopsy

## DIFFERENTIAL DIAGNOSIS
- HIV
- Interstitial lung disease
- Lymphoma
- Mycobacterial infection
- Parathyroid disease

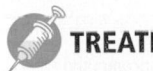 TREATMENT

### PRE-HOSPITAL
Provide supplemental oxygen.

### INITIAL STABILIZATION/THERAPY
- Provide supplemental oxygen.
- Monitor for dysrhythmias.

### ED TREATMENT/PROCEDURES
- Patients should be observed without therapy, if possible, owing to potential for spontaneous improvement.
- Initiate steroids in patients demonstrating one of the following:
  - Symptomatic or progressive stage II pulmonary disease
  - Stage III pulmonary disease Malignant hypercalcemia
  - Severe ocular disease
  - Neurologic sequelae
  - Nasopharyngeal/laryngeal involvement
  - Evidence of hepatic infiltration/disease

- Consider topical corticosteroids and cycloplegic agents for anterior uveitis or dermatologic manifestations.

### MEDICATION
Prednisone: 10–80 mg (peds: 0.5–2 mg/kg) PO qd
- Lower doses for hypercalcemic nephropathy and mild to moderate disease
- Higher doses for neurosarcoidosis

 FOLLOW-UP

### DISPOSITION
*Admission Criteria*
- Hypoxia/hypoxemia
- Patients with moderate to severe respiratory symptoms
- Significant cardiac conduction delays
- Severe thrombocytopenia

*Discharge Criteria*
Follow-up is established.

*Issues for Referral*
- Rheumatology:
  - For routine care and follow-up
    - ~q2mo for patients with active disease on steroids, q3–4mo for asymptomatic patients
- Pulmonary Medicine:
  - For formal pulmonary function testing (to monitor for progression of restrictive lung disease) with spirometry and DLCO
- Ophthalmology:
  - Within 48 hr for acute uveitis

### FOLLOW-UP RECOMMENDATIONS
- Restrict excess calcium from the diet
- Monitor for complications related to chronic steroid therapy

## PEARLS AND PITFALLS
- Evaluate patients with chest radiographs to determine stage and progression of disease.
- Prednisone is treatment of choice for exacerbations of disease.
- Monitor for signs of hypercalcemia and related complications.
- Be aware of acute neurologic and ocular sequelae.

## ADDITIONAL READING
- American Thoracic Society. Statement on sarcoidosis. *Am J Crit Care Med*. 1999;160:736–755.
- Baughman, RP. Pulmonary sarcoidosis. *Clin Chest Med*. 2004;25:521.
- Iannuzzi M, Rybicki B, Teirstein A. Sarcoidosis. *N Engl J Med*. 2007;357:2153–2165.
- Swierzewski S. Sarcoidosis. Pulmonology Channel. Updated December 4, 2007. Available at: http://www.pulmonologychannel.com/sarcoidosis. Accessed November 16, 2009.
- Author. Sarcoidosis. In: DS Basow, ed., *UpToDate*. Waltham, MA: UpToDate, 2009.

### See Also (Topic, Algorithm, Electronic Media Element)
- Dyspnea
- HIV/AIDS
- Hyperparathyroidism
- Tuberculosis

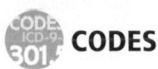 CODES

ICD9
135 Sarcoidosis

S

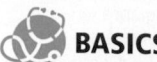 **SCABIES**
James Hwang

## 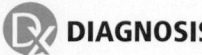 BASICS

### DESCRIPTION
- Mites mate on skin surface and gravid female burrows into stratum corneum to lay eggs:
  - Animal scabies burrow but cannot reproduce.
- Symptoms result from delayed type IV hypersensitivity reaction to mite, eggs, saliva, and feces:
  - Inflammatory reaction is responsible for intense pruritus, which is the hallmark of the disease.
  - Crusted Norwegian scabies is characterized by large numbers of mites and is seen in disabled, immunocompromised, and institutionalized patients:
    - More infectious than ordinary scabies due to high mite count.
- Despite >2,500 yr existence, an effective way to prevent scabies is still not known.
- Secondary infection is common and, as such, the morbidity associated with scabies is underestimated.
- Scabies is a major global health problem in many indigenous and resource-poor communities.
- Infestations become secondarily infected and epidemic acute poststreptococcal glomerulonephritis and rheumatic heart disease are often associated with endemic scabies.

#### Pediatric Considerations
- Scabies manifests itself in various forms in children and differs from that in adults.
- Highest prevalence is in children <2 yr old.

### ETIOLOGY
- Epidemiology:
  - Over the past 2 decades, the number of patients with scabies is increasing.
- Produced by the human scabies mite, *Sarcoptes scabiei* var. *hominis*, or from animal mites.
- It is transmitted by prolonged direct skin-to-skin contact or, less frequently, by infested bedding or clothing:
  - It is a disease of overcrowding and poverty, rather than a reflection of poor hygiene.
  - Probability of being infected is related to number of mites on infected person and length of contact.
- Mites subsist on a diet of dissolved human tissue (do not feed on blood) and can live up to 4 days off a host's body.
- On average, the number of mites on a host at any time is ~5–15:
  - Main differences between crusted Norwegian scabies and ordinary scabies is the number of mites present on the host: Patients with crusted Norwegian scabies are infected with thousands or up to a million mites.

## DIAGNOSIS

### SIGNS AND SYMPTOMS
Generalized and intense itching that is worse at night and usually spares the head and face.

#### History
- Site, severity, duration, and timing of itch
- History should include family members and close contacts.
- Generalized, intensely pruritic eruption:
  - Pruritus is intensified at night.
- Onset 10–30 days after exposure and infestation; reinfestation provokes immediate (within 1–4 days) pruritus:
  - Patients with Norwegian scabies are usually immunocompromised, have a decreased inflammatory response, and have less pruritus.

#### Physical Exam
- Often minimal cutaneous findings
- Primary lesion: Linear, elevated, white-gray burrow (up to 1-cm long, width of a human hair) with small vesicle containing black dot at the end (mites barely visible to naked eye):
  - Found symmetrically in web spaces of fingers, flexor surfaces of wrists and elbows, waistline, periumbilical skin, axillary folds, buttocks, penis, scrotum, vulva, and areola.
  - Head and neck rarely affected in adults but more commonly in infants and children.
- Secondary lesions: Crusted papules, nodules, excoriations, or secondary impetigo or folliculitis seen on back, shoulders, axilla, waist, buttocks, and flexor aspects of elbows:
  - Secondary lesions are usually more numerous and prominent than burrows but also may be few if topical steroids used.
  - Longstanding infestation results in chronic excoriation, eczematization, and hyperpigmented and lichenified skin.
- Crusted Norwegian scabies produce gross scaling with hyperkeratotic plaques on hands, feet, scalp, and pressure-bearing areas.

#### Pediatric Considerations
- Eruption may be seen from head to toe.
- Distribution typically involves the proximal 1/2 of the foot and heel.
- Vesicles are often found in infants due to their predisposition for vesicle formation.
- Neonatal scabies is associated with poor feeding, poor weight gain, and frequent super infection.

### ESSENTIAL WORKUP
- Careful history and skin exam for characteristic lesions
- The diagnosis is easily missed and should be considered in any patient with persistent generalized pruritus.

### DIAGNOSTIC TESTS & INTERPRETATION
#### Lab
- May be indicated in immunocompromised patients or in patients with systemic infection.
- New diagnostic laboratory studies are being developed (circulating IgE levels, PCR, ELISA, and DNA finger printing).
- When endemic, empiric treatment may be more cost effective than lab testing.

#### Imaging
Epiluminescence microscopy and noncomputed dermoscopy are noninvasive, simple, accurate, and rapid imaging techniques.

#### Diagnostic Procedures/Surgery
- Scrape skin with no. 15 blade and mineral oil (adheres scraped material to blade) and observe under low-power microscope for mites, eggs, or fecal material.
- A negative scraping does not exclude infestation due to low number of parasites:
  - Sensitivity <50% and is affected by number of sites sampled and sampler's experience.

### DIFFERENTIAL DIAGNOSIS
- Atopic dermatitis
- Dermatitis herpetiformis
- Papular urticaria
- Folliculitis
- Lichen planus.
- Pruritic urticarial papules and plaques of pregnancy.
- Adult linear IgA bullous dermatosis.
- Syphilis
- Pediculosis
- Pityriasis rosea
- Impetigo
- Seborrheic dermatitis
- Lymphoma
- Flea bites and bedbugs.

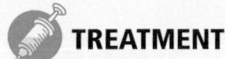

# TREATMENT

## PRE-HOSPITAL
Maintain universal precautions.

## INITIAL STABILIZATION/THERAPY
No specific stabilization necessary in routine cases.

## ED TREATMENT/PROCEDURES
- Treatment should not be empiric for patients with generalized itching but reserved for patients with a history of exposure, a typical eruption, or both.
- Treat patient and all persons in immediate contact with topical scabicide:
  - Treat all contacts at the same time, regardless of the presence of symptoms.
- Permethrin is 89–92% effective, and is the best tolerated:
  - <2% of permethrin is absorbed into the skin, making its potential toxicity low:
    ○ For children ≥2 mo older
- Crotamiton is 50–60% effective and used when other scabicides are not tolerated.
- Ivermectin administered orally for 2 doses 14 days apart has shown excellent results (similar efficacy as permethrin):
  - Effective in patients unable to tolerate topical scabietics or in patients with resistant or crusted Norwegian scabies.
- Lindane is slightly less effective and is potentially toxic to the CNS:
  - Lindane absorption (through skin, lung or intestinal mucosa, or mucous membranes) is about 10%.
  - Side effects include: Nausea, headache, vertigo, amblyopia, irritability, and seizure.
  - Do not use in pediatric patients.
  - Prohibited in states such as California.
- Sulfur is the oldest known treatment of scabies, and is the drug of choice for infants <2 mo and for pregnant or lactating women.
- Crusted Norwegian scabies 1st requires removal of hyperkeratotic scale with 6% salicylic acid in petroleum jelly to facilitate entry of the scabicide.
- Treatment failures:
  - Treatment failures are frequent in crusted Norwegian scabies, and use of multiple agents including oral medications is often necessary.
  - Machine wash and dry in hot cycles (60°C) or dry clean all clothes and bedding worn within 2 days of treatment; vacuum household floors, carpets, mattresses, and furniture.
  - Emphasize that itching may continue for 1–4 wk after mites are killed due to skin inflammatory reaction.
  - Topical steroids and oral antihistamines can reduce pruritic symptoms.
  - Relapses can occur from untreated areas such as the scalp and subungual regions.
  - Treatment failures tend to arise from poor patient understanding and inadequate patient education.

## MEDICATION
- Scabicides:
  - Crotamiton 10% lotion or cream: Apply topically from neck down in adults and entire skin surface in children q.h.s. for 2 nights, then rinse off 48 hr after last application.
  - Ivermectin 3 mg tablets: 1st PO dose of 200 μg/kg should be followed by 2nd PO dose of 200 μg/kg 14 days later (pregnancy category C).
  - Lindane 1% lotion or cream: Apply topically from neck down and rinse off after 8–12 hr; contraindicated in infants, pregnancy, lactation, excessive excoriations, or seizure disorder.
  - Permethrin 5% cream (Elimite): Apply topically from neck down in adults and entire skin in children q.h.s., rinse off after 8–14 hr (pregnancy class B, unknown safety in breast-feeding)
  - Sulfur 5–10% precipitated in petrolatum: Apply topically nightly for 3 consecutive nights and then wash off 24 hr later.
- Antipruritics:
  - Low sedating/selective antihistamines:
    ○ Cetirizine (Zyrtec): Adults and peds >6 yr: 5–10 mg/d PO; 6–12 mo: 2.5 mg/dPO; 12–24 mo: 2.5 mg/d PO to b.i.d.; 2–6 yr: 2.5–5 mg/d PO
    ○ Fexofenadine (Allegra): Adult and peds >12 yr: 180 mg/d PO or 60 mg PO b.i.d.; 6 mo–5 yr: 15–30 mg PO b.i.d.; 6–11 yr: 30 mg PO b.i.d.
    ○ Loratadine (Claritin): Adults and peds >6 yr: 10 mg/d PO; 2–5 yr: 5 mg/d PO
  - Sedating/nonselective antihistamines:
    ○ Diphenhydramine (Benadryl): Adults and peds >12 yr: 25–50 mg PO q4–6h; 2–6 yr: 6.25 mg PO q4–6h; 6–12 yr: 12.5–25 mg PO q4–6h
    ○ Doxepin: 25–50 mg PO b.i.d., peds: Dosing currently unavailable
    ○ Hydroxyzine HCl (Atarax): Adults and peds >12 yr: 25–100 mg PO q6–8h; <6 yr: 2 mg/kg/d PO divided q6–8h; 6–12 yr: 12.5–25 mg PO q6–8h

### First Line
Permethrin 5% cream

### Second Line
Crotamiton or PO Ivermectin

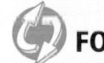

# FOLLOW-UP

## DISPOSITION

### Admission Criteria
Patients with severe topical or systemic super infection

### Discharge Criteria
Nontoxic appearing patients with routine symptoms

### Issues for Referral
Refractory or relapsing cases

## FOLLOW-UP RECOMMENDATIONS
Re-evaluate after 1–4 wk for recurrence:
- Retreat if live mites are found.

## PEARLS AND PITFALLS

- Scabies is a common parasitic infection that is transmitted by prolonged direct skin-to-skin contact.
- Scabies in children can differ from that in adults.
- Crusted Norwegian scabies is characterized by a large number of mites, and is seen in immunocompromised or institutionalized patients:
  - Follow-up is recommended and treatment failure is common:
    ○ Proper patient education can decrease treatment failures.

## ADDITIONAL READING

- Burkhart CG, Burkhart CN, Burkhart K. An epidemiologic and therapeutic reassessment of scabies. *Cutis*. 2000;65:233–240.
- Chosidow O. Scabies. *N Engl J Med* 2006;354: 1718–1727.
- Scabies. Atlanta. Centers for Disease Control and Prevention, 2008. Accessed at http://www.cdc.gov/scabies/.
- Walton SF, Currie BJ. Problems in diagnosing scabies, a global disease in human and animal populations. *Clin Microbiol Rev*. 2007;20:268–279.

### See Also (Topic, Algorithm, Electronic Media Element)
- Pediculosis
- Pityriasis rosea

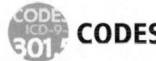 CODES

**ICD9**
133.0 Scabies

S

# SCAPHOID FRACTURE

*Davut J. Savaser*
*Robyn Heister Girard*

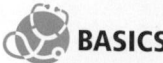 **BASICS**

## DESCRIPTION
- The scaphoid is the most commonly fractured carpal bone.
- This bone is the stabilizer between the distal and proximal carpal rows.
- Injury may result in arthritis, avascular necrosis, or malunion.
- Classified as:
  – Proximal 3rd (10–20%)
  – Middle 3rd (the waist, 70–80%)
  – Distal 3rd (the tuberosity)
  – Tubercle fractures
- Fractures are missed on initial radiographs 10–15% of the time, and delayed diagnosis greatly increases risk of complications.
- The blood supply to the scaphoid enters distally; the more proximal the fracture, the higher the risk for avascular necrosis.
- The more proximal the fracture, the higher the likelihood for avascular necrosis
- As the wrist is forcibly hyperextended, the volar aspect of the scaphoid fails in tension and the dorsal aspect fails in compression resulting in a fracture.

## ETIOLOGY
Generally results from a fall on an outstretched (dorsiflexed) hand (FOOSH injury).

 **DIAGNOSIS**

## SIGNS AND SYMPTOMS
### History
FOOSH injury

### Physical Exam
- Maximal pain and tenderness in the anatomic snuffbox (may be elicited with direct palpation or axial loading of the thumb)
- Dorsal wrist pain distal to the radial styloid and decreased range of motion of the wrist and thumb
- Rarely, incidental damage to the superficial branches of the radial nerve results in sensory changes.
- Palpate the scaphoid tubercle for tenderness by radially deviating the wrist and palpating over the palmar aspect of the scaphoid.

### Pediatric Considerations
- Carpal fractures are rare in children (and the elderly), as the distal radius usually fails 1st.
- If present, carefully evaluate mechanism.

## DIAGNOSTIC TESTS & INTERPRETATION
### Imaging
- Radiographic imaging should include 3 views of the wrist: PA, lateral, oblique, and scaphoid view (wrist prone and in ulnar deviation).
- Pay special attention to the middle 3rd, or waist, of the bone: 70% of injuries occur here.
- Fracture may be identified by subtle findings such as a displaced fat pad.
- 10–15% of all fractures are not visible on radiographs at the time of injury.
- Bone scintigraphy or MRI as early as 3 days postinjury can rule out fracture and allow for earlier rehabilitation:
  – CT is not as reliable.

### Diagnostic Procedures/Surgery
- If fracture is open or associated injuries are identified, urgent surgical intervention may be indicated.
- Associated injuries with scaphoid fracture:
  – Scapholunate dissociation
  – Distal radial fracture
  – Lunate fracture/dislocation
  – Bennett's fracture of thumb
  – Radiocarpal joint dislocation
  – Proximal and distal carpal bone joint dislocation

## DIFFERENTIAL DIAGNOSIS
- Bennett fracture
- Rolando fracture
- Extra-articular fracture at the base of the thumb metacarpal
- Gamekeeper thumb
- DE Quervain tenosynovitis
- Perilunate dislocation
- Scapholunate dissociation
- Lunate fracture or dislocation

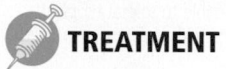 **TREATMENT**

## PRE-HOSPITAL
Splint as appropriate.

## INITIAL STABILIZATION/THERAPY
- Evaluate patient for other injuries.
- Dress open wounds.
- Immobilize with thumb in neutral position, ice, and elevate.

## ED TREATMENT/PROCEDURES

- Assess mechanism of injury and point of maximal tenderness.
- Exam with special attention to skin integrity and neurovascular status.
- If snuffbox tenderness is present, place in thumb spica splint.
- Counsel patient regarding risk of malunion and avascular necrosis.
- Clinically suspected scaphoid fractures without radiographic evidence:
  - Should be treated as a nondisplaced scaphoid fracture
  - Spica splint thumb in a position as if the patient was embracing a wine glass.
  - Repeat physical/radiographic exam in 7–10 days.
- Nondisplaced scaphoid fractures:
  - Thumb spica splint
- Displaced scaphoid fractures:
  - Nonunion rate of 50%
  - Often an indication for internal fixation

## MEDICATION

Pain control with NSAIDs or narcotics as needed

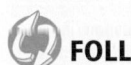 **FOLLOW-UP**

## DISPOSITION

### Admission Criteria

Open fracture or presence of other more serious injuries

### Discharge Criteria

- Closed injuries, with 72-hr orthopedic follow-up
- Patients with splints for nondisplaced fractures may be allowed to return to full work or activity of work/sport if the cast does not interfere with the exercises of work or specific sport activities.

### Issues for Referral

- If fracture is angulated or displaced >1 mm, immediate orthopaedic referral is indicated.
- All scaphoid or suspected scaphoid injuries must be referred to orthopaedics.
- If no radiographic abnormalities found on initial radiograph, after placing in thumb spica splint, refer to orthopaedics or primary care in 7–10 days with repeat radiographs at that time.

## PEARLS AND PITFALLS

- Perfusion enters scaphoid bone distally.
- Avascular necrosis (especially with proximal 3rd fractures), occurs with inadequately reduced or immobilized fractures.

## ADDITIONAL READING

- Eisenhauer MA. Wrist & Forearm. In: Rosen P, et al., eds. *Emergency Medicine: Concepts and Clinical Practice*, 5th ed. St. Louis, MO: Mosby-Year Book, 2002:535–539.
- Simon RR, Sherman SC, Koenignecht SJ. *Emergency Orthopedics: The Extremities*, 5th ed. New York: McGraw-Hill, 2007;189–193.
- Kumar S, O'Connor A, Dsespois M, et al. Use of early magnetic resonance imaging in the diagnosis of occult scaphoid fractures: The CAST Study. *N Z Med J.* 2005;11;118(1209):U1296.
- Perron AD, Brady WJ, Keats TE, et al. Orthopedic pitfalls in the ED: Scaphoid fracture. *Am J Emerg Med.* 2001;19(4):310–316.
- Pillai A, Jain M. Management of clinical fractures of the scaphoid: Results of an audit and literature review. *Euro J Emerg Med.* 2005;12(2):47–51.
- Plancher KD. Methods of imaging the scaphoid. *Hand Clinics.* 2001;17(4):703–721.
- Rockwood CA Jr, Green DP, Bucholz RW, et al. eds. *Fractures in Adults*, 4th ed. Philadelphia: Lippincott Raven, 1996.
- Uehara DT. The hand in emergency medicine. *Emerg Clin North Am.* 1993;11(3):781–796.

### See Also (Topic, Algorithm, Electronic Media Element)

Lunate Fracture and Dislocations

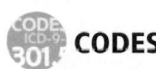 **CODES**

### ICD9

814.01 Closed fracture of navicular (scaphoid) bone of wrist

# SCHIZOPHRENIA

Joshua L. Roffman
Donald C. Goff

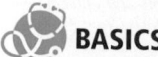 **BASICS**

## DESCRIPTION
- A chronic psychotic disorder characterized by delusions, hallucinations, disorganization, negative symptoms, and cognitive deficits
- Onset typically early in adulthood
- Comorbid substance abuse (alcohol, cannabis, and stimulants) is common.
- ~10% of patients commit suicide.
- Violence may result from impaired judgment, paranoia, and command hallucinations.
- Patients with schizophrenia can have abnormally high pain thresholds that can complicate the detection of medical illness.
- Premorbid phase:
  – Development of negative symptoms with deterioration of personal, social, and intellectual functioning
- Active phase:
  – May be precipitated by a stressful event
  – Development of active delusions, hallucinations, and bizarre behavior
- Residual phase:
  – Patients are left with impaired social and cognitive ability

## ETIOLOGY
- Genetic component (concordance rate of 50% in monozygotic twins)
- Specific genes uncertain
- Stressors during pregnancy may increase risk.
- Influenza during second trimester
- Birth complications

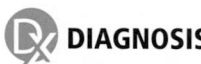 **DIAGNOSIS**

## SIGNS AND SYMPTOMS
Criteria of the *Diagnostic and Statistical Manual of Mental Disorders* (*DSM*) require the presence of at least 2 of the following symptoms for more than 6 mo:
- Delusions (fixed, false beliefs):
  – Bizarre, paranoid, or grandiose
  – Often involve the conviction that others are tampering with one's mind or body
- Hallucinations:
  – Typically hearing voices
  – May involve any sensory modality
- Thought disorder:
  – Disorganized speech ranging from odd, idiosyncratic logic to incoherence
- Grossly disorganized or catatonic behavior
- Negative symptoms:
  – Apathy
  – Flat affect
  – Social isolation
  – Anhedonia

## ESSENTIAL WORKUP
- Obtain history from additional sources:
  – Friends or family
  – Assists in establishing the diagnosis
- Evaluate potential dangerousness to self or others:
  – The content of delusions and the nature of auditory hallucinations should be explored to assess safety.
- Medical and neurologic screening
- Assessment for drug-induced psychosis (see Psychosis, Medical vs. Psychiatric)
- Rule out affective psychosis (bipolar disorder, psychotic depression)
- Evaluate for delirium or dementia:
  – Schizophrenia does not affect orientation.

## DIAGNOSTIC TESTS & INTERPRETATION
### Lab
- Toxicology screen
- Electrolytes, BUN, creatinine, glucose, calcium
- Thyroid panel (see Psychosis, Medical vs. Psychiatric)
- If warranted by clinical history and presentation, consider lumbar puncture (occult CNS infection), EEG (occult seizure), or karyotype (eg, 22q11 deletion).

### Imaging
Head imaging only with suspicion of neurologic etiology

## DIFFERENTIAL DIAGNOSIS
- Delirium
- Drug-induced psychosis
- Huntington disease
- Temporal lobe epilepsy
- Bipolar (manic depressive) disorder
- Psychotic depression
- Delusional disorder
- Schizotypal personality
- Brief psychotic episode
  – Similar symptoms that occur with duration of <1 mo
- Schizophreniform disorder:
  – Similar symptoms that occur with duration between 1 and 6 mo

 **TREATMENT**

## PRE-HOSPITAL
- Prehospital personnel must protect themselves from harm.
- Patients can display unpredictable and violent behavior toward themselves and others.
- Patients may require restraints to protect themselves or emergency medical services crew.
- Know local laws as they apply to involuntary restraint.

## INITIAL STABILIZATION/THERAPY
- Safety of health care workers and patient is paramount.
- Patient may require a quiet room.
- Presence of security staff may be needed.
- Physical or chemical restraints as appropriate
- Agitation may be treated with a high-potency antipsychotic and benzodiazepine:
  – IM haloperidol combined with lorazepam is synergistic.
  – Ziprasidone or olanzapine may also be administered IM for agitation.
- Negative symptoms tend to be less responsive to pharmacotherapy than psychotic symptoms.

## ED TREATMENT/PROCEDURES
- Psychiatric consultation after medical evaluation is completed
- High-potency conventional antipsychotic agents (haloperidol, fluphenazine):
  – Minimal cardiovascular effects (droperidol and thioridazine affect QT interval)
  – Oral and IM administration can produce extrapyramidal symptoms:
    ○ Dystonia
    ○ Parkinsonism
    ○ Akathisia (restlessness of lower extremities)
  – IV haloperidol associated with fewer extrapyramidal symptoms

- Low-potency conventional agents (chlorpromazine, thioridazine):
  – Fewer extrapyramidal symptoms
  – More sedating
  – Orthostatic hypotension
  – Anticholinergic side effects
- Atypical antipsychotic agents (risperidone, olanzapine, quetiapine, ziprasidone, aripiprazole, paliperidone, iloperidone, asenapine):
  – Better tolerated with fewer extrapyramidal symptoms
  – Risperidone, iloperidone, and quetiapine can cause orthostatic hypotension
  – Ziprasidone and iloperidone delay cardiac repolarization (QT interval)
  – Clozapine is the only agent that is clearly more effective for psychotic symptoms:
    ○ Requires weekly monitoring of WBCs due to agranulocytosis.
    ○ Highly sedating, anticholinergic, hypotensive
- Risperidone microspheres (Consta), paliperidone palmitate (Sustenna), haloperidol decanoate, and fluphenazine decanoate are long-acting depot preparations.
- If a high-potency conventional antipsychotic agent is administered, patients younger than age 40 should be started on benztropine (Cogentin) 2 mg b.i.d. for 10 days to reduce the risk of dystonic reactions.

## MEDICATION

- Aripiprazole (Abilify): 5–30 mg/d
- Olanzapine (Zyprexa): 10–20 mg/d
- Risperidoxe (Risperdal): 4–8 mg/d
- Thioridazine (Mellaril): 300–800 mg/d
- Chlorpromazine (Thorazine): 300–800 mg/d
- Clozapine (Clozaril): 200–900 mq/d
- Fluphenazine (Prolixin): 5–20 mg/d
- Haloperidol (Haldol): 5–20 mg/d, acute agitation; 5–20 mg IV/IM, repeat q30–60min
- Lorazepam (Ativan): acute agitation, 2–4 mg IV/IM, repeat q30–60min
- Quetiapine (Seroquel): 250–750 mg/d

- Ziprasidone (Geodon): 80–160 mg/d
- Paliperidone (Invega): 6–12 mg/d
- Asenapine (Saphris) 5–10 mg bid (sublinqual)
- Iloperidone (Fanapt) 6–12 mg b.i.d. (requires initial titration starting at 1 mg b.i.d.)
- Perphenazine (Trilafon): 12–32 mg/d

### Geriatric Considerations
Elderly patients with dementia-related psychoses treated with antipsychotic drugs are at increased risk of death.

 FOLLOW-UP

### DISPOSITION
#### Admission Criteria
- Admit if patient is a danger to self or others or is gravely disabled.
- Criteria for involuntary hospitalization vary by state.
- Patients with new-onset psychosis should also be admitted for evaluation and stabilization.

#### Discharge Criteria
- Patient is not a danger to self or others and able to perform activities of daily living.
- Psychiatric follow-up is arranged.
- Psychotic symptoms may persist at time of discharge.

### FOLLOW-UP RECOMMENDATIONS
- Outpatient psychopharmacologic follow-up should occur within one week of discharge.
- Patients taking antipsychotics (especially atypicals) should be monitored for obesity and related metabolic syndromes.
- Adjunctive cognitive behavioral therapy and other psychosocial treatments can help patients manage psychotic symptoms.

## PEARLS AND PITFALLS

- Visual, olfactory, gustatory, or tactile hallucinations should prompt medical workup for secondary causes of psychosis, as should atypical age of onset (>30 years old).
- Early treatment with antipsychotic medications has consistently been associated with better outcomes in schizophrenia.

## ADDITIONAL READING

- Freudenreich O, Holt DJ, Cather C, Goff D. The evaluation and management of patients with first-episode schizophrenia: A selective, clinical review of diagnosis, treatment, and prognosis. *Harv Rev Psychiatry*. 2007;15:189–211.
- Goff D, Heckers S, Freudenreich O. Schizophrenia. In: Nemeroff C, ed. *Med Clin North Am*. 2001;85: 663–689.

### See Also (Topic, Algorithm, Electronic Media Element)
Psychosis, acute

 CODES

**ICD9**
295.90 Unspecified type schizophrenia, unspecified state

**S**

# SCIATICA/HERNIATED DISC
*Ruth Granlund*

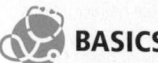

## BASICS

### DESCRIPTION
- Pain that radiates from the back into buttocks and lower extremity distal to knee, with or without sensory or motor deficits:
- 95% sensitive, 88% specific for herniated disc (HD)
- Peaks fourth to fifth decade
- 2%–10% of low back pain
- 95% L5 or S1 nerve root
- 50%–80% improve with conservative management
- 5%–10% require surgery

### ETIOLOGY
- Protrusion of colloidal gel (*nucleus pulposus*) through weakened surrounding fibrous capsule (*annulus fibrosis*)
- Risk factors:
  - Smoking
  - Repetitive lifting/twisting
  - Vehicular/machinery vibration
  - Obesity
  - Sedentary lifestyle

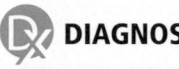

## DIAGNOSIS

### SIGNS AND SYMPTOMS
*History*
- Low back pain precedes onset of leg pain.
- Leg pain predominates with time.
- Sharp, well localized, radiates distal to knee
- Exacerbated by activities that increase intradiscal pressure:
- Valsalva maneuver
- Cough
- Nerve-root tension (sitting, straight leg raise)
- Relieved by decreasing pressure/tension:
- Lying supine
- Walking

*Physical Exam*
- Neurologic exam (motor, sensory, deep tendon reflexes)
- L4 root/L3–4 disc:
  - Knee extension/hip adduction
  - Anteromedial leg/knee/medial malleolus
  - Patellar reflex
- L5 root/L4–5 disc:
  - Great toe and foot dorsiflexion
  - Dorsomedial foot/first web space
  - No reflex

- S1 root/L5–S1 disc:
  - Foot plantarflexion
  - Posterior leg/lateral malleolus/dorsolateral foot
  - Achilles' reflex
  - Rectal exam (tone, sensation)
- Straight leg raise:
- Elevate ipsilateral leg by heel 30–60 degrees with or without dorsiflexing foot.
- Reproduces radicular pain past knee
- 80% sensitive for HD
- Crossed straight leg raise test (pathognomonic):
- Elevate contralateral leg
- Pain in involved leg
- Less sensitive but very specific for HD

### ESSENTIAL WORKUP
- Complete history and physical exam
- See below for test indications.

### DIAGNOSTIC TESTS & INTERPRETATION
*Lab*
- Indicated if clinical suspicion for differential diagnoses (DDX), not limited to:
- CBC
- ESR/CRP
- UA

*Imaging*
**PA/Lateral of LS spine**
- Helps to rule out some DDX
- Indications:
  - Extremes of age (<20, >55 yr)
  - Unresolved back pain (>4–6 wk) despite conservative treatment
  - Red flags on history and physical exam:
    ○ Trauma
    ○ Constitutional symptoms (fever, unexplained weight loss, malaise)
    ○ History of cancer
    ○ Immunocompromised
    ○ IV drug abuse
    ○ Recent bacterial infection
    ○ Worse at night/wakes patient from sleep
    ○ Fever
    ○ Midline point tenderness
    ○ Neurologic deficits

**MRI (Criterion Standard)**
- Indications:
- Acute, severe neurologic deficits (order from ED)
- Suspicion of infectious etiology of back pain:
  - Epidural abscess
  - Osteomyelitis
  - Discitis
- 6 wk failed conservative therapy (order on outpatient basis)
- Disc disease (>25%):
- Incidental finding on MRI in asymptomatic patients
- No relationship between extent of protrusion and degree of symptoms

**CT Myelogram**
- Rarely used alternative for MRI
- CT better at bone details

### Diagnostic Procedures/Surgery
- Postvoid residual (PVR):
  - Overflow incontinence = PVR >100 mL, suspect cauda equina syndrome

### DIFFERENTIAL DIAGNOSIS
- Sciatica
- Lumbosacral strain
- Degenerative joint disease
- Spondylolisthesis
- Hip/sacroiliac joint (infection, fracture, bursitis)
- Pneumonia, pulmonary embolus
- Pancreatitis
- Pyelonephritis, renal calculi
- Ectopic pregnancy, pelvic inflammatory disease
- Abdominal aortic aneurysm (AAA)
- Peripheral vascular disease (claudication)
- Herpes zoster
- Psychologic: functional or secondary gain (drug seeking, disability)
- Irritating lesion affecting a lumbosacral nerve anywhere along its route:
- Brain:
  - Thalamic or spinothalamic tumor, hemorrhage
- Spinal cord (*myelopathy*):
  - spinal stenosis, tumor, hematoma, infection (epidural abscess, discitis, osteomyelitis)

- Root (*radiculopathy*):
  – Intradural: tumor, infection
  – Extradural: HD, lumbar spine/foraminal stenosis (pseudoclaudication), spondylolisthesis, cyst, tumor, infection
- Plexus (*plexopathy*):
  – tumor, AAA, infection (iliopsoas abscess), hematoma (retroperitoneal)
- Peripheral nerve (*neuropathy*):
  -toxic/metabolic/nutritional, infection, trauma, ischemia, infiltration, compression, entrapment

### Pediatric Considerations
- Usually secondary to trauma or serious underlying medical disease (eg, leukemia); consider complete workup
- <10 yr
- Infection
- Tumor
- Arteriovenous malformation
- ≥10 yr
- Traumatic HD
- Spondylolisthesis
- Scheuermann disease
- Tumor

### Pregnancy Considerations
- Ectopic pregnancy
- Labor
- Pyelonephritis
- Musculoskeletal

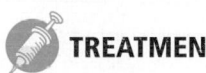

## TREATMENT

### PRE-HOSPITAL
Full spine precautions for trauma victims

### INITIAL STABILIZATION/THERAPY
Evaluate for neurosurgical emergency

### ED TREATMENT/PROCEDURES
Pain relief:
- NSAIDs first line
- Muscles relaxants, opioids as needed in acute phase

### MEDICATION
- NSAIDs:
  – Ibuprofen (Motrin, Advil): 600–800 mg (peds: 5–10 mg/kg per dose) PO t.i.d.–q.i.d.
  – Naproxen (Naprosyn, Aleve): 500 mg PO b.i.d.
- Muscle relaxants (short term):
  – Cyclobenzaprine (Flexeril): 10–20 mg PO t.i.d.
  – Diazepam (Valium): 2–10 mg (peds: 0.1 mg/kg per dose) PO t.i.d.–q.i.d.
  – Methocarbamol (Robaxin): 1,000–1,500 mg PO q.i.d.

- Opioids (short term):
  – Hydromorphone (Dilaudid): 2–4 mg PO/0.5–2 mg IM/IV q4–6h PRN
  – Morphine sulfate: 2–10 mg (peds: 0.1 mg/kg per dose) IM/IV q2–4h PRN
  – Tylenol #3: 1–2 PO q4–6h PRN
  – Vicodin: 1–2 PO q4–6h PRN

 ## FOLLOW-UP

### DISPOSITION
#### Admission Criteria
- Severe neurologic deficit (cauda equina syndrome, inability to walk)
- Progressive neurologic deficit
- Multiple root involvement
- Unstable fracture, infection, neoplasm
- Inability to manage as outpatient (social situation/pain)

#### Discharge Criteria
Patient able to ambulate, follow instructions, has reliable home situation and planned follow-up

#### Issues for Referral
Abnormal workup that does not warrant immediate admission. Where and when depend on results (large DDX).

### FOLLOW-UP RECOMMENDATIONS
- Consultant (orthopedic spine surgeon or neurosurgeon) or PCP within 1 week
- Conservative treatment (4–6 wk):
- Medication as noted
- Avoid complete bed rest, 2 days at most
- Limited activity in acute phase but gradually increase activity/exercise as tolerated
- Avoid movements that load lower back or exacerbate pain:
  – Heavy lifting, twisting, bending, stooping, bodily vibration
- Therapies of unproven benefit:
- Chiropractic care
- OTranscutaneous electrical nerve stimulation (TENS)
- Traction
- Back brace/corset
- Ultrasound
- Diathermy
- Acupuncture, acupressure
- Massage

## ADDITIONAL READING
- Van der Windt DA, Simons E, Riphagen II, et al. Physical examination for lumbar radiculopathy due to disc herniation in patients with low-back pain. *Cochrane Database Syst Rev.* 2010;2:CD007431.
- Della-Giustina DA. Emergency department evaluation and treatment of back pain. *Emerg Med Clin North Am.* 1999;17(4):877–893.
- Deyo RA, Weinstein JN. Low back pain. *N Engl J Med.* 2001;344(5):363–370.
- Haas M, Sharma R, Stano M. Cost-effectiveness of medical and chiropractic care for acute and chronic low back pain. *J Manip Physiol Ther.* 2005;28(8): 555–563.
- Herkowitz HN, Garfin SR, Balderston RA, et al. *Rothman-Simone: The Spine,* 4th ed. Philadelphia: Saunders, 1999.
- Roh JS. Degenerative disorders of the lumbar and cervical spine. *Orthop Clin North Am.* 2005;36(3): 255–262.
- Wheeler AH. Diagnosis and management of low back pain and sciatica. *Am Fam Physician.* 1995;52(5):1333–1341.

 ## CODES

### ICD9
- 722.2 Displacement of intervertebral disc, site unspecified, without myelopathy
- 722.10 Displacement of lumbar intervertebral disc without myelopathy

S

# SEBORRHEIC DERMATITIS

*Ian Glen Ferguson*

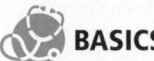 **BASICS**

## DESCRIPTION
- A common, chronic relapsing, inflammatory skin disorder, varying from mild dandruff to extensive adherent scale
- Erythematous, greasy, yellow, scaly, and crusting papulosquamous lesions
- Affects areas of high sebaceous gland concentration
- Periods of remission and exacerbation frequent in adults

## ETIOLOGY
- Multifactorial with genetic, environmental, and hormonal influences
- Strong association with *Malassezia* yeasts
- Complex physiologic response:
  - Immunologic
  - Inflammatory
  - Hyperproliferation
- Disease flares are common with physical and emotional stress or illness.
- Factors predisposing patients to develop seborrheic dermatitis and more severe or refractory disease:
  - Parkinson disease
  - Paralysis
  - AIDS
  - Mood disorders
  - CHF
  - Immunosuppression of premature infants
- Medications reported to induce or aggravate the condition include:
  - Buspirone
  - Carbamazepine
  - Chlorpromazine
  - Cimetidine
  - Gold
  - Griseofulvin
  - Haloperidol
  - Interferon-α
  - Lithium
  - Methyldopa
  - Phenothiazines
  - Phenytoin
  - Primidone
  - Psoralen
  - Stanozolol
  - Thiothixene

## DIAGNOSIS

### SIGNS AND SYMPTOMS
*Infants*
- Onset is typically at 1 mo of age and usually resolves by 12 mo.
- Flexural fold involvement may appear as diaper dermatitis:
  - Frequently develops a bacterial or fungal superinfection.
- Cradle cap:
  - Thick greasy, adherent scale on the vertex of the scalp
  - Affects up to 70% of newborns during the first 3 months of life
  - May be accompanied by inflammation or secondary infection

*Young Children*
Blepharitis:
- White scale adherent to eyelashes and eyelid margins with erythema
- Resistant to treatment and persistent
- May result in blepharoconjunctivitis

*Adolescents and Adults*
- Classic seborrheic dermatitis:
  - Minor itching with greasy, fine, dry, white scaling overlying red, inflamed skin
- Exacerbated by avoidance of washing
- Usually bilateral and symmetrical:
  - Scalp, forehead, eyebrows, eyelids
  - Areas of facial hair
  - External ear canals, posterior auricular folds
  - Nasolabial folds
  - Posterior neck
  - Presternal, naval, and body folds:
    ○ Axillary, inframammary
    ○ Groin, and anogenital
    ○ May cause areas of hypopigmentation in dark skinned individuals

### ESSENTIAL WORKUP
Diagnosis is based on clinical history and physical examination.

### DIAGNOSTIC TESTS & INTERPRETATION
*Lab*
- Potassium hydroxide preparations of skin scrapings may suggest yeast involvement.
- Fungal culture may help to exclude dermatophytosis as an alternate diagnosis.

*Imaging*
None required

*Diagnostic Procedures/Surgery*
Skin biopsy (rarely required):
- May help to exclude other diagnoses
- Consider, if the diagnosis remains unclear or the condition fails to respond to treatment

### DIFFERENTIAL DIAGNOSIS
- Atopic dermatitis:
  - Later onset in infants (usually > 3 months)
  - Characteristically affects antecubital and popliteal fossa in adults:
  - Pruritus, oozing, and weeping support the diagnosis of atopic dermatitis.
  - Family history of atopy (asthma or allergic rhinitis) favors diagnosis of atopic dermatitis.
  - Axillary involvement favors the diagnosis of seborrheic dermatitis.
- Contact dermatitis:
  - Polymorphous:
    ○ Erythema, edema, and vessicles
  - Tends to spare skin folds
  - May complicate seborrheic dermatitis as an unwanted reaction to treatment agents.

- Cutaneous candidiasis:
  - Primary or secondary infection of the skin by *Candida* fungus
  - May affect any bodyarea
  - Pruritis, erythema, mild scaling, and occasional blistering
  - Often associated with diabetes, obesity, or other illness
  - Common in infants
  - Presence of pseudohyphae on cytologic examination with potassium hydroxide does not exclude seborrheic dermatitis.
- Dermatophytosis:
  - Generally distributed asymmetrically
  - Scalp–Tinea capitis
  - Body–Tinea corporis
  - Groin–Tinea cruris
  - Can be very difficult to distinguish from seborrheic dermatitis
  - Hyphae on cytologic examination with potassium hydroxide is suggestive of tinea
- Langerhans cell histiocytosis:
  - Systemic signs such as fever and adenopathy
  - Infants affected may display scaling.
  - Reddish-brown papules or vesicles
  - Associated splenomegaly
  - Purpuric lesions
- Leiner disease:
  - Prevalent in infant females
  - Rapid onset in second to fourth month of life
  - Complement dysfunction
  - Severe generalized erythematous, and exfoliative seborrheic dermatitis
  - Severe diarrhea and failure to thrive
- Lupus:
  - Erythematous malar rash of the nose and malar eminences
  - Chronic or discoid lupus:
    ○ Discrete erythematous papules or plaques
    ○ Thick adherent scale
    ○ When removed reveals a "carpet tack" appearance
- Psoriasis:
  - Thicker plaques with silvery white scales
  - Less likely confined to scalp
- Rosacea:
  - Usually with central facial erythema or forehead involvement
- Tinea versicolor (pityriasis versicolor):
  - A chronic superficial fungal disease usually located on the upper trunk, neck, or upper arms
  - Characterized by hypopigmented or hyperpigmented, fine, scaly coalescing macules.
  - Usually asymptomatic
  - Also associated with *Malassezia* yeast
    ○ Not a dermatophyte
  - Short, thick hyphae with spores (spaghetti-and-meatball pattern) seen on cytologic examination with potassium hydroxide.

### Pediatric Considerations

Infants with seborrheic dermatitis and cradle cap may present with concurrent atopic dermatitis.

#### ALERT
Seborrheic dermatitis is one of many conditions that may cause erythroderma (generalized exfoliative dermatitis):
- Severe scaling erythematous dermatitis involving 90% or more of the body

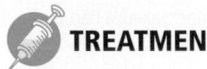 **TREATMENT**

**PRE-HOSPITAL**
None required

**INITIAL STABILIZATION/THERAPY**
None required

**ED TREATMENT/PROCEDURES**
- Seborrheic dermatitis is a chronic condition:
  - Emergent treatment is not required unless secondary infection is present.
- Patient education:
  - Early treatment when condition flares
  - Emphasize hygiene and demonstrate proper cleansing of scaly lesions.
  - Increase frequency of showering.
  - Wash all affected areas.
  - Moderate exposure to sunlight may be beneficial as UV-A and UV-B light inhibit the growth of *Malassezia* yeasts.

**MEDICATION**
- Pharmacologic options are often utilized in a multifaceted approach.
- Therapy is directed at decreasing the reservoir of lipophilic yeast and the sebum that supports its growth, thus reducing inflammation and improving hygiene.
- Severe cases may require removing scales and cornified nonviable epithelium to facilitate further treatment.
- Scales may be softened by applying mineral oil (overnight if necessary) prior to washing.
- Gentle brushing with a soft brush (toothbrush) or fine-tooth comb after washing may help remove stubborn scales.

#### First Line
- Topical antifungal preparations:
  - Ketoconazole cream or shampoo 2%
- Topical low-potency corticosteroids:
  - Effective anti-inflammatory action
  - Add if not responding to antifungal alone
  - Apply to skin and scalp
    - Hydrocortisone 1%, 2%, 2.5%

- Antidandruff shampoo:
  - Use daily to decrease scaling and itching
  - Pyrithione zinc:
    - Head and Shoulders
    - Denorex Daily Protection
  - Selenium sulfide:
    - Dandrex
    - Selsun Blue
- Keratolytics:
  - Removes cornified epithelium:
  - Salicylic acid
    - Denorex Extra Strength Protection
    - Neutrogena T/Sal
  - Salicylic acid and sulfur
    - Sebulex
- Coal tar:
  - Antibacterial
  - Antipruritic properties
  - Slows epidermal cell production
  - May soften thick scalp scales
    - Denorex Therapeutic Protection
    - DHS Tar Gel
    - Neutrogena T/Gel
    - Pentrax
- Blepharitis/blepharoconjunctivitis:
  - Daily cleansing of lashes with baby shampoo
  - Sodium sulfacetamide ophthalmic ointment or solution may be applied to the eye.

#### Second Line
- Moderate and high-potency corticosteroids:
  - Indicated only for conditions refractory to less potent agents.
  - Use only briefly.
  - Use only on torso and extremities.
  - Do not use on delicate skin, such as the face, genitals, or flexures.
    May cause cutaneous atrophy and telangiectasias
  - Frequent use may hasten recurrence of lesions and foster dependence from rebound effect.
- Moderate potency:
  - Triamcinolone acetonide
  - Fluocinolone acetonide
- High potency:
  - Clobetasol propionate
  - Betamethasone dipropionate

 **FOLLOW-UP**

**DISPOSITION**

**Admission Criteria**
Admission unlikely to be required unless severe secondary infection or erythroderma is present.

**Discharge Criteria**
Patients may be discharged with recommended medications and follow-up.

### Issues for Referral
- Refer patients to primary care physician when considering underlying illness or comorbidities.
- Consider referral to a qualified dermatologist when the diagnosis remains elusive or the condition fails to respond to therapy.

**FOLLOW-UP RECOMMENDATIONS**
- Improvement should be seen within 7–10 days but may take months to resolve completely and may recur.
- Adolescent and adult forms may persist as a chronic dermatitis.
- Provide return precautions for signs of secondary bacterial or fungal infections:
  - Fever, erythema, tenderness, or ulceration

## PEARLS AND PITFALLS
- Severe and sudden attacks of seborrheic dermatitis may be the initial presentation of an immunocompromised patient.
- Admission may be warranted for further evaluation of the underlying disease process.

## ADDITIONAL READING
- Elewski BF. Safe and effective treatment of seborrheic dermatitis. *Cutis*. 2009;83:333–338.
- Gupta AK, Madzia SE, Batra R. Etiology and management of seborrheic dermatitis. *Dermatology*. 2004;208:89–93.
- Hurwitz S. *Clinical Pediatric Dermatology*, 3rd ed. Philadelphia: Elsevier Saunders, 2006.
- Naldi L, Rebora A. Clinical practice. Seborrheic dermatitis. *N Engl J Med*. 2009;360:387–396.

 **CODES**

**ICD9**
- 690.10 Seborrheic dermatitis, unspecified
- 690.11 Seborrhea capitis
- 690.12 Seborrheic infantile dermatitis

# SEIZURE, ADULT

*Atul Gupta*
*Rebecca Smith-Coggins*

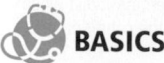

## BASICS

### DESCRIPTION
- Generalized seizures:
  - Classically tonic–clonic (grand mal)
  - Begin as myoclonic jerks followed by loss of consciousness
  - Sustained generalized skeletal muscle contractions
  - Nonconvulsive generalized seizures:
    ○ Absence seizures (petit mal); alteration in mental status without significant convulsions or motor activity
- Partial seizures:
  - Simple:
    ○ Brief sensory or motor symptoms without loss of consciousness (ie, jacksonian)
  - Complex:
    ○ Mental and psychological symptoms
    ○ Affect changes
    ○ Confusion
    ○ Automatisms
    ○ Hallucinations
    ○ Associated with impaired consciousness
  - Status epilepticus
  - Variable definitions:
    ○ Seizure lasting longer than 30 min
    ○ Recurrent seizures without return to baseline mental status between events
    ○ Some prefer a definition of a seizure lasting longer than 5–10 min
  - Life-threatening emergency with mortality rate of 10%–12%
  - Highest incidence in those <1 yr and >60 yr of age
  - At least half of patients presenting to the ED in status do not have a history of seizures.
- Alcohol withdrawal seizures ("rum fits"):
  - Peak within 24 hr of last drink
  - Rarely progress to status epilepticus
- Patients with a single seizure have a 35% risk of recurrent seizure within 5 yr.

### Pediatric Considerations
Febrile seizure is a generalized seizure occurring between 3 mo and 5 yr of age:
- Typically lasts <15 min
- Associated with a rapid rise in temperature
- Without evidence of CNS infection or other definitive cause

### ETIOLOGY
- Hypoxia
- Hypertensive encephalopathy
- Eclampsia
- Infection:
  - Meningitis
  - Abscess
  - Encephalitis
- Vascular
  - Ischemic stroke
  - Hemorrhagic stroke
  - Subdural hematoma
  - Epidural hematoma
  - Subarachnoid hemorrhage
  - Arteriovenous malformation
- Structure:
  - Primary or metastatic neoplasm
  - Degenerative disease (eg, multiple sclerosis)
  - Scar from previous trauma
- Metabolic:
  - Electrolytes
  - Hypernatremia
  - Hyponatremia
  - Hypocalcemia
  - Hypo/hyperglycemia
  - Uremia
- Toxins/Drugs:
  - Lidocaine
  - Tricyclic antidepressants
  - Salicylates
  - Isoniazid
  - Cocaine
  - Alcohol withdrawal
  - Benzodiazepine withdrawal
- Congenital abnormalities
- Idiopathic
- Trauma

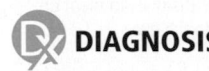

## DIAGNOSIS

### SIGNS AND SYMPTOMS
- Altered level of consciousness
- Involuntary repetitive muscle movements:
  - Tonic posturing or clonic jerking
- Seizures of abrupt onset:
  - Aura may precede a focal seizure
- Duration usually 90–120 sec:
  - Impaired memory of the event
  - Postictal state is a brief period of confusion and somnolence following a seizure.
- Evidence of recent seizure activity:
  - Confusion or somnolence
  - Acute intraoral injury
  - Urinary incontinence
  - Posterior shoulder dislocation
  - Temporary paralysis (Todd paralysis)
- Other findings may suggest etiology of seizure:
  - Fever and nuchal rigidity (CNS infection)
  - Needle tracks; stigmata of liver disease (drugs and alcohol)
  - Head trauma:
    ○ Papilledema (increased intracranial pressure)
    ○ Lateralized weakness, sensory loss, or asymmetric reflexes

### History
- History of seizures:
  - Medication compliance
- Recent illness
- Head trauma
- Headaches
- Anticoagulation therapy
- Fever
- Neck stiffness

### Physical Exam
- Complete neurologic exam:
  - Todd paralysis
- Complete secondary and tertiary survey to evaluate for any trauma secondary to seizure or potential cause for seizure

### ESSENTIAL WORKUP
- A thorough history is the most valuable part of the workup:
  - Witness accounts
  - History of prior seizures
  - Presence of acute illnesses
  - Past medical problems
  - History of substance use
- Patients with chronic seizure disorder and typical seizure pattern may need to have only serum glucose and anticonvulsant levels checked.
- New-onset seizure mandates workup:
  - Electrolytes including calcium, phosphorus
  - Head CT
  - Toxicology screen
  - Pregnancy test if woman is of childbearing age
  - Search for specific underlying cause
  - Patient's condition and resources for follow-up determine whether all these tests must be done in the ED.

### Pediatric Considerations
- A child with a first febrile seizure should receive fever workup as dictated by clinical condition.
- Frequently there is a family history of febrile seizure.
- Labs and radiographs as needed to determine source of fever
- Lumbar puncture for first febrile seizure:
  - Consider strongly if age <1 yr
  - Lethargy or poor feeding
  - Exam difficult
  - Unreliable follow-up

### DIAGNOSTIC TESTS & INTERPRETATION
#### Lab
- Serum anticonvulsant levels
- Blood alcohol level
- Toxicology screen
- CBC:
  - WBC often elevated
- Chemistry panel
- Bicarbonate often low
- Lactate may be elevated
- CSF:
  - May have transient increase in WBC to $20/\mu L$

### Imaging
- Noncontrast head CT:
  - Persistent or progressive alteration of mental status
  - Focal neurologic deficits
  - Seizure associated with trauma
- CT scan with contrast should be obtained in HIV-positive patients to rule out toxoplasmosis.
- MRI is sensitive for low-grade tumors, small vascular lesions, early inflammation, and early cerebral infarcts:
  - Consider electively in new-onset seizures

### Diagnostic Procedures/Surgery
- EEG may be arranged with neurology on an outpatient basis.
- Bedside EEG may be performed in ED if there is suspicion of nonconvulsive status epilepticus or psychogenic seizures.

## DIFFERENTIAL DIAGNOSIS
- Syncope (may also have incontinence, twitching, and jerking)
- Hyperventilation syndrome
- Psychogenic seizures
- Transient ischemic attacks
- Sleep disorders
- Delirium tremens
- Hypoglycemia

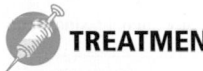 

## TREATMENT

### PRE-HOSPITAL
Anticonvulsant as per local protocol

## INITIAL STABILIZATION/THERAPY
- Airway management as indicated
- Pulse oximetry, oxygen with suction available:
  - C-spine precautions
  - Rapid sequence intubation if patient cannot protect airway or with hypoxia or major head trauma
  - IV access, rapid determination of serum glucose
    - If hypoglycemic, give IV dextrose 1 amp
  - Lorazepam or diazepam for active seizures
  - Naloxone if concern for narcotic overdose

## ED TREATMENT/PROCEDURES
- First-time seizure:
  - No structural lesions
  - Normal head CT if performed
  - Return to baseline with normal neuro exam
    - Discharge with close follow-up with PCP and/or neurologist
- First-time seizure:
  - Structural lesion on CT or MRI
    - Start antiepileptic drug (AED) in consultation with PCP and/or neurologist
  - Recurrent seizure not on AED
    - Start AED in consultation with PCP and/or neurologist
  - Recurrent seizure with subtherapeutic AED level
    - IV and/or PO load current AED
- Recurrent seizure with therapeutic AED level:
  - Need careful evaluation for cause of seizures, new lesions, etc.
    - Adjust and/or add AED in consultation with neurologist

- Seizure in a pregnant patient:
  - Evaluate as other seizure patients
  - Strongly consider eclampsia if >20 wk gestation
- Seizures related to alcohol:
  - Determine if seizure is caused by withdrawal (typically 6–48 hr after cessation of drinking) or another cause
  - Management of withdrawal seizures is benzodiazepines

### Pediatric Considerations
- Fever control with acetaminophen and ibuprofen
- Anticonvulsants not needed for febrile seizures
- Anticonvulsants should be prescribed in conjunction with neurologist.

## MEDICATION
- Acetaminophen: 10–15 mg/kg PO or PR
- Diazepam: 0.2 mg/kg IV per dose; 0.5 mg/kg PR
- Fosphenytoin: 15–20 mg/kg phenytoin equivalents (PE) at rate of 100–150 mg/min IV/IM
- Ibuprofen: 5–10 mg/kg PO
- Lorazepam: 0.1 mg/kg IV per dose (max. 10 mg)
- Naloxone: 0.4–2 mg IV/IM/SQ (peds: 0.1 mg/kg IV/IM/SQ)
- Phenobarbital: 15–20 mg/kg IV at rate of 1 mg/kg/min (plan to protect airway)
- Phenytoin: 15–20 mg/kg IV at rate of 40–50 mg/min (peds: use rate of 0.5–1.0 mg/kg/min)
- Propofol: 5–50 $\mu$g/kg/min IV, titrate to effect (plan to protect airway)
- Valproate sodium: 10–20 mg/kg

### First Line
Benzodiazepines

### Second Line
- Fosphenytoin
- Phenobarbital
- Phenytoin
- Propofol
- Valproate sodium

## FOLLOW-UP

### DISPOSITION

### Admission Criteria
- Patients with status epilepticus should be admitted to the ICU.
- Patients with seizures secondary to underlying disease (eg, meningitis, intracranial lesion) must be admitted for appropriate treatment and monitoring.
- Patients with poorly controlled repetitive seizures should be admitted for monitoring.
- Delirium tremens

### Discharge Criteria
- Patient with normal workup and appropriate neurology follow-up
- Uncomplicated seizure in patient with chronic seizure disorder
- Seizure secondary to reversible cause:
  - Hypoglycemia if blood sugar has stabilized
  - Alcohol withdrawal if baseline mental status and no further seizures
- Simple febrile seizure

### Issues for Referral
- Consider early neurology follow up
- Anticonvulsant drug level monitoring

## FOLLOW-UP RECOMMENDATIONS
No driving until seizures are under control

## PEARLS AND PITFALLS
- Most common cause of recurrent seizure is subtherapeutic anticonvulsant drug level
- Benzodiazepines are the first-line treatment to stop seizure activity
- Treat the underlying cause if identifiable

## ADDITIONAL READING
- ACEP Clinical Policies Committee Clinical Policies Subcommittee on Seizures. Clinical policy: Critical issues in the evaluation and management of adult patients presenting to the emergency department with seizures. *Ann Emerg Med*. 2004;43:605–625.
- French JA, Pedley TA. Initial management of epilepsy. *N Engl J Med*. 2008;359:166–176.
- Krumholz A, Wiebe S, Gronseth G, et al. Evaluating an apparent unprovoked first seizure in adults (an evidence based review): Report of the Quality Standards Subcommittee of the American Academy of Neurology and the American Epilepsy Society. *Neurology*. 2007;69:1996–2007.
- Wolfson AB, Hendey GW, Ling LJ, et al, eds. *Harwood Nuss' Clinical Practice of Emergency Medicine*, 5th ed. Philadelphia: Lippincott, 2010.

### See Also (Topic, Algorithm, Electronic Media Element)
- Headaches
- Hypertensive Emergencies
- Intracerebral Hemorrhage
- Preeclampsia/Eclampsia
- Seizure, febrile
- Seizure, pediatric

## CODES

### ICD9
- 345.50 Partial epilepsy, without mention of impairment of consciousness, without mention of intractable epilepsy
- 345.90 Epilepsy, unspecified, without mention of intractable epilepsy
- 780.39 Other convulsions

# SEIZURE, FEBRILE

*John P. Santamaria*

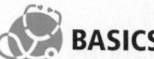 **BASICS**

## DESCRIPTION

- Occurs between 6 mo and 5 yr of age associated with fever:
  - No evidence of intracranial infection or other defined CNS primary cause
  - Average age of onset is 18–22 mo
  - Children with previous nonfebrile seizures excluded
- Most common pediatric convulsive disorder:
  - Affects 2%–4% of young children in the U.S.
- Occurs in normal children with a systemic viral illness
- High-risk children:
  - History of febrile seizure in immediate family members
  - Delayed neurologic development
  - Males
- Subgroups:
  - Simple febrile seizures:
    - Brief, self-limited lasting <10–15 min, resolve spontaneously
    - Generalized without any focal features
  - Complex febrile seizures:
    - Duration >15 min
    - Focal features
    - More than one seizure within a 24-hr period
- Risk of recurrence:
  - One third of cases
  - Early age of onset, history of febrile or afebrile seizures in first-degree relatives, and temperature <40°C during initial seizure increase the likelihood of recurrence.
- Risk of subsequent epilepsy:
  - Greatest for those with prior abnormal neurologic development, a complex first febrile seizure, or a family history of afebrile seizures
  - Only slightly greater than the general population if first febrile seizure is simple and neurologic development normal
  - Not affected by the use of prophylactic medications

## ALERT

Because this is usually self-limited, intervention must be individualized in relation to airway, breathing, and seizure management.

## ETIOLOGY

Common childhood infections:
- Upper respiratory illnesses
- Otitis media
- Roseola
- Gastrointestinal infections
- *Shigella* gastroenteritis

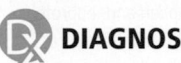 **DIAGNOSIS**

## SIGNS AND SYMPTOMS
- Fever
- Seizure may occur concurrent with recognition of the febrile illness.
- Seizure
- Generalized tonic–clonic seizure most common:
  - Tonic phase:
    - Muscular rigidity
    - Apnea and incontinence
    - Self-limited and last only a few minutes
  - Other seizure types:
    - Staring with stiffness
    - Limpness
    - Jerking movements without prior stiffening

### History
- Careful history and physical exam help confirm diagnosis and rule out other etiologies
- Symptoms/Evidence of infectious illness
- Duration of fever
- Medication exposure/toxin
- Trauma/Occult trauma
- Developmental level
- Family history of seizures
- Complete description of seizure
- Presence of meningismus, tense/bulging fontanelle, preexisting altered mental status
- Evidence of focal deficits or increased intracranial pressure

### Physical Exam
See History.

## DIAGNOSTIC TESTS & INTERPRETATION
### Lab
- Routine laboratory studies not indicated.
- Evaluate for a source of fever if serious bacterial infection is suspected:
  - WBC
  - UA
  - Blood and urine cultures
- Electrolytes and bedside glucose in infants and children with vomiting or diarrhea

### Imaging
- Chest radiograph only in patients with significant respiratory symptoms or pertinent findings on physical exam
- Head CT:
  - Indicated with traumatic injuries, focal neurologic findings, or inability to exclude elevated intracranial pressure
- Lumbar puncture:
  - Not routinely indicated
  - Indications 12–18 mo of age:
    - History or irritability, decreased feeding, lethargy
    - Physical signs of meningitis
    - Complex seizure
    - Prolonged postictal state
    - Antibiotics altering presentation
    - Abnormal mentation after postictal state
  - Indications >18 mo old:
    - Signs/Symptoms of CNS infection present
- EEG:
  - Not helpful in the initial evaluation of febrile seizure
  - May be indicated if developmental delay, underlying neurologic abnormality, or focal seizure
  - Does not help predict recurrences or risk for later epilepsy
- Anticonvulsant levels
- Toxicology studies of blood and urine if history and physical exam suggestive

## DIFFERENTIAL DIAGNOSIS
- Febrile delirium
- Febrile shivering with pallor and perioral cyanosis
- Breath-holding spell during febrile event
- Acute life-threatening event
- Other causes of seizure:
  - Afebrile seizure occurring during febrile event
  - Sudden discontinuance of anticonvulsants
  - Infection:
    - Meningitis/Encephalitis
    - Acute gastroenteritis, often with dehydration
  - Head trauma
  - Toxicologic:
    - Anticholinergics
    - Sympathomimetics
    - Other
  - Hypoxia
  - Metabolic disease
  - Intracranial masses
  - CNS vascular lesions

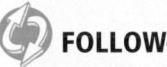 **TREATMENT**

### PRE-HOSPITAL
- Protect the airway
- Oxygen
- Support breathing as needed
- Cautions:
  - Keep child from incurring injury while actively convulsing.
  - Respiratory insufficiency and apnea occur secondary to overaggressive treatment with benzodiazepines.
  - Simple febrile seizures are self-limited and generally require no anticonvulsant therapy or ventilatory support.

### INITIAL STABILIZATION/THERAPY
- Support the airway and breathing.
- Benzodiazepines rarely needed:
  - Prolonged seizures or compromised patients
  - Lorazepam, diazepam, or midazolam
  - Rectal diazepam or nasal midazolam may be easily administered with good efficacy.

### ED TREATMENT/PROCEDURES
- Rarely is pharmacologic intervention required; usually self-limited.
- Seizures refractory to benzodiazepines:
  - Phenytoin or fosphenytoin
  - Phenobarbital
  - Work up to exclude other etiologies
- Administer antipyretics acutely and routinely for at least the next 24 hr:
  - Acetaminophen or ibuprofen (may use both)
- Appropriate antibiotic treatment for specific bacterial disease if identified

### MEDICATION
- Acetaminophen: 15 mg/kg PO, PR
- Diazepam: 0.2 mg/kg IV (max 10 mg); 0.2–0.5 mg/kg PR (max 20 mg)
- Fosphenytoin: 20 mg/kg IV over 20 min
- Ibuprofen: 10 mg/kg PO
- Lorazepam: 0.1 mg/kg IV (max 5 mg)
- Midazolam: 0.1 mg/kg IV, 0.2 mg/kg buccal/IN/IM (max 7.5 mg)
- Phenobarbital: 20 mg/kg IV over 20 min or IM
- Phenytoin: 20 mg/kg IV over 30–45 min

 **FOLLOW-UP**

### DISPOSITION
#### Admission Criteria
- Recurrent or prolonged seizures
- Fever with source not appropriately treated as outpatient

#### Discharge Criteria
- Simple febrile seizures:
  - Normal neurologic examination
  - Source of fever is appropriately treated as outpatient
- Reassurance to parents

### FOLLOW-UP RECOMMENDATIONS
Schedule follow-up with primary care physician.

## PEARLS AND PITFALLS
- Although aggressive treatment of fever with antipyretics is often recommended, there is no evidence that this reduces seizure recurrence.
- Oral diazepam during febrile illness may reduce risk of recurrence; prophylactic anticonvulsants with other anticonvulsants rarely indicated—such treatment is controversial and to be considered only after extensive discussion.

### ADDITIONAL READING
- American Academy of Pediatrics, Steering Committee on Quality Improvement and Management Subcommittee on Febrile Seizures. Febrile seizures: Clinical practice guideline for the long-term management of the child with simple febrile seizures. *Pediatrics.* 2008;121(6): 1281–1286.
- Barata I. Pediatric seizures. *Crit Decisions Emerg Med.* 2005;19(6):1–21.
- Blumstein M, Friedman M. Childhood seizures. *Emerg Med Clin North Am.* 2007;25:061–1086.
- Hirabayashi Y, Okumura A, Kondo T, et al. Efficacy of a diazepam suppository at preventing febrile seizure recurrence during a single febrile seizure. *Brain Dev.* 2009;31:414–418.
- Strengell T, Uhari M, Tarkka R. Antipyretic agents for preventing recurrences of febrile seizures. *Arch Pediatr Adolesc Med.* 2009;63(9):799–804.

### See Also (Topic, Algorithm, Electronic Media Element)
Anticholinergic Poisoning; Seizures, Pediatric

**CODES**

#### ICD9
- 780.31 Febrile convulsions (simple), unspecified
- 780.32 Complex febrile convulsions

# SEIZURE, PEDIATRIC

*John P. Santamaria*

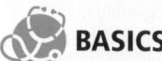

## BASICS

### DESCRIPTION
Sudden, abnormal discharges of neurons resulting in a change in behavior or function

### ETIOLOGY
- Febrile seizures
- Infection
- Idiopathic
- Trauma
- Toxicologic:
  - Ingestion
  - Drug action
  - Drug withdrawal
- Metabolic:
  - Hypoglycemia
  - Hypocalcemia
  - Hypo/Hypernatremia
  - Inborn errors of metabolism
- Perinatal hypoxia
- Intracranial hemorrhage
- CNS structural anomaly or malformation
- Degenerative disease

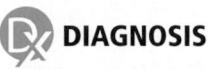

## DIAGNOSIS

### SIGNS AND SYMPTOMS
#### Neonates
- Subtle abnormal repetitive motor activity:
  - Facial movements
  - Eye deviations
  - Eyelid fluttering
  - Lip smacking/sucking
- Respiratory alterations
- Apnea
- Seizure activity:
  - Focal or generalized tonic seizures
  - Focal or multifocal clonic seizure
  - Myoclonic movements
- Generalized problems (metabolic, infection, etc.) may present with focal seizures.

#### Older Infants and Children
- Generalized seizures:
  - Tonic–clonic
  - Tonic
  - Clonic
  - Myoclonic
  - Atonic ("drop")
  - Absence
- Partial or focal seizures:
  - Simple:
    - Consciousness maintained
  - Simple partial seizures:
    - Motor, sensory, and/or cognitive symptoms
    - Motor activity focal: one part or side
    - Paresthesias, metallic tastes, and visual or auditory hallucinations

- Complex:
  - Consciousness impaired
  - Complex partial seizure
- Simple partial seizure progresses with impaired consciousness:
  - Aura precedes altered consciousness; auditory, olfactory, or visual hallucination
  - May generalize
- Status epilepticus:
  - Generalized is most common
  - Sustained partial seizures
  - Absence seizures
  - Persistent confusion; postictal period

### History
- Determine whether seizures are febrile or afebrile
- Determine type of seizure:
  - Partial versus generalized
  - Presence of eye findings, aura, movements, cyanosis
  - Duration
  - State of consciousness, postictal state
  - Predisposing conditions/history/family history (syndromes with a genetic component)

### Physical Exam
- Vital signs, including temperature
- Careful neurologic exam, including state of consciousness
- Eye, including fundoscopic exam
- Skin examination to identify neruocutaneous diseases such as tuberous sclerosis

### DIAGNOSTIC TESTS & INTERPRETATION
#### Lab
- Bedside glucose test
- Performed in young infants and those in status epilepticus
- Select studies in other children reflecting history and physical examination:
  - Electrolytes
  - Blood urea nitrogen
  - Creatinine
  - Glucose
  - Calcium
  - Magnesium
  - CBC
  - Toxicology screen
- Patients on anticonvulsant therapy:
  - Drug levels
- Febrile seizure:
  - Laboratory studies to evaluate for a serious underlying bacterial infection if suspected

#### Imaging
- Head CT:
  - Focal seizure
  - New focal neurologic abnormality
  - Suspected intracranial hemorrhage or mass lesion
  - New-onset status epilepticus without identifiable cause
  - Not routinely indicated for first afebrile seizure
- Lumbar puncture:
  - Suspicion of meningitis or encephalitis
  - CT first if suspect increased intracranial pressure
- MRI:
  - Rarely urgently indicated for seizures
- EEG:
  - Generally indicated in children with an afebrile seizure as a predictor of risk of recurrence and classify the seizure type/epilepsy syndrome
  - Postictal slowing seen within 24–48 hr of a seizure and may be transient; delay EEG if possible
  - Rarely helpful in the acute setting

### DIFFERENTIAL DIAGNOSIS
- Neonates:
  - Apnea due to other causes
  - Jitters or tremors
  - Gastroesophageal reflux
- Infants and toddlers:
  - Breath-holding spells
  - Night terrors
- Children and adolescents:
  - Migraine headache
  - Syncope
  - Tics
  - Pseudoseizures
  - Hysteria

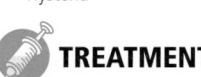

## TREATMENT

### PRE-HOSPITAL
Cautions:
- Many conditions may be mistaken for seizures (see Differential Diagnosis, below).
- Immobilize cervical spine if trauma suspected.
- Check fingerstick glucose or administer dextrose as appropriate.

## INITIAL STABILIZATION/THERAPY
- ABC support if actively seizing
- Airway:
  - Oxygen/Monitor pulse oximetry.
  - Nasopharyngeal airway preferred over oral airway
  - Bag valve–mask support if hypoventilating or persistently hypoxic
  - Intubation if seizures are refractory and bag valve–mask support is unsuccessful
- IV access:
  - If hypoglycemic, give dextrose
- Maintain spine precautions if trauma suspected

### ALERT
Airway and breathing must be stabilized concurrent with management of ongoing seizures if present.

## ED TREATMENT/PROCEDURES
### Status Epilepticus
- Benzodiazepine:
  - Lorazepam is preferred due to its longer duration of action.
  - Valium is acceptable.
  - If IV access is not available:
    o Diazepam may be given per rectum; use a TB syringe or 14-gauge Angiocath or feeding tube for IV solution or preformed rectal gel suppository
    o Midazolam intranasal/buccal/IM also effective
- Phenytoin:
  - If benzodiazepines fail
  - For longer-term control
  - Fosphenytoin easier to administer
- Phenobarbital:
  - Use if benzodiazepines and phenytoin fail to break the seizure.
  - Risk of respiratory depression greatly increases if a benzodiazepine has also been given.
- Alternative therapies in the event of refractory status epilepticus
- Consultation appropriate:
  - Paraldehyde (per rectum)
  - Barbiturate coma:
    o Barbiturate (pentobarbital) coma requires intubation and EEG monitoring to be sure the seizure is suppressed
    o Associated hypotension
  - General anesthesia:
    o A final resort
    o Continuous EEG is needed to be sure the seizure is abolished.

- Neonates:
  - Penobarbital is acceptable first-line therapy.
  - Preferred maintenance drug

### ALERT
Note: Aggregate response to second- and third-line agents is <10%.

## MEDICATION
- $D_{10}$: 5 mL/kg IV for neonates
- $D_{25}$: 2 mL/kg IV for children
- Diazepam: 0.2mg/kg IV (max 10 mg); 0.2–0.5 mg/kg PR (max 20 mg)
- Fosphenytoin: 20 mg/kg IV over 20 minutes
- Lorazepam: 0.1 mg/kg IV (max 5 mg)
- Midazolam: 0.1 mg/kg IV, 0.2 mg/kg buccal/IN/IM (max 7.5 mg)
- Pentobarbital: 10–15 mg/kg IV over 1–2 hr; maintenance: 1–3 mg/kg/h IV
- Penobarbital: 20 mg/kg IV over 20 min
- Phenytoin: 20 mg/kg IV slowly over 30–45 min

 **FOLLOW-UP**

## DISPOSITION
### Admission Criteria
- ICU:
  - Active status epilepticus, intubated, or persistent mental status changes
  - Repetitive seizures in narrow time frame
- Inpatient unit:
  - Status epilepticus resolved in the ED
  - Underlying cause of seizure unresolved, uncontrolled, or poorly understood
  - Intracranial hemorrhage
  - Mass lesion
  - Meningitis/Encephalitis
    Drug
  - Toxin ingestions

### Discharge Criteria
- The child is alert with normal mental status and neurologic exam.
- No evidence of an underlying cause requiring hospitalization
- Reliable parent or caregiver
- Home telephone

### Issues for Referral
Unresponsive or repetitive seizures

## FOLLOW-UP RECOMMENDATIONS
- Provide seizure precautions and aftercare instructions
- Follow-up with PCP or pediatric neurologist

## PEARLS AND PITFALLS
- Phenobarbital is the preferred treatment for theophylline-induced seizures, poor response to benzodiazepines and phenytoin
- Consider intranasal or buccal midazolam if no IV access

## ADDITIONAL READING
- Abend N, Huh J, Helfaer M, Dlugos D, Anticonvulsant medication in the pediatric emergency room and intensive care unit. *Pediatr Emerg Care*. 2008;24(10):705–718.
- Barata I, Pediatric seizures. *Crit Decisions Emerg Med*. 2005;19:1–10.
- Blumstein M, Friedman M. Childhood seizures. *Emerg Med Clin North Am*. 2007;25:1061–1086.
- Yoshikawa, H, First-line therapy for theophylline-associated seizures. *Acta Neurol Scand*. 2007;115:57–61.

### See Also (Topic, Algorithm, Electronic Media Element)
Seizures, Febrile

 **CODES**

### ICD9
- 345.90 Epilepsy, unspecified, without mention of intractable epilepsy
- 780.31 Febrile convulsions (simple), unspecified
- 780.39 Other convulsions

S

# SEPSIS

*Richard E. Wolfe*
*Nathan Shapiro*

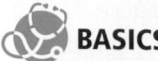 **BASICS**

## DESCRIPTION

- Presence of an infection with an associated systemic inflammatory response
- Derived from the ancient Greek word for rotten flesh and putrefaction
- The Systemic Inflammatory Response Syndrome (SIRS) is comprised of 4 criteria:
  - Temperature >38°C or <36°C
  - Heart rate >90 bpm
  - Respiratory rate >20/min or $PaCO_2$ <32 mm Hg
  - WBC >12,000/mm$^3$, <4,000/mm$^3$, or >10% band forms
- Sepsis = Infection with ≥2 SIRS criteria:
  - During sepsis, release of chemical messengers by the inflammatory response causes dysfunction.
  - Macrocirculatory failure through decreased cardiac output or decreased perfusion pressure (often due to decreased peripheral resistance)
  - Microcirculatory failure through impaired vascular autoregulatory mechanisms and functional shunting of oxygen
  - Cytopathic hypoxia and mitochondrial dysfunction
- Hemodynamic changes result from the inflammatory response:
  - Elevated cardiac output in response to vasodilatation
  - Later myocardial depression:
    ○ Due to injury at the cellular level or mediators acting on the heart
- Multiple organ dysfunction syndrome (MODS):
  - Adult respiratory distress syndrome (ARDS)
  - Acute tubular necrosis and kidney failure
  - Hepatic injury and failure
  - Disseminated intravascular coagulation
- Sepsis should be viewed as a continuum of severity from a proinflammatory response to organ dysfunction and tissue hypoperfusion:
  - Severe sepsis: Sepsis with at least 1 of the following organ dysfunctions:
    ○ Acidosis
    ○ Renal dysfunction
    ○ Acute change in mental status
    ○ Pulmonary dysfunction
    ○ Hypotension
    ○ Thrombocytopenia or coagulopathy
    ○ Liver dysfunction
  - Septic shock: Sepsis-induced hypotension despite fluid resuscitation:
    ○ Systolic blood pressure (BP) <90 mm Hg or reduction of >40 mm Hg from baseline
- Sepsis is the 10th leading cause of death in the U.S.:
  - In-hospital mortality for septic shock is ~30%

## ETIOLOGY

- Gram-negative bacteria most common:
  - *Escherichia coli*
  - *Pseudomonas aeruginosa*
  - Rickettsiae
  - *Legionella* spp.

- Gram-positive bacteria:
  - *Enterococcus* spp.
  - *Staphylococcus aureus*
  - *Streptococcus pneumoniae*
- Fungi (*Candida* species)
- Viruses

### Pediatric Considerations
- Children with a minor infection may have many of the findings of SIRS.
- Major causes of pediatric bacterial sepsis:
  - *Neisseria* meningitis
  - Streptococcal pneumonia
  - *Haemophilus influenzae*

 **DIAGNOSIS**

## SIGNS AND SYMPTOMS
### History
- Question for signs of infection and a systemic inflammatory response:
  - Fever
  - Dyspnea
  - Altered mental status:
    ○ Change in mental status
    ○ Confusion
    ○ Delirium
  - Nausea and vomiting
- Look for a source of the infection:
  - Cough, shortness of breath
  - Abdominal pain
  - Diarrhea
  - Dysuria/frequency
- Past history should highlight risk factors and immunosuppressive states:
  - Underlying terminal illness
  - Recent chemotherapy
  - Malignancy
  - History of a splenectomy
  - HIV
  - Diabetes
  - Nursing home resident

### Physical Exam
- An elevated respiratory rate is an early warning sign of sepsis and occurs without underlying pulmonary pathology or acidosis.
- Blood pressure is often normal early in sepsis.
- Hypotension when septic shock occurs
- Extremities are often warmed and flushed despite hypotension.
- Look for a source of the infection:
  - Abdominal exam:
    ○ Diffuse tenderness suggests peritonitis
    ○ Localized to right upper quadrant (liver or gallbladder)
    ○ Right lower quadrant (appendicitis with or without abscess)
    ○ Suprapubic area or lower quadrants (urinary tract or pelvic source or diverticulitis)
    ○ Flank pain suggests pyelonephritis or retroperitoneal abscess

  - Rectal exam to assess for an abscess
  - Chest exam for signs of pneumonia
  - Any rash is important:
    ○ Localized erythema with lymphangitis (streptococcal or staphylococcal cellulitis)
    ○ Rash involving palms of hands and soles of feet (rickettsial infection)
    ○ Petechiae scattered on the torso and extremities (meningococcemia)
    ○ Ecthyma gangrenosum (pseudomonas septicemia)
    ○ Round, indurated, painless lesion with surrounding erythema and central necrotic black eschar
  - Decubitus ulcers
  - Indwelling catheter:
    ○ Surrounding skin erythematous with or without purulent drainage
- CNS infections:
  - Coma
  - Neck stiffness (meningitis)

## ESSENTIAL WORKUP
- Serum lactate should be done early in the course to assess severity and need for goal-directed therapy.
- Blood cultures prior to antibiotics:
  - Serial lactate levels may be used to assess the progression of the disease and the effect of therapy.
- Broad spectrum of laboratory tests and imaging studies to locate the source of the infection and assess for MOF.
- Placement of a central line with an $ScvO_2$ catheter may be used to adjust therapy.

## DIAGNOSTIC TESTS & INTERPRETATION
### Lab
- Serum lactate:
  - >4 mmol/L defines severe sepsis
- CBC with differential:
  - Leukocytosis is insensitive and nonspecific
  - Neutrophil count <500 cells/mm$^3$ should prompt isolation and empiric IV antibiotics in chemotherapy patients.
  - >5% bands on a peripheral smear is an imperfect indicator of infection.
  - Hematocrit:
    ○ Patients should be maintained with a hematocrit >30% and hemoglobin >10 g/dL.
  - Platelets:
    ○ May be elevated in the presence of infection or sepsis-induced volume depletion
    ○ Low platelet count is a significant predictor of bacteremia and death.
- Electrolytes, BUN, creatinine, glucose:
- Ca, Mg, pH
- C-reactive protein
- Cortisol level
- INR/prothrombin time/partial thromboplastin time
- Liver function tests
- ABG:
  - Mixed acid–base abnormalities: Respiratory alkalosis with metabolic acidosis

- Blood cultures:
  - From 2 different sites
  - 1 may be drawn through an indwelling central line (ie, Broviac).
- Urine analysis and culture

### Imaging
- CXR:
  - Determine whether pneumonia is the infectious source.
  - Fluffy, bilateral infiltrates may indicate that ARDS is already present.
  - Free air under the diaphragm indicates the source of the infection in intraperitoneal and a surgical intervention is mandatory.
- Soft-tissue plain films:
  - Indicated if extremity erythema or severe pain
  - Air in the soft tissues associated with necrotizing or gas-forming infection
- Imaging studies to locate the source of the infection based on the presentation:
  - CT scan of the abdomen and pelvis
  - Abdominal US for gallbladder disease
  - Transesophageal ECG
  - MRI

### Diagnostic Procedures/Surgery
- Lumbar puncture:
  - For meningeal signs or altered mental status
- Central venous access:
  - Central venous pressure (CVP) and ongoing measurement of central venous oximetry.

### DIFFERENTIAL DIAGNOSIS
- Pancreatitis
- Trauma
- Toxic shock syndrome
- Anaphylaxis
- Adrenal insufficiency
- Drug or toxin reactions
- Heavy metal poisoning
- Hepatic insufficiency
- Neurogenic shock

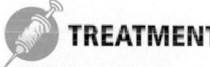

## TREATMENT

### PRE-HOSPITAL
Aggressive fluid resuscitation for hypotension

### INITIAL STABILIZATION/THERAPY
- ABCs
- Supplemental oxygen to maintain $PaO_2$ >60 mm Hg
- Intubation and mechanical ventilation if shock or hypoxia are present
- Administer 0.9% NS IV.

### ED TREATMENT/PROCEDURES
- Early goal directed therapy:
  - 500 cc boluses of 0.9% saline up to 1–2 L empirically
  - Place central line.
  - Continue 500 cc saline boluses until CVP >8 cm $H_2O$.
  - If the mean arterial pressure <65 mm Hg and CVP >8, then initiate pressors:
    ○ Dopamine or norepinephrine to raise blood pressure
    ○ Norepinephrine is preferred if tachycardia or dysrhythmias are present.

○ Epinephrine for cases where shock is refractory to other pressors
○ If the $ScvO_2$ <70 and HCT <30, transfuse 2 units PRBCs.
○ If $ScvO_2$ >70 and HCT >30 and MAP > 60, then add dobutamine.
- Administer antibiotics early, based on the most likely organisms or site of infection.
- If source identified, or highly suspected, treat the most likely organisms:
  - Pulmonary source:
    ○ 2nd- or 3rd-generation cephalosporin and gentamicin, and possibly erythromycin
  - Intra-abdominal source:
    ○ Ampicillin and metronidazole and gentamicin
    ○ Cefoxitin and gentamicin
  - Urinary tract source:
    ○ Ampicillin or piperacillin and gentamicin or levofloxacin

### Pediatric Considerations
- Antibiotic therapy based on age:
  - <3 mo (2 drugs): Ampicillin and gentamicin or cefotaxime (50–180 mg/kg/d div. q4–6h)
  - ≥3 mo: Cefotaxime or ceftriaxone (50–100 mg/kg/d div. q12–24h)
- Initiate vasopressors after no response to 60 mL/kg IV fluid.
- Avoid hyponatremia and hypoglycemia.
- Dexamethasone for children with bacterial meningitis:
  - 0.15 mg/kg q6h for 4 days

### MEDICATION
- Ampicillin: 1–2 g (peds: 50–200 mg/kg/24 h) IV q4–6h
- Cefoxitin: 1–2 g (peds: 100–160 mg/kg/24 h) IV q6–8h
- Ceftazidime: 1–2 g (peds: 100–150 mg/kg/24 h) IV q8–12h
- Dopamine: 1–5 μg/kg/min (renal dose); 5–10 μg/kg/min (pressor dose)
- Gentamicin: 1–1.5 mg/kg (peds: 2–2.5 mg/kg q8h) IV q8h
- Metronidazole: Load with 1 g (peds: 15 mg/kg) IV, then 500 mg (peds: 7.5 mg/kg q6h)
- Nafcillin: 1–2 g IV q4h (peds: 50 mg/kg/24 h div. q4–6h)
- Norepinephrine: 2–8 μg/min
- Piperacillin: 3–4 g IV q4–6h
- Vancomycin: 500 mg (peds: 10 mg/kg) IV q6h

### First Line
- Normal immune function without an identifiable source:
  - 2nd- or 3rd-generation cephalosporin and gentamicin
  - Nafcillin and gentamicin
  - Add vancomycin if there is a history of methicillin-resistant *S. aureus,* or the patient resides in a nursing facility, or there is a history of recent hospitalizations.

### Second Line
Immunocompromised host without an identifiable source:
- Piperacillin and gentamicin
- Ceftazidime and either nafcillin or vancomycin and gentamicin

 FOLLOW-UP

### DISPOSITION
#### Admission Criteria
Sepsis almost always requires inpatient care.

#### Discharge Criteria
Patients with less severe infections (eg, strep pharyngitis) meeting the criteria for sepsis with stabilized vital signs

#### Issues for Referral
Sepsis with toxicity, septicemia, or septic shock requires admission, generally to an ICU.

## PEARLS AND PITFALLS
- Start antibiotics as soon as sepsis is suspected.
- Failure to recognize multiorgan failure and initiate aggressive fluid resuscitation in the initial presentation of sepsis is a pitfall.

## ADDITIONAL READING
- Barochia AV, Cui X, Vitberg D, et al. Bundled care for septic shock: An analysis of clinical trials. *Crit Care Med.* 2010;38:668–678.
- Martin JB, Wheeler AP. Approach to the patient with sepsis. *Clin Chest Med.* 2009;30:1–16.
- Pope JV, Jones AE, Gaieski DF, et al. Multicenter study of central venous oxygen saturation (ScvO2) as a predictor of mortality in patients with sepsis. *Annals Emerg Med.* 2010;55(1):40–46.
- Rivers E, Nguyen B, Havstad S, et al. Early goal-directed therapy in the treatment of severe sepsis and septic shock. *N Engl J Med.* 2001;345(19):1368–1377.
- Shapiro NI, Wolfe RE, Moore RB, et al. Mortality in Emergency Department Sepsis (MEDS) score: A prospectively derived and validated clinical prediction rule. *Crit Care Med.* 2003;31(3):670–676.

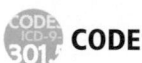 CODES

### ICD9
- 038.9 Unspecified septicemia
- 995.91 Sepsis
- 995.92 Severe sepsis

# SERUM SICKNESS

*Kelly Corrigan*

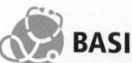 **BASICS**

## DESCRIPTION
- Type III hypersensitivity reaction
- When a foreign protein or drug (the antigen) is injected, the body's immune system responds by forming antibodies to the foreign material and subsequently forms complexes composed of the antigen, antibody, and complement.
- These complexes then deposit in tissue, inciting an inflammatory response:
  – C3a and C5a act as anaphylatoxins.
  – C5a is strongly chemotactic for neutrophils.
  – The neutrophils then infiltrate the vessel wall at the site of the immune complex deposition and release enzymes, such as collagenase and elastase, that damage vessel walls.
- Typically, symptoms arise 6–21 days after the primary exposure to the antigen.
- Symptoms can start 1–4 days after exposure if there has been an initial immunizing exposure.
- Symptoms typically last 1–2 wk before spontaneously resolving.

## ETIOLOGY
- Serum sickness:
  – Vaccines containing foreign protein or serum such as pneumococcal vaccine or rabies.
  – Antivenom and tetanus inoculations made with horse protein
- Serum sickness–like reaction:
  – Caused by nonprotein drugs, mostly antibiotics:
    ○ Penicillins, amoxicillin
    ○ Cephalosporins (ie, Cefaclor)
    ○ Sulfonamides (ie, Bactrim)
    ○ Thiazides
    ○ Gold
    ○ Thiouracils
    ○ Hydantoins
    ○ Phenylbutazone
    ○ Aspirin
    ○ Streptomycin

## DIAGNOSIS

### SIGNS AND SYMPTOMS
Classic presentation is fever, rash, arthralgias, and lymphadenopathy.

### History
- Fever
- Rash (urticarial, morbilliform, scarlantiform)
- Arthralgias
- Myalgias
- Lymphadenopathy
- Facial and neck edema
- Chest pain
- Shortness of breath

### Physical Exam
- Fever
- Rash
- Lymphadenopathy
- Arthritis
- Edema
- Splenomegaly
- Peripheral neuritis
- Myocarditis/pericarditis
- Anaphylaxis

## ESSENTIAL WORKUP
- History of a possible offending agent and time course of 6–21 days before onset of symptoms
- Physical exam revealing rash as well as joint, muscular, cardiac, neurologic, or renal insult from vasculitic type process

## DIAGNOSTIC TESTS & INTERPRETATION
### Lab
- Decreased complement levels
- CBC, possible eosinophilia
- Elevated ESR
- Hypergammaglobulinemia
- Urine with proteinuria or hematuria

### Imaging
Consider CXR.

### Diagnostic Procedures/Surgery
Biopsy is the only means of definitive diagnosis.

## DIFFERENTIAL DIAGNOSIS
- Vasculitides (eg, polyarteritis nodosa, Goodpasture, Wegener)
- Rashes (eg, erythema multiforme, toxic epidermal necrolysis)
- Immunologic (eg, systematic lupus erythematosus, polymyositis, anaphylaxis)
- Infectious (eg, tickborne disease, Rocky Mountain spotted fever, mononucleosis)

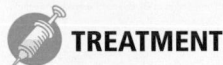 TREATMENT

**PRE-HOSPITAL**
- ABC stabilization
- Anaphylaxis treatment as indicated.

**INITIAL STABILIZATION/THERAPY**
ABCs if a severe systemic reaction is present

**ED TREATMENT/PROCEDURES**
- Symptomatic relief until the disease spontaneously resolves in 1–13 wk
- Antihistamines
- Antipyretics
- NSAIDs
- Prednisone is controversial

**MEDICATION**
- Acetaminophen: 325–650 mg PO/PR (peds: 10–15 mg/kg) q4–6h
- Diphenhydramine: 50–100 mg (peds: 5 mg/kg/d, divided) q6–8h
- Ibuprofen: 200–800 mg PO (peds >6 mo: 5–10 mg/kg) q6–8h
- Prednisone: 0.052 mg/kg/day PO (peds: 12 mg/kg/day), 2-wk taper

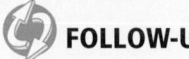 FOLLOW-UP

**DISPOSITION**
*Admission Criteria*
- Involvement of the airway
- Relapse of symptoms and signs after initial steroids
- Immunosuppression
- Concomitant serious disease
- Sociologic considerations

*Discharge Criteria*
Stable; most cases are self-limiting.

*Issues for Referral*
Skin testing with heterologous antisera is performed routinely to avoid anaphylaxis to future administration of heterologous serum.

**FOLLOW-UP RECOMMENDATIONS**
Primary care follow-up

## PEARLS AND PITFALLS

- Identification and cessation of the offending antigen is crucial in the treatment of serum sickness.
- Significant morbidity comes from a failure to diagnose when the serum sickness is not considered on the differential.

## ADDITIONAL READING

- Chen S. Serum sickness (emergency medicine). Emedicine. Emedicine.medscape.com/article/756444-overview.
- Gamarra RM, et al. Serum sickness-like reactions in patients receiving IV Infliximab. *J Emerg Med*. 1999;34:615–619.
- Piessens WF. Systemic immune complex disease. In: Ruddy S, ed. *Kelley's Textbook of Rheumatology*, 6th ed. Philadelphia: Saunders, 2001.
- Pilettey C, et al. Serum sickness-like syndrome after omalizumab therapy fro asthma. *J Allergy Clin Immunol*. 2007;120(4):972–793.

**See Also (Topic, Algorithm, Electronic Media Element)**
- Anaphylaxis
- Vasculitis

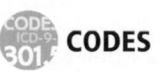 CODES

**ICD9**
999.5 Other serum reaction, not elsewhere classified

S

# SEXUAL ASSAULT
*Lauren M. Smith*

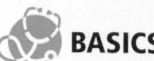 **BASICS**

## DESCRIPTION
Specific legal definition varies from state to state:
- Nonconsensual completed or attempted penetration between the penis and vulva or penis and anus
- Nonconsensual contact between the mouth and the penis, vulva, or anus
- Nonconsensual penetration of the anal or genital opening with a finger, hand, or object
- Nonconsensual intentional touching, directly or through clothing, of the genitalia, vagina, anus, groin, inner thigh, or buttocks

## ETIOLOGY
- 72% of female rape victims are raped by someone they know.
- Men are primarily raped and physically assaulted by strangers and acquaintances, not intimate partners.
- Nearly 25% of women and 7% of men have been raped or sexually assaulted by a current or former partner.
- ~54% of rapes of women occur before the age of 18.

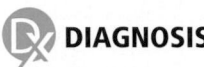 **DIAGNOSIS**

## SIGNS AND SYMPTOMS
- Victims might not disclose assault:
  - Most will reveal history only in response to direct questions.
- Tachycardia or pounding heart beat
- Headaches
- Nausea
- Back pain
- Skin problems
- Menstrual symptoms
- Sudden weight change
- Sleeping disorders
- Abdominal pain
- Trouble breathing
- Associated injuries:
  - Of those with injuries, 70% report no injury at presentation.
  - Lacerations of perineum
  - Vulvar trauma
  - Laceration of vaginal wall (more common in younger patients, near introitus)
  - Multiple contusions
  - Abrasions
  - Human bite
  - Lacerations or puncture wound to extremity
  - Burns
  - Depressed skull fracture

### Pediatric Considerations
- Must follow state laws regarding child abuse
- Most of the physical exams in child sexual abuse cases are normal
- In prepubertal children, an exam will most likely not require a speculum exam. If a speculum exam is warranted, it should be done under sedation; consider involving a sexual assault examiner.
- In interviewing the child, ask open-ended questions.
- Use toys and dolls to have the child explain what happened.
- Early psychiatric intervention is necessary.

### History
- Obtain complete history even if patient does not wish to file charges, including:
  - Time and place of assault
  - Physical description of assailants
  - Number of assailants
  - Types of penetration: vaginal, oral, rectal
  - Assailant ejaculation: ask if assailant used condom
  - Any bodily fluid exchange
  - Use of force, weapons, restraints, drugs, or alcohol
  - Ask if victim has memory loss or lost consciousness
  - Victim's activity since assault:
    ○ Changed clothes
    ○ Douched
    ○ Bathed
    ○ Urinated
    ○ Defecated
    ○ Ate
    ○ Tampon use
  - Full gynecologic history
  - Last voluntary intercourse
  - Sperm may be mobile up to 5 days in cervix and 12 hr in vagina
- Address all physical complaints.

### Physical Exam
- Use local evidence kit even if victim unsure of reporting to police.
- Female chaperone required if male physician
- If clothes soiled, photograph prior to undressing, with patient's consent.
- Note emotional state of victim.
- Note general appearance of clothes:
  - Staining
  - Tears
  - Mud
  - Leaves
  - Wood lamp for seminal stains
  - Have patient disrobe while standing on sheet and place all clothes in paper bag.

- Plastic causes mold and increases bacterial counts.
- Only the patient should handle the clothing.
- Arrange for change of clothes.
- Complete physical should be done with emphasis on:
  - Abrasions
  - Lacerations
  - Bites
  - Scratches
  - Foreign bodies
  - Ecchymosis
  - Dried semen on skin
- Forensic collection:
  - Fingernail scrapings
  - Scalp or pubic hair samples
  - If oral penetration, swab between teeth for acid phosphatase (assay for semen) and sperm.
  - Throat culture for *Gonococcus* and *Chlamydia* if oral sex
- Gynecologic exam:
  - Explain all steps and allow patient to pace exam.
  - Comb and collect pubic hair per local protocol.
  - Lubricate speculum with water (not lubricant).
  - Look for genital trauma even in asymptomatic patients.
  - May use toluidine blue to identify small pelvic lacerations from traumatic intercourse:
    ○ Best applied to vaginal mucosa at introitus
  - Special attention to hymen as one of most common places for trauma
  - Lacerations to vaginal wall near introitus more common in younger patients
  - Aspirate secretions pooled in posterior fornix and place in sterile container to be examined for sperm and acid phosphates:
    ○ If no secretions in posterior fornix, wipe with cotton tip.
    ○ Swab and microscopically examine for sperm and acid phosphates.
  - Swab for *Gonococcus* and *Chlamydia*:
    ○ Controversial; evidence can be used by defense to show promiscuity.
  - Colposcope allows visualization of small lesions and enables photography of findings.
  - Rectal exam and cultures for *Gonococcus* and *Chlamydia* if there was penetration or attempted penetration

## ESSENTIAL WORKUP
- Obtain written consent prior to any exam, test, or treatment.
- Allow patient to pause and proceed at comfortable pace.
- Allow advocate to stay with patient during exam with patient's consent.

## DIAGNOSTIC TESTS & INTERPRETATION
### Lab
- Syphilis serology
- Hepatitis band C panel
- HIV testing and counseling
- Drug testing (if suspect victim was drugged, can be used against victim if other agents detected)
- Blood type
- Pregnancy test
- *Gonococcus* culture
- *Chlamydia* culture
- Other labs as needed based on injuries

### Imaging
As indicated by injuries

### Diagnostic Procedures/Surgery
As indicated by injuries

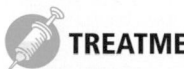 TREATMENT

### PRE-HOSPITAL
- Treat patient in a kind, nonjudgmental manner.
- C-spine immobilization for patients with head/neck trauma

### INITIAL STABILIZATION/THERAPY
Treat life-threatening injuries.

### ED TREATMENT/PROCEDURES
- Place patient in quiet, private room.
- Assure patient of confidentiality regarding name and reason for visit.
- Regularly assure patient of safety.
- Enforce nonjudgmental behavior by staff.
- Designate nursing and medical provider for entire stay who is familiar with evidence collection kit.
- Have sexual assault nurse examiner (SANE) perform exam if available.
- Contact community or in-hospital advocate to stay with patient while in ED.
- Alert hospital security to possibility of assailant presenting to ED.
- Contact police if patient consents or local law requires.

- Collect evidence as outlined above and according to local law.
- Offer pregnancy prophylaxis if not currently pregnant:
  – Estimated risk of pregnancy is 2%–4% if woman not using contraceptives.
  – Administer prophylactic therapy for *Gonococcus, Chlamydia, Trichomonas*.
  – Consider prophylactic HIV treatment.
  – Consider prophylactic therapy or vaccine for hepatitis B.

### MEDICATION
#### Pregnancy Prophylaxis
Hormonal therapy **if within 72 hr**:
- Levonorgestrel 0.75 mg PO stat and repeat in 12 hr (preferred) or
- Levonorgestrel 1.5 g PO, 1 dose
- Ethinyl estradiol 100 $\mu$g PO stat and repeat in 12 hr

#### STI Prophylaxis
- Ceftriaxone 125 mg IM (*Gonococcus*)
- Doxycycline 100 mg PO b.i.d. for 7–10 days *or* azithromycin 1 g PO, 1 dose (*Chlamydia*)
- Metronidazole (Flagyl) 2 g PO, 1 dose (*Trichomonas*)

#### HIV Prophylaxis
- Lopinavir/ritonavir (Kaletra) 200 mg/50 mg 2 tablets twice daily plus emtricitabine/tenofovir (Truvada) 200 mg/300 mg once daily for **high-risk exposures** (source known to be HIV+ or is an intravenous drug user [IVDU], or MSM)
- Emtricitabine/tenofovir (Truvada) 200 mg/300 mg once daily for exposures from persons other than those noted above.

 FOLLOW-UP

### DISPOSITION
#### Admission Criteria
Serious traumatic injury

#### Discharge Criteria
- Medical follow-up for culture and HIV test results
- Safe place for patient to go to

#### Issues for Referral
- Mental health services and counseling
- For all pediatric cases, the Department of Children and Family Services should be contacted.

### FOLLOW-UP RECOMMENDATIONS
Follow-up should be provided for repeat HIV testing at 6 wk, 3 mo, and 6 mo.

## PEARLS AND PITFALLS
- ~70% of rape victims do not tell their doctors.
- Women who are disabled, pregnant, or attempting to leave their abusers are at increased risk of intimate partner rape.
- Most of pediatric exams in alleged sexual assault cases will be normal (80–96%)
- If HIV prophylaxis medications are started, baseline CBC, BMP, and LFTs should be obtained.

## ADDITIONAL READING
- Burgess AW, Fawcett J. The comprehensive sexual assault assessment tool. *Nurse Pract*. 1996;21:66.
- Dunn SFM, Gilchrist VJ. Sexual assault. *Primary Care*. 1993;20:359–373.
- Dupre AR, Hampton HL, Morrison H, et al. Sexual assault. *Obstet Gynecol Surv*. 1993;45:640–648.
- Levine DL, Kaufman LE. Rape and sexual violence: The adult and adolescent female victim. In: Bernstein E, Bernstein J, eds. *Case Studies in Emergency Medicine and the Health of the Public*. Boston: Jones & Bartlett, 1996:100–112.
- Tjaden P, Thoennes N. *Full Report of the Prevalence, Incidence, and Consequences of Violence Against Women*. Washington, DC: National Institute of Justice and the Centers for Disease Control and Prevention, 2000.

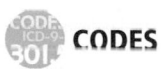 CODES

### ICD9
- 995.03 Adult sexual abuse
- V71.5 Observation following alleged rape or seduction

S

# SHOCK

Nathan Shapiro
Christopher Fischer

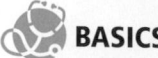

## BASICS

### DESCRIPTION

- Inadequate supply of blood flow to tissues to meet the demands of the tissues
- Tissue oxygen requirements are not fulfilled.
- Toxic metabolites are not removed.
- If untreated, inevitable progression from inadequate perfusion to organ dysfunction and ultimately to death.
- Major categories of shock:
  - Hypovolemic shock:
    ○ Decreased blood volume
    ○ Suspect hemorrhage if acute onset
    ○ Severe dehydration if progressive onset and elevated hematocrit, blood urea nitrogen, and creatinine
  - Obstructive (cardiogenic) shock:
    ○ Decreased cardiac output and tissue hypoxia with adequate intravascular volume and myocardial dysfunction
    ○ Venous congestion with increase in central venous pressure
    ○ Compensatory increase in SVR
    ○ May be caused by cardiac dysfunction, obstruction to inflow of blood to the heart, or obstruction to outflow of blood from the heart
  - Septic shock:
    ○ An initial infectious insult overwhelms the immune system.
    ○ Biochemical messengers (cytokines, leukotrienes, histamines, prostaglandins) cause vessel dilatation.
    ○ Capillary endothelium becomes disrupted and the vessels leak.
    ○ Drop in SVR leads to inadequate tissue perfusion.
    ○ Secondarily, decreased cardiac output from "cardiac stun" resulting in cold septic shock
  - Neurogenic shock:
    ○ Spinal cord insults disrupt sympathetic stimulation to vessels.
    ○ Loss of sympathetic tone causes arteriodilating and vasodilatation.
    ○ Lesions proximal to T4 disrupt sympathetic, spares vagal innervation causing bradycardia.
  - Anaphylactic shock:
    ○ An antigen stimulates the allergic reaction.
    ○ Mast cells degranulate.
    ○ Histamine releases, along with autocoids, stimulate an anaphylaxis cascade.
    ○ Vascular smooth muscle relaxes.
    ○ Capillary endothelium leaks.
    ○ Drop in SVR leads to inadequate tissue perfusion.
  - Pharmacologic agents may cause shock through smooth muscle dilation or myocardial depression.

### ETIOLOGY

- Hypovolemic shock:
  - Abdominal trauma, blunt or penetrating
  - Abortion—complete, partial, or inevitable
  - Anemia—chronic or acute
  - Aneurysms—abdominal, thoracic, dissecting
  - Aortogastric fistula
  - Arteriovenous malformations
  - Blunt trauma
  - Burns
  - Diabetes
  - Diarrhea
  - Diuretics
  - Ruptured ectopic pregnancy
  - Epistaxis
  - Fractures (especially long bones)
  - Hemoptysis
  - GI bleed
  - Mallory-Weiss tear
  - Penetrating trauma
  - Placenta previa
  - Postpartum hemorrhage
  - Retroperitoneal bleed
  - Severe ascites
  - Splenic rupture
- Toxic epidermal necrolysis:
  - Vascular injuries
  - Vomiting
- Cardiogenic shock:
  - Cardiomyopathy
  - Conduction abnormalities and arrhythmias
  - MI
  - Myocardial contusion
  - Myocarditis
  - Pericardial tamponade
  - Pulmonary embolus
  - Tension pneumothorax
  - Valvular insufficiency
  - Ventricular septal defect
- Vasogenic shock:
  - Acute respiratory distress syndrome
  - Bacterial infection
  - Bowel perforation
  - Cellulitis
  - Cholangitis
  - Cholecystitis
  - Endocarditis
  - Endometritis
  - Fungemia
  - Infected indwelling prosthetic device
  - Intraabdominal infection or abscess
  - Mediastinitis
  - Meningitis
  - Myometritis
  - Pelvic inflammatory disease
  - Peritonitis
  - Pyelonephritis
  - Pharyngitis
  - Pneumonia
  - Septic arthritis
  - Thrombophlebitis
  - Tubo-ovarian abscess
  - Urosepsis

- Anaphylactic:
  - Drug reaction (most commonly to aspirin, $\beta$-lactam antibiotics)
  - Exercise (rare)
  - Food allergy (peanuts, tree nuts, shellfish, fish, milk, eggs, soy, and wheat account for 90% of food related anaphylaxis)
  - Insect sting
  - Latex
  - Radiographic contrast materials
  - Synthetic products
- Pharmacologic:
  - Antihypertensives
  - Antidepressants
  - Benzodiazepines
  - Cholinergics
  - Digoxin
  - Narcotics
  - Nitrates
- Neurogenic:
  - Spinal cord injury

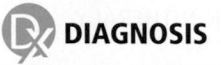

## DIAGNOSIS

### SIGNS AND SYMPTOMS

Generalized shock:

- Hypotension
- Decreased peripheral pulses
- Tachycardia
- Tachypnea
- Decreased urine output
- Diaphoresis
- Obtundation
- Lethargy

### History

Standard medical history with a goal of deducing the etiology of the shock and important precipitating factors

### Physical Exam

- Standard physical exam to assist in determining the etiology (eg, wounds, cardiac exam signs of cellulitis and urticarial rash, etc.)
- Targeted physical exam to focus on the type of shock state:
  - Hypovolemic (classic symptoms):
    ○ Neck veins are flat.
    ○ Mucous membranes are dry.
    ○ Extremities are cold.
  - Cardiogenic shock (classic symptoms):
    ○ Jugular venous distension is present.
    ○ Mucous membranes are moist.
    ○ Extremities are cold.
  - Early septic shock (classic symptoms):
    ○ Neck veins are flat.
    ○ Mucous membranes are dry.
    ○ Extremities are warm.
    ○ During late shock, extremities may become cold and mottled.

## ESSENTIAL WORKUP
- Identify type or types of shock present.
- Identify underlying cause of shock.

## DIAGNOSTIC TESTS & INTERPRETATION
### Lab
- Hemoglobin/hematocrit
- WBC:
  - High: Nonspecific marker of infection
  - Low: Neutropenic infections
- Electrolytes
- Blood glucose:
  - High: Diabetic ketoacidosis or septic shock
  - Low: Pediatric sepsis
- Prothrombin time/partial thromboplastin time
- Cardiac enzymes
- Urinalysis
- $\beta$-Human chorionic gonadotropin
- Lactic acid level:
  - Good surrogate marker of shock state

### Imaging
- CXR
- ECG
- Abdominal US
- CT abdomen:
  - Requires that the patient 1st be stabilized
  - In the setting of abdominal trauma and in search for suspicion of abdominal infection

### Diagnostic Procedures/Surgery
EKG:
- Assess for ischemia and other disorders of cardiac muscle:
- Electrical alternans or low voltage with cardiac tamponade
- Right-heart strain with pulmonary embolism

## TREATMENT

### PRE-HOSPITAL
- ABCs per standard protocol
- Fluid resuscitation as warranted

### INITIAL STABILIZATION/THERAPY
- Large-bore IV access:
  - When possible, central venous access and monitoring
- Fluid resuscitation in noncardiogenic shock patients
- Control bleeding with direct pressure measures.
- Stabilization of a fractured pelvis with sheet or commercial device or external fixation

### ED TREATMENT/PROCEDURES
- Hypovolemic shock:
  - Identify source of volume depletion
  - Aggressive fluid resuscitation keeping systolic blood pressure (SBP) >100 mm Hg until definitive treatment
  - 2–3 L crystalloid initially
  - Packed RBCs if 2–3 L crystalloids do not improve SBP
  - Identify source of bleeding and rapidly move toward definitive treatment.
  - Thoracotomy and aortic cross-clamping in refractory shock with penetrating torso trauma

- Cardiogenic shock:
  - Ease work of breathing with intubation
  - Insult-specific therapy (eg, thrombolytics for MI, pericardiocentesis for pericardial tamponade)
  - Treat dysrhythmias.
- Septic shock:
  - Aggressive crystalloid fluid resuscitation
  - Titrate fluid to urine output >30 cc/hr
  - Blood product transfusion to maintain HCT 30–35%
  - Early antimicrobial therapy
  - Inotropic support as needed
  - Dopamine and/or norepinephrine infusion
- Anaphylactic shock:
  - Intubation for airway compromise
  - Epinephrine
  - Subcutaneous in noncritical settings
  - IV drip for immediate life threats or refractory hypotension
  - H-1 blockers (diphenhydramine)
  - H-2 blockers (cimetidine)
  - Corticosteroids (hydrocortisone or methylprednisolone)
  - Nebulized $\beta_2$-antagonists for bronchospasm
  - Patients taking $\beta$-blockers may be more likely to experience severe symptoms of anaphylaxis
- Pharmacologic shock:
- Supportive therapy:
  - Decontamination of overdoses with charcoal
  - Inotropic agents as needed
  - Drug specific antidotes
- Neurogenic shock:
  - Supportive therapy
  - Traction and fracture stabilization
  - Corticosteroids

## MEDICATION
- Albuterol: 2.5 mg/2.5 cc nebulizer PRN
- Calcium gluconate: 100–1,000 mg IV
- Cimetidine: 300 mg IV
- Diphenhydramine: 50–100 mg IV over 3 min
- Dobutamine: 5–40 $\mu$g/kg/min IV:
  - Dopaminergic: 1–3 $\mu$g/kg/min IV
  - $\beta$-Effects: 3–10 $\mu$g/kg/min IV
  - $\alpha/\beta$ Effects: 10–20 $\mu$g/kg/min IV
  - $\alpha$-Effects: 20 $\mu$g/kg/min IV
- Epinephrine:
  - 1–4 $\mu$g/min IV infusion
  - SQ/IM 1:1,000 0.1–0.3 mg repeat q5–20min × 3 p.r.n.
  - IV 1:10,000 10 mL (1 mg) over 10 min IV
- Glucagon: 1–5 mg IV bolus initial, then 1–20 mg/h infusion
- Hydrocortisone: 5–10 mg/kg IV
- Methylprednisolone: 1–2 mg/kg IV
- Naloxone: 0.01 mg/kg IV initial, titrate to effect
- Norepinephrine: Start 2–4 $\mu$g/min IV, titrate up to 1–2 $\mu$g/kg/min IV
- Phenylephrine: 40–180 $\mu$g/kg/min IV

 FOLLOW-UP

### DISPOSITION
### Admission Criteria
- All patients in shock need to be admitted.
- ICU criteria:
  - All patients with persistent shock need ICU monitoring.
- Patients with shock definitively reversed may be admitted to non-ICU setting (eg, tension pneumothorax that has been decompressed and chest tube placed).

### Discharge Criteria
Patients who are in shock should not be discharged home from the ED.

### Issues for Referral
- Traumatic hypovolemic shock (hemorrhagic shock) patients may require a trauma center.
- Patients with cardiogenic shock due to MI may require cardiac catheterization or additional cardiac surgery support.
- Septic shock due to necrotizing fasciitis may require advanced surgical support.
- Neurogenic shock with spinal cord injury will require neurosurgical care.

## PEARLS AND PITFALLS
- Identify the etiology of shock.
- Aggressively resuscitate the patient, 1st with intravenous fluids and next with vasopressor support to minimize hypoxic exposure.

## ADDITIONAL READING
- Kline JA. Shock. In: Marx J, et al., eds., *Rosen's emergency medicine: Concepts and clinical practice.* St. Louis: Mosby Year Book, 2002:33–47.
- Rivers E, Nguyen B, Havstad S, et al. Early goal directed therapy in the treatment of severe sepsis and septic shock. *N Engl J Med.* 2001;345: 1368–1377.
- Shapiro NI, Howell M, Talmor D. A blueprint for a sepsis protocol. *Acad Emerg Med.* 2005;12:4: 352–359.

 CODES

### ICD9
- 785.50 Shock, unspecified
- 785.51 Cardiogenic shock
- 785.52 Septic shock

# SHOULDER DISLOCATION

*Doodnauth Hiraman*
*Wallace A. Carter*

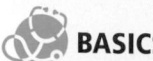 **BASICS**

## DESCRIPTION

- Shoulder is a very dynamic joint, prone to injury.
- Anterior dislocation (90–96%):
  - Injury is from direct or indirect forces on the abducted and externally rotated arm.
  - Injury may also result from a direct blow to posterior lateral aspect of shoulder.
- Posterior dislocation:
  - Often missed
  - Forces on the adducted and internally rotated arm result in posterior dislocation of humeral head in relation to glenoid fossa.
  - Most common mechanism is seizure and sudden contraction of all the posterior muscle groups.
  - Other mechanisms include electrocution and direct blow to anterior shoulder.
- Inferior dislocation (rare):
  - Luxatio erecta
  - Hyperabduction of arm, tear of rotator cuff, and rotation of arm 180° above head
  - Commonly seen after a fall from a height:
    - Arm has struck object on descent and is thrust above the head.
  - Often accompanied by neurovascular injury and fracture

### Pediatric Considerations
Dislocation is rare in children: Epiphysial fractures must be suspected.

### Geriatric Considerations
Dislocation is often accompanied by fracture.

## ETIOLOGY

- Falls from height
- Impact injuries
- Distraction injuries of upper arm
- Seizures
- Electrocution

 **DIAGNOSIS**

## SIGNS AND SYMPTOMS

- Severe pain in the affected shoulder
- Anterior dislocation:
  - Shoulder is squared off.
  - Prominent acromion process and palpable anterior fullness
  - Arm is held in slight abduction and external rotation.
- Posterior dislocation:
  - Coracoid process is prominent, with a palpable posterior bulge.
  - Arm is held in slight adduction and internal rotation.
- Inferior dislocation (luxatio erecta):
  - Rare but easy to identify
  - Arm is shortened and fixed above head as if raised to ask a question.
- Head of humerus may be palpable on the lateral chest wall.

## ESSENTIAL WORKUP

- Evaluate neurovascular status of distal arm.
- Retest neurovascular status after any manipulation.
- Dislocation requires prompt treatment:
  - Incidence of posttraumatic arthritis increases with time dislocation is untreated.
  - Plain films of the shoulder should be obtained immediately.
  - Even in clinically obvious cases, films should be obtained before manipulation, unless a significant delay will result.
  - An impacted humeral head fracture may be converted to a displaced humeral head fracture if manipulated.

## DIAGNOSTIC TESTS & INTERPRETATION
### Imaging

- At least 2 views should be obtained:
  - Anteroposterior (AP):
    - To visualize dislocation or fracture
  - Trans-scapular Y or axillary view:
    - To visualize if anterior or posterior
- Anterior dislocation:
  - Posterolateral compression fracture of the humeral head (Hills-Sachs deformity)
  - Corresponding lesion on anterior glenoid rim is the Bankart lesion:
    - These do not require treatment.
  - Fractures of the greater tuberosity of the humeral head are seen in 15–35%:
    - If there is >1 cm displacement after reduction, surgical intervention may be necessary.
- Posterior dislocation:
  - Often missed on AP film
- Degree of overlap on radiographic film is smaller and displaced superiorly, producing the meniscus sign.
- Rotated humerus yields "light bulb on a stick" finding on AP view:
  - Reverse Hill-Sachs deformity from compression fracture of the anterior medial humeral head may also be seen.

## DIFFERENTIAL DIAGNOSIS

- Fracture of the humeral head
- Fracture of the humeral shaft
- Acromioclavicular injury
- Septic shoulder joint
- Hemarthrosis in shoulder joint
- Scapular fracture
- Cervical spine injury

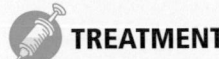

# TREATMENT

## PRE-HOSPITAL
Neurovascular injury should be identified and the arm splinted in the position of most comfort.

## INITIAL STABILIZATION/THERAPY
- Airway management and resuscitate as indicated.
- Exclude more serious injuries, especially in multitrauma patient.
- Ensure no injury to axillary nerve or vessels.

## ED TREATMENT/PROCEDURES
- Adequate analgesia and muscle relaxation are essential for successful reduction:
  - Procedural sedation with a short-acting opioid and a benzodiazepine OR
  - Methohexital or etomidate alone
  - In the cooperative patient, intra-articular block only (20 cc of lidocaine 1% or bupivacaine 0.5%) into shoulder joint
- Anterior dislocation reduction techniques:
  - Scapular manipulation:
    ○ Patient seated, traction to arm in horizontal plane, countertraction with other hand on clavicle
    ○ 2nd person adducts tip of scapula medially, moving glenoid fossa
  - Stimson:
    ○ Patient in prone position with arm dangling over side, hang 10–15 lb around wrist; muscle fatigued over 20–30 min
    ○ Can concurrently use scapular manipulation
    ○ Only 1 person required
  - Traction/countertraction:
    ○ Patient in supine position with continuous longitudinal traction to affected arm
    ○ Countertraction from sheet wrapped around chest
    ○ Arm internally or externally rotated if unsuccessful after several minutes
  - External rotation:
    ○ Patient supine; elbow at 90°; gentle, slow external rotation of arm
    ○ Should be done slowly and with cooperative patient

- Posterior dislocation reduction techniques:
  - May use Stimson or traction/countertraction techniques with manipulation of humeral head anteriorly
- Inferior dislocation (luxatio erecta) reduction techniques:
  - Patient in supine position; gentle longitudinal traction to distract humeral head
  - Gentle countertraction with sheet draped over trapezius and chest
  - Arm slowly rotated from 180–0°
- Postreduction care:
  - Post reduction films
  - Place in sling and swath or shoulder immobilizer immediately after reduction.
  - Shoulder should remain immobilized for 2–3 wk in young patients.
  - Immobilization time should be less in older patients to avoid frozen shoulder.

## MEDICATION
- Bupivacaine 0.5%: 20 cc intra-articular to shoulder
- Diazepam: 5–10 mg IV (peds: 0.2 mg/kg)
- Etomidate: 0.2 mg/kg IV (adult and peds)
- Fentanyl: 50–100 μg IV (peds: 2–4 μg/kg)
- Lidocaine 1%: 20 cc intra-articular to shoulder
- Methohexital: 1–1.5 mg/kg IV (peds: Not routinely used)
- Midazolam: 2–5 mg IV (peds: 0.035–0.1 mg/kg)
- Morphine: 2–8 mg IV (peds: 0.1 mg/kg)
- Propofol: 1–2 mg/kg IV

# FOLLOW-UP

## DISPOSITION
### Admission Criteria
- Failure to reduce shoulder may require admission for reduction under general anesthesia or open reduction.
- Patients with neurovascular compromise

### Discharge Criteria
Patients with successful reductions, confirmed by plain films, may be discharged with shoulder in appropriate immobilizer and with orthopaedic follow-up.

- Recurrent dislocation may require elective surgery.
- Patients with residual neurapraxia from injury or manipulation may be safely discharged with instructions that most symptoms will resolve, but should have neurology follow-up.

### Issues for Referral
- Patients with residual neurapraxia should be advised to see a neurologist.
- Routine orthopaedic consultation should be advised with all successful reductions.

## PEARLS AND PITFALLS
Make sure to document sensory exam of axillary nerve prior to reduction.

## ADDITIONAL READING
- Hendey GW. Necessity of radiographs in the emergency department management of shoulder dislocations. *Ann Emerg Med.* 2000;36(2):108–113.
- Kahn J. The role of post-reduction x-rays after dislocation. *Acad Emerg Med.* 2001;8(5):521.
- McNamara RM. Reduction of anterior shoulder dislocations by scapular manipulation. *Ann Emerg Med.* 1993;22(7):1140–1144.
- Perrron AD, et al. Acute complications associated with shoulder dislocation at an academic emergency department. *J Emerg Med.* 2003;24(2):141–145.
- Quillen DM, et al. Acute shoulder injuries. *Am Family Physician.* 2004;70(10):1947–954.
- Sileo MJ, Joseph S, Nelson CO, et al. Management of acute glenohumeral dislocations. *Am J Orthop (Belle Mead NJ).* 2009;38(6):282–290.
- Ufberg JW, et al. Anterior shoulder dislocations: Beyond traction countertraction. *J Emerg Med.* 2004;27(3):301–306.

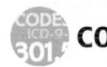

# CODES

## ICD9
831.00 Closed dislocation of shoulder, unspecified site

# SICK SINUS SYNDROME

*David F. M. Brown*
*Arjun K. Venkatesh*

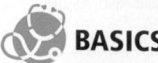 BASICS

## DESCRIPTION
- Collective term used to describe dysfunction in the sinus node's automaticity and impulse generation
- Mechanism:
  - Caused by progressive degeneration of the intrinsic functions of the SA node
  - Characterized by periods of unexplained sinus node dysfunction leading to bradyarrhythmias, often without appropriate atrial or junctional escape rhythms
- Syndrome includes:
  - Chronic sinoatrial (SA) nodal dysfunction
  - Frequently depressed pacemakers
  - Arteriovenous nodal conduction disturbances
  - Sluggish return of SA nodal activity after DC cardioversion

## ETIOLOGY
- Intrinsic causes:
  - Idiopathic degenerative fibrosis of Sinus node is the most common cause.
  - Coronary artery or SA nodal artery disease
  - Cardiomyopathy
  - Leukemia and metastatic disease
  - Infiltrative cardiac or collagen vascular disease, including amyloidosis
  - Surgical trauma
- Inflammatory diseases:
  - Rheumatic heart disease
  - Chagas disease
  - Pericarditis and myocarditis
- Extrinsic causes:
  - Drugs:
    - $\beta$-Blockers, calcium channel blockers, clonidine
    - Digoxin, amiodarone
    - Lithium, phenytoin
  - Autonomically mediated syndromes (cholinesterase deficiency)
  - Hyperkalemia/hypokalemia
  - Hypothyroidism
  - Hypothermia
  - Hypoglycemia
  - Sepsis/infection

### Pediatric Considerations
Associated with congenital abnormalities and subsequent surgical repair, as well as with congenital sinoatrial nodal artery deficiency

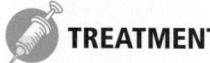 DIAGNOSIS

## SIGNS AND SYMPTOMS
Symptoms represent CNS hypoperfusion from bradydysrhythmia, traditional cardiovascular presentations

### History
- Asymptomatic
- Palpitations/fatigue
- Syncope/presyncope/dizziness
- Anginal equivalents (chest pain/SOB)

### Physical Exam
- Bradycardia
- Alternating bradycardia and atrial tachycardia
- Altered mental status
- Cyanosis
- Transient ischemic attack/stroke

## ESSENTIAL WORKUP
- Ascertaining etiology
- 12-lead EKG
- CXR

## DIAGNOSTIC TESTS & INTERPRETATION
### Lab
- Serum electrolytes (including magnesium and calcium)
- Cardiac markers
- Digoxin level, if appropriate
- Thyroid function testing

### Imaging
EKG:
- Inappropriate sinus bradycardia
- Sinus pauses or sinoatrial block
- Atrial fibrillation with slow ventricular response
- Prolonged pauses after cardioversion or carotid massage
- Bradyarrhythmias may alternate with supraventricular tachydysrhythmia.
- Tachy-Brady syndrome: Bursts of atrial tachycardia interspersed with bradycardia

### Diagnostic Procedures/Surgery
Most electrophysiological studies are no longer recommended due to poor sensitivity and specificity.

## DIFFERENTIAL DIAGNOSIS
- Other bradydysrhythmias
- Other tachyarrhythmias: In particular, be careful to distinguish SSS from atrial fibrillation, because DC cardioversion or the use of nodal agents in presumed Afib can be harmful if SA node dysfunction coexists.
- Electrolyte derangements
- Medication toxicity: $\beta$-Blockers, calcium channel blockers, clonidine, digoxin
- Excessive vagal tone

## TREATMENT

### PRE-HOSPITAL
- Advanced life support transport
- Oxygen supplementation
- Cardiac monitoring
- Atropine if bradycardic and hemodynamically unstable
- Transcutaneous pacing for unstable patients

### INITIAL STABILIZATION/THERAPY
- Atropine if a bradydysrhythmia is causing unstable signs/symptoms: Angina, mental confusion, or hypotension
- Transcutaneous pacing if atropine unsuccessful
- If this fails, emergent transvenous pacing

### ED TREATMENT/PROCEDURES
Supraventricular tachydysrhythmia alternating with bradycardia
- Unstable:
  - Cardiovert
  - Anticipate subsequent profound bradycardia
- Stable patients:
  - Cardiac monitoring
- Digoxin, diltiazem, verapamil, or magnesium can be used for tachydysrhythmia
- Any medication may cause profound bradycardia

- Bradycardia:
  - Discontinuation of medications that alter sinus node function
  - Correct reversible causes of SA nodal depression: $O_2$, warming, glucose

### ALERT
Rewarming is critical in hypothermia as atropine may cause myocardial instability

- Anticoagulate patients with atrial fibrillation and tachy-brady syndrome.

### MEDICATION
- Atropine: 0.5–1.0 mg IV/ET:
  - Repeat q5min as necessary, max. dose of 0.04 mg/kg (peds: 0.02 mg/kg, minimum, 0.1 mg)
- Diltiazem: 0.25 mg/kg IV over 2 min followed in 15 min by 0.35 mg/kg IV over 2 min
- Verapamil: 2.5–5 mg IV bolus over 2 min:
  - May repeat with 5–10 mg q15–30min max. 20 mg
  - Peds: <1 yr: 0.1–0.2 mg/kg over 2 min; repeat q30min 1–15 yr: 0.1–0.3 mg/kg over 2 min, max. dose 5 mg/dose, can repeat once.
- Digoxin: 0.5 mg IV initially then 0.25 mg IV q4h until desired effect (max. 1 mg IV)
- Isoproterenol: 2–3 $\mu$g/min IV, titrate to goal heart rate/BP, max. 10 $\mu$g/min (peds: 0.1 $\mu$g/kg/min)—do *not* co-administer with epinephrine and *only* use in unstable patient
- Epinephrine: 1 mg IV (peds: 0.01 mg/kg IV): For cardiac arrest
- Glucagon: 0.05–0.15 mg/kg IV (peds: 0.05–0.10 mg/kg)
- Heparin: Load 80 IU/kg IV; infusion at 18 IU/kg/h
- Magnesium: 1–2 g IV

### First Line
1st-line definitive therapy is a permanent demand pacemaker to provide a "floor" to bradydysrhythmia:
- Patients with additional tachydysrhythmias will require additional nodal agents.

### Second Line
No clear evidence to distinguish between 1st- and 2nd-line treatment.

 FOLLOW-UP

### DISPOSITION
#### Admission Criteria
- New onset
- Symptomatic: CHF, syncope, chest pain, dizziness
- Persistent bradyarrhythmia or tachydysrhythmia .
- Advanced age; >60 yr
- Patients should be admitted to a telemetry floor with cardiology consultation.
- Most will require permanent pacing.

#### Discharge Criteria
- Asymptomatic, otherwise healthy patients can be evaluated as outpatients.
- Holter monitoring

#### Issues for Referral
- Need for formal cardiac electrophysiology evaluation
- Need for permanent pacemaker placement

### FOLLOW-UP RECOMMENDATIONS
#### Geriatric Considerations
- High incidence of CAD is present in patients with sick sinus syndrome, so a complete cardiovascular risk-factor evaluation and prevention is needed.
- Patient with atrial fibrillation and tachy-brady syndrome need long-term anticoagulation.
- All patients require evaluation by a cardiologist or EP specialist for permanent pacemaker.

### PEARLS AND PITFALLS
- Patients who are asymptomatic on ED arrival may have normal EKGs. Consider obtaining a rhythm strip or Holter monitor if clinical suspicion remains high.
- Use of any nodal agents (BB, CCB, or digoxin) in patients with SSS related tachydysrhythmia risks SA block or SA arrest and should only be administered when prepared for transcutaneous pacing.

### ADDITIONAL READING
- Adan V, Crown LA. Diagnosis and treatment of sick sinus syndrome. *Am Fam Phys*. 2003;67(8): 1725–1732.
- Brady W, Harrigan R. Evaluation and management of bradyarrhythmias in the emergency department. *Emerg Med Clin North Am*. 1998;16(2):361–388.
- Kaushuk V, Leon A, Forrester J, et al. Bradyarrhythmias, temporary and permanent pacing. *Crit Care Med*. 2000;28:N121–N128.
- Mangrum J, DiMarco M. Primary care: The evaluation and management of bradycardia. *N Engl J Med*. 2000;342:703–709.
- Rubenstein JJ, Schulman CI, Yurchak PM, et al. Clinical spectrum of the sick sinus syndrome. *Circulation*. 1972;46:513.
- Ufberg JW, Clarfk JS. Bradydysrhythmias and atrioventricular conduction blocks. *Emerg Med Clin North Am*. 2006;24:1–9.

### See Also (Topic, Algorithm, Electronic Media Element)
Bradydysrhythmia

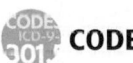 CODES

ICD9
427.81 Sinoatrial node dysfunction

# SICKLE CELL DISEASE

*Steven H. Bowman*
*Jeanette Haslett*

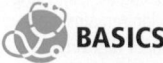 **BASICS**

## DESCRIPTION

- Sickle cell disease (SCD) caused by abnormal hemoglobin (hemoglobin S), which polymerizes under stress and deforms RBCs, resulting in hemolysis, vasoocclusion, tissue ischemia, and infarction.
- Affects multiple organ systems
- Inherited autosomal recessive disorder caused by a single amino acid substitution in hemoglobin gene
- Occurs in people of African, Mediterranean, Middle Eastern, and Indian descent
- Severity variable even among the same phenotype
- Vasoocclusion, ischemia, and infarction crises occur in essentially all organ systems:
  - Bone/Joint crises:
    - Vasoocclusion of bone microvasculature causes infarction.
    - Long bones, ribs, sternum, spine and pelvis affected.
    - Dactylitis, or "hand–foot syndrome," occurs at ages 6–24 mo.
  - Chest crisis or syndrome:
    - Vasoocclusion of pulmonary vasculature with infarcts
    - Fat embolism, viral and bacterial infections may contribute
    - High mortality (2%–14%)
    - 50% of sickle cell patients will experience one episode of acute chest syndrome.
    - Radiographic pulmonary infiltrate with fever and respiratory symptoms
    - Difficult to distinguish from pneumonia
    - More common in children
  - Splenic sequestration:
    - Splenic sinusoids become congested with sickled RBCs, obstructing outflow.
    - High mortality (12%–20%)
    - May be rapidly fatal due to circulatory collapse
    - More common in children <5 yr; rare in adults
  - Aplastic crisis:
    - Bone marrow suppression usually occurs secondary to viral infection, most commonly Parvovirus B19.
    - Increased baseline hemolysis in patients with SCD requires maximum erythropoiesis.
    - Decrease in hematocrit may be severe.
    - Generally self-limited
    - More common in children
  - Cerebrovascular accident/transient ischemic attack (TIA):
    - Secondary to infarction in children; hemorrhage in adults
    - Peak incidence between ages 9 and 15 yr; prevalence 5%–20%
    - Often preceded by TIAs
  - Bacterial infection:
    - Sepsis is the leading cause of death in patients with SCD.
    - Ability to fight encapsulated organisms is impaired secondary to decreased splenic function.
    - Children <5 yr of age have 400-fold increase in pneumococcal infections.

- *Streptococcus pneumoniae, Haemophilus influenzae, Staphylococcus aureus, Escherichia coli,* and *Salmonella* are leading organisms.
    - Sites: lung, CNS, bone, kidney
  - Priapism
    - Painful failure of detumescence
    - Low-flow (ischemic) priapism more common than high-flow (nonischemic)
    - Low flow associated with stasis, acidosis, and ischemia

## RISK FACTORS
### Genetics
Genotypes/phenotypes/severity/incidence in African Americans:

- SS, SCD, marked severity, 0.3%
- SC, SC disease, mild to moderate severity, 0.1%
- S β-thalassemia, β-thalassemia, mild to moderate severity, <0.1%
- AS, sickle cell trait, no manifestation of disease, 8%

## ETIOLOGY
Common crisis precipitants:
- Infection (bacterial and viral)
- Dehydration
- Hypoxemia
- Acidosis
- Surgery/Trauma
- Weather changes
- Pregnancy
- Toxins

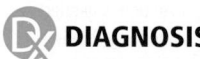 **DIAGNOSIS**

## SIGNS AND SYMPTOMS
- May present with either:
  - Painful episode
  - Complications of the disease
  - Combination of above
- May not demonstrate usually autonomic signs of acute pain
- Sickle cell crisis:
  - Bone/Joint crisis:
    - Pain in extremities, back, sternum, or joints
    - Variable swelling, warmth
    - Variable joint effusion
    - Hand–foot syndrome in infants; swelling in hands and feet and a reluctance to walk or use hands
  - Abdominal crisis:
    - Abdominal pain without peritonitis
    - Variable nausea, vomiting, diarrhea
  - Priapism—prolonged painful erection
- Complications/Progression of disease
  - Chest crisis (or syndrome):
    - Pleuritic chest pain
    - Cough with variable hemoptysis
    - Dyspnea
    - Tachypnea
    - Rales

- Splenic sequestration crisis:
    - Abdominal pain
    - Splenomegaly
    - Variable nausea, vomiting
    - Fatigue, lethargy
    - Pallor
    - Tachycardia
    - Hypotension, syncope, shock
  - Aplastic crisis:
    - Variable fever, headache, nausea, vomiting
    - Fatigue
    - Pallor
    - Tachycardia
  - Cerebrovascular accident/TIA
    - Focal neurologic deficit
    - Mental status changes
    - Seizure
  - Infections:
    - Fever
    - Localizing signs

### Pediatric Considerations
- Acute sickle cell complications in children carry high morbidity and should be screened for aggressively.
- Infections commonly precipitate crisis.
- Patient's immunization history (pneumococcal and *H. influenzae*) must be confirmed.
- Determine if child is receiving prophylactic penicillin, normally indicated in children ≤5.
- Overwhelming infection highest in children <3 yr of age.

### Pregnancy Considerations
- Increased rates of asymptomatic bacterial infection, UTI, and pyelonephritis leading to septicemia
- Increased risk of miscarriage and preterm labor
- Increased risk of placental abruption
- Anemia is more profound.

### History
- Onset of current symptoms
- Genotype
- Previous and recent crises events
- Immunizations
- Determine typical vs. atypical crisis

### Physical Exam
- Conduct a thorough physical exam:
  - Vital signs: BP, HR, Temp, $O_2$ sat
  - Pulmonary exam
    - Rales, wheezing, tachypnea
  - Abdominal exam
    - Organomegaly, tenderness, peritonitis,
  - Musculoskeletal exam
    - Edema or erythema on extremities
    - Warm, swollen hands and feet in children
  - Neurologic exam
    - Focal neurologic impairment
    - Cranial nerve palsy

## ESSENTIAL WORKUP

Conduct a thorough physical exam, with focus on signs of infection or ischemia.

## DIAGNOSTIC TESTS & INTERPRETATION

### Lab

- CBC:
  - Anemia may be profound. Compare with prior values if available.
  - For major sequestration HgB ≤6 g/dL or 3 g/dL less than baseline
  - Leukocytosis is common and does not necessarily indicate infection.
- Reticulocyte count:
  - Generally elevated >5.0% in SS individuals
  - A low count (≤3% or lower than the patient's normal value) may indicate an aplastic crisis.
- Consider the following if indicated:
  - UA
    - ○ Asymptomatic hematuria is common.
    - ○ Urinary tract infection may precipitate pain crisis and requires aggressive treatment.
  - Electrolytes, BUN/creatinine, glucose
  - Blood cultures
  - Urine culture
  - Type and screen (or cross)
  - Urine pregnancy test in women

### Imaging

- Radiographs should be directed to confirm diagnosis:
  - Chest radiograph if pneumonia or chest syndrome suspected
  - Extremities if osteomyelitis suspected
- IV contrast may exacerbate or precipitate a crisis.
- Head CT/MRI to evaluate stroke

### Diagnostic Procedures/Surgery

Lumbar puncture if CNS infection or subarachnoid hemorrhage is suspected

## DIFFERENTIAL DIAGNOSIS

- Sickle cell crises may mimic or obscure more serious underlying pathology (eg, acute abdomen, MI, PE, nephrolithiasis)
- Suspect other diagnoses if pain is more severe or atypical.

 TREATMENT

## INITIAL STABILIZATION/THERAPY

- Identify and treat high morbidity complications:
  - Sepsis
  - Splenic sequestration
  - Chest crisis
  - Central venous access
- Assess pain and initiate therapy.

## ED TREATMENT/PROCEDURES

- Analgesia:
  - Choice of analgesic agent depends on patient, severity of episode, and prior agents.
  - Evaluate patient frequently and titrate medications accordingly for relief of pain.

- Hydration:
  - 1.5–2 times maintenance after correction of deficits
  - Oral hydration if patient can tolerate fluids by mouth
  - Parenteral IV solution 0.45% NS for adults and children or 0.2% NS for infants
  - Monitor fluids closely.
- Complication-specific therapy:
  - Oxygen, bronchodilators: chest syndrome, pneumonia
  - Antibiotics: sepsis, pneumonia, osteomyelitis
  - Acute simple transfusion: sequestration crisis, blood loss, accelerated hemolysis
  - Exchange transfusion may be required for more severe complications: CVA
- Bladder catheterization for priapism and urinary retention
- Consultations:
  - Hematology for splenic sequestration, aplastic crisis and CNS events if exchange transfusion required
  - Neurology/Neurosurgery for acute CNS events
  - Urology for priapism

## MEDICATION

- Severe/moderate pain:
  - Hydrocodone: 0.15/mg/kg/dose PO q4h
  - Hydromorphone: 0.01–0.02 mg/kg/dose IV q3h–q4h or 0.04–0.06 mg/kg/dose PO q4h
  - Morphine: 0.1–0.15 mg/kg/dose IV q3h–q4h or 0.3–0.6 mg/kg/dose PO q4h
  - Ketorolac: 30 mg IV initially, then 15–30 mg q6h–q8h
  - Meperidine: 0.75–1.5 mg/kg/dose IV q2h–q4h
- Mild pain:
  - Acetaminophen: 1 g (peds: 15 mg/kg/dose) PO q4h
  - Codeine: 0.5–1 mg/kg/dose PO
  - Ibuprofen: 800 mg (peds: 5–10 mg/kg/dose) PO q8h
- Antibiotics select appropriate agents based on pathogens described above

 FOLLOW-UP

## DISPOSITION

### Admission Criteria

- Refractory pain crisis
- Signs of bacterial infection or fever of undetermined etiology
- Chest syndrome
- Sequestration crisis
- Aplastic crisis
- CVA or TIA
- Refractory priapism
- Symptomatic anemia

### Discharge Criteria

- Resolution of pain crisis
- No indications for admission

### Issues for Referral

Meticulous primary care can limit the frequency and severity of pain crises.

## FOLLOW-UP RECOMMENDATIONS

If discharged, patient should see PCP or hematologist in 1–2 days.

## PEARLS AND PITFALLS

- Distinguish typical sickle cell crisis from more acute life-threatening complications.
- Promptly recognize and treat high-morbidity complications.
- Treat pain aggressively with appropriately selected and administered analgesic agents.
- Patients with a history of chronic pain syndromes such as SCD may not demonstrate the usual autonomic signs of acute pain, such as tachycardia or diaphoresis.

## ADDITIONAL READING

- Fuh B. Sickle cell disease emergencies in children. *Pediatr Emerg Med Rep.* 2009.
- Hassell K. Pregnancy and sickle cell disease. *Hematol Oncol Clin North Am.* 2005;19:903–916.
- Montalembert M. Management of sickle cell disease. *BMJ* 2008;337(a1397):626–630.
- Stephens C. Sickle cell disease: A review of the state-of-the-art emergency management and outcome-effective therapy. *Emerg Med Rep.* 1999;20(18):183.
- Stuart MJ, Nagel RL. Sickle cell disease. *Lancet.* 2004;364(9442):1343–1360.
- Wang W, et al. Sickle cell anemia and other sickling syndromes. In: Greer J, et al, eds. *Wintrobe's Clinical Hematology*, 12th ed. Philadelphia: Lippincott Williams & Wilkins, 2009:1038–1082.

## See Also (Topic, Algorithm, Electronic Media Element)

Anemia

 CODES

### ICD9

- 282.5 Sickle-cell trait
- 282.60 Sickle-cell disease, unspecified
- 282.61 Hb-ss disease without crisis

S

# SINUSITIS

*Erica Douglass*
*Maria E. Moreira*

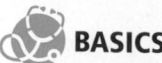 **BASICS**

## DESCRIPTION

- Inflammation of the mucous membranes lining the paranasal sinuses
- Classifications:
  - Acute: signs and symptoms last <4 weeks.
  - Subacute: signs and symptoms last 4–8 weeks.
  - Chronic: signs and symptoms last >8 weeks in spite of antibiotic treatment.
  - Recurrent: 3 or more episodes per year
- Nosocomial sinusitis is associated with nasogastric and nasotracheal tubes.
- Viral sinusitis is 20–200 times more common than bacterial sinusitis.
  - Complication of simple viral upper respiratory tract infection or allergic rhinitis
- Pathophysiology:
  - As mucous membranes become inflamed, sinus ostia narrow and block drainage.
  - Air is absorbed and negative pressure develops, resulting in transudate formation.
  - Bacteria are trapped and multiply, resulting in suppuration and converting the viral infection to a bacterial infection.
  - Foreign bodies, nasal polyps, tumors, or traumatic fractures can lead to obstruction of ostia.
- Immunocompromised patients and patients with impaired mucociliary movement are also predisposed to sinusitis.
- GERD has been suggested as a cause of sinusitis.

## ETIOLOGY

- Acute sinusitis:
  - *Haemophilus influenzae*
  - *Streptococcus pneumoniae*
  - *Moraxella catarrhalis*
  - *Staphylococcus aureus*
  - Anaerobes
  - Viruses (rhinovirus most common)
- Chronic sinusitis:
  - Same as acute, with increasing incidence of anaerobes and gram negatives
  - Often polymicrobial
  - Also more common:
    - *Staphylococcus aureus*
    - *Peptostreptococcus*
    - *Fusobacterium*
    - *Bacteroides*
    - *Aspergillus*
- Nosocomial sinusitis:
  - *S. aureus*
  - Streptococcal species
  - *Pseudomonas*
  - *Klebsiella*
- Immunocompromised patients with sinusitis:
  - The usual bacterial pathogens
  - Fungal pathogens (*Aspergillus*)

### Pediatric Considerations
- Ethmoid and maxillary sinuses are present at birth.
- Frontal and sphenoid sinuses do not emerge until age 6–7 yr
- Sinusitis is more common in children than adults.
- Periorbital/orbital cellulitis is a common complication of ethmoid sinusitis in children.
  - Periorbital swelling, fever, ptosis, proptosis, and painful or decreased extraocular movements

 **DIAGNOSIS**

## SIGNS AND SYMPTOMS
### History
- Facial–dental pain
- Headache
- Halitosis
- Cough
- Purulent nasal discharge and blockages
- Postnasal discharge
- Hyposmia
- Fever
- Frontal sinusitis:
  - Pain of the lower forehead
  - Pain worsened when lying on the back; improves when upright.
- Maxillary sinusitis:
  - Malar facial pain
  - Maxillary dental pain
  - Referred ear pain
  - Pain worsens with head upright or bending forward and improves with reclining.
- Ethmoid sinusitis:
  - Retroorbital pain
  - Periorbital edema
- Sphenoid sinusitis (very uncommon):
  - Pain over the occiput or mastoid
  - Pain worse when lying on back or bending forward.
- Recent history of nasotracheal intubation suggests nosocomial sinusitis:
  - Involves atypical pathogens such as *Pseudomonas* and gram-negative organisms
- Rhinocerebral mucormycosis:
  - Rare but rapidly progressive fungal infection
  - Occurs in diabetic and other immunocompromised patients
  - Orbital and facial pain out of proportion to physical signs
  - Lethargy, headache in a systemically ill-appearing patient
  - Black eschar or pale area on the palate or nasal mucosa

### Physical Exam
- Edema of the nasal mucous membranes
- Pus in the nares or posterior pharynx
- Warmth, tenderness, and possibly cellulitis over the affected sinus
- Sinus tenderness on palpation
- Periorbital edema

## ESSENTIAL WORKUP
- Clinical diagnosis based on history and physical exam

## DIAGNOSTIC TESTS & INTERPRETATION
### Lab
Laboratory studies are not helpful for diagnosis or management.

### Imaging
- Imaging is unnecessary in uncomplicated cases.
- Plain-film radiography:
  - Normal plain films do not rule out bacterial involvement.
  - A Waters view may help in the diagnosis of maxillary sinusitis.
  - Opacification or air/fluid level in involved sinus
- CT:
  - Preferred if imaging is necessary
  - May assist in diagnosing complications
  - IV contrast if concern for osteomyelitis or abscess

### Diagnostic Procedures/Surgery
- Sinus aspirate culture:
  - Gold standard for making a microbial diagnosis
  - Not used in routine medical practice
- Functional endoscopic sinus surgery (FESS):
  - Restores physiologic sinus ventilation and drainage

### Pediatric Considerations
FESS is a safe and effective treatment in children.

## DIFFERENTIAL DIAGNOSIS
- Uncomplicated viral or allergic rhinits
- Otitis media
- Dacrocystits
- Migraine and cluster headache
- Dental pain
- Trigeminal neuralgia
- Temporomandibular joint disorders
- Giant cell arteritis/Temporal arteritis
- Rhinitis medicamentosa (decongestants, beta blockers, antihypertensives, birth control pills)
- Nasal polyp, tumor, or foreign body
- CNS infection
- Granulomatous or ciliary disease
- Aspergillosis

### Pregnancy Considerations
- Pregnancy rhinitis:
  - Nasal congestion during last 6 or more weeks of pregnancy
  - Disappears within 2 weeks after delivery

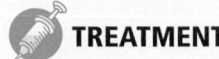 **TREATMENT**

**PRE-HOSPITAL**
No special considerations

**INITIAL STABILIZATION/THERAPY**
Toxic-appearing patients may require airway management and fluid resuscitation:

**ED TREATMENT/PROCEDURES**
- Cost-effective approach favors appropriate antibiotic therapy and no testing.
- Establish good drainage with topical or oral decongestants and *Mucor* evacuants.
- Reduce edema with topical corticosteroids in chronic sinusitis.
- Humidification and saline spray are beneficial adjuncts to pharmacologic therapy.
- Reserve antibiotics for patients with:
  - Pain and discharge for more than 10 days in spite of decongestant and analgesic treatment
  - Severe symptoms
- Acute sinusitis—antibiotic choices if no antibiotic treatment in the previous month:
  - Amoxicillin, amoxicillin–clavulanate, cefpodoxime
- Acute sinusitis—antibiotic choices if antibiotic treatment in the previous month (>30% risk of drug resistant *S. pneumoniae*):
  - Amoxicillin–clavulanate, ciprofloxacin (adult), levofloxacin (adult), moxifloxacin (adult)
- Acute sinusitis—clinical failure after 3 days of antibiotic treatment:
  - Amoxicillin–clavulanate or cefpodoxime (mild to moderate disease)
  - Gatifloxacin, levofloxacin, moxifloxacin (severe disease in adults)
- Acute sinusitis—patient with penicillin or cephalosporin allergy:
  - Clarithromycin, azithromycin, trimethoprim–sulfamethoxazole, doxycycline, levofloxacin, moxifloxacin, or trimethoprim–sulfamethoxazole
- Acute sinusitis—aspergillosis:
  - Ear-nose-throat (ENT) consultation
- Chronic sinusitis:
  - 3–6 week course of antibiotics (controversial), douche, and topical steroids
  - ENT consultation

**MEDICATION**
- Antibiotics:
  - Amoxicillin:500–1500 mg PO t.i.d. (peds: 40 mg/kg/day PO t.i.d.)
  - Amoxicillin–clavulanate: 250–500 mg PO t.i.d. or 875 mg PO b.i.d. (peds: 40 mg/kg/day, based on the amoxicillin component, PO t.i.d.)
  - Azithromycin: 500 mg PO once then 250 mg PO per day for 4 days per day or 2 g x 1 dose (peds: 10 mg/kg on day 1 and then 5 mg/kg on days 2–5)
  - Cefpodoxime: 200–400 mg PO b.i.d. (peds: 10 mg/kg/d PO b.i.d.)
  - Cefuroxime: 250–500 mg PO b.i.d. (peds: 15 mg/kg/day PO b.i.d.)
  - Clarithromycin: 500 mg PO b.i.d. (peds: 7.5 mg/kg/day PO b.i.d.)
  - Doxycycline: 100 mg PO b.i.d.
  - Levofloxacin: 500 mg PO per day (adult)

- Moxifloxacin: 400 mg PO per day (adult)
- Trimethoprim–sulfamethoxazole: 1 double-strength tablet PO b.i.d. (peds: 8–12 mg/kg/day, based on the trimethoprim component, PO b.i.d.)
- If signs and symptoms not improved after 3 to 5 days of one antibiotic, switch to another antibiotic.
- Decongestants:
  - Nasal saline sprays and irrigants
  - Topical: not to be used for more than 3 days
  - Oxymetazoline hydrochloride 0.05%: 2–3 gtt or sprays per nostril b.i.d.
  - Phenylephrine hydrochloride 0.5%: 2–3 sprays per nostril q3–4h; oral: if longer than 3 days of treatment
  - Pseudoephedrine: 60 mg PO q4h–q6
  - Other agents:
  - Pain control
  - Antihistamines
  - Allergy treatment
- *Mucor* evacuants:
  - Guaifenesi: 5–20 mL PO q4h (peds: 5–10 mL per dose if 6–12 yr old, 2.5–5 mL if 2–6 yr old)
- Corticosteroids for chronic sinusitis:
  - Beclomethasone dipropionate: 1 spray per nostril q.d./b.i.d./t.i.d.
  - Dexamethasone sodium phosphate: 2 sprays per nostril b.i.d./t.i.d.

**First Line**
- Decongestants
- *Mucor* expectants

**Second Line**
Antibiotics

 **FOLLOW-UP**

**DISPOSITION**

**Admission Criteria**
- Evidence of spread of infection beyond the sinus cavity
- Toxic-appearing patients
- Immunocompromised/Diabetic patients with extensive infection
- Multiple sinus involvement
- Frontal sinus involvement
- Extremes of age
- Severe comorbidity
- ENT evaluation and aspiration if patient is severely ill, immunocompromised, or has pansinusitis and is ill-appearing

**Discharge Criteria**
- Most cases of uncomplicated sinusitis may be managed on an outpatient basis.
- Follow-up with primary care physician or ENT specialist if symptoms persist >7 days.

**Issues for Referral**
- Complications of acute infection
- Immunocompromised patients
- Nasal polyps
- Chronic rhinosinusitis
- Concerns for osteomyelitis, CNS infection, or abscess

**FOLLOW-UP RECOMMENDATIONS**
If no relief with initial treatment with decongestants and *Mucor*-expectants, follow-up with PCP or ENT.

**PEARLS AND PITFALLS**
- Term *rhinosinusitis* preferred, since inflammation of sinuses rarely occurs without inflammation of the nasal mucosa
- Plain films and CT do not distinguish between viral and bacterial etiologies
- Patients presenting with <10 days of symptoms should be treated with supportive care:
  - Viral is sinusitis expected to resolve within 10 days.
  - Bacterial sinusitis may resolve spontaneously within first 10 days.

**ADDITIONAL READING**
- Ah-See K. Sinusitis and its management. *BMJ*. 2007;334:358.
- Ahovuo-Saloranta A, Borisenko OV, Kovanen N, et al. Antibiotics for acute maxillary sinusitis. *Cochrane Database Syst Rev*. 2008;CD000243.
- Cherry WB, Li JT. Chronic rhinosinusitis in adults. *Am J Med*. 2008;121:185.
- Falgas ME, Giannopoulou KP, Vardakas KZ, et al. Comparison of antibiotics with placebo for treatment of acute sinusitis: A meta-analysis of randomized controlled trials. *Lancet Infect Dis*. 2008;8:543.
- Hamilos DL. Approach to the evaluation and medical management of chronic rhinosinusitis. *Clin Allergy Immunol*. 2007;20:299.
- Harvey R, Hannan SA, Badia L, et al. Nasal saline irrigations for the symptoms of chronic rhinosinusitis. *Cochrane Database Syst Rev*. 2007;CD006394.
- Morris P, Leach A. Antibiotics for persistent nasal discharge (rhinosinusitis) in children. *Cochrane Database Syst Rev*. 2002;CD001094.
- Piccirillo JF. Clinical practice: Acute bacterial sinusitis. *N Engl J Med*. 2004;351:902.
- Rosenfeld RM, Andes D, Bhattacharyya N, et al. Clinical practice guideline: Adult sinusitis. *Otolaryngol Head Neck Surg*. 2007;137:S1.
- Young J, De Sutter A, Merenstein D, et al. Antibiotics for adults with clinically diagnosed acute rhinosinusitis: A meta-analysis of individual patient data. *Lancet*. 2008;371:908.
- Zalmanovici A, Yaphe J. Steroids for acute sinusitis. *Cochrane Database Syst Rev*. 2007;CD005149.

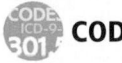 **CODES**

**ICD9**
- 461.9 Acute sinusitis, unspecified
- 473.9 Unspecified sinusitis (chronic)

S

# SKIN CANCER

*Adam Z. Barkin*
*Michael K. Doney*

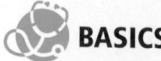 **BASICS**

## DESCRIPTION

- Most common cancer in the U.S.
- Increasing incidence
- 1 in 6 will have skin cancer during their lifetime.
- Nonmelanoma skin cancer:
- Rarely fatal
- Fast-growing
- May be destructive if left untreated:
  - Basal cell carcinoma (BCC):
    - Cells arise from epidermis.
    - Most common skin cancer
    - Account for 75% of all nonmelanoma skin cancers
    - Male > Female, 3:2
    - Most important risk factor is sun exposure.
    - Locally invasive without risk of distant metastasis
    - More common in fair-skinned patients
    - Most lesions are on the head and neck.
  - Squamous cell carcinoma (SCC):
    - 2nd most common skin cancer
    - 20% of cases of skin cancer
    - Most arise from precancerous actinic keratosis lesions.
    - Male > Female
    - Most important risk factor is sun exposure, especially sunburn.
    - 70% occur on head and neck
    - More common in older, fair-skinned patients
    - Risk of regional lymph node and distant metastasis
    - SCC lesions of mucosal surfaces are more aggressive
  - Actinic keratosis:
    - Thickened scaly growth caused by sunlight or other artificial light source
    - Premalignant lesions
    - 0.1–10% may transform into SCC
    - Found on areas of body with sun exposure

- Melanoma:
  - 5% of all diagnosed skin cancer in the U.S.
  - 62,000 new cases in 2008
  - 15% are fatal
  - 75% of skin cancer deaths
  - Arises from melanin-producing cells
  - Most important risk factor is sun exposure, especially sunburn.
  - Additional risk factors:
    - Fair skin; blond/red hair
    - Multiple common melanocytic nevi
    - Atypical nevi
    - Immunosuppression
    - Positive family history
    - History of nonmelanoma skin cancer (basal cell or squamous cell carcinoma)
    - ≥5 sunburns in early life doubles the risk for malignant melanoma
  - Risk of regional lymph node and distant metastasis

## ETIOLOGY

- UV irradiation:
  - Both UVA and UVB rays
  - Sun exposure
  - Tanning beds
- SCC often associated with human papilloma virus (HPV)
- Immunosuppression may predispose to SCC
- Vitamin D metabolism may play a role

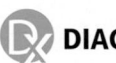 **DIAGNOSIS**

## SIGNS AND SYMPTOMS

- BCC:
  - May be single or multiple
  - Usually painless
  - Usually appears in sun-exposed areas of skin
  - Nodular BCC:
    - Most common
    - Waxy or pearly papule
    - Well-demarcated borders
    - May have central ulceration
  - Pigmented BCC:
    - Similar to nodular BCC with dark pigment
    - Often mistaken for melanoma

- Cystic BCC:
  - Bluish/gray cystic nodules
  - May be mistaken for benign cysts
- Superficial BCC:
  - Scaly patch-like or papule
  - Pink, red or brown
- Micronodular BCC:
  - Well-defined border
  - Aggressive
  - Rarely with ulceration
- Morpheaform BCC:
  - Poorly defined borders
  - May appear "scar-like"
  - Aggressive
  - Ulceration and bleeding are rare
- SCC:
  - Characteristic lesion is raised, firm, keratotic papule or plaque.
  - Often enlarging
  - Usually asymptomatic but may be ulcerated and painful
  - Ulcers often crust and ooze
  - Cranial nerve involvement may indicate an aggressive tumor with perineural invasion:
    - Facial numbness, asymmetry, weakness or pain
- Actinic keratosis:
  - Rough, pink, circumscribed lesions <1 cm in diameter
- Melanoma:
  - Pigmented skin lesion
    - 2% will be amelanotic
  - Features suggestive of melanoma (the *ABCDs* of melanoma):
    - *A*symmetry (not regularly round or oval)
    - *B*order irregularity (notched or poorly defined)
    - *B*leeding (spontaneous)
    - *C*olor variegation (shades or combinations of brown, tan, red, white, or blue-black)
    - *D*iameter >6 mm
  - Lesions rarely symptomatic unless ulcerated
  - Superficial spreading melanoma:
    - 70% of all malignant melanomas
    - May have a wide variety of colors
    - Often arise from dysplastic nevus
    - Usually <3 cm
    - Slight elevation and induration is common
    - Often have satellite lesions

- Nodular melanoma:
  - 10–15% of melanomas
  - The most symmetric of the different melanomas.
  - Dark brown or black
  - Often exophytic
- Lentigo maligna melanomas:
  - Premalignant lesion
  - 10% of melanomas
  - Often are large with areas of hypopigmentation
- Acral lentiginous melanoma:
  - Equal among black and white patients
  - Occur on palms, soles, and subungual region
  - May be mistaken for subungual hematoma
- Mucosal lentiginous melanoma:
  - Develops from mucosal epithelium in respiratory, GI, and GU tracts
  - 3% of all melanomas
  - Often diagnosed at a later stage of disease
- Malignant melanoma:
  - Presentation related to affected organ system
  - Lymphangitic spread with local to regional lymphadenopathy
  - Typical visceral sites of hematogenous spread include liver, lung, bone, and brain.

## ESSENTIAL WORKUP
Suspicious lesions require biopsy, a procedure rarely done in ED.

## DIAGNOSTIC TESTS & INTERPRETATION
### Lab
- No specific testing is required.
- Tests of liver enzymes and function are ordered if suspicion of metastatic melanoma exists.

### Imaging
- CXR may show pulmonary involvement by metastatic melanoma.
- Head or body CT scan may show visceral involvement by metastatic melanoma.

### Diagnostic Procedures/Surgery
Biopsy usually performed by consultant

## DIFFERENTIAL DIAGNOSIS
- For BCC:
  - SCC
  - Bowen disease
    Actinic keratosis
  - Paget disease
  - Benign nevus
  - Melanoma

- For SCC:
  - Actinic keratosis
  - BCC
  - Keratoacanthoma
  - Melanoma
  - Wart
- For melanoma:
  - Atypical nevus
    Common nevus
  - Actinic keratosis
  - Pigmented basal cell carcinoma
  - SCC

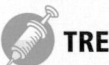 TREATMENT

### PRE-HOSPITAL
No specific pre-hospital care is required.

### INITIAL STABILIZATION/THERAPY
No specific stabilization is usually required beyond basic wound care.

### ED TREATMENT/PROCEDURES
- No specific ED treatment
- Treat complications of visceral involvement by metastatic melanoma or locally invasive BCC.

 FOLLOW-UP

### DISPOSITION
#### Admission Criteria
- Usually admission occurs only because of visceral involvement or invasive spread.
- Admission is rarely required because of the lesions themselves.

#### Discharge Criteria
Patients are generally discharged with instructions on obtaining biopsy and/or further evaluation.

#### Issues for Referral
Discharged patients should be advised to consult a dermatologist or experienced primary care physician.

## FOLLOW-UP RECOMMENDATIONS
- Biopsy is required for diagnosis of skin cancer.
- Urgent follow-up with dermatologist or primary care physician is advised.
- Patients with nonmelanoma skin cancer have a 30–50% chance of developing additional skin cancer within 5 yr.

## PEARLS AND PITFALLS
- Advise patient to obtain urgent follow-up for any suspicious lesion.
- 1 in 6 people will have skin cancer during their lifetime.
- Protection from UVA and UVB rays is key to preventing skin cancer.

## ADDITIONAL READING
- Arora A, Attwod J. Common skin cancers and their precursors. *Surg Clin N Am.* 2009;89:703–712.
- Califano K, Nance M. Malignant melanoma. *Facial Plast Surg Clin N Am.* 2009;17:337–348.
- Lee DA, Miller SJ. Nonmelanoma skin cancer. *Facial Plast Surg Clin N Am.* 2009;17:309–324.
- Ricotti C, Bouzari N, Agadi A, et al. Malignant skin neoplasms. *Med Clin N Am.* 2009;93:1241–1264.
- Rubin AI, Chen EH, Ratner D. Basal-cell carcinoma. *N Engl J Med.* 2005;353:2262–2269.

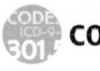 CODES

### ICD9
- 172.9 Melanoma of skin, site unspecified
- 173.9 Other malignant neoplasm of skin, site unspecified

S

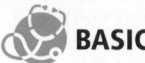 **SLEEP APNEA**

*Ajay Bhatt*

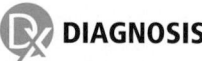 **BASICS**

## DESCRIPTION

- Disorder characterized by cessation of breathing during sleep:
  - Defined as apneic episodes greater than 10 sec with brief EEG arousals or greater than 3% oxygenation desaturation
- Risk factors:
  - Obesity
  - Male
  - >40 yr of age
  - Upper airway anomalies
  - Myxedema (hypothyroidism)
  - Alcohol/Sedative abuse
  - Smoking
- Associated illness:
  - Various dysrhythmias, particularly atrial fibrillation and bradyarrhythmia
  - Right and left heart failure
  - MI
  - Stroke
  - Motor vehicle accidents
  - Hypertension poorly controlled by medical therapies

## EPIDEMIOLOGY

- Affects about 9% of middle-aged men and 4% of middle-aged women
- 80% of moderate or severe cases undiagnosed in middle-aged adults

## ETIOLOGY

3 classifications of sleep apnea:

- Obstructive (84%) is due to upper airway closure despite intact respiratory drive:
  - Also known as Pickwickian syndrome
  - Pharyngeal airway is narrowed
- Central (0.4%) is due to lack of respiratory effort despite patent upper airway.
- Complex (15%) is due to a combination of obstructive and central sleep apnea.

**DIAGNOSIS**

## SIGNS AND SYMPTOMS

- Excessive daytime sleepiness
- Snoring
- Irritability

### History

- Significant other apnea report
- Difficulty sleeping
- Decreased attention/concentration
- Depression
- Decreased libido/impotence

### Physical Exam

- Hypertension, hypoxemia
- Obesity
- Craniofacial anomalies
- Macroglossia
- Enlarged tonsils
- Elevated jugular veins (secondary to pulmonary hypertension)
- Large neck circumference

## ESSENTIAL WORKUP

- Pulse oximetry
- ECG
- Chest radiograph

## DIAGNOSTIC TESTS & INTERPRETATION

### Lab

ABG is the best test to demonstrate hypercarbia and hypoxemia.

### Imaging

- Consider lateral neck soft tissue radiograph to rule out other etiologies of upper airway obstruction.
- Chest radiograph to assess other etiologies of hypoxemia
- Chest CT rarely indicated

### Diagnostic Procedures/Surgery

Polysomnogram (PSG) is required for diagnosis:

- >5 apneic episodes per hour
- Not a consideration for ED management

## DIFFERENTIAL DIAGNOSIS

- Asthma
- Cheyne–Stokes breathing
- COPD
- Diaphragmatic paralysis
- High altitude–induced periodic breathing
- Hypothyroidism
- Left heart failure
- Narcolepsy
- Obesity hyperventilation syndrome
- Primary pulmonary hypertension

**TREATMENT**

## PRE-HOSPITAL

Caution not to overventilate patient with chronic CO retention

## INITIAL STABILIZATION/THERAPY

Chin lift/jaw thrust maneuver, oxygen as needed, oral or nasal airway devices

## ED TREATMENT/PROCEDURES

- Proper technique is required for airway management:
  - Supplemental oxygen as needed
  - Bag-mask-valve ventilation may be difficult
    ○ Consider use of nasal and oral airways
    ○ 2-person technique to ensure a good seal.
- Continuous positive airway pressure (CPAP) is the standard of treatment:
  - Acts as a pneumatic splint by maintaining upper airway patency
  - BiPAP is an alternative for patients requiring high pressures or with comorbid breathing disorders.
  - Long-term CPAP therapy decreases blood pressure, insulin resistance, and risk of cardiovascular disease.

### ALERT

**Endotracheal intubation**

- Higher prevalence of difficult intubation:
  - Patients frequently have higher Mallampati scores.
  - Excess pharyngeal tissue in lateral walls often obstructs airway visualization.
  - Patients have overall lower arterial oxygen saturation.
- Plan and consider several methods of definitive airway control:
  - Have alternative devices (laryngeal mask airway, bougie) available.
  - Be prepared to perform cricothyroidotomy if necessary.
- Use neuromuscular blockade only if successful oral intubation is reasonably likely and bag-mask ventilation is easy.
- Positive end-expiratory pressure for ventilated patients

## MEDICATION

- Insufficient evidence to recommend any medication for treatment
- See Airway Management for details on induction agents and neuromuscular blockade.
- Wakefulness-promoting agents (modafinil and armodafonil) are approved as an adjunct to CPAP patients with excessive sleepiness.

### ALERT

Avoid sedative use.

- Relaxes the upper airway and worsens airway obstruction and snoring

### *Long-Term Management*

- Surgical considerations:
  - Most intend to reduce or bypass the excessive pharyngeal/airway resistance that occurs during sleep.
  - Efficacy is unpredictable; no good randomized trials
  - Not a consideration for ED management
- Dental devices:
  - Currently recommended by the American Academy of Sleep Medicine (AASM)
  - Available appliances include tongue repositioning and mandibular devices or soft palate lifters.

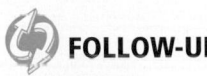 FOLLOW-UP

### DISPOSITION

### *Admission Criteria*

- Ventilatory failure, especially if intubation is necessary
- Hemodynamic Instability

### *Discharge Criteria*

- Maintenance of $O_2$ saturation >85% for several hours using oxygenation or ventilation equipment available to the patient at home
- Very low likelihood of decompensation overnight
- Patients with sleep apnea who present after motor vehicle crashes:
  - Manage initially like other blunt trauma patients.
  - Later, consider the increased risk with sleep apnea and intervene to prevent future accidents.

### FOLLOW-UP RECOMMENDATIONS

- PCP referral for sleep apnea and associated comorbidities
- Referral of patients with suspected sleep apnea to a pulmonologist
- Encourage weight loss and diet control.
- Cardiology referral is appropriate when sleep apnea is complicated by heart failure or dysrhythmias.

## PEARLS AND PITFALLS

- Sleep apnea increases risk of cardiovascular disease, stroke, and diabetes mellitus.
- CPAP is the standard of treatment.
- Avoid the use of sedatives.
- Preparation is essential, as sleep apnea increases intubation complications.
- Primary care referral and CPAP compliance education improve therapy.

## ADDITIONAL READING

- Buchner NJ, Sanner BM, Borgel J, Rump LC. Continuous positive airway pressure treatment of mild to moderate obstructive sleep apnea reduces cardiovascular risk. *Am J Respir Crit Care Med*. 2007;176(12):1274–1280.
- Caples SM, Gami AS, Somers VK. Obstructive sleep apnea. *Ann Intern Med*. 2005;142(3):187–197.

- Epstein LJ, Kristo D, Strollo PJ Jr, et al. Clinical guideline for the evaluation, management and long-term care of obstructive sleep apnea in adults. *J Clin Sleep Med*. 2009;5(3):263–276.
- Mulgrew AT, Fox N, Ayas NT, Ryan CF. Diagnosis and initial management of obstructive sleep apnea without polysomnography: A randomized validation study. *Ann Intern Med*. 2007;146(3):157–166.
- Rosenberg R, Doghramji P. Optimal treatment of obstructive sleep apnea and excessive sleepiness. *Adv Ther*. 2009;26:295–312.
- Young T, Skatrud J, Peppard PE. Risk factors for obstructive sleep apnea in adults. *JAMA*. 2004;291(16):2013–2016.

### See Also (Topic, Algorithm, Electronic Media Element)

- Airway Management
- Dyspnea

The author gratefully acknowledges Mark Sagarin for his previous edition of this chapter.

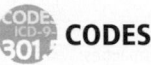 CODES

### ICD9

- 327.21 Primary central sleep apnea
- 327.23 Obstructive sleep apnea (adult) (pediatric)
- 780.57 Unspecified sleep apnea

S

# SLIPPED CAPITAL FEMORAL EPIPHYSIS

*Judd L. Glasser*

 **BASICS**

## DESCRIPTION
- Femoral epiphysis translates, or "slips," relative to the femoral head/neck.
- Classified:
  - Degree of displacement:
    - (Mild, grade 1) <1/3 translation
    - (Moderate, grade 2) 1/3–1/2 translation
    - (Severe, grade 3) >1/2 translation
  - Temporal:
    - Acute (<3 wk of symptoms)
    - Chronic (>3 wk of symptoms)
    - Peak age at onset 13–15 yr for boys and 11–13 yr for girls
    - Most patients are obese.
    - Male > Female (8:3).
    - ~20% of cases involve bilateral joint.

## ETIOLOGY
- True etiology remains elusive.
- Association with endocrine abnormalities:
  - Especially hypothyroidism and treatment with growth hormone

 **DIAGNOSIS**

## SIGNS AND SYMPTOMS
- Presents with limp or exertional limp
- Pain in the knee, thigh, groin, or hip (referral of pain along the obturator nerve):
  - Vague and dull for weeks in chronic slipped capital femoral epiphysis (SCFE)
  - Severe and sudden onset in an acute SCFE
- Commonly presents with the leg externally rotated
- Flexion is restricted (cannot touch thigh to abdomen).

## History
- May present with chronic hip pain with exertion
- May have acute pain following minor trauma
- May acute on top of chronic pain

## Physical Exam
- Observe resting position of the leg.
- If the patient refuses to ambulate, do not allow further ambulation attempts

## ESSENTIAL WORKUP
- Plain radiographs:
  - Further imaging should be done with direction from consultant
- Orthopedic consultation

## DIAGNOSTIC TESTS & INTERPRETATION
### Lab
- Without diagnostic radiographic abnormality, the practitioner should consider the following tests to help risk stratify possible alternative diagnoses:
- CBC with differential
- Sedimentation rate
- C-reactive protein

### Imaging
- Anteroposterior and frog-leg lateral radiograph films of *both* hips should be obtained:
  - Widened or irregular physis
  - Bird's beak appearance of the actual slipping of the epiphysis off of the femoral head
- Klein line (line drawn parallel lateral femoral neck does not transect epiphysis)

### Diagnostic Procedures/Surgery
If septic hip is suspected, aspiration and fluid analysis may be needed to exclude.

## DIFFERENTIAL DIAGNOSIS
- Legg-Calve-Perthes:
  - Typically seen in 4–9-yr-old age range
- Septic arthritis of hip
- Osteomyelitis
- Toxic synovitis
- Femur or pelvic fractures
- Inguinal or femoral hernia

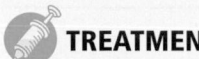 **TREATMENT**

### PRE-HOSPITAL
Patient should be immobilized for transport, as with suspected hip fracture or dislocation.

### INITIAL STABILIZATION/THERAPY
- Immobilize hip.
- Keep non–weight-bearing.
- Do not attempt reduction.

### ED TREATMENT/PROCEDURES
- SCFE is an urgent orthopaedic condition; delay in diagnosis may lead to chronic irreversible hip joint disability.
- Consult orthopaedics immediately for definitive immobilization or operative intervention.

### MEDICATION
Pain management is appropriate; avoid PO medications, as acute SCFE often may be managed with emergent surgical fixation.

 **FOLLOW-UP**

### DISPOSITION
*Admission Criteria*
- Patients with acute or acute or chronic (unstable) SCFE require orthopaedic admission for urgent operative fixation (usually single central pinning).
- Chronic SCFE may be managed with delayed operative fixation.

*Discharge Criteria*
- None
- It is too difficult to achieve complete non–weight-bearing status, which is required to prevent further slippage, avascular necrosis, and chondrolysis

### FOLLOW-UP RECOMMENDATIONS
Should be arranged by orthopedic specialist

## PEARLS AND PITFALLS
- Klein line can be a helpful tool in picking up the abnormality on plain radiograph.
- Remember to examine the hip when a child presents with knee or thigh pain.
- 1 in 5 cases will present with bilateral findings.

## ADDITIONAL READING
- Aronsson DD, Loder RT, Breur GJ, et al. Slipped capital femoral epiphysis: Current concepts. *J Am Acad Ortho Surg.* 2006;14(12):666–679.
- Loder RT. Controversies in slipped capital femoral. *Orthopedic Clin North Am.* 2006;37(2):211–221.
- Uglow MG, Clarke NMP. The management of slipped capital femoral epiphysis. *J Bone Joint Sur.* 2004;86-B:631–635.

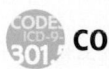 **CODES**

### ICD9
732.2 Nontraumatic slipped upper femoral epiphysis

S

# SMALL-BOWEL INJURY

*Barry J. Knapp, II*

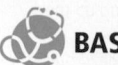

## BASICS

### DESCRIPTION
2 general causes:
- Blunt visceral trauma
- Penetrating: Visceral injury (96% of gunshot wounds, 50% of stabbings)—serosal tear, bowel wall hematoma, perforation, bowel transection, mesenteric hematoma/vascular injury

### ETIOLOGY
- Blunt:
  - 3rd most commonly injured organ (5–10% of all blunt trauma victims)
  - Motor vehicle accidents
  - Nonvehicular trauma: Abuse/assault, bicycle handlebars, large-animal kick
  - Blast victims
- Mortality rate from small-bowel injury is 33%.
- Mesenteric tears may initially be asymptomatic:
  - Deceleration injury at fixed points (eg, ligament of Treitz)
  - Shearing mechanisms near fixed points (eg, ileocecal junction, adhesions)
  - Compressive force against anterior spine
  - Bursting or "blowout" at antimesenteric margin from sudden closed-loop intraluminal pressure rise
- Associated injuries:
  - Liver and splenic lacerations; thoracic and pelvic fractures
  - Seatbelt syndrome: Abdominal wall ecchymosis, small-bowel injury; chance fracture of L1, L3
- Penetrating:
  - Small bowel is the 2nd most commonly injured organ (32%) in anterior abdominal stabbing.
  - Small-bowel injury is most common in gunshot wounds (49%).

#### Pediatric Considerations
- Blunt:
  - Less common in children (1–8% of all blunt pediatric trauma)
  - Lower chance of intestinal injury in vehicular accidents when both shoulder and lap belts are worn.
  - Be cautious of nonpenetrating trauma: Air-gun accidents at close range (<10 feet)
  - Consider the possibility of nonaccidental trauma.

## DIAGNOSIS

### SIGNS AND SYMPTOMS
- Delays in diagnosis are common.
- Presence of a "seatbelt sign" doubles the risk for small-bowel injury.
- Initial presentation may be mild:
  - Uniformly, patients will progress to serious signs/symptoms.
- Delays in diagnosis add to morbidity and mortality:
  - Mortality is 2% when diagnosis is made within 8 hr, 31% when made after 24 hr.

#### History
- History of blunt or penetrating abdominal trauma
- Must consider in ill children without a definite history of trauma (child abuse)

#### Physical Exam
- In awake, alert patients look for:
  - Abdominal tenderness (87–98%)
  - Abdominal pain (85%)
  - Peritoneal signs (67%)
- Many patients will have:
  - Abdominal wall bruising (54%)
  - Hypotension (38%)
  - Guaiac-positive rectal exam (5%)
- Small-bowel injury may initially be obscured by abnormal mental status, severe associated injuries.
- Small-bowel injury not initially apparent may be indicated by:
  - Progressive abdominal pain
  - Intestinal obstruction
  - Decreased urine output
  - Tachycardia

### ESSENTIAL WORKUP
- Initial physical exam should note all wounds and areas of tenderness.
- CT for all medically stable patients
- Serial abdominal exam and vital signs even after "negative" CT
- For medically unstable patients, diagnostic peritoneal lavage (DPL) is superior to US in determining presence of a hollow viscus injury.

### DIAGNOSTIC TESTS & INTERPRETATION
#### Lab
- No diagnostic test has proven highly sensitive in the prediction of small-bowel injury.
- Serum amylase, lipase, and liver function tests have poor sensitivity for acute injury.

#### Imaging
- Plain radiography of chest/abdomen:
  - Not useful for small-bowel injury
  - Incidence of pneumoperitoneum visible on plain radiograph is only 8%.
- CT:
  - Diagnostic standard for solid-organ injury and head trauma but is less sensitive for hollow viscous injuries
  - Newest-generation helical CT scanners have a sensitivity of 88% and a specificity of 99%.
  - The benefits of oral contrast are controversial.
  - Blunt trauma:
    - Used in stable patients
    - Indications in blunt trauma include abdominal distention, absent bowel sounds, blood in the nasogastric tube, abdominal abrasions or contusions, gross hematuria, lap belt injury, assault/abuse as mechanism, abdominal tenderness, trauma score <12.
    - Specific signs for small-bowel injury on CT are pneumoperitoneum (sensitivity 50–75%) and extravasation of contrast (sensitivity 12%).
    - Signs on CT suggestive of small-bowel injury include unexplained free intraperitoneal fluid (most sensitive 73%), thickened bowel wall >3 mm (61% sensitive), intramural hematomas (75–88% sensitive), interloop fluid, mesenteric streaking.
  - Penetrating: CT is not recommended because sensitivity is only 14%; false-negative result rate is 18%.
- US: Not sensitive in hollow viscous injury because air in bowel makes visualization difficult

#### Diagnostic Procedures/Surgery
- DPL:
  - Invasive but may helpful in unstable patients or in patients with clinically suspicious but nondiagnostic abdominal CT
  - Sensitive for hemoperitoneum but not source of bleeding
  - Positive if RBC count of >100,000/mm³
  - Lavage amylase >20 IU/L and leukocyte count >500/mm³ (late markers of small-bowel injury)
  - Lavage microscopy for succus/vegetable matter/feces is specific for small-bowel injury but not sensitive.
  - Lavage alkaline phosphatase (>3 IU/L) is reported to be a useful immediate marker of small-bowel injury.
- Laparoscopy: Plays a key role in diagnosing small-bowel injury in stable patients with progressive signs or symptoms

## DIFFERENTIAL DIAGNOSIS

- Hemoperitoneum owing to vascular insult
- Solid visceral organ injury or gastric/colon/rectum perforation
- Vertebral injury and associated ileus

### Pediatric Considerations

Delay in diagnosis of 1–2 days is common and increases morbidity.

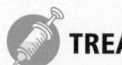

## TREATMENT

### PRE-HOSPITAL

#### ALERT

- Patients should be transported to the nearest trauma center.
- Do not attempt to replace eviscerated abdominal contents; cover with moist gauze, blanket, and transport.
- Do not remove impaled objects in the abdomen; stabilize the object with gauze and tape and transport.

### INITIAL STABILIZATION/THERAPY

- Standard advanced trauma life support protocols, including airway, breathing, and circulation management
- Aggressive fluid resuscitation, central line suggested with pressure infusion of warmed IV fluid (lactated Ringer solution or normal saline)
- Cover eviscerated small bowel with moist gauze; do not remove impaled foreign body in ED.

### ED TREATMENT/PROCEDURES

- Immediate transfer to OR is required for patients with an indication for laparotomy:
  - Evisceration
    Abdominal pain with hypotension
  - Positive diagnostic peritoneal lavage or abdominal CT
  - Thoracic abdominal herniation visualized on chest radiograph
  - Impaled foreign body
  - Penetrating gunshot wound to the abdomen
  - Tetanus and antibiotic prophylaxis should be given for penetrating abdominal wounds and blunt injury requiring surgical exploration.

- Local wound exploration is safe for abdominal stab wounds.
- Serial abdominal exams and observation for otherwise stable patients
- Judicious analgesia as BP permits after diagnosis is established

### MEDICATION

- Cefotetan (Cefotan): 1–2 g (peds: 20 mg/kg) IV or
- Cefoxitin (Mefoxin): 1–2 g (peds: 40 mg/kg) IV or
- Ceftizoxime (Cefizox): 1–2 g (peds: 50 mg/kg) IV plus
- Flagyl: 500 mg (peds: 7.5 mg/kg) IV

## FOLLOW-UP

### DISPOSITION

#### Admission Criteria

- Indication for laparotomy
- Abnormal mental status/intoxication with abdominal injury
- Presence of abdominal pain, tenderness (even with a negative workup) mandates admission for observation and serial exams
- Stab and gunshot wounds that violate the abdominal fascia, positive DPL, or worsening findings on clinical exam

#### Discharge Criteria

- Minimal mechanism blunt trauma in a sober patient with normal exam result who has no abdominal pain and will receive adequate follow-up
- Explicit discharge instructions to return for worsening signs/symptoms are important to identify those with unsuspected injury.
- Penetrating wounds that do not violate abdominal fascia

### FOLLOW-UP RECOMMENDATIONS

Discharged patients who develop abdominal complaints should return promptly to the ED.

## PEARLS AND PITFALLS

- Small bowel injury should be considered in any blunt/penetrating abdominal trauma victim.
- Initial presentation of patients with small-bowel injuries may be unimpressive.
- Presence of a "seatbelt sign" doubles the risk for small-bowel injury.

- CT scanning may miss a significant percentage of small-bowel injuries.
- Observation and serial exams are an important aspect of detecting occult injuries.

## ADDITIONAL READING

- ACEP Policies Committee. Critical Issues in the evaluation of adult patients presenting to the emergency department with acute blunt abdominal trauma. *Ann Emerg Med.* 2004;43(2):278–290.
- Avarello JT, Cantor RM. Pediatric major trauma: An approach to evaluation and management. *Emerg Med Clin North Am.* 2007:25(3).
- CDC Fact Sheet "Blast Injuries: Abdominal Blast Injuries" 2009. Available at www.emergency.cdc. gov/Blastinjuries
- Cordle R, Cantor R. Pediatric trauma. In: Rosen P, et al., eds., *Rosen's emergency medicine: Concepts and clinical practice*, 7th ed. St. Louis: CV Mosby, 2009.
- Fakhry SM, Brownstein M, Watts DD, et al. Relatively short diagnostic delays (<8 hours) produce morbidity and mortality in blunt small bowel injury: An analysis of time to operative intervention in 198 patients from a multicenter experience. *J Trauma.* 2000;48:408–415.
- Gross E, Martel M. Multiple trauma. In: Rosen P, et al., eds., *Rosen's emergency medicine: Concepts and clinical practice*, 7th ed. St. Louis: CV Mosby, 2009.
- Hanks PW, Brody JM. Blunt injury to mesentery and small bowel: CT evaluation. *Rad Clin North Am.* 2003;41(6):1171–1182.
- Herr S, Fallat ME. Abusive abdominal and thoracic trauma. *Clin Ped Emerg Med.* 2006;7:149–152.
- Sikka R. Unsuspected internal organ traumatic injuries. *Emerg Med Clin North Am.* 2004;22(4): 1067–1180.

## CODES

### ICD9

- 863.20 Injury to small intestine, unspecified site, without open wound into cavity
- 863.30 Injury to small intestine, unspecified site, with open wound into cavity

# SMOKE INHALATION

*Trevonne M. Thompson*

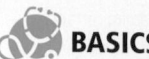 **BASICS**

## DESCRIPTION
- Suspect smoke inhalation in anyone involved in a fire within a closed space or with a history of loss of consciousness.
- May cause direct injury to the upper (supraglottic) airway structures
- May cause chemical/irritant effect to lower airway structures
- May cause systemic toxicity from inhaled substances

## ETIOLOGY
- Direct heat injury from heated gases/smoke:
  - Limited to supraglottic structures because of the heat-dissipating properties of the upper airway
- Irritant effect from smoke components
- Systemic toxicity from inhaled cellular toxins:
  - Carbon monoxide
  - Hydrogen cyanide

### ALERT
Inhalation of steam can be rapidly fatal:
- Steam has approximately 4,000 times the heat-carrying capacity of hot air.
- Can rapidly cause obstructive glottic edema, thermally induced tracheitis, and hemorrhagic edema of the bronchial mucosa

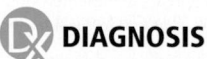 **DIAGNOSIS**

## SIGNS AND SYMPTOMS
### History
- Exposure to a fire or heavy smoke
- Typically in a confined space
- Maintain high index of suspicion with history of loss of consciousness

### Physical Exam
- May have a normal physical examination with symptoms developing during the 24-hr interval following exposure
- Upper airway (supraglottic):
  - Nasopharyngeal irritation
  - Hoarseness
  - Stridor
  - Cough
- Lower airway:
  - Chest discomfort
  - Hemoptysis
  - Bronchospasm
  - Bronchorrhea
- May have symptoms and signs of carbon monoxide and/or cyanide toxicity

### ALERT
The following signs are suggestive of significant inhalation injury:
- Facial and upper cervical burns
- Carbonaceous sputum
- Singed eyebrows and nasal vibrissae

## ESSENTIAL WORKUP
- Pulse oximetry:
  - May be falsely elevated in cases of carbon monoxide exposure
- ABG measurement:
  - Hypoxia
  - Metabolic acidosis in cases of carbon monoxide or hydrogen cyanide
- Chest radiography:
  - Initial radiograph typically normal
  - May show signs of pulmonary injury over the next 24 hr

## DIAGNOSTIC TESTS & INTERPRETATION
### Lab
- Electrolytes, BUN, creatinine, glucose
- CBC
- Coagulation profile
- Creatine phosphokinase when indicated in burn patients
- Carboxyhemoglobin to evaluate for potential carbon monoxide exposure
- Cyanide level:
  - In suspected cases of cyanide exposure, do not wait for the level before initiating therapy.
  - May send lactate level as a marker of cyanide toxicity
- Pregnancy test

### Diagnostic Procedures/Surgery
- Peak expiratory flow rate:
  - Low peak flow associated with more severe injury
- $PaO_2/FiO_2$ ratio:
  - A ratio of <300 after initial resuscitation is associated with the development of respiratory failure.

## DIFFERENTIAL DIAGNOSIS
- Irritant gas exposure
- Asphyxiant gas exposure
- Cardiogenic pulmonary edema
- COPD exacerbation
- Asthma exacerbation
- Pneumonia

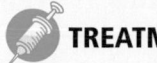 **TREATMENT**

**PRE-HOSPITAL**
- 100% oxygen by face mask
- Intubation for patients with agonal breathing
- Rapid transport to ED for those with stridor:
  - May need advanced airway management
- Albuterol nebulizer therapy for bronchospasm

**INITIAL STABILIZATION/THERAPY**
- 100% oxygen via face mask
- Intubation:
  - Respiratory distress:
- Drooling
- Stridor:
  - Refractory hypoxia
  - CNS depression
  - Significant facial/upper airway burns
- Establish IV access.

**ED TREATMENT/PROCEDURES**
- Inhaled or nebulized albuterol as needed for bronchospasm
- Corticosteroids as needed for patients with history of asthma or COPD
- Intubated patients:
  - Low endotracheal tube cuff pressure
  - Frequent suctioning
  - Positive end-expiratory pressure
- If indicated, treat for carbon monoxide toxicity:
  - 100% oxygen
  - Hyperbaric oxygen in appropriate cases when available
- If indicated, treat for cyanide toxicity:
  - 100% oxygen
  - Sodium nitrite
- Use with caution in cases of significant carbon monoxide exposure:
  - Sodium thiosulfate
  - Hydroxycobalamin

**MEDICATION**
- Albuterol nebulization: 2.5–5 mg in 2.5 mL of normal saline q20min:
  - Alternatively, 15 mg nebulizer treatment continuous over 1 hr
- Methylprednisolone 125 mg IV (peds: 1–2 mg/kg)
- Prednisone: 40–60 mg PO (peds: 1–2 mg/kg)
- Sodium thiosulfate 12.5 g (50 mL of 25% solution) slow IV infusion (peds: 412.5 mg/kg or 1.65 mL/kg of 25% solution)
- Hydroxycobalamin 5 g IV infused over 15 min (peds: 70 mg/kg)

 **FOLLOW-UP**

**DISPOSITION**
*Admission Criteria*
- Intubated
- Significant associated burns
- Persistent dyspnea, hoarseness, odynophagia, carbonaceous sputum
- Persistent cough
- Asthma/COPD with bronchospasm
- Significant carbon monoxide or cyanide exposure
- Comorbid medical illnesses

*Discharge Criteria*
- Minimal exposure history
- Asymptomatic
- Significant exposure history, asymptomatic after 4–6 hr observation

*Issues for Referral*
- In cases of significant associated burn injuries, transfer to burn facility as appropriate.
- In cases of significant carbon monoxide toxicity, transfer to hyperbaric oxygen facility as appropriate.

**FOLLOW-UP RECOMMENDATIONS**
Burn follow-up for patients with associated burns.

## PEARLS AND PITFALLS

- In suspected cases of cyanide exposure, do not wait for the level before initiating therapy.
- Order carboxyhemoglobin to evaluate for potential carbon monoxide exposure.

## ADDITIONAL READING

- American Burn Association. Inhalation injury: Diagnosis. *J Am Coll Surg*. 2003;196(2):307–312.
- Lee-chiong TL. Smoke inhalation injury. *Postgrad Med*. 1999;105(2):55–62.
- Miller K, Chang A. Acute inhalation injury. *Emerg Med Clin North Am*. 2003;21(2):533–557.

**See Also (Topic, Algorithm, Electronic Media Element)**
- Carbon Monoxide
- Cyanide
- Hyperbaric Oxygen

 **CODES**

**ICD9**
987.9 Toxic effect of unspecified gas, fume, or vapor

S

# SNAKE ENVENOMATION

Adam Black
Timothy B. Erickson

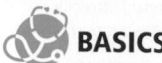 **BASICS**

## DESCRIPTION
- Pit viper venom:
  - Mixture of proteolytic enzymes and thrombin-like esterases:
    - Enzymes cause local muscle and subcutaneous tissue necrosis.
    - Esterases have anticoagulant effect, leading to disseminated intravascular coagulation (DIC) in severe envenomations.
- Bite location:
  - Head or trunk bite more severe than bite on extremities
  - Lower extremity bites may have delayed presentation.
- Severe envenomation:
  - Direct bite into artery or vein
  - All coral snake venom (primarily neurotoxic)
- Bite mark significance:
  - Venomous snake: classically includes one or two puncture marks
  - Nonvenomous snake: horseshoe-shaped row of multiple teeth marks
- 25% of all pit viper bites are dry and do not result in envenomation.

## ETIOLOGY
### Venomous snakes indigenous to the U.S.
- Pit vipers:
  - Account for 95% of all envenomations
- Rattlesnakes, cottonmouths, and copperheads
- Coral snakes (Elapidae):
  - More severe envenomations
  - Western coral snakes, found in Arizona and New Mexico
  - More venomous eastern coral snakes, found in Carolinas and Gulf states

### International exotic venomous snakes
North American bites occur in zoos owing to illegal importation/smuggling

### Pediatric Considerations
- Small children are the most likely targets for snake envenomations.
- Those who freeze with fear in response to snake are also more susceptible to multiple envenomations.
- Because of their low body weight, smaller children and infants are more vulnerable to severe envenomation.

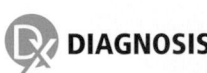 **DIAGNOSIS**

## SIGNS AND SYMPTOMS
- Local:
  - Classic skin changes:
    - One or two puncture wounds
    - Pain and swelling at site
  - Swelling and edema of involved extremity:
    - Within 1 hr in severe envenomations
    - Tender proximal lymph nodes
  - Ecchymosis, petechiae, and hemorrhagic vesicles develop within several hours.

- Systemic:
  - Weakness
  - Diaphoresis
  - Dizziness
  - Nausea
  - Scalp paresthesias
  - Periorbital fasciculations
  - Metallic taste
  - Severe bites can lead to:
    - Coagulopathies and DIC
    - Hypotension
    - Shock
    - Pulmonary edema
    - Hematuria
    - Rhabdomyolysis
    - Renal failure
    - Cardiac dysfunction
    - Thrombocytopenia
  - Potential compartment syndrome in involved extremity
  - Coral snake venom:
    - Primarily neurotoxic, leading to weakness, diplopia, confusion, delayed respiratory depression
    - Local effects may be deceivingly minimal.

### History
- Description of snake
- Geographic location of bite

### Physical Exam
Search for manifestations of bites as described above.

## ESSENTIAL WORKUP
- Careful exam of wound site and involved extremity:
  - Essential in judging severity of envenomation
- Assess for anaphylactic reactions

## DIAGNOSTIC TESTS & INTERPRETATION
### Lab
- CBC
- PT/PTT
- DIC panel
- Electrolytes, BUN/creatinine, glucose
- Creatine phosphokinase (CPK)
- UA
- Type and cross-match with moderate to severe envenomation.

### Imaging
Plain radiographs if foreign body suspected

## DIFFERENTIAL DIAGNOSIS
- Nonpoisonous snakes:
  - Smooth, tapered body
  - Narrow head
  - Round pupils
  - No rattles
- Pit vipers:
  - Triangular or arrow-shaped head
  - Vertical or elliptical pupils
  - Rattles

- Coral snakes (applies only in the U.S., not internationally):
  - "Red on yellow—kill a fellow"
  - "Red on black—venom lack"

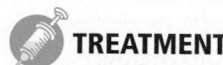 **TREATMENT**

## PRE-HOSPITAL
- Retreat well beyond striking range of snake.
- Immobilize extremity in functional position at level of heart.
- Keep physical activity minimal.
- Remove rings, watches, and all constrictive clothing.
- If snake is killed, transport in closed container:
  - If snake is indigenous to region, positive identification not essential.
  - Even severed head can envenomate.
- Controversies:
  - Incision and suction of bite wound is not recommended:
    - Can lead to further wound contamination with human mouth flora.
    - Incision attempts by inexperienced can lead to severe tendon, nerve, and vascular damage.
  - Tourniquets, cryotherapy, and electrocautery:
    - Contraindicated owing to tissue damage
  - Although mechanical suction devices do exist, no clinical trials support their use.

### Pediatric Considerations
- Increased urgency in transport to hospital setting is indicated:
- Envenomation more likely to be severe
- Severity due to relatively low body weight of small child

## INITIAL STABILIZATION/THERAPY
- Airway, breathing, and circulation management (ABCs)
- Vigorous hydration with 0.9% normal saline (NS) to maintain intravascular volume and renal blood flow
- Monitor
- Immobilize bitten extremity

## ED TREATMENT/PROCEDURES
- Supportive care
- Monitor for compartment syndrome:
  - Repeated measurements of extremity circumference every 15–20 min until local progression/swelling subsides.
  - A true compartment syndrome is unlikely following rattlesnake envenomation.
  - Prophylactic fasciotomy and digital dermatomy rarely indicated.
  - Surgical therapy considered only in cases where elevated compartment pressures have been documented despite aggressive antivenom therapy.

- Analgesia
- Tetanus prophylaxis if needed
- Broad-spectrum antibiotics for moderate to severe envenomations
- Steroids not indicated except for reactions to antivenin (see below)
- Wound severity:
  - Minimal:
    ○ Local swelling and tenderness
  - Moderate:
    ○ Extremity swelling
    ○ Evidence of systemic toxicity
  - Severe:
    ○ Obvious toxicity
    ○ Unstable vital signs
    ○ Coagulopathy
    ○ Coral snake, Mojave rattlesnake
    ○ Lab abnormalities

### Antivenom
- Indications for Crotalid antivenom therapy:
  - Significant extremity swelling
  - Clinical signs of systemic toxicity
  - Unstable vital signs
  - Lab evidence of coagulopathy
- CroFab:
  - Fundamental treatment for pit viper envenomation
  - High-affinity purified ovine Fab antibody fragment antivenin
  - Minimizes hypersensitivity reactions
  - Dosing: four to six vials regardless of patient size; may require two to four additional vials if symptoms persist
  - CroFab vials dissolved in 250–500 mL 0.9% NS, infused over 30–60 min
  - Crotaline Fab equally effective and safer than the older polyvalent antivenin product, resulting in reduced rates of allergic reaction.
    ○ In the event that Fab antivenom is not available, treat with traditional Crotalidae antivenin equine formulation (below)
- Crotalidae antivenin:
  - Second-line treatment for pit viper envenomation
  - Effective for rattlesnakes, cottonmouths, and copperheads
  - Most effective if given within 4–6 hr of bite
  - Skin test with diluted horse serum (in antivenin kit) before antivenin administration suggested
  - Treatment complications include anaphylaxis and serum sickness.
  - Dosage (each vial contains 10 mL of antivenin) by wound severity:
    ○ Minimal/moderate: 10 vials
    ○ Severe: 15–20 vials
  - Victims of severe envenomations who develop positive skin test:
    ○ May still receive antivenin
    ○ Pretreat with diphenhydramine and corticosteroids.
    ○ Monitor closely for anaphylaxis with epinephrine at bedside.

- Coral snake antivenin:
  - Effective against more toxic eastern coral snake but not against western coral snakes
  - After proper skin testing, 3–5 vials of antivenin recommended.
  - Treatment complications include anaphylaxis and serum sickness.
  - Coral snake venom is are neurotoxic; watch for respiratory depression, control airway
- International exotic venomous snakes:
  - Specific antivenins may be available at local zoos.

### Treatment Assistance
- Contact local poison control center 800-222-1222, local zoo, or regional herpetologist.
- Call Antivenom Index at 602-626-6016 in Tucson, Arizona, for assistance in treatment of exotic snakes not indigenous to the U.S.

### Pediatric Considerations
- Proportionally more antivenin per body weight
- Standard adult doses often required

### Pregnancy Considerations
- If mother has systemic signs of envenomation toxicity, fetus is also at risk; timely antivenom therapy is still indicated.
- Consult obstetrical specialist.

 FOLLOW-UP

### DISPOSITION
#### Admission Criteria
- 24-hr observation for patients requiring antivenin administration after pit viper bites or Mojave rattlesnake envenomations
- ICU admission for:
  - Evidence of moderate to severe envenomation, especially in children
  - All victims of coral snake bites, symptomatic exotic snake envenomations

#### Discharge Criteria
Suspicious bite that shows no signs or symptoms of envenomation for 6–8 hr and has normal lab panel:
- Discharge with follow-up in 24 hr.
- Observe lower extremity bites for up to 12 hr because of possible delayed toxicity.
- Coral snake and Mojave rattlesnake bites may require 24-hr observation period.
- Dry bites occur in up to 25% of pit viper bites.

### FOLLOW-UP RECOMMENDATIONS
PCP or Toxicology follow up 1 wk after antivenom therapy to assess for possible serum sickness or envenomation wound infection.

## PEARLS AND PITFALLS
- Avoid overly aggressive prehospital care interventions; best to rapidly transport to closest medical center.
- Be sure to administer proper dose of antivenom in a timely fashion when clinically indicated.

## ADDITIONAL READING
- Corneille MG, Larson S, Stewet R, et al. A large single-center experience with treatment of patients with crotalid envenomations: Outcomes with an evolution of antivenom therapy. *Am J Surg.* 2006;192:848–852.
- Cox M, Reeves J, Smith K. Concepts in Crotalidae snake envenomation management. *Orthopedics.* 2006;29(12)1083–1087.
- Dart RC, McNally J. Efficacy, safety, and use of snake antivenoms in the United States. *Ann Emerg Med.* 2001;37:181–188.
- Fezelat J, Teperman S, Tougher M. Recurrent hemorrhage after western diamondback rattlesnake envenomation treated with crotalidae polyvalent immune fab (ovine). *Clin Toxicol.* 2008;46(9): 823–827.
- Lavonas EJ, Gerardo CJ, O'Malley G, et al. Safety and efficacy of Crotalidae polyvalent immune Fab in pediatric crotaline envenomations. *Acad Emerg Med.* 2007;14:373–376.
- Offerman SR, Barry JD, Richardson WH, et al. Subcutaneous crotalidine Fab antivenom for the treatment of rattlesnake envenomation in a porcine model. *Clin Toxicol.* 2009;47(1):61–68.
- Simpson ID, Jacobsen IM. Antisnake venom production crisis—Who told us it was uneconomic and unsustainable? *Wild Environ Med.* 2009;20(2):144–155
- Soghoian SE, Olsen D, Hatall BA, et al. Subcutaneous crotaline Fab administration in a model of rattlesnake envenomation. *Clin Toxicol.* 2009;47(6):605.

 CODES

### ICD9
989.5 Toxic effect of venom

# SPIDER BITE, BLACK WIDOW
*Tarlan Hedayati*

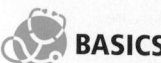 **BASICS**

## DESCRIPTION
- Syndromes caused by envenomation by black widow spider bite
- Mechanism of toxicity:
  - Females are responsible for human envenomations
  - Venom contains potent neurotoxin, $\alpha$-latrotoxin:
    - Causes cation-channel opening presynaptically, resulting in increased neurotransmitter release into synapses and neuromuscular junctions.
    - Increased neurotransmitter release causes increased neurologic, motor, and autonomic effects.
- Morbidity and mortality are dose dependent.
- Severity of envenomation depends on:
  - Premorbid health of victim:
    - HTN or cardiovascular disease increase risk
  - Size and age of victim:
    - Children (ie, smaller size for a given dose of venom) are at greater risk of morbidity and mortality.
  - Number of bites
  - Location of bite wounds
  - Size and condition of spider
- Rarely fatal

## ETIOLOGY
Black widow spider features:
- Appearance:
  - Glossy black with red markings shaped like an hourglass or a pair of spots on the ventral aspect of the globular abdomen
  - Females have 25–50-mm leg spans and 15-mm-long bodies.
- Found throughout North America, except the far north and Alaska
- Prefer dark sheltered hideaways such as garages, barns, outhouses, woodpiles, and low-lying foliage
- Most bites occur during the warmer months when spiders are defending their webs and egg clutches.

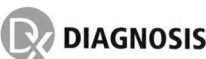 **DIAGNOSIS**

## SIGNS AND SYMPTOMS
### History
- History of spider bite very unreliable and species usually not identified
- Bite:
  - Described as a pinprick or pinch, if felt at all
- Local complaints (within minutes of bite)
  - Pain:
    - Sharp, burning at the bite site
    - Usually resolves spontaneously within minutes or hours
    - May become worse and spread proximally from the bite

- Systemic complaints (within 15–60 min):
  - Cardiac:
    - Palpitations
    - Chest pain or tightness
  - Pulmonary:
    - Shortness of breath
    - Cough
  - Neuromuscular:
    - Headache
    - Dizziness
    - Painful regional muscle cramps and spasms
    - Cramping may progress to larger muscle groups
    - Arm bites may lead to arm and chest muscle tightness and dyspnea
    - Leg bites may lead to abdominal pain and leg spasms
    - Cutaneous dysesthesias and hyperesthesias
    - Localized or diffuse diaphoresis
  - GI:
    - Nausea, vomiting
    - Abdominal pain
  - Genitourinary:
    - Painful persistent erection
  - Gynecologic:
    - Pregnant patients may develop uterine contractions and preterm labor
  - Skin:
    - Pruritus
  - Psychiatric:
    - Anxiety
    - Sense of impending doom

### Physical Exam
- Vital signs may be abnormal:
  - HTN or hypotension
  - Tachycardia or bradycardia
  - Fever
  - Tachypnea
- Cardiac:
  - Dysrhythmias
  - Myocarditis
- Pulmonary:
  - Bronchorrhea
  - Pulmonary edema
  - Respiratory failure:
    - Usually due to respiratory muscle weakness
- Abdomen:
  - Rigidity
- Genitourinary:
  - Priapism
- Neurologic findings:
  - Tetanic contractions, fasciculations or tremors of extremities
  - Spasm and rigidity in large muscle groups
  - Autonomic instability
  - Seizure
- Skin:
  - Local
    - 2 pinpricks from the spider's fangs
    - Tender and blanched skin with surrounding erythema ("target lesion")
    - Swelling
    - Localized sweating

- Diffuse:
  - Urticaria
  - Piloerection
  - Generalized diaphoresis
- Psychiatric:
  - Acute toxic psychosis
  - Agitation or restlessness

## ESSENTIAL WORKUP
Diagnosis is based on:
- Clinical presentation
- Careful inquiry to elicit spider bite history
- Identification of spider (if possible)

## DIAGNOSTIC TESTS & INTERPRETATION
### Lab
- No specific blood tests for black widow spider venom
- CBC:
  - WBC may be mildly
- Electrolytes, calcium,
- BUN, creatinine
- Lipase, LFTs
- Creatine kinase:
  - Elevated in patients with significant muscle spasm
- Cardiac enzymes
- Pregnancy test
- Urinalysis:
  - May demonstrate albuminuria
- ABGs in rare cases with pulmonary edema
- ECG and cardiac monitoring for:
  - Patients with known cardiac disease
  - Patients with chest pain, unstable vital signs or dysrhythmias
  - May show digitalis effect transiently

### Imaging
- CXR for respiratory complaints
- Abdominal imaging to rule out other causes of pain

## DIFFERENTIAL DIAGNOSIS
- Acute surgical abdomen (eg, appendicitis, cholecystitis, pancreatitis, AAA)
- Ureterolithiasis/nephrolithiasis
- Sympathomimetics (eg, cocaine, amphetamines)
- Hypocalcemia
- Tetanus
- Muscular injury or strain
- Hypertensive emergency
- MI/acute coronary syndrome
- Anxiety disorder
- Allergic reaction

**TREATMENT**

### PRE-HOSPITAL
- ABCs/ACLS
- Immobilize the wound site and apply cool compresses or ice for comfort during transport to hospital.
- Supportive measures (analgesics, anxiolytics) may be required for patients with systemic symptoms.
- Negative-pressure venom extraction devices have not been recommended for widow spider bites
- Every effort should be made by caregivers at the scene to find and bring in the responsible spider for identification.

### INITIAL STABILIZATION/THERAPY
- ABCs
- ACLS as needed
- Fetal monitoring for pregnant patients

### ED TREATMENT/PROCEDURES
- Clean the bite site thoroughly
- Tetanus prophylaxis
- Antiemetics for nausea and vomiting
- Analgesics
- Antihistamines
- Benzodiazepines for agitation and restlessness
- Muscle cramps/spasm therapy:
  - Benzodiazepines
  - Narcotics
- Antihypertensive agents for symptomatic HTN
- Antivenin:
  - Elicit history of allergy to horse or horse serum
  - Indications:
    - Moderate to severe symptoms that do not respond to symptomatic measures
    - Significant HTN
    - Respiratory distress
    - Symptomatic and pregnant
    - Priapism
    - Severe rhabdomyolysis
    - Compartment syndrome
    - Seizures
  - Perform a skin test for sensitivity to horse serum prior to antivenin administration (test kit included in the antivenin package).
  - Watch for type I immediate hypersensitivity reaction in 1st 20 min:
    - Occurs in up to 25% of recipients
    - Consider pretreatment with antihistamines or SC epinephrine 1:1,000
    - Treat anaphylactic reactions with steroids, antihistamines, epinephrine, and cardiopulmonary support
  - Due to the small quantity of antivenin used, if serum sickness reactions occur, they are usually mild.
  - Effectiveness is usually apparent within 2 hr of the 1st treatment and repeated doses are rarely necessary.
  - Antivenin may help prevent persistent neuropathic symptoms

### MEDICATION
- Antivenin: 1 ampule (2.5 mL) diluted into 50–250 mL NS (peds: Same dose) IV over 1 hr
- Diphenhydramine: 10–50 mg IV or IM q6–8h (peds: 5 mg/kg/day divided q.i.d.)
- Lorazepam: 1–2 mg IV or IM (peds 0.01 mg/kg IV or IM)
- Morphine sulfate: 2–10 mg (peds: 0.1 mg/kg) IV or IM PRN (titrate to patient response)
- Sodium nitroprusside: 0.5–10 mcg/kg/min if diastolic >120 mm Hg
- Tetanus prophylaxis

 **FOLLOW-UP**

### DISPOSITION
#### Admission Criteria
- Pediatric, elderly, pregnant or symptomatic patients
- Significant cardiovascular symptoms and signs, or severe HTN, particularly in presence of premorbid cardiac disease or chronic HTN
- Respiratory distress or pulmonary edema
- Persistent symptoms not responding to aggressive management and specific antivenin

#### Discharge Criteria
- Asymptomatic patients with no positive identification of a black widow spider can be released after observation for 1–2 hr.
- Asymptomatic patients with no comorbid illness with a positive identification of the black widow spider should be observed for a minimum of 4–6 hr and discharged if their condition does not change.
- All discharged patients must be instructed to watch for the following symptoms and to seek appropriate follow up:
  - Hematuria
  - Rash
  - Joint pain
  - Lymphadenopathy
  - Shortness of breath
  - Signs of infection
- Discharged patients who received antivenin should be instructed to watch for signs of serum sickness:
  - Type III delayed hypersensitivity
  - Uncommon
    Occurs 5 days–3 wk post treatment
  - Treat with antihistamines and steroids

#### Issues for Referral
Toxicology consult for patients requiring admission or antivenin administration

### FOLLOW-UP RECOMMENDATIONS
- In most untreated patients, symptoms peak after 2–3 hr and then begin to resolve, occasionally recurring episodically over the following few days.
- In otherwise healthy adults, complete resolution of symptoms occurs within 2–3 days
- Neurology follow-up if:
  - If persistent neurologic symptoms last weeks to months:
    - Fatigue
    - Generalized weakness or myalgias
    - Paresthesias
    - Headache
    - Insomnia
    - Impotence
    - Polyneuritis

## PEARLS AND PITFALLS
- Widow bites in infants may present as intractable crying
- A high fever and WBC count should prompt consideration of alternatives to spider bites (eg, infection)

## ADDITIONAL READING
- Boyer LV, Binford GJ, McNally JT. Spider bites. In: Auerbach, ed. *Wilderness Medicine*, 5th ed. Philadelphia: Mosby; 2007.
- Clark RF, Wethern-Kestner S, Vance MV, et al. Clinical presentation and treatment of black widow spider envenomation: A review of 163 cases. *Ann Emerg Med*. 1992;21(7):782–787.
- Otten EJ. Venomous animal injuries. In: Marx JA, Hockenberger RS, Walls RM, et al., eds. *Rosen's Emergency Medicine*, 7th ed. Philadelphia. Mosby; 2009.
- Weinstein SA, Dart R, Staples A, et al. Envenomations: An overview of clinical toxicology for the primary care physician. *Am Fam Physician*. 2009;80(8):793–802.

### See Also (Topic, Algorithm, Electronic Media Element)
Spider Bite, Brown Recluse

**CODE ICD-9-301** **CODES**

ICD9
989.5 Toxic effect of venom

**S**

# SPIDER BITE, BROWN RECLUSE
*Tarlan Hedayati*

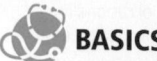 **BASICS**

## DESCRIPTION
Local or systemic illness caused by brown recluse spider bite envenomation

## ETIOLOGY
- Brown recluse spider (also known as fiddleback spiders) features:
  - Appearance:
    ○ Delicate body and legs spanning 10–25 mm
    ○ Tan- to dark-brown with darker violin-shaped marking visible on the upper aspect of the head
    ○ 3 pairs of eyes
  - Found widely throughout the south-central part of the U.S.
  - Habitat: Typically warm and dry locations indoors or outdoors such as wood piles, bundles of rags, cellars, under rocks, or in attics
  - Bites are typically defensive
- Mechanism of toxicity:
  - Venom is a complex cocktail of enzymes and peptides that:
    ○ Binds to RBC and causes hemolysis
    ○ Causes prostaglandin release and activates complement cascade
    ○ Causes lipolysis and tissue necrosis
    ○ Triggers platelet aggregation and thrombosis
    ○ Triggers allergic response to venom antigenic properties
    ○ May lead to shock and DIC in rare cases
  - Toxicity proportional to:
    ○ The amount of venom relative to the size of patient
    ○ Location of envenomation on the body

### Pediatric Considerations
- Children are more vulnerable to a given amount of venom than healthy adults
- Fatality more common in children due to severe intravascular hemolysis

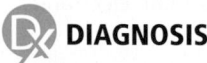 **DIAGNOSIS**

## SIGNS AND SYMPTOMS
Diagnosis is based not only on the clinical presentation but also on a reliable history of a spider bite.

### History
- An isolated cutaneous lesion is the most common presentation
- Bite sites are usually located in areas under clothing where spider gets trapped between clothing and skin

- Local wound symptom onset:
  - Bite onset is usually asymptomatic, but some may report burning or stinging sensation
  - 1–24 hr later, patients may report aching or pruritis locally
- Systemic features:
  - Rare complication
  - More common in children than adults
  - Develop during the 1st 1–3 days postenvenomation.
  - Patient may report:
    ○ Fever, chills
    ○ Weakness, malaise
    ○ Nausea, vomiting, diarrhea
    ○ Dyspnea
    ○ Myalgias, muscle cramps, arthralgias
    ○ Jaundice
    ○ Petechial or urticarial rash
    ○ Generalized pruritic rash
    ○ Hematuria or dark urine

### Physical Exam
- Bite wound:
  - Usually no visible injury if examined within 1st 1–3 days
  - There may be a pinprick lesion, local blanching and induration, or erythema.
  - Tissue injury may develop at bite site:
    ○ Initially, bite mark may be surrounded by edema
    ○ Next, an erythematous border will develop around a purple center with a thin ring of ischemia between the 2
    ○ Serous or hemorrhagic bullae may form in the center after 24–72 hr.
    ○ Blister may gradually enlarge and darken with the development of and eschar of skin and subcutaneous fat necrosis over 3–4 days.
    ○ Eschar sloughs off 2–5 wk later leaving an ulcer in its place
    ○ Necrosis develops most extensively where subcutaneous fat is greatest.
    ○ Lower extremity blisters may spread distally under the influence of gravity.
    ○ Local response is not dependent on the extent of envenomation and cannot be used to predict the likelihood or severity of subsequent systemic illness.
- Skin:
  - Jaundice
  - Petechia
  - Urticaria
  - Generalized maculopapular rash

## ESSENTIAL WORKUP
- Careful inquiry required to elicit the spider bite history
- Routine laboratory testing not necessary unless systemic toxicity present.

## DIAGNOSTIC TESTS & INTERPRETATION
### Lab
- Spider venom can be detected in skin lesions, but widespread clinical testing is not available yet.
- CBC
  - Hemolytic anemia
  - Thombocytopenia, particularly with DIC
  - Leukocytosis
- Electrolytes
  - Hyperkalemia or acidosis in renal failure
- BUN, creatinine
- Prothrombin time/partial thromboplastin test may be prolonged in DIC
- D-Dimer and fibrin degradation products may be elevated in DIC
- Fibrinogen may be decreased in DIC
- Urinalysis
  - Hemoglobinuria
  - Proteinuria

### Imaging
- CXR in systemic toxicity
- Soft-tissue radiograph of bite site

## DIFFERENTIAL DIAGNOSIS
- Angioedema
- Bacterial soft-tissue infection; MRSA
- Burn
- Cutaneous anthrax
- Diabetic ulcer
- Decubitus ulcer
- Erythema nodosum
- Fungal infection
- Gonococcal hemorrhagic lesion
- Herpes simplex
- Intravenous drug use or "skin popping"
- Vascular insufficiency with secondary ulcer
- Lyme disease
- Neoplastic lesion
- Other arachnid envenomation
- Poison ivy or oak
- Pyoderma gangrenosum
- Sporotrichosis
- Stevens-Johnson syndrome
- Thrombosis
- Vasculitis
- Warfarin use

**TREATMENT**

## PRE-HOSPITAL
- Loosely immobilize wound site.
- Elevate the affected extremity
- Cover bite with cool compresses.
- Transport to hospital when patient experiences immediate onset of symptoms.
- Supportive measures for patients with systemic symptoms

### ALERT
Every effort should be made by caregivers at the scene to find and bring in the responsible spider for identification.

## INITIAL STABILIZATION/THERAPY
IV fluids, oxygen, cardiac monitoring if the patient is experiencing signs of systemic collapse

## ED TREATMENT/PROCEDURES
- Cleanse the bite site thoroughly
- Tetanus prophylaxis
- Analgesics
- Antibiotics:
  - Appropriate if wound appears infected
  - Not indicated prophylactically
  - Antistaphylococcal
- Dapsone:
  - Controversial: Consider for severe toxicity.
  - Screen for G6PD deficiency before initiating
  - Monitor for methemoglobinemia, hemolysis, and leukopenia during therapy.
- Excision of necrotic wound:
  - Not indicated in the 1st 8 wk because may cause more severe ulcer formation
- Hemoglobinuria:
  - Treated with IV fluids and alkalinization
  - Monitor renal, fluid, and electrolyte status
- Dialysis for renal failure
- Pressors for shock state
- Specific antivenin:
  - Not commercially available
  - Not FDA approved for use in the U.S.
- Therapies requiring further investigation:
  - Topical or systemic steroids
  - Hyperbaric therapy (has been shown to decrease wound size in animal model)
  - Topical nitroglycerin
  - Negative pressure wound therapy, or vacuum-assisted closure

## MEDICATION
- Antibiotics
  - Clindamycin: 150–300 mg PO q6h (peds: 8–16 mg/kg/day PO divided QID)
  - Severe skin infections:
    - Vancomycin: 1g IVPB q12h (peds: 10 mg/kg q6h)
- Dapsone: Progressive dosage of 50–200 mg/day (peds: 2 mg/kg/24 h PO)
- Methylprednisolone: 125 mg IV bolus followed by prednisone 30–50 mg/d for 5 days (peds: methylprednisolone 1–2 mg/kg IV, prednisone 1–2 mg/kg PO)
- Morphine sulfate: 2–10 mg (peds: 0.1 mg/kg) IV or IM PRN

### Pediatric Considerations
- Use dapsone only in severe cases because of increased potential for side effects such as:
  - Hepatitis
  - Methemoglobinemia
  - Hemolytic anemia
  - Leukopenia

 **FOLLOW-UP**

## DISPOSITION
### Admission Criteria
- Significant local reaction or signs of systemic toxicity
- Lower threshold for children, patients with significant comorbidities

### Discharge Criteria
- No evidence of systemic toxicity or severe progression of local wound necrosis after envenomation
- Daily reassessment by primary physician, including blood work, until 3–4 days after envenomation to evaluate for systemic toxicity.
- Patients should be advised about prolonged course for skin healing with consideration for surgical excision after 8 wk.
- Patients should be advised about potential for extensive scarring, infection, and recurrent ulceration.

### Pediatric Considerations
Longer observation period or admission because of the higher mortality in this population

### Issues for Referral
Consider consultation with:
- General surgery or plastic surgery for wound management
- Hyperbaric specialist for wound management
- Toxicologist
- Nephrologist for cases of renal failure
- Intensivist in cases of shock or DIC

## FOLLOW-UP RECOMMENDATIONS
- Primary care physician for continued evaluation of wound
- General surgery or plastic surgery for management of complicated wounds
- Hyperbaric specialist for wound management

## PEARLS AND PITFALLS
- Remember the limited range of brown recluse spiders and the rarity of arachnidism as a cause of necrotic skin wounds.
- In the absence of a reliable spider bite by history, other diagnoses must be carefully sought and excluded.
- Be sure to screen for G6PD deficiency in as it causes methemoglobinemia and hemolysis in patients receiving dapsone.
- Have a low threshold for admitting pediatric patients, adults with systemic symptoms, or anyone with a large, painful, or infected wound.

## ADDITIONAL READING
- Furbee BR, et al. Brown recluse spider envenomation. *Clin Lab Med.* 2006;26(1):211–226.
- Mold JW, Thompson DM. Management of Brown Recluse Spider Bites in Primary Care. *J Am Board Fam Pract.* 2004;17:347–352.
- Swanson DL, Vetter RS. Bites of Brown Recluse Spiders and Suspected Necrotic Arachnidism. *New Eng J Med.* 2005;352:700–707.
- Wong SC, et al. Loxoscelism and negative pressure wound therapy (vacuum-assisted closure): a clinical case series. *American Surgeon.* 2009;75(11). 1128–1131.

### See Also (Topic, Algorithm, Electronic Media Element)
Spider Bite, Black Widow

**CODES**

ICD9
989.5 Toxic effect of venom

S

# SPINAL CORD SYNDROMES
*Judd L. Glasser*

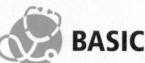

## BASICS

### DESCRIPTION
- Anterior cord syndrome:
  - Results from flexion or axial loading mechanism or direct cord compression from vertebral fractures, dislocations, disc herniation, tumor, or abscess
  - Rarely caused by laceration or thrombosis to the anterior spinal artery
- Brown-Séquard syndrome:
  - Hemisection of the spinal cord, classically as a result of a penetrating wound
  - Rarely unilateral cord compression
- Central cord syndrome:
  - Most commonly occurs in elderly patients who have preexisting cervical spondylosis and stenosis
  - Forced hyperextension causes buckling of the ligamentum flavum, creating a shearing injury to the central portion of the spinal cord.
- Dorsal cord syndrome:
  - Associated with hyperextension injuries
- Complete cord syndrome:
  - Blunt or penetrating trauma that results in complete disruption of spinal cord
  - Symptoms that remain >24 hr generally are permanent.

### ETIOLOGY
- Spinal cord syndromes result from localized disruption of neurotransmission and exhibit mixed motor and sensory deficits. The most common mechanism is trauma.
- Patients with arthritis, osteoporosis, metastatic disease, or other chronic spinal disorders are at risk of developing spinal injuries as the result of even minor trauma.

## DIAGNOSIS

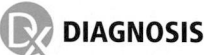

### SIGNS AND SYMPTOMS
#### History
Acute loss of motor and or sensory function usually following a traumatic event

#### Physical Exam
- Anterior cord syndrome:
  - Bilateral spastic paralysis and loss of pain and temperature sensation below the level of the lesion
  - Preservation of dorsal column function (proprioception and position sense)
- Brown-Séquard syndrome (lateral cord syndrome):
  - Ipsilateral spastic paresis and loss of dorsal column function (proprioception and position sense)
  - Contralateral loss of pain and temperature sensation
  - Deficits usually begin 2 levels below the injury.

- Central cord syndrome:
  - Loss of motor function affects upper extremities more severely than lower extremities.
  - Most profound deficits occur in the distal upper extremities.
  - Sensory loss is more variable.
- Dorsal cord syndrome:
  - Loss of proprioception, position sensation, and coordination below the level of the lesion
- Complete cord syndrome:
  - Flaccid paresis below the level of the injury
  - Low BP and heart rate, flushed skin, priapism may be present (loss of sympathetic tone).
- Sensory deficit levels:
  - C2: Occiput
  - C4: Clavicular region
  - C6: Thumb
  - C8: Little finger
  - T4: Nipple line
  - T10: Umbilicus
  - L1: Inguinal region
  - L5: Dorsum of the foot
  - S5: Perianal area
- Motor deficit levels:
  - C5: Elbow flexion
  - C7: Elbow extension
  - C8: Finger flexion
  - T1: Finger abduction
  - L2: Hip flexion
  - L3: Knee extension
  - L4: Ankle dorsiflexion
  - S1: Ankle plantar flexion

### ESSENTIAL WORKUP
- Detailed neurologic exam, focused on determining if any deficit exists and attempting to define the level of injury
- A neurosurgical consultation if deficit exists is recommended in most cases

### DIAGNOSTIC TESTS & INTERPRETATION
#### Lab
- Basic preoperative laboratory studies are indicated.
- Consider sedimentation rate and C-reactive protein to risk-stratify other potential diagnoses.

#### Imaging
All areas of clinical suspicion should be imaged with plain radiographs.

##### Geriatric Considerations
In cases in which plain radiographs may be difficult to interpret due to severe DJD, the use of CT may be more appropriate.
- CT of the spine when plain films are normal or ambiguous:
  - CT allows assessment of the spinal canal and any impingement by bone fragments.
- MRI is the imaging modality of choice for detection of spinal cord damage; in the acute setting, the indications for MRI are:
  - Neurologic deficits not explained by plain films or CT
  - Clinical progression of a spinal cord lesion
  - Determination of acute surgical candidacy
  - Disadvantages of MRI include
    - The inability to adequately monitor the patient while undergoing the study
    - The incompatibility with certain metal devices
    - The time to complete the exam

#### Diagnostic Procedures/Surgery
- Myelography is used with CT when MRI is not available or cannot be performed.
- A lumbar puncture may be required if considering Guillain-Barré, multiple sclerosis, or transverse myelitis.

### DIFFERENTIAL DIAGNOSIS
- Dorsal root injury
- Peripheral nerve injury
- Guillain-Barré syndrome
- Multiple sclerosis
- Transverse myelitis
- Epidural abscess
- Cerebral vascular accident

## TREATMENT

### PRE-HOSPITAL
- Full spinal immobilization
- IV access should be established for fluid resuscitation in the setting of neurogenic shock.
- Patients should be transported to the nearest trauma center:
  - Prompt evaluation and neurosurgical intervention may lead to a better outcome.

### Pediatric Considerations
Cervical collars must be the appropriate size for the child; splinting the head and body with towels and tape is a reasonable alternative.

### INITIAL STABILIZATION/THERAPY
- Spinal immobilization must be maintained at all times.
- Intubation must proceed with in-line spinal immobilization.
- IV fluids should be administered at maintenance levels unless shock is present:
  - Spinal trauma may cause hypotension due to loss of sympathetic tone; fluid administration is 1st-line treatment.
  - Other causes of hypotension (eg, hemorrhage) should be sought before being attributed to spinal cord injury (SCI).
  - Generally, hypovolemic shock causes tachycardia, whereas neurogenic shock results in bradycardia.
  - If BP does not improve after a fluid challenge and no other cause for hypotension can be found, vasopressor use may be necessary; $\alpha$-agonist is preferred.

### ED TREATMENT/PROCEDURES
- Other injuries must be treated as indicated.
- Level of SCI should be determined as a baseline to follow for improvement or deterioration.

- A neurosurgeon must be consulted once an SCI is suspected, even when plain films are normal; early surgical decompression or immobilization may reduce morbidity.
- The patient with an SCI should be managed at an appropriate regional trauma or spinal center:
  - If necessary, transfer should occur as soon as management of other injuries allow.
- IV antibiotics and tetanus prophylaxis are given to patients with a penetrating injury.
- IV vasopressor support may be required to treat neurogenic shock.

### MEDICATION
- Phenylephrine: 0.5–2 $\mu$g/kg bolus then 50–100 $\mu$g/min drip
- Ephedrine: 10 mg bolus, will last for up to 3–4 hr
- Ancef: 1,000 mg q8h

### ALERT
In the early 1990s, the use of high-dose methylprednisolone infusion was widely adopted as standard of care following the reports of the Second and Third National Acute Spinal Cord Injury Study (NASCIS II, NASCIS III); however, extensive systematic review of this therapy and the evidence to support it has demonstrated that this therapy is not recommended for routine use in SCI.

## FOLLOW-UP

### DISPOSITION
#### Admission Criteria
All patients with spinal cord syndrome must be admitted to an ICU setting.

#### Discharge Criteria
No patient with symptoms suggestive of SCI should be discharged.

## PEARLS AND PITFALLS
- A detailed neurological exam and attempt to document the spinal level of neurological symptoms is critical.
- Involve neurosurgical consultants early, as outcome is time-dependent in many cases.
- EM physicians should not feel compelled to start methylprednisolone treatment for acute SCI.

## ADDITIONAL READING
- Bracken MB, et al. A randomized controlled trial of methylprednisolone or naloxone in the treatment of acute spinal cord injury. *N Engl J Med*. 1990;322(20):1405–1411.
- Cass D. Steroids in acute spinal cord injury. *J Can Assoc Emerg Physicians*. 2003;5(1):7.
- Gerling MC, Davis DP, Hamilton RS, et al. Effects of cervical spine immobilization technique and laryngoscope blade selection on an unstable cervical spine in a cadaver model of intubation. *Ann Emerg Med*. 2000;36(4):293–300.
- Sayer FT, Kronvall E, Nilsson OG. Methylprednisolone treatment in acute spinal cord injury: The myth challenged through a structured analysis of published literature. *Spine J*. 2006;6(3):335–343.
- Hockberger RS, Kirshenbaum KJ. Spinal trauma. In: Marx JA, et al., eds. *Rosen's emergency medicine: Concepts and clinical practice*, 5th ed. St. Louis: CV Mosby, 2002:329–370.
- Hurlbert RJ. The role of steroids in acute spinal cord injury: An evidence-based analysis. *Spine*. 2001;26(24S):39–46.

## CODES

### ICD9
- 952.02 C1-c4 level with anterior cord syndrome
- 952.07 C5-c7 level with anterior cord syndrome
- 952.12 T1-t6 level with anterior cord syndrome

S

# SPINE INJURY: CERVICAL, ADULT

*Gary M. Vilke*

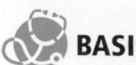

## BASICS

### DESCRIPTION
- Injury to the neck that results in injury to the spinal cord, cervical spine, or ligaments supporting the cervical spine
- May have more than one mechanism concurrently
- Flexion injuries:
  - Simple wedge fracture: Usually a stable fracture
  - Anterior subluxation: Disruption of the posterior ligament complex without bony injury; potentially unstable injury
  - Clay shoveler's fracture: avulsion fracture of the spinous process of C7, C6, or T1; stable fracture
  - Flexion teardrop fracture: Extremely unstable fracture; may be associated with acute anterior cervical cord syndrome
  - Atlanto-occipital dislocation: Unstable injury
  - Bilateral facet dislocation: Can occur from C2–C7; unstable injury
- Flexion/rotation injuries:
  - Unilateral facet dislocation "locked" vertebra: Stable injury
  - Rotary atlantoaxial dislocation: Unstable injury
- Extension injuries:
  - Extension teardrop fracture: An avulsion fracture of the anteroinferior corner of the involved vertebral body; unstable in extension and stable in flexion
  - Posterior arch of C1 fracture: Arch is compressed between the occiput and the spinous process of the axis during hyperextension; unstable fracture
  - Avulsion fracture of the anterior arch of the atlas: Horizontal fracture of C1 and prevertebral soft-tissue swelling on the lateral C-spine
  - Hangman's fracture: Traumatic spondylolisthesis of the axis involving the pedicles of C2; unstable fracture
  - Hyperextension dislocation: Described as the syndrome of the paralyzed patient with a radiographically normal-appearing C-spine
- Extension–rotation injury:
  - Pillar fracture: Generally stable fracture
- Vertical compression (axial loading) injuries:
  - Jefferson fracture: Burst fracture of both the anterior and posterior arch of C1; extremely unstable fracture
  - Burst fracture: A comminuted fracture of the vertebral body with variable retropulsion of the posterior body fragments into the spinal canal

### ETIOLOGY
- Blunt trauma is the major cause of neck injuries:
  - Automobile accidents account for >50%.
  - Falls account for approximately 20%.
  - Sporting accidents account for 15%.
  - Minor trauma in patients with severe arthritis may result in cervical injuries.
- Penetrating trauma

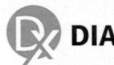

## DIAGNOSIS

### SIGNS AND SYMPTOMS
- Neck pain, tenderness on palpation
- Numbness, weakness, paresthesias of upper or lower extremities
- Always assume a C-spine injury in any patient with:
  - Altered mental status (unconscious, intoxicated, on drugs, or hypoxic) following trauma or if events are unknown but trauma is likely
  - Inability to communicate (mentally retarded, language barrier, or intubated) following trauma or if events are unknown but trauma is likely
  - Distracting injury
  - Blunt trauma involving head or neck
- Incomplete cervical cord syndromes (see separate chapter):
  - Brown-Séquard syndrome: Hemisection of cord from penetrating injury (ipsilateral motor paralysis/contralateral sensory hypesthesia)
  - Anterior cord syndrome: Cervical flexion injury causing cord contusion (paralysis/hypesthesia with sparing of position/touch/vibratory sensations)
  - Central cord syndrome: Patients with cervical degenerative arthritis with forced hyperflexion (deficits greater in upper extremities relative to lower extremities)

### History
- Obtain history of head or neck trauma.
- Identify history of ankylosing spondylitis or other brittle bone diseases.
- Specific symptoms:
  - Neck pain
  - Weakness
  - Numbness or tingling
  - Stinger

### Physical Exam
- Direct visualization of neck for bruising or deformity
- Palpation over the spinous processes
- Motor, sensory, and reflex examination of upper and lower extremities

### ESSENTIAL WORKUP
Complete physical examination and radiographic imaging if clinically indicated

### DIAGNOSTIC TESTS & INTERPRETATION
#### Imaging
- Standard radiographs include three separate views: lateral, anteroposterior, and open-mouth views of the odontoid while still immobilized.
- Lateral radiograph must include C1-T1; a swimmer's view may be necessary to view lower levels.
- Supine oblique views may help in identifying subtle rotational injuries.
- CT should be obtained when C-spine fractures, dislocations, or soft tissue swelling is seen on plain films or for unexplained neck pain/neurologic deficit with normal radiograph.
- CT (helical) is considered a good alternative to plain films and is favored in certain patients, including intubated victims of blunt trauma.
- Flexion–extension views may be needed to evaluate for dynamic ligamentous injuries if static radiographs are negative and the alert, cooperative patient still complains of pain.
- MRI has become a valuable tool in evaluating of patients with neurologic deficits, including spinal cord injury without radiographic abnormality.

### DIFFERENTIAL DIAGNOSIS
- Cervical muscle strain injury (whiplash)
- C-spine dislocation
- Cervical fracture dislocation
- Complex or simple cervical fractures

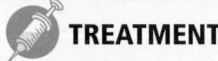 **TREATMENT**

**PRE-HOSPITAL**
- If C-spine injury suspected, immobilize with a hard collar, neck pads, and backboard.
- Immobilized patients require constant observation in case of vomiting.
- Immobilize C-spine in patients with penetrating neck wounds only if a neurologic deficit is present.
- If the weapon is still embedded, immobilize the neck to avoid further injury and do not remove the impaling object unless it directly impedes breathing.

**INITIAL STABILIZATION/THERAPY**
- Immobilize the spine using a rigid collar and backboard plus tape/towels or lightweight foam pads along the side of the neck.
- Stabilize the airway, establish IV access, and support circulation:
  - Preferred method is careful orotracheal rapid sequence intubation with in-line spinal immobilization.
  - Fiberoptic intubation set should be at the bedside and considered if available.

**ED TREATMENT/PROCEDURES**
- Assess patient for other injuries; remember that the abdominal exam in a C-spine–injured patient is unreliable and further objective testing is indicated.
- Patients with ankylosing spondylitis or other brittle bone diseases are at risk for fracture and cord injury with even trivial mechanisms.
- Patients may be clinically cleared and do not require C-spine radiograph (based on NEXUS) if they:
  - Have no altered level of alertness
    Are not intoxicated
  - Have no tenderness in the posterior midline cervical spine
  - Have no distracting painful injury
  - Have no focal neurologic deficit

- If a neurologic deficit is present, consult neurosurgery.
- If the radiographs or CT is abnormal, consult neurosurgery or the orthopedic spine service.
- If the radiographs are normal but the alert and cooperative patient is having severe neck pain, consider flexion–extension films, CT, or MRI; if abnormal, consult neurosurgery.

**MEDICATION**
High-dose steroid protocol for patients with neurologic deficits due to fractures or dislocations.

*First Line*
Methylprednisolone: 30 mg/kg IV bolus then 5.4 mg/kg/hr over the next 23 hr; begin within 8 hr of injury

 **FOLLOW-UP**

**DISPOSITION**
*Admission Criteria*
- C-spine fractures or dislocations associated with a neurologic deficit or any unstable fracture or dislocation should be admitted to the ICU or a monitored setting.
- Stable C-spine fractures or dislocations should be admitted.
- Isolated spinous process fractures that are not associated with any neurologic deficit or instability on plain films.
- Simple cervical wedge fractures with no neurologic deficit.

*Discharge Criteria*
- Patients with acute cervical strain "whiplash"
- Musculoskeletal injuries that are associated with mild to moderate pain, no neurologic deficit, and normal radiographs

*Issues for Referral*
The patient with a radiographically normal C-spine but continuous pain may be discharged with a hard collar and appropriate orthopedic follow-up.

**FOLLOW-UP RECOMMENDATIONS**
Return to ED for evaluation if pain increases or numbness, weakness, stingers, or other clinical changes develop

**PEARLS AND PITFALLS**
- Trivial neck injuries in patient with ankylosing spondylitis or other brittle bone diseases may result in significant injuries.
- All the NEXUS criteria need to be applied to safely rule out a clinically significant spinal fracture without imaging.

**ADDITIONAL READING**
- Hoffman JR, Mower WR, Wolfson AB, et al. Validity of a set of clinical criteria to rule out injury to the cervical spine in patients with blunt trauma. *N Engl J Med*. 2000;343:94–99.
- Richards PJ. Cervical spine clearance: A review. *Injury Int J Care inured*. 2005;36:248–269.
- Stiell IG, Clement CM, McKnight RD, et al. The Canadian C-spine rule versus the NEXUS low-risk criteria in patients with trauma. *N Engl J Med*. 2003;349(26):2510–2518.
- Van Goethem JW, Maes M, Ozsarlak O, et al. Imaging in spinal trauma. *Eur Radiol*. 2005;15:582–590.

**See Also (Topic, Algorithm, Electronic Media Element)**
- Ankylosing Spondylitis
- Head Trauma, Blunt
- Spinal Cord Syndromes

 **CODES**

ICD9
- 805.00 Closed fracture of cervical vertebra, unspecified level
- 805.10 Open fracture of cervical vertebra, unspecified level
- 806.00 Closed fracture of c1-c4 level with unspecified spinal cord injury

S

# SPINE INJURY: CERVICAL, PEDIATRIC

*Steven T. Riley*

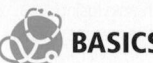 **BASICS**

## DESCRIPTION

- Accounts for 2% of pediatric trauma-caused hospital admissions in the U.S.
- Children <8 yr of age:
  - Anatomic differences lead to predominance of C1-3 injuries.
  - Relatively larger head
  - Weaker cervical musculature
  - Ligamentous laxity
  - Horizontally oriented facets
- Children 8–12 yr of age:
  - Increased incidence of pancervical injuries
- Children >12 yr of age:
  - Injury patterns consistent with those of adults
  - Lower cervical spine injuries more common
  - Evident radiographically
- Spinal cord injury without radiographic abnormality (SCIWORA):
  - Occurs in ~20% of pediatric cervical spine injuries
  - More common in children <8 yr of age
  - Symptoms may be transient and have resolved by time of evaluation:
    ○ Paresthesias
    ○ Burning sensation down spine
    ○ Weakness
  - Symptoms often occur immediately after injury but may have delayed onset (ie, minutes to days).

## ETIOLOGY

- Motor vehicle and pedestrian accidents
- Falls
- Sports injuries

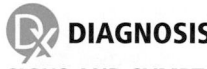 **DIAGNOSIS**

## SIGNS AND SYMPTOMS

- Cervical spine pain
- Limited range of motion
- Neurologic deficit that may be transient
- May be masked by altered mental status or distracting injury
- General signs:
  - Hypotension
  - Bradycardia
  - Hypoventilation or apnea
- Neck signs:
  - Tender to palpation over cervical spine
  - Limited range of motion
  - Torticollis

- Respiratory signs:
  - Diaphragmatic breathing
- Abdominal signs:
  - Ileus
  - Fecal incontinence
  - Absent rectal tone
- Genitourinary signs:
  - Priapism
  - Urinary retention
- Neurologic signs:
  - Paresthesias or sensory deficit
  - Focal weakness
- Paralysis:
  - Partial cord syndromes
  - Quadriplegia
  - Absent reflexes
- Preverbal child may be unable to express symptoms and may not cooperate during exam.

## ESSENTIAL WORKUP

- Obtain cervical spine radiographs for:
  - Cervical spine tenderness
  - Altered mental status
  - Neurologic deficit (even if transient)
  - Distracting injury or mechanism of injury (ie, in preverbal child)
- Remember, the National Emergency X-Radiography Utilization Study C-spine decision rule does not apply to children.
- Additional imaging studies (CT, MRI) may be indicated if plain radiographs are inconclusive and clinical examination suggests injury. May also be indicated if head CT being done to evaluate intracranial injury to expedite evaluation.

## DIAGNOSTIC TESTS & INTERPRETATION
### Imaging

- Cervical spine radiographs:
  - Standard initial views: anteroposterior, lateral, and odontoid
  - Identifies approximately 80% of fractures, dislocations, and subluxations
  - Need to visualize all seven cervical vertebrae
  - Space between anterior arch of C1 and anterior aspect of odontoid process:
    ○ 5 mm or smaller in children and 3 mm in adults
  - Thickening of prevertebral soft tissue:
    ○ Suggests underlying fracture or ligamentous injury
    ○ Also occurs with neck flexion, expiration, swallowing
    ○ Too much variability exists for measurements to be highly sensitive.
    ○ Soft tissue below the glottis should be approximately twice as thick as above the glottis.

- Pseudosubluxation of C2:
  ○ Normal variant
  ○ A result of ligamentous laxity and often resolves by age of 8 yr
  ○ C2 anteriorly displaced on C3
  ○ Posterior cervical line retains normal relationships.
  ○ Line drawn between anterior aspect of spinous processes of C1 and C3 should pass within 2 mm of anterior aspect of spinous process of C2.
  ○ Larger than 2-mm space suggests underlying hangman fracture.
  ○ Can be applied only at C1-3
  - Anterior vertebral wedging of C3 and C4:
    ○ May be mistaken for compression fracture
  - Epiphysial growth plates may resemble fractures:
    ○ Posterior arch of C1 fuses by 4 yr of age.
    ○ Anterior arch of C fuses by 10 yr of age.
    ○ Base of odontoid fuses with body of C2 by 7 yr of age.
  - Flexion and extension views:
    ○ Limited use
    ○ May be useful if suspected occult ligamentous injury
    ○ Negative cervical spine films
    ○ No neurologic abnormalities
- CT scan:
  - If fracture suspected despite negative plain radiographs
  - For further definition of fracture identified on plain radiographs
  - If need for differentiating between synchondrosis and fracture
- MRI:
  - Suspected spinal cord injury with or without abnormalities found on plain radiographs or CT

## DIFFERENTIAL DIAGNOSIS

- Cervical muscle strain
- Torticollis
- Cervical adenitis
- Retropharyngeal abscess
- Meningitis

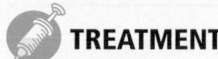
# TREATMENT

## PRE-HOSPITAL
- Immobilize all infants and children with potential cervical spine injuries:
- Appropriate size cervical collar
- Tape, towels, padding in combination with car seat or spine board if formal collar not available
- Larger head creates cervical flexion.
- Place padding under neck, shoulders, and back.
- Align external auditory meatus with shoulder.

## INITIAL STABILIZATION/THERAPY
- Maintain cervical spine immobilization:
- Logroll patient.
- One person must be devoted to in-line cervical spine immobilization if intubation is required.

## ED TREATMENT/PROCEDURES
- Any trauma patient with neurologic deficit consistent with spinal cord injury should have req methylprednisolone considered.
- Neurosurgical consultation:
  - True subluxation
  - Fracture
  - Transient or persistent neurologic deficit

## MEDICATION
### First Line
Methylprednisolone: loading dose 30 mg/kg IV over 1 hr; maintenance infusion 5.4 mg/kg/hr over next 23 hr; initiate within 8 hr of injury

# FOLLOW-UP

## DISPOSITION
### Admission Criteria
- Altered mental status
- Signs/symptoms of spinal cord injury
- Fracture
- Obtain appropriate consultation:
  - Neurosurgery
  - Orthopedic Spine

### Discharge Criteria
- Completely normal mental status
- No radiographic abnormalities
- No transient or persistent neurologic deficit
- Educate parents:
  - SCIWORA can present with delayed onset of symptoms.
  - Patient should return to hospital if paresthesias, weakness, or paralysis is present.

## FOLLOW-UP RECOMMENDATIONS
- Follow up with orthopedic surgeon or neurosurgeon as directed
- If concussion suspected, follow-up suggested
- Children with significant trauma should have psychological follow-up.

# PEARLS AND PITFALLS

- Maintain appropriate immobilization during evaluation.
- In most cases plain radiographs can be used as initial screening tool.
- Be aware of unique features of pediatric cervical spine.
- Symptoms of SCIWORA can be transient or delayed.

# ADDITIONAL READING

- Ehrlich P, Wee C, Drongowski R, et al. Canadian C-spine Rule and the National Emergency X-radiography Utilization Low-Risk Criteria for c-spine radiography in young trauma patients. *J Pediatr Surg.* 2009;44:987–991.

- Egloff A, Kadom N, Vezina G, et al. Pediatric cervical spine trauma imaging: A practical approach. *Pediatr Radiol.* 2009;39:447–456.
- Pieretti-Vanmarcke R, Velmahos G, Nance M, et al. Clinical clearance of the cervical spine in blunt trauma patients younger than 3 years: A multi-center study of the American Association for the Surgery of Trauma. *J Trauma.* 2009;67:543–549.
- Polk-Williams A, Carr B, Blinman T, et al. Cervical spine injury in young children: A National Trauma Data Bank review. *J Pediatr Surg.* 2008;43:1718–1721.
- Swischuk LE. *Imaging of the Cervical Spine in Children.* New York: Springer-Verlag; 2004.

## See Also (Topic, Algorithm, Electronic Media Element)
Head Injury

# CODES

## ICD9
- 805.00 Closed fracture of cervical vertebra, unspecified level
- 805.10 Open fracture of cervical vertebra, unspecified level
- 806.00 Closed fracture of c1-c4 level with unspecified spinal cord injury

S

# SPINE INJURY: COCCYX

*Gary Schwartz*

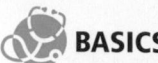

## BASICS

### DESCRIPTION
- Usually results from a fall that ends with the victim in sitting position
- Fall usually occurs from standing height.
- Can occur during childbirth
- More common in women

### ETIOLOGY
See "Description."

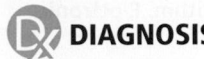

## DIAGNOSIS

### SIGNS AND SYMPTOMS
- Tenderness localized over the coccyx
- Ecchymosis over the gluteal fold
- Pain with sitting, especially when leaning forward, and with defecation

### History
Patient or witness to provide full history of accident including any earlier events that might influence mechanism of fall or insult

### Physical Exam
A full physical examination:
- Including rectal exam to assess tenderness or mobility of coccyx
- No evidence of neurologic deficit should be found in isolated coccygeal fractures.

### ESSENTIAL WORKUP
Most often isolated injury, but if other spinal injury of concern, spinal immobilization should be instituted.

### DIAGNOSTIC TESTS & INTERPRETATION
### Imaging
Routine radiographic imaging unnecessary:
- Concern about unnecessary radiation to gonads when diagnosis can be made clinically
- Imaging is indicated if concern for other spine injuries.
- Radiographs can be hard to interpret because coccyx has normal variant positions that can be confused with fracture.
- Lateral radiograph is best view for fracture and dislocation.

### DIFFERENTIAL DIAGNOSIS
- Coccygodynia
- Levator ani syndrome
- Pilonidal cyst
- Perirectal abscess

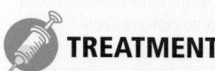

## TREATMENT

### PRE-HOSPITAL
Pain management
Assess for other injuries

### INITIAL STABILIZATION/THERAPY
- Usually none required; if patient unstable, consider other diagnoses.
- Medicate for pain.

### ED TREATMENT/PROCEDURES
- Pain medication
- Reduction of displaced coccygeal fracture, but rarely necessary.

## TREATMENT-GENERAL-MEASURES
Recommend donut-shaped seat cushion for comfort.

## MEDICATION
- Medication for pain if and as needed
- Stool softener

## SURGERY/OTHER PROCEDURES
Reduction may be attempted if displaced coccygeal fracture evident, but rarely needed or successful.

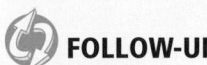 **FOLLOW-UP**

## DISPOSITION
### Admission Criteria
Admission is generally not required.

### Discharge Criteria
Coccygeal fracture can be managed on an outpatient basis unless other intercurrent injury makes admission necessary.

## ADDITIONAL READING

- Cwinn AA. Pelvis. In: Marx J. *Rosen's Emergency Medicine: Concepts and Clinical Practice*. 5th ed. St. Louis: Mosby; 2002:632–633.
- Gutierrez PR, Mas Martinez JJ, Arenas J. Salter-Harris type I fracture of the sacro-coccygeal joint. *Pediatr Radiol*. 1998;28:734.
- Traub S, Glaser J, Manino B. *Coccygectomy for the treatment of therapy-resistant coccygodynia. J Surg Orthop Adv*. 2009;18(3):147–149.

 **CODES**

### ICD9
- 805.6 Closed fracture of sacrum and coccyx without mention of spinal cord injury
- 806.60 Closed fracture of sacrum and coccyx with unspecified spinal cord injury

### ICD10
S39.9

S

# SPINAL INJURY: LUMBAR

*Bret E. Ginther*

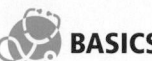

## BASICS

### DESCRIPTION
- Flexion compression fracture:
  - Wedge compression:
    - If <50% anterior compression of the vertebral body, injury considered stable
    - No ligamentous injury
    - No neurologic deficit
  - Burst fracture:
    - Vertebral body fracture with retropulsion of bone into the neural canal
    - Kyphosis evident on lateral radiograph
    - Posterior ligamentous injury
    - Anterior compression, lower extremities, calcaneal fractures
    - Possible neurologic deficit
- Flexion distraction (lap belt injury):
  - Abdominal injuries likely
  - Chance fracture:
    - Purely bony injury; fracture line through spinous process, pedicles, and vertebral body
    - No kyphosis evident on lateral radiograph
    - Often no neurologic deficit
  - Facet dislocation:
    - Mostly soft-tissue injury; no fracture
    - Complete disruption of posterior ligaments and intervertebral disc
    - Neurologic deficit may be present.
- Flexion rotation:
  - Unstable injury
  - Neurologic deficit often present
- Extension:
  - Unstable, uncommon
  - Disruption of anterior longitudinal ligament and intervertebral disc
  - Neurologic sequelae rare but possible
- Shear injuries (translational injuries):
  - Anterior, posterior, or lateral translation of superior vertebral segment over the inferior segment
  - Complete ligamentous disruption
  - Neurologic deficit present
- Simple fractures:
  - Isolated spinous process fracture:
    - Ligamentous disruption
    - No neurologic deficit
  - Isolated transverse process fracture:
    - Ligamentous disruption
    - Neurologic deficit possible; rare isolated root injury

### ETIOLOGY
- Blunt trauma with axial distraction, axial compression, or translational forces applied to lumbar region
- Fall from height landing on the feet (associated calcaneal fractures) or on the buttocks
- Motor vehicle accidents (MVA)

### Pediatric Considerations
- Rare reports of child abuse presenting as lower extremity flaccid paralysis owing to lumbar spine fracture
- Spinal cord terminates at L3 in newborn and recedes to T12 by adulthood; direct cord damage possible in children with high lumbar fractures.
- End plate avulsion fractures: Adolescent injury usually at L4–L5 or L5–S1 level; ligament pulls off vertebral body end plate; associated neurologic findings; usually resolves with excision of end plate fracture

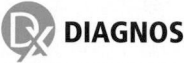

## DIAGNOSIS

### SIGNS AND SYMPTOMS
- Pain or localized tenderness to palpation in lumbar midline
- Ecchymosis or deformity overlying lumbar region; palpable deformity; paraspinal muscle spasm
- Increased interspinous distance by palpation
- Step-off (anterior or posterior displacement of spinous process) by palpation
- Neurologic deficits referable to lumbar spinal nerves:
  - Loss of bladder control
  - Motor: Hip flexion (L1–L4), leg extension (L3, L4), ankle dorsiflexion (L4, L5), toe extension (L5)
  - Sensory: Inguinal crease (L1), medial thigh (L2–L3), knee (L4), lateral calf (L5)
  - Reflexes: Knee jerk (L2–L4)
- Pain may be masked by associated distracting injuries (eg, pelvis, calcaneal fractures).
- Patients with multiple injuries and altered mental status have an unreliable clinical exam and require imaging evaluation.

### History
Mechanism to suggest forces applied to lumbar region:
- MVA
- Fall
- Direct impact to lumbar region

### Physical Exam
- Midline lumbar tenderness or deformity
- Neurologic findings involving lumbar spinal nerves

### Geriatric Considerations
- Consider abuse in cases of uncertain mechanism.
- Increase suspicion of bleeding consequences, such as spinal hematomas, in patients taking Coumadin or other blood thinners.

### ESSENTIAL WORKUP
Following criteria associated with higher risk of thoracolumbar (TL) spine injuries and should be imaged:
- TL pain or tenderness to palpation
- Decreased level of consciousness (Glasgow Coma Scale <14)
- Drug intoxication
- Neurologic deficits (described above)
- Painful, distracting injuries
- Severe injury mechanism (eg, rollover MVA, auto vs. pedestrian, fall >10 feet)
- Lumbar radiographs (described under Imaging)
- Careful neurologic exam including:
  - Assessment of rectal tone
  - Bulbocavernosus and cremasteric reflexes

### DIAGNOSTIC TESTS & INTERPRETATION
#### Lab
- Standard trauma labs, as indicated:
- CBC
- Chemistry panel
- Coagulation studies
- Urinalysis

#### Imaging
- Lumbar radiography with minimum of anteroposterior and lateral views. Characteristics of *unstable* fractures include:
  - Widening of interspinous, interlaminar, or interpedicular distance
  - Kyphosis >20°
  - Translation >2 mm
  - Vertebral body height loss >50%
  - Articular process fracture
- Radiographs may not identify burst fractures in 25% of cases.
- If a fracture is identified, entire spine should be imaged to evaluate potential associated spinal injuries.
- Spinous process fracture, transverse process fracture, or simple transverse sacral fracture require lumbar flexion-extension films if patient is neurologically intact and there is no evidence of unstable injury.
- CT or MRI should be performed for further evaluation of suspected fractures or fractures identified on plain films to assess spinal cord integrity.

#### Diagnostic Procedures/Surgery
Consider postvoid residual urinary catheterization to identify/characterize urinary retention.

## DIFFERENTIAL DIAGNOSIS

- Contusion
- Pathologic fracture (metastatic cancer)
- Osteoporosis
- Pelvic fracture
- Traumatic herniated disc
- Low posterior rib fracture
- Tuberculous spondylitis (Pott disease)
- Ankylosing spondylitis
- Osteogenesis imperfecta (pediatric)
- Congenital scoliosis with hemivertebra (mistaken for lateral wedge fracture)
- Child abuse
- Spinal hematoma
- Epidural abscess

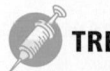 TREATMENT

### PRE-HOSPITAL
It is difficult to determine whether an injury is stable in the field; any patients with suspected spinal injuries should be immobilized to prevent further injury.

### INITIAL STABILIZATION/THERAPY
- Immobilization while tending to immediate life-threatening conditions
- Airway, breathing, and circulation management

### ED TREATMENT/PROCEDURES
- Maintain spinal immobilization.
- High-dose methylprednisolone protocol for any neurologic deficit (best in concert with specialist consultation)
- Consultation with orthopaedic spine or neurosurgery service
- Appropriate analgesia
- The following stable injuries may be treated conservatively if CT confirms stability of injury and patient is neurologically intact:
  - Isolated spinous process, transverse process fracture
  - Chance fracture
  - Anterior wedge compression (<50%) fracture
  - Stable burst fracture
- Total contact orthotic devices may be useful; limited activities; sleep prone; avoid pillows and soft mattresses, which may worsen deformity.

### MEDICATION
- Narcotic pain medication in absence of contraindications
- High-dose steroid protocol: Methylprednisolone: 30 mg/kg IV load over 1 hr, then 5.4 mg/kg/hr for the next 23 hr; initiate in ED within 8 hr of injury if possible.

### First Line
- Tylenol: 1g (peds: 15 mg/kg) PO q 4h p.r.n.
- Motrin: 400–800 mg (peds: 10 mg/kg) PO q6h p.r.n.
- Dilaudid: 1–2 mg (peds: 0.015 mg/kg) IV/IM q3h p.r.n.
- Morphine: 2–10 mg (peds: 0.1–0.2 mg/kg) IV/IM q3h p.r.n.
- Toradol: 30 mg IV or 60 mg IM (peds 0.5 mg/kg IV or 1 mg/kg IM) q6h p.r.n.
  - Use half Toradol dose for patients >65

### Second Line
- Flexeril: 5–10 mg PO q8h p.r.n.
- Soma: 350 mg PO q8h p.r.n.
- Zofran: 4–8 mg IV/PO (peds >4y, 4mg IV/PO) q8h p.r.n.
- Compazine: 5–10 mg IV/IM/PO (peds 2.5 mg PR/PO) q8h p.r.n.
- Phenergan: 12.5–25 mg IM/PO/IV (peds 0.5–1 mg/kg IM/PR) q8h p.r.n.
  - IV Phenergan NOT recommended due to reports of tissue necrosis

 FOLLOW-UP

### DISPOSITION

### Admission Criteria
Patients with traumatic lumbar fractures should be admitted for stabilization procedures, parenteral pain control, management of possible ileus, and evaluation for associated injuries.

### Discharge Criteria
- Neurologically intact patients with stable injuries evaluated in conjunction with a spine surgeon
- Patients with simple compression (wedge) fractures with no neurologic deficit may be considered for outpatient management if adequate pain control and appropriate follow-up can be arranged.
- Simple transverse sacral fracture, isolated spinous process fracture, and isolated transverse process fracture may also be considered for outpatient management.
- The patient must be neurologically intact with a stable living situation; CT scan and flexion-extension films must confirm fracture stability.

### Issues for Referral
Patients discharged with stable injuries should have primary care or orthopedic appointment in 1 wk to monitor for recovery and evaluate for potential complications.

### FOLLOW-UP RECOMMENDATIONS
Return to ED for new neurologic symptoms or pain not controlled by discharge medications. Otherwise, follow up as described above.

## PEARLS AND PITFALLS

- Lumbar fractures are rare in pediatrics. Aggressively pursue causative factor if mechanism is not evident.
- Older individuals may have underlying medical cause of lumbar pathology. Pursue alternative causes of pain, such as hematomas and infections. Be wary of patients on blood thinners.
- CT should follow compression fractures seen on plain films to assess for stability and potential canal involvement.
- Otherwise healthy, ambulatory patients with simple post MVA low back pain may be safely discharged without imaging if the exam is otherwise reassuring.

## ADDITIONAL READING

- Denis F. Spinal instability as defined by the 3-column spine concept in acute spinal trauma. *Clin Orthop.* 1984;189:65–76.
- Gabos P, Tuten H, Leet A, et al. Fracture-dislocation of the lumbar spine in an abused child. *Pediatrics.* 1998;101:473–477.
- Hanck J, Muñiz A. Cervical spondylodiscitis, osteomyelitis, and epidural abscess mimicking a vertebral fracture. *J Emerg Med.* 2009; in press.
- Holmes J, Panacek E, Miller P, et al. Prospective evaluation criteria for obtaining thoracolumbar radiographs in trauma patients. *J Emerg Med.* 2003;24:1–7.
- Institute for Safe Medical Practices Newsletter. Action needed to prevent serious injury with IV promethazine. August 10, 2006 accessed 12/2009 at www.ismp.org/Newsletters/acutecare/articles/20060810.asp
- Krueger MA, Green DA, Hoyt D, et al. Overlooked spine injuries associated with lumbar process fractures. *Clin Orthop.* 1996;327:191–195.
- Petersilge C, Emery S. Thoracolumbar burst fracture: Evaluating stability. *Semin Ultrasound CT MR.* 1996;17:105–113.
- Savitsky E, Votey S. Emergency department approach to acute thoracolumbar spine injury. *J Emerg Med.* 1997;15:49–60.
- Tamir E, Anekstein Y, Mirovsky Y, et al. Thoracic and lumbar spine radiographs for walking trauma patients: Is it necessary? *J Emerg Med.* 2006;31:403–405.

### See Also (Topic, Algorithm, Electronic Media Element)
- Pediatric Trauma
- Spinal Cord Syndromes
- Trauma, Multiple

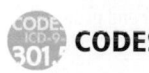 CODES

### ICD9
- 805.4 Closed fracture of lumbar vertebra without mention of spinal cord injury
- 805.5 Open fracture of lumbar vertebra without mention of spinal cord injury
- 952.2 Lumbar spinal cord injury without spinal bone injury

# SPINE INJURY: THORACIC

*Richard D. Zane*

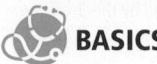

## BASICS

### DESCRIPTION
- The following forces account for most thoracic fractures and dislocations:
  - Axial compression
  - Flexion–rotation
  - Shear
  - Flexion–distraction
  - Extension
- 3 anatomically distinct columns; if 2 of the 3 columns are disrupted, the spinal column is unstable:
  - Posterior column: Posterior bony arch and interconnecting ligamentous structures
  - Middle column: Posterior aspects of the vertebral bodies, posterior annulus fibrosis, and posterior longitudinal ligament
  - Anterior column: Anterior longitudinal ligament, anterior annulus fibrosis, and anterior vertebral body
- Major vs minor fractures:
  - Minor:
    - Isolated articular fracture
    - Transverse process fracture
    - Spinous process fracture
    - Pars interarticularis fracture
  - Major:
    - Compression fracture
    - Burst fracture
    - Seat belt injury
    - Fracture–dislocation
- Compression fracture (anterior or lateral flexion):
  - Fracture of anterior portion of vertebral body with intact middle column
  - May be posterior column disruption
  - Type A: Fracture through both end plates
  - Type B: Fracture through superior end plate
  - Type C: Fracture through inferior end plate
  - Type D: Both end plates intact
- Burst fracture (axial loading):
  - Fracture through middle column of spine
  - May have spreading of posterior elements and laminar fractures with possible retropulsion into the spinal canal and potential neurologic compromise
  - Type A: Fracture through both end plates
  - Type B: Fracture through superior end plate
  - Type C: Fracture through inferior end plate
  - Type D: Burst in middle column with rotational injury leading to subluxation
  - Type E: Burst in middle column with asymmetric compression of anterior column
- Seat belt injury (flexion–distraction):
  - Distraction of posterior and middle columns with anterior column intact
  - Typically caused by lap belts used without shoulder harness
  - Type A: Through bone
  - Type B: Primarily ligamentous
  - Type C: Disruption of bone through middle column
  - Type D: Through ligaments and disc with no middle column fracture

- Fracture–dislocations:
  - Failure of all three columns following compression, tension, rotation, or shear forces
  - Type A: Flexion–rotation; fall from height
  - Type B: Shear—violent force across long axis of trunk
  - Type C: Flexion-distraction; bilateral facet dislocation

### ETIOLOGY
- Thoracic spine is rigid owing to the support of the rib cage and the costovertebral articulations:
  - The spinal canal is narrowest in the thoracic spine.
- Traumatic thoracic spine fractures require enormous forces. Motor-vehicle and motorcycle collisions, pedestrians struck, and falls (particularly from height >10 ft) account for most fractures:
  - A small percentage are caused by penetrating injuries (see "Spinal Cord Syndromes").
  - 50% of all spinal fractures and 40% of all spinal cord injuries occur at the thoracolumbar junction (T11-L2).

#### Pediatric Considerations
- Suspect child abuse if thoracic spine injury without clear history of motor vehicle trauma.
- Posterior rib fractures raise index of suspicion for abuse and require closer survey of thoracic spine and entire body for occult injury.

#### Geriatric Considerations
Increased brittleness of bones in eldery (>65 yr) predispose to fractures with less severe mechanism, falls from lesser height.

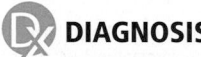

## DIAGNOSIS

### SIGNS AND SYMPTOMS
- Significant force is required to produce thoracic vertebral fractures.
- Pain at the fracture site or impingement of nearby structures by bone fragments
- Because of the stabilizing influence of the rib cage, a tremendous amount of force is needed to cause thoracic spine dislocations:
  - Concomitant internal injury should be suspected.
  - Thoracic spine fracture–dislocation is less common than thoracolumbar fracture–dislocation but has higher incidence of neurologic impairment.
  - Spinal injury at another anatomic level should heighten suspicion for thoracic injury and vice versa.
- Common signs and symptoms:
  - Localized soft tissue defect
  - Ecchymosis or hematoma
    - Scapular contusions
  - Step-offs, deformity, or widening of disc space (more specific)
  - Pain or tenderness (more sensitive)
    - Localized—pain and tenderness over spinous process
    - Referred—paraspinal, anterior chest, or abdomen

- Paraspinal muscle spasm
- Paresthesia or dysesthesia
- Weakness (focal or global)
- Distal areflexia, flaccid plegia
- Bowel or bladder incontinence
- Priapism
- Loss of temperature control
- Spinal shock—hypotension with bradycardia

#### History
- Mechanism of injury
- Comorbidities

### ESSENTIAL WORKUP
- Rapid evaluation of ABCs
- Primary and secondary trauma survey
- Detailed neurologic exam, including rectal tone and perianal sensation
- Thorough spine exam for deformity or tenderness
- Any midline tenderness elicited on examination, distracting injury, altered mental status or intoxication with concerning mechanism mandates plain film spine radiography.
- If fracture present, determine whether it is stable or unstable.
- Assess for bulbocavernous reflex in spinal shock.

### DIAGNOSTIC TESTS & INTERPRETATION
#### Imaging
- Midline pain or tenderness, significant motor-vehicle accident, or falls from height are indications for screening with anteroposterior and lateral plain film views of the spine.
- Thin-cut CT scanning is indicated in any patient with evidence of spinal fracture on plain films to assess spinal canal integrity or in patients with normal plain films and significant pain or tenderness and mechanism for severe injury.
- Any finding of a fracture anywhere in the thoracic spine mandate imaging of the entire spine with plain radiographs at a minimum.
- Data from CT of chest/abdomen/pelvis are increasing being reformatted to clear the thoracolumbar spine in trauma patients:
  - More sensitive than plain radiographs without additional cost or radiation
- MRI for further evaluation of suspected spinal cord injury, compression, or ligamentous tear

### DIFFERENTIAL DIAGNOSIS
- Arthritis (degenerative and rheumatoid)
- Ankylosing spondylitis
- Spina bifida
- Congenital malformation
- Degenerative disc disease
- Neoplasm
- Pathologic fracture:
  - Osteoporosis
  - Benign or malignant bone tumors

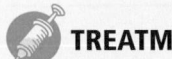 **TREATMENT**

**PRE-HOSPITAL**
- If the patient's positioning initially prevents placement of a long spinal board, a short board should be placed until the patient is fully extricated.
- Patients with neurologic deficit should be transported directly to a trauma center.

**INITIAL STABILIZATION/THERAPY**
- Manage airway and resuscitate as indicated:
  - Airway intervention should be done with in-line cervical immobilization.
  - Identify hypotension that may be secondary to hemorrhage vs neurogenic.
  - Consider fluid resuscitation with crystalloid followed by blood products if indicated.
- Preserve residual spinal cord function and prevent further injury by stabilizing the spine.

**ED TREATMENT/PROCEDURES**
- Perform all needed resuscitation and diagnostic tests with the patient in full spinal immobilization.
- If spinal cord injury is suspected, consider the administration of high-dose steroids and consult a spine surgeon.
- If spinal fracture or ligamentous injury is suspected without neurologic impairment, arrange CT or MRI scanning while consulting. neurosurgery or orthopaedic surgery.
- Pain control should be administered as soon as possible; NSAIDs, opiates, and benzodiazepines are the mainstays of treatment.
- Neurogenic hypotension presents with bradycardia or normal heart rate, rather than the tachycardia seen with hypovolemic shock:
  - Neurogenic hypotension should be treated with crystalloid bolus but may require vasopressors.

**MEDICATION**
- High-dose steroid administration is rapidly falling out of favor due to lack of evidence supporting use and risk of untoward effects of steroids.
- Strong consideration should be given to eliminating from protocols.
- If given, must be within 8 hr of injury as indicated by regional/hospital protocol.

- Methylprednisolone: 30 mg/kg IV bolus over 15 min followed 45 min later by a maintenance infusion of 5.4 mg/kg/hr for the next 23 hr if started within 3 hr of injury; consider continuing for 48 hr if started 3–8 hr after injury.
- High-dose steroid treatment not recommended >8 hr after injury.

 **FOLLOW-UP**

**DISPOSITION**
*Admission Criteria*
- Patients with significant spinal cord or column injury should be treated at a regional trauma center.
- Unstable spinal column injury
- Spinal cord or root injury
- Ileus
- Pain control
- Concomitant traumatic injury
- ICU-level care based on severity of injuries

*Discharge Criteria*
Stable minor fractures after orthopedic or neurosurgical evaluation.

**FOLLOW-UP RECOMMENDATIONS**
Outpatient neurosurgical or orthopedic follow-up as indicated after appropriate ED or inpatient evaluation and treatment.

**PEARLS AND PITFALLS**
- Suspect and evaluate for thoracic spine injury in any trauma patient.
- CT evaluation is indicated for any patient with significant mechanism, pain, or tenderness; distracting injury or injury at another spinal level; intoxication or altered mental status.
- Maintain spinal immobilization until cleared by radiologic and clinical exam.
- Early consultation with spine surgeon if presence of fracture, neurologic deficit or instability.
- Treatment with high-dose steroids is currently an area of controversy. Begin treatment within 8 hr of injury if initiating high-dose steroid protocol.

**ADDITIONAL READING**

- Bagley LJ, et al. Imaging of spinal trauma. *Radiol Clin North Am.* 2006;44(1):1–12, vii.
- Bracken MB. Steriods for acute spinal cord injury. *Cochrane Database Syst Rev.* 2009;4. CD:001046.
- Block BE, et al. Thoracic and lumbar spine injuries in children. *Contemp Orthop.* 1994;29(4):243–555.
- Brandser EA, El-Khoury GY. Thoracic and lumbar spine trauma. *Radiol Clin North Am.* 1997;35(3): 533–557.
- Chiles BW III, Cooper PR. Acute spinal injury. *N Engl J Med.* 1996;334(8):514–520.
- El-Khoury GY, Whitten CG. Trauma to the upper thoracic spine: anatomy, biomechanics, and unique imaging features. *Am J Roentgenol.* 1993;160: 95–102.
- Hockberger RS, et al. Spine. In: Rosen P, et al, eds. *Emergency Medicine: Concepts and Clinical Practice,* 5th ed. St. Louis: Mosby, 2002:329–369.
- Hockberger RS, et al. Spinal injuries. In: Marx JA, et al, eds. *Rosen's Emergency Medicine: Concepts and Clinical Practice,* 7th ed. Philadelphia: Mosby, 2010:337–375.
- Inaba K, et al. Visceral torso computed tomography for clearance of the thoracolumbar spine in trauma: A review of the literature. *J Trauma.* 2006;60: 915–920.
- Rivas LA, et al. Multislice CT in thoracic trauma. *Radiol Clin North Am.* 2003;41(3):599–616.

 **CODES**

**ICD9**
- 805.2 Closed fracture of dorsal (thoracic) vertebra without mention of spinal cord injury
- 805.3 Open fracture of dorsal (thoracic) vertebra without mention of spinal cord injury
- 806.20 Closed fracture of t1-t6 level with unspecified spinal cord injury

S

# SPLENIC INJURY

*Albert Jin*

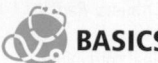

## BASICS

### DESCRIPTION
- The spleen is formed by reticular and lymphatic tissue and is the largest lymph organ.
- The spleen lies in the left upper quadrant (LUQ) between the fundus of the stomach and the diaphragm.

### ETIOLOGY
- The spleen is the most commonly injured intra-abdominal organ:
  - In nearly 2/3 of cases, it is the only damaged intraperitoneal structure
- Motor-vehicle accidents (auto–auto, pedestrian–auto) are the major cause (50–75%), followed by blows to the abdomen (15%) and falls (6–9%)
- Mechanism of injury and kinematics are important factors in evaluating patients for possible splenic injury.
- Splenic injuries are graded by type and severity of injury:
  - Grade I:
    - Hematoma: Subcapsular, <10% surface area
    - Laceration: Capsular tear, <1 cm in parenchymal depth
  - Grade II:
    - Hematoma: Subcapsular, 10–50% surface area; intraparenchymal, <5 cm in diameter
    - Laceration: Capsular tear, 1–3 cm in parenchymal depth and not involving a trabecular vessel
  - Grade III:
    - Hematoma: Subcapsular, >50% surface area or expanding, ruptured subcapsular or parenchymal hematoma; intraparenchymal hematoma, ≥5 cm or expanding
    - Laceration: >3 cm in parenchymal depth or involving the trabecular vessels
  - Grade IV:
    - Laceration: Involving the segmental or hilar vessels and producing major devascularization (>25% of spleen)
  - Grade V:
    - Laceration: Completely shattered spleen
    - Vascular: Hilar vascular injury that devascularizes the spleen

### Pediatric Considerations
- Poorly developed musculature and relatively smaller anteroposterior diameter increase the vulnerability of abdominal contents to compressive forces.
- Rib cage is extremely compliant and less prone to fracture in children but provides only partial protection against splenic injury.
- Splenic capsule in children is relatively thicker than that of an adult; parenchyma of spleen seems to contain more smooth muscle than in adults.
- Significant abdominal injury occurs in only about 5% of child abuse cases but is the 2nd most common cause of death after head injury.

## DIAGNOSIS

### SIGNS AND SYMPTOMS
#### History
- In blunt trauma, note the type and direction (horizontal or vertical) of any deceleration or compressive forces:
  - Injuries are caused by compression of the spleen between the anterior abdominal wall and the posterior thoracic cage or vertebra (eg, lap-belt restraints).
- In penetrating trauma, note the characteristic of the weapon (type and caliber), distance from the weapon, or the type and length of knife or impaling object:
  - Injuries result from a combination of the kinetic energy and shear forces of penetration.

#### Physical Exam
- Systemic signs from acute blood loss:
  - Syncope, dizziness, weakness, confusion
  - Hypotension or shock
- Local signs:
  - LUQ abdominal tenderness
  - Palpable tender mass in LUQ (Balance sign)
  - Referred pain to the left shoulder (Kehr sign)
  - Abdominal distention, rigidity, rebound tenderness, involuntary guarding
- Contusions, abrasions, or penetrating wounds to the chest, flank, or abdomen may indicate underlying spleen injury.
- Fractures of lower left ribs are commonly seen in association with splenic injuries.

### Pediatric Considerations
Age-related difficulties in communication, fear-induced uncooperative behavior, or a concomitant head injury make clinical exam less reliable.

### ESSENTIAL WORKUP
- Physical exam is neither specific nor sensitive for splenic injury.
- Adjunctive imaging studies are required.

### DIAGNOSTIC TESTS & INTERPRETATION
#### Lab
- No hematologic laboratory studies are specific for diagnosis of injury to the spleen.
- Obtain baseline hemoglobin, type and cross-match, and chemistries.

#### Imaging
- Plain abdominal radiographs:
  - Too nonspecific to be of value
  - CXR findings suggestive for splenic injury include left lower rib fracture(s), elevation of left hemidiaphragm, or left pleural effusion
- Ultrasound (US; FAST exam):
  - Can be done at bedside, especially if the patient is too unstable to go to CT
  - Primary role is detecting free intraperitoneal blood, which may suggest splenic injury
  - Does not image solid parenchymal damage well
  - Technically compromised by uncooperative patient, obesity, substantial bowel gas, and SC air
- CT scan:
  - Procedure of choice in stable patient
  - Depicts the presence and extent of splenic injury and adjacent organs, including the retroperitoneum
  - Provides the most specific information in patients stable enough to go to the CT scanner
- Angiography:
  - Has been added to the diagnostic and treatment options for selected cases

#### Diagnostic Procedures/Surgery
Diagnostic peritoneal lavage (DPL):
- Extremely sensitive for the presence of hemoperitoneum although nonspecific for source of bleeding and does not evaluate retroperitoneum

### DIFFERENTIAL DIAGNOSIS
- Intraperitoneal organ injury, especially liver
- Injury to retroperitoneal structures
- Thoracic injury

**TREATMENT**

**PRE-HOSPITAL**
- Obtain details of injury from prehospital providers.
- Insert 2 large-bore IVs.
- Penetrating wounds or evisceration should be covered with moist, sterile dressings.

**INITIAL STABILIZATION/THERAPY**
- Airway management (including C-spine immobilization)
- Standard trauma resuscitation measures:
  - Adequate IV access, including central lines and cutdowns, as dictated by the patient's hemodynamic status
  - Fluid resuscitation, initially with 2 L of crystalloid (NS or lactated Ringer solution), followed by blood products as needed

**ED TREATMENT/PROCEDURES**
- Immediate laparotomy may be appropriate in the acutely injured patient who is hemodynamically unstable with presumed hemoperitoneum and splenic injury.
- Most patients with acute splenic injury either are hemodynamically stable or stabilize rapidly with relatively small amounts of fluid resuscitation.
- Adjunctive diagnostic procedures supplementing the physical exam should be performed early in the evaluation, followed by laparotomy when indicated by positive diagnostic findings.
- Gunshot wounds to the anterior abdomen are routinely explored in the OR.
- Stab wounds can be managed by local wound exploration, followed by US or DPL when intraperitoneal penetration is suspected.

- Operative vs. nonoperative management:
  - Patients with signs and symptoms of intraperitoneal hemorrhage, those with operative indications based on imaging/diagnostic procedures, and those who fail nonoperative management should undergo laparotomy.
  - Splenectomy vs. splenic salvage depends on the grade of splenic injury.
  - >70% of all stable patients are currently being treated via nonoperative management:
    ○ Hemodynamic stability
    ○ Negative abdominal exam
    ○ Absence of contrast extravasation on CT
    ○ Absence of other clear indications for exploratory laparotomy
    ○ Absence of associated health conditions that carry an increased risk for bleeding (eg, coagulopathy, hepatic failure, anticoagulant use, coagulation factor deficiency)
    ○ Injury grade I–III
  - Option for angiographic embolization in hemodynamically stable patient

*Geriatric Considerations*
Patients >55 yr should be considered for operative management due to decreased physical tolerance to traumatic insult and reduced physiologic reserve.

*Pediatric Considerations*
Nonoperative management of splenic injuries is considered safe:
- Concerns for overwhelming postsplenectomy infection/sepsis

 **FOLLOW-UP**

**DISPOSITION**
*Admission Criteria*
All patients with splenic injury require hospitalization for definitive laparotomy or observation with serial abdominal exams, serial hematocrit determinations, and bed rest.

*Discharge Criteria*
Only asymptomatic patients objectively demonstrated not to have splenic or other traumatic injury may be discharged.

## ADDITIONAL READING

- Beauchamp RD, et al. The Spleen. *Sabiston textbook of surgery*, 18th ed. Philadelphia: Saunders Elsevier, 2008.
- Harbrecht B. Is anything new in adult blunt splenic trauma? *Am J Surg*. 2005;190(2):273–278.
- Izu, BS et al. Impact of splenic injury guidelines on hospital stay and charges in patients with isolated splenic injury. *Surgery*. 2009;146(4):787–791.
- Marx J. Abdominal trauma. In: Rosen P, et al, eds. *Emergency medicine: Concepts and clinical practice*, 5th ed. St. Louis: CV Mosby, 2002:415–436.
- Richardson, JD. Changes in the management of injuries to the liver and spleen. *J Am C Surg*. 2005;200(5):648–669.

 **CODES**

**ICD9**
- 865.00 Unspecified injury to spleen without mention of open wound into cavity
- 865.10 Unspecified injury to spleen with open wound into cavity

S

# SPONDYLOLYSIS/SPONDYLOLISTHESIS

Lisa G. Lowe Hiller

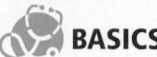 **BASICS**

## DESCRIPTION

- Spondylolysis:
  - Bony defect at the pars interarticularis (the isthmus of bone between the superior and inferior facets)
  - Can be unilateral or bilateral
  - Bilateral form has a much higher likelihood of slippage or spondylolisthesis than the unilateral form
- Spondylolisthesis:
  - The slipping forward of one vertebra upon another
  - Spondylolysis can contribute to spondylolisthesis, which is noted in ~5% of the population. It is 2–4 times more common in males.
  - Of those with spondylolysis, 50% will have some degree of spondylolisthesis develop during their lifetime, and 50% of those will be symptomatic:
    ○ Literature does not associate athletic activity with increased slippage.
  - Spondylolisthesis predisposes to nerve root impingement and frequently sciatica.
- Classification:
  - Type 1—dysplastic: Congenital defect of the neural arch or intra-articular facets is often associated with spina bifida occulta.
  - Type 2—isthmic: Stress fracture from repetitive microtrauma through the neural arch
  - Type 3—degenerative: Long-standing segmental instability
  - Type 4—traumatic
  - Type 5—pathologic: Leneralized or focal bone disease.
  - Spondylolisthesis is divided into four grades based on degree of slippage (Meyerding grading system):
    ○ Grade I: Up to 25% of the vertebral body width
    ○ Grade II: 26%–50% of vertebral body width
    ○ Grade III: 51%–75% of vertebral body width
    ○ Grade IV: 76%–100% of vertebral body width
  - The most common location for spondylolisthesis is L5 displaced on the sacrum (85%–95%), followed by L4 on L5.

### Pediatric Considerations
- Spondylolysis is one of the most common causes of serious low back pain in children, although it is most often asymptomatic.
- Symptoms most often present during adolescent growth spurt from age 10–15 yr.
- Seen commonly in athletic teens; particularly in sports involving back hyperextension (eg, gymnastics, diving, football).
- Acute symptoms are related to trauma.

## ETIOLOGY
Unknown; theories include congenital pars anomalies, alterations in bone density, and recurrent subclinical stress injury.

 **DIAGNOSIS**

## SIGNS AND SYMPTOMS
### History
- Onset often gradual, unless traumatic
- Often associated with feeling of stiffness or spasm in paravertebral muscles
- Pain in the back and proximal legs aggravated by standing and walking
- Sitting or forward bending relieves pain.
- Pain occurs after varying amounts of exercise, with standing, or with coughing:
  - Aggravating factors can include repetitive hyperextending movements.
  - Alleviating factors can include rest, although the course is variable and slow and usually requires sitting or stooping positions.
- Systemic/neurologic symptoms: minimal, unless there is significant trauma or "slip."

### Physical Exam
- Hyperlordotic posture:
  - Trunk may appear shortened.
  - Rib cage approaches iliac crests.
- Hamstring tightness:
  - Knees flexed to allow patient to stand upright
- Only "typical" finding is one-legged hyperextension:
  - Standing on one leg and leaning backward reproduces pain on ipsilateral side.
- Palpation may reveal step-off with a prominent spinous process of L5 in significant spondylolisthesis.
- Neurologic exam is usually normal:
  - If abnormal, pain and sensorimotor loss is in a dermatomal distribution.
  - Consider herniation or spondylolisthesis.

### Pediatric Considerations
- Spondylolysis in a child <10 yr is rare; these patients should be watched for:
- Constant pain lasting several weeks
- Pain occurring spontaneously at night
- Pain that interferes repeatedly with school, play, or sports
- Pain associated with marked stiffness, limitation of motion, fever, or neurologic signs
- Pain at the lumbosacral junction

## DIAGNOSTIC TESTS & INTERPRETATION
### Lab
There are no required laboratory studies.

### Imaging
- Lumbosacral spine radiographs:
  - Lateral and oblique radiographs of spine most helpful.
  - Spondylolysis will manifest as a radiolucent defect in the pars interarticularis, visible as a "collar" or "broken neck" on the oblique view "Scottie dog":
  - Secondary radiographic signs may include sclerosis of the contralateral pedicle and spina bifida occulta at the level of the spondylolysis.
  - Majority (80%–95%) found at L5–S1 level, 15% at L4–L5.
  - Spondylolisthesis will manifest as forward slipping of one vertebral body on another (seen on lateral view).
- Single photon emission computed tomography (SPECT)—better specificity for linking back pain to spondylolysis.
- CT scan:
  - Pathology more clearly demonstrated than on plain films
  - Can identify other spinal pathology
  - Plays an important role for orthopedics in management decisions through identification of new stress fractures and healing of old stress fractures.
  - If a CT scan is obtained in the ED, sagittal reconstructions should be performed and the CT scanner should be at minimum a 16-slice scanner.
  - Outpatient evaluation unless history of recent trauma.
- MRI—exact role not yet clarified in literature:
  - Useful for defining root impingement and foraminal narrowing.
  - May be useful in the assessment of acuity of abnormality.
  - Can identify alternate pathologic diagnoses.

### Pediatric Considerations
- Lower threshold for ordering imaging studies.
- Progressive slipping more likely to occur than in adults.

### DIFFERENTIAL DIAGNOSIS
- Tuberculosis (Pott disease)
- Discitis
- Bone or spinal cord tumor
- Pyelonephritis
- Retroperitoneal infection
- Injury to muscles or joints of back
- Congenital hip dislocation
- Rickets
- Ruptured intervertebral disc
- Vascular claudication
- Osteomyelitis
- Osteoid osteoma

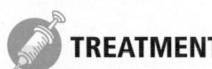

## TREATMENT

### PRE-HOSPITAL
Spinal precautions are not needed unless there is a history of recent trauma.

### INITIAL STABILIZATION/THERAPY
Vigorous attempts at traction should not be pursued.

### ED TREATMENT/PROCEDURES
- Pain control and muscle relaxants as clinically needed
- Supportive therapy if symptoms are mild
- Restrict activities if repetitive trauma is likely aggravating cause (eg, sports) for 3–6 wk, followed by reintroduction of activity when asymptomatic.
- Consider antilordotic braces (controversial) or physical therapy.
- Orthopedic consult or referral if symptoms are moderate to severe or unresponsive to supportive care
- Surgical intervention typically consists of spinal fusion in the flexed position:
  – 50% of symptomatic patients with spondylolisthesis may require surgery.
- All symptomatic patients with grade III or IV spondylolisthesis should probably undergo surgery.
- Exercises are not of proven benefit.

### Pediatric Considerations
- Activity restriction is not necessary if minimal or no symptoms.
- Literature suggests good outcome for young athletes with conservative treatment.

### MEDICATION
- Muscle relaxants:
  – Example—methocarbamol: 1,000–1,500 mg PO q.i.d. (peds: safety and effectiveness for children <12 yr of age not established)
  – Diazepam: 2–10 mg PO t.i.d. – q.i.d.
  – Cyclobenzaprine: 5–10 mg PO t.i.d. (peds: safe for ages >15 yr old)
- NSAIDs:
  – Example—ibuprofen: 200–800 mg PO t.i.d.–q.i.d. (peds: 5–10 mg/kg PO q6h)
- Opioids (doses can vary on oral medications):
  – Example—morphine sulfate: 0.1 mg/kg up to 2- to 4-mg increments IV.
  – Acetaminophen/hydrocodone: 5/500 mg 1–2 tabs PO q.i.d.
  – Acetaminophen/oxycodone: 5/325 mg 1–2 tabs PO q.i.d.
  – Acetaminophen/codeine: 300/30 mg 1–2 tabs PO q.i.d. (peds: 0.5–1 mg/kg codeine PO q4–6h; max 60 mg per dose codeine; 1g per dose, 75 mg/kg/day up to 4 g/day >3 yr old)

## FOLLOW-UP

### DISPOSITION
#### Admission Criteria
- Inability to walk
- Inability to cope at home due to pain or social situation
- New or progressive neurologic deficit

#### Discharge Criteria
- Orthopedic follow-up arranged
- Social support system in place
- Pain control
- Patient education

#### Pediatric Considerations
Close follow-up is mandatory.

## ADDITIONAL READING

- Castillo M, Mukherji S. Spinal imaging: Overview and update. *Neuroimaging Clin N Am*. 2007;7(1):92–93.
- Congeni J, McCulloch J, Swanson K. Lumbar spondylolysis. A study of natural progression in athletes. *Am J Sports Med*. 1997;25(2):248–253.
- Debnath UK, Freeman BJ, et al. Clinical outcome and return to sport after the surgical treatment of spondylolysis in young athletes. *J Bone Joint Surg*. 2003;85(2);244.
- Iwamoto J, Takeda T, Wakano K. Returning athletes with severe low back pain and spondylolysis to original sporting activities with conservative treatment. *Scand J Med Sci Sports*. 2004;14(6):337.
- Miller SF, Congeni J, Swanson K. Long-term functional and anatomical follow-up of early detected spondylolysis in young athletes. *Am J Sports Med*. 2004;32(4):928.
- Nachemson A. Newest knowledge of low back pain. *Clin Orthop*. 1992;279:8.
- Satndaert CJ. Spondylolysis. *Phys Med Rehab Clin North Am*. 2000;11(4):785–801.
- Skinner H. Disorders, diseases and injuries of the spine. In: *Current Diagnosis and Treatment in Orthopedics*. Norwalk, CT: Appleton & Lange, 1995:206–211.
- Vitek G. Spine conference spondylolysis and spondylolisthesis. *Ortho News Mag*. May 1995. Available at: www.nmis.com/onm/html/sponconf-spon.htm.
- Weinstein J, Wiesel S. Lumbar and lumbosacral spondylolisthesis In: *The Lumbar Spine: The International Society for the Study of the Lumbar Spine*. Philadelphia: Saunders, 1990:471–545.

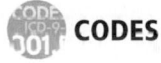

## CODES

### ICD9
- 738.4 Acquired spondylolisthesis
- 756.11 Congenital spondylolysis, lumbosacral region
- 756.12 Spondylolisthesis, congenital

S

# SPONTANEOUS BACTERIAL PERITONITIS

Michael Schmidt
Lucas C. Rosiere

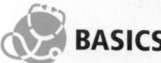

## BASICS

### DESCRIPTION
- Infection of ascites fluid without an evident intra-abdominal surgically treatable source:
  – Ascites polymorphonuclear leukocyte count >250/mL with a positive bacterial ascites culture
- Must be distinguished from secondary bacterial peritonitis:
  – Nonsurgical management of secondary bacterial peritonitis carries 100% mortality.
  – Surgical management of spontaneous bacterial peritonitis (SBP) carries 80% mortality.

### ETIOLOGY
- Mechanism:
  – Portal hypertension causes translocation of overgrown bacteria through edematous gut mucosa to lymph nodes to the peritoneal cavity.
  – Transient bacteremia with low serum complement
  – Impaired activity of reticuloendothelial system phagocytosis and opsonization
  – Can also seed ascitic fluid via bacteremia from infections outside of the gut
- Usually seen in the setting of cirrhosis:
  – Rare in other conditions causing ascites (nephrotic syndrome or CHF)
- Predominant organisms:
  – 65% aerobic gram-negative (50% of which are *E. coli*)
  – 35% gram-positive (74% streptococci)
- Gram-positives account for 50% of cases in patients who are on prophylactic therapy with fluoroquinolones.

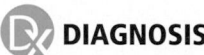

## DIAGNOSIS

### SIGNS AND SYMPTOMS
13% of patients with SBP have no signs or symptoms of infection.

#### History
- Abdominal pain: diffuse, constant, often very mild
- Fever, chills
- Diarrhea from bacterial overgrowth
- Worsening ascites
- Altered mental status
- Fatigue, myalgias

#### Physical Exam
- Fever is the most common sign:
  – A lower threshold for fever (>37.8°C or >100.0°F) is maintained for cirrhotic patients owing to baseline hypothermia
- Altered mental status
- Ascites
- Abdominal tenderness:
  – Development of a rigid abdomen does not occur because of the separation of visceral and parietal pleura due to ascites.

### ESSENTIAL WORKUP
- Paracentesis is the mainstay of diagnosis unless patient has peritoneal dialysis:
- Procedure:
  – Coagulopathy does not have be corrected before the procedure (except for platelets <20,000)
  – Location (with patient supine):
    ○ 3 cm cephalad and medial to anterosuperior iliac spine OR
    ○ 2 cm caudad to the umbilicus (ensure bladder emptying beforehand)
  – 40 mL should be aspirated, then change needles to avoid contamination:
    ○ 10 mL for each culture bottle
    ○ 10 mL for cell count, chemistries, Gram's stain (lithium–heparin tube, EDTA tube, and sterile container)
  – Inoculate culture bottles with ascitic fluid immediately at the bedside.

### DIAGNOSTIC TESTS & INTERPRETATION
#### Lab
- Routine ascites fluid assays:
  – Cell count and differential
    ○ Include bands as PMNs
  – Total protein
  – Albumin
  – Culture
  – Gram's stain
  – Optional fluid assays
    ○ Glucose
    ○ LDH (from lysed PMNs)
    ○ Amylase

- Characteristics of ascitic fluid consistent with SBP:
  – PMNs >250/mL
  – total protein <1 g/dL
  – Normal amylase
  – Positive culture
  – Positive Gram's stain
  – Glucose >50 mg/dL
  – LDH >63 mU/mL
  – Serum–ascites albumin gradient >1.1 g/dL consistent with portal hypertension
- Blood tests (usually reflect underlying disease):
  – CBC with differential
  – Basic metabolic panel
  – PT/PTT
  – LFTs (including albumin)
  – Blood cultures
  – UA and culture

#### Imaging
- Abdominal ultrasound:
  – Confirms presence of ascites
  – Helps guide paracentesis
- Chest radiograph
- Abdominal radiographs: flat-plate and upright to evaluate for perforation or obstruction
- Water-soluble contrast CT if likely secondary bacterial peritonitis with negative x-rays

#### Diagnostic Procedures/Surgery
Exploratory laparotomy if free air on x-ray or extravasation of contrast on CT

### DIFFERENTIAL DIAGNOSIS
- Alcohol hepatitis:
  – Fever, leukocytosis, abdominal pain ± ascites
  – Ascites PMNs <250/mm$^3$
- Secondary bacterial peritonitis:
  – Due to perforation or abscess
  – Polymicrobial Gram's stain or 2 of following
    ○ Ascites total protein >1 g/dL
    ○ Ascites glucose <50 mg/dL
    ○ Ascites LDH >1/2 upper limit of normal serum LDH
  – Orange ascites with bilirubin >6 mg/dL suggests ruptured gallbladder
- Culture-negative neutrocytic ascites:
  – Ascites PMNs >250/mL, culture negative

- Monomicrobial nonneutrocytic bacterascites:
  - Due to colonization phase of SBP
  - Ascites PMNs <250/mL, monomicrobial culture
  - Treated like SBP if symptomatic
- Polymicrobial bacterascites:
  - Due to accidental gut perforation (1 in 1,000 paracenteses)
  - Ascites PMNs <250/mL, polymicrobial culture
- Pancreatitis:
  - Elevated ascites amylase
- Peritoneal carcinomatosis or tuberculous peritonitis:
  - Secondary bacterial peritonitis criteria with non-PMN predominance and no fever

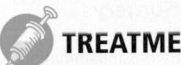

## TREATMENT

### PRE-HOSPITAL
- IV fluids for hypotension
- Accucheck for altered mental status

### INITIAL STABILIZATION/THERAPY
- ABCs
- Aggressive IV fluid resuscitation
- Prompt antibiotic treatment for septic shock

### ED TREATMENT/PROCEDURES
- Administer platelets before paracentesis only if <20,000
- Give empiric antibiotics immediately after paracentesis for otherwise unexplained:
  - Ascites PMNs >250/mL or
  - Temperature >37.8°C or
  - Altered mental status or
  - Abdominal pain/tenderness
- Antibiotic options:
  - 1st choice: 3rd-generation cephalosporin
    2nd choice: Ampicillin–sulbactam or aztreonam
    Avoid aminoglycosides, fluoroquinolones
  - Add metronidazole for secondary bacterial peritonitis
- IV albumin is helpful in preventing renal impairment and reducing mortality in diagnosed SBP.

### Prognosis
- In-hospital noninfection–related mortality is 20%
- 1- and 2-yr mortality rates after an episode of SBP are 70%–80%, respectively.

## MEDICATION
- Albumin: 1.5 g/kg IV on day 1
- Ampicillin-sulbactam 1.5–3 g IM/IV q6h
- Aztreonam: 0.5–2 g IM/IV q6–12h
- Cefotaxime: 2 g IV q8h
- Ceftriaxone: 2 g IV q8h

 FOLLOW-UP

### DISPOSITION
#### Admission Criteria
- Admit all patients for IV antibiotics and Gastroenterology consultation
- ICU admission for septic shock or severe hepatic encephalopathy

#### Discharge Criteria
If patient refuses admission and has no shock, encephalopathy, azotemia or GI bleeding, a dose of IV ceftriaxone and a course of oral fluoroquinolones followed by close follow-up may be appropriate.

#### Issues for Referral
Hepatology or Gastroenterology referral may be indicated.

### ALERT
Infections related to continuous abdominal peritoneal dialysis

- Symptoms: cloudy peritoneal fluid (90%), abdominal pain (80%), and fever (50%)
- Signs: abdominal tenderness, 70%
- Diagnosis: peritoneal WBCs >100/mL with positive Gram's stain or culture
- Microbiology:
  - >50% of cases are due to gram-positives, most commonly staphylococci.
    *E. coli* is an *uncommon* cause of peritonitis in patients with chronic ambulant peritoneal dialysis.
- Treatment:
  - Antibiotics are given through the intraperitoneal (IP) route.
  - 1st choice: cefazolin (1 g IP per day) + ceftazidime (1 g IP per day)
  - Vancomycin (2 g IP every week) is alternative to cefazolin.
  - Amikacin 2 mg/kg/d IP

## FOLLOW-UP RECOMMENDATIONS
GI specialty or PCP follow-up for patients with SBP

## PEARLS AND PITFALLS
- One must rule our secondary bacterial peritonitis first.
- Bedside inoculation of blood culture bottles with ascitic fluid increases culture yield.
- Maintain high suspicion for SBP, since many patients may be asymptomatic.

## ADDITIONAL READING
- Grabeau CM, Crago SF, Hoff LK, et al. Performance standards for therapeutic abdominal paracentesis. *Hepatology*. 2004;40:484.
- Such J, Runyon BA. Spontaneous bacterial peritonitis. *Clin Infect Dis*. 1998;27:669.
- Wong CL, Holroyd-Leduc J, Thorpe KE, Straus SE. Does this patient have bacterial peritonitis or portal hypertension? How do I perform a paracentesis and analyze the results? *JAMA*. 2008;299:1166.

### See Also (Topic, Algorithm, Electronic Media Element)
- GI Bleeding
- Hepatitis
- Hepatorenal Syndrome

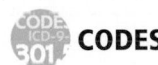 CODES

ICD9
567.23 Spontaneous bacterial peritonitis

S

# SPOROTRICHOSIS
*Maggie Ferng*

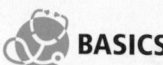 **BASICS**

## DESCRIPTION
- Lymphocutaneous:
  - Most common form
  - Inoculation of fungus (*Sporothrix schenckii*) into skin/soft tissue
  - Disease with or without hematogenous spread after traumatic inoculation with soil or plant material
  - Secondary to animal bites/scratches, trauma
  - Increased risk: farmers, gardeners, forestry workers
- Pulmonary:
  - Inhalation of conidia aerosolized from soil/plant decay
  - Increased risk: alcoholics, diabetics, COPD, steroid users
- Multifocal extracutaneous:
  - Cutaneous inoculation or hematologic spread
  - Increased risk: HIV/immunosuppressed patients

## ETIOLOGY
- Fungal infection caused by *S. schenckii*:
- Dimorphic fungus
- Occurs as mold on decaying vegetation, moss, and soil in temperate and tropical environments
- Animal vectors, notably cats and armadillos

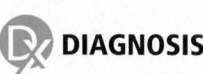 **DIAGNOSIS**

## SIGNS AND SYMPTOMS
- Several clinical manifestations/syndromes
- Determined by mode of inoculation and host factors
- Lymphocutaneous:
  - Initial lesions appear days to weeks after inoculation
  - Begin as papules, become nodular, often ulcerate
    - Distal extremities more commonly involved
    - Size: millimeters to 4 cm
    - Pain absent or mild
    - Drainage is nonpurulent
  - Systemic symptoms usually absent
  - Secondary nodular lesions develop along lymphatics draining original site.
  - May wax and wane over years if untreated

- Fixed cutaneous:
  - Plaquelike or verrucous lesion at site of inoculation (typically face and extremities)
  - Ulceration uncommon
  - Do not manifest lymphangitic progression
- Extracutaneous:
  - Osteoarticular
    - Secondary to local or hematologic inoculation
    - Septic arthritis more common than osteoarthritis
    - Joint inflammation, effusion, and pain
    - Single or multiple joint involvement of extremities
    - Indolent onset, few systemic symptoms
    - Tenosynovitis, septic arthritis, bursitis, nerve entrapment syndrome
    - Usually poor outcome due to delayed diagnosis
- Pulmonary:
  - Syndrome resembles mycobacterial infection.
  - Fever, weight loss, fatigue
  - Productive cough, hemoptysis
- Multifocal extracutaneous (disseminated):
  - Low-grade fever, weight loss
  - Diffuse cutaneous lesions
  - Arthritis/osteolytic lesions/parenchymal involvement
  - Chronic lymphocytic meningitis
  - Ocular adnexa, endophthalmitis
  - Genitourinary, sinuses
  - Can be fatal if untreated
  - Often occurs in immunocompromised host

## History
- Activity with exposure to soil, moss or organic material
- Fixed cutaneous or lymphocutaneous: Healthy host
- Disseminated/extracutaneous: Diabetics, COPD, HIV/AIDS

## Physical Exam
- Fixed cutaneous/lymphocutaneous: Lesions found on exam
- Disseminated: Nonspecific findings

## ESSENTIAL WORKUP
Diagnosis dependent on isolation *S. schenckii* from site of infection:
- Culture from aspirated material, tissue biopsy, or sputum

## DIAGNOSTIC TESTS & INTERPRETATION
### Lab
- Blood tests not indicated with cutaneous disease
- Cultures of sputum, synovial fluid, CSF, blood as indicated by extracutaneous manifestations
- No reliable serologic assays available

### Imaging
- Pulmonary:
  - Chest radiograph reveals cavitary lesions
- Extracutaneous/disseminated:
  - Consider bone scan in immunocompromised host.

### Diagnostic Procedures/Surgery
- Lymphocutaneous/fixed cutaneous:
  - Biopsy reveals pyogranulomatous inflammation, 3–5-mm cigar-shaped yeast
- Pulmonary:
  - Gram's stain of sputum may yield yeast; sputum cultures often positive
- Extracutaneous/disseminated:
  - CSF reveals lymphocytic meningitis, increased protein/decreased glucose

## DIFFERENTIAL DIAGNOSIS
- Lymphocutaneous:
  - Leishmaniasis
  - Nocardiosis
  - Mycobacterium marinum
  - Tularemia
- Fixed cutaneous:
  - Bacterial pyoderma
  - Foreign-body granuloma
  - Inflammatory dermatophyte infections
  - Blastomycosis
  - Mycobacteria
- Osteoarticular:
  - Rheumatoid arthritis
  - Gout
  - Tuberculosis
  - Bacterial arthritis
  - Pigmented villonodular synovitis
- Pulmonary and meningitis:
  - Histoplasmosis
  - Coccidioidomycosis
  - Cryptococcal disease
  - Mycobacterial infections

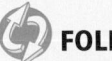 **TREATMENT**

### INITIAL STABILIZATION/THERAPY
Airway/hemodynamic stabilization for severely ill patients with extracutaneous manifestations

### ED TREATMENT/PROCEDURES
- Lymphocutaneous/fixed cutaneous:
  - Itraconazole (drug of choice): Better tolerated but more expensive and potential for hepatotoxicity
  - Saturated solution of potassium iodide (SSKI): Less expensive but bitter taste and side effects (anorexia, nausea, diarrhea) lead to limited acceptability
  - Local heat therapy for cutaneous disease (>35°C) inhibits fungal growth, use in pregnant patients or others who cannot tolerate medication, therapy may take 3–6 mo
- Pulmonary:
  - Itraconazole or amphotericin B in early disease, effective in ~30% of cases
  - More advanced disease often requires resection plus amphotericin B
- Osteoarticular:
  - Itraconazole: First line, therapy more than 1 yr, amphotericin B if refractory
- Disseminated:
  - Amphotericin initially
  - Itraconazole in stable, immunocompetent patients
  - HIV and sporotrichosis: Suppressive therapy with itraconazole is recommended after initial infection

### MEDICATION
- Amphotericin B: Lipid form 2–3 mg/kg daily, if using deoxychelate form (no risk of renal dysfunction) 0.7–1 mg/kg q.d.
- Itraconazole: Lymphocutaneous: 200 mg PO per day for 6 mo, pulmonary/osteoarticular 200 mg PO b.i.d.
- SSKI: 5 gtt in water or juice t.i.d.; increase by 5 gtt per dose each week up to a max 40–50 gtt t.i.d. as tolerated, for 6–12 wk or until lesions resolve

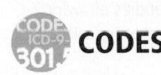 **FOLLOW-UP**

### DISPOSITION
#### Admission Criteria
- Systemic signs/symptoms
- Pulmonary, CNS, multifocal disease
- Immunosuppressed host with disseminated disease

#### Discharge Criteria
Lymphocutaneous/fixed cutaneous form, nontoxic

#### Issues for Referral
Infectious disease consultant as appropriate

### FOLLOW-UP RECOMMENDATIONS
Infectious disease specialist, Dermatology, appropriate specialist given disease involvement (Orthopedics, Neurology)

## PEARLS AND PITFALLS

Fixed cutaneous, lymphocutaneous, pulmonary, extracutaneous/disseminated disease secondary to *S. schenckii*:

- Innoculation with soil, moss or organic material (skin break or inhalation)
- Healthy hosts develop fixed cutaneous/lymphocutaneous disease, immunocompromised hosts develop extracutaneous/disseminated disease
- Disseminated disease presents with nonspecific symptoms that often result in delayed diagnosis and poor outcome.
- Oral itraconazole is first-line therapy except for disseminated disease, where amphotericin is used initially

## ADDITIONAL READING

- Bustamante B, Campos PE. Endemic sporotrichosis. *Curr Opin Infect Dis*. 2001;14(2):145–149.
- da Rosa AC, Scroferneker ML, Vettorato R, et al. Epidemiology of sporotrichosis: A study of 304 cases in Brazil. *J Am Acad Dermatol*. 2005;52:451.
- Kauffman CA, Bustamante B, Chapman SW, Pappas PG. Clinical practice guidelines for the management of sportrichosis: 2007 update by the Infectious Diseases Society of America. *Clin Infect Dis*. 2007;45:1255.
- Rex JH, Okhuysen PC. *Sporothrix schenckii*. In: Mandel GL, Douglas RG, Bennett JE, eds. *Principles and Practice of Infectious Diseases*, 5th ed. New York: Churchill Livingstone, 2000:2695–2699.

**CODES**

### ICD9
117.1 Sporotrichosis

**S**

# STAPHYLOCOCCAL SCALDED SKIN SYNDROME

Tala R. Elia
Peter L. Hulsey

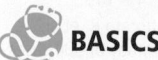 **BASICS**

## DESCRIPTION

- Results from the actions of a soluble epidermolytic exotoxin produced by *Staphylococcus aureus:*
  - Produced at a distant site of infection or colonization
  - Disseminates hematogenously
  - Lyses desmosomes of granular cells in the superficial epidermis
  - Results in generalized intradermal exfoliation
- Typically affects infants and children <6 yr of age:
  - Adults have specific staph antibodies allowing them to localize, metabolize, and excrete the staph toxins.
  - Infants and children are unable to metabolize and excrete toxin efficiently.
  - Immunocompromised adults and those with severe renal dysfunction are also susceptible
- Presentation determined by age and extent of rash:
  - Classic staphylococcal scalded skin syndrome
  - Pemphigus neonatorum
  - Bullous impetigo
- Typically, coagulase-positive phage group II *Staphylococcus:*
  - Phage groups I and III also implicated

## ETIOLOGY

- Colonization often without overt infection
- Concurrent infection or break of skin barrier:
  - Nasopharynx
  - Urinary tract
  - Minor skin abrasions
  - Circumcision site
  - Conjunctivitis
  - Umbilicus/omphalitis
  - Impetigo
  - Endocarditis and septicemia
- Often no focus identified

## DIAGNOSIS

## SIGNS AND SYMPTOMS

- Constitutional symptoms:
  - Malaise
  - Fever
  - Irritability
  - Child may appear well, ill or overtly toxic
  - Abrupt onset
- Scarlatiniform erythematous rash (sandpaperlike) resembling a "sunburn"— erythroderma
- Exquisitely tender skin
- Areas of prominence:
  - Around the flexor areas of the neck
  - Intertriginous areas, especially axilla and groin
  - Near the eyes and mouth
  - Increased erythema in skin creases
- Facial edema with radial crusting fissures around the eyes, nose, and mouth
- Flaccid bullae:
  - Within 1–3 days after onset of rash
  - Initially over flexures (axillae, groin, body orifices)
  - Bullae migrate through epidermis with light lateral pressure; epidermis separates with minor pressure (Nikolsky sign).
  - Rupture within hours
  - Epidermis separates with minor trauma.
  - Epidermis is shed in sheets.
  - Denuded areas are moist, sensitive, and painful.
  - Complete healing within 2 wk, no scarring
- Purulent conjunctivitis
- Mucous membranes not affected
- Complications rare:
  - Hypothermia
  - Fluid and electrolyte imbalance
  - Secondary infection
  - Pneumonia
  - Septicemia
  - Cellulitis
  - Osteomyelitis

## ESSENTIAL WORKUP

- Clinical presentation is diagnostic.
- Determine location/source of toxin producing *Staphylococcus.*
- Assess systemic nature of infection.

## DIAGNOSTIC TESTS & INTERPRETATION

### Lab

- CBC and urinalysis:
  - Assess for sepsis if source not obvious.
- Electrolytes:
  - Indicated if signs of dehydration or extensive rash
- Blood cultures (rarely positive)

### Imaging

Indicated as need to determine location/source of infection

### Diagnostic Procedures/Surgery

- Fluid aspirated from bullae:
  - Sterile in staphylococcal scalded skin syndrome
  - Consistent with hematogenous dissemination of the toxin
- Isolation of staphylococci from a site other than the blisters:
  - Commonly conjunctivae, nasopharynx, or blood
- Skin biopsy or frozen histologic section:
  - Determine level of epidermal/dermal separation (cleavage is in granular layer of dermis).
  - Indicated for children on medications, those >6 yr, and in cases of mixed presentation

## DIFFERENTIAL DIAGNOSIS

- Infection:
  - Scarlet fever:
    - Involves the mucous membranes
    - Strawberry tongue:
    - Painful desquamation does not occur.
  - Bullous impetigo:
    - Turbid or cloudy bullous fluid
  - Bullous varicella:
    - Tzanck prep or viral base reveals giant cells.
    - 5 days after the onset of varicella
  - Toxic shock syndrome:
    - Rapid development of clinical signs and symptoms
    - Mucous membrane and multiorgan involvement

- Toxic epidermal necrolysis or drug eruption:
  - Much more common in adults
  - Severely afflicted mucous membranes
  - Full-thickness epidermal necrosis
- Dermatologic:
  - Erythema multiforme
  - Epidermolysis hyperkeratosis
  - Epidermolysis bullosa
  - Pemphigus vulgaris
- Scald injury
- Secondary rash of an underlying disorder:
  - Lymphoma
  - Aspergillosis
  - Irradiation
  - Graft-versus-host reaction
  - Kawasaki disease

 **TREATMENT**

**PRE-HOSPITAL**
- 9% NS fluid bolus if dehydration present
- Initial burn treatment

**INITIAL STABILIZATION/THERAPY**
- Management is similar to an extensive 2nd-degree burn:
  - Involvement of large body-surface area will require IV fluids.
- Provide adequate analgesia.
- Undress and place child on sterile linen.
- Limit handling of child.
- Apply moist sterile dressings.
- Avoid excess heat loss.

**ED TREATMENT/PROCEDURES**
- Topical burn creams are of no proven benefit.
- Steroids are contraindicated.
- IV antibiotics effective against penicillinase-resistant *S. aureus:*
  - Cefazolin
  - Nafcillin
  - Vancomycin if methicillin-resistant *S. aureus* (MRSA) suspected
- Oral antibiotics for mild involvement:
  - Dicloxacillin
  - Erythromycin
  - Cephalexin

**MEDICATION**
- Cefazolin: 50–100 mg/kg/24 hr IV div. q.i.d.
- Cephalexin: 25–100 mg/kg/24 hr PO div. q.i.d.
- Dicloxacillin: 12–25 mg/kg/24 hr PO div. q.i.d.
- Erythromycin: 30–50 mg/kg/24 hr PO div. q.i.d.
- Nafcillin: 1–2 g IV q6h (peds: newborns, 50–100 mg/kg/24 h IV div. q6h; children, 100–200 mg/kg/24 h IV div. q6h)
- Vancomycin 40–60 mg/kg div. q.i.d.

 **FOLLOW-UP**

**DISPOSITION**
*Admission Criteria*
- Children <1 yr
- All toxic-appearing children
- Widespread skin involvement
- Dehydration and/or electrolyte derangement

*Discharge Criteria*
- Older, well-appearing children with mild involvement
- Oral antibiotics for 7 days
- Follow-up within 48 hr

*Issues for Referral*
- Infectious disease consultant
- Surgeon if source needs excision/drainage

## ADDITIONAL READING

- Blyth M, Estela C, Young AE. Severe staphylococcal scalded skin syndrome in children. *Burns* 2008;34:98–103.
- Freedberg IM, et al. *Fitzpatrick's Dermatology in General Medicine,* 6th ed. New York: McGraw-Hill, 2003: ch 195.
- Ladhani L. Recent developments in staphylococcal scalded skin syndrome. *Clin Microbiol Infect.* 2001;7(6):301–307.
- Stanley JR, Amagai A. *N Engl J Med.* 2006; 355(17):1800–1810.

 **CODES**

**ICD9**
695.81 Ritter's disease

S

# STERNOCLAVICULAR JOINT INJURY

Christopher Tedeschi
Wallace A. Carter

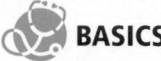
## BASICS

### DESCRIPTION
- Sternoclavicular joint (SCJ) is the only joint that connects the upper limb to the trunk.
- Among the least frequently injured joints in the body
- Trauma from vehicular or athletic injuries through direct or indirect mechanism
- Congenital or spontaneous dislocation and subluxation are rarely seen
- SCJ stability depends on ligamentous attachments, primarily anterior and posterior sternoclavicular ligaments, interclavicular ligament, and costoclavicular ligament

### ETIOLOGY
- Injury to the SCJ can be from sprains, subluxations, and dislocations.
- The SCJ can dislocate anteriorly or posteriorly.
- Direction of dislocation depends on the shoulder position:
  - Anterior dislocation more likely when the acromion is posterior to the manubrium.
  - Posterior dislocation more likely when the acromion is anterior to the manubrium.
- Anterior dislocation is more common (95–98% of dislocations):
  - Caused by a posteriorly directed force to the anterolateral aspect of the shoulder
  - Reciprocal anterior displacement of the medial clavicle
  - May be associated with pneumothorax, hemothorax, pulmonary contusion, and rib fractures
  - Subluxation and dislocation may occur spontaneously.
- Posterior dislocation results from:
  - Anterior-to-posterior blow to the medial clavicle
  - Anteriorly directed force to the posterolateral aspect of the shoulder
  - Reciprocal posterior displacement of the medial clavicle
- Posterior dislocation is a surgical emergency:
  - Indications for immediate reduction:
    - Compression or tear of trachea, esophagus, or great vessels
    - Recurrent laryngeal nerve injury

### Pediatric Considerations
- The medial epiphyseal growth plates of the clavicles are last to ossify and fuse between ages 22 and 25:
  - Until fusion, growth plate is the weakest part of the joint
- Fractures through the medial epiphysis mimic SCJ dislocations:
  - Classified as Salter-Harris type I or II fractures
  - True dislocations of the SCJ are extremely rare in children because of strong ligamentous attachments.

## DIAGNOSIS

### SIGNS AND SYMPTOMS
- Pain and swelling localized to the medial clavicle and SCJ
- Affected arm supported across the chest by the contralateral arm
- Neck may be angled toward dislocated side to avoid tension of the sternocleidomastoid.
- Inability to abduct or externally rotate arm
- If the SCJ is dislocated, shoulder appears shortened:
  - Head tilts toward injured side due to sternocleidomastoid muscle spasm
- In anterior dislocation, medial end of the clavicle is visibly prominent and palpable.
- In posterior dislocation, there may be a sulcus of the SCJ area through which the lateral border of the manubrium may be palpated:
  - Dislocation may be masked by significant swelling over the sternoclavicular region, or may mimic anterior dislocation.
- Posterior dislocation may be accompanied by signs of vascular compromise or damage to mediastinal structures:
  - Signs of shock
  - Venous congestion in the neck or upper extremities
  - Asymmetric upper extremity pulses
  - Neurapraxia
  - Shortness of breath, hoarseness, dysphagia
- If subluxed or sprained, the SCJ is tender on direct palpation and with shoulder movement:
  - No deformity or significant AP mobility

### History
- High-energy direct blow, most often from athletic injuries or motor vehicle collisions
- Sprains and subluxations may be associated with other injuries of the shoulder girdle.

### Physical Exam
For any concern of posterior dislocation, a thorough neurovascular assessment is warranted:
- Palpate pulses in upper extremities
- Hoarseness may signify injury to the recurrent laryngeal nerve.
- Upper extremity neurologic exam
- Assess venous return in upper extremities.
- Dysphagia or respiratory distress may signify compression or disruption of trachea or esophagus.

### ESSENTIAL WORKUP
- Complete trauma evaluation and resuscitation for other life-threatening injuries
- Special attention to respiratory, neurologic, and vascular status
- A posterior dislocation implies a substantial mechanism of injury; other life-threatening injuries must be ruled out.
- Appropriate analgesia for patient comfort

### DIAGNOSTIC TESTS & INTERPRETATION
#### Imaging
- Difficult to assess SCJ injury with routine radiographs:
  - May demonstrate asymmetry of the SCJ compared with contralateral side
  - More useful to assess coexisting bony, pulmonary, and mediastinal injury
- US can reliably demonstrate SCJ dislocations:
  - Noninvasive, portable, and simple to use
  - May be useful in the initial ED evaluation of unstable patients with chest trauma
  - Use high-frequency linear probe
  - In anterior dislocation, medial clavicle seen anterior relative to manubrium compared to contralateral side
- CT scan is best to evaluate the SCJ:
  - Useful when plain films are inconclusive
  - Accurately differentiates fractures from dislocations
  - Demonstrates the position of the medial end of the clavicle
  - Shows detailed anatomy of the thoracic outlet and mediastinum
  - Contrast CT can show related vascular injuries and is the imaging modality of choice.
- MRI can be useful in demonstrating ligamentous and soft tissue SCJ injuries:
  - The articular disc is the most vulnerable soft-tissue structure in SCJ injury.
  - Can demonstrate particular ligamentous injuries in the setting of joint subluxation
  - Better suited for after the initial period of diagnosis and treatment

### DIFFERENTIAL DIAGNOSIS
- Sternoclavicular sprain, subluxation or dislocation
- Medial clavicle fracture
- Septic arthritis
- Osteomyelitis of medial clavicle
- Osteoarthritis

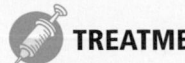

# TREATMENT

## PRE-HOSPITAL
- Attention to airway and vital signs, and neurovascular status of the affected extremity
- The affected arm should be splinted in the position of comfort before transport to the ED.

## INITIAL STABILIZATION/THERAPY
- Endotracheal intubation for signs of airway compromise or as needed in the trauma patient:
  - Then immediate medial clavicular reduction
- Emergent SCJ reduction for:
  - Hoarseness
  - Dysphagia
  - Neurovascular compromise:
    - Upper extremity weakness
    - Paresthesia
    - Diminished pulses
    - Signs of shock
    - Analgesia and sedation as needed

## ED TREATMENT/PROCEDURES
- *Anterior dislocations* may be reduced in the ED:
  - Procedural sedation for adequate pain control and muscle relaxation
  - Rolled towel placed between the shoulder blades in the supine position:
    - Longitudinal traction applied to the extended arm with shoulder abducted 90°
    - Assistant applies gentle pressure over the displaced end of the clavicle.
    - After reduction, immobilize with a well-padded figure-of-8 dressing.
  - Many anterior dislocations remain unstable after reduction.
  - Surgery rarely indicated, as deformity is mainly cosmetic
- *Posterior dislocations* require urgent reduction best achieved in the OR under general anesthesia:
  - Orthopedic and thoracic surgery consults
  - Closed reduction is preferred but may not be possible in injuries > 48 hr.
  - If surgeon not immediately available, emergent reduction in the ED may be necessary:
    - Relieve serious airway, neurologic, or vascular compromise.
    - A sterile towel clamp used to grasp medial clavicular head and gentle anterior traction applied to reduce the dislocation.
    - Adequate sedation is key.

## MEDICATION
Procedural sedation:
- Atropine: Used in pediatric patients in conjunction with ketamine to reduce secretions (peds: 0.02 mg/kg IV, minimum dose of 0.1 mg)
- Etomidate: 0.1 mg/kg IV
- Fentanyl: 1–2 μg/kg IV
- Ketamine: Peds: 1 mg/kg IV – up to 2 additional doses of 0.5 mg/kg IV prn
- Midazolam: 0.01 mg/kg (peds: 0.05–0.1 mg/kg) IV q2–3min
- Propofol: Initial bolus 1 mg/kg IV, then 0.5 mg/kg q3min as needed (adults and peds)

# FOLLOW-UP

## DISPOSITION
### Admission Criteria
- Posterior dislocations of the SCJ require admission for possible reduction in the OR and evaluation for potential intra-thoracic complications.
- Co-existing injury significant enough to warrant hospitalization

### Discharge Criteria
- SCJ sprains
- Anterior dislocations of the SCJ without neurovascular compromise or other significant injury
- Appropriate outpatient orthopedic follow-up arranged

### Issues for Referral
Outpatient referral to an orthopedist should be recommended for patients with any significant SCJ injuries.

## FOLLOW-UP RECOMMENDATIONS
- It is difficult to achieve long-term stability after closed reduction of dislocations, so close orthopedic follow-up is advisable.
- Repeat MR or CT imaging may be beneficial.
- Even for mild sprains and subluxations, high-risk activity should be avoided for up to 3 mo.

## PEARLS AND PITFALLS
- Since the SCJ is rarely injured, this potentially life-threatening injury may be missed during ED evaluation and resuscitation.
- Posterior dislocations mandate early thoracic and cardiothoracic surgery consultation.
- Posterior dislocation may be mistaken for anterior due to marked swelling over the joint.
- In the pediatric population, a Salter-Harris fracture may mimic a dislocation.

## ADDITIONAL READING
- Benitez CL, Mintz DN, Potter HG. MR imaging of the sternoclavicular joint following trauma. *J Clin Imaging*. 2004;28:59–63.
- Buckley BJ, Hayden SR. Posterior sternoclavicular dislocation. *J Emer Med*. 2008;34:331–332.
- Chakarun CJ, Wolfson N. Images in emergency medicine: Posterior sternoclavicular joint dislocation. *Ann Emerg Med*. 2009;53:714.
- Ferri M, Finlay K, et al. Sonographic exam of the acromioclavicular and sternoclavicular joints. *J Clin Ultrasound*. 2005;33:345–355.
- Jaggard MK, Gupte CM, Gulati V, et al. A comprehensive review of trauma and disruption to the sternoclavicular joint with the proposal of a new classification system. *J Trauma*. 2009;66:576–584.
- Miner JR, Burton JH. Clinical practice advisory: Emergency department procedural sedation with propofol. *Ann Emer Med*. 2007;50:182–187.
- Robinson CM, Jenkins PJ, et al. Disorders of the sternoclavicular joint. *J Bone Joint Surg (Br)*. 2008;90-B:685–696.

### See Also (Topic, Algorithm, Electronic Media Element)
- Acromioclavicular Joint Injury
- Arthritis, Septic
- Clavicle Fracture
- Trauma, Multiple

# CODES

## ICD9
- 839.61 Closed dislocation, sternum
- 848.41 Sternoclavicular (joint) (ligament) sprain

# STEVENS–JOHNSON SYNDROME

*James Comes*
*Herbert G. Bivins*

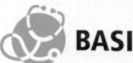 **BASICS**

## DESCRIPTION
- Stevens–Johnson syndrome (SJS) is an idiosyncratic, severe mucocutaneous disease:
  - Blistering of less than 10% of the body surface area
  - 95% of patients have mucous membrane lesions.
    ○ Usually at 2 or more sites
  - 85% have conjunctival lesions.
  - Lesions often involving face, neck, and central trunk regions become confluent over hours to days.
- Erythema multiforme (EM), SJS, and toxic epidermal necrolysis (TEN) may be considered variants of the same disease.

## ETIOLOGY
- The most common causes include medications and infections:
  - Damage to the skin is thought to be mediated by cytotoxic T lymphocytes and mononuclear cells aimed at keratinocytes expressing (drug-related) antigens.
  - Cytokines from activated mononuclear cells probably contribute to cell destruction and systemic manifestations.
- Causative medications:
  - Antibiotics (eg, penicillin, sulfonamide)
  - Anticonvulsants
  - Oxicams
  - NSAIDs
  - Allopurinol
- Infections:
  - *Mycoplasma pneumoniae*
  - Herpes simplex

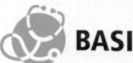 **DIAGNOSIS**

## SIGNS AND SYMPTOMS
### History
- Prodrome:
  - Fever
  - Headache
  - General malaise
  - Upper respiratory infection (URI) symptoms,
  - Arthritis, arthralgias, and myalgias prior to mucocutaneous lesions
- Skin: mild to moderate skin tenderness followed by skin pain, burning sensation, and paresthesias
- Eye: conjunctival burning or itching
- Mucous membranes: Painful micturition, painful swallowing
- Drug exposure precedes symptoms usually by 2 wk. Reexposure may result in onset of symptoms within 48 hr
- Risk factors include HIV, genetic factors, viral infections, and underlying immunologic diseases.

### Physical Exam
- Rash: target lesions, erythematous or purpuric macules with or without confluence, and raised flaccid blisters or bullae with skin detachment that spread with lateral pressure (Nikolsky sign) on erythematous areas
- Mucous membrane: erythematous tender erosions of the mouth, pharynx, trachea, genitalia, or anus; possibly pseudomembrane formation
- Eye: mild to severe conjunctivitis with possible formation of pseudomembranes and corneal ulcers

## ESSENTIAL WORKUP
A complete history and physical examination with careful attention to mucous membranes, percentage of blistering, and identification of likely etiology

## DIAGNOSTIC TESTS & INTERPRETATION
### Lab
- Electrolytes
- Liver enzymes may be mildly elevated
- CBC:
  - Anemia and lymphopenia are common
- UA

### Imaging
Chest radiography if pneumonia is a consideration

### Diagnostic Procedures/Surgery
Skin biopsy of lesions and mucous membranes demonstrates necrosis of the entire epidermal layer with formation of subepidermal split above basement membrane.

## DIFFERENTIAL DIAGNOSIS
- EM major:
  - Overlapping SJS and TEN (skin detachment between 10% and 30% of the body surface area plus widespread macules or flat atypical target lesions)
- Toxic epidermal necrolysis (skin detachment greater than 30% of the body surface area plus widespread macules or flat atypical targets)
- Thermal burns
- Phototoxic reactions
- Exfoliative dermatitis
- Pustular drug eruptions
- Bullous fixed drug eruptions
- Paraneoplastic pemphigus
- Graft-versus-host disease in bone marrow transplant patients

### Pediatric Considerations
Staphylococcal scalded skin syndrome is in the pediatric differential diagnosis of severe blistering mucocutaneous diseases.

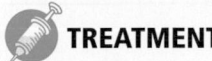

## TREATMENT

### PRE-HOSPITAL
- ABCs
- Observe universal precautions
- IV access if indicated

### INITIAL STABILIZATION/THERAPY
- Endotracheal intubation and ventilatory support may be required for impending respiratory failure (more commonly associated with TEN).
- IV fluids

### ED TREATMENT/PROCEDURES
- Fluid replacement:
  - Fluid losses may be significant.
- Recognize and treat underlying infections:
  - Sepsis is the primary cause of death, frequently from gram-negative pneumonia.
  - Secondarily infected cutaneous lesions can be treated with debridement of blisters, compresses, and systemic antibiotics.
- Corticosteroids are controversial.
- Prophylactic antibiotics may be indicated if systemic steroids are given.
- Intravenous immunoglobulin (IVIG) may be beneficial
- Mild systemic symptoms may be treated with acetaminophen or NSAIDs provided they are not the cause of the mucocutaneous reaction.
- Mucous membrane lesions are extremely painful and may require parenteral analgesics.
- Large extensive bullae should be debrided, ideally in a burn unit.

### MEDICATION
- Acetaminophen: 650–975 mg PO/PR (peds: 15 mg/kg per dose)
- Acyclovir: 5–10 mg/kg IV q8h (for herpes simplex virus infections)
- Ibuprofen: 300–800 mg PO (peds: 5–10 mg/kg per dose)
- Morphine sulfate: 0.1 mg/kg per dose IV

### First Line
- Fluid replacement
- Treat underlying etiology
- Treat secondary infections
- Analgesia

### Second Line
- IVIG
- Corticosteroids

## FOLLOW-UP

### DISPOSITION

#### Admission Criteria
- Patients with SJS should be admitted to the hospital.
- Patients with extensive epidermal detachment should be admitted to a burn center or a specialized intensive care unit.

#### Discharge Criteria
Patients with erythema multiforme minor may be discharged with appropriate and timely follow-up.

#### Issues for Referral
Patients must be made aware of the likely offending drug (and its class) and that it must never be administered to them again.

### FOLLOW-UP RECOMMENDATIONS
Follow-up with PCP and/or dermatologist

## PEARLS AND PITFALLS
- SJS may begin like an influenza illness. Lesions appear 1–3 days after the prodrome.
- The diagnosis is clinical and biopsy is supportive.
- *M. pneumoniae* and herpes simplex are more common triggers in children than in adults.

## ADDITIONAL READING

- Stella M, Clemente A, Bollero D, et al. Toxic epidermal necrolysis (TEN) and Stevens-Johnson syndrome (SJS): Experience with high-dose intravenous immunogobulins and topical conservative approach. A retrospective analysis. *Burns.* 2007;33:452–459.
- James JD, Berger TG, Elston DM. *Andrew's Clinical Dermatology,* 10th ed. Philadelphia: Saunders, 2006.
- Levi N, Bastuji-Garin S, Mockenhaupt M, et al. Medications as risk factors of Stevens-Johnson syndrome and toxic epidermal necrolysis in children: A pooled analysis. *Pediatrics.* 2009;123:e297–e304.
- Wolff K, Johnson RA, Suurmond D. Stevens-Johnson syndrome and toxic epidermal necrolysis. In: *Fitzpatrick's Color Atlas & Synopsis of Clinical Dermatology,* 5th ed. New York: McGraw-Hill, 2005: 144–147.

### See Also (Topic, Algorithm, Electronic Media Element)
- Erythema Multiforme
- Toxic Epidermal Necrolysis

 ## CODES

### ICD9
- 695.13 Stevens-Johnson syndrome
- 695.14 Stevens-Johnson syndrome-toxic epidermal necrolysis overlap syndrome

S

# STING, BEE

*Daniel T. Wu*

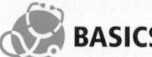

## BASICS

### DESCRIPTION
- Injection of hymenoptera venom causes:
  - Release of biologic amines
  - Local or systemic allergic reactions
- Reactions are:
  - Usually IgE-mediated type I hypersensitivity reactions
  - Rarely type III (Arthus) hypersensitivity reactions

### ETIOLOGY
- Hymenoptera—order of the phylum Arthropoda
- Includes bees (Aspidae family), wasps and hornets (Vespidae family), fire ants (Formicidae family)

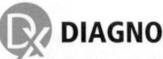

## DIAGNOSIS

### SIGNS AND SYMPTOMS
**History**
History and physical exam—keys to diagnosis

**Physical Exam**
5 Types of Reactions to Stings
- Local reaction:
  - Most common type of reaction
  - Local pain, erythema, and edema at sting site
  - Symptoms occur immediately and resolve within 1–2 hr
- Large local reaction:
  - Similar to local reaction but affects larger area or entire limbs
  - Peaks at 48 hr and can last several days
  - Mild to moderate fever
- Systemic reaction:
  - Includes anaphylaxis
  - Can be fatal (usually owing to respiratory failure)
  - Respiratory:
    - Wheezing
    - Coughing
    - Stridor
    - Shortness of breath
    - Hoarseness
    - Angioedema
  - Gastrointestinal:
    - Nausea
    - Vomiting
    - Diarrhea
    - Abdominal pain

- Cardiovascular:
  - Hypotension
  - Chest pain
  - Tachycardia
  - Shock
- Other:
  - Urticaria
  - Pruritus
  - Flushing
- Symptoms occur within 15–20 min and last ≤72 hr
- Toxic reaction:
  - Result of multiple stings and large doses of venom
  - Symptoms similar to anaphylaxis
- Unusual reactions:
  - Owing to unusual immune response
  - Vasculitis
  - Nephrosis
  - Serum sickness
  - Neuritis
  - Encephalitis
  - Reaction delayed (days to weeks after sting)

### ESSENTIAL WORKUP
- History and physical key to diagnosis
- No radiologic or laboratory test will confirm hymenoptera envenomation or anaphylaxis.

### DIAGNOSTIC TESTS & INTERPRETATION
**Lab**
CBC, electrolytes, BUN, creatinine, glucose, arterial blood gases (ABGs):
- Not routine
- Consider when significant systemic effects present

**Diagnostic Procedures/Surgery**
ECG:
- When significant systemic effects in patients at risk for cardiovascular disease

### DIFFERENTIAL DIAGNOSIS
- Insect bites sometimes cause pain; stings always cause pain.
- Cellulitis:
  - Difficult to distinguish between large local reactions and cellulitis
  - Infections of Hymenoptera envenomations are rare and usually caused by wasp envenomations.
  - Local reaction can resemble periorbital cellulitis.
- Gout
- Soft tissue trauma
- Systemic/toxic reactions:
  - Pulmonary embolus
  - Anaphylaxis from different agent
  - Hyperventilatory syndrome/anxiety
  - Acute coronary syndrome

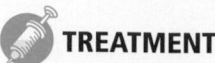

## TREATMENT

### PRE-HOSPITAL
Most deaths occur within first hr owing to either respiratory obstruction or anaphylaxis causing cardiovascular and respiratory collapse.

### INITIAL STABILIZATION/THERAPY
**Acute Severe Systemic Reaction/Anaphylaxis**
- ABCs:
  - Intubation/ventilation with rapidly increasing signs of laryngeal compromise
  - Oxygen
  - 0.9% normal saline (NS) IV access
- Epinephrine SC/IV
- Antihistamines IV
- When signs of systemic reactions:
  - Assess for patent airway.
  - Establish IV access.

### ED TREATMENT/PROCEDURES
- Systemic reactions:
  - Epinephrine for respiratory symptoms/hypotension
  - Antihistamines—$H_1$ (diphenhydramine) and $H_2$ (cimetidine, ranitidine, or famotidine) blockers
  - Steroids (prednisone, methylprednisolone, or dexamethasone)
  - Inhaled $\beta$-agonist for wheezing/shortness of breath
  - For persistent hypotension:
    - 0.9% NS IV fluid resuscitation
    - Vasopressor (epinephrine/$\alpha$-adrenergic) for hypotension resistant to IV fluids
- Removal of remnants of stinger at site of envenomation (bees may leave stingers with venom sacs) by scraping, not squeezing
- Local reactions:
  - Cool compress
  - Elevation
  - Remove constrictive clothing or jewelry
  - Topical antihistamine/topical steroidal cream as needed
  - Oral antihistamine or steroids as needed

## MEDICATION

- Albuterol, $\beta$-agonist (inhaled): 3 mg in 5 mL solvent (peds: 0.1 mg/kg of 5 mg/mL concentration) via nebulization
- Cimetidine: 300 mg (peds: 5 mg/kg) IV/IM/PO
- Ranitidine: 50 mg IV/IM (peds 2–4 mg/kg/day div q 6–8 hr IV/IM)
- Famotidine: 40 mg IV (peds 1 mg/kg/day div b.i.d. IV)
- Diphenhydramine:
  - 50–100 mg (peds: 1 mg/kg) IV for severe reactions
  - 25–50 mg (peds: 1 mg/kg) PO q.i.d. for severe local reactions
- Epinephrine:
  - 0.1 mg: 1 mL of 1:10,000 dilution (peds: 0.01 mg/kg 0.1 mL/kg of 1:10,000 dilution up to 1 mL) IV over 5 min for shock
  - 0.3–0.5 mg (0.3 mL–0.5 mL of 1:1,000 dilution; peds: 0.01 mg/kg up to 0.5 mg) SC for severe reactions but not in shock
- Methylprednisolone: 125 mg (peds: 1–2 mg/kg) IV
- Norepinephrine: 4–12 $\mu$g/min (peds: 0.1 $\mu$g/kg/min) titrated continuous infusion
- Prednisone: 60 mg (peds: 1–2 mg/kg) PO

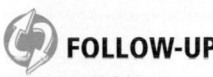 **FOLLOW-UP**

## DISPOSITION

### Admission Criteria
- Worsening symptoms, airway compromise
- Persistent unstable vital signs require ICU admission.
- Life-threatening reaction requires 24-hr observation.
- Systemic reaction requires minimum of 6 hr of observation.

### Discharge Criteria
- Minimal isolated local reaction
- Systemic reactions that resolve and do not recur during 6-hr observation period

### Issues for Referral
Follow-up:
- Provide patients with life-threatening reactions emergency anaphylaxis kits (EpiPen ; peds: EpiPen Jr. if <15 kg) and medical identification bracelets (Medi-Alert).
- Systemic reaction requires follow-up for possible immunotherapy.

## FOLLOW-UP RECOMMENDATIONS
Allergist follow-up for patients with systemic reactions.

## PEARLS AND PITFALLS

- Treat patients who present with systemic reactions to bee stings aggressively.
- Provide prescriptions for EpiPen to patients discharged after presenting with life-threatening reactions to bee stings.

## ADDITIONAL READING

- Bahna SL. Insect sting allergy: A matter of life and death. *Pediatr Ann*. 2000;29:753–758.
- Freeman T. Stings of Hymenoptera insects: Reaction types and acute management. UpToDate, Sept 25, 2009.
- McDougle L, Klein G, Hoehler FK. Management of Hymenoptera sting anaphylaxis: A preventive medicine survey. *J Emerg Med*. 1995;13:9–13.
- Moffitt JE. Stinging insect hypersensitivity: A practice parameter update. *J Allergy Clin Immunol*. 2004;114:869–886.
- Reisman R. Insect stings. *N Engl J Med*. 1994;331:523–527.
- Reisman RE. Stinging insect allergy. *Clin Allergy*. 1992;76:863–893.

### See Also (Topic, Algorithm, Electronic Media Element)
Anaphylaxis

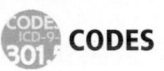 **CODES**

**ICD9**
989.5 Toxic effect of venom

S

# STING, SCORPION
*Frank LoVecchio*

 **BASICS**

## DESCRIPTION
- Scorpion venom is neurotoxic:
  - Sodium channels opening
  - Prolonged firing of neurons
- Autonomic, somatic, and cranial nerve excitation occurs.
- Symptoms begin within minutes of bite.
- Symptoms persist 1–72 hr.

## ETIOLOGY
- *Centuroides* species found in southern U.S., Mexico, Central America, and Caribbean
- Many other species in Asia, Africa, Israel, South America, and Middle East

### Pediatric Considerations
- Can be misdiagnosed as seizures, amphetamine poisoning, or meningitis
- Higher mortality and severity of illness

 **DIAGNOSIS**

## SIGNS AND SYMPTOMS
- Onset within minutes, progressing to max severity in ~1–2 hr but may persist ≤48–72 hr.
- Scorpion species determines symptomatology (*Centuroides sculpturatus*, aka *Centuroides exilicauda* or bark scorpion, is the only species in the U.S. causing symptoms).
- Local tissue effects:
  - No erythema
  - Pain
  - Hyperesthesia
- Autonomic effects:
  - Sympathetic symptoms:
    ○ Tachycardia
    ○ Hypertension
    ○ Hyperthermia
    ○ Pulmonary edema
    ○ Agitation
    ○ Perspiration
  - Parasympathetic effects:
    ○ Hypotension
    ○ Bradycardia
    ○ Hypersalivation
- Somatic effects:
  - Involuntary muscle contractions
  - Restlessness
- Cranial nerve effects:
  - Roving eye movements
  - Blurred vision
  - Nystagmus
  - Tongue fasciculations
  - Loss of pharyngeal muscle control

## ESSENTIAL WORKUP
- Identification of scorpion species not needed if scorpion is native to U.S. (see above).
- High clinical suspicion in endemic areas
- Grade severity of envenomation:
  - Grade I: Local pain and/or paresthesias at site
  - Grade II: Local pain and pain and/or paresthesias at a remote site
  - Grade III: Either cranial/autonomic *or* somatic skeletal neuromuscular dysfunction
  - Grade IV: Both cranial/autonomic *and* somatic skeletal muscle dysfunction

## DIAGNOSTIC TESTS & INTERPRETATION
### Lab
- Grade I and II envenomations:
  - None
- Grade III and IV envenomations:
  - BUN, creatinine
  - Electrolytes
  - UA
  - CBC
- Severely agitated patients:
  - Creatine kinase
  - Urine myoglobin
- Severe respiratory distress:
  - ABGs

### Imaging
- Chest radiograph for respiratory symptoms
- ECG for tachycardia

## DIFFERENTIAL DIAGNOSIS
- Snake, spider, insect envenomation
- Tetanus
- Diphtheria
- Botulism
- Overdose/dystonic reaction
- Seizures
- Infections

 **TREATMENT**

## PRE-HOSPITAL
- Evaluate ABCs
- IV access

## INITIAL STABILIZATION/THERAPY
- ABCs
- Endotracheal intubation if necessary
- IV
- O₂
- Monitor

## ED TREATMENT/PROCEDURES

- Mild envenomations—grade I and II:
  - Oral analgesics
  - Tetanus prophylaxis
- Severe envenomations—grade III and IV:
  - Antivenom (no longer available in U.S. but available in Mexico)
  - FAB antivenom undergoing trials in U.S.; available at participating institutions
  - Tetanus prophylaxis
  - Hypertensive urgencies/emergencies:
    ○ Standard therapy such as labetalol
  - Hypotension:
    ○ IV fluid resuscitation and pressor therapy with dopamine
  - Severe agitation:
    ○ Midazolam
  - Treatment for rhabdomyolysis if present

## MEDICATION

- Antivenom: Trial under way for new FAB product
- Dopamine: 2–5 $\mu$g/kg/min IV; increase in 5–10 $\mu$g/kg/min as needed
- Midazolam: 1–2 mg (peds: 0.01–0.05 mg/kg) IV
- Labetalol: 20 mg (peds: 0.3–1.0 mg/kg/dose) q10min
- Fentanyl: 50–150 $\mu$g (peds: 1–5 $\mu$g/kg) IV
- Tetanus toxoid: 0.5 mL IM (peds: same dose)

### Pediatric Considerations

Antivenom doses are the same in children because dosage is based on venom burden.

## FOLLOW-UP

### DISPOSITION

### Admission Criteria

- Grade III and IV envenomations require admission to ICU.
- If antivenom is given with resolution of symptoms, observe for 1–2 hr if asymptomatic.

### Discharge Criteria

- Grade I and II envenomations after a short observation period (3–4 hr after sting occurred) for progression of symptoms
- Grade III and IV envenomations given antivenom with resolution of symptoms can be discharged.
- If patient received antivenom, discuss signs and symptoms of delayed serum sickness.
- Discuss possibility of persistence of pain and paresthesias at site.
- Encourage patient to return for progression of symptoms.

### Pediatric Considerations

Toddlers are more likely to have early airway involvement.

### FOLLOW-UP RECOMMENDATIONS

Primary care follow-up if antivenin given.

## PEARLS AND PITFALLS

Maintain high index of suspicion for scorpion stings in endemic areas when patients present with typical symptoms.

## ADDITIONAL READING

- LoVecchio F, McBride C. Scorpion envenomations in young children in central Arizona. *J Toxicol Clin Toxicol.* 2003;41(7):937–940.
- Sofer S. Scorpion envenomation. *Intens Care Med.* 1995;21(8):626–628.
- Walter GE, Bilden EF, Gibly RL. Envenomations. *Crit Care Clin.* 1999;15(2):353–386.
- Boyer LV, Theodorou AA, Berg RA, et al. Antivenom for critically ill children with neurotoxicity from scorpion stings. *N Engl J Med.* 2009;360(20): 2090–2098.

## See Also (Topic, Algorithm, Electronic Media Element)

- Botulism
- Rhabdomyolysis
- Seizures
- Spider Bite, Black Widow
- Tetanus

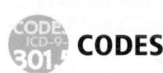 CODES

ICD9
989.5 Toxic effect of venom

S

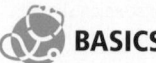

# STREPTOCOCCAL DISEASE
*Scott C. Sherman*

## BASICS

### DESCRIPTION
- Increase in frequency of aggressive streptococcal necrotizing skin infection noted in 1980s and dubbed "flesh-eating bacteria."
- Affects otherwise healthy patients aged 20–50 yr who did not have underlying predisposing diseases.
- Rapid progression of shock and multiorgan dysfunction, with death occurring within 1–2 days
- Invasive infections caused by group A *Streptococcus* (GAS) include:
  - Necrotizing fasciitis (NF)
    - Progressive, rapidly spreading soft tissue infection located within the deep fascia and subcutaneous fat
  - Streptococcal toxic shock syndrome (STSS).
    - May occur in patients with GAS associated NF
    - Portals of entry for streptococci include vagina, pharynx, mucosa, and skin. Unknown in 50% of cases
  - "Other" invasive disease defined as isolation of GAS from a normally sterile body site (ie, sepsis, bacteremic pneumonia, septic arthritis, etc.)
- Approximately 9,400 cases of invasive GAS occurred in 1999; 6% were necrotizing fasciitis and 3% were STSS.
- Occur sporadically, with occasional outbreaks in long-term care facilities and hospitals.
- Rate of invasive GAS disease ~6 times the annual incidence of meningococcal disease.

### STSS Case Definition
- Isolation of GAS from sterile or nonsterile body site
- Hypotension
- 2 or more of the following:
  - Renal impairment
  - Coagulopathy
  - Liver abnormalities
  - Acute respiratory distress
  - Extensive tissue necrosis (necrotizing fasciitis)
  - Erythematous rash

### ETIOLOGY
- Necrotizing fasciitis:
  - GAS is causative in 10% of cases. Blunt trauma is risk factor.
  - Mixed anaerobic and aerobic organisms are found in 70% of cases.
  - *Staphylococcus aureus*, *Clostridium* species, and other enteric organisms

- Streptoccoccal toxic shock syndrome:
  - Occurs when susceptible host is infected with virulent strain
  - M protein types 1, 3, and 28 are most common.
  - Pyrogenic exotoxins (eg, A, B, and C) produce fever and shock via activation of tumor necrosis factor and interleukins.
  - Nonsteroidal anti-inflammatory drugs appear to mask or predispose patients.
  - Risk factors:
    - Age <10 or >60 yr
    - Cancer
    - Renal failure
    - Leukemia
    - Severe burns
    - Corticosteroids

## DIAGNOSIS

### SIGNS AND SYMPTOMS
#### History
*Pain* is the most common initial symptom of necrotizing fasciitis and is out of proportion to physical findings:
- Often abrupt in onset and severe
- Occurs in 85% of cases
- Often requires palliative IV narcotics
- Usually involves an extremity
- May mimic peritonitis, pelvic inflammatory disease, pneumonia, acute MI, or pericarditis

#### Physical Exam
- *Fever* most common sign:
  - Can present with hypothermia, especially if patient is in shock
- *Altered mental status* present in 55% of cases
- *Soft tissue infection* (erythema and swelling) present in 80%:
  - Indistinct borders, blisters, bullae
  - No lymphangitis or lymphadenopathy
- Influenzalike syndrome in 20%:
  - Fever
  - Chills
  - Myalgias
  - Nausea, vomiting
  - Diarrhea

- Shock:
  - Present at admission or within 4–8 hr in *all* patients
  - Frequently persists despite fluids, antibiotics, and vasopressors
- Renal failure:
  - Precedes onset of shock in many cases
  - Dialysis often necessary
  - Kidney function returns to normal within 4–6 wk in survivors.
- ARDS:
  - Occurs in 55% of patients

### ESSENTIAL WORKUP
- Suspect necrotizing fasciitis when pain is out of proportion to examination.
- Obtain plain films to search for presence of air in soft tissues.
- Blood cultures should be obtained.

### DIAGNOSTIC TESTS & INTERPRETATION
#### Lab
- CBC with differential:
  - Mild leukocytosis with left shift initially
- Electrolytes, BUN, and creatinine
- Calcium level:
  - Hypocalcemia in association with fat necrosis from necrotizing fasciitis
- Urinalysis:
  - Hemoglobinuria if renal involvement
- Serum creatine phosphokinase:
  - An elevated or rising level correlates with necrotizing fasciitis or myositis.
- Aerobic and anaerobic blood cultures
- Wound cultures
- PT/PTT/INR/DIC panel

## Imaging

- Plain films:
  - Gas in soft tissues in 25%–75% of cases of necrotizing fasciitis
  - Not commonly associated with group A beta-hemolytic streptococcal infection
  - More common in mixed anaerobic infections
- CT scan:
  - Asymmetric thickening of deep fascia
  - Gas
- MRI:
  - High signal intensity of the fascia in T2-weighted images associated with NF

## Diagnostic Procedures/Surgery

Aspiration of involved areas with Gram stain and culture may be useful

## DIFFERENTIAL DIAGNOSIS

- Sepsis
- Cellulitis
- Erysipelas
- Necrotizing fasciitis/myositis secondary to infection by another pathogen

 TREATMENT

## PRE-HOSPITAL

Stabilize as appropriate

## INITIAL STABILIZATION/THERAPY

- Maintain ABCs.
- Treat shock with fluids and vasopressors as needed:
  - Hypotension is often intractable, and up to 10–20 L/day may be required.
- Intubation and mechanical ventilation for:
  - ARDS
  - Severe shock
  - Ventilatory failure

## ED TREATMENT/PROCEDURES

- Broad-spectrum antibiotics immediately after cultures until the presence of GAS has been confirmed:
  - Clindamycin is a potent suppressor of GAS bacterial toxin synthesis and inhibits M-protein synthesis
- Early surgical consultation. Most patients will require an operative procedure (eg, fasciotomy, surgical debridement, exploratory laparotomy, intraocular aspiration, amputation, or hysterectomy):
  - Immediate surgery is indicated if there is:
    - ○ Extensive necrosis or gas
    - ○ Compartment syndrome
    - ○ Profound systemic toxicity
- Droplet precautions for the first 24 hr of antibiotic therapy
- Reports of successful use of IV immunoglobulin
- Hyperbaric oxygen therapy still controversial

## MEDICATION

- NF due to invasive streptococcal disease (NOTE: In the ED, empiric treatment should be initiated until monomicrobial NF caused by GAS has been confirmed):
  - Clindamycin: 900 mg IV (peds: 40 mg/kg per day), and
  - Penicillin G: 4 million IU IV (peds: 250,000 IU per day), or
  - Vancomycin: 15 mg/kg IV (peds: 10 mg/kg q6h) if patient has penicillin allergy
- Empiric treatment of NF from all causes (C. perfringens, GAS, methicillin-resistant S. aureus [MRSA], mixed anaerobes/aerobes):
  - Piperacillin/tazobactam 3.5 g IV and Clindamycin 900 mg IV and
  - Vancomycin 1 g IV
  - For patients with a penicillin allergy treat with aztreonam 2 g IV, clindamycin 900 mg IV, vancomycin 1 g IV, and metronidazole 500 mg IV

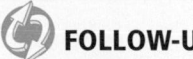 FOLLOW-UP

## DISPOSITION

### Admission Criteria

ICU admission required for all patients with suspected invasive streptococcal infection. Mortality from GAS NF ~20%, but with both NF and STSS, mortality rate increases to 70%.

### Discharge Criteria

None

## PEARLS AND PITFALLS

- Hypotension and shock may require large amounts of IV fluids and vasopressors.
- Broad-spectrum antibiotics should be administered until the presence of GAS can be confirmed.
- Surgical consultation should be obtained for debridement.

## ADDITIONAL READING

- Martin JM, Green M. Group A streptococcus. *Semin Pediatr Infect Dis.* 2006;17:140–148.
- Nuwayhid ZB, Aronoff DM, Mulla ZD. Blunt trauma is a risk factor for group A streptococcal necrotizing fasciitis. *Ann Epidemiol.* 2007;17:878–881.
- Ahmed S, Ayoub E. Severe, invasive group A streptococcal disease and toxic shock. *Pediatr Ann.* 1998;27:287–292.
- Stevens DL. The flesh eating bacterium. What's next? *J Infect Dis.* 1999;179:(Suppl 2)S366–374.

 CODES

### ICD9

- 038.0 Streptococcal septicemia
- 041.00 Streptococcus infection in conditions classified elsewhere and of unspecified site, streptococcus, unspecified
- 041.01 Streptococcus infection in conditions classified elsewhere and of unspecified site, streptococcus, group A

S

# STRIDOR
*Gregory Ciottone*

 **BASICS**

## DESCRIPTION
Impedance of air movement through the upper airway, which causes high-pitched audible wheezing and vibratory harsh sounds evident on auscultation over larynx during inspiration

## ETIOLOGY
- Congenital:
  - Laryngomalacia
- Ectopic thyroid:
  - Laryngeal webs/rings
  - Vocal cord dysfunction
- Infection:
  - Bacterial tracheitis
  - Epiglottitis
  - Viral croup
  - Peritonsillar abscess
  - Retropharyngeal abscess
  - Supraglottitis
  - Uvulitis (eg, Quincke disease)
  - Ludwig angina
  - Diphtheria
  - Tetanus
- Extrinsic compression:
  - Trauma
  - Hematoma
  - Vascular anomalies (eg, rings)
- Intraluminal obstruction of the trachea:
  - Foreign body
  - Cyst
  - Invasive tumors
  - Squamous cell
  - Lymphomas
  - Thyroid carcinomas
  - Laryngeal or tracheal papilloma
- Subglottic stenosis:
  - Postoperative scarring
  - After radiation therapy
- Angioedema
- Vocal cord dysfunction:
  - Congenital
  - Surgical injury
  - Postintubation trauma
  - Thyroid malignancy
  - Mediastinal mass

 **DIAGNOSIS**

## SIGNS AND SYMPTOMS
- Anxiety
- Audible wheezing or grunting with inspiration
- Increased respiratory rate
- Feeding difficulties in infants
- Effort required for inspiration:
  - Nasal flaring
  - Use of accessory muscles
- Intercostal retractions
- Paradoxic diaphragmatic movement (late finding)
- Dyspnea
- Cough
- Fever
- Drooling
- Sore throat
- "Hot potato" voice in adults
- Trismus:
  - Peritonsillar abscess, retropharyngeal abscess, Ludwig angina
- Respiratory distress:
  - Agitation
  - Diaphoresis
  - Cyanosis
  - Decreased respiratory rate
  - Somnolence

### History
- Respiratory distress, worse with agitation
- Audible stridor
- Cyanosis
- Feeding difficulties

### Physical Exam
- Tachypnea
- Respiratory distress, worse with agitation
- Audible stridor
- Cyanosis

## ESSENTIAL WORKUP
- Visualization of the upper airway:
  - Radiographic if symptoms very mild; be careful!
- Direct visualization in OR with a surgeon prepared to perform a cricothyrotomy or tracheostomy is the safest approach.

## DIAGNOSTIC TESTS & INTERPRETATION
### Lab
These tests are not helpful and thus avoidable; may upset a child even more.

### Imaging
Radiograph of lateral neck:
- Not essential
- Only done in extremely mild cases

### Diagnostic Procedures/Surgery
- Fiberoptic laryngoscopy:
  - Should be performed with an intubating fiberoptic laryngoscope in a setting where a rapid surgical airway can be obtained
- Direct laryngoscopy:
  - Diagnostic study of choice
  - Should be performed in a setting where a rapid surgical airway can be obtained

## DIFFERENTIAL DIAGNOSIS
- Bronchospasm
- Malingering (patient breathing against a closed glottis)

**TREATMENT**

## PRE-HOSPITAL
- Keep child calm, with mother if possible.
- Supply blow-by oxygen.
- Maintain adequate airway.
- Use bag-valve mask (BVM) if respiratory status deteriorates.
- Intubate if BVM ineffective.
- Provide rapid transport with ED notification.

## INITIAL STABILIZATION/THERAPY
- In children: Avoid agitation. Supply blow-by oxygen.
- Use 100% nonrebreathing-type face mask

### Pediatric Considerations
- Avoid agitating child.
- Watch for rapid deterioration of respiratory status.

## ED TREATMENT/PROCEDURES
- Airway management:
  - Stridor comprises a difficult airway passage:
    - Be prepared to create an airway surgically before intubation.
    - If time permits, perform intubation in OR with surgeon and pediatric anesthesiologist present.
    - Intubate with tube 1 or 2 sizes smaller than would be normally used.
- Oral awake intubation:
  - Ketamine induction
  - Patient is sedated but continues to ventilate during procedure.
- Avoid blind nasotracheal intubation.
- Provide surgical airway if intubation fails or sudden deterioration in respiratory status occurs.
- Postintubation ceftriaxone in cases of infectious cause
- Sedation/paralysis for duration of intubated status after airway is secured.

## MEDICATION
- Atropine: 0.02 mg/kg IV
- Ceftriaxone: 1–2 g IV
- Diazepam: 2–10 mg IV (peds: 0.2–0.3 mg/kg)
- Etomidate: 0.3 mg/kg IV
- Fentanyl: 3 $\mu$g/kg IV
- Ketamine: 1–2 mg/kg IV or 4–7 mg/kg IM
- Lidocaine: 1.5 mg/kg IV
- Midazolam: 1–5 mg IV (0.07–0.30 mg/kg for induction)
- Vecuronium: 0.1 mg/kg IV
- Controversies:
  - Heliox therapy
  - Racemic epinephrine therapy
  - Early intubation

 FOLLOW-UP

## DISPOSITION
### Admission Criteria
All cases of stridor that are not completely resolved during the ED course mandate admission of patient to hospital.

### Discharge Criteria
None

### Issues for Referral
Consultation with an otolaryngologist or a pediatric surgeon prior to airway visualization

## PEARLS AND PITFALLS
Attempting visualization of the airway without the back-up needed for an emergency tracheostomy is a pitfall.

## ADDITIONAL READING
- Beckman DB. Diagnostic dilemma: Vocal cord dysfunction. *Am J Med.* 2001;110:731–741.
- Chang AB. A review of cough in children. *J Asthma.* 2001;38:299–309.
- Gupta VK. Heliox administration in the pediatric intensive care unit: An evidence based review. *Pediatri Crit Care Med.* 2005;6(2):204–211.
- Konarzewski W. Adult epiglottitis: An under-recognized, life threatening condition. *Br J Anaesth.* 2001;86:456–457.
- Levy RJ. Pediatric airway issues. *Crit Care Clin.* 2000;16:489–504.
- McGahey-Oakland PR. A wheezing toddler. *J Pediatr Healthcare.* 2005;19(3):176–177.
- Mellis C. Respiratory noises: How useful are they clinically? *Pediatr Clin North Am.* 2009;56(1): 1–17, ix.
- Nakamura H. Acute epiglottitis: A review of 80 patients. *J Laryngol Otol.* 2001;115:31–34.
- Verghese ST. Pediatric otolaryngologic emergencies. *Anesthesiol Clin North Am.* 2001;19:237–256.
- Walaschek C. Vocal cord dysfunction without end? *Klin Padiatr.* 2010;222(2):84–85.

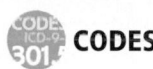 CODES

### ICD9
- 748.3 Other congenital anomalies of larynx, trachea, and bronchus
- 786.1 Stridor

S

# SUBARACHNOID HEMORRHAGE
*Alfred Joshua*

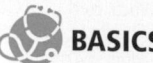 **BASICS**

## DESCRIPTION
- Bleeding into the subarachnoid space and CSF:
  - Spontaneous
    - Most often results from cerebral aneurysm rupture
    - Aneurysms that occur are more likely to rupture (>25 mm).
  - Traumatic
    - Represents severe head injury

## EPIDEMIOLOGY
- Incidence is 6–16 per 100,000 individuals.
- Affects 21,000 in United States annually
- Associated mortality in 30%–50% of patients
- Uncommon prior to third decade; incidence peaks in sixth decade

## RISK FACTORS
- Previous ruptured aneurysm who have other aneurysms
- Family history
- Hypertension
- Smoking
- Alcohol abuse
- Sympathomimetic drugs:
  - Cocaine, methamphetamine, and ecstasy (MDMA) use
- Gender (female : male 1.6:1)

### Genetics
- 3–7-fold increased risk with first degree relatives with subarachnoid hemorrhage (SAH)
- Strongest genetic association only represents only 2% of SAH patients:
  - Autosomal dominant polycystic kidney disease, Ehlers–Danlos Type IV, familial intracranial aneurysms

### Pediatric Considerations
- Most often due to arteriovenous malformation in children
- Although rare in children, SAH is a leading cause of pediatric stroke.

## ETIOLOGY
- "Congenital," saccular, or Berry aneurysm rupture (80%–90%):
  - Occur at bifurcations of major arteries
  - Incidence increases with age.
  - Aneurysms may be multiple in 20%–30%.
- Nonaneurysmal perimesencephalic hemorrhage (10%)
- Remaining 5% of causes include:
  - Mycotic (septic) aneurysm due to syphilis or endocarditis
  - Arteriovenous malformations
  - Vertebral or carotid artery dissection
  - Intracranial neoplasm
  - Pituitary apoplexy
- Severe closed head injury

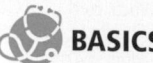 **DIAGNOSIS**

## SIGNS AND SYMPTOMS
### History
- Classically a severe, sudden headache:
  - Often described as "thunderclap" or "worst headache of life"
  - Headache is often occipital or nuchal, but may be unilateral.
  - Usually develops within seconds and peaks within minutes
  - Distinct from prior headaches
  - Headache often maximal at onset
- Sentinel headaches and minor bleeding occur in 20%–50%:
  - May occur days to weeks prior to presentation and diagnosis
- Seizures, transient loss of consciousness, or altered level of consciousness occur in more than 50% of patients.
- Vomiting occurs in 70%.
- Syncope, diplopia, and seizure are particularly high-risk features for SAH.

### Physical Exam
- Focal neurologic deficits occur at the same time as the headache in 33% of patients:
  - Third cranial nerve (CN III) palsy (the "down and out" eye) occurs in 10%–15%.
  - Isolated CN VI palsy or papillary dilation may also occur.
- Nuchal rigidity develops in 25%–70%.
- Retinal hemorrhage may be only clue in comatose patient.

## ESSENTIAL WORKUP
- Complete neurologic examination and fundoscopic exam
- Emergent noncontrast head CT scan:
  - Diagnoses 93%–98% of SAH if performed within 12 hr
  - Thin cuts (3 mm) through base of brain improve diagnostic yield.
  - CT is less sensitive after 24 hr or if hemoglobin <10 g/L.
- Lumbar puncture (LP) and CSF analysis must be performed if CT negative and history suggests possibility of SAH.

### Pregnancy Considerations
- Incidence slightly increased in pregnancy
- Workup should include CT and LP.

## DIAGNOSTIC TESTS & INTERPRETATION
### Lab
- Baseline CBC and differential
- Electrolytes, renal function tests
- Coagulation studies
- Cardiac markers:
  - Troponin-I elevated in 10%–40%
- CSF analysis (see below)

### Imaging
- Chest radiograph for pulmonary edema:
  - Occurs in up to 40% with severe neurologic deficit
- Traditional gold standard: Four-vessel digital subtraction cerebral angiography
- Spiral CT angiography:
  - Useful for operative planning
  - Quite sensitive for detection of aneurysms >4 mm, less with smaller aneurysms
- MR angiography:
  - MRI is less sensitive for hemorrhage.
  - Quite sensitive for detection of aneurysms >4 mm, less with smaller aneurysms
- Transcranial Doppler ultrasound:
  - May be useful in detecting vasospasm.

### Diagnostic Procedures/Surgery
- Lumbar puncture:
  - Presence of erythrocytes in CSF indicates SAH or traumatic tap:
    - If traumatic tap suspected, LP should be performed one interspace higher.
    - Diminishing erythrocyte count in successive tubes suggests but does not firmly establish a traumatic tap.
    - Xanthochromia is diagnostic of SAH if performed 12 hours after onset.
  - An elevated opening pressure may indicate SAH, cerebral venous sinus thrombosis, or pseudotumor cerebri.
- ECG:
  - ST-segment elevation or depression
  - QT prolongation
  - T-wave abnormalities
  - Often mimics ischemia or infarction
  - Symptomatic bradycardia, ventricular tachycardia, and ventricular fibrillation

## DIFFERENTIAL DIAGNOSIS
- Neoplasm
- Arterial dissection
- Aneurysm (unruptured)
- Arteriovenous malformation
- Migraine
- Pseudotumor cerebri
- Meningitis
- Encephalitis
- Hypertensive encephalopathy
- Hyperglycemia or hypoglycemia
- Temporal arteritis
- Acute glaucoma
- Subdural hematoma
- Epidural hematoma
- Intracerebral hemorrhage
- Thromboembolic stroke
- Sinusitis
- Seizure disorder
- Cerebral venous sinus thrombosis
- Cavernous sinus thrombosis

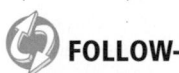

# TREATMENT

## PRE-HOSPITAL

- Initial assessment and history:
  - Level of consciousness
  - Glasgow Coma Scale score
  - Gross motor deficits
  - Other focal deficits
- Patients with SAH may need emergent intubation for rapidly deteriorating level of consciousness.
- IV access should be established.
- Provide supplemental oxygen.
- Monitor cardiac rhythm.
- Patients should be transported to a hospital with emergent CT and ICU capability.

## INITIAL STABILIZATION/THERAPY

- Manage airway, resuscitate as indicated:
  - Rapid sequence intubation
  - Pretreat with lidocaine and defasciculating dose of nondepolarizing paralytic to blunt increase in intracranial pressure (ICP) during intubation.
  - Cardiac monitoring and pulse oximetry
  - Establish adequate IV access.
- Obtain urgent neurosurgical consultation.

## ED TREATMENT/PROCEDURES

- Prevent rebleeding:
  - Risk of rebleeding highest in the first few hr after aneurysmal rupture
- Manage intracranial pressure (ICP):
  - Elevate head of bed to 30 degrees.
  - Prevent increases in ICP from vomiting and defecation with antiemetics and stool softeners.
  - Treat increased ICP with controlled ventilation and mannitol.
  - Maintain central venous pressure > 8 mm Hg and urine output >50 mL/hr
- Blood pressure (BP) control:
  - Balance HTN-induced rebleeding vs cerebral hypoperfusion
  - Goal mean arterial pressure 100–120 mm Hg, systolic BP <160
    - Labetalol, hydralazine, nitroprusside, or nicardipine for hypertension
  - Correct hypovolemia:
    - Should start within 96 hr of SAH
    - Treat hypotension with volume expansion.
- Cerebral vasospasm:
  - May cause secondary ischemia and infarction after SAH:
  - Oral nimodipine improves functional outcome.
    - Discuss with neurosurgeon prior to administration
  - Monitor with transcranial Doppler.
- Adequately treat pain.
- Seizures:
  - Manage with IV benzodiazepine
  - Consider prophylactic anticonvulsants in immediate posthemorrhagic period
- Correct temperature, electrolyte, glucose, or pH abnormalities.
- Treat coagulopathy, thrombocytopenia, and severe anemia.

- Monitor for and correct pulmonary edema and cardiac arrhythmias.
- Antifibrinolytic therapies:
  - Discuss with neurosurgeon prior to initiation
  - Consider administration immediately after aneurysmal rupture in patients at high risk of rebleeding when this is combined with treatment of aneurysm and monitoring for hypotension.
- When patient is stable, expedited transfer to hospital with neurosurgical capabilities is mandatory.

## MEDICATION

- Diazepam: 5–10 mg (peds: 0.2–0.3 mg/kg) IV/IM q10–1 min PRN; max 30 mg (peds: 10 mg)
- Fentanyl: 1–3 $\mu$g/kg (adults and peds) IV q1–4h PRN
- Fosphenytoin: 15–20 phenytoin equivalents (PE) per kg (adults and peds) IV × 1; maintenance 4–6 mg/kg/day IV
- Hydralazine: 10–20 mg (peds: 0.1–0.5 mg/kg IV) q30min–q4h PRN
- Labetalol: 20 mg IV bolus, then 40–80 mg q10min; max 300 mg; follow with IV continuous infusion 0.5–2 mg/min (peds: 0.4–1 mg/kg/hr IV continuous infusion; max 3 mg/kg/hr)
- Lidocaine: 1–1.5 mg/kg IV × 1 (adults and peds)
- Lorazepam: 2–4 mg (peds: 0.03–0.05 mg/kg per dose; max. 4 mg per dose) IV q15min PRN
- Midazolam: 1–2 mg (peds: 0.15 mg/kg IV × 1) IV q10min PRN
- Morphine: 2–10 mg (peds: 0.05–0.2 mg/kg IV) q2h–q4h PRN
- Nicardipine: 5–15 mg/hr IV continuous infusion (peds: safety not established)
- Nimodipine: 60 mg PO/NGT q4h; (peds: safety not established)
- Nitroprusside: 0.25–10 $\mu$g/kg/min IV continuous infusion (adults and peds)
- Ondansetron: 4–8 mg (peds: 0.1–0.15 mg/kg max 4 mg) PO/IM/IV t.i.d. PRN
- Phenytoin: 15–20 mg/kg IV load at max. 50 mg/min; max 1.5 g; maintenance 4–6 mg/kg/day IV; (adult and pediatric)
- Promethazine: 12.5–25 mg (peds >2 yr old: 0.25–1 mg/kg; max 25 mg per dose) PO/IM/IV q4–6h hr PRN

## SURGERY/OTHER PROCEDURES

- Per neurosurgical consultant
- Early operative or endovascular intervention may prevent vasospasm and improve outcome.

# FOLLOW-UP

## DISPOSITION

### Admission Criteria

- All patients with SAH should be admitted to an ICU.
- Patients with negative CT findings and equivocal LP findings should be admitted.

### Discharge Criteria

- Patients with negative CT and LP findings and onset of symptoms <2 wk
- Outpatient follow-up for headache treatment and further evaluation

### Issues for Referral

Early referral to center with access to neurosurgeons and endovascular specialists (if none at practicing institution)

## PROGNOSIS

- Mortality is 12% before arrival to hospital.
- Ultimately fatal in more than 50%.
- In cases of "sentinel bleed" or early detection of aneurysmal rupture, outcomes are improved with early surgical or interventional approaches.

## PEARLS AND PITFALLS

- Failure to consider SAH in differential diagnosis for new, acute headache
- Failure to assess previous headache workup as complete (CT and LP)

## ADDITIONAL READING

- Armin SS, Colohan AR, Zhang JH. Traumatic subarachnoid hemorrhage: Our current understanding and its evolution over the past half century. Neurol Res. 2006;28(4):445–452.
- Bederson JB, Connolly ES Jr., et al. Guidelines for the management of aneurysmal subarachnoid hemorrhage: A statement for healthcare professionals from a special writing group of the Stroke Council, American Heart Association. Stroke. 2009;40:994–1025.
- Edlow JA, Malek AM, Ogilvy CS. Aneurysmal subarachnoid hemorrhage: Update for emergency physicians. J Emerg Med. 2008;34(3):237–251.
- Rabinstein AA. The AHA Guidelines for the Management of SAH. What we know and so much we need to learn. Neurocrit Care. 2009;10(3):414–417.
- Uysal E, Yanbuloglu B, Erturk M, et al. Spiral CT angiography in diagnosis of cerebral aneurysms of cases with acute subarachnoid hemorrhage. Diagn Intervent Radiol. 2005;11(2):77–82.
- Wolfson A, et al. Blunt neck trauma. In: Harwood-Nuss' Clinical Practice of Emergency Medicine. Philadelphia: Lippincott Williams & Wilkins, 2005.

# CODES

## ICD9

- 430 Subarachnoid hemorrhage
- 852.00 Subarachnoid hemorrhage following injury, without mention of open intracranial wound, with state of consciousness unspecified

S

# SUBDURAL HEMATOMA
*Colleen Campbell*

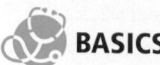 **BASICS**

## DESCRIPTION
- Classification of subdural hematoma (SDH):
  - Acute: Diagnosis within the 1st 3 days
  - Subacute: Diagnosis 3 days–3 wk
  - Chronic: Diagnosis after 3 wk
- CT description:
  - Rarely crosses midline
  - Does cross suture lines
  - Inner margins are often seen to be irregular.
- Acute:
  - Most commonly due to acceleration-deceleration forces and less commonly from direct trauma
  - Sagittal movement of the head causes stretch of parasagittal bridging veins.
  - Other bleeding sites include:
    ○ Laceration of dura
    ○ Venous sinus injury
    ○ Cortical arteries
    ○ Nontraumatic injuries: Intracerebral aneurysm rupture, arteriovenous malformation, coagulation disorder, arterial HTN, drug or alcohol abuse
- Chronic:
  - Encapsulated hematoma most likely caused by repeated small hemorrhages of bridging veins.

## ETIOLOGY
- Acute:
  - Most common type of intracranial hematoma (66–70%)
  - Occurs most commonly at cerebral complexities > falx cerebri > tentorium cerebelli
  - Peak incidence 15–24 yr, 2nd peak >75 yr
  - Represents 26–63% of blunt head injury
  - Motor vehicle crash (MVC) is most common cause overall.
  - Falls and assault more commonly result in isolated SDH (72%) than do MVCs (24%).
  - Elderly patients and those with seizure disorders are at increased risk.
  - Mortality is related to presenting signs and symptoms as well as comorbidities:
    ○ Mortality is 50% for age >70
    ○ Less than 1/2 present as *simple extra-axial collection* (22% mortality rate)
    ○ ~40% of patients will have *complicated SDH*: Parenchymal laceration or intracerebral hematoma (mortality rate >50%)
    ○ Third group *associated with contusion* (30% mortality rate with functional recovery of 20%)
- Chronic:
  - Most common in babies or elderly with atrophy:
    ○ Associated with infarction in underlying brain
  - 75% of patients are >50.
  - <50% have history of trauma.
  - 50% are alcoholic.
  - Epilepsy, shunting procedures, and coagulopathy are also associated.

### Pediatric Considerations
- May occur secondary to trauma at birth
- Nonaccidental trauma more common

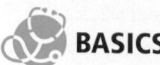 **DIAGNOSIS**

## SIGNS AND SYMPTOMS
- Acute:
  - 1/5 have diagnosis discovered at autopsy.
  - Most commonly misdiagnosed as intoxication or cerebrovascular accident (CVA)
  - Headache and altered mental status:
    ○ 50% unconscious at discovery
- Subacute/chronic:
  - Headaches, nausea, vomiting, and seizures are frequent symptoms.
  - Presentation varied:
    ○ Fluctuating mental status
    ○ Unsteady gait
    ○ Slow progression of deficits

### Pediatric Considerations
Imaging is necessary in infants with persistent vomiting, new seizures, lethargy, irritability, bulging or tense fontanels.

### Physical Exam
- Acute:
  - Headache and altered mental status
  - Most common clinical signs are hemiparesis or hemiplegia:
    ○ Seen in 40–65%
    ○ SDH opposite motor deficit in 60–85%
  - Pupillary abnormality seen in 28–79%:
    ○ SDH will be on same side of pupillary abnormality in 70–90%.
  - Seizures may be seen in ~10% initially.
  - Papilledema in <1/3
- Chronic:
  - Presentation is varied and mimics other diseases.

## ESSENTIAL WORKUP
Obtain directed history:
- Mechanism of injury kinetics
- Neurologic status: Baseline and at-scene
- Complicating factors:
  - Past medical history, medications
  - Allergies, drug use
  - Rapid neurologic assessment:
- Glasgow Coma scale ([GCS] after fluid resuscitation most important)
- Brainstem reflexes:
  - Anisocoria
  - Pupillary light reflex
  - Corneal, gag, oculocephalic/oculovestibular
  - Head imaging

## DIAGNOSTIC TESTS & INTERPRETATION
### Lab
- ABG, CBC, electrolytes with glucose, prothrombin time (PT), partial thromboplastin time (PTT)
- Blood ethyl alcohol, drug screen

### Imaging
- Head CT in coordination with other necessary trauma workup
- Acute:
  - Characteristic CT finding is crescent-shaped clot overlying hemispheric convexity.
  - May have irregular medial border of hematoma
  - Mixed density of clot may represent active bleeding
  - Most (60%) associated with other intracranial lesions
  - Intracranial volume of hematoma >2% predicts poor prognosis
- Chronic:
  - MRI is a better choice, as lesion may be isodense on CT from 2–3 wk.
  - MRI volume in diffusion-weighted images correlates with Rankin disability score.
  - CT may show hypodense lesion after 3 wk.
  - Spinal radiographs

### Pediatric Considerations
US can be used to visualize cerebral structures if fontanelles are patent.

## DIFFERENTIAL DIAGNOSIS
- Acute:
  - Diffuse axonal injury
  - Cerebral contusion
  - Intracerebral bleed
  - Subdural hygroma
  - Epidural hematoma
  - Shaken baby/battered child syndrome
- Chronic:
  - Pseudotumor cerebri
  - Brain tumor
  - Dementia
  - Meningitis
  - CVA/transient ischemic attack
  - Cerebral atherosclerosis
  - Toxic, metabolic, respiratory, or circulatory causes

**TREATMENT**

## INITIAL STABILIZATION/THERAPY
- Manage airway and resuscitate as indicated:
  - Hypoxia is a strong predictor of outcome.
  - Maintain $SAO_2$ >95%.
  - Rapid-sequence intubation (RSI) is indicated for GCS <9 or for evidence of increased intracranial pressure (ICP).
  - RSI for $PaCO_2$ >45, anisocoria, drop of GCS by 3, loss of gag reflex, C-spine injury
- Routine hyperventilation is no longer recommended due to resultant diminished cerebral perfusion pressure.
- Controlled ventilation to maintain $PCO_2$ 35–40 mm Hg:
  - NS to maintain mean arterial pressure (MAP) 100–110 is necessary:
    - A single episode of systolic BP <90 is associated with poor outcome.
  - Spine precautions
  - Elevate head of bed 20–30° (only after adequate fluid resuscitation to avoid resultant decrease in cerebral blood flow [CBF]).
- Not considered helpful:
  - Steroids
  - Antibiotic prophylaxis
  - Hyperventilation (unless herniation is imminent)
  - Fluid restriction
  - Calcium-channel blockers
  - Hypothermia not proven
  - NACL 3% not yet proven helpful

## ED TREATMENT/PROCEDURES
- Acute:
- Early neurosurgical intervention (<4 hr) in comatose patients shows reduced mortality:
  - Burr holes may be used as temporizing measure in deteriorating patients.
  - ICP monitoring is indicated for patients with abnormal CT who are intubated.
- Nonoperative treatment may be indicated for small SDH:
  - <20 mL of blood, <1 cm, midline shift <5 mm, no mass effect, no neurologic deficit This requires frequent neurologic reassessment
  - 10% go on to require operative intervention.
- Maintain euvolemic state with isotonic fluids:
  - Arterial line placement to monitor MAP, $PO_2$, and $PCO_2$
  - Foley Catheter to monitor I/O status

- Control ICP:
  - Prevent pain, posturing, and increased respiratory effort
    - Sedation with benzodiazepines
    - Neuromuscular blockade with vecuronium or pancuronium in intubated patients
    - Etomidate is a good induction agent.
  - Mannitol may be used once euvolemic:
    - Shown to increase MAP > cerebral perfusion pressure and CBF as well as decrease ICP
  - Keep osmolality between 295 and 310.
  - Use furosemide (Lasix) as an adjunct only if normovolemic.
  - Treat HTN:
    - Labetalol, nicardipine, or hydralazine
  - Treat hyperglycemia if present:
    - Associated with increased mortality in traumatic brain injury
  - Treat and prevent seizures:
    - Diazepam and phenytoin (Dilantin): Prophylactic anticonvulsants not indicated

## MEDICATION
- Diazepam: 5–10 mg (peds: 0.2–0.3 mg/kg) IV/IM q10–15min PRN; maximum, 30 mg (peds: 10 mg)
- Dilantin: Adults and peds: Load 18 mg/kg at 25–50 mg/min
- Etomidate: 0.3 mg/kg IV for induction of RSI
- Fentanyl: 2–4 ug/kg
- Hydralazine: 10–20 mg (peds: 0.1–0.5 mg/kg IV) q30–4h PRN
- Labetalol: 20 mg IV bolus, then 40–80 mg q10min; max. 300 mg; follow with IV continuous infusion 0.5–2 mg/min; (peds: 0.4–1 mg/kg/h IV continuous infusion; max. 3 mg/kg/h)
- Lasix: Adults and peds: 0.5 mg/kg IV
- Lidocaine: As preinduction agent, 1.5 mg/kg IV
- Mannitol: Adults and peds: 0.25–0.5 g/kg IV q4h
- Midazolam: 1–2 mg (peds: 0.15 mg/kg IV × 1) IV q10min PRN
- Nicardipine: 5–15 mg/hr IV continuous infusion (peds: Safety not established)
- Pentobarbital: 1–5 mg IV q6h
- Rocuronium: 1 mg/kg for induction
- Thiopental: As induction agent, 20 mg/kg IV

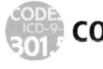 **FOLLOW-UP**

## DISPOSITION
### Admission Criteria
- Acute SDH patients should be admitted to the operating room or ICU by the neurosurgical service.
- Subacute subdurals should be admitted to a monitored setting.

### Discharge Criteria
Patients with chronic SDH often can be managed as outpatients in conjunction with neurosurgery, adequate home resources, and appropriate follow-up.

### Issues for Referral
All patients need neurosurgical evaluation immediately.

## PEARLS AND PITFALLS
The following factors predict prognosis:
- GCS on admission
- Time to treatment
- Pupil abnormalities
- CT volume of hematoma and presence of midline shift
- Midline shift > hematoma volume

## ADDITIONAL READING
- Chestnut RM. Care of CNS injuries. *Surg Clin N Am.* 2007;87(1):119–156.
- Classification and prediction of outcome based on computed tomography imaging. *J Int Med Res.* 2009;37(4):983–985.
- Reslow LA, Licht DJ, et al. Predictors of outcome in childhood intracerebral hemorrhage: A prospective cohort study. *Stroke.* 2010;41(2):313–318.
- Heegaard W, Biros M. Traumatic brain injury. *Em Med Clin N Am.* 2007;22593:655–678, viiii.
- Juj JW, Raghupathi R. New concepts in treatment of pediatric traumatic brain injury. *Anesth Clin.* 2009;27(2):213–240.
- Provenzale J. CT and MRI imaging of acute cranial trauma. *Emerg Radiol.* 2007;14(1):1–12. Epub Feb 22.

**CODES**

### ICD9
852.20 Subdural hemorrhage following injury, without mention of open intracranial wound, with state of consciousness unspecified

# SUDDEN INFANT DEATH SYNDROME (SIDS)

*Thea James*
*Roger M. Barkin*

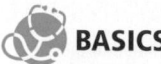 **BASICS**

## DESCRIPTION

- Sudden, unexpected death of an infant <1 yr old who was typically well before being placed down to sleep
- Death remains unexplained after being thoroughly investigated by autopsy, examination of the death scene, investigation of the circumstances, and review of the family and infant medical histories.
- The major cause of death in infants from 1 month to 1 yr of age; the incidence has declined markedly since the initiation of the "Back to Sleep" program in 1994:
  - 1983–1991: 5,000–6,000 deaths/yr in the U.S.
  - 1999: 2,648 deaths in the U.S.
- Peak occurrence of SIDS at 2–4 mo of age:
  - 88% occur <5.5 mo of age
  - 2% occur >12 mo of age
- 60:40 male-to-female ratio
- 2003 rates per 100,000 live births: All populations, 52.9; non-Hispanic white, 50.5; non-Hispanic black, 100.8; American Indian/Alaska Natives, 124.0; Asian American or Pacific Islander, 27.7
- Higher incidence reported in fall and winter
- Recent respiratory infection common
- Sleeping on back (supine) reduces incidence significantly ("Back to Sleep"). Practice of infants sleeping on their backs began earlier in Europe than in the U.S., resulting in lower incidence.
- Use of pacifiers has been associated with lower risk of SIDS.
- Cosleeping/bed sharing with parents increases risk of SIDS.

## ETIOLOGY

- Most likely multifactorial
- Many researchers suggest that SIDS infants have predisposing conditions that make them more vulnerable to normal internal and external stresses of infant life.
- Proposed and unproven hypotheses: dysrhythmias, hyperthyroidism, mast cell activation, infection, anemia, mineral and electrolyte abnormalities/imbalances, airway obstruction, suffocation, congenital diseases, neurologic events, occult trauma
- Associations/risk factors for SIDS appear to be environmental and behavioral, including maternal, prenatal, and postnatal.
- Maternal influences prevalent in SIDS infants:
  - Prenatal cigarette smoking
  - Maternal age <20 years during first pregnancy
  - Maternal low weight gain
  - Illicit drug use
  - Short intervals between pregnancies
  - Prenatal illness, sexually transmitted diseases, urinary tract infections

- Other possible risk factors and associations:
  - Intrauterine growth retardation
  - Low birth weight
  - Exposure to environmental smoking
  - Gastroesophageal reflux (GER)
  - Hyperthermia, including heavy bed linens, blankets
  - Bed sharing
  - Infant gastrointestinal illnesses and listlessness have been reported in proximity to SIDS deaths.

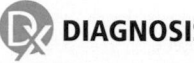 **DIAGNOSIS**

## SIGNS AND SYMPTOMS

### History

- No significant preexisting signs or symptoms to alert caretakers
- Unpredictable, unpreventable
- Most infants appear normal when put to bed and are subsequently found dead.
- Death occurs quickly while the infant is sleeping.
- Typically the event is silent; no signs of suffering.
- No clinical or pathologic explanation for death
- Apparent life-threatening episode (ALTE):
  - Prolonged period of apnea (>20 sec), lasting long enough to cause changes in skin color—cyanosis, pallor, and occasionally erythema
  - Limpness, choking, gagging
  - Appears well when evaluated by clinicians after recovery from ALTE; infant should be transported to hospital for evaluation, admission, and monitoring.
  - Link with SIDS has been suggested

### Physical Exam

- The infant is seemingly healthy and well-appearing, well developed, and well nourished prior to the event; often appears well when evaluated after the episode if that event was brief and self-limited.
- Survivors may experience complications of pulmonary edema, aspiration pneumonia, and neurologic sequelae secondary to hypoxia, including seizures.

## ESSENTIAL WORKUP

- SIDS is a diagnosis of exclusion. An evaluation for other primary or contributing conditions is mandatory.
- A diagnosis of SIDS is preceded by the multifactorial workup.
- Thorough investigation of the death scene:
  - Where the infant slept and conditions in sleeping space (temperature, bedding, bed sharing)
  - Position in which infant was sleeping; what (if anything) it was doing
  - Interview the parents, family members, caregivers
  - Collect and examine potentially relevant items from the death scene
  - Maintain sensitivity toward family; investigation could be difficult for them.

- Investigate infant and family histories:
  - History related to infant: prenatal, perinatal, and postbirth medical history
  - Family medical and social history, particularly mother
  - Family is very vulnerable at the time of the investigation; ultimately, it may help them through the grieving process.
  - Could reveal a preventable cause:
    - Could reveal no preventable cause; could help family to realize that there was nothing they could have done to prevent the death
  - Investigate other possible risk factors

## DIAGNOSTIC TESTS & INTERPRETATION

### Lab

- Selective studies reflecting nature of episode and patient condition
- Arterial blood gas
- CBC
- Electrolytes, including calcium, magnesium, and phosphorous
- LFTs
- Toxicology screen
- Blood culture and other sepsis workup as indicated
- UA and culture
- ECG
- EEG

### Imaging

- Chest radiograph if ongoing resuscitation or to exclude pulmonary disease
- Radiologic skeletal survey to exclude abuse (often done by pathologist)
- If child survives, CT; consider upper GI to exclude reflux

### Diagnostic Procedures/Surgery

- Autopsy:
  - Some states require an autopsy in all SIDS cases
  - Important that postmortem examination be done, especially because SIDS is a diagnosis of exclusion
  - Involves microscopic examination of vital organs through tissue samples as well as gross examination
  - Some postmortem findings in SIDS cases that might establish alternative cause of death:
    - Congenital cardiomyopathies
    - Cardiac rhabdomyomas
    - Tuberous sclerosis
    - Rare genetic diseases
    - Viral myocarditis
    - Intracranial arteriovenous malformations
    - ECG of surviving family members may suggest family disorder, such as prolonged-QT syndrome.

## DIFFERENTIAL DIAGNOSIS

- Cardiovascular:
  - Dysrhythmia
  - Myocarditis
  - Tuberous sclerosis
  - Cardiomyopathy
  - Congenital heart disease

- Respiratory:
  - Asphyxiation
  - Drowning
  - Gastroesophageal reflux
- Infection
- Overwhelming infection:
  - Bronchiolitis/Respiratory syncytial virus
  - Bronchopneumonia
  - Pertussis
  - Tracheobronchitis
- CNS:
  - Cerebral edema
  - Subdural hematoma
  - Meningitis
  - Encephalitis
  - Arteriovenous malformation
- Gastrointestinal:
  - Enterocolitis with diarrhea
- Pancreas:
  - Cystic fibrosis
  - Islet cell hyperplasia
  - Hypertrophy or neoplasm
- Endocrine:
  - Congenital adrenal hyperplasia/hypoplasia
- Systemic:
  - Dehydration
  - Sepsis
  - Intoxication, overdose
  - Hyperthermia
  - Intoxication
  - Infantile apnea

 **TREATMENT**

- Initiate optimal resuscitation at the scene; transport infant to ED and continue the protocols en route.
- On rare occasion and under medical direction, resuscitations have been aborted and child pronounced at the scene; consideration must be given to the emotional, social, and clinical circumstances.

### PRE-HOSPITAL

- Resuscitation procedures supplemented by support for the family
- Evaluate setting; determine if suspicion of abuse

### INITIAL STABILIZATION/THERAPY

- Assess and support ABCs (bedside).
- Administer appropriate medications per protocols by endotracheal tube if other IV access unobtainable (lidocaine, epinephrine, atropine, and naloxone).
- Monitor vital signs: BP, heart rate, respirations, and oxygen saturation continuously.
- Conduct a thorough physical examination; look for accidental as well as intentional trauma.
- Assess the scene and family members.

### ED TREATMENT/PROCEDURES

- Resuscitate patient per established protocols, seamlessly continuing efforts initiated by prehospital personnel.
- If resuscitation unsuccessful and no obvious diagnosis found, parents should not be told that SIDS is the cause of death:
  - In speaking with the parents, SIDS may be included among the possible causes of death.
  - A diagnosis cannot be made until completion of an autopsy, investigation of circumstances and death scene, and exploration of the medical histories of the infant and family.
- Family support:
  - If resuscitation unsuccessful, attention should then focus on the family; if resuscitation ongoing, communication and support of family is essential.
  - All family members and caregivers are affected; they experience grief, guilt, failure, and inadequacy.
  - Some parents want to spend quiet time holding their infants after an unsuccessful resuscitation.
  - Family is defined variably among different cultures and could be more extensive than nuclear or traditional extended family; ED personnel should attempt to be sensitive to cultural needs and expectations of the family.
  - Family should be offered support in the ED and supplied with resources of support for beyond the day of the infant's death; local, state, and national SIDS Foundation resources should be made available.
  - Support may be obtained from Sudden Infant Death Syndrome Alliance/First Candle, 1314 Bedford Avenue, Suite 210, Baltimore, MD 21208 (800-221-7437) or local SIDS support organization.
- Emergency personnel support.
  - ED debriefing should be conducted for all staff who were involved in the infant's care, including EMS personnel; this can be important to allow people to express their feelings and freely process the event in a supportive setting.
  - The child's PCP should be involved in follow-up and support of family.

 **FOLLOW-UP**

### DISPOSITION

*Admission Criteria*

Admit all infants who have ALTE for evaluation and monitoring after initial resuscitation and stabilization.

*Discharge Criteria*

None

*Issues for Referral*

- All survivors should have a pediatric consultation.
- Autopsy required for those who have died.
- Families may need support.

## PEARLS AND PITFALLS

SIDS or ALTE require aggressive resuscitative efforts when appropriate, combined with family support.

## ADDITIONAL READING

- American Academy of Pediatrics, Task Force on Infant Sleep Position and Sudden Infant Death Syndrome. Changing concepts of sudden infant death syndrome: Implications for infant sleeping environment and sleep position. *Pediatrics.* 2000;24:650–656.
- Carroll-Pankhurst C, Mortimer EA Jr. Sudden infant death syndrome, bed sharing, parental weight, and age at death. *Pediatrics.* 2001;108:1239–1240.
- Fu Ly, Colson ER, Corwin MJ, et al. Infant sleep location: Associated material and infant characteristics with sudden infant death syndrome. Prevention recommendations. *J Pediatr.* 2008;153:503–508.
- Hauck FR, Omojokun OO, Siadaty MS. Do pacifiers reduce the risk of sudden infant death syndrome? *Pediatrics.* 2005;116:16–23.
- Krous HF, Beckwith B, Byard RW, et al. Sudden infant death syndrome and unclassified sudden infant deaths: A definitional and diagnostic approach. *Pediatrics.* 2004;114:234.
- Paris CA, Remler R, Daling JR. Risk factors for sudden infant death syndrome: Changes associated with sleep position recommendations. *J Pediatr.* 2001;139:771.

### See Also (Topic, Algorithm, Electronic Media Element)

- Abuse, Child
- Resuscitation, Neonatal; Resuscitation, Pediatric

 **CODES**

**ICD9**
798.0 Sudden infant death syndrome

# SUICIDE, RISK EVALUATION

*Lawrence T. Park*
*Jennifer M. Park*

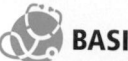 **BASICS**

## DESCRIPTION

- The intentional taking of one's own life
- Suicidal ideation:
  - Passive: No real plan or intent
  - Active: With plan and intent to die
- Suicidal gesture: Self-injurious behavior not intended to cause death (eg, superficial cutting, cigarette burns, head banging)
- Reckless behavior: Not taking prescribed medications, taking too much of prescribed medications, running into traffic
- Risk-to-rescue ratio—lethality of plan compared with likelihood of rescue:
  - High risk-to-rescue ratio indicates increased severity of attempt.

## ETIOLOGY

- 33,300 suicides in United States (CDC 2006)
- 12–25 attempts per every completed suicide
- 17.7 per 100,000 males (WHO 2005)
- 4.5 per 100,000 females
- 11.1 per 100,000 general population
- Two peaks in age group most at risk for suicide:
  - Age 15–24 yr (third leading cause of death in this age group)
  - Age >60 yr (highest rates of any age group, increasing incidence with age)

### Risk Factors for Suicidal Behavior

- Depression (bipolar or unipolar)
- Alcohol or drug abuse
- History of physical or sexual abuse
- History of head injury or neurologic disorder
- Firearms in the home
- Cigarette smoking
- Positive family history of suicide attempt
- Other psychiatric or medical diagnosis:
  - Anxiety/panic disorders
  - Schizophrenia
  - Personality disorders
  - Chronic severe medical illness
  - Epilepsy
  - AIDS
  - Huntington disease
  - Stroke
  - Traumatic brain injury
  - Cancer
  - Multiple sclerosis
  - Spinal cord injuries
  - HTN
  - Cardiopulmonary disease
  - Peptic ulcer disease
  - Chronic renal failure
  - Cushing disease
  - Rheumatoid arthritis
  - Porphyria

- Gender:
  - Women 3 times more likely to attempt suicide.
  - Men 3 times more likely to complete suicide.
- Psychological:
  - Impulsivity/aggression
  - Depression
  - Anxiety
  - Hopelessness
  - Self-consciousness/social disengagement
  - Poor problem-solving abilities
  - Social
  - Widowed
  - Divorced
  - Separated
  - Lack of social supports
  - Recent loss of relationship
  - Anniversary of loss
- Environmental
- Rural areas:
  - Access to firearms
  - Poverty
  - Unemployment

### Risk Factors for Completed Suicide

- Male
- Age >60 yr
- White or Native American
- Widowed/divorced
- Living alone
- Unemployment/poverty
- Past suicide attempt

### Methods of Suicide

- Firearms (most common among men and women, 3 of 5 completed suicides)
- Overdose (second most common among women); most common means of suicide attempt (70% of failed attempts are by overdose)
- Hanging (second most common among men)

### Populations at Highest Risk for Completing Suicide

- >90% of patients who commit suicide have a psychiatric diagnosis.
- Depression—especially psychotic depression
- Anxiety and panic disorder
- Alcohol or drug intoxication
- Schizophrenia
- Adolescents

### Others at Risk for Completing Suicide

- Recent discharge from psychiatric facility
- History of suicidal ideation or suicide attempt
- Serious physical illness present in up to 70% of all suicides, particularly in elderly patients.
- History of incarceration
- Physicians
- Victims of violence/abuse

### Decreased Risk for Suicide

- Patients with mood disorders (major depression and bipolar disorder) treated with lithium
- Patient with major depression treated with electroconvulsive therapy
- Patients with schizophrenia treated with clozapine
- **NOT** shown to decrease suicide rates: treatment with selective serotonin reuptake inhibitors (SSRIs) for major depression

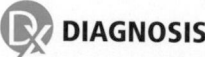 **DIAGNOSIS**

## SIGNS AND SYMPTOMS

- Depressed mood
- Verbalization of suicidal ideation
- Hopelessness
- Helplessness
- Anger/aggression
- Impulsivity
- Psychotic symptoms (ie, paranoia, command auditory hallucinations)

### History

- Obtain history to assess risk:
  - Asking about suicide does not increase risk for attempt
- Degree of suicidal ideation
- Plan: immediate risk of self-injury?:
  - Means available to complete plan
  - Activity toward initiating plan
  - Patient's expectations of lethality of plan
- Intent: Reasons, goal
- Risk-to-rescue ratio
- Plan or intent to harm others?
- Presence of acute precipitants:
  - Recent losses, lack of social supports
- Risk factors:
  - History of past suicide attempts
  - Psychiatric review of symptoms: depression, psychosis, panic/anxiety
  - Chronic medical illness
  - Alcohol or drug abuse
- Serial assessment of mental status, consistency of responses
- Factors preventing suicide

### Physical Exam

- As needed to address acute medical issues
- Look for evidence of injuries and signs of self-neglect.

## ESSENTIAL WORKUP

- Collateral information from outpatient treaters, family, friends
- Safety plan:
  - Would the patient immediately seek help if suicidal ideation recurred?
  - Elimination of means of suicide
  - Access to other means of suicide
  - Support and supervision in the outpatient setting
  - Prompt outpatient follow-up with psychiatric therapy
  - Patient investment in not attempting suicide
  - Identifying reasons for living
  - Safety contracts are no guarantee that individuals will not attempt suicide.

## DIAGNOSTIC TESTS & INTERPRETATION
### Lab

- Blood alcohol level
- Serum toxicology screen: aspirin, acetaminophen, and other medications
- Urine drug screen:
  - Many psychiatric facilities require toxicology screen before placement.
- Carbon monoxide (as indicated)

*Imaging*
Not routinely indicated

*Diagnostic Procedures/Surgery*
ECG – as indicated

## DIFFERENTIAL DIAGNOSIS
- Normal despondency
- Bereavement
- Adjustment disorder with depressed mood
- Major depressive disorder
- Bipolar disorder
- Organic mental disorder (head injury, dementia, delirium)
- Schizophrenia
- Panic and anxiety disorders
- Alcohol or drug abuse
- Borderline personality disorder
- Antisocial personality disorder
- Accidental death
- Attempted homicide

*Pediatric Considerations*
- Suicide is third leading cause of death among young people 15–24 yr of age.
- More than 5,000 adolescents commit suicide every year.
- Rapidly increasing in young black males ages 10–14 yr
- Less evidence available to link suicide in youth to overt psychiatric illness
- Stresses:
  - Prior attempts
  - Family disruption
  - History of psychiatric disorder
  - Depression
  - Disciplinary crisis
  - Broken romance
  - School difficulties
  - Bereavement
  - Rejection
  - History of physical or sexual abuse
- Early warning signs:
  - Progressive declining schoolwork
  - Multiple physical complaints
  - Substance abuse
  - Disrupted family relations

*Geriatric Considerations*
- Suicide rates highest in age >65 years
- Completed suicide: 83% men
- Risk factors: divorced, widowed, male, social isolation
- Tend to use more lethal methods
- Lower ratio of attempts to completions

##  TREATMENT

### PRE-HOSPITAL
- For potentially dangerous patient who refuses transport to treatment facility; involve police and impose restraint.
- Risk to medics on the scene in cases of firearms or other weapons
- Know state and local laws, availability of mobile crisis units, and when to involve the police.

### INITIAL STABILIZATION/THERAPY
- Prevent ability to elope
- Ensure patient safety:
  - Remove sharp objects, belts, shoelaces, and other articles that could be use for self-injury
- Provide safe environment
- Appropriate supervision

### ED TREATMENT/PROCEDURES
- Confer with patient's outpatient therapist or physician if possible
- Voluntary admission to psychiatric facility
- Involuntary admission if patient refuses voluntary
- For involuntary psychiatric admission, patient must have psychiatric disorder and one of the following:
  - Risk for danger to self
  - Risk for danger to others
  - Inability to care for self owing to extremely poor judgment

### MEDICATION
Treat underlying psychiatric disorder.

## 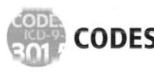 FOLLOW-UP

### DISPOSITION

*Admission Criteria*
- If patient endorses suicidal ideation with plan and intent, admission may be needed for safety
- If impulsivity, anger, or aggression hinder ability to control behavior

*Discharge Criteria*
- Patient has no suicidal ideation.
- Patient agrees to return to ED immediately or seek psychiatric help if suicidal ideation recurs.
- Patient has passive suicidal ideation without plan or intent.
- Patient has good support network or placement in appropriate crisis housing
- Appropriate outpatient psychiatric follow-up is ensured.
- In some cases, patients who express suicidal ideation while intoxicated may be discharged if no longer suicidal once they are sober.
- Some patients with borderline personality disorder and chronic suicidal ideation are discharged after careful psychiatric evaluation in consultation with long-term outpatient caregivers.

### FOLLOW-UP RECOMMENDATIONS
Close psychiatric follow-up for those with acute illness who do not require admission

## PEARLS AND PITFALLS
- A careful history will identify risk factors for suicide.
- Access collateral sources of information about patient's recent thoughts and behavior.
- Maintain patient safety during evaluation.
- Hospital admission may be required if patient endorses suicidal ideation and plan.

## ADDITIONAL READING

- Ali A, Hassiotis A. Deliberate self harm and assessing suicidal risk. *Br J Hosp Med (Lond)*. 2006;67(11):M212–M213.
- Cooper JB, Lawlor MP, Hiroeh U, et al. Factors that influence emergency department doctors' assessment of suicide risk in deliberate self-harm patients. *Eur J Emerg Med*. 2003;10(4):283–287.
- Moscicki EK. Epidemiology of completed and attempted suicide: Toward a framework for prevention. *Clin Neurosci Res*. 2001;1:310–323.
- National Institute of Mental Health. Suicide in the U.S. 2009. http://www.nimh.nih.gov/health/publications/suicide-in-the-us-statistics and prevention/index.shtml
- Nock MK, Borges G, Bromet LJ, et al. Suicide and suicidal behavior. *Epidemiol Rev*. 2008;30:133–154.

**See Also (Topic, Algorithm, Electronic Media Element)**
Depression

## 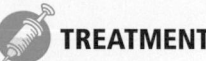 CODES

ICD9
V62.84 Suicidal ideation

S

# SUPRAVENTRICULAR TACHYCARDIA

*James Adams*
*Matthew J. Pirotte*

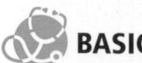 **BASICS**

## DESCRIPTION
- Rhythm that originates ectopically above the His bundle
- Heart rate of 100 bpm or greater
- Irregular narrow complex supraventricular tachycardia (SVT):
  - Atrial fibrillation (AF):
    ○ Most common form of SVT seen in the ED
    ○ 10% of people >75 yr of age have AF.
  - Atrial flutter with variable block
  - Multifocal atrial tachycardia
- Regular narrow complex SVT:
  - Atrial flutter
  - Arteriovenous nodal re-entry:
    ○ 60% of SVT
    ○ Typically present age 30–40 yr
    ○ 70% are women.
  - AV reentry involving an accessory pathway
- Wide complex SVT:
  - Aberrant conduction or a bundle branch block is present.
  - Conduction is outside of the normal His-Purkinje system.
  - More common in younger patients without structural disease
  - Always suspect a ventricular rhythm with a wide complex rhythm
  - Treat as VT unless absolutely certain of SVT

## ETIOLOGY
- Atrial tachycardia:
  - Precipitated by a premature atrial or ventricular contraction
  - Electrolyte disturbances
  - Drug toxicity
  - Hypoxia
- Junctional tachycardia:
  - AV nodal reentry
  - Myocardial ischemia
  - Structural heart disease
  - Preexcitation syndromes:
- Wolff-Parkinson-White (WPW) syndrome:
  - Drug and alcohol toxicity
- AF:
  - HTN
  - Coronary artery disease
  - Hypothyroidism
  - Heavy alcohol intake
  - Mitral valve disease
  - Chronic pulmonary disease
  - Pulmonary embolus
  - WPW syndrome
  - Hypoxia
  - Digoxin toxicity
  - Chronic pericarditis
  - Idiopathic AF
- Atrial flutter:
  - Ischemic heart disease
  - Valvular heart diseases
  - CHF
  - Myocarditis
  - Cardiomyopathies
  - Pulmonary embolus
  - Other pulmonary disease

## DIAGNOSIS

### SIGNS AND SYMPTOMS
- Palpitations (most common)
- Lightheadedness, pressure in the head
- Dyspnea
- Diaphoresis
- Dizziness
- Weakness
- Chest discomfort
- Syncope
- Prominent neck veins "frog sign"
- Signs of instability:
  - Mental status changes
  - Chest pain/ischemia
  - Acute pulmonary edema
  - Hypotension

### History
- Abrupt onset of palpitations, lightheadedness, weakness, chest pain:
  - Current symptoms
  - Previous episodes
- Insidious onset of generalized weakness and malaise
- Prior cardiac history
- Medications:
  - Over-the-counter, decongestants
- Illicit drug use

### Physical Exam
- Vital signs:
  - Tachycardia
  - BP normal or hypotensive
  - Respiratory rate normal or tachypneic
- Cardiac:
  - Regular or irregularly irregular rhythm
  - JVD may be present in setting of heart failure
- Pulmonary:
  - Rales may be present in setting of heart failure.

### ESSENTIAL WORKUP
- ABCs, assess stable vs. unstable
- History
- EKG

### DIAGNOSTIC TESTS & INTERPRETATION
#### Lab
Studies are indicated when underlying metabolic abnormalities or ischemia is considered:
- CBC
- Electrolytes
- Cardiac enzymes
- Thyroid function (usually low yield)

#### Imaging
- CXR:
  - Assess cardiac size
  - Evaluate for pulmonary process
  - More useful in AF/flutter

### Diagnostic Procedures/Surgery
- EKG:
  - Atrial flutter:
    ○ Regular atrial rate usually >300
    ○ Beat-to-beat uniformity of cycle length, polarity, and amplitude
    ○ Sawtooth flutter waves directed superiorly and most visible in leads II, III, aVF
    ○ AV block, usually 2:1, but occasionally greater or irregular
  - Multifocal atrial tachycardia:
    ○ 3 distinctly different P waves with varying pulse rate intervals
  - Atrial tachycardia:
    ○ Rate of 100–200 bpm
    ○ P wave precedes QRS and is morphologically different from the sinus P wave.
  - Junctional tachycardia:
    ○ Usually 1:1 conduction, with ventricular rates equaling the atrial rate.
    ○ May be either paroxysmal or sustained
    ○ Ventricular rates >200 bpm in an adult suggest an accessory pathway syndrome such as WPW syndrome.
    ○ Absence of preceding P waves
    ○ Often retrograde P waves buried in the QRS
    ○ Paroxysmal junctional tachycardia rates range from 120–200 bpm.
    ○ Nonparoxysmal junctional tachycardia rates rarely exceed 130 bpm.

### DIFFERENTIAL DIAGNOSIS
- Sinus tachycardia:
  - Sepsis
  - Hypovolemia
  - Pericardial tamponade
  - Acute MI
  - Drug intoxication
- Wide complex tachycardias:
  - Distinguish between supraventricular with aberrancy or ventricular origins.

 **TREATMENT**

### PRE-HOSPITAL
- Supplemental oxygen
- IV access
- Monitor

### INITIAL STABILIZATION/THERAPY
- IV access
- Oxygen
- Monitor
- Determination of unstable vs. stable patient made by determining whether the patient has organ perfusion (see above).

### ED TREATMENT/PROCEDURES

- AF:
  - Most likely diagnosis when the rhythm is irregular
  - When unstable, then immediate cardioversion
  - When stable, rate control is a priority:
    - $\beta$-Blockers or calcium channel blockers, amiodarone, and digoxin
    - Cardioversion in stable patients should not be attempted unless the dysrhythmia is known to be acute (<24 hr in duration), otherwise anticoagulation is the 1st step.
- WPW syndrome:
  - Consider direct current cardioversion or amiodarone, flecainide, or procainamide.
  - Avoid adenosine, $\beta$-blockers, calcium channel blockers, and digoxin.
- In regular narrow complex SVTs:
  - Vagal maneuvers will occasionally terminate the dysrhythmia:
    - Carotid massage (although beware of carotid disease, especially in elderly)
    - Ice to face in children (mammalian diving reflex)
    - Valsalva maneuver
  - If this is unsuccessful, adenosine is the drug of choice
  - Adenosine 6 mg will convert 60–80% of SVT
- Wide complex SVT:
  - Try to determine whether ventricular tachycardia or SVT with aberrancy:
  - If in doubt must be treated as VT:
  - Brugada criteria may help identify VT (See Ventricular Tachycardia)
  - Verapamil is absolutely contraindicated.
  - Adenosine should be reserved for SVT with aberrancy and is rarely indicated.
  - Electrical cardioversion:
    - Fewer potential complications than anti-arrhythmic drugs when mechanism unknown
  - Antidysrhythmic drugs:
    - IV procainamide and IV amiodarone
    - Lidocaine is less effective, although sometimes more readily available.
    - Bretylium lacks any evidence of efficacy.

#### Pediatric Considerations

- Synchronized cardioversion for unstable patient 0.5–1 J/kg
- SVT is the most common dysrhythmia seen in young adults and children without underlying heart disease:
  - Initial vagal maneuvers:
    - Infants: Ice/water bag to forehead x 15 seconds
    - Children: Valsalva: "Blow into straw"
- Aberrant conduction:
  - WPW syndrome and atrioventricular nodal reentry tachycardia are the 2 most common forms of SVT seen in children.
- Use verapamil only >1 yr of age.

#### Pregnancy Considerations

- Adenosine considered safe
- 2nd-line agents IV propranolol or metoprolol
- Avoid verapamil (maternal hypotension)
- Cardioversion is safe.

### MEDICATION

- Adenosine: 6 mg (peds: 0.1 mg/kg up to 6 mg) rapid IVP; if no response after 1–2 min, then 12 mg (peds: 0.2 mg/kg up to 12 mg), may repeat 12 mg (0.2 mg/kg)
- Amiodarone: Load with 15 mg/min IV over 10 min (peds: 5 mg/kg over 20–60 min), then 1 mg/min IV for 6 hr
- Digoxin: 0.5 mg IV initially, then 0.25 mg IV q4h
- Diltiazem: 0.25 mg/kg IV (usually 10–20 mg) over 2 min, followed in 15 min by 0.35 mg/kg IV over 2 min
- Esmolol: 0.5 mg/kg IV over 1 min; maintenance infusion, 0.05 mg/kg/min IV over 4 min, then 0.1–0.2 mg/kg/min IV continuously
- Lidocaine: 100 mg IV
- Metoprolol: 5–15 mg slow IV push at 5-min intervals to total of 15 mg
- Procainamide: 20–30 mg/min IV up to 17 mg/kg, may increase to 50 mg/min for more urgent situations
- Propranolol: 0.1 mg/kg div. into equal doses at 2–3-min intervals
- Sotalol: Load 10 mg/min IV up to 1.0–1.5 mg/kg body weight
- Verapamil: 2.5–5.0 mg IV bolus over 2 min; may repeat with 5–10 mg q15–30 min to max. of 20 mg

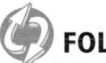 **FOLLOW-UP**

#### DISPOSITION

##### Admission Criteria
- Possible cardiac ischemic event
- Persistent supraventricular tachycardia
- Possible pre-excitation syndrome
- Other underlying metabolic abnormalities

##### Discharge Criteria
Terminated rhythm without organ hypoperfusion

##### Issues for Referral
If there are no concerns for underlying cardiac disease or metabolic derangement, a patient with uncomplicated SVT that is successfully treated may be discharged to follow-up with a primary doctor or cardiologist.

#### FOLLOW-UP RECOMMENDATIONS
The patient should return to the ED if feeling faint, dizzy, numbness or weakness of the face or limbs, or trouble seeing or speaking.

### PEARLS AND PITFALLS

- Valsalva maneuvers should, ideally, be attempted with the patient lying flat. Despite the modest likelihood of success, the maneuver is simple and efficient.

- The most worrisome heart rhythm in a patient with an accessory pathway, such as WPW, is atrial fibrillation. At high ventricular rates, the a-fib can appear deceptively regular, but should not be mistaken for benign SVT.
- When adenosine has no apparent effect, an escalating dose beyond 12 mg, to 18 mg, is sometimes used. However, if any lower adenosine dose transiently slows the heart rhythm, but the fast rate quickly resumes, then an increased dose is not warranted and an alternative medication should be used
- A wide complex tachycardia of uncertain etiology should be treated as ventricular tachycardia, typically with amiodarone and potentially with procainamide if an accessory pathway is possible.
- Since procainamide can be administered at a maximal rate of 50 mg/min, it takes a minimum of 20 min to administer 1 g, or 30 min to administer 1.5 g. Therefore, request the medicine promptly to optimize timing of administration. If QRS widening or hypotension occur, slow the rate of administration or discontinue the medication.

### ADDITIONAL READING

- Atkins DL, Dorian P, Gonzalez ER, et al. Treatment of tachyarrhythmias. *Ann Emerg Med*. 2001;37:S91–S109.
- Chauhan VS, Krahn AD, Klein GJ, et al. Supraventricular tachycardia. *Med Clin North Am*. 2001;85(2):193–223.
- Connors S, Dorian P. Management of supraventricular tachycardia in the emergency department. *Can J Cardiol*. 1997;13(Suppl A): 19A–24A.
- Delacretz E. Supraventricular tachycardia. *NEJM*. 2006;354.1039–1051.
- Gupta AK, Thakur RK. Wide QRS complex tachycardias. *Med Clin North Am*. 2001;85(2): 245–266, ixx.
- Joglar JA, Page RL. Treatment of cardiac arrhythmias during pregnancy: Safety considerations. *Drug Saf*. 1999;20:85–94
- Mioara M, Saladino R. Emergency department management of the pediatric patient with supraventricular tachycardia. *Ped Emerg Care*. 2007;23:176–189.

**See Also (Topic, Algorithm, Electronic Media Element)**
Ventricular Tachycardia

 **CODES**

#### ICD9
- 427.0 Paroxysmal supraventricular tachycardia
- 427.31 Atrial fibrillation
- 427.89 Other specified cardiac dysrhythmias

# SYMPATHOMIMETIC POISONING

Sean Patrick Nordt
James W. Rhee

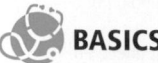 **BASICS**

## DESCRIPTION

- Direct or indirect stimulation of adrenergic receptors in sympathetic and central nervous systems
- Often no correlation between dosage and degree of toxicity
- Cocaine may also block sodium channels of cardiac myocytes, leading to "tricyclic" or class 1a–type dysrhythmias.

### Pediatric Considerations

- Sympathomimetic poisoning in children may present similarly to meningitis or other systemic illness.
- Urinary toxicology screening may be only way to discover sympathomimetic poisoning in children presenting with altered mental status.
- Methylphenidate (Ritalin, Concerta) and other sympathomimetics used for ADHD may cross-react with altered mental status.

## ETIOLOGY

- Sympathomimetic toxicity can result from use of any sympathetically active drug, including:
  - All amphetamines, methamphetamines, and derivatives (ecstasy, MDMA)
  - Cocaine
  - Phencyclidine (PCP)
  - Lysergic acid diethylamide (LSD)
  - Decongestants (rare)
- Drug delivery routes: Inhalation, injection, snorting, or ingestion

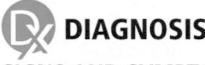 **DIAGNOSIS**

## SIGNS AND SYMPTOMS

- Vital signs:
  - Tachycardia:
    - Bradycardia possible for cocaine and some other decongestants
  - Increased BP:
    - Severely intoxicated patients may be hypotensive.
  - Tachypnea
  - Hyperthermia:
    - Often present, may be severe, and is often overlooked
- CNS:
  - Anxiety
  - Headache
  - Agitation
  - Altered mentation
  - Diaphoresis
  - Seizures
  - Stroke
  - Dystonia (rare)
- Cardiovascular:
  - Palpitations
  - Chest pain
  - Myocardial ischemia or infarction
  - Tachydysrhythmias
  - Cardiovascular collapse
  - Murmur (eg, endocarditis)

- Other:
  - Dilated pupils
  - Dry mucous membranes
  - Urinary retention may cause enlarged bladder.
  - Needle track marks or abscesses on extremities should be sought.
  - Increased or decreased bowel sounds
  - The presence of diaphoresis and bowel sounds may help to differentiate sympathomimetic toxicity from anticholinergic poisoning.

### History

- Assess history for possible sympathomimetic agents:
  - Cold preparations
  - Prescription amphetamines
  - Recreational drug use
- Assess for possible coingestions
- Evaluate for symptoms of end organ injury:
  - Chest pain
  - Shortness of breath
  - Headache, confusion and vomiting

### Physical Exam

- Common findings include:
  - Agitation
  - Tachycardia
  - Diaphoresis
  - Mydriasis
- Severe intoxication characterized by:
  - Tachycardia
  - Hypertension
  - Hyperthermia
  - Agitated delirium
  - Seizures
  - Diaphoresis
- Hypotension and respiratory distress may precede cardiovascular collapse
- Evaluate for associated conditions;
  - Cellulitis and soft tissue infections
  - Diastolic cardiac murmurs or unequal pulses
  - Examine carefully for trauma
  - Pneumothorax from inhalation injury
  - Focal neurological deficits

## ESSENTIAL WORKUP

- Monitor vital signs:
  - Increased temperature (>40°C possible):
    - Core temperature recording essential
    - Peripheral temperature may be cool.
    - Indication for urgent cooling
    - Ominous prognostic sign
  - BP:
    - Severe hypertension can lead to cardiac and neurologic abnormalities.
    - Late in course, hypotension may supervene.
- ECG:
  - Signs of cardiac ischemia
  - Ventricular tachydysrhythmias
  - Reflex bradycardia

## DIAGNOSTIC TESTS & INTERPRETATION

### Lab

- Urinalysis for:
  - Blood
  - Myoglobin
- Electrolytes, BUN/creatinine, glucose:
  - Hypoglycemia may contribute to altered mental status.
  - Acidosis may accompany severe toxicity.
  - Rhabdomyolysis may cause renal failure.
  - Hyperkalemia—life-threatening consequence of acute renal failure
- Coagulation profile to monitor for potential disseminated intravascular coagulation (DIC):
  - INR, PT, PTT, platelets
- Creatine phosphokinase (CPK):
  - Markedly elevated in rhabdomyolysis
- Urine toxicology screen:
  - For other toxins with similar effects (eg, cocaine)
  - Some amphetaminelike substances (eg, methcathinone) may not be detected.
- Aspirin and acetaminophen levels if suicide attempt a possibility
- Arterial blood gas (ABG)

### Imaging

- CXR:
  - Adult respiratory distress syndrome
  - Noncardiogenic pulmonary edema
- Head CT for:
  - Significant headache
  - Altered mental status
  - Focal neurologic signs
  - Subarachnoid hemorrhage, intracerebral bleed

### Diagnostic Procedures/Surgery

Lumbar puncture for:

- Suspected meningitis (headache, altered mental status, hyperpyrexia)
- Suspected subarachnoid hemorrhage and CT normal

## DIFFERENTIAL DIAGNOSIS

- Sepsis
- Thyroid storm
- Serotonin syndrome
- Neuroleptic malignant syndrome
- Pheochromocytoma
- Subarachnoid hemorrhage
- Drugs that cause delirium:
  - Anticholinergics:
    - Belladonna alkaloids
    - Antihistamines
  - Tricyclic antidepressants
  - Cocaine
  - Ethanol withdrawal
  - Sedative/hypnotic withdrawal
  - Hallucinogens
  - Phencyclidine

- Drugs that cause hypertension and tachycardia:
  - Sympathomimetics
  - Anticholinergics
  - Ethanol withdrawal
  - Phencyclidine
  - Caffeine
  - Phenylpropanolamine
  - Ephedrine
    Monoamine oxidase inhibitors
  - Theophylline
  - Nicotine
- Drugs that cause seizures:
  - Anticholinergics
  - Camphor
  - Carbamazepine
  - Carbon monoxide
  - Chlorinated hydrocarbons
  - Cholinergics (organophosphate insecticides)
  - Cocaine
  - Cyanide
  - Ethanol withdrawal
  - Hypoglycemics
  - Isoniazid
  - Lead
  - Lithium
  - Local anesthetics
  - Phencyclidine
  - Phenothiazines
  - Phenytoin
  - Propoxyphene
  - Salicylates
  - Sedative/hypnotic withdrawal
  - Strychnine
  - Theophylline

 TREATMENT

### PRE-HOSPITAL
- Patient may be uncooperative or violent
- Secure IV access.
- Protect from self-induced trauma.

### INITIAL STABILIZATION/THERAPY
- ABCs
- Establish IV 0.9% NS access.
- Cardiac monitor
- Naloxone, dextrose (or Accu-Chek), and thiamine if altered mental status

### ED TREATMENT/PROCEDURES
- Decontamination:
  - Gastric lavage:
    o Consider if recent (within 1 hr) or life-threatening ingestion
    o Instill activated charcoal through large-bore orogastric tube both before and after lavage.
  - Administer activated charcoal with sorbitol.
    o Consider if recent ingestion
  - Whole-bowel irrigation with polyethylene glycol solution for body packers
- Hypertensive crisis:
  - Initially administer benzodiazepines if agitated.
  - $\alpha$-blocker (phentolamine) as second-line agent
  - Nitroprusside for severe, unresponsive HTN
  - Avoid $\beta$-blockers, which may exacerbate HTN.

- Agitation, acute psychosis:
  - Administer benzodiazepines.
  - Use butyrophenones (eg, haloperidol) *with caution* to manage agitation:
    o May lower seizure thresholds and may prolong QT duration
- Dysrhythmias:
  - Sodium bicarbonate is treatment of choice for ventricular dysrhythmias and heart blocks indicative of sodium channel blocking effects with cocaine poisoning (eg, widened QRS complex on electrocardiography).
  - Lidocaine for ventricular dysrhythmias refractory to alkalinization, benzodiazepines, and supportive care
- Hyperthermia:
  - Benzodiazepines if agitated
  - Active cooling if temperature >40°C:
    o Tepid water mist
    o Evaporate with fan.
- Paralysis:
  - Indicated if muscle rigidity and hyperactivity contributing to persistent hyperthermia
- Rhabdomyolysis:
  - Administer benzodiazepines.
  - Hydrate with 0.9% NS.
    Maintain urine output at 1–2 mL/min
  - Hemodialysis (if acute renal failure and hyperkalemia occur)
- Seizures:
  - Maintain airway
    Administer benzodiazepines
  - Phenobarbital if unresponsive to benzodiazepines
  - Phenytoin contraindicated

### MEDICATION
- Activated charcoal: 1–2 g/kg up to 100 g PO
- Dextrose: D$_{50}$W one amp: 50 mL or 25 g (peds. D$_{25}$W 2–4 mL/kg) IV
- Diazepam (benzodiazepine): 5–10 mg (peds. 0.2–0.5 mg/kg) IV
- Lorazepam (benzodiazepine): 2–6 mg (peds: 0.03–0.05 mg/kg) IV
- Nitroprusside: 1–8 $\mu$g/kg/min IV (titrated to blood pressure)
- Phenobarbital: 15–20 mg/kg at 25–50 mg/min until cessation of seizure activity
- Phentolamine: 1–5 mg IV over 5 minutes (titrated to BP)
- Sodium bicarbonate: 1 or 2 amps (peds: 1–2 mEq/kg) IV push
- Sorbitol: 1–2 g/kg to max. of 100 g PO mixed in activated charcoal slurry (peds: >1-yr-old: 1–1.5 g/kg as 35% solution to max. of 50 g); avoid repeat doses of sorbitol

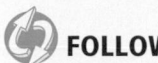 FOLLOW-UP

### DISPOSITION
*Admission Criteria*
- Admit all body packers or stuffers to hospital.
- Severe manifestations of toxicity to monitored bed:
  - Seizures
  - Dysrhythmias
  - Hyperthermia
  - Rhabdomyolysis
  - Severe hypertension
  - Altered mental status
- Ischemic chest pain

*Discharge Criteria*
Mildly intoxicated patients can be observed and treated in ED until resolution of clinical manifestations.

### FOLLOW-UP RECOMMENDATIONS
Patients may need referral for chemical dependency rehab and detoxification

## PEARLS AND PITFALLS
- Admit patients with severe or persistent symptoms
- Monitor core temperature
  - Hyperthermia above 40°C may be life threatening
  - Treat with aggressive sedation and active cooling
- Recognize rhabdomyolysis and hyperkalemia
- Avoid physical restraints in agitated patients if possible
- Consider associated emergency conditions:
  - Patients with chest pain should be evaluated for acute coronary syndromes and treated accordingly
  - Consider infection in altered patients with fevers and history of IV drug use
  - Methamphetamine abuse frequently associated with traumatic injury
- Benzodiazepines are first-line therapy in symptomatic sympathomimetic intoxication

## ADDITIONAL READING
- Albertson TE, Derlet RW, Van Hoozen BF. Methamphetamine and the expanding complications of amphetamines. *West J Med*. 1999;170:214–219.
- Callaway CW, Clark RF. Hyperthermia in psychostimulant overdose. *Ann Emerg Med*. 1994;24:68–76.
- Gray SD, Fatovich DM, McCoubrie DL, Daly FF. Amphetamine-related presentations to and inner-city tertiary emergency department: A prospective evaluation. *Med J Aust* 2007;186:336.
- Richards CF, Clark RF, Holbrook T, et al. The effects of cocaine and amphetamines on vital signs in trauma patients. *J Emerg Med*. 1995;13:59–63.

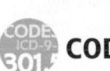 CODES

### ICD9
971.2 Poisoning by sympathomimetics (adrenergics)

# SYNCOPE

*Jarrod Mosier*
*Samuel A. Keim*

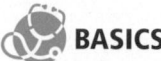 **BASICS**

## DESCRIPTION

- Transient loss of consciousness associated with loss of postural tone
- Ultimately, it is the lack of oxygen to the brainstem reticular-activating system that results in a loss of consciousness and postural tone.
- Most commonly, an inciting event causes a drop in cardiac output.
- Cerebral perfusion is reestablished by autonomic regulation, as well as by the reclined posture, which results from the event.
- Accounts for 3% of ED visits
- All-cause death rate at 30 days after ED visit for syncope is 1.4%

### ALERT
Suspected cardiac syncope must be admitted to monitored bed

### Geriatric Considerations
- Elderly with highest incidence, as well as increased morbidity
- >1/3 will have numerous potential causes.

## ETIOLOGY
- Neurally mediated syncope:
  - Reflex response causing vasodilatation and bradycardia with resulting cerebral hypoperfusion
  - Vasovagal (common faint):
    ○ Often incited by pain or fear
    ○ Prodromal findings are usually present.
    ○ Typically lasts <20 sec
    ○ Tilt-table testing is the gold standard to diagnose
  - Carotid sinus syncope:
    ○ Cough, sneeze
    ○ GI stimulation (eg, defecation)
    ○ Micturition
- Orthostatic:
  - Positional changes cause abrupt drop in venous return to heart
  - Volume depletion:
    ○ Severe dehydration (eg, vomiting, diarrhea, diuretics)
- Hemorrhage (see Hemorrhagic Shock):
  - Autonomic failure
    ○ Diabetic or amyloid neuropathy
    ○ Parkinson disease
    ○ Drugs (eg, β-blockers) and alcohol
- Cardiac arrhythmias:
  - Typically sudden and without prodromal symptoms
  - Tachydysrhythmia or bradydysrhythmia
  - Inherited syndromes (eg, long QT syndrome, Brugada syndrome)
  - Pacemaker/implantable cardioverter defibrillator malfunction

- Structural cardiac or cardiopulmonary disease:
  - Valvular disease (especially aortic stenosis)
  - Hypertrophic cardiomyopathy
  - Acute MI
  - Aortic dissection
  - Pericardial tamponade
- Pulmonary embolus
- Neurologic:
  - Transient spike in intracranial pressure that exceeds cerebral perfusion pressure
  - Postsyncopal headache is almost universal.
  - May be presentation of a subarachnoid hemorrhage
- Cerebrovascular steal syndromes

### Pregnancy Considerations
- Pregnant patients frequently experience presyncope or syncope from various causes. 5% of patients experience syncope, 28% experience presyncope throughout their pregnancy.
- Placenta acts as an AV malformation, causing decreased SVR that potentiates orthostatic symptoms.
- Fetus lying on IVC can lead to neurogenic and hypovolemic syncope.
- Pregnant patients at higher risk of DVT/PE, urinary tract infections, seizures (preeclampsia), valvular incompetencies. Must consider these diagnoses in ED evaluation.

 **DIAGNOSIS**

## SIGNS AND SYMPTOMS
### History
- Prodromal symptoms:
  - Lightheadedness
  - Diaphoresis
  - Dimming vision
  - Nausea
  - Weakness
- The following findings suggest an underlying life threat:
  - Sudden event without warning
  - Chest pain or palpitations
- 6 Ps of a syncope history:
- Preprodrome activities
- Prodrome symptoms: Visual symptoms, nausea
- Predisposing factors: Age, chronic disease, family history of sudden death
- Precipitating factors: Stress, postural symptoms
- Passerby witness: What did they see?
- Postictal phase, if any: Suggests seizure

### Physical Exam
- Evaluate for trauma.
- Orthostatic vital signs
- Check for difference in BP in both arms, suggesting aortic dissection or subclavian steal syndrome.
- Careful cardiovascular exam, including murmurs, bruits, and dysrhythmias
- Rectal exam to check for GI bleeding
- Urine pregnancy test in reproductive-age female
- Careful neurologic exam

### Pediatric Considerations
- Warning signs of a potential serious underlying disease:
  - Syncope during exertion
  - Syncope to loud noise, fright, extreme stress
  - Syncope while supine
  - Family history of sudden death at young age (<30 yr)

## ESSENTIAL WORKUP
- EKG immediately upon arrival to check for:
  - Ischemia
  - Dysrhythmias
  - Block
  - Long QT interval
  - Brugada Syndrome
  - Wolff-Parkinson-White syndrome
- Detailed history and physical exam will determine diagnosis in 85% of those who eventually obtain a diagnosis.

## DIAGNOSTIC TESTS & INTERPRETATION
### Lab
- Driven by history and physical exam
- CBC in suspected occult hemorrhage
- Serum bicarbonate:
  - Normal with most syncopal events
  - Marked decreased bicarbonate obtained <1 hr after the event:
    ○ Suggestive of a grand mal seizure rather than syncope
    ○ If due to seizure, should normalize 1 hr after the event
- Cardiac enzymes in suspected ischemia
- Pregnancy test in reproductive-age female
- Electrolytes in patients with profound dehydration or diuretic use

### Imaging
- EKG and monitoring until cardiac etiology ruled out
- CXR +/− CT angiography if CHF, dissection, or massive pulmonary embolism suspected
- Head CT if abnormal neurologic exam or transient ischemic attack suspected
- ECG if concern for structural defects

## DIFFERENTIAL DIAGNOSIS

- Seizure is most commonly mistaken for syncope:
  - Key differentiating factor is postictal confusion.
  - Brief tonic movements and urinary incontinence may be seen with syncope.
- Metabolic disorders (eg, hypoxemia, hyperventilation, hypoglycemia)
- Toxicologic
- Stroke
- Psychogenic syncope
- Malingering
- Breath-holding spells in children

 **TREATMENT**

### PRE-HOSPITAL

- Oxygen
- Cardiac monitoring
- IV access

### INITIAL STABILIZATION/THERAPY

- Advanced cardiac life support (ACLS) interventions for unstable patients
- Oxygen
- Cardiac monitoring
- IV access with normal saline fluid bolus in suspected hypovolemia
- Consider coma cocktail: Dextrose, thiamine, and naloxone for persistent altered mental status

### ED TREATMENT/PROCEDURES

- ACLS interventions for dysrhythmias
- Standard regimens for acute MI
- Control BP for subarachnoid hemorrhage and aortic dissection
- Consider thrombolytics for submassive pulmonary embolism.

### MEDICATION

- Dextrose: $D_{50}W$ 1 amp (50 mL or 25 g) IV (peds: $D_{25}W$ 2–4 mL/kg IV)
- Naloxone: 2 mg IV or IM (peds: 0.1 mg/kg)
- Thiamine: 100 mg IV or IM (peds: 50 mg)

 **FOLLOW-UP**

### DISPOSITION

#### Admission Criteria

- San Francisco Syncope Rule identifies patients at high risk for serious 7-day outcomes ("CHESS") (Sensitivity ~90%):
  - History of **C**HF
  - **H**ematocrit <30%
  - Abnormal **E**CG
  - Patient complaint of **s**hortness of breath
  - **S**ystolic BP <90
- ROSE Rule for 1-mo serious outcomes (Sensitivity ~ 87%):
  - BNP >300 pg/mL
  - Positive fecal blood
  - Hemoglobin <9 g/dL
  - Oxygen saturation <94%
  - Q-wave on EKG
- Other recommendations:
  - Suspected cardiac syncope must be admitted to monitored bed.
  - GI bleeds: Consider ICU bed
  - Admit elderly patients with syncope.

#### Discharge Criteria

- Neurally mediated syncope or orthostatic syncope from volume depletion may be evaluated on outpatient basis with close follow-up, if patient is reliable and has a good social structure.
- Driving restrictions until cleared

#### Issues for Referral

All syncope patients should follow-up, typically with primary care, unless specific diagnosis is known or strongly suspected.

### FOLLOW-UP RECOMMENDATIONS

The patient should be instructed to seek medical help immediately if any of the following occur:

- Recurrent loss of consciousness in the next 6 mo
- New chest pain, pressure, squeezing, tightness, a rapid heartbeat or palpitations
- Shaking chills, or a fever >102°F
- New or worsening difficulty breathing
- Abdominal pain, vomiting, black or bloody stool
- Severe headache, dizziness, confusion or change in behavior

## PEARLS AND PITFALLS

- Always inquire about presyncopal symptoms.
- If in doubt, admit for observation.

## ADDITIONAL READING

- Brignole M, et al. Task force report: Guidelines on management (diagnosis and treatment) of syncope. *Eur Heart J.* 2001;22(15):1256–1306.
- Brignole M, et al. ESC Guidelines on management (diagnosis and treatment) of syncope—Update 2004. *Eur Heart J.* 2004;25(22):2054–2072.
- Hayes OW. Evaluation of syncope in the emergency department. *Emerg Med Clin North Am.* 1998;16(3): 601–615.
- Massin M, et al. Syncope in pediatric patients presenting to an emergency department. *J Pediatr.* 2004;145(2):223–228.
- Meyer MD. Evaluation of the patient with syncope: An evidence based approach. *Emerg Med Clin North Am.* 1999;17(1):189–201.
- Reed MJ, et al. The ROSE (risk stratification of syncope in the emergency department) study. *J Am Coll Cardiol.* 2010;55(8):722–724.
- Sun BC, et al. External validation of the San Francisco Syncope Rule. *Ann Emerg Med.* 2007;50(6):742–743.
- Quinn J, et al. Derivation of the San Francisco Syncope Rule to predict patients with short-term serious outcomes. *Ann Emerg Med.* 2004;43(2): 224–232.
- Yarlagadda S, Poma PA, Green LS, Katz V. Syncope during pregnancy. *Obstet Gynecol.* 2010;115(2): 377–380.

### See Also (Topic, Algorithm, Electronic Media Element)

Hemorrhagic Shock

## CODES

### ICD9

- 337.01 Carotid sinus syndrome
- 780.2 Syncope and collapse

S

# SYNDROME OF INAPPROPRIATE ANTIDIURETIC HORMONE SECRETION (SIADH)

*Matthew D. Bitner*

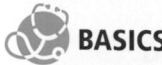

## BASICS

### DESCRIPTION
- Most common cause of hyponatremia in hospitalized patients
- More of a problem of *water balance* than one of sodium balance
- Normal regulation of water balance:
  - Antidiuretic hormone (ADH):
    - Integral part of the homeostatic mechanism that controls water balance
    - Increases water permeability of the kidney collecting tubules, resulting in free water reabsorption in the renal medulla
    - Synthesized by hypothalamus but secreted by posterior pituitary
  - Water deprivation (increased plasma osmolality) stimulates secretion as sensed by:
    - Osmoreceptors
    - Left atrial stretch receptors
    - Carotid baroreceptors
    - Aortic arch
    - Pulmonary veins
- Hyponatremia:
  - *Mild*: Serum sodium <135 mEq/L
  - *Moderate*: Serum sodium <130 mEq/L
  - *Severe*: Serum sodium <125 mEq/L
  - Excess extracellular water *relative* to sodium
  - Depletional hyponatremia:
    - Sodium depletion can be caused by diet, gastrointestinal losses, diuretic use, renal or adrenal disease.
    - Often accompanied by extracellular fluid volume depletion
    - Hyponatremia associated with clinical signs of hypovolemia
    - Increased hematocrit, BUN, creatinine
    - Urinary sodium excretion <20 mEq/L
  - Dilutional hyponatremia:
    - Increased extracellular water in presence of normal or increased total body sodium
    - Can be caused by increased fluid intake (oral, IV), drugs or medical conditions that cause water retention
    - Euvolemia with edema
    - Normal or decreased hematocrit, BUN, creatinine
    - Urinary sodium excretion >20 mEq/L
    - Inappropriate ADH secretion is a form of dilutional hyponatremia.
- Definition of SIADH:
  - ADH secretion in absence of hyperosmolality or hypovolemia
- Criteria for definition:
  - Essential features:
    - *Hyponatremia*—despite correction for hyperglycemia, hyperproteinemia, or hyperlipidemia
    - *Euvolemia*—no clinical signs of volume depletion (orthostasis, tachycardia) or volume overload (edema, ascites)
    - *Hyposmolality* of the plasma—<275 mOsm/kg of water
    - Normal renal, adrenal, and thyroid function
    - No recent diuretic use
    - Urine osmolality >100 mOsm/kg of water
  - Supplemental features:
    - Plasma uric acid <4 mg/dL
    - BUN <10 mg/dL
    - FENa >1%
    - Failure to correct hyponatremia after an infusion of normal saline (0.9%)

### ETIOLOGY
- **Malignant disorders:**
  - ADH-producing tumors
  - Small-cell lung cancer
  - Pancreatic cancer
  - Prostate cancer
  - Pituitary tumor
  - Thymoma
  - Lymphoma
- **Pulmonary disorders:**
  - Pneumonia
  - TB
  - Lung abscess
  - COPD
- **CNS disorders:**
  - Meningitis
  - Encephalitis
  - CVA
  - Head trauma
- **Medications:**
  - Chlorpropamide
  - Vincristine
  - Anticonvulsants (carbamazepine)
  - Tricyclic antidepressants
  - Antipsychotics
  - SSRIs (fluoxetine)
  - Narcotics
  - Nicotine
  - NSAIDs
  - Ecstasy (MDMA)
  - Vasopressin analogs (DDAVP, oxytocin, vasopressin)
- **Transient:**
  - Endurance exercise
  - General anesthesia
  - Pain
  - Nausea
  - Stress
- **Other:**
  - Hereditary
  - Positive-pressure ventilation
  - AIDS
  - Idiopathic

## ALERT
Cerebral salt-wasting syndrome (CSWS) can mimic SIADH.
- Seen in patients with cerebral tumors or Subarachnoid hemorrhage and in transphenoidal pituitary postoperative patients
- Etiology unclear
- Represents appropriate water resorption in the face of salt wasting
- Fluid restriction can help differentiate the two.
  - In SIADH: Hypouricemia will correct
  - In CSWS: Hypouricemia will persist
- Treatment of CSWS may differ from that of SIADH
  - Infusion of normal saline
  - May benefit from fludrocortisones therapy

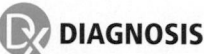

## DIAGNOSIS

### SIGNS AND SYMPTOMS
- Serum sodium <135 mEq/L:
  - May be asymptomatic
- Serum sodium <130 mEq/L:
  - Weakness
  - Lethargy
  - Weight gain
  - Headache
  - Anorexia
- Sodium serum <120 mEq/L:
  - Altered mental status
  - Seizure
  - Coma
- Chronic hyponatremia: 50% asymptomatic
- High mortality when hyponatremia develops acutely

### History
- Thorough medication history
- Course of illness (acute, subacute, or chronic)

### Physical Exam
- Volume status
- Stigmata of malignancy

### ESSENTIAL WORKUP
- Diagnosis is one of exclusion, need to evaluate for other causes of:
  - Depletional hyponatremia
  - Dilutional hyponatremia
- Electrolytes, BUN, creatinine, glucose, protein, lipids:
  - Hyponatremia (serum sodium <135 mmol/L)
  - Serum hyposmolality (serum osmolality <275 mOsm/kg)
- Urine osmolality:
  - Inability to excrete a dilute urine
  - Urine osmolality >100 mOsm/kg
- Urine sodium:
  - Continued urinary excretion of sodium
  - Urinary sodium >20 mEq/L

## DIAGNOSTIC TESTS & INTERPRETATION

### Lab
- Serum protein levels
- Lipid levels
- Glucose levels
- Serum osmolality
- LFT and thyroid function test
- Morning cortisol level

### Imaging
Chest radiograph and CT of the head to screen for pathology causing SIADH

## DIFFERENTIAL DIAGNOSIS

### Causes of Hyponatremia
- See etiologies above
- Increased extracellular fluid (dilutional hyponatremia):
  - Renal failure/insufficiency
  - CHF
  - End-stage liver disease
- Normal extracellular fluid (dilutional hyponatremia):
  - SIADH
  - Physical and emotional stress
  - Myxedema
  - Sheehan syndrome (postpartum hypopituitarism)
  - Reset osmostat syndromes (dilute urine at lower than normal sodium levels)
- Decreased extracellular fluid (depletional hyponatremia):
  - Increased losses
    - Excessive sweating
    - Vomiting
    - Diarrhea
  - Third-space sequestration
  - Diuretic use
  - Aldosterone deficiency:
    - Addison disease
  - Salt-losing nephropathies:
    - Renal tubular acidosis
- Pseudohyponatremia:
  - Hyperglycemia
  - Hyperproteinemia
  - Hyperlipidemia

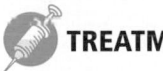 **TREATMENT**

## PRE-HOSPITAL
- In patients with altered mental status, maintenance and protection of the airway are paramount.
- When hypovolemia is suspected, appropriate fluid resuscitation should be initiated.
- Rapid patient evaluation and transport are essential.

## INITIAL STABILIZATION/THERAPY
- Severe symptomatic hyponatremia with CNS manifestations
- Endotracheal intubation for patients in need of airway protection:
  - IV access
  - Identify/treat other causes:
    - Naloxone
    - Thiamine/Dextrose (or point-of-care glucose measurement)
  - Treat seizures with benzodiazepines
- Proceed to hyponatremia treatment

## ED TREATMENT/PROCEDURES
- Most effective treatment of SIADH is successful *eradication of the underlying cause*.
- Initial treatment of hyponatremia caused by SIADH is the same for all causes of euvolemic/hypervolemic hyponatremia.

### Mildly symptomatic hyponatremia, chronic hyponatremia with minimal symptoms, asymptomatic hyponatremia
- Serum sodium usually >125 mEq/L
- Fluid restriction 800–1000 mL/day alone (if no response, possibly restrict to 500–600 mL/day) or in conjunction with:
  - 0.9% NS infusion
  - IV furosemide
- Correct serum sodium by no more than 0.5 mEq/L/hr (5-6 mEq/day):
  - Too rapid correction of serum sodium levels can induce *central pontine myelinolysis*, associated with development of bulbar palsy, quadriplegia, seizures coma, and death.

### Severe hyponatremia:
- Symptomatic patient, serum sodium <125 mEq/L
- Increase serum sodium by no more than 12 mEq/L in first 24 hr at rate of 1 mEq/L/hr (8–12 mEq/day when serum sodium below 125 mEq/L and slow to 5–6 mEq/day when serum sodium rises to 125 mEq/L).
- Target level: 125 mEq/L
- Treat patients with significant neurologic symptoms with 3% saline solution.
- Serum sodium laboratory testing every 1–2 hr

### Acute life-threatening hyponatremia:
- Serum sodium usually <120 mEq/L
- Associated with seizures or coma
- Clinical goal: Stop seizure and improve neurologic status
- Therapeutic goal: Same as for severe hyponatremia
- Administer hypertonic saline solution (3%) for significant neurologic symptoms.
- Stop hypertonic saline when symptoms (ie, seizures) resolve and transition to normal saline.
- IV furosemide to promote diuresis and induce a negative fluid balance.
- Once serum sodium = 125 mEq/L, further IV fluid should be in form of 0.9% saline solution.
- Restoration of serum sodium to normal levels should take place over ≥48 hr.
- Drugs that inhibit the secretion or the renal effect of ADH:
  - Indicated when SIADH not self-limited and cause cannot be removed
  - Demeclocycline (blocks renal effect of ADH)

## MEDICATION
- Demeclocycline: 300 mg PO b.i.d.–q.i.d.
- Hypertonic saline solution (3% NaCl): 250–500 mL (max initial dose 5mL/kg):
  - 25–100 mL/hr
  - Limit rate in rise of serum sodium to 0.5–1.0 mEq/L/hr.
  - Discontinue when a resolution in hyponatremic seizure is obtained, or serum sodium of 125 mEq/L is reached.
  - Rise in serum sodium by 4–6 mEq/L is usually sufficient to stop seizures.
- Normal saline solution (0.9% NS): standard maintenance rates
- Lasix: 1 mg/kg up to 20–40 mg IV

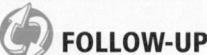 **FOLLOW-UP**

## DISPOSITION

### Admission Criteria
- Severe life-threatening hyponatremia
- Symptomatic hyponatremia
- Serum sodium <125 mEq/L regardless of symptoms
- New-onset SIADH in which underlying cause must be diagnosed and treated
- Complications secondary to the underlying cause of SIADH
- Patient's compliance an issue

### Discharge Criteria
- Asymptomatic chronic hyponatremia
- Serum sodium >125 mEq/L
- No unstable comorbid factors
- Known diagnosis of SIADH

## FOLLOW-UP RECOMMENDATIONS
All patients with hyponatremia that meet discharge criteria still require follow-up to check for resolution, monitoring, and/or diagnosis of the underlying cause of the SIADH/hyponatremia.

## PEARLS AND PITFALLS
- SIADH is a diagnosis of exclusion.
- Must evaluate for other causes as well as renal, thyroid, adrenal, cardiac, and hepatic dysfunction.
- Take a thorough medication history.

## ADDITIONAL READING
- Balasubramanian A, Flareau B, Sourberr J. Syndrome of inappropriate antidiuretic hormone secretion. *Hospital Physician.* 2007;39:33–36.
- Brimioulle S, Orellana-Jimenez C, Aminian A, et al. Hyponatremia in neurological patients: Cerebral salt wasting versus inappropriate antidiuretic hormone secretion. *Intens Care Med.* 2008;34:125–131.
- Ellison D, Berl T. The syndrome of Inappropriate Antidiuresis. *N Engl J Med.* 2007;356(20):2064–2072.
- Fried LF, Palevsky PM. Hyponatremia and hypernatremia. *Med Clin North Am.* 1997;81(3):585–609.
- Miller M. Syndrome of excess antidiuretic hormone release. *Crit Care Clin.* 2001;17(1):1123.

### See Also (Topic, Algorithm, Electronic Media Element)
- Hyponatremia

The author gratefully acknowledges the contribution of Arunachalam Einstein on the previous edition of this chapter.

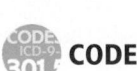 **CODES**

**ICD9**
253.6 Other disorders of neurohypophysis

# SYNOVITIS, TOXIC

*Ian R. Grover*

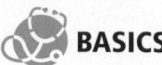

## BASICS

### DESCRIPTION
- Nonspecific inflammation and hypertrophy of the synovium with an effusion of the hip joint in children
- It can affect any joint but most commonly affects the hip.
- Disease process is self-limiting.
- Most common cause of acute hip pain and a limp in children aged 3–10.
- Also referred to as acute transient synovitis and irritable hip syndrome.
- Age group most affected is 3–6 yr.
- Male > Female (2:1)
- Right hip > left

### ETIOLOGY
- Cause of toxic synovitis is unknown.
- Infectious etiology is suspected, because an upper respiratory infection precedes the symptoms of transient synovitis in ~50% of cases.

## DIAGNOSIS

### SIGNS AND SYMPTOMS
- Unilateral hip pain
- Pain in the anteromedial thigh and knee
- Pain with weight-bearing
- Limp
- Low-grade fever
- Decreased range of motion (ROM) of the affected hip
- Pain with ROM of the affected hip

### History
- Acute onset of unilateral hip pain
- No history of trauma
- Pain with ambulation
- Recent upper respiratory infection

### Physical Exam
- Low-grade fever, usually <38.5°C (101.3°F)
- Nontoxic appearing
- Limited hip ROM due to pain
- Hip is usually held in the flexed and externally rotated position for maximal comfort.

### ESSENTIAL WORKUP
- Hip x-rays
- AP pelvis
- CBC, C-reactive protein (CRP), ESR if concerned for septic arthritis

### DIAGNOSTIC TESTS & INTERPRETATION
#### Lab
CBC, CRP, ESR:
- May be normal or elevated
- An elevated white blood cell count, CRP, or ESR alone does not differentiate toxic synovitis from septic arthritis or osteomyelitis.
- If white blood cell count, CRP, and ESR are normal, more serious causes of hip pain are less likely.

#### Imaging
- Plain hip films (anteroposterior and frog-leg view):
  - Usually normal
  - May detect an effusion or other causes of hip pain
- US to rule out joint effusion and to guide hip joint aspiration if required
- MRI (rarely indicated):
  - Very useful in diagnosing Legg-Calvé-Perthes (LCP) disease
- Bone scan:
  - Used to differentiate LCP disease from toxic synovitis
  - Can detect osteomyelitis
  - The increased radiation is usually reserved for recurrent cases or cases in which the diagnosis is still in question.

### Diagnostic Procedures/Surgery
Joint aspiration:
- Not necessary if the patient is afebrile with a normal WBC count, CRP, and ESR
- Abnormal joint fluid analysis indicates SA (see "Arthritis, Septic")

### DIFFERENTIAL DIAGNOSIS
- SA
- Osteomyelitis
- Soft-tissue infection
- LCP disease
- Slipped capital femoral epiphysis
- Juvenile rheumatoid arthritis
- Rheumatic fever
- Chondrolysis
- Gaucher disease
- Osteosarcoma
- Ewing sarcoma
- Osteoid osteoma
- Leukemia
- Tuberculosis of the hip
- Fracture
- Lyme disease
- Psoas abscess
- Sickle cell crisis

### Pediatric Considerations
- 4–17% of children have a recurrent episode.
- 10% of recurrent cases may be the presenting feature of a chronic inflammatory condition.
- 2–10% of patients with toxic synovitis later develop LCP disease:
  - Suggested that toxic synovitis may represent an early stage of LCP disease.

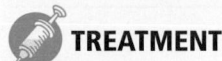

# TREATMENT

## PRE-HOSPITAL
- Keep leg in position of comfort.
- Treat with NSAIDs.

## ED TREATMENT/PROCEDURES
- Conservative treatment
- Bed rest in position of comfort: Flexion and external rotation
- Initiate NSAIDs.
- Apply heat to the area.
- Antibiotics and steroids are not indicated.
- Some authors recommend no weight-bearing for 7–10 days following improvement and return of normal hip function, citing increased risk for recurrence.
- Close follow-up is essential, with repeat radiographs due to association with LCP.

## MEDICATION

### First Line
- Ibuprofen: 200–600 mg (peds >6 mo old: 5–10 mg/kg/dose) PO q6h p.r.n.
- Naproxen: 250–500 mg (peds >6 mo old: 5-10 mg/kg/dose) PO b.i.d. p.r.n.

### Second Line
Acetaminophen: 325–650 mg (peds: 10–15 mg/kg/dose) PO/PR q4–6h p.r.n.

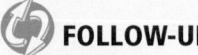

# FOLLOW-UP

## DISPOSITION

### Admission Criteria
Patients with severe joint pain or a large effusion may require hospitalization for bed rest and analgesics.

### Discharge Criteria
All patients who have had more serious causes of hip pain excluded and have been diagnosed with toxic synovitis can be discharged from the hospital with good follow-up.

### Issues for Referral
Follow-up with an orthopedic surgeon in 1–2 wk for close follow up.

## FOLLOW-UP RECOMMENDATIONS
- Return to the ED immediately for worsening pain in the hip or increasing fever.
- Follow-up with pediatric orthopedic surgeon in 1–2 wk for close monitoring.
- Patients should have repeat x-rays done in 6 mo to exclude LCP disease.

# PEARLS AND PITFALLS

- Most cases are diagnosed by history and physical exam alone.
- ~50% of children have a history of a preceding viral illness.
- NSAIDs help treat the pain and shorten the course of the illness.
- Nearly all children recover from toxic synovitis within 2 wk and without sequelae.
- ~1–3% of children with toxic synovitis develop LCP disease.

# ADDITIONAL READING

- Caird MS, Flynn JM, Leung YL, et al. Factors distinguishing septic arthritis from transient synovitis of the hip in children. A prospective study. *J Bone Joint Surg Am*. 2006;88:1251–1257.
- Della-Giustina K, Della-Giustina D. Emergency department evaluation and treatment of pediatric orthopedic injuries. *Emerg Med Clin North Am*. 1999;17(4):895–922.
- Kermond S, Fink M, Graham K, et al. A randomized clinical trial: Should the child with transient synovitis of the hip be treated with nonsteroidal anti-inflammatory drugs? *Ann Emerg Med*. 2002;40(3):294–299.
- Kocher MS, Mandiga R, Zurakowski D, et al. Validation of a clinical prediction rule for the differentiation between septic arthritis and transient synovitis of the hip in children. *J Bone Joint Surg*. 2004;86:1629–1635.
- McCarthy JJ, Noonan KJ. Toxic synovitis. *Skeletal Radiol*. 2008;37:963–965.
- Taekema HC, Landham PR, Maconochie I. Distinguishing between transient synovitis and septic arthritis in the limping child: How useful are clinical prediction tools? *Arch Dis Child*. 2009;94:167–168.

## See Also (Topic, Algorithm, Electronic Media Element)
- Arthritis, Septic
- Hip Injury
- Legg-Calve-Perthes Disease

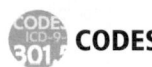

# CODES

## ICD9
- 727.00 Synovitis and tenosynovitis, unspecified
- 727.09 Other synovitis and tenosynovitis

# SYPHILIS
*Jessica Freedman*

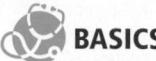

## BASICS

### DESCRIPTION
- Sexually transmitted disease
- 12 million new cases diagnosed annually worldwide
- Acquired via mucous membranes/disrupted skin
- Divided into 3 stages:
  - Primary syphilis:
    ○ Painless chancre or ulcer
  - Secondary syphilis:
    ○ Replication and hematogenous spread
    ○ Begins 3–6 wk after primary lesion
    ○ Late latent secondary phase
  - Tertiary or late syphilis:
    ○ Very uncommon
    ○ Cardiovascular and neurologic symptoms

### ETIOLOGY
Treponema pallidum:
- Spirochete bacteria

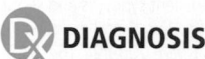

## DIAGNOSIS

### SIGNS AND SYMPTOMS
#### Primary (Early) Syphilis
- 21-day incubation period
- No constitutional symptoms
- Chancre:
  - *Painless* papule at site of inoculation
  - Clean-based, circular, sharply defined borders:
    ○ Solitary lesions
    ○ Commonly on penis, vulva, and rectum
    ○ Bilateral regional lymphadenopathy
  - Heals spontaneously in 3–6 wk
- Rectal chancre:
  - Painful or painless
  - Rectal irritation/discharge
  - Painless enlargement of lymph nodes

#### Secondary (Early) Syphilis
- Occurs 3–6 wk after primary lesion.
- Disseminated stage
- Rash (most common):
  - Symmetric, diffuse, polymorphous, papular or maculopapular rash
  - Rash may be diverse and not fit a pattern
  - Starts on trunk and flexor extremities
  - Spreads to involve palms and soles:
    ○ Discrete, red/reddish-brown
    ○ 0.5–2 cm in diameter
- Condyloma lata:
  - Large raised gray/white lesions, painless, moist
  - Mucous membranes:
    ○ Oral cavity and perineum
    ○ Very contagious
    ○ Intertriginous areas
    ○ Flat rectal warts

- Systemic symptoms:
  - Fever, headache, malaise, anorexia, sore throat, myalgias, and weight loss
- Diffuse lymphadenopathy:
  - Palpable nodes at inguinal, axillary, posterior cervical, femoral, and/or epitrochlear regions
  - Painless, firm, and rubbery
- Less common:
  - "Moth-eaten" alopecia
  - Syphilitic meningitis
  - Scleritis
- Loss of lateral third of eyebrows
- Painless mucosal lesions (mucous patches)
- Secondary stage resolves spontaneously in 1–2 months

#### Latent Secondary Syphilis
- Period of no symptoms but positive serology:
  - Cerebrospinal fluid (CSF) normal
- Late latent stage *not* infectious except for fetal transmission in pregnant women
- Persists for lifetime or develops into tertiary syphilis

#### Tertiary (Late) Syphilis
- Occurs in 1/3 of patients with untreated latent secondary syphilis
- Neurologic and cardiovascular involvement
  - Destructive stages of disease
- Neurosyphilis (most common):
  - Asymptomatic:
    ○ Positive CSF– Venereal Disease Research Laboratories (VDRL)
    ○ CSF pleocytosis (10–100 lymphocytes)
    ○ Elevated CSF protein at 50–100 mg/dL
  - Meningitis:
    ○ Aseptic; CSF with positive VDRL, higher protein, and lower glucose (compared with above)
    ○ Cranial nerve palsy, including isolated eighth nerve palsy
  - General paresis:
    ○ Loss of cortical function
    ○ Argyll Robertson pupils (small fixed pupils that do *not* react to strong light, but do react to accommodative convergence)
  - Tabes dorsalis (peripheral neuropathy)
- Degeneration of posterior columns/posterior or dorsal roots of spinal cord
- Dementia
- Paresthesias, abnormal gait, and lightning (sudden, severe) pain of extremities/trunk
- Progressive loss of reflexes, vibratory/position sensation
- Positive Romberg sign
- Vision: optic atrophy
- Pupils: Argyll Robertson pupils
- Urinary incontinence

- Gummas:
  - Late benign syphilis of cutaneous skin/viscera:
    ○ Bone, brain, abdominal viscera, etc.
- Granulomatous, cellular hypersensitivity reaction:
  - Round, irregular, or serpiginous shape
  - "Great pox"
- Cardiovascular:
  - Thoracic aortic aneurysm (ascending most common):
    ○ Dilated aorta and aortic valve regurgitation
    ○ Aortic valve insufficiency
    ○ Coronary thrombosis
    ○ Destructive lesions of skeletal structures or skin
- HIV-infected:
  - Strong association with syphilis
- Increased incidence of neurosyphilis

#### Congenital Syphilis
- In utero infection:
  - Age <2 yr:
    ○ Hepatosplenomegaly, rash, condyloma lata, rhinitis (snuffles), jaundice (nonviral hepatitis), osteochondritis
- Older children (syphilis stigmata):
  - Interstitial keratitis, nerve deafness, anterior bowing of shins, frontal bossing, mulberry molars, Hutchinson teeth, saddle nose, etc.

### ESSENTIAL WORKUP
Rapid plasma reagin (RPR)

### DIAGNOSTIC TESTS & INTERPRETATION
#### Lab
- Serology:
- Nontreponemal test:
- RPR
- VDRL
- Positive 14 days after chancre appears
- Early false negatives, especially ≤7 days after primary chancre
- Repeat negative test in 2 wk and correlate with disease activity
- False positives in 1%–2% of general population
- Fourfold change in titer clinically significant
- 100% sensitivity in secondary syphilis
- Nonreactive after successful treatment
- Treponemal antibody test
- Fluorescent treponemal antibody absorption (FTA–ABS)
- Hemagglutination assay for antibody to *T. pallidum* (MHA–TP)
- More sensitive and specific
- 1% false-positive rate
- Confirmatory test

- Reactive for patient's lifetime
- More costly and harder to perform
- Dark-field microscopy
- Identifies treponemes from primary and secondary lesions:
- Suspicious early lesions with negative serology (early primary syphilis)
- False negatives with ointments, creams
- Oral specimen unsuitable
- CSF analysis for tertiary neurosyphilis:
- Tertiary syphilis:
- Positive VDRL/RPR
- Lymphocytes >5/mL
- Protein >45 mg/dL
- Decreased glucose

## DIFFERENTIAL DIAGNOSIS
- Genital ulcer:
  - Chancroid (painful)
  - Genital herpes:
    ○ Vesicular, multiple lesions
  - Lymphogranuloma venereum
  - Granuloma inguinale
  - Superficial fungal infection
  - Carcinoma
- Secondary and tertiary syphilis:
    Pityriasis rosea
  - Drug-induced rash
  - Acute febrile exanthems
  - Psoriasis
  - Lichen planus
  - Scabies
  - Infectious mononucleosis
  - Viral illness
  - Bacteremia
  - Tertiary syphilis:
  - Psychosis
  - Dementia
  - Multiple sclerosis
  - Meningitis
  - Encephalitis
  - Delirium
  - Unknown overdose

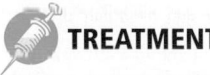

## TREATMENT

### INITIAL STABILIZATION/THERAPY
Lower BP and establish IV access for aortic dissection.

### ED TREATMENT/PROCEDURES
- Treatment other than penicillin with increased relapse rate:
  - Desensitize those allergic to penicillin.
- Pregnancy:
  - Treat with penicillin even in latent syphilis. If patient allergic to penicillin, admit for desensitization.

- Jarisch–Herxheimer reaction:
  - Transient febrile reaction to therapy
  - May be owing to antigen liberation from spirochetes or activation of complement cascade
  - Peaks at 8 hr, resolves in 24 hr
  - Symptoms:
    ○ Fever, headache, malaise, worsening rash
  - Treat with antipyretics.
  - No serious sequelae
- Recommended testing:
  - Sexual partners
  - Concomitant sexually transmitted diseases including HIV
  - Repeat serology test in 6 and 12 mo.

## MEDICATION
- Early primary, secondary, early latent (<1 yr):
  - Benzathine penicillin G: 2.4 million U IM
  - Doxycycline: 100 mg PO b.i.d. for 14 days
  - Tetracycline: 500 mg PO q.i.d. for 14 days
- Late latent (>1 yr) except neurosyphilis:
  - Benzathine penicillin G: 2.4 million U IM 3 times over 2 wk on days 0, 7, and 14
  - Doxycycline: 100 mg PO b.i.d. for 4 wk
  - Tetracycline: 500 mg PO q.i.d. for 4 wk
- Neurosyphilis:
  - Penicillin G: 3–4 million U IV q4h for 10–14 days
  - Procaine penicillin: 2.4 million U IM daily *plus*
  - Probenecid: 500 mg PO q.i.d. for 10–14 days
- Congenital syphilis:
  - Penicillin G: 50,000 $\mu$g/kg IM q8–12h for 10–14 days *or*
  - Procaine penicillin: 50,000 $\mu$g/kg IM daily for 10–14 days

 **FOLLOW-UP**

### DISPOSITION
#### Admission Criteria
- Neurosyphilis requires IV antibiotics
- Pregnant women allergic to penicillin requiring desensitization

#### Discharge Criteria
Follow-up care:
- Measure for falling titers in 6 mo and 1 yr after treatment.
- Tertiary/latent (>1 yr):
  - Measure for falling titers in 3, 6, 12, and 24 mo after treatment.

### *Issues for Referral*
Infectious disease consultation for secondary and tertiary syphilis as well as congenital and neurosyphilis

### FOLLOW-UP RECOMMENDATIONS
Titers must be monitored.

## PEARLS AND PITFALLS
- Syphilis is known as the "great imitator."
- In patients presenting with unknown rash, think of syphilis and ask about history of genital lesions.
- Be sure to examine mucous membranes of all patients presenting with rash.
- Think of tertiary syphilis with neurologic symptoms of unknown etiology.

## ADDITIONAL READING
- Hook EW. Syphilis control: a continuing challenge. *N Engl J Med.* 2004;351:122.
- Domantay-Apostol GP et al. Syphilis: The international challenge of the great imitator. *Dermatol Clin.* 2008;26(2):191v–201v.
- Mandell GL, Bennett JE, Dolin R. *Treponema pallidum* (syphilis). In: *Mandell, Douglas, and Bennett's Principles and Practice of Infectious Diseases*, 7th ed. Philadelphia: Churchill Livingstone, 2009, chapter 238.
- McKinzie J. Sexually transmitted disease. *Emerg Med Clin North Am.* 2001;19:723–743.
- Centers for Disease Control and Prevention (CDC). Primary and secondary syphilis in United States, 2002. *MMWR* 2003;52:1117.
- Schacter J. Classification of latent syphilis. *Sex Transm Dis.* 2005;32:143.
- Timmermans M. Neurosyphilis in the modern era. *J Neurol Neurosurg Psychiatry.* 2004;75:1727.

 **CODES**

### ICD9
- 091.2 Other primary syphilis
- 091.9 Unspecified secondary syphilis
- 097.9 Syphilis, unspecified

# SYSTEMIC LUPUS ERYTHEMATOSUS
*Steven Furer*

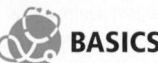 **BASICS**

## DESCRIPTION
- Chronic autoimmune disease; peak onset between ages 15–40 yr; characterized by flares and remissions
- Multisystem disease with diverse clinical manifestations:
  - Mucocutaneous
    ○ Most commonly involved system
    ○ 4 specific skin rashes
  - Arthritis
  - Cardiac:
    ○ Endocarditis
    ○ Myocarditis
    ○ CHF
    ○ Conduction abnormalities
    ○ Atherosclerosis
    ○ MI
  - Renal:
    ○ Glomerulonephritis
    ○ Renal failure
  - Pulmonary:
    ○ Pleural effusion (usually exudative)
    ○ Pneumonitis
    ○ Pulmonary hemorrhage
    ○ Pulmonary embolism
    ○ Pneumonia
    ○ Pleuritis
    ○ Pulmonary edema
    ○ Pulmonary hypertension
  - Neurologic:
    ○ Lupus cerebritis
  - Vascular:
    ○ Vasculitis
    ○ Thrombosis
    ○ Atherosclerosis
  - Gastrointestinal:
    ○ Peritonitis
    ○ Mesenteric vasculitis and ischemia
    ○ Pancreatitis

### Pediatric Considerations
- Neonatal lupus may occur when maternal autoantibodies cross the placenta.
- Congenital heart block is the most serious complication.

### Geriatric Considerations
- 10 times greater risk of MI due to atherosclerosis
- High incidence of osteoporosis related to chronic steroid use

## RISK FACTORS
### Genetics
- More common in females than males (9:1 ratio)
- More common in African Americans
- Higher frequency of systematic lupus erythematosus and other autoimmune diseases among first-degree relatives

## ETIOLOGY
- Autoantibody production against cell nucleus and cytoplasmic structures, leading to inflammatory changes, vasculitis, and immune complex deposition in multiple organ systems
- A significant percentage of patients have an associated antiphospholipid syndrome:
  - Characterized by antibodies against cellular phospholipid components
  - Tendency toward recurrent vascular thrombosis
- Lupus is a chronic disease with several exacerbating factors:
  - Infection
  - Sun exposure
  - Trauma
  - Medications
    ○ Sulfonamides, commonly
  - Stress
  - Diet
- Drug-induced lupus is a milder disease that eventually resolves once the drug is discontinued. Common medications include:
  - Chlorpromazine
  - Methyldopa
  - Procainamide
  - Hydralazine
  - Isoniazid
  - Quinidine

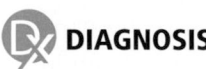 **DIAGNOSIS**

- 4 of the 11 criteria in the following list are needed to make the diagnosis:
  - Malar rash
  - Discoid rash
  - Photosensitivity rash
  - Oral ulcers
  - Arthritis
  - Serositis
  - Neurologic disorders
  - Hematologic disorders
  - Immunologic disorders
  - Renal disorders
  - Antinuclear antibodies

## SIGNS AND SYMPTOMS
- Systemic:
  - Fatigue
  - Fever
  - Weight loss
  - Dyspnea
- Skin:
  - Malar rash (butterfly facial)
  - Discoid rash (raised red patches)
  - Photosensitivity rash (subacute cutaneous lupus)
- Musculoskeletal:
  - Myalgias
  - Joint pain
  - Arthritis:
    ○ Defined as two or more peripheral joints
    ○ Polyarthritis, symmetric, or migratory
- Heart:
  - Chest pain
  - Pericardial rub
  - Murmur
- Vascular:
  - Vasculitis
  - Thrombosis
  - Atherosclerosis
  - Peripheral vascular disease
- Lungs:
  - Dyspnea
  - Tachypnea
  - Pleural rub
  - Rales
- Nervous system:
  - Psychosis
  - Depression
  - Headache
  - Seizures
  - Peripheral neuropathies
  - Stroke
  - Cranial nerve deficits
- Gastrointestinal:
  - Painless oral ulcers
  - Abdominal pain
  - Guarding or rebound tenderness
  - Positive stool guaiac suggests mesenteric ischemia.

### History
- Symptoms commonly accumulate and exacerbate over years, with flares and remissions. A history of fatigue, rashes, and joint pain may point to the diagnosis.
- Patients describe arthralgias out of proportion to physical findings.

### Physical Exam
- Check for fever.
- Carefully evaluate skin for rashes and vasculitis.

## ESSENTIAL WORKUP
- Thorough history and physical exam needed to distinguish between major and minor flare-ups
- Major flare-ups:
  - CBC
  - Electrolytes, BUN, creatinine, glucose
  - UA
  - ESR
  - Chest radiograph, ECG, and pulse oximetry for cardiorespiratory symptoms

## DIAGNOSTIC TESTS & INTERPRETATION
### Lab
- CBC:
  - Leukopenia, thrombocytopenia
  - Degree of hematologic disorders suggests degree of disease activity.
- ESR:
  - May be elevated during acute exacerbations
  - Not a good indicator of active disease

- CRP may also be elevated; marked elevation may be a sign of infection.
- PTT:
  - May be elevated in patients with lupus anticoagulant
- UA:
  - Protein
  - Casts
  - Hematuria
  - WBCs
- Amylase is elevated in mesenteric ischemia and pancreatitis.
- Send antinuclear antibody, rheumatoid factor (RF), anti-streptolysin O (ASO) titer if diagnosis unclear.
- Anti-Sm and anti-dsDNA are diagnostic.
- A false-positive Venereal Disease Research Laboratory (VDRL) test is supportive of the diagnosis.
- Joint aspirate typically shows fluid with fewer than 3,000 WBCs.

### Imaging
- CXR:
  - Pneumonitis
  - Pneumonias
  - Pleural effusion
  - Cardiomegaly
- ECG
- Echocardiogram
- CT chest
  - Pulmonary embolus
  - Pulmonary hemorrhage
  - Diffuse alveolar hemorrhage

### Pregnancy Considerations
- Pregnancy is not recommended during active disease owing to the high risk of spontaneous abortion.
- The effect of pregnancy on disease activity is variable.

### DIFFERENTIAL DIAGNOSIS
- Hypotension in the known lupus patient may be due to shock from a major flare-up, secondary to acute steroid withdrawal, or the result of sepsis.
- Other autoimmune diseases:
  - Rheumatic fever
  - Rheumatoid arthritis
  - Dermatomyositis
  - Overlap syndromes
- Skin changes:
  - Urticaria
  - Erythema multiforme
- Idiopathic thrombocytopenic purpura
- Multiple sclerosis
- Epilepsy

##  TREATMENT

### INITIAL STABILIZATION/THERAPY
ABCs

### ED TREATMENT/PROCEDURES
- Mainstays include NSAIDs, antimalarials, corticosteroids, and immunosuppressive drugs.
- Special attention must be given to CNS and renal involvement as well as infections; these are the main determinants of morbidity:
  - Atherosclerosis is a leading cause of death in the older lupus patient.
- Mild flare-ups—arthralgias, myalgias, and fatigue; rash:
  - NSAIDs, acetyl salicylic acid (ASA), topical steroids for rash, sunscreen
  - COX-2 inhibitors if no sulfa allergy
  - If not sufficient, begin low-dose prednisone.
- Major flare-ups—life- or organ-threatening:
  - Methylprednisolone
  - Anticoagulation for thrombosis; give blood products early if needed.
  - Psychotropics for neuropsychiatric symptoms
  - Anticonvulsants for seizures
  - If poor response, consult rheumatology before starting cytotoxic medications such as azathioprine or cyclophosphamide.
- Chronically:
  - Prednisone ; taper
  - NSAIDs
  - Rheumatologist initiated:
    - Antimalarials; quinacrine, chloroquine
    - Cyclophosphamide
    - Azathioprine
    - Methotrexate
  - Hormonal therapy, thalidomide, and monoclonal antibodies are under investigation.

### MEDICATION
- Methylprednisolone: 15 mg/kg/d IV up to 1 g; consult rheumatologist for peds dosing
- Prednisone 5–30 mg (peds: <0.5 mg/kg) PO daily for minor flare
- Prednisone 1–2 mg/kg/d PO for major flares in adults
- Ibuprofen 800 mg (peds: 5–10 mg/kg) PO t.i.d.
- Celecoxib 100 mg PO b.i.d.

##  FOLLOW-UP

### DISPOSITION
#### Admission Criteria
- Patients who have end-organ disease such as renal or CNS involvement, pericarditis, pancreatitis, or GI symptoms
- Those with severe end-organ or life-threatening manifestations should be admitted to the ICU.
- Patients with lupus should be treated as immunocompromised and suspected or diagnosed infections should be treated aggressively.

#### Discharge Criteria
- Patients may be discharged home with mild flare-ups if afebrile, well hydrated, and not ill-appearing.
- ESR should not be used as disposition criterion as it may be elevated long after a flare-up has subsided.

### Issues for Referral
- Because lupus is a chronic disease, a rheumatologist or knowledgeable PCP must follow the patient adequately.

### FOLLOW-UP RECOMMENDATIONS
PCPs must educate patients regarding sun protection, immunizations, and lowering risks of atherosclerosis.

## PEARLS AND PITFALLS

- The diagnosis of SLE is complicated and requires a thorough history and physical supported by appropriate lab testing.
- Chronic steroid therapy leads to immunosuppression.
- Renal involvement confers a poor prognosis.
- All patients with SLE should be offered annual seasonal influenza vaccinations and be sure that pneumococcal vaccination is up to date.
- VDRL may be falsely positive

## ADDITIONAL READING

- Buyon JP. Systemic lupus erythematosus: Clinical and laboratory features. In: Klippel JH, ed. *Primer on the rheumatic diseases*, 13th ed. Atlanta: Arthritis Foundation, 2008: 303–318.
- Ruiz-Irastorza G, Khamashta MA. Systemic lupus erythematosus. *Lancet*. 2001;357:1027–1032.
- Schur PH, et al. Overview of the therapy and prognosis of systemic lupus erythematosus in adults. UptoDate.com. http://utdol.com/
- Tseng CE, Buyon JP, et al. The effect of moderate-dose corticosteroids in preventing severe flares in patients with serologically active, but clinically stable, systemic lupus erythematosus: Findings of a prospective, randomized, double-blind, placebo-controlled trial. *Arthritis Rheum.* 2006;54:3623–3632.

## CODES

### ICD9
710.0 Systemic lupus erythematosus

# TACHYDYSRHYTHMIAS

*James Adams*
*Matthew J. Pirotte*

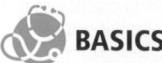 **BASICS**

## DESCRIPTION

- Any disturbance of the heart's rhythm resulting in a rate >100 bpm
- Reentry is the most common underlying mechanism for tachydysrhythmia:
- Sinus tachycardia:
  - Narrow complex regular rhythm at a rate of 100–150 bpm
  - Infants and young children can obtain rates of 170–225 bpm.
  - Functional response to physiologic stress caused by increased catecholamine tone or decreased vagal stimulation
- Supraventricular tachycardia (SVT):
  - A narrow complex tachycardia that originates above the His bundle
- Irregular SVT:
  - Atrial fibrillation (AF)
  - Atrial flutter
  - Multifocal atrial tachycardia
- Regular SVT:
  - Atrial tachycardia
  - Any rapid dysrhythmia from a nonsinus focus above the AV node
  - Junctional tachycardia:
    - Regular tachycardia without preceding depolarization waves
- Ventricular tachycardia (VT):
  - ≥3 consecutive ventricular ectopic beats at a rate of 100 bpm
  - Most common initiating rhythm in sudden death in patients with previous MI
- Torsades de pointes:
  - Paroxysmal form of VT with undulating axis and prolonged baseline QT interval
  - Secondary to either congenital or acquired abnormalities of ventricular repolarization
  - Often the result of drug therapy or electrolyte disturbances
- VF:
  - Oscillations without evidence of discrete QRST morphology
  - Accounts for 80–85% of sudden cardiac deaths
  - Frequently results from degeneration of sustained VT

## RISK FACTORS
### Genetics
Rare cases of autosomal dominant atrial tachycardias without structural heart disorders

## ETIOLOGY
- Sinus tachycardia:
  - Acute MI
  - Anemia
  - Anxiety
  - CHF
  - Drug intoxication
  - Hyperthyroidism
  - Hypovolemia
  - Hypoxia
  - Infection
  - Pain
  - Pericardial tamponade
  - Pulmonary embolus

- Atrial tachycardia:
  - Precipitated by a premature atrial or ventricular contraction
  - Electrolyte disturbances
  - Drug toxicity
  - Hypoxia
- Junctional tachycardia:
  - AV nodal reentry
  - Myocardial ischemia
  - Structural heart disease
  - Preexcitation syndromes
  - Drug and alcohol toxicity
- AF:
  - HTN
  - Coronary artery disease
  - Hypothyroidism
  - Alcohol intake
  - Mitral valve disease
  - Chronic obstructive pulmonary disease
  - Pulmonary embolus
  - Wolf-Parkinson-White (WPW) syndrome
  - Hypoxia
  - Digoxin toxicity
  - Chronic pericarditis
  - Idiopathic atrial fibrillation
- Atrial flutter:
  - Ischemic heart disease
  - Valvular heart disease
  - CHF
  - Myocarditis
  - Cardiomyopathies
  - Pulmonary embolus
  - Electrolyte abnormalities
  - Recent cardiac surgery
- Multifocal atrial tachycardia:
  - Hypoxic effects of chronic lung disease
  - Theophylline toxicity
- VT:
  - Dilated cardiomyopathy
  - Cardiac ischemia
  - Hypoxia
  - Cardiac scarring/fibrosis
  - After cardiac surgery or congenital anomaly repair
  - Digoxin toxicity
  - Long QT syndrome
  - Electrolyte abnormalities
- Torsades de pointes (polymorphic VT):
  - Drug toxicity (antiarrhythmic class IA and IC agents)
  - Hypokalemia
  - Hypomagnesemia
  - Congenital QT prolongation
- VF:
  - Acute MI (most common)
  - Chronic ischemic heart disease
  - Hypoxia
  - Acidosis
  - Anaphylaxis
  - Electrocution
  - Shock
  - Hypokalemia
  - Initiation of quinidine therapy
  - Massive hemorrhage

 **DIAGNOSIS**

## SIGNS AND SYMPTOMS
- Asymptomatic:
- Palpitations
- Lightheadedness
- Dyspnea
- Diaphoresis
- Dizziness
- Weakness
- Chest discomfort
- Angina
- Syncope
- Prominent neck veins
- Signs of instability:
  - Hypotension
  - Pulmonary edema
  - Chest pain
  - Mental status changes

### History
- Acute onset of palpitations, lightheadedness, generalized weakness, or shortness of breath
- Sudden collapse, often preceded for minutes-hours by chest pain
- Prior history of cardiac disease common (ischemia, CHF)

### Physical Exam
Determine if the patient is hemodynamically stable:
- Assess mental status.
- Assess heart rate.
- Assess BP: Normal or hypotensive
- Cardiac exam

## ESSENTIAL WORKUP
- ABCs
- Determination of unstable vs. stable patient
- Detailed history
- 12-lead EKG and rhythm strip to categorize the tachycardia:

## DIAGNOSTIC TESTS & INTERPRETATION
### Lab
Studies should be ordered based on the presentation to evaluate underlying metabolic abnormalities or ischemia.

### Diagnostic Procedures/Surgery
EKG:
- SVT:
  - Narrow-complex, rate usually 130–160
  - Uniformity of polarity and amplitude
  - No P waves visible
- AF:
  - Irregular, narrow quasi-random signal (QRS) complexes, rate 110–130

- Atrial flutter:
  - Regular atrial rate, usually >300
  - Beat-to-beat uniformity of cycle length, polarity, and amplitude
  - Sawtooth flutter waves directed superiorly and most visible in leads II, III, aVF
  - AV block usually 2:1, but occasionally greater or irregular
- Multifocal atrial tachycardia:
  - Three distinctly different conducted P waves with varying pulse rate intervals
- VT:
  - QRS is usually 0.12 sec and often 0.14 sec.
- Torsades de pointes:
  - Ventricular rate >200 bpm
  - QRS structure displays an undulating axis, with the polarity of the complexes appearing to shift around the baseline.
  - Occurrence is often in short episodes of <90 sec.
- VF:
  - EKG shows oscillations without evidence of discrete QRST morphology.
  - Oscillations are usually irregular and occur at a rate of 150–300 bpm.
  - When the amplitude of most oscillations is 1 mm, the term "coarse" is used.
  - "Fine" VF is used for oscillations <1 mm.

## TREATMENT

### PRE-HOSPITAL
Cardiopulmonary resuscitation if pulseless

### INITIAL STABILIZATION/THERAPY
- IV access
- Oxygen
- Cardiac monitor
- Determine rhythm.

### ED TREATMENT/PROCEDURES
- Irregular narrow complex (A fib):
  - Rate control
  - β-Blockers or calcium channel blockers
  - Anticoagulation if onset is >24 hr
  - Cardioversion for *severe* hemodynamic compromise
- Regular narrow complex tachydysrhythmia:
  - Vagal maneuvers occasionally terminate the dysrhythmia:
    - Beware of carotid disease in elderly.
  - Adenosine:
    - May be diagnostic, revealing underlying AF/atrial flutter
- Stable wide complex tachycardia:
  - Determine whether VT or SVT with aberrancy
  - Administration of AV nodal-blocking agents (verapamil, adenosine) may result in VF:
    - With WPW, use amiodarone, flecainide, procainamide, or DC cardioversion.
  - Electrical cardioversion should be utilized when mechanism unknown.
  - Antidysrhythmic drugs include procainamide and amiodarone.

- Torsades de pointes:
  - Magnesium, overdrive pacing, amiodarone
  - Correct underlying abnormal electrolytes.
  - Consider repletion of serum K to 4.5.
- Polymorphic VT:
  - Ejection fraction (EF) normal:
    - β-Blockers, lidocaine, amiodarone, or procainamide
  - EF abnormal:
    - Amiodarone or lidocaine; then synchronized cardioversion
  - Treat ischemia and correct electrolytes.
- Monomorphic VT:
  - EF normal:
    - Procainamide preferred to amiodarone, sotalol, lidocaine; synchronized cardioversion
  - EF abnormal:
    - Amiodarone or lidocaine
    - Procainamide with caution as may cause hypotension; synchronized cardioversion
- VF or pulseless VT:
  - Treatment per ACLS protocol

### MEDICATION
- Adenosine: 6 mg (peds: 0.1 mg/kg up to 6 mg) rapid IV push; if no response after 1–2 min, then 12 mg (peds: 0.2 mg/kg up to 12 mg), may repeat 12 mg (0.2 mg/kg)
- Amiodarone:
  - *VT/SVT:* 15 mg/min (peds: 5 mg/kg IV over 20–60 min, max. 15 mg/kg/d IV) IV over 10 min, followed by 1 mg/min IV over the next 6 hr and then 0.5 mg/min over 18 hr
  - *VF/pulseless VT:* 300 mg (peds: 0.5 mg/kg) IV push; may give 150 mg IV push 3–5 min after if no response, max. 2.2 g in 24 hr
- Epinephrine: 1 mg (peds: 0.01 mg/kg) IV push q3–5min; 2.5 mg (peds: 0.1 mg/kg) endotracheally q3–5min
- Lidocaine: 1–1.5 mg/kg (100 mg) (peds: 1 mg/kg) IV push, may repeat q5–10min, max. dose 3 mg/kg
- Magnesium sulfate: 2 mg IV push over 2 min (peds: 25–50 mg/kg, max. 2 g, IV over 10–20 min)
- Procainamide:
  - *VF/pulseless VT:* 30 mg/min (peds: Not recommended) IV load until rhythm resolves, hypotension, QRS widens >50% or max. 17 mg/kg, then 1–4 mg/min IV
  - *Perfusing VT:* 20 mg/min (peds: 15 mg/kg IV over 30–60 min) IV load until rhythm resolves, hypotension, QRS widens >50% or max. 17 mg/kg, then 1–4 mg/min IV
  - *SVT:* 15–17 mg/kg IV at 20–30 mg/min *or* 100 mg IV q5min slow IV push until rhythm resolves or max. dose 1,000 mg (peds: 3–6 mg/kg IV over 5 min, max. 100 mg/dose, may repeat q5–10min as needed to total dose 15 mg/kg)
- Vasopressin: 40 units (peds: Not recommended) IV push once

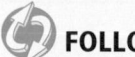 **FOLLOW-UP**

### DISPOSITION
#### *Admission Criteria*
- VT or VF
- Possible cardiac ischemic event
- Persistent SVT
- Underlying metabolic abnormalities

#### *Discharge Criteria*
Terminated supraventricular rhythm without organ hypoperfusion

#### *Issues for Referral*
Electrophysiologic testing:
- Diagnostic but not required emergently
- Determines therapy for accessory pathways

## PEARLS AND PITFALLS
- Always suspect a ventricular rhythm with a wide complex rhythm, especially in the older patient.
- Antidysrhythmic administration may increase success rate of cardioversion.
- Rapid, uninterrupted chest compressions may increase the success rate of defibrillation for a patient with a pulseless rhythm.

## ADDITIONAL READING
- American Heart Association. ACLS guidelines. 2000.
- American Heart Association. Guidelines for Management of Patients with Ventricular Arrythmias. 2006.
- Atkins DL, Dorian P, Gonzalez ER. Treatment of tachyarrhythmias. *Ann Emerg Med.* 2001;37: S91–S109.
- Connors S, Dorian P. Management of supraventricular tachycardia in the emergency department. *Can J Cardiol.* 1997;13(Suppl A): 19A–24A.
- Dagres N, Gutersohn A, Wieneke H, et al. A new hereditary form of ectopic atrial tachycardia with autosomal dominant inheritance. *Int J Cardiol.* 2004;93(2–3):311–313.
- Obel OA, Camm AJ. Supraventricular tachycardia: ECG diagnosis and anatomy. *Eur Heart J.* 1997;18(Suppl C):C2–C11.

### See Also (Topic, Algorithm, Electronic Media Element)
- Atrial Fibrillation
- Supraventricular Tachycardia
- Ventricular Tachycardia

 **CODES**

### ICD9
- 427.89 Other specified cardiac dysrhythmias
- 427.9 Cardiac dysrhythmia, unspecified
- 785.0 Tachycardia, unspecified

T

# TASER INJURIES

*Christian M. Sloane*

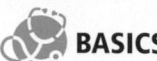

## BASICS

### DESCRIPTION

- Tasers are part of a class of less lethal weapons referred to as conducted energy weapons (CEWs).
- Most common in the U.S. are those made by Taser International; these include the M-26 and X-26, although others exist.
- These devices use a high-voltage low-amperage current to override the subject's ability to control the peripheral nervous system; they cause pain so as to induce subject compliance.
- Handheld devices such as stun guns require the application of 2 exposed probes to the skin (or close to the skin) to cause a localized response.
- Other devices, such as the M-26 and X-26, have barbed probes attached to thin wires that can be shot up to 35 ft to deliver current from a distance.
- Needle lengths of Taser barbs are 0.35 for the regular cartridge and up to 0.52 inches for the XP cartridge.
- The effects of CEWs vary depending on the type of device being used, location, placement, and distance between the probes on the subject's body. If probe spread on the body is less than 5 cm, effectiveness is less.
- Skin effects
  - May leave marks at site of probe contact, called csignature marksd
  - Small puncture wound from barbs
- Skeletal effects
  - Fractures may result from falls.
  - Vertebral compression fractures have been reported as a result of a Taser discharge.
  - Barbs may penetrate bone.
- Muscle effects
  - Strains possible
  - Rhabdomyolysis possible with repeated prolonged use, though more likely could result from the underlying cause leading to use of the Taser (e.g., excited delirium syndrome, or ExDS)

- Cardiovascular effects
  - Theoretically could cause ventricular fibrillation if a charge were delivered over the heart during a vulnerable part of the cardiac cycle.
  - A case of atrial fibrillation has been reported following Taser use.
  - No significant effects in otherwise healthy subjects. Does not cause changes in ECG or troponin I.
  - Unclear how device would affect pacemakers/automatic internal cardiac defibrillators (AICDs). Energy is low; theoretically should not cause damage. Could cause an AICD to deliver a shock if electrical activity of the CEW is misinterpreted as a dysrhythmia.
- Nervous system effects
  - There have been case reports of skull penetration and seizure.
- Respiratory effects
  - Initial concerns that the CEWs would disrupt ventilation proved unfounded. Research has shown that subjects actually increase ventilation during an application.

### ETIOLOGY
The devices are commonly used in law enforcement but may also be used in self-defense, by those wishing to commit a crime, or an accidental discharge of a weapon on to law enforcement personnel.

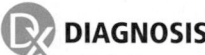

## DIAGNOSIS

### SIGNS AND SYMPTOMS

> **ALERT**
> Subjects on whom a device has been used may be in a state of ExDS.

### History
- A history of the use of a device is usually obtained. Important factors are:
- The type of device
- The mode used (probe or drive stun)
- The number of cycles discharged
- The duration of cycles applied
- Location of contact on the body

### Physical Exam
- Pay particular attention to the location of barb strike. Barbs in the skin, though unlikely, may cause injury to underlying structures:
- Eye
- Face
- Neck
- Groin
- Genitals
  - Secondary injuries do occur
    ○ From fall
    ○ From aspiration if device is deployed in the water
    ○ From tetanic muscle contraction
    ○ From barb penetration

### ESSENTIAL WORKUP
- All persons who have been exposed to CEW activation should receive a medical evaluation. The scope of that evaluation should depend on the type of use and state of the subject.
- For a subject who subsequently becomes compliant, is alert, and is acting appropriately and/or had CEW darts hit areas that are not medically sensitive, the darts may be removed and an evaluation done at intake to a detention facility.
- Given the risk to a subject who is in a state of ExDS regardless of CEW use, such a person requires an ED evaluation.

### Geriatric Considerations
The above groups warrant a medical evaluation, given that there are so few data to guide any definitive statements about their use.

### DIAGNOSTIC TESTS & INTERPRETATION
Labs should be directed at the underlying reason the person was "tasered." No labs are required simply because the person was tasered.

### Lab
If ExDS is present:
- CBC
- Chemistry panel
- Creatine kinase
- UTOX
- VBG to check for acidosis
- Lactate

## Imaging

- Not routine
- If altered level of consciousness with no clear cause, then head CT
- X-ray if Taser barb penetrated bone; this is most likely if it hit a digit or where bone is close to skin (eg, tibia, nose).
- US if individual is pregnant
- Other Imaging guided by suspicion of traumatic/secondary injury

## Diagnostic Procedures/Surgery

- Pacemaker interrogation if patient has pacemaker or AICD, since the device may have been damaged or have delivered a shock.
- ECG if there is underlying significant heart disease
- Women who are pregnant >20 wk should have fetal monitoring.

## DIFFERENTIAL DIAGNOSIS

Usually not unclear if device used.

 TREATMENT

### PRE-HOSPITAL

- If patient is acting normally, has normal vital signs, and AO × 3 appropriate, no special intervention is needed. Depending on jurisdiction, barb may be removed if not in sensitive area (face, eye, groin, neck, genitals). Otherwise, stabilize barb and transport patient to hospital for removal.
- If patient is agitated, treatment as per agitation/ExDS.
- If cardiac dysrthymia is present, initiate cardiac monitoring, IV access, oxygen.
- Treat any secondary traumatic injuries.

## INITIAL STABILIZATION/THERAPY

If ExDS, then treat per guidelines, including medications.

## ED TREATMENT/PROCEDURES

Initial treatment is steered toward underlying injuries.

- If patient acting normally, normal vital signs, AO × 4 appropriate, and no complaints of secondary injury, no special intervention needed.
- Update tetanus status as needed.
- Taser barb removal: Using 2 fingers of nondominant hand, stabilize skin around the barb by holding it down. Use dominant hand to grasp barb shaft and pull barb out.
- Treat the puncture wound like any other.
- Approach secondary traumatic injuries per trauma protocols.
- Treat dysrhthymias per protocol.

## MEDICATION

- Tetanus vaccination, dT or dTaP: 0.5 mL IM
- Midazolam (Versed) 5 mg IM/IV for agitation
- Haloperidol (Haldol) 5mg IM/IV for agitation

 FOLLOW-UP

### DISPOSITION

#### Admission Criteria

- Admit for signs of:
  - Cardiac instability
  - Excited delirium syndrome
  - Serious secondary injury

#### Pregnancy Considerations

Any female who is pregnant should undergo a medical evaluation of the pregnancy; if viable, she should undergo fetal monitoring at an appropriate facility.

## Discharge Criteria

Patient acting normally, normal vital signs, AO × 4 appropriate, and no complaints of secondary injury, or secondary injuries treated and stable for discharge

### Issues for Referral

Wound care, injury follow-up

## PEARLS AND PITFALLS

- These patients may be suffering from ExDS, hence law enforcement became involved or Taser was used. Failure to aggressively treat this life-threatening condition will result in untoward outcome.
- Always screen for possible secondary injury.
- Stable, alert, appropriate subjects do not need much more than simple barb removal (if necessary), a tetanus vaccination update, and wound care.

## ADDITIONAL READING

- Robb M, Close B, Furyk J, et al. Review article: Emergency Department implications of the TASER. *Emerg Med Australas.* 2009;21(4):250–258.
- Vilke GM, Sloane CM, Suffecool A, et al. Physiologic effects of the TASER after exercise. *Acad Emerg Med.* 2009;16(8):704–710. Epub 2009; July 10.

### See Also (Topic, Algorithm, Electronic Media Element)

Excited Delirium Syndrome, Puncture Wounds

T

# TEMPORAL-MANDIBULAR JOINT INJURY/SYNDROME

Ben Osborne
Yalonda L Phillipps

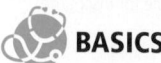 **BASICS**

## DESCRIPTION

- Myofascial pain causing temporomandibular joint (TMJ) dysfunction
- Prevalence of 40–75% of one sign of TMJ disorder
- Most common in 20–50-yr-olds
- Females seek treatment more frequently
- 40% have symptoms that resolve spontaneously.
- TMJ is a synovial joint:
  - Allows for hinge and sliding movements
- Articular disorders:
  - Congenital or developmental
  - Degenerative joint disorders:
    - Inflammatory
    - Non-inflammatory (osteoarthritis)
  - Trauma
  - TMJ hypermobility:
    - Laxity
    - Dislocation
    - Subluxation
  - TMJ hypomobility:
    - Trismus
    - Fibrosis
  - Infection
  - Neoplasm
- Masticatory muscle disorders:
  - Local myalgias
  - Myositis
  - Muscle spasm
  - Contracture
  - Myofascial pain disorder
- TMJ clicking:
  - May be normal finding; present as a transient finding in 40–60% of the population
- TMJ motion:
  - Typical range is 35–55 mm (maxillary to mandible incisors).
  - Limited by adhesions within the joint or disk displacement or trismus from muscle spasm

- Intra-articular disk disorder:
  - Anterior displacement with reduction:
    - Displacement in closed mouth position
    - Often with a click and variable pain with opening mouth
    - May worsen over time
  - Anterior disk displacement without reduction:
    - Disk is a mechanical obstruction to opening mouth
    - Maximal opening may be 20–25 mm.
    - Often difficult to correct

## ETIOLOGY

TMJ dysfunction is poorly understood:
- Multifactorial:
  - Bruxism (teeth grinding)
  - Trauma
  - Malocclusion
- Onset may be related to stress.

 **DIAGNOSIS**

## SIGNS AND SYMPTOMS
### History
- Preauricular pain:
  - Constant
  - Dull and aching
  - May be referred to the ipsilateral ear, head, or neck
  - Exacerbated by mandibular movement (pathognomonic)
  - More conspicuous at night and may cause insomnia
  - Often worsens through the day
- Tongue, lip, or cheek biting
- Ear pain
- Ear fullness
- Tinnitus
- Dizziness
- Neck pain
- Headache

### Physical Exam
- Joint sounds:
  - Popping or clicking sensation with TMJ articulation
  - A palpable or audible click with opening and closing
- Malalignment and limited range of motion:
  - Dentoskeletal malocclusion or lateral deviation
  - Open or closed locking of the jaw
- Tenderness over the muscles of mastication and TMJ:
  - Masseter muscle most commonly painful

## ESSENTIAL WORKUP
- Diagnosis based on clinical presentation
- Exclude other causes of headache and facial pain.

## DIAGNOSTIC TESTS & INTERPRETATION
### Lab
No specific laboratory tests are indicated unless there is concern for other disease process.

### Imaging
- Panorex is the screening radiograph of choice:
  - May demonstrate fracture or intra-articular pathology (ie, tumor or degenerative joint disease) but usually unremarkable
- CT: Best for evaluating bony structures for fractures, dislocations, etc.
- MRI: Best imaging for nonreducing displaced disks: Allows for better visualization of joints simultaneously

## DIFFERENTIAL DIAGNOSIS
- Acute coronary syndrome
- Carotid artery dissection
- Intracranial hemorrhage (subarachnoid hemorrhage)
- Inflammatory diseases:
  - Giant cell (temporal) arteritis
  - Rheumatoid arthritis
- Trigeminal or glossopharyngeal neuralgia
- Vascular headache
- Intraoral and dental pathology
- Herpes zoster
- Salivary gland disorder
- Otitis media
- Sinusitis
- Elongated styloid process pain

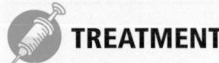 **TREATMENT**

**PRE-HOSPITAL**
Provide comfort and reassurance

**INITIAL STABILIZATION/THERAPY**
Make sure airway is patent.

**ED TREATMENT/PROCEDURES**
- Acute therapeutic options:
  - Patient reassurance and education—"usually mild and self-limited"
  - Rest
  - Heat
  - Analgesics and anxiolytics
  - Urgent reduction of open or closed locking TMJ; may require procedural sedation
  - Reduction of TMJ dislocation:
    ○ Often requires procedural sedation
    ○ Monitor airway.
    ○ May face the patient or perform from behind patient
    ○ Protect thumbs with gauze and/or tongue depressors.
    ○ Thumbs rest on intraoral surface of mandible.
    ○ Fingers wrap around jaw.
    ○ Firm, progressive downward pressure as jaw is guided first in a caudal direction and then posteriorly
  - Physical therapy—moist heat or ice packs
  - Pain site injections with mixture of steroids/lidocaine
- Outpatient management:
  - Combination pharmacotherapy:
    ○ NSAIDs
    ○ Muscle relaxants
    ○ Antidepressants
    ○ Sedative hypnotics
  - Home physical therapy—moist heat or ice packs and mechanically soft diet
  - Occlusal appliance worn during sleep
  - Referral to dentist or oral–maxillofacial surgeon

**MEDICATION**
*First Line*
- Acetaminophen: 325–1,000 mg (peds 15 mg/kg) PO q6h
- Cyclobenzaprine: 5–10 mg PO t.i.d. (peds: 5–10 mg PO t.i.d. if >15 yr old); caution with hepatic impairment
- Diazepam: 2–10 mg PO b.i.d.–t.i.d. (peds: <12 yr old 0.12–0.8 mg/kg/day PO div q6–8h)
- Ibuprofen: 600 mg (peds: 10 mg/kg) PO q8h

*Second Line*
- Nortriptyline: 10–50 mg PO qhs
- Narcotic analgesic
- Sedative hypnotics

 **FOLLOW-UP**

**DISPOSITION**
*Admission Criteria*
TMJ syndrome can be managed on an outpatient basis unless a locked or dislocated joint cannot be reduced.

*Discharge Criteria*
Treat as outpatient with pain medication, muscle relaxants, and warm compresses.

**FOLLOW-UP RECOMMENDATIONS**
Patients with TMJ syndrome may need referral to ENT, oral surgeon, or dentist for further care.

**PEARLS AND PITFALLS**
- TMJ locking must be addressed urgently.
- NSAIDs, rest, and heat are first-line therapy.

**ADDITIONAL READING**
- Buescher JJ. Temporomandibular joint disorders. *Am Fam Physician*. 2007;76:1477–1482.
- Lewis EL, Dolwick MF, Abramowicz S, et al. Contemporary imaging of the temporomandibular joint. *Dent Clin North Am*. 2008;52:875–890.
- Marx JA, Hockberger RS, Walls RM, et al. *Rosen's Emergency Medicine: Concepts and Clinical Practice*, 7th ed. St. Louis: Mosby; 2009.
- Scrivani SJ, Keith DA, Kaban LB. Temporomandibular disorders. *N Engl J Med*. 2008;359:2693–2705.

 **CODES**

ICD9
- 524.60 Temporomandibular joint disorders, unspecified
- 524.61 Temporomandibular joint disorders, adhesions and ankylosis (bony or fibrous)
- 524.62 Temporomandibular joint disorders, arthralgia of temporomandibular joint

T

# TENDON LACERATION
*Nicholle D. Bromley*

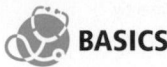
## BASICS

### ALERT
Tendons near lacerations must be explored through *complete range of motion* to rule out injury.

### DESCRIPTION
- Based on mechanism
- External trauma:
  - Penetrating trauma:
    - Gunshot wounds
    - Glass
    - Knives
    - Foreign bodies
  - Blunt trauma:
    - Crushing force or avulsion from hyperextension of a joint
- Internal trauma:
  - Entrapment/laceration from bony fracture (rare)

### ETIOLOGY
Tendon injuries grossly categorized into those affecting upper versus lower extremities:
- Upper-extremity injuries frequently related to the workplace, home, an assault, or attempted suicide
- Lower-extremity injuries most often associated with work or motor vehicle accident

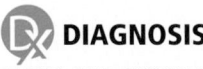
## DIAGNOSIS

### SIGNS AND SYMPTOMS
- Pain is the cardinal symptom.
- Functional deficit
- Soft-tissue damage:
  - Swelling
  - Ecchymosis
  - Lacerations
  - Hemorrhage
- Abnormal resting position of the extremity or large joint instability increases suspicion for tendon injury.

### ESSENTIAL WORKUP
- A careful history:
  - Mechanism, time of injury
  - Hand position during injury
  - Hand dominance
  - Drug allergies
  - Medications
  - Past medical history
  - Tetanus vaccination status
- Physical exam:
  - Examine resting position of hand.
  - Examine the wound in position of initial injury.
  - Perform neurovascular exam before local anesthesia is instilled.
  - Examine each digit separately.
  - Test strength against resistance.
  - Examine tendon with direct visualization through full range of motion.

- Flexor digitorum profundus injuries:
  - Present with inability to flex the distal interphalangeal (IP) joint
  - Exam involves stabilizing the proximal IP joint in full extension while the patient attempts to flex distal IP joint.
- Flexor digitorum superficialis injuries:
  - Present with inability to flex the proximal IP joint of a digit
  - Usually established by means of standard superficialis tendon test:
    - While holding the uninjured digits in full extension, the patient attempts to flex the affected finger at the proximal IP joint.
    - False negative if profundus is functional.
  - The distal IP joint extension test:
    - May make this diagnosis more apparent
    - Patient is asked to make a precision pinch between thumb and the injured finger.
    - Then asked to flex the proximal IP joint so that the distal IP joint is hyperextended
    - Confirms the integrity of the flexor digitorum superficialis
- Forearm and wrist flexor injuries:
  - Present with inability to flex ulnar or radial side of wrist or to flex the wrist while opposing the thumb to the little finger
- Extensor tendon injuries:
  - Found by weakness or lack of extension of the distal phalanx against resistant
  - Indicates partial or complete disruption
  - Best determined with patient placing palm on flat surface and asking the patient to attempt to extend the fingers individually
  - Palpate each tendon.
  - Loss of normal tension indicates injury.
- Further explore tendons and wounds after local anesthesia (1% lidocaine or 0.5% bupivacaine) in a bloodless, well-lit surgical field:
  - Tendons near lacerations must be explored through complete range of motion.
  - Best elucidates tendon injuries distal or proximal to a skin wound

### Pediatric Considerations
- More difficult to get an adequate exam
- The healing process is usually quicker and more often associated with complete return to preinjury function.

### DIAGNOSTIC TESTS & INTERPRETATION
#### Lab
Wounds 1st examined >12 hr after injury or wounds with evident infection should be cultured.

#### Imaging
- Radiographs are frequently needed to identify radiopaque foreign bodies or fractures.
- High-frequency US can be used to identify complete tendon lacerations:
  - Partial tendon lacerations difficult to image
  - A water bath may help when attempting to image a painful extremity.
- US guidance may help to guide removal of foreign bodies.

### DIFFERENTIAL DIAGNOSIS
- Always rule out an associated foreign body or fracture.
- Partial lacerations are common but more difficult to diagnosis than complete disruptions because they may demonstrate intact function:
  - Alterations of the normal resting hand position may indicate partial laceration.
- Lacerations over the metacarpophalangeal joint should be considered the result of a human bite until proven otherwise:
  - Look for associated extensor tendon injury while metacarpophalangeal joint flexed.
- Lacerations over the proximal IP joint may involve the lateral bands or the central slip of the extensor mechanism:
  - Boutonnière deformity from improper repair
- Disruption of the extensor tendon distal to the central slip results in a mallet finger deformity.
- "Jersey finger" is a closed traumatic injury with avulsion of the flexor digitorum profundus, seen when a football player grabs the jersey of another player and his finger gets stuck.
- Avulsion of the flexor digitorum superficialis distally may be present with or without an associated avulsion fracture:
  - Suspect when a grasping finger is hit by a fast-moving object (jammed finger).

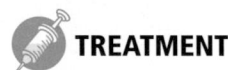
## TREATMENT

### PRE-HOSPITAL
- Do not remove foreign matter from the patient in the field.
- Immobilize and transport patient.
- Apply direct pressure to control hemorrhage.
- Assess distal neurovascular status for signs of compromise.
- Contact medical control before any attempted reduction.

### INITIAL STABILIZATION/THERAPY

- Evaluate extremity and control hemorrhage with direct pressure.
- Remove all jewelry or constricting bands.

### ED TREATMENT/PROCEDURES

- Pain control as required
- Administer tetanus toxoid as needed.
- Copious irrigation with 1 L NS
- Broad-spectrum antibiotic, such as a 1st-generation cephalosporin (Cefazolin)
- Tendon lacerations associated with human bites:
  - Must be copiously irrigated
  - Place on IV antibiotics with coverage of oral anaerobes (ampicillin/sulbactam).
  - Immobilize and elevate the hand.
- Remove all foreign bodies and provide debridement of avascular tissue.
- Partial tendon lacerations that involve >20% of the cross-sectional area of the tendon must be repaired.
- Simple extensor tendon lacerations may be repaired in the ED:
  - Use a 4-0 or 5-0 nonabsorbable suture in a figure-of-8 or a modified Kessler stitch.
- *All* suspected flexor tendon, wrist, and distal forearm tendon lacerations require consultation by a hand surgeon, ideally within 12 hr.
- Tendon lacerations over the proximal IP joint may result in a boutonnière deformity:
  - Refer to a hand surgeon.
- The superficial nature of multiple tendons, nerves, and vessels on the volar aspect of the wrist renders them easily vulnerable to penetrating trauma:
- "Spaghetti wrist" or "full house":
  - Volar wrist laceration with at least 10 structures involved
  - Requires prompt consultation with a hand surgeon
- Tendon lacerations associated with fractures require referral for operative repair.
- If a surgeon is not promptly available:
  - Irrigate copiously.
  - Close skin without repair of tendon.
  - Immobilize injured hand with a bulky volar dressing and splint.
  - Wrist in 20–30° of flexion
  - Metacarpal joint in 60–70° of flexion
  - IP joints in 10–15° of flexion

### MEDICATION

- Ampicillin/sulbactam: 3 g IV q6 (peds: 200 mg/kg/d IM or IV divided q6h)
- Cefazolin: 1 g IV piggyback (peds: 100 mg/kg/d IM or IV divided q6h, followed by 40 mg/kg/d PO q.i.d. for 5–7 days)
- Tetanus toxoid: 0.5 mL IM (peds: <7 yr—diphtheria-pertussis-tetanus vaccine preferred; in those >7 yr, adult dose tetanus toxoid if immunization series not completed), tetanus immune globulin, as required, 250 IU administered IM

## FOLLOW-UP

### DISPOSITION

*Admission Criteria*

- Patients with infected tendon lacerations must be admitted for operative debridement.
- Any patients with tendon injury secondary to human bite must be admitted for operative debridement and IV antibiotics.
- Any patients with significant flexor tendon laceration may be admitted for timely operative repair or transferred to the nearest hand surgeon.

*Discharge Criteria*

- Patients with an extensor tendon laceration that is not infected, nor associated with other significant injury or underlying fracture, which was repaired by the ED physician and is now properly splinted, may be discharged with timely surgical follow-up.
- Patients with an extensor tendon laceration requiring surgeon referral for repair (wrist, forearm, proximal IP joint), which has been properly treated and splinted, with the patient placed on antibiotics, may be discharged for timely surgical follow-up.

## PEARLS AND PITFALLS

It is very important to test strength because tendon injuries with up to a 90% full-thickness laceration can have normal range of motion. Therefore, test strength against resistance.

### ADDITIONAL READING

- Blaivas M, Lyon M, Brannam L, et al. Water bath evaluation technique for emergency ultrasound of painful superficial structures. *Am J Emerg Med.* 2004;22:589–593.
- Dogan T, Celebiler O, Gorungluoglu R, et al. A new test for superficialis flexor tendon function. *Ann Plast Surg.* 2000;45:93–96.
- Finlay K, Friendman L. Common tendon and muscle injuries: Upper extremities. *Ultrasound Clin.* 2007;2:4:577–594.
- Hudson DA, de Jager LT. The spaghetti wrist: Simultaneous laceration of the median and ulnar nerves with flexor tendons at the wrist. *J Hand Surg (Br).* 1993;18:171–173.
- Jackimczyk K. Hand injuries. In: Wolfson A, et al, eds., *Clinical practice of emergency medicine.* Philadelphia: Lippincott Williams & Wilkins; 2010, 41;278–286.
- Jozsa LG, Kannus P. *Human tendons: Anatomy, physiology and pathology.* Champaign, IL: Human Kinetic; 1997.
- Lee DH, Robbin ML, Galliott R, et al. Ultrasound evaluation of flexor tendon lacerations. *J Hand Surg (Am).* 2000;25:236–241.
- Perron AD, Brady WJ, Keats TE, et al. Orthopedic pitfalls in the emergency department. Closed tendon injuries of the hand. *Am J Emerg Med.* 2001; 19:76–80.
- Stahl S, Kaufman T, Bialik V. Partial lacerations of flexor tendons in children: Primary repair versus conservative treatment. *J Hand Surg (Br).* 1997;22B:377–380.

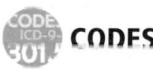

## CODES

ICD9

- 880.23 Open wound of upper arm, with tendon involvement
- 881.22 Open wound of wrist, with tendon involvement
- 882.2 Open wound of hand except fingers alone, with tendon involvement

# TENDONITIS

*James P. Killeen*

## BASICS

### DESCRIPTION
- The term "tendinitis" has been used to describe chronic painful tendon injuries before the underlying pathology was understood. This term has led to confusion about the cause, chronicity, and treatment of the underlying disorder. The terms "tendinosis" or "tendinopathy" should be used to describe chronic tendon disorders.
- Overuse syndrome:
  – Clinical syndrome of chronic pain and tendon thickening
  – Synovial cells increase in thickness
  – Excess synovial fluid collection
  – Constant irritation
- If no further injury occurs, the acute process may last from 48 hr to 2 wk.
- Tendinopathy as the presence of fibrosis without inflammatory cells and with symptoms that persist >3 mo.

### ETIOLOGY
- Mechanical overload or repetitive microtrauma to the musculotendinous unit:
  – Intrinsic factors:
    ○ Inflexibility
    ○ Muscle weakness or imbalance
  – Extrinsic factors:
    ○ Excessive deviation, frequency, or activity
  – In tendinopathies, the collagen is in a state of disrepair, with proliferation and chronic irritation of neurovascular repair tissue in the tendon and its linings.
- Chemotactive and vasoactive chemical mediators are released:
  – Vasodilatation and cellular edema increase the number and activity of polumorphonuclear cells (PMNs).

## DIAGNOSIS

### SIGNS AND SYMPTOMS
#### History
- The patient's history should explain what movement led to the injury.
- Repetitive stress and mechanical overload
- The classic inflammatory signs include pain, warmth, erythema, and swelling.
- Pain will resolve quickly after initial movement, only to become a throbbing pain after exercise.

#### Physical Exam
- Defined as inflammation of the tendon only
- There is a poor distinction between tendonitis and tenosynovitis (degree of inflammation). These are now called tendonopathies.
- Clinical findings:
  – Warmth
  – Presence of an effusion
  – Decreased range of motion
  – Instability
  – Pain on motion
  – Tenderness over tendon site

### Specific Conditions Supraspinatus Tendonopathy
Supraspinatus and other rotator cuff tendons:
- Compressed between humerus and acromion
- Overuse of the extremity may lead to microtrauma of the tendons fibers.
- Neer classification:
  – Stage 1:
    ○ Age <25
    ○ Involved in sports requiring repetitive overhead motion (eg, swimmers or pitchers)
    ○ Edema and hemorrhage of the tendon
    ○ Flexion–abduction motion will elicit pain.
    ○ "Dull aches"
  – Stage 2:
    ○ Age 25–40
    ○ Pain is constant and worsens at night.
    ○ Active motion is limited by pain.
    ○ Passive range of motion is preserved.
    ○ Diffuse, intense pain
    ○ Fibrosis and thickening of the tendon
  – Stage 3:
    ○ Partial or complete tendon tears
    ○ Raising the humerus in a forced forward flexion while preserving scapular rotation causes impingement.

### Calcific Tendonitis
- Age >40 years with unknown etiology.
- Any tendon of the rotator cuff can be affected, but there is a predisposition for the supraspinatus.
- Most cases are asymptomatic and are found on routine radiographs.
- Calcium is deposited within the tendon over time; it then undergoes spontaneous resorption, causing pain.
- Acute attacks may develop from crystal release.

### Bicipital Tendonopathy
- Pain to the anterior shoulder, which radiates down the radius
- Discomfort when rolling on the shoulder or trying to reach a hip pocket or back zipper
- Focal tenderness is between the greater and lesser tuberosities of the humerus.
- Yergason test:
  – Elbow is flexed at 90 degrees and arm held against the body.
  – Pain increases with resisted supination of the wrist.
- Speeds test:
  – Pain along the bicipital groove with resisted forward flexion and forearm supination

### Lateral Epicondylitis (Tennis Elbow)
- Rotational repetitive motion causes pain.
- Dull ache on the outside of the elbow that increases with grasping and twisting
- Inflammation at the insertion of the common extensor tendon at lateral epicondyle of humerus
- Resisted active dorsiflexion of the wrist on extension of the middle finger against resistance can reproduce pain with the elbow extended.
- Inflammation at site of insertion of the flexor carpi radialis on the medial epicondyle:
  – Bowlers, golfers, pitchers
  – Active flexing of the wrist against resistance causes pain.

### Wrist/Hand
- Inflammatory changes of the synovial lining between tendons and the retinaculum
- De Quervain tenosynovitis:
  – Inflammation of the abductor pollicis longus and extensor pollicis brevis
  – Finkelstein's test:
    ○ Patient makes fist with thumb curled in palm.
    ○ Wrist is deviated in the direction of the ulna.
    ○ Pain occurs in first extensor compartment.
  – Osteoarthritis of the carpometacarpal joints or gonococcal tenosynovitis causes the same pain.

### Trigger Finger
- Proximal portion of the palmar flexor tendon sheath becomes stenosed and catches as the finger is moved.
- Symptoms vary from pain to locking in flexion.

### Ankle
- Achilles' tendonopathy:
  – Overuse injury commonly seen in males
  – Trauma or systemic disease causing inflammation
  – With repeated stress, scar tissue formation and degeneration of the tendon will occur.
  – Patient will have pain, reduced range of motion, or morning stiffness.
- Achilles' tendon rupture
  – Seen more commonly in 30- to 40-yr-old recreational athletes
  – "Popping sensation"
  – Acute weakness, inability to continue activity
  – Feels like being kicked or hit in back of leg
  – May initially have a gap by palpation, followed by ecchymosis and a boggy sensation
  – Inability to plantarflex the foot with complete rupture
  – Thompson test:
    ○ Patient lies prone with the feet hanging over edge of bed.
    ○ Physician squeezes calf muscles and looks for plantarflexion.
    ○ 20–30% of Achilles' tendon ruptures are missed at the initial visit because the clinician was falsely reassured by the patient's ability to plantarflex or walk.
    ○ The Matles, the patient lies prone with knees flexed to 90 degrees. Observe whether the affected foot is dorsiflexed or neutral (both are abnormal) compared to the uninjured side, where the foot should appear plantarflexed.

## Pediatric Considerations

- Apophysitis occurs in children at an ossification center subject to traction:
  - Little League elbow at the medial epicondyle
  - Osgood–Schlatter syndrome at tibial tubercle
- Avascular necrosis (AVN):
  - Presents with pain and swelling around a joint
  - Can occur at various locations
  - Well-recognized sites:
    - Capitellum of the humerus
    - Head of the femur
    - Tarsal navicular
    - Metatarsal head
    - Diagnosis is made by plain radiographs.
    - Radiographs are often required to rule out fracture, AVN, osteochondritis dissecans, and bony tumor.

## ESSENTIAL WORKUP

Physical examination

## DIAGNOSTIC TESTS & INTERPRETATION

### Lab

CBC, C-reactive protein (CRP), ESR only if more serious infection suspected

### Imaging

- Radiographs:
  - Extra-articular from articular etiologies
  - "SECONDS":
    - Soft tissue swelling
    - Erosions
    - Calcifications
    - Osteoporosis
    - Narrowing
    - Deformity
    - Separation
- US:
  - Evaluate joint effusions
  - More sensitive than MRI
  - Limited use in the emergency setting
  - Focal tendon thickening
  - Focal hypoechoic areas
  - Irregular and ill-defined borders
  - Peritendinous edema
- MRI:
  - Internal morphology of the tendon and surrounding structures
  - Helps diagnose retrocalcaneal bursitis and insertional tendonitis
  - Reveals tendon thickening and increased signal with chronic tendon abnormalities
- Scintigraphy:
  - 99m-Technetium pertechnetate phosphate (binds with plasma protein) and concentrates in joint space (bursitis)

## DIFFERENTIAL DIAGNOSIS

- Septic arthritis
- Fracture
- Osteoarthritis

 TREATMENT

### PRE-HOSPITAL

Immobilize injured extremity as indicated.

### INITIAL STABILIZATION/THERAPY

Ice and immobilization pending workup

### ED TREATMENT/PROCEDURES

- General:
  - Rest
  - NSAIDs
  - Ice (10- to 20-min intervals)
  - Range of motion exercises
  - Eccentric exercise is the application of a load (ie, muscular exertion) to a lengthening muscle.
  - Local injection for pain control
  - Outpatient management
  - Admit only for surgery or severe disability.
  - Allow 6–12 wk to heal.
  - Recent studies have described successful investigational therapies.
  - Prolotherapy, an US-guided injection of dextrose and lidocaine to stimulate repair.
  - Sclerotherapy injections of polidocanol, a sclerosing substance to reduce neovascularity
  - Aprotinin, a broad-spectrum protease and matrix metalloproteinase (MMP) inhibitor, injected peritendinously
- Calcific tendonitis:
  - Therapy with low-energy radio shock waves has recently been shown to bring significant pain relief:
    - Thought to increase the resorption of calcium
  - Cimetidine has been used to decrease pain and calcium deposits.
- Trigger finger:
  - Conservative treatments such as rest, splinting (thumb spica) and NSAIDs for most
  - Some physicians suggest cortisone injections (84–91% cure rate).
  - Surgical release of A-1 pulley may be required.
- De Quervain tenosynovitis:
  - Rest, ice, NSAIDs
  - Thumb spica splint for 3–5 days often helps.

- Achilles' tendonitis:
  - Rest, ice, NSAIDs
  - Orthotics or heel wedges
  - Cryotherapy has been shown to be useful in controlling inflammation.
  - Achilles' rupture should be splinted posteriorly in slight plantarflexion:
    - Refer to orthopedics, as patients often need surgery.

### MEDICATION

Ibuprofen: 400–800 mg PO q6–8h (max 2,400 mg/day); peds: 5–10 mg/kg per dose PO q4–6h (max 50 mg/kg/day)

 FOLLOW-UP

### DISPOSITION

#### Admission Criteria

Admit patients requiring surgery or having other more serious illness/injury.

#### Discharge Criteria

Most patients may be managed as outpatients with appropriate referral.

## ADDITIONAL READING

- Wilder RP, Sethi S. Overuse injuries: Tendinopathies, stress fractures, compartment syndrome, and shin splints. *Clin Sports Med*. 2004;23:55–81, 61.
- Woodley BL, Newsham-West RJ, Baxter GD. Chronic tendinopathy: Effectiveness of eccentric exercise. *Br J Sports Med*. 2007;41:188.
- Manias P, Stasinopoulos D. A controlled clinical pilot trial to study the effectiveness of ice as a supplement to the exercise programme for the management of lateral elbow tendinopathy. *Br J Sports Med*. 2006;40:81.
- Paoloni JA, Appleyard RC, Nelson J, et al. Topical glyceryl trinitrate treatment of chronic noninsertional Achilles tendinopathy. A randomized, double-blind, placebo-controlled trial. *J Bone Joint Surg Am*. 2004;86-A:916.
- Scarpone M, Rabago DP, Zgierska A, et al. The efficacy of prolotherapy for lateral epicondylosis: A pilot study. *Clin J Sport Med*. 2008;18:248.

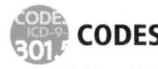 CODES

### ICD9

726.90 Enthesopathy of unspecified site

# TENOSYNOVITIS
*James P. Killeen*

## 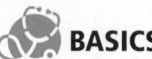 BASICS

### DESCRIPTION
- Definition:
  - Inflammation of the tendon and tendon sheath
- Caused by inflammation, overuse, or infection
- Synovial sheaths cover tendons as they pass through osseofibrous tunnels:
  - Visceral and parietal layers of the synovium lubricate and nourish the tendons.
  - Infection can be introduced into tendon sheath.
- Skin wound
- Hematogenous spread
- Flexor tenosynovitis (FTS) of hand:
  - Typically infectious etiology
  - Penetrating injury, especially at flexion creases of the finger is most common mechanism.
  - High-pressure "injection" injury to fingers
- Air tools
- Paint sprayers
- Hydraulic equipment
- May appear minor on the surface but are associated with high incidence of FTS.

### ETIOLOGY
- De Quervain tenosynovitis:
  - Caused by overuse
  - Inflammatory in nature
- Gonococcal (GN) tenosynovitis:
  - *Neisseria gonorrhoeae*
- Non-GN infectious tenosynovitis:
  - *Staphylococcus aureus* and streptococci are most common in penetrating injuries.
  - *Pasteurella multocida* is common with cat bites.
  - *Eikenella corrodens* is common with human bites.
  - *Pseudomonas* is seen in patients with diabetes or marine-associated injuries.
  - *Mycobacterium* species may occur in immunocompromised patients.
  - Fungal tenosynovitis may occur from puncture wounds due to thorns or woody plants.

## 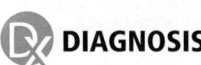 DIAGNOSIS

### SIGNS AND SYMPTOMS
- Kanavel signs of FTS include:
  - Tenderness and symmetric swelling along flexor tendon sheath (sausage digit)
- Flexed position of the digit
- Pain with passive extension of the finger

### Hand
- De Quervain tenosynovitis:
  - Repetitive pinching motion of thumb and fingers
- Assembly-line workers
- Carpenters
- Gardeners (landscaping or weeding):
  - Pain in the radial aspect of the wrist becomes worse with activity and better with rest.
  - Pain occurs on palpation along the radial aspect of the wrist.
  - Pain occurs with passive range of motion of the thumb.
  - Finkelstein test:
    ○ Pain occurs with ulnar deviation of the wrist with the thumb cupped in a closed fist.
- GN tenosynovitis:
  - Most commonly affects teenagers, young adults
  - Seen in the ankle, hand, or wrist
  - More commonly seen in women
  - Vaginal or penile discharge usually absent
  - Fever, chills, polyarthralgia common
  - Erythema, tenderness to palpation, and painful range of motion of the involved tendon
  - Dermatitis may be present.
  - Hemorrhagic macules or papules on the distal extremities or trunk

### Forearm
Traumatic tenosynovitis is seen after a direct blow to the lower portion of the forearm.

### Ankle
- Stenosing tenosynovitis:
  - Commonly seen at the inferior retinaculum of the peroneus tendon
  - Patients are usually >40 yr old and have some predisposing trauma.
  - Motion increases the pain.
- Rheumatoid tenosynovitis:
  - Medially, the posterior tibial and flexor hallucis longus tendons are commonly involved.
  - Laterally, the peronei are involved.
  - Anteriorly, the anterior tibial tendon is involved.
  - Motion increases the pain.
  - Spontaneous rupture may occur.

### History
- Assess for infectious etiology:
  - History of sexually transmitted disease exposure, penile or vaginal discharge
- Obtain history of mechanism:
  - High-pressure injections
  - Puncture wounds, bites
  - Environmental exposures
- Assess tetanus status and comorbid factors (eg, diabetes and immunocompromise).

### Physical Exam
- Assess Kanavel signs.
- Document neurovascular status.
- Identify signs and symptoms of systemic illness as well as other potential sites of infection.

### ESSENTIAL WORKUP
Thorough history and physical examination will often lead to appropriate diagnosis.

### DIAGNOSTIC TESTS & INTERPRETATION
#### Lab
- CBC, ESR:
  - May be of assistance in infectious etiology
- GN cultures (urethra, cervix, rectum, pharynx) may be useful.
- LFTs may be elevated with disseminated *N. gonorrhoeae* infection.

#### Imaging
- Radiographs are of low yield unless a radiopaque foreign body is suspected to be retained in soft tissue.
- MRI has proved accurate in assisting the diagnosis of tenosynovitis:
  - Generally unnecessary in the ED

### DIFFERENTIAL DIAGNOSIS
- Ankle, soft tissue injuries
- Bursitis
- Carpal tunnel syndrome
- Cellulitis
- Compartment syndrome
- Endocarditis
- Felon
- Gonorrhea
- Gout and pseudogout
- Hand infections
- High-pressure hand injuries
- Soft-tissue hand injuries
- Soft-tissue knee injuries
- Reiter syndrome
- Rheumatic fever
- Rheumatoid arthritis

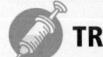 **TREATMENT**

**PRE-HOSPITAL**

- Delay in definitive treatment leads to significant increased morbidity and loss of function.
- The affected extremity should be elevated and immobilized.

**INITIAL STABILIZATION/THERAPY**

- Manageme airway and resuscitate as indicated:
  - Septic shock
- Elevation, immobilization of affected extremity
- IV access
- Tetanus status
- Procedure:
  - Diagnostic arthrocentesis is indicated if joint effusion is present with tenosynovitis:
    o Most patients with disseminated GC infection have coexisting septic arthritis.
    o Cultures are negative in 50% of patients.
    o 25% GC arthritis is polyarticular.
    o Joint fluid glucose is normal.
    o WBCs usually < 50,000; Gram's stain positive in 25% of the patients.

**ED TREATMENT/PROCEDURES**

*Hand*

- High-pressure injection injuries to hand:
  - Surgical emergency
  - Immediate hand surgery consultation
  - Pain management
- Infectious FTS of hand:
  - Immediate hand surgery consultation
  - Broad-spectrum antibiotic coverage
- De Quervain tenosynovitis:
  - Rest, NSAIDs, and thumb spica splint
  - Consider lidocaine/corticosteroid injection if condition is unresponsive
- GC tenosynovitis:
  - Admit for IV antibiotic therapy.
  - Penicillin or first-generation cephalosporin for initial therapy
  - Second-generation cephalosporin as an alternative
  - Surgical drainage may be indicated if antibiotics do not improve the condition.
  - Pain management

- Non-GN infectious tenosynovitis:
  - If diagnosis is equivocal, the patient should receive IV antibiotic therapy and consultation with a hand surgeon.
  - Cover for *Staphylococcus* and *Streptococcus* as well as anaerobic bacterial infection.
  - Consider coverage for *Pseudomonas* for the diabetic or immunocompromised patient.
  - Aminoglycosides may be added for double coverage.
  - Pain management

*Forearm*

Traumatic tenosynovitis:

- Rest, ice, elevation, immobilization
- NSAIDs

*Ankle*

- Stenosing tenosynovitis:
  - Rest, ice, elevation, immobilization
  - NSAIDs
- Rheumatoid tenosynovitis:
  - Rest, ice, elevation, immobilization
  - NSAIDs

**MEDICATION**

- Cefazolin: 1–2 g IV q8h (peds: 50–100 mg/kg/day IV div q8h)
- Cefotetan: 1–2 g IV q12h (peds: 50–100 mg/kg/day IV div q12h)
- Cefoxitin: 1–2 g IV q8h (peds: 80–160 mg/kg/day IV div q6–8h)
- Ceftriaxone: 1–2 g IV q12h (peds: 50–100 mg/kg/day IV div q12h)
- Clindamycin: 600–900 mg IV q8h (peds: 20–40 mg/kg/day div q8h)
- Penicillin G: 12–24 mIU IV div. q4–6h (peds: 100,000–400,000 IU/kg/day IV div q4–6h)
- Timentin: 3.1 g IV q6h (peds: 200–300 mg/kg/day IV div q4–6h)
- Tobramycin: 1 mg/kg IV q8h or 5 mg/kg IV q24h (peds: 2–2.5 mg/kg IV q8h)
- Zosyn: 3.375 g IV q6h (peds: 200–400 mg/kg/day IV div q6–8h)

 **FOLLOW-UP**

**DISPOSITION**

- Patients with FTS require immediate consultation with a hand specialist and admission.
- Patients presenting within 24–48 hr may have more conservative therapy to include immobilization, elevation IV antibiotics, and close observation.
- Surgical debridement is indicated if patient is not improved within the first 24 hr or physical findings are not resolved within 48 hr.
- Patients presenting >48 hr require surgical debridement in the operating room.
- The hand surgeon may attempt continuous catheter irrigation of the tendon sheath.

*Admission Criteria*

Patients with infectious or high-pressure etiologies for tenosynovitis should be admitted.

*Discharge Criteria*

Patients with inflammatory etiologies can be managed as outpatients with appropriate referral.

**ADDITIONAL READING**

- *Emergency Orthopedics, The Extremities,* 3rd ed. Norwalk, CT: Appleton & Lange, 1995.
- Hausman MR, Lisser SP. Hand infections. *Orthop Clinic N Am.* 1992;23(1):171–185.
- Richie CA, Briner WW. Corticosteroid injection for treatment of de Quervain's tenosynovitis: A pooled quantitative literature evaluation. *J Am Board Fam Pract.* 2003;16(2):102–106.
- White PH. Regional problems of the arm and leg in children. In: Maddison PJ, et al., eds. *Oxford Textbook of Rheumatology,* vol. 1. New York: Oxford University Press, 1993:80–84.
- Wilder RP, Sethi S. Overuse injuries: Tendinopathies, stress fractures, compartment syndrome, and shin splints. *Clin Sports Med.* 2004;23:55–81, 61.
- Zarin M, Ahmad I. Surgical treatment of de Quervain's disease. *J Coll Physicians Surg Pak.* 2003;13(3):157–158.
- Baskar S, Mann JS, Thomas AP, et al. Plant thorn tenosynovitis. *J Clin Rheumatol.* 2006;12:137.

 **CODES**

**ICD9**

727.00 Synovitis and tenosynovitis, unspecified

T

# TESTICULAR TORSION
*Edward Newton*

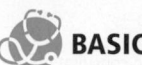

## BASICS

### DESCRIPTION
- Rotation of the testicle around the spermatic cord and vascular pedicle
- Rotation often occurs medially (two thirds of cases):
  - Ranges from incomplete (90°–180°) to complete (360°–1080°) torsion
  - Depending on the degree of torsion:
    - Vascular occlusion occurs
    - Infarction of the testicle after more than 6 hr of warm ischemia
- Testicular salvage:
  - 73–100% with less than 6 hr of ischemia
  - 50–70% at 6–12 hr
  - Less than 20% after 12 hr
  - It is still worthwhile to attempt to salvage the testicle up to 24 hr after the onset.
- Testicular infarction leads to atrophy and may ultimately decrease fertility.

### EPIDEMIOLOGY
Bimodal distribution of torsion:
- Peak incidences in infancy and adolescence
- 85% of cases of occur between ages 12 and 18 yr, with a mean of 13 yr.
- Torsion is rare after age 30 but still possible.

### ETIOLOGY
- Congenital abnormality of the genitalia:
  - High insertion of the tunica vaginalis on the spermatic cord
  - Redundant mesorchium
  - Permits increased mobility and twisting of the testicle on its vascular pedicle
- The anatomic abnormality is bilateral in 12%, so both testicles are susceptible to torsion.

## DIAGNOSIS

### SIGNS AND SYMPTOMS
#### History
- Sudden onset of unilateral testicular pain
- Scrotal swelling and erythema
- Less commonly, torsion may present with pain in the inguinal or lower abdominal area.
- Up to 40% of patients may describe previous similar episodes that remitted spontaneously:
  - Represents spontaneous torsion and detorsion
- Nausea and vomiting occur in 50% of cases.
- Low-grade fever occurs in 25%.
- There is often a history of minor trauma to the testicle preceding the onset of pain.
- Symptoms of urinary infection (dysuria, frequency, and urgency) are absent.

#### Physical Exam
- In distinguishing torsion from epididymitis, localized tenderness is helpful early; however, once significant scrotal swelling occurs, the anatomy becomes indistinct.
- The affected testicle may lie transversely as opposed to the normal vertical lie.
- Cremasteric reflex is frequently absent on the affected side with testicular torsion.
- Sensitivity 96%; specificity 66%
- Prehn sign:
  - Relief of pain on elevation of the testicle in epididymitis
  - Worsening or no change in the pain with torsion
  - Considered unreliable

### ESSENTIAL WORKUP
- The presentation of an "acute scrotum" in a child or adolescent requires rapid assessment and immediate consultation with a urologist.
- These patients require noninvasive flow studies or surgical exploration to confirm torsion.
- 25–30% of these patients ultimately prove to have testicular torsion.

## DIAGNOSTIC TESTS & INTERPRETATION
### Lab
- Elevated WBC count with a left shift is present in 50% of cases.
- Urinalysis is usually normal, but up to 20% of cases of torsion include pyuria.
- There are no laboratory tests specific for testicular torsion.

### Imaging

#### ALERT
- There are limitations of all flow studies:
  - Reflect only the current state of perfusion
  - Spontaneously detorsed testicle may show normal or even increased flow.
  - Still at high risk for recurrent torsion

- Traditional criterion standard has been technetium-99m radionuclide scans:
  - Decreased flow in the torsed testicle compared with the unaffected side
  - Frequent time delays in obtaining scans
- Doppler ultrasound:
  - Assess testicular blood flow and visualize the torsed spermatic cord directly.
  - Has replaced nuclear scanning:
    - Less invasive
    - More readily available test
    - Comparable results
  - Overall sensitivity and specificity of 98% and 100%, respectively for torsion but lower in distinguishing between testicular torsion and torsion of the appendix testis.
  - Epididymitis will reveal increased flow due to inflammation.
  - Torsion will reveal decreased or no blood flow.
  - Color-flow Doppler is the most commonly available.
  - Use of Doppler contrast material may enhance the accuracy.

### Pediatric Considerations
- All imaging techniques have technical limitations in infants:
  - Testicular vessels are very small.
  - Amount of blood flow to the testicle under normal conditions is minimal.
- Scrotal exploration may be required.

### Diagnostic Procedures/Surgery
- Scrotal exploration can be done rapidly under local anesthesia to diagnose and treat torsion.
- The "bell-clapper" deformity of both testicles should be corrected by orchiopexy.

## DIFFERENTIAL DIAGNOSIS
- Acute hydrocele
- Epididymitis/orchitis
- Henoch–Schönlein purpura
- Incarcerated inguinal hernia
- Testicular neoplasm
- Testicular trauma or rupture of the testicle
- Testicular tumor
- Torsion of the appendix testis (31–70% of acute scrotum cases)
- Other intra-abdominal conditions:
  - Appendicitis
  - Pancreatitis
  - Renal colic

 TREATMENT

### PRE-HOSPITAL
- There is no definitive treatment that can be rendered in the field.
- Prehospital personnel must recognize the urgency of acute testicular pain in young patients.
- These patients should be transported to the ED immediately.

### INITIAL STABILIZATION/THERAPY
- IV fluid, analgesics as appropriate

### ED TREATMENT/PROCEDURES
- Examination of testicle to exclude primary neoplasm
- Establish the diagnosis and mobilize appropriate urologic care.
- Applying an ice pack to the scrotum relieves pain:
  - May prolong the viability of the ischemic testicle
- If definitive care is likely to be delayed beyond 4–5 hr from the onset of torsion, manual detorsion may be attempted (26.5–80% successful).
  - Externally rotate the affected testicle opposite the usual medial direction of torsion.
  - Continue until pain is relieved, normal anatomy is restored, or Doppler US shows return of flow.
  - All patients who undergo manual detorsion must be surgically explored.

### MEDICATION
Analgesia

 FOLLOW-UP

### DISPOSITION
#### Admission Criteria
- Patients with confirmed torsion must be admitted for scrotal exploration and bilateral orchiopexy.
- Flow studies that are inconclusive and technical failures mandate further investigation by surgical exploration of the scrotum.
- Admission for urgent surgical exploration of an acute scrotum is mandatory if there is any potential delay in obtaining a flow study:
  - Patients in whom apparent spontaneous detorsion has occurred should undergo exploration for bilateral orchiopexy.

#### Discharge Criteria
- Patients with negative scrotal exploration and those with normal flow studies can be discharged with appropriate urologic follow-up.
- Parameters for return to ED must be discussed because of the possibility of recurrent torsion.
- Patients with an obvious diagnosis other than testicular torsion can be referred for care.

## PEARLS AND PITFALLS
- Testicular torsion can mimic acute appendicitis in children.
- Remember that "time is testicle"; emergent workup and consultation are required.
- Maintain a high index of suspicion for testicular torsion in all age groups even though peak incidence is in adolescents and neonates.
- If testicular torsion is diagnosed early, a near 100% salvage rate for the testicle is possible. Orchiopexy is not a guarantee against future torsion, although it does reduce the odds.

## ADDITIONAL READING
- Baldisseroto M. Scrotal emergencies. *Pediatr Radiol*. 2009;39:516–521.
- Gatti JM, Murphy JP. Acute testicular disorders. *Pediatr Rev*. 2008;29:235–241.
- Leslie JA, Cain MP. Pediatric urologic emergencies and urgencies. *Pediatr Clin North Am*. 2006;53:513–527.
- Lin EP, Bhatt S, Rubens DJ, et al. Testicular torsion: Twists and turns. *Semin Ultrasound CT MRI*. 2007;28:317–328.
- Scmitz D, Safranek S. How useful is the physical exam in diagnosing testicular torsion? *J Fam Pract*. 2009;58:433–434.

### See Also (Topic, Algorithm, Electronic Media Element)
- Epididymitis/Orchitis
- Hydrocele

 CODES

ICD9

608.20 Torsion of testis, unspecified

# TETANUS
*Daniel T. Wu*

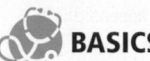 **BASICS**

## DESCRIPTION
- Rare disease in the U.S. but still prevalent in third-world countries
- About 40 cases per year in the U.S.
- 500,000–1,000,000 cases worldwide
- Incubation period:
  - Inoculation to the appearance of the first symptoms:
    ○ 48 hr to 3 wk or more
  - Period of onset:
    ○ <7 days—poor prognosis
    ○ Very poor prognosis if <48 hr from first symptom to first reflex spasm
- Neonatal tetanus:
  - Due to infected umbilical stump
  - Symptom onset in second week of life when maternal antibodies decrease
  - Rare in U.S. but common in third-world countries
  - Worldwide, accounts for over half of all tetanus infections
- Mortality rates as high as 20%

## ETIOLOGY
- *Clostridium tetani*:
  - Slender, motile, heat-sensitive, anaerobic gram-positive rod with a terminal spherical spore
  - Spore characteristics
  - Resistant to oxygen, moisture, temperature extremes
  - Can survive indefinitely until it germinates
  - Ubiquitous in soil and feces
- When inoculated into a wound or devitalized tissue or injected IV as a contaminant of street drugs, the spores germinate under anaerobic conditions and produce two toxins.
- Toxins:
  - Tetanolysin:
    ○ Damages tissue
    ○ Does not cause clinical manifestations of tetanus infection
  - Tetanospasmin:
    ○ Powerful neurotoxin
    ○ Disrupts the release of neurotransmitters such as gamma-aminobutyric acid (GABA)
    ○ Responsible for the clinical manifestations
- Muscle spasms
- Autonomic instability
- Uncontrolled motor activity

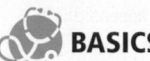 **DIAGNOSIS**

## SIGNS AND SYMPTOMS
### Generalized
- Most common type accounting for about 80% of all cases
- Initial presentation:
  - Muscle stiffness and pain
  - Trismus (initial)
  - Risus sardonicus (characteristic facial appearance)
- Systemic symptoms:
  - Irritability
  - Restlessness
  - Diaphoresis
- Later manifestations:
  - Muscle group rigidity
  - Sudden burst of tonic contractions of muscle groups causing:
    ○ Opisthotonos
    ○ Flexion and adduction of the arms
    ○ Clenching of fists
    ○ Extension of the lower extremities
  - Diaphragmatic spasm or paralysis:
    ○ May compromise respiration
- Hypersympathetic state (most common cause of death):
  - Begins in the second week
  - Dysrhythmias
  - BP changes
  - Diaphoresis
  - Hyperthermia

### Local
- Less common form of disease, accounting for about 17% of all cases
- Typical localized spasms around area of initial infection may:
  - Be mild
  - Persist for months before resolving
  - Evolve to generalized form (13%)

### Cephalic
- Rare variant of disease
- Follows head injury or otitis media
- Spasm of lower cranial and facial muscles:
  - Cranial nerve palsies, CN VII most common
- May progress to generalized tetanus

### Neonatal
- Generalized form of tetanus occurring during the first weeks of life
- Often caused by infection of umbilical stump
- Clinical manifestations:
  - Irritability
  - Poor suck
  - Facial grimacing
  - Muscle spasms with touch
- Very high mortality rate (50%–100%)
- Incubation period 1–2 wk

### History
- Investigate source of infection.
- Acute skin wound not necessary to contract infection
- >25% of infections occurred in the absence of known acute trauma.
- Infections can occur from abscesses, ulcers, and gangrene.
- Elicit tetanus immunization status.

## ESSENTIAL WORKUP
- Perform complete physical examination focusing on cardiovascular and respiratory status, neurologic and cranial nerve exam.
- Diagnosis of tetanus is clinical:
  - Suspect in all cases of trismus
  - No wound recalled in one fifth of cases
  - Full tetanus immunization almost eliminates diagnosis.

## DIAGNOSTIC TESTS & INTERPRETATION
Often of limited or no benefit for diagnosis but useful for ruling out other etiologies or assessing complications of disease

### Lab
- CBC
- Electrolytes, BUN, creatinine, glucose, calcium:
  - For hypocalcemia
- Strychnine level
- ABG, pulse oximetry:
  - For oxygenation status
- Wound culture for *C. tetani*:
  - Positive only about 30% of time
- *C. tetani* titers:
  - Will be useful only after the fact
- CSF analysis:
  - Normal with tetanus
  - Exclude meningitis/encephalitis

### Imaging
CT brain for altered mental status:
- Normal

## DIFFERENTIAL DIAGNOSIS
- Strychnine poisoning
- Jaw muscles usually spared or not involved early in strychnine poisonings
- Dystonic reaction to dopamine blockade
- Infection:
  - Meningitis
  - Rabies
  - Encephalitis
  - Peritonitis
  - Alveolar abscess
- Tetany/hyperventilation syndrome
- Hysteria
- Dislocated mandible/temporomandibular joint syndrome
- Bell palsy (cephalic form, before trismus)

 ## TREATMENT

### PRE-HOSPITAL
- Evaluate airway carefully:
  - Endotracheal intubation complicated by trismus, vocal cord paralysis, and facial/neck rigidity
- Avoid excessive stimulation because it may provoke tetany of musculature.

### INITIAL STABILIZATION/THERAPY
- ABCs:
  - Prophylactic intubation
  - Require neuromuscular blockade due to trismus
  - Establish IV 0.9% NS
  - Monitor BP and cardiac rhythm (autonomic instability).
- Administer benztropine or, diphenhydramine to exclude dystonic reaction.

### ED TREATMENT/PROCEDURES
- Focuses on three goals:
  - Stabilizing the patient and supportive care
  - Neutralizing the toxin
  - Removing any remaining organism
- Stabilization and supportive care:
  - Secure airway:
    - Prophylactic intubation may be necessary.
  - Paralytic agent may be needed in the setting of trismus:
    - Succinylcholine should be used with caution due to the risk of hyperkalemia from upregulation of acetylcholine receptors.
  - Treat muscle spasms with benzodiazepines; if large doses fail, can administer dantrolene.

- Autonomic instability therapy:
  - Occurs days to weeks after the onset of symptoms
  - Tachydysrhythmia and hypertension:
    - No treatment universally effective
    - Alpha and beta blockers can be tried but may cause worsening of symptoms (labetalol has been used for its alpha- and beta-blocking effects).
    - Clonidine, magnesium, morphine, fentanyl, and epidural anesthesia may be tried.
  - Hypotension:
    - Rule out septicemia and hypovolemia.
    - Initiate dopamine or dobutamine when low cardiac output.
    - Neutralization of the toxin
- Human tetanus immune globulin (TIG):
  - 3,000–6,000 U IM for both adults and children
  - Administer before debridement of wound.
  - Neutralizes unbound toxins
  - No effect on toxin already bound in CNS
- Removal of remaining organism:
  - Limits the severity of the infection
  - Debridement removes any necrotic tissue.
  - Antibiotics are effective in eliminating *C. tetani*:
    - Metronidazole is the antibiotic of choice.
    - Penicillin is a viable alternative.
- Prevention:
  - Primary vaccination series should be completed by age 18 mo; children receive the booster at ages 4, 11, and then every 10 yr after.
  - Diphtheria, pertussis, and tetanus vaccine for children <7 yr
  - Tetanus diphtheria (Td) can be used for children >7 yr and adults.
  - Clinical tetanus does not confer immunity.
  - For clean, minor wounds:
    - Td should be given if unknown prior vaccination history or greater than 10 yr since last booster.
  - For tetanus-prone wounds:
    - Td should be given if unknown vaccination history or >5 years since last booster.
    - TIG should be given if unknown vaccination or patient has never received the primary series.

### MEDICATION
- Benztropine: 1–2 mg IV
- Chlorpromazine: 10–50 mg IM
- Diazepam (benzodiazepine): 5–10 mg (peds: 0.2–0.4 mg/kg) IV
- Diphenhydramine: 50 mg IV
- Dobutamine: 2.5–15 μg/kg/min IV
- Dopamine: 2–20 μg/kg/min IV
- Doxycycline: 100 mg IV q12h
- Erythromycin: 500 mg IV q6h

- Labetalol: 20 mg (peds: 0.3–1 mg/kg per dose) IV q10min up to 300 mg PRN—start infusion 2 mg/min (peds: 0.4–1 mg/kg/hr max 3 mg/kg/hr as needed)
- Metronidazole: 1.0 g (peds: 15 mg/kg) load, followed by 500 mg (7.5 mg/kg) IV q6h
- Penicillin G potassium: 1.2 mIU (peds: 100,000 IU/kg/24 h) IV q6h for 10 days
- Propranolol 0.5–1 mg (peds: 0.01–0.1 mg/kg) IV
- TIG:
  - 250 IU IM
  - Administer in separate site from Td toxoid
  - For unimmunized or incompletely immunized in presence of tetanus prone wound
- Td 0.5 mL IM

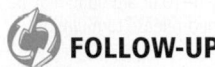 ## FOLLOW-UP

### DISPOSITION
**Admission Criteria**
All patients should be admitted to an ICU.

**Discharge Criteria**
None for suspected generalized tetanus

## PEARLS AND PITFALLS
Aggressive management is indicated for tetanus-prone wounds.

## ADDITIONAL READING

- American Academy of Pediatrics. *Red Book 1009 Report of the Committee on Infectious Disease.* Elk Grove, IL: AAP; 2009.
- CDC Tetanus Surveillance—United States 1998–2000, *MMWR.* 2003;52(ss-3):1–7.
- Centers for Disease Control and Prevention. *Tetanus. Epidemiology and prevention of Vaccine—Preventable Diseases,* 8th ed. Washington, DC: CDC ("The Pink Book").
- Hsu SS, Tetanus in the emergency department: A current review. *J Emerg Med.* 2001;20:357–365.
- McQuillan GM. Serologic immunity to diphtheria and tetanus in the United States. *Ann Intern Med.* 2002;136:660–666.
- Pickering L, ed. *Report of the Committee on Infectious Diseases,* 26th ed. Elk Grove, IL: American Academy of Pediatrics; 2003.
- Thawaites CL. Preventing and treating tetanus. *BMJ.* 2003;326:117–118.

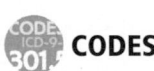 ## CODES

**ICD9**
037 Tetanus

T

# THEOPHYLLINE POISONING
*Harry C. Karydes*

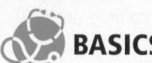 **BASICS**

## DESCRIPTION
- Theophylline causes:
  - Release of endogenous catecholamines resulting in stimulation of $\beta_1$ and $\beta_2$ receptors
  - Adenosine antagonism
  - Inhibition of phosphodiesterase (at supratherapeutic levels)
- Available in immediate and sustained-release formulations
- Peak absorption generally 6–10 hr although may be twice as long with sustained-release formulation
- *Acute overdose*:
  - Ingestion within 8-hr interval in patient with no prior theophylline use
- *Acute-on-chronic overdose*:
  - Single excessive dose in patient previously receiving usual therapeutic doses for $\geq$24 hr
- *Chronic intoxication*:
  - Accumulation of theophylline >20 mg/L associated with prior therapeutic use for $\geq$24 hr secondary to:
    - Drug–drug, drug–diet, or drug–disease interactions
  - Use of serial excessive doses

## ETIOLOGY
- Acute ingestions require larger concentrations to achieve specific toxic effects compared with acute-on-chronic or chronic overdoses.
- Drug–drug interactions:
  - Inhibiting theophylline metabolism:
    - $H_2$-receptor antagonists
    - Macrolide antibiotics
    - Fluoroquinolones
    - Allopurinol
    - Influenza vaccine
    - Interferons
  - Enhances theophylline metabolism (leads to toxicity when discontinued):
    - Carbamazepine
    - Barbiturates
    - Smoking
    - Rifampin
- Chronic theophylline accumulation:
  - Uncontrolled CHF
  - Liver disease (cirrhosis or severe hepatitis)
  - Acute viral infections

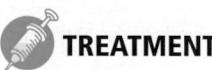 **DIAGNOSIS**

## SIGNS AND SYMPTOMS
- Cardiovascular:
  - Sinus or supraventricular tachycardias:
    - Multifocal atrial tachycardia
    - Atrial fibrillation
    - Caused by beta$_1$-receptor stimulation and adenosine antagonism
  - Hypotension:
    - Associated with theophylline >100 $\mu$g/mL (acute ingestion)
    - Due to vasodilatation induced by beta$_2$-receptor stimulation
    - May be refractory to fluids, positioning, and conventional vasopressors
- Central nervous system:
  - Tremor
  - Mental status changes
  - Seizures:
    - 14% of chronic intoxications
    - 5% of acute intoxications
- Gastrointestinal:
  - Nausea, vomiting:
    - Protracted and may be refractory to antiemetics at usual doses
  - Abdominal pain
  - Pharmacobezoar:
    - From sustained-release dosage forms in acute ingestions
    - Delays peak concentrations
- Metabolic:
  - Hypokalemia:
    - As low as 1.5 mEq/L
    - Due to beta-receptor stimulation
  - Hyperglycemia
  - Leukocytosis
  - Hypercalcemia, hypophosphatemia, hypomagnesemia
  - Metabolic acidosis

## ESSENTIAL WORKUP
- Serum theophylline concentration:
  - Finding of $\geq$20 $\mu$g/mL confirms diagnosis.
- ECG and cardiac monitoring
- Detailed history to differentiate acute from acute-on-chronic from chronic intoxication

## DIAGNOSTIC TESTS & INTERPRETATION
### Lab
- Serum theophylline level:
  - Repeat every 2 hr until decreasing to confirm immediate absorption is complete and peak value has occurred.
  - Serious morbidity in acute overdose if $\geq$100 $\mu$g/mL
- CBC
- Electrolytes:
  - Transient hypokalemia
- Serum acetaminophen level (for intentional ingestions)

### Imaging
- KUB (kidneys, ureters, bladder):
  - Undissolved sustained-release tablets or pharmacobezoars may appear as radiopacities.
  - Bead-filled capsules may appear as radiolucencies.
- US of stomach may detect intact sustained-release dosage forms.

## DIFFERENTIAL DIAGNOSIS
- Caffeine/beta-agonist bronchodilator overdose
- Amphetamines
- Sympathomimetics
- Anticholinergic agents
- Drug withdrawal syndromes
- Pheochromocytoma
- Thyrotoxicosis

**TREATMENT**

## PRE-HOSPITAL
Bring pill bottles/pill samples in suspected overdose.

## INITIAL STABILIZATION/THERAPY
- ABCs:
  - Cardiac monitor
  - Isotonic crystalloids as needed for hypotension
- Naloxone, thiamine, and dextrose (D$_{50}$W) as indicated for altered mental status
- Cardiovascular:
  - Initiate beta blockers or calcium channel blockers for rate control with supraventricular tachyarrhythmia
  - Adenosine is antagonized by theophylline and may not be effective

– Administer isotonic crystalloid intravenous fluid resuscitation for hypotension:
  ○ With treatment failure, consider beta blocker to reverse theophylline-induced beta$_2$-receptor–stimulated vasodilation.
  ○ If vasopressors are needed, choose vasopressor that is not a beta agonist, such as phenylephrine.
– Treat ventricular dysrhythmias conventionally.
• Seizures:
  – Administer benzodiazepines.
  – Phenytoin is contraindicated; it is usually ineffective and may paradoxically worsen seizures in theophylline intoxications.

### ED TREATMENT/PROCEDURES
#### Decontamination
• Administer activated charcoal
• Multidose activated charcoal:
  – Especially with sustained-release products
  – Binds theophylline, which back-diffuses to small intestine
  – For mild to moderate toxicity
  – 25 g q2h until theophylline level ≤20 $\mu$g/mL
• Initiate whole-bowel irrigation with sustained-release products:
  – Administer until a clear, colorless rectal effluent or serum theophylline <20 $\mu$g/mL
  – 1–2 L/h of polyethylene glycol until clear rectal effluent
• Treat protracted vomiting with metoclopramide or 5-HT$^3$-receptor antagonists.
• Avoid syrup of ipecac.

#### Electrolyte Disturbances
• Treat hypokalemia in acute ingestions cautiously:
  – Relative hypokalemia owing to beta-receptor–mediated intracellular shift of extracellular potassium
  – Aggressive correction leads to potentially serious hyperkalemia as theophylline concentrations decrease.
• Most electrolyte imbalances respond to beta-blocker therapy:
  – Generally not indicated because of absence of associated morbidity and potential for beta blocker–induced bronchospasm in pulmonary patients

#### Extracorporeal Elimination
Initiate hemodialysis or hemoperfusion if theophylline level:
• ≥90 $\mu$g/mL and symptomatic in acute ingestions
• ≥40 $\mu$g/mL and:
  – Seizures or
  – HTN unresponsive to intravenous fluid or
  – Ventricular dysrhythmias

### MEDICATION
• Activated charcoal: 1 g/kg PO, if dose ingested is known, 10 g/1 g theophylline ingested, no one dose >100 g
• Diazepam: 0.1 mg/kg IV q5–10min until seizures controlled, up to 30 mg
• Diltiazem: 0.25 mg/kg IV bolus; may repeat after 15 min, then 5–15 mg/h infusion for control of heart rate in patients with contraindication to beta blockade
• Esmolol: 500 $\mu$g/kg IV bolus, followed by 50 $\mu$g/kg/min infusion; increase by 50 $\mu$g/kg/min increments to max of 200 $\mu$g/kg/min
• Metoclopramide: 10 mg IV bolus; may repeat to max of 1 mg/kg
• Ondansetron: 0.15 mg/kg IV bolus up to max of 32 mg total
• Polyethylene glycol (high molecular weight): 1–2 L/h via nasogastric tube

 **FOLLOW-UP**

### DISPOSITION
#### Admission Criteria
• Acute overdoses with serum theophylline concentrations >100 ≥ g/mL
• Acute-on-chronic or chronic theophylline with either serum concentration >60 $\mu$g/mL or patient >60 yr old
• Seizures or fluid and vasopressor refractory hypotension in patient with serum theophylline concentration >40 $\mu$g/mL

#### Discharge Criteria
• Two consecutive (≥2 hr apart) decreasing serum theophylline concentrations with most recent concentration <30 $\mu$g/mL
• Mildly symptomatic or asymptomatic patient meeting above criterion and no evidence of suicidal intention

### FOLLOW-UP RECOMMENDATIONS
• Follow up with medical toxicologist or primary care doctor
• If patient is on chronic theophylline, dosing regimen may have to be adjusted.

## PEARLS AND PITFALLS

• Seizures are a major complication.
• Tachydysrhythmias are common in overdose.
• Multiple-dose activated charcoal is beneficial in theophylline overdose.

*A special thanks to Dr. Gerald Maloney who contributed to previous edition.*

## ADDITIONAL READING

• Hoffman RJ. Methylxanthines and selective $\beta_2$-adrenergic agonists. In: Flomenbaum NE, Goldfrank LR, Hoffman RS, et al., eds. *Goldfranks's Toxicologic Emergencies*, 8th ed. New York: McGraw-Hill; 2006.
• Henderson A, Wright DM, Pond SM. Management of theophylline overdose patients in the intensive care unit. *Anaesth Intens Care*. 1992;20:56–62.
• Shannon MW. Comparative efficacy of hemodialysis and hemoperfusion in severe theophylline intoxication. *Acad Emerg Med*. 1997;4:674–678.
• Shannon MW. Life-threatening events after theophylline overdose. *Arch Intern Med*. 1999;159:989–994.

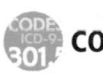 **CODES**

ICD9
974.1 Poisoning by purine derivative diuretics

# THORACIC OUTLET SYNDROME

*Erin R. Horn*
*Daniel C. McGillicuddy*

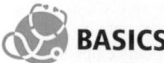 **BASICS**

## DESCRIPTION

- The symptoms of thoracic outlet syndrome (TOS) are produced by compression of the brachial plexus, subclavian vein, or subclavian artery during their passage from the cervical area toward the axilla and proximal arm.
- Subdivided into 3 categories depending on the predominant symptoms:
  - Neurogenic thoracic outlet syndrome (NTOS):
    - Comprises 90–95% of adult patients
    - Female > Male
    - True (1–3%): Those with objective findings
    - Disputed (90%): Those with no or limited objective findings
  - Venous thoracic outlet syndrome (VTOS):
    - 4% of patients
  - Arterial thoracic outlet syndrome (ATOS):
    - Least common, <1%
    - Male = Female
- Vascular manifestations are more common in adolescents, seen in >50% of teens with TOS.
- Right extremity is more commonly affected.

## ETIOLOGY

- Anatomic anomalies:
  - Bony anomalies include cervical rib, 1st thoracic rib, or clavicular abnormalities:
    - Cervical ribs occur in <1% of the population, ~70% in women, and most are asymptomatic.
    - Fracture of the clavicle and trauma to the sternoclavicular and costoclavicular joints
  - Congenital bands or anomalous muscles
  - May play a role in neurologic and venous types but is almost always implicated in arterial type
- Neurogenic:
  - Often have a history of neck trauma, such as whiplash (hyperextension injuries)
- Venous:
  - May be preceded by excessive activity, especially in adolescent athletes
  - Caused by acute thrombosis of the subclavian vein (also called Paget-Schrötter disease) or by venous impingement

- Arterial:
  - Often develop spontaneously
  - Unrelated to trauma or work
  - Almost always have a complete cervical rib or an anomalous 1st rib
  - Caused by subclavian artery aneurysm or subclavian/axillary artery impingement:
    - Arterial emboli that arise from either mural thrombus in the subclavian artery aneurysm or from thrombus forming distal to subclavian artery stenosis
- Descent of the shoulder girdle and sagging musculature can also predispose to TOS:
  - Aging
  - Obesity
  - Heavy breasts

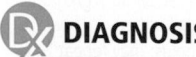 **DIAGNOSIS**

## SIGNS AND SYMPTOMS

- Neurogenic:
  - Classically, pain, paresthesia, and weakness of the hand, arm, and shoulder
  - May see wasting of the thenar eminence, also known as Gilliatt-Sumner hand
  - May also see Raynaud phenomenon, hand coldness, color change:
    - Not caused by ischemia, rather due to overactive sympathetic fibers that run on the circumference of the lower trunks of the brachial plexus
    - Similar symptoms can be seen in arterial TOS, so the 2 must be differentiated by evaluating for other signs and symptoms.
- Venous:
  - Swelling of the arm and cyanosis:
    - NTOS and ATOS do not exhibit arm swelling.
  - May see pain, aching of the arm
  - Hand paresthesia:
    - May be due to swelling as opposed to nerve compression
- Arterial:
  - Digital ischemia, claudication, pallor, coldness, paresthesia, and pain of the hand
  - Usually spares the shoulder and neck
  - Pallor and coldness are due to ischemia and not Raynaud
  - Aneurysmal:
    - Painless pulsating mass

## History

- May be positional or exacerbated by repetitive use (ie, working overhead)
- Usually insidious in onset and progressive
- Can occur or worsen suddenly after trauma

## Physical Exam

Provocative maneuvers can reveal NTOS (VTOS and ATOS often diagnosed with history and symptoms only):

- Elevated arm stress test (EAST):
  - Arms abducted 90 degrees from the thorax and elbows flexed at 90 degrees
  - Shoulders braced slightly back of the frontal plane
  - Fists are open and closed for 3 min.
  - Early heaviness and fatigue of the arm
  - Gradual onset of hand numbness
  - Progressive aching through the arm and top of shoulder
- Adson test:
  - Arm down, patient rotates head toward extremity, looks up, and inhales.
  - Positive result is the alteration or obliteration of the radial pulse or change in the BP.
  - Not a reliable test, as many patients with NTOS have a negative test and many control patients have a positive test.
- Neither test is very sensitive nor specific.

## ESSENTIAL WORKUP

- Careful history and physical exam
- EKG to rule out cardiac ischemia

## DIAGNOSTIC TESTS & INTERPRETATION

### Lab
Consider a coagulation workup for either venous or arterial TOS.

### Imaging
- Perform as outpatient except in case of limb-threatening ischemia and/or suspicion of venous thrombus
- CXR:
  - Assess for anatomic abnormalities: 1st rib, cervical rib, clavicle deformity:
    - Without an abnormality, ATOS is very unlikely.
  - Pulmonary disease
- Cervical spine series:
  - Fracture
  - Scoliosis

- US can diagnose venous thrombosis
- Duplex scanning is the best way to screen for subclavian artery aneurysm or stenosis, which, if present, can lead to arteriography
- Arteriogram:
  - Usually used to help a surgeon plan reconstruction
  - Indications include:
    - Decreased radial pulse
    - BP is 20 mm Hg less than the opposite limb.
    - Suspected subclavian stenosis
    - Bruit or abnormal supraclavicular pulsations or pulsating mass
    - Peripheral emboli in the upper extremity
- Venography:
  - Indicated if edema, peripheral unilateral cyanosis, or distended thoracic and extremity veins
- Neurogenic TOS:
  - No gold standard test: Diagnosis remains mostly clinical.
  - Electromyography and nerve conduction velocity tests are often normal.
- MRI may be required to assess for spinal cord disease or a herniated cervical disk.

## DIFFERENTIAL DIAGNOSIS

- Cardiac ischemia
- Cervical spondylosis or disk disease
- Carpal tunnel syndrome or nerve entrapments
- Pancoast tumor; other neck/mediastinum malignancies
- Neuritis
- Myositis
- Raynaud disease
- Multiple sclerosis or degenerative spinal cord disease
- Shoulder inflammatory diseases: Arthritis, rotator cuff injury, bicipital tendonitis
- Atherosclerotic or thromboembolic disease

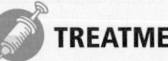

## TREATMENT

### ED TREATMENT/PROCEDURES

- Heparinization if signs of arterial or venous thrombosis
- Vascular surgery consult for signs of ischemia and for catheter directed thrombolysis if needed:
  - Anticoagulation and thrombolysis followed by surgical decompression is required for thrombosis
- Initial management:
  - The majority improve with conservative treatment consisting of physical therapy and medications for symptomatic relief.
- Surgery reserved for failure of medical therapy:
  - Often required for vascular forms
  - People with NTOS often undergo more extensive evaluation and medical management prior to surgical intervention
  - 70–90% of patients experience some to complete relief postoperatively.

### MEDICATION

- Cyclobenzaprine (Flexeril): 10 mg PO t.i.d.
- Diazepam: 5 mg PO t.i.d.
- Ibuprofen: 800 mg PO t.i.d.
- Methocarbamol (Robaxin): 1,000–1,500 mg PO t.i.d.
- Soothing liniments or ointments

## FOLLOW-UP

### DISPOSITION

#### Admission Criteria

- Ischemia
- Venous thrombosis
- Arterial thrombosis
- Arterial aneurysm or stenosis
- Intractable pain

#### Discharge Criteria

- Non–limb-threatening neurologic findings
- Absence of arterial or venous thrombosis

### FOLLOW-UP RECOMMENDATIONS

Vascular, neurological, or orthopedic consultation is indicated according to the pathologic condition.

## PEARLS AND PITFALLS

- 3 types of TOS: Neurogenic, arterial and venous:
  - Neurogenic is the most common in adults.
  - Arterial and venous TOS are the more common types in children and adolescents.
- Venous TOS is the only type that has arm swelling and edema.
- Both neurogenic and arterial TOS have hand coldness and pallor, but for different reasons.
- May have a history of repetitive use or trauma
- Exam or imaging may reveal a congenital abnormality such as a cervical rib.

## ADDITIONAL READING

- Arthur LG, Teich S, et al. Pediatric thoracic outlet syndrome: A disorder with serious vascular complications. *J Pediatr Surg.* 2008;43:1089–1094.
- Atasoy E. Thoracic outlet compression syndrome. *Orthop Clin North Am.* 1996;27:265–303.
- Huang JH, Zager EL, et al. Thoracic outlet syndrome. *Neurosurg.* 2004;55(4):897–902.
- Mackinnon SE, Novak CB. Thoracic outlet syndrome. *Curr Probl Surg.* 2002;39(11):1070–1145.
- Maru S, Dosluoglu H, et al. Thoracic outlet syndrome in children and young adults. *Eur J Vasc Endovasc Surg.* 2009;38:560–564.

### See Also (Topic, Algorithm, Electronic Media Element)

www.ninds.nih.gov

## CODES

**ICD9**
353.0 Brachial plexus lesions

### Acknowledgements

Thank you to prior author Anna cheh.

T

# THROMBOTIC THROMBOCYTOPENIC PURPURA

*Hany Y. Atallah*

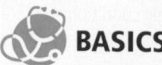 **BASICS**

## DESCRIPTION

- Thrombotic thrombocytopenic purpura (TTP) is a severe disorder of abnormal clotting affecting multiple organ systems.
- Classically characterized by pentad of:
  - Thrombocytopenia
  - Hemolytic anemia
  - Mild renal dysfunction
  - Neurologic signs
  - Fever
- Uncommon to see all 5 features in one patient; if present, severe end-organ damage or ischemia has likely taken place.
- Thrombocytopenia and hemolytic anemia are the most common features.
- Associated with acquired or congenital deficiency of plasma von Willebrand factor–cleaving protease (VWFcp)

### Classic Course

- Acute onset
- Fulminant course lasting days to a few months
- Nearly always fatal without treatment:
  - Greater than 90% mortality without treatment
  - Reverses to >90% survival with modern treatment
- Clinical presentations include:
  - Idiopathic
  - Familial, chronic or relapsing
  - Drug-induced:
    - Allergic or immune mediated (quinine, ticlopidine, clopidogrel)
    - Dose-related toxicity (mitomycin C, cyclosporine)
  - Pregnancy, postpartum associated:
    - 10–25% of cases
  - Bone marrow transplantation associated
  - Infection
- More common in the 3rd–6th decades of life
- Uncommon in pediatric or geriatric populations
- Women affected about twice as frequently as men

## ETIOLOGY

- Unknown primary stimulant; possibly systemic endothelial cell damage results inactivation of coagulation pathway
- Platelet aggregation and fibrin deposition occurring in arterioles and capillaries leading to microthrombi and obstruction to blood flow
- Platelet aggregation leads to:
  - Consumption of platelets
  - Widespread microvascular hyaline thrombotic lesions
- Microvasculature obstruction with platelet aggregates leads to:
  - Red cell hemolysis
  - Accumulation of heme breakdown products
  - Anemia
- End-organ ischemia results from diffuse thrombosis in small vessels:
  - Most common in heart, brain, kidney, pancreas, and adrenal glands
  - Lungs and liver relatively spared
- Deficiency of vWF cp causes failure of control of coagulation pathway.

## RISK FACTORS

### Genetics

- Some cases are genetic/familial.
- VWFcp was recently identified as new member of ADAMTS family and designated ADAMTS13.
- Mutations in ADAMTS13 gene cause autosomal recessive form of chronic relapsing TTP.

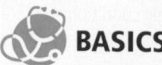 **DIAGNOSIS**

## SIGNS AND SYMPTOMS

Five Major Clinical Features: Classic Pentad

- Thrombocytopenia:
  - Platelet count <20,000/mm$^3$
- Microangiopathic and hemolytic anemia:
  - Hb <10 g/dL (<6 g/dL in 40%)
- Neurologic symptoms:
  - Presenting complaint in 60%, occur in 90%
  - Typically fluctuating
  - Headache
  - Altered mentation (confusion, stupor, coma)
  - Behavioral or personality changes
  - Focal sensory or motor deficits or aphasia
  - Seizures
  - Spontaneous intracranial hemorrhage
- Renal insufficiency:
  - Usually mild
  - Creatinine <3.0 mg/dL
- Fever:
  - Occurs in acute episodes and prodromal syndromes
  - Fever is the least common feature

### History

- General:
  - Weakness
  - Fatigue
  - Fever
  - Malaise
- Hemorrhage:
  - Easy bruising
  - Epistaxis
  - Menorrhagia
  - GI bleeding
  - Loss or change in vision
- GI complaints:
  - Nausea
  - Anorexia
  - Diarrhea
  - Abdominal pain
- Neurologic:
  - Headache
  - Confusion
  - Seizure
  - Behavioral or personality changes
  - Focal sensory or motor deficits or aphasia
- Changes in vision or blindness

### Physical Exam

- Purpura
- GI hemorrhage
- Epistaxis
- Jaundice
- Shock
- Altered mental status
- Focal sensory or motor deficits
- Pulmonary infiltrates and edema
- Alteration of vision, retinal hemorrhage/detachment.
- Abnormalities of cardiac conduction

## ESSENTIAL WORKUP

### Clinical Diagnosis

- Because of success of treatment, base diagnosis on:
  - Identification of two major findings:
    - Thrombocytopenia
    - Microangiopathic hemolytic anemia
  - Exclude other major differential diagnoses.
- Comprehensive history and physical exam with directed laboratory testing
- Identify possible drug-associated disease and avoid re-exposure.

## DIAGNOSTIC TESTS & INTERPRETATION

### Lab

- CBC/platelet count/reticulocyte count:
  - Anemia: Hemoglobin <10 g/dL
  - Thrombocytopenia <20,000/mm$^3$
  - Increased reticulocyte count
- Coagulation studies:
  - Normal
- Peripheral blood smear:
  - Macroangiopathic changes
  - Schistocytes
  - Helmet cells
  - Nucleated RBCs
- Coombs test:
  - Negative direct Coombs test
- Electrolytes, BUN, creatinine, glucose:
  - Mild elevation of BUN, creatinine
  - Hyperkalemia owing to RBC lysis
- Lactate dehydrogenase (LDH):
  - Elevated 5 to 10 times due to hemolysis and tissue ischemia
- Bilirubin:
  - Increased unconjugated bilirubin
- Urinalysis:
  - Hematuria (microscopic to gross)
- ADAMTS13 assay may be used to distinguish chronic recurring TTP, TTP secondary to presence of ADAMTS13 inhibitor, and hemolytic-uremic syndrome (HUS):
  - ADAMTS13 deficiency does not detect all patients who may respond to plasma exchange transfusions.

### Imaging

CT head:

- To rule out intracranial hemorrhage

### Diagnostic Procedures/Surgery

- Biopsy:
  - Confirms diagnosis
  - Reveals hyaline lesions in small vessels
  - Contraindicated during fulminant presentation (hemorrhage risk)
- EEG:
  - To predict need for anticonvulsant therapy

## DIFFERENTIAL DIAGNOSIS

- Hemolytic uremic syndrome (HUS):
  - Triad of thrombocytopenia, schistocytosis, and renal dysfunction
  - Neurologic symptoms unusual
  - Often preceded by infectious prodrome and diarrhea
- Disseminated intravascular coagulation (DIC):
  - Causes deposition of fibrin in microvasculature and not hyaline
  - Coagulation studies abnormal
- Idiopathic thrombocytopenic purpura (ITP):
  - No evidence of hemolysis
  - LDH and bilirubin normal
- Pregnancy-related thrombocytopenia:
  - Pre-eclampsia, eclampsia
  - Pregnancy-associated hemolysis
  - HELLP (hemolysis, elevated liver enzymes, and low platelets)
- Evans syndrome:
  - Autoimmune hemolytic anemia
  - Prominence of microspherocytes rather than schistocytes
  - Positive direct Coombs test
- Malignant hypertension
- Bacterial sepsis
- Subacute bacterial endocarditis
- Autoimmune disorders (e.g., systemic lupus erythematosus [SLE])
- Disseminated malignancy
- Heparin-associated thrombocytopenia
- Prosthetic valves or severely calcified aortic stenosis

## TREATMENT

### PRE-HOSPITAL

- ABCs
- Evaluate for other possible causes of altered mental status (hypoglycemia, overdose)

### INITIAL STABILIZATION/THERAPY

- ABCs
- 0.9% normal saline (NS) IV fluid resuscitation for shock or GI hemorrhage
- RBC transfusions:
  - For significant anemia or bleeding complications
- Platelet transfusions:
  - Reserve for life-threatening hemorrhage (eg, CNS bleeds) or required invasive procedures
  - May aggravate the thrombotic, microvascular obstructive process and worsen the end-organ ischemia and shock

## ED TREATMENT/PROCEDURES

- *Fresh frozen plasma* (FFP) or fresh unfrozen plasma:
  - Initiated as bridge to exchange transfusions on diagnosis of TTP
  - Success rate approaching 64%
  - Provides a platelet-antiaggregating factor absent or diminished in patient's own serum
  - Used prophylactically to prevent recurrence in chronic relapsing variant
- Plasma exchange transfusions:
  - Most important component of treatment
  - Combination of plasmapheresis and FFP infusion
  - Plasmapheresis removes:
    ○ Immune complexes responsible for endothelial damage and initiation of TTP
    ○ Circulating proaggregation factors promoting platelet aggregation
  - Perform daily until:
    ○ Platelet count normalizes
    ○ Neurologic symptoms improve
    ○ LDH normalizes
  - Improvement of renal function may lag behind other findings.
  - Taper frequency based on empiric judgment of response; may need to resume if relapse occurs.
  - Complications include:
    ○ Allergy or serum sickness
    ○ Secondary infection
    ○ Hypotension
- Corticosteroids:
  - Unproven therapeutic benefit
  - May limit immunologically mediated endothelial damage and decrease splenic sequestration of platelets and damaged RBCs
  - Supportive benefit if adrenal glands damaged through hemorrhage or ischemia
- Antiplatelet or immunosuppressive drugs:
  - Aspirin and dipyridamole most commonly used
  - Use of Sulfapyrazine, dextran, and vincristine has been reported.
  - Used with variable effectiveness
  - Can worsen bleeding complications
  - Heparin is ineffective.
- Splenectomy:
  - Historically recommended
  - Of uncertain efficacy
- Dialysis:
  - For renal failure

## MEDICATION

- Aspirin: 325–650 mg PO q4–6h
- Dipyridamole: 75–100 mg PO q.i.d.
- FFP:
  - Plasma infusion: 30 mL/kg/d (75–100 mL/h)
  - Plasma exchange transfusion: 3–4 L/day
- Methylprednisolone: 0.75 mg/kg q12h
- Prednisone: 1–2 mg/kg/day (high dose up to 200 mg/day)
- Rituximab: 375 mg/m$^2$ IV once per wk for 4–8 doses
- Vincristine: 2 mg IV q4–7d for 4 doses

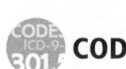 FOLLOW-UP

### DISPOSITION

**Admission Criteria**

- Newly diagnosed serious platelet disorder, especially with bleeding complications or altered mental status or renal dysfunction
- ICU admission for TTP with active bleeding or neurologic findings:
  - Transport to tertiary care center with appropriate specialty care facilities.

### FOLLOW-UP RECOMMENDATIONS

Patients with known disease and found to be stable may follow up with a hematologist.

## PEARLS AND PITFALLS

- TTP can be confused with HELLP syndrome in pregnant females.
- Because of the high mortality of untreated TTP, recognition of the disease and initiation of treatment is key.

## ADDITIONAL READING

- George JN. Clinical practice. Thrombotic thrombocytopenic purpura. *N Engl J Med.* 2006;354:1927.
- George JN, Woodson RD, Kiss JE, et al. Rituximab therapy for thrombotic thrombocytopenic purpura: A proposed study of the Transfusion Medicine/ Hemostasis Clinical Trials Network with a systematic review of rituximab therapy for immune-mediated disorders. *J Clin Apher.* 2006;21:49.
- Kremer Hovinga JA, Meyer SC. Current management of thrombotic thrombocytopenic purpura. *Curr Opin Hematol.* 2008;15(5):445–450.
- Stella CL, Dacus I, Guzman E, et al. The diagnostic dilemma of thrombotic thrombocytopenic purpura/hemolytic uremic syndrome in the obstetric triage and emergency department: Lessons from 4 tertiary hospitals. *Am J Obstet Gynecol.* 2009; 200(4):381.e1–e6.

### See Also (Topic, Algorithm, Electronic Media Element)

- Disseminated Intravascular Coagulation
- HELLP Syndrome
- Idiopathic Thrombocytopenia
- Renal Failure

## CODES

**ICD9**
446.6 Thrombotic microangiopathy

# THUMB FRACTURE

Leslie C. Oyama
John MacKay, Jr.

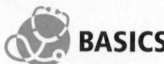 **BASICS**

## DESCRIPTION
- Distal phalangeal fractures:
  - Blunt trauma, hyperextension of the thumb, axial loading of the thumb
  - *Tuft fracture* is a similar fracture in other digits, in which the distal phalanx is crushed and fragmented.
  - It may be open or closed and associated with nail bed injury.
  - It is treated as a soft-tissue injury.
- Proximal phalangeal fractures and thumb metacarpal fractures:
  - Blunt trauma to the thumb:
    - ○ Axial loading of the thumb with the metacarpophalangeal (MP) joint flexed, hand closed or the thumb MP joint otherwise stabilized
  - Bennett fracture:
    - ○ Oblique intra-articular fracture of the ulnar aspect of the base of the thumb metacarpal with the larger distal fragment displaced
  - Rolando fracture:
    - ○ Comminuted Y-shaped intra-articular fracture of the ulnar base of the thumb metacarpal with the large distal fragment displaced

## ETIOLOGY
- Falls
- Motor vehicle accidents
- Sports, especially downhill or alpine skiing
- Basketball
- Baseball
- Football
- Rugby

 **DIAGNOSIS**

## SIGNS AND SYMPTOMS
- Pain, swelling, and deformity of the thumb
- Exam should include the thenar eminence for pain or deformity.
- The thumb may be rotated distal to the fracture site.
- The base of the thumb may appear radially deviated relative to the rest of the hand in the resting position.
- Occasionally, there may be damage to the thumb digital nerves.

### Pediatric Considerations
- Fractures to the thumb sometimes occur in children.
- Consider nonaccidental trauma.
- Do not neglect appropriate pain management in children.

### Physical Exam
Immobilize thumb pending definitive evaluation.

## ESSENTIAL WORKUP
Radiography as noted below

## DIAGNOSTIC TESTS & INTERPRETATION
### Imaging
- Plain radiography of affected areas
- Avoid testing stress of thumb MP joint, as in testing for gamekeeper thumb, until all plain radiography is complete.

## DIFFERENTIAL DIAGNOSIS
- Extra-articular fracture of the base of the thumb metacarpal
- Scaphoid fracture
- Gamekeeper thumb

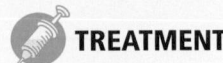 **TREATMENT**

**PRE-HOSPITAL**
- Dress open wounds.
- Immobilize in neutral position.
- Elevate and apply cold to reduce swelling.
- Age-appropriate social management

**INITIAL STABILIZATION/THERAPY**
Immobilize thumb pending definitive evaluation.

**ED TREATMENT/PROCEDURES**
- Thumb spica splint with the thumb in neutral position, as if holding a beverage can
- Splint instructions should be provided to patient.

**MEDICATION**
Pain control with oral analgesic preparations

 **FOLLOW-UP**

**DISPOSITION**
*Admission Criteria*
Open fracture, presence of multiple trauma, or other more serious injuries

*Discharge Criteria*
- Counsel patient that there is a strong likelihood of the need for operative repair.
- Closed injuries, referral, and explain frequent need for operative fixation

*Issues for Referral*
72-hr orthopedic referral

## PEARLS AND PITFALLS

Due to tendon insertions, fractures at the base of thumb are often unstable.

## ADDITIONAL READING

- American Society for Surgery of the Hand. *The Hand: Primary Care of Common Problems,* 2nd ed. New York: Churchill Livingstone; 1990.
- Antosia RE, Lyn E. Hand. In: Marx J, et al. *Rosen's Emergency Medicine: Concepts and Clinical Practice,* 5th ed. St. Louis, MO: Mosby-Year Book; 2002;493–506.

- Chaffin TH. Phalangeal fractures. In: Hart RG, Uehara DT, Wagner MJ, et al., eds. *Emergency and primary care of the hand*. Dallas: ACEP; 2001; 111–122.
- Carlsen BT, Moran SL. Thumb trauma: Bennett fractures, Rolando fractures, and ulnar collateral ligament injuries. *J Hand Surg Am*. 2009;34(5): 945–952.
- Sullivan JH, Tsonis GD. Metacarpal fractures. In: Hart RG, Uehara DT, Wagner MJ, et al., eds. *Emergency and Primary Care of the Hand*. Dallas: ACEP; 2001; 99–110.

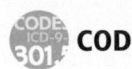 **CODES**

**ICD9**
- 816.00 Closed fracture of phalanx or phalanges of hand, unspecified
- 816.01 Closed fracture of middle or proximal phalanx or phalanges of hand
- 816.02 Closed fracture of distal phalanx or phalanges of hand

T

# TIBIAL PLATEAU FRACTURE

Binh T. Ly
Leslie C. Oyama

## 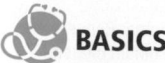 BASICS

### DESCRIPTION
- Synonym: Tibial condylar fracture
- Fracture or depression of the proximal tibial articulating surface
- Valgus or varus force applied in combination with axial loading:
  - *Lateral* plateau fractures:
    - Occurs classically after pedestrian struck by a vehicle bumper
    - Lateral aspect of the knee with a medially directed force
  - *Medial* plateau fractures are much less common and require significant force.
- Younger patients are more resistant to depressed plateau fractures.
- Elderly patients are more prone to depression-type fractures.

### Schatzker Classification of Plateau Fractures
- Type 1:
  - Split fracture of the *lateral* tibial plateau *without* depression of the plateau
  - Occurs in younger patients
  - Cancellous bone of the plateau resists depression.
  - Usually occurs from a valgus force in combination with axial load
- Type 2:
  - Combination of split fracture *and* depression of *lateral* plateau
  - The mechanism is similar to type 1 injury.
  - Patients tend to be in their fourth decade of life or older.
  - Have weaker subchondral bone
- Type 3:
  - Local depression of the *lateral* plateau
  - Injuries may be unstable.
- Type 4:
  - Fracture/depression of the *medial* plateau
  - Requires much more force (varus and axial loading)
  - Be suspicious for associated injuries.
  - Damage to other structures:
    - Popliteal artery
    - Peroneal nerve
    - Lateral collateral ligament
    - Medial meniscus
    - Cruciate ligaments
- Type 5:
  - Bicondylar fracture
  - High-energy injury
  - Associated injuries:
    - Popliteal vessel injury
    - Peroneal nerve injury
    - Compartment syndrome
- Type 6:
  - *Bicondylar,* grossly comminuted fracture of the plateau
  - Diaphyseal–metaphyseal dissociation
  - Violent force, usually a fall from a height
  - Associated neurovascular injuries and compartment syndrome

## ETIOLOGY
- Mechanism of injury:
  - Fall from a height, causing impact of femoral condyles on tibial surface
  - Vehicle bumper injury (forces directed lateral to medial)
  - Violent twisting force (eg, skiing)
- Associated injuries include:
  - Ligamentous (collaterals, cruciates)
  - Meniscal
  - Neurovascular (peroneal nerve and popliteal vessels)

### Pediatric Considerations
- Tibial plateau fractures are rare in children.
- Dense cancellous bone of the tibial plateau

## 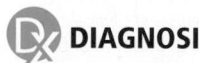 DIAGNOSIS

### SIGNS AND SYMPTOMS
- Painful swollen knee
- Inability to bear weight
- Knee effusion (hemarthrosis)
- Limited active and passive range of motion of the knee
- Tenderness along the proximal tibia and joint line
- Possible varus or valgus deformity of the knee
- Possible joint instability due to associated ligamentous injury

### History
- Hit in lateral knee by a car bumper
- Fall from a height with axial load
- Twisting injury

### Physical Exam
- Decision aids for the use of radiography:
  - Ottawa knee rule—knee radiographs are indicated if any of the following are present:
    - Age >55 yr
    - Tenderness of the fibular head
    - Isolated patellar tenderness
    - Inability to flex to 90 degrees
    - Inability to transfer weight for 4 steps both immediately after the injury and in the ED
    - Limping is allowed.
  - Pittsburgh knee rule—knee radiographs are indicated in fall or blunt trauma when the following are present:
    - Age <12 or >55 yr
    - Pittsburgh knee rule should be applied with caution to patients <18 yr old.
    - Inability to bear weight fully for 4 steps on both toe pads and heel pads of each foot
    - Limping is *not* allowed.

- Neurovascular examination:
  - High-energy mechanism carries risk for neurovascular injury and compartment syndrome.
  - Check popliteal, posterior tibial, and dorsalis pedis pulses.
  - Check integrity of peroneal nerve:
    - Ankle and great toe dorsiflexion
    - Sensation in dorsal web space between great and second toes
- Plain radiography:
  - Anteroposterior (AP) and cross-table lateral views of the knee and proximal tibia
  - Cross-table lateral view may demonstrate lipohemarthrosis (fat–fluid level).
  - Oblique views may identify fractures not apparent on other films.
  - Pay attention to areas of ligamentous attachment where avulsion fractures may take place:
    - Medial and lateral femoral condyles
    - Tibial spine (intercondylar eminence)
    - Fibular head

### DIAGNOSTIC TESTS & INTERPRETATION
#### Imaging
- Tibial plateau view:
  - AP view with the knee in 10–15 degrees of flexion helps visualize depressions.
- Sunrise view of the patella:
  - Useful in identifying fractures of the patella not visualized on AP or lateral views
- CT scan may reveal occult fractures not seen on plain radiographs:
  - Further delineates extent of fractures
- MRI can be used to better elucidate soft tissue injuries.
- Arteriography is indicated if:
  - High-energy mechanism
  - Schatzker type 4, 5, or 6 fracture
  - Alteration in distal pulses
  - Expanding hematoma
  - Bruit
  - Injury to anatomically related nerves

#### Diagnostic Procedures/Surgery
- Arthrocentesis to look for fat globules:
  - If mechanism strongly suggests fracture
  - Effusion present without fracture on plain radiographs
- Compartment pressure measurements are indicated if:
  - Pain not over fracture site
  - Pain on passive stretch
  - Paresthesias
  - Abnormality of pulses
  - Intracompartmental pressures >30 mm Hg are an indication for emergent orthopedic consultation.

## DIFFERENTIAL DIAGNOSIS

- Knee dislocation
- Proximal fibular fracture
- Femoral condyle fracture
- Patellar fracture
- Tibial subcondylar fracture
- Tibial tuberosity fracture
- Tibial spine fracture
- Cruciate ligament tears
- Collateral ligament tears
- Meniscal tears

### Pediatric Considerations

Include oblique views as part of routine radiography.

 TREATMENT

### PRE-HOSPITAL

Cautions:

- In high-energy mechanisms, associated major injuries take precedence.
- Immobilize to prevent further neurologic or vascular injury.

### INITIAL STABILIZATION/THERAPY

- Stabilization of the multiple-injury trauma patient
- Long-leg splint
- Ice
- Elevation
- Frank dislocations with vascular compromise may need immediate reduction in ED.

### ED TREATMENT/PROCEDURES

- No weight bearing
- Pain control
- Nondisplaced fractures or minimally displaced (<8 mm) *lateral* plateau fractures without ligamentous injury:
  - Aspiration of hemarthrosis and injection of local anesthetic
  - Examination for ligamentous instability
  - If knee is *stable:*
    - Compressive dressing
    - Ice and elevation for 48 hr
    - No weight bearing/crutches
  - If knee is *unstable,* then urgent orthopedic consultation is warranted.

- Open fractures:
  - Remove contaminants.
  - Apply moist sterile dressing.
  - Assess tetanus immunity.
  - Antibiotics
  - Emergent orthopedic consultation

### MEDICATION

Open fractures

- Cefazolin: 2 g IV (peds: 50 mg/kg)
- Gentamicin: 2–5 mg/kg IV (peds: 2.5 mg/kg)
- Tetanus toxoid if indicated
- Vancomycin: 1 g IV loading dose (peds: 10 mg/kg) if penicillin-allergic

 FOLLOW-UP

### DISPOSITION

#### Admission Criteria

- Open fractures for debridement, irrigation, and IV antibiotics
- Comminuted, bicondylar fractures for traction
- High-energy mechanisms for observation of neurovascular status and development of compartment syndrome
- Pain control

#### Discharge Criteria

Nondisplaced or minimally displaced, stable fractures of the lateral plateau

### FOLLOW-UP RECOMMENDATIONS

Orthopedic follow-up.

- Long leg splint with ice, elevation and non-weight-bearing status of affected joint

## PEARLS AND PITFALLS

Lipohemarthrosis (blood and fat globules) on arthrocentesis, as seen on CT or US (multilayered fluid collection in the subquadricipital recess) is pathognomonic for intra-articular knee fracture.

## ADDITIONAL READING

- Bonnefoy O, Diris B, Moinard M, et al. Acute knee trauma: Role of ultrasound. *Eur Radiol.* 2006; 16:2542–2254.
- Emparanza JI, Aginaga JR. Validation of the Ottawa Knee Rules. *Ann Emerg Med.* 2001;38(4):364–368.
- Seaberg DC, Yealy DM, Lukens T, et al. Multicenter comparison of two clinical decision rules for the use of radiography in acute, high-risk knee injuries. *Ann Emerg Med.* 1998;32:813.
- Simon RR, Koenigsknecht SJ. *Emergency Orthopedics: The Extremities,* 4th ed. New York: McGraw-Hill; 2001.
- Stiell IG, Greenberg GH, Wells GA, et al. Prospective validation of a decision rule for the use of radiography in acute knee injuries. *JAMA.* 1996;275(8):611–615.
- Watson JT, Wiss DA. Fractures of the proximal tibia and fibula. In: Bucholz RW, Heckman JD, eds. *Rockwood and Green's Fractures in Adults,* 5th ed. Philadelphia: Lippincott Williams & Wilkins; 2001: 1801–1838.

 CODES

### ICD9

823.00 Closed fracture of upper end of tibia

# TIBIAL/FIBULAR SHAFT FRACTURE
*Colleen Campbell*

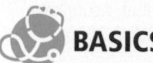 **BASICS**

## DESCRIPTION
### Fracture Description
**Tibia**
- 80% have associated fibular fractures
- Open vs. closed
- Extent of soft tissue damage
- Gustilo–Anderson classification of open fractures:
  - Type I:
    - Wound <1 cm
    - Little soft tissue damage
    - No crush injury
  - Type II:
    - Wound >1 cm
    - Moderate soft tissue damage
    - Little or no devitalized soft tissue
  - Type III—severe soft tissue injury:
    - A—adequate soft tissue coverage of bone
    - B—tissue loss/periosteal stripping
    - C—neurovascular injury requiring surgery
- Anatomic location:
  - Proximal, middle, or distal third
  - Articular extension
- Displacement
- Degree of shortening
- Angulation
- Configuration:
  - Spiral, transverse, or oblique
  - Comminuted, with butterfly fragment or multiple fragments

**Fibula**
- Proximal:
  - Associated with peroneal nerve injury
  - Disruption of ankle syndesmosis (Maisonneuve fracture)
- Middle
- Distal

### Pediatric Considerations
- Third most common long bone fracture in children
- Second most common long bone fracture in nonaccidental trauma (usually apophyseal or metaphyseal corner)
- Nonphyseal fracture patterns:
  - Compression (torus)
  - Incomplete tension–compression (greenstick)
  - Plastic/bowing deformity of fibula may occur.
  - Complete fractures
- Physeal fracture patterns:
  - Tibial shaft fractures may extend to the physis in Salter–Harris II pattern.

## ETIOLOGY
- High- vs. low-energy injury
- Amount of soft tissue injury is prognostic and determined by the degree of energy involved.
- Indirect force—frequently low-energy trauma:
  - Rotary and compressive forces often result in oblique and spiral fractures.
- Skiing, fall, child abuse
- Direct force—high-energy trauma:
  - Direct blow to leg often results in transverse and comminuted fractures.
- Pedestrian vs. auto, motor vehicle crash (MVC):
  - Bending force over a fulcrum often produces comminution with a wedge-shaped butterfly fragment.
- Skier's boot top, football tackle, MVC

### Pediatric Considerations
- Bicycle spoke injury:
  - Foot and lower leg get caught between frame and wheel spoke
  - Crush injury is the primary problem.
  - Initial benign appearance of the soft tissues is often deceiving:
    - Full-thickness skin loss can occur in days.
  - Orthopedic surgery consultation should be obtained for all spoke-injury patients with associated fractures.
- Toddler fracture:
  - Spiral fracture involving the distal third of the tibia with intact fibula secondary to rotational force (turning on planted foot)
  - Age range is 9 mo–6 yr, most often when learning to walk.
  - Fractures in midshaft or more transverse are suggestive of nonaccidental trauma.

 **DIAGNOSIS**

## SIGNS AND SYMPTOMS
### History
- History of trauma
- Pain is usually immediate, severe, and well localized to the fracture site.

### Physical Exam
- Visible or palpable deformity at the fracture site
- Significant soft tissue damage with high-energy trauma
- Inability to bear weight if tibia involved:
  - May be able to walk if isolated fibular fracture
- Foot drop on affected leg from injury to the peroneal nerve as it wraps around the fibular head
- Compartment syndrome

### Pediatric Considerations
- Rely on parents for historical information.
- Child may present limping with no obvious deformity.

## ESSENTIAL WORKUP
- Careful assessment of soft tissues
- Careful neurovascular examination (compare with contralateral side)
- Examine for associated injuries.
- Completely expose patient and put into gown.
- Assessment for compartment syndrome

## ALERT
- Compartment syndrome
- Occurs in 8% of diaphyseal fractures, more common in younger patients
- Relatively common complication of tibial fractures and may not appear until 24 hr after injury
- Pain disproportionate to that expected
- Patient may have swollen, tight compartment, but does not always have pain on palpation of compartment.
- Pain on passive stretch of foot, toes
- Sensory deficit
- Motor weakness is a late finding.
- Pulselessness is not a sign of compartment syndrome:
  - Palpable pulses are almost always present in compartment syndrome unless there is underlying arterial injury.
- 4 leg compartments: Anterior, lateral, deep posterior, and superficial posterior
- Anterior compartment:
  - Deep peroneal nerve
  - Sensation of first web space
  - Ankle and toe dorsiflexion
  - Anterior tibial artery feeds dorsalis pedis artery
- Lateral compartment:
  - Superficial peroneal nerve
  - Sensation of dorsum of foot
  - Foot eversion
- Deep posterior compartment:
  - Tibial nerve
  - Sensation to sole of foot
  - Ankle and toe plantarflexion
  - Posterior tibial and peroneal arteries
- Superficial posterior compartment:
  - Branch of sural cutaneous nerve
  - Sensation to lateral foot

## DIAGNOSTIC TESTS & INTERPRETATION
### Lab
Include creatine phosphokinase levels if concerned about compartment syndrome

### Imaging
- Anteroposterior and lateral views of the leg, knee, and ankle
- Bone scan at 1–4 days for toddler fracture and stress fractures if radiographs unrevealing
- CT scan for complex fracture pattern to evaluate for rotational malalignment
- CT or MRI for pathologic fracture
- MRI for stress fractures may be necessary.

### Diagnostic Procedures/Surgery
Compartment pressures:
- Pressures >30 mm Hg are an indication for orthopedic consultation and fasciotomy.
- Delta p or difference between diastolic BP and compartment pressure <20 is indicative of compartment syndrome
- Repeated pressure measurements over time, taken within 5 cm of fracture site, are necessary.

### *Pediatric Considerations*
Oblique radiograph to detect nondisplaced fractures

### DIFFERENTIAL DIAGNOSIS
- Stress fracture
- Pathologic fracture
- Osteomyelitis

### *Pediatric Considerations*
- Sarcoma
- Pathologic fracture
- Osteomyelitis
- Nonaccidental trauma

 TREATMENT

### PRE-HOSPITAL
- Look for associated injuries in high-energy mechanisms.
- Assess for neurologic or vascular compromise.
- Adequate immobilization is essential to prevent further injury.

### INITIAL STABILIZATION/THERAPY
- Manage airway and resuscitate as indicated.
- Life-threatening injuries take precedence.
- Immobilize extremity.
- Apply ice.
- Strict NPO
- Pain control

### ED TREATMENT/PROCEDURES
- Closed fractures:
  - Gentle attempt at reduction if fracture is displaced (do not attempt multiple reductions).
  - Immobilization:
    o Well-padded long leg posterior splint
    o Knee in 10–20 degrees of flexion
  - Avoid circumferential cast.
  - If pain persists after immobilization, suspect:
    o Compartment syndrome
    o Avoid elevation of leg in suspected compartment syndrome; it lowers perfusion to the extremity.
    o Nerve compression
  - Crutches
- Open fractures:
  - Remove contaminants and cover wound with moist, sterile dressing.
  - Antibiotics
  - Tetanus prophylaxis
  - Immobilization with well-padded long leg posterior splint
  - Immediate orthopedic surgery consultation for debridement and fracture fixation

- Isolated fibular fracture:
  - Usually treated symptomatically:
    o Padded splint
    o Elevation
    o Ice
    o No weight bearing until swelling resolves
  - Crutches if not bearing weight

### MEDICATION
- Gram-positive cocci coverage for open fractures: Cefazolin 2 g loading dose then 1 g (peds: 50 mg/kg/day) IV/IM q8h
- Gustilo–Anderson type III, add gram-negative rod coverage: Gentamicin 3–5 mg/kg (peds: 2.5 mg/kg) IV q8h
- Farming accident, add *Clostridium* spp coverage: Penicillin G 10 million IU (peds: 250,000–400,000 IU/kg/day) IV q6h
- Tetanus toxoid 0.5 mL IM and tetanus immune globulin 250 U IM as indicated by the type of wound and the number of primary immunizations
- If penicillin-allergic: Vancomycin 1 g (peds: 10 mg/kg) IV q12h

 FOLLOW-UP

### DISPOSITION
#### *Admission Criteria*
- Multiple trauma
- High-energy mechanism
- Soft tissue involvement
- Risk for compartment syndrome
- All open fractures
- Displaced, angulated, transverse, shortened, comminuted, and otherwise unstable fractures
- Intra-articular involvement
- Neurovascular compromise
- Inadequate pain control
- Pathologic fracture
- Nonaccidental trauma in children

#### *Discharge Criteria*
- Minimally displaced fracture with low-energy injury mechanism
- Close orthopedic follow-up
- Return parameters for compartment syndrome in a reliable patient
- If fracture is >48 hr old, compartment syndrome is unlikely to develop; if it has not occurred, discharge criteria may be more liberal.

### FOLLOW-UP RECOMMENDATIONS
- Most pediatric fractures are treated with long leg cast for 4–6 wk.
- Nondisplaced and miminally displaced fractures in adults may be treated with long leg cast and closed reduction.
- Open contaminated fractures may be treated with external fixation and debridements.
- Treatment with Intramedullary nail allows for early mobilization and weight bearing as tolerated.
- Kirschner wires are sometimes used in treatment.

### PEARLS AND PITFALLS
- High incidence of associated injuries in high energy trauma:
  - Associated injuries commonly include:
    o Femoral fractures ("floating knee injury")
    o Head trauma
    o Spine fractures
  - Deep venous thrombosis occurs in 10%–25% of patients following tibial fracture.

### ADDITIONAL READING
- Browner. Fractures of the tibial shaft. In: *Skeletal Trauma*, 4th ed. 2008.
- Green and Swiontkowski. *Fractures of the Tibia and Fibula: Skeletal Trauma in Children*. 2008.
- Newton EJ: Emergency department management of select orthopedic injuries. *Emerg Med Clin N Am*. 2007;3:763–793, lx–x.
- Park S, Ahn J, Gee AO, et al. Compartment syndrome in tibial fractures. *J Orthop Trauma*. 2009;7:514–518.

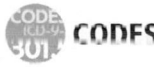 CODES

#### ICD9
- 823.20 Closed fracture of shaft of tibia
- 823.21 Closed fracture of shaft of fibula
- 823.22 Closed fracture of shaft of fibula with tibia

# TICK BITE

Jonathan A. Edlow

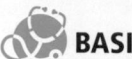 **BASICS**

## DESCRIPTION
Tick bite patient concerns:
- Tick removal
- Local effect of the bite
- Possibility of acquiring a tickborne illness:
  - Often fear contracting Lyme disease
  - Want to be tested or treated for Lyme

## ETIOLOGY
- Specific tickborne infections are discussed in other chapters.
- Tick bite can be from different species of ticks of two major types:
  - Soft ticks (Ornithodoros):
    - Cause tickborne relapsing fever
    - Only feed for minutes and therefore almost never provoke a visit to the ED
  - Hard ticks—especially *Ixodes* and *Dermacentor*:
    - Feed for several days to a week and therefore may lead to an ED visit
- Lyme disease transmission:
  - Species of tick, stage of development, duration of attachment, and geography may all play a role in the possibility of developing Lyme disease.
  - Most cases of Lyme are associated with bites from nymphal *I. scapularis* ticks.
  - Most cases are transmitted only after the tick has been attached for 24–48 hr:
    - Degree of engorgement is a marker for duration of attachment.

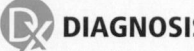 **DIAGNOSIS**

## SIGNS AND SYMPTOMS
Tick is attached to skin.

### History
- The patient has usually made the diagnosis themselves, although sometimes they mistake the tick for skin tags or other skin lesions.
- Ask regarding duration of tick attachment, as this may influence the decision to prescribe antibiotic prophylaxis.

### Physical Exam
Directly examine the skin and the tick:
- Try to identify the tick species.
- Estimate degree of engorgement.

### ALERT
- Some of the tickborne infections are potentially fatal and must be diagnosed based on history, physical and epidemiological context.
- Because the drug of choice for some of these infections—doxycycline—is not usually prescribed for empiric therapy for acutely ill febrile patients, ask about the potential for tick bites in the history of febrile patients and consider using this drug in the appropriate settings.

## ESSENTIAL WORKUP
Accurate history and physical exam searching for presence of tick

## DIAGNOSTIC TESTS & INTERPRETATION
### Lab
- Testing for Lyme disease is *not* indicated:
  - Such antibody testing would only reflect prior exposure to *Borrelia burgdorferi*
  - No treatment implications whatsoever for the current bite

### Diagnostic Procedures/Surgery
- Testing of the tick itself is not recommended.
- See treatment for tick removal.

## DIFFERENTIAL DIAGNOSIS
- Tickborne diseases in North America:
  - Lyme disease
  - Babesiosis
  - Ehrlichiosis
  - Rocky Mountain spotted fever
  - Relapsing fever
  - Tularemia
  - Colorado Tick fever
  - Q-fever
  - Tickborne encephalitis (Powassan fever)
  - Tick paralysis
- Additional tickborne diseases found in Europe:
  - Tickborne encephalitis
  - Boutonneuse fever (*R. connori*)
  - Other spotted fever rickettsiae

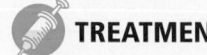

## TREATMENT

### INITIAL STABILIZATION/THERAPY
Remove tick:
- Early removal reduces the likelihood of transmission of tickborne infections.

### ED TREATMENT/PROCEDURES
- Tick removal method:
  - Grasp the tick with very fine forceps, as close to the skin as possible, and gently lift up over 30–120 sec.
  - Most ticks will come out.
  - Do not to squeeze the tick, which could inject infectious materials.
  - If mouthparts are left in the skin, although this could lead to local infection or foreign body reaction, it has no implications for transmission of tickborne diseases.
- Another described method:
  - Inject an intradermal wheal of lidocaine with epinephrine beneath the tick.
  - Tick may crawl out of its own accord.
- Methods *not* to use include:
  - Burning the tick with a match Covering it with petroleum jelly or other noxious agents
- Lyme disease prophylaxis:
  - Indicated if the tick is an engorged *I. scapularis* nymph, or if the physician decides to prophylax
  - Doxycycline 200 mg for 1 dose
  - For children, there is no studied single dose regimen:
    - Prescribe amoxicillin (25–50 mg/kg) for 10 days in divided doses.
    - No data support prophylactic antibiotics for other tickborne diseases.

### Pediatric Considerations
- Several studies used 10 days of amoxicillin in children for prevention of Lyme disease.
- No patients in the treated groups developed Lyme or seroconverted.

### Pregnancy Considerations
Although there are no high quality data on antibiotic prophylaxis for Lyme disease in pregnant women, some authors recommend having a very low threshold for treating pregnant women with tick bites (using amoxicillin).

### MEDICATION
- Amoxicillin: 25–50 mg/kg in divided doses t.i.d. for 14–21 days
- Doxycycline: 200 mg PO for 1 dose

## FOLLOW-UP

### DISPOSITION

#### Admission Criteria
- Tick bite and symptoms or signs of tick paralysis
- Tick bite leading to a soft-tissue infection sufficiently severe to require admission

#### Discharge Criteria
All other patients, the vast majority, are safely discharged.

### FOLLOW-UP RECOMMENDATIONS
- Follow-up with primary care physicians if there are issues regarding local bacterial infection from the bite (cellulitis) or subsequent symptoms and signs of 1 of the tickborne infections listed above.
- Seek medical attention in the event of a febrile illness and to report the history of the tick bite to that physician.

## PEARLS AND PITFALLS
- Early tick removal reduces the likelihood of transmission of tickborne infections.
- Lyme disease prophylaxis is indicated if the tick is an engorged *I. scapularis* nymph.

## ADDITIONAL READING
- Edlow JA. Erythema migrans. *Med Clin North Am*. 2002;86:239–260.
- Edlow JA. Introduction to tick-borne diseases. *Emergency Medicine On-Line Textbook*. Boston: Medical Publishing Corporation; 1997, updated 2005.
- Fix AD, Strickland T, and Grant J. Tick bites and Lyme disease in an endemic setting. *JAMA*. 1998;279: 206–210.
- Nadelman RB, et al. Prophylaxis with single dose doxycycline for the prevention of Lyme disease after an Ixodes scapularis tick bite. *N Engl J Med*. 2001; 245:79–84.
- Needham GR. Evaluation of five popular methods for tick removal. *Pediatrics*. 1985;75:997–1002.
- Sood SK, et al. Duration of tick attachment as a predictor of the risk of Lyme disease in an area in which Lyme disease is endemic. *J Infect Dis*. 1997; 175:996–999.

### See Also (Topic, Algorithm, Electronic Media Element)
- Lyme Disease
- Rocky Mountain Spotted Fever

## CODES

### ICD9
919.4 Insect bite, nonvenomous, of other, multiple, and unspecified sites, without mention of infection

T

# TINEA INFECTIONS, CUTANEOUS

*Heather D. Torrez*
*Mark Richmond*

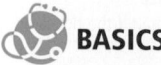

## BASICS

### DESCRIPTION
- Superficial fungal infections of the hair, skin, or nails:
  - Usually confined to the stratum corneum layer
- Tinea requires keratin for growth, so does not involve mucosa.

### ETIOLOGY
- Dermatophytes:
  - *Microsporum*
  - *Trichophyton*
  - *Epidermophyton*
  - *Malassezia furfur*, a yeast, is the etiologic agent of tinea versicolor (not a true tinea).
- Trauma or maceration of the skin may allow fungal entry into skin.
- Transmission may be person to person, animal to person, or soil to person.

### Pediatric Considerations
- Fungi can be spread from toys and brushes.
- Tinea unguium is rare in children; it is associated with Down syndrome, immunosuppression, and tinea pedis or capitis.

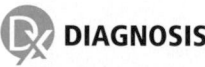

## DIAGNOSIS

### SIGNS AND SYMPTOMS
- Tinea capitis:
  - Children are predominately affected.
  - Most contagious dermatophytosis
  - Alopecia, dandrufflike scaling
  - Kerion:
    - Boggy, inflammatory mass that exudes pus and causes cervical lymphadenopathy
  - "Black dots" from infected hairs broken off at the scalp
- Tinea corporis ("ringworm"):
  - Arms, legs, and trunk
  - Sharply marginated, annular lesion with raised margins and central clearing
  - Hair follicle involvement may produce indurated papules and pustules.
  - Lesions may be single, multiple, or concentric.
  - Pets are often a vector.
- Tinea cruris ("jock itch"):
  - Erythematous, scaly, marginated patches involving the perineum, thighs, and buttocks
  - Associated with heat, humidity, and tight-fitting undergarments
  - Unlike the case in candidiasis, the scrotum and penis are spared.
- Tinea pedis ("athlete's foot"):
  - Scaling, maceration, fissuring between the toes
  - Risk factors:
    - Advanced age
    - Immunocompromised status
    - Hot, humid climates
    - Infrequent changing of socks
  - More common in adults than children
  - Most common tinea infection in the U.S.
  - "Trichophytid" reaction:
    - Vesicular eruption remote from the infection
    - Involving hands, mimics dyshidrotic eczema

- Tinea unguium:
  - One type of onychomycosis
  - Yellow or brown discoloration with thickening and debris under the nails
  - Onycholysis: Loosening of the nail from its bed
  - May involve the plantar surface of the foot
- Tinea versicolor:
  - Most common in warm months
  - Round or oval superficial brown, yellow, or hypopigmented macules that may coalesce
  - Upper trunk, arms, and neck
  - Facial involvement is common in children.

### ALERT
Cellulitis is a frequent complication of tinea pedis.

### History
- Time of onset from inoculation to visible skin changes is about 2 wk.
- Main symptom is itching:
  - Hair loss with tinea capitis
- Participation in contact sports or contacts with similar skin disease

### Physical Exam
- Tinea capitis: Alopecia, broken hairs at scalp surface
- Tinea corporis: Areas of exposed skin typically involved with annular scaly plaques, raised edges, may have pustules and vesicles
- Tinea cruris: Erythematous lesions on groin and pubic region with central clearing and raised edges
- Tinea pedis: Scaling, maceration, and fissuring of toe webs, often only one foot affected
- Tinea unguium: Separation of nail plate from nail bed with thickened, discolored, broken nails

### ESSENTIAL WORKUP
- Diagnose by clinical exam.
- If diagnosis is in doubt, confirm with microscopy before starting oral antifungals because of possible side effects.

### DIAGNOSTIC TESTS & INTERPRETATION
#### Lab
Fungal cultures are slow-growing and should not be routinely done.

#### Imaging
Generally not indicated

#### Diagnostic Procedures/Surgery
- Wood lamp is insensitive:
  - Not all fungi fluoresce
  - *Trichophyton*, the most common cause of tinea infections, does not fluoresce.
  - *Microsporum* fluoresces green
  - *Malassezia* (tinea versicolor) fluoresces yellow to yellow-green.
  - Erythrasma (nontinea corynebacterial infection) will fluoresce coral red.
- Microscopy:
  - Cleanse area with 70% ethanol.
  - Scrape active margin of lesion with #10 or #15 scalpel blades.
  - Place scrapings on a glass slide, add a drop of 10–20% potassium hydroxide solution, and cover with a coverslip.
  - The presence of septate hyphae confirms dermatophyte infection.
  - Budding yeasts and short hyphae ("spaghetti and meatballs") confirms *Malassezia*.

### Pediatric Considerations
Methods to obtain fungal elements for culture or microscopy:
- Brushing the hair with a toothbrush
- Rolling a moistened cotton swab
- Collecting skin cells with transparent tape

### DIFFERENTIAL DIAGNOSIS
- Tinea capitis: Impetigo, pediculosis, alopecia areata, seborrheic dermatitis, atopic dermatitis, and psoriasis
- Tinea corporis: Impetigo, herpes simplex, Lyme disease, verruca vulgaris, psoriasis, nummular eczema, granuloma annulare, herald patch of pityriasis rosea, erythema multiforme, urticaria, seborrheic dermatitis, and secondary syphilis
- Tinea cruris: Impetigo, seborrheic dermatitis, psoriasis, candidal infection, irritant and allergic contact dermatitis, and erythrasma
- Tinea pedis: Scabies, erythrasma, *Candida*, allergic and contact dermatitis, and psoriasis
- Tinea unguium: Psoriasis, dermatitis, lichen planus, and congenital nail dystrophy
- Tinea versicolor: Vitiligo, secondary syphilis

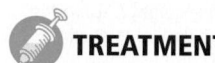

## TREATMENT

### PRE-HOSPITAL
Maintain universal precautions.

### INITIAL STABILIZATION/THERAPY
None required except in immunocompromised or septic patients

### ED TREATMENT/PROCEDURES
- Improvement usually occurs within 1–2 wk of treatment; hair and nail tinea require longer treatment of 3–6 mo.
- Topical antifungals do not penetrate hair or nails:
  - Use in conjunction with systemic agent for tinea capitis or unguium.
- Tinea capitis:
  - Griseofulvin has traditionally been first-line therapy.
  - Newer oral antifungals, including terbinafine, itraconazole, and fluconazole, are preferred:
    - Retained in tissues longer
    - Allows for shorter treatment courses without a decrease in efficacy
    - Improved compliance
  - Terbinafine is now considered the drug of choice by most:
    - Pill form may be crushed in food.
  - Selenium sulfide or ketoconazole shampoo reduces transmissibility.
  - Kerion may respond more rapidly with addition of prednisone.
- Tinea corporis, cruris, and pedis:
  - Topical terbinafine or imidazoles (ketoconazole, miconazole, and clotrimazole) are first-line agents:
    - Topicalterbinafine has been shown to be as effective as or more effective than the imidazoles, with a shorter course.
  - Oral therapy may be necessary for cases resistant to topical treatment or for immunocompromised patients.
  - Keep the area dry (talc powders) and frequently change socks and underclothes.

- Tinea unguium:
  - Requires oral therapy and longer course than other tinea infections
  - Terbinafine had a slightly higher cure rate than imidazoles (ketoconazole, miconazole, and clotrimazole) or griseofulvin in a meta-analysis.
  - Ciclopirox 8% nail lacquer approved for treatment but has low cure rates:
    ○ May enhance oral therapy
- Tinea versicolor:
  - Topicals are first-line therapy:
    ○ Selenium sulfide 2.5% shampoo was as effective as topical ketoconazole.
  - Oral ketoconazole, itraconazole, or fluconazole have been used with cure rates up to 97% but are not as safe as topicals.

### ALERT

Terbinafine may be less effective than griseofulvin against *Microsporum* species causing tinea capitis; however, *Trichophyton* species are the predominant causative organism in children.

### MEDICATION

- Ciclopirox 8% nail lacquer: Apply to affected nails daily, max 48 wk; remove with alcohol every 7 days (peds: same).
- Clotrimazole: Apply 1% cream to affected area b.i.d. for 2–4 wk (peds: same).
- Fluconazole: Tinea unguium—150–300 mg/wk pulse therapy for 3–6 mo for fingernails, 6–12 mo for toenails; tinea corporis, cruris, and pedis: 150 mg PO weekly for 2–4 wk; tinea versicolor: 400 mg PO single dose (peds: 6 mg/kg/day for 3–6 wk for tinea capitis)
- Griseofulvin: Tinea capitis, corporis, cruris—500 mg PO qd for 4–6 wk (peds: 10–20 mg/kg up to 500 mg PO qd until hair regrows, usually 6–8 wk)
- Itraconazole: Tinea capitis: Adults and peds: 3–5 mg/kg PO qd for 2–4 wk; tinea unguium: 200 mg PO qd for 3 mo; tinea versicolor: 400 mg PO qd for 3–7 days; contraindicated in CHF
- Ketoconazole: 2% topical cream qd for 2 wk; tinea capitis, corporis, cruris, pedis—200 mg PO qd for 4 wk (peds: 3.3–6.6 mg/kg PO qd for 4 wk); tinea versicolor—400 mg PO × 1 or 200 mg qd for 7 days (contraindicated with terfenadine and astemizole); soda increases absorption 65%
- Miconazole: Apply cream to affected area b.i.d. for 2–4 wk (peds: same).
- Prednisone: Adults—none (peds: 1 mg/kg PO qd for 2 wk)
- Selenium sulfide: 2.5% shampoo to affected area for 10 min for 1–2 wk (peds: same).
- Terbinafine: 1% topical cream b.i.d. for 2–3 wk for tinea pedis, qd for tinea corporis and tinea cruris; tinea unguium—250 mg PO qd for 6 wk for fingernails, 12 wk for toenails (peds: <20 kg, 67.5 mg/day; 20–40 kg, 125 mg/day; >40 kg, 250 mg/day at same interval as adult; tinea pedis: 250 mg PO per day for 2 wk; tinea capitis: 250 mg/day for 4 wk [dose by weight as for tinea unguium for 4 wk])

- Tolnaftate: Apply 1% cream/powder/solution to affected area b.i.d. for 2–3 wk (peds: same)

### ALERT
The oral antifungals may rarely cause hepatotoxicity:
- Consider checking liver transaminases prior to initiating therapy.

### Pediatric Considerations
Topical preparations are preferred when possible.

### Pregnancy Considerations
- There are few studies addressing the use of antifungal medications during pregnancy in humans.
- Some of the imidazoles have shown adverse effects in animals—class C (fluconazole, itraconazole, ketoconazole).
- Risk:benefit ratio must be considered; elective antifungal therapy is generally not recommended in pregnancy.
- Topical clotrimazole may be used:
  - Clotrimazole, miconazole, and terbinafine are class B drugs.

### First Line
- Tinea capitis: Terbinafine
- Tinea corporis, cruris, pedis: Topical terbinafine or imidazoles (ketoconazole, miconazole, and clotrimazole)
- Tinea versicolor: Selenium sulfide shampoo and topical ketoconazole

 FOLLOW-UP

### DISPOSITION
#### Admission Criteria
- Invasive disease in immunocompromised host
- Kerion with secondary bacterial infection

#### Discharge Criteria
- Most patients may be managed as outpatients.
- Children may return to school once appropriate treatment has been initiated.

### Issues for Referral
Patients started on oral antifungals should be referred for follow-up to monitor therapy and advised regarding symptoms of hepatitis.

### FOLLOW-UP RECOMMENDATIONS
Monitor for complications such as bacterial superinfection, cellulitis, generalized invasive infection:
- Especially in immunocompromised (diabetics, HIV patients)

## PEARLS AND PITFALLS
- Tinea capitis is the most common pediatric dermatophyte infection.
- Itching is the main symptom in most forms of tinea, with associated hair loss in tinea capitis.
- History may reveal participation in contact sports, etc., or contact with other infected persons or pets.

## ADDITIONAL READING
- Fleece D, Gaughan J, Aronoff S. Griseofulvin versus terbinafine in the treatment of tinea capitis: A meta-analysis of randomized clinical trials. *Pediatrics*. 2004;114:1312–1315.
- González U, Seaton T, Bergus G, et al. Systemic antifungal therapy for tinea capitis in children. *Cochrane Database Syst Rev*. 2007;4:CD004685. DOI: 10.1002/14651858.CD004685.pub2.
- Rashid RM, Miller AC, Silverberg, MA. Tinea. May 12, 2009. Available at http://emedicine.medscape. com/article/787217-overview
- Sladden MJ, Johnston GA. Common skin infections in children. *BMJ*. 2004;329:95–99.
- Zhang AY, Camp WL, Elewski BE. Advances in topical and systemic antifungal. *Dermatol Clin*. 2007;25:165–183.

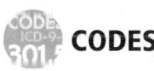 CODES

### ICD9
- 110.0 Dermatophytosis of scalp and beard
- 110.1 Dermatophytosis of nail
- 110.2 Dermatophytosis of hand

T

# TOLUENE POISONING
*Matthew Valento*

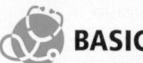 **BASICS**

## DESCRIPTION
Volatile hydrocarbon

## ETIOLOGY
- Abused for its euphoric effect
- Occupational exposures
- Used as organic solvent found in:
  - Oil paints and stains
  - Paint thinners
  - Glues, inks, dyes
  - Coolants
  - Petroleum products
  - Aerosolized household products
  - Correction fluid

### Pediatric Considerations
- Prevalent in adolescent age group:
  - Inexpensive "high" with readily available sources
  - Many psychosocial problems
- May develop chronic neurologic dysfunction
- Mechanism:
  - Rapidly absorbed by inhalation
  - Readily crosses blood–brain barrier, reaching high concentrations in brain
  - May sensitize myocardium to arrhythmogenic effect of catecholamines
  - Alveolar excretion and liver metabolism
- Methods of intoxication:
  - Sniffing: Simple inhalation of substance directly from container
  - Huffing: Vapors inhaled through cloth saturated with substance
  - Bagging: Vapors inhaled from bag containing substance
- Toxic range:
  - 100 ppm: Impairment of psychomotor and perceptual performance
  - 500–800 ppm: Headache, drowsiness, nausea, weakness, and confusion
  - >800 ppm: Convulsions, ataxia, staggering gait for several days
  - 10,000–30,000 ppm: Anesthesia within 1 min

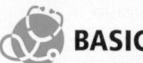 **DIAGNOSIS**

## SIGNS AND SYMPTOMS
- Acute:
  - Neurologic:
    - Depression
    - Euphoria
    - Ataxia
    - Dizziness
    - Seizures
  - Cardiac:
    - Fatal dysrhythmias
  - Pulmonary:
    - Chemical pneumonitis
    - Pulmonary edema
  - Electrolytes:
    - Hypokalemia
    - Hypocalcemia
    - Hyperchloremic metabolic acidosis, likely from hippuric acid
  - Gastrointestinal:
    - Abdominal pain
    - Nausea, vomiting
    - Hematemesis
  - Renal:
    - Renal tubular acidosis
    - Hematuria
    - Proteinuria
  - Musculoskeletal:
    - Diffuse weakness
- Chronic:
  - Neurologic:
    - Peripheral neuropathy
    - Encephalopathy
    - Cerebral/cerebellar atrophy
    - Optic atrophy
    - Cognitive/neurobehavioral abnormalities
  - Cardiac:
    - Dysrhythmias
    - Dilated cardiomyopathy
  - Renal:
    - Distal renal tubular acidosis
    - Renal failure
    - Fanconi syndrome
  - Musculoskeletal:
    - Rhabdomyolysis
  - Psychiatric:
    - Addiction/withdrawal

### Pregnancy Considerations
Microcephaly reported from mothers who chronically abused toluene while pregnant

### History
- Detailed history of sniffing, huffing, bagging, or other abuse of paints/solvents
- Occupational exposures

### Physical Exam
- Presence of agent on lips, nose, or clothes (metallic paint has highest concentration)
- Perioral eczematous dermatitis from chronic huffing or bagging
- Odor of agents

## ESSENTIAL WORKUP
- Detailed physical exam
- CXR for suspected pneumonitis

## DIAGNOSTIC TESTS & INTERPRETATION
### Lab
- Electrolytes, BUN, creatinine, glucose:
  - Hypokalemia
  - Normal or high anion gap metabolic acidosis
  - Hyperchloremia
  - Impaired renal function
  - Severe hypocalcemia/hypophosphatemia
- Urinalysis:
  - Check for myoglobin (rhabdomyolysis)
  - Hematuria and protein often present
- Creatinine kinase if suspect rhabdomyolysis
- Alcohol level—often coingestant
- Liver enzymes, prothrombin time (PT), partial thromboplastin time (PTT), INR, if hepatic dysfunction suspected
- Urine for hippuric acid (metabolite of toluene):
  - Confirms exposure but does not correlate with systemic effects

### Imaging
- EKG:
  - For atrial and ventricular dysrhythmias
- CXR:
  - Indicated if dyspnea or low oxygen saturation
  - Chemical pneumonitis
- CT:
  - For altered mental status/chronic exposure
  - Cerebral/cerebellar atrophy

### Diagnostic Procedures/Surgery

- Serum levels only detectable for short time after exposure
- Urine hippuric acid may confirm exposure to toluene.

## DIFFERENTIAL DIAGNOSIS

- Alcohol intoxication
- Other hydrocarbon abuse
- Nitrous oxide abuse
- Methanol
- Ethylene glycol
- Salicylate
- Heavy metal exposure
- Guillain-Barré syndrome
- Metabolic abnormalities

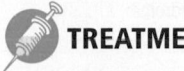 TREATMENT

### PRE-HOSPITAL

- Rapid onset of toxicity
- Death possible with sudden cardiac dysrhythmias (sudden sniffing death), often from catecholamine surge (eg, eluding police)
- Decontamination for occupational exposures
- Forced emesis is not indicated:
  - Decreased level of consciousness may lead to aspiration.

### INITIAL STABILIZATION/THERAPY

- ABCs
- Supplemental oxygen
- Cardiac monitor
- 0.9% NS IV access
- Naloxone, thiamine, and check glucose if altered mental status

## ED TREATMENT/PROCEDURES

- Treat cardiac dysrhythmias in standard fashion:
  - Consider $\beta$-blocker for tachydysrhythmia.
- Monitor respiratory status with CXR, pulse oximetry, and ABG if significant inhalation.
- Steroids not recommended for pneumonitis.
- Correct metabolic abnormalities:
  - Potassium
  - Calcium
  - Phosphate
- Acidosis resolves with IV fluids.
- If rhabdomyolysis, maintain high urine output.
- Gastric decontamination for oral ingestion:
  - Charcoal does not bind hydrocarbons well and stomach distention may predispose to vomiting and aspiration.

### MEDICATION

- Dextrose: $D_{50}W$, 1 amp: 50 mL or 25 g (peds: $D_{25}W$, 2–4 mL/kg) IV
- Naloxone (Narcan): 2 mg (peds: 0.1 mg/kg) IV or IM initial dose
- Thiamine (vitamin $B_1$): 100 mg (peds: 50 mg) IV or IM

 FOLLOW-UP

### DISPOSITION

### Admission Criteria

- Altered mental status
- Dysrhythmias
- Hepatic dysfunction
- Renal failure
- Rhabdomyolysis
- Severe metabolic derangements
- Refractory hypokalemia

### Discharge Criteria

After 4–6 hr of observation:

- Mental status at baseline
- No evidence of cardiac, metabolic, or neurologic derangement

## FOLLOW-UP RECOMMENDATIONS

Psychiatry referral for intentional/repeated ingestions

## PEARLS AND PITFALLS

- Myocardial sensitization to catecholamines:
  - Possibility of sudden dysrhythmia/death
- Monitor and replete electrolyte abnormalities.

## ADDITIONAL READING

- Baskerville JR, Tichenor GA, Rosen PB. Toluene induced hypokalemia: Case report and literature review. *Emerg Med J.* 2001;18(6):514–516.
- Filley C, Kleinschmidt-Demasters B. Toxic leukoencephalopathy. *N Engl J Med.* 2001;345: 425–432.
- Horowitz R. Aromatic hydrocarbons. In: Ford MD, Delaney KA, Ling LJ, et al., eds. *Clinical Toxicology.* Philadelphia: WB Saunders; 2001;803–812.
- Leikin J, Paloucek F. *Leikin and Paloucek's Poisoning and Toxicology Handbook*, 3rd ed. Hudson, OH: Lexi-Comp; 2002;1195–1196.
- Tang HL, Chu KH, Cheuk A, et al. Renal tubular acidosis and severe hypophosphatasemia due to toluene inhalation. *Hong Kong Med J.* 2005;11(1): 50–53.

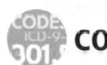 CODES

### ICD9

982.0 Toxic effect of benzene and homologues

# TOOTHACHE
*Franklin D. Friedman*

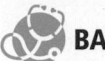 **BASICS**

## DESCRIPTION
- Tooth pain is caused by irritation of the root nerves located in pulpal tissue (the pulp is the tooth's center and its neurovascular supply).
- Other etiologies may cause oral pain.

## ETIOLOGY
- Dental:
  - Dental caries (hard structures demineralized by bacteria)
  - Pulpitis (inflamed pulp secondary to infection)
  - Reversible pulpitis is mild inflammation of the tooth pulp caused by caries encroaching on the pulp.
  - Irreversible pulpitis is the result of an untreated carious lesion causing severe inflammation of the pulp and severe, persistent, poorly localized discomfort.
  - Periapical abscess (necrotic pulp and subsequent abscess)
  - Postextraction pain (dry socket, infection)
  - Cracked-tooth syndrome (pain, cold sensitivity, crack difficult to visualize)
- Periodontal disease:
  - Gingivitis and periodontitis (gingivitis with loss of periodontal ligament attachment)
  - Periodontal abscess (gum boil)
  - Pericoronitis (gingival inflammation from malerupted tooth)
  - Acute necrotizing ulcerative gingivitis (gingival pain, ulcers with/without pseudomembranes)
  - Denture stomatitis
  - Herpetic gingivostomatitis
  - Aphthous ulcers (canker sores)
  - Traumatic ulcers

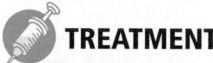 **DIAGNOSIS**

## SIGNS AND SYMPTOMS
### History
- Tooth pain:
  - May be referred to jaw, ear, face, eye, and neck (sensory distribution of fifth cranial nerve)
  - Pain often associated with chewing, changes in temperature, and recumbency.
- Malodorous breath
- Fever and chills
- Foul taste in mouth
- Associated symptoms
- Duration of symptoms
- Treatments that have already been tried

### Physical Exam
- Dental caries
- Facial swelling or erythema
- Trismus:
  - Decreased maximal interincisal opening (normal opening, 35–50 mm)
- Inspect and palpate lips, salivary glands, floor of the mouth, lymph nodes of the neck.
- Assess voice changes.
- Identify periodontal abscess.
- Evaluate for deep-space infection.
- Examine face for swelling, redness, tenderness, and increased warmth.
- Examine neck for adenopathy and stiffness.
- Teeth should be percussed for tenderness and mobility.
- Teeth should be examined for fracture and missing teeth.
- Dental numeric system used in adults:
  - Maxillary: Right to left 1–16; mandibular: left to right 17–32 (peds: A–J and K–T)
  - Alternatively identification of teeth by their location is also appropriate (ie, left rearmost, upper molar, or right center lower incisor).

## ESSENTIAL WORKUP
- Obtain full medical and dental history.
- Ask about drug allergies, especially antibiotics and analgesics.
- Assess need for predental procedure antibiotic prophylaxis:
  - Rheumatic fever
  - Cardiac valve replacements
  - Orthopedic joint replacements
  - Mitral valve prolapse or valvular heart disease
- If physical exam conflicts with patient's history and intraoral source of pain is not apparent consider other sources of pain:
  - Nonodontogenic etiologies of pain
  - Factitious pain/drug-seeking behavior

## DIAGNOSTIC TESTS & INTERPRETATION
### Lab
- No lab tests needed except in patients with signs of systemic toxicity and those patients with perceptible deep-space infection.
- As with any other infection with symptoms of systemic toxicity, consider CBC, blood cultures, markers of inflammation like ESR or CRP.

### Imaging
- Panoramic and periapical radiograph views if suspicion exists about dental infection or fracture
- CT or MRI to evaluate deeper infections

### Diagnostic Procedures/Surgery
A local or regional dental nerve block may sometimes offer both therapeutic and diagnostic benefit.

## DIFFERENTIAL DIAGNOSIS
- Sinusitis
- Otitis media
- Pharyngitis
- Peritonsillar abscess
- Temporomandibular joint syndrome:
  - Usually presents with pain around the ear
- Trigeminal neuralgia
- Vascular headache
- Herpes zoster
- Cardiac ischemia

### Pediatric Considerations
- Tooth eruption in a child or infant may cause oral pain, irritability, low-grade fever, diarrhea, and decreased food intake.
- Facial swelling with fever and leukocytes >15,000/mm$^3$ suggests a nonodontogenic source.
- Children have a maximum of 20 deciduous teeth, 10 upper and 10 lower.

**TREATMENT**

## PRE-HOSPITAL
- Maintain patent airway in patients with severe facial swelling or trismus.
- The patient should be kept in a sitting position if possible.

## INITIAL STABILIZATION/THERAPY
- Airway management for deep-space infection and airway compromise
- Early pain management as indicated

## ED TREATMENT/PROCEDURES

- Appropriate analgesia
- NSAIDs are *first-line* therapy for uncomplicated dental pain.
- Opiate analgesics are an alternative therapy.
- Dental anesthetic field block:
  - Injected along the buccal surface of the affected tooth
  - Specific nerve block for multiple teeth
  - Long-acting anesthetic (eg, bupivacaine)
- Antibiotics if dental infection is present:
  - *Penicillin is the antibiotic of choice* if patient is not allergic.
  - Clindamycin for patients with penicillin allergy or for predominance of anaerobes
- Localized periapical and periodontal abscesses should be incised, drained, and irrigated:
  - Drain may be placed for 24 hr.
- Saline rinses at home four times a day and dental referral in 24 hr

## MEDICATION

- Antibiotics:
  - Clindamycin: 150–450 mg PO q6h (peds: 15–30 mg/kg/24 hr [max 2 g] q6h):
    - IV dose 300–900 mg (peds: 25–40 mg/kg/24 hr div q6–8h)
  - Penicillin VK: 500 mg PO q6h (peds: 25–50 mg/kg/24 h [max. 3 g] q6h)
  - Penicillin G potassium aqueous: 4 mU IM/IV q4h (peds: 250,000–400,000 U/kg/day IM/IV div q4–6h, max 24 mU/day)
- Analgesics:
  - Acetaminophen: 650–1,000 mg PO q4h (peds: 15 mg/kg/dose q4h)
  - Acetaminophen and codeine #3: 1–2 tablets PO q4–6h (peds: elixir—codeine 12 mg/5 mL)
  - Acetaminophen and oxycodone: 1 or 2 tablets PO q6h (peds: 0.05–0.15 mg/kg per dose [max 10 mg])
  - Ibuprofen: 400–800 mg PO q8h (peds: 10 mg/kg PO q6h)
  - Ketorolac: 30 mg IV, 60 mg IM q6h (peds: 1 mg/kg per dose IM)
  - Morphine sulfate: 2–8 mg SC or IV q2h (peds: 0.1 mg/kg per dose SC or IV q2h)

### Pediatric Considerations

Teething infants may be helped by over-the-counter topical anesthetics and oral analgesics.

 **FOLLOW-UP**

## DISPOSITION

### Admission Criteria

- Suspicion of deep-space infections (eg, Ludwig angina, retropharyngeal abscess)
- Facial cellulitis proximal to the eye
- Extensive trismus
- Inability to maintain nutrition and hydration
- Evidence of systemic toxicity

### Discharge Criteria

Patients with toothache and localized dental infections can be discharged from the ED.

### Issues for Referral

Patients treated in the ED should be referred to a dentist or dental surgeon promptly.

## FOLLOW-UP RECOMMENDATIONS

Regular and routine dental evaluations

## PEARLS AND PITFALLS

- Mistaking a deep infection for local infection
- Failing to identify source of referred pain to the mouth

## ADDITIONAL READING

- Annino DJ, Goguen LA. Pain from the oral cavity. *Otolaryngol Clin North Am.* 2003;6;1127–1135.
- Douglass AB. Common dental emergencies. *Am Fam Physician.* 2003;67;511–516.
- Roberts JR, Hedges JR, Chanmugan AS, et al. eds. *Clinical Procedures in Emergency Medicine,* 4th ed. Philadelphia: Saunders; 2004.
- Rodriguez DS, Sarlani E. Decision making for the patient who presents with acute dental pain. *AACN Clin Issues.* 2005;16;359–372.
- Van Meter MW, Dave AK. Nerve block, oral. *Emedicine.* http://emedicine.medscape.com/article/82850-overview. Accessed November 12, 2009.

### See Also (Topic, Algorithm, Electronic Media Element)

- Aphthous Ulcer
- Facial Fracture
- Periodontal Abscess
- Peritonsillar Abscess
- Retropharyngeal Abscess
- Temporal-Mandibular Joint Injury/Syndrome

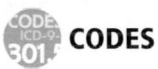 **CODES**

### ICD9

525.9 Unspecified disorder of the teeth and supporting structures

# TORTICOLLIS

*Andrew K. Chang*
*Michelle Davitt*

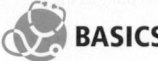 **BASICS**

## DESCRIPTION
- "Twisted neck" (L. *tortus*, twisted + *collum*, neck)
- A fixed or dynamic posturing of the head and neck
- Synonym(s): Cervical dystonia, wry neck

## ETIOLOGY
### Local
- Acute wry neck:
  - Develops overnight without provocation
  - Most prevalent
  - Self-limited, symptoms resolve in 1 to 2 weeks
  - Cervical spine disease
  - Fracture
  - Dislocation, subluxation
  - Infections
  - Spondylosis
  - Tumor
  - Scar tissue–producing injuries
  - Ligamentous laxity in atlantoaxial region
- Inflammatory disease causing muscular damage:
  - Myositis
  - Lymphadenitis
  - Tuberculosis
  - Myasthenia gravis
- Infections of surrounding soft tissues:
  - Nasopharyngeal abscess
  - Retropharyngeal abscess
  - Cervical adenitis
  - Tonsillitis
  - Meningitis
  - Mastoiditis
  - Sinusitis

### Compensatory
- Tilt with essential head tremor (patient tilts head to suppress tremor)
- Ocular muscle palsy

### Central
- Idiopathic spasmodic torticollis:
  - Female > Male
  - Onset 31–60 years old
- Dystonias:
  - Torsion dystonia
  - Generalized tardive dystonia
  - Wilson disease
  - λ-Dopa therapy
  - Acute (neuroleptic drugs)
  - Strychnine poisoning

## Pediatric Considerations
### Local
- Congenital:
  - Odontoid hypoplasia
  - Hemivertebrae
  - Spina bifida
  - Arnold–Chiari syndrome
  - Pseudotumor of infancy
  - Hypertrophy or absence of cervical musculature
- Otolaryngologic:
  - Vestibular dysfunction
  - Otitis media
  - Cervical adenitis
  - Pharyngitis
  - Retropharyngeal abscess
  - Pharyngitis
  - Mastoiditis
  - Esophageal reflux
  - Syrinx with spinal cord tumor
- Trauma:
  - Cervical fracture/dislocation
  - Clavicular fractures
  - Pneumomediastinum
- Juvenile rheumatoid arthritis

### Compensatory
- Strabismus (fourth cranial nerve paresis)
- Congenital nystagmus
- Posterior fossa tumor

### Central
Dystonias:
- Torsion dystonia
- Drug induced
- Cerebral palsy

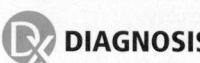 **DIAGNOSIS**

## SIGNS AND SYMPTOMS
- Intermittent painful spasms of sternocleidomastoid (SCM), trapezius, and other neck muscles
- Head is rotated and twisted to one direction.
- Pure flexion (anterocollis) or extension (retrocollis) is *rare:*
  - Represents symmetric involvement of muscles
- Symptoms usually aggravated by standing, walking, or stressful situations
- Usually does not occur with sleep

### History
- Intermittent painful spasms of SCM, trapezius, and other neck muscles
- Obtain a complete medication history.
- The majority of antipsychotic medication–induced dystonic reactions occur between 12 and 23 hr.
- Obtain a complete trauma history.

### Physical Exam
- Head is rotated and twisted to one direction.
- Neck movements vary from jerking to smooth.
- The presence of fever supports an infectious or inflammatory etiology.
- If the neurologic exam is focal, consider spinal cord or CNS disease.
- Congenital form:
  - A firm, nontender enlargement of the SCM muscle visible at birth.

## ESSENTIAL WORKUP

- Geared toward diagnosing life-threatening etiologies above
- Distinguish torticollis from other causes of neck stiffness (meningismus).
- Cervical spine films to evaluate for fracture except patients with chronic paroxysmal episodes

## DIAGNOSTIC TESTS & INTERPRETATION

### Lab

No specific tests helpful

### Imaging

CT or MRI of cervical spine if retropharyngeal abscess or tumor suspected

### Diagnostic Procedures/Surgery

- Consider administering an anticholinergic medication if drug-induced etiology is suspected.
- Consider performing the Tensilon test if myasthenia gravis is a consideration.

## DIFFERENTIAL DIAGNOSIS

- CNS infections
- Tumors of soft tissue or bone
- Basal ganglia disease
- Abscess of cervical glands
- Myositis of cervical muscles
- Cervical disk lesions
- Myasthenia gravis

 TREATMENT

## PRE-HOSPITAL

- Ensure patent airway
- Cervical spine precautions for any history of trauma
- Support head

## INITIAL STABILIZATION/THERAPY

- Cervical spine immobilization if fracture is suspected
- If airway management is necessary, rapid sequence intubation is the method of choice.

## ED TREATMENT/PROCEDURES

- Drug (eg, phenothiazine) induced:
  - Diphenhydramine or benztropine
- Acquired:
  - Soft collar and rest
  - Physical therapy
  - Massage
  - Local heat
  - Analgesics

## MEDICATION

- Benztropine (for drug-related dystonia): 1–2 mg IM or slow IV, followed by 3–5 days PO
- Clonazepam (second-line drug): 0.5 mg PO t.i.d.
- Diphenhydramine (for drug-related dystonia): 25–50 mg IV or IM followed by 3–5 days PO q6-8h; (peds: 5 mg/kg/24 hr div q6h IV, IM, or PO)
- Trihexyphenidyl (a first-line drug): 2–5 mg/day PO, advance to 30 mg/day
- Valium: 2–5 mg IV, 2–10 mg PO t.i.d. (peds: 0.1–0.2 mg/kg per dose IV or PO q6h)
- Botulinum toxin is first line agent for treating non-drug-induced torticollis, though this is not typically administered in the ED setting.

 FOLLOW-UP

## DISPOSITION

### Admission Criteria

- Cervical spine fracture
- Diagnosis in doubt
- Infectious causes
- Toxic appearance
- Inability to maintain adequate fluid intake
- Lack of support system

### Issues for Referral

- Some patients who fail medical treatment may benefit from surgical treatment, such as accessory nerve ablation or deep brain stimulation.

## FOLLOW-UP RECOMMENDATIONS

- Outpatient referral to an orthopedist, neurologist, or neurosurgeon who uses botulinum toxin in his or her practice
- Return to ED for weakness or worsening symptoms.

## PEARLS AND PITFALLS

Exclude infectious, inflammatory, traumatic, spinal cord and CNS causes of torticollis.

## ADDITIONAL READING

- Shanker V, Bressman S. What's new in dystonia? *Curr Neurol Neurosci Rep.* 2009;9:278–284.
- Simpson D, Blitzer B, Brashear A, et al. Assessment: Botulinum neurotoxin for the treatment of movement disorders (an evidence-based review): Report of the Therapeutics and Technology Assessment Subcommittee of the American Academy of Neurology. *Neurology.* 2008;70: 1699–1706.
- Ropper AH, Samuels MA, eds. *Adams and Victor's Principles of Neurology,* 9th ed. New York: McGraw-Hill; 2009.

 CODES

### ICD9

723.5 Torticollis, unspecified

# TOXIC EPIDERMAL NECROLYSIS

*Andrew K. Chang*
*Purvi D. Shah*

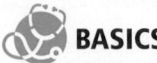 **BASICS**

## DESCRIPTION

- One of the most fulminant and potentially fatal of all dermatologic disorders
- Skin sloughing at the dermal–epidermal interface results in the equivalent of a second-degree burn.
- Can affect up to 100% of total body surface area.
- May extend to involve:
  - Gastrointestinal (GI) mucosa (esophagitis, GI bleeding)
  - Respiratory mucosa (dyspnea, bronchial hypersecretion, respiratory failure)
  - Renal epithelium (glomerulonephritis)
- Hypothesized to be a type IV hypersensitivity reaction
- Current classification system proposes three categories within the spectrum of Stevens–Johnson syndrome (SJS) and toxic epidermal necrolysis (TEN) based on percentage of total body surface area (BSA):
  - SJS: Less than 10% of BSA
  - Overlap SJS–TEN: 10–30% of BSA
  - TEN: more than 30% of BSA
- More common in older patients (more medications), HIV patients (more medications, immunocompromised), systematic lupus erythematosus patients, and bone marrow transplant recipients
- Mortality rate is about 30%, usually due to secondary sepsis from *Staphylococcus aureus* and *Pseudomonas aeruginosa*.
- Synonym(s):
  - Lyell syndrome
  - Fixed drug necrolysis
  - Epidermolysis necroticans combustiformis
  - Epidermolysis bullosa

## ETIOLOGY

- Dose-independent drug reactions are the usual cause of TEN:
  - Drugs introduced within previous 1–3 wk are most likely candidates.
  - Frequently implicated drugs include:
    - Sulfonamide antibiotics
    - Anticonvulsants (phenytoin, phenobarbital, carbamazepine, lamotrigine)
    - NSAIDs (oxicams, pyrazolones, sulindac),
    - Allopurinol
    - Antiretroviral drug nevirapine.
- Other causes: Severe mycoplasmal infections, graft-versus-host disease, idiopathic cases (combined less than 4%)

 **DIAGNOSIS**

## SIGNS AND SYMPTOMS
### History

- Prodrome: 1 to several days of fever, conjunctivitis, pharyngitis, cough, malaise, pruritus, cutaneous tenderness, erythema, anorexia, myalgias, arthralgias, dysuria, vomiting, or diarrhea
- Mucous membranes are commonly affected 1–3 days before skin lesions appear (oropharynx, eyes, genitalia, anus, esophageal and intestinal mucosa, respiratory epithelium).

### Physical Exam
- Skin:
  - Rash usually begins on face (scalp usually spared) and trunk as erythematous macules, irregular targetlike bullae, or diffuse, ill-defined erythema.
  - Widespread epidermolysis, denuding of skin surfaces, flaccid bullae, and sheetlike sloughing of epidermis generally progress over 3–4 days but can progress rapidly over hours.
  - Nikolsky sign: With lateral pressure, the skin denudes and sloughs from separation of epidermis from dermis.
- Oral mucosa: Initial swelling and erythema followed by blistering and ulceration of the lips and oral mucosa
- Ocular lesions (pseudomembranes, synechiae or adhesions, keratitis, corneal erosions)

## ESSENTIAL WORKUP
- Diagnosis is made clinically:
  - Based on history and characteristic skin and mucous membrane lesions
- Ophthalmology consultation is required for eye involvement (evaluation and removal of pseudomembranes and adhesions).

## DIAGNOSTIC TESTS & INTERPRETATION
### Lab
- No confirmatory laboratory tests exist.
- CBC: Normocytic anemia, leukocytosis, lymphopenia/neutropenia, and thrombocytopenia may be present.
- ESR may be elevated as a result of systemic inflammation.
- Serum chemistry: Electrolyte derangements if extensive fluid losses:
  - Prerenal azotemia
- UA may show hematuria (urethral mucosal erosion, glomerulonephritis) or casts (acute tubular necrosis).
- Bacterial sampling of skin; and blood cultures

### Imaging
Chest radiograph should be obtained if pneumonitis or *Mycoplasma pneumoniae* is suspected.

### Diagnostic Procedures/Surgery
- SCORTEN (severity of illness score for TEN): Each risk factor earns one point, a higher score means a poorer prognosis:
  - Age >40 yr
  - Malignancy
  - Tachycardia >120/min
  - Initial percentage of epidermal detachment >10%
  - BUN >27 mg/dL
  - Serum glucose level >252 mg/dL
  - Serum bicarbonate level <20 mEq/
- Biopsy may be performed by consulting dermatologist to rule out autoimmune bullous diseases, staphylococcal scalded skin syndrome, and other diagnoses:
  - Results not immediately available to ED physician.

## DIFFERENTIAL DIAGNOSIS
- SJS
- Erythema multiforme major (EMM):
  - Differentiation of TEN from EMM
  - *Etiology:* TEN is mainly drug-induced; EMM occurs mainly after herpes simplex virus (HSV) infection
  - Lesions:
    - TEN: Widely distributed, mainly on the trunk and face, nonspecific, target like lesions that often are confluent and too numerous to count
    - EMM: Limited in number, symmetric and acral distribution, typical target type (at least three concentric rings) with or without blisters
  - *Prognosis:* EMM is usually benign; recurrence of disease is common (30%); therapeutic prevention of EMM due to HSV is prevention of HSV recurrence.
- Staphylococcal scalded skin syndrome (SSSS):
  - Differentiation of TEN from SSSS:
  - *Age:* TEN: primarily adults (but may occur in children); SSSS: primarily affects children.
  - Etiology:
    - TEN most often represents an idiosyncratic, drug-induced, dose-independent reaction and hence does not require treatment with antibiotics.
    - SSSS results from infection and requires antibiotics.
  - *Pain:* TEN, painful; SSSS, painless
  - *Mucous membranes:* Involved with TEN; usually spared with SSSS
  - *Skin cleavage:* Dermal–epidermal junction in TEN; intraepidermally in SSSS (both can produce a positive Nikolsky sign).

- Autoimmune bullous diseases (pemphigus vulgaris, bullous pemphigoid)
- Scarlet fever
- Toxic shock syndrome
- Chemical or thermal scalds
- Kawasaki syndrome

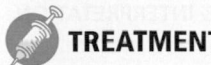 TREATMENT

### PRE-HOSPITAL
- Transport to facility with burn center.
- Care during transport should be gentle to avoid skin trauma.
- IV catheter should be avoided for short transport if hemodynamically stable (more sterile conditions in ED).
- Avoid using adhesive materials.

### INITIAL STABILIZATION/THERAPY
- If intubation is required, gentle technique must be used to minimize mucosal damage.
- Meticulous sterile technique
- Peripheral IV line is preferred over central line to decrease risk of sepsis.
- Cardiac monitor, pulse oximeter, nasogastric tube, Foley catheter

### ED TREATMENT/PROCEDURES
- Identify and stop any causative medication.
- Aggressive fluid resuscitation with lactated Ringer solution as in burn care (Parkland formula):
  - Urine output should be maintained at a rate of at least 0.5 mL/kg/hr.
- Warming measures and frequent core temperature evaluation are important.
- If available, cover with biologic dressings (eg, Biobrane):
  - Reduces pain, decreases caloric and evaporative losses, and facilitates healing
- Antibiotic drops for eyes
- Petroleum jelly application to lips
- Prevention of peptic stress ulcers
- Topical antibiotics are unproven but may be applied with the exception of silver sulfadiazine (sulfonamide derivative).
- Timely admission to burn unit/ICU

### MEDICATION
There are no established treatment regimens; however, there are several suggested guidelines:
- Pain should be controlled with IV opiates.
- Antibiotics should be used when documented signs of sepsis are present or for sudden deterioration in the clinical setting.
- Antihistamines can be used for pruritus.
- Anticoagulation should be considered while patients are nonambulatory for prevention of thromboembolic events.
- Systemic corticosteroids continue to be controversial:
  - Retrospective studies show no benefit and suggest greater risk of death from infection.
- IVIG should be started 48–72 hr after bulla formation but can be helpful after 72 hr.
- The following experimental therapies are under investigation:
  - Cyclosporine: 3 mg/kg/day
  - Cyclophosphamide: 300 mg/day
  - Anti-TNF-$\alpha$ antibodies: Infliximab 5 mg/kg per dose

 FOLLOW-UP

### DISPOSITION
#### Admission Criteria
All patients with suspected toxic epidermal necrolysis should be admitted to a burn unit (if burn unit is unavailable and transfer is not possible, then admit to intensive care unit).

#### Issues for Referral
- Transfer to facility with burn unit has been shown to improve patient outcome.
- Dermatology should be called to help confirm the diagnosis.
- Ophthalmology should be called to evaluate and prevent corneal ulcerations and adhesions.
- Surgery or Plastic Surgery should evaluate the need for wound debridement.
- Respiratory Therapy should initiate pulmonary toilet in the setting of pulmonary mucosal sloughing.

### PEARLS AND PITFALLS
- Burn units and ICUs offer the best management settings.
- Remember to educate patients on medications (including combinations medications and structurally similar medications).
- Aggressive fluid hydration is essential.

### ADDITIONAL READING
- Mistry RD, Schwab SH, Treat JR. Stevens–Johnson syndrome and toxic epidermal necrolysis. *Pediatr Emerg Care.* 2009;25:519–522.
- Dorafshar A, Dickie SR, Cohn AB, et al. Antishear therapy for toxic epidermal necrolysis: An alternative approach. *Plast Reconstr Surg.* 2008;122:151–160.
- Arif H, Buchsbaum R, Weintraub D, et al. Comparison and predictors of rash associated with 15 antiepileptic drugs. *Neurology.* 2007;6:1701–1709.
- Bachot N, Roujeau JC. Differential diagnosis of severe cutaneous drug eruptions. *Am J Clin Dermatol.* 2003;4:561–572.
- Paquet P, Pierard GE, Quatresooz P. Novel treatments for drug-induced toxic epidermal necrolysis (Lyell's syndrome). *Int Arch Allergy Immunol.* 2005;136;205–216.

### See Also (Topic, Algorithm, Electronic Media Element)
Burns

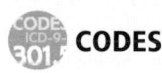 CODES

#### ICD9
- 695.13 Stevens-Johnson syndrome
- 695.14 Stevens-Johnson syndrome-toxic epidermal necrolysis overlap syndrome
- 695.15 Toxic epidermal necrolysis

T

# TOXIC SHOCK SYNDROME

*Michelle Sergel*

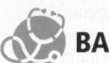 **BASICS**

## DESCRIPTION

- Toxic shock syndrome (TSS) is a severe, acute life-threatening illness caused by toxin-producing strains of *Staphylococcus aureus* or, to a lesser extent, by group A streptococcus (GAS, streptococcal TSS).
- *S. aureus* produces an exotoxin, TSS toxin (TSST-1):
  - Produced by 20% of *S. aureus* isolates
- GAS produces pyrogenic exotoxins—most commonly exotoxins A (SPEA) and B (SPEB).
- The exotoxins are superantigens, a significant factor in the production of symptoms associated with TSS.
- Biologic properties of superantigens include the ability to:
  - Activate up to 20% of T cells at one time resulting in massive cytokine production
  - Induce fever directly on the hypothalamus or indirectly via interleukin-1 (IL-1) and tumor necrosis factor (TNF) production
  - Enhance delayed hypersensitivity
  - Suppress neutrophil migration and immunoglobulin
  - Enhance host susceptibility to endotoxins
- Massive vasodilation occurs:
  - Causes rapid movement of serum proteins and fluids from the intravascular to the extravascular space, causing hypotension.

## ETIOLOGY

- Initially TSS was a disease of young, healthy menstruating females due to highly absorbent tampons:
  - Changes were made to reduce the absorbency and composition of tampons.
- Approximately one half of reported TSS cases are nonmenstrual, including:
  - Surgical wounds
  - Postpartum wound infections
  - Mastitis
  - Septorhinoplasty
  - Sinusitis
  - Osteomyelitis
  - Arthritis
  - Burns
  - Nasal packing (nasal tampons)
  - Cutaneous and subcutaneous lesions
- 30–50% of healthy adults and children carry *S. aureus* in the nasal vestibule, vagina, and rectum and/or on the skin.
- GAS infections often begin within 24–72 hr at the site of minor trauma, often without a visible break in the skin or from a viral infection (eg, varicella, influenza).

 **DIAGNOSIS**

## SIGNS AND SYMPTOMS

- Criteria for diagnosis for staphylococcal TSS—CDC case definition:
  - Fever >38.9°C (102.0°F)
  - Hypotension (systolic BP <90 mm Hg) or shock
  - Diffuse, blanching nonpruritic macular erythroderma rash
  - Subsequent desquamation 1–2 wk after the onset of illness (particularly involving palms and soles)
  - Multisystem involvement—*at least three* of the following should be present:
    ○ Gastrointestinal: Profuse diarrhea or vomiting at onset of illness
    ○ Musculoskeletal: Severe myalgias or greater than a twofold increase in creatine phosphokinase (CPK)
    ○ Mucosal inflammation: Conjunctival, vaginal, or pharyngeal hyperemia
    ○ Renal: Increase in blood urea nitrogen (BUN) or creatinine greater than 2 times normal upper limit or sterile pyuria without evidence of infection
    ○ Hepatic: Total bilirubin or transaminases greater than 2 times normal upper limit
    ○ Hematologic: Thrombocytopenia <100,000/mm$^3$
    ○ CNS: Disorientation, confusion, or hallucinations
  - Negative results on the following tests, if obtained: throat, or CSF cultures, rise in titer to Rocky Mountain spotted fever (RMSF), leptospirosis, or rubeola
- Criteria for diagnosis for GAS TSS:
  - Isolation of GAS from a normally sterile site
  - Hypotension
  - Plus 2 or more of the following:
    ○ Renal impairment (creatinine >2)
    ○ Coagulopathy
    ○ Liver involvement (>2 times the upper limit of normal for transaminases or bilirubin)
    ○ ARDS
    ○ Erythematous macular rash, may desquamate
    ○ Soft tissue necrosis
- Other:
  - Tachycardia frequently present
  - Can rapidly progress to multisystem dysfunction (ARDS or DIC)
  - Most common initial symptom of strep TSS is diffuse or localized pain—abrupt in onset, severe, and usually precedes physical findings
  - Approximately 80% of patients with strep TSS have clinical signs of soft tissue infection.

## ESSENTIAL WORKUP

- Clinical diagnosis using diagnostic criteria with the absence of other causes of illness
- A thorough history and physical examination

## DIAGNOSTIC TESTS & INTERPRETATION

### Lab

- CBC:
  - Leukocytosis or leukopenia, marked bandemia common
- Electrolytes, BUN, creatinine, glucose:
  - Elevated BUN and creatinine common
- Calcium, magnesium:
  - Hypocalcemia/hypomagnesemia often present
- Urinalysis:
  - Normal or sterile pyuria without evidence of infection
- CPK:
  - Two-fold increase
- Hepatic function:
  - Elevated total bilirubin, AST, ALT
- Prothrombin time (PT), partial thromboplastin time (PTT), platelets:
  - Thrombocytopenia <100,000 platelets/mm$^3$
- Culture the site of injury/infection if possible.
- Blood, urine, throat, and CSF cultures as indicated:
  - The case definition does not require a positive blood culture for *S. aureus*, but does for *Streptococcus* organisms.
- Serology for RMSF, rubeola, and leptospirosis
- Hepatitis B surface antigen

### Imaging

- Chest radiograph to rule out other sources of systemic illness
- Consider radiograph or CT scan of involved soft tissue if localized pain to rule out abscess or necrotic tissue.

## DIFFERENTIAL DIAGNOSIS

- Staphylococcal scalded skin syndrome:
  - In children <5 yr of age
  - Initial macular rash followed by the formation of ill-defined bullae that can be rubbed off revealing a shiny, moist epidermis (positive Nikolsky sign)
- Scarlet fever:
  - Preceding streptococcal pharyngitis
  - Rash begins on the upper chest, neck, and back spreading to the remainder of the trunk, sparing the palms and soles.
  - Hypotension absent

- Kawasaki disease:
  - Fever, conjunctival hyperemia, and erythema of the mucous membranes
  - Not associated with renal failure, hypotension, or thrombocytopenia
- Stevens–Johnson syndrome:
  - Severe multisystem involvement
  - Mucosal involvement prominent with involvement of the mouth, conjunctivae, vagina, anus, and urethral meatus
- Leptospirosis:
  - Transmitted through contact with infected animals
  - Fever, headache, severe myalgias, and conjunctival suffusion
  - Truncal rash that only desquamates in children
- RMSF:
  - Rash is pink and macular, beginning on the wrists, palms, ankles, and soles spreading to the trunk and face.
  - Petechiae appear after 4 days.
- Meningococcemia:
  - Meningitis present
  - Rash is petechial

 TREATMENT

### PRE-HOSPITAL
- ABCs
- Hemodynamic support:
  - May need massive amounts of IV fluids

### INITIAL STABILIZATION/THERAPY
- ABCs
- Aggressive management of circulatory shock with IV fluids and pressors

### ED TREATMENT/PROCEDURES
- Hypotension:
  - Aggressive fluid replacement:
    - During the first 24 hr, may require 4–20 L of crystalloid and/or fresh-frozen plasma (colloid)
    - Caution: Large amounts of IV fluids and pressor agents used to treat refractory hypotension can result in the rapid onset of pulmonary edema.
    - Pressors (dopamine) if fluid correction fails to restore normal arterial pressure
- Infection management:
  - Search for and treat the focus of infection.
  - Remove the source of infection (eg, tampon, nasal or wound packing).
  - Early surgical/gynecologic consultation if drainage or debridement of infectious sites necessary

- Antibiotics:
  - It is not clear whether antibiotics alter the course in acute TSS, however there appears to be a more favorable outcome with antibiotics in GAS infections.
  - Clindamycin is a potent suppresser of bacterial toxin synthesis.
    - Clindamycin plus vancomycin for TSS
  - If TSS due to known methicillin-susceptible S. aureus then clindamycin plus oxacillin or nafcillin
  - Clindamycin plus imipenem or merepenem or ticarcillin–clavulanate or pipercillin–tazobactam for GAS TSS
- IV immunoglobulin (IVIG) treatment:
  - May be efficacious in streptococcal toxic shock, but no controlled trials have proven efficacy in staphylococcal TSS.
  - May initiate if no response to fluids, pressors, and antibiotics in patients with pulmonary edema and hypotension

### MEDICATION
- Clindamycin: 600–900 mg (peds: 20–40 mg/kg/24 hr) IV q6–8h
- Vancomycin: 30 mg/kg qd IV divided in two doses (peds: 40 mg/kg qd IV divided in 4 doses)
- Imipenem: 500 mg q6h
- Meropenem: 1 g q8h
- Ticarcillin–clavulanate: 3.1 g q4h
- Pipercillin–tazobactam: 4.5 g q6h
- Dopamine: 2–20 $\mu$g/kg/min IV, titrate to BP
- For staphylococcal TSS: IVIG, 400 mg/kg over several hours
- For streptococcal TSS: IVIG 1 g/kg on day 1 then 0.5 g/kg on days 2 and 3
- Nafcillin: 1.5 g (peds: 100 mg/kg/24 hr) IV q4h
- Oxacillin: 1–2 g (peds: 50–100 mg/kg/24 hr) IV q4h

 FOLLOW-UP

### DISPOSITION
#### Admission Criteria
- Most cases require admission.
- ICU admission for critically ill or those in shock

#### Discharge Criteria
None

#### Issues for Referral
Early surgical/gynecologic consultation if drainage or debridement of an infectious site is necessary.

### FOLLOW-UP RECOMMENDATIONS
- Patients who are bacteremic are treated for a minimum of 14 days:
  - Depending on the clinical course
  - Continue treatment for 14 days from the last positive culture.
- Screening for S. aureus nasal carriage in patient with S. aureus TSS and eradication of the carrier state with mupirocin

## PEARLS AND PITFALLS
- One must consider the diagnoses of staphylococcal TSS and GAS TSS.
- The mainstay for treatment for TSS is supportive while hypotension is present.
- Prompt and aggressive exploration and debridement of suspected deep-seated infection is recommended.
- Empiric therapy with broad-spectrum antibiotics including clindamycin is recommended.

## ADDITIONAL READING
- Durenbert J, Ihendyane N, Sjolin J, et al. Intravenous immunoglobulin G therapy in streptococcal toxic shock syndrome: A European randomized double-blind placebo controlled trial. Clin Infect Dis. 200;37:333.
- Hauser AR. Another toxic shock syndrome: Streptococcal infection is even more dangerous than the staphylococcal form. Postgrad Med. 1998;104: 31–43.
- Keller MA, Stiehm ER. Passive immunity in prevention and treatment of infectious diseases. Clin Microbiol Rev. 2000,13.602.
- Stevens, DL. The toxic shock syndromes. Infect Dis Clin North Am. 1996;10:727.

### See Also (Topic, Algorithm, Electronic Media Element)
- Streptococcal Infections
- Kawasaki Disease

## CODES

ICD9
040.82 Toxic shock syndrome

# TOXOPLASMOSIS

*Roger M. Barkin*
*Ann M. Buchanan*

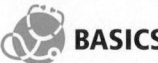 **BASICS**

## DESCRIPTION

- *Toxoplasma gondii*—intracellular protozoan parasite:
  - Three forms:
    - Tachyzoite: Asexual invasive form
    - Tissue cyst: Persists in tissues of infected hosts during chronic phase
    - Oocyst: Contains sporozoites and produced during sexual cycle in cat intestine
- Transmission:
  - Ingesting tissue cysts or oocysts:
    - Ingesting undercooked meat
    - Vegetables contaminated with oocysts
    - Contact with cat feces, through cat or soil
  - Transplacental
  - Blood product
  - Organ transplantation

## ETIOLOGY

- 70% of adults seropositive
- Asymptomatic in most immunocompetent patients
- Worldwide; cats are common host
- Incubation is 7 days with range of 4–21 days

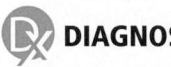 **DIAGNOSIS**

## SIGNS AND SYMPTOMS

Four types of infection

### Immunocompromised Host

- CNS:
  - Subacute presentation (90%)
  - Encephalitis
  - Headache
  - Altered mental status
  - Fever
  - Seizures
  - Cranial nerve palsies
  - Spinal cord lesions
  - Cerebellar signs
  - Meningitislike symptoms
  - Movement disorders
  - Neuropsychological symptoms:
    - Psychosis
    - Paranoia
    - Dementia
    - Anxiety
    - Agitation
- Pulmonary:
  - Pneumonitis
  - Prolonged febrile illness
  - Nonproductive cough
  - Dyspnea

### Immunocompetent Host

- 90% are asymptomatic
- Lymphadenopathy, usually cervical
- Fever
- Malaise
- Mononucleosislike syndrome with macular rash and hepatosplenomegaly
- Headache
- Sore throat
- Night sweats
- Maculopapular rash
- Urticaria
- Usually, self-limited process; resolves in 2–12 mo
- Rarely presents with pneumonitis or encephalitis

### Ocular Toxoplasmosis

- Blurred vision
- Scotoma
- Pain
- Photophobia
- Retina:
  - Small clusters of yellow–white cottonlike patches
  - Chorioretinitis; affects 85% of young adults with untreated congenital infection

### Congenital Toxoplasmosis

- Results from an asymptomatic acute infection during pregnancy
- First trimester:
  - Spontaneous abortion
  - Stillbirth
  - Severe disease up to 25% of the time
- Second or third trimester:
  - 50–60% chance of acquiring congenital toxoplasmosis
  - 2% fatal
- Most asymptomatic at birth
- Delayed onset. 70–90% asymptomatic at birth:
  - CNS disease
  - Ocular disease (blindness months to years later)
  - Lymphadenopathy
  - Hepatosplenomegaly
  - At birth, may have maculopapular rash, lymphadenopathy, hepatomegaly, splenomegaly, jaundice, thrombocytopenia

## ESSENTIAL WORKUP

- Diagnose via:
  - Isolation of organism:
    - Blood
    - CSF for encephalitis
    - Bronchoalveolar lavage for pneumonitis
    - Amniotic fluid
    - Aqueous humor
  - Detection of tachyzoites in tissues or body fluids
  - Demonstrating characteristic lymph node pathology
- Thorough ocular examination:
  - Retinal examination
  - Visual acuity

## DIAGNOSTIC TESTS & INTERPRETATION

### Lab

- LDH >600/UL associated with toxoplasmosis
- CBC:
  - Atypical lymphocytes
- ABG/pulse oximetry for pulmonary symptoms
- IgG antibodies:
  - High number of false-positive and false-negative results
  - Common tests:
    - Sabin–Feldman dye test
    - Indirect fluorescent antibody
    - Agglutination
    - Enzyme-linked immunosorbent assay test
- Immunoglobulin M (IgM) antibodies:
  - Absence excludes diagnosis in immunocompetent host
  - Reference laboratories may be helpful, such as Remington Lab (www.pamf.org/serology)
  - Diagnoses acute infection
  - Appear in 5 days
  - Disappear in weeks to months
  - Neonatal testing differentiates from maternal infection

### Imaging

- Chest radiograph for pulmonary symptoms:
  - Pneumonitis associated with reticulonodular pattern
- CT head with contrast:
  - Multiple bilateral hypodense ring enhancing lesions
- MRI brain:
  - High signal abnormalities on T2-weighted images
- Serial fetal ultrasonography can be useful in exploring congenital infection of the CNS or other signs.

### Diagnostic Procedures/Surgery
- Brain biopsy for encephalitis—definitive diagnosis

## DIFFERENTIAL DIAGNOSIS
- Cryptococcal meningitis
- CNS lymphoma
- *Pneumocystis carinii* pneumonia
- Cytomegalovirus retinitis

## TREATMENT

### INITIAL STABILIZATION/THERAPY
- Treat seizures in standard fashion with diazepam and phenytoin.
- Initiate oxygen if hypoxia due to pneumonitis.

### ED TREATMENT/PROCEDURES
#### Immunocompetent
Toxoplasmic lymphadenitis:

- No antibiotics unless symptoms severe and persistent
- Treat symptomatic patients with pyrimethamine and folinic acid plus sulfadiazine or clindamycin for 2–4 wk.
- Clindamycin may be a useful alternative to sulfadiazine because of the side effects of the latter.
- Pyrimethamine and sulfadiazine (Eon Labs 800-526 0225) is available as a combination drug.
- Corticosteroids may be useful for ocular complications and CNS disease.
- Reassess to determine if longer therapy needed.

#### Immunocompromised
- Confirmed acute infection by serology/symptoms:
  - Treat with pyrimethamine and folinic acid plus sulfadiazine or clindamycin for 4–6 wk after resolution of symptoms.
  - Alternative medications:
    ○ Trimethoprim–sulfamethoxazole
    ○ Pyrimethamine and folinic acid plus dapsone
- CNS symptoms plus a lesion on CT or MRI:
  - Treat empirically with pyrimethamine and folinic acid plus sulfadiazine or clindamycin.
  - Brain biopsy or CSF to confirm diagnosis
  - Administer anticonvulsants only if confirmed prior seizures:
    ○ Poorer outcome for patients on anticonvulsants

- Chronic asymptomatic infection:
  - No therapy required
  - Prophylaxis options for toxoplasmosis in AIDS and immunosuppressed patients:
    ○ Trimethoprim–sulfamethoxazole; lifelong prophylaxis should be considered in HIV patients after consultation.
    ○ Pyrimethamine (75 mg/wk) and dapsone (200 mg/wk)

#### Ocular
- Treat with pyrimethamine and sulfadiazine for 1 month.
- May add clindamycin
- Administer systemic steroids with macular or optic nerve involvement.

#### Acute Acquired Infection in Pregnancy
- Initially treat with spiramycin pending confirmatory tests and consultation (FDA, Division of Special Pathograns and Transplant Drug Products 301-796-1600).
- After the infection is documented, initiate treatment after consultation:
  - Spiramycin in the first 17 wk
  - Pyrimethamine and sulfadiazine after 17 wk
- Spiramycin may reduce congenital transmission but does not treat fetus if infection is in placenta; maternal therapy may decrease severity of congenital disease.
- Treat congenital infection with sulfadiazine, pyrimethamine, and folinic acid for 12 mo.
- Prevention of exposure in seronegative pregnant women is important when contacting cats or their excrement.

### MEDICATION
- Clindamycin:
  - 600 mg (peds: 20–40 mg/kg/24 hr) IV q6h
  - 300 mg (peds: 8–20 mg/kg/24 hr) PO q6h
- Dapsone: 100 mg PO per day (child >1 mo 2 mg/kg PO per day)
- Folinic acid: 5–10 mg PO daily in conjunction with pyrimethamine
- Pyrimethamine: 100 mg b.i.d. on first day loading dose, then 25–50 mg PO per day then 0.5—1 mg/kg/24 hr)
- Spiramycin: FDA authorization required
- Sulfadiazine: 500 mg–2 g (peds: 100–200 mg/kg/24 hr) PO q6h
- Trimethoprim–sulfamethoxazole: 5 mg/kg of trimethoprim component IV or PO q6h

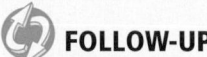 FOLLOW-UP

### DISPOSITION
#### Admission Criteria
- Acute infection with severe systemic symptoms
- Immunocompromised patients with:
  - Toxoplasmosis encephalitis
  - Pneumonitis
  - Sepsis

#### Discharge Criteria
- Immunocompetent patients with:
  - Mild symptoms
  - Ocular
- Maternal/congenital infection with mild symptoms

#### Issues for Referral
Infectious disease consultant

## ADDITIONAL READING
- American Academy of Pediatrics. *Red Book 2009 Report of the Committee on Infectious Diseases*. Elk Grove, IL: AAP; 2009.
- Centers for Disease Control and Prevention. Guidelines for prevention and treatment of opportunistic infections in HIV infected adults and adolescents. *MMWR*. 1009;58:1–207. http://www.cdc.gov/mmwr/pdf/rr/rr58e324.pdf
- Rodriguez JC, Martinez MM, et al. Evaluation of different techniques in the diagnosis of *Toxoplasma* encephalitis. *J Med Microbiol*. 1997;46:597–601.
- Sciammarella J. Toxoplasmosis. July 6, 2002. http://www.emedicine.com/emerg/topic601.htm

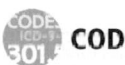 CODES

### ICD9
130.9 Toxoplasmosis, unspecified

T

# TRANSFUSION COMPLICATIONS

*Jason J. Prystowsky*

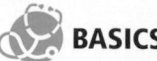 **BASICS**

## EPIDEMIOLOGY

- Some type of transfusion reaction occurs in 2% of units given during or within 24 hr of use.
- Noninfectious complications:
  - Febrile nonhemolytic reaction: RBCs 1 in 500 transfusions, platelets 1 in 900
  - Allergic reaction (nonanaphylactic): 1 in 3 to 1 in 300
  - Anaphylaxis: 1 in 20,000 to 1 in 50,000
  - Acute hemolytic reaction: 1 in 38,000 to 1 in 70,000
  - Delayed hemolytic reaction: 1 in 4,000 to 1 in 11,000
  - Transfusion-associated circulatory overload (TACO): 1 in 100, but as high as 10% in susceptible populations
  - Alloimmunization: 1 in 10 to 1 in 100
  - Graft-versus-host disease: 1 in 400,000; rare but has >90% mortality.
  - TRALI (transfusion-related lung injury): 1 in 5,000 to 1 in 190,000; represents 13% of reported transfusion-related deaths
  - Iron overload: Unknown incidence, depends on volume of blood, often occurs after >100 RBC units
  - Hypocalcemia: Unknown incidence, depends on volume of blood; due to citrate toxicity
  - Hyperkalemia: Unknown incidence, depends on volume of blood, rate of transfusion, and duration of blood storage prior to transfusion.
- Infectious complications:
  - Bacterial contamination: RBCs 1 in 65,000 to 1 in 500,000; platelets 1 in 1,000 to 1 in 10,000:
    - ○ Most common bacterial agents: *Yersinia enterocolitica*, *Psuedomonas spp*, *Serratia spp*.
    - ○ Leading cause of mortality among infectious complications; 17% to 22% of all cases
  - Hepatitis C: 1 in 1.6 million
  - Hepatitis B: 1 in 100,000 to 1 in 400,000
  - HTLV I and II: 1 in 500,000 to 1 in 3 million
  - HIV: 1 in 1.4 million to 4.7 million
  - HAV: 1 in 1,000,000
  - B19 Parvovirus: 1 in 40,000; posttransfusion anemia rare with scattered case reports
  - Parasites: *Babesia* and malaria: <1 in 1 million
  - Parasites: *Trypanosoma cruzi*: 1 in 42,000
  - Case reports of Epstein–Barr virus, Lyme disease, brucellosis, human herpesvirus, Creutzfeld–Jacob disease

## Acute Intravascular Hemolytic Transfusion Reaction

- Mortality and morbidity correlate with amount of incompatible blood transfused (symptoms can occur with exposure to as little as 5–20 mL)
- Occurs immediately from:
  - ABO incompatibility
  - Blood type identification error
  - Incompatible transfused cells immediately destroyed by antibodies

- Intravascular hemolysis causing activation of coagulation system, leading to inflammation, shock, and DIC
- Mediators (cytokines) released during inflammatory response
- Renal failure:
  - Cytokines cause local release of endothelin in kidney, causing vasoconstriction.
  - Leads to parenchymal ischemia and acute renal failure
- Respiratory failure owing to pulmonary edema/adult ARDS:
  - Free hemoglobin (Hb) causes vasoconstriction in pulmonary vasculature.

## Other Transfusion-Related Complications

- Hemolysis because of Rh incompatibility:
  - Mild, self-limiting
  - 1:200 units transfused
- Febrile nonhemolytic transfusions reaction:
  - Most common transfusion reaction
  - Temperature increases at least 1°C with chills within 6 hr
  - Antigen–antibody reaction to transfused blood components (WBCs, platelets, plasma)
  - Usually mild
  - Occurs more often with multiparous women or multiple transfusions
  - Recurs in 15% of patients
  - Febrile nonhemolytic transfusion reaction is a diagnosis of exclusion.
  - Acetaminophen may be used prophylactically; its use as premedication is controversial, though not harmful.
- Allergic transfusion reaction:
  - Occurs in 1% of transfusions
  - Usually seen with immunoglobulin A (IgA)–deficient patients
  - Urticaria alone is not a reason to stop transfusion.
  - Antihistamine may be used as therapy or prophylactically.
- Premedicating transfusions with acetaminophen and diphenhydramine found to have no effect on incidence of transfusion reaction compared with placebo in some trials.

## Delayed Reactions

- Infection:
  - HIV, hepatitis B, hepatitis C
    - ○ Blood screened for viruses
    - ○ Blood treated to inactivate viruses
    - ○ Blood donors with recent history of travel or poor health are deferred from donating.
- Delayed extravascular hemolytic reaction:
  - Occurs 7–10 days after transfusion
  - Antigen–antibody reaction that develops after transfusion
  - Coombs test positive
  - Usually asymptomatic
  - Blood bank analysis detects antibody.

- Electrolyte imbalance:
  - Hypocalcemia: Calcium binds to citrate
  - Hyper/hypokalemia: Citrate metabolized to bicarbonate, which drives potassium intracellularly; prolonged storage of blood may cause hemolysis and hyperkalemia
- Graft-versus-host disease:
  - Fatal in >90%
  - Immunologically competent lymphocytes transfused into immunocompetent host
  - Host unable to destroy new WBCs
  - Donor WBCs recognize host as foreign and attack host's tissues.
- Anaphylactic reaction:
  - Can occur with <10 mL of exposure
  - Generalized flushing, urticaria, laryngeal edema, bronchospasm, profound hypotension, shock, or cardiac arrest all possible
  - Treat with subcutaneous epinephrine, supportive hemodynamic and respiratory care.
- Transfusion-related lung injury (TRALI):
  - Symptoms typically begin with 6 hr of transfusion.
  - Acute onset of respiratory distress, bilateral pulmonary edema, fever, tachycardia, hypotension, with normal cardiac function
  - 3rd most common cause of fatal transfusion
  - Difficult to distinguish from ARDS and TACO; often misdiagnosed and underreported
  - Provide supportive care.
  - Disease is typically self-limited within 96 hr.
  - Mortality is 5–10%.
  - Diuretics contraindicated

### Pediatric Considerations

Blood can be transfused through 22-gauge peripheral catheter under pressure (but less than 300 mm Hg) with minimal hemolysis.

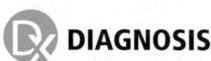 **DIAGNOSIS**

## SIGNS AND SYMPTOMS

- General:
  - Fevers
  - Chills
  - Burning at infusion site
  - Urticaria/pruritus/skin erythema
- Pulmonary:
  - Dyspnea
  - Bronchospasm
  - Respiratory distress/failure
- Cardiovascular:
  - Tachycardia
  - Hypotension
  - Substernal chest pain/tightness
- GI:
  - Nausea
  - Vomiting
  - Diarrhea

- Hematologic:
  - Bleeding
  - Hemoglobinuria
  - Oozing from surgical wounds
  - Jaundice
  - DIC
- Miscellaneous:
  - Low back pain
  - Renal failure (oliguria/anuria)
  - Classic triad of fever, flank pain, and red–brown urine of acute hemolytic reactions is rarely seen.

## ESSENTIAL WORKUP
- Recognize clinical findings of transfusion reaction.
- Recheck identifying information of blood and patient compatibility.
- Recognize evidence of hypotension/shock, severe respiratory distress, sepsis, fever, and urticaria; intervene appropriately.

## DIAGNOSTIC TESTS & INTERPRETATION
### Lab
- CBC
- Electrolytes, BUN, creatinine, glucose:
  - For electrolyte abnormalities
- PT, PTT
- Serum calcium
- Fibrinogen, fibrin degradation products
- Bilirubin (direct/indirect)
- Coombs test
- Hemoglobinemia:
  - Pink or red supernatant of plasma or serum indicates hemolysis.
- Urinalysis:
  - Hemoglobinuria: Dipstick-positive blood without RBCs on micro
- Lab findings indicating hemolysis:
  Thrombocytopenia (<100,000)
  - Fibrinogenopenia (<150 mg/L)
  - Fibrin degradation products
  - Prolonged activated PTT (aPTT)
  - Spherocytosis
- Lab findings indicating hemolysis due to Rh incompatibility:
  - Positive Coombs test
  - Elevated indirect bilirubin
  - Posttransfusion hemoglobin/hematocrit not showing expected rise

### Imaging
Chest radiograph: Diffuse patchy infiltrates without cardiomegaly if TRALI.

### Diagnostic Procedures/Surgery
ECG for dysrhythmia, sign of electrolyte abnormality

## DIFFERENTIAL DIAGNOSIS
- Sepsis
- Anaphylaxis/allergic reaction to medication

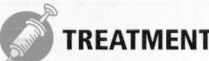 TREATMENT

### PRE-HOSPITAL
Routine stabilization

### INITIAL STABILIZATION/THERAPY
- Immediately stop infusion:
  - Severity of reaction proportional to amount of blood transfused
- ABCs
- Supplemental oxygen—intubation and mechanical ventilation if needed
- Recheck blood-identifying information—patient's bracelet, blood labels, call blood bank

### ED TREATMENT/PROCEDURES
- Hypotension:
  - 0.9% normal saline (NS) hydration with two large-bore IVs
  - Avoid Ringer lactate or solutions containing dextrose.
  - Trendelenburg position
  - Dopamine
- Prevention of renal failure:
  - Maintain urine output of 1 mL/kg/hr
  - Adequate hydration
    Furosemide or mannitol if oliguric
  - Dopamine infusion at 2 μg/kg/min
- Febrile reactions:
  - Antipyretics (acetaminophen/nonsteroidal anti-inflammatory drugs [NSAIDs])
  - Antihistamine (diphenhydramine + ranitidine) IV
  - Steroids (methylprednisolone)
- Allergic reactions:
  - Antihistamine (diphenhydramine + ranitidine) IV
  - Epinephrine for respiratory symptoms
  - Steroids (methylprednisolone)
- Redraw blood sample for repeat ABO/Rh typing, direct antiglobulin testing
- Foley catheter to monitor urine output
- Replenish calcium if hypocalcemia develops.
- Treat DIC.

### MEDICATION
- Calcium gluconate: 10 mL of 10% (peds. 100 mg/kg/dose) solution slow IV push
- Dopamine: 2–20 μg/kg/min IV
- Diphenhydramine: 25–50 mg (peds: 1.25 mg/kg) IV or PO
- Ranitidine: 50 mg IV (peds: 1–2 mg/kg per dose max 50 mg)
- Epinephrine (1 in 1,000): 0.3–0.5 mL (peds: 0.01 mL/kg) SC
- Methylprednisolone: 125 mg (peds: 2 mg/kg) IV

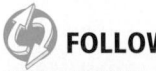 FOLLOW-UP

### DISPOSITION
#### Admission Criteria
- Acute hemolytic transfusion reaction, pulmonary complications, anaphylaxis, sepsis:
  - Require ICU monitoring
- Delayed hemolytic transfusion reactions for evaluation/treatment
- Electrolyte abnormalities requiring cardiac monitoring

#### Discharge Criteria
Uncomplicated febrile or allergic reaction

## PEARLS AND PITFALLS
- Blood transfusion is substantially overutilized and has significant associated risk, such as transfusion reactions, transmission of pathogens, and immune suppression.
- Maintaining body temperature during massive transfusion is crucial to correcting coagulopathy.
- Failure to properly compare patient identification to labeling on blood or failure to wait for fully cross-matched blood carries significant risks.
- Suspect acute intravascular hemolysis if patient develops hypotension, dark urine, or oozing from IV or other puncture sites.

## ADDITIONAL READING
- Bakdash D, Yazer M. What every physician should know about transfusion reactions. *CMAJ*. 2007;177:141–147.
- Kennedy LD, Case LD, Hurd DD, et al. A prospective, randomized, double-blind controlled trial of acetaminophen and diphenhydramine pretransfusion medication versus placebo for the prevention of transfusion reactions. *Transfusion*. 2008;48(11):2285–2291.
- Kuriyan M, Carson J. Blood transfusion risks in the intensive care unit. *Crit Care Clin*. 2004;20: 237–253.
- Shander A, Goodnaugh LT. Why an alternative to blood transfusion. *Crit Care Clin*. 2009;25:261–277.
- Tobian AA, King KE, Ness PM. Transfusion premedications: A growing practice not based on evidence. *Transfusion*. 2007;47:1089.

### See Also (Topic, Algorithm, Electronic Media Element)
- Allergic Reaction
- Anaphylaxis
- Disseminated Intravascular Coagulation
- Sepsis

 CODES

#### ICD9
- 999.6 Abo incompatibility reaction, not elsewhere classified
- 999.7 Rh incompatibility reaction, not elsewhere classified
- 999.89 Other transfusion reaction

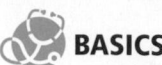

## BASICS

### DESCRIPTION
- Transient global amnesia (TGA) has the following features:
  - Episode of amnesia with abrupt onset
  - No focal neurologic signs or symptoms
  - Temporary, severe, anterograde amnesia:
    - Acute inability to form new memories
    - Permanent memory gap after the episode
  - Temporary long-ranging retrograde amnesia:
    - More recent memories at more risk
    - Previously encoded memories unavailable only temporarily
  - Gradually shrinks until only remaining memory deficit is the memory gap induced by the anterograde amnesia
- Incidence between 3.4 and 10 per 100,000 people:
  - 23.5 per 100,000 in people >50 yr of age
- Average age 61 yr:
  - TGA rare <40 yr
- Most attacks last between 1 and 8 hr (range 15 min–7 days).

### ETIOLOGY
- The exact etiology of TGA is unknown; speculation is controversial.
- Multimodal MRI, SPECT, and PET have shown some abnormalities of regional blood flow in selectively vulnerable hippocampal structures.
- Speculated causes:
  - Vasoconstriction due to hyperventilation:
    - Psychogenic hyperventilation in setting of age-related cerebrovascular autoregulatory dysfunction
  - Venous congestion with Valsalva:
    - Ultrasonography has suggested internal jugular vein incompetence
  - Migraine (in younger patients)
- No clear correlation between TGA and thromboembolic cerebrovascular disease has been found.

## DIAGNOSIS

### SIGNS AND SYMPTOMS
Diagnostic criteria:
- Attack must be witnessed.
- Acute onset of anterograde amnesia
- No alteration in consciousness
- No cognitive impairment except amnesia
- No loss of personal information (eg, name, birth date, address, etc.)
- No focal neurologic symptoms
- No epileptic features
- No recent history of head trauma or seizures
- Attack must resolve within 24 hr.
- Other causes of amnesia excluded.

### *History*
- Often precipitated by stressful condition:
  - Cough, Valsalva
  - Physical exertion
  - Sexual intercourse
  - Extreme fright or shock
  - Intense heat or cold
- Patient will likely feel that something is wrong:
  - May ask "how did I get here?"
  - Will be generally aware of attack
- May have other subtle transient symptoms at onset, such as headache, dizziness, nausea
- Historical features helpful in excluding other diagnoses are:
  - Onset of attack witnessed, with no seizure activity or epileptiform features noted
  - No history of seizures in prior 2 mo
  - No history of recent traumatic brain injury
  - Acute anterograde amnesia with relatively preserved remote memory

### *Physical Exam*
- Marked anterograde amnesia
- Most cases (≤90% in case series) will demonstrate repetitive questioning.
- Neurologic and general exam normal
- TGA patient will not have findings of an acute confusional state or dementia and will not:
  - Be somnolent, inattentive, or globally confused
  - Confabulate
  - Be disoriented to name, birth date, address, phone number, date
  - Have problems performing complex tasks and following complex commands
- Aphasia, apraxia, and agnosia are not findings consistent with TGA.

### ESSENTIAL WORKUP
- True TGA can be diagnosed with a careful history and physical alone.
- If clinical diagnosis is certain, no other workup is essential.

### DIAGNOSTIC TESTS & INTERPRETATION
Testing indicated only when the diagnosis is uncertain.

#### *Lab*
- CBC, comprehensive chemistries including glucose, LFTs, NH3, thyroid studies, and UA for organic metabolic etiologies where implicated
- Tox screen, alcohol level for tox etiologies where suspected

#### *Imaging*
- Consider MRI if indicated.
- Head CT for intracranial mass if indicated

#### *Diagnostic Procedures/Surgery*
- EEG for seizure if suspected
- Lumbar puncture and CSF analysis for encephalitis if suspected

### DIFFERENTIAL DIAGNOSIS
- Since TGA is a unique and very characteristic entity, there is little in the way of a differential diagnosis to consider.
- Other entities may present somewhat similarly but will have historical or exam features that readily distinguish them from TGA:
  - Acute confusional state/Korsakoff syndrome/metabolic disorder:
    - Alcohol, medication, or toxin ingestion
    - Decreased attention or other findings of an encephalopathy
    - Impairment with serial 7's or spelling "world" backwards
    - Able to lay down new memory if allowed time to encode
  - Complex partial seizures/epileptic amnestic attacks:
    - Witnessed epileptiform activity or features (eg, blank stares, automatisms)
    - Short duration (typically <30 min; TGA lasts hours)
    - No repetitive questioning
    - Frequent and rapid recurrences

- Psychogenic amnesia:
  ○ Younger patient with a known psychiatric stressor
  ○ Psychiatric history or history of personality changes
  ○ Typically no anterograde amnesia (only a retrograde gap)
  ○ Psychogenic memory loss for personal identification, name, birth date, etc.
- Temporal lobe brain lesion or encephalitis affecting the temporal lobe:
  ○ Typically with other associated neurologic symptoms (eg, visual field cut)
  ○ Progressive and permanent amnesia
- Previously unrecognized Alzheimer dementia:
  ○ Memory loss for personal information such as date, phone number, address
  ○ Signs of additional global cognitive impairment

 **TREATMENT**

**PRE-HOSPITAL**
There are no considerations in true TGA that are specific to the prehospital environment.

**INITIAL STABILIZATION/THERAPY**
There is no known effective therapy for TGA.

**ED TREATMENT/PROCEDURES**
- TGA is a self-limited, relatively benign entity.
- Observe the patient for improvement.
- Assuming a true diagnosis of TGA, no acute treatment beyond reassurance of patient and family is indicated.

**MEDICATION**
*First Line*
Not applicable

*Second Line*
Not applicable

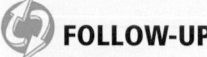 **FOLLOW-UP**

**DISPOSITION**
*Admission Criteria*
- Admission for further observation for patients without significant improvement at the time of disposition
- Patients with uncertain diagnosis
- Patients showing a trend toward resolution but who have suboptimal social support at home

*Discharge Criteria*
- A clear diagnosis of TGA
- Resolving or resolved amnesia
- Good social support

*Issues for Referral*
Refer patients with recurrent episodes of TGA to a neurologist:
- Recurrence rate of TGA is extremely low.
- Selected case series have revealed that patients in this subgroup have a different prognosis:
  - May have sustained focal cerebral blood flow abnormalities on specialized imaging
  - More likely to go on to develop clinical epilepsy

**FOLLOW-UP RECOMMENDATIONS**
Given median age of TGA patients (60 years), follow-up with primary care provider for general cardiovascular risk factor modification may be beneficial.
- No follow-up specific to TGA is indicated.
- See "Issues for Referral" for patient with recurrent episode of TGA.

**PEARLS AND PITFALLS**
- TGA is a distinct and relatively benign entity:
  - Acute onset of isolated anterograde amnesia
  - Resolves spontaneously

- Be aware of subtle features that may suggest a more pathologic alternative diagnosis:
  - Short, recurrent episodes or automatisms in epilepsy
  - Cognitive impairment with encephalopathy
  - Subtle neurologic signs in encephalitis
- If there is uncertainty regarding the diagnosis, the highest-yield tests may be MRI and EEG.

## ADDITIONAL READING

- Harrison M, Williams M. The diagnosis and management of transient global amnesia in the emergency department. *Emerg Med J.* 2007;24: 444–445.
- Owen D, Paranandi B, Sivakumar R, et al. Classical diseases revisited: Transient global amnesia. *Postgrad Med J.* 2007;83:236–239.
- Quinette P, Guillery-Girard B, Dayan J, et al. What does transient global amnesia really mean? Review of the literature and thorough study of 142 cases. *Brain.* 2006;129(Pt 7):1640–1658.
- Sander K, Sander D. New insights into transient global amnesia: Recent imaging and clinical findings. *Lancet Neurol.* 2005;4:437–444.
- Schreiber SJ, Doepp F, Klingebiel R, et al. Internal jugular vein incompetence and intracranial venous anatomy in transient global amnesia. *J Neurol Neurosurg Psychiatry.* 2005;76:509–513.

**See Also (Topic, Algorithm, Electronic Media Element)**
- Delirium
- Dementia

 **CODES**

**ICD9**
437.7 Transient global amnesia

# TRANSIENT ISCHEMIC ATTACK

Alexander Blau
Rebecca Smith-Coggins

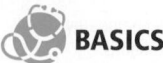 **BASICS**

## DESCRIPTION

- Classically a temporary neurologic deficit that resolves within 24 hr due to transient decrease in blood supply:
  - 80%, however, resolve in <30 min.
- Current definition tissue-based, not time-based:
  - Infarction can occur independent of symptom duration
  - Tissue injury established by neuroimaging
- Contrasts with other ischemic neurologic conditions:
  - Stroke in evolution—neurologic deficits that continue to worsen over minutes to hours
  - Completed stroke—persistent deficit after 3 wk despite improvement

## ETIOLOGY

Mechanism

- Transient cerebral hypoperfusion from:
  - Low flow state from atherosclerotic lesions of large arteries (eg, internal carotid origin, middle cerebral artery stem, junction of vertebral and basilar artery)
  - Embolus from extracranial circulation
  - Local thrombus formation
  - Vasculopathy (eg, carotid or vertebral dissection, Takayasu, Moyamoya)
  - Decreased perfusion pressure or hyperviscosity

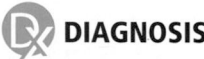 **DIAGNOSIS**

## SIGNS AND SYMPTOMS

- The vessel and extent of involvement dictate neurologic deficits.
- Carotid artery (anterior circulation):
  - Manifests signs and symptoms of both anterior cerebral artery (ACA) and middle cerebral artery (MCA) involvement
- ACA:
  - Motor and sensory—contralateral leg > arm, ± face
  - Verbal—anarthria (speechlessness), dysarthria, perseveration
  - Visual—amaurosis fugax, blurred vision on one side of field of vision of both eyes opposite to side of diseased artery
  - Contralateral neglect
  - Frontal release signs, altered behavior
- MCA:
  - Motor and sensory—contralateral arm and face > lower extremity
  - Visual—homonymous hemianopsia, gaze preference to side of infarct
  - Dominant—receptive and/or expressive aphasia
  - Non-dominant—inattention, neglect, apraxia

- Vertebrobasilar system (posterior circulation):
  - Crossed deficits
  - Visual—diplopia/gaze palsy, homonymous field defect, nystagmus
  - Vestibulocerebellar—dizziness, vertigo, ataxia
  - "Top of the Basilar" syndrome—hallucination, altered alertness and memory, gaze palsy
  - Wallenberg syndrome—ipsilateral cranial nerve deficits, contralateral motor weakness, gait and limb ataxia, and incomplete Horner syndrome (anhydrosis usually absent)
  - "Drop attack"—sudden onset of inability to walk, often with vertigo, headache, neck pain, and nausea/vomiting
- Lacunes/subcortical areas:
  - Classically with stepwise/progressive onset
  - Pure motor or sensory deficits
  - Motor deficit is unilateral and equal in face/arm/leg.
  - Ataxic hemiparesis
  - Clumsy hand–dysarthria syndrome

## History

- Timing—establishing time of onset, duration, and tempo of symptoms is critical to management, risk stratification and building a differential diagnosis
- Prior TIAs:
  - Patient high-risk if crescendo symptoms or recurrent episodes despite medical therapy
  - History of recurrent symptoms that vary by vascular territory suggests cardioembolic phenomena
- Identification of risk factors for vascular and heart disease:
  - Risk assessment may impact ED disposition

## ESSENTIAL WORKUP

- Neurologic evaluation assessing level of consciousness, mentation, vision, ICP, cranial nerves, motor and sensory function, coordination, speech, and signs of neglect
- Noncontrast head CT to rule out hemorrhage
- ECG and cardiac monitoring to diagnose atrial fibrillation, myocardial infarction, or other cardiac abnormalities
- Glucose level

## DIAGNOSTIC TESTS & INTERPRETATION
### Lab

- CBC: Assess for anemia or signs of hyperviscosity (elevated hematocrit or thrombocytosis).
- Electrolytes: Evaluate for hyponatremia or other abnormalities that can mimic stroke
- Finger stick glucose: Rule out hypoglycemia
- Coagulation studies ± thrombophilic studies:
  - Investigate for hypercoagulable state, establish baseline for possible anticoagulation therapy.
- Toxicologic screen:
  - Cocaine- or amphetamine-induced ischemia
  - Especially in younger patients
- Arterial blood gases
- Cardiac enzymes
- Lipid panel
- Blood cultures and ESR if endocarditis suspected

## Imaging

- Noncontrast head CT:
  - Primarily to assess for hemorrhage
  - Sensitivity >90% for subarachnoid bleed
  - Ischemic evidence on CT often does not appear until >6 hr after symptom onset.
- MRI—identifies and distinguishes ischemia and infarcts earlier than CT but is less sensitive for hemorrhage:
  - Diffusion-weighted imaging (DWI) scans are sensitive for infarct within the 1st few hours of symptom onset
  - Better modality for posterior circulation (magnetic resonance angiography)
  - Improved detection of posterior bleeding
- Carotid duplex scan:
  - Indicated with crescendo TIAs or when a high-grade carotid obstruction is suspected
  - Can detect stenosis of >60% but cannot distinguish 95% from 100% occlusion
  - Positive findings would suggest candidacy for urgent CEA or anticoagulation.
- Echo—may demonstrate cardioembolic source (mural thrombus, tumor, or valvular vegetation)
- Angiography—gold standard for detection of both stenosis and aneurysm of cerebral vasculature:
  - Cost, availability, and invasiveness may preclude its use.

## Diagnostic Procedures/Surgery

- ECG/cardiac monitoring—to evaluate for cardiac activity that may predispose to embolism or low-perfusion states

## DIFFERENTIAL DIAGNOSIS

- Subarachnoid/intracerebral hemorrhage
- Subdural/epidural hematoma
- Brain aneurysm or arteriovenous malformation
- Giant cell arteritis
- Air embolism
- Migraine headache
- Todd's paralysis
- Ménière disease
- Benign positional vertigo
- Vestibular neuronitis
- Seizures/epilepsy
- Brain tumor/mass
- Syncope
- Peripheral nerve or nerve root compression
- Dementia
- Hepatic/renal/hypertensive encephalopathy
- Wernicke encephalopathy
- Carotid dissection after neck trauma
- Hypoglycemia
- Diabetic ketoacidosis/hyperosmolar coma
- Multiple sclerosis
- Hyperventilation
- Hysteria or other psychiatric disease

### Pediatric Considerations

- Severe dehydration with associated hypernatremia
- Congenital heart disease
- Sickle cell anemia
- Meningitis
- Acute and congenital hemiplegia of childhood
- Moyamoya disease:
  - Rare primary vascular disease defined by diffuse cerebral arterial narrowing that manifests as reoccurring TIAs

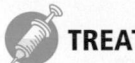 TREATMENT

## PRE-HOSPITAL

- Cautions:
  - Initial assessment of neurologic deficits crucial as they may resolve prior to ED arrival
  - Avoid glucose-containing fluids, except with confirmed hypoglycemia

## INITIAL STABILIZATION/THERAPY

- Airway: support as needed
- Breathing: oxygen
- Circulation: careful hydration with avoidance of cerebral edema and decreased cerebral blood flow (CBF)

## ED TREATMENT/PROCEDURES

- Early evaluation to prevent transient ischemia from converting to infarct
- Neurology consultation:
  Evaluation by neurology within 24 hr of symptom onset has been shown to reduce short-term risk of stroke.
- Antiplatelet therapy with aspirin
  - 30–325 mg of aspirin daily reduces risk of stroke by 20% after prior stroke or TIA.
- Full anticoagulation with heparin may be indicated with atrial fibrillation or following neurology consultation if patient is having recurrent symptoms or minor stroke.
  - Transition to warfarin with target INR of 2.5 for patients with atrial fibrillation
- Patients with aspirin failure can be started on clopidogrel, ticlopidine, or aspirin-dipyridamole.
- HTN:
  - Only patients suspected to have neurologic findings from HTN (eg, hypertensive encephalopathy) should be treated acutely with agents such as nitroprusside, nicardipine, or labetalol.
  - Avoid aggressive BP reduction, as stroke treatment requires maintained perfusion to the brain.
- Patients with TIA and high-grade carotid stenosis (>70%) benefit from carotid endarterectomy within 2 wk of symptom onset.

## MEDICATION

- Aspirin: 50–325 mg PO daily
- Aspirin-dipyridamole: 25/200 mg PO BID
- Clopidogrel: 75 mg PO daily

- Heparin: 5000 IU SC q8h–q12h, or 5,000–7,500 IU IV bolus; 1,000 IU/h infusion
- Labetalol 20 mg/min IV bolus, then 20–80 mg q10min; max. 300 mg; infusion 0.5–2 mg/min IV
- Nicardipine: 5 mg/h IV infusion, increase by 2.5 mg/h q5min–q15min; max. 15 mg/h, pediatric dosing unavailable
- Nitroprusside (adults and peds): 0.25–10 $\mu$g/kg/min IV
- Ticlopidine: 250 mg PO BID

 FOLLOW-UP

## DISPOSITION

### Admission Criteria

- Controversial, disposition decisions are best made in conjunction with neurology.
- Consider admission when:
  - Recurrent TIA and taking aspirin, clopidogrel, aspirin-dipyridamole, ticlopidine, or warfarin
  - Known hypercoagulable state
  - Vertebrobasilar TIA
  - Possible cardioembolic source (eg, atrial fibrillation, infective endocarditis)
  - Symptomatic internal carotid stenosis >50%
  - "Crescendo" TIAs (>3 ischemic events in a 72-hr period that increase in frequency, duration, or severity of symptoms)
  - Event within 72 hr and ABCD2 score >= 3
    - Age ≥60 = 1 point
    - BP ≥140/90 = 1 point
    - Clinical features (unilateral weakness = 2 points; isolated speech disturbance = 1 point)
    - Duration of symptoms (≥60 min = 2 points; 10–59 min = 1 point)
    - Diabetes = 1 point

### Discharge Criteria

- Completely asymptomatic patients with extensively investigated condition or patients presenting with TIAs >1 wk before ED visit may be discharged as long as appropriate follow-up is ensured.
- Absence of high-risk features:
  - Vertebrobasilar TIA
  - High-grade carotid stenosis (>50%)
  - "Crescendo" TIAs
  - Recurrent TIA on maximal antiplatelet therapy
  - Suspected cardioembolic source
- Patients with contraindications to antiplatelet therapy or surgery may be discharged if stable.
- ABCD2 score of 0–2 and ability to complete outpatient workup within 2 days of discharge.
- Prognosis:
  - Overall 4% risk of stroke at 2 days
  - Overall 9% risk of stroke at 90 days
  - 1.0% risk of stroke at 2 days for ABCD2 <4
  - 8.1% risk of stroke at 2 days for ABCD2 >5
  - Overall 5-yr risk of stroke after TIA is ~25%

### Pediatric Considerations

All children with TIA require admission for close monitoring of BP, fluid status, and neurologic status in pediatric intensive care.

## FOLLOW-UP RECOMMENDATIONS

- Primary MD follow-up is essential for long-term medication management and counseling regarding appropriate lifestyle modification.
- Vascular surgery consultation within 1 wk and CEA within 2 wk for patients with significant carotid artery stenosis.
- Cardiology follow-up for patients with underlying arrhythmia, cardiomyopathy, valvular disease, or CAD.

## PEARLS AND PITFALLS

- Failure to identify a carotid stenosis prior to discharging a patient with anterior circulation TIA.
- Failure to recognize an emergent alternate diagnosis (eg, intracranial hemorrhage, hypoglycemia).
- Neurology consultation should be obtained prior to ED discharge as stroke risk–reduction has been demonstrated with early evaluation.

## ADDITIONAL READING

- Easton JD, Saver JL, Albers GW, et al. Definition and Evaluation of Transient Ischemic Attack: A Scientific Statement for Healthcare Professionals From the American Heart Association/American Stroke Association Stroke Council; Council on Cardiovascular Surgery and Anesthesia; Council on Cardiovascular Radiology and Intervention; Council on Cardiovascular Nursing; and the Interdisciplinary Council on Peripheral Vascular Disease. *Stroke.* 2009;40:2276–2293.
- Thacker EL, Wiggins KL, Rice KM, et al. Short-Term and Long-Term Risk of Incident Ischemic Stroke After Transient Ischemic Attack. *Stroke.* 2010;41: 239–243.
- Shah KH, Metz HA, Edlow JA. Clinical prediction rules to stratify short-term risk of stroke among patients diagnosed in the emergency department with a transient ischemic attack. *Ann Emerg Med.* 2009;53:662–673.
- Carpenter CR, Keim SM, Crossley J, et al. Post transient ischemic attack early stroke stratification: the ABCD(2) prognostic aid. *J Emerg Med.* 2009;36:194–198.

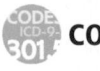 CODES

**ICD9**
435.9 Unspecified transient cerebral ischemia

T

# TRANSPLANT REJECTION

*Tarina Lee Kang*

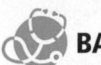 **BASICS**

## DESCRIPTION
- A transplant recipient's immune response to a graft's genetically dissimilar antigens resulting in rejection of the transplanted organ
- HLA incompatibility:
  – Most common cause of rejection
  – Rejection of solid organ transplants
- Antibodies blood group incompatibility:
  – Much less of a risk to graft survival than HLA incompatibility
  – May result in hyperacute rejection of primarily vascularized grafts, such as kidney and heart
- 3 phases of rejection:
  – Hyperacute:
    ○ Occurs in the immediate postoperative period
    ○ Antibody reaction to red cells or HLA antigens
    ○ Endothelial damage
    ○ Platelets accumulate, thrombi develop, and tissue necrosis occurs.
    ○ Rare with careful donor–recipient matching
  – Acute:
    ○ Usually occurs within the 1st months after transplantation but may happen at any time if immunosuppressant medication is stopped
    ○ T cell-dependent process whereby inflammatory cells infiltrate the allograft releasing cellular and humoral factors that destroy the graft
    ○ Presents with constitutional symptoms and signs of transplant organ insufficiency
  – Chronic:
    ○ Occurs over years
    ○ Results in the gradual failure of the transplanted organ

## ETIOLOGY
- Reduction or noncompliance with medication:
  – Medication interactions with cyclosporine, tacrolimus, or sirolimus
  – Phenobarbital, phenytoin, carbamazepine, rifampin, isoniazid
- Kidney transplant rejection:
  – Early rejection caused by T and B lymphocytes, which attack microvasculature and impair graft perfusion; volume depletion, hypotension, infection
  – Chronic rejection caused by progressive nephrosclerosis of renal vessels, infection
- Cardiac transplant rejection:
  – Acute rejection occurs in 75–85% of patients within the 1st 3–6 mo.
  – Acute rejection due to T-cell–mediated response
  – Accelerated atherosclerosis is the hallmark of chronic rejection and presents as CHF, ventricular dysrhythmias, hypotension, syncope, or sudden death.
- Lung transplant rejection:
  – Rejection develops early.
  – 25–40% develop chronic rejection.
  – Rejection caused by endothelial, vascular, and lymphocyte inflammation, recurrent acute rejection
- Liver transplant rejection:
  – Commonly follows reduction in the immunosuppression regimen

- Bone marrow transplant rejection:
  – Acute graft-versus-host disease (immune attack of donor marrow on lung tissue)
  – Chronic graft-versus-host disease (incidence, 25–50% of patients)
  – Marrow rejection:
    ○ Most frequent in patients with aplastic anemia who do not receive total body radiotherapy or in patients receiving mismatched or unrelated transplants

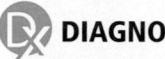 **DIAGNOSIS**

## SIGNS AND SYMPTOMS
- Renal transplant rejection:
  – Progressive systemic HTN
  – Decreased urine output
  – Swelling, fever, and tenderness:
    ○ Uncommon with immunosuppressive therapy
- Heart transplant rejection:
  – Fever
  – Dyspnea
  – Syncope, near-syncope
  – Nausea, vomiting
  – Chest pain
  – Hypotension or poorly controlled HTN
  – Palpitations
  – Can be asymptomatic
- Lung transplant rejection:
  – Cough
  – Dyspnea
  – Fever
  – Rales
  – Rhonchi
- Liver transplant rejection:
  – Fever
  – Right upper quadrant pain
  – Jaundice
- Bone marrow transplant rejection:
  – Fever
  – Generalized wasting
  – Dyspnea
  – Cough
  – Hypoxia
  – Chest pain
  – Rash
  – Mucositis
  – Keratoconjunctivitis
  – Dysphagia
  – Abdominal pain
  – Diarrhea
  – Jaundice
  – Encephalopathy
  – Seizures

## ESSENTIAL WORKUP
- Careful history of changes in medication
- Low threshold for screening labs and imaging for transplant rejection even with minimal signs and symptoms

## DIAGNOSTIC TESTS & INTERPRETATION
### Lab
- CBC
- Blood levels of immunosuppressant medications:
  – Levels may not represent trough if patient took medication prior to ED visit.
- Blood cultures
- Renal transplant rejection:
  – Electrolytes, BUN, creatinine
  – Urinalysis:
    ○ Presence of leukocytes may be seen during rejection as well as with infection.
    ○ Fractional excretion of sodium to help differentiate rejection from iatrogenic causes
- Heart transplant rejection:
  – Cardiac troponin T
- Lung transplant rejection:
  – ABG
- Liver transplant rejection:
  – Liver function tests
  – Late acute rejection presents with elevated bilirubin and transaminases.
- Bone marrow transplant rejection:
  – ABG
  – Liver function tests

### Imaging
- CXR:
  – Diffuse infiltrates are seen in early acute lung rejection, but when rejection occurs >1 mo after transplantation, radiographs may be normal or unchanged.
  – Bone marrow transplant rejection:
    ○ Interstitial infiltrates, pleural effusion, pulmonary edema
- Renal US:
  – Indicated for suspicion of renal transplant rejection:
    ○ Demonstration of hydronephrosis implies obstructive uropathy and warrants urgent percutaneous nephrostomy.
- ECG:
  – Assess for changes in cardiac output in patients at risk for rejection of a heart transplant.
- Suspicion of liver transplant rejection:
  – Hepatic US
  – CT abdomen

### Diagnostic Procedures/Surgery
- EKG:
  – Heart transplant rejection:
    ○ Commonly demonstrates 2 P waves because the native sinus node is left in place
    ○ Decreased quasi-random signal voltage, new S3, or new CHF or atrial arrhythmias suggest rejection.
- Renal transplant rejection:
  – Allograft biopsy
- Heart transplant rejection:
  – Endomyocardial biopsy
- Lung transplant rejection:
  – Pulmonary function tests
  – Bronchoscopy/biopsy

## DIFFERENTIAL DIAGNOSIS
- Infections:
  - Wide variety of bacterial, mycobacterial, fungal, viral, and parasitic pathogens can cause opportunistic infections in transplant patients.
- Immunosuppressant toxicity
- Drug interactions with immunosuppressant medication
- Renal transplant rejection:
  - Any disorder that can affect the native kidneys can also occur in the transplant recipient.
  - Iatrogenic nephrotoxicity:
    - Cyclosporine, tacrolimus
    - May be exacerbated by other medication
  - Urinary tract infection/pyelonephritis:
    - Classic organisms as with native kidney infections
    - Tubulointerstitial nephritis caused by the BK-polyoma virus (incidence 3–5%)
  - Acute occlusion of the transplant renal artery or vein:
    - Acute occlusion usually occurs within the 1st posttransplant week (incidence 0.5–8%) and causes oligoanuria and acute renal failure.
  - Peritransplant hematoma
  - Urinary leak
  - Lymphocele
  - Obstructive uropathy
  - Bleeding after renal graft biopsy
- Lung transplant rejection:
  - Cytomegalovirus pneumonia is the most common pathogen in transplanted lungs.
  - Aspergillus is the most common fungal infection.
  - Upper respiratory infection or bronchitis:
    - Mimic chronic lung rejection
  - Medication-induced pneumonitis
- Liver transplant rejection:
  - Ascending cholangitis:
    - Occurs because the biliary stent is left in place for months after surgery and can be colonized
  - Cholestatic hepatitis from azathioprine
  - Methotrexate-induced hepatotoxicity

## TREATMENT

### PRE-HOSPITAL
Avoid aggressive fluid resuscitation.

### INITIAL STABILIZATION/THERAPY
- ABCs
- Shock state treated with IV fluids and pressor agents
- Treat hypertensive crisis like other hypertensive emergencies.

### ED TREATMENT/PROCEDURES
- For kidney, heart, lung, and liver rejection, administer IV methylprednisolone:
  - Stress-dose corticosteroid coverage is also indicated in any ill-appearing transplant patient.
- Avoid blood transfusions because these need special screening to prevent transmission of disease.

- Heart transplant rejection:
  - Pressors and inotropics work as usual in the transplanted heart.
  - Atropine will have no effect on bradycardia because there is no vagal innervation.
  - Use dopamine, epinephrine drips, or external pacing to increase heart rate if bradycardia is symptomatic.
- Common immunosuppressive regimens are cyclosporine, prednisone, and azathioprine or tacrolimus (formerly known as FK506), and prednisone.
- Mycophenolate mofetil:
  - May reduce incidence of chronic allograft nephropathy, with less HTN and hyperuricemia than earlier regimens

### MEDICATION
- Cyclosporine: 5–6 mg/kg PO q12h; maintenance dose determined by blood level: 250–400 ng/mL (initial) 125–200 ng/mL (long term)
- Cyclosporine microemulsion: 4–5 mg/kg PO q12h; maintenance dose determined by blood level: 250–400 ng/mL (initial) 125–200 ng/mL (long term)
- Tacrolimus: 0.1 mg/kg PO q12h; maintenance dose determined by blood level 10–20 ng/mL (initial) 5–10 ng/mL (long term)
- Azathioprine: 1.5–2.5 mg/kg PO per day (adjusted for blood counts); blood-level monitoring not used in clinical practice
- Mycophenolate mofetil: 1.0–1.5 g PO q12h (adjusted according to GI adverse effects and blood counts); blood-level monitoring not used in clinical practice
- Prednisone: 0.5 mg/kg/d (initial) 0.1 mg/kg/d (long term)
- Sirolimus: 2–5 mg/d PO (adjusted according to level); blood level:10–20 ng/mL (initial) 5–15 ng/mL (long term)

 FOLLOW-UP

### DISPOSITION
#### Admission Criteria
- Admit transplant recipients with fever, shortness of breath, signs or symptoms of rejection, abdominal pain, or other signs of organ infection.
- Admit to the ICU patients who are septic or have cardiopulmonary compromise.

#### Discharge Criteria
Nontoxic patients in whom rejection or serious infection has been excluded may be discharged with close follow-up.

#### Issues for Referral
Treatment decisions should be made in consultation with the patient's oncologist, transplant surgeon, or organ specialist.

### FOLLOW-UP RECOMMENDATIONS
The patient's transplant team should actively participate in the follow-up plan:
- All attempts at verbal communication with the covering transplant physician should be made while the patient is in the ED with any symptoms suggestive of rejection.

## PEARLS AND PITFALLS
- Transplant patients presenting with minor complaints are at high risk for rejection and require an in-depth assessment in the ED, in conjunction with their transplant team.
- Patients with signs of possible transplant rejection should also be considered for infection and drug toxicity.

## ADDITIONAL READING
- Andrews PA. Renal transplantation. *Br Med J.* 2002;324:530–534.
- Buckley RH. Transplantation immunology: Organ and bone marrow. *J Allerg Clin Immunol.* 2003;111(2).
- Deng MC. Cardiac transplantation. *Heart.* 2002; 87:177–184.
- Jain A, Khanna A, Molmenti EP, et al. Immunosuppressive therapy. *Surg Clin North Am.* 1999;79:59–76.
- Noble-Jamieson G, Barnes N. Diagnosis and management of late complications after liver transplantation. *Arch Dis Child.* 1999;81:446–451.
- Sternbach GL, et al. Emergency department presentation and care of heart and heart/lung transplant recipients. *Ann Emerg Med.* 1992;21: 1140.
- Suthanthiran M, Strom TB. Mechanisms and management of acute renal allograft rejection. *Surg Clin North Am.* 1998;78:77–94.
- Venkat KK, Venkat A. Care of the renal transplant recipient in the emergency department. *Ann Emerg Med.* 2004;44(4):330–341.
- Yen KT. Pulmonary complications in bone marrow transplantation: A practical approach to diagnosis and treatment. *Clin Chest Med.* 2004;25(1): 189–201.

 CODES

ICD9
- 996.80 Complications of unspecified transplanted organ
- 996.81 Complications of transplanted kidney
- 996.82 Complications of transplanted liver

T

# TRAUMA, MULTIPLE
*Daniel Davis*

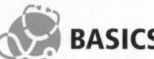 **BASICS**

## DESCRIPTION
- Standardized approach for rapid assessment of the trauma patient
- Although presented as a sequential method for gathering information, many of these steps can be performed simultaneously.
- Life-threatening injuries must be immediately addressed and treated before going on to the next level of care.
- With any change in the patient's status, the primary survey should be repeated.

## ETIOLOGY
Variety of causes such as:
- Motor vehicle/motorcycle crashes
- Falls from heights
- Assault
- Airplane crashes
- Train derailments
- Results of mass-casualty weapons
- Terrorism

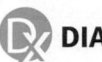 **DIAGNOSIS**

- Triage to a major trauma center is determined by local protocols.
- Injured patients with a need for surgical, neurosurgical, or orthopedic intervention should be transported to a major trauma center.
- Recent recommendations from the American College of Surgeons suggest that trauma victims with unstable vital signs should be taken to a Level I trauma center, where a larger volume of critically injured patients are seen.
- Primary survey should be performed at the scene and en route.

## SIGNS AND SYMPTOMS
- Primary survey (ABCDE):
  - Airway, cervical spine:
    - Look, listen, and palpate from nose/mouth to trachea/bronchial tree.
    - Assess airway patency.
    - Evaluate gag reflex.
    - Cervical spine must be immobilized with significant mechanism of injury and either altered mental status or distracting injuries or with signs and symptoms suggestive of neck injury.

- Ability to speak or effective movement of air with respiration indicates patency.
- Gurgling, stridor, wheezing, snoring, choking, or absence of air movement requires immediate intervention.
- Manage airway compromise before next step in primary survey.
  - Breathing:
    - Awake, alert patient with normal speech and good air movement suggests effective breathing.
    - Symmetric chest wall rise/fall, equal breath sounds, normal respiratory rate, and oxygen saturation at 95% or more suggest effective breathing.
    - Asymmetric chest movement, unequal breath sounds, abnormal respiratory rate, decreased oxygen saturation, inadequate air movement, or an obtunded patient suggests ineffective breathing.
    - Decreased unilateral breath sounds, tracheal shift, hyperexpansion, hyperresonance to percussion, subcutaneous air, hypoxia, or hemodynamic compromise raises concerns about tension pneumothorax.
    - Decreased breath sounds with dullness to percussion suggest hemothorax.
    - Manage patients immediately with needle thoracostomy followed by tube thoracostomy.
  - Circulation:
    - Adequate circulating blood volume must be maintained.
    - Primary assessment includes BP, heart rate, pulse quality, and end-organ function (eg, mentation, urine output, capillary refill).
    - Tachycardia and oliguria indicate early shock; hypotension is a late finding.
  - Disability:
    - Assess level of consciousness, gross motor function, and pupillary size/reactivity.
    - Glasgow Coma Scale is most commonly used; score of ≤8 indicates severe head injury/coma.
    - Spinal cord injuries are grossly assessed by observing movement of all extremities.
    - Pupillary size and reactivity to light measure brainstem function.
  - Exposure:
    - Patient should be undressed completely.
- Secondary survey:
  - After the primary survey has been completed
  - Patient stabilized at each level
  - Complete physical exam from head to toe is performed.
  - "Tubes and fingers in every body cavity"

## History
The mechanism of injury, initial clinical presentation, suspected injuries, and treatment rendered should be elicited from EMS personnel.

## Physical Exam
Initial stabilization should begin simultaneously with essential workup.

## ESSENTIAL WORKUP
- Primary and secondary survey
- Cervical spine and chest radiographs are mandatory for *victims of major trauma.*
- Pelvic radiographs should be performed with clinical suspicion of pelvic trauma or with hemodynamic instability.
- Hemoglobin/hematocrit, ABG, blood type
- Urine dip for blood
- UA if dip shows positive result
- Urine-based pregnancy test for any female patient of childbearing age

## DIAGNOSTIC TESTS & INTERPRETATION
### Lab
Baseline coagulation and chemistry studies with massive injury or hemorrhage

### Imaging
- Loss of consciousness, posttraumatic amnesia (anterograde or retrograde), or persistent altered level of consciousness is indication for head CT.
- Significant blunt and penetrating chest trauma requires objective evaluation of the heart and great vessels with echocardiography, CT scan, angiography, or direct visualization.
- Blunt abdominal trauma requires objective evaluation using US, abdominal CT, or diagnostic peritoneal lavage, depending on patient's condition:
  - Hemodynamically stable patients should have an abdominal CT with IV contrast.
  - Unstable patients should have an abdominal ultrasound (FAST exam) or diagnostic peritoneal lavage.
  - Many centers now doing "Pan CT scan," including head, neck, chest, abdomen/pelvis in a single pass with IV contrast
  - Pan CT lowers missed injury rate but involves significant radiation exposure
- Extremity injury:
  - Radiographs
  - Suspected vascular damage requires angiography or duplex ultrasound.

## DIFFERENTIAL DIAGNOSIS
Some level of clinical suspicion should be maintained for other medical conditions leading to trauma (eg, seizures, dysrhythmias).

**TREATMENT**

**INITIAL STABILIZATION/THERAPY**

- The initial treatment should parallel the primary survey with injuries treated before addressing the next assessment level.
- Airway with cervical spine control:
  Jaw thrust, suctioning, and oropharyngeal or nasopharyngeal airways provide initial airway support.
- Rapid sequence intubation is the airway management option of choice for multiple trauma patients:
  - Insertion of an extraglottic airway (eg, Combitube, laryngeal tube, or laryngeal mask airway) or cricothyroidotomy may be necessary.
- Breathing:
  - 100% oxygen and respiratory monitoring
  - Tension pneumothorax should be diagnosed clinically and decompressed on an emergency basis with a needle thoracostomy below the axilla or above the second rib in the midclavicular line.
- Tube thoracostomy should follow.
  - Open chest wounds should be covered with an adherent dressing and a tube thoracostomy performed.
  - Respiratory distress from flail segment or pulmonary contusion should prompt early intubation with mechanical ventilation and positive end expiratory pressure.
  - Hyperventilation should be avoided except with impending herniation or intracranial HTN resistant to other therapies; end-tidal carbon dioxide monitoring should be used.
- Circulation:
  Two large-bore IV lines with constant hemodynamic and cardiac monitoring should be placed.
- Alternatives include central lines, venous cut-downs (eg, saphenous or femoral), or intraosseous lines.
  - Aggressive fluid replacement with 3 parts fluid for every 1 part circulatory volume loss remains the standard of care; adjust fluids based on ongoing assessment.
    ○ 2 L initial bolus in adults, 20 mL/kg in children
    ○ Whole blood or autotransfused blood for hemorrhagic shock or uncontrolled bleeding

- Pericardial tamponade requires emergent pericardiocentesis/pericardial window.
- External bleeding should be managed with direct pressure.
- Disability:
  - Head injury with Glasgow Coma Scale score of ≤8 should initiate treatment for elevated intracranial pressure with mannitol or hypertonic saline, rapid-sequence intubation, oxygenation, and controlled ventilation to a $Pco_2$ of 35 mm Hg.
  - Elevate head 20–30°, maintaining spine immobilization.

**ED TREATMENT/PROCEDURES**

- Definitive treatment is often surgical.
- Prompt stabilization, early recognition of the need for operative intervention, and appropriate trauma surgical consultation are paramount.

**MEDICATION**

Dictated by need for specific interventions

*Pediatric Considerations*

Intraosseous lines are an alternative to IV lines for fluids and medications.

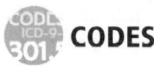 **FOLLOW-UP**

**DISPOSITION**

*Admission Criteria*

- Most major trauma patients should be admitted for observation, monitoring, and further evaluation.
- Patients with significant injuries or hemodynamic instability should be admitted to an ICU.
- Patients requiring frequent assessments should be admitted to a monitored setting.

*Discharge Criteria*

Patients with minor trauma and negative objective workup/imaging may be observed in the ED for several hours and then discharged.

*Issues for Referral*

The main indications for referral concern the availability of subspecialists, such as neurosurgeons, orthopedists/hand surgeons, otolaryngologists, plastic surgeons, or intensivists

**FOLLOW-UP RECOMMENDATIONS**

Follow-up should be driven by the types of injuries and subspecialty care required.

**PEARLS AND PITFALLS**

- The ABCs of trauma remain the standard approach to guide the initial assessment and treatment of trauma patients.
- A high index of suspicion for occult injuries should be maintained, with a low threshold for obtaining objective imaging.
- Trauma systems are defined by an organized approach to accessing quality trauma and subspecialty care.

**ADDITIONAL READING**

- Committee on Trauma, American College of Surgeons. *Resources for Optimal care of the Injured Patient*. St. Louis: Mosby; 2006.
- Gin Shaw SL, Jordan RC. Multiple traumas. In: Marx J, et al., eds. *Rosen's Emergency Medicine: Concepts and Clinical Practice*, 5th ed. St. Louis: Mosby; 2002:242–255.
- Krantz BE. Initial assessment. In: Feliciano DV, et al., eds. *Trauma*. Stamford, CT: Appleton & Lange; 1996:123.

**See Also (Topic, Algorithm, Electronic Media Element)**

Specific anatomic injuries, shock, airway management.

**CODES**

**ICD9**

959.8 Other and unspecified injury to other specified sites, including multiple

T

# TRICHOMONAS
*Herbert Neil Wigder*

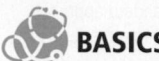

## BASICS

### DESCRIPTION
- Sexually transmitted disease
- Causes urogenital infections
- Sequelae:
  - May cause premature rupture of membranes or preterm labor in pregnancy
  - May cause low birth weight newborns
  - May facilitate transmission of HIV
- Prevalence:
  - 7.4 million cases per year in the U.S.
  - 28% of women treated in STD clinics
  - Overall prevalence 2.3%:
    - Prevalence in black women 10.5%
- Incubation 4–28 days

### ETIOLOGY
*Trichomonas vaginalis*:
- Flagellated protozoan:
  - Commonly found in urethra, bladder, and Skene gland

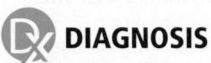

## DIAGNOSIS

### SIGNS AND SYMPTOMS
*OTHER*
- Vaginitis:
  - Vaginal discharge:
    - Frothy yellow/green to gray/white
  - Vulvar itching and irritation
  - Vaginal odor
  - Symptoms same as with bacterial vaginosis (caused by *Gardnerella vaginalis*) and vulvovaginal candidiasis (caused by *Candida albicans*)
  - Dysuria and urinary urgency
  - Painful sexual intercourse
  - Often asymptomatic (25%)
- Cervix:
  - Diffuse erythema (10%–33%)
  - Punctate hemorrhage—colpitis macularis or strawberry cervix (2%)
- Abdominal pain uncommon

*Male*
- Often asymptomatic (90%)
- Nongonococcal urethritis:
  - 20% of nonspecific urethritis
  - Scant discharge
  - Dysuria and urinary urgency
- Prostatitis
- Epididymitis
- Reversible sterility

*Physical Exam*
- Female:
  - Vaginal discharge:
    - Frothy yellow/green to gray/white
  - Odor
  - Red ulcerations—vaginal wall and cervix
- Male:
  - Scant discharge

### ESSENTIAL WORKUP
- Females: "Hanging-drop" slide test:
  - 60–70% sensitive in symptomatic patients
  - Saline wet mount from cervical/vaginal vault smear:
    - Requires immediate evaluation of slide
    - Many polymorphonuclear leukocytes (PMNs)
    - Motile, pear-shaped, flagellated trichomonads (slightly larger than leukocytes; seen in 60%)
    - Specimen from spun urine less sensitive
  - Absence of trichomonads does not rule out *T. vaginalis* infection
  - Many EDs not equipped to perform hanging-drop slide test
- Elevated vaginal pH (>4.5) common:
  - Not specific
- Males: Wet preparation slide test insensitive

### DIAGNOSTIC TESTS & INTERPRETATION
*Lab*
- Culture:
  - 95% sensitivity:
    - Prostate massage before collection increases sensitivity in males.
  - Do culture when trichomonads suspected but not confirmed by wet-mount microscopy
- Point-of-care tests:
  - Sensitivity >83%, specificity >97%
  - OSOM Trichomonas Rapid Test
  - Affirm VP III:
    - Also tests for for *G. vaginalis* and *C. albicans*
- Polymerase chain reaction (PCR):
  - Expensive

### DIFFERENTIAL DIAGNOSIS
- UTI
- Gonorrhea
- *Chlamydia*
- Bacterial vaginosis
- Candidal vaginitis
- Nonspecific vaginitis

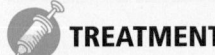 **TREATMENT**

### ED TREATMENT/PROCEDURES

- Female:
  - Metronidazole 2 g PO once:
    - 90–95% cure rate
  - Tinidazole 2 g PO once:
    - 86–100% cure rate
  - Metronidazole-resistant infections 2–5%
  - Treatment of infections resistant to single-dose metronidazole:
    - Metronidazole 500 mg PO b.i.d. for 7 days *or*
    - Tinidazole 2 g PO once
  - Metronidazole gel, less effective:
    - Not recommended
- Pregnant:
  - Metronidazole FDA category B
- Males (urethritis):
  - Metronidazole 2 g PO once
  - Tinidazole 2 g po once
  - Metronidazole 500 mg PO b.i.d. for 7 days
- Avoid concomitant alcohol use with metronidazole:
  - No alcohol for 24 hr after last metronidazole
  - Precipitates Antabuse reaction
  - Treat sex partners to prevent reinfection:
    - Avoid sex until partners are cured.
    - Cured if patient and partner asymptomatic after completion of therapy
- Advise using latex condoms
- Consider testing for concomitant STDs including gonorrhea, *Chlamydia*, syphilis, and HIV.
- Typical treatment for nongonococcal urethritis (eg, azithromycine, doxycycline) does not treat *Trichomonas vaginalis*.

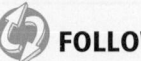 **FOLLOW-UP**

### DISPOSITION
***Discharge Criteria***
All patients

## PEARLS AND PITFALLS

- Vaginitis in females not responding to treatment for bacterial vaginosis might be due to *Trichomonas* infection.
- Nongonococcal urethritis in males not responding to azithromycin or doxycycline might be due to *Trichomonas*.

## ADDITIONAL READING

- Centers for Disease Control and Prevention. Sexually transmitted diseases treatment guidelines 2006. http://www.cdc.gov/std/treatment/2006/vagina-discharge.htm. Accessed November 1, 2009.

- Centers for Disease Control and Prevention. Trichomonas Infection (Trichomoniasis). http://www.cdc.gov/ncidod/dpd/parasites/trichomonas/factsht_trichomonas.htm. Accessed November 1, 2009.
- Miller WC, Swygard H, Hobbs MM, et al. The prevalence of trichomoniasis in young adults in the United States. *Sex Trans Dis*. 2005;32(10):593–598.
- Wendel KA, Workowski KA. Trichomoniasis: Challenges to appropriate management. *Clin Infect Dis*. 2007;44:S123–S129.

**See Also (Topic, Algorithm, Electronic Media Element)**
Urethritis

 **CODES**

### ICD9
- 131.00 Urogenital trichomoniasis, unspecified
- 131.01 Trichomonal vulvovaginitis
- 131.02 Trichomonal urethritis

T

# TRICYCLIC ANTIDEPRESSANT, POISONING

*Steven Aks*

## BASICS

### DESCRIPTION
- Primary mechanism of tricyclic antidepressant (TCA) toxicity:
  - Sodium channel blocking effect (quinidinelike effect)
  - Inhibition of norepinephrine reuptake
  - Alpha blockade
  - Anticholinergic effect
- Selective serotonin reuptake inhibitors (SSRIs):
  - Wider margin of safety than TCA
  - Less CNS/cardiovascular toxicity
- Nonselective serotonin reuptake inhibitors:
  - Serotonin and norepinephrine reuptake inhibitors (SNRIs)
  - Can cause cardiac dysrhythmias or seizures
  - Venlafaxine (Effexor)
  - See "Antidepressants, Poisoning."

### ETIOLOGY
- Tricyclic antidepressants:
  - Amitriptyline
  - Nortriptyline
  - Imipramine
  - Doxepin
- Newer-generation antidepressants (nontricyclic):
  - Have different toxic profile than TCAs
  - See "Antidepressants, Poisoning."

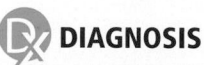

## DIAGNOSIS

### SIGNS AND SYMPTOMS
- Rapid deterioration may occur.
- Classic TCA compounds (imipramine, amitriptyline, nortriptyline)—greatest cardiovascular toxicity
- Newer agents (serotonergic agents)—less overall toxicity in overdose
- CNS:
  - Stimulation or depression
  - Stimulation:
    - Tremulousness
    - Agitation
    - Fasciculation
    - Seizures (resulting acidemia may lead to worsening cardiovascular toxicity)
  - Depression:
    - Drowsiness
    - Lethargy
    - Coma
- Cardiovascular system:
  - Hypotension
  - Tachycardia:
    - Early; owing to blockade of norepinephrine reuptake and anticholinergic effects
  - Bradycardia:
    - Late; owing to catecholamine depletion state
  - ECG changes:
    - QRS widening (>100–120 ms)
    - Rightward shift in terminal 40 ms in frontal plane axis (r wave >3 mm in aVR)
  - Dysrhythmias:
    - Supraventricular tachycardia (SVT)
    - Ventricular arrhythmias

- Anticholinergic effects (less common):
  - Dilated pupils
  - Decreased bowel sounds
  - Urinary retention

### History
Substance ingestion in patient with access to TCA

### Physical Exam
- CNS:
  - Stimulation or depression
- Cardiovascular:
  - Tachycardia
  - Mydriasis or midrange pupils
  - Decreased bowel sounds
  - Urinary retention (rare)

### ESSENTIAL WORKUP
- ECG: Factors associated with TCA poisoning:
  - Sinus tachycardia (almost always present at some time after poisoning)
  - QRS widening:
    - Greater than 100 ms associated with seizure
    - Greater than 160 ms associated with ventricular dysrhythmia
  - QT prolongation
  - PR prolongation
  - Rightward shifting of terminal 40 ms QRS axis
  - R-wave amplitude in aVR >3 mm
- Continuous cardiac monitor

### DIAGNOSTIC TESTS & INTERPRETATION
#### Lab
- CBC
- Electrolytes, BUN, creatinine, glucose
- ABG
- Urine toxicology screen:
  - Rule out other toxins.
- TCA levels:
  - Not useful
  - Do not correlate well with degree of toxicity
  - Qualitative screen appropriate to confirm ingestion if necessary

#### Imaging
Chest radiograph for aspiration pneumonia/pulmonary edema

### DIFFERENTIAL DIAGNOSIS
- Drugs that cause coma:
  - Alcohols
  - Alcohol withdrawal
  - Anticholinergics
  - Lithium
  - Phencyclidine (PCP)
  - Opioids
  - Phenothiazines
  - Sedative hypnotics
  - Salicylates

- Cardiotoxic drugs:
  - Antidysrhythmics (category IA)
  - Digoxin toxicity
  - Sympathomimetics
  - Anticholinergics
- Drugs that cause seizures:
  - Alcohol withdrawal
  - Anticholinergics
  - Camphor
  - Isoniazid
  - Lindane
  - Lithium
  - Phenothiazines
  - Sympathomimetics
  - Toxic alcohols

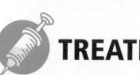

## TREATMENT

### PRE-HOSPITAL
- Do not be lulled into false sense of security with well-appearing patient:
  - Rapid onset of altered mental status, seizures, and dysrhythmias occur.
- Perform endotracheal intubation if any evidence of compromise.
- Secure IV access.
- Administer sodium bicarbonate if any evidence of QRS widening (>100–120 ms):
  - One ampule in adults
  - 1–2 mEq/kg in children
- Ipecac contraindicated (risk for aspiration with development of depressed mental status or seizure)

### INITIAL STABILIZATION/THERAPY
- ABCs:
  - Low threshold to intubate patients with altered mental status
- IV 0.9% normal saline (NS)
- Oxygen
- Cardiac monitor:
  - For wide complex rhythm (QRS >100–120 ms) bolus sodium bicarbonate
- Naloxone, thiamine, glucose (Accu-Chek) for altered mental status
- Flumazenil contraindicated in combined TCA/benzodiazepine overdose

## ED TREATMENT/PROCEDURES
### Cardiac Toxicity
- Initiate therapy for cardiac toxicity aggressively to prevent deterioration.
- QRS widening (>100–120 ms):
  – Bolus with 1 amp (peds: 1–2 mEq/kg) of sodium bicarbonate; repeat if sudden increase in QRS width
  – Maintain arterial pH of 7.45–7.5 with hyperventilation.
  – Initiate sodium bicarbonate infusion if hyperventilation alone does not reach target pH.
- Dysrhythmia:
  – Sinus tachycardia requires no treatment.
  – Bolus 1–2 amps of sodium bicarbonate (1–2 mEq/kg in children) for sudden change in rhythm
  – Follow advanced cardiac life support (ACLS) protocol with addition of sodium bicarbonate boluses:
    ○ Lidocaine is second-line agent after sodium bicarbonate.
  – Use of class IA (procainamide) and IC agents and physostigmine contraindicated

### Hypotension
- 0.9% NS fluid bolus
- Norepinephrine:
  – Preferred pressor (over dopamine)
  – Counters alpha blockade better
  – Dopamine requires higher doses.

### Decontamination
- Gastric lavage:
  – For recent ingestion (<1–2 hr)
  – Performed when airway has been secured in lethargic patient
- Administer activated charcoal with sorbitol.
- Ipecac contraindicated

### Seizure
- Diazepam first line followed by Phenobarbital
- Neuromuscular paralysis with short-acting agent (rocuronium/vecuronium) for refractory seizures (monitor EEG)
- Sodium bicarbonate bolus to prevent acidosis

## MEDICATION
### First Line
- Sodium bicarbonate: 1–2 amps IV push (peds: 1–2 mEq/kg); drip—add 3 amps to 1 L of D$_5$W (efficacy of drip is unknown)
- Activated charcoal slurry: 1–2 g/kg up to 90 g PO
- Sorbitol: 1–2 g/kg to max of 150 g (peds: >1 year old: 1–1.5 g/kg as 35% solution to max of 50 g) PO mixed in activated charcoal slurry this is unnecessary

### Second Line
- Dextrose: D$_{50}$W, one amp: 50 mL or 25 g (peds: D$_{25}$W, 2–4 mL/kg) IV
- Diazepam (benzodiazepine): 5–10 mg (peds: 0.2–0.5 mg/kg) IV
- Dopamine: 2–20 μg/kg/min IV infusion titrated to desired effect
- Lorazepam (benzodiazepine): 2–6 mg (peds: 0.03–0.05 mg/kg) IV
- Naloxone (Narcan): 2 mg (peds: 0.1 mg/kg) IV or IM initial dose
- Norepinephrine: 4–12 μg/min (peds: 0.05–0.1 μg/kg/min) IV infusion titrated to desired effect

 **FOLLOW-UP**

### DISPOSITION
### Admission Criteria
- Symptomatic patients observed >6 hr
- Altered mental status
- Dysrhythmia or conduction delay
- Seizure
- Heart rate >100 beats per min 6 hr after ingestion
- Coingestion requiring prolonged observation

### Discharge Criteria
- Asymptomatic after 6 hr observation
- No alteration in mental status
- Normal ECG with heart rate <100 beats per min
- Active bowel sounds; tolerated activated charcoal
- Psychiatry clearance if there has been suicide attempt or gesture

### Issues for Referral
Toxicology or poison center consultation for significant ingestions

### FOLLOW-UP RECOMMENDATIONS
Psychiatry for suicide attempts

## PEARLS AND PITFALLS
- The hallmark of TCA poisoning is rapid clinical deterioration.
- Vigilant monitoring for QRS widening beyond 120 ms is essential.
- Achieve target pH with hyperventilation in the intubated TCA overdose patient.
- Treat acute widening of the QRS beyond 120 ms with bolus bicarbonate.

## ADDITIONAL READING

- Geis GL, Bond GR. Antidepressant overdose: Tricyclics, selective serotonin reuptake inhibitors, and atypical antidepressants. In: Erickson TB, Ahrens W, Aks SE, et al., eds. Pediatric Toxicology. New York: McGraw-Hill; 2004:297–302.
- Liebelt EL, Francis PD, Woolf AD. ECG lead aVR versus QRS interval in predicting seizures and arrhythmias in acute tricyclic antidepressant toxicity. Ann Emerg Med. 1995;26:195–201.
- Reilly TH, Kirk MA. Atypical antipsychotics and newer antidepressants. Emerg Med Clin North Am. 2007;25:477–497.
- Woolf AD, Erdman AR, Nelson LS, et al. Tricyclic antidepressant poisoning: An evidence-based guideline for out-of-hospital management. Clin Toxicol. 2007;45:203–233.

### See Also (Topic, Algorithm, Electronic Media Element)
Antidepressant Poisoning

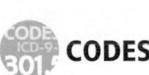 **CODES**

ICD9
969.05 Poisoning by tricyclic antidepressants

# TRIGEMINAL NEURALGIA

*James M. Leaming*
*Spencer A. Adoff*

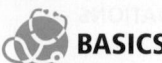 **BASICS**

## DESCRIPTION

- The trigeminal nerve (cranial nerve V) innervates the face, oral mucosa, nasal mucosa, and cornea with its sensory fibers.
- Trigeminal neuralgia is also known as tic douloureux.
- Usually occurs in patients >50 yr of age
- Facial pain syndrome recognizable by history alone
- Classical vs. symptomatic:
  - Classical:
    - Recurrent attacks of unilateral (uncommonly bilateral) of superficial, sharp, or stabbing pain
    - Lasts for <1 sec–2 min
    - Episodes are stereotyped in each individual.
    - No clinically evident neurologic deficit
    - Not caused by another disorder
  - Symptomatic:
    - Same as above but a causative lesion (not vascular compression) is identified

## ETIOLOGY

- Mechanism of pain production remains controversial; accepted theory suggests:
  - Demyelination of cranial nerve, leading to ectopic stimulation and pain:
    - Demyelination caused by tortuous or aberrant vascular compression of nerve root
- Secondary causes:
  - Herpes zoster
  - Multiple sclerosis
  - Space-occupying lesions:
    - Cerebropontine angle tumor
    - Aneurysm
    - Arteriovenous malformation

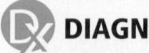 **DIAGNOSIS**

## SIGNS AND SYMPTOMS

- Brief, intense, recurrent sharp pain
- Unilateral in the distribution of a branch of the trigeminal nerve:
  - Can occur in all 3 nerves: Maxillary > mandibular > ophthalmic
- More common on right side of face
- May occur without provocation, but triggers can be produced by talking, smiling, chewing, brushing teeth, shaving, or touching the face
- Can occur infrequently or hundreds of times per day
- No pain between episodes, although chronic cases may complain of a continuous ache

### History

- Rule out possible symptomatic causes with the following atypical features:
  - Abnormal neurologic exam
  - Abnormal oral/dental exam
  - Abnormal ear exam or hearing loss
  - Symptoms of dizziness, vertigo, visual changes, or numbness
  - Pain lasting >2 min
  - Not in trigeminal nerve distribution
- Most common age group is 60–70
- Females > Males

### Physical Exam

- Physical examination findings are normal; if abnormality found, consider other cause.
- Carefully examine head and neck, with emphasis on cranial nerves.
- Patient's report of pain following stimulation of a trigger point is pathognomonic.

## ESSENTIAL WORKUP

Diagnosis is made clinically.

## DIAGNOSTIC TESTS & INTERPRETATION

### Lab

No specific laboratory tests apply.

### Imaging

- Patients with characteristic history and normal neurologic examination may be treated without further workup.
- If dental problems are suggested, dental radiographs may be useful.
- MRI brain/CT head may be useful if multiple sclerosis or tumor is suggested:
  - May be useful in initial presentation

## DIFFERENTIAL DIAGNOSIS

- Multiple sclerosis
- Temporomandibular joint syndrome
- Glossopharyngeal neuralgia
- Compression of trigeminal root by tumors
- Dental problems/pain
- Cluster headache
- Postherpetic neuralgia
- Sinusitis
- Otitis media
- Temporal arteritis

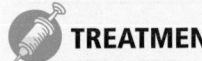

## TREATMENT

### ED TREATMENT/PROCEDURES
- Appropriate pain relief
- Medical therapy:
  - Carbamazepine most commonly used
  - Other antiepileptics show some support as adjuvants for refractory pain.
- May need neurosurgical evaluation for treatment and/or exploration

### MEDICATION

#### First Line
Carbamazepine: 200–800 mg/day PO b.i.d.

#### Second Line
- Gabapentin: Start 300 mg PO qd
- Lamictal: Start 25 mg PO qd
- Oxcarbazepine: 450–1,200 mg PO b.i.d.; start 300 mg PO b.i.d.
- Phenytoin: 300–400 mg/d div qd–t.i.d.
- Valproic acid: Start 250 mg PO b.i.d.

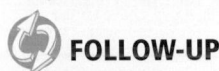

## FOLLOW-UP

### DISPOSITION

#### Admission Criteria
- Trigeminal neuralgia with presence of other focal neurologic findings
- Positive CT or MRI studies may require emergent neurologic or neurosurgical consultation.
- Refractory or recurrent trigeminal neuralgia not responding to outpatient pain management or anticonvulsant therapy:
  - May require admission for surgical intervention and ablation of the trigeminal nerve

### Discharge Criteria
Patients without any focal neurologic findings and improved pain control in the ED may be managed as outpatients.

### Issues for Referral
Referral to a pain management center may be helpful in cases of refractory pain:
- Anesthetic blocks of the trigeminal ganglion may be helpful.

### FOLLOW-UP RECOMMENDATIONS
- Follow up with PCP or neurologist for treatment.
- Referral to a neurosurgeon may be indicated for refractory pain:
  - Percutaneous vs. open surgical treatment

## PEARLS AND PITFALLS

- Unilateral, paroxysmal, and sharp/stabbing facial pain, following a portion of CN V distribution
- Trigger points are pathognomonic.
- Do not miss an alternate (nonvascular) cause of nerve compression, such as CNS mass or aneurysm.
- Carbamazepine is the most common treatment.

## ADDITIONAL READING

- Kraft RM. Trigeminal neuralgia. *Am Fam Physician*. 2008;77:1291–1296.
- Siqueira S, Teixeira M, Siqueira J. Clinical characteristics of patients with trigeminal neuralgia referred to neurosurgery. *Eur J Dent*. 2009;3: 207–212.
- Wolfson AB, Hendey GW, Ling LJ, et al., eds. *Harwood-Nuss' Clinical Practice of Emergency Medicine*, 5th ed. Philadelphia: Lippincott Williams & Wilkins; 2010.

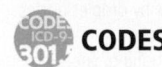

## CODES

### ICD9
- 053.12 Postherpetic trigeminal neuralgia
- 350.1 Trigeminal neuralgia

T

# TUBERCULOSIS

*Vittorio J. Raho*

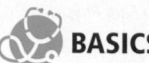

## BASICS

### DESCRIPTION
- Infection with *Mycobacterium tuberculosis,* an aerobic acid-fast bacillus, resulting in disease
- Tuberculosis (TB) is an infectious disease with protean manifestations, causing significant global morbidity and mortality.

### Mechanism
- Most common route of infection is by droplet nuclei inhaled through the respiratory tract,
- Bacteria are dispersed through coughing, sneezing, speaking, singing.
- Primary TB/latent TB infection (LTBI):
  – Initial infection occurs when organisms enter the alveoli, become engulfed by macrophages, and spread via regional lymph nodes to the bloodstream.
  – Patients are usually asymptomatic.
  – May be progressive/fatal in immunocompromised hosts
  – Positive reaction to purified protein derivative (PPD) indicates past exposure or infection.
  – May progress to active TB
- Reactivation TB:
  – Latent infection becomes active tuberculosis.
  – Systemic (15%) and pulmonary (85%) symptoms
- Tuberculosis affects about one third of the world's population (90 million new cases in the past decade worldwide, with about 30 million deaths).
- Centers for Disease Control and Prevention (CDC) statistics from 2007 show TB in the U.S. at an all-time low.
- TB rates in the U.S. have continued to decline since 1993, although rate of decline is slowing.
- Increase in U.S. foreign-born cases
- Still an estimated 10–15 million people are infected in the U.S. alone.

### ETIOLOGY
- *M. tuberculosis,* a slow-growing bacterium
- Humans are the only known reservoir.
- Recent TB epidemics:
  – HIV-infected patients
  – Multidrug-resistant TB (MDR-TB)
  – Extensively drug-resistant TB (XDR-TB):
    ○ High mortality, few effective drugs

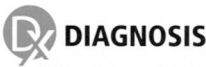

## DIAGNOSIS

### SIGNS AND SYMPTOMS
- Depending upon site of infection; all human tissues have potential for infection.
- Pulmonary tuberculosis:
  – Cough
  – Fever
  – Malaise
  – Weight loss
  – Night sweats
  – Hemoptysis
  – Pleuritic chest pain
  – Shortness of breath

- Extrapulmonary TB:
  – CNS infections:
    ○ Meningismus
    ○ Cranial nerve defects
    ○ Malaise
    ○ Intermittent headache
    ○ Low-grade fever
    ○ Confusion
    ○ Diplopia
    ○ Hyponatremia (due to syndrome of inappropriate anti-diuretic hormone)
    ○ Acute ischemic stroke
  – Pericarditis:
    ○ Pleuritic chest pain increased with recumbency
  – Renal infection:
    ○ Fever
    ○ Flank pain
    ○ Sterile pyuria
  – Spinal TB (Potts disease):
    ○ Back pain/stiffness
    ○ Fever
    ○ Point tenderness
    ○ Decreased range of motion
  – Cervical lymphadenitis:
    ○ Unilateral, painless
    ○ Known as scrofula
    ○ Draining sinus tracts may form
  – Miliary TB:
    ○ Multi–organ system involvement
    ○ Diffuse adenopathy
    ○ Hepatomegaly
    ○ Splenomegaly
    ○ Weight loss
    ○ Fever

### History
Predisposing factors and conditions for TB:
- HIV infection and other immunocompromised states (organ transplant, renal failure, diabetes)
- Drug and alcohol abuse
- Poverty
- Homelessness (living in shelters)
- Institutionalization (nursing homes, prisons)
- Immigration from an endemic area
- Positive PPD test/previous infection

### Physical Exam
- Fever
- Tachycardia
- Hypoxia
- Cachexia
- Abnormal breath sounds
- Cervical lymphadenopathy

### ESSENTIAL WORKUP
- Diagnosis difficult due to the variety of clinical presentations
- Chest radiography:
  – Most valuable test for diagnosing active pulmonary TB
- Skin testing: PPD

## DIAGNOSTIC TESTS & INTERPRETATION
### Lab
- CBC
- Electrolytes, BUN, creatinine, glucose, LFTs
- ABGs for oxygenation/ventilation assessment
- Sputum staining for acid-fast bacilli (Ziehl–Neelsen stain):
  – Provides a quick presumptive diagnosis
- Sputum, CSF, blood, urine, or peritoneal fluid culture:
  – Gold standard for diagnosis of TB
  – Average time for positive culture is 3–6 wk.
  – DNA polymerase chain reaction (PCR) testing more rapid
- Lumbar puncture with CSF analysis:
  – For suspected TB meningitis
  – Elevated WBCs with lymphocyte predominance
  – Elevated protein
  – Low to normal glucose

### Imaging
- Chest radiograph:
  – May be normal
  – In primary disease, parenchymal infiltrates with unilateral hilar adenopathy are the classic findings.
  – Reactivation TB typically appears as cavitary lesions with or without calcification, usually in upper lung segments.
  – Miliary tuberculosis shows bilateral disseminated 2-mm nodules throughout lungs.
  – Chest radiograph may be nondefinitive in AIDS/immunocompromised patients.
  – Unilateral pleural effusion in both primary and reactivation tuberculosis
  – Tracheal deviation with scarring or atelectasis
  – Ghon focus—calcified scar/healed primary focus of infection
  – Ghon complex—primary infiltrate with associated unilateral hilar adenopathy
- Spine radiographs for Potts disease:
  – May be normal
  – Anterior wedging of two involved vertebral bodies and destruction of disk
- CT chest:
  – Better defines extent of disease

### Diagnostic Procedures/Surgery
Skin testing:
- Inject 0.1 mL of PPD intradermally in the forearm.
- Positive test indicates prior or current infection with *M. tuberculosis.*
- Test results are read between 48 and 72 hr after administration.
- Interpretation of positive: >5 mm induration:
  – Close contacts with TB patients
  – Positive chest radiographs for TB
  – HIV-positive
  – Organ transplant or other immunosuppression

- >10-mm induration:
  - IV drug users
  - Immigrants from high-prevalence countries (within 5 yr)
  - Underlying disease (diabetes, renal failure, malignancies)
  - Health care workers
  - Prison inmates
  - Institutionalized (nursing home, homeless shelters)
- >15-mm induration:
  - Low-risk individuals

## DIFFERENTIAL DIAGNOSIS
- Bacterial pneumonia
- Bronchiectasis
- Coccidiomycosis
- Histoplasmosis
- Lung abscess
- Lung carcinoma
- Lymphoma
- *Pneumocystis carinii* pneumonia
- Pulmonary embolism
- Sarcoidosis

 TREATMENT

### PRE-HOSPITAL
- Place patient in respiratory isolation (negative flow).
- Place a mask on the patient to prevent respiratory spread of the disease.
- Initiate treatment with an IV, oxygen, and pulse oximetry.
- Endotracheal intubation may be required in patients with severe hemoptysis or respiratory compromise.
- Providers should wear submicron particulate filter masks (N-95 designation).
- Inform close contacts.

### INITIAL STABILIZATION/THERAPY
- ABCs:
  - Control airway as needed.
  - Administer oxygen as needed.
  - Place on patient cardiac monitor and pulse oximetry.
  - Establish IV access with 0.9% normal saline
- Isolate patients in negative pressure rooms with at least six air exchanges per hr.
- Protection for health care workers (N-95 masks)

### ED TREATMENT/PROCEDURES
- *Isolation* and strict respiratory precautions
- Treatment is augmented due to increasing multidrug resistance.
- Any regimen must contain at least 2 drugs to which the TB bacillus is susceptible.
- CDC currently recommends initial therapy that includes 4 first-line drugs.
- Initial treatment is continued for 2 mo and then tailored depending on culture susceptibilities.
- Final treatment continues at least 4 mo more after susceptibility testing.
- LTBI with normal chest x-ray given isoniazid (INH) for 9 mo

- Consult infectious disease specialists when treating HIV patients on antiretroviral therapies.
- Add dexamethasone for TB meningitis.
- Surgical drainage for TB empyema may be necessary; consult thoracic surgeon.
- Directly observed therapy (DOT) may be necessary to ensure compliance in certain populations.
- Intermittent (biweekly) regimen may demonstrate higher patient compliance.

## MEDICATION
### First Line
- Isoniazid (INH): 5 mg/kg, max 300 mg (peds: 10–15 mg/kg, max. 300 mg) PO/IM per day:
  - Refractory seizures in overdose, treat with pyridoxine 5 g IV over 5 min
  - Caution with alcohol coingestion, hepatitis
- Rifampin (RIF): 10 mg/kg, max 600 mg (peds: 10–20 mg/kg, max 600 mg) PO/IV per day
- Pyrazinamide (PZA): 20–25 mg/kg/day max 2 g (peds: 15–30 mg/kg/day) or:
  - <55 kg: 1 g PO per day
  - 56–75 kg: 1.5 g PO per day
  - >75 kg: 2 g PO per day
  - Not recommended in pregnancy
- Ethambutol (ETB): 15–20 mg/kg, max 1,600 mg (peds: 15–30 mg/kg, max 1 g) PO per day
  - Not recommended <13 yr old, requires visual testing

### Second Line
- Streptomycin: 15 mg/kg/d, max 1 g (peds: 20–40 mg/kg/day) IM/IV per day:
  - Teratogenicity, contraindicated in pregnancy
- Ethionamide: 0.5–1 g (peds: 15–20 mg/kg/day) PO divided q.i.d.
- Rifabutin: 5 mg/kg, max 300 mg (peds: unknown) PO per day
- Levaquin: 750 mg (peds: contraindicated) PO/IV per day
- Capreomycin: 15 mg/kg/day, max. 1 g (peds: 15 mg/kg/day) IM/IV per day
- Amikacin/kanamycin: 15 mg/kg/day, max. 1 g (peds: 15–30 mg/kg/day) IM/IV per day

 FOLLOW-UP

### DISPOSITION
### Admission Criteria
- Respiratory compromise
- Suspicion of diagnosis
- Inability to comply with outpatient therapy
- Unavailable outpatient resources (no PCP)
- Involuntary admission for noncompliant outpatients occurs:
  - Be aware of respective state laws concerning involuntary admission (consult infectious disease specialist).

### Discharge Criteria
- Without respiratory compromise
- Home isolation procedure compliance
- Ability and willingness to comply with long-term therapy
- Appropriate outpatient follow-up and treatment available
- Notification of the public health authorities is mandatory.

### Issues for Referral
Referral to Department of Public Health for DOT

### FOLLOW-UP RECOMMENDATIONS
- Sputum analysis periodically to document clearance
- Medication toxicity monitoring:
  - INH, RIF, PZA: Monitor liver function tests for hepatitis
  - PZA: Check uric acid levels
  - ETB: Eye testing for color blindness

## PEARLS AND PITFALLS
- Early isolation and respiratory precautions
- Careful history to establish risk factors
- The chest x-ray and PPD are great diagnostic aids.
- Initial 4-drug regimen for active disease
- Nonadherent, active TB patients are considered a public health hazard:
  - Specific state laws are applicable in numerous areas.

## ADDITIONAL READING
- American Thoracic Society, CDC, Infectious Disease Society of America. Treatment of tuberculosis. *Am J Respir Care Med.* 2003;167:603–662.
- Centers for Disease Control and Prevention. Treatment of Tuberculosis, American Thoracic Society, CDC, and Infectious Diseases Society of America. *MMWR.* 2003;52(RR11):1–77.
- Centers for Disease Control and Prevention. *MMWR.* 2005;54(RR15):1–37.
- Centers for Disease Control and Prevention. *MMWR.* 2005;54(RR12):1–81.
- http://www.cdc.gov/tb/publications/factsheets/. Accessed December 21, 2009.
- http://www.who.int/tb/publications/global_report/en/index.html, accessed 12/12/2009
- Moran GJ, Talan DA. Tuberculosis. In: Wolfson AB et al., eds. *Harwood-Nuss' Clinical Practice of Emergency Medicine*, 4th ed. Philadelphia: Lippincott Williams & Wilkins, 2005:751–756.

### See Also (Topic, Algorithm, Electronic Media Element)
- Pneumonia, Adult
- Bronchiectasis
- Coccidiomycosis
- Histoplasmosis
- Lymphoma
- *Pneumocystis carinii* Pneumonia
- Pulmonary Embolism
- Sarcoidosis

 CODES

### ICD9
- 011.90 Unspecified pulmonary tuberculosis, confirmation unspecified
- 795.5 Nonspecific reaction to tuberculin skin test without active tuberculosis

T

# TULAREMIA

*Ian Greenwald*
*Roger M. Barkin*

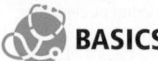 **BASICS**

## DESCRIPTION

- Tularemia is an acute febrile illness caused by the small aerobic gram-negative intracellular coccobacillus *Francisella tularensis*:
  – Organism is highly infectious.
  – Person-to-person transmission has not been reported.
- Humans become infected through different environmental exposures:
  – Wounds inflicted by infected arthropods
  – Direct contact with infectious animal tissue or fluid
  – Being bitten by infected tick, deerfly, or other infected insect
  – Contact with or ingestion of contaminated food, water, or soil
  – Inhalation of infected aerosols (eg, cutting grass with power mowers, which may aerolize the organism)
- The 4 major strains of the bacterium have different virulence and geographic location:
  – The North American strain is the most virulent.
- Natural hosts:
  – Lagomorphs and other rodents
  – Found in species wild animals (insects, rabbits, hares, ticks, flies, muskrats, beavers), domestic animals (sheep, cattle, cats), ticks, and water and soil contaminated by infected animals
- Natural vectors:
  – Ticks
  – Biting flies
  – Mosquitoes
  – Wild rabbits
- Weaponization of tularemia was accomplished during the Cold War:
  – Because of its infectivity and ability to be aerosolized, it remains a potential biological agent for mass destruction.
- Laboratory technicians handling culture specimens are at high risk:
  – *F. tularensis* cultures should be manipulated only in a biosafety level 3 facility.

## ETIOLOGY

- Individuals who spend time outdoors in endemic areas are at higher risk:
  – Farmers
  – Hunters
  – Forest workers
  – Those who handle animal carcasses are at highest risk (taxidermists and butchers).
  – Two thirds of cases occur in males.
- Although tularemia can occur worldwide, it is endemic in the northern hemisphere:
  – Reported nationwide except in Hawaii
  – States with the highest incidence include Missouri, Arkansas, South Dakota, and Oklahoma.
  – Few hundred cases annually in the U.S., although probably underreported
  – Peak season is June–October.
- Mortality is 5–15%. Appropriately treated patients have mortality as low as 1%.

### Pediatric Considerations
- Children who spend time outdoors in endemic rural areas are at risk.
- There is a recent case report of a U.S. child who developed tularemia from a commercially purchased pet hamster after sustaining a superficial bite.

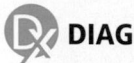 **DIAGNOSIS**

## SIGNS AND SYMPTOMS
- Tularemia has different presentations based on route of entry:
  – Primary route of entry is through skin; most often a cutaneous ulcer develops.
- Incubation is 3–5 days, range 1–14 days. Lesion usually begins as papule, often with fever.
- 6 forms of illness:
  – Ulceroglandular:
    ○ Most common presentation (70–80% of cases)
    ○ Inoculated cutaneously (scratch, abrasion, insect bite) with as few as 50 organisms
    ○ Initially, a local cutaneous papule at point of entry
    ○ Followed by tender regional adenopathy and constitutional symptoms to include fever, chills, myalgias, and headaches
  – Glandular:
    ○ Rare form
    ○ Gains access to lymphatic system or bloodstream through inapparent abrasion
    ○ Tender regional lymphadenopathy with no local lesions
  – Oculoglandular:
    ○ Rare form
    ○ Organism enters through a splash of infected blood/fluid to the eye or is introduced by eye rubbing after handling infectious materials (eg, rabbit carcass).
    ○ Edema, conjunctivitis, injection, chemosis with periauricular, submandibular, or cervical lymphadenopathy
  – Pharyngeal:
    ○ Rare form
    ○ From ingestion of contaminated food or water
    ○ Severe throat pain with exudative pharyngitis and regional lymphadenitis
  – Typhoidal (aka septicemic):
    ○ Unapparent point of entry
    ○ Fever develops, along with severe diarrhea, bowel necrosis, and pneumonia.
    ○ Occurs in 10–15% of cases and is most lethal if not recognized early and treated with antibiotics.
  – Pneumonic:
    ○ Secondary to inhalation
    ○ Seen in sheep shearers, farmers, landscapers, and lab technicians
    ○ Fever, dry cough, and pleuritic chest pain develop.
    ○ Pneumonia can occur in 10–15% of patients with ulceroglandular tularemia and up to 50% of patients with typhoidal tularemia.

### History
- Exposure and epidemiologic risk factors can be helpful.
- Sudden fever, chills, headaches
- Progression of components of signs and symptoms may be useful in defining form of illness.

### Physical Exam
- Fever
- Tender, well-demarcated cutaneous ulcer
- Tender regional lymphadenopathy; lymph nodes can develop fluctuance and spontaneously drain.
- Exudative pharyngitis (with pharyngeal tularemia)
- Ulcerations of the conjunctiva with pronounced chemosis (with oculoglandular tularemia)

## DIAGNOSTIC TESTS & INTERPRETATION
### Lab
- No rapid diagnostic test available
- Routine lab studies nonspecific:
  – CBC can be normal.
  – ESR might be slightly elevated.
  – UA: 25% have pyuria
  – CSF: May have increased protein or mild pleocytosis
  – LFTs are often abnormal.
- Gram's stain, cultures, and tissue biopsies:
  – Often negative
- Blood cultures usually negative because of specific growth requirements
- Enzyme-linked immunosorbent assay and polymerase chain reaction are available through reference laboratories.
- Serum antibody titers:
  – Typically do not reach diagnostic levels until ≥10 days after the onset of illness
  – A single titer of at least 1:160 for tube agglutination is diagnostic for *F. tularensis* infection.
  – May not be elevated before day 11 of illness and generally are diagnostic after 16th day.

### Imaging
- Chest radiograph for:
  – Consolidative process, pleural effusions, and hilar adenopathy
- CT scan of chest for:
  – Severe pulmonary symptoms
  – Other possible etiologies of atypical pneumonia

## DIFFERENTIAL DIAGNOSIS
- Ulceroglandular tularemia mimics include:
  – Tuberculosis
  – Cat-scratch disease
  – Syphilis
  – Chancroid
  – Lymphogranuloma venereum
  – Toxoplasmosis
  – Sporotrichosis
  – Rat-bite fever
  – Anthrax

- Oculoglandular tularemia mimics include:
  - Adenoviral infection
- Pharyngeal tularemia mimics include:
  - Diphtheria
  - Bacterial pharyngitis
  - Infectious mononucleosis
  - Adenoviral infection
- Typhoidal tularemia mimics include:
  - Salmonellosis
  - Brucellosis
  - Legionnaire's disease
  - Q fever
  - Malaria
  - Disseminated fungal or mycobacterial infections
- Pulmonary tularemia mimics include:
  - Mycoplasmal infection
  - Legionnaire's disease
  - Chlamydial infection
  - Tuberculosis

 TREATMENT

### PRE-HOSPITAL
- Universal precautions
- Management of ABCs
- Treat dehydration/hypotension with boluses of normal saline.

### INITIAL STABILIZATION/THERAPY
- ABCs
- Supplemental oxygen for hypoxia
- Fluid resuscitation with normal saline for intravascular volume depletion or septic shock
- Central line access for unstable patients
- Vasopressors for persistent hypotension

### ED TREATMENT/PROCEDURES
- Fever control with acetaminophen
- Early administration of antibiotic therapy after obtaining cultures
- Antibiotic options:
  - First-line agents: Streptomycin or gentamicin continued for 10 days
  - Ciprofloxacin if community-acquired pneumonia is in the differential diagnosis of patients ≥18 yr of age

- Tetracycline or doxycycline in those >8 yr of age; or chloramphenicol:
  - Continue for 14 days, since these drugs are only bacteriostatic.
  - Associated with a higher rate of treatment failures than the previously mentioned antibiotics
  - Third tier of treatment, since they are static

### Pediatric Considerations
Streptomycin and gentamicin are recommended as first-line agents.

### MEDICATION
#### First Line
- Gentamicin: 5 mg/kg IV or IM q24h (peds: 2.5 mg/kg IV or IM q8h)
- Streptomycin: 1 g IM (peds: 15 mg/kg, not to exceed 2 g/d) q12h

#### Second Line
- Ciprofloxacin: 400 mg (peds: 15 mg/kg) IV q12h
- Chloramphenicol: 15 mg/kg IV q6h (adult and peds)
- Doxycycline: 100 mg (peds: if weight ≥45 kg, 100 mg; if weight ≤45 kg, 2.2 mg/kg) IV q12h

 FOLLOW-UP

### DISPOSITION
#### Admission Criteria
- ICU admission for advanced age, neutropenia, severe hypoxemia, hemodynamic instability, or patients presenting with typhoidal tularemia
- Inpatient floor bed admission for mild to moderate illness:
  - Isolation bed required only for the purpose of ruling out other etiology (eg, tuberculosis)

#### Discharge Criteria
Outpatient therapy oral or IM therapy for mild illness with close follow-up

#### Issues for Referral
Critical care and infectious disease consultation to assist in assessment of differential considerations and manage life-threatening complications

### FOLLOW-UP RECOMMENDATIONS
Infectious disease consultation to manage ongoing treatment and reduce subsequent exposures

### PEARLS AND PITFALLS
- Patients presenting with high fever and regional lymphadenopathy, especially if there is an ulcer or conjunctivitis, should have tularemia in the differential.
- Epidemiology may be useful in pointing to this diagnosis.
- Diagnosis ultimately based upon serology.
- Vaccine currently under review by FDA, not currently available in the U.S.
- Also known as "rabbit fever" or "deer-fly fever"
- Currently listed as category A (critical agent of concern) bioterrorism agent because of pathogenicity. It can be disseminated via dispersal in food, water, or air.

### ADDITIONAL READING

- American Academy of Pediatrics. *Red Book 2009 Report of the Committee on Infectious Diseases*. Elk Grove, IL: AAP; 2009.
- Centers for Disease Control and Prevention. Brief report: Tularemia associated with a hamster bite—Colorado, 2004. *MMWR*. 2005;53: 1202–1203.
- Centers for Disease Control and Prevention. Tularemia—United States, 1990–2000. *MMWR*. 2002;51:181–184.
- Dennis DT, Inglesby TV, et al. Tularemia as a biological weapon. *JAMA*. 2001;285:2763–2773.
- Eliasson H, Broman T, Forsman M. Tularemia: Current epidemiology and disease management. *Infect Dis Clin North Am*. 2006;20:289–311.
- Ellis J, Oyston PC, Green M, et al. Tularemia. *J Clin Microbiol Rev*. 2002;15:631–634. *Francisella tularensis* in the United States. *EID Journal*. 2005;11(12):1834–1841.

 CODES

#### ICD9
- 021.0 Ulceroglandular tularemia
- 021.1 Enteric tularemia
- 021.2 Pulmonary tularemia

# TUMOR COMPRESSION SYNDROMES
*Hany Y. Atallah*

## 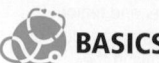 BASICS

### DESCRIPTION
- Complications arising from the compression of neural or vascular structures by solid tumors or their direct infiltration of such structures
- Spinal cord compression:
  - Affects over 20,000 patients each year
  - Occurs in 5–14% of cancer patients
  - More than 50% of cases are metastases from lung, breast, or prostate cancer.
  - Vertebral metastases are far more common than epidural spinal cord compression (ESCC).
  - Approximately 20% of cases of ESCC represent the initial manifestation of malignancy.
- Other neurologic tumor compression:
  - Brachial plexus
  - Recurrent laryngeal nerve compression by mediastinal lymph nodes
- Superior vena cava syndrome (SVC):
  - Obstruction of returning blood flow in the superior vena cave by compression, infiltration, or thrombosis
  - Venous hypertension within the area ordinarily drained by the SVC
  - In severe cases, gradual elevation of the intracranial pressure (ICP), with altered mental status and coma
  - 60–85% caused by malignancy

### ETIOLOGY
- Spinal cord compression:
  - Prostate cancer
  - Breast cancer
  - Lung cancer
  - Renal cell carcinoma
  - Multiple myeloma
  - Melanoma
  - Thyroid cancer
  - Lymphoma
  - Sarcoma
- Brachial plexus compression:
  - 0.4% of cancers
  - 2–5% of those who receive radiation treatment
  - Lung cancer
  - Breast cancer
- SVC syndrome from tumor compression:
  - Lung cancer (most common):
    ○ Small cell lung cancer primarily
  - Postirradiation fibrosis
  - Lymphoma
  - Breast cancer
  - Testicular cancer
  - See differential diagnosis for nontumoral causes of the SVC syndrome.

### Pediatric Considerations
In children with spinal cord compression, common causes are sarcoma, neuroblastoma, germ cell tumors, and lymphoma.

##  DIAGNOSIS

### SIGNS AND SYMPTOMS
#### History
- Spinal cord compression:
  - History of malignancy
  - Back or neck pain:
    ○ Prolonged
    ○ Worse with rest
    ○ Most commonly affects the thoracic spine
  - Paresthesias
  - Difficulty ambulating
  - Constipation
  - Urinary retention
  - Urinary or fecal incontinence
  - Weight loss
- Brachial plexus compression:
  - Neuropathic pain involving the medial aspect of the upper extremity
- Intrathoracic vagal nerve compression:
  - Ipsilateral aching facial pain around the ear
- SVC syndrome:
  - Orthopnea
  - Dyspnea
  - Tightness of the shirt collar
  - Cough
  - Chest pain
  - Headache
  - Facial swelling
  - Head fullness
  - Blurred vision
  - Dizziness
  - Syncope

#### Physical Exam
- Spinal cord compression:
  - Loss of rectal tone
  - Loss of anal wink
  - Weakness in 60–85% of patients
  - Sensory findings less common
- Laryngeal nerve compression:
  - Hoarseness
  - Vocal cord paralysis
- Brachial plexus:
  - Ulnar paresthesias
  - Weakness and wasting of intrinsic hand muscles
  - Pan-plexopathy
  - Horner syndrome
- SVC syndrome:
  - Periorbital edema
  - Conjunctival suffusion
  - Facial swelling
  - Facial plethora
  - Upper extremity edema
  - Findings exacerbated by recumbent or stooped-over position
  - Usually worse in the early morning hours
  - ICP may be elevated in severe cases:
    ○ Altered mental status
    ○ Coma
    ○ Papilledema

## DIAGNOSTIC TESTS & INTERPRETATION
### Imaging
- Chest radiograph:
  - Spinal cord compression:
    ○ May identify a primary lung tumor
    ○ Helpful in excluding tuberculous spondylitis
  - SVC compression:
    ○ Mass present in 10%
    ○ Pleural effusion in 25%
    ○ Plain spinal radiography
  - Will show 85% of metastases causing compression
  - A normal spine (or one showing just degenerative changes) on plain radiology does not exclude the diagnosis of possible cord compression.
- CT:
  - Contrast CT is more sensitive and specific than plain radiography and radionucleotide imaging in distinguishing benign from malignant disease in spinal compression syndrome
  - May identify mass and impingement in vena cava obstruction
- MRI:
  - Study of choice for spinal cord compression
  - Indicated in patients with back or neck pain and:
    ○ History of cancer
    ○ Bowel or bladder dysfunction
    ○ Lower extremity weakness
    ○ Sensory loss

### Diagnostic Procedures/Surgery
- CT myelography:
  - Indicated for spinal cord compression when MRI is unavailable or contraindicated (pacemaker, metallic implants, severe claustrophobia)
- Minimally invasive techniques can often be used to establish a tissue diagnosis in cases of SVC syndrome.
- Occasionally an invasive procedure is required to obtain a tumor biopsy in patients with SVC syndrome:
  - Bronchoscopy
  - Mediastinoscopy
  - Scalene node biopsy
  - Limited thoracotomy
- Radiation therapy (RT) can be done to shrink the tumor:
  - Should be done after tissue diagnosis is made, as RT can obscure tissue and make definitive diagnosis difficult.
- Endovascular stents can be used to achieve more rapid relief than can be achieved using radiation therapy.

## DIFFERENTIAL DIAGNOSIS
### Spinal Cord Compression
- Amyotrophic lateral sclerosis
- Arteriovenous malformations
- Epidural abscess
- Intervertebral disk disease
- Multiple sclerosis
- Neurologic diseases
- Osteoporotic vertebral fractures
- Primary bone tumors
- Spinal infarction
- Spondylitis
- Spondylosis
- Transverse myelitis

### Superior Vena Cava Syndrome
- Pericardial tamponade
- Nephrotic syndrome
- Cor pulmonale
- Cirrhosis
- Nonmalignant etiologies of SVC syndrome:
  - Goiter
  - Pericardial constriction
  - Primary thrombosis
  - Idiopathic sclerosing aortitis
  - Tuberculous mediastinitis
  - Fibrosing mediastinitis
  - Histoplasmosis
  - Indwelling central venous catheters

 **TREATMENT**

### INITIAL STABILIZATION/THERAPY
- Early diagnosis and treatment are the keys to an improved outcome.
- Level of neurologic dysfunction on presentation is a key factor in the prognosis for spinal cord compression.
- Avoid IV line placement in upper extremities if severe SVC compression is present.

## ED TREATMENT/PROCEDURES
### Spinal Cord Compression
- Corticosteroids (dexamethasone):
  - Administer in ED.
  - Higher doses alleviate the pain more rapidly, but studies indicate no significant difference in outcome with regard to sphincter function or ambulation between the dose schedules.
- Radiotherapy:
  - Definitive treatment modality
  - Pain medication with narcotics
  - Oncology, radiotherapy, and neurosurgical consultation for further management of tumor/malignancy
  - Consider empiric broad-spectrum antibiotics prior to the MRI if an epidural abscess is being considered.

### SVC Compression
- Manage the underlying malignancy with either radiotherapy or chemotherapy.
- Elevation of the head of the bed.
- Judicious use of diuretics will transiently improve symptoms.
- Administer steroids if there is respiratory compromise.
- Urgent oncology referral
- Intravascular stents may relieve the obstruction more rapidly.

### MEDICATION
- Dexamethasone: 1 mg/kg loading dose, followed by 4–24 mg q6h
- Furosemide (Lasix): No prior use—40 mg IVP; prior use—double 24 hr dose (80–180 mg IV)
- Hydrocodone/acetaminophen: 5/500 mg PO q4h–q6h
- Oxycodone/acetaminophen: 5/500 mg PO q4h–q6h

 **FOLLOW-UP**

### DISPOSITION
#### Admission Criteria
- Admission is advisable for all patients presenting with a tumor compression syndrome.
- Transfer to a center with neurosurgical capabilities may be needed for patients with spinal cord compression.

#### Discharge Criteria
None

#### Issues for Referral
- Radiation oncology should be consulted for patients presenting with tumor compression.
- Early neurosurgical consultation for patients with spinal cord compression

## PEARLS AND PITFALLS
- Average life expectancy among patients who present with malignancy-associated SVC syndrome is approximately 6 months.
- Presentations may be subtle and compression syndromes should always be considered in patients with known malignancy and unexplained complaints.

## ADDITIONAL READING
- Cole JS, Patchell RA. Metastatic epidural spinal cord compression. *Lancet Neurol.* 2008;7(5):459–466.
- Graham PH, Capp A, Delaney G, et al. A pilot randomised comparison of dexamethasone 96 mg vs 16 mg per day for malignant spinal-cord compression treated by radiotherapy: TROG 01.05 Superdex study. *Clin Oncol (R Coll Radiol).* 2006;18:70.
- Lanciego C, Pangua C, Chacón JI, et al. Endovascular stenting as the first step in the overall management of malignant superior vena cava syndrome. *AJR Am J Roentgenol.* 2009;193(2):549–558.
- Wilson LD, Detterbeck FC, Yahalom J. Clinical practice. Superior vena cava syndrome with malignant causes. *N Engl J Med.* 2007;356:1862.

The author gratefully acknowledges the contributions of Richard Wolfe and Martin J. Carey to the previous editions of this chapter.

 **CODES**

ICD9
- 344.60 Cauda equina syndrome without mention of neurogenic bladder
- 459.2 Compression of vein

# TYMPANIC MEMBRANE PERFORATION

*Andrew K. Chang*
*Hong K. Choi*

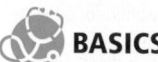 **BASICS**

## DESCRIPTION

Perforations can be classified in several ways:

- Duration:
  - Acute (<3 mo)
  - Chronic (>3 mo)
- Site:
  - Pars tensa
  - Pars flaccida
- Extent:
  - Limited to one quadrant (<25%)
  - Two or more quadrants
  - Total perforation

## ETIOLOGY

- Infection (acute otitis media):
  - Most common cause of an acute perforation
- Blunt trauma (slap to the ear)
- Penetrating trauma (Q-tip)
- Extrusion of tympanostomy tubes
- Rapid pressure change (diving, flying):
  - Rupture usually occurs between 100 and 400 mm Hg (at a depth of 2.6 ft, there is a pressure differential of 60 mm Hg).
- Extreme noise (blast)
- Lightning
- Acute necrotic myringitis (beta-hemolytic streptococcus)
- Slag burns (welding or metalworking)
- Complications of surgical procedures:
  - Myringotomy, tympanoplasty, tympanostomy tube insertion

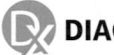 **DIAGNOSIS**

## SIGNS AND SYMPTOMS

### History

- Ear pain (mild)
- Severe pain or complete hearing loss in the affected ear suggests additional injuries.
- Tinnitus
- Vertigo (especially if perforation occurs in water)

### Physical Exam

- Loss of hearing (partial)
- Purulent or bloody discharge from ear canal
- Insufflation via pneumatic otoscope:
  - Small perforations may be evident only as an immobile tympanic membrane.
  - Holding pressure for 15 sec (the fistula test) may cause nystagmus or vertigo if the pressure is transmitted through the middle ear and into a labyrinthine fistula.
- Weber test (tuning fork on midline bone):
  - Sound should be equal or louder in the injured ear, consistent with decreased conduction.
  - Sound localizing to the opposite side of injury indicates possible otic nerve injury.
- Rinne test (tuning fork on mastoid process):
  - Usually normal (air conduction detected after bone conduction fades) or shows a small conductive loss

## ESSENTIAL WORKUP

Clinical examination:

- Direct visualization of tympanic membrane with otoscope
- Test hearing in both ears.
- Note any nystagmus with changes of position or pressure on the tragus occluding the canal (fistula sign).

## DIAGNOSTIC TESTS & INTERPRETATION

### Lab

If an aural drainage is present, it may be desirable to culture the drainage.

### Imaging

Cranial CT:

- Obtain if clinically indicated to rule out temporal bone fracture

## DIFFERENTIAL DIAGNOSIS

- Temporal bone fracture
- Serous otitis media
- Infectious otitis media
- Otitis externa
- Cerumen impaction
- Barotrauma
- Acoustic trauma
- Foreign body
- Child abuse

**TREATMENT**

## INITIAL STABILIZATION/THERAPY

ABCs of trauma care:

- Immobilize cervical spine and investigate for intracranial injury when indicated.

## ED TREATMENT/PROCEDURES

- Remove debris from the ear canal:
  - Do not irrigate because this may force more debris into the middle ear.
  - If the tympanic membrane is not visible because of impacted cerumen and suspicion for perforation is high, remove cerumen by manual disimpaction or suctioning.
- If clinically indicated, obtain CT scan to rule out temporal bone fracture.
- Prophylactic antibiotics are not indicated.
- Prescribe antibiotics if there is evidence of infection or if water or contaminants may have entered the ear canal:
  - Amoxicillin
  - Augmentin
  - Cefixime, Ceftriaxone
  - Azithromycin
  - Clindamycin
- Analgesics if needed for pain
- With the exception of fluoroquinolones, the use of ototopical medication is controversial because of the risk of ototoxicity:
  - Most advocate an antibiotic–cortisone otic medication whenever a discharge is present because this may treat or prevent an external canal infection and hasten the resolution of the middle-ear infection.
  - Ototopical antibiotics provide a high concentration of antibiotic in the middle ear, potentially exceeding the MIC of organisms.
  - Ototopical fluoroquinolones are the first-line therapy for chronic suppurative otitis media and in traumatic TM perforation with suspected entry of water into the middle ear (SCUBA, bathing, etc.).
- Urgent ENT consultation (indications):
  - Vertigo
  - Sensorineural hearing loss
  - Severe tinnitus
  - Active and significant bleeding
  - Facial paralysis

## MEDICATION

- Amoxicillin: 500 mg PO t.i.d. (peds: 80–90 mg/kg/24 hr) PO b.i.d. for 7–10 days.
- Augmentin: 875 mg (peds: 90 mg/kg/24 hr) PO b.i.d. for 7–10 days.
- Cefixime: 400 mg (peds: 8 mg/kg/24 hr) PO q.d. for 7–10 days.
- Ceftriaxone: 1–2 g IV/IM (peds 50 mg/kg IM, max 1g) × 1 dose.
- Azithromycin: 2 g (peds 30 mg/kg, max 1500 mg) PO × 1 dose.
- Clindamycin: 150–450 mg (peds 30 mg/kg/24 hr) PO q.i.d. for 7–10 days.
- Ciprofloxacin/dexamethasone otic: 4 drops b.i.d. for 7–10 days.

### First Line

- Amoxicillin and Augmentin are the primary antibiotic choices for acute
- titis media with subsequent tympanic membrane perforation.
  - Augmentin should be selected for patients with recurrent infections or those who have used antibiotics within 1 month.
  - Ciprofloxacin with dexamethasone otic drops are the medications of choice for chronic suppurative otitis media and traumatic tympanic membrane perforation with suspicion of water or contaminant entry into the middle ear (SCUBA, bathing, Q-tip).

### Second Line

- Penicillin-allergic patients may be prescribed cephalosporins. Ceftriaxone IM may be preferred in patients with vomiting or compliance issues.
- Azithromycin or clindamycin may be used for patients with hypersensitivity type I allergic reaction to penicillin.

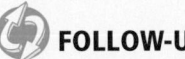 **FOLLOW-UP**

## DISPOSITION

### Admission Criteria

- Associated injuries requiring admission
- Severe vertigo impairing ambulation

### Discharge Criteria

- Almost all patients will be discharged.

### Issues for Referral

- Arrange outpatient ENT follow-up within 1 wk:
  - After detailed examination and formal audiometric tests, most otolaryngologists practice "watchful waiting" because most tympanic membrane perforations heal spontaneously.
  - Operative repair (patch or tympanoplasty) is reserved for the 10%–20% that do not heal spontaneously.

## FOLLOW-UP RECOMMENDATIONS

- Provide detailed discharge instructions:
  - Occlude the ear canal with cotton coated in petroleum jelly or antibiotic ointment when showering to prevent entry of water into the middle ear, which can be painful and may cause further infection.
  - Swim only with fitted earplugs.
  - Avoid forceful blowing of the nose.
- Expected outcome:
  - Most perforations heal spontaneously in a few days to several months; in one study of children, 70% closed within 1 wk and 94% closed within 1 mo.
  - Perforations caused by molten metal or electrical burns are less likely to heal spontaneously.
    - Complications include infection, dislocation of ossicles, perilymph leak, and cholesteatoma.

## PEARLS AND PITFALLS

- Acute otitis media is the most common cause of tympanic membrane perforation.
  - Small tympanic membrane perforations may be diagnosed only through insufflation by pneumatic otoscope.

- Debris, cerumen, or discharge should be suctioned or manually removed; irrigation is contraindicated in cases of suspected tympanic membrane perforation.
- Ototopical fluoroquinolones are the antibiotics of choice for chronic suppurative otitis media and traumatic tympanic membrane perforation with suspected penetration by foreign body, water, or contaminant.
- Most perforations heal spontaneously; however, care must be exercised to prevent further introduction of infectious agents into the open middle ear.

## ADDITIONAL READING

- Kristensen S. Spontaneous healing of traumatic tympanic membrane perforations in man: A century of experience. *J Laryngol Otol*. 1992;106:1037–1050.
- Macfadyen CA. Systemic antibiotics versus topical treatments for chronically discharging ears with underlying eardrum perforations. *Cochrane Database Syst Rev*. 2005(4):CD004618.
- Haynes DS. Ototoxicity of ototopical drops: An update. *Otolaryngol Clin North Am*. 2007;40(3):669–683, xi.
- Ramakrishnan K. Diagnosis and treatment of otitis media. *Am Fam Physician*. 2007;76(11):1650–1658.
- Wright D. Treatment of otitis media with perforated tympanic membrane. *Am Fam Physician*. 2009;79(8):653–654.

### See Also (Topic, Algorithm, Electronic Media Element)

- Barotrauma
- Otitis Media

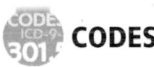 **CODES**

### ICD9

384.20 Perforation of tympanic membrane, unspecified

T

# ULTRAVIOLET KERATITIS

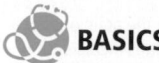

Yasuharu Okuda
Nicholas Genes

## BASICS

### DESCRIPTION
- Corneal epithelial damage caused by direct exposure to ultraviolet (UV) light.
- Also known as photokeratitis, UV conjunctivitis, snow blindness, and welder's flash.

### ETIOLOGY
- Work-related exposures seen in welders, electricians, and mechanics
- Recreational exposures, including tanning booths and high-altitude sports
- Occurs with corneal absorption of UV-B light at wavelengths of 290–310 nm.
- UV-B penetrates to the epithelia nocireceptor terminal axons, destroying them and triggering stimulation of the subendothelial nerves, which causes the pain.
- Related both to intensity and duration of exposure

## DIAGNOSIS

### SIGNS AND SYMPTOMS
- Patients will present with bilateral eye pain, photophobia, redness, and tearing.
- No purulent discharge will be present.
- Associated facial edema, lid edema, and erythema may be present.

### History
- Elicit history of exposure to UV light 6–12 hr prior to complaint of pain.
- Complaints may include:
  - Severe pain
  - Photophobia
  - Tearing
  - Foreign-body sensation

### Physical Exam
- Visual acuity may be mildly diminished.
- Eye exam reveals chemosis, injection, tearing.
- Slit-lamp exam with topical ophthalmic anesthetics and flourescein:
  - Multiple superficial punctate corneal lesions
  - Otherwise unremarkable

### ESSENTIAL WORKUP
- Accurate history including:
  - Type of exposure
  - Timing and duration of exposure
- Visual acuity
- Complete ocular examination including:
  - Extraocular movements
  - Exam of conjunctiva/sclera/cornea with fluorescein
  - Anterior chamber checking for cell and flare
  - Eversion of lids to check for foreign bodies

### DIAGNOSTIC TESTS & INTERPRETATION
#### Lab
Blood testing will not be necessary unless widespread severe sunburn is present.

#### Imaging
A careful history should obviate need for orbital US/CT/MRI for foreign body.

### DIFFERENTIAL DIAGNOSIS
- Infection:
  - Bacterial or viral conjunctivitis
  - Corneal ulcers
- Allergic conjunctivitis
- Corneal abrasion
- Traumatic iritis
- Foreign bodies
- Chemical burns:
  - Acid
  - Alkali
- Thermal burns

## TREATMENT

### PRE-HOSPITAL
Pressure patching or applying mild pressure to eyes with closed lids may provide some temporary relief in cases where diagnosis is already unambiguously established.

### INITIAL STABILIZATION/THERAPY
Apply topical anesthetic agents for pain relief and to obtain more thorough physical exam.

### ED TREATMENT/PROCEDURES
- Topical anesthetic to facilitate slit-lamp exam
- Provide adequate oral analgesia as needed.
- Apply topical antibiotic ointment.
- Initiate short-acting cycloplegic agent.
- May apply eye patching for comfort:
  - Soft double patching with mild pressure for patient comfort
  - If both eyes involved, either patch both eyes or patch the eye that is more severely affected.
  - Patching has not been shown to accelerate healing.

## MEDICATION

- Topical anesthetic agent (for ED only):
  - Tetracaine hydrochlorideophthalmic solution 0.5%:, 1 or 2 drops into affected eye
    - Do not prescribe for outpatient as it may decrease healing and increase corneal ulcer formation.
- Oral analgesics:
  - Ibuprofen 10 mg/kg t.i.d. with meals
  - Acetaminophen with oxycodone 500 mg/5 mg, q4–6h PRN for breakthrough pain
- Topical antibiotic ointment:
  - Erythromycin ophthalmic ointment 0.5%, apply to affected eye q.i.d.
- Cycloplegic agent:
  - Scopolamine hydrobromideophthalmic solution 0.25%:, 1 or 2 drops into affected eye q6–q8h
  - Cyclopentolate hydrochlorideophthalmic solution 0.5%:, 1 or 2 drops into affected eye q6–8h

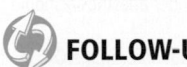 **FOLLOW-UP**

## DISPOSITION

### Admission Criteria
Consider admission for patients with severe decreased visual acuity, who require bilateral patching, or whose social circumstances make self-care and follow-up difficult.

### Discharge Criteria
Nearly all patients may be discharged from the ED following treatment with oral analgesics, topical antibiotics, cycloplegics, and/or patching:
- Lesions should heal completely within 24–72 hr.

### FOLLOW-UP RECOMMENDATIONS
- Follow up with ophthalmologist within 24–48 hr to monitor healing and symptom resolution.
- Long-term UV damage to eye may result in pterygium and some forms of corneal degeneration, though association with UV keratitis episodes has not been demonstrated.

## PEARLS AND PITFALLS

- Determining UV exposure 6–12 hours prior is the key to diagnosis and prevention:
  - The patient may not be aware of exposure
- Supportive care is all that is necessary.
- Those at risk for occupational exposure must wear UV safety goggles, not glasses or lenses.
- This exquisitely painful injury is self-limited, but risks from repeated exposures are not well defined.

## ADDITIONAL READING

- Marx JA, et al. *Rosen's Emergency Medicine: Concepts and Clinical Practice*, 6th ed. St. Louis: Mosby, 2009.
- Jacobs DS. Photokeratitis. In: Basow DS, ed. *UpToDate*. Waltham, MA: UpToDate, 2009.
- Yen Y, Lin Hs, Lin Hu, et al. Photokeratoconjunctivitis caused by different light sources. *Am J Emerg Med*. 2004;22:511–515.
- Young R. Family of sunlight-related eye diseases. *Optom Vision Sci*. 1994;71(2):128–144.

### See Also (Topic, Algorithm, Electronic Media Element)
- Conjunctivitis
- Corneal Burn
- Red Eye

 **CODES**

ICD9
370.8 Other forms of keratitis

U

# URETHRAL TRAUMA

*Amanda J. Lamond*

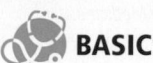 **BASICS**

## DESCRIPTION

- Blood at the urethral meatus, a palpable full bladder, inability to void, and/or gross hematuria are common findings with urethral trauma.
- Found in 14% of pelvic fractures
- High association with bilateral pubic rami fractures (aka, straddle fractures)
- Females: Urethral injuries are rare likely due to short, unexposed, and mobile urethras.
- Girls <17 yr: Higher injury rate likely from a more flexible pelvic ring
- Bladder neck most commonly injured location.
- Males: The urethra is divided into 2 sections.
- Posterior urethra:
  – More commonly injured (~90%)
  – Prostatic portion
  – Membranous
- Anterior urethra:
  – Injuries are rare
  – Bulbar
  – Penile
- Posterior urethra injuries comprise up to 90% of trauma and have the classification scheme detailed below:
  – Type 1: Urethra stretched but not ruptured
  – Type 2: Prostatic/membranous portions disrupted (either partially or completely); urogenital diaphragm intact
  – Type 3: Urethral disruption both proximal and distal to the genitourinary diaphragm

## ETIOLOGY

- Females:
  – Straddle injuries
  – Rare with pelvic fractures
  – Childbirth or vaginal surgery
  – Sexual trauma/abuse
- Males:
  – Pelvic fractures: Especially straddle injuries
  – Penetrating trauma, mutilation
  – Sexual activity/instrumentation

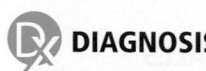 **DIAGNOSIS**

## SIGNS AND SYMPTOMS

- Males:
  – Blood at the urethral meatus or gross hematuria
- Females:
  – Blood in the vaginal vault or gross hematuria

### History
Trauma

### Physical Exam

- Examination of the torso and pelvis during the secondary survey may elicit pelvic pain.
- Triad of blood at the urethral meatus, inability to urinate, and a palpably full bladder
- Blood at the meatus found in 50% of cases.
- Urologic injury can be indicated by gross hematuria (any color to the urine other than clear or yellow)
- Digital rectal exam: "High-riding prostate" has a sensitivity of <50%. Do not rely on this finding to rule out urethral trauma if suspected.
- Bedside US: FAST exam, suprapubic views may reveal blood surrounding the bladder.

## ESSENTIAL WORKUP

- Females:
  – Perform a detailed vaginal exam to exclude vaginal laceration or other etiologies of bleeding.
  – If trauma is suspected, radiological evaluation of urethra should be performed.
  – If this is not possible, suprapubic aspiration or cystostomy should be done.
- Male:
  – Radiographic evaluation of urethral integrity should be performed before urinary catheter placement if injury is suspected.
  – If not possible, suprapubic aspiration or cystostomy should be performed.

### Pediatric Considerations

- If an exam of the male or female genitals cannot easily be performed, exam under anesthesia should occur.
- An exam with procedural sedation or in the OR, in addition to being better tolerated by the patient, allows the physician to rule out sexual abuse and to confirm that the injury is consistent with the history.

## DIAGNOSTIC TESTS & INTERPRETATION
### Lab
Urinalysis, hematocrit, BUN, creatinine

### Imaging

- Retrograde urethrography (RUG):
  – Water-soluble contrast is injected via a catheter-tipped syringe at the urethral meatus.
  – Extravasation of contrast and its relation to the prevesical space and urogenital diaphragm should be noted.
  – Proximity of the extravasation to the meatus and the bladder should be appreciated.
  – If the urethral tear is complete, there will be no contrast within the bladder and marked extravasation will occur.
  – A partial tear will demonstrate contrast material within the bladder with varying amounts of extravasation.

- Excretory urethrography to define proximal urethral tears.
- Cystography
- 40% of urethral injuries have concomitant bladder injuries.

### Diagnostic Procedures/Surgery
Urethral trauma warrants urgent urological consultation.

### DIFFERENTIAL DIAGNOSIS
- Perineal and vaginal trauma
- Bladder injury
- Ureter or kidney trauma

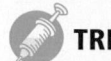 **TREATMENT**

### PRE-HOSPITAL
Prehospital trauma protocols

### INITIAL STABILIZATION/THERAPY
Stabilization of multiple traumas takes precedence.

### ED TREATMENT/PROCEDURES
- Urethral contusions, lacerations, and avulsions are best managed by an experienced urologist.
- Bladder decompression is an important initial intervention. If urethral Foley catheter placement is not possible, suprapubic aspiration/cystostomy may need to be performed.

### MEDICATION
Appropriate analgesia

### First Line
Opioids:

- Morphine, Dilaudid, fentanyl, as needed per trauma protocols for pain

 **FOLLOW-UP**

### DISPOSITION
### Admission Criteria
- Concurrent traumatic injuries
- Need for emergent operative management of urethral, penile, or bladder injuries
- Partial lacerations:
  - Managed with urethral or suprapubic drainage
- Complete lacerations:
  - Managed surgically or with suprapubic drainage alone:
    - Repaired with end-to-end anastomosis

### Discharge Criteria
Isolated urethral injuries frequently may be managed in the outpatient setting after appropriate urinary catheterization or suprapubic cystostomy with next-day urologic follow-up.

### Issues for Referral
Urologic follow-up is necessary if patient is discharged from ED.

### FOLLOW-UP RECOMMENDATIONS
Urologic follow-up is necessary for all patients with urethral injuries.

## PEARLS AND PITFALLS

- Consult urology before attempting to insert a Foley in a trauma patient in whom urethral injury is highly suspected.
- Passing a Foley catheter against resistance could convert a partial tear to a complete tear.
- Failure to recognize a urethral injury can result in urinary incontinence and sexual dysfunction.

## ADDITIONAL READING

- Goldman SM, Sandler CM, Corriere JN Jr. , et al. Blunt urethral trauma: A unified, anatomical mechanical classification. *J Urology.* 1997;157: 85–89.
- Marx JA, Hockberger RS, Walls RM, et al. *Rosen's emergency medicine: Concepts and clinical practice,* 7th edition. Philadelphia: Mosby Elsevier, 2010.
- Rosenstein D, McAninch J. Urological emergencies. *Med Clinics of North Am.* 2004;88(2).
- Smith J, Denney P. Imaging of renal trauma. *Radiologic Clinics of North Am.* 2003;41(4).
- Walsh P. et al. *Campbell's urology,* 9th ed. New York: Saunders, 2007.

### See Also (Topic, Algorithm, Electronic Media Element)
Pelvic Trauma

 **CODES**

**ICD9**
867.0 Injury to bladder and urethra without mention of open wound into cavity

U

# URETHRITIS

*Hany Y. Atallah*

##  BASICS

### DESCRIPTION
- Urethritis is inflammation of the urethra from any cause (usually infection).
- Associated with urethral discharge and dysuria
- Urethritis may develop after exposure to a partner with an STD, bacterial vaginosis, or UTI.
- Urethritis may also develop after orogenital contact.

### ETIOLOGY
- STD; the most common causes are:
  - *Neisseria gonorrhoeae* (35%)
  - *Chlamydia trachomatis* (25%–50%)
  - *Mycoplasma genitalium* and *Ureaplasma urealyticum* (30%)
- Rarer causes:
  - *Trichomonas vaginalis*
  - Candidal species
  - Herpes simplex virus
  - Adenovirus
  - Genital warts
  - Enteric bacteria (in the setting of insertive anal sex)
  - Alcohol
  - Systemic illnesses
  - Urethral foreign bodies

## 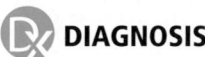 DIAGNOSIS

- Symptoms usually develop 1–2 wk after exposure but can take up to 4–6 wk.
- Initially minimal or absent in many patients

### SIGNS AND SYMPTOMS
- Urethral discharge, dysuria
- Cloudy first portion of urine
- Pyuria
- Inguinal adenopathy may be present.

### History
- Color, consistency, and quantity of urethral discharge.
- Associated symptoms of dysuria, urgency, frequency, hematuria, and hematospermia
- Risk factors for STDs:
  - Recent new partner or multiple sexual partners
  - Symptoms of partner
  - Anal/oral practices
  - Young age
  - Lower socioeconomic status

### Physical Exam
- Urethral discharge
- Staining on undergarments
- Meatal crusting
- Genital lesions
- Lymphadenopathy
- Palpate testes, epididymis, and spermatic cord:
  - Masses or tenderness

### ESSENTIAL WORKUP
- Urethral swabs for *N. gonorrhoeae* and *Chlamydia* species will confirm the diagnosis.
- DNA amplification, DNA probe, and testing of urine specimens via polymerase chain reaction (PCR) have shown good sensitivity and are acceptable tests
- A rapid plasma regain (RPR) or Venereal Disease Research Laboratory (VDRL) should be drawn because STDs frequently occur together.

### DIAGNOSTIC TESTS & INTERPRETATION
### Lab
- Gram's stain and cultures from urethral swabs should be reviewed when the patient is re-evaluated by his or her physician after treatment.
- DNA amplification (ligase chain reaction [LCR] or PCR) can be used on first-void urine or urethral swab:
  - Equal efficacy for diagnosing *N. gonorrhoeae* and *Chlamydia* species
- UA should be performed after urethral swabs to identify UTIs.

### DIFFERENTIAL DIAGNOSIS
- Chemical irritation from soaps or spermicides
- Epididymitis
- Orchitis
- Pelvic inflammatory disease
- Prostatitis
- Reactive arthritis (formerly Reiter syndrome)
- Urethral chancre (from syphilis)
- UTI

### Pediatric Considerations
- Urethritis in children should arouse suspicion of child abuse.
- Because *N. gonorrhoeae* infects the entire vaginal vault in prepubescents, a speculum examination is not required:
  - External examination and cultures are sufficient.
- Potential complications:
  - Recurrent infections
  - Ascending UTIs, including pelvic inflammatory disease and epididymoorchitis
  - Fallopian tube damage and infertility
  - Arthritis
  - Conjunctivitis, uveitis, and blindness

## 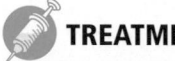 TREATMENT

### INITIAL STABILIZATION/THERAPY
Most patients will not require significant stabilization.

### ED TREATMENT/PROCEDURES
- Treatment may be given empirically based on probable etiology.
- Patients should be treated for both *N. gonorrhoeae* and *C. trachomatis*.

### MEDICATION
- Gonorrhea:
  - Azithromycin 2 g orally once
  - Cefixime 400 mg PO once
  - Cefotaxime 500 mg IM once (administered with probenicid 1 g orally once)
  - Cefoxitin 2 g IM once (administered with probenicid 1 g orally once)
  - Cefpodoxime 400 mg PO once
  - Ceftizoxime 500 mg IM once
  - Ceftriaxone 125 mg (peds: 25–50 mg/kg) IM/IV once
  - Cefuroxime 1 g orally once
  - Ciprofloxacin 500 mg PO once
  - Gatifloxacin 400 mg PO once
  - Levofloxacin 250 mg PO once
  - Ofloxacin 400 mg PO once
  - Spectinomycin 2 g IM once

- *Chlamydia*:
  - Azithromycin 1 g (peds: 10 mg/kg/day 1, 5 mg/kg days 2 through 5) PO once
  - Doxycycline 100 mg PO b.i.d. for 7 days
  - Erythromycin base 500 mg (peds: 40 mg/kg/day div. q.i.d.) PO q.i.d. for 7 days
  - Erythromycin ethyl succinate 800 mg (peds: 30–50 mg/kg/day div. q.i.d.) PO q.i.d. for 7 days
  - Levofloxacin 500 mg PO q.d. for 7 days
  - Ofloxacin: 300 mg PO b.i.d. for 7 days

### Pregnancy Considerations
- Fluoroquinolones and doxycycline are contraindicated in pregnancy
- Azithromycin is safe and effective
- Repeat testing 3 wk after treatment is recommended to ensure cure.

### ALERT
Increasing incidence of quinolone-resistant *N. gonorrhoeae* nationwide.

 FOLLOW-UP

## DISPOSITION
### Admission Criteria
Patients should not require admission for urethritis unless there are other complaints or infections.

### Discharge Criteria
All patients should be discharged with follow-up arranged at an outside clinic or with PCP.

### Issues for Referral
- If child abuse is suspected, child protective services must be involved; the child should be admitted if a safe home situation cannot be ensured.
- Sexual partners should be evaluated.
- In many states, STDs require reporting.

## FOLLOW-UP RECOMMENDATIONS
- All patients should follow up with primary care to ensure adequate treatment of the infection.
- All patients with suspected or confirmed urethritis should be referred for HIV testing.
- Patients should be given information regarding safe sexual practices.

## PEARLS AND PITFALLS

- Always treat for both *N. gonorrhoeae* and *C. trachomatis* in suspected urethritis.
- There is increasing evidence suggesting that patients with recurrent urethritis should be evaluated for infection with other atypical organisms.
- Always consider other STDs in patients with urethritis.
- Ensure that patients will inform their sexual partners so that they can be treated as well.

## ADDITIONAL READING

- Centers for Disease Control and Prevention. *Sexually Transmitted Disease Surveillance, 2006.* Atlanta: U.S. Department of Health and Human Services, 2007.
- Mandell GL, Bennett JE, Dolin R, eds. *Principles and Practice of Infectious Diseases*, 6th ed. Philadelphia: Churchill Livingstone, 2004.
- Merchant RC, Depalo DM, Stein MD, Rich JD. Adequacy of testing, empiric treatment, and referral for adult male emergency department patients with possible chlamydia and/or gonorrhea urethritis. *Int J STD AIDS*. 2009;20(8):534–539.

- Takahashi S, Matsukawa M, Kurimura Y, et al. Clinical efficacy of azithromycin for male nongonococcal urethritis. *J Infect Chemother*. 2008;14(6):409–412.
- Workowski KA, Berman SM. Sexually transmitted diseases treatment guidelines, 2006. *MMWR Recomm Rep*. 2006;55:1.

### See Also (Topic, Algorithm, Electronic Media Element)
- Chancroid
- Epididymitis/Orchitis
- Gonococcal Disease
- Herpes, Genital
- Lymphogranuloma Venereum
- Pelvic Inflammatory Disease
- Prostatitis
- Syphilis
- Urinary Tract Infections, Adult
- Urinary Tract Infections, Pediatric
- Vaginal Discharge/Vaginitis

 CODES

### ICD9
- 099.49 Other nongonococcal urethritis, other specified organism
- 597.80 Urethritis, unspecified

U

# URINARY RETENTION
*Denise S. Lawe*

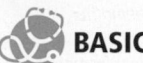 **BASICS**

## DESCRIPTION
- Acute urinary retention (AUR):
  - Sudden inability to void spontaneously
  - Occurs most frequently in men >60 yr old
  - Most common cause of AUR in the ED is benign prostatic hyperplasia (BPH).
- Atonic bladder:
  - More common in women
  - Decompensated bladder that has resulted from years of infrequent voiding
  - Destruction of sensory nerve fibers from the bladder to spinal cord that prevents transmission of stretch signals and prevents micturition reflex contractions
  - Loss of bladder control occurs despite intact neurogenic connections to the brain.
  - Bladder fills to capacity and overflows a few drops at a time (overflow incontinence).
- Automatic bladder:
  - From damage of the spinal cord above the level of S2–S3
  - Micturition inhibited due to "spinal shock" from the sudden loss of facilitatory impulse from the brainstem and cerebrum
  - Intermittent straight catheterization facilitates the return of the excitability of micturition reflex by preventing physical bladder injury.
- Neurogenic bladder:
  - From partial damage to spinal cord or brainstem that interrupts inhibition
  - Sacral centers are in a constant state of excitation, so that even a small quantity of urine results in frequent and relatively uncontrollable micturition.

## ETIOLOGY
- Anatomic:
  - Penis:
    - Phimosis
    - Paraphimosis
    - Meatal stenosis
    - Foreign-body constriction
  - Urethra:
    - Tumor
    - Pelvic masses
    - Prolapse of pelvic organs
    - Foreign body
    - Calculus
    - Urethritis
    - Stricture
    - Meatal stenosis (female)
    - Hematoma
    - Vulvar edema after vaginal delivery

- Prostate gland
  - Benign prostatic hypertrophy
  - Carcinoma
  - Prostatitis
  - Contracture of bladder neck
  - Prostatic infarction
- Neurologic causes:
  - Motor/paralytic
    - Spinal shock
    - Spinal cord syndromes
  - Sensory/paralytic
    - Diabetes
    - Multiple sclerosis
    - Spinal cord syndromes
- Drugs:
  - Antihistamines
  - Anticholinergics
  - Antispasmodics
  - Tricyclic antidepressants
  - Alpha-adrenergic stimulators
  - Narcotics
  - NSAIDs

 **DIAGNOSIS**

## SIGNS AND SYMPTOMS
- Lower abdominal or suprapubic discomfort
- Patients may appear restless or in distress
- Chronic urinary retention usually painless

### History
- Past medical history:
  - History of urinary retention?
  - History of BPH or prostate cancer?
  - History of other cancer?
  - History of radiation treatment?
  - History of pelvic trauma?
- Any signs or symptoms of urinary tract infection, pyelonephritis, or calculus?
- Any neurologic symptoms?
- History of or current IV drug abuse?
- Back pain?
- Complete list of all medications

### Physical Exam
- Abdominal palpation
- Rectal examination
- Pelvic exam in all women
- Thorough neurologic exam
- In the trauma patient, evaluate for evidence of uretheral injury.

## ESSENTIAL WORKUP
- Thorough history and physical examination
- UA

## DIAGNOSTIC TESTS & INTERPRETATION
### Lab
- Basic chemistry to assess renal function only if concerned for acute renal insufficiency (this usually does not occur in AUR)
- No benefit to PSA test; usually elevated in setting of AUR

### Imaging
- Pelvic US or CT scan if concerned for a new or worsening mass or malignancy
- MRI spine if there is concern for an acute neurologic process

### Diagnostic Procedures/Surgery
Postvoid residual: more than 200 mL is abnormal.

## DIFFERENTIAL DIAGNOSIS
- Chronic urinary retention
- UTI

 **TREATMENT**

### PRE-HOSPITAL
If there is septic shock, support unstable vital signs as appropriate.

### INITIAL STABILIZATION/THERAPY
- Prompt bladder decompression:
  - Immediate placement of 14F–18F Foley catheter
  - If obstruction does not allow passage of 14F–18F Foley and there is a history of prior transurethral procedure or known stricture, downsize to a 10F–12F.
  - In men with no prior instrumentation, a 20F–22F catheter with a Coude tip is indicated.
  - If unable to pass a Foley, then either suprapubic aspiration as a temporizing measure or placement of suprapubic catheter is indicated.
- Defer catheterization of the ureter in the trauma patient suspected of having a ureteral injury (gross hematuria, high-riding prostate on rectal exam, blood at the meatus) until a retrograde urethrogram has been done.

## ED TREATMENT/PROCEDURES

- Drain bladder and monitor urine output:
  - Rapid decompression following catheter placement may result in transient gross hematuria, rarely clinically significant.
  - Postobstructive diuresis:
    - ○ Can be a complication of AUR in the catheterized patient
    - ○ No randomized trials comparing rapid and intermittent bladder decompression
    - ○ It is generally now felt that rapid bladder decompression is safe provided that supportive care is available if hypotension develops.
- Probably best to observe for 2–3 hr after bladder decompression to ensure that a postobstructive diuresis does not cause clinical deterioration.
- Place leg Foley bag before discharge if Foley is to remain indwelling.
- Educate patient and family on Foley care.
- Although commonly used, prophylactic antibiotics are not indicated for patients with an indwelling urinary catheter and no evidence of infection.
- Start patients with BPH on an alpha blocker.

## MEDICATION

- Prazosin HCl (Minipress) for treatment of BPH: initially 1 mg PO b.i.d. to t.i.d., slowly increase to 20 mg/day in divided doses
- Tamsulosin (Flomax) is an alpha-1 antagonist used to treat BPH: 0.4 mg PO qd initially; may increase to 0.8 mg PO qd
- Alfuzosin (Uroxatral) is an alpha blocker used to treat BPH: 2.5 mg PO t.i.d.
- Terazosin (Hytrin) facilitates urinary flow in the presence of BPH: start 1 mg PO q.h.s., max 20 mg/day

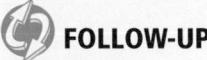 **FOLLOW-UP**

### DISPOSITION

*Admission Criteria*

- Significant postobstructive diuresis requiring IV fluids or pressors
- Urosepsis
- Obstruction related to spinal cord compression
- Consider in patient with obstruction due to malignancy or mass

*Discharge Criteria*

Most patients can be discharged

*Issues for Referral*

Due to the risk of cancer, all obstructions should be referred for the work-up of etiology.

### FOLLOW-UP RECOMMENDATIONS

Mandatory urologic follow-up

- In men with BPH, the urinary catheter is sometimes left in for 1–2 wk.

## PEARLS AND PITFALLS

- Carefully evaluate for evidence of a mass or malignancy as the cause of AUR.
- Carefully evaluate for evidence of spinal cord compression as the cause of AUR.
- Take a thorough drug history including over-the-counter medications, especially if no other clear reason for AUR.

## ADDITIONAL READING

- Acute Urinary Retention. www.uptodate.com. October 14, 2009.
- Marx J, Hockenberger R, Walls R. Acute urinary retention. In: *Rosen's Emergency Medicine,* 7th ed. Philadelphia: Elsevier, 2009.
- Brunicardi FC, Andersen DK, Billiar TL, et al. Acute urinary retention. In: *Schwartz's Principles of Surgery.* New York: McGraw-Hill, 2009.

### See Also (Topic, Algorithm, Electronic Media Element)

Urinary Tract Infections

 **CODES**

ICD9
788.20 Retention of urine, unspecified

U

# URINARY TRACT FISTULA

*Denise S. Lawe*

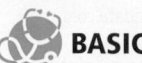 **BASICS**

## DESCRIPTION

Urinary tract fistulas can form between any part of the urinary tract and structures in the thoracic cavity, the abdominal cavity, the pelvis, and the skin.

## ETIOLOGY

- Colovesical fistula:
  - Complication of primary gastrointestinal disease
    - Diverticular disease, most common
    - Crohn's disease
    - Bladder/colon carcinoma
    - Pelvic trauma
    - Radiation exposure
  - More common in males
- Vesicovaginal, urethrovaginal, and ureterovaginal fistulas:
  - Vesicovaginal fistula is the most common acquired fistula of the urinary tract
  - Etiology varies with geography (developed vs developing countries)
    - In developed countries it is usually iatrogenic due to injury to the structures during gynecologic, urologic, or other pelvic surgery.
    - In developing countries it is usually due to obstructed labor and obstetric trauma.

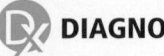 **DIAGNOSIS**

## SIGNS AND SYMPTOMS

- Colovesical fistula:
  - Chronic or recurrent UTIs
  - Suprapubic pain
  - Abnormal urine: pneumaturia, fecaluria, hematuria, malodorous urine, debris in the urine (food particles)
  - Diarrhea
- Vesicovaginal fistula:
  - If due to radiation therapy, may not present for months to years
  - If after surgical procedure, may present on removal of Foley or 1–3 wk postprocedure
  - Usually painless
  - Constant urine leakage from the vagina
  - Perineal skin irritation due to urine leakage
- Urethrovaginal fistula:
  - Symptoms largely dependent on size and location of fistula
  - May be asymptomatic or with continuous vaginal urine drainage
- Ureterovaginal fistula:
  - Postoperativel, abdominal/flank pain and/or low-grade fever likely due to urinoma or renal obstruction
  - Subsequently, constant urine drainage through vagina 1–4 wk postprocedure

## History

- A thorough past medical, surgical, and obstetric history to determine risk factors
- Description and timing of presumed urinary discharge: intermittent or positional usually due to ureterovesical fistula; continuous flow more likely to be from vesicovaginal fistula.
- Characteristics of presumed urinary discharge
- Associated symptoms

## Physical Exam

- Colovesical fistula:
  - There might be findings consistent with the primary gastrointestinal disease; otherwise physical exam is frequently unremarkable
- Vesicovaginal, urethrovaginal, ureterovaginal fistula:
  - Speculum exam may reveal a small reddened area of granulomatous tissue at site of the fistula opening.

## ESSENTIAL WORKUP

Must evaluate for associated urinary infection, renal obstruction, or acute emergencies related to primary disease processes (eg, complications from a malignancy or Crohn's disease).

## DIAGNOSTIC TESTS & INTERPRETATION

### Lab

- Urinalysis:
  - Colovesical fistula:
    - WBCs, bacteria, and debris
  - Vesicovaginal, urethrovaginal, and ureterovaginal fistula:
    - WBCs, bacteria
- BUN and creatinine:
  - If renal obstruction is present, might be abnormal.

### Imaging

- Colovesical fistula:
  - CT of the abdomen/pelvis with contrast
- Vesicovaginal fistula:
  - Cystoscopy or voiding cystourethrography
- Ureterovaginal fistula:
  - Cystoscopy and intravenous pyelogram
- Urethrovaginal fistula:
  - Voiding cystourethrography

### Diagnostic Procedures/Surgery
- Colovesical fistula:
  - Oral administration of activated charcoal will result in black particles in urine, which can be diagnostic.
- Vesicovaginal, urethrovaginal, ureterovaginal fistula:
  - Double-dye test: (1) tampon is placed in vagina, (2) oral phenazopyridine is administered, (3) methylene blue or indigo carmine is instilled into the bladder, (4). if, after an hour, tampon is yellow-orange at the top, ureterovaginal fistula is suggested. Midportion blue discoloration suggests vesicovaginal fistula. Distal blue discoloration suggests urethrovaginal fistula.

## DIFFERENTIAL DIAGNOSIS
- Colovesical fistula:
  - Recurrent UTI
  - Other causes of pneumaturia
    - UTI with gas-forming organism such as clostridia
    - Fermentation of diabetic urine
    - Recent urinary tract instrumentation
- Vesicovaginal, urethrovaginal, and ureterovaginal fistulas:
  - Urinary incontinence
  - Normal vaginal discharge
  - Vaginitis

 TREATMENT

### INITIAL STABILIZATION/THERAPY
Treat urosepsis (rare) with IV fluid bolus, pressors, and IV antibiotics as appropriate.

### ED TREATMENT/PROCEDURES
- Colovesical fistula:
  - Evaluate for complications from patient's primary disease.
  - Obtain cultures if there are signs of UTI.
  - Initiate broad spectrum antibiotic if infection is found.
  - Urgent urologic referral for further management and possible surgical treatment

- Vesicovaginal, urethrovaginal, and ureterovaginal fistula:
  - Place Foley catheter
  - Initiate broad-spectrum antibiotics if a UTI is present.
  - Urgent referral to urologist and gynecologist for further care

 FOLLOW-UP

### DISPOSITION
#### Admission Criteria
- Sepsis
- Inability to take oral antibiotics
- Acute emergencies from primary gastrointestinal disease or malignancies

#### Discharge Criteria
- No evidence of sepsis
- Able to tolerate oral antibiotics if urinary tract infection present

### FOLLOW-UP RECOMMENDATIONS
Urogenital specialist (Urology or Gynecology) follow-up is required.

## PEARLS AND PITFALLS
- Suspect a urinary tract fistula in the patient with the appropriate risk factors and recurrent UTIs
- In the presence of urinary tract fistula, malignancy is always an important diagnostic consideration.

## ADDITIONAL READING
- Basler J. Colovesical fistula. *eMedicine*. August 2004.
- Katz. Urinary fistula. In: *Comprehensive Gynecology*, 5th ed. St Louis: Mosby, 2007.
- Acute diverticulitis complicated by fistula formation. In: Basow DS, ed., *UpToDate*. Waltham, MA.
- Vesicovaginal, urethrovaginal and ureterovaginal fistulas. In: Basow DS, ed., *UpToDate*. Waltham, MA.
- Wein. Urinary tract fistula. In: *Campbell-Walsh Urology*, 9th ed. Philadelphia: Saunders, 2007.

### See Also (Topic, Algorithm, Electronic Media Element)
Urinary Tract Infections, Adult

 CODES

### ICD9
- 599.1 Urethral fistula
- 619.0 Urinary-genital tract fistula, female

U

# URINARY TRACT INFECTIONS, ADULT

Paul A. Szucs
Barnet Eskin

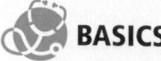 **BASICS**

## DESCRIPTION
- Colonization of urine with uropathogens and invasion of genitourinary tract (GU)
- Defined as urinary symptoms with $\geq 10^2$ to $10^5$ CFU/ml of uropathogen and $\geq 10$ WBC/mm$^3$
- Lifetime risk of UTI in women is >50%
- Uncomplicated cystitis:
  - Females aged 13–50
  - Symptoms <2–3 days
  - Not pregnant
  - Afebrile (temperature <38°C)
  - No flank pain
  - No costovertebral angle tenderness (CVAT)
  - Fewer than 4 urinary tract infections (UTI) in past year
  - No recent instrumentation or previous GU surgery
  - No functional/structural GU abnormality
  - Not immunocompromised
  - Neurologically intact
- Complicated cystitis:
  - Do not meet above criteria
  - Male gender
  - Patients with anatomic, functional, or metabolic abnormalities of GU tract
  - Postvoid residual urine
  - Catheters
  - Resistant pathogens
  - Recent antimicrobial use
- Uncomplicated pyelonephritis:
  - Renal parenchymal infection
  - Dysuria, frequency, urgency
  - Fever, chills, myalgias
  - Flank, back or abdominal pain
  - CVA tenderness
  - Nausea, vomiting
  - Leukocytosis (common)
- Complicated pyelonephritis:
  - Renal parenchymal infection
  - Temperature >40°C
  - Urosepsis with septic shock
  - Intractable nausea, vomiting
  - Diabetes, other immunosuppression
  - Pregnancy (especially later half)
  - Concomitant obstruction or stone
  - Asymptomatic (occult)

## ETIOLOGY
- Mechanism:
  - Organisms colonize periurethral area and subsequently infect the GU tract.
- Risk factors:
  - Population:
    - Newborn, prepubertal girls, young boys
    - Sexually active young woman
    - Postmenopausal woman, elderly males
  - Behavior:
    - Sexual intercourse, spermicides, diaphragms
    - Elderly females/postmenopausal state:
- Less efficient bladder emptying, bladder prolapse, alteration of bladder defenses

- Increased vaginal pH
- Contamination due to urinary or fecal incontinence (Enterobacteriaceae)
- Instrumentation:
  - Elderly males due to prostatic hypertrophy and instrumentation
- Organisms:
  - *Escherichia coli* (80–85%)
  - *Staphylococcus saprophyticus* (10%)
  - Other (10%): Klebsiella, *Proteus mirabilis*, Enterobacter spp., *Pseudomonas aeruginosa*, group D streptococci

 **DIAGNOSIS**

## SIGNS AND SYMPTOMS
- Lower tract infection (UTI): Cystitis:
  - Dysuria, frequency, urgency
  - Hesitancy
  - Suprapubic pain
  - Hematuria
- Upper tract infection: Pyelonephritis:
  - Symptoms of cystitis:
    - Fever, chills
    - Flank pain and/or tenderness
    - Nausea, vomiting, anorexia
  - Leukocytosis
  - Up to 50% of patients with cystitis may actually have pyelonephritis:
    - Symptom duration >5 days, homelessness, and recent UTI are risk factors for upper tract infection
  - Elderly or frail patients:
    - Altered mental status
    - Anorexia
    - Decreased social interaction
    - Abdominal pain
    - Nocturia
    - Incontinence
    - Syncope or dizziness

## ESSENTIAL WORKUP
- Urinalysis (dipstick test, microscopy)
- Females: Pregnancy test
- Females: Rule out urethritis, vaginitis, pelvic inflammatory disease (PID)
- Males: Rule out urethritis, epididymitis, prostatitis.
- Males: Inquire about anal intercourse and HIV.
- Urologic evaluation in young healthy males with 1st UTI is *not* routinely recommended.

## DIAGNOSTIC TESTS & INTERPRETATION
### Lab
- Rapid Urine Screen:
  - Dipstick (leukocyte esterase + nitrite) most effective when urine contains $10^5$ CFU/mL
  - Laboratory specimen unnecessary if pyuria and bacteriuria confirmed by dipstick
    - Leukocyte esterase: positive likelihood ratio (LR+) $\sim$5, negative likelihood ratio (LR-) $\sim$0.3
  - Nitrite: LR+ $\sim$30, LR- $\sim$0.5

- Urinalysis/microscopy:
  - Obtain if rapid urine screen is unavailable or negative in patients with presumed UTI.
  - 10 WBC/mm$^3$ in clean catch midstream urine indicates infection.
  - Bacteria detected in unspun urine indicates >10$^5$ CFU/ml. (LR+ $\sim$20, LR- $\sim$0.1)
- Indications for urine culture:
  - Complicated UTIs
  - Negative rapid urine screen or microscopy in patients with presumed UTI
  - Persistent signs and symptoms after 2–3 days of treatment
  - Recurrence (relapse versus reinfection)
  - Recently hospitalized patients
  - Nosocomial infections
  - Pyelonephritis
  - Additional labs dictated by clinical setting

### Geriatric Considerations
Asymptomatic bacteriuria (including positive cultures) occurs in 20% of women >65 yr, 50% of women >80 yr and generally should *not* be treated.

### Imaging
- Indicated for complicated upper tract disease (see Pyelonephritis)
- Helical CT, IV pyelogram or renal ultrasound if concomitant stone or obstruction suspected

### Diagnostic Procedures/Surgery
Patients with significant hematuria, recurrent UTI with same uropathogen, or symptoms of obstruction *need* urologic evaluation to identify structural or functional abnormality.

## DIFFERENTIAL DIAGNOSIS
- Appendicitis
- Diverticulitis
- Epididymitis
- Nephrolithiasis
- PID/cervicitis
- Prostatitis
- Pyelonephritis
- Urethritis
- Vulvovaginitis

 **TREATMENT**

## INITIAL STABILIZATION/THERAPY
Urosepsis/septic shock:
- Manage airway and resuscitate as indicated
- IV crystalloid
- Vasopressors as needed

## ED TREATMENT/PROCEDURES
### Stable Patients
- For uncomplicated UTIs in women for most antibiotics, 3 days of therapy:
  - more effective than single dose
  - clinically as effective as 5–10 day course with fewer side effects

- Resistance varies by place and changes over time:
  - In North America, 40–50% of *E. coli* are resistant to ampicillin; <10% to fluoroquinolones.
  - Resistance to trimethoprim-sulfamethoxazole (TMP/SMX) is increasing (up to 30%).
  - Nitrofurantoin: In some studies, nitrofurantoin resistance is less than for other more widely used antibiotics
  - Culture resistance may not correlate at all with clinical effect because urine antibiotic concentrations are much higher than those used in laboratory testing. However, symptom resolution may be delayed a few days in patients with resistant bacteria.
- Antibiotics of choice:
  - TMP/SMX
  - Nitrofurantoin
  - Fluoroquinolones first-line treatment in women:
    ○ Sulfonamide intolerance
    ○ All quinolones equally effective (~95% susceptibility rates) but side effects vary
    ○ High frequency of antimicrobial resistance related to recent treatment
    ○ Live in areas with unknown or significant resistance to TMP/SMX (>10–20%)
  - 2nd- or 3rd-generation oral cephalosporins (cefuroxime, cefixime) may be reasonable alternatives in specific circumstances.
    ○ Require 7-day treatment regimens Amoxicillin-clavulanate not as effective as ciprofloxacin, probably due to failure to eradicate vaginal *E. coli*
  - Diabetic women have increased risk of bacteriuria with *Klebsiella* spp.
  - Treat dysuria with phenazopyridine.
  - Treat pain with appropriate analgesics.
- Cranberry juice or tablets:
  - Lowers the UTI recurrence rate, especially in women with history of recurrent UTIs, but there is no good evidence for using it for treatment
  - Prevents *E. coli* from adhering to uroepithelial cells
- Treatment of upper tract disease—*rule of 2s*:
  - 2 L of IV fluid
  - 2 tablets of Tylenol #3
  - 2 g of ceftriaxone or 2 mg/kg of gentamicin If fever drops by 2°C and patient can retain 2 glasses of water
  - Discharge with fluoroquinolone for 2 wk.
  - Follow up in 2 days.

## Pregnancy Considerations
- Asymptomatic bacteriuria in pregnancy
- Treat with 3–7-day course of antibiotics:
  - Cephalexin
  - TMP/SMX:
    ○ SMX should not be used late in pregnancy as kernicterus can result.
  - Amoxicillin (but has high rate of resistance)
  - Fosfomycin also safe and effective in pregnancy
  - Nitrofurantoin (contraindicated if patient G6PD-deficient)
  - Quinolones not recommended during pregnancy:
    ○ CNS reactions
    ○ Blood dyscrasias
    ○ Effects on collagen formation

## MEDICATION
- Amoxicillin: 500 or 875 mg PO q12h
- Cefixime: 400 mg/day PO or 200 mg PO q12h
- Ceftazidime: 1–2 g IV q8h–q12h
- Ceftriaxone: 1–2 g IV/IM q24h
- Cefuroxime: 250–500 mg PO q12h
- Cephalexin: 250–500 mg PO q6h
- Ciprofloxacin: 100–500 mg PO q12h
- Doripenem: 500 mg IV q8h
- Fosfomycin: 3 g single dose
- Gentamicin: 2 mg/kg IV or IM q8h
- Levofloxacin: 250 mg PO q24h
- Nitrofurantoin macrocrystals 100 mg PO q12h
- Norfloxacin: 800 mg PO daily in 1 or 2 divided doses
- Ofloxacin: 200 mg PO q12h or 400 mg IV q12h
- Phenazopyridine: 200 mg PO t.i.d. for 2 days:
  - For symptomatic treatment of dysuria
  - May turn urine and contact lenses orange
- TMP/SMX: 160 mg/800 mg PO q12h or q8h–q10h mg/kg IV q12h

# FOLLOW-UP

## DISPOSITION
### Admission Criteria
- Inability to comply with oral therapy
- Unstable vital signs
- Toxic appearance
- Pyelonephritis:
  - Intractable symptoms
  - Extremes of age
  - Immunosuppression
  - Urinary obstruction
  - Consider if coexisting urolithiasis
  - Significant comorbid disease
  - Outpatient treatment failure
  - Late in pregnancy

### Discharge Criteria
- Well appearing
- Stable vital signs
- Can maintain oral hydration
- Can comply with oral therapy
- No significant comorbid disease
- Adequate follow-up (48–72 hr) as needed
- Healthy patients with uncomplicated pyelonephritis who respond to treatment in ED according to rule of 2s
- Pyelonephritis in early pregnancy with good follow-up may be treated as outpatients

### Issues for Referral
Recurrent UTIs require work-up for underlying pathology.

## FOLLOW-UP RECOMMENDATIONS
Follow-up for UTIs should start with primary care physician.

## PEARLS AND PITFALLS
- For women who have more than two episodes of acute cystitis in 6 mo or 3 episodes in 1 yr, consider long-term (6–12 months) prophylactic antibiotics or postcoital prophylaxis
- Pregnant women should be screened and treated for asymptomatic bacteriuria (ASB) because 20–40% of women with ASB progress to pyelonephritis.
- ASB should also be treated when it occurs in renal transplant recipients, patients who have recently undergone a urologic procedure, and patients with neutropenia.
- Risk factors for acute cystitis in men include increased age, lack of circumcision, HIV infection (especially with lower CD4 counts), anatomic abnormalities such as benign prostatic hypertrophy or urethral strictures, and sexual activity (especially insertive anal intercourse). 30% of young men with bacteriuria have an anatomic abnormality
- 25% of male genitourinary complaints are attributable to prostatitis.
- In patients with indwelling catheters, pyuria is less strongly correlated with UTI than in patients without catheters.

## ADDITIONAL READING
- Hooton TM. Practice guidelines for urinary tract infection in the era of managed care. *Int J Antimicrob Agents*. 1999;11:241–245.
- Hooton TM, Stamm WE. Diagnosis and treatment of uncomplicated urinary tract infection. *Infect Dis Clin North Am*. 1997;11(3):551–581.
- McLaughlin SP, Carson CC. Urinary tract infections in women. *Med Clin North Am*. March 2004;88(2): 417–429.
- St. John A, Boyd JC, Lowes AJ, et al. The use of urinary dipstick tests to exclude urinary tract infection. *Am J Clin Pathol* 2006;126:428–36.
- Stamm WE, Hooton TM. Management of urinary tract infections in adults. *N Engl J Med*. 1993; 329(18):1328–1334.
- Warren JW, Abrutyn F, Hebel JR, et al. Guidelines for antimicrobial treatment of uncomplicated acute bacterial cystitis and acute pyelonephritis in women. *Clin Infect Dis*. 1999;103(4):843–852.

### See Also (Topic, Algorithm, Electronic Media Element)
- Pyelonephritis
- Urinary Tract Infection, Pediatric

 CODES

ICD9
- 595.0 Acute cystitis
- 595.9 Cystitis, unspecified
- 599.0 Urinary tract infection, site not specified

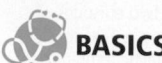 **BASICS**

## DESCRIPTION
- Bacteria colonize via retrograde contamination of rectal or perineal flora:
  - Infants—often hematogenous spread
  - Older children—vesicoureteral reflux major risk
- UTI is defined by culture with organisms of >10,000/mL on a catheterized or suprapubic specimen. Other collection techniques are not routinely used in young children for definitive diagnosis.
- In infants 0–3 months old, UTI is associated with a 30% incidence of sepsis.
- Predisposing factors:
  - Poor perineal hygiene
  - Short urethra of female
  - Female > male
  - Infrequent voiding
  - Constipation
  - Sexual activity
  - Circumcision probably reduces risk

## ETIOLOGY
- UTI found in 4%–7% of febrile infants
- Bacterial agents:
  - *Escherichia coli* accounts for 90%
  - *Klebsiella pneumoniae*
  - *Staphylococcus aureus*
  - *Enterobacter* species
  - *Proteus* species
  - *Pseudomonas aeruginosa*
  - *Enterococcus* species

**Dx DIAGNOSIS**

### ALERT
UTIs in children may be difficult to diagnosis without laboratory confirmation.

## SIGNS AND SYMPTOMS
- Often nonspecific
- Neonates:
  - Manifestations of sepsis
  - Feeding difficulties
  - Irritability, listlessness
  - Fever, hypothermia
- 1 mo–3 yr of age:
  - Fever
  - Irritability
  - Vomiting, diarrhea
  - Abdominal pain
  - Poor feeding, failure to thrive

- Hematuria
- In girls <2 yr, an increased risk is associated with those having ≥3 factors (<12 mo old, white, temp ≥39°C, absence of other source of fever, fever ≥2 days)
- >3 yr of age:
  - Dysuria
  - Frequency
  - Enuresis
  - Pain: abdominal, suprapubic, back, costovertebral (CVA)
  - Fever
  - Hematuria
  - Malodorous cloudy urine
  - Systemic toxicity: high fever and chills with CVA tenderness
- Complications:
  - Recurrent UTI
  - Pyelonephritis
  - Chronic renal failure:
    - Scarring probably may be reduced by early detection and intervention
  - Perinephric abscess
  - Bacteremia/sepsis
  - Urolithiasis

## ESSENTIAL WORKUP
- UA with microscopic RBC and WBC counts and Gram's stain for bacteria:
  - UA alone has low diagnostic sensitivity in infants.
  - Causes of pyuria besides UTI include chemical (bubble bath) or physical (masturbation) irritation, dehydration, renal tuberculosis, trauma, acute glomerulonephritis, respiratory infections, appendicitis, pelvic infection, and gastroenteritis.
  - Leukocyte esterase correlates with presence of pyuria.
  - Positive nitrite test indicates presence of bacteria capable of fixing nitrate.
  - Gram's stain of urinary sediment is more reliable than dipstick methods of diagnosis and superior to traditional UA.
  - Up to 80% of UAs in neonates with documented UTIs may be normal.
- Urine culture:
  - Specimen should be cultured within 30 min or refrigerated.
  - False-negative results may be caused by dilution, improper culture medium, recent antimicrobial therapy, fastidious organisms, bacteriostatic agent in urine, and complete obstruction of ureter.

- Urine collection methods:
  - Clean-catch in cooperative male children
  - Plastic bag collection adequate for UA (70% contamination rate)
  - Clean the perineum (females) and glans (males) before application.
  - Can be used to rule out an infection if patient is not placed on antibiotics empirically and follow-up culture possible if the initial assessment is suggestive of infection.
- Positive culture usually must be confirmed by suprapubic or catheterized specimen because contamination using other techniques is common:
  - Bladder catheterization:
    - Acceptable in all infants
    - Higher success rate than suprapubic aspiration
    - Aseptic technique essential
    - Discarding the first 1–2 mL of urine before collecting specimen reduces contamination.
  - Suprapubic aspiration:
    - Most useful in infants
    - Full bladder optimal
    - Less commonly used than catheter
    - Ultrasound may be useful adjunctive measure to improve yield.

## DIAGNOSTIC TESTS & INTERPRETATION
### Lab
- CBC and blood culture for young children with fever or nonspecific symptoms and no source on exam. Consider additional evaluation as appropriate.
- Electrolytes, BUN, creatinine:
  - Check if there is dehydration, pyelonephritis, or recurrent infection.

### Imaging
- Children requiring radiologic evaluation:
  - Infants <3 mo of age
  - Males (increased association with anomaly) with first UTI
  - Clinical signs and symptoms consistent with pyelonephritis
  - Clinical evidence of renal disease
  - Some suggest that girls <3 yr of age with a first UTI should be studied.
  - Females >3 yr of age
  - First UTI in patients who have a family history of UTIs, abnormal voiding pattern, poor growth, HTN, urinary tract anomalies, or failure to respond promptly to therapy
  - Second UTI

- Voiding cystoureterogram (VCUG) and US:
  - UTI is often associated with vesicoureteral reflux and other genitourinary abnormalities.
  - Ultrasonography is useful in excluding obstructive lesion and identifying children with solitary/ectopic kidney and some patients with moderate renal damage/scarring.
  - Nuclear cystogram is often substituted for VCUG in females.
  - Further evaluation with nuclear medicine studies depends upon the grade of vesicoureteral reflux and response to treatment

## DIFFERENTIAL DIAGNOSIS
- Infection:
  - Volvovaginitis
  - Viral cystitis
  - Urethritis (*Neisseria gonorrhea* or *Chlamydia trachomatis*)
  - Glomerulonephritis
  - Appendicitis
- Trauma:
  - Chemical irritation
  - Perineal
  - Sexual abuse
  - Genitourinary
  - Masturbation
  - Foreign body
- Nephrolithiasis
- Diabetes

 ## TREATMENT

### INITIAL STABILIZATION/THERAPY
- Treat infants <3 mo old presumptively for sepsis if febrile and/or toxic until blood and other appropriate cultures are final.
- Airway intervention for septic/acidotic infants with depressed respiratory drive
- Bolus of 20 mL/kg 0.9% NS for dehydration, hypovolemia, or sepsis; may repeat

### ED TREATMENT/PROCEDURES
- Initiate IV antibiotics in all febrile infants <3 mo with UTI:
  - Ampicillin and gentamicin in neonates
  - Cephalosporins after 4–8 wk of age
- Outpatient oral antibiotic for 7–10 days for children discharged:
  - Amoxicillin
  - Amoxicillin/clavulanate
  - Ampicillin
  - Cephalexin
  - Nitrofurantoin
  - Trimethoprim–sulfamethoxazole (TMP–SMX)

## MEDICATION
### First Line
- Amoxicillin: 40 mg/kg/24 h PO q8h
- Amoxicillin/clavulanate: 40 mg/kg/24 h PO q8h
- Ampicillin: 100 mg/kg/24 h IV q6h
- Cefotaxime: 100 mg/kg/24 h IV or IM q6–8h
- Ceftriaxone: 50 mg/kg/24 h q12h–q24h IV or IM
- Cephalexin: 50 mg/kg/24 h PO q6h–q12h
- Gentamicin: 2.5 mg/kg/dose IV q8h if full-term and age >7 days; 2.5 mg/kg/dose IV q12h if full-term and age 0–7 days (special dosing regimens in infants <36 wk s postconceptual age)
- Nitrofurantoin: 5–7 mg/kg/24 hr PO q6h
- TMP–SMX (BactrimSeptrasuspension): 5 mL liquid (of 40/200 per 5 mL) per 10-kg per dose PO b.i.d.

 ## FOLLOW-UP

### DISPOSITION
#### Admission Criteria
- Infants <3 mo
- Dehydration
- Ill appearance/toxicity/sepsis
- Suspected pyelonephritis
- Urinary obstruction
- Vomiting, inability to retain medications
- Immunocompromised patient
- Renal insufficiency
- Foreign body (indwelling catheter)
- Pregnant patient

#### Discharge Criteria
- Sufficiently hydrated
- Low risk for sepsis or meningitis
- Able to take oral antibiotics; compliant

#### Issues for Referral
- Patients needing admission often require a pediatrician, urologist, or infectious disease consultant.
- Good follow-up is mandatory.

### FOLLOW-UP RECOMMENDATIONS
Monitoring of urine for sterility, further evaluation for underlying pathology, and following growth pattern

## PEARLS AND PITFALLS
- UTI may require laboratory confirmation of clinical suspicion. Signs and symptoms are often nonspecific.
- Febrile infants with UTI may be bacteremic.
- Neonates with UTI may have normal urinalysis.

## ADDITIONAL READING
- American Academy of Pediatrics, Subcommittee on Urinary Tract Infection. Practice parameter: the diagnosis, treatment and evaluation of the initial urinary tract infection in febrile infants and young children. *Pediatrics*. 1999;103:843.
- Dayan PS, Bennett J, Best R, et al. Test characteristics of urine gram stain in infants ≤60 days of age with fever. *Pediatr Emerg Care*. 2002;18:12.
- Gorelick MH, Hoberman A, Kearney D, et al.*Pediatr Emerg Care*. 2003;19:162–164
- Peniakov M, Antonelli J, Naor O, et al. Reduction of contamination of urine samples obtained by in-out catheterization by culturing the later urine stream. *Pediatr Emerg Care*. 2004;6:418.
- Sahsi RS, Carpenter CR. Does this children have a urinary tract infection? *Ann Emerg Med* 2009: 53:680–684.
- Smeilie JM, Jodal U, Lax H. Outcome of 10 years of severe vesicoureteral reflux managed medically. *J Pediatr*. 2001;139:656.
- Wald E. Urinary tract infections in infants and children: A comprehensive overview. *Curr Opin Pediatr*. 2004;16:85–88.

### See Also (Topic, Algorithm, Electronic Media Element)
Urinary Tract Infection, Adult

 ## CODES

### ICD9
599.0 Urinary tract infection, site not specified

U

# URTICARIA
*Fred Severyn*

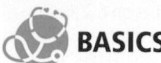

## BASICS

### DESCRIPTION
- Skin mast cell release of inflammatory mediators, primarily histamine:
  - Increased vascular permeability and pruritus
- Edema of the epidermis as well as the upper and middle dermis
- 40% of patients with uritcaria have angioedema:
  - Affects deeper subdermal and/or submucosal sites
  - Acute urticaria
  - Duration of <6 wk
  - More common in children and young adults
  - Chronic urticaria
  - More common in adults
  - More common in women (60%) than men (40%)

### Pediatric Considerations
- Urticaria often the result of reactions to foods.
- Swelling of distal extremities and acrocyanosis may be prominent in infants.
- Bullae may form in the center of the wheal, especially on legs and buttocks.

### ETIOLOGY
#### Acute
- Drugs:
  - Penicillin
  - Sulfa
  - NSAID
  - ACE inhibitors
- Foods or additives
- Herbal medications, vaccines, opiates
- Insect bites, stings
- Connective tissue
- Endocrine disorders, especially Hashimoto thyroiditis
- Cancers, especially lymphoproliferative
- Pregnancy, menstrual cycle, extraneous estrogens
- Infections:
  - Viral (including hepatitis, HIV)
  - Bacterial
  - Fungal
  - Parasitic
- Inhaled or contact allergen
- Emotional stress
- Physical urticaria—<20 identified types, including:
  - Dermographism:
    - Most common form
    - Reaction to skin pressure
    - Linear wheals under tight clothing
    - Areas scratched with a firm object
  - Cholinergic:
    - Monomorphic wheals 2–3 mm
    - Bright red flare and intense pruritus
  - A response to elevated core temperature:
    - Hot bath
    - Fever
    - Exercise

- Other rare forms:
  - Cold-induced (may be fatal in cold immersions)
  - Delayed pressure
  - Sun exposure
  - Aquagenic
  - Vibratory

#### Chronic
- 75% idiopathic
- Autoimmune
- Immune complex–induced
- Often an unrecognized recurring physical urticaria
- May be due to occult or subclinical infection or systemic disease

## DIAGNOSIS

### SIGNS AND SYMPTOMS
#### History
- Prior history
- Familial history
- Alleviating or aggravating factors
- Time course of presentation:
  - Often helpful to circle lesions to document their duration
  - Fever
  - Arthritis/arthralgias
  - Weight loss
  - lymphadenopathy
  - Hypotension
  - Flushing
  - Headache
  - Dizziness
  - Swelling of face and tongue
  - Respiratory distress
    - May be part of an anaphylactic reaction

#### Physical Exam
- Focus on signs of systemic involvement or infection.
- Airway—angioedema, airway narrowing, ability to handle secretions, abnormal phonation, stridor
- Breathing—wheezing
- Circulation—systemic signs of anaphylaxis, such as hypotension
- Abdomen—hepatosplenomegaly, pregnancy
- Dermal—associated edema, associated petechiae or purpura:
  - Generalized, transient, pruritic, well-circumscribed skin eruptions
  - May include palms or soles
  - Erythematous or white
  - Nonpitting
  - Edematous plaques (wheals)
  - May be surrounded by white or red ring (flare)
  - May have clear center
  - Intense swelling
  - May include bullae or purpuric lesions
  - Lesions are of various sizes and shapes, haphazard in distribution, and may become confluent.
  - Wheals usually resolve in 3–4 hr.
  - New lesions evolve as old ones resolve
  - *Acute:* <6 wk
  - *Chronic:* >6 wk

- Lymphadenopathy
- Dermographism:
  - Scratch skin with a tongue blade; observe for linear wheal.
- Cholinergic:
  - Exercise challenge to raise core temp or induce sweating
- Expose to sunlight.
- Cold-induced:
  - Place an ice cube on skin for 5 min.
- Aquagenic:
  - Apply tap water at differing temperatures.
- Significant mucosal edema:
  - Suspect angioedema
  - Severe reaction with hypotension
  - Suspect anaphylaxis
- Prolonged, painful, or nonblanching lesions:
  - Suspect vasculitis

### ESSENTIAL WORKUP
- Complete history and physical exam:
- Lesion appearance, location, timing, duration
- Acute vs chronic
- Associated symptoms, triggers
- Coexisting diseases, allergies, medications
- Environment, exposures, and new foods
- Characteristics and location of hives
- Evaluate for sources of infection and signs of systemic diseases.

### DIAGNOSTIC TESTS & INTERPRETATION
#### Lab
- Acute cases: not needed
- Chronic cases:
  - Evaluate for infection or systemic disease:
    - CBC with differential, ESR
    - Thyroid-stimulating hormone and thyroid functions
    - Urinalysis, liver function tests
- Skin biopsy if urticarial vasculitis suspected (not done in ED)

#### Imaging
- Acute cases: not needed
- Chronic cases:
  - Directed at search for occult infection

#### Diagnostic Procedures/Surgery
Skin biopsy—for chronic urticaria or existence of petechiae/purpura.

### DIFFERENTIAL DIAGNOSIS
- Angioedema:
  - Usually presents with abdominal symptoms
  - Life-threatening
  - Hereditary or acquired
- Cutaneuous vasculitis
- Serum sickness
- Erythema multiforme
- Bullous pemphigoid
- Juvenile rheumatoid arthritis
- Erythema marginatum
- Dermatitis herpetiformis
- Systemic mastocytosis

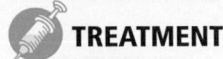 **TREATMENT**

### PRE-HOSPITAL
- Cautions:
  - Patients with severe allergic reactions can progress rapidly to respiratory failure.
- Severe reaction:
  - Manage airway, oxygen.
  - IM/SQ epinephrine
  - Parenteral or inhaled beta agonist
  - IV crystalloid
  - Vasopressors as needed

### INITIAL STABILIZATION/THERAPY
Remove offending agent if possible.

### ED TREATMENT/PROCEDURES
- Largely symptomatic except in severe reactions
- Avoid offending agent.
- Beta agonist (parenteral or inhaled):
  - Severe hives, angioedema, systemic features
- $H_1$-receptor antagonist (first or second generation):
  - Mainstay of treatment
- $H_2$-receptor antagonist:
  - May be beneficial as adjunct to $H_1$ blocker when no response to $H_1$ blocker alone
- Corticosteroid (oral):
  - Severe or refractory cases
- Tricyclic antidepressants:
  - Potent histamine blockers
- Avoid NSAIDs and opiates:
  - May exacerbate condition
- Concurrent use of ketoconazole or macrolides alters hepatic metabolism of antihistamine; use with caution.
- Chronic urticaria unresponsive to antihistamines may respond to colchicine or dapsone; topical steroids are not effective.

### MEDICATION
- Beta agonists
  - Albuterol (0.5% solution): 0.5 mL nebulized q20min PRN (peds: 0.01–0.05 mL/kg per dose [max. 0.5 mL/dose] nebulized q20min PRN)
  - Epinephrine (1:1000 solution): 0.1–0.5 mg SC or IM q10–5min PRN (peds: 0.01 mg/kg, SC [max single dose not to exceed 0.3 mg] q15min PRN)
  - IV Epinephrine 0.1–0.25 mg (1:10,000 sol) IV over 5–10 min q 5–15 min then 1–4 $\mu$g/min IV if anaphylactic shock.
  - Terbutaline: 0.25 mg SC q15min–q30min PRN (max 0.5 mg q4h); (peds: <12 yr old; 0.005–0.01 mg/kg [max 0.4 mg/dose] SC q15–20min × 3 PRN)
- $H_1$-receptor antagonist (first generation—sedating)
  - Diphenhydramine: 25–50 mg PO, IV, or IM q6h (peds: 1 mg/kg q6h [max 300 mg/24 hr])
  - Hydroxyzine: 25–50 mg PO or IM q6h (peds: 2 mg/kg/24 hr PO div q8h or 0.5–1 mg/kg IM q4–6h PRN)

- $H_1$-receptor antagonist (second generation—less sedating, not as effective):
  - Cetirizine: adult and peds ≥6 yr old: 5–10 mg PO qd (peds 2–6 yr old: 2.5 mg qd to b.i.d.)
  - Loratadine: 10 mg PO b.i.d. (peds 2–6 yr old: 5 mg PO qd
  - Fexofenadine: 60 mg PO b.i.d. or 180 mg PO per day (peds 6–12 yr old: 30 mg PO b.i.d.)
- $H_2$-receptor antagonist (suggested dosage):
  - Famotidine: 20 mg IV q12h or 20–40 mg PO q.h.s. (peds: 1 mg/kg/day div q.i.d. [max 40 mg/24 hr])
  - Ranitidine: 150 mg PO b.i.d. (peds: neonate: 2–4 mg/kg/24 hr PO div q8–12h or 2 mg/kg/24 hr IV div q6–8h; infants and children 4–5 mg/kg/24 hr PO div q8–12h or 2–4 mg/kg/24 hr IV or IM div q6–8h)
- Corticosteroid:
  - Methyprednisolone: 125 mg IV (peds: start at 2 mg/kg × 1)
  - Prednisolone: 50 mg PO qdy for 3 days (peds: 0.5–2 mg/kg/24h [max. 80 mg/24 hr] div. qd to b.i.d for 3–5 days)
  - Prednisone: 40 mg PO per day or 20 mg PO b.i.d. for 3–5 days (peds: 1–2 mg/kg/24 hr [max 80 mg/24 hr] div. qd to b.i.d for 3–5 days)
- Topical therapy:
  - Calamine/pramoxine Hcl: apply b.i.d.
- Antileukotrienes:
  - Montelukast: 10 mg PO qd
  - Zafirlukast: 20 mg PO b.i.d.

### First Line
- $H_1$-receptor antagonist, first generation
- Corticosteroids
- Beta agonists:
  - Albuterol if mild reaction
  - Epinephrine if severe

### Second Line
- Antileukotrienes
- $H_1$-receptor antagonist, second generation

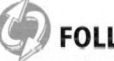 **FOLLOW-UP**

### DISPOSITION
#### Admission Criteria
- Respiratory distress or failure
- Refractory hypotension or shock
- Severe refractory cases requiring IV medications
- Other systemic disease or infection

### Discharge Criteria
- Normal ventilation and oxygenation
- Normal BP
- Absence of other condition requiring admission
- Symptoms controlled
- Adequate ability of caregivers at home to monitor for further exacerbations

### FOLLOW-UP RECOMMENDATIONS
Follow with PCP, especially if lasting >6 wk.

## PEARLS AND PITFALLS
- If severe, there is often a biphasic course. Rebound may occur in 4–6 hr
- Chronic urticaria often has a systemic cause.

## ADDITIONAL READING
- Amar SM, Dreskin SC. Urticaria. *Prim Care Clin Office Pract.* 2008;35:141–157.
- Dibbern D. Urticaria: Selected highlights and recent advances. *Med Clin North Am.* 2006;90:187–209.
- Lack G. Food allergy. *N Engl J Med.* 2008;359: 1252–1260.
- Muller B. Urticaria and angioedema: A practical approach. *Am Fam Physician.* 2004;69:1123–1128.
- Kaplan A. Chronic Urticaria and angioedema. *N Engl J Med.* 2002;346:175–9
- Wolfson AB, Hendey GW, Ling LJ, et al., eds. *Harwood Nuss' Clinical Practice of Emergency Medicine,* 5th ed. Philadelphia: Lippincott Williams & Wilkins, 2010.
- Zuraw BL. Hereditary angioedema. *N Engl J Med.* 2008;359:1027–1036.

### See Also (Topic, Algorithm, Electronic Media Element)
- Angioedema
- Erythema Multiforme
- Vasculitis

 **CODES**

### ICD9
- 708.8 Other specified urticaria
- 708.9 Unspecified urticaria

U

# VAGINAL BLEEDING
*Carla C. Valentine*

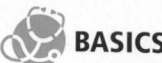 **BASICS**

## DESCRIPTION
- Common presenting complaint in EDs
- Most cases have benign etiology.
- Some patients may have potentially life-threatening conditions.
- Most important principles in evaluating women with vaginal bleeding:
  - Any woman capable of childbearing might be
  - pregnant.
  - Menstrual and sexual histories do not rule out
  - pregnancy.

## ETIOLOGY
- PREGNANCY-RELATED
- Early pregnancy:
  - Ectopic pregnancy (occurs in 2% of
  - pregnancies)
  - Abortion:
    - Threatened, incomplete, complete, missed, inevitable, septic
  - Molar pregnancy
  - Trauma
- Later pregnancy:
  - Placenta previa
  - Placental abruption
  - Molar pregnancy
  - Labor
  - Trauma
- Immediate postpartum period:
  - Postpartum hemorrhage
  - Uterine inversion
  - Retained placenta
  - Endometritis
- NONPREGNANT PATIENTS
- Dysfunctional uterine bleeding
- Structural abnormalities
- Uterine fibroids
- Cervical/endometrial polyps
- Pelvic tumors
- Atrophic endometrium:
  - Most common cause of postmenopausal bleeding
- Rare for systemic disorders to present solely with vaginal bleeding:
  - Von Willebrand disease
  - Idiopathic thrombocytopenic purpura
- Trauma
- Foreign bodies
- Infections

## DIAGNOSIS

### SIGNS AND SYMPTOMS
*History*
- Light-headedness
- Fatigue
- Weakness
- Thirst
- Duration of bleeding
- Quantity
  - Average tampon holds approximately 5 mL of blood
  - Average pad holds approximately 5–15 mL of blood
- Last menstrual period
- Home pregnancy tests
- Prior ectopic pregnancy
- Passage of clots or tissue
- Menstrual history
- Family history
- Trauma

*Physical Exam*
- Vitals signs
- Cardiopulmonary examination
- Abdominal examination (gravid uterus,
- masses)
- Pelvic examination
  - Source of bleeding
  - Evidence of trauma
  - Cervical os open or closed
- Change in mental status may occur with significant blood loss and/or hypotension.

### ESSENTIAL WORKUP
- Qualitative pregnancy test:
  - Point-of-care urine-based pregnancy test preferred
- Pelvic examination:
  - Essential for all women with vaginal bleeding
  - Speculum/bimanual exam
  - Assess whether cervical os open or closed.
  - Delay pelvic examination pending US result in late pregnancy:
    - Evaluate for placenta previa as the etiology of vaginal bleeding.
  - Defer exam if patient is near term with possible rupture of fetal membranes.
- Pregnancy test mandatory for all patients with childbearing potential.
- Early pregnancy:
  - Blood type and Rh
  - Ultrasound to confirm intrauterine pregnancy (IUP)
  - Quantitative beta-human chorionic gonadotropin (HCG)
  - Hematocrit
  - Type and cross-match:
    - Ectopic pregnancy
    - Low hematocrit levels
    - Hemodynamic instability
  - UA
- Later pregnancy:
  - Type and Rh
  - Fetal heart tones
  - US indications:
    - No fetal heart tones
    - No documented intrauterine pregnancy
    - Unknown placental lie
  - Hematocrit if significant bleeding
  - Type and cross-match if placenta previa/abruption or low hematocrit levels
  - DIC panel if placental abruption:
    - Platelets, (PT, PTT
    - Fibrinogen, fibrin split products
- Early postpartum:
  - US for retained products
  - Hematocrit
  - Beta-HCG if concerned about retained tissue

## DIAGNOSTIC TESTS & INTERPRETATION
*Lab*
- Hematocrit for women with significant
- bleeding
- Type and Rh
- Platelet count for suspected thrombocytopenia
- PT/PTT for suspected coagulopathy
- Send any passed tissue or clot for pathology evaluation.
- Endometrial sampling required if patient > 35–40 yr:
  - Risk of endometrial cancer

*Imaging*
- Bedside US may be indicated based on presentation, pregnancy status, and other considerations.

## DIFFERENTIAL DIAGNOSIS
- Dysfunctional uterine bleeding
- Ectopic pregnancy
- Menorrhagia
- Menometrorrhagia
- Threatened miscarriage
- Placental abruption
- Placenta previa
- Postpartum hemorrhage
- Leiomyoma
- Pelvic masses and tumors
- Postcoital bleeding
- Traumatic injury
- Thyroid dysfunction
- Bleeding disorders

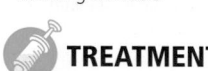 **TREATMENT**

### PRE-HOSPITAL
- Establish IV 0.9% NS with 1–2 L fluid bolus for significant bleeding or hypotension.
- Administer high-flow oxygen in pregnant or unstable patients.
- In later pregnancy:
  - Place patient in left lateral recumbent position to prevent occlusion.

### INITIAL STABILIZATION/THERAPY
- Manage airway and resuscitate as indicated.
- Place cardiac/pulse oximeter monitors.
- Oxygen for significant bleeding or unstable patient
- Establish 2 large-bore IV lines and initiate fluid bolus (1–2 L) for hypotensive patients:
- Type and cross-match
  - Transfuse blood if continued hypotension from blood losses despite IV fluid resuscitation
  - Conjugated estrogens (Premarin) 25 mg IV slowly over 10–15 min q4–6h until bleeding stops for uncontrolled menorrhagia
    - Not to exceed four doses

## ED TREATMENT/PROCEDURES

- If unstable with surgical condition, arrange for transfer of the patient to the OR as soon as possible.
- RhoGAM for vaginal bleeding, pregnancy, and Rh-negative mother:

EARLY PREGNANCY

- If ultrasound reveals an ectopic pregnancy:
  - Methotrexate according to standards at treating institution
  - Definitive treatment is surgery.
- If US reveals an intrauterine pregnancy (IUP) without concerns of heterotopic pregnancy (1/2,600–1/30,000):
  - Discharge patient with arranged obstetric follow-up with precautions for a threatened miscarriage.
- US indeterminate for IUP or ectopic with beta-HCG greater than institutional discriminatory zone:
  - Cannot exclude ectopic pregnancy
  - If hemodynamically stable with little bleeding, repeat measurement of beta-HCG and outpatient obstetric follow-up within 48 hr
  - Strict return parameters
- US indeterminate for IUP or ectopic with beta-HCG level less than institutional discriminatory zone:
  - Patient stable with low risk for ectopic pregnancy may be discharged.
  - Repeat measurement of beta-HCG level and obstetric follow-up within 48 hr
  - Patient may still have an ectopic pregnancy
- Complete abortion:
  - Discharge patient if stable without significant ongoing bleeding
- Incomplete abortion:
  - Obstetric consultation is required.
  - Dilation and curettage versus expectant management
- Missed abortion:
  - Expectant management initially
- Septic abortion:
  - IV antibiotics and admission
- Molar pregnancy:
  - Chemotherapy
  - Very responsive in early stages of disease

LATER PREGNANCY:

- Placenta previa:
  - Obstetric consultation for possible admission
- Placental abruption:
  - Induction of labor if large
  - Can lead to fetal/maternal death
  - May require cesarean section

IMMEDIATE POSTPARTUM

- Uterine inversion:
  - Prevent by avoiding strong traction on umbilical cord after delivery.
  - Replace uterus immediately.
  - Occasionally requires operative management
- Postpartum hemorrhage:
  - Extraction of placenta if retained
  - Hysterectomy if uncontrolled life-threatening bleeding

EARLY POSTPARTUM:

- Retained tissue:
  - Dilation and curettage
- Endometritis:
  - IV antibiotics

NONPREGNANT

- Menses:
  - NSAID and supportive care
- Dysfunctional uterine bleeding (DUB)
  - < 35–40 yr of age:
    - If known anovulatory DUB:
    - Medroxyprogesterone (Provera)—Warn patient about withdrawal bleeding
    - Oral contraceptive pill daily for 7 days
  - Patients >35–40 yr of age:
    - US for any masses palpated during physical exam
    - Gynecologic referral
    - Uterine sampling necessary before initiation of hormonal treatment:
    - Evaluate for endometrial cancer

STRUCTURAL ABNORMALITIES

- Pap smear/biopsy for cervical lesions
- Ultrasound for workup of pelvic masses
- Fibroids or uterine tumors
- Conservative management or lumpectomy/
- hysterectomy

## MEDICATION

- Conjugated estrogens 25 mg IV slowly over 10–15 min
- q4–6h until bleeding stops (not to exceed 4 doses)
- Known anovulatory DUB:
- Medroxyprogesterone 10 mg PO per day for first 10 days of menstrual cycle (warn patient about withdrawal bleeding)
- Norethindrone and ethinyl estradiol (Ortho-Novum) 1/50 q.i.d. for 7 days
- RhoGAM 300 μg IM if >13 wk pregnant
- MICRhoGAM 50 μg IM if <13 wk pregnant

 **FOLLOW-UP**

### DISPOSITION
#### Admission Criteria
- Ectopic pregnancy not meeting methotrexate discharge criteria:
- Uterine inversion
- Septic abortion
- Placental abruption
- Postpartum hemorrhage
- Endometritis
- Unstable dysfunctional uterine bleeding:
- Newly diagnosed molar pregnancy

#### Discharge Criteria
- Stable vital signs
- Confirmed IUP
- Ectopic pregnancy meeting institutional methotrexate discharge criteria
- Pregnant patient with low risk for ectopic pregnancy:
  - No findings of IUP on ultrasound
  - Levels of beta-HCG below discriminatory zone
- Nonpregnant patients with vaginal bleeding that are hemodynamically stable

### Issues for Referral
- Obstetric/gynecologic referral

### FOLLOW-UP RECOMMENDATIONS
- Obstetric referral within 48 hr for first-trimester vaginal bleeding without identified IUP
- OB/GYN referral for patients with menorrhagia for continued evaluation, workup, and treatment

### PATIENT EDUCATION
- *Ectopic precautions:* Patients should return to the ED immediately for increasing abdominal pain, vaginal bleeding more than 1 pad per hr for 3–4 hr, fever >100.4°F, syncope, or dizziness. Patients should not be left alone until the diagnosis of ectopic pregnancy can be safely ruled out. Family and friends should also be instructed on the warning signs and symptoms of ruptured/bleeding ectopic pregnancies.

## PEARLS AND PITFALLS

- Pregnancy test for all women of reproductive age
- If there is first-trimester vaginal bleeding, evaluate for ectopic pregnancy.

## ADDITIONAL READING

- Casablanca Y. Management of dysfunctional uterine bleeding. *Obstet Gynecol Clin North Am.* 2008;35: 219–234.
- McWilliams GDE, Hill MJ, Dietrich CS. Gynecologic emergencies. *Surg Clin North Am.* 2008;88: 265–283.
- Munro MG, Mainor N, Basu R, et al. Oral medroxyprogesterone acetate and combination oral contraceptives for acute uterine bleeding: A randomized controlled trial. *Obstet Gynecol.* 2006; 108:924.
- Oyelese Y, Scorza WE, Mastrolia R, et al. Postpartum hemorrhage. *Obstet Gynecol Clin North Am.* 2007;34:421–441.
- Sakornbut E, Leeman L, Fontaine P. Late pregnancy bleeding. *Am Fam Physician.* 2007;75:1119–206.
- Wolfson AB, Hendey GW, Ling LJ, et al, eds. *Harwood-Nuss' Clinical Practice of Emergency Medicine,* 5th ed. Philadelphia: Lippincott Williams & Wilkins, 2010.

### See Also (Topic, Algorithm, Electronic Media Element)
- Vaginal Bleeding In Pregnancy
- Threatened Abortion
- Placental Abruption
- Placenta Previa
- Ectopic Pregnancy

 **CODES**

ICD9
623.8 Other specified noninflammatory disorders of vagina

**V**

# VAGINAL BLEEDING IN PREGNANCY

*Paul Ishimine*

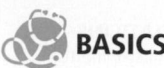 **BASICS**

## DESCRIPTION
- Leading cause of maternal/fetal morbidity and mortality
- Early pregnancy hemorrhage (≤20 wk):
  - Occurs in 30% of all pregnancies
  - 50% lead to spontaneous abortion.
- Late pregnancy hemorrhage (>20 wk):
  - Occurs in 3%–5% of all pregnancies
- Risk factors:
  - Risk factors differ for each underlying cause:
    - Advanced maternal age
    - Substance abuse (e.g., cocaine, tobacco)
    - Pelvic inflammatory disease (PID)
    - Previous cesarean section
    - Previous termination of pregnancy
    - Previous dilation and curettage (D&C)
    - Previous ectopic pregnancy
    - Increased parity
    - Multiple gestation
    - Pre-eclampsia
    - HTN
    - Trauma
- Genetics
  - 50%–60% of miscarriages due to chromosomal abnormalities

## ETIOLOGY
- Vaginal
- Cervical
- Uterine
- Uterine–placental interface
- Hematologic dysfunction

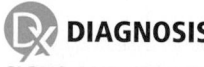 **DIAGNOSIS**

## SIGNS AND SYMPTOMS
### History
- Intensity and duration of bleeding:
  - Amount
  - Color (dark or bright red)
  - Painful or painless
  - Watery, blood-tinged mucus, clots or tissue:
  - Life-threatening conditions may present with only minimal vaginal bleeding
- Last menstrual period
- Estimated duration of gestation
- Gravidity/parity
- Fever
- Last intercourse
- Intrauterine device use
- Previous obstetric–gynecologic complications
- Spontaneous abortion: classically crampy, diffuse pelvic pain
- Ectopic pregnancy: classically sharp pelvic pain with lateralization
- Placenta previa: classically painless bright red hemorrhage
- Placental abruption: classically painful dark red hemorrhage

### Physical Exam
- Vital signs:
  - Tachycardia
  - Hypotension
  - Orthostatic changes in pulse or BP
  - Signs of hemodynamic instability may be absent due to pregnancy-related physiologic increase in blood volume.
- Fetal heart tones:
  - Fetal cardiac activity seen on transvaginal ultrasound at 6.5 wk
  - Auscultated with Doppler past 10 wk gestation
- Abdominal examination:
  - Uterine size
  - Peritoneal signs
  - Firm or tender uterus in late pregnancy suggests abruption
- Pelvic exam—only in early pregnancy:
  - Evaluate source and intensity of bleeding.
  - Determine patency of cervical os (perform this with a finger and only in the first trimester):
    - Threatened abortion: os closed
    - Inevitable abortion: os open
    - Incomplete abortion: os open or closed
    - Complete abortion: os closed
    - Embryonic demise (missed abortion): os closed
  - Products of conception may be noted in incomplete or completed abortion:
    - Products of conception in the cervical os can result in profuse bleeding.
  - Evaluate uterine size, tenderness.
  - Evaluate for uterine fibroids or adnexal masses.
  - Late pregnancy: Do not perform pelvic exam unless in controlled OR setting:
    - Severe hemorrhage may ensue.
    - Placenta previa or vasa previa must be ruled out by sonography prior to pelvic exam.

## ESSENTIAL WORKUP
- CBC
- Type and screen
- Quantitative HCG in early pregnancy
- Urinalysis
- US:
  - Transvaginal US provides more information than transabdominal US, especially early pregnancy.

## DIAGNOSTIC TESTS & INTERPRETATION
### Lab
- CBC:
  - Dilutional "anemia" is a normal physiologic change in pregnancy:
    - Blood volume expands by 45%
- Qualitative beta-human chorionic gonadotropin (beta-hCG):
  - Rapid, bedside confirmation of pregnancy
- Quantitative beta-hCG:
  - Useful to correlate with ultrasound findings
  - Detectable 9–11 days following ovulation
- Blood typing and Rh typing
  - Cross-match if significant bleeding
- Prothrombin time, partial thromboplastin time, and DIC panel in embryonic demise, placental abruption
- Blood cultures with septic abortion
- Suspected products of conception to lab for identification of chorionic villi

### Imaging
- US:
  - Essential for the evaluation of bleeding in pregnancy
  - Transvaginal US is more helpful than transabdominal US in early pregnancy bleeding.
    - Confirms intrauterine pregnancy (IUP)
    - Detects gestational sac at 5 wk or beta-hCG = 1000–2000 IU, yolk sac at 6 wk, and cardiac activity at 5–6 wk of gestation.
    - Essentially rules out ectopic pregnancy by showing IUP (except in women at high risk for heterotopic pregnancy).
    - Proves ectopic pregnancy by showing fetal pole outside uterus
    - Suggests ectopic pregnancy by detecting free fluid in cul-de-sac or adnexal mass
    - Detects retained products of conception
    - Demonstrates "snowstorm" appearance within uterus with gestational trophoblastic disease

### Diagnostic Procedures/Surgery
- Culdocentesis:
  - Limited use with ultrasound available
  - Identifies free fluid in cul-de-sac
- D&C or vacuum aspiration
  - Indicated if suspected incomplete or septic abortion or embryonic demise, gestational trophoblastic disease, or anembryonic gestation to evacuate retained products of conception
- Laparoscopy/laparotomy
  - Indicated for unstable patients not responsive to resuscitation maneuvers
  - Definitive diagnosis and treatment of ectopic pregnancy

## DIFFERENTIAL DIAGNOSIS
- Early pregnancy (<20 wk):
  - Implantation bleeding
  - Threatened abortion
  - Complete, incomplete, inevitable, embryonic demise (missed abortion), and septic abortion
  - Ectopic pregnancy
  - Heterotopic pregnancy
  - Gestational trophoblastic disease (molar pregnancy)
  - Subchorionic hemorrhage
  - Infection (e.g., cervicitis)
  - Trauma
  - Cervical and vaginal lesions (e.g., polyps, ectropion, carcinoma)
- Anembryonic gestation (blighted ovum)
  - Bleeding disorders
- Late pregnancy (>20 wk):
  - Placental abruption (30%)
  - Placenta previa (20%)
  - Bloody show (associated with cervical insufficiency or labor)
  - Vasa previa
  - Cervical/vaginal trauma or pathology
  - Uterine rupture (uncommon)
  - Bleeding disorders

 **TREATMENT**

**PRE-HOSPITAL**
- Unstable vital signs warrant aggressive resuscitation and continuous cardiac monitoring.
- In late pregnancy, position patient on left side to decrease uterine compression of vena cava.
- Consider preferential transport of a woman greater than 23–24 wk gestation with vaginal bleeding to a facility with obstetric capabilities.

**INITIAL STABILIZATION/THERAPY**
- Airway management, resuscitation as indicated
- Oxygen
- Pulse oximetry
- Cardiac monitor
- Two large-bore IV lines with normal saline or lactated Ringer solution infusion
- Blood transfusion as indicated
- Continuous fetal monitoring in later pregnancy

**ED TREATMENT/PROCEDURES**
- All women with early pregnancy vaginal bleeding must be evaluated for ectopic pregnancy, (preferably by transvaginal ultrasound).
- Administer Anti-Rh$_0$ (D) immune globulin if patient is Rh negative.
- Suspected ectopic pregnancy:
  - Unstable: consider bedside US with emergent OB/GYN consultation for laparoscopy/laparotomy
  - Stable: perform US;
    - If confirmatory or suggestive of ectopic pregnancy, obtain OB/GYN consultation for surgery or methotrexate therapy
    - If inconclusive, obtain OB/GYN consultation and arrange for repeat beta-hCG testing in two days
- Threatened abortion:
  - Emergent OB/GYN consultation for heavy/uncontrolled bleeding
  - Arrange OB/GYN follow-up for minimal bleeding
- Inevitable/incomplete/missed (embryonic demise) abortion:
  - Products of conception in the cervical os can result in profuse bleeding:
    If products of conception cannot be removed with gentle traction, obtain emergent OB/GYN consultation.
  - Arrange follow-up with OB/GYN if bleeding minimal
- Complete abortion:
  - Emergent OB/GYN consultation for heavy/uncontrolled bleeding
  - Arrange follow-up with OB/GYN if bleeding minimal.
- Septic abortion:
  - Initiate broad-spectrum antibiotic therapy.
  - Emergent OB/GYN consultation for D&C
- Late pregnancy vaginal bleeding:
  - Hemodynamic stabilization:
    - Fluid resuscitation
    - Positioning of patient onto left side or displacement of uterus laterally to relieve compression of the inferior vena cava

- DIC:
  - Associated with late pregnancy bleeding
  - Especially with placental abruption
  - Treated with blood, coagulation factors, and platelets
  - Immediate obstetric consultation and rapid transfer to obstetric unit

**MEDICATION**
*First Line*
- Anti-Rh$_0$ (D) immune globulin: <12 weeks—50 $\mu$g IM; >12 weeks—300 $\mu$g IM
- Methotrexate
  - Variable dosing regimens
  - Only recommended for hemodynamically stable women with unruptured ectopic pregnancy with low beta-hCG
- Antibiotics for septic abortion:
  - Multiple acceptable antibiotic regimens
  - Must provide polymicrobial coverage

*Second Line*
- Misoprostol has been used in completed abortion to facilitate uterine evacuation in completed miscarriage

 **FOLLOW-UP**

**DISPOSITION**
*Admission Criteria*
- Early pregnancy vaginal bleeding with:
  - Unstable vital signs or significant hemorrhage
  - Ruptured ectopic pregnancy
  - Incomplete abortion (open os)
  - Septic abortion
- All patients with late pregnancy vaginal bleeding need to be admitted to a labor and delivery unit.

*Discharge Criteria*
- Threatened abortion (closed os) with stable symptoms
- Complete abortion, embryonic demise, anembryonic gestation with stable vital signs
- Asymptomatic, hemodynamically stable patient with small, unruptured ectopic (or suspected ectopic) pregnancy after OB consultation
- Controlled bleeding from local vaginal/cervical source

*Issues for Referral*
- Patients with embryonic demise, anembryonic gestation, or gestational trophoblastic disease need to be referred for uterine evacuation if D&C not performed in ED.
- Women with threatened, inevitable, complete, or missed (embryonic demise) abortion should have OB/GYN follow-up within 24–48 hr.

**FOLLOW-UP RECOMMENDATIONS**
- Discharge instructions
  - No strenuous activity, tampon use, douching, or intercourse
  - Seek medical advice for increased pain, bleeding, fever, or passage of tissue
- All pregnant women with vaginal bleeding during pregnancy who are discharged from the ED require follow-up care.
- Women with threatened abortions require serial beta-hCG testing and repeat examination in 48 hr
- Women with known ectopic pregnancy or in whom ectopic pregnancy is suspected need to have beta-HCG levels checked in 48 hr.

## PEARLS AND PITFALLS

- Failure to check Rh status in pregnant women with vaginal bleeding
- Failure to give Anti-Rh$_0$ (D) immune globulin in Rh negative pregnant women with vaginal bleeding
- Placenta previa or vasa previa must be ruled out by sonography prior to pelvic exam.

## ADDITIONAL READING

- Deutchman M, Tanner Tubay A, Turok DK. First trimester bleeding. *Am Fam Physician*. 2009;79: 985–992, 993–994.
- Haljenisu PJ, Mol F, Mol BWJ, et al. Interventions for tubal ectopic pregnancy. *Cochrane Database Syst Rev*. 2007;1:CD000324.
- Sakornbut E, Leeman L, Fontaine P. Late pregnancy bleeding. *Am Fam Physician*. 2007;75:1199–1206.
- Seeber BE, Barnhart KT. Suspected ectopic pregnancy. *Obstet Gynecol*. 2006;107(2 Pt 1): 399–413.

### See Also (Topic, Algorithm, Electronic Media Element)
- Abortion, Spontaneous;; Ectopic Pregnancy, Hydatidiform Mole; Placental abruption; Placenta Previa; Postpartum Hemorrhage

 **CODES**

ICD9
- 640.90 Unspecified hemorrhage in early pregnancy, unspecified as to episode of care
- 641.90 Unspecified antepartum hemorrhage, unspecified as to episode of care

V

# VAGINAL DISCHARGE/VAGINITIS

*Carrie Tibbles*

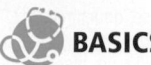

## BASICS

### DESCRIPTION
- Abnormal discharge from the vagina as defined by an increased amount or change in color
- Vaginitis is vaginal discharge or vulvovaginal discomfort.
- Some amount of vaginal discharge is normal.
- Glands in the cervix produce a clear mucus that may turn white or yellow when exposed to air.

### ETIOLOGY
- Bacterial vaginosis:
  – The most common cause
  – Loss of normal *Lactobacillus* (eg, antibiotics)
  – Inability to maintain normal vaginal pH (<4.5) resulting in proliferation of normally present pathogens
  – Overgrowth of normally present bacteria such as *Gardnerella vaginalis*, *Mycoplasma hominis*, *Mobiluncus sp.*, *Prevotella sp.*, and Peptostreptococcal
- Introduction of an infective pathogen:
  – Trichomoniasis
  – Candidiasis
  – Group A strep; *S. aureus*
- Fungal infections:
  – Often underlying immune dysfunction:
    ○ Diabetes
    ○ HIV
- Chemical irritants
- Foreign body
- Atrophic vaginitis
- Hypersensitivity
- Collagen vascular disease
- Herpes simplex virus (HSV):
  – Vulvovaginitis
  – Cervicitis
- Lichens sclerosis (atrophic)
- Fistula

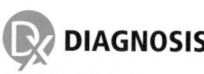

## DIAGNOSIS

### SIGNS AND SYMPTOMS
- Abnormal discharge
- Vulvovaginitis
- Localized pain
- Erythema
- Edema
- Dysuria
- Pruritus
- Asymptomatic
- Excoriations
- Abnormal odor

### History
- Description and duration of symptoms
- Description of discharge if any
- Timing with regard to menses
- Sexual history of patient and partners if possible
- Sexual practices
- Hygienic practices
- Use of oral contraceptives and/or antibiotics
- Likelihood of pregnancy
- Other symptoms (ie, abdominal pain; rule out pelvic inflammatory disease [PID])

### Physical Exam
- Abdominal exam to assess for tenderness
- Inspection of vulva, vaginal os, perineal area
- Speculum and bimanual exam

### ESSENTIAL WORKUP
- Pelvic exam
- Saline and KOH wet prep of vaginal discharge

### DIAGNOSTIC TESTS & INTERPRETATION
### Lab
- $\beta$-Human chorionic gonadotropin ($\beta$-hCG)
- pH of discharge with Nitrazine paper (normal in premenopausal adults is between 3.5 and 4.1)
- Saline wet prep exam of discharge at 400×: Clue cells (bacterial vaginosis), motile trichomonads (*Trichomonas* spp.), budding yeast/pseudohyphae, presence of polymorphonuclear leukocytes (PMNs)
- Potassium hydroxide (KOH) wet prep exam of discharge for pseudohyphae (*Candida* spp.)
- KOH prep: "Whiff" test (bacterial vaginosis)
- Endocervical swab for gonorrhea (culture-Thayer-Martin media; DNA probe; amplification techniques—PCR/LCR) and chlamydia (DNA probe or amplification techniques—PCR/LCR),
- Trichomonas Rapid Test (point-of-care test using immunochromatographic technology)
- Nucleic acid probe test for *Trichomonas*, *G. vaginalis*, and *C. albicans* (point-of-care test)
- Viral cultures for HSV, DFA, or Tzanck smear for multinucleated giant cells if ulcers or vesicles are present
- Gram stain for infectious pathogens and to evaluate ratio of gram-positive to gram-negative rods
- Consider vaginal C & S (rule out staph/strep)
- Urinalysis/urine culture: (If c/o dysuria)
- Rule out sexually transmitted infections:
  – GC/Chlamydia testing
  – Consider RPR to rule out syphilis.
  – Discuss HIV testing.

### Imaging
N/A unless fistula is suspected.

### DIFFERENTIAL DIAGNOSIS
- UTI
- PID
- Dermatitis
- Discharge from cervicitis can be mistaken for vaginitis
- Chlamydia trachomatis
- *Neisseria gonorrhoeae*

## TREATMENT

### ED TREATMENT/PROCEDURES
- Bacterial vaginosis:
  – Vaginal metronidazole gel for 5 days *or* metronidazole 500 mg PO for 7 days *or* vaginal clindamycin cream to 7 days *or* clindamycin PO for 7 days *or* clindamycin ovules PV 3 days
  – Rx before certain gynecologic procedures
  – Advise no alcohol intake if taking metronidazole up to 24 hr after treatment.
  – Routine treatment of male sex partner: No
  – *Lactobacillus* not found to be more effective than placebo
- Candidiasis: Single oral dose fluconazole *or* 3–7 days of intravaginal imidazole drug
  – Routine treatment of male sex partner: No
- Chemical irritant:
  – Avoid irritant
  – Use sitz baths, cotton underwear.
- Foreign body: Removal of foreign body; may necessitate sedation for removal and appropriate antibiotics if infection present
- Chlamydia cervicitis:
  – 1 dose azithromycin (for cervicitis, not adequate for PID) vs. 7 days of doxycycline, ofloxacin, levofloxacin, or erythromycin
  – Treat for presumed concurrent gonococcal infections.
  – Routine treatment of male sex partners: Yes
- Gonococcal cervicitis:
  – 1-dose treatment with ceftriaxone or cefixime vs. spectinomycin
  – In some locations, quinolone-resistant gonorrhea exists and is on the rise and should not be 1st-line treatment.
  – Treat for presumed concurrent chlamydial infection.
  – Routine treatment of male sex partners

- HSV:
  - Acyclovir, famciclovir, or valacyclovir for 7–10 days for initial attack; 5 days for recurrences
  - Lidocaine jelly for topical relief
  - Rule out other causes of genital ulcers. Offer RPR, HIV testing and counseling
  - Routine treatment of male sex partners: Only if symptomatic; however, patient and partner may shed virus asymptomatically.
- Lichen sclerosis:
  - Referral to gynecologist for estrogen cream and further treatment
- Trichomoniasis:
  - Metronidazole 2 g PO once *or*
  - Tinidazole 2 g PO *or*
  - Metronidazole 500 mg PO b.i.d. for 7 days. (avoid ethyl alcohol)
  - Routine treatment of male sex partners: Yes
- All sexually transmitted causes:
  - Advise patient to avoid sexual contact with partner until partner is evaluated and treated when appropriate.
  - Educate regarding STDs/safer sex/HIV/hepatitis vaccines

### *Pregnancy Considerations*
- Bacterial vaginosis:
  Rx symptomatic woman and asymptomatic pregnant women with history of preterm birth with oral metronidazole
- Chlamydia cerviditis:
  - Azithromycin is the 1st-line choice for treating chlamydia in pregnant patients
  - Do not treat with doxycycline, ofloxacin, or levofloxacin.

### *Pediatric Considerations*
- Ask about new irritants: Bubble bath, soap, and laundry detergent.
- Consider sexual assault/abuse

### MEDICATION
- Acyclovir: 200 mg PO 5 times per day for 10 days or 400 PO t.i.d. for 10 days (for initial attack); 200 mg PO 5 times per day for 5 days or 400 PO t.i.d. for 5 days (for recurrent attack)
- Azithromycin: 1 g PO × 1
- Butoconazole 2% cream: 5 g PV for 3 days
- Butoconazole SR 2% cream: 5 g PV × 1
- Ceftriaxone: 125 mg IM or 250 mg IM × 1
- Cefixime: 400 mg PO × 1
- Ciprofloxacin: 500 mg PO × 1

- Clindamycin 2% cream: 1 applicator PV q.h.s. for 7 days
- Clindamycin: 300 mg PO b.i.d. × 7 days
- Clotrimazole 1% cream: 5 g intravaginally for 7–14 days; 100 mg vaginal tablet × 7 days; 2–100 mg vaginal tablet for 7 days
- Doxycycline: 100 mg PO b.i.d. for 7 days (class D)
- Erythromycin ethyl succinate: 800 mg PO q.i.d. for 7 days
- Erythromycin base: 500 mg PO q.i.d. for 7 days
- Famciclovir: 250 mg PO t.i.d. × 7–10 days (for initial attack); 125 mg PO b.i.d. × 5 days (for recurrent infection)
- Fluconazole: 150 mg PO × 1
- Levofloxacin: 500 mg PO per day × 7 days
- Metronidazole: 500 mg PO b.i.d. for 7 days
- Metronidazole 0.75% gel: PV once daily for 5 days
- Miconazole: 1,200 mg PV × 1
- Miconazole: 200 mg PV q.h.s. for 3 days
- Miconazole: 5 g 2% cream PV q.h.s. for 7 days or 100 mg supp. PV q.h.s. for 7 days
- Nystatin 100,000 unit vaginal tablet: Every day for 14 days
- Spectinomycin: 2 g IM × 1
- Terconazole: 80 mg supp q.h.s. for 3 days or 5 g of 0.8% cream PV q.h.s. for 3 days or 5 g of 0.4% cream PV for 7 days
- Tinidazole: 2 g PO once
- Tioconazole: 5 g of 6.5% cream PV × 1
- Valacyclovir: 1 g PO b.i.d. × 7–10 days (for initial attack); 500 mg PO b.i.d. × 3–5 days or 1 g PO per day × 5 days (for recurrent attack)

 **FOLLOW-UP**

### DISPOSITION
#### Admission Criteria
- Disseminated gonococcal infection
- Sepsis secondary to foreign body
- PID toxicity
- Pain control, consequent inability to urinate or pass stool (HSV)

#### Discharge Criteria
Most can be discharged; follow-up in ~1 wk is suggested.

### *Issues for Referral*
- Vaginal discharge and vaginitis can be safely managed as an outpatient by the patient's primary physician or gynecologist:
  - Suggested follow-up in 1 wk

### FOLLOW-UP RECOMMENDATIONS
- Recommend good hygiene
- Eating yogurt rich in lactobacillus can help prevent vaginal yeast infections.
- Advise patient to return to the ED or see her doctor if:
  - Symptoms do not resolve in 3–5 days
  - Abdominal pain or cramping
  - Fever or chills
  - Pain during sexual intercourse
  - Lower back or flank pain
  - Difficulty urinating, or urinary frequency

## PEARLS AND PITFALLS
- pH of bacterial vaginosis is often >4.5
- Candidiasis often presents right before menses and can be precipitated by antibiotic use, DM, and immunosuppression.
- Trichomoniasis often presents after menses and has similar risk factors as other sexually transmitted diseases, including number of sexual partners and sexual practices.

## ADDITIONAL READING
- Anderson MR, Klink K, Cohrssen A. Evaluation of vaginal complaints. *JAMA* 2004;291(11): 1368–1379.
- Botash AS. Vaginitis. *Emedicine*. November 3, 2009.
- Centers for Disease Control and Prevention Sexually Transmitted Diseases Treatment Guidelines. 2006.
- Egan ME, Lipsky MS. Diagnosis of vaginitis. *Am Fam Physician*. 2000;62(5):1095–1104.
- Quan M. Vaginitis: Meeting the clinical challenge. *Clin Cornerstone*. 2000;3(2):36–37.

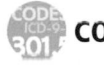 **CODES**

### ICD9
- 616.10 Vaginitis and vulvovaginitis, unspecified
- 623.5 Leukorrhea, not specified as infective

**V**

# VALVULAR HEART DISEASE

*Liudvikas Jagminas*

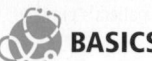

## BASICS

### DESCRIPTION
- Mitral stenosis:
  - Obstruction of diastolic blood flow into the left ventricle (LV)
- Mitral regurgitation:
  - Inadequate closure of the leaflets allows retrograde blood flow into the left atrium (LA).
  - Acute: Pressure overload in LA and pulmonary veins causing acute pulmonary edema
  - Chronic: LV volume overload with dilatation and hypertrophy with LA enlargement
- Aortic stenosis:
  - Obstruction of LV outflow with increased systolic gradient
  - Progressive increase in LV systolic pressure and concentric hypertrophy
- Aortic regurgitation:
  - Acute LV pressure and volume overload leading to left-heart failure and pulmonary edema
  - Chronic volume overload with LV dilation and hypertrophy

### Pregnancy Considerations
Pregnancy is associated with significant hemodynamic changes that can aggravate valvular heart disease and increase the risk of thromboembolic events.

### Geriatric Considerations
- Degenerative valvular disease is most common (aortic stenosis and mitral regurgitation)
- Aortic valve replacement is most common surgical procedure

### ETIOLOGY
- Mitral stenosis:
  - Rheumatic fever
  - Cardiac tumors
  - Rheumatologic disorders (lupus, rheumatoid arthritis)
  - Myxoma
  - Congenital defects: Parachute valve
- Mitral regurgitation (acute):
  - Ruptured papillary muscle (infarction, trauma)
  - Papillary muscle dysfunction (ischemia)
  - Ruptured chordae tendineae (trauma, endocarditis, myxomatous)
  - Valve perforation (endocarditis)
  - Weight-loss medications (fenfluramine, dexfenfluramine)
- Aortic stenosis:
  - Congenital aortic stenosis: Male > Female (4:1)
  - Congenital bicuspid valve (1–2%)
  - Rheumatic aortic stenosis
  - Calcific aortic stenosis
- Aortic regurgitation:
  - Infective endocarditis
  - Rupture of sinus of Valsalva
  - Acute aortic dissection
  - Chest trauma

- Following valve surgery
- Bicuspid aortic valve
- Rheumatic fever
- Weight-loss medications (fenfluramine, dexfenfluramine)
- Collagen vascular or connective-tissue diseases
- Systematic lupus erythematosus
- Marfan syndrome
- Pseudoxanthoma elasticum
- Ankylosing spondylitis
- Ehlers-Danlos syndrome
- Polymyalgia rheumatica

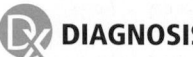

## DIAGNOSIS

### SIGNS AND SYMPTOMS
- Mitral stenosis:
  - Malar flush ("mitral facies")
  - Prominent jugular A waves
  - Right ventricular lift
  - Loud S1
  - Opening snap
  - Low-pitched diastolic rumble
  - Exertional dyspnea
  - Fatigue
  - Palpitations
  - Paroxysmal nocturnal dyspnea
  - Orthopnea
  - Hemoptysis
  - Systemic emboli
  - Pulmonary edema
- Mitral regurgitation:
  - Acute pulmonary edema
  - Jugular venous pressure (JVP) exhibits cannon A waves and giant V waves.
  - Harsh blowing apical crescendo-decrescendo murmur radiating to the axilla
  - Palpable thrill at apex
  - S3 and S4
  - Palpitations
  - Atrial fibrillation
  - Dyspnea
  - Orthopnea
  - Nocturnal paroxysmal dyspnea
  - Peripheral edema
  - Systemic emboli
  - Normal JVP
  - Left ventricular hypertrophy (LVH)
  - Apical high-pitched pansystolic murmur
  - Decreased or obscured S1
  - Widely split S2
  - S3
- Aortic stenosis:
  - Exertional angina
  - Syncope (during exercise)
  - CHF (initially diastolic failure, then systolic)
  - Sudden death secondary to ventricular fibrillation
  - Harsh crescendo-decrescendo (diamond-shaped) systolic murmur at aortic focus radiating to carotids

- Absent aortic component of S2
- Delayed upstroke in peripheral pulse (pulsus parvus et tardus)
- S4 gallop
- Ejection click
- Aortic regurgitation:
  - Fatigue
  - Dyspnea on exertion
  - Paroxysmal nocturnal dyspnea
  - Orthopnea
  - Syncope
  - Acute pulmonary edema
  - High-pitched blowing decrescendo diastolic murmur at aortic area
  - Accentuated A2 heart sound
  - Wide pulse pressure
  - Corrigan pulse (collapsing pulse)
  - Duroziez sign (to-and-fro murmur)
  - De Musset sign (head bobbing with systole)
  - Quincke pulse (nail bed pulsations)
  - Austin Flint murmur (soft diastolic rumble)

### ESSENTIAL WORKUP
- History and symptoms
- Thorough cardiopulmonary exam
- ECG

### DIAGNOSTIC TESTS & INTERPRETATION
#### Lab
- Blood cultures:
- Presumed endocarditis
- CBC:
  - Anemia

#### Imaging
- CXR:
  - Mitral stenosis:
    - Enlarged LA
    - Pulmonary vascular congestion (Kerley B lines)
    - Prominent pulmonary arteries
  - Mitral regurgitation:
    - LV and LA enlargement in chronic cases
    - Pulmonary edema and normal LV and LA dimensions in acute cases
  - Aortic stenosis:
    - LVH
    - Aortic calcification
    - Dilation of ascending aorta
    - Pulmonary congestion and cardiomegaly
  - Aortic regurgitation:
    - Acute = normal cardiac silhouette and pulmonary edema
    - Chronic = enlarged LV and dilated aorta
- ECG:
  - Quality assessment of valvular structures
  - Measurements of flow through valves
  - Identification of regurgitation
  - Ventricular dilatation or hypertrophy
- Spiral CT scan:
  - To exclude aortic dissection with acute aortic regurgitation

### Diagnostic Procedures/Surgery

EKG:

- Mitral stenosis:
  - Left atrium enlargement (broad notched P waves)
  - RV hypertrophy
  - Right axis deviation
  - Atrial fibrillation
- Acute mitral regurgitation:
  - Left atrial enlargement
  - LVH
  - Left axis deviation
- Aortic stenosis:
  - LVH most common
  - Atrial fibrillation
  - Interventricular conduction delay
  - Complete AV block
- Aortic regurgitation:
  - Acute = LV strain
  - Chronic = LVH and strain

### DIFFERENTIAL DIAGNOSIS

See "Etiology."

##  TREATMENT

### PRE-HOSPITAL

Avoid vasodilators in aortic stenosis.

### INITIAL STABILIZATION/THERAPY

- ABCs
- Administer oxygen.
- Monitor and measure pulse oximetry.
- IV access

### ED TREATMENT/PROCEDURES

- Mitral stenosis:
  - Treat symptoms of CHF.
  - Rate control if in atrial fibrillation
  - Digoxin
  - β-Blockers
  - Heparin (if new-onset atrial fibrillation)
  - Diuretics
  - Endocarditis prophylaxis/education
- Mitral regurgitation:
  - Differentiate between acute and chronic MR:
  - Acute:
    ○ Afterload reduction (nitroglycerin, morphine, or sodium nitroprusside)
    ○ Diuresis
    ○ Intra-aortic balloon pump (temporizing for urgent surgery)
  - Chronic:
    ○ Diuresis
    ○ Nitrates
    ○ Hydralazine
    ○ ACE inhibitor
    ○ Digoxin
    ○ β-Adrenergic blocker (ventricular rate control)
    ○ Calcium antagonist (ventricular rate control)
    ○ Heparin (if atrial fibrillation)
    ○ Endocarditis prophylaxis/education

- Aortic stenosis:
  - Gentle diuresis if CHF
  - Mild hydration if hypotensive and not in CHF
  - Avoid nitrates and afterload reduction.
  - Digoxin
  - Intra-aortic balloon pump (temporize for surgery)
  - Endocarditis prophylaxis/education
- Aortic regurgitation:
  - Chronic:
    ○ Preload and afterload reduction
    ○ Digoxin
    ○ Diuretics
    ○ Endocarditis prophylaxis/education
  - Acute:
    ○ Preload and afterload reduction
    ○ Intra-aortic balloon pump
    ○ Urgent surgery

### MEDICATION

- Atenolol: 0.3–2 mg/kg/d PO, max. 2 mg/kg/d (peds: 1–2 mg/kg/dose PO daily suggested)
- Digoxin: 0.5 mg bolus IV, then 0.25 mg IV q2h up to 1 mg; 0.125–0.375 mg/d PO
- Diltiazem: 0.25 mg/kg IV over 2 min (repeat in 15 min PRN with 0.35 mg/kg) then 5–15 mg/h
- Enalapril: 1.25 mg IV q6h; PO 2.5–10 mg b.i.d. (peds: 0.1–0.5 mg/kg/d PO div. q12–24h; max: 0.58 mg/kg/d or 40 mg/d
- Esmolol: IV: 500 μg bolus, then 50–400 μg/kg/min
- Furosemide: 20–80 mg/d PO/IV/IM; titrate up to 600 mg/d for severe edematous states (peds: 1 mg/kg IV/IM slowly under close supervision; not to exceed 6 mg/kg)
- Heparin: 80 IU/kg IV bolus, then 18 IU/kg/hr drip, adjust to maintain partial thromboplastin time 1.5–2 × control (INR 2–3)
- Hydralazine: 10–25 mg IV q2–4h (peds: 0.1–0.5 mg/kg IM/IV q4–6h; max. 20 mg/dose)
- Metoprolol: 5 mg IV q2min × 3 doses; then 50 mg PO q6h × 48 hr
- Nitroglycerin: Start at 20 mcg/min IV and titrate to effect (up to 300 mcg/min); SL 0.3–0.6 mg p.r.n.; Topical 1–2 inches of 2% q6h (peds: 0.25–0.5 μg/kg/min IV, increase by 0.5–1 mg/kg/min; max. 20 μg/kg/min)
- Phentolamine: 5 mg bolus IV, then 1–2 mg/min IV infusion
- Propranolol IV: 1–3 mg at 1 mg/min
- Sodium nitroprusside IV: 0.5 μg/kg/min; increase in increments of 0.5 to 1.0 μg/kg/min q5–10min up to 10 μg/kg/min
- Amoxicillin: 2 g PO 1h before the procedure; alternatively, 3 g PO 1h before the procedure, followed by 1.5 g PO 6h after the initial dose:
  - Pediatric dose: 50 mg/kg PO 1h before procedure
- Ampicillin: 2 g IV/IM 30 min before the procedure (peds: 50 mg/kg IV/IM 30 min before the procedure)
- Clindamycin: 600 mg PO 1h before procedure (peds: 20 mg/kg PO 1h before procedure; not to exceed 600 mg)

## 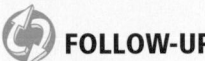 FOLLOW-UP

### DISPOSITION

#### Admission Criteria

- New onset atrial fibrillation
- CHF/pulmonary edema
- Hemodynamically unstable
- Acute mitral or aortic regurgitation
- Cardiac ischemia
- Angina
- Syncope
- Arrhythmias

#### Discharge Criteria

- Hemodynamic stability
- Unchanged ECG
- Resolution of CHF symptoms with diuresis
- Chronic mitral regurgitation

#### Issues for Referral

For patients who are candidates for outpatient management, close follow-up with a cardiologist to assess severity of valvular disease and need for cardiac surgery

Educate patient about risks of valvular heart disease and need for antibiotic prophylaxis with dental and medical procedures.

### PEARLS AND PITFALLS

In patients with chest pain and aortic stenosis, nitrates are contraindicated.

### ADDITIONAL READING

- Bonow RO, Cheitlin MD, Crawford MH, et al. Task Force 3: Valvular heart disease. *J Am Coll Cardiol*. 2005;45(8):1334–1340.
- Carabello BA, Crawford FA. Valvular heart disease. *N Engl J Med*. 1997;337(1):32–41. [published erratum appears in *N Engl J Med*. 1997;337:507].
- Elkayam U, Bitar F. Valvular heart disease and pregnancy part I: Native valves. *J Am Coll Cardiol* 2005;46:223–230.
- Roldan CA, Shively BK, Crawford MH. Value of the cardiovascular examination for detecting valvular heart disease in asymptomatic subjects. *Am J Cardiol*. 1996;77:1327–1331.

## 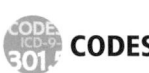 CODES

#### ICD9

- 424.0 Mitral valve disorders
- 424.1 Aortic valve disorders
- 424.2 Tricuspid valve disorders, specified as nonrheumatic

**V**

# VARICELLA

*H. Samuel Ko*
*Mark Richmond*

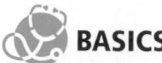 **BASICS**

## DESCRIPTION
- Commonly known as chickenpox
- Classic viral illness of childhood
- Most common in late winter and early spring; epidemics tend to occur every 2–5 yr.
- In the prevaccine era, 90% of children were infected by 15 yr of age and virtually all persons acquired varicella by adulthood:
  - Vaccine has reduced incidence by 85%.
- Adults have a 15 times greater risk for death from varicella than children.

## ETIOLOGY
- DNA virus
  - Latency in cranial nerve ganglia, dorsal root ganglia, and autonomic ganglia; periodic reactivation:
  - Presents as herpes zoster or shingles decades after primary infection
  - Virus is transmitted by respiratory route and direct contact with skin lesions.
  - Humans are only known reservoir.

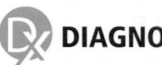 **DIAGNOSIS**

## SIGNS AND SYMPTOMS
- Varicella causes a spectrum of disease.
- Classic childhood Illness
  - Usually affects children ages 1–9
  - Low-grade fever (100–103°F), headache and malaise:
    - Concurrent or precedes rash by 1–2 days
  - Classic exanthem:
    - Lesions begin on the face, spreading to the trunk and extremities.
    - Vesicles, pustules, and small scabs on erythematous base
    - Lesions in varying stages of evolution
    - "Dewdrop on rose petal"
    - Round or oval, 0.5–1.0 cm in diameter
    - Duration of vesicle formation 3–5 days
    - Pruritus, anorexia, and listlessness
    - 10- to 21-day incubation period; average is 14 days
    - Infectious from 48 hr before vesicle formation until all vesicles are crusted (typically 4–5 days)
    - May involve conjunctival, oropharyngeal, or vaginal mucosa
    - Bacterial superinfection of the skin develops in 1%–4% of otherwise healthy children.
- Neonates
  - Congenital varicella syndrome:
    - Occasionally follows maternal zoster infection
    - Cicatricial skin lesions
    - Limb hypoplasia or paresis
    - Microcephaly
    - Ophthalmic lesions, congenital cataracts, chorioretinitis

- Adolescents and adults
  - Presents similarly to disease in children but generally of greater severity:
    - Extracutaneous manifestations in 5%–50%
- Immunocompromised patients
  - HIV, transplant patients, leukemia patients are the highest risk for disseminated form.
  - Patients on chemotherapy, immunosuppresants, and long-term corticosteroid therapy
  - Absolute neutrophil counts and absolute lymphocyte counts <500 are the best predictors of complicated disease.
  - More numerous lesions that may have hemorrhagic base
  - Healing may take longer
  - Extracutaneous manifestations, especially pneumonia, common
- Pregnant patients
  - Prevalent in young expectant women
  - Produces a more severe disease presentation:
    - Risk to the fetus of congenital varicella syndrome greatest in first half of pregnancy
    - Maternal disease severity greatest if infection in second half of pregnancy
  - Perinatal disease occurs in mother from 5 days predelivery to 48 hr postdelivery.
- Extracutaneous manifestations
  - Pneumonitis:
    - 25 times more common in adults
    - Most common in adult smokers and immunocompromised children
    - Occurs 3–5 days after onset of rash
    - Early signs: continued eruption of new lesions, cough, new-onset cough
    - Tachypnea, dyspnea, cyanosis, pleuritic chest pain, and hemoptysis
  - Cerebellar ataxia:
    - May develop 5 days after rash
    - Ataxia, vomiting, slurred speech, fever, vertigo, tremor
  - Cerebritis:
    - Develops 3–8 days after appearance of rash:
    - Duration about 2 wk
    - Progressive malaise
    - Headache, meningismus, vomiting, fever, delirium, seizures
  - Reye syndrome

### Geriatric Considerations
- Increased risk of extracutaneous manifestations
- Lower immunity allows for reactivation as herpes zoster

### Pediatric Considerations
- Do not use aspirin for treatment of fever associated with Reye syndrome. Acetaminophen is recommended antipyretic.
- Parents need to be cautioned regarding risk for secondary bacterial infection and possible progression to sepsis.

### Pregnancy Considerations
- Pregnant women with no childhood history of varicella and no antibodies to varicella zoster virus (VZV) require varicella zoster immunoglobulin (VZIG).
- Varicella pneumonia in pregnancy is regarded as a medical emergency and is associated with life-threatening respiratory compromise and death (mortality can be 10%–45%).
- More likely to occur in third trimester.

### History
- Thorough history:
  - Fever, systemic symptoms
  - Immunization history
  - Immunocompetent vs immunocompromised

### Physical Exam
- Thorough physical exam
  - Characterize rash spread and extent
  - Evaluate for any extracutaneous manifestations

## ESSENTIAL WORKUP
- History and physical are sufficient in uncomplicated cases.
- Pneumonitis:
  - Chest radiographs classically demonstrates 2- to 5-mm peripheral densities, may coalesce and persist for weeks
- Reye syndrome:
  - Ammonia level peaks early.
  - LFTs will be elevated
  - PT, PTT
- Cerebritis:
  - Lumbar puncture demonstrates lymphocytic pleocytosis and elevated levels of protein.

## DIAGNOSTIC TESTS & INTERPRETATION
### Lab
- Viral culture (3–5 days), polymerase chain reaction (PCR), or rapid antigen testing with enzyme-linked immunosorbent assay (ELISA). Use skin scrapings from crust or base of lesion.
- Serologic tests for varicella antibodies
- Fluorescent antibody to membrane antigen (FAMA) test is regarded as gold standard but is demanding and time-consuming.

### Imaging
- Not generally indicated unless there is concern for extracutaneous manifestations

### Diagnostic Procedures/Surgery
- Liver biopsy definitive test for Reye syndrome

## DIFFERENTIAL DIAGNOSIS
- Impetigo
- Disseminated herpes
- Disseminated coxsackievirus
- Measles
- Rickettsial disease
- Insect bites
- Scabies
- Erythema multiforme
- Drug eruption (especially Stevens–Johnson syndrome)

**TREATMENT**

### PRE-HOSPITAL

- Nonimmune transport personnel must avoid respiratory or physical contact with patients.
- Transport personnel with varicella or herpes zoster should not come in contact with immunocompromised or pregnant patients.

### INITIAL STABILIZATION/THERAPY

- Airway management and resuscitate as indicated:
  - Protect airway if obtunded.

### ED TREATMENT/PROCEDURES

- Generally, acetaminophen and antipruritics are all that is needed for classic childhood illness.
- Closely cropped nails and good hygiene help prevent secondary bacterial infection.
- Neonatal:
  - VZIG for infants if maternal varicella develops <5 days before delivery or ≤48 hr after delivery
  - Of the infants who receive VZIG, 50% will develop varicella and should be kept in strict isolation for the incubation period.
  - IV acyclovir indicated in neonates:
    - Chickenpox and unwell-appearing (poor feeding and tachypnea)
    - High-risk neonate who did not receive VZIG
    - Immunocompromised or premature neonate
- Infants/children ≤12 yr of age
  - Acyclovir
  - Normally not needed for uncomplicated patients
  - Must be initiated within 24 hr of disease onset to be efficacious
  - Reduces total lesions by 25% and fever by 1 day
  - May be considered in children taking corticosteroids, long-term salicylate therapy, or with chronic cutaneous or pulmonary diseases
  - Prophylaxis with VZIG
  - Indicated in susceptible individuals:
    - Immunocompromised children at high risk for complication with a significant exposure
    - Living in same household as a person with active chickenpox or herpes zoster
    - Playmate contact >1 hr with person infected with chickenpox or zoster
  - 72 hr postexposure for maximal effect
  - May provide benefit ≥96 hr postexposure for immunocompromised patients
  - Ineffective once clinical illness is established
- Adolescents/adults:
  - Symptomatic with antipyretics and antipruritics
  - Acyclovir initiated within 24 hr decreases progression to disseminated disease
- Pregnant women:
  - Pregnant women with no childhood history of varicella and no antibodies to VZV require VZIG.
  - Acyclovir, when initiated during incubation period or ≤24 hr of onset of rash:
    - Prophylaxis after exposure is 84% protective
    - Currently regarded as safe during pregnancy (category B)
  - IV acyclovir for pneumonitis/other complications:
    - Respiratory, neurologic, hemorrhagic rash, or continued fever >6 days

- Immunocompromised patients:
  - Acyclovir recommended, shortens course
  - Must be initiated ≤72 hr of onset
  - Decreases progression to disseminated disease
  - Foscarnet for acyclovir-resistant disease
  - Interferon
  - Prophylaxis with VZIG for the susceptible immunocompromised patient
- Extracutaneous:
  - IV acyclovir or foscarnet if viral resistance
- Vaccine
  - Children:
    - Routine vaccination at 12–18 mo
    - Recommended for all susceptible children by age 13
  - Adolescents and adults:
    - Persons >13 yr old without history of varicella
    - Two doses separated by 4–8 wk
    - Recommended in high-risk groups: health care workers, family member of immunocompromised person, susceptible women of childbearing age, teachers, military, international travelers
    - Currently no indications for elderly patients, although recent evidence suggests the vaccine decreases morbidity from herpes zoster and postherpetic neuralgia
  - Postexposure prophylaxis:
    - Effectiveness of 70%–100% if given ≤72 hr of exposure
    - Not effective if >5 days but will produce immunity if not infected
  - Immunocompromised persons:
    - Most immunocompromised persons should not be immunized.

### MEDICATION

- Acyclovir:
  - Uncomplicated: 800 mg PO 5 times a day for 7 days; adolescents (13–18 yr old): 20 mg/kg per dose q.i.d. for 7 days (peds: 20 mg/kg suspension PO q.i.d. for 5 days [max 800 mg PO q.i.d.])
  - Immunocompromised: 10 mg/kg IV q8h infused over 1 hr *or* 800 mg PO 5 times a day for 7 days (peds: 10–12 mg/kg IV q8h infused over 1 hr *or* 500 mg/m²/day IV q8h)
- Diphenhydramine: 25–50 mg IV, IM, or PO q4h (peds: 5 mg/kg/day elixir 12.5 mg/5 mL)
- Famciclovir: 500 mg PO t.i.d.
- Foscarnet: 40 mg/kg q8h over 1 hr for ≥10 days (peds: same)
- Hydroxyzine: 25–50 mg IM or PO q4–6h (peds: 0.5 mg/kg q4–6h suspension 10 and 25 mg/5 mL)
- Valacyclovir: 1,000 mg PO t.i.d. for 5–7 days
- VZIG: 625 IU IM (peds: 1 vial per 10 kg IM to a max of 5 vials [each vial contains 125 IU])

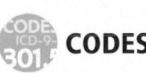 **FOLLOW-UP**

### DISPOSITION

#### Admission Criteria

- Patients with pneumonia require admission:
  - ICU for respiratory observation or support
- Immunocompromised patients: ICU vs ward, depending on severity of illness
- Neonates require admission for IV acyclovir.
- All admitted patients must be kept in isolation.

#### Discharge Criteria

- Immunocompetent children without evidence of Reye syndrome or secondary bacterial infection
- Adults with no evidence of extracutaneous disease

### FOLLOW-UP RECOMMENDATIONS

- Patients who are discharged need close follow-up with PCP to assure resolution without complications.

## PEARLS AND PITFALLS

- Patient with varicella are infectious from 48 hr before vesicle formation until all vesicles are crusted
- Varicella vaccine has reduced the incidence of disease by 85%.
- Varicella pneumonia in pregnancy is a medical emergency.

## ADDITIONAL READING

- American Academy of Pediatrics. Varicella zoster infections. Pickering L, ed. *Red Book: 2003 Report of the Committee on Infectious Diseases*, 26th ed. Elk Grove Village, IL: American Academy of Pediatrics, 2003: 672–686.
- Gilden D. Varicella zoster virus and central nervous system syndromes. *Herpes*. 2004;11(Suppl 2): 89A–94A.
- Heininger U, Seward J. Varicella. *Lancet*. 2006;368: 1365–1376.
- Kempf W, et al. Swiss recommendations for the management of varicella zoster infections. *Swiss Med Wkly*. 2007;137:239–2351.
- Mohsen AH, McKendrick M. Varicella pneumonia in adults. *Eur Respir J*. 2003;21:886–891.
- Mueller NH, et al. varicella zoster virus infection: Clinical features, molecular pathogenesis of disease, and latency. *Neurol Clin*. 2008;26:675–697.
- Sauerbrei A, Wutzler P. Herpes simplex and varicella zoster virus infections during pregnancy: Current concepts of prevention, diagnosis and therapy. Part 2: Varicella-zoster virus infections. *Med Microbiol Immunol*. 2007;196:95–102.

### See Also (Topic, Algorithm, Electronic Media Element)

- Herpes Zoster

## CODES

### ICD9

052.9 Varicella without mention of complication

# VARICES

*John Bailitz*
*Tamara Espinoza*

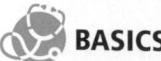

## BASICS

### DESCRIPTION
- Increased portal venous pressure results in portal–systemic shunts.
- Shunts at gastroesophageal junction result in fragile submucosal esophageal varices.

### ETIOLOGY
- 10%–30% of all cases of upper gastrointestinal (GI) bleeding
- 90% of upper GI bleeding in patients with cirrhosis
- Variceal hemorrhage occurs in 30% of patients with cirrhosis: Only 50% will stop bleeding spontaneously
  - 30% mortality per episode
  - 70% have recurrent bleeding.
- In adults:
  - Cirrhosis due to alcoholism or chronic hepatitis
  - Storage disease: Wilson or hemochromatosis
  - Middle East: Schistosomiasis
- In children:
  - Intrahepatic obstruction from biliary cirrhosis
  - Biliary atresia
  - Cystic fibrosis
  - Beta-antitrypsin deficiency
  - Hepatitis

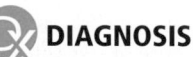

## DIAGNOSIS

### SIGNS AND SYMPTOMS
- General
  - Weakness and fatigue
  - Tachycardia
  - Tachypnea
  - Hypotension
  - Cool, clammy skin; prolonged capillary refill
- Abdominal
  - Significant active upper GI bleeding:
    ○ Hematemesis
    ○ Hematochezia
    ○ Melena
    ○ 20%–40% of total blood volume loss possible
  - Abdominal pain
- Stigmata of severe hepatic dysfunction:
  - Jaundice
  - Spider angiomata
  - Palmar erythema
  - Pedal edema
  - Hepatosplenomegaly
  - Ascites
- History of portal hypertension:
  - Most commonly alcoholic cirrhosis
  - Others, including:
    ○ Primary biliary cirrhosis
    ○ Schistosomiasis
    ○ Budd–Chiari syndrome
    ○ Severe CHF
    ○ Sarcoidosis

- Cardiovascular
  - Chest pain/shortness of breath
- CNS
  - Syncope
  - Confusion and agitation initially
  - Lethargy and obtundation later

### Pediatric Considerations
- Massive hematemesis: typical initial presentation:
  - Hypotension may be a late finding.

### History
- Gastroesophageal varices are present in 50% of patients with cirrhosis and correlate with severity of disease.
- Most important predictor of hemorrhage is size of varux. Other factors include number of varices, severity of hepatic disease and endoscopic findings.
- Patients with PBC develop varices and variceal hemorrhage early in their course of disease, even prior to development of cirrhosis.

### Physical Exam
- Vitals signs may be normal or may show tachycardia (early) and hypotension (late).
- Altered mental status with encephalopathy or poor perfusion
- Active hematemsis
- Stigmata of alcoholic liver disease
  - Ascites
  - General edema
  - Jaundice

### ESSENTIAL WORKUP
- Gastric tube placement:
  - Determines whether patient is actively bleeding
  - Decompresses stomach which may aid in hemostasis. Possible role in reducing aspiration risk
  - Facilitates endoscopic exam
  - Will not increase or cause esophageal variceal bleeding
- Emergent endoscopy

### DIAGNOSTIC TESTS & INTERPRETATION
#### Lab
- Type and cross-match 6–8 units:
  - Significant transfusion requirements
- ABG for:
  - Acidosis
  - Hypoxemia
- CBC:
  - Hematocrit is an unreliable indicator of early rapid blood loss.
  - Perform serial CBCs to follow blood loss.
- Electrolytes, BUN, creatinine, glucose:
  - Evaluate renal function.
  - BUN:creatinine ratio >30 suggest significant blood in GI tract.
- PT/PTT/INR and platelets:
  - Coagulopathy
  - Prolonged bleeding times
  - Thrombocytopenia

#### Imaging
- Chest radiograph (portable) for aspiration/perforation
- ECG for myocardial ischemia

### DIFFERENTIAL DIAGNOSIS
- Bleeding/perforated peptic ulcer
- Erosive gastritis
- Mallory–Weiss syndrome
- Boerhaave syndrome
- Aortoenteric fistula
- Gastric varices
- Gastric vascular ectasia

## TREATMENT

### PRE-HOSPITAL
- Airway stabilization
- Treat hypotension 0.9% normal saline infusion bolus through 2 large-bore 16-gauge or large IV lines.
- Cardiac and pulse oximetry monitoring

### INITIAL STABILIZATION/THERAPY
- ABCs with early aggressive airway control/intubation:
  - Early intubation = easier intubation
  - For AMS or massive hemoptysis
  - Facilitates emergency endoscopy
- Establish central IV access with invasive intravascular monitoring for hypotension not responsive to initial fluid bolus.
- Replace lost blood as soon as possible:
  - Initiate with O-negative blood until type-specific blood available.
  - 10 mL/kg bolus in children
  - Fresh-frozen plasma and platelets may be required.
- Place gastric tube nasally (awake) or orally (intubated)
- Controversy:
  - Overly aggressive volume expansion may lead to rebound portal HTN, rebleeding, and pulmonary edema.
  - Transfusion goal is Hb = 8.
  - rFVIIa may decrease hemostasis failure rates in Child–Pugh class B/C patients

### Pediatric Considerations
- Initiate intraosseous access if peripheral access unsuccessful in unstable patient.
- Most bleeding in children stops spontaneously.
- Vital signs changes may be a late finding in children:
  - Subtle changes in mental status, capillary refill, mild tachycardia, or orthostatic changes may indicate significant blood loss.
  - Overaggressive correction in infants can quickly lead to significant electrolyte abnormalities.

## ED TREATMENT/PROCEDURES

- Emergent endoscopy required for active bleeding
  - Use pharmacologic and tamponade devices as temporizing measures.
- **Endoscopy**
  - Emergent with active bleeding in nasogastric tube
  - Procedure of choice in acute esophageal bleeding
  - Esophageal band ligation equivalent to sclerotherapy with fewer complications:
    o May be difficult to visualize in cases of massive bleeding
  - Sclerotherapy with massive bleeding
  - Gastric varices are not amenable to endoscopic repair due to high rebleeding rate.
    o Treat pharmacologically.
  - Administer antibiotics at time of procedure to decrease risk for spontaneous bacterial peritonitis:
    o Fluoroquinolone or ceftriaxone
- **Pharmacological Therapy**
  - Octreotide is first-line therapy:
    o Complications include hyperglycemia and abdominal cramping.
  - Vasopressin replaced by octreotide secondary to high incidence of vascular ischemia
- **Balloon Tamponade**
  - Initiate in massive uncontrollable bleed.
  - Sengstaken–Blakemore and Minnesota tubes
  - Applies direct pressure but risks esophageal perforation and ulceration
  - Temporary benefit only with massive uncontrolled bleeding in hands of experienced clinician
- **Refractory Bleeding Therapy**
  - Interventional radiology:
    o Transjugular intrahepatic portosystemic shunt procedure. Recommended for refractory gastric varices or for patients who are poor surgical candidates
  - Surgical options:
    o Portacaval shunt
    o Variceal transection
    o Stomach devascularization
    o Liver transplantation

## MEDICATION

- Cefotaxime: 2 g (peds: 50–180 mg/kg/24 h) IV q8h
- Norfloxacin 400 mg PO q12 or Ciprofloxacin 500 mg IV q12 if cannot tolerate PO (contraindicated in peds)
- Ceftriaxone: 2 g (peds: 50–75 mg/kg/24 hr) IV q24h in Child–Pugh class B/C or in quinolone-resistant areas
- Octreotide: 50 $\mu$g bolus, then 50 $\mu$g/hr infusion for 5 days
- Erythromycin 250 mg IV
  - Shown to aid in gastric clearing for better visualization during endoscopy

### First Line
- Octreotide
- Norfloxacin PO or ciprofloxacin IV

### Second Line
- Erythromycin
- Ceftriaxone

 **FOLLOW-UP**

### DISPOSITION
#### Admission Criteria
- ICU admission for actively bleeding varices
- Recent history of variceal bleeding
- High risk for early rebleeding:
  - Age >60 yr, renal failure, initial hemoglobin count <8

#### Discharge Criteria
- Nonbleeding varices

#### Issues for Referral
- Continued hemorrhage requiring surgery or higher level of care
- Liver transplant

### FOLLOW-UP RECOMMENDATIONS
- Timely outpatient GI follow-up
  - Will need annual surveillance endoscopies
- Medication and lifestyle modifications

## PEARLS AND PITFALLS

- Intubate early, especially in patients with hepatic encephalopathy or hemodynamic instability.
- Begin prophylactic antibiotics prior to endoscopy. Improves survival
- In the U.S., octreotide has replaced vasopressin owing to better side-effect profile. If vasopressin is required, use IV nitroglycerin infusion concomitantly to reduce end-organ ischemia.
- Control the airway prior to placement of balloon tamponade device, which provides only a temporizing measure prior to surgery or TIPS
- Hematochezia in a hemodynamically unstable patient is an upper GI bleed until proven otherwise.
- Consult your GI specialists early, since endoscopy is the first line diagnostic and therapeutic procedure.

## ADDITIONAL READING

- Harry R, Wendon J. Management of variceal bleeding. *Curr Opin Crit Care.* 2002;8:164–170.
- Nevens F. Review article: A critical comparison of drug therapies in currently used therapeutic strategies for variceal haemorrhage. *Aliment Pharmacol Ther.* 2004;20(Suppl 3):18–22.
- Witting MD. "You wanna do what?" Modern indications for nasogastric intubation. *J Emer Med.* 2007;33:61–64.
- Garcia-Tsao G, Sanyal AJ, Grace ND, Carey WD. Prevention and management of gastroesophageal varices and variceal hemorrhage in cirrhosis. *Am J Gastroenterol.* 2007;102:2086–102.
- Sass DA, Chopra KB. Portal hypertension and variceal hemorrhage. *Med Clin N Am.* 2009;93:837–853.

### See Also (Topic, Algorithm, Electronic Media Element)
- Cirrhosis
- Gastrointestinal Bleeding

 **CODES**

### ICD9
- 456.0 Esophageal varices with bleeding
- 456.1 Esophageal varices without mention of bleeding
- 456.8 Varices of other sites

V

# VASCULITIS

*Richard E. Wolfe*
*Andrew Milstein*

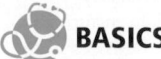 **BASICS**

## DESCRIPTION

- Injury to the walls of blood vessels from inflammation:
  - Ischemia and necrosis
  - Aneurysms and hemorrhage
  - Immunopathologic mechanisms:
    - Deposition of circulating antigen–antibody complex
    - Cell-mediated hypersensitivity
    - Granulomatous tissue reaction from persistent inflammation and formation of epithelioid and giant cells
    - May be immune complex-mediated or associated with antineutrophil cytoplasmic antibodies
- The vasculitides represent a wide group of disorders:
  - Multisystem disease with constitutional symptoms and inflammatory laboratory indices
  - Secondary to another disorder or trigger, or primary if vasculitis is the principal feature and the cause is unknown
  - Multiple factors determine presentation:
    - The size of the affected blood vessels
    - The specific distribution, severity, and duration of the inflammation
    - Degree of permeability or occlusion of the affected vessels
  - Association with other disorders:
    - Classification caries based on vessel size, histopathology, or dominant organ involved
- 1 out of 2,000 adults has some form of vasculitis

## ETIOLOGY

- Temporal (giant cell) arteritis:
  - Granulomatous arteritis of the aorta and its major branches often involving the temporal artery
  - Patients >50 yr
- Takayasu arteritis:
  - Granulomatous inflammation of the aorta and its major branches
  - Usually occurs in patients <50 yr
- Polyarteritis nodosa (PAN):
  - Small- and medium-sized arteritis
  - Common distribution includes vessels supplying the muscles, joints, intestines, nerves, kidneys, and skin
  - Most common in middle-age
- Kawasaki disease:
  - Associated with the mucocutaneous lymph node syndrome
  - Coronary arteries are often involved and involves large-, medium-, and small-sized arteries
  - Usually occurs in children
- Wegener granulomatosis:
  - Necrotizing vasculitis affecting small- to medium-sized vessels
  - Commonly, a granulomatous inflammation involving the respiratory tract and necrotizing glomerulonephritis

- Microscopic polyangiitis:
  - Necrotizing affecting small vessels
  - Necrotizing glomerulonephritis is very common.
  - Pulmonary capillaritis often occurs.
- Churg-Strauss syndrome (allergic granulomatosis):
  - Small- and medium-sized arteries
  - Mainly lungs, GI, and nerves
  - Can also involve heart, skin, and kidney
- Buerger disease (thromboangiitis obliterans):
  - Recurring inflammation and thrombosis of small and medium arteries and veins of the hands and feet
  - Typically between 20 and 40 yr and male
- Henoch-Schönlein purpura
- Hypersensitivity vasculitis
- Leukocytoclastic vasculitis
- Behçet disease
- Isolated CNS vasculitis
- Secondary vasculitides:
  - Bacterial infections:
    - Streptococcal, tuberculous, staphylococcal, Lyme disease, leprosy
  - Viral infections:
    - Hepatitis B or C, cytomegalovirus, herpes zoster, HIV)
  - Rickettsial infections
  - Drug-related
  - Connective tissue disease:
    - Systemic lupus erythematosus
    - Sjögren syndrome
    - Rheumatoid arthritis
    - Scleroderma
    - Dermatomyositis
  - Malignancy:
    - Hairy cell leukemia
    - Lymphoma
    - Solid organ tumors
  - Reiter syndrome and ankylosing spondylitis
  - Familial Mediterranean fever
  - Mixed cryoglobulinemia
  - Goodpasture syndrome
  - Erythema nodosum
  - Serum sickness

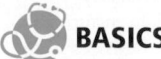 **DIAGNOSIS**

## SIGNS AND SYMPTOMS

- Systemic complaints are common early in the presentation of vasculitis, before vascular-related complications occur:
  - Fever, fatigue, weight loss, diffuse aches and pains
- Signs of arterial insufficiency:
  - Ischemic pain:
    - Angina, abdominal angina, claudication
  - Neurologic ischemia:
    - Headache, TIA, stroke, visual and sensorineural hearing loss, visual hallucinations, neuropathy
  - Renal ischemia:
    - Severe or resistant HTN

- Dermatologic ischemia:
  - Classic skin findings include nodular lesions, ulcers, livedo reticularis, and digital ischemia
  - Purpura, hair loss, nail-fold infarcts, papules, may also be seen
- Nondestructive oligoarthritis
- Ocular ischemia:
  - Posturally dependent visual blurring, diplopia, splinter or retinal hemorrhages, Roth spots, scleritis, and episcleritis
- Respiratory tract:
  - Sinusitis, epistaxis, nasal and oral ulcerations, strawberry gums, stridor from subglottic stenosis
- GI ischemia:
  - Hematochezia, melena, hematemesis, peritonitis, hepatitis
- Cardiac:
  - Syncope, postural dizziness, pericarditis, CHF

### History

- Suspect vasculitis with general systems and signs of arterial insufficiency:
  - Claudication, angina, abdominal angina, or TIA, in a young patient
  - Prolonged systemic illness with multiorgan dysfunction
  - History of glomerulonephritis, peripheral neuropathy, or autoimmune disease
- Diagnostic clues to the etiology:
  - Age, gender, ethnicity, travel history
  - Specific complaints that suggest the size of the involved vessel and organs
  - Recent infections
  - Connective-tissue disorders
  - Medications that may cause vasculitis
    - Penicillin, sulfa, phenytoin, allopurinol, gold, thiazide, NSAIDs, furosemide, quinidine, thiouracils, mefloquine, anthrax vaccination

### Physical Exam

Classify vasculitis:

- Large arteries:
  - Diminished pulses and bruits over several large arteries
  - BP discrepancy >10 mm Hg between left and right limbs
  - Pulse discrepancy >30 mm Hg between the left and right limbs
  - Cool extremities due to claudication and ulceration
- Medium and small arteries:
  - Palpable purpura (nodules, ulcers, livedo papules)
  - Skin ulcers
  - Digital ischemia

## ESSENTIAL WORKUP

- History and physical exam
- CBC, ESR, urinalysis, BUN, creatinine

## DIAGNOSTIC TESTS & INTERPRETATION

### Lab
- CBC:
  - Mild leukocytosis
  - Anemia
- ESR >20 mm/h
- ANA and ANCA titers
- Urinalysis:
  - Proteinuria and hematuria

### Imaging
- CXR:
  - PAN usually has a nonspecific patchy alveolar infiltration.
- Look for complications or alternate diagnoses
- CT scan:
  - Sinus CT for cases of Wegener granulomatosis
- MRI and MRA:
  - Positron emission tomography (PET scan) for suspected Takayasu arteritis
- ECG:
  - Indications:
    ○ Suspected Takayasu arteritis
    ○ Aortic regurgitation
- US
- Arteriography

### Diagnostic Procedures/Surgery
- EKG:
  - Pericarditis, conduction disturbances
- Endoscopy, sigmoidoscopy, and colonoscopy for GI tract involvement
- Positive tissue biopsy
- Polyarteritis nodosa:
  - 3 of the following 10 criteria are needed for the diagnosis:
    ○ Weight loss >4 kg
    ○ Livedo reticularis
    ○ Testicular pain or tenderness
    ○ Myalgias or weakness
    ○ Mononeuropathy or polyneuropathy.
    ○ Diastolic BP >90 mm Hg
    ○ Elevated kidney blood
    ○ Hepatitis B virus tests positive (for surface antigen or antibody).
    ○ Arteriogram (angiogram) showing the arteries that are dilated (aneurysms) or constricted by the blood vessel inflammation.

## DIFFERENTIAL DIAGNOSIS
- Thrombosis
- Malignancy
- Sepsis
- Drug toxicity
- Coagulopathy
- Renal failure
- Arthritis
- CHF
- Scurvy
- Antiphospholipid antibody syndrome
- Thrombocythemia
- Polycythemia vera
- Pernicious anemia
- Disseminated intravascular coagulation
- Cryofibrinogenemia
- Cholesterol emboli
- Calciphylaxis lesions

# TREATMENT

## INITIAL STABILIZATION/THERAPY
Initial stabilization of cardiac complications

## ED TREATMENT/PROCEDURES
- Treatment for vasculitis is determined by the underlying cause or the specific disease and is best initiated by rheumatology.
- PAN: Steroids, cyclophosphamide
- Takayasu arteritis: Corticosteroids, methotrexate, azathioprine, cyclophosphamide
- Wegner granulomatosis: Corticosteroids:
  - Cyclophosphamide, azathioprine may be substituted
  - Plasma exchange may be helpful in severe disease.

## MEDICATION
- Azathioprine: 2 mg/kg/d
- Captopril (Capoten): 12.5–25 mg PO t.i.d. initially (peds: 0.5–1 mg/kg/d in 3 doses, max. 6 mg/kg/d)
- Cyclophosphamide:
  - IV: 0.5–1 $g/m^2$ body surface area
  - PO: 2 mg/kg/d (up to 4 mg/kg) (ped dose as per consultant)
- Furosemide: 40–100 mg IV (peds: 1 mg/kg IV)
- Lamivudine: 100 mg/d
- Methylprednisolone: 0.25–1 mg IV t.i.d
- Methotrexate: 0.3 mg/kg/wk up to 25 mg/kg/wk
- Prednisolone: 1 mg/kg/d PO
- Prednisone: 40–60 mg/d (peds: 1–2 mg/kg/d)

# FOLLOW-UP

## DISPOSITION

### Admission Criteria
- Patients with evidence of severe disease and end-organ dysfunction should be admitted.
- Consult for procedures to revascularize ischemic organs.

### Discharge Criteria
Less-symptomatic patients without evidence of end-organ involvement

### Issues for Referral
- Any patient suspected of vasculitis and being managed as an outpatient should be referred as soon as possible to a rheumatologist for the definitive diagnosis and treatment.
- Consult appropriate specialties based on the severity of the end-organ damage.

## FOLLOW-UP RECOMMENDATIONS
Stress the need for close follow up with general symptoms to confirm the diagnosis and initiate therapy that will be life-saving on a long-term basis.

## PEARLS AND PITFALLS
- Temporal (giant cell) arteritis does not occur before age 50 yr.
- Nodular lesions are the skin changes most likely to yield a diagnosis of vasculitis.

## ADDITIONAL READING

- Allen NB, Bressler PB. Diagnosis and treatment of the systemic and cutaneous necrotizing vasculitis syndromes. *Med Clin North Am*. 1997;81(1): 243–259.
- Langford CA. Vasculitis. *J Allerg Clin Immunol*. 2010;125(2 Suppl 2):S216–225.
- Semple D, Keogh J, Forni L, et al. Clinical review: Vasculitis on the intensive care unit-part 1: Diagnosis. *Critical Care*. 2005;9(1):92–97.
- Semple D, Keogh J, Forni L, et al. Clinical review: Vasculitis on the intensive care unit-part 2: Treatment and prognosis. *Critical Care*. 2005;9(2): 193–197.
- Stone JH. Vasculitis: A collection of pearls and myths. *Rheum Dis Clin N Am*. 2007;33:691–739.

### See Also (Topic, Algorithm, Electronic Media Element)
- Erythema Nodosum
- Henoch-Schönlein Purpura
- Hepatitis
- Reiter Syndrome
- Systemic Lupus Erythematosus

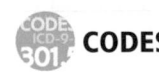 CODES

### ICD9
- 446.5 Giant cell arteritis
- 446.7 Takayasu's disease
- 447.6 Arteritis, unspecified

V

# VENOUS INSUFFICIENCY

Gudrun T. Hoskuldsdottir
Bo E. Madsen

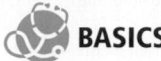 **BASICS**

## DESCRIPTION

- Inadequacy of the venous valves that causes impaired venous drainage and thus edema of the extremities
- A chronic condition of lower extremity vascular incompetence
- Normal blood flow in the venous system is unidirectional from the superficial veins to the deep veins.
- This flow is maintained by contraction of muscles and by valves in the veins.
- Damage to the valves, for example following DVT, causes them to become rigid and they lose their ability to prevent retrograde blood flow properly.
- This causes increased pressure distally and distention of the veins, which in turn causes seperation of the valve leaflets.
- As the increased pressure is transmitted into the dermal microcirculation extravasation of macromolecules and red blood cells occurs.
- This serves as a stimulus for inflammatory injury and starts a cascade of inflammatory events that causes ulcer formation and poor ulcer healing.
- The superficial veins swell because of regurgitation and edema, and skin changes occur.
- Other than DVT and genetics, other predisposing factors have not been proven but older age, standing occupation, and previous injury have been mentioned.

## ETIOLOGY

- Primary vascular incompetence (most common): Deep vein thrombosis (DVT)

 **DIAGNOSIS**

## SIGNS AND SYMPTOMS

### History

- Asymptomatic phase:
  - Venous dilation ranging from venous flares to small varicosities
- Symptomatic phase:
  - Ankle and calf swelling
  - Itching
  - Profuse bleeding
  - Hyperpigmentation
  - Lipodermatosclerosis
  - Ulcer formation
  - Ankle and calf swelling
  - Dull ache in the legs:
    - Worsened by prolonged standing
    - Resolves with leg elevation

- Itching
- Burning sensation
- Pain
- Night cramps
- Skin discoloration/hyperpigmentation
- Ulcer formation
- Varicose veins
- Lipodermatosclerosis

### Physical Exam

- Varicose veins
- Telangiectasias
- Phlebectasias
- Reticular veins
- Ankle and calf edema
- Ulcers, situated over the malleoli or medial portion of calf
- Red, purple discoloration of skin
- Stasis dermatitis
- Brownish hyperpigmentation
- Atrophie blanche
  - Sclerosis and atrophy of skinVaricosities
  - Dependent ankle/calf edema
- Skin changes:
  - Induration
  - Sclerosis
- Venous ulcers:
  - Over either malleoli or medial portion of the calf with preserved peripheral pulses
- Bacterial infection:
  - Surrounding cellulitis
  - Rapidly growing ulcer
  - Increased pain
  - Lymphangitis
- Leg edema and ulcers with ascites, periorbital edema, orthopnea, or an abnormal cardiac exam suggest other etiologies.

## ESSENTIAL WORKUP

The physical exam is essential to the diagnosis.

## DIAGNOSTIC TESTS & INTERPRETATION

### Lab

- Lab tests add little to the physical exam unless other causes need to be excluded.
- Cardiac markers, brain natriuretic, albumin, and tests of renal function can be sent if considering other causes of leg edema.

### Imaging

- Doppler auscultation (DopA):
  - Used to estimate blood flow, as well as the presence or absence of reflux in a given vein.
  - Indications are diameter >3 mm, signs/symptoms of chronic venous insufficiency and the presence of a painful vessel.
- Duplex US (DUS):
  - Combines Doppler and gray-scale imaging and shows vascular anatomy, soft-tissue features, detection and quantification of reflux and the source of it.
  - Can be used for diagnosis, as part of the treatment (dupex-guided sclerotherapy and endovenous ablation) and for postoperative evaluation.
- Photophletysmography (PPG):
  - Assesses venous hemodynamics and venous refilling time with and without leg muscle contraction.
  - Used to measure vein outflow and inflow, as well as muscle pump adequacy.
- Duplex US:
  - Assess for DVT or valvular incompetence.
- Venography:
  - Gold standard
  - Expensive and invasive

### Diagnostic Procedures/Surgery

Ankle-brachial index:

- Should be measured if arterial insufficiency is suspected

## DIFFERENTIAL DIAGNOSIS

- Arterial insufficiency
- Lymphatic disorders
- Soft-tissue infection
- Pyoderma gangrenosum
- Leg edema:
  - CHF
  - Nephrotic syndrome
  - Liver failure
  - Lymphatic obstruction
- Leg ulcers:
  - Arterial insufficiency
  - Soft-tissue infection
  - Polyarteritis
  - Pyoderma gangrenosum

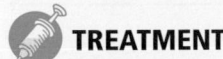 **TREATMENT**

### INITIAL STABILIZATION/THERAPY
- Leg elevation
- Control bleeding with direct pressure.

### ED TREATMENT/PROCEDURES
- Leg elevation
- Compression stockings
- Anticoagulants if confirmed DVT
- Antibiotics if signs of infection
- Aspirin
- Antihistamines for pruritus
- Compression stockings
- Anticoagulants for confirmed DVT
- Steroids for stasis dermatitis
- Aspirin
- Antibiotics for signs of infection
- Astringents:
  - Domeboro solution
- Antihistamines for pruritus

### MEDICATION
- Aspirin: 325 mg/d PO
- Augmentin: 875 mg b.i.d. PO
- Benadryl: 12.5–25 mg q.i.d. PO
- Cephalexin: 500 mg q.i.d. PO
- Dicloxacillin: 500 mg q.i.d. PO
- Coumadin: Dose per prothrombin time/INR
- Lovenox: 1 mg/kg SC b.i.d.

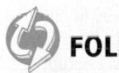 **FOLLOW-UP**

### DISPOSITION
#### Admission Criteria
- Evidence of cellulitis, lymphangitis, or osteomyelitis may require admission.
- DVT requiring IV heparin rather than outpatient Lovenox

#### Discharge Criteria
- Bleeding is under control.
- DVT has been ruled out.
- No evidence of bacterial infection requiring admission
- Appropriate follow-up/referral arranged
- Home services for dressing changes

#### Issues for Referral
The patient should be referred to their primary care physician or a vascular surgeon.

### FOLLOW-UP RECOMMENDATIONS
- Home service for ulcer management
- Immediate surgical procedures are not required for varicose veins.
- Vein stripping, vein ligation, and sclerotherapy are options for cases refractory to medical management:
  - Does not improve healing but reduces ulcer recurrence
  - Sclerotherapy: Causes irreversible occlusion of the vein.
- Endovenous thermal ablation:
  - A procedure by which thermal energy is endovenously delivered to the lumen of the vein causing occlusion of the vein.

## PEARLS AND PITFALLS

In patients with extremity pain or ulcerations, ensure arterial insufficiency is not the underlying cause before assuming venous insufficiency.

## ADDITIONAL READING

- Barwell JR, Davies CE, Deacon J, et al. Comparison of surgery and compression with compression alone in chronic venous ulceration (ESCHAR study): Randomised controlled trial. *Lancet.* 2004, 363(9424):1854–1859.
- Beebee-Dimmer JL, Pfeifer JR, Engle JS, et al. The epidemiology of chronic venous insufficiency and varicose veins. *Ann Epidemiol.* 2005;15:175–184.
- Guyton AC, Hall JE. *Textbook of medical physiology,* 10th ed. Philadelphia: WB Saunders, 2000: 158–159.
- Kasper DL, Fauci AS, Longo DL, et al., eds., *Harrison's principles of internal medicine,* 16th ed. McGraw-Hill, 2005:1493.
- Kundu S, Grassi CJ, et al. Multi-disciplinary quality improvement guidelines for the treatment of lower extremity superficial venous insufficiency with ambulatory phlebectomy from the Society of Interventional Radiological Society of Europe, American College of Phlebology and Canadian Interventional Radiology Association. *J Vasc Interv Radiol.* 2010;21:19–31.
- Nguyen TH. Evaluation of venous insufficiency. *Semin Cutan Med Surg* 2005;24:162–174.
- Pappas PJ, Lal BK, Padberg FT, et al. *Pathophysiology of chronic venous insufficiency. The vein book.* Boston: Elsevier, 2006:89–101.
- Marx JA, Hockberger RS, Walls RM. *Rosen's emergency medicine: Concepts and clinical practice.* St. Louis: Mosby, 2002:1228.
- Tintinalli JE, Kelen GD, Stapczynski JS. *Emergency medicine: A comprehensive study guide.* New York: McGraw-Hill, 2004:1529–1530.

### See Also (Topic, Algorithm, Electronic Media Element)
Deep Venous Thrombosis

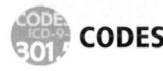 **CODES**

**ICD9**
459.81 Venous (peripheral) insufficiency, unspecified

# VENTILATOR MANAGEMENT

*Owen Lander*

## BASICS

### DESCRIPTION
- Mechanical positive-pressure ventilation to generate a controlled flow of gas into a patient's airways to substitute for normal respiratory physiologic function
- Modern ventilators are capable of combining various elements of the following delivery modes:
- Delivery modes:
  - Pressure-cycled:
    - Each breath at the set rate is delivered to set a maximum pressure.
    - Markedly reduces the risk of barotrauma
    - May see markedly variable tidal volumes and minute ventilation as a result of changes in patient's chest wall and lung compliance and spontaneous respiratory efforts
  - Volume-cycled:
    - Each breath at the set rate is delivered to a set volume.
    - Provides consistent and reliable minute ventilation, appealing in the initial management setting
    - Can generate excessive peak pressures, particularly if patient's chest wall or lung compliance decreases
    - In most cases, can be limited by protective peak pressure cut-off limits
- Support modes:
  - Control mode:
    - Each breath, triggered or preset, is delivered as a "full breath," whether volume- or pressure-cycled.
  - Support mode:
    - Relies solely on supplying set support pressure to patient initiated breaths, terminating when expiratory effort is detected
  - Continuous mandatory ventilation (CMV):
    - A control mode that delivers breaths only at the set respiratory rate.
    - Rarely used because it frequently results in severe air hunger and asynchrony between the patient and the ventilator
    - In the paralyzed or apneic patient, assist control (AC) is equivalent to CMV.
  - Assist control (AC):
    - Delivers a full breath at the preset respiratory rate
    - In addition, any inspiratory effort by the patient will also trigger the delivery of full breath at the set volume or pressure.
    - Ensures adequate minute ventilation while avoiding asynchrony in the nonapneic patient.
    - Can result in overventilation, hypocarbia, and alkalosis in patients with significant spontaneous respiratory effort secondary to pain or agitation
    - Can result in excessive peak pressures, barotrauma, and breath stacking, particularly in patients with COPD, requiring prolonged exhalation phases
  - Intermittent mandatory ventilation (IMV):
    - Delivers full breaths at the set respiratory rate
    - Spontaneous respirations by the patient are allowed but not supported.

- Rarely used owing to the subjective discomfort of mixing fully supported breaths with unsupported breaths against the resistance of ventilator tubing and the possibility of delivering a full breath to a patient who has already spontaneously inhaled or is trying to exhale
  - Synchronous intermittent mandatory ventilation (SIMV):
    - Designed to fit a set number of full breaths per minute around any spontaneous respirations of the patient
    - Will not deliver a preset full breath when the patient is actively breathing
    - Spontaneous respirations are aided by an adjustable amount of pressure support.
    - Has replaced IMV owing to marked increase in patient comfort and synchrony with the ventilator as well as reduced risk of barotrauma
  - Pressure support ventilation (PSV):
    - Provides a set amount of pressure support whenever inspiratory effort is detected, terminating when the flow rate of delivered air drops below a certain point, indicating that the patient is ready to exhale
    - Comfortable for the patient, allowing the patient to breathe as much and as often as desired with sufficient support
    - Requires a nonapneic patient who has an adequate and appropriate respiratory drive
    - May be augmented on some ventilators with a fail-safe set IMV rate if the patient becomes apneic
- High-frequency oscillating ventilation
  - Very small tidal volumes at very high respiratory rates, up to 180/min, primarily used in neonatal and adult refractory acute respiratory distress syndrome (ARDS)
- Noninvasive positive-pressure ventilation (NIPPV):
  - Increasingly available
  - Tight-fitting mask delivers respiratory support without intubation.
  - Essentially a PSV mode of ventilation with variable positive end-expiratory pressure (PEEP)
  - May avoid intubation in mild to moderate reversible respiratory failure
    - CHF
    - COPD
  - An awake, responsive patient is mandatory.
  - Adequate respiratory drive required
  - Titrated to the same goals as full mechanical ventilation

## DIAGNOSIS

### SIGNS AND SYMPTOMS
- Indications for mechanical ventilation:
  - Apnea
  - Respiratory distress with altered mentation
  - Inadequate oxygenation/ventilation
  - Clinically significant increased work of breathing
  - Obtundation requiring airway control
- Controlled hyperventilation considered:
  - Head injury
  - Overdose of tricyclic drug
  - Metabolic acidosis
  - Severe circulatory shock

### History
- Focused on primary etiology of indication for intubation and respiratory support
  - Identification of underlying respiratory/pulmonary disease critical

### Physical Exam
- Focused on 3 primary organ systems
  - Pulmonary
    - Lung sounds
    - Air entry
    - Assessment of work of breathing
  - Cardiovascular
    - Volume status
    - Blood pressure
    - Anticipated effects of positive-pressure ventilation and hemodynamic effects
  - Mental status
    - Ability to protect and maintain airway
    - Ability of respiratory drive to match physiologic needs

### DIAGNOSTIC TESTS & INTERPRETATION
#### Lab
- ABG:
  - Within 15 min of initial intubation
  - Repeat as clinically indicated:
    - Changes in clinical status
    - Changes in ventilator settings
    - Significant changes of or inability to obtain noninvasive $SaO_2$ or $ETCO_2$ values
  - $PaO_2$ >60 mm Hg and saturation >90%
  - pH should be 7.20–7.5 initially:
    - Avoid overly rapid changes in pH via abrupt changes in ventilation.
    - Acutely pH is most easily managed via changes in the $PaCO_2$.
- Serum bicarbonate level
  - Asses for chronic $CO_2$ retention

#### Imaging
- Chest radiograph:
  - Confirmation of correct placement of endotracheal tube
  - Evaluation for primary pulmonary etiology/complications

### DIFFERENTIAL DIAGNOSIS
- Problems in providing effective mechanical ventilation:
  - Abdominal distention
  - Bronchospasm
  - Decreased venous return
  - Hyperinflation
  - Mucous plugging/secretions
  - Patient asynchrony
  - Pneumothorax
  - Pulmonary edema
  - Ventilator problems

## TREATMENT

### PRE-HOSPITAL
- Respiratory support per local EMS protocol

### INITIAL STABILIZATION/THERAPY
- Cardiac monitor
- Blood pressure monitoring
- Pulse oximetry to ensure $SaO_2$ >90%

- Continuous core temperature via esophageal or rectal probe if available:
  - Critically ill patients because of the risk of hypothermia (especially if paralyzed)
- End-tidal $CO_2$ monitoring when available:
  - Can reduce the frequency of serial ABG measurements

### ED TREATMENT/PROCEDURES

- Ventilator settings should be adjusted to the patient's specific requirements:
- Mode:
  - Volume-cycled modes are the first choice, pressure cycled modes are rarely used except in PSV.
  - SIMV or AC are the initial modes of choice in the emergently intubated patient.
  - PSV can be considered in patients with less severe respiratory failure and a robust respiratory drive or mixed-mode ventilators.
- Respiratory rate:
  - Initial rate of 8–14 breaths per min
  - Higher rates for increased ventilation must be balanced against increased risk of air trapping and barotrauma
  - Rates as low as 4–6 breaths per min may be required in severe asthma to allow for exhalation.
- Tidal volume:
  - Traditional volumes of 10–12 mL/kg are based on maintaining normal pH in patients with normal lung parenchyma.
  - Increasing evidence of negative effects of higher volumes, especially in patients with primary lung pathology, support an initial volume of 8–10 mL/kg.
  - Lower volumes of 5–8 mL/kg are indicated in patients with severe asthma/COPD or the presence of ARDS
- PEEP:
  - 3–5 cm $H_2O$
- Positive inspiratory pressure (PIP):
  - Should be set if possible, or monitored, to ensure it remains at or below 35 cm $H_2O$
- All patients should be adequately sedated to tolerate mechanical ventilation:
  - Benzodiazepines are the drug of choice owing to their muscle relaxing, amnestic, and anxiolytic effects.
- Always provide analgesia, optimally morphine or fentanyl.
- Continued paralysis postintubation may be required:
  - Can complicate management; avoid unless necessary for nonphysiologic ventilator settings
  - Reduce the work of breathing in severe shock.
  - Tolerance of hypercapnia and prolonged I:E ratios in severe obstructive lung disease
- Bronchodilators should be used in patients with obstructive lung disease.

### Meeting the Goals of Ventilation

- Oxygenation:
  - Titrate $FIO_2$ to maintain $SaO_2$ >90% and $PaO_2$ >60 mm Hg
  - Patients with high metabolic demand may benefit from slightly increased oxygenation.
  - $PaO_2$ >110 using $FIO_2$ >0.50 offers no significant benefit and increases the risk of oxygen toxicity.

---

- $FIO_2$ 1.0 refractory hypoxia:
  - Incremental increase in PEEP
  - 1–2 cm $H_2O$ at a time
  - Maximum 10 cm $H_2O$
  - Increased risk of hyperinflation, barotrauma, decreased venous return
- Ventilation:
  - Titrate minute ventilation (RR × TV) to achieve pH >7.20 and <7.55
  - $PaCO_2$ >35 mm Hg and <50 mm Hg (or patient baseline) as feasible within goal pH range
  - Max respiratory rate no higher than allows for complete exhalation on each breath
  - Max tidal volume limited by PIP and plateau pressures <35 cm $H_2O$

### Acute Changes

- Often manifested by abrupt decrease in oxygen saturation and increase in PIP
- Patient intolerance/asynchrony is a diagnosis of exclusion.
- Delineate ventilator source from patient etiology.
- Check tube placement.
- Deep suction
- Stat portable chest radiograph
- Stat ABG if noninvasive values in doubt
- Lung exam:
  - Wheezes, decreased air movement → consider bronchospasm.
  - Crackles → consider pulmonary edema.
  - Absent breath sounds → consider pneumothorax.
  - Prolonged expiratory phase → consider breath stacking, hyperinflation.
- Disconnect patient from ventilator, allow for full exhalation, and bag valve with 100% oxygen:
  - Patient bags easily and saturation corrects quickly:
    - Ventilator problem
    - Inappropriate ventilator mode
    - Inadequate sedation
  - Patient is difficult to bag ventilate and oxygenate:
    - Tension p
    - Bronchospasm
    - Hyperinflation
    - Mucous plug
    - Extubation or mainstem intubation
  - Patient is relatively easy to bag ventilate, difficult to oxygenate:
    - Pulmonary edema
    - Pneumothorax
    - Pulmonary embolus

### MEDICATION

- Midazolam: 0.03–0.05 mg/kg IV q5–10min, titrate to sedation
- Lorazepam: 0.03–0.05 mg/kg IV q5–10min, titrate to sedation
- Propofol: 0.3–0.5 mg/kg IV loading dose, maintenance initiated at 10 $\mu$g/kg/min IV infusion. Increase 5–10 $\mu$g/kg/min to adequate sedation.
- Morphine: 0.02–0.05 mg/kg IV q15–20min PRN
- Fentanyl: 0.5–1 $\mu$g/kg IV q10–15min PRN
- Albuterol: 2.5–5 mg/5 mL saline q20–30min via in-line endotracheal delivery
- Ipratropium bromide: 0.5 mg/2.5 saline q4h vial in-line endotracheal delivery
- Ketamine: 0.5–3 mg/kg/hr (peds: 0.25–1 mg/kg/hr) IV infusion

---

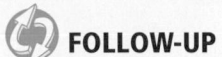 **FOLLOW-UP**

### DISPOSITION

#### Admission Criteria

- ICU admission for all intubated patients

### PEARLS AND PITFALLS

- Assess patient's metabolic and physiologic needs/efforts preintubation and aim to support with ventilator strategy.
- Do not employ postintubation paralysis for convenience—paralyzed patients cannot exhibit response to current ongoing oxygenation/ventilation needs.
- Follow up all interventions/ventilator changes with ABG or accurate noninvasive measurements of $SaO_2$ and $EtCO_2$.
- Investigate all acute changes in patient status systematically to identify source.
- Patient asynchrony or ventilator intolerance is a diagnosis of exclusion.
- Enlist the support of your admitting intensivist for unclear or refractory ventilation/oxygenation issues.
- Include ventilator setting evaluation in assessing hemodynamic changes.

### ADDITIONAL READING

- Oakes DF, Shortall SP. *Oakes' Ventilator Management 2009: A Bedside Reference Guide.* Orono, ME: Health Educator Publications, 2008.
- Tobin MJ. *Principles and Practice of Mechanical Ventilation.* New York: McGraw Hill, 2006.
- MacIntyre N, Branson R. *Mechanical Ventilation.* Philadelphia: Saunders, 2000.
- Anderson ML, Younger JG. Mechanical ventilation and noninvasive ventilatory support. In: JA Marx, RS Hockberger, RM Walls, et al, eds. *Rosen's Emergency Medicine Concepts and Clinical Practice,* 7th ed. St. Louis: Mosby, 2009.

#### See Also (Topic, Algorithm, Electronic Media Element)

- Dyspnea
- Respiratory Distress

 **CODES**

#### ICD9

- V46.11 Dependence on respirator, status
- V46.14 Mechanical complication of respirator (ventilator)

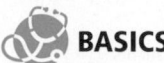

# VENTRICULAR FIBRILLATION

*Richard E. Wolfe*
*Ra'ed A. Hijazi*

## BASICS

### DESCRIPTION
- Ventricular fibrillation (VF) is completely disorganized depolarization and contraction of small areas of the ventricle without effective cardiac output.
- Cardiac monitor displays absence of quasi-random signal (QRS) complexes and T waves with the presence of high-frequency, irregular undulations that are variable in both amplitude and periodicity.

### ETIOLOGY
- Damaged myocardium creates sites for re-entrant circuits
- Myocardial damage may be caused by multiple factors including ischemia, necrosis, reperfusion, healing, and scar formation
- Initial rhythm in approximately 5%–70% of patients sustaining sudden cardiac death in the prehospital setting:
- Most often a result of severe myocardial ischemia
  - 7% of patients with STEMI develop sustained VF
    - 80%–85% occur in the first 24 hr
    - Patients who survive the 1st month after primary VF have a similar prognosis to patients with ST-elevation myocardial infarction (STEMI) without VF
- Complication of cardiomyopathy:
  - Up to 50% of patients with dilated cardiomyopathy suffer an episode of VF.
  - In hypertrophic cardiomyopathy, unexpected sudden death occurs with reported frequency of up to 3%/yr.
- Other less common causes of VF:
  - Blunt chest trauma
  - Hypothermia
  - Iatrogenic myocardial irritation form pacemaker placement or pulmonary artery catheter
- VF is often preceded by ventricular tachycardia (VT). Conditions predisposing to VT:
  - Drug toxicities (cyclic antidepressants, digitalis)
  - Congenital and acquired prolonged QT syndromes.
  - Short QT syndrome
  - Brugada syndrome
  - Idiopathic VF (5%–10%)

### Pediatric Considerations
- Primary ventricular dysrhythmias are extremely rare in children.
- VF usually results from a respiratory arrest, hypothermia, or near drowning.

## DIAGNOSIS

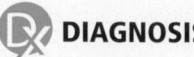

### SIGNS AND SYMPTOMS
- Loss of consciousness, seizure, transient gasping followed by apnea
- Absent pulse and heart sounds
- Death if the rhythm remains untreated

### ESSENTIAL WORKUP
- Cardiac monitor

### DIAGNOSTIC TESTS & INTERPRETATION
#### Lab
- Laboratory tests are not useful during resuscitation.
- After successful resuscitation, electrolytes including calcium and magnesium, cardiac enzymes, troponin, and toxicology screen

### DIFFERENTIAL DIAGNOSIS
- Asystole: Fine VF may mimic asystole in a single lead. Check rhythm in another lead for fine fibrillations.

## TREATMENT

### ALERT
- Early defibrillation of VF is the most important determinant of survival, and each minute without defibrillation reduces survival by 7%–10%.
- Supraventricular tachycardia or VT with a pulse may degenerate into VF if cardioverted without synchronization.
- In a hypothermic cardiac arrest (core temperature <30°C), if the patient remains in VF after the delivery of the first 3 shocks, rewarm the patient first before further attempts of defibrillation.
- Do not defibrillate any conscious patient.

### Controversies
- Biphasic automatic external defibrillation (AED):
  - Biphasic is now recommended in the 2005 guidelines because less energy is required
- Escalating biphasic energy levels have been shown to improve conversion of ventricular fibrillation
- Lidocaine has shown inconsistent evidence of benefit and some evidence of increased mortality, which challenges its routine prophylactic use.

### PRE-HOSPITAL
- ABCs
- Follow initial stabilization according to respective prehospital policies and procedures.

### INITIAL STABILIZATION/THERAPY
- AED or manual defibrillator confirms shockable rhythm
- Initiate SCREAM acronym
- **Shock**
  - Perform defibrillation as quickly as possible.
  - 360 J monophasic for 1st and subsequent shocks
  - 2005 guidelines recommend a single initial defibrillatory shock instead of the 3-shock sequence.
  - Biphasic energy level is device-dependent, follow manufacturer's recommendations.
    - If unknown, use 200 J for 1st shock and the same or higher energy for subsequent shocks.
  - May repeat q2min until rhythm changes
- **CPR**
  - After shock, immediately begin chest compressions followed by respirations and airway management.
    - 30:2 ratio for 2 min
- **Rhythm**
  - Rhythm check after every 2 min of CPR
- Secondary ABCD survey to try and determine underlying cause while resuscitation in progress
- Epinephrine
  - May start during CPR before or after shocking
  - 1mg IV/IO q3–5min
  - May use vasopressin 40 U IV/IO in place of the 1st or 2nd dose of epinephrine
- Establish IV access.
- **Antiarrhythmic Medications**
  - Amiodarone, lidocaine
  - Magnesium for torsade des pointes
  - Procainamide
- Epinephrine can be initiated 10–20 min after vasopressin.
- If the patient is successfully resuscitated, start a continuous infusion of the last antiarrhythmic agent administered.

- If the patient was successfully resuscitated prior to antiarrhythmic administration, give:
  - Amiodarone 150 mg in 100 mL D$_5$W over 10 min followed by a maintenance infusion *or*
  - Lidocaine 1–1.5 mg/kg IV bolus followed by a maintenance infusion
- Consider buffers for hyperkalemia, acidosis, and drug overdoses
  - Sodium bicarbonate
- Begin an evaluation for the cause of the VF arrest recognizing that the most likely cause is myocardial ischemia.

### Pediatric Considerations
Defibrillation sequence: monophasic 2 J/kg, 2–4 J/kg, 4 J/kg

## MEDICATION

- Vasopressin: 40 units IV bolus single dose
- Epinephrine —1:10,000 concentration; 1 mg IV bolus, repeat dose q3–5min:
  - Epinephrine via ETT: 1:1,000 concentration; 2–2.5 mg diluted in 10 mL NS via ETT
- Amiodarone —300 mg in 20–30 mL NS/D$_5$W IV bolus, repeat 150 mg in 20–30 mL NS/D$_5$W IV bolus q3–5min:
  - Amiodarone infusion: 1 mg/min for first 6 hr then 0.5 mg/min for 18 hr, additional 150 mg in 100 mL D$_5$W over 10 min; repeat q10min as needed. Max cumulative dose 2.2 g/24 hr
- Lidocaine: 1–1.5 mg/kg IV bolus, repeat 0.5–.75 mg/kg IV bolus. Max IV bolus dose is 3 mg/kg:
  - Lidocaine via ETT: 2–4 mg/kg
  - Lidocaine infusion: 1–4 mg/min (30 to 50 µg/kg/min)
- Magnesium sulfate: 1–2 g in 10 mL D$_5$W IV bolus
- Procainamide: 20–50 mg/min until arrhythmia suppressed, hypotension, QRS widens by 50%, or a total of 17 mg/kg is reached.
  - Procainamide infusion: 1–4 mg/min
- Sodium bicarbonate: 1 mEq/kg IV bolus
- Follow each medication with a 20 mL NS flush.

### Pediatric Considerations
- Epinephrine: 0.01 mg/kg (0.1 mL/kg of 1:10,000) IV/IO repeat with same dose q3–5min *or* give 0.1–0.02 mg/kg (or 0.1–0.02 mL/kg of 1:1,000):
  - Epinephrine via ETT: 0.1 mg/kg (0.1 mL/kg of 1:1,000)
- Amiodarone: 5 mg/kg IV/IO, may repeat 5 mg/kg; ma. cumulative dose 15 mg/kg/day
- Lidocaine: 1 mg/kg IV/IO:
  - Lidocaine infusion 20–50 µg/kg/min
- Magnesium sulfate: 25–50 mg/kg IV/IO up to 2 g
- Follow each medication with a 3–5 mL NS flush.

 **FOLLOW-UP**

## DISPOSITION
### Admission Criteria
- All patients who survive need admission to the ICU/CCU.

### Discharge Criteria
- No patient who suffers a VF arrest may be discharged from the ED.

### Issues for Referral
- Patients with episodes of VF occurring >48 hr post-MI may need referral to electrophysiology.

## PEARLS AND PITFALLS

- ACC/AHA guidelines recommend that patients with an acute myocardial infarction should have their serum potassium maintained above 4.0 meq/L to prevent ventricular dysrhtyhmias

## ADDITIONAL READING

- De Jong JS, et al. Prognosis among survivors of primary ventricular fibrillation in the percutaneous coronary intervention era. *Am Heart J.* 2009;158: 467–472.
- Guidelines 2005 for cardiopulmonary resuscitation and emergency cardiovascular care. Part 4: Advanced life support. *Circulation.* 2005;112: 111–125.
- Stiehl IG, et al., BIPHASIC Trial: A randomized comparison of fixed lower versus escalating higher energy levels for defibrillation in out-of-hospital cardiac arrest. *Circulation.* 2007;115:1511–1517.
- Ewy GA. Cardiocerebral rResuscitation: The new cardiopulmonary resuscitation. *Circulation.* 2005;111:2134–2142.
- Vilke GM, et al. The three-phase model of cardiac arrest as applied to ventricular fibrillation in a large, urban emergency medical services system. *Resuscitation.* 2005;64(3):341–346.

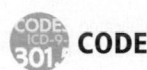 **CODES**

**ICD9**
427.41 Ventricular fibrillation

V

*Richard S. Krause*

 **BASICS**

## DESCRIPTION

- Ventricular peritoneal (VP) shunts are usually placed for hydrocephalus.
  - Conduit between cerebrospinal fluid (CSF) and peritoneal cavity
- *Obstruction:* Shunt malfunction impairs drainage of CSF:
  - Increases intracranial pressure (ICP)
  - Rate of increase in ICP determines severity.
- *Overdrainage* syndrome:
  - Upright posture increases CSF outflow
  - Decreases ICP
  - Produces headache, as after lumbar puncture
- *Infection:*
  - Shunt is a foreign body.
  - *Staphylococcus epidermidis* and other Staph. species in 75% of infections
  - Gram-negative organisms also implicated
  - Multidrug-resistant *Staph. aureus* (MRSA) has been reported.
  - Most occur within weeks of placement
- *Slit ventricle syndrome:*
  - Prolonged overdrainage causes decreased ventricular size.
  - Intermittent increases in ICP occur owing to proximal obstruction.

### Pediatric Considerations

- Complications more common in children, especially neonates
- If cranial sutures are open, CSF may accumulate without much ICP increase.
- Produces relatively nonspecific signs and symptoms
  - Drowsiness, headache, and vomiting are the commonest symptoms

## ETIOLOGY

- Shunt may be needed to treat increased ICP due to:
  - Congenital malformations
  - Idiopathic intracranial hypertension (pseudotumor cerebri)
  - After stroke
  - Tumor or other mass lesions
  - After head trauma
  - Subarachnoid hemorrhage
  - Scarring at base of brain after bacterial meningitis

**DIAGNOSIS**

## SIGNS AND SYMPTOMS

- Shunt obstruction:
  - Headache, nausea
  - Malaise, general weakness, irritability
  - Decreased level of consciousness
  - Increased head size or bulging fontanelle
  - Seizures: New-onset or increased frequency
  - Autonomic instability
  - Decreased upward gaze
  - Apnea
  - Papilledema: Rare
- Overdrainage syndrome:
  - Headache, focal neurologic signs, malaise, seizures, coma
  - Signs and symptoms often postural
- Rapid overdrainage may cause upward shift of the brainstem, leading to signs and symptoms of herniation: Apnea, bradycardia, decreased level of consciousness (LOC)
- Shunt infections:
  - Fever (may be absent)
  - Meningeal signs
  - Local signs of infection (erythema, swelling, tenderness)
  - Peritonitis (can cause retrograde CSF infection)
  - Infections usually occur soon after shunt placement (about 80% ≤ 6 mo).
- Slit ventricle syndrome:
  - Episodic headache
  - Alternating periods of normal behavior and lethargy
  - Headache, nausea, and vomiting

### History

- Timing of shunt placement
- Reason for shunt
- Recent instrumentation/revision

### Physical Exam

- Altered mental status
- Focal neurologic deficit
- Fever
- Erythema or tender shunt

## ESSENTIAL WORKUP

- Suspected shunt malfunction:
  - Manipulation of the pumping chamber:
    - Chamber should compress easily and refill within 3 sec.
    - Failure to compress easily implies distal obstruction.
    - Failure to fill implies proximal obstruction.
    - Up to 40% of malfunctioning shunts compress/fill normally.
  - Head CT
  - Shunt series:
    - Radiographs of skull, chest, abdomen
    - Aids in diagnosis of disconnection, malposition, or kinking of shunt components
- Suspected infection:
  - Aspiration of CSF from shunt reservoir (in consultation with neurosurgeon):
    - May be performed using sterile technique and 23-gauge butterfly needle
    - Slowly aspirate 5–10 mL CSF for the studies noted in the next section.

## DIAGNOSTIC TESTS & INTERPRETATION
### Lab

- Electrolytes, renal function, and glucose
- Anticonvulsant levels
- CBC
- Suspected infection:
  - Analysis of CSF from the shunt reservoir:
    - Send for culture, cell count, Gram's stain, glucose, and protein levels.
    - CSF analysis may have normal early result, especially with prior antibiotic treatment.
  - Blood cultures

### Imaging

- Cranial CT: To compare ventricular size and evaluate catheter position
  - Enlarged ventricles: Shunt malfunction
  - Smaller ventricles: Overdrainage
  - Most useful when compared with previous scan
  - Diagnose subdural hematoma
- US: Used in children with open fontanelle to evaluate position of shunt tip and assess ventricular size
- If symptoms of shunt malfunction are present but scan is not diagnostic, shunt tap is next test.
  - Shunt manometry: High pressure >20 cm $H_2O$ implies distal shunt obstruction

### Diagnostic Procedures/Surgery

- If symptoms of shunt malfunction present but scan not diagnostic shunt tap is next test.
  - Shunt manometry: High pressure >20 cm $H_2O$ implies distal shunt obstruction.
  - Also used to evaluate CNS infection

## DIFFERENTIAL DIAGNOSIS

- Seizure disorder (idiopathic, toxic, metabolic)
- Infections:
  - CNS Infection not related to the shunt
  - Systemic infections
- Metabolic abnormalities:
  - Hypoglycemia
  - Hyponatremia
  - Hypoxia
- Intoxication/poisoning
- Head trauma

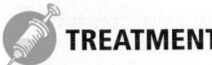

## TREATMENT

### PRE-HOSPITAL

- Patients with shunt malfunction are at risk for apnea and respiratory arrest.
- Oxygen should be applied with close monitoring of respiratory status.
- If increased ICP is suspected, transport patient with head elevated to 30 degrees.

### INITIAL STABILIZATION/THERAPY

- Signs of impending herniation:
  - Rapid sequence intubation and controlled ventilation to $P_{CO_2}$ ~35 mm Hg
  - Consider pretreatment with lidocaine (pediatric: plus atropine).
  - Thiopental or etomidate for induction
  - Succinylcholine may increase ICP a few mm Hg, although this may not be clinically significant.
  - Use only pretreatment dose of nondepolarizing agent if depolarizing agent chosen.
  - Nondepolarizing agent (rocuronium) may be preferable.
- Forced pumping of shunt chamber:
  - Flush the device with 1 mL of saline solution to remove distal obstruction.
  - Allow slow drainage of CSF from the reservoir to achieve pressure <20 cm $H_2O$.

- IV mannitol to lower ICP
- *Ventricular puncture* and CSF drainage is a procedure of last resort if less invasive procedures unsuccessful and neurosurgeon unavailable.
- *Status epilepticus*: treated with benzodiazepines (lorazepam).

## ED TREATMENT/PROCEDURES

- Early neurosurgeon consultation
- Shunt malfunction:
  - Elevate head of bed to 30 degrees.
  - Medical management with diuretics (mannitol, furosemide) may be appropriate in certain mild cases.
- Overdrainage syndrome:
  - Maintain patient's supine position.
  - Correct volume depletion.
- Shunt infection:
  - Systemic antibiotics:
    - Vancomycin *plus* cefotaxime *or* gentamicin if gram-negative suspected

## MEDICATION

- Adult and pediatric doses:
  - Atropine: 0.02 mg/kg IV (minimum 0.1 mg)
  - Cefotaxime: 1–2 g (peds: 50 mg/kg) IV/IM q 8–12h
  - Furosemide: 1 mg/kg IV
  - Gentamicin: 2–5 mg/kg IV
  - Lidocaine: 1 mg/kg IV
  - Mannitol: 1 g/kg IV
  - Rocuronium: 1 mg/kg IV
  - Succinylcholine: 1.5 mg/kg IV
  - Vancomycin: 1 g q12h (peds: 10–15 mg/kg q6–8h) IV
  - Vecuronium: 0.1–0.3 mg/kg IV

## FOLLOW-UP

### DISPOSITION

#### Admission Criteria

- Patients with shunt complications usually require neurosurgical consultation and admission. An ICU or other monitored setting is often needed.

### Discharge Criteria

- If shunt malfunction is ruled out, disposition depends on alternate diagnosis and patient condition.

## PEARLS AND PITFALLS

- Shunt malfunction is relatively uncommon.
  - Avoid "tunnel vision" in a patient with a shunt and consider other causes for the presentation.
  - Severe constipation may cause increased intra-abdominal pressure.
- Decreased CSF drainage through the shunt may then occur and result in increased ICP.
- Treatment of constipation may ameliorate the apparent "shunt malfunction."

## ADDITIONAL READING

- Barnes NP, et al. Ventriculoperitoneal shunt block: What are the best predictive clinical indicators? *Arch Dis Child.* 2002;87:198–201.
- Madsen MA. Emergency department management of ventriculoperitoneal cerebrospinal fluid shunts. *Ann Emerg Med.* 1986;15:1330–1343.
- Martínez-Lage JF et al. Severe constipation: An under-appreciated cause of VP shunt malfunction: A case-based update. *Childs Nerv Syst.* 2008;24: 431–435.
- Moza K, McMenomey SO, Delashaw JB Jr. Indications for cerebrospinal fluid drainage and avoidance of complications. *Otolaryngol Clin N Am.* 2005;38:577–582.

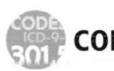 CODES

### ICD9

- 996.2 Mechanical complication of nervous system device, implant, and graft
- V45.2 Postsurgical presence of cerebrospinal fluid drainage device

# VENTRICULAR TACHYCARDIA

*Shannon Straszewski*
*Daniel C. McGillicuddy*

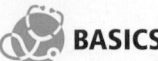 **BASICS**

## DESCRIPTION
- A wide-complex tachydysrhythmia with a quasi-random signal (QRS) >120 and a rate >100
- Rapid and regular depolarization of the ventricles independent of the atria and the normal conduction system
- Reentry:
  - Structural heart disease most common
  - Seen in dilated cardiomyopathy, ischemia, and infiltrative heart disease, previous MI, scarring
  - May be pharmacologically induced
  - Usually produces a regular and monomorphic rhythm
- Triggered automaticity:
  - Minority of ventricular tachycardia (VT)
  - Caused by repetitive firing of a ventricular focus
- Torsades de pointes:
  - Polymorphic form of VT
  - Alternating electrical polarity and amplitude
  - Prolongation in repolarization necessary
  - Usually pharmacologically induced
- Regardless of the mechanism, all VT may degenerate to ventricular fibrillation (VF).

## ETIOLOGY
- Wide complex tachycardia:
  - 80% likelihood of being VT
  - 20% supraventricular tachycardia (SVT) with a baseline left bundle branch block (LBBB) or aberrancy
- Wide complex tachycardia and a history of MI:
  - >98% likelihood of being VT
  - Age >35: 80% risk of VT
  - Age <35: 75% risk of SVT
- Incidence of nonsustained VT:
  - 0–4% in the general population
  - Up to 60% of patients with dilated cardiomyopathy
- Associated with increased risk for sudden cardiac death (SCD)

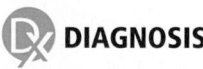 **DIAGNOSIS**

## SIGNS AND SYMPTOMS
### History
- Asymptomatic
- Syncope/near syncope
- Lightheadedness/dizziness
- Shortness of breath
- Palpitations
- Chest discomfort/pain
- Diaphoresis
- Cannon A waves
- Hypotension
- CHF
- Beat-to-beat variability of systolic BP
- Variability in heart tones, especially S1

### Physical Exam
- Establish presence of pulses, mental status and vital sign abnormalities.
- Auscultation of heart will reveal tachycardia.

## ESSENTIAL WORKUP
- EKG:
  - Most important initial test to differentiate VT from SVT with aberrancy or LBBB
- VT:
  - ≥3 consecutive QRS complexes with a ventricular rate over 100 bpm and a QRS duration >120 msec
- Torsades de pointes:
  - Polymorphic VT that rotates its axis every 10–20 beats
- Criterion to determine VT:
  - Atrial ventricular (AV) dissociation (present in 60–75%)
  - Fusion beats (P wave partially activates ventricle in advance of next VT cycle), capture beats (P wave totally activates ventricle)
  - Uniform morphology (except in the case of torsades)
  - Extreme axis deviation (−90 to + 180 degrees)
  - QRS >140 msec, with right bundle branch block (RBBB) morphology; or QRS >160 msec, with LBBB morphology, but >160 suggests VT regardless of bunch branch morphology
  - QRS concordance in the precordial leads
  - RBBB pattern V1 with R > R′ is VT 50:1.
  - LBBB pattern with Q or QS pattern in V 6 is VT 50:1.
  - Brugada's criteria defines VT in wide complex tachycardia:
    - 99% sensitivity, 97% specificity
    - AV dissociation
    - R-S interval absent in all precordial leads
    - QRS onset to the nadir of S >100 msec in any precordial lead
    - V-1 R wave >30 msec; R-S interval >70 msec, slurred, notched S
    - Wide QRS with LBBB in precordium
  - Indicators of SVT with aberrancy include:
    - Normal-axis QRS <140 msec
    - Absence of Q waves
    - RBBB in V1 with rsR′ triphasic pattern
    - AV Nodal Blockade: Slowing of impulse conduction velocity seen with antiarrhythmic drugs is more pronounced at faster rates, so may result in wide-complex SVT (SVT with aberrancy)

## DIAGNOSTIC TESTS & INTERPRETATION
### Lab
- Cardiac enzymes
- Electrolytes, BUN, creatinine, glucose
- Magnesium level
- Calcium level
- Digoxin level if toxicity suspected

### Imaging
CXR:
- Cardiomegaly or other cardiac anomalies may be apparent.

### Diagnostic Procedures/Surgery
Esophageal pacing catheters:
- May be able to detect atrial activity to establish AV dissociation and therefore diagnose VT
- Catheters can then be used to overdrive pace if needed.

## DIFFERENTIAL DIAGNOSIS
- SVT with aberrancy or baseline LBBB
- Proarrhythmia secondary to antidysrhythmia medications; suspect if:
  - VT morphology is different than previous episodes of VT
  - Medications have recently been started or changed
  - QT interval is >440 msec.
  - Torsades de pointes
  - If VT continues to recur after cardioversion

 **TREATMENT**

## PRE-HOSPITAL
- Cautions:
  - Transport stable patients suspected of being in VT without attempting to convert them.
  - *Synchronized* cardioversion for unstable patients with a pulse
  - Defibrillation for pulseless VT
- Controversies:
  - Lidocaine:
    - No benefit in the prevention of VT in patients with isolated premature ventricular contractions, regardless of the frequency

## INITIAL STABILIZATION/THERAPY
Pulseless VT: Defibrillate immediately and follow the ventricular fibrillation treatment plan.

## ED TREATMENT/PROCEDURES

- Unstable patient:
  - Definition:
    - Chest pain
    - Hypotension
    - Evidence of worsening heart failure
  - Initiate immediate synchronized cardioversion with 100 J, quickly progressing to 200 J, 300 J, and 360 J if no response.
    - If the VT is polymorphic, begin cardioversion at 200 J.
  - Sedate the patient before cardioversion if at all possible.
  - If unable to terminate the VT, administer lidocaine and repeat the cardioversion.
  - Antitachycardia overdrive pacing if torsades
  - After successful return of sinus rhythm, begin amiodarone.
- Stable patient, monomorphic VT:
  - Normal cardiac function at baseline:
    - Procainamide or sotalol; may also consider amiodarone or lidocaine
  - Impaired cardiac function at baseline:
    - Amiodarone bolus, then infusion or lidocaine, then synchronized cardioversion
- Stable patient, polymorphic VT:
  - Normal QT interval at baseline:
    - Correct electrolyte abnormalities.
    - Treat ischemia if present.
    - Then begin 1 of the following: b2-blockers, lidocaine, amiodarone, procainamide, or sotalol.
  - Prolonged QT Torsades de pointes:
    - Correct electrolytes.
    - Magnesium sulfate or overdrive pacing or 1 of the following: Isoproterenol, phenytoin, lidocaine
    - Isoproterenol is used to overdrive the tachycardia if the patient has no history of coronary artery disease.
    - Temporizing measure until external pacing available
  - Impaired cardiac function at baseline
  - Amiodarone bolus or lidocaine bolus then synchronized cardioversion

### Pediatric Considerations

- Primary cardiac arrest and VT are rare in children.
- Usually secondary to hypoxia and acidosis
- VT is tolerated for longer periods in children than adults and is less likely to degenerate to VF.
- Infants in VT most commonly present with CHF.

- VT in children results from:
  - Cardiomyopathy
  - Congenital structural heart disease
  - Congenital prolonged QT syndromes
  - Coronary artery disease secondary to vasculitis
  - Toxins, poisons, drugs
  - Severe electrolyte imbalances, especially of potassium

## MEDICATION

### First Line

- Procainamide: 20–30 mg/min until converted or for a total max. dose of 17 mg/kg; maintenance infusion 1–4 mg/min
- Amiodarone: 150 mg IV bolus over 10 minutes, may repeat; arrest dose is 300 mg IV/IO max. cumulative dose 2.2 g IV/24 h; infusion 540 mg IV over 18 hr (0.5 mg/min) (peds: 5 mg/kg IV or IO over 20–60 minutes, max. 15 mg/kg/d)
- $MgSO_4$: 2 g in $D_5W$ over 5–10 min followed by infusion of 0.5–1.0 g/h IV, titrate to control torsades

### Second Line

- Lidocaine: 1–1.5 mg/kg bolus IV push 1st dose, 0.5–0.75 mg/kg 2nd dose, and q5–10min for a max. of 3 mg/kg; tracheal administration 2–4 mg/kg; maintenance infusion 1–4 mg/min if converted. Not recommended for ACS induced VT(peds: 1 mg/kg bolus with infusion 20–50 bcg/kg/min)
- Adenosine: 6 mg IV push followed by 12 mg IV push if needed in 1–2 minutes (peds: 1 mg/kg, max. 6 mg; note: Does not convert VT, no longer ACLS protocol)
- Isoproterenol: 2–10 bcg/min, titrate to heart rate (peds: 0.1 bcg/kg/min); note: Do not give with epinephrine, may precipitate VT/VF(no longer part of ACLS protocol)

 **FOLLOW-UP**

### DISPOSITION

#### Admission Criteria

- Admit sustained VT to a critical care setting.
- Admit nonsustained VT and a history of MI or dilated cardiomyopathy for electrophysiologic studies.

#### Discharge Criteria

- Rare patients with nonsustained VT and a previous evaluation that revealed no structural heart disease can be discharged:
  - At low risk for SCD
- Patients with automatic internal cardiac defibrillators that are well functioning can also be discharged.

### Issues for Referral

All patients discharged with VT should be followed by a cardiologist within 48 hr.

### FOLLOW-UP RECOMMENDATIONS

Patients should follow-up with a cardiologist.

## PEARLS AND PITFALLS

- Search for contributing factors such as toxins, metabolic abnormalities, trauma, hypothermia, thrombosis.
- Unstable VT requires early defibrillation.
- Administer postresuscitation maintenance medications to prevent recurrence.
- Watch for bradycardia and GI toxicity after amiodarone administration.
- Discontinue any proarrhythmic drugs
- Consider b2-blockade for ischemia-induced VT and polymorphic VT.

## ADDITIONAL READING

- Connolly SJ, Dorian P, Roberts RS, et al. Comparison of beta-blocker, amiodarone plus beta-blockers, or sotalol for prevention of shocks from implantable cardioverter defibrillators: The OPTIC Study: A randomized trial. *JAMA*. 2006;295:165–71.
- Saliba WI, Natale A. Ventricular tachycardia syndromes. *Med Clin North Am*. 2001;85(2): 267–304.
- Zipes DP, Camm AJ, Borggrefe M, et al. ACC/AHA ESC 2006 Guidelines for management of patients with ventricular arrhythmias and the prevention of sudden cardiac death executive summary. *J Am Coll Cardiol*. 2006;48:1064.

### See Also (Topic, Algorithm, Electronic Media Element)

2005–2006 ACLS guidelines

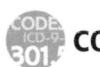 **CODES**

### ICD9

427.1 Paroxysmal ventricular tachycardia

### Acknowledgment

Thank you to the prior author on this chapter, Jennifer Audi

**V**

# VERTEBROBASILAR INSUFFICIENCY

*Leo Kobayashi*

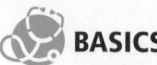 **BASICS**

## DESCRIPTION

- Inadequate perfusion of vertebrobasilar (VB) arterial circulation from thrombotic, embolic, or low-flow states
- Vertebral arteries (VA) derive from subclavian arteries and give rise to the anterior spinal artery and the basilar artery.
- Arteries supplying the brainstem and cerebellum originate from the VB system before it branches into the two posterior cerebral arteries (PCA), such that a wide variety of focal neurological deficits arise from VB circulatory dysfunction.

## ETIOLOGY

- Mechanism
  - Thrombosis:
    - VB ischemia due to underlying VB atherosclerosis and clot formation
  - Embolus:
    - VB ischemia due to embolization of clot from proximal location
  - Low-flow states:
    - Hypoperfusion of VB system from systemic (e.g., cardiogenic shock) or localized (e.g., subclavian steal) reduction in blood flow
  - Less common etiologies:
    - Fibromuscular dysplasia
    - Hypercoagulable states
- Ischemic mechanisms causing VB insufficiency can herald and lead to VB territory infarcts.
- Severe episodes of VB hypoperfusion or loss of circulation can lead to:
  - "Locked-in" syndrome:
    - Quadriplegia with intact consciousness
  - "Top-of-basilar" syndrome:
    - Pontine and cerebellar dysfunction with diminished level of consciousness

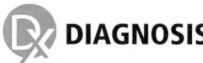 **DIAGNOSIS**

## SIGNS AND SYMPTOMS

- All history and physical exam items may present intermittently.

### History

- Dizziness/vertigo ("mild," "nonviolent"; may be isolated finding)
- "Drop attack"
- Headache
- Mental status changes
- Nausea/vomiting
- Paresis/paresthesia
- Seizure
- Syncope
- Visual changes

### Physical Exam

- Brainstem:
  - "Crossed" findings (i.e., ipsilateral facial and contralateral body deficits)
  - Altered mental status or responsiveness
  - Decreased respiratory drive
  - Horner syndrome (enophthalmos, ptosis, miosis, anhidrosis)
  - Internuclear ophthalmoplegia
  - Nystagmus (especially nonfatigable, vertical/rotatory)
  - Paresis/paresthesias
- Cranial nerves:
  - Extraocular muscle paresis (e.g., diplopia)
  - Pupillary abnormalities
  - Facial paresthesia
  - Facial muscle paresis
  - Hearing abnormalities
  - Dysphagia
  - Dysarthria
- Cerebral cortex (PCA circulation):
  - Visual disturbances (e.g., homonymous hemianopsia)
- Cerebellar:
  - Ataxia
  - Dysmetria
  - Gait abnormality
- Cardiovascular:
  - Carotid/VA bruit
  - Irregular/asymmetric/weak pulses

## ESSENTIAL WORKUP

- Emergent head CT (noncontrast) to evaluate for hemorrhage (parenchymal, subarachnoid, traumatic), large acute infarcts, prior pathology
- Thorough neurologic and cardiac exam
- 12-lead ECG for arrhythmias and myocardial ischemia

## DIAGNOSTIC TESTS & INTERPRETATION

### Lab

- CBC:
  - Anemia, thrombocytopenia; polycythemia, thrombocytosis
- Coagulation studies (PT/PTT)
  - Hypo- and hypercoagulable states; baseline values for anticoagulant and fibrinolytic therapies
- Electrolytes, BUN/creatinine, glucose
- Cardiac markers for concurrent myocardial ischemia
- Urinalysis
- ESR for systemic vasculitides
- Rapid plasma reagin
- Thyroid stimulating hormone
- Lipid profile

### Imaging

- Emergent head CT (noncontrast); consider head and neck CT angiogram (CTA) for possible acute vascular intervention
- Chest radiograph; consider chest CTA for cardiopulmonary and great vessel pathology
- MRI/magnetic resonance angiography (MRA) for improved characterization of ischemic lesion and cerebrovascular circulation (e.g., congenital VB anomalies, exclusion of VA dissection)
- Echocardiography for intracardiac embolic source
- Cervical Doppler ultrasound
- Transcranial Doppler ultrasound

### Diagnostic Procedures/Surgery

- Neuroangiography for diagnosis
- Directed intra-arterial thrombolytic therapy/angioplasty/stenting/embolectomy are still under investigation)

## DIFFERENTIAL DIAGNOSIS

- CNS:
  - CVA (hemorrhagic or ischemic):
    - Cerebral
    - Cerebellar
    - Brainstem
  - Multiple sclerosis
  - Migraine syndromes
  - Seizure (focal)
  - Traumatic injury/postconcussive
  - Tumor
  - Vascular malformation hemorrhage (arteriovenous malformation, subarachnoid)
  - Brainstem herniation
- Peripheral nervous system:
  - Vestibular neuronitis
- Ear, nose, throat:
  - Cerebellopontine angle tumor
  - Ear canal pathology (foreign body, tumor)
  - Labyrinthitis/otitis media
  - Ménière disease
  - Paroxysmal positional vertigo
- Cardiovascular:
  - Arrhythmia
  - Myocardial ischemia/infarct
  - Aneurysm/dissection (VA, basilar artery, subclavian artery, aorta)
  - Hypovolemia
  - Vasculitides
- Endocrine:
  - Adrenal insufficiency
  - Hypothyroidism
- Hematologic:
  - Anemia
  - Coagulopathy/hypercoagulable state

- Infectious:
  - Encephalitis/meningitis
  - Otitis media/mastoiditis
  - Septic shock
  - Syphilis
- Metabolic:
  - Hypoglycemia; hyperglycemia
  - Electrolyte imbalance
- Toxicologic:
    Ataxia: alcohols, lithium, phenytoin
  - Salicylism
  - Serotonin syndrome
  - Iatrogenic

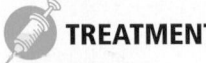 **TREATMENT**

### PRE-HOSPITAL
- ABCs
- Fingerstick glucose measurement
- Naloxone if indicated
- Notification:
  - Urgent contact with receiving facility if airway compromise or hemodynamic instability

### INITIAL STABILIZATION/THERAPY
- ABCs
- Administer oxygen.
- Place on cardiac monitor and pulse oximeter.
- Establish IV access with 0.9% normal saline.

### ED TREATMENT/PROCEDURES
- Cerebrovascular perfusion management:
  - Supportive care
  - Supine position
  - Antiplatelet agent if no hemorrhagic source
  - Anticoagulation:
    - Consider in consultation with neurology if significant risk factors for embolic source, unstable or progressive ischemic symptoms.
  - Ideal BP targets not well defined: maintain BPs within patient's expected range (i.e., account for chronic hypertension).
- If hypotensive: Fluid resuscitation; vasopressors or blood as indicated
- If hypertensive: Administer titratable antihypertensive medications for severe HTN (mean arterial pressure >140 mm Hg, systolic BP >220 mm Hg, diastolic BP >130 mm Hg) or hemorrhage/aneurysm/dissection, myocardial or other end-organ dysfunction
- Gastrointestinal:
  - NPO (rehydrate with IV fluids; maintain normoglycemia)
  - Antiemetics
- Consultation:
  - Neurology
  - Vascular interventional radiology for neuroangiography

### MEDICATION
- Aspirin: 325 mg PO
- Clopidogrel: 75 mg PO
- Coumarin (dose for atrial fibrillation): 2–5 mg PO loading dose
- Heparin (dose for atrial fibrillation): 50–60 units/kg IV bolus, then IV infusion at 12–18 units/kg for target PTT 50–70 sec
- Labetalol: 20–40 mg IV over 2 min, then 40–80 mg IV q10min (max. 300 mg IV)
- Meclizine: 25 mg PO q8–12h
- Naloxone: 0.4–2 mg IM/IV q2–3min PRN
- Nitroprusside: 0.25–10 mg/kg/min IV infusion (max. 10 mg/kg/min IV)
- Ondansetron: 4 mg IV
- Promethazine: 12.5–25 mg PO/PR/IV q6–8h
- Ticlopidine: 250 mg PO

 **FOLLOW-UP**

### DISPOSITION
#### Admission Criteria
- ICU admission for:
  - Altered mental status with airway issues
  - Concurrent hemodynamic instability
  - Malignant cardiac arrhythmias
- Admit to hospital to identify or exclude etiologies of VB ischemia and to prevent recurrence or progression to VB circulation cerebrovascular accident, especially in the following populations:
  - Elderly
  - Inability to ambulate
  - Inability to tolerate oral intake
  - Inability to arrange (expeditious) outpatient follow-up
  - New or changing neurologic deficit Persistent dizziness
  - Syncope
  - Vascular risk factors

#### Discharge Criteria
- Consider discharge with outpatient follow-up in populations with the following:
  - None of above indications to consider admission
  - Alternative explanation for symptomatology

#### Issues for Referral
- VB ischemia-related referrals as arranged/recommended by admitting team
- Arrange expeditious referrals with PCP or appropriate specialist (e.g., neurology, otorhinolaryngology, vascular surgery) as indicated for alternative explanation for symptomatology.

### FOLLOW-UP RECOMMENDATIONS
- VB ischemia-related follow-up as arranged/recommended by admitting team
- Urgency and nature of other follow-up as determined by alternative explanation of symptomatology

## PEARLS AND PITFALLS
- Always consider VB insufficiency for dizziness, vertigo, mental status changes, syncope, and overlapping/atypical neurologic presentations.
- Start antithrombotic/antiembolic treatments for VB insufficiency in absence of contraindications.

## ADDITIONAL READING

- Caplan LR. Vertebrobasilar disease. In: HJM Barnett, J. Bogousslavsky, H Meldrium, eds. *Advances in Neurology*. Philadelphia: Lippincott Williams & Wilkins, 2003;92:131–140.
- Lang E, Afilalo M. Vertebrobasilar atherothrombotic disease. *eMedicine*. Updated June 2008. Available at http://emedicine.medscape.com/article/794678-overview Accessed Nov. 15, 2009
- Love BB, Biller J. Neurovascular system. In: CG Goetz, ed. *Textbook of Clinical Neurology*, 3rd ed. Philadelphia: Elsevier, 2007: 405–434.
- Marquardt L, Kuker W, Chandratheva A, et al. Incidence and prognosis of > or </drug> 50% symptomatic vertebral or basilar artery stenosis: Prospective population-based study. *Brain*. 2009;134:982–988.
- Savitz SI, Caplan LR. Vertebrobasilar disease. *N Engl J Med*. 2005;352:2618–2626.

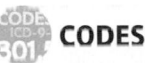 **CODES**

**ICD9**
435.3 Vertebrobasilar artery syndrome

V

# VERTIGO
*Jonathan S. Olshaker*

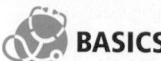 **BASICS**

## DESCRIPTION

- "Dizzy" describes a variety of experiences, including:
  - Sensations of motion
  - Weakness, fainting
  - Lightheadedness
  - Unsteadiness
  - Depression
- True vertigo:
  - Sensation of disorientation in space combined with a sensation of motion
  - Hallucination of movement either of the self or the external environment
  - Most patients have an organic basis for these symptoms.
- Maintenance of equilibrium depends on interaction of 3 systems:
  - Visual
  - Proprioceptive
  - Vestibular
- Any disease that interrupts the integrity of above systems may give rise to vertigo.
- Peripheral vertigo:
  - Sudden onset
  - Severe symptoms
  - Intermittent episodes lasting seconds to minutes, occasionally hours
  - Horizontal or horizontorotary nystagmus (also positional, fatigues, and suppressed by fixation)
  - Normal neurologic exam
  - Sometimes associated hearing loss or tinnitus
- Central vertigo:
  - Gradual onset
  - Usually mild continuous symptoms
  - Can be seconds to minutes with vascular causes
  - All varieties of nystagmus (horizontal, vertical, rotatory)
  - Absence of hearing loss
  - No positional association
  - Presence of neurologic findings most of the time

## ETIOLOGY
### Peripheral

- Benign paroxysmal positional:
  - Probable cause is loose particles in semicircular canals
  - Dependent on head position
  - Fatigue
- Acute labyrinthitis:
  - Associated with hearing deficit
  - Sudden onset
  - May be serous, acute suppurative, toxic, or chronic

- Ototoxic drugs:
  - Aminoglycosides
  - Antimalarials
  - Erythromycin
  - Furosemide
- Ménière disease:
  - Episodic vertigo, hearing loss, and tinnitus
- Vestibular neuronitis:
  - Severe vertigo and symptoms resolving over days to weeks
  - No hearing deficits
  - Highest incidence in 3rd–5th decade
- Acoustic neuroma:
  - Tumor of Schwann cells enveloping the 8th cranial nerve (CN VIII)
  - Develops into central cause
  - Progressive unilateral hearing deficits and tinnitus
  - May also involve CN V, VII, or X
- Trauma:
  - Rupture of tympanic membrane, round window, labyrinthine concussion, or development of perilymphatic fistula can all have severe symptoms.
- Otitis media and serous otitis with effusion
- Foreign body in ear canal

### Central
- Cerebellar hemorrhage:
  - Neurosurgical emergency
  - Sudden onset of headache, vertigo, vomiting, and ataxia
  - Visual paralysis to affected side
  - Ipsilateral CN VI paralysis
- Vertebrobasilar artery insufficiency:
  - Dysarthria
  - Ataxia
  - Numbness of the face
  - Hemiparesis, headache
  - Diplopia/visual disturbances
  - Disturbances may be transient or exacerbated by movement of the neck.
  - Consider in elderly patients with isolated new-onset vertigo without an obvious cause.
  - Can sometimes rapidly progress in the 1st 24–72 hr
- Cerebellar infarction:
  - Nausea
  - Vomiting
  - Ipsilateral nystagmus
  - Ataxia
- Trauma:
  - Vertiginous symptoms common after whiplash injury
  - Postconcussive syndrome or damage to labyrinth or CN VIII secondary to basilar skull fracture
  - Vertebral artery injury has been seen after chiropractic manipulation.

- Temporal lobe epilepsy:
  - Associated with hallucinations, aphasia, trancelike states, or convulsions
  - More common in younger patients
- Vertebrobasilar migraines:
  - Prodrome of vertigo, dysarthria, ataxia, visual disturbances, or paresthesias followed by headache
  - Often a family history of migraines or similar attacks
- Tumor
- Multiple sclerosis:
  - Onset between 20–40 yr
  - All forms of nystagmus
  - May have abrupt onset of severe vertigo and vomiting
  - History of other vague and varying neurologic signs or symptoms
- Subclavian steal syndrome:
  - Exercise of an arm causing shunting of blood from vertebral and basilar arteries into the subclavian artery, resulting in vertigo or syncope
  - Secondary to a stenotic subclavian artery
  - Diminished unilateral radial pulse or differential systolic BP between arms
- Hypoglycemia:
  - Suspect in diabetic patient or any other patient with unexplained symptoms or mental status change

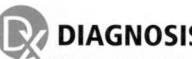 **DIAGNOSIS**

## SIGNS AND SYMPTOMS
Sensation of motion, spinning, disorientation in space, or disequilibrium

### History
- Does true vertigo exist?
- Time of onset and the duration of vertigo
- Are auditory symptoms present?
- Are there associated neurologic symptoms?
- Has there been head or neck trauma?
- Past medical history
- Medication history

### Physical Exam
- Auscultation of the carotid and vertebral arteries for bruits
- Pulses and pressures in both arms
- Inspection of the ears:
  - Evaluation of hearing (Weber and Rinne tests)
- Ocular assessment (pupils, fundi, visual acuity, nystagmus)
- Cardiac auscultation
- Full neurologic exam

## ESSENTIAL WORKUP
- Ask patient to describe the sensation without using the word "dizzy."
- Determine whether the cause is a peripheral or a central process using patient's clinical presentation (see above).

## DIAGNOSTIC TESTS & INTERPRETATION
### Lab
Electrolytes, BUN, creatinine, glucose

### Imaging
- EKG for any suspicion of cardiac etiology
- Head CT/MRI for evaluation of suspected tumor, central cause, or posttraumatic cause
- MRI or angiography for suspected vertebrobasilar insufficiency

### Diagnostic Procedures/Surgery
Audiology or electronystagmography often helpful in outpatient follow-up

## DIFFERENTIAL DIAGNOSIS
More likely other cause when "dizziness" actually is lightheadedness or malaise:
- DM
- Hypothyroidism
- Drugs (eg, alcohol, barbiturates, salicylates)
- Hyperventilation
- Cardiac (ie, arrhythmia, MI, or other etiologies of syncope); peripheral vascular disease (ie, HTN, orthostatic hypotension, vasovagal)
- Infection/sepsis

## TREATMENT
### PRE-HOSPITAL
- ABCs
- Medication per EMS protocol

### INITIAL STABILIZATION/THERAPY
- ABCs
- IV access for dehydration/vomiting
- Monitor
- Trauma evaluations as indicated
- Finger-stick blood glucose

## ED TREATMENT/PROCEDURES
- Based on accurate diagnosis:
  - Central etiologies require more aggressive workup than peripheral.
  - Neurosurgical intervention for cerebellar bleed
  - Symptomatic treatment for peripheral vertigo with appropriate follow-up
- Administer medication to control vertiginous symptoms—options:
  - Diphenhydramine
  - Meclizine
  - Promethazine
  - Diazepam
- Initiate IV antibiotics for acute bacterial labyrinthitis.
- Epley and Semont maneuvers can be successful in ED with BPPV.

## MEDICATION
- Diazepam (Valium): 2.5–5 mg IV q8h or 2–10 mg PO q8h
- Diphenhydramine (Benadryl): 25–50 mg IV, IM, or PO q6h
- Meclizine (Antivert): 25 mg PO q6h p.r.n.
- Promethazine (Phenergan): 12.5 mg IV q6h or 25–50 mg IM, PO, or PR q6h

 FOLLOW-UP

### DISPOSITION
### Admission Criteria
- Cerebellar infarct/hemorrhage
- Vertebrobasilar insufficiency
- Acute suppurative labyrinthitis
- Intractable nausea/vomiting
- Inability to ambulate

### Discharge Criteria
Patient with peripheral etiology and stable

### Issues for Referral
Otolaryngology follow-up for suspected acoustic neuroma or perilymphatic fistula

### FOLLOW-UP RECOMMENDATIONS
- Primary care, neurology, or otolaryngology follow-up for all
- Epley and Semont maneuvers are extremely effective in treating BPPV.

## PEARLS AND PITFALLS
- Isolated vertigo can be sole symptoms of stroke or bleed.
- Central causes are usually continuous, but vertigo can last seconds or minutes with vascular causes.

## ADDITIONAL READING
- Baloh RW. Dizziness: Neurological emergencies. *Neurol Clin North Am*. 1998;16:305.
- Chawla N, Olshaker JS. Diagnosis and management of dizziness and vertigo. *Med Clin North Am*. 2006;90(2):291–304.
- Herr R, Zun L, Mathews JJ. A directed approach to the dizzy patient. *Ann Emerg Med*. 1989;18(6): 664–672.
- Kerber KA, Brown DL, Lisabeth LD, et al. Stroke among patients with dizziness, vertigo and imbalance in the Emergency Department. A population based study. *STROKE*. 2006;37(10): 2484–2487.
- Kerber KA, Meurer WJ, West BT, et al. Dizziness presentation in US Emergency Departments 1995-2004. *Acad Emerg Med*. 2008;15(8): 744–750.
- Olshaker S. Vertigo. In: Marx J, et al., eds. *Rosen's emergency medicine: Concepts and clinical practice*. St. Louis: CV Mosby, 2010:93–100.
- Prokopakis EP, Chimona T, Tsagournisakis M, et al. Benign paroxysmal positional vertigo: 10 year experience in treating 592 patients with canalek repositioning procedures. *Laryngoscope*. 2005;115(9):1667–71.

### See Also (Topic, Algorithm, Electronic Media Element)
Dizziness; Labyrinthitis

 CODES

### ICD9
- 386.2 Vertigo of central origin
- 386.10 Peripheral vertigo, unspecified
- 780.4 Dizziness and giddiness

V

# VIOLENCE, MANAGEMENT OF

*Richard E. Wolfe*
*Robert Vissers*

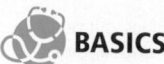 **BASICS**

## DESCRIPTION
- Managing violent and agitated patients is an everyday challenge for emergency providers.
- The ED is the site in the hospital where violence toward staff members is most likely to occur:
  – The emergency medicine treatment and active labor act (EMTALA) mandates the medical evaluation for all patient presenting to the ED.
  – The ED is the easiest site for patients to access care, pain control, and shelter 24-hr/day.
  – Many patients with a potential for violence are brought to the ED against their will.
- High prevalence of intoxicated patients and psychiatric patients
- Risk factors for substance-related violence:
  – Male gender
  – Younger age
  – Lower income
  – History of violence
  – Past juvenile detention
  – History of parental physical abuse
  – Drug abuse
  – Comorbid mental health and substance disorders
  – Victimization in the past year
  – Unemployed and looking for work in the past
- No difference exists in:
  – Ethnicity
  – Language
  – Age
  – Education
  – Medical diagnosis

## ETIOLOGY
- Functional:
  – Schizophrenia
  – Affective
  – Antisocial
  – Borderline
  – Paranoid
  – Adjustment disorders
  – Antisocial behavior
- Organic:
  – CNS:
    ○ Delirium
    ○ Dementia
    ○ Infection
    ○ Seizures
    ○ Cerebrovascular accident
    ○ Head injury
  – Metabolic:
    ○ Hypoglycemia
    ○ Hypoxia
    ○ Hypothermia or hyperthermia
  – Endocrine disorders:
    ○ Drugs
    ○ Alcohol and sedatives (withdrawal, intoxication)
    ○ Cocaine
    ○ LSD
    ○ Phencyclidine
    ○ Anticholinergics
    ○ Steroids

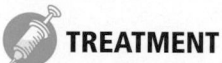 **DIAGNOSIS**

## ALERT
- Restrain potentially violent patients.
- Seek police aid in control of violent or dangerous patients.

## SIGNS AND SYMPTOMS
Behaviors suggesting impending violence:
- Provocative behavior
- Anger
- Pacing
- Loud speech
- Tense posture
- Pounding, clenching of fists

### History
- Historical context of violent behavior
- Previous threats and violence
- Psychiatric history
- Substance abuse
- Self-mutilation
- Verbal threats
- Plans of violence
- Identification of a possible organic cause for the violent behavior:
  – Age >40 without a history of psychiatric disease or substance abuse
  – Rapid onset of the violent behavior
  – History of visual-olfactory-tactile hallucinations
  – Morning headaches
  – Seizures
- Recent head trauma
- Underlying disorder in the past medical history that may predispose to altered mental status:
  – Diabetes
  – Hyperthyroidism
  – Brain tumors, particularly in the limbic and hypothalamic areas
  – CNS infection
  – AIDS

### Physical Exam
- Signs suggesting an organic cause for the violent behavior:
  – Abnormal vital signs
  – Focal neurological findings
  – Seizure activity
  – Speech or gait deficits without evidence of alcohol or substance abuse

## ESSENTIAL WORKUP
- Identify prodromes of violence:
  – Begins with anxiety
  – Then defensiveness
  – Then physical aggression
- Pay careful attention to findings during neurologic and mental status exams and note vital signs.
- Must often be performed with the patient under restraints

## DIAGNOSTIC TESTS & INTERPRETATION
### Lab
- CBC if suspected infectious cause for behavior.
- Electrolytes, BUN, creatinine, glucose if metabolic or toxic etiology suspected.
- Drug screen if ingestion likely.

### Imaging
CT head for altered mental status or head trauma

**TREATMENT**

## PRE-HOSPITAL
Restrain violent patients and seek police assistance if necessary.

## INITIAL STABILIZATION/THERAPY
- Prevention of violence:
  – Deterrence:
    ○ Signs stating weapons not permitted
    ○ Visible security personnel
    ○ Metal detectors
    ○ Secure single public entrance
    ○ Tracking system alerting providers to patients with a past history of violence in the ED
  – Triage to an appropriate assessment room:
    ○ Sparse, solid walls
    ○ Lockable
    ○ Visible
    ○ Exits clear of obstruction
    ○ Equipment free
    ○ Panic button
  – Never underestimate the potential for violence.
  – ED protocols for violent situations
  – Educate staff on preventing, recognizing, and dealing with potentially violent situations.
- Approaching the potentially violent patient:
  – Immediately assess safety.
  – Call security and employ physical or chemical restraint if the patient is violent or threatening, or if there is an immediate perceived danger.
  – Search and undress:
    ○ Preferably done voluntarily
    ○ If involuntary, ensure careful documentation of reasons to undress and search in terms of risk to patient and providers

- Remove any potential weapons before interview.
- Maintain open exit for patient and physician.
- Maintain distance of 6–8 ft.
- Allow patient to ventilate.
- Develop therapeutic alliance.
- Be nonjudgmental; make peace offering.
- Use submissive posture:
  ○ Avoid eye contact.
- Leave immediately and initiate seclusion or restraint if there is any destabilization of situation or patient behavior.

## ED TREATMENT/PROCEDURES

- Verbal deescalation:
  - Situation can be verbally controlled, particularly if situational precipitant can be identified.
- Isolation:
  - Temporarily isolate patient in an appropriate room before more definitive restraint, or to prevent leaving.
- Physical restraints:
  - Required for patient's safety, the safety of others, and to allow physical exam
  - Performed by several trained personnel, by protocol, with clear documentation of indications and rechecks
- Chemical restraint:
  - Least restrictive and potentially therapeutic
  - Before applying physical restraints, patients should be offered voluntary chemical sedation.
  - Cooperative patients should receive a combination of an oral benzodiazepine (lorazepam) and an oral antipsychotic (risperidone).
  - If uncooperative, patients often require physical restraint 1st.
  - The IM route is preferred in patients without IV access:
    ○ Oral medication should not be attempted in involuntary use of chemical restraints because of the risk of human bites.
  - A number of options are available for monotherapy.
  - Benzodiazepines (lorazepam, midazolam):
    ○ Optimal class of agents for cocaine intoxication, other adrenergic, and anticholinergic overdose
    ○ Avoid in pregnant patients and in patients with alcohol intoxication

- Conventional antipsychotic (droperidol, haloperidol):
  ○ Optimal class of agents for psychiatric illness
  ○ Decrease the dose in elderly patients
  ○ Avoid in patients with a history of Parkinson disease, anticholinergic drug intoxication, prolonged QT syndrome, and neuroleptic malignant syndrome
  ○ Consider droperidol instead of haloperidol if rapid sedation desired.
  ○ Dystonic reactions (treat with diphenhydramine or benztropine)
  ○ Neuroleptic malignant syndrome (rare)
  ○ QT prolongation and torsades de pointes (rare)
- May use combination if single agent ineffective
- Administer q15–30min until desired effect reached.
- Duty to warn:
  - Doctor can owe a duty to warn a 3rd party when that 3rd party is in danger because of the medical or psychologic condition of the patient.

## MEDICATION

- Benztropine: 2 mg IM or IV
- Diphenhydramine: 50 mg IV, IM, or PO
- Droperidol: 2.5–5 mg IV or IM
- Haloperidol: 5–10 mg IV or IM; 0.5–2 mg for elderly
- Lorazepam: 1–2 mg IV, IM, or PO
- Midazolam: 1–2 mg IV, IM, or PO
- Risperdal: 1 mg PO

 **FOLLOW-UP**

## DISPOSITION

### Admission Criteria

- Violence secondary to an associated organic cause that is not temporary or reversible in the ED
- Psychiatric admission:
  - Patient is considered to be a danger to either self or others.
  - Involuntary commitment if uncooperative

### Discharge Criteria

- Violent behavior was caused by a temporary, reversible organic cause (drug or alcohol intoxication), and the patient is now deemed to be in control, competent, and not a danger to self or others.
- Psychiatric consultation before discharge recommended
- If violent act is owing to antisocial behavior, rather than an organic or psychiatric condition, patient may be discharged into police custody, with the warning that the patient may be a danger to self or others.

## ADDITIONAL TREATMENT

### Issues for Referral

- Violent psychiatric patients require psychiatric consultation.
- Other consultation may be indicated with organic causes of violent behavior based on the underlying etiology.

## FOLLOW-UP RECOMMENDATIONS

- Follow-up instructions for patients in police custody should be communicated to the providers responsible for caring for the patient while in custody:
  - Do not provide incarcerated patients with the time and date for return visits to the hospital because of potential escape risk.
- Instructions about the signs and symptoms of a dystonic reaction for patients treated with neuroleptic agents
- Consider instituting a formal security plan in the hospital if 1 does not exist.

## PEARLS AND PITFALLS

- Assuming that violent behavior is either psychiatric or alcohol-induced and not recognizing treatable organic causes is a pitfall.
- Aggressive analgesia can decrease the likelihood of a patient with a painful condition physically acting out.
- Failure to document the initial and continued need for patient restraint is a pitfall.

## ADDITIONAL READING

- Coburn VA, Mycyk MB. Physical and chemical restraints. *Emerg Med Clin N Am.* 2009;27: 655–667.
- Hill S, Petit J. The violent patient. *Emerg Med Clin North Am.* 2000;18:301–315.
- Lukens TW, Wolf SJ, Edlow JA, et al. Clinical policy: Critical issues in the diagnosis and management of the adult psychiatric patient in the emergency department. *Ann Emerg Med.* 2006;47(1):79–99.
- Rossi J, Swan MC, Isaacs ED. The violent or agitated patient. *Emerg Med Clin N Am* 2010;28:235–256.
- Spivak HR, Prothrow-Stith D. Addressing violence in the emergency department. *Clin Pediatr Emerg Med.* 2003;4(2):135–140.

## See Also (Topic, Algorithm, Electronic Media Element)

Psychosis, Acute

V

# VISUAL LOSS
*Jason Hoppe*

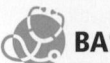 **BASICS**

## DESCRIPTION
- Decrease in visual function (i.e., visual acuity, visual fields, blurry vision)
- Visual loss has many etiologies and can be caused by multiple body systems.

## ETIOLOGY
- Ophthalmologic:
  - Eyelid or tear film abnormality
  - Anterior segment (cornea, anterior chamber, iris, lens)
  - Posterior segment (vitreous, retina, optic nerve)
  - Posterior to the eye (optic nerve, chiasm, radiations)
- Traumatic:
  - Corneal abrasion
  - Hyphema
  - Lens dislocation
  - Ruptured globe
  - Commotio retinae
  - Retinal detachment
  - Retinal/vitreous hemorrhage
  - Retrobulbar hemorrhage
- Neurologic:
  - Cerebral (cerebrovascular accident [CVA]) or intracranial pathology (mass lesion)
  - Multiple sclerosis
  - Optic neuritis
  - Migraine
- Cardiovascular system:
  - Embolic
  - Thrombotic
  - Ischemic
  - Hypertensive events
- Immunologic system:
  - Uveitis
  - Giant cell arteritis
- Infection:
  - Orbital cellulitis/abscess
  - Cavernous sinus thrombosis
  - HIV optic neuropathy or cytomegalovirus (CMV) retinitis
- Endocrine:
  - Diabetic retinopathy
  - Thyroid disease may cause diplopia (muscle hypertrophy) or corneal erosions
- Toxic:
  - Methanol (acute severe loss, subacute optic atrophy)
  - Licorice (transient loss, self-limited)
  - Digitalis (flashing lights, color changes)
  - Amiodarone (rare cause of optic neuropathy)

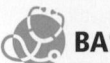 **DIAGNOSIS**

- Categorize visual loss by the properties associated with the decrease in visual function.
- Transient (<24 hr):
  - Min:
    - Transient ischemic attack = amaurosis fugax (unilateral)
    - Vertebrobasilar artery insufficiency (bilateral)
  - Min to hr:
    - Migraine
    - Sudden BP changes

- Persistent (>24 hr):
  - Painless: Sudden
    - Retinal artery or vein occlusion
    - Vitreous hemorrhage
    - Retinal detachment
    - Optic neuritis
    - Temporal arteritis/giant cell arteritis
    - Cerebral infarct
  - Painless: Gradual (wk to yr)
    - Cataract
    - Presbyopia
    - Refraction errors
    - Open-angle glaucoma
    - Chronic retinal disease
    - Macular degeneration
    - Diabetic retinopathy
    - CMV retinopathy
    - CNS tumor
  - Painful:
    - Corneal abrasion, ulcer, burn or foreign body
    - Angle closure glaucoma
    - Optic neuritis
    - Iritis/uveitis/endophthalmitis
    - Keratoconus with hydrops
    - Orbital cellulitis/abscess
- Monocular: pathology anterior to optic chiasm
- Binocular: pathology posterior to optic chiasm
- Associated with systemic neurologic symptoms of visual field defects:
  - CVA (especially posterior or occipital circulation)
  - Mass lesion (pituitary adenomas, aneurysm, meningioma, other tumors)
- Malingering/hysteria

## SIGNS AND SYMPTOMS
### History
- Decreased vision
  - Loss of vision
  - Blurry vision
  - Double vision
    - Horizontal or vertical
- History of trauma
- Use of corrective lenses:
  - Contacts
  - Glasses
- Prior eye surgery or problems
- Eye pain
- Conjunctival redness or discharge
- New floaters
- Flashing lights
- Pain with eye movement
- Key elements to determine:
  - Acute or gradual onset?
  - Length of symptoms?
  - Transient vision loss or permanent?
  - Binocular or monocular?
  - Degree of vision loss?
  - Painful or painless?
  - Other comorbidities

### Physical Exam
- Ophthalmologic:
  - Visual acuity
  - Pupil exam
  - Afferent papillary defect
  - Confrontational visual field exam
  - Extraocular muscle function
  - Slit-lamp examination
  - Fundoscopy
    - Optic nerve heal swelling
    - Pale retina with a cherry-red spot
  - Tonometry
- Cardiovascular:
  - Murmurs
  - Carotid bruits
  - Temporal artery tenderness
- Neurologic exam:
  - Complete exam for other deficits
  - Optic chiasm and intracerebral lesions
  - Occipital and posterior circulation lesions
- General:
  - Signs of immune, endocrine, or toxic disorders

## ESSENTIAL WORKUP
- Thorough history and physical examination

## DIAGNOSTIC TESTS & INTERPRETATION
### Lab
- May be obtained to determine extent of other comorbidities in association with vision loss (i.e., diabetes, cardiovascular disease)
- Erythrocyte sedimentation rate if giant cell arteritis is suspected

### Imaging
- Tests should be directed toward the suspected etiology of visual loss.
- Dilated fundus exam may be performed to assess for posterior segment disease.
- Temporal artery biopsy may be obtained if temporal arteritis is suspected.
- Brain CT, MRI, MRA, and transcranial Doppler may be used to evaluate neurologic symptoms and vertebrobasilar artery.
- Urgent cardiac and carotid ultrasound if a retinal artery occlusion is diagnosed.
- Facial CT may be used to evaluate extent of traumatic injuries.

## DIFFERENTIAL DIAGNOSIS
- Trauma
- Neurologic lesion
- Infectious
- Cardiovascular
- Toxic/metabolic
- Autoimmune

# TREATMENT

## PRE-HOSPITAL
- Chemical burns
  - Begin copious irrigation with water or saline

## ED TREATMENT/PROCEDURES
- Direct therapy toward cause of visual loss.
- Ophthalmology consultation for visual loss with an uncertain diagnosis
- Three conditions for which identification and treatment must begin within minutes:
  - Central retinal artery occlusion
  - Chemical burn
  - Acute angle-closure glaucoma

### Central Retinal Artery Occlusion
- Clinical criteria:
  - Unilateral, painless, dramatic vision loss
  - Afferent pupillary defect
  - Pale fundus with a cherry-red spot (macula)
  - Counting fingers to light perception in 94% of patients
- Therapy:
  - Immediate ophthalmology consultation
  - Maneuvers and medications to lower intraocular pressure, allowing the embolus to move to the periphery
    - Ocular massage: direct pressure to eye for 5–15 sec then sudden release, repeat for 15 min
    - Acetazolamide: 500 mg IV or PO
    - Topical beta blocker
    - Anterior chamber paracentesis by an ophthalmologist
  - Referral for cardiac and carotid artery workup
  - Rule out giant cell arteritis

### Chemical Burn
- Clinical criteria:
  - Alkali worse than acids
  - White eye (vessels have already sloughed) worse than red eye (vessels are intact)
  - Treat mace, cements, plasters, solvents
- Therapy:
  - Topical anesthetic
  - Copious irrigation of the eyes with LR or NS (nonsterile water is acceptable if others not available); minimum of 30 min
  - Goal: neutral pH 5–10 min after ending irrigation
  - Do not try to neutralize acids with alkalis or vice versa
  - Evert lids and use moist cotton-tipped applicator to sweep furnaces of residual chemical precipitants
  - Dilate with cycloplegic (atropine, cyclopentolate, tropicamide)
  - Do not use phenylephrine; it will vasoconstrict already ischemic conjunctival blood vessels
  - Erythromycin ointment q1–2h
  - Artificial tears q1hr
  - Check intraocular pressure

### Acute Angle-Closure Glaucoma
- Signs and symptoms:
  - Unilateral, painful vision loss
  - Nausea, vomiting, headache
  - Cornea injected, edematous
  - Middilated, sluggish pupil
  - Swollen, "steamy" lens
  - Cell, flare in shallow anterior chamber
  - Increased intraocular pressure
- Therapy:
  - Topical beta blocker
  - Topical prostaglandin analog
  - Acetazolamide
  - Topical alpha-2 agonist
  - Pilocarpine
  - Mannitol: if no decrease in IOP after 1 hr

## MEDICATION
- Antibiotic drops:
  - Ciprofloxacin 0.3%: 1–2 gtt q1–6h
  - Gentamicin 0.3%: 1–2 gtt q4h
  - Ofloxacin 0.3%: 1–2 gtt q1–6h
  - Levofloxacin 0.5%: 1–2 gtt q2h
  - Polymyxin (Polytrim) 1 gtt q3–6h
  - Sulfacetamide 10%, 0.3%: 1–2 gtt q2–6h
  - Tobramycin 0.3%: 1–2 gtt q1–4h
  - Trifluridine 1%: 1 gtt q2–4h
- Antibiotic ointments:
  - Bacitracin 500 units/g 1/2-in. ribbon q3–6h
  - Ciprofloxacin 0.3%: 1/2-in. ribbon q6–q8h
  - Erythromycin 0.5%: 1/2-in. ribbon q3–6h
  - Gentamicin 0.3%: 1/2-in. ribbon q3–4h
  - Neosporin 1/2-in. ribbon q3–4h
  - Polysporin 1/2-in. ribbon q3–4h
  - Sulfacetamide 10%: 1/2-in. ribbon q3–8h
  - Tobramycin 0.3%: 1/2-in. ribbon q3–4h
  - Vidarabine 1/2-in. ribbon 5 times per day
- Mydriatics and cycloplegics:
  - Atropine 1%, 2%: 1–2 gtt/day to q.i.d.
  - Cyclopentolate 0.5%, 1%, 2%: 1–2 gtt PRN
  - Homatropine 2%: 1–2 gtt b.i.d.–t.i.d.
  - Phenylephrine 0.12%, 2.5%, 10%: 1–2 gtt t.i.d.–q.i.d.
  - Tropicamide 0.5%, 1%: 1–2 gtt PRN dilation
- Corticosteroid–antibiotic combination drops (with ophthalmology consultation):
  - Prednisolone (Blephamide) 1–2 gtt q1–8h
  - Hydrocortisone/neomycin/bacitracin/polymyxin B (Cortisporin) 1–2 gtt q3–4h
  - Dexamethasone/neomycin/polymyxin B (Maxitrol) 1–2 gtt q1–8h
  - Prednisolone/gentamicin (Pred-G) 1–2 gtt q1–8h
  - Dexamethasone/tobramycin/chlorobutanol (TobraDex) 1–2 gtt q2–26h
- Glaucoma agents (always with ophthalmology consultation):
  - Alpha-2 agonists
    - Brimonidine 1% 1 gtt t.i.d.
    - Apraclonidine 1% 1 gtt t.i.d.
  - Beta blocker
    - Betaxolol 0.25%, 0.5%: 1–2 gtt b.i.d.
    - Carteolol 1% 1 gtt b.i.d.
    - Levobunolol 0.25%, 0.5%: 1 gtt q.d.–b.i.d.
  - Carbonic anhydrase inhibitor
    - Acetazolamide 500 mg PO/IV q.d.–q.i.d.
  - Miotic (parasympathomimetic)
    - Pilocarpine 0.25%, 0.5%, 1%, 2%, 3%, 4%, 6%, 8%, 10%: 1–2 gtt t.i.d.–q.i.d.
  - Osmotic agent
    - Mannitol 1–2 g/kg IV over 45 min
  - Prostaglandin analog
    - Latanoprost 0.005% 1 gtt q.d.
- Only if mechanical closure is ruled out
  - Timolol 0.25%, 0.5%: 1 gtt b.i.d.

# FOLLOW-UP

## DISPOSITION
### Admission Criteria
- Ruptured globe
- Hyphema (depending on severity)
- Orbital cellulitis/abscess
- Cavernous sinus thrombosis
- Significant cardiac, carotid, or neurologic disease
- Unexplained, progressive vision loss

### Discharge Criteria
- If the diagnosis is certain and visual loss will not progress

## FOLLOW-UP RECOMMENDATIONS
- Follow-up should be discussed with ophthalmology for emergent or urgent issues
- Referral for cardiac and carotid workup in embolic disease

## PEARLS AND PITFALLS
- Document visual acuity for all eye complaints
- Topical anesthesia will aid in diagnosis as well as facilitating a proper eye exam.
- Consider ocular issues and a detailed eye exam with headache complaints.

## ADDITIONAL READING
- Khare GD, Symons RC, Do DV. Common ophthalmic emergencies, *Int J Clin Pract*. 2008;62:1776–1784.
- Kunimoto DY, Kanitkar KD, Makar MS. *The Wills Eye Manual: Office and Emergency Room Diagnosis and Treatment of Eye Disease*, 4th ed. Philadelphia: Lippincott Williams & Wilkins, 2004. Website: www.eyeatlas.com
- Mahmood AR, Narang AT. Diagnosis and management of the acute red eye. *Emerg Med Clin N Am*. 2008;26:35–55.
- Vortmann M, Schneider JI. Acute Monocular Visual Loss. *Emerg Med Clin N Am*. 2008;26:73–96.

### See Also (Topic, Algorithm, Electronic Media Element)
- Chalazion, Conjunctivitis, Corneal Abrasion, Corneal Burn, Corneal Foreign Body, Dacryocystitis, Giant Cell Arteritis, Globe Rupture, Hordeolum, Hyphema, Iritis, Red Eye, Optic Artery Occlusion, Optic Neuritis, Orbital Cellulitis, Ultraviolet Keratitis, Vitreous Hemorrhage

# CODES

### ICD9
- 369.00 Blindness of both eyes, impairment level not further specified
- 369.3 Unqualified visual loss, both eyes
- 369.20 Low vision, both eyes, not otherwise specified

V

# VITREOUS HEMORRHAGE

*Jessa Williams*
*Carl G. Skinner*

 **BASICS**

## DESCRIPTION
Vitreous hemorrhage is a secondary diagnosis; identification of a specific cause is necessary for successful treatment:
- Retinal vessel tear secondary to vitreous separation
- Sudden tearing of vessels owing to trauma
- Spontaneous bleeding owing to neovascularization

## ETIOLOGY
- Blunt or penetrating trauma
- Retinal break/tear/detachment
- Any proliferative retinopathy
- Diabetes mellitus
- Sickle cell disease
- Retinal vein occlusion
- Eales disease
- Senile macular degeneration
- Retinal angiomatosis
- Retinal telangiectasia
- Peripheral uveitis
- Subarachnoid or subdural hemorrhage:
  – Terson Syndrome
- Intra-ocular tumor

### Pediatric Considerations
- Prematurity
- Congenital retinoschisis
- Pars planitis
- Child abuse:
  – Shaken-baby syndrome

 **DIAGNOSIS**

## SIGNS AND SYMPTOMS
- Sudden, painless unilateral loss or decrease in vision
- Appearance of dark spots (floaters), cobwebs, or haze in visual axis:
  – Above findings sometimes accompanied by flashing lights; floaters move with head movements
- Blurred vision, decreased visual acuity
- Loss of red reflex
- Inability to visualize fundus
- Mild afferent papillary defect

### History
- Ocular or systemic diseases
- Trauma

### Physical Exam
Fundoscopic exam:
- Absent red reflex
- No view of the fundus
- Acute:
  – RBCs in anterior vitreous
- Chronic:
  – Yellow appearance from hemoglobin breakdown

## ESSENTIAL WORKUP
- History with special attention to pre-existing systemic disease and trauma
- Complete ocular exam including:
  – Slit lamp
  – Tonometry
  – Dilated fundoscopic exam

## DIAGNOSTIC TESTS & INTERPRETATION
### Lab
- CBC
- PT/PTT/INR if indicated
- Electrolytes, BUN, creatinine, glucose

### Imaging
- B-scan US when no direct retinal view is possible to rule out retinal detachment or intraocular tumor
- Fluorescein angiography to define the cause
- CT scan/anteroposterior/lateral orbital films to rule out intraocular foreign body

### Diagnostic Procedures/Surgery
If nontraumatic, scleral depression

## DIFFERENTIAL DIAGNOSIS
- Vitreitis (leukocytes in the vitreous):
  – May include anterior or posterior uveitis
- Retinal detachment without hemorrhage
- Central retinal venous occlusion (CRVO)
- Central retinal artery occlusion (CRVA)

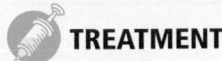

# TREATMENT

## PRE-HOSPITAL
Protect the eye from trauma or pressure:
- Monitor blood pressure

## INITIAL STABILIZATION/THERAPY
- Bed rest with head of bed elevated
- No activity resembling Valsalva maneuver (lifting, stooping, or heavy exertion)
- Avoid NSAIDs and other anticlotting agents.

## ED TREATMENT/PROCEDURES
- Urgent ophthalmologic consultation is needed with treatment based on the cause of the hemorrhage; an examination is carried out by the consultant:
  - Laser photocoagulation or cryotherapy for proliferative retinal vascular diseases
  - Repair of retinal detachments
- Surgical vitrectomy is needed for:
  - Blood that does not clear with time
  - VH from retinal detachement
  - Associated neovascularization
  - Hemolytic or ghost-cell glaucoma

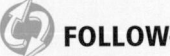

# FOLLOW-UP

## DISPOSITION
### Admission Criteria
Retinal break or detachment

### Discharge Criteria
Retinal break or retinal detachment must be excluded as cause of hemorrhage.

## FOLLOW-UP RECOMMENDATIONS
Re-evaluation daily for 2–3 days; if etiology is still unknown, B-scan US every 1–3 weeks.

# PEARLS AND PITFALLS

- Be sure to consider alternate diagnoses of CRVO or CRAO.
- Consider retinal detachment.
- Get history of trauma and use of blood thinners.
- Even minor bleeds require urgent ophthalmology consultation.

# ADDITIONAL READING

- Ehler JP, Shah CP. *The Wills Eye Manual: Office and Emergency Room Diagnosis and Treatment of Eye Disease*, 5th ed. Philadelphia: Lippincott Williams & Wilkins; 2008.
- Leveque T. Approach to the patient with acute visual loss. In: DS Basow, ed. *UpToDate*. Waltham, MA: UpToDate; 2009.
- Levin AV. Retinal hemorrhages: Advances in understanding. *Pediatr Clin N Am*. 2009;56(2): 333–344.
- Pelletier AL, Thomas J, Shaw FR. Vision loss in older persons. *Am Fam Physician*. 2009;79(11):963–970.
- Sumit S, Ventura AACM, Waheed N. Vitreoretinal disorders. *Ultrasound Clin*. 2008;3(2):217–228.
- Vortman M, Schneider JI. Acute monocular vision loss. *Emerg Med Clin N Am*. 2008;26:73–96.

## See Also (Topic, Algorithm, Electronic Media Element)
- Central Retinal Artery Occlusion (CRVA)
- Central Retinal Venous Occlusion (CRVO)
- Retinal Detachment
- Visual Loss

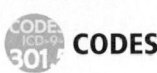 # CODES

### ICD9
379.23 Vitreous hemorrhage

# VOLVULUS

*Ronald E. Kim*

## BASICS

### DESCRIPTION
- Axial twist of a portion of the gastrointestinal (GI) tract around its mesentery causing partial or complete obstruction of the bowel
- Anatomic predisposition: redundant/freely mobile segment, with close approximation of points of fixation of bowel
- Precipitated by pathologic distention of the colon
- Blood supply compromised by venous congestion and eventual arterial inflow obstruction, leading to gangrene of the bowel and potential infarction

### ETIOLOGY
- Third most common cause of colonic obstruction (10%–15%) following tumor and diverticular disease
- Sigmoid (75%):
  - Due to redundant sigmoid colon with narrow mesocolon base
  - Most common in:
    ○ Elderly
    ○ Institutionalized
    ○ Chronic bowel motility disorders
    ○ Psychiatric diseases
  - Associated with chronic constipation and concomitant laxative use
- Cecal volvulus (22%):
  - More common in young adults
  - Due to improper congenital fusion of the mesentery with the posterior parietal peritoneum, causing the cecum to be freely mobile in varying degrees
  - Associated with increased gas production (malabsorption and pseudoobstruction)
  - Can be seen in pregnancy and after colonoscopy
- Transverse colon and splenic flexure (3%)
- Gastric volvulus (rare) associated with diaphragmatic defects

### Pediatric Considerations
- Midgut volvulus:
  - Due to congenital *malrotation* in which the midgut fails to rotate properly in utero as it enters the abdomen
  - Entire midgut from the descending duodenum to the transverse colon rotates around its mesenteric stalk, including the superior mesenteric artery.
  - Common in neonates (80% <1 month old, often in first week; 6%–20% >1 year old)
  - Males > females, 2:1
  - Sudden onset of bilious emesis (97%) with abdominal pain
  - May have previous episodes of feeding problems/bilious emesis
  - In children >1 year old, associated with failure to thrive, alleged intolerance to feedings, chronic intermittent vomiting, bloody diarrhea
  - Constipation
  - Mild distention, since obstruction higher in GI tract
  - May not appear toxic based on degree of ischemia

## DIAGNOSIS

### SIGNS AND SYMPTOMS
#### History
- 80% present with chronic symptoms
- Bowel obstruction:
  - Colicky, cramping abdominal pain (90%)
  - Abdominal distention (80%)
  - Obstipation (60%)
  - Nausea and vomiting (28%)
- Cecal volvulus:
  - Sudden onset of pain and distention
  - Asymmetric abdominal distention
- Sigmoid volvulus:
  - More insidious onset
- Gastric volvulus:
  - Triad of Brochard: severe epigastric distension, intractable retching, inability to pass nasogastric tube (NGT, 30% of patients)

#### Physical Exam
- Presence of gangrenous bowel:
  - Increased pain
  - Peritoneal signs: guarding, rebound, and rigidity
  - Fever
  - Blood on digital rectal exam
  - Tachycardia and hypovolemia
- Cecal volvulus:
  - Often a palpable mass in the left upper quadrant/midabdomen

#### Pediatric Considerations
- Child will appear well with normal exam early in clinical course
- 40% of neonates with bilious vomiting will require a surgical intervention
- Hematochezia, abdominal distention or pain, and shock indicate ischemia/necrosis
- 70% present with chronic symptoms

### ESSENTIAL WORKUP
- Plain abdominal radiograph:
  - Suggestive but often inconclusive
  - Diagnostic finding present in <70% of cases
  - Sigmoid volvulus: inverted U-shaped loop of dilated colon arising from the pelvis
  - Cecal volvulus—dilated and displaced:
    ○ Cecum in the left abdomen (kidney-shaped), often with dilated loops of small bowel

### DIAGNOSTIC TESTS & INTERPRETATION
#### Lab
- May give clues as to the presence of gangrenous bowel, but normal laboratory values do not exclude the diagnosis
- CBC:
  - Leukocytosis (WBC >20,000) suggests strangulation with infection/peritonitis.
- Electrolytes, blood urea nitrogen, creatinine, glucose:
  - Anion gap acidosis due to lactic acidosis
  - Prerenal azotemia due to dehydration
- Urinalysis:
  - Elevated specific gravity and ketones

#### Imaging
- Barium enema
  - "Bird's beak" deformity at the site of torsion
  - Perform cautiously owing to perforation risk.
  - May be therapeutic
- Upper GI series:
  - Abrupt ending or corkscrew tapering of contrast seen
- CT scan:
  - "Whirl" sign in cecal volvulus
  - May be useful in sigmoid volvulus to determine extent of obstruction
- Ultrasound:
  - Abnormal position of the superior mesenteric vein
  - "Whirlpool" sign of volvulus: vessels twirled around the base of the mesentery

#### Pediatric Considerations
- Diagnosis of midgut volvulus:
  - Duodenum lies entirely to the right of the spine on plain films.
  - "Double-bubble" sign on an upright film due to distended stomach and proximal duodenal loop
  - Established by upper-GI swallow: coiled spring/corkscrew appearance of jejunum in the right upper quadrant
  - Plain x-ray normal or equivocal in 20% of cases

### ALERT
- Evaluate any child with signs/symptoms of obstruction (including bilious vomiting and abdominal pain) for malrotation, even if he or she appears nontoxic.
- Delay in diagnosis >1–2 hr results in gangrenous bowel, necessitating large resection and leading to permanent parenteral nutrition with its associated complications.

#### Diagnostic Procedures/Surgery
- Endoscopic decompression with rectal tube placement
  - Successful in 78% of patients with sigmoid volvulus; less effective for cecal volvulus
  - Recurrence is common
  - Elective surgical treatment after endoscopic detorsion

### DIFFERENTIAL DIAGNOSIS
- Obstruction due to colonic tumor or diverticulitis
- Small bowel obstruction
- Ileus
- Intussusception
- Appendicitis
- Pelvic inflammatory disease and salpingitis, especially for cecal volvuli
- Ovarian torsion

#### Pediatric Considerations
- Meconium ileus
- Hirschsprung's disease
- Duodenal atresia
- Meckel's diverticulum
- Necrotizing enterocolitis

- Intussusception
- Appendicitis
- Medical conditions:
  - Colic
  - Henoch-Schönlein purpura
  - Inborn errors of metabolism
  - Trauma
  - Gastroesophageal reflux
  - Pyelonephritis
  - Meningitis

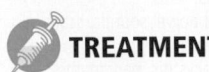

## TREATMENT

### PRE-HOSPITAL
- Establish IV assess
- NPO

### INITIAL STABILIZATION/THERAPY
- ABCs
- Aggressive fluid resuscitation with 0.9% NS bolus of 20 mL/kg (peds) or 2-L bolus (adult)
- NGT
- Foley catheter

### ED TREATMENT/PROCEDURES
- Obtain surgical consultation.
- Prepare patient for the OR.
- Correct hypovolemia and electrolyte abnormalities.
- Preoperative broad-spectrum antibiotics if suspected sepsis or perforation

### *Definitive Therapy*
**Sigmoid Volvulus**
- Nontoxic patient.
  - Reduce volvulus nonoperatively with sigmoidoscopy:
    - 60%–80% successful
    - 40%–50% recurrence
  - Follow with elective sigmoid resection and primary anastomosis (<3% recurrence)
- Toxic patient:
  - Emergent resection of sigmoid and any gangrenous bowel, with placement of end-colostomy

**Cecal Volvulus**
- Emergent operative reduction followed by cecectomy and primary anastomosis (preferred), or cecopexy if the cecum is still viable (higher recurrence).

### *Pediatric Considerations*
- Laparotomy within 1–2 hr to reduce risk for ischemia
- Surgical detorsion of bowel with resection of gangrenous bowel and a Ladd procedure is performed to prevent recurrent volvulus.

### MEDICATION
- Ampicillin sulbactam (Unasyn): 3 g (peds: 100–200 mg/kg/24 hr) IV q6h
- Cefoxitin (Mefoxin): 2 g (peds: 80–160 mg/kg/24 hr) IV q6h

## FOLLOW-UP

### DISPOSITION
**Admission Criteria**
- Admit with a surgical consult all suspected of having a volvulus.

### *Discharge Criteria*
- None

### *Issues for Referral*
- Surgical consultation necessary
- Atypical malrotation: asymptomatic or symptoms of gastroesophageal reflux
  - Close observation with repeat contrast study
  - Defer surgery

### FOLLOW-UP RECOMMENDATIONS
- Surgical follow postoperatively.

## PEARLS AND PITFALLS

- Consider volvulus in any child <1 mo old presenting with vomiting
  - Bilious vomiting is due to mechanical intestinal obstruction until proven otherwise.
- Delayed diagnosis leads to increased morbidity, more often with adults than children.
  - 70% adults not diagnosed until >6 mo from initial presentation; most present with chronic abdominal symptoms.
  - If gangrene present, mortality = 25%–80%

- Operative repair for all adult patients
- Contrast upper GI series ideal for children vs CT for adults; similar diagnostic accuracy

## ADDITIONAL READING

- American Society for Gastrointestinal Endoscopy. The role of endoscopy in the management of patients with known and suspected colonic obstruction and pseudo-obstruction. *Gastrointest Endosc.* 2010;71(4):669–679.
- Cappell MS, Batke M. Mechanical obstruction of the small bowel and colon. *Med Clin N Am.* 2008;92: 575—597.
- Durkin ET, et al. Age-related differences in diagnosis and morbidity of intestinal malrotation. *J Am Coll Surg.* 2008;206(4):658–663.
- Louie JP. Essential diagnosis of abdominal emergencies in the first year of life. *Emerg Med Clin N Am.* 2007;25:1009–1040.
- Madiba TE, Thomson SR. The management of cecal volvulus. *Dis Colon Rectum.* 2002;45(2):264–267.
- Rolandelli RH, Roslyn JJ. Colon and rectum. In: Townsend CM Jr, ed. *Sabiston Textbook of Surgery*, 18th ed. Philadelphia: Saunders, 2007;1369–1371.

### See Also (Topic, Algorithm, Electronic Media Element)
- Bowel Obstruction

 **CODES**

**ICD9**
560.2 Volvulus

V

# VOMITING, ADULT
*Scott G. Weiner*

 **BASICS**

## DESCRIPTION
- 3 phases:
  - Nausea: Unpleasant sensation prior to vomiting
  - Retching: Rhythmic contractions of diaphragm, abdominal muscles, intercostals that bring gastric contents up the esophagus
- Vomiting: Forceful retrograde expulsion of gastric contents through the mouth
- Vomiting center in medulla coordinates vomiting through vagus, phrenic, spinal nerves
- Irritated by impulses from the GI tract, pharynx, vestibular system, heart, genitalia, or via stimulation of chemoreceptor trigger zone (CTZ) in the area postrema of the brain by medications or toxins in circulation
- CTZ response mediated by dopamine $D_2$, serotonin (5-HT3), cholinergic, and histamine receptors:
- Medications providing symptomatic treatment of vomiting antagonize these receptors

## ETIOLOGY
- GI:
  - Appendicitis
  - Boerhaave syndrome
  - Bowel obstruction or ischemia
  - Cholecystitis, biliary colic
  - Gastric outlet obstruction, gastroparesis
  - Gastritis, gastroenteritis
  - GI bleeding
  - Hepatitis
  - Inflammatory bowel disease
  - Pancreatitis
  - Peptic ulcer disease, dyspepsia
  - Peritonitis
  - Ruptured viscus
- Neurologic:
  - Elevated ICP
  - Intracranial blood
  - Labyrinthitis, vertigo
  - Meningitis
  - Migraine
  - Stroke
  - Tumor
- Endocrine:
  - Adrenal insufficiency
  - DKA
  - Hypoparathyroid, hyperparathyroid
  - Hypothyroid, hyperthyroid
  - Uremia
- Pregnancy:
  - Hyperemesis gravidarum
  - Nausea/vomiting of pregnancy

- Drug toxicity:
  - Acetaminophen
  - Aspirin
  - Digoxin
  - Theophylline
- Therapeutic medication use:
  - Antibiotics
  - Aspirin
  - Chemotherapy
  - Ibuprofen
- Drugs of abuse:
  - Narcotics/narcotic withdrawal
  - Alcohols
- Genitourinary:
  - Gonadal torsion
  - Nephrolithiasis
  - UTI/pyelonephritis
- Miscellaneous:
  - Carbon monoxide poisoning
  - Electrolyte disorders
  - Glaucoma
  - Motion sickness
  - MI
  - Post-procedural (after anesthesia)
  - Self-induced (eating disorders)
  - Sepsis

 **DIAGNOSIS**

## SIGNS AND SYMPTOMS
### History
- Symptom duration, frequency, severity
- Characteristics of vomiting: Timing, description, content of vomitus
- Associated symptoms: Pain, fever, diarrhea, neurologic
- Past surgical or GI history
- Medication and drugs use
- Last menstrual period
- Complete past medical history

### Physical Exam
- Vital signs:
  - Fever: Appendicitis, gastroenteritis, cholecystitis, hepatitis, bowel perforation
  - Tachycardia: Dehydration

- Head, ears, eyes, nose, throat:
  - Abnormal anterior chamber: Glaucoma
  - Dry mucous membranes: Dehydration
  - Nystagmus: Labyrinthitis, stroke, intracranial hemorrhage
  - Papilledema: Elevated intracranial pressure (ICP)
- Abdomen:
  - Blood in stool: Peptic ulcer
  - Decreased bowel sounds: Ileus
  - Distention, high-pitched bowel sounds, scars or hernias: Intestinal obstruction
  - Pain: Appendicitis, cholecystitis, pancreatitis, perforated viscus, ovarian torsion
  - Testicular pain: Torsion
- Neurologic:
  - Abnormal mental status, cerebellar test abnormalities, cranial nerve abnormalities: CNS pathology

## ESSENTIAL WORKUP
The workup is also aimed at determining the underlying cause of vomiting and excluding dangerous sequelae.

## DIAGNOSTIC TESTS & INTERPRETATION
### Lab
- CBC:
  - Elevated WBC: Infectious process (eg, appendicitis, gastroenteritis)
  - Elevated hematocrit: Dehydration
  - Decreased hematocrit: GI bleed from ulcer
- Electrolytes:
  - Prolonged vomiting may cause hypochloremia, hypokalemia.
  - Blood urea nitrogen/creatinine ratio >20 may indicate dehydration.
- Liver function tests:
  - Amylase/lipase elevation: Pancreatitis
  - AST/ALT elevation: Hepatitis
  - Alkaline phosphatase elevation: Cholecystic etiology
- Urine analysis:
  - WBC, nitrites, leukocyte esterase, bacteria: UTI
  - Ketones: Dehydration, diabetic ketoacidosis (DKA)
  - Pregnancy test in women of childbearing age
- Toxicology screen/drug levels:
  - Indicated in suspected drug toxicity or overdose

## Imaging

- Abdominal series (kidney, ureter, bladder/upright):
  - Suspected bowel obstruction or perforated viscus
- CT abdomen/pelvis:
  - Suspected appendicitis, obstruction, nephrolithiasis
- CT/MRI head:
  - Suspected intracranial etiology
- US:
  - Suspected biliary disease, gonadal torsion, nephrolithiasis

## Diagnostic Procedures/Surgery

- EKG:
  - Suspected MI
- Endoscopy:
  - Peptic ulcer disease leading to significant GI bleed

 TREATMENT

### PRE-HOSPITAL

- Aimed at stabilizing patient until arrival in the ED, where antiemetics can be administered and the workup of underlying cause of vomiting can proceed:
- Placement of IV, oxygen, cardiac monitor
- Begin administration of isotonic fluids in suspected dehydration.
- Fingerstick glucose in mental status change
- Specific protocols may permit antiemetics for motion sickness or other etiologies of vomiting.

### INITIAL STABILIZATION/THERAPY

- Address ABCs.
- Urgent fluid resuscitation if vomiting has led to hypovolemic shock
- Urgent antiemetic therapy for patient comfort
- Urgent analgesic therapy if indicated

### ED TREATMENT/PROCEDURES

- 3 principles of ED treatment:
  - Correct fluid, electrolyte, and nutritional deficiencies as a result of vomiting.
  - Identify and treat underlying cause.
  - Suppress or eliminate symptoms.
- Antibiotics if indicated: UTI, appendicitis, bacterial gastroenteritis
- Medications:
  - Serotonin antagonists becoming 1st line treatment:
    - Ondansetron, dolasetron, granisetron
    - Excellent safety profile, including in children
    - Useful in chemotherapy-induced nausea
    - Ondansetron available as an oral dissolving tablet for patients who cannot tolerate pills
  - Dopamine $D_2$ antagonists also useful in most types of nausea:
    - Prochlorperazine, promethazine, metoclopramide, droperidol
    - Side effects (eg, akathisia, dystonia) more common than in serotonin antagonists
    - Note black box warnings on use of droperidol (potential QT prolongation and/or torsades de pointes) and promethazine (tissue injury with IV administration)

- Anticholinergic and antihistamine agents useful in labyrinthitis, positional vertigo, and motion sickness:
  - Meclizine, diphenhydramine, scopolamine
- Consultation with surgery, neurology, gastroenterology, urology, or obstetrics depending on underlying etiology

### MEDICATION

- Diphenhydramine: 25–50 mg IM/IV/PO
- Dolasetron: 12.5 mg IV
- Droperidol: 0.625–1.25 mg IM/IV
- Granisetron: 1 mg IV or 2 mg PO
- Hydroxyzine: 25–100 mg IM
- Meclizine: 25–50 mg PO
- Metoclopramide: 10 mg IM/IV/PO
- Ondansetron: 4–8 mg IM/IV/PO
- Prochlorperazine: 5–10 mg IM/IV/PO or 25 mg PR
- Promethazine: 12.5–25 mg PO/PR/deep IM
- Scopolamine: 1 patch 4 hr prior to travel

### Geriatric Considerations

- Dopamine-antagonizing antiemetics have potential cardiac side effects:
  - The doses of these medications should be reduced in the elderly.
- Serotonin antagonists are safer in this population.

### Pregnancy Considerations

- Vomiting occurs in 25–55% of pregnancies
- Phenothiazine (promethazine, chlorpromazine, metoclopramide) or serotonin–antagonizing antiemetics (granisetron, ondansetron) most commonly used

### First Line

- Serotonin antagonists
- Dopamine $D_2$ antagonists

### Second Line

- Anticholinergics
- Antihistamines
- Benzodiazepines
- Glucocorticoids

 FOLLOW UP

### DISPOSITION

#### Admission Criteria

- Significant underlying disease or symptoms necessitating close observation or surgical procedure
- Uncontrolled emesis resulting in inability to tolerate food or liquids by mouth
- Severe dehydration requiring continued IV fluids
- Significant electrolyte disturbances
- Unknown etiology of vomiting with inadequate outpatient follow-up

### Discharge Criteria

- Significant underlying pathology is excluded.
- Patient is sufficiently hydrated.
- Emesis is controlled.
- Close follow-up is arranged (preferably within 24–36 hr)

### FOLLOW-UP RECOMMENDATIONS

- All patients who are unable to tolerate fluids at home should return to the ED.
- Patients in whom the etiology of vomiting is unknown or who had electrolyte disturbances should follow-up.

## PEARLS AND PITFALLS

- Vomiting is a symptom and not a diagnosis:
  - It is important to be familiar with the broad differential diagnoses and exclude dangerous etiologies.
- Many antiemetics have notable side effects, ranging from dystonia to cardiac arrhythmias.
  - Know contraindications and treatment of adverse reactions before using these agents.
- Oral dissolving tablets and suppositories useful to avoid IV and for home care

## ADDITIONAL READING

- Longstreth GF. Approach to the adult patient with nausea and vomiting. Up to Date on-line text. www.uptodate.com. June 2009.
- Malagelada JR, Malagelada C. Nausea and vomiting. In: Feldman M, et al., eds. *Sleisenger and Fordtran's gastrointestinal and liver diseases*, 8th ed. Philadelphia: Saunders, 2006.
- Zun LS, Singh A. Nausea and vomiting. In: Marx JA, et al., eds. *Rosen's emergency medicine: Concepts and clinical practice*, 7th ed. St. Louis: Mosby, 2009.

### See Also (Topic, Algorithm, Electronic Media Element)

Vomiting, Pediatric

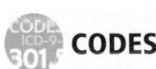 CODES

ICD9
787.03 Vomiting alone

V

# VOMITING, PEDIATRIC
*Mark A. Hostetler*

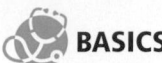 **BASICS**

## DESCRIPTION
- Forceful retrograde expulsion of gastric contents through the mouth; characterized by nausea, retching, and emesis; no gastric contents are expelled during retching.
- Emesis results from sustained contraction of abdominal muscles and diaphragm; at the same time, the pylorus and antrum contract.

## ETIOLOGY
Mechanism:

- Gastrointestinal (GI)/mechanical: Gastroesophageal reflux (GER), meconium ileus, necrotizing enterocolitis, hypertrophic pyloric stenosis, intussusception, malrotation with midgut volvulus, Hirschsprung disease, congenital obstructions (atresias, stenoses, and webs), hernia, foreign body/bezoar, paralytic ileus
- Metabolic/endocrine: Inborn errors of metabolism (amino acidurias, fatty acid oxidation disorders, urea cycle defects), uremia, congenital adrenal hyperplasia, kernicterus
- Neurologic: CNS bleeding (often due to trauma), tumor, hydrocephalus
- Infectious: Otitis media, urinary tract infection (UTI), pneumonia, sepsis, meningitis/encephalitis
- Feeding problems: Chalasia, improper technique (overfeeding, improper position), milk allergy
- Other: Toxicologic, nonaccidental trauma

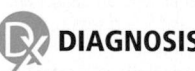 **DIAGNOSIS**

## SIGNS AND SYMPTOMS
- General:
  - Appearance variable depending on the underlying cause
  - Signs of dehydration, including tachycardia, tachypnea, pallor, decreased perfusion, and shock
  - Altered mental status may occur secondary to shock, hypoglycemia, or extra-abdominal conditions (sepsis, inborn error of metabolism, increased intracranial pressure, toxicologic poisoning).
- Vomiting characteristics:
  - Assess color, composition, onset, progression, and relationship to intake and position.
  - Nonbilious emesis is caused by a lesion proximal to the pylorus.
  - Bilious (green) emesis indicates obstruction below the ampulla of Vater; in infants, bilious emesis is associated with a more serious underlying condition (malrotation, volvulus, intussusception, bowel obstruction); may also be due to adynamic ileus or sepsis.

- Bloody emesis involves a lesion proximal to the ligament of Treitz; bright red bloody emesis has little or no contact with gastric juices due to an active bleeding site at or above cardia.
- "Coffee-grounds" emesis results from reduction of heme by gastric juices.
- Feculent odor suggests lower obstruction or peritonitis.
- Undigested food in emesis suggests an esophageal lesion or one at or above the cardia.
- GER: Begins shortly after birth, remains relatively constant, usually with normal weight gain
- Hypertrophic pyloric stenosis: Begins insidiously at 2–4 wk of age and progresses, becoming increasingly forceful (projectile) after feedings
- Obstruction and/or ischemic bowel (malrotation with midgut volvulus, intussusception, necrotizing enterocolitis): Sudden onset associated with rapid progression to appearing ill out of proportion to the duration of illness; abdomen distended and tender.
- Abdominal:
  - Distention suggests obstruction.
  - Peritoneal signs suggest inflammation and possible perforation.
- Complications:
  - Aspiration
  - Mallory–Weiss tear
  - Boerhaave syndrome

## History
- Constitutional:
  - Fever
- Vomiting characterics:
  - Timing, duration
  - Bilious?
  - Bloody?
- Associated symptoms:
  - Diarrhea
  - Abdominal pain
  - Dysuria
  - Inguinal swelling
- PMHx:
  - History of similar
  - Past surgical history

## Physical Exam
- General:
  - General appearance, vital signs
- Cardiovascular:
  - Quality heart tones
  - Pulses, perfusion
- Abdominal:
  - Tenderness, distention, mass
  - Bowel sounds
- Genitourinary:
  - Scrotal swelling, tenderness, mass
- Rectal:
  - Presence of blood, mass, tenderness

## ESSENTIAL WORKUP
Exclude life-threatening causes of vomiting.

## DIAGNOSTIC TESTS & INTERPRETATION
### Lab
As indicated by differential considerations:
- Metabolic assessment (glucose, electrolytes)
- Infection assessment (CBC, culture—urine)
- Pregnancy tests for females of childbearing age

### Imaging
- Evaluation/treatment of hypovolemia and hypoglycemia
- As indicated by differential considerations
- Abdominal radiographs (flat plate, upright, and decubitus) helpful for evaluation of obstruction or perforation
- Pelvic and abdominal US for evaluation of hypertrophic pyloric stenosis, appendicitis as well as pelvic or scrotal pathology
- Abdominal CT scan helpful for evaluation of appendicitis, mass/tumor often requiring contrast

### Diagnostic Procedures/Surgery
Nasogastric tube:
- Location, character, and severity of gastric bleeding

## DIFFERENTIAL DIAGNOSIS
- Neonate/infant:
  - GI/mechanical: GER, meconium ileus, necrotizing enterocolitis, hypertrophic pyloric stenosis, intussusception, malrotation with midgut volvulus, Hirschsprung disease, congenital obstructions (atresias, stenoses, and webs), hernia, foreign body/bezoar, paralytic ileus
  - Metabolic/endocrine: Inborn errors of metabolism (amino acidurias, fatty acid oxidation disorders, urea cycle defects), uremia, congenital adrenal hyperplasia, kernicterus
  - Neurologic: CNS bleeding (often due to trauma), tumor, hydrocephalus
  - Infectious: Otitis media, UTI, pneumonia, sepsis, meningitis/encephalitis
  - Feeding problems: Chalasia, improper technique (overfeeding, improper position), milk allergy
  - Other: Toxicologic, nonaccidental trauma
- Child/adolescent:
  - GI: Gastroenteritis, obstruction (hernia, adhesions, intussusception, foreign body, bezoar), pancreatitis, appendicitis, peritonitis, paralytic ileus, trauma (duodenal hematoma)
  - Metabolic/endocrine: Diabetic ketoacidosis, uremia, adrenal insufficiency
  - Infectious: Gastroenteritis, UTI, sinusitis, upper respiratory infection, sepsis, meningitis, encephalitis, pneumonia, hepatitis
  - Neurologic: CNS mass/tumor, CNS bleeding (often due to trauma), cerebral edema, concussion, migraine, kernicterus
  - Other: Toxicologic, (nonaccidental) trauma, pregnancy, bulimia

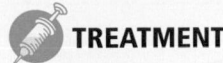 TREATMENT

### PRE-HOSPITAL
Not applicable

### INITIAL STABILIZATION/THERAPY
- Fluid resuscitation with 0.9% NS IV; caution if concern about increased intracranial pressure
- Determine bedside fingerstick glucose.

### ED TREATMENT/PROCEDURES
- Continue fluid resuscitation and correction of electrolyte imbalance if present.
- Decompress stomach with nasogastric or orogastric tube if abdomen distended or vomiting persistent.
- Continue evaluation for underlying cause.
- Consider antiemetic medications.
- Surgical consultation if acute abdomen; antibiotics if peritonitis or other systemic infection present

### MEDICATION
Antiemetics may be helpful once the underlying cause of vomiting has been determined.

#### First Line
Ondansetron: 4–8 mg (peds: 0.1 mg/kg per dose) IV q6h

#### Second Line
- Metoclopramide: 10 mg (peds: 0.1 mg/kg per dose) PO q6h
- Prochlorperazine: 2.5–5 mg (peds: 0.1 mg/kg per dose) IV, IM, or PR q6h
- Promethazine: 12.5–25 mg (peds: 0.25 mg/kg per dose) PO, PR, or IM q6h

 FOLLOW-UP

### DISPOSITION

#### Admission Criteria
- Unstable vital signs, including persistent tachycardia or other evidence of hypovolemia
- Serious etiologic condition
- Inability to exclude serious etiologic conditions
- Intractable vomiting or inability to take oral fluids
- Inadequate social situation or follow-up

#### Discharge Criteria
- Stable; able to tolerate oral fluids
- Benign etiology considered most likely
- Serious or potentially important etiologies excluded
- Parental understanding of instructions to advance clear liquids slowly and return for continued vomiting, abdominal distention, decreased urination, fever, lethargy, or unusual behavior

#### Issues for Referral
Chronic or recurrent episodes of vomiting or abdominal pain:
- Pediatric gastroenterology

### FOLLOW-UP RECOMMENDATIONS
PCP in 1–2 days

## PEARLS AND PITFALLS

- Determine presence or absence of bile or blood in emesis.
- Bilious vomiting in the neonate is malrotation until proven otherwise.
- Consider causes of vomiting other than just gastrointestinal (see Differential Diagnosis).

## ADDITIONAL READING

- Hostetler MA. Gastrointestinal disorders. In: Marx JA, Hockerberger RS, Walls RM, et al., eds. *Emergency Medicine: Concepts and Clinical Practice,* 7th ed. St. Louis: Mosby; 2010:2168–2187.
- Hostetler MA, Schulman M. Necrotizing enterocolitis presenting in the emergency department: Case report and review of differential considerations for vomiting in the neonate. *J Emerg Med.* 2001;21(2):165–170.
- Irish MS, Pearl RH, Caty MG, et al. The approach to common abdominal diagnoses in infants and children. *Pediatr Clin North Am.* 1998;45(4): 729–772.
- Kimura K, Loening-Baucke V. Bilious vomiting in the newborn: Rapid diagnosis of intestinal obstruction. *Am Fam Physician.* 2000;61(9):2791–2798.
- Pearl RH, Irish MS, Caty MG, et al. The approach to common abdominal diagnoses in infants and children. Part II. *Pediatr Clin N Am.* 1998;45(6): 1287–1326.

 CODES

### ICD9
787.03 Vomiting alone

V

# VON WILLEBRAND DISEASE

*Matthew A. Wheatley*

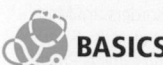 **BASICS**

## DESCRIPTION

- Coagulopathy caused by deficiency or dysfunction of von Willebrand Factor (vWF)
- vWF functions:
  - Mediates platelet-endothelial cell adhesion
  - Carrier protein for factor VIII
- Genetics:
  - Most cases inherited—multiple genetic defects identified
  - Type 1—quantitative defect of vWF:
    - 70% of cases
    - Autosomal dominant
    - vWF deficiency results from decreased synthesis and increased clearance of protein.
    - Manifestation ranges from asymptomatic to moderate bleeding.
  - Type 2—qualitative defect of vWF:
    - 10–15% of cases
    - Divided into types 2A, 2B, 2M, 2N—all are autosomal dominant except 2N.
    - Decrease in intermediate- and high-molecular-weight multimer
    - 2N—decreased binding to factor VIII
    - Leads to decreased levels of VIII and thus more serious coagulopathy
  - Type 3—absent or severe deficiency in amount of vWF:
    - Rare disease—1 per million cases
    - Autosomal dominant
    - Severe coagulopathy
  - vWD genetically associated with sickle cell disease, hemophilia A, factor XII deficiency, hereditary hemorrhagic telangiectasia, and thrombocytopenia

## ETIOLOGY

- In addition to genetic causes, acquired forms exist.
- Multiple mechanisms:
  - vWF antibody production
  - Decreased synthesis
  - Proteolysis
  - Increased clearance from binding to tumor cells
- Seen in association with the following:
  - Malignancy:
    - Wilms tumor
    - Multiple myeloma
    - Chronic lymphocytic leukemia
    - Non-Hodgkin lymphoma
    - Chronic myelogenous leukemia
    - Waldenstrom macroglobulinemia
    - Monoclonal gammopathy of uncertain significance
  - Immunologic:
    - Systematic lupus erythematosus
    - Rheumatoid arthritis
  - Medication-induced:
    - Valproic acid
    - Ciprofloxacin
    - Hetastarch
    - Griseofulvin
  - Miscellaneous:
    - Hypothyroidism
    - Uremia
    - Hemoglobinopathies
    - Cirrhosis
    - congenital heart disease
    - Disseminated intravascular coagulation

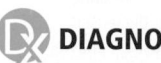 **DIAGNOSIS**

## SIGNS AND SYMPTOMS

- Symptoms vary depending on type of disease.
- Many type 1 and some type 2 are asymptomatic, severe type 2 and type 3 are symptomatic:
  - Easy bruising
  - Menorrhagia
  - Recurrent epistaxis
  - Gum bleeding
  - Gastrointestinal bleeding
  - Soft tissue bleeds and hemarthroses
  - Prolonged or excessive procedural bleeding

### Pregnancy Considerations

- Pregnancy causes increased vWF levels in patients with types 1 and 2 disease.
- Pregnancy, labor, and delivery are usually uncomplicated.
- vWF levels fall quickly after delivery:
  - Patients may suffer postpartum bleeding 10–28 days after delivery.

### History

- Most often diagnosed in pediatric and adolescent populations
- Family history
- Minor/moderate recurrent mucosal bleeding most common historical clue
- Heavy menses

### Physical Exam

- Most will have normal exam.
- Multiple large bruises
- Deep-tissue hematomas, hemarthroses

## ESSENTIAL WORKUP

- Screen and refer for testing if historical concerns or consistent physical findings.
- For type 1 diagnosis, patient must have significant mucocutaneous bleeding, laboratory confirmation, and family history of type 1 disease.

## DIAGNOSTIC TESTS & INTERPRETATION
### Lab

- CBC: Normal platelet count and morphology
- PT: Normal
- PTT:
  - Mildly prolonged in 50%
  - Due to low factor VIII levels or coexistent factor deficiency
- Measurement of vWF level and activity:
  - vWF ristocetin cofactor activity (vWF:RCo):
    - Uses platelet agglutination to determine vWF function
  - vWF antigen—tests for vWF level in serum using rabbit antibodies
- Bleeding time:
  - May be normal in type 1 (50%); prolonged in types 2 and 3
  - Not specific and hard to reproduce; has fallen out of favor for diagnosis

## DIFFERENTIAL DIAGNOSIS

- Hemophilia A, B
- Platelet defects
- Use of antiplatelet drugs—NSAIDs
- Platelet-type pseudo vWD
- Bernard–Soulier syndrome

 **TREATMENT**

### PRE-HOSPITAL
Direct pressure for control of hemorrhage

### INITIAL STABILIZATION/THERAPY
Resuscitation with crystalloid and packed RBCs as needed

### ED TREATMENT/PROCEDURES

- 3 treatment strategies:
  - Increase endogenous vWF
  - Replacement of vWF
  - Agents that generally promote hemostasis but do not alter levels of vWF

- Desmopressin acetate (DDAVP):
  - Promotes release of vWF from endothelial cells, increases factor VIII levels
  - Maximal levels obtained at 30–60 min, with duration of 6–8 hr
  - Effective for type 1; variable effectiveness for type 2; not indicated for type 3
  - Patients may use intranasal spray at home before menses or minor procedures.
- vWF replacement therapy:
  - Humate–P factor VIII concentrate with vWF:
    - Treated to reduce virus transmission risks
    - Indicated for type 3 vWD and severe bleeding in all types
    - Doses, length of treatment depend on severity of bleeding.
    - Fresh frozen plasma, cryoprecipitate:
    - Less desirable because they carry infection risk
- Antifibrinolytic therapy:
  - Aminocaproic acid (Amicar) and trasexamic acid (Cyklokapron)
  - Block plasmin formation to prevent clot degradation
- Topical agents—applied directly to bleeding site:
  - Gelfoam or Surgicel soaked in thrombin Micronized collagen
  - Fibrin sealant
- Avoid antiplatelet agents.

## MEDICATION

- Aminocaproic acid: 50–60 mg/kg PO/IV q4h–q6h
- Cryoprecipitate: 10–12 units initial dose or 2–4 bags/10 kg
- Desmopressin (DDAVP):
  - 0.3 $\mu$g/kg IV, max 20 $\mu$g
  - 0.3 $\mu$g/kg SQ, max 20 $\mu$g
  - 300 $\mu$g intranasal
  - Peds: <50 kg—150 $\mu$g intranasal

- Fresh frozen plasma (FFP)—10–20 mL/kg IV
- Antihemophilic factor/vWF complex, human (Humate-P): 40–80 IU/kg IV
- Tranexamic acid: 20–25 mg/kg PO, IV q8h

### First Line

- Minor bleeding (epistaxis, oropharyngeal, soft tissue):
  - IV or intranasal desmopressin
- Major bleeding (intracranial, retroperitoneal):
  - Replace vWF and factor VIII so activity level is at least 100 IU/dL.

### Second Line

Minor bleeding:

- vWF concentrate:
  - Given if desmopressin is ineffective
  - Should be given in consultation with a hematologoist

 **FOLLOW-UP**

## DISPOSITION

### Admission Criteria

- Patients with significant bleeding requiring further IV medical management
- Observation after major trauma for types 2 and 3 vWD
- Consider transferring patients with major bleeding events to a center with round-the-clock laboratory capability, and a care team that includes a hematologist and a surgeon skilled in management of bleeding disorders.

### Discharge Criteria

- Control of hemorrhage
- Adequate follow-up and access to medical therapy

## FOLLOW-UP RECOMMENDATIONS

Hematology:

- Severe, difficult-to-manage bleeding
- Prior to elective/semielective procedures
- Definitive workup of suspected cases

## PEARLS AND PITFALLS

Patients may not know their type of hemophilia:

- Consider FFP for the patient with unknown type of hemophilia in the setting of trauma or bleeding.

## ADDITIONAL READING

- Federici A, Mannucci P. Advances in the genetics and treatment of von Willebrand disease. *Curr Opin Pediatr.* 2002;14:23–33.
- Greer J, Foerster J. *Wintrobe's Clinical Hematology,* 11th ed. Philadelphia: Lippincott Williams & Wilkins; 2004.
- Hoffman R, Benz E, Shattil S, et al, eds. *Hematology: Basic Principles and Practice,* 4th ed. Philadelphia: Churchill Livingstone; 2005.
- Mannucci P. Treatment of von Willebrand disease. *N Engl J Med.* 2004;351:683.
- Nichols WL, Hultin MB, James AH, et al. Von Willebrand disease (vWD): Evidence-based diagnosis and management guidelines, the National Heart, Lung and Blood Institute (NHLBI) Expert Panel report (USA). *Haemophilia.* 2008;14:171–232.
- *The Diagnosis, Evaluation and Management of von Willebrand Disease. National Heart, Lung and Blood Institute.* http://www.nhlbi.nih.gov/guidelines/vwd/. Accessed November 11, 2009.

## See Also (Topic, Algorithm, Electronic Media Element)

Hemophilia

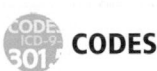 **CODES**

**ICD9**
286.4 Von Willebrand's disease

# WARFARIN/COUMADIN OVERDOSE

*John Bailitz*
*Joanne C. Witsil*

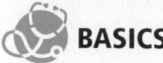 **BASICS**

## DESCRIPTION
Most commonly prescribed oral anticoagulant:
- Inhibits regeneration of vitamin K cofactor required for hepatic carboxylation of factors II, VII, IX, and X
- Blocks the coagulation cascade's extrinsic system and common pathway
- Commonly used for venous thromboembolism and prevention of embolism with prosthetic heart valves or atrial fibrillation
- Adjustments based on the international normalization ratio (INR)
  - Typical therapeutic range 2.0–3.0
  - 2.5–3.5 for mechanical valves and antiphospholipid syndromes:
- Contraindications include any condition in which the risk of hemorrhage or adverse reaction outweighs clinical benefit.
  - Prior hypersensitivity
  - Skin reactions
  - Recent surgeries
  - Active or potential gastrointestinal (GI), intracerebral, or genitourinary (GU) bleeding
  - Fall risk

## ETIOLOGY
- Many factors including age, other drugs, diet, and comorbidities affect INR/bleeding versus thromboembolism:
  - Increase INR:
    - Multiple antibiotics
    - NSAIDs
    - Amiodarone
    - Propranolol
    - Prednisone
    - Cimetidine
    - Influenza vaccine
    - Grapefruit
    - Mango
    - Gingko biloba
    - Garlic
    - Alcohol (if concomitant liver disease)
    - Hypermetabolic states produced by fever
    - Hyperthyroidism
    - Cancer
    - Collagen vascular disease
    - Congestive heart failure
    - Age
    - Liver disease
  - Decrease INR:
    - Carbamazepine
    - Barbituates
    - Rifampin
    - Haloperidol
    - St. John Wart
    - High vitamin K foods
    - Hereditary Coumadin resistance
    - Hyperlipidemia

- Bleeding complications:
  - 15% of patients have bleeding complications/year
    - 4.9% major
    - Up to 0.8% fatal, most commonly intracranial hemorrhage (ICH):
- Bleeding risk:
  - Directly related to INR
    - Increases dramatically above 4.0
  - Inversely related to time spent in therapeutic range:
  - Risk factors for bleeding:
    - Age >75 yr
    - Past GI bleeding
    - Hypertension, cerebrovascular disease, severe heart disease
    - Diabetes
    - Renal insufficiency
    - Alcoholism or liver disease
    - Occult GI and GU malignancies
    - Genetic polymorphism of the cytochrome P450 CYP2C9

### Pregnancy Considerations
Warfarin:
- Pregnancy class X
- Crosses the placenta causing spontaneous abortion and birth defects

 **DIAGNOSIS**

## SIGNS AND SYMPTOMS
- Presentation may be occult or dramatic:
  - High index of suspicion required to detect potentially life-threatening complications
- Subtherapeutic/Low INR: Breakthrough thrombosis
- Therapeutic and supratherapeutic: GI, CNS, retroperitoneal bleeding
- Skin necrosis and limb gangrene:
  - Classic lesions of Coumadin skin necrosis and limb gangrene begin on the third to eighth day of therapy resulting from capillary thrombosis in subcutaneous fat (skin necrosis) and obstruction of venous circulation of the limb (limb gangrene).
  - Associated with protein C deficiency, but may occur with protein S deficiency and in patients with normal levels
  - Eschar in center differentiates lesions from ecchymosis due to excess Coumadin therapy

## ESSENTIAL WORKUP
- Thorough history:
  - Many chief complaints are complicated by anticoagulation.
    - Reason for anticoagulation, recent dose changes, compliance, recent INR testing, other prescriptions, over the counter, and alternative medicines
    - Subtle changes in mental status, recent "minor falls," or bleeding

- Check for vital sign abnormalities:
  - Early hemorrhagic shock
  - Hypertension and bradycardia may be secondary to Cushing response in ICH.
  - Cardiac meds often mask important changes in vital signs.
- Examine carefully for:
  - Pallor, contusions, abrasions, ecchymosis, palpable pulses in affected extremity and skin lesions
  - Check stool for blood.

## DIAGNOSTIC TESTS & INTERPRETATION
### Lab
- Prothrombin time/partial thromboplastin time/INR:
  - Significant bleeding may occur even in INR therapeutic range.
  - PTT also elevated with toxicity
- CBC:
  - Initial HCT inaccurate measure of acute rapid bleeding
  - Platelets
    - Aspirin and ADP inhibitors/Plavix result in normal platelet levels but qualitative deficits.
- Electrolytes, blood urea nitrogen (BUN), creatinine, glucose:
  - Evaluate renal function.
  - Elevated BUN may indicate blood in GI tract.
- Type and cross-match

### Imaging
- Low threshold for CT imaging to detect occult but life threatening bleeding:
- Head CT:
  - Minor mechanisms of blunt head trauma without loss of consciousness
  - Detect ICH presenting with only mild symptoms of headache and nausea before the classic gradual progression of symptoms to focal deficits and coma
- Abdominal CT:
  - Blunt abdominal trauma without significant tenderness
  - For retroperitoneal hemorrhage

## DIFFERENTIAL DIAGNOSIS
- All causes of bleeding:
  - GI, retroperitoneal, CNS, and traumatic
- Skin lesions—hemorrhagic skin disorders:
  - Hemostatic deficits such as platelet disorders
  - Vascular purpuras including glucocorticoid use, vitamin C deficiency, purpura fulimnans, disseminated intravascular coagulation, Henoch-Schönlein purpura, protein C deficiency

# TREATMENT

## PRE-HOSPITAL
- ABCs
- Treat hypotension with two large-bore IV lines and 0.9% NS infusion.
- Cardiac and pulse oximetry monitoring

## INITIAL STABILIZATION/THERAPY
- Establish central IV access for hypotension not responsive to initial fluid bolus:
  - Compressible sites only
- Replace lost blood as soon as possible:
  - Initiate with O-negative blood until type-specific blood available.
  - 10 mL/kg bolus in children

## ED TREATMENT/PROCEDURES
- Specific management depends on the INR, presence of bleeding, reason for anticoagulation, and reliability of patient:
  - INR <5 without bleeding:
    - Lower or omit next dose.
    - Recheck INR in 24 hr.
  - INR ≥5–<9 without bleeding:
    - Omit next 1 or 2 doses or omit 1 dose and give 1–2.5 mg PO vitamin K.
    - If at increased risk for bleeding or pre-op, then administer vitamin K 1–≤5 mg PO, INR will be lowered in 24 hr.
    - Recheck INR in 24 hr.
  - INR ≥9 without significant bleeding:
    - Hold Coumadin and give vitamin K 2.5–5 mg PO; INR will be substantially lowered in 24–48 hr
  - INR >20 with minor or life-threatening bleeding regardless of INR:
    - Hold Coumadin
    - Vitamin K 10 mg by slow IV infusion
    - Fresh frozen plasma (FFP) 3–4 units, or prothrombin complex concentrate or recombinant factor VIIa depending on volume status and availability
- In the setting of controlled bleeding, maintain the INR at the lower level of therapeutic efficacy:
  - 1.5–2.0 for atrial fibrillation
  - 2.0–2.5 with a mechanical heart valves

## MEDICATION
- Vitamin K1 phytonadione:
  - Side effects:
    - Anaphylaxis with IV > IM or PO
    - SC absorption unpredictable
    - IM administration may result in hematoma formation.
    - Breakthrough thromboembolism with complete correction
    - High-dose vitamin K1 risks prolonged warfarin resistance and may precipitate thromboembolism for up to 1 wk
  - 10 mg IV infusion over 10–30 min is recommended for life threatening active bleeding with effects beginning in 1–2 hr
- Fresh frozen plasma (FFP):
  - Traditionally 3–4 units of FFP (1 L) are given to control continued bleeding in the short term without excessive risk of thromboembolism.

- Patient response is variable and may not correlate with correction of the INR.
- Side effects:
  - Virus transmission
  - Fluid overload
- Prothrombin complex concentrate (PCC):
  - PCC is a fractionation product of FFP containing equal amounts of factors II, VII, IX, and X.
  - Long shelf life and easy reconstitution into a highly concentrated volume (500–1,000 U/20 ml versus 1 L of FFP per dose)
  - Rapid and quick reversal without volume overload where available
  - Side effects:
    - Thrombosis
    - Less virus transmission then FFP
  - For patients with an INR of 2.0–3.9, administer 25 U/kg, 4.0–5.9, 35 U/kg, and >6.0, 50 U/kg
  - Not available for use in the United States
- Recombinant factor VIIa:
  - Produces a rapid "thrombin burst" reducing INR and bleeding
  - No risk of virus transmission
  - Small volume
  - Single bolus of 15–90 μg/kg bodyweight
  - Side effects:
    - Thrombosis rare
    - Expensive
    - Available for use in the U.S.
    - Not approved indication

# FOLLOW-UP

## DISPOSITION

### Admission Criteria
- Active GI, retroperitoneal, or CNS bleeding
- Anticoagulated trauma patient with evidence of active bleeding requires:
  - Reversal of anticoagulation and blood replacement
  - Early surgical consultation for operative intervention
  - Transport to a level one-trauma center after initial stabilization for definitive care.
- Skin necrosis and limb gangrene requires admission for anticoagulation with alternative agents in consultation with a hematologist.
- Subtherapeutic patient may require adequate anticoagulation with inpatient heparin or low molecular weight heparin to prevent a breakthrough thromboembolism:
  - Outpatient Lovenox therapy followed by increased coumadin with close follow-up prevents unnecessary hospitalization
  - Daily average risk or thromboembolism low for most indications

### Discharge Criteria
- Asymptomatic reliable patient with a supratherapeutic INR after consideration of:
  - Indication for anticoagulation, reason for supratherapeutic level, underlying comorbidities, overall risk of bleeding, fall risk, social situation, reliability, and availability of follow up
- Asymptomatic anticoagulated patient with minor trauma, therapeutic INR, stable hemoglobin, normal imaging studies, and reliable caretakers, can be discharged with close follow up.

### Issues for Referral
Patient should follow up with primary care physician or specialist within 24-48 hours of discharge for INR check and further coumadin adjustments.

### FOLLOW-UP RECOMMENDATIONS
Educate patient on monitoring for signs and symptoms of excessive bleeding and/or new thrombotic event.

## PEARLS AND PITFALLS
- Maintain a low threshhold for imaging trauma patients on warfarin.
- Just hold the next dose of warfarin for an INR <5 without bleeding.
- Vitamin K1 IV may result in fatal anaphylaxis:
  - Use only in patients with INR > 20 with minor bleeding, or patients with life threatening bleeding
    - Administer PO for everyone else.
- For rapid reversal, FFP is still considered first line agent:
  - Administer recombinant factor VIIa if it is available and patient unable to tolerate the excess fluid volume from the amount of FFP to be given for correction.

## ADDITIONAL READING
- Ansell J, Hirsh J, Hylek E, et al. Pharmacology and management of the vitamin K antagonists. *Chest.* 2008;133:160S–198S.
- Crowther MA, Ageno W, Garcia D, et al. Oral vitamin K versus placebo to correct excessive anticoagulation in patients receiving warfarin. *Ann Intern Med.* 2009;150:293–300.
- Denas G, Marzot F, Offelli P, et al. Effectiveness and safety of a management protocol to correct over-anticoagulation with oral vitamin K: a retrospective study of 1,043 cases. *J Thromb Thrombolysis.* 2009;27(3):340–347.
- Schulman S, Beyth RJ, Kearon C, et al. Hemorrhagic complications of anticoagulant and thrombolytic treatment. *Chest.* 2008;133:257S–298S.
- Wiedermann CJ, Stockner I. Warfarin-induced bleeding complications-clinical presentation and therapeutic options. *Thromb Res.* 2008;122 (Suppl 2):S13–S18.

## CODES

### ICD9
964.2 Poisoning by anticoagulants

W

# WARTS

*Gary M. Vilke*

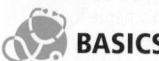 **BASICS**

## DESCRIPTION

- Warts are caused by the human papillomaviruses (HPV).
- Causes cellular proliferation and vascular growth
- Lesions are typically verrucous and hyperkeratotic.
- Lesions resolve spontaneously in most cases:
  - 1/3 within 6 mo
  - 2/3 within 2 yr
  - 90% within 5 yr
  - Likely due to cell-mediated immune response
- Cutaneous warts:
  - Verrucae vulgaris (common warts):
    - Dorsum of hands
    - Sides of fingers
    - Adjacent to nails
    - Usually asymptomatic
  - Verrucae plantaris (plantar warts):
    - Weight bearing parts of sole: Heels, metatarsal heads
    - Often symptomatic and painful
    - More common in adolescents and young adults
  - Flat (juvenile) warts:
    - Primarily on light exposed areas
    - Head, face, neck, legs, dorsum of hands
    - Small in size
    - Range from a few to hundreds
- Anogenital warts:
  - Known as condyloma acuminata or venereal warts
  - Most are asymptomatic and may go unrecognized
  - HPV types 6 and 11 account for 90% of anogenital warts
- HPV types 16 and 18 account for 70% of cervical cancers

## ETIOLOGY

- HPV is host-specific to humans.
  - Cause infection of epithelial tissues and mucous membranes
  - Infects the basal layer of skin or mucosa
- There are >100 types of HPV that variably infect different body sites.
- HPV transmission is:
  - Direct: Skin to skin
  - Indirect: Contaminated surface to skin
  - Autoinoculation: Scratching, sucking (especially in young children)
- Incubation period can range from weeks to >1 yr

### Pediatric Considerations

- 10–20% of children will have warts
- Peak incidence between 12 and 16 yr
- May produce laryngeal papillomatosis in infants from viral exposure at birth
- Must consider sexual abuse in children with anogenital warts

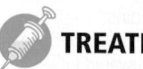 **DIAGNOSIS**

## SIGNS AND SYMPTOMS

### History

- Complete sexual history
- Prior history of warts and treatment
- HIV status
- Cutaneous warts:
  - Common warts:
    - Usually asymptomatic unless on a pressure point
    - May present with bleeding secondary to minor trauma
  - Plantar warts:
    - Often painful with weight-bearing
  - Flat (or juvenile) warts:
    - On light-exposed areas of skin
    - May spread with shaving face, neck, legs
- Anogenital warts:
  - In men, usually on glans penis, shaft, scrotum, or anus
  - In women, found on labia, vagina, cervix, or anus
  - May extend into urethra, bladder, or rectum:
    - Dysuria
    - Pain, itching, and/or bleeding with bowel movements
  - May have symptoms involving mouth or throat if oral sexual contact

### Physical Exam

- Cutaneous warts:
  - Common warts:
    - Hard, rough, raised, dome-shaped lesions
    - Obscure normal skin markings
    - Hypervascular and may bleed with minor trauma
  - Plantar warts:
    - Soles of the feet
    - Obscure normal skin markings
    - Hypervascular and may bleed with gentle scraping
  - Flat (or juvenile warts):
    - Flesh-colored
    - Flat-top and smooth
    - Small: Range from pinpoint to size of pencil eraser
- Anogenital warts:
  - Pedunculated growths often with cauliflower-like appearance
  - Lesions are soft and usually present in multiples.
  - Flesh-colored to slightly pigmented or red

## ESSENTIAL WORKUP

Diagnosis made by characteristic appearance of lesions

## DIAGNOSTIC TESTS & INTERPRETATION

### Lab

- Pregnancy test for females
- Biopsy and viral typing not recommended for typical lesions.
- If difficult to see, add acetic acid to suspected area, which will cause infected areas to whiten and become more visible.
- Screen for other sexually transmitted diseases.

### Diagnostic Procedures/Surgery

Biopsy indicated if failing therapy, patient immunocompromised, or warts are pigmented, indurated, fixed, or ulcerated

## DIFFERENTIAL DIAGNOSIS

- Cutaneous warts:
  - Common wart
    - Callus; will not bleed
  - Plantar wart:
    - Callus, corn, bunion
  - Flat (or juvenile) wart:
    - Moles, skin tag, lichen planus
- Anogenital wart:
  - Condyloma latum (secondary syphilis)
  - Herpes simplex
  - Prominent glands around head of penis
  - Benign or malignant neoplasm
  - Molluscum contagiosum

**TREATMENT**

## INITIAL STABILIZATION/THERAPY

None required

## ED TREATMENT/PROCEDURES

- Cutaneous warts:
  - Occlusion with duct tape:
    - Least invasive
    - Maintain on wart for 6 days
    - Gentle debridement with pumice stone or nail file on day 7
    - Minimal side effects
    - Good for young children
    - May also enhance other topical treatments
  - Salicylic acid:
    - Inexpensive, mild side effects
    - OTC is 17% salicylic acid
    - Prescription strength has up to 70% salicylic acid
    - Soak wart in warm water for 10–20 min.
    - Apply salicylic acid overnight.
    - Gently debride in morning.
    - Patches are also available.
    - Resolution may take weeks to months.

- Anogenital warts:
  - May use imiquimod, podofilox, podophyllin, trichloroacetic acid, or alternative therapies listed below.
  - Nonintervention may be best course in children, as treatment has not been well studied.
- Alternative treatments:
  - Cryotherapy with liquid nitrogen or dry ice
  - Electrocautery
  - Laser therapy
  - Surgical excision
  - Interferon for use by subspecialists
- Provide appropriate referral.

## MEDICATION

- Topical medications:
  - Imiquimod cream: Apply 3 times/wk for up to 16 wk:
    ○ Cream may weaken diaphragms and condoms.
  - Podofilox 0.5% gel or solution:
    ○ Apply b.i.d. for 3 days, then rest 4 days; may repeat for 4 cycles
    ○ Do not use on perianal, rectal, urethral, or vaginal lesions.
  - Podophyllin 15–25% in benzoin: Weekly topical application:
    ○ Protect surrounding normal tissue with petroleum jelly.
    ○ Wash off 1–4 hr later
    ○ Do not use in pregnancy: Highly toxic and teratogenic.
    ○ Do not use on cervix, vagina, or anal canal as may cause dysplastic changes.
  - Salicylic acid:
    ○ Wash off 6–10 hr later.
    ○ May be repeated weekly
- Vaccine:
  - Gardasil: Targets HPV types 6, 11, 16, 18:
    ○ Recommended for girls >9 yr
    ○ 3-shot series over 6 mo
    ○ For the prevention of cervical cancer, vulvar and vaginal cancer, genital warts, and other low-grade cervical lesions
  - Cervarix: Targets HPV types 16, 18:
    ○ 3 shots over 6 mo
  - Universal vaccination may provide significant reduction of cervical cancer in developing countries without well established screening.
  - Both vaccines are 96% effective.
  - There are still controversies surrounding routine use and acceptance.

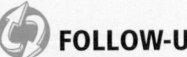

# FOLLOW-UP

## DISPOSITION
### Admission Criteria
Disseminated cases in immunocompromised patients may require admission.

### Discharge Criteria
Most patients can be treated as outpatients.

### Issues for Referral
- All medication-based therapies require follow-up and subsequent dosing. Should not initiate treatment unless follow-up can be secured.
- For treatment failures, referral to PMD or dermatology should be made for alternative treatment options.
- Refer sexually active teenage girls to pediatrician or primary care for HPV vaccination.

## FOLLOW-UP RECOMMENDATIONS
- Pain, burning, redness, or other changes in symptoms require prompt reevaluation.
- Arrange follow-up with appropriate provider: Pediatrician, gynecologist, dermatologist, primary care physician.

## PEARLS AND PITFALLS

- Pregnancy test must done before initiation of medical therapy.
- HPV vaccine does not protect from all forms of HPV, just those most commonly associated with cervical cancer.
- Consider sexual assault in children with anogenital warts.

## ADDITIONAL READING

- Centers for Disease Control and Prevention, Workowski KA, Berman SM. Sexually transmitted diseases treatment guidelines, 2006. *MMWR Recomm Rep*. 2006;55(RR-11):1–94.

- Gilson R, Ross J, Maw R, et al. A multi-centre, randomised, double-blind, placebo-controlled study of cryotherapy versus cryotherapy and podophyllotoxin cream as treatment for external anogenital warts. *Sex Transm Infect*. 2009 Aug 20. [Epub ahead of print]
- Herman BE, Corneli HM. A practical approach to warts in the emergency department. *Pediatr Emerg Care*. 2008;24:246–251.
- Hsueh PR. Human papillomavirus, genital warts and vaccines. *J Microbiol Immunol Infect*. 2009;42: 101–106.
- Hutchinson DJ, Klein KC. Human papillomavirus disease and vaccines. *Am J Health-Syst Pharm*. 2008;65:2105–2112.
- Kodner CM, Nasraty S. Management of genital warts. *Am Fam Physician*. 2004;70:2335–2342.
- Markowitz LE, Dunne EF, Saraiya M, et al. Centers for Disease Control and Prevention (CDC); Advisory Committee on Immunization Practices (ACIP). Quadrivalent Human Papillomavirus Vaccine: Recommendations of the Advisory Committee on Immunization Practices (ACIP). *MMWR Recomm Rep*. 2007

## See Also (Topic, Algorithm, Electronic Media Element)
- Herpes, Genital
- HIV/AIDS
- Molluscum Contagiosum

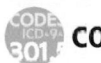 CODES

### ICD9
- 078.10 Viral warts, unspecified
- 078.11 Condyloma acuminatum
- 078.12 Plantar wart

W

# WEARNESS

Kathryn A. Volz
Jason Imperato

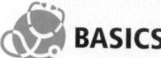 **BASICS**

## DESCRIPTION
- Defined as a decrease in physical strength or energy
- Often multifactorial
- Distinguish neuromuscular disorder vs. non-neuromuscular disorder
- Categories of neuromuscular disorders:
  - Upper motor neuron (UMN) lesions:
    - Deep tendon reflexes (DTR) increased
    - Plantar reflexes upgoing
    - Increased muscle tone
    - Muscle atrophy absent
  - Lower motor neuron (LMN) lesions:
    - DTRs decreased to absent
    - Plantar reflexes absent or normal
    - Decreased muscle tone
    - Muscle atrophy present
    - Fasciculations
  - Neuromuscular junction (NMJ) lesions:
    - DTRs normal
    - Plantar reflexes normal or absent
    - Decreased muscle tone
- Categories of non-neuromuscular disorders:
  - Infectious
  - Endocrine
  - Metabolic
  - Cardiac
  - Rheumatologic
  - Toxic
  - Psychiatric

## ETIOLOGY
- Neuromuscular disorders:
  - UMN lesions:
    - Multiple sclerosis
    - Amyotrophic lateral sclerosis
    - Transverse myelitis
    - Poliomyelitis
  - LMN lesions:
    - Guillain-Barré syndrome
    - Toxic neuropathies
    - Impingement syndromes
    - Diphtheria
    - Porphyria
    - Seafood toxins

- NMJ lesions:
  - Myasthenia gravis
  - Lambert-Eaton syndrome
  - Botulism
  - Periodic paralysis
  - Tick paralysis
  - Electrolyte imbalances
- Nonneuromuscular disorders:
  - Dehydration
  - Anemia
  - Malignancy
  - Cerebrovascular accident
  - Head or neck trauma
  - Myocardial ischemia
  - Infection/sepsis:
    - Urinary tract infection
    - Pneumonia
    - Meningitis
    - Mononucleosis
    - HIV
    - Arboviruses
  - Endocrine abnormalities:
    - Hypothyroidism
    - Adrenal crisis
    - Periodic paralyses
  - Rheumatologic disorders:
    - Systemic lupus erythematosus
    - Polymyalgia rheumatica
  - Toxins:
    - Medications
    - Environmental
    - Carbon monoxide poisoning
    - Cocaine
    - Alcohol

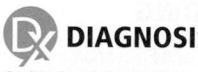 **DIAGNOSIS**

## SIGNS AND SYMPTOMS
- Altered physical strength:
  - Assessment of strength:
    - 1: No contraction
    - 2: Active movement with gravity eliminated
    - 3: Active movement against gravity
    - 4: Active movement against gravity and resistance
    - 5: Normal power
  - Change in muscle tone:
    - Flaccidity
    - Spasticity
    - Rigidity
  - Abnormal DTRs
  - Abnormal plantar reflexes
  - Muscle atrophy:
    - Difference of >1 cm in the leg and thigh and >0.5 cm in the forearm and arm

- Systemic findings:
  - Weakness
  - Fatigue
  - Dizziness
  - Paresis
  - Paresthesias
  - Hoarse voice
  - Dysphagia
  - Visual changes
  - Confusion
  - Associated symptoms:
    - Fever
    - Chest pain
    - Dyspnea
    - Cough
    - Weight loss
    - Rash
    - Dysuria
    - Upper respiratory infection symptoms

## ESSENTIAL WORKUP
- Clinical suspicion gathered through history and physical exam guides further testing:
- Generalized vs. focal
- Acute vs. chronic
- Proximal vs. distal
- Ascending vs. descending
- Symmetric vs. asymmetric
- Improved vs. worsened with activity

## DIAGNOSTIC TESTS & INTERPRETATION
Diagnostic testing should be broad unless history and physical exam identify the cause of weakness.

### Lab
- Serum glucose
- CBC
- Electrolytes
- BUN/creatinine
- Toxin screen
- Urinalysis
- Thyroid function tests (rule out hypothyroidism)
- ESR (rule out rheumatologic cause)
- Carboxyhemoglobin (rule out CO poisoning)
- Troponin/CK-MB (rule out cardiac ischemia)
- Digoxin level (rule out digoxin toxicity)

### Imaging
- EKG (rule out ACS/arrhythmia)
- CXR (rule out pneumonia)
- CT head or MRI head (rule out intracranial pathology)

### Diagnostic Procedures/Surgery

- Bedside spirometry:
  - Forced vital capacity, negative inspiratory force, peak expiratory flow rate
  - May identify those with impending ventilatory failure
- Lumbar puncture:
  - In suspected Guillain-Barré syndrome:
    - Albumin-cytologic dissociation in cerebrospinal fluid (protein > 400, WBC <10) is virtually diagnostic.
- Tensilon test:
  - Distinguishes myasthenic crisis from cholinergic crisis in myasthenia gravis

### DIFFERENTIAL DIAGNOSIS

- Physiologic causes of weakness:
  - Simple fatigue:
    - Excessive physical activity
    - Inadequate rest
    - Excessive or inadequate diet
    - Pregnancy
- Psychiatric causes of weakness:
  - Anxiety
  - Depression
  - Dependent personality
  - Hypochondriasis
  - Chronic fatigue syndrome
  - Fibromyalgia
  - Malingering

 **TREATMENT**

Treatment is geared to the underlying cause of weakness.

### PRE-HOSPITAL

- Supplemental oxygen
- IV access
- Fingerstick glucose determination
- Consider endotracheal intubation in patients with severe respiratory distress.

## INITIAL STABILIZATION/THERAPY

- Supplemental oxygen
- IV access
- Endotracheal intubation for impending ventilatory failure

## ED TREATMENT/PROCEDURES

- Neurology consult if needed
- When the diagnosis is determined, specific therapies can be applied:
  - Plasma exchange and/or IV immunoglobulin (IVIG) for Guillain-Barré syndrome
  - Hydrocortisone for adrenal insufficiency
  - Potassium supplementation for hypokalemia
  - Dextrose for hypoglycemia
  - Antibiotics for infectious etiologies
  - Specific antidotes for botulism and diphtheria
  - Digibind for digoxin toxicity

 **FOLLOW-UP**

### DISPOSITION

#### Admission Criteria

- All patients with new-onset neuromuscular disorders should be admitted for definitive diagnosis.
- Any evidence of impending ventilatory or circulatory compromise warrants ICU admission.

#### Discharge Criteria

- Resolution of symptoms
- Stable vital signs
- Definitive diagnosis and correction of abnormality

## FOLLOW-UP RECOMMENDATIONS

- Discharged patients with non-neurologic etiologies should have follow-up with their PCP.
- Discharged patients with neurologic etiologies should have urgent neurology follow-up.

## PEARLS AND PITFALLS

- Identify early and aggressively treat patients at risk for respiratory compromise due to Guillain-Barré, botulism, myasthenia gravis.
- Identify elderly patients with acute coronary syndrome or infection presenting as weakness.
- Consider endocrine causes of weakness, including adrenal insufficiency and hypothyroidism.

## ADDITIONAL READING

- Chew WM, Birnbaumer DM. Evaluation of the elderly patient with weakness: An evidence based approach. *Emerg Med Clin N Am*. 1999;17(1): 265–278.
- LoVecchio F, Jacobson S. Approach to generalized weakness and peripheral neuromuscular disease. *Emerg Med Clin N Am*. 1997;15(3):605–623.
- Losman E. Weakness. In Marx J, et al., eds., *Rosen's emergency medicine: Concepts and clinical practice*, 7th ed. St. Louis: Mosby, 2009:87–92.

 **CODES**

### ICD9

- 728.87 Muscle weakness (generalized)
- 780.79 Other malaise and fatigue

W

# WEST NILE VIRUS

*Roger M. Barkin*
*Marnta Malik*

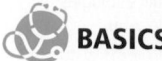

## BASICS

### DESCRIPTION
Infectious agent is an arbovirus, a member of the Flaviviridae family.

### ETIOLOGY
- Vector-borne virus
- Transmitted by infected mosquitoes in late summer/early fall
- Wild birds are primary reservoir hosts; human is infected by cross-feeding mosquitoes.
- Introduced to Western Hemisphere 1999; became more widespread owing to vector of *Culex* mosquito
- Infection after blood transfusion and solid-organ transplant can occur.
- There are case reports of occupational exposure and infection of lab workers via percutaneous inoculation.

#### Pregnancy Considerations
Infection via transplacental transmission and breast-feeding has been reported.

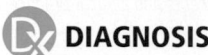

## DIAGNOSIS

### SIGNS AND SYMPTOMS
- Variable severity of illness:
  - 80% asymptomatic
  - 20% mild symptoms, flulike illness
  - Approximately 1/150 with CNS involvement (encephalitis, meningitis)
- Incubation period is usually 2–6 days but can be up to 14 days in average patient and up to 21 days in immunocompromised patient.
- Symptoms have a sudden onset and last <1 wk with mild infection.
- Mortality rate in severe cases is estimated at 7%.
- Severity of illness is related to degree of CNS invasion by virus.
- Immunocompromised patients have prolonged viremia, delayed development of antibody, and increased likelihood of severe disease.

#### Geriatric Considerations
- Patients >60 yr, if infected, at higher risk for developing more severe disease and neurologic consequences.
- Advanced age is most important risk factor for death.

### History
- General:
  - Fever
  - Malaise
  - Anorexia
  - Headache
  - Acute phase resolves within several days but fatigue and weakness may persist for wks
- Neurologic:
  - Altered mental status (change in level of consciousness, confusion, agitation, irritability)
  - Severe, diffuse muscle weakness; may be asymmetric and involve the face
  - Flaccid paralysis, which may resemble poliomyelitislike syndrome, associated with anterior horn cell injury. Cranial nerve and bulbar abnormalities have been reported
  - May resemble Guillain–Barré syndrome
  - Seizures
- Gastrointestinal:
  - Nausea, vomiting, diarrhea
  - Abdominal pain
- Musculoskeletal:
  - Myalgia
  - Arthralgia
- Respiratory:
  - Cough
  - Sore throat
- Ophthalmologic:
  - Photophobia
  - Eye pain

### Physical Exam
- General:
  - Temperature >38°C (>100°F)
  - Transient maculopapular rash
- Neurologic:
  - Altered mental status
  - Hyporeflexia, areflexia
  - Ataxia
  - Extrapyramidal signs
  - Cranial nerve palsies, paresis
  - Myoclonus
  - Profound motor weakness
- Gastrointestinal:
  - Hepatosplenomegaly
- Musculoskeletal:
  - Nuchal rigidity
- Hematologic:
  - Lymphadenopathy
- Dermatologic:
  - Rash (maculopapular or morbilliform on neck, trunk, extremities)
- Cardiovascular:
  - Myocarditis (rare)
- Ophthalmologic:
  - Optic neuritis
  - Vitritis
  - Chorioretinitis

### ESSENTIAL WORKUP
- Most sensitive screening test is serologic testing of CSF and serum for IgM antibody-capture enzyme-linked immunosorbent assay (ELISA) and culture.
- Centers for Disease Control and Prevention (970-221-6400)
- Can be detected during first 4 days of illness, nearly all tests are positive by day 7–8; may remain positive up to 1 yr after infection
- Procedures for submitting samples vary by state.
- Refer to local public health department for guidelines.

### DIAGNOSTIC TESTS & INTERPRETATION
**Lab**
- CSF:
  - Pleocytosis with lymphocyte predominance
  - Elevated protein
  - Normal glucose
- CBC:
  - WBCs may be mildly elevated (50%) or normal.
  - Leukopenia may be present (15%).
  - Anemia can occur.
- Chemistry:
  - Hyponatremia sometimes seen:
    - Cause uncertain, possibly syndrome of inappropriate antidiuretic hormone (SIADH) when CNS involvement exists
  - Pancreatitis (rare)
  - Fulminant hepatitis (rare)

*Imaging*
- CT head usually normal
- MRI can be useful to identify CNS inflammation:
  - One third of patients show abnormality.
  - Imaging findings generally nonspecific but may include enhancement of leptomeninges and/or periventricular white matter or can mimic demyelinating process.

*Diagnostic Procedures/Surgery*
Lumbar puncture

## DIFFERENTIAL DIAGNOSIS
- Other causes of meningitis:
  - Bacterial
  - Viral
  - Tuberculous
  - Fungal
- Other causes of viral encephalitis:
  - Other arboviruses, especially St. Louis encephalitis virus
  - Enterovirus, particularly in patients ≤16 yr of age
  - Herpes simplex virus (HSV)
  - Cytomegalovirus (CMV)
  - Epstein–Barr virus (EBV)
  - Mumps virus
  - Varicella zoster virus
  - Rabies virus
- Intracranial abscess
- CNS vasculitis
- Nonspecific viral syndrome
- Gastroenteritis

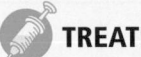 TREATMENT

### INITIAL STABILIZATION/THERAPY
- ABCs
- Seizure precautions

### ED TREATMENT/PROCEDURES
- Supportive care
- IV fluids for signs of dehydration
- For signs of meningitis, administer antibiotics pending results of CSF.
- Consider acyclovir if index of suspicion for the only treatable cause of viral encephalitis, HSV, is high.
- Administer antipyretics and pain medications.
- No known effective antiviral therapy or vaccine
- No controlled studies proving effectiveness of interferon-α2b, ribavirin, corticosteroids, anticonvulsants, or osmotic agents

 FOLLOW-UP

### DISPOSITION
*Admission Criteria*
- Neurologic symptoms
- Dehydration
- Concerning risk factors (advanced age, immunocompromise)

*Discharge Criteria*
- No signs of CNS involvement (encephalitis, meningitis)
- Able to tolerate oral solutions

### FOLLOW-UP RECOMMENDATIONS
Neurologist to monitor for potential ongoing residual.

## PEARLS AND PITFALLS
Consider HSV in differential, since HSV is treatable.

## ADDITIONAL READING

- Centers for Disease Control and Prevention: Interim guidelines for the evaluation of infants born to mothers infected with West Nile Virus during pregnancy. *MMWR*. 2004;53:154–157.
- Hayes EB, O'Leary DR. West Nile virus infection: A pediatric perspective. *Pediatrics*. 2004;113: 1375–1381.
- Nash D, Mostashari F, Fine A, et al. The outbreak of West Nile virus infection in the New York City area in 1999. *N Engl J Med*. 2001;344:1807–1814.
- Petersen LR, Marfin AA, Gubler DJ. West Nile virus. *JAMA*. 2003;290:524–528.
- Ravindra KV, Freifeld AG, et al. West Nile virus–associated encephalitis in recipients of renal and pancreas transplants: Case series and literature review. *Clin Infect Dis*. 2004;38:1257–1260. Epub 2004 Apr 14.
- Solomon T, Ooi MH, et al. West Nile encephalitis. *Br Med J*. 2003;326:865–869. *West Nile Virus: Information and Guidance for Clinicians*. Available at http://www.cdc.gov/ncidod/dvbid/westnile/clinicians.
- Zak I, Altinok D, et al. West Nile virus infection. *AJR Am J Roentgenol*. 2005;184(3):957–961. Review

### See Also (Topic, Algorithm, Electronic Media Element)
Meningitis; Encephalitis, HSV

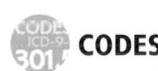 CODES

**ICD9**
066.40 West nile fever, unspecified

W

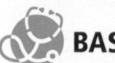

# WHEEZING
*Stephen K. Epstein*

## BASICS

### DESCRIPTION
- Result of turbulent airflow:
  - High-pitched sound with dominant frequency at 400 Hz:
    - Gas flowing through constricted airways analogous to a vibrating reed
  - Resonant vibration of the bronchial walls when airflow velocity reaches critical values
- Caused by airway narrowing between 2–5 mm:
  - Wheezing is very low pitched with airway diameters of 5 mm.
  - Airways of <2 mm are unable to transmit sound because the energy is lost as friction heat.
- Airway narrowing is caused by a combination of ≥1 of the following:
  - Constriction (as with reactive airway disease)
  - Peribronchial interstitial edema
  - Inflammation
  - Obstruction

### ETIOLOGY
- Pulmonary (small airway):
  - Asthma
  - Acute respiratory distress syndrome
  - Anaphylaxis
  - Aspiration pneumonia:
    - Wheezing occurs early in the disease due to intense bronchospasm following the event.
  - Byssinosis:
    - Occupational lung disease of textile workers exposed to cotton dust
  - Drugs:
    - Can precipitate angioedema or allergic reaction
    - ACE inhibitors
    - $\beta$-Blockers
    - Aspirin and NSAIDs
  - Forced exhalation in normal patients
  - Hyperventilation
  - Chronic obstructive pulmonary disease
  - Chronic cor pulmonale
  - Chemical pneumonitis
  - Carcinoid tumors
  - Paroxysmal nocturnal dyspnea
  - Pulmonary edema
  - Pulmonary embolism:
    - Rarely associated with wheezing
    - Focal
  - Pneumonia
  - Sleep apnea
- Pulmonary (large airway):
  - Vocal cord dysfunction (paralysis, paradoxical movement)
  - Foreign body
  - Epiglottitis:
    - Wheezing associated with stridor in 10% of cases
  - Diphtheria
  - Smoke inhalation
  - Bronchial tumor
  - Tracheal tumor

### Pediatric Considerations
- Viral bronchiolitis in patients <3 yr of age
- Asthma
- Croup
- Foreign-body aspiration
- Congenital abnormalities:
  - Tracheomalacia
  - Tracheal stenosis
- Cystic fibrosis
- CHF

## DIAGNOSIS

### SIGNS AND SYMPTOMS
- A whistling sound made while breathing:
  - Diffuse:
    - As with reactive airway disease or pulmonary edema
  - Focal:
    - As with pneumonia or pulmonary embolism
- Dyspnea
- Respiratory distress
- Chest pain
- Cough
- Sputum production:
  - Frothy (pulmonary edema)
- Stridor
- Fever
- Cyanosis
- Tachypnea
- Tachycardia

### History
- Current URI:
  - Rhinoviruses implicated in reactive airways
- Recent exercise:
  - Exercise-induced asthma, vocal cord dysfunction

### Physical Exam
- Mental status:
  - Lethargy, confusion, and fatigue in the setting of respiratory distress is the primary reason for airway management.
- Presence of muscle retractions
- Lung auscultation

### ESSENTIAL WORKUP
- Pulse oximetry:
  - Useful for assessing severity, but not for predicting hospital admission
- Peak flow:
  - Useful in assessing need for hospitalization
- CXR

### DIAGNOSTIC TESTS & INTERPRETATION
### Lab
- ABG:
  - Sometimes used to determine whether patient is fatiguing by noting falling oxygenation, rising $CO_2$, and acidosis
  - Clinical assessment is a more reliable indicator of the need for airway management.
- WBC:
  - Elevated WBC does not distinguish infection from other disorders, as stress causes demargination.
  - WBC is also elevated in noninfected patients taking steroids.
  - A normal WBC does not rule out an underlying pneumonia.

### Imaging
- Peak expiratory flow (PEF):
  - To assess function of small airways
  - Use to determine severity and track the progress of therapy in patients with reactive airway disease.
- CXR:
  - Assess for diagnosis of pulmonary conditions:
    - Pneumonia
    - Foreign-body aspiration
  - Assess for pulmonary edema.
- EKG:
  - Useful when patient is at risk for cardiac ischemia
  - Indicated in all cases in which wheezing is caused by pulmonary edema
- Soft-tissue neck:
  - Used to assess for foreign body or obstructing mass

### Diagnostic Procedures/Surgery
Bronchoscopy:
- Indicated when obstruction is thought to be causal
- Used to retrieve an inhaled foreign body or diagnose an underlying tumor

### DIFFERENTIAL DIAGNOSIS
See "Etiologies."

## TREATMENT

### PRE-HOSPITAL
- Supplemental oxygen
- Initiate pulse oximetry and cardiac monitoring.
- Initiate therapy for underlying condition when indicated:
  - Asthma
  - Pulmonary edema
- Intubate for respiratory failure or anticipated respiratory failure.

## INITIAL STABILIZATION/THERAPY
- ABCs
- Intubation for impending airway failure:
  – Prepare for possible foreign body in airway.
  – Anticipate difficult airway.

## ED TREATMENT/PROCEDURES
- Correct hypoxemia: Supplemental oxygen
- Initial assessment of severity:
  – PEF >40%: Mild–moderate
  – PEF <40%: Severe
- Treat the underlying condition.
- Rapid reversal of airflow obstruction:
  – Bronchodilators:
    ○ Reversibility following the use of short-acting β-agonists such as albuterol or terbutaline suggests reactive airway disease.
  – Anticholinergics: Ipratropium bromide:
    ○ Add to β-agonist therapy for severe disease
- Reduce likelihood of relapse:
  – Trial of steroids indicated if wheezing is caused by bronchospasm or noninfectious inflammation.
- Adjunctive agents
  – Heliox:
    ○ Less dense than air or oxygen alone
    ○ Decreases work of breathing
    ○ More efficacious in large-airway disease
    ○ Not as effective for small-airway disease
  – Magnesium sulfate:
    ○ Evidence for benefit only in moderate to severe asthmatics
  – Ketamine:
    ○ For intubation of the asthmatic patient

## MEDICATION
### First Line
- Albuterol: 2.5–5 mg in 2.5 mL NS q20min inhaled × 3 doses (peds: 0.15 mg/kg/dose q20min × 3 doses, min. dose 2.5 mg)
- Levalbuterol: 1.25–2.5 mg q20 minutes × 3 doses (peds: 0.075 mg/kg (minimum dose 1.25 mg) q20 minutes × 3 doses)
- Prednisone: 40–80 mg PO (peds: 1 mg/kg/d in 2 div. doses; max. 60 mg/d)
- Prednisolone: Peds 1 mg/kg/d in 2 div. doses; max. 60 mg/d
- Racemic epinephrine: Peds: 0.25–0.5 mL nebulized for croup

### Second Line
- Ipratropium bromide: 0.5 mg q20min x 3 doses (peds: 0.25–0.5 mg q20min × 3 doses); may mix with albuterol
- Methylprednisolone: 40–80 mg IV (peds:× 1–2 mg/kg/dose IV or PO div. q12h for 24 hr) for patients who cannot tolerate PO
- Terbutaline: 0.25 mg SC q0.5h for 2 doses (peds: 0.01 mg/kg up to 0.3 mg SC):
  – No proven advantage over aerosol therapy
- Magnesium sulfate

##  FOLLOW-UP

### DISPOSITION
#### Admission Criteria
- Hypoxia
- Persistent or worsening wheezing
- Underlying condition requires hospital admission

#### Discharge Criteria
- Improvement or resolution of wheezing
- PEF >70% predicted
- Adequate oxygenation

#### Issues for Referral
Asthma:
- Referral should be made for a written asthma action plan.

### FOLLOW-UP RECOMMENDATIONS
The patient should be instructed to return to the ED with shortness of breath, fever, hemoptysis, or chest pain.

## PEARLS AND PITFALLS

Be prepared to manage the airway if administering an anxiolytic.

## ADDITIONAL READING

- Boushey HA, Corry DB, Fahy JV. Asthma. In: Murray JF, Nadel JA, eds., *Textbook of respiratory medicine*, 3rd ed. Philadelphia: WB Saunders, 2000:1247–1288.
- *Dorland's illustrated medical dictionary*, 28th ed. Philadelphia: WB Saunders, 1994.
- Fiz JA, et al. Detection of wheezing during maximal forced exhalation in patients with obstructed airways. *Chest*. 2000;122(1):186–191.
- Krieger BP. When wheezing may not mean asthma. *Postgrad Med*. 2002;112(2):101–111.
- Mellis. Respiratory noises: How useful are they clinically? *Pediatr Clin North Am*. 2009;56(1):1–17, ix.
- National Heart, Lung, and Blood Institute, National Asthma Education and Prevention Program, Expert Panel Report 3: Guidelines for the Diagnosis and Management of Asthma. US Department of Health and Human Serives, 2007. Available at http://www.nhlbi.nih.gov/guidelines/asthma/asthgdln.htm
- Weinberger M, Abu-Hasan M. Pseudo-asthma: When cough, wheezing, and dyspnea are not asthma. *Pediatrics*. 2007;120(4):855–864.
- White MV. Differential diagnosis in the difficult asthmatic. *Immunol Allergy Clin North Am*. 2001;21(3).

### See Also (Topic, Algorithm, Electronic Media Element)
- Asthma, Adult
- Asthma, Pediatric

##  CODES

ICD9
786.07 Wheezing

W

# WITHDRAWAL, ALCOHOL
*Trevonne M. Thompson*

## BASICS

### DESCRIPTION
- Alcohol withdrawal is the most common withdrawal syndrome encountered in the emergency department
- Neuroexcitation is the hallmark of alcohol withdrawal
- Alcohol withdrawal may be life-threatening.
- More severe symptoms and signs are seen in patients with prior episodes of withdrawal, a process called kindling
- Alcoholism is not uncommon among older adults.
- Age-related increase in alcohol sensitivity
- Alcohol-related problems may be misdiagnosed as normal consequences of aging.

### ETIOLOGY
- Chronic alcohol use downregulates GABA (inhibitory) receptors, upregulates NMDA (excitatior) receptors.
- Abstinence or reduction in use leads to increased adrenergic activity because of these receptor adaptations
- 4 components to alcohol withdrawal
  - Early withdrawal
  - Withdrawal seizures
  - Alcoholic hallucinosis
  - Delirium tremens (DTs)
- DTs occur in 5% of patients experiencing alcohol withdrawal
- DTs have a 5–15% mortality rate

## DIAGNOSIS

### SIGNS AND SYMPTOMS
- Early withdrawal:
  - Typically occurs 6–8 hr after the last drink
  - Typically lasts 1–2 days
    - Tremulousness
    - Anxiety
    - Palpitations
    - Nausea
    - Anorexia
- Withdrawal seizures:
  - Typically occur 6–48 hr after the last drink
  - Typically last 2–3 days
    - Generalized seizures, generally brie
- Alcoholic hallucinosis:
  - Typically occurs 12–48 hr after the last drink
  - Typically lasts 1–2 days
    - Visual hallucinations (most common)
    - Tactile hallucinations
    - Auditory hallucinations
    - Sensorium typically otherwise clear
- Delirium tremens:
  - Typically occurs 48–96 hr after the last drink
  - Can last up to 5 days
  - Not necessarily preceded by hallucinosis or seizures
    - Tachycardia
    - HTN
    - Diaphoresis
    - Delirium
    - Agitation
    - Sensorium typically not clear

### History
Obtain substance abuse history
- Time of last substance use
- History of previous withdrawal and how severe

### Physical Exam
A thorough physical examination is necessary

### ESSENTIAL WORKUP
Thorough history and physical examination with attention to the vital signs

### DIAGNOSTIC TESTS & INTERPRETATION
#### Lab
- Electrolytes, BUN, creatinine, glucose, magnesium
- CBC
- Alcohol level
- Urine drug screening rarely alters management
- Urinalysis
- Blood/urine culture:
  - For suspected infection

#### Imaging
- Not necessary if early withdrawal is clearly the presenting issue
- CT head:
  - For altered mental status or if the clinical situation is not straightforward
- CXR:
  - If secondary infection (eg, aspiration pneumonia) is suspected.

*Diagnostic Procedures/Surgery*
ECG when clinically warranted

## DIFFERENTIAL DIAGNOSIS

- Benzodiazepine withdrawal
- Barbiturate withdrawal
- Intracerebral hemorrhage
- CNS infection
- Epilepsy
- Hypoglycemia
- Hyperthyroidism
- Sepsis
- Drug intoxication
- Psychosis
- Electrolyte disorder

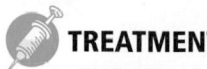 **TREATMENT**

### PRE-HOSPITAL
- Assess vital signs
- Assess capillary glucose

### INITIAL STABILIZATION/THERAPY
- Attention to the ABCs
- Obtain IV access
- IV fluid administration
- Cardiopulmonary monitoring

### ED TREATMENT/PROCEDURES
- Aggressive supportive care
- Benzodiazepines:
  - The standard therapy
  - No single benzodiazepine is more effective than another
  - High doses are often required to control symptoms and signs
- Barbiturates may be used as an alternate or adjunct to benzodiazepines.
- Propofol may also be used in severe cases.

## MEDICATION

- Chlordiazepoxide: 25–100 mg PO for mild symptoms and signs; 25 mg IV in repeated doses as necessary for severe symptoms and signs
- Diazepam: 5–20 mg PO for mild symptoms and signs; 5–10 mg IV; repeat for severe symptoms and signs
- Lorazepam: 2 mg PO, repeat q2h–q4h as needed for mild symptoms and signs; 2 mg IV in repeated doses as necessary for severe symptoms and signs
- Phenobarbital: 30–60 mg PO for mild symptoms and signs; 15–20 mg/kg slow intravenous administration for severe symptoms or status epilepticus
- Propofol: Start with 25–75 mcg/kg/min, then titrate as necessary

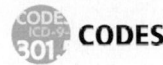 **FOLLOW-UP**

## DISPOSITION

### Admission Criteria
- Moderate-to-severe symptoms
- Persistent symptoms despite treatment
- DTs or impending DTs
- Co-morbid medical illness

### Discharge Criteria
Mild symptoms and signs responsive to therapy

## FOLLOW-UP RECOMMENDATIONS
Referral to detox program or facility

## PEARLS AND PITFALLS

- Misdiagnosis of medical disease as withdrawal syndrome
- Misunderstanding the relationship between withdrawal syndromes and co-morbid medical illness
- Administer sufficient quantities of benzodiazepines to control symptoms.

## ADDITIONAL READING

- DeBellis R, et al. Management of delirium tremens. *J Intensive Care Med.* 2005;20:164–173.
- McKeon A, Frye MA, Delanty N. The alcohol withdrawal syndrome. *J Neurol Neurosurg Psych.* 2008;79:854–862.
- Rathlev NK, et al. Alcohol-related seizures. *J Emerg Med.* 2006;31:157–163.
- Tetrault JM, O'Connor PG. Substance abuse and withdrawal in the critical care setting. *Crit Care Clin.* 2008;24:767–788.

### See Also (Topic, Algorithm, Electronic Media Element)
Withdrawal, Drug

## CODES

ICD9
- 291.0 Alcohol withdrawal delirium
- 291.81 Alcohol withdrawal

W

# WITHDRAWAL, DRUG

*Trevonne M. Thompson*

 **BASICS**

## DESCRIPTION
- Neuroexcitation is the hallmark of benzodiazepine, barbiturate, and opiate withdrawal
- Benzodiazepine and barbiturate withdrawal can be life-threatening
- Opiate withdrawal can be extremely uncomfortable but is not typically life-threatening
- Cocaine and amphetamine withdrawal are similarly not life-threatening

## ETIOLOGY
- Chronic exposure to certain drugs cause adaptive changes in the CNS
- Withdrawal syndromes occur when the constant presence of drug is removed or reduced and the adaptive changes persist
- Tolerance occurs when increasing amounts of drug are required to achieve a given response
- Withdrawal and tolerance are distinct entities

 **DIAGNOSIS**

## SIGNS AND SYMPTOMS
- Benzodiazepines and barbiturates:
  - Anxiety
  - Agitation
  - Irritability
  - Tremor
  - Sleep disturbance
  - Tachycardia
  - Hypertension
  - Hyperthermia
  - Autonomic instability
  - Seizures
- Opiates:
  - Restlessness
  - Irritability
  - Drug craving
  - Yawning
  - Piloerection
  - Mydriasis
  - Nausea
  - Vomiting
  - Diarrhea
  - Abdominal pain
  - Tachycardia
  - HTN
- Cocaine:
  - Depressed mood
  - Fatigue
  - Vivid dreams
  - Sleep disturbance
  - Psychomotor retardation or agitation
- Amphetamines:
  - Fatigue
  - Irritability
  - Sleep disturbance
  - Anxiety

### History
Obtain substance abuse history
- Time of last substance use
- History of previous withdrawal

### Physical Exam
A thorough physical examination is necessary

## ESSENTIAL WORKUP
Thorough history and physical examination with attention to the vital signs

## DIAGNOSTIC TESTS & INTERPRETATION
### Lab
- Electrolytes, BUN, creatinine, glucose
- Urine drug screening rarely alters management

### Imaging
Not necessary if withdrawal is clearly the presenting issue.
- If the clinical situation is not straightforward for withdrawal, CNS imaging may be indicated

## DIFFERENTIAL DIAGNOSIS

- Ethanol withdrawal
- Intracerebral hemorrhage
- CNS infection
- Encephalopathy
- Hypoglycemia
- Hyperthyroidism
- Sepsis
- Psychosis
- Electrolyte disorder
- Drug intoxication

 **TREATMENT**

### PRE-HOSPITAL

- Assess vital signs
- Assess capillary glucose

### INITIAL STABILIZATION/THERAPY

- Attention to ABCs
- Obtain IV access
- IV fluid administration
- Cardiopulmonary monitoring

### ED TREATMENT/PROCEDURES

- Benzodiazepine and barbiturate withdrawal:
  - Aggressive supportive care
  - Begin long-acting agent of the same class causing the withdrawal
- Opiate withdrawal:
  Supportive care
  - Antiemetics for nausea and vomiting
  - Clonidine to reduce severity of signs and symptoms
  - Opiate therapy if withdrawal is complicating other disease states
- Cocaine and amphetamine withdrawal:
  - Supportive care

## MEDICATION

- Chlordiazepoxide: 25–100 mg PO for mild symptoms and signs; 25 mg IV in repeated doses as necessary for severe symptoms and signs
- Clonidine: 0.1–0.3 mg PO q4–6h
- Diazepam: 5–20 mg PO for mild signs and symptoms; 5–10 mg IV in repeated doses as necessary for severe symptoms and signs
- Lorazepam: 1–2 mg PO for mild symptoms and signs; 2 mg IV In repeated doses as necessary for severe symptoms and signs
- Phenobarbital: 30–60 mg PO for mild symptoms and signs; 15–20 mg/kg slow IV administration for severe symptoms or status epilepticus.
- Ondansetron 4–8 mg PO/IV

 **FOLLOW-UP**

### DISPOSITION

#### Admission Criteria

- Moderate to severe withdrawal symptoms
- Persistent withdrawal symptoms
- Psychosis with withdrawal
- Autonomic instability
- Concomitant medical condition that may complicate withdrawal
- Suicidal ideation or otherwise psychiatrically unstable

#### Discharge Criteria

- Mild symptoms responsive to therapy
- Psychiatrically stable

### FOLLOW-UP RECOMMENDATIONS

Referral to detox program or facility

## PEARLS AND PITFALLS

- Misdiagnosis of medical disease as withdrawal syndrome
- Misunderstanding the relationship between withdrawal syndromes and co-morbid medical illness
- Important to administer sufficient quantities of benzodiazepines for patient in benzodiazepine withdrawal states.

## ADDITIONAL READING

- Hamilton RJ. Withdrawal Principles. In Flomenbaum NE, et al, eds. *Goldfrank's Toxicologic Emergencies,* 8th ed. New York: McGraw-Hill, 2006.
- Olmedo R, Hoffman RS. Withdrawal syndromes. *Emerg Med Clin North Am.* 2000;18:273–288.
- Tetrault JM, O'Connor PG. Substance abuse and withdrawal in the critical care setting. *Crit Care Clin.* 2008;24:767–788.

### See Also (Topic, Algorithm, Electronic Media Element)

Withdrawal, Alcohol

 **CODES**

**ICD9**
292.0 Drug withdrawal

W

# WOLFF-PARKINSON-WHITE SYNDROME

Mitchell Adelstein
Richard M. Wolfe

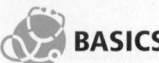

## BASICS

### DESCRIPTION
- Syndrome caused by tachydysrhythmias resulting from the presence of an abnormal accessory atrioventricular (AV) pathway
- Wolff-Parkinson-White (WPW) abnormality or pattern is defined as the presence of preexcitation on the EKG:
  - The abnormality is present in 1.5–3% of the population.
- WPW syndrome requires that the abnormality is present and that paroxysms of tachycardia occur.
- Accessory pathways:
  - Small bands of tissue that failed to separate during development:
    ○ Left lateral (free wall) accessory pathway is the most common
    ○ The posteroseptal region of the AV groove is the 2nd most common location
    ○ Right free wall
    ○ Anteroseptal
- Conduction in WPW may be anterograde, retrograde, or both.
- Anterograde is the most common (70%):
  - Also described as Type A or orthodromic
  - Impulse travels from the atria down the AV node to the ventricle and then up the retrograde pathway.
  - A circuit is created that potentiates reentrant tachycardia.
- Retrograde is less common (30%):
  - Also described as Type B or antidromic
  - The circuit operates in the opposite direction.
- Sudden death occurs in 1 per 1,000 patient-years in persons with known ventricular preexcitation.

### ETIOLOGY
- Idiopathic:
  - Unknown mechanism in most cases, with familial predisposition
- Rarely inherited as an autosomal dominant trait
- Associated in rare cases with a familial hypertrophic cardiomyopathy

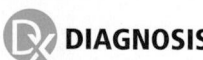

## DIAGNOSIS

### SIGNS AND SYMPTOMS
#### History
- Asymptomatic
- Palpitations:
  - Fast or irregular
- Chest pain
- Dyspnea
- Dizziness
- Nausea
- Diaphoresis
- Syncope

#### Physical Exam
- Tachycardia:
  - Rapid and regular:
    ○ Supraventricular tachycardia
    ○ Atrial flutter
  - Irregular:
    ○ Atrial fibrillation
- Signs of instability:
  - Chest pain
  - Hypotension
  - Change in mental status
  - Rales
  - Cyanosis

### ESSENTIAL WORKUP
- WPW syndrome should be considered the underlying etiology in all cases of tachydysrhythmia.
- The diagnosis should be based on the characteristic EKG findings once the patient has converted to a sinus rhythm.

### DIAGNOSTIC TESTS & INTERPRETATION
#### Lab
- Cardiac enzymes only if signs of ischemia
- Consider electrolytes

#### Diagnostic Procedures/Surgery
- EKG
- Preexcitation:
  - Short pulse rate, <0.12 seconds
  - Delta wave: Small slurred upstroke at the beginning of the QRS
  - Prolonged quasi-random signal (QRS), >0.10 seconds with variable morphology linked to specific accessory pathway
- Left lateral pathway:
  - Positive Δ-waves
  - Q waves with negative to isoelectric deflections in V1 and in the inferior leads:
    ○ May suggest a former high lateral MI and right axis deviation
- Posteroseptal accessory pathway:
  - Negative deflecting Δ-waves
  - QRS complexes in the inferior leads:
    ○ Often mistaken for prior inferior MI
- Tachydysrhythmias:
  - Orthodromic atrioventricular reentrant tachycardia (OAVRT):
    ○ The pathway that conducts the impulse to the ventricle is the AV node/His-Purkinje system
    ○ Narrow QRS complex tachycardia
    ○ However, this may be associated with a wide QRS complex in the presence of a preexisting or rate-related functional bundle branch block.
    ○ P wave following the QRS
    ○ Rate between 150–250 bpm
    ○ The Δ-wave seen during sinus rhythm is lost since antegrade conduction is not via the accessory pathway

- Antidromic AVRT:
  ○ Regular
  ○ Wide QRS complex
  ○ The antegrade limb is usually the accessory pathway.
- Atrial fibrillation:
  ○ Irregular
  ○ Wide complex with variable QRS morphologies

### DIFFERENTIAL DIAGNOSIS
- Preexcitation:
  - Inferior MI
- Narrow complex supraventricular tachycardias without an accessory pathway:
  - AV nodal reentry tachycardia
- Wide complex tachycardia:
  - Atrial fibrillation with intraventricular conduction delay
  - Ventricular tachycardia

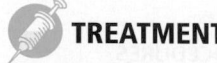

## TREATMENT

### PRE-HOSPITAL
- Supplemental oxygen
- Monitor
- Synchronized cardioversion:
  - Signs of instability
  - Atrial fibrillation with WPW; wide complex tachycardia
- Prehospital use of adenosine:
  - Stable patients do not require emergent conversion.
  - Unstable patients should undergo cardioversion not adenosine.

### INITIAL STABILIZATION/THERAPY
- Unstable patients:
  - Synchronized cardioversion starting with 50 J-min
  - Increase incrementally until sinus rhythm is restored.
- Stable patients with wide complex tachycardia:
  - Amiodarone
  - Procainamide
  - Avoid lidocaine, calcium channel blockers, β-blockers, and digoxin in patients with wide complex tachycardia

### ED TREATMENT/PROCEDURES
- Stable patients:
  - Vagal maneuvers such as a Valsalva:
    ○ Right carotid artery massage for no more than 10 seconds
    ○ Auscultate the artery 1st for a bruit that would contraindicate this procedure
  - Fluid replacement and Trendelenburg if the patient has mild hypotension
  - Pharmacologic conversion if carotid massage fails

- Orthodromic AVRT:
  - Adenosine or verapamil when narrow complex
- Antidromic AVRT:
  - Procainamide is the drug of choice
  - Although verapamil and β-blockers can be used when the diagnosis is certain, their administration is dangerous in ventricular tachycardia and WPW with atrial fibrillation, which can be hard to distinguish from this dysrhythmia.
- Irregular wide complex tachycardia:
  - WPW syndrome with atrial fibrillation
  - Amiodarone or procainamide.

### Pediatric Considerations
- Children may develop ventricular rates up to 320 bpm that are poorly tolerated.
- Cardiovert unstable children with 0.5–2 J/kg.
- Vagal maneuvers and adenosine are safe in stable children.

### MEDICATION
- Adenosine: 6 mg rapid IV bolus over 1–2 seconds; if ineffective, repeat with 12 mg (peds: 0.1 mg/kg rapid IV push, repeat with 0.2 mg/kg)
- Amiodarone: 150 mg IV over 10 minutes, 360 mg over the next 6 hr
- Magnesium: 2 g IV bolus
- Procainamide: 6–13 mg/kg IV at 0.2–0.5 mg/kg/min until either arrhythmia controlled, QRS widens 50%, or hypotension, then 2–6 mg/min, max. of 1,000 mg

### First Line
- Amiodarone for wide complex tachycardias
- Adenosine for narrow complex tachycardias

### Second Line
- Procainamide for wide complex tachycardias
- Procainamide, verapamil, or esmolol can be considered as 2nd line agents for patients with WPW presenting with regular narrow complex tachycardias

## FOLLOW-UP

### DISPOSITION
#### Admission Criteria
- Patients with signs of instability require admission to a monitored bed.
- Failure of outpatient therapy for continuous pharmacologic control or ablation

#### Discharge Criteria
- Most patients will be stable and can be discharged once converted to sinus rhythm.
- Follow-up should be arranged with a cardiologist.

#### Issues for Referral
Electrophysiology studies to assess for radioablation or surgery may be performed on outpatient basis.

### FOLLOW-UP RECOMMENDATIONS
The patient should be instructed to return to the ED with any symptoms suggestive of a tachydysrhythmia:
- Palpitations
- Dizziness
- Chest pain
- Feeling faint

## PEARLS AND PITFALLS

Never use calcium channel blockers, β-blockers, or digoxin in patients with preexcitation with atrial fibrillation or wide complex tachycardia:
- These medications prolong the refractory period of the AV node, increasing the rate of transmission through the accessory pathway, and may result in fatal ventricular dysrhythmias.

## ADDITIONAL READING

- Al-Khatib SM, Pritchett EL. Clinical features of Wolff-Parkinson-White syndrome. *Am Heart J.* 1999;(3 Pt 1):403–413.
- Keating L. Electrocardiographic features of Wolff-Parkinson-White syndrome. *Emerg Med J.* 2003;20(5):491–493.
- Mark DG, Brady WJ, Pines JM. Preexcitation syndrome: Diagnostic considerations in the ED. *Am J Emerg Med.* 2009;27:878–888.
- Rosner MH. Electrocardiography in the patient with Wolff Parkinson White syndrome: Diagnostic and initial therapeutic issues. *Am J Emer Med.* 1999;17(7):705–714.
- Shah CP. Clinical approach to wide QRS complex tachycardias. *Emerg Med Clin North Am.* 1998,16.331–360.
- Xie B, Thakur RK, Shah C, et al. Emergency management of cardiac arrhythmias: Clinical differentiation of narrow QRS complex tachycardias. *Emerg Clin North Am.* 1998;16:295–330.
- Zipes DP. Specific arrhythmias: Diagnosis and treatment. In: Braunwald E, ed. *Heart disease: A textbook of cardiovascular medicine.* 5th ed. Philadelphia: WB Saunders, 1997:667–675.

### See Also (Topic, Algorithm, Electronic Media Element)
Preexcitation Syndrome

 **CODES**

#### ICD9
426.7 Anomalous atrioventricular excitation

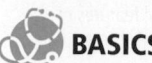 **WOUND BALLISTICS**

*Brian K. Snyder*

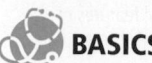

## BASICS

### DESCRIPTION
The physical forces that determine the wounding potential of gunshot and other penetrating wounds

### ETIOLOGY
- Wounding potential of bullet is determined by mass and velocity.
- The type and severity of a wound is determined by:
  – Wounding potential
  – Construction and shape of the bullet
  – Orientation upon striking body
  – Deformity or fragmentation
  – What tissues the bullet traverses
- Traditional distinction between low and high muzzle *velocity* does not differentiate kind and severity of wounding:
  – A civilian hunting rifle or a large-caliber handgun with a hollow-point bullet may produce a more severe wound than a round with a full metal jacket from a "high-velocity" military rifle.
- Bullets wound by two main mechanisms—**crush** and **stretch:**
  – Sonic pressure wave that precedes bullet has no role in wounding.
  – Bullet crushes tissue it directly passes through, forming a *permanent cavity.*
  – *Stretch* is produced by radial energy transferred from bullet as it slows down in tissue, forming *temporary cavity.*
  – A bullet is stabilized in flight by *spin* transmitted from rifling in the barrel.
  – Spin minimizes *yaw,* which is the angle between the long axis of the bullet and its flight vector.
  – Without spin, a bullet would yaw to its most stable flight configuration, which is base and center of mass forward:
    ○ Not aerodynamically efficient
  – As bullet enters tissue, spin of bullet is reduced and bullet will yaw.
  – When yaw is 90 degrees, a bullet crushes maximal amount of tissue, slows down the most, and maximal stretch injury occurs.
- Bullets designed to deform in tissue (soft point, hollow point) will expand on impact:
  – Increases amount of crush injury
  – Moves bullet center of mass forward
- Jacketed bullets prevent lead stripping in the barrel, which occurs at high muzzle velocities:
  – Jacketed bullets do not deform but may fragment.
  – Fragmentation increases surface area and crush injury.

- Bullets striking bone often fragment and may cause bone fragments to become secondary projectiles.
- Severity of wound also depends upon *tissue composition and thickness:*
  – Minimally elastic tissues, near-water-density tissue (brain, liver), fluid-filled (heart, bowel) and dense organs (bone) may be injured by the temporary cavity.
  – More elastic tissue, such as lung and skeletal muscle, may absorb the energy from temporary cavity formation and sustain minimal damage.
  – Extremities are often not thick enough for the bullet to fully yaw:
    ○ Temporary cavity formation is minimal.
    ○ Most damage is caused by direct crush injury of the bullet, its fragments, or secondary projectiles.
- Short-range shotgun blasts produce severe wounds with compromise of the blood supply:
  – In short-range shotgun injuries, pellets may be greatly scattered in tissue secondary to the pellets striking each other.
- Stab wounds with knives and other sharp instruments are low-energy wounds with tissue injury from direct weapon contact.

 **DIAGNOSIS**

### SIGNS AND SYMPTOMS
- Severe underlying tissue damage and life-threatening injury may occur with even small entrance wounds.
- A knowledge of how different kinds of weapons and bullets wound, the trajectory of the bullet through the body, and the effect on different body tissues will allow the physician to carefully evaluate gunshot and stab wounds and their potential morbidity and mortality.

### History
- Field personnel can provide information about weapon type and size, distance, and angle between the weapon and victim:
- This information may not be available or may be inaccurate.

### Physical Exam
- Evaluate for entrance and exit wounds:
- May estimate trajectory and potential for tissue damage
- Exit wounds are often stellate and larger than entranced wounds unless energy is dissipated at skin surface by special bullet type (hollow point, etc.).
- With high-velocity projectiles, exit wound may be much more extensive than entrance wound.
- Because of the elasticity of the skin, bullet can often be palpated subcutaneously.
- It is not always possible to differentiate entrance from exit wounds; clinicians do this poorly, so wounds should be described fully only in the medical record; classification as entrance or exit wounds should be avoided.

### ESSENTIAL WORKUP
- ABCs must be stabilized prior to any workup.
- All injury tracts must be accounted for.
- Place markers at wound sites.
- Examine all areas of the body for wounds (remember the perineum, axillae, and scalp).

### DIAGNOSTIC TESTS & INTERPRETATION
#### Lab
Initial laboratory tests are not especially helpful in diagnosis but may be helpful in guiding resuscitation.

#### Imaging
- Anteroposterior and lateral radiographs help localize bullet:
  – With placement of markers at wound sites, wound trajectory can be estimated
  – Fragments, fractures, pneumothoraces, or hemothoraces can be identified.
- US:
  – A positive FAST scan is highly predictive of a therapeutic laparotomy. A negative FAST scan does not exclude significant intra-abdominal injury.
- CT scanning:
  – Identify location of projectile.
  – Location and amount of tissue damage (especially to the head and brain)
  – Abdominal CT is increasingly used in the evaluation of stable patients with penetrating back/flank or abdominal trauma.
  – In penetrating trauma of the thorax, an initial negative CT scan of the thorax obviates the usual practice of repeated chest radiographs.
- Angiography may be necessary if patient has potential vascular injury and surgical exploration is not otherwise warranted.

### *Diagnostic Procedures/Surgery*
- Local wound exploration with clear delineation of the base of the wound tract that does not penetrate deep structures may be sufficient to evaluate stab wounds.
- Abdominal wounds that encroach the posterior fascia require further evaluation, either diagnostic peritoneal lavage or surgical exploration.
- Extent of tissue injury often apparent only on surgical exploration.

## DIFFERENTIAL DIAGNOSIS
Organs at risk of damage can be inferred from weapon type, distance, locations of entrance and exits wounds, or projectiles on imaging.

- Tissues surrounding the projectile tract are also at risk of injury (ie, from temporary cavity).
- Projectiles may fragment and create multiple injury tracts.

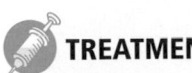 TREATMENT

### PRE-HOSPITAL
- Gunshot and stab wounds to chest with unstable vital signs warrant a needle thoracostomy in the side of the chest with the entrance wound:
  - Relieves tension pneumothorax
  - If no improvement, a needle thoracostomy should be placed in the contralateral hemithorax.
- Impaled objects or projectiles should not be removed:
  - Immobilize with tape and gauze and transport.
- Clothing should be preserved if possible:
  - Clothing should be cut around holes made by the projectiles to preserve evidence.
- Patient should be transported to the closest trauma center.
- Hypotensive patient may be taken directly to the OR.

### INITIAL STABILIZATION/THERAPY
Stabilize airway, breathing, and circulation. Secure adequate IV access.

## ED TREATMENT/PROCEDURES
- Impaled objects should be removed only in the OR.
- In the ED, estimate tissue injury based on the above principles.
- Wound care includes appropriate exploration, irrigation, and debridement of devitalized tissue.
- All bullets are contaminated with bacteria and are **not** sterilized by being fired:
  - All nongrazing bullet wounds warrant empiric antibiotics.
- Early trauma, orthopedic, and vascular surgery consultation is necessary.

## MEDICATION
Prophylactic antistaphylococcal antibiotics should be prescribed for several days:

- Cefazolin 1 g IV q6h
- Cephalexin 500 mg PO q6–8h
- For penicillin-allergic patients or patients at risk for methicillin-resistant *S. aureus* then vancomycin 1 g IV q12h or clindamycin 300 mg IV/PO q6h can be prescribed
- Intra-abdominal wounds require broader coverage (many regimens available) such as cefotetan 1 g IV q6h, piperacillin/tazobactam 3.75 mg IV q6h, or the combination of ciprofloxacin 500 mg IV q12h with metronidazole 500 mg IV q8h

 FOLLOW-UP

### DISPOSITION
#### *Admission Criteria*
- Patients with neurovascular compromise and extensive tissue damage must be admitted for appropriate surgical intervention.
- Patients with nontrivial injury to the head, neck, torso, or abdomen should be admitted.
- Patients with injury from high-velocity projectiles or gunshot wounds should be admitted to a monitored setting for observation of neurovascular status.

#### *Discharge Criteria*
Patients with minor penetrating extremity trauma or stabbing victims found not to have significant injury may be discharged with appropriate follow-up.

#### *Issues for Referral*
Emergent consultation of appropriate surgical specialists should be obtained for patients with potential injuries to vascular or nervous structures.

### FOLLOW-UP RECOMMENDATIONS
Patients not admitted to the hospital should have scheduled follow-up with a trauma surgeon or an appropriate surgical specialist (eg, orthopedist for extremity trauma).

## PEARLS AND PITFALLS

- Do not underestimate the extent of underlying tissue damage or injury to critical structures given the size or location of entrance or exit wounds.
- Account for all projectiles and all injury tracts.
- Gunshot and stab wounds are usually reportable to local law enforcement.

## ADDITIONAL READING

- Fackler ML. Gunshot wound review. *Ann Emerg Med*. 1996;28:194–203.
- Ramirez RM, Cureton EL, et al. Single-contrast computed tomography for the triage of patients with penetrating torso trauma. *J Trauma*. 2009;67:583–588.
- Santucci RA, Chang Y. Ballistics for physicians: Myths about wound ballistics and gunshot injuries. *J Urol*. 2004;171:1408–1414.
- Swan KG, Swan RC. Principles of ballistics applicable to the treatment of gunshot wounds. *Surg Clin Am*. 1991;71:221–239.

W

# Emergency Medications

| Drug | Adult | Pediatric (Pediatric dose should not generally exceed adult dose) |
|------|-------|------------------------------------------------------------------|
| Abciximab (ReoPro) | 0.25 mg/kg IV, then 0.125 mg/kg/min infusion | N/A |
| Adenosine (Adenocard) (3 mg/mL) | 6 mg IV (rapid) Give 12 mg IV; if no response after 2 min, may repeat 12 mg IV if needed | 0.1 mg/kg IV (rapid); give 0.2 mg/kg if no response after 2 min |
| Albuterol (Ventolin, Proventil) (0.5% soln: 5 mg/mL) | 2.5 mg (0.5 mL) by inhalation; may repeat or give continuously; MDI available. | 0.03 mL (0.15 mg/kg/dose) by inhalation; may repeat or give continuously |
| Alteplase (rt-PA, Activase) | *Stroke*: 0.9 mg/kg (max 90 mg). Give 10% of the total dose IV bolus over 1 min followed by remaining total dose over 1 hr *Pulmonary embolus*: 100 mg IV over 2 hr | N/A |
| Amiodarone | *Cardiac arrest*: 300 mg IV push *Wide complex tachycardia*: 150 mg IV over 10 min | *Cardiac arrest*: 5 mg/kg IV push *Wide complex tachycardia*: 5/mg/kg IV over 20–60 min |
| Amrinone, inamrinone | 0.75 mg/kg over 10–15 min; *Infusion*: 5–10 $\mu$g/kg/min | 0.75 mg/kg over 10–15 min; *Infusion*: infants and children: 5–10 $\mu$g/kg/min; neonates 3–5 $\mu$g/kg/min |
| Atenolol | 5 mg IV q5min to 10 mg total | N/A |
| Atropine (0.1, 0.4, 1 mg/mL) | 0.5–1.0 mg IV/ET | 0.02 mg/kg IV/ET (min 0.1 mg/dose) |
| Bicarbonate, sodium 44, 50 mEq/50 mL | 1 mEq/kg/dose IV q10min PRN (per ABG) | 1 mEq/kg/dose IV q10min PRN (per ABG); dilute |
| Calcium chloride (10% soln: 100 mg/mL, 1.36 mEq Ca $\mu$/mL | 500 mg/dose IV slowly q10min PRN | 20 mg/kg/dose IV slowly q10min PRN |
| Calcium gluconate (10% soln: 100 mg/mL, 0.46 mEq/mL) | Hyperkalemia: 1–2 g IV over 5–10 min | |
| Crystalloid (0.9% NS, LR) | *Flush*: 1–2 L IV over 20–30 min; may repeat | Flush: 20 mL/kg IV over 20–30 min; may repeat |
| Defibrillation | 200 J/dose; double for subsequent dose; synchronized: 50–100 J | 2 J/kg/dose; double for subsequent dose; synchronized: 0.5–1.0 J/kg/dose |
| Dexamethasone (Decadron) (4, 24 mg/mL) | 5–10 mg IM/IV | 0.15–0.60 mg/kg/dose IM/IV |
| Dextrose (D50W: 25 g/50 mL) | 25–50 g IV | 0.5–1.0 g (2–4 mL D25W)/kg/dose IV |
| Diazepam (Valium) (5 mg/mL) | 5–10 mg IV | 0.2–0.3 mg/kg/dose IV q2–5min slowly; 0.2–0.5 mg/kg/dose PR q5min |
| Digibind (40-mg vial binds 0.6 mg dig) | 3–5 vials for chronicoverdose; 10–20 vials for acute overdose | Dose (in no. of vials) = [(serum digitoxin concentration in ng/mL) (weight in kg)] ÷ 100 |
| Digoxin | *Load*: 0.5 mg IV initially followed by 0.25 mg q6h × 2 Adjust loading dose by 50% in end stage renal disease | *Initial IV loading dose:* <2 yr: 15–25 $\mu$g/kg 2–5 yr: 10–15 $\mu$g/kg 5–10 yr: 7–15 $\mu$g/kg |
| Diltiazem | 15–20 mg (0.25 mg/kg) IV over 2 min; may repeat IV bolus dose in 15 min with 25–30 mg (0.35 mg/kg) over 2 min infusion: 5–15 mg/hr | N/A |

# Emergency Medications (*Continued*)

| Drug | Adult | Pediatric (Pediatric dose should not generally exceed adult dose) |
|---|---|---|
| Dobutamine (Dobutrex) (250 mg/vial) | 2–20 $\mu$g/kg/min IV drip max 40 $\mu$g/kg/min | 2–15 $\mu$g/kg/min IV drip |
| Dopamine (40, 80, 160 mg/mL) | 5–20 $\mu$g/kg/min IV drip | 5–20 $\mu$g/kg/min IV drip |
| Enalapril (enalaprilat) | 0.625–1.25 mg IV over 5 min then 1.25–5 mg IV q6h | N/A |
| Enoxaparin (Lovenox) | 1 mg/kg | N/A |
| Epinephrine | *Asystole:* 1 mg IV q3–5min<br>*Anaphylaxis/allergy:* 0.3 mg (1:1,000) SC q15–20min PRN | *Asystole:* 0.01 mg/kg/dose (1:10,000) IV q3–5min PRN. ET, IO and subsequent IV doses, (0.1 mg)/kg/dose (1:1,000) q3–5min PRN<br>*Anaphylaxis/allergy:* 0.01 mg/kg (1:1,000) SC, q15–20min PRN |
| Epinephrine, racemic (Vaponefrin) (2.25% soln) | 0.5–0.75 mL/dose by inhalation; may repeat | 0.25–0.75 mL/dose by inhalation; may repeat |
| Eptifibatide (Integrilin) | 180 $\mu$g/kg (max: 22.6 mg) IV, then 2 $\mu$g/kg/min (max 15 mg/hr) infusion | N/A |
| Esmolol | *Load:* 500 $\mu$g/kg over 1 min<br>*Infusion:* 50–200 $\mu$g/kg/min to max 0.3 mg/kg/min (max 300 mg total dose) | *Load:* 100–500 $\mu$g/kg IV over 1 min<br>*Infusion:* 25–100 $\mu$g/kg/min |
| Fentanyl (Sublimaze) (50 $\mu$g/mL) | 0.5–1 $\mu$g/kg/dose slow IV up to 50–100 $\mu$g/dose | 1–2 $\mu$g/kg/dose slow IV up to 4 mg/kg/dose |
| Flumazenil | 0.2 mg IV, then 0.3 mg followed by 0.5 mg/min up to 3 mg | 0.01 mg/kg IV to max of 0.2 mg |
| Fosphenytoin | 15–20 mg phenytoin equivalents (PE)/kg over 20 min for IV or give IM | 15–20 mg phenytoin equivalents/kg IV/IM |
| Furosemide (Lasix) (10 mg/mL) | 20–40 mg IV | 1 mg/kg IV |
| Glucagon | 1 mg q5min, max 5 mg | 0.03–0.1 mg/kg IV/IM/SC q5–20min, max 1 mg |
| Heparin | 60–80 IU/kg IV, then 15–18 IU/kg/hr | 50–75 IU/kg then 15–25 IU/kg/hr |
| Hydralazine (Apresoline) (20 mg/mL) | 10–20 mg IM/IV | 0.1–0.2 mg/kg/dose IV/IM; max 20 mg |
| Insulin, regular | DKA: 2–10 units/hr IV | DKA: 0.05–0.2 units/kg/hr IV drip |
| Isoproterenol (200 $\mu$g/mL) | 2–10 $\mu$g/min | 0.05–2 $\mu$g/kg/min IV drip |
| Labetalol (Normodyne) (5 mg/mL) | *Load:* 20 mg/dose IV q10min up to 300 mg<br>*Maintenance:* 0.5–2 mg/min | *Load:* 0.25–1.0 mg/kg/dose IV slow push; may repeat<br>Infusion: 0.4–1 mg/kg/hr, max 3 mg/kg/hr |
| Lidocaine (Xylocaine) (10, 20 mg/mL) | *Load:* 1–1.5 mg/kg/dose IV (or ET) q5–10min PRN up to 3–5 mg/kg max 3 mg/kg<br>*Maintenance:* 1–4 mg/min IV drip | *Load:* 1 mg/kg/dose IV (or ET) q5–10min PRN up to 3–5 mg/kg<br>*Maintenance:* 20 $\mu$g/kg/min IV drip |
| Lorazepam (Ativan) (2, 4 mg/mL) | 0.5–2 mg IV/IM/PO up to 5 mg | 0.05–0.15 mg/kg/dose IV/IM |
| Magnesium sulfate | Severe asthma: 1–2 g IV over 5–10 min<br>Pre-eclampsia: 4 g | 25–50 mg/kg over 10 min |
| Mannitol (200, 250 mg/mL) | *Load:* 0.5–1 g/kg IV<br>*Maintenance:* 0.25–0.5 g/kg IV | *Load:* 0.5–1 g/kg IV<br>*Maintenance:* 0.25–0.5 g/kg IV |
| Metoprolol | 5 mg IV q5min to 15 mg total | N/A |

(*continued*)

# Emergency Medications (*Continued*)

| Drug | Adult | Pediatric (Pediatric dose should not generally exceed adult dose) |
|---|---|---|
| Midazolam (Versed) (1 mg/mL) | 1–2.5 mg, max 2.5–5 mg IV | 0.05–0.1 mg/kg/dose IV |
| Morphine (8, 10, 15 mg/mL) | 0.1–0.2 mg/kg/dose IV/IM up to 15 mg | 0.1–0.2 mg/kg/dose IV/IM |
| Naloxone (Narcan) (0.4, 1 mg/mL) | 1–2 mg IV, IM, ET | 0.1 mg/kg/dose IV, ET |
| Nicardipine (Cardene IV) (Concentration of premade bags will depend on institution) | No bolus, start infusion at 2.5–5 mg/hr, may increase rate by 2.5 mg/hr q10–15min to a max of 15 mg/hr | |
| Nitroglycerin (Tridil) (0.5 mg, 0.8 mg, 5 mg, 10 mg/mL) | 5 $\mu$g/min IV drip, titrate up as needed to 300 $\mu$g/min | 0.25–0.5 $\mu$g/kg/min IV drip, titrate up as needed |
| Nitroprusside | 0.10 $\mu$g/kg/min up to 5.0 $\mu$g/kg/min | 0.10 $\mu$g/kg/min up to 5.0 $\mu$g/kg/min IV |
| Norepinephrine | 0.5 $\mu$g/min IV up to 20 $\mu$g/min | 0.05–0.1 $\mu$g/kg/min IV and titrate max 1–2 $\mu$g/kg/min |
| Pancuronium (Pavulon) (1, 2 mg/mL) | 0.1–0.15 mg/kg/dose IV q30–60min | 0.04–0.1 mg/kg/dose IV q30–60min |
| Phenobarbital (65, 130 mg/mL) | *Load:* 15–20 mg/kg/dose IV (<5–50 mg/min) | *Load:* 15–20 mg/kg/dose IV (<1 mg/kg/min) |
| Phenytoin (Dilantin) (50 mg/mL) | *Seizure load:* 10–20 mg/kg/dose IV (<40 mg/min) up to 1,000 mg; fosphenytoin (Cerebyx) permits more rapid administration, also | *Seizure load:* 10–20 mg/kg/dose IV (<0.5 mg/kg/min); fosphenytoin alternative |
| Procainamide | *Load:* 20 mg/min IV to max dose 17 mg/kg *Infusion:* 1–4 mg/min | *Load:* 2–6 mg/kg/dose over 5 min (max dose: 100 mg/dose); repeat dose q5–10min PRN up to a total max of 15 mg/kg; do not exceed 500 mg in 30 min *Maintenance:* 20–80 $\mu$g/kg/min by continuous infusion |
| Propranolol (Inderal) (1 mg/mL) | 1 mg IV over 10 min q5min to total dose 5 mg | 0.01–0.1 mg/kg/dose low IV over 10 min; max 1 mg |
| Reteplase (Retavase) | 10 IU IV over 2 min, repeat in 30 min | N/A |
| Succinylcholine (Anectine) (20 mg/mL) | 1–1.5 mg/kg/dose IV up to 150 mg | 1–1.5 mg/kg/dose IV |
| Tenecteplase (TNKase) | 30–50 mg IV bolus | N/A |
| Terbutaline | 0.25 mg SC × 1 | 0.01 mL/kg/dose SC *Nebulized:* 0.01–0.03 mg/kg/dose in 2 mL saline |
| Thiopental | 3–5 mg/kg IV | 2–5 mg/kg IV |
| Tirofiban (Aggrastat) | 0.4 $\mu$g/kg/min for 30 min then 0.1 $\mu$g/kg/min | N/A |
| Vasopressin | Pulseless Vt/VF: 40 U IV × 1 dose | N/A |
| Vecuronium (Norcuron) (10 mg/mL) | 0.1 mg/kg/dose IV | 0.1 mg/kg/dose IV |
| Verapamil | 2.5–5.0 mg IV; then 5–10 mg IV | N/A |